THE UFAW HANDBOOK ON

The Care and Management of Laboratory and Other Research Animals

The Universities Federation for Animal Welfare

UFAW, founded 1926, is an internationally recognised, independent, scientific and educational animal welfare charity (Registered in England Charity No. 207996) concerned with promoting high standards of welfare for farm, companion, laboratory and captive wild animals, and for those animals with which we interact in the wild.

It works to improve animals' lives by:

- promoting and supporting developments in the science and technology that underpin advances in animal welfare;
- promoting education in animal care and welfare;
- providing information, organising meetings and publishing books, videos, articles, technical reports and the journal *Animal Welfare*;
- providing expert advice to government departments and other bodies and helping to draft and amend laws and guidelines;
- enlisting the energies of animal keepers, scientists, veterinarians, lawyers and others who care about animals.

'Improvements in the care of animals are not now likely to come of their own accord, merely by wishing them: there must be research . . . and it is in sponsoring research of this kind, and making its results widely known, that UFAW performs one of its most valuable services.'

Sir Peter Medawar CBE FRS, 8th May 1957
Nobel Laureate (1960), Chairman of the UFAW Scientific Advisory Committee (1951–1962)
UFAW relies on the generosity of the public through legacies and donations to carry out its work improving the welfare of animal now and in the future. For further information about UFAW and how you can help promote and support its work, please contact us at the address below.

Universities Federation for Animal Welfare
The Old School, Brewhouse Hill, Wheathampstead, Herts AL4 8AN, UK
Tel: 01582 831818 Fax: 01582 831414 Website: www.ufaw.org.uk
Email: ufaw@ufaw.org.uk

THE UFAW HANDBOOK ON

The Care and Management of Laboratory and Other Research Animals

Eighth Edition

Edited by Robert Hubrecht and James Kirkwood

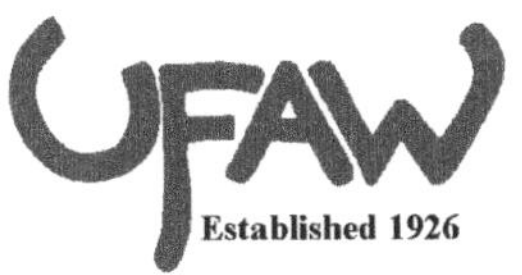

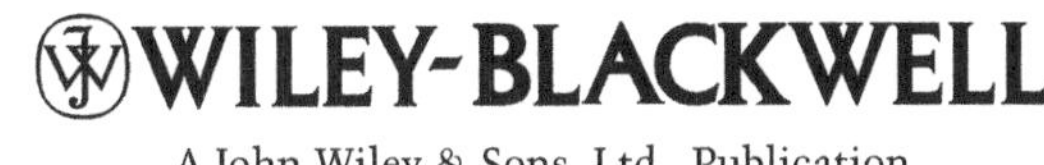

A John Wiley & Sons, Ltd., Publication

This edition first published 2010
Seventh edition published 1999
Sixth edition published 1987; Fifth edition published 1976; Fourth edition published 1972; Third edition published 1959; Second edition published 1957 (all by Longman Group Ltd)
First edition published 1947

Blackwell Publishing was acquired by John Wiley & Sons in February 2007. Blackwell's publishing programme has been merged with Wiley's global Scientific, Technical, and Medical business to form Wiley-Blackwell.

Registered office
John Wiley & Sons Ltd, The Atrium, Southern Gate, Chichester, West Sussex, PO19 8SQ, United Kingdom

Editorial offices
9600 Garsington Road, Oxford, OX4 2DQ, United Kingdom
2121 State Avenue, Ames, Iowa 50014-8300, USA

For details of our global editorial offices, for customer services and for information about how to apply for permission to reuse the copyright material in this book please see our website at www.wiley.com/wiley-blackwell.

Library of Congress Cataloging-in-Publication Data

The UFAW handbook on the care and management of laboratory and other research animals. – 8th ed. / edited for UFAW by Robert Hubrecht and James Kirkwood.
p. ; cm.
Rev. ed. of: The UFAW handbook on the care and management of laboratory animals / edited for UFAW by Trevor Poole. 7th ed. 1999.
Includes bibliographical references and index.
ISBN 978-1-4051-7523-4 (hardback : alk. paper) 1. Laboratory animals–Handbooks, manuals, etc. I. Hubrecht, R. II. Kirkwood, James K. III. Universities Federation for Animal Welfare. IV. UFAW handbook on the care and management of laboratory animals. V. Title: Handbook on the care and management of laboratory and other research animals.
[DNLM: 1. Animals, Laboratory–Handbooks. 2. Animal Welfare–Handbooks. QY 39 U23 2010]
SF406.U55 2010
636.088′5–dc22 2009031825

A catalogue record for this book is available from the British Library.

Set in 9 on 11 pt Palatino by Toppan Best-set Premedia Limited

2 2012

Contents

Contributors

Christian R. Abee
University of Texas, M.D. Anderson Cancer Center, Michale E. Keeling Center for Comparative Medicine and Research, Department of Veterinary Sciences, 650 Cool Water Dr, Bastrop, TX 78602, USA

James R. Anderson
Department of Psychology, University of Stirling, Stirling FK9 4LA, UK

Lucy Asher
Royal Veterinary College, North Mimms, Hertfordshire AL9 7TA, UK

Melissa Bateson
Centre for Behaviour and Evolution, Newcastle University, Newcastle upon Tyne NE2 4HH, UK

Vera Baumans
Department Animals in Science and Society, Division Laboratory Animal Science, Utrecht University, PO Box 80.166, 3508 TD Utrecht, The Netherlands

Kathryn Bayne
Global Director, AAALAC International, 5283 Corporate Dr., Suite #203, Frederick, MD 21703, USA

Darin C. Bennett
Avian Research Centre, Faculty of Land and Food Systems, University of British Columbia, Vancouver, BC V6T 1Z4, Canada

Iain Berrill
Institute of Aquaculture, University of Stirling, Stirling FK9 4LA, UK

Alan G. Brady
University of Texas, M.D. Anderson Cancer Center, Michale E. Keeling Center for Comparative Medicine and Research, Department of Veterinary Sciences, Bastrop, TX, USA

Hannah M. Buchanan-Smith
Behaviour and Evolution Research Group, Department of Psychology, University of Stirling, Stirling FK9 4LA, UK

Bernd U. Budelmann
Department of Neuroscience & Cell Biology, University of Texas Medical Branch, 301 University Boulevard, Galveston, TX 77555-1069, USA

Kimberly M. Cheng
Avian Research Centre, Faculty of Land and Food Systems, University of British Columbia, Vancouver, BC V6T 1Z4, Canada

Sonja T. Chou
Charles River, Inc., 251 Ballardvale Street, Wilmington, MA 01887, USA

Silke Corbach-Söhle
Clinical Neurobiology Laboratory, German Primate Center, Leibniz Institute for Primate Research, Göttingen, Germany; current address: Comparative Biology Centre, Medical School, Newcastle NE2 4HH, UK

Jonathan J. Cooper
Department of Biological Sciences, University of Lincoln, Riseholme Park, Riseholme, Lincoln LN2 2LG, UK

John E. Cooper
Department of Veterinary Medicine, University of Cambridge, Madingley Road, Cambridge CB3 0ES, UK

Mike Dennis
Health Protection Agency, Porton Down, Salisbury, Wiltshire SP4 0JG, UK

Ian J.H. Duncan,
The Campbell Centre for the Study of Animal Welfare, University of Guelph, Guelph, Ontario N1G 2W1, Canada

Therese Edström
AstraZeneca R & D Mölndal, Pepparedsleden 1, SE-431 83 Mölndal, Sweden

Roger Ewbank
c/o UFAW, The Old School, Brewhouse Hill, Wheathampstead, Herts, AL4 8AN, UK

Michael F.W. Festing
c/o Understanding Animal Research, 25 Shaftsbury Avenue, London W1D 7EG, UK

Malcolm P. France
Laboratory Animal Services, University of Sydney, NSW 2006, Australia

Roger Francis
c/o Institute of Animal Technology, 5 South Parade, Summertown, Oxford OX2 7JL, UK

Eberhard Fuchs
Clinical Neurobiology Laboratory, German Primate Center, Leibniz Institute for Primate Research, Göttingen, Germany

Hilary Gates
MRC, Mammalian Genetics Unit, Harwell OX11 0RD, UK

Colin L. Gilbert
The Babraham Institute, Babraham Hall, Cambridge CB22 3AT, UK

Mark Haselgrove
School of Psychology, University of Nottingham, University Park, Nottingham NG7 2RD, UK

Barbara Holgate
Biological Services, King's College London, Room 1.12, Hodgkin Building, Guys Campus, London SE1 1UL, UK

Wolfgang Holtz
Department of Animal Science, Georg-August-University, Albrecht-Thaer-Weg 3, 37075 Goettingen, Germany

Bryan Howard
(formerly of) University of Sheffield, Sheffield, UK*

Robert Hubrecht
UFAW, The Old School, Brewhouse Hill, Wheathampstead, Hertfordshire AL4 8AN, UK

Anne Hudson
Food and Environment Research Agency, York YO41 1LZ, UK

Ian R. Inglis
Food and Environment Research Agency, York YO41 1LZ, UK

Sylvia Kaiser
Department of Behavioural Biology, University of Muenster, Badestasse 9, D 48149 Muenster, Germany

Keith M. Kendrick
Cognitive and Systems Neuroscience, The Babraham Institute, Babraham, Cambridge CB22 3AT, UK

James Kirkwood
UFAW, The Old School, Brewhouse Hill, Wheathampstead, Hertfordshire AL4 8AN, UK

Carl B. Kole
Kole Aviation and Special Cargoes Consulting, 3519 Highcrest Road, Rockford, IL 61107-1305, USA

*Any communication to the author should be sent to Universities Federation for Animal Welfare, The Old School, Brewhouse Hill, Wheathampstead, Hertfordshire. AL4 8AN, UK

Jaap M. Koolhaas
Department of Behavioral Physiology, University Groningen, P.O. Box 14, 6750 AA Haren, The Netherlands

Christine Krüger
Central Animal Laboratory, University Clinic of Essen, Hufelandstraße 55, D-45122 Essen, Germany

Susan P. Lambeth
Department of Veterinary Sciences, Michale E. Keeling Center for Comparative Medicine and Research, The University of Texas M.D. Anderson Center, Bastrop, TX, USA

Julie M. Lane
Food and Environment Research Agency, Sand Hutton, York YO41 1LZ, UK

Naomi Latham
Department of Zoology, University of Oxford OX1 3PS, UK

Gail Laule
Active Environments, Inc, 7651 Santos Rd., Lompoc, CA 93436, USA

Graham Law
Division of Ecology & Evolutionary Biology, Faculty of Biomedical and Life Sciences, University of Glasgow, Glasgow G12 8QQ, UK

Lena Lidfors
Department of Animal Environment and Health, Swedish University of Agricultural Sciences, P.O. Box 234, SE-532 23 Skara, Sweden

Maggie Lloyd
Red Kite Veterinary Consultants, PO Box 306, Wallingford OX10 1DF, UK

Cathleen Lutz
Associate Director, Genetic Resource Sciences; Mouse Repository, The Jackson Laboratory, 600 Main Street, Bar Harbor, Maine 04609, USA

Judy MacArthur Clark
Animals Scientific Procedures Inspectorate, Home Office, Marsham Street, London SW1 4DF, UK

Fiona Mathews
School of Biosciences, University of Exeter, Exeter EX4 4PS, UK.

Sandra McCune
WALTHAM® Centre for Pet Nutrition, Freeby Lane, Waltham-on-the-Wolds, Melton Mowbray, Leics LE14 4RT, UK

Robbie A. McDonald
Food and Environment Research Agency, Sand Hutton, York YO41 1LZ, UK

Anthony McGregor
Department of Psychology, Durham University, South Road, Durham DH1 3LE, UK

Fernando Montesso
Animal Health Trust, Lanwades Park, Kentford, Newmarket CB8 7UU, UK

Timothy H. Morris
The School of Veterinary Medicine and Science, The University of Nottingham, Sutton Bonington Campus, Sutton Bonington, Leicestershire LE12 5RD, UK

Ruedi G. Nager
Division of Ecology & Evolutionary Biology, Faculty of Biomedical and Life Sciences, University of Glasgow, Glasgow G12 8QQ, UK

Timo Nevalainen
NLAC, University of Kuopio, Finland

Michael Plant
Harlan Laboratories UK Ltd, Shaw's Farm, Blackthorn, Bicester, Oxon OX25 1TP, UK

C. Jane Pomeroy
Biological Services, Royal Veterinary College, Royal College Street, London NW1 0TU, UK

Jan-Bas Prins
Leiden University Medical Center, Leiden, The Netherlands

Jon Richmond
Home Office, PO Box 6779, Dundee DD1 9WN, UK

Merel Ritskes-Hoitinga
Head Central Animal Laboratory, 231 Centraal Dierenlaboratorium (CDL), Universitair Medisch Centrum (UMC) St Radboud, PO Box 9101, NL-6500 HB Nijmegen, The Netherlands

Norbert Sachser
Department of Behavioural Biology, University of Muenster, Badestr. 9, D-48149 Muenster, Germany

Bart Savenije
3R Research Center, Central Animal Laboratory, Radboud University Nijmegen Medical Center, The Netherlands

Steven J. Schapiro
Department of Veterinary Sciences, Michale E. Keeling Center for Comparative Medicine and Research, The University of Texas M. D. Anderson Center, Bastrop, TX, USA

Chris Sherwin
Department of Clinical Veterinary Science, University of Bristol, UK

Jan Strubbe
Department of Neuro-Endocrinology, Laboratory of Animal Physiology, University of Groningen, The Netherlands

Roy Sutcliffe
Charles River Inc., Research Models and Services UK, Manston Road, Margate, Kent CT9 4LT, UK

Richard Tinsley
School of Biological Sciences, University of Bristol, Woodland Road, Bristol BS8 1UG, UK

Simon Tonge
Whitley Wildlife Conservation Trust, Paignton Zoo Environmental Park, Totnes Road, Paignton, Devon TQ4 7EU, UK

James F. Turnbull
Institute of Aquaculture, University of Stirling, Stirling FK9 4LA, UK

John L. VandeBerg
Southwest National Primate Research Center and Department of Genetics, Southwest Foundation for Biomedical Research, P.O. Box 760549, San Antonio, TX 78245-0549, USA

Elisabetta Visalberghi
Istituto di Scienze e Tecnologie della Cognizione, Consiglio Nazionale delle Ricerche, Rome, Italy

Eva Waiblinger
Swiss Animal Protection SAP, Rainstrasse 53, CH-8706 Meilen, Switzerland

Rikke Westh Thon
PixieGene A/S, Axelborg, Copenhagen, Denmark.

William J. White
Charles River Inc., 251 Ballardvale Street, Wilmington, MA 01887, USA

David Whittaker
Huntingdon Life Sciences, Woolley Road, Alconbury, Huntingdon, Cambridgeshire PE28 4 HS, UK

Lawrence E. Williams
University of Texas, M.D. Anderson Cancer Center, Michale E. Keeling Center for Comparative Medicine and Research, Department of Veterinary Sciences, Bastrop, TX, USA

Sarah Williams-Blangero
Department of Genetics, Southwest Foundation for Biomedical Research, P.O. Box 760549, San Antonio, TX 78245-0549, USA

Sarah Wolfensohn
Veterinary Services, University of Oxford, Parks Road, Oxford OX1 3PT, UK

Foreword

The UFAW Handbook on the Care and Management of Laboratory and Other Research Animals is now here again in an 8th edition.

When I was contacted by Robert Hubrecht earlier this year and asked if I would like to write a foreword to this new edition I jumped at the chance. This book has formed an important part of the laboratory research environment throughout the last 50 years and it is a real privilege to able to make some contribution, albeit a very small contribution, to the 8th edition.

It is important to see this hugely authoritative work in the context of UFAW itself, and the sustained contribution to the improvement of laboratory animal welfare that this organisation has made since its inception. *The Universities Federation for Animal Welfare* was created formally in 1936, although its origins can be traced back farther than that to 1926, when the body from which it evolved, the *University of London Animal Welfare Society*, was founded by Major Charles Hume. It was Hume who laid the foundations for future developments by making it clear that animal welfare must be closely associated with science, and with human and veterinary medicine, but that importantly policy should be based on facts rather than sentimentality. It is still the vision that progress in this area will be best served by ensuring that there is close alignment between scientific progress and animal welfare, so that opportunities to exploit scientific and technical know-how for delivering real improvements are realised quickly and effectively.

Under the guidance of Hume, UFAW led the way in improving animal welfare, among their stated aims being the promotion, by educational and other methods, of interest in the welfare of animals, and enlisting the influence of University 'men and women' on behalf of animals. William Russell, the late and greatly lamented polymath, then came on to the scene, and joined UFAW from Oxford University in 1954. Some short time later Russell was joined by Rex Burch, and as they say, the rest is history. In 1959 Russell and Burch published their influential book *The Principles of Humane Experimental Technique*, and this year (2009) has seen many appreciations and celebrations of the 50th anniversary of this truly groundbreaking event in the evolution of experimental research.

However, let it not be forgotten, that some 12 years before the Russell and Burch book was published there was another seminal literary event. In 1947 there appeared the first edition of the UFAW handbook, edited by Alastair Worden. That book, which ran to some 368 pages, was also hugely influential and provided a template for best practice for the use of animals in research. From those important beginnings, and through a series of succeeding editions, has evolved this current *tour de force*. This 8th edition is a magnificent achievement and represents a truly comprehensive and authoritative work embracing in 50 very detailed chapters all aspects of animal care and husbandry.

This book, which will serve to inform and guide practice for years to come, is a timely reminder of what UFAW has achieved. The many authors that have contributed to this work, and in particular the editors who have undertaken the Herculean task of producing a volume of such quality, are to be warmly congratulated.

This is an important job well done.

Professor Ian Kimber
Professor of Toxicology
University of Manchester
Faculty of Life Sciences
Manchester, UK

1 Introduction

Robert Hubrecht and James Kirkwood

It is widely accepted, and implicit in the legislation of many countries, that animals used in research should be kept as far as possible in a state of good welfare. This duty of care is not only a legal and ethical obligation but is also very often necessary to achieve high-quality science. Animals housed in conditions that meet their needs are much less likely to be stressed, a state which can bias results or result in increased variation between animals as they attempt to cope with the stressor. Therefore, it is often said that good animal welfare is in both the animals' and the scientists' best interests. From the very first edition of the Handbook in 1947, the UFAW Laboratory Animal Handbook has promoted the importance of high standards of care for animals used in research. Indeed, the 1947 edition was the first manual on laboratory animal care and housing ever to be published and was instrumental in stimulating the development of laboratory animal care as a fundamental component of laboratory animal science. Since then, it has remained an internationally valued resource that has helped to refine laboratory animal use and to advance the Three Rs (3 Rs – replacement, reduction and refinement), originally described in 1959 by the UFAW scholars Russell and Burch in the *Principles of Humane Experimental Technique*, and now generally accepted as the key ethical principles under which animal experimentation should be carried out.

Professor, Sir Harold Himsworth, Honorary Physician to the Queen and a prominent scientist in the study of diabetes, stated in a foreword to the 3rd edition in 1959 that, '*Good intentions and wishful thinking are never enough when faced with natural problems. Knowledge and yet more knowledge is needed.*' Yet it is not always easy to acquire this knowledge. It is hard to shake off the biases of anthropomorphism and anthropocentrism to establish the real requirements of animals. Nonetheless, since the publication of the previous 7th edition, there have been considerable scientific developments in the field of laboratory animal welfare that fully justify the production of this updated volume.

We have included in this edition 10 new chapters on implementing the Three Rs in research, addressing areas that have developed considerably since the last edition and drawing attention to some important general principles. There has been a dramatic increase in the numbers of genetically altered animals used in research, mainly mice, and so we have included a chapter on phenotyping to draw attention to techniques that can be used to better characterise these animals and identify welfare issues. Good experimental design, which has implications on the numbers of animals used, needs to take account of genetic status and sometimes of housing conditions. Given the importance of these considerations, a general introduction to experimental design is included that we hope will be of use, not only to animal care staff, but also to researchers and those involved in ethical review. The implications of research on wild animals, often not within a closely controlled laboratory environment and in some cases in the field, are not always well understood, and so we have included chapters to address issues relating to these animals. This edition also includes a chapter on the use of non-traditional laboratory animals – those not commonly used in biomedical research.

Since the 7th edition there have been considerable developments in animal welfare research relating to both the methodology of assessing animal welfare and the use of new techniques to judge the importance of environmental provisions aimed at allowing animals to express strongly motivated behaviours. These advances are reflected within the husbandry sections of individual chapters, and in the chapters on assessing welfare and the provision of enrichment. Finally, we have included chapters on: legislation and the oversight of animal experiments – at both local and national level; on training and competence assessment; and on euthanasia.

We have also made other changes. The previous edition was published as two volumes but this time we have reverted to a single volume, which we believe will be more convenient as a source of information. It is not possible to cover all the species used in research around the world but we have provided chapters on the most commonly used species or groups of species. Fish are becoming increasingly used in research, and we have provided updated information in a chapter on general issues common to marine and freshwater fish.

We have endeavoured as editors to ensure that the chapters reflect UFAW's approach to the care and husbandry of animals used in research, however the chapters are the individual authors' work and the views they have expressed should not be taken as UFAW's official opinions. We have included a chapter on chimpanzees although not all countries use or permit their use. As with other species, their inclusion in this book is not meant to imply approval of their use, but is to encourage implementation of high standards of care.

It is very important to us that The UFAW Handbook should be an international resource, so we have tried to ensure that the text is not overly biased towards the European situation. However, at the time of writing there has been a recent review of European standards of housing (Appendix A to Council of Europe ETS 123 and Annex II to European Directive 86/609). In addition, changes to the European legislation (European Directive 86/609) are being debated that might affect both its scope and the regulation of animal care. Many chapters make reference to these changes to draw attention to recent views on minimum appropriate standards and possible future legal obligations. It is, of course, the responsibility of those working with animals to ensure that the practices they adopt comply with national legislation relating to health and safety and animal welfare.

It has been our goal to produce an authoritative resource in the tradition of previous editions of the Laboratory Handbook. The best information about animals' needs and how these can be met, is based on well planned and executed animal welfare science studies published in the refereed scientific literature. However, many aspects of animal husbandry have not yet received such detailed scientific investigation and are based on practices that are considered through practical experience to be suitable. To help us to ensure that as far as possible the chapters reflect good current practice and are a guide for future developments, all the chapters in the Handbook have been peer reviewed by anonymous referees. We are enormously grateful to all those who have undertaken these reviews, for their time and expertise and for their advice which has been of great assistance to both editors and authors.

We are also extremely grateful to the authors for their time and energy in distilling the research literature and their practical experiences into concise and valuable chapters, to AstraZeneca for a generous donation towards the production costs, and to Laboratory Animals Limited for their help in promoting this volume. We hope that this Handbook will be a useful resource for all those caring for and working with animals used in science, and that it will help promote good animal welfare and good science.

PART 1
IMPLEMENTING THE THREE Rs IN RESEARCH USING ANIMALS

2 The Three Rs

Jon Richmond

Opening remarks

The Universities Federation for Animal Welfare (UFAW) promotes the welfare of animals bred, kept and used for experimental and other scientific purposes by:

- adopting a scientific approach to animal welfare, providing evidence-based insights into *'what is meaningful to the animal'*; and
- advocating that *'best welfare is indeed best science'* and that we must *'... aim at well-being rather than at mere absence of distress'* (Russell & Burch 1959).

In 1954 UFAW commissioned work by William Russell and Rex Burch which led to the publication in 1959 of *The Principles of Humane Experimental Technique* (Russell & Burch 1959). Russell and Burch demonstrated that high standards of animal welfare underpin good science, indeed that better welfare facilitates better science, arguing that *'... humanity can be promoted without prejudice to scientific and medical aims'* and *'... the humanest possible treatment of experimental animals ... is actually a prerequisite for successful animal experiments'*. They advised that:

> *... If we are to use a criterion for choosing experiments to perform, the criterion of humanity is the best we could possibly invent ... The greatest scientific experiments have always been the most humane and most aesthetically attractive, conveying that sense of beauty and which is the essence of science at its most successful. ...*

That is, the Three Rs (3Rs) are part of mainstream science, not something separate from it.

This chapter provides an overview to the Three Rs of humane experimental technique as they have evolved in the half-century since Russell and Burch's landmark publication, focusing on general principles, as a prelude to the more detailed and context-specific material contained in later chapters.

Introduction

The use of animals for scientific purposes is an emotive and sensitive issue, and must be conducted with care and compassion. Whilst there are national and cultural differences in the precise language used, and the protection offered, it is now generally accepted that some animals, such as the vertebrates, are likely to be able to experience pain, suffering and distress. All of those involved in the care and use of live animals for scientific or other experimental purposes have a moral, and in many cases a legal, obligation to minimise any justifiable suffering caused.

It is generally accepted that animal studies should only be undertaken when all of the following conditions are met:

- the scientific objectives are timely, of sufficient importance and attainable;
- there is no non-sentient replacement alternative;
- all relevant and practical reduction and refinement strategies have been implemented;
- the design and conduct of the study minimises the animal welfare cost as reflected in the total pain, suffering and distress that may be produced, and not simply the number of animals used;
- the scientific and societal benefits are maximised.

Animal welfare is a complex issue: it comprises not only the health of an animal, but also its state of well-being. It has both physical and psychological dimensions and can be compromised not only by the infliction of that which is unpleasant, but also by the denial of that which is pleasurable.

Implementing humane experimental technique requires: knowledge and understanding of behaviours and findings in normal animals; the impact of care systems and scientific procedures; how welfare can be evaluated; and the development and application of informed, practical solutions.

The acceptance of the principles of humane experimental technique established by Russell and Burch (1959) led to a period of reducing animal use and significant welfare gains, at a time of increasing investment and rapid advances in the biomedical sciences. However, the use of animals for experimental and other scientific purposes is again increasing, primarily due to the production and use of genetically altered animals (Home Office 2007). The established principles of humane experimental technique are, nevertheless, sufficiently wide-ranging and flexible to be applicable to this class of animal use not foreseen at the time of Russell and Burch's publication.

There is a need to ensure, as new technologies and trends emerge and new and revised regulatory requirements are introduced, that the principles of humane experimental technique inform strategic thinking, regulatory frameworks and scientific and husbandry practices.

Model systems

Early scientific use of animals was generally curiosity-driven, and involved demonstrating biological phenomena without necessarily having practical applications in mind (Barley 1999). The imperative subsequently shifted towards understanding the underlying mechanisms and regulation of observed phenomena. We are now largely in the era of 'deductive science': formulating and testing hypotheses with practical applications, with the results being widely published. These differing approaches to science are still reflected in the types of studies undertaken and animal models used (Festing 2000):

- exploratory models generate knowledge without necessarily being relevant to any immediate practical application;
- explanatory models elucidate the mechanisms;
- predictive models allow problem solving and decision making.

The high-fidelity fallacy

For the most part, animals in science are now used to model complex and dynamic biological systems. Both animal and non-animal models mimic only limited aspects of the human condition or other system of interest (Sams-Dodd 2006) and this must be kept in mind when the most appropriate model is selected, and findings analysed, interpreted, generalised and extrapolated.

Russell and Burch (1959) warned of the 'high-fidelity fallacy': the false assumption that high fidelity (the closeness in biological terms of a model system to the actual system of interest) equates to a sound model system. Non-human primates can be considered to be high-fidelity models of man as *'in their general physiological and pharmacological properties'* they are *'more consistently like us than are other organisms'*. However, any instinctive preference for high-fidelity models *'ignores all the advantages of correlation'*, whereby *'the responses of two utterly different systems may be correlated with perfect regularity'*. High-fidelity models are not necessarily required in practice as what is essential is not that a model system 'looks like' the system of interest, but that it behaves like it. High-discrimination models are the required scientific tools. This is a key concept. The essential quality of a good model system is high discrimination: its ability, in the context of a defined biological process or outcome, to produce responses which correlate with the response of the system which they model.

Replacement alternatives (for example isolated tissues, cell cultures and computer models) are high discrimination but, inevitably, low fidelity. They *'reproduce one particular property of the original, in which we happen to be interested'*. The Limulus Amoebocyte Lysate test (Levin & Bang 1964), used to detect the presence of Gram-negative endotoxins in a range of materials used in clinical practice, is an example of a low-fidelity/high-discrimination model. It does not use mammalian tissue; does not rely on reproducing the pyrexia and other systemic adverse effects seen when Gram-negative endotoxins interact with mammalian systems; but instead reliably demonstrates the presence of Gram-negative endotoxins by a specific change in the haemolymph of horseshoe crabs.

The Three Rs

The concepts of replacement, reduction and refinement in relation to the use of animals in science can be traced back to Victorian Britain (Richmond 2000). An 1839 London Medical Gazette editorial advised that live animals should not be used:

> ... *till it is sufficiently clear that the fact pursued neither is, nor can be proved by any other evidence which is within reach, nor by any more mode of enquiry.* (Anon. 1839)

The principles of humane experimental technique also feature in Marshall Hall's publications from the same period. In an 1847 Lancet article he wrote:

> *We should never have recourse to experiment in cases which observation can afford us the information required; No experiment should be performed without a distinct and definite object and without the persuasion that the object will be attained and produce a real and uncomplicated result; We should not needlessly repeat experiments and cause the least possible suffering, using the lowest order of animals and avoiding the infliction of pain; We should try to secure due observation so as to avoid the necessity of repetition.* (Hall 1847)

Russell and Burch (1959) subsequently provided a conceptual framework where humane animal care and use was set in the context of the need, whilst safeguarding or enhancing the quality of the science undertaken. This framework requires the implementation of all reasonable and practical means available to replace sentient animals; the reduction to the necessary minimum of the numbers used; the refinement of their production, care and use to minimise the suffering caused; and the promotion of research relevant to replacement, reduction and refinement.

They referred to replacement, reduction and refinement as the principles of humane experimental technique, but not as 'alternative methods' or the '3 Rs'. The earliest reference to replacement, reduction and refinement as the *'Three Rs'* is in David Smyth's book *Alternatives to Living Animals* (Smyth 1978).

Russell and Burch (1959) defined:

- replacement as *'any scientific method employing non-sentient material which may in the history of animal experimentation replace methods which use conscious living vertebrates'*;
- reduction as means of minimising, other than by replacement, *'the number of animals used to obtain information of a given amount and precision'*;
- refinement as measures leading to a *'decrease in the incidence or severity of inhumane procedures applied to those animals which have to be used'*.

Progress with the Three Rs is not solely, or even primarily, driven by a desire to improve animal welfare. Methodological improvements are required to overcome the limitations of existing animal models and open up new lines of scientific enquiry. In practice, 'alternative' methods are generally more technically 'advanced', cost effective, reliable, easily scalable and scientifically valid than those traditionally used.

Thus the case for the Three Rs can be made simultaneously on three grounds:

- better animal welfare;
- better science in terms of quality and rate of progress;
- logistics and economics.

A holistic approach

A holistic, rather than sequential, approach to the Three Rs is required, particularly with respect to reduction and refinement where tensions can exist, balances may have to be struck and synergies exploited. In all cases decisions must be taken on a case-by-case basis in the context of the specific scientific objectives being pursued.

Simple words: complex meanings

The commonly used definitions of replacement, reduction and refinement are deceptively simple, and the use of these everyday words conceals subtleties of meaning that must be carefully considered and fully understood in order to appreciate the power and relevance of the Three Rs. Even the term 'alternatives' can mislead by creating the false impression that only replacement is relevant; and that alternative methods simply substitute for, but retain the scope and limitations of, the original animal models.

Replacement methods are not just substitutes for animal models: they are often better science, more powerful and versatile and the tools of choice. For example the use of robotics and *in vitro* replacement systems for high-throughput screening of potential novel pharmaceuticals allows rates of progress not previously possible using animal models.

Reduction is best considered as minimisation or optimisation of animal numbers. The intention is to minimise the number of animals required to provide suitably robust data: using more is wasteful; using fewer at best requires that work is repeated and at worst results in misleading conclusions being drawn from the available data. There are occasions when the original estimates of the number of animals required prove on examination to be too few to meet the scientific objective, and on these occasions applying the principles of reduction will result in the intentional use of more animals than originally estimated.

The total number of animals used annually for experimental and other scientific purposes is determined by a range of factors, including the level of spending on science (which is increasing in real terms), strategic funding priorities (for example better understanding of gene function and control), the availability of new technologies (such as the ability to produce genetically altered animals) and changes in regulations to protect man and the environment (for example the European Union REACH legislation). Because of such drivers, progress with replacement and reduction cannot be judged simply on the basis of the total number of animals used for experimental and other scientific purposes. However, there are specific classes of animal use where replacement and reduction have had a demonstrable impact; for example improved tissue culture systems have effectively ended the use of animals to produce monoclonal antibodies by the ascites method; and the use of the Limulus Amoebocyte Lysate test has reduced the use of rabbits for pyrogen testing.

In some cases, to minimise welfare costs, balances have to be struck between reduction and refinement. More aggressive protocols, the intensive re-use of animals and less refined endpoints may allow scientific objectives to be attained using fewer animals, but at a disproportionate welfare cost. On other occasions, there may be a choice to be made between the use of asymptomatic large-animal models which will not experience significant pain, suffering or distress; and symptomatic small-animal models which will. Experience and expert judgment may be required to determine which option is both scientifically satisfactory and minimises the overall likely suffering. In all cases, the correct and most humane principle that can be applied is to minimise the total suffering that might be caused, without compromising the scientific objective, and without imposing an unreasonable welfare cost on any experimental subject (Richmond 1999).

Despite the tremendous progress that has been made with refinement, as evidenced by numerous practical instances detailed elsewhere in this book, it has proved difficult to date to capture and publish definitive data, other than case studies, which objectively demonstrate the resulting aggregate welfare gains.

Scientific validation and regulatory acceptance

The adoption of new and improved research technologies depends on the publication and acceptance of technical progress. However, in many cases little or no prominence is given to progress with the Three Rs in mainstream core-science journals, and, although there are specialist publications and websites dedicated to the Three Rs, this literature may be unfamiliar to many scientists.

Formal scientific validation of alternative methods with respect to their relevance and reliability for their stated purpose, is required if non-animal tests, and more refined animal tests, are to gain regulatory acceptance. Scientific validation addresses test optimisation and definition, within-laboratory variability, transferability between laboratories, between-laboratory variability, predictive capacity, applicability domain and minimum performance standards (Balls *et al.* 1995). Although these can be addressed in a sequential process, *'modular'* approaches (Hartung *et al.* 2004) have been developed to take account the non-sequential development of alternatives; as have *'weight-of-evidence'*

(Balls *et al.* 2006) and 'catch-up' schemes to cope more efficiently with variations on existing methods.

The scientific validation of replacement, reduction and refinement alternatives is fraught with problems.

Although the most appropriate means to assess the validity of any replacement or more refined method would seem to be a direct comparison of its performance against reliable human (or other target species) data, this is seldom possible. Where animal test data is available the inherent variability, indeed unreliability, of some existing animal models presents difficulties. Available animal data tends to be of variable quality, generated using test systems not themselves fully standardised or scientifically validated, and which imperfectly reproduce the human response. An improved alternative test that has greater specificity or sensitivity, although better science and more reliable, will therefore give different results to the established animal model. The inability to reproduce strictly the results obtained with imperfect but established test methods can delay the validation and acceptance of new and improved test systems. In addition there is still no efficient global mechanism for the rapid regulatory acceptance and use of newly validated test methods.

Training and teamwork

The ability to review that which has already been reported and to make new connections, or offer new insights, is common to success in many walks of life. It should be regarded as a core competence of all of those involved in the care and use of animals for scientific purposes. A scientific training and continuing professional development should instil and maintain the knowledge, mindset and practices that place the Three Rs at the heart of animal-based research and testing. The objective is not only to equip individuals with factual knowledge and technical skills relating to their immediate area of scientific interest, but also to develop the other competencies required to plan, conduct, assess and report high-quality, humane research and to keep abreast of technical progress.

This includes awareness and acceptance that expert input from others is required, as it is no longer possible for any one person to have all of the necessary knowledge and skills; and even the largest research teams may at times have to seek expert advice. For example, with the relentless increase in information available in both peer-reviewed journals and the internet, accessing and assessing relevant information increasingly needs specialist training and skills, requiring either the training of scientists to do this better, or placing reliance on information specialists. In addition, it is no more reasonable to expect a short training course in statistics to turn a biological scientist into a competent statistician, than it would be to expect an equally short training in the biological sciences to turn a statistician into a competent biological scientist.

For these reasons many research organisations provide institutional-level expert support with elements of animal care and use, experimental design, laboratory animal science and veterinary medicine.

Replacement

Although we do not currently have the means to replace all forms of animal use without slowing or halting scientific progress in many areas of research and testing, replacement is relevant to fundamental and applied biomedical research, regulatory testing and the use of animals for education and training. Replacement alternatives offer a range of benefits over the animal models they supersede, often allowing more rapid progress than was possible using animal models and in some cases providing scientific insights not possible using animal models.

Russell and Burch (1959) defined replacement as *'any scientific method employing non-sentient material which may in the history of animal experimentation replace methods which use conscious living vertebrates'*, distinguishing between 'absolute' replacement, with no sentient animal use (for example computer models), and 'relative' replacement, using animals in non-painful procedures (for example humane killing to obtain tissue, or the use of immature forms incapable of experiencing pain, suffering or distress).

Replacement alternatives must be based on good science and produce responses that correlate with those of biological systems which they model. Their development requires an understanding of the underlying biological mechanisms and their responses; and is often dependent on the availability (or *de novo* generation) of reliable animal or human reference data, and appropriate non-animal technologies.

Progress with replacement models has, to date, been largely with single-stage processes involving biological effects mediated by clearly understood single-event mechanisms, and for which there is high-quality human or relevant animal data. Devising non-animal models of more dynamic and complex biological interactions is more difficult; although a 2007 NC3Rs workshop has indicated that even with processes as complex as emesis there are signs that non-sentient test systems are possible and perhaps even within reach.

The range of replacement options can be deceptively wide and may include:

- strategies avoiding the need to generate new animal-based data;
- systems allowing elements of evidence gathering, analysis or decision making to be undertaken without live animal use;
- methods and models providing the required insights without causing procedure-related pain, suffering or distress to sentient animals.

Replacement strategies and systems

In some instances, scientific objectives can be achieved without the need for additional animal use. Examples include:

- Amending regulatory requirements and provisions to dispense with inessential tests: for example the Abnormal Toxicity Test (Schwanig *et al.* 1997) is no longer required for the evaluation of a range of products used in clinical practice.

- Harmonising international validation processes, regulatory testing requirements and decision making to eliminate the need to use animals in different protocols to inform multiple regulators about a single toxicological endpoint.
- Reformulating scientific objectives to allow relevant insights to be gained using existing data or new non-animal data.
- Reviewing published work to ensure that relevant existing data is not overlooked and animal experiments inadvertently replicated. There is, however, an important distinction to make between unnecessary duplication (the unintended repetition of studies that have already been completed and reported) and justified, intentional replication. This latter class of animal use may be necessary when introducing new model systems, evaluating procedural changes, restarting programmes of work after periods of inactivity or changing laboratories or key personnel.
- Data sharing where previous relevant findings have not been published – for example accessing data generated for in-house decision making or contained in regulatory submissions.

Replacement methods and models

Where additional data are required, a wide range of replacement methods and models can be considered:

- The use of physico-chemical properties to predict biological effects to screen or fully evaluate test materials. Examples include the use of pH and buffer capacity to predict potential severe ocular irritation or corrosion; and the use of computer models, generally strictly limited in scope and heavily dependent on reliable *in vivo* data, allowing molecular structure to be correlated with specific biological activities.
- The use of non-sentient organisms. Examples include the use of bacteria to assess genotoxic potential (Ames *et al.* 1973).
- The use of immature forms of sentient species incapable of experiencing pain, suffering or distress; for example fish larvae to evaluate aquatic toxicity.
- The use of *ex vivo* and *in vitro* systems, of animal or human origin, at the level of the organ, tissue slice, cell culture/suspension or sub-cellular component. These may be absolute replacements (for example non-primary cell cultures that do not require to be maintained using foetal calf serum), or relative replacements (for example animal primary-cell cultures, or other cell culture systems requiring the use of foetal calf serum).
- Human studies, subject to appropriate ethical safeguards. Data may be gathered in the course of volunteer, clinical-trial, post-marketing surveillance or epidemiological studies. New technologies (for example improved methods of diagnostic imaging, and pre-clinical markers of biological effects) can offer new opportunities to work with human subjects.
- A wide range of replacement alternatives can be used in education and training to demonstrate biological phenomena, processes and interactions; train participants in manual skills; and develop problem-solving skills. These include models, films and videotapes of procedures, interactive software simulations, courseware on compact discs and interactive laser discs, and virtual reality systems. See, for example, the Interniche website[1].

Reduction

Russell and Burch (1959) defined reduction as *'reduction in the number of animals used to obtain information of a given amount and precision'* other than by replacement, stressing the imperative to use the right number rather than too many or too few.

Reduction can be considered to comprise any strategy or method which:

- other than by replacement reduces the need for animal studies; or
- minimises the number of animals required to achieve a defined scientific objective; or
- permits more data or product to be obtained from the animals that must still be used.

Reduction and refinement must always be considered simultaneously. Focusing purely on decreasing numbers can lead to solutions that reduce the numbers used, but produce a disproportionate increase in the pain and distress caused to the animals that are used (Richmond 1999).

Whilst statistical elements of experimental design such as sample size, power, variation, precision and the proper application of appropriate statistical methods are important means of determining the number of animals required and interpreting the data that is generated (Festing & Altman 2002), there are equally important non-statistical reduction considerations such as selection of suitable experimental subjects, husbandry and care systems, procedural details and other means of controlling and minimising unwanted stressors and unnecessary variables (see Chapters 3–16).

It is important to be aware of the full range of reduction options and opportunities.

- The sequence in which objectives are pursued and experiments are carried out are important considerations.
- One of the most effective means of minimising the numbers of animals required for a programme of work is to apply tiered and hierarchical approaches to enable the early identification and discarding of materials (and hypothesis) not destined for further development, thus obviating the need for inessential animal studies. Taking the assessment of the ocular safety of materials as an example (Gallegos Saliner & Worth 2007): considering physicochemical properties; considering *in vitro* test results; conducting dermal safety tests; and identifying strong skin irritants and corrosive materials, enable a reliable evaluation to be made of likely ocular safety without the need to undertake tests on live animals. When ocular safety tests on live animals are

[1] http://www.interniche.org/

still required, testing first on a single animal can reduce the number of animals used as materials giving strong positives in a single animal do not require confirmatory testing using additional animals. These examples also link to refinement, dispensing with the need to use animals to test materials most likely to cause the greatest degrees of pain, suffering, distress and lasting harm. In other contexts, small proof-of-concept studies, if they fail to demonstrate the expected outcomes, obviate the need for failed large-scale definitive studies.

 - Preliminary *in vitro* data can reduce the number of animals required for definitive studies.
 - Although no single *in vitro* test, indeed no battery of such tests, has yet been scientifically validated as a full replacement for the live rabbit ocular safety test, a positive test result for some classes of test materials in some *in vitro* test systems can be accepted as evidence of ocular corrosive or severe irritant potential, requiring that only materials testing negative in the *in vitro* systems are further characterised using live animals (Gallegos Saliner & Worth 2007). This example again links to refinement.
 - Preliminary cytotoxicity data is now used to reduce the number of animals used in acute toxicity studies by determining the appropriate doses of test materials to be used in the animal studies (ICCVAM 2001).

- Sometimes definitive studies can only be planned in detail once preliminary animal data are available:
  - Pilot experiments are small-scale preliminary studies to examine the logistics of proposed definitive studies (see Chapter 3). In many cases the results will not be published, but will be used to design improved definitive studies. Procedural improvements can include insights into: likely inter-individual variation and the number of animals required to obtain robust scientific results; the most appropriate dosing and sampling regimens; the nature, incidence, severity and timing of possible physiological, behavioural changes and adverse effects; and how they can best be avoided, elucidated or managed. Importantly, they may identify and remedy unexpected, extraneous experimental variables before larger-scale studies are undertaken.
- The number of animals required to meet the scientific objectives reflects the required degree of precision and certainty; thus the number of animals required should be no more than is necessary to meet the scientific objective:
  - There may be opportunities for reducing the number of animals required by taking account of prevalence of the outcome of interest (Hoffmann & Hartung 2006): it may require less data to identify candidate test materials with a common property, than with an uncommon property.
  - Where test materials are only to be assigned to general categories, requiring only an estimate of their biological properties, smaller numbers of animals may be sufficient rather than the larger numbers required to calculate the more precise or absolute values necessary to place test materials in rank order.
- Making appropriate use of control groups and data:
  - A negative control is known to give a negative result, acting as a means of demonstrating the baseline result obtained when a test was conducted, and confirming that the basic conditions of the test system were able to produce appropriate negative results even if the experiment does not produce a negative result.
  - A positive control is treated to produce a positive result under normal conditions, confirming that the basic conditions of the test system were able to produce appropriate positive results even if the experiment does not produce a positive result.
  - Control and other experimental groups are in all other respects exposed to identical conditions, observations and investigations.
  - Control groups can be used as standards for comparison, making conclusions about the relevance and significance of the results more robust by demonstrating that the test system is appropriately responsive; eliminating alternative explanations of experimental results (the possibility that the experimental subjects were prone to, or incapable of, giving appropriate positive or negative results); and taking account of other potential confounding variables within the test system (for example the chance that some unrecognised intercurrent problem influenced the responses observed).
  - In cases where the experiment causes substantial suffering it may be possible to reduce the numbers of animals in the treatment group but increase the numbers in the control group (by more than the numbers reduced in the treatment group). This technique results in the same statistical power, but fewer animals suffering in the treatment group. This example illustrates the need for taking informed decisions when refinement, in the sense of the total suffering that may be caused, must be balanced against outcomes requiring the use of larger numbers of animals.
  - When there is a need for control data, the number of animals might, in some circumstances, be minimised by the use of a single concurrent control to evaluate simultaneously a range of test materials for the same biological property, or by the use of historical controls. Both of these are relevant, for example, when animals are used to evaluate the skin sensitisation potential of test materials. In these studies a single control group may suffice when a number of test materials are tested in the same laboratory on the same day. Moreover, the routine use of concurrent positive controls, to demonstrate that the test method as applied in a laboratory can produce an appropriate positive response, is generally unnecessary if the routine testing programme itself regularly produces both positive and negative results.
- In some circumstances, a disproportionately large amount of additional information can be gained from

the use of small additional satellite groups to pursue more than one scientific objective within a single experiment. For example, toxicokinetic data can be gathered in the course of single-dose toxicity studies (ICH 1994).

- The degree of uniformity/lack of variability within and between experimental subjects is an important determinant of the number of experimental subjects required, and all reasonable efforts should be made to control relevant genetic and epigenetic factors and promote uniformity. In this context there are many synergies between reduction and refinement:
  - The use of purpose-bred animals permits varying degrees of control of genetic variability and microbiological status, and for many of the commonly used species the availability of inbred and isogenic strains allows the use of smaller group sizes than is possible with outbred or random-bred animals (see Chapter 4). In some instances the use of genetically identical animals allows scientific progress to be made that would otherwise be impossible (Festing & Fisher 2000).
  - Variability can be further reduced by providing a controlled and standardised environment, with the most uniform populations and results being produced when the environment is optimal for the animals' well-being (Chance 1957; Chance & Russell 1997). Variation (and therefore sample size) is reduced, not simply by ensuring a uniform environment, but by providing specific environmental conditions.
  - Stressed animals have different baseline behaviours, physiological findings and range of responses to experimental interventions, from unstressed animals. Therefore, all reasonable efforts should be made to identify and remove or minimise unnecessary stressors (Poole 1997).
- Even when the number of animals required for a given experiment cannot be reduced, there may be some scope to reduce the number of animals required for a programme of work by the responsible re-use of animals:
  - ○ Re-use may be defined as the second or subsequent scientific use of an animal that has already completed a series of procedures for a defined scientific purpose when the use of a naïve, unused animal would have also been scientifically satisfactory.
  - ○ Whilst re-use may reduce the total of number of animals required for programmes of work, it has to be balanced against the resulting increased, cumulative suffering experienced by the individual re-used animals.
  - ○ Re-use should only be considered when the following conditions are met:
    1. The first use has not compromised the suitability of the animal for the second or subsequent use (for example animals which have been exposed to a pathogen or immunogen will not give a naïve response if subsequently re-exposed).
    2. Animals experienced only minimal pain, suffering and distress, and no lasting harm, from their earlier use.
    3. The animals have been shown on a case-by-case basis by a competent person, after completion of the first use, to have been restored to a normal state of well-being.

    Examples include the re-use of rabbits which have given negative results in skin irritation tests for a single ocular safety study; the use of animals as blood donors; and, subject to suitable recovery periods, the re-use of dogs or non-human primates in pharmacokinetic studies.
- Matching the production of animals and the availability of animal tissues to known or likely demand avoids waste. Common examples include cryo-preservation of genetically altered animal lines (Glenister & Rall 2000) rather than maintaining 'tick-over' colonies, and through in-house tissue-sharing schemes finding scientific uses for tissue harvested when breeding stock are humanely killed.
- Retrospective analyses of results may show that the number of animals needed could in future be reduced without loss of precision. This has been found to be the case with some vaccine potency assays (Hendriksen & Steen 2000).

Synergies and conflicts

It is clear from the above that reduction and refinement are interrelated and must be considered concurrently.

In addition there are technologies that involve initial surgical preparation but which then reduce the total number of animals required, minimise the stress animals subsequently experience and improve the quality of the findings. For example, there is a range of implantable telemetery devices (Kramer & Kinter 2003) that allow the remote capture of intermittent or continuous streams of 'physiological data' whilst animals undertake normal activities unstressed by disturbances to the social group, sedation, handling or restraint. These technologies may permit the numbers of animals per study to be reduced by the capture of serial data and the re-use of telemeterised animals.

In such cases there are trade-offs to be made between the welfare costs of the initial surgical preparation, the reduction in the number of animals required to give meaningful results, the procedural stresses that can be avoided after recovery from surgery and the improved nature and quality of the data that can be gathered (Brockway *et al.* 1993; Schnell & Gerber 1997), illustrating the interaction between the Three Rs, and the need to take a holistic rather than a sequential approach when putting humane experimental technique into practice.

Refinement

Russell and Burch (1959) defined refinement as measures leading to a '*decrease in the incidence or severity of inhumane procedures applied to those animals which have to be used*'.

Refinement is not just a matter of minimising the incidence of adverse effects, or the number of animals used; it is minimising the total pain, suffering, distress and lasting harm that may be caused. A higher incidence of findings not indicative of a high welfare cost, such as reduced weight gain, may be preferable to a lower incidence of endpoints clearly indicative of higher levels of suffering.

The significance of refinement

Refinement improves the quality of life of every animal bred, kept and used for experimental and other scientific purposes, and benefits every programme of work using live animals.

Consideration of refinement starts the moment there is an intention to breed or keep an animal for experimental or other scientific purposes; continues throughout the scientific use of the animal until it is humanely killed or otherwise disposed of; and does not end until the lessons learned are incorporated into future practice.

If research findings are to be considered meaningful then, before the scientific procedures are applied, the animals will ideally have physiological parameters and behaviours within the normal range. More refined systems of care and use, or rather the higher welfare state they produce, impact on experimental findings (Poole 1997; Bayne 2005). A key concept is that the impact of refinement on research findings must be seen as a stimulus rather than a barrier to developing and accepting more refined methods – as refinement, high standards of welfare, normal experimental subjects and good science go hand-in-hand. The possible limitations and inadequacies of data sets and conclusions obtained with less refined practices, rather than constituting a criticism of the scientific validity of data obtained by more refined methods, are an indictment of the reliability of the less refined methods. The fact that more refined methods might influence results is thus a powerful reason to accept, rather than resist, progress and change.

Staff competencies and responsibilities

Animals in captivity are totally dependent on man for their well-being, and the attitudes and skills of those responsible for their care and use are the most important factors in achieving high welfare standards and conducting sound science. In addition to being technically competent, it is important that all staff develop and display an appropriate 'culture of care'.

The best and most refined use of animals in science requires a multidisciplinary, team approach. Laboratory animal veterinarians, laboratory animal scientists and animal care staff must play an active and expert part in refining animal care and use. Staff must be trained to recognise both normal behaviours and signs of pain and distress, both to improve all aspects of animal care and facilitate the recognition of experimental effects.

Those responsible for assessing animal welfare must be empowered to make the best provision for their housing, care and use; and to take prompt action when scientific and welfare endpoints are approached or reached. They must be aware of contingency plans to deal with unexpected adverse effects.

Assessing well-being

To make proper provision for animal welfare it is essential to understand and recognise what is *'meaningful to the animal'* and to do *'what is right for the animals'* (Russell & Burch 1959). Recognition of an abnormal state depends on an awareness of, and familiarity with, normality in the species and individual under observation. In the absence of evidence to the contrary, it is to be assumed that any stimulus, experience or pathology that produces pain and discomfort in man, also does so in sentient animals (Home Office 1965).

The behavioural and physiological responses of animals to adverse effects are not uniform between species, strains, individuals of the same species and strain, or even in the same individual at different times (Scharmann 1999). Thus assessment of welfare takes place at the level of the individual animal.

Welfare is assessed by taking into account behavioural, physiological, clinical and laboratory findings (see Chapter 6). Of these, behavioural findings and changes are often the earliest, most sensitive and most meaningful indicators.

Confidence in indices of welfare is best placed in findings which:

- occur in an appropriate context;
- progress with the nature and severity of the insult;
- are predictive of the ultimate welfare, clinical or pathological outcomes;
- can be controlled with appropriate specific, supportive or symptomatic measures or treatments.

For example, signs considered to be indicative of pain should occur in contexts where there is reason to believe pain may be present, and should abate with prompt, effective analgesic administration. However, it is important to recognise that:

- animals may be distressed, though not in pain, and therefore display signs which analgesics will not alleviate – this may be seen for example in animals with locomotor impairments due to neurological damage;
- analgesics can have direct pharmacological effects unrelated to pain relief producing behavioural changes and altering clinical findings (Roughan & Flecknell 2000);
- identifying and managing chronic pain and distress, where the signs can be insidious, pose particular difficulties (Flecknell & Roughan 2004).

As the judgement of animal well-being ultimately rests with humans a degree of critical anthropomorphism is perhaps inevitable. 'Critical' in this context implies empathy tempered with objective knowledge of the animal, its needs and normal behaviours; preceding events; and the significance of any signs which may be seen.

Expert judgement can be required to understand the scope, limitations, possible interpretations and significance of even seemingly objective measures. Pitfalls to be borne in mind include:

- demonstrating behavioural or physiological differences contingent upon changes to an animal's environment. Otherwise, the procedures applied may not clearly indicate which represents the lesser welfare cost or higher welfare state;
- preference testing (Kirkden & Pajor 2006) may only identify the least objectionable rather than the optimum option, and short-term preferences may not be indicative of long-term preferences, needs and benefits;
- although technology is improving, measuring even basic physiological phenomena and behaviours sometimes requires additional interventions that add welfare costs or alter the parameters being measured.

Severity scoring systems

A number of disturbance indices and severity scoring systems (see, for example, Hendriksen & Morton 1999) have been developed to assist with the assessment of the welfare of animals used for experimental purposes, to identify protocols with high welfare costs where work on replacement or refinement might most usefully be commissioned, and to evaluate the impact of potential refinement measures (see Chapter 6).

Such systems are based upon discrete and continuous indices of welfare, with continuous variables categorised to reflect what we understand to be meaningful differences in levels of significance and suffering. Combinations of signs tend to be more significant than the occurrence of any sign in isolation. Although they must be contextualised and adapted to reflect the research objectives, models and protocols, they are valid whether impaired welfare is due to the immediate or delayed, local or systemic, or primary, secondary or tertiary effects of the procedural interventions.

They encourage the use of standard documentation, and plain non-technical language with a limited range of keywords to identify, describe and record findings. These simplify staff training, provide a systematic approach to evaluating welfare and facilitate communication within and between research groups.

Refinement: contingent and direct costs

The welfare costs to animals bred, kept and used for experimental and other scientific purposes have two distinct components (Russell & Burch 1959):

- 'contingent' welfare costs (harms), comprising the welfare-negative aspects of animal production and care whether caused by acts of commission or omission;
- 'direct' costs (harms) resulting form the experimental procedures applied.

Refinement: contingent harms

Animal facilities and care practices must facilitate high standards of animal welfare and high-quality research by eliminating, or controlling and minimising, unwanted variables whilst making the best possible, appropriate provision for the physiological, social and behavioural needs of the animals (see Chapters 9–12).

The physical environment, husbandry, accommodation and care

Many elements of accommodation and care affect the welfare of animals and their response to experimental interventions (Poole 1997; Bayne 2005). These can affect both the validity and reproducibility of findings to an extent that experimental results may only be valid for, and reproducible within, the conditions under which they were obtained.

Ideally, standards of animal care and accommodation would be based on objective evidence of what is required to make best provision for animal welfare. At present much of the evidence required to derive and support such standards does not exist, with guidelines and regulations being based on a combination of the results of welfare research, field research, existing good practice and only making provision for the minimum expected or acceptable standards of care and accommodation (Council of Europe 2006).

Pair- and group-housing

It has been shown in many species that housing with one or more socially compatible conspecific significantly reduces stress, and that being kept singly in isolation compromises both an animal's welfare and its suitability as an experimental subject (Poole 1997). Animals, other than those which are naturally solitary, should be socially housed in stable groups of compatible individuals. Nevertheless, care is required to ensure that pair- and group-housed animals are socially compatible, and it must be remembered that population density and group size influence the physiological and psychological state of the animal and affect experimental responses.

There will be some circumstances, for example the use of a single instrumented animal, when the companion animals will not be experimental subjects yet will be exposed to any contingent harms.

Animals should be singly housed only on veterinary or other welfare grounds, or justified scientific need; in which case animal care and veterinary staff should be involved, and appropriate additional resources targeted at animal welfare.

Space: requirements and structure

The key considerations are the animals' physical and behavioural needs, and how provision for these is best made within the context of their production, care and use.

Basic physiological and ethological needs (such as freedom of movement, appropriate social contact and the ability to withdraw from social conflict; the performance of meaningful activities; and access to food and water) should never be restricted without good cause, and then only to the justifiable minima.

Animals should be provided with a sufficiently spacious and complex environment to facilitate a wide range of normal activities and behaviours, taking account of their physiological and ethological needs. The preferred systems will vary according to species, strain, age, physiological condition, stocking density and group size, and whether animals are kept as stock, for breeding or experiments.

Environmental enrichment

Environmental enrichment (see Chapter 10) covers a wide range of provisions with which a captive animal can interact to promote its physical and psychological well-being. Enrichment can achieve this by allowing and maintaining the expression of normal species-appropriate (and in some cases strain-specific) social interactions, and physical, behavioural and mental activities; or preventing or reducing abnormal physical findings and behaviours.

The laboratory environment can never reproduce the complexity of an animal's natural environment, and the intention is generally to mimic critical natural environmental factors so that normal, strongly motivated behaviours can be expressed, reinforced and maintained (Blanchard & Blanchard 2003). Not all natural behaviours are appropriate in the laboratory setting (Fraser 1993): natural behaviours may represent what the animal needs or wants to, would not normally choose to do (for example, responding to or coping with environmental stressors), or will only choose to do when the opportunity or need arises.

Environmental enrichment options can be categorised as:

- Social enrichment: housing with compatible conspecifics complemented by space of sufficient volume and complexity to permit an appropriate range of species-specific interactions and interaction with man. In many circumstances, social enrichment is both more effective than inanimate physical enrichment, and a prerequisite for the effectiveness of physical enrichment. Appropriate early social experience can be essential for the development of a normal behavioural repertoire; thus conditions at breeding and rearing facilities play a large part in determining the subsequent suitability of animals as experimental subjects or future breeding stock.
- Physical enrichment: including the provision of an adequate amount of suitably structured space, materials to manipulate, sensory stimuli and a varied diet. To prevent or reduce stress-induced behaviours animals should be given a degree of control over their environment by encouraging species-appropriate physical exercise, foraging, manipulative and cognitive activities.

A creative and critical approach is required. Not all changes are beneficial; and if one form of enrichment is chosen others may have to be excluded.

It is important that appropriate options are identified and critically evaluated in terms of immediate and long-term impact on the animals' well-being and on the research objectives (Bayne 2005; Benefiel *et al.* 2005). Assessing the impact of potential environmental enrichments depends on the ability of staff to interpret and draw informed inferences about the animal's state of mind and welfare state. Measures of success can include:

- normalisation of the frequency and duration of appropriate normal activities;
- greater control over the spatial, physical and social environment;
- reduced frequency of abnormal behaviours;
- increased, appropriate and purposeful use of the environment;
- increased ability to adapt to and cope with changes and challenges;
- more robust scientific results.

It cannot be overemphasised that the most important resources required to devise and evaluate environmental enrichment opportunities are competent and caring staff.

Restraint

During the course of a variety of husbandry and scientific procedures, animals may be restrained to minimise the risk of injury to the subject and handler, and facilitate the performance of the procedures. Restraint can be stressful, producing changes in physiological parameters and behaviours depending on the nature, duration and degree of restraint, particularly when the restrained animal is also removed from its enclosure or social group. Appropriate restraint procedures will depend on the species and the nature and duration of the procedure for which the animal is being restrained, with the most refined method of restraint being that which causes the least stress to the animal and its social group.

Training to accept reasonable restraint procedures is possible in a range of species, and has been shown to reduce the resulting physiological and behavioural changes (Wolfensohn & Honess 2005). Consideration should always to the use of procedural training to encourage animals to allow the safe performance of routine procedures without the need for restraint (see Chapter 16).

Marking and identification of animals

Individual animals bred, kept and used for experimental and other scientific purposes need to identifiable. This is generally achieved by marking individual animals rather than identification based on natural physical characteristics. Faced with a choice of effective identification and marking methods, the preferred means is that which causes the least pain, suffering or distress to the animal.

Transport of animals

The transport of animals, between or within establishments, indeed even within a room, can be stressful. All reasonable efforts must be made to avoid or minimise any stress that may be caused, and to ensure that animals are acclimatised to a new environment before being used for scientific purposes (see Chapter 13). Journey times should be minimised, the least stressful modes of transport used, and appropriate contingency plans should be in place.

The subsequent acclimatisation period will vary with the stresses imposed by transportation; the differences in the housing and care systems; and the species, strain and the condition of individual animals. It may be necessary to take expert advice to determine the appropriate minimum period for recovery and acclimatisation, and to confirm that animals have recovered before being used for scientific purposes.

In some cases, welfare costs can be minimised by transporting ova or embryos rather than live animals – and this is also a means of disease control when acquiring animals from facilities of different or unknown microbiological status.

Humane killing

The majority of animals produced and used for scientific purpose are humanely killed as part of, or at the end of, their scientific use – as are surplus stock.

Humane methods of killing (AVMA 2001; Close *et al.* 1996, 1997), when properly applied, typically ensure rapid loss of consciousness without producing signs of pain or distress, and result in the death of an animal with a minimum of physical and mental suffering. They should also be aesthetically acceptable, and must incorporate careful and compassionate animal handling routines that avoid or minimise the stress due to any necessary restraint or the need to remove the animal from its enclosure or social group (see Chapter 17). All require expertise which can only be developed by appropriate training, and the provision and maintenance of appropriate equipment.

After a humane killing method is applied, in all cases death should be confirmed before removing tissues or disposing of cadavers.

Refinement: direct harms

A number of procedures applied to animals for experimental purposes impose welfare costs. The welfare costs tend to vary in proportion to:

- the degree of sentience and needs of the individual experimental subject;
- the nature, duration, intensity and frequency of the challenge;
- the biological systems and mechanisms involved;
- other factors which aggravate or ameliorate the suffering experienced by an individual experimental subject.

Choice of experimental subjects

Animals produced and used for experimental and other scientific purposes should to all intents and purposes be normal, with any departure from their normal state being directly and intentionally attributable to the scientific procedures applied. Standardisation of experimental subjects requires an understanding and control of factors including the animal's genotype; environmental conditions; other elements of animal husbandry, accommodation and care; and microbiological status.

The choice of species is thus relevant to refinement. Some species:

- are afforded special legal protection;
- are believed to have a greater capacity to experience pain and distress (sometimes referred to as 'neurophysiological sensitivity');
- have specific, complex husbandry requirements difficult to provide in the research context.

Choosing the species whose needs can best be catered for in the laboratory setting may constitute refinement.

In addition, where there is flexibility in the interpretation and implementation of regulatory testing requirements, selection of the 'lowest' appropriate species should be on scientific considerations, not custom and practice or availability.

Animal models of disease, animals expressing harmful natural genetic mutations and some lines of genetically altered animals (Wells *et al.* 2006) have specific problems and needs in addition to, or different from, those of normal animals. These special needs must be considered, identified and met when such animals are bred, kept or used for scientific purposes.

Wild-caught animals

Such are the environmental, ethical, welfare and scientific benefits of using purpose-bred animals, that the use of non-purpose bred, and in particular wild-caught, animals requires special and specific justification. Where the use of wild-caught animals can be justified, capture should be by competent persons using humane methods, minimising the impact of capture both on the captured animals and the remaining wildlife and habitat (see Chapter 7). Animals in poor health should be examined promptly by a competent person, and appropriate action taken.

Proper provision must be made for the acclimatisation, quarantine, housing, transportation, husbandry and care of wild-caught animals, mindful that their behaviours and needs are likely to be different to those of animals bred in captivity. The eventual fate of wild-caught animals should be given due consideration before work begins.

Experimental models

Always consider whether the scientific objective might be achieved by the use of animal models where pre-clinical endpoints can be set. The murine local lymph node assay for skin sensitisation (Kimber *et al.* 1990) is a case in point. It relies on subclinical changes caused by the induction phase of the sensitisation process; whereas the traditional guinea pig maximisation test relies on the clinical changes and gross pathology of the acute dermatitis seen as a result of the subsequent full-blown allergic response.

Procedural training

Training using positive reinforcement (see Chapter 16) to encourage co-operation during procedures (from weighing animals, through common methods of dosing and sampling, to sophisticated behavioural testing), can be beneficial to the animals, their handlers and the programme of work (Wolfensohn & Honess 2005) by:

- reducing the procedure-related stress;
- dispensing with the need for animals to be forcibly restrained;
- fostering human/animal socialisation;
- enabling those handling the animals to become familiar with individual animals' normal behaviours;
- reducing the time taken to perform the procedures.

Reward vs punishment

Behavioural testing often requires that experimental subjects remain interested in performing prescribed tasks. Various means have been devised to better motivate experimental subjects to undertake such tasks on demand or for longer periods.

Methods of motivating test subjects may be based upon rewards/positive reinforcement (for example, access to a preferred food or drink as a reward for displaying the desired behaviours) or punishment/negative reinforcement (for example, exposure to an air-puff or mild electric shock to discourage other behaviours). In some cases, the reward may be made more desirable by a period of deprivation (for example, access to fluid after a period of enforced fluid deprivation).

The most refined and ethically justifiable paradigms are those that rely solely on reward/positive reinforcement systems without prior deprivations, with punishment/negative reinforcement regimens requiring specific justification.

Dosing

Research protocols commonly require that animals are dosed with test materials, and detailed advice on limit volumes and practical issues is available elsewhere (Diehl *et al.* 2001). Refinement is relevant to consideration of:

- The dose or exposure:
  - if the intention is to mimic natural exposure, to attain or maintain a particular level at a target site, or to produce a specific effect (and not to produce unwanted effects) pilot studies may be required to identify the appropriate dose/exposure parameters.
- The route of administration:
  - With oral administration admixing the test material with food or water (providing palatability is not a problem) or administration in liquid, tablet or capsule form, may be more refined than gavage-dosing. When gavage-dosing is used staff must be sufficiently well trained and experienced to avoid misdosing or accidental injury; and the timing of the doses, and volumes administered, must neither compromise the animals' normal food and fluid intake, nor cause discomfort or other volume-related effects.
  - Test materials may be administered parenterally by injection or cannula. Other than administration directly into the circulation, this can lead to varying rates of uptake depending principally on the injection site, the general condition of the animal and the volume and formulation used. Administration by intraperitoneal injection is a special case: it results in the test material being taken up simultaneously into the systemic circulation and hepatic portal circulation (where it may be metabolised by the liver before it enters the systemic circulation). How test materials partition between the portal and systemic circulations depends on the nature and volume of the test material, varies from subject to subject, and in the same subject from day to day.
  - Topical application of test materials to skin or mucous membranes may require some form of restraint, or other measures, to ensure the test material remains in place and is not ingested by the animal or its cage mates.
- The frequency and duration of dosing:
  - These are generally determined by the properties of the test material (for example, its bioavailability and biological effects), its interaction with the experimental subject (for example, how it is metabolised, where it accumulates and how it is excreted) and the study objective.
- The equipment used:
  - For injection procedures the smallest bore needle capable of delivering the volume required in an acceptable time should be used.
  - The need for multiple injections, and the associated restraint procedures, may be dispensed with by the placement and use of cannulae to permit repeated (or continuous) administration. These potential *refinement* gains must be balanced against the welfare costs of the procedures to insert the cannulae, the restraint and other cannula-care procedures that may be required, and the possible cannula-related problems.
- The volumes to be administered:
  - For intravascular administration the volume and the time over which materials are administered should avoid unwanted volume-related effects, and should not produce any biological changes due to the nature and volume of the vehicle used. Advice on limit volumes (which should always be considered the justifiable maxima rather than the norm) can be found elsewhere (Diehl *et al.* 2001).
  - For injection into closed spaces (for example, intramuscular or intradermal injection) the volumes and rates of administration should avoid adverse effects due to pressure effects or over-stretching of tissues.
- The formulations to be administered:
  - The formulation and volume of test materials used are generally determined by the frequency of administration, the required accuracy of dosing, the nature and solubility of the test material, the required dose and preferred concentration.
  - In general, for parenteral administration the closer the osmolarity, pH, buffer capacity, viscosity and temperature of the test material to normal body fluids the greater the biocompatibility and the less discomfort and stress will be caused.

In many cases the most refined options to meet the scientific objective can only be determined by pilot studies.

Blood sampling

Blood sampling is one of the most common procedures used in animal research, and advice on limit volumes (which should always be considered the justifiable maxima rather than the norm) and other practical issues is available elsewhere (Diehl *et al.* 2001).

Refinement is relevant to:

- The nature of the sample:
  - In many species venous blood can be obtained from superficial veins by venepuncture or venesection.
  - Arterial blood is generally obtained by direct arterial puncture or closed cardiac puncture (the insertion of a needle directly though the chest wall into the left ventricle of the heart under general anaesthesia). Cardiac puncture is best suited to sampling under general anaesthesia from which the animals are not allowed to recover.
  - Blood obtained by retro-orbital puncture is not a physiological fluid: such samples comprise admixed capillary and venous blood, contaminated with other tissue fluids, in which a variety of clotting factors have been activated. Its haematological and biochemical parameters are neither physiological nor representative of blood anywhere in the systemic circulation.
- The frequency of sampling and the volumes required:
  - The volumes, rates of withdrawal and frequency of sampling must be designed to prevent hypovolaemia and anaemia. Average blood volumes and limit sampling volumes are generally calculated on the basis of body weight (Joint Working Group on Refinement (JWGR) 1993; Wolfensohn & Lloyd 2003), but must be interpreted in the knowledge that the safe sampling limits are typically lower in animals with welfare problems.
  - If frequent samples are required, consider cannulation as a means of minimising the stress of sampling.

Up-to-date information and detailed advice on contemporary good practice can be found at the NC3Rs web site[2].

Non-invasive sampling

A range of biochemical parameters can be measured without the need to obtain blood samples. A number of hormones and metabolites can be measured in urine and faeces, allowing estimates to be made of recent circulating levels in unrestrained animals, mindful that there is a time lag between their production, release and excretion. Procedural training has been used to ensure animals deposit excreta in suitable receptacles without being restrained.

Although physiological responses to instantaneous stressors cannot be measured in urine or faeces, for some materials determination of salivary levels can provide a minimally invasive means for measurement of short-term responses and for detecting and quantifying other metabolites and biomarkers (Chiappin *et al.* 2007).

Anaesthesia and analgesia

A detailed review of current best practice in the use of anaesthetics and analgesics is beyond the scope of this chapter, and authoritative information can be found elsewhere (see, for example, Flecknell 2009; Flecknell & Waterman-Pearson 2000) and in the species-specific chapters, but there are a few general principles particularly relevant to refinement.

General anaesthetic agents affect many physiological parameters, and care must be taken to ensure this does not compromise experimental data or animal welfare. Appropriate steps should be taken to monitor and maintain the circulation, respiratory function and the body temperature of the anaesthetised subject within normal physiological limits throughout surgery and until the effects of general anaesthesia have worn off.

Recovery from general anaesthesia can be hazardous, and animals should not be left unattended until the effects of general anaesthesia have worn off, any necessary specific, symptomatic or supportive treatments have been given and their effectiveness determined. Consideration should be given to administering the first dose of analgesia before recovery from anaesthesia as total post-operative analgesic requirements are reduced when the initial dose of analgesic precedes the animal's ability to feel pain.

Post-operative analgesia should be the norm, and it should be administered as required to control pain and speed the restoration of normal behaviours, such as food and water intake, thus shortening the post-surgery catabolic phase. This requires appropriate observation schedules, and that the treatments given are based on the findings in, and needs of, individual animals.

Surgery

Surgical procedures must only be carried out by competent persons; using the best available surgical and animal care techniques; and the anaesthetic and analgesic regimens best suited to the species, the nature and duration of the procedure and the scientific objective. Recovery surgery should be performed using aseptic technique in areas designed for and dedicated to this purpose.

The availability of trained, competent staff to take responsibility for the care of animals during the post-operative period must be determined before surgery is scheduled. To make best provision for post-operative care it is recommended that complex surgical procedures are carried out as early in the working week, and working day, as possible.

Observation schedules

Arrangements must be made to check animals under study at appropriate times to gather data and safeguard their welfare. All animals should be checked at least once a day by a competent person capable of recognising and remedy-

[2] http://www.nc3rs.org.uk/bloodsamplingmicrosite/page.asp?id=426

ing welfare problems. The frequency of checks should be intensified when problems are likely, or have occurred.

Good communication and teamwork are essential. Positive findings, the action taken and the animal's response should be recorded.

Humane endpoints

Humane endpoints, minimising the direct welfare costs of justifiable animal-based research, are essential components of humane experimental technique, and a cornerstone of refinement (Richmond 1999). Humane endpoints incorporate all reasonable and practical steps that can be taken to minimise justifiable suffering by avoiding, or promptly recognising and remedying, unnecessary adverse effects arising during scientific procedures.

To some the term 'humane endpoint' merely represents '*the earliest indicator in an animal experiment of severe pain, severe distress, suffering, or impending death*' (OECD 2000). That is a dangerous misconception.

Contrary to the narrow OECD definition, humane endpoints are often particularly appropriate when levels of pain and distress being experienced are not high and death is not imminent. Indeed, early indicators are often the most meaningful with respect to welfare problems and scientific outcomes, and avoid unwanted later changes due to unnecessary secondary or tertiary effects.

Humane endpoints in practice

Humane endpoints must be objective and evidence-based in order to:

- avoid the needless culling of animals whose welfare is less compromised than believed, or before the scientific objective has been achieved;
- prevent evidence indicative of significant suffering being missed;
- inform judgments about the severity of different procedures and models;
- evaluate potential refinements.

Although they must be contextualised to the project, the experiment and the experimental group, they are best thought of as being applied to the individual animal.

Humane endpoints take account of legal, ethical, welfare and scientific considerations, and must cater for a number of eventualities including:

- having achieved the experimental objective (or when it is recognised it cannot be achieved), even if there is no immediate welfare problem; indeed in some cases preclinical endpoints can be set and implemented;
- experimental subjects experiencing pain, suffering, distress or lasting harm beyond that which is required or can be justified; again such endpoints are often invoked at low levels of suffering – for example reduced weight gain can often be accepted as an early indication of overt toxicity;
- when intercurrent problems, for example a subclinical background infection, compromise the quality of the data or product, even when they may not have compromised the well-being of the animals – for example mice known to be carrying the mouse hepatitis virus may have no overt welfare problem, but will have atypical immune responses.

When an endpoint is recognised, the action taken may take several forms including:

- the animal ceasing to be an experimental subject;
- adjusting the protocol to reduce or remove the immediate cause of the adverse effect to allow the animal to recover;
- the administration of specific, symptomatic or supportive treatments;
- humane killing.

Humane endpoints must be described in meaningful terms and be promptly recognised and acted on by those entrusted with the welfare of the animals. There should be no delay between their detection and appropriate action being taken.

Planning of humane endpoints

Before animal use begins, humane endpoints should be defined; minimum observation schedules determined; and arrangements for the provision or withholding of specific, symptomatic and supportive treatments, and other remedial measures, established. This requires an understanding and consideration of likely adverse effects (immediate and delayed: primary, secondary and tertiary), and how they will be avoided, recognised and remedied. The critical periods, training needs and resource implications should be identified before work starts. Thought must also be given to how unforeseen outcomes will be identified, interpreted, reported and managed. Particular care may be required to recognise transient pharmacological effects not indicative of true welfare problems. Pilot studies can inform the timing of observations and how the adverse effects should be identified and managed, minimising the welfare costs of definitive studies.

An understanding of relevant biological mechanisms and likely clinical findings allows appropriate symptomatic and supportive therapies to be delivered, permitting the processes of interest to continue whilst minimising or eliminating unnecessary suffering. In practice, primary changes are often subtle in nature and, even when symptomatic and supportive treatments are given, are overshadowed by less specific secondary (for example anorexia) or tertiary (for example weight loss or dehydration) changes. Untreated secondary and tertiary effects compromise both science and welfare: therefore you do not need a reason to give supportive or symptomatic treatment, rather you need good reason not to do so.

In some cases scientific judgements can be made on the basis of what might otherwise have been assumed to be general, non-specific changes (eg, behaviour, appearance, body weight, food or water intake, or body temperature). Examples include the use of the HID50 (hypothermia-induced dose 50) as an indicator of impending overwhelming infection as an alternative to the significant morbidity and mortality associated with traditional LD50 or PD50 studies to establish bacteriological virulence (Soothill *et al.* 1992).

Death should seldom, if ever, be set or accepted as a required scientific endpoint. As procedure-related death is often the result of secondary or tertiary changes, it may be that lethal endpoints are not consistent with good science and could be replaced by earlier humane killing and autopsy, or be avoided by improved observation schedules and supportive or symptomatic treatments.

The humane endpoints and associated actions must be communicated to, and understood and implemented, by the staff involved. The documentation and verbal descriptors should use plain language and be understood by the staff checking the animals; should read across to other studies involving the same research team and establishment; and be meaningful to those working elsewhere in the same field of research to allow comparison with similar work performed by others, to define best practice and further raise standards.

Staff must be properly trained to recognise, and empowered to promptly implement, the endpoints. Welfare is not protected by systems that necessitate that decisions and action require lengthy internal notifications or consultations.

Recognition and implementation

All animals should be checked at least once a day by trained staff, and the schedules intensified as required to ensure the prompt recognition and alleviation of significant welfare problems. All instances where animals are killed *in extremis* or found dead should be reviewed and the endpoints and observational schedules revised as necessary. These events may indicate that opportunities for refinement have been missed, and require that additional animals are used.

Once work is underway and insights are being gained into the likely welfare costs and scientific outcomes of procedures, those involved should again ask whether the specific experimental objective and findings to date justify the levels of suffering being produced, and whether the objective and/or methods can be adjusted to provide equally useful data at a lower welfare cost.

Review and lessons learned

Completed studies should be reviewed to determine whether all of the likely clinical manifestations of the pathologies produced were detected, and if the scientific objectives could have been achieved if earlier endpoints were applied. This information should be taken into account when future studies are planned.

Published work should describe how endpoints were determined and implemented and summarise the welfare problems encountered. Russell and Burch offered sound advice in this area: the objective is not just to enable others to 'do what you did', but to allow them to 'see what you saw'.

Responsibility for the Three Rs

The Three Rs of replacement, reduction and refinement are now accepted, sustained and implemented at international, national, institutional and individual level.

International activity

International acceptance of the Three Rs plays an important part in ensuring that the principles of humane experimental technique are implemented. Examples of where only international collaboration is, and will remain, essential are discussed in the following paragraphs.

Legislative provision

Both the European Union and the Council of Europe have made provision for the care and use of animals for experimental and other scientific purposes that reflect the Three Rs.

Regulatory requirements

The development of new and revised international regulatory requirements increasingly reflects the Three Rs. Harmonisation of regulatory requirements can ensure that a single test is sufficient to satisfy international regulators about a single toxicological endpoint.

The mutual acceptance of data and data-sharing prevent unnecessary duplication of animal tests.

Scientific validation

This is expensive and time consuming, and increasingly takes place at the international level in order to set agreed priorities, reduce the time required, pool available resources and ensure international acceptance of the outcomes. Organisations such as the European Centre for the Validation of Alternative Methods[3], the USA's National Toxicology Program Interagency Center for the Evaluation of Alternative Toxicological Methods Interagency Coordination Committee on the Validation of Alternative Methods[4] and Japanese Centre for the Validation of Alternative Methods[5] not only support validation within their own geographical regions, but actively collaborate to make the best use of available resources to ensure that:

- as far as possible their validation processes are consistent;
- multiple centres from around the world contribute to validation studies;

[3]http://ecvam.jrc.it/
[4]http://iccvam.niehs.nih.gov/
[5]http://altweb.jhsph.edu/wc6/paper483.pdf

- processes are in place to ensure that the validation studies of the other centres can be quickly reviewed and, if appropriate, endorsed by the others.

International meetings

Science is international, and international meetings focusing on the Three Rs such as the World Congresses on Alternatives and Animal Use in the Life Sciences, and societies such the Middle European Society for Alternative Methods to Animal Testing[6], and various international laboratory animal science associations provide opportunities to showcase progress with the Three Rs at the international level.

Nevertheless, much remains to be done at the international level:

- There are still significant differences between, and in some cases within, economic regions in the legislative provision made for the protection of animals used for experimental and other scientific purposes.
- Regulatory requirements are still imperfectly harmonised and can be slow to adopt technical progress.
- Scientific validation remains a time-consuming process and, despite the increasing co-operation between the validation centres, there is still the potential for different centres coming to different conclusions about the same data sets.
- The international meetings and societies are high quality and well attended, but tend to attract those already active in, and familiar with, the Three Rs.

National activity

Much can be, and is being, done at national level. Clearly national legislative provision for the protection of animals used for experimental and other scientific purposes is important to ensure that the Three Rs are given due consideration. National support for the Three Rs is also expressed in other significant ways:

- Government funding for work on the Three Rs. The amounts involved can be difficult to determine as funding primarily to improve methodologies is not necessarily premised on animal welfare considerations and may not be readily identifiable as direct support for the Three Rs.
- The establishment of national centres to champion the development and acceptance of alternative methods – for example the National Centre for the Three Rs in the UK, ZEBET in Germany, the Canadian Council for Animal Care in Canada, the Center for Alternatives to Animal Testing in the USA and the Norwegian Reference Centre for Laboratory Animal Science and Alternatives in Norway. These act as focal points for the discussion and dissemination of good practice.
- For a comprehensive listing of professional, industrial, academic and other non-governmental organisations specifically involved with developing and promoting alternative methods see the AltTox website[7].

[6]http://www.zet.or.at/node,185,de,megat.php
[7]http://www.alttox.org/ttrc/resources/organizations.html

Institutional activity

There is a number of institutions that play an active part in the promotion and uptake of humane experimental technique.

Funding bodies

Funding bodies should ensure that the Three Rs are given due consideration before programmes of work are funded, and that progress with the Three Rs made in the course of funded work is published.

Research journals

Research journals should ensure that published work takes account of the Three Rs, and that progress with the Three Rs is published.

Animal users and breeders

Establishments that breed, keep and use animals for scientific purposes play a central role. Institutional support extends far beyond simply providing suitable physical facilities and typically includes the provision of:

- expert advice on accommodation and care, statistics and other elements of experimental design, veterinary care and laboratory animal science;
- animal facilities and standards of accommodation which meet or surpass published provisions and recommendations;
- systematic education, training and continued professional development to develop and maintain both the necessary technical competencies and the required culture of care;
- processes which encourage innovation and continuous improvement.

Individual activity

There is no doubt that the factors that are most important to promote the development and application of humane experimental technique and the Three Rs are the expertise and culture of those responsible for the production, care and use of animals – both their individual contributions and their ability recognise and capitalise on the expertise of others. Each individual involved must take responsibility for their own personal development and personal effectiveness, mindful that competence can be attained by experience, qualification and training. This requires ensuring that individuals:

- obtain appropriate training and continued professional development (including periodic revalidation of existing skills), keep abreast of good practice by involvement with appropriate professional societies and scientific bodies and seek opportunities to visit and benchmark against other establishments;
- make timely contributions to the planning and performance of animal production and use;

- confirm that others with responsibility for the animal welfare are both competent and effective;
- make sure that only high-quality science is undertaken;
- ensure that best practice is being followed;
- require that outcomes are reviewed, lessons learned incorporated into future practice and technical improvements communicated to others;
- network with others, both to share their own expertise and capitalise on the knowledge and experience of others.

Concluding remarks

In addition to considering the principles set out above, and applying the practices set out in later chapters, it is hoped that readers will in due course be able to capitalise on, and communicate to others, their own new insights and practical examples of how the principles of replacement, reduction and refinement can further contribute to both animal welfare and high-quality science.

References

Ames, B.N., Lee, F.D. and Durston, W.E. (1973) An improved bacterial test system for the detection and classification of mutagens and carcinogens. *Proceedings of the National Academy of Sciences USA*, **70**, 782–786

Anon (1839) Editorial. *London Medical Gazette*, 24 May 1839, 212–215

AVMA (2001) 2000 Report of the American Veterinary Medical Association Panel on Euthanasia. *Journal of the American Veterinary Medical Association*, **218**, 669–696

Balls, M., Blaauboer, B.J., Fentem, J.H. *et al.* (1995) Practical aspects of the validation of toxicity test procedures. The report and recommendations of ECVAM workshop 5. *Alternatives to Laboratory Animals*, **23**, 129–147

Balls, M., Amcof, P., Bremer, S. *et al.* (2006) The principles of weight of evidence validation of test methods and test strategies. *Alternatives to Laboratory Animals*, **34**, 603–620

Barley, J.B. (1999) Animal experimentation, the scientist and ethics. *Animal Technology*, **50**, 1–10

Bayne, K. (2005) Potential for unintended consequences of environmental enrichment for laboratory animals and research results. *Institute for Laboratory Animal Research Journal*, **46**, 129–139

Benefiel, A.C., Dong W.K. and Greenough, W.T. (2005) Mandatory 'enriched' housing of laboratory animals: the need for evidence-based evaluation. *Institute of Laboratory Animal Research Journal*, **46**, 95–105

Blanchard, R.J. and Blanchard, D.C. (2003) Bringing natural behaviors into the laboratory: a tribute to Paul MacLean. *Physiololgy & Behaviour*, **79**, 515–524

Brockway, B.P., Hassler, C.R. and Hicks, N. (1993) Minimizing stress during physiological monitoring. In: *Refinement and Reduction in Animal Testing*. Eds Niemi, S.M. and Willson, J.E., pp. 569. Scientists Center for Animal Welfare, Bethesda

Chance, M.R.A. (1957) The contribution of environment to uniformity: variance control, refinement in pharmacology. *Laboratory Animals Bureau, Collected Papers*, **6**, 59–73

Chance, M.R.A. and Russell, W.M.S. (1997) The benefits of giving experimental animals the best possible environment. In: *Comfortable Quarters for Laboratory Animals*, 8th edn. Ed. Reinhardt, V., pp. 12–14. Animal Welfare Institute, Washington, DC

Chiappin, S., Antonelli, G., Gatti, R. *et al.* (2007) Saliva specimen: a new laboratory tool for diagnostic and basic investigation. *Clinica Chemica Acta*, **383**, 30–40

Close, B., Banister, K., Baumans, V. *et al.* (1996) Recommendations for euthanasia of experimental animals: Part 1. DGXI of the European Commission. *Laboratory Animals*, **30**, 293–316

Close, B., Banister, K., Baumans, V. *et al.* (1997) Recommendations for euthanasia of experimental animals: Part 2. DGXI of the European Commission. *Laboratory Animals*, **31**, 1–32

Council of Europe (2006) Multilateral Consultation of Parties to the European Convention for the Protection of Vertebrate Animals used for Experimental and other Scientific Purposes (ETS 123) Appendix A. *Cons 123 (2006) 3*. Available from URL: http://www.coe.int/t/e/legal_affairs/legal_co-operation/biological_safety,_use_of_animals/laboratory_animals/2006/Cons123(2006)3AppendixA_en.pdf (accessed 24 November 2008)

Diehl, K.H., Hull, R., Morton, D. *et al.* (European Federation of Pharmaceutical Industries Association and European Centre for the Validation of Alternative Methods) (2001) A good practice guide to the administration of substances and removal of blood, including routes and volumes. *Journal of Applied Toxicology*, **21**, 15–23

Festing, M. (2000) Doing better animal experiments; together with notes on genetic nomenclature of laboratory animals. *ANZCCART News*, **13**, Insert

Festing, M.F.W. and Fisher, E.M.C. (2000) Mighty mice. *Nature*, **404**, 815

Festing, M.F. & Altman, D.G. (2002) Guidelines for the design and statistical analysis of experiments using laboratory animals. *Institute for Laboratory Animal Research Journal*, **43**, 244–258

Flecknell, P.A. (2009) *Laboratory Animal Anaesthesia*, 3rd edn. Academic Press, London

Flecknell, P. and Waterman-Pearson, A. (2000) *Pain Management in Animals*. W.B. Saunders, Harcourt Health Sciences, London

Flecknell, P.A. and Roughan, J.V. (2004) Assessing pain in animals – putting research into practice. *Animal Welfare*, **13**, S71–S75

Fraser, D. (1993) Assessing animal well-being: common sense, uncommon science. Food Animal Well-Being 1993 – Conference Proceedings and Deliberations, Purdue University

Gallegos Saliner, A. and Worth, A. (2007) Testing strategies for the prediction of skin and eye irritation and corrosion for regulatory purposes. EUR 22881 EN, JRC 37853 (available at http://ecb.jrc.ec.europa.eu/documents/qsar/eur_22881_en.pdf) (accessed 24 November 2008)

Glenister, P.H. and Rall, W.F. (2000) Cryopreservation and rederivation of embryos and gametes. In: *Mouse Genetics and Transgenics – a Practical Approach*. Eds Jackson, I.J. and Abbott, C.M., pp. 27–59. Oxford University Press, Oxford

Hall, M. (1847) On experiments in physiology as a question of medical ethics. *The Lancet*, **1847**, 58–60

Hartung, T., Bremer, S., Casati, S. *et al.* (2004) A modular approach to the ECVAM principles on test validity. *Alternatives to Laboratory Animals*, **32**, 467–472

Hendriksen, C.F.M. and Morton, D.B. (eds) (1999) Humane Endpoints in Animal Experimentation for Biomedical Research. In: Proceedings of the International Conference, 22–25 November 1998, Zeist, The Netherlands. The Royal Society of Medicine Press, London

Hendriksen, C.F.M. and Steen, B. (2000) Humane endpoints for animals used in biomedical research and testing refinement of vaccine potency testing with the use of humane endpoints. *Institute for Laboratory Animal Research Journal*, **V41**, 105–113

Hoffmann, S. and Hartung, T. (2006) Toward an evidence-based toxicology. *Human & Experimental Toxicology*, **25**, 497–513

Home Office (1965) *Report of the Departmental Committee on Experiments on Animals*. (The Littlewood Report). Her Majesty's Stationery Office, London

Home Office (2007) *Statistics of Scientific Procedures on Living Animals, Great Britain 2006*. The Stationery Office, London

Interagency Coordinating Committee on the Validation of Alternative Methods (ICCVAM) (2001) Guidance document on using in vitro data to estimate in vivo starting doses for acute toxicity. NIH publication no. 01-4500. http://iccvam.niehs.nih.gov/ (accessed 24 November 2008)

International Conference on Harmonisation of Technical Requirements for Registration of Pharmaceuticals for Human Use (ICH) (1994) ICH harmonised tripartite guideline: note for guidance on toxicokinetics: the assessment of systemic exposure in toxicity studies, S3A. Available at: http://www.ich.org/lob/media495.pdf (accessed 24 November 2008)

Joint Working Group on Refinement (1993) Removal of blood from laboratory mammals and birds. First Report of the BVA/FRAME/RSPCA/UFAW Joint Working Group on Refinement. *Laboratory Animals*, **27**, 1–22

Kimber, I., Hilton, J. and Botham, P.A. (1990) Identification of contact allergens using the murine local lymph node assay. Comparisons with the Buehler Occluded Patch Test in Guinea Pigs. *Journal of Applied Toxicocology*, **10**, 173–180

Kirkden, R. and Pajor, E. (2006) Using preference, motivation and aversion tests to ask specific questions about animals' feelings. *Applied Animal Behaviour*, **100**, 29–47

Kramer, K. and Kinter, L. (2003) Evaluation and applications of radiotelemetry in small laboratory animals. *Physiological Genomics*, **13**, 197–205

Levin, J. and Bang, F.B. (1964) The role of endotoxin in the extracellular coagulation of limulus blood. *Bulletin of the Johns Hopkins Hospital*, **115**, 265–274

Organisation for Economic Co-operation and Development (OECD) (2000) *Guidance Document on the Recognition, Assessment, and Use of Clinical Signs as Humane Endpoints for Experimental Animals Used in Safety Evaluation*. Environmental Health and Safety Publications, Series on Testing and Assessment, No. 19 http://www.oecd.org/ehs/ (accessed 24 November 2008)

Poole, T. (1997) Happy animals make good science. *Laboratory Animals*, **31**, 116–124

Richmond, J. (1999) Criteria for humane endpoints. In: Humane Endpoints in Animal Experiments for Biomedical Research: Proceedings of the International Conference, 22–25 November 1998, Zeist, The Netherlands. Eds Hendriksen, C.F.M. and Morton, D.B., pp. 26–32. Royal Society of Medicine Press, London

Richmond, J. (2000) The Three Rs: a journey or a destination? *Alternatives to Living Animals*, **28**, 761–773

Roughan, J.V. and Flecknell, P.A. (2000) Effects of surgery and analgesic administration on spontaneous behaviour in singly housed rats. *Research in Veterinary Science*, **69**, 283–288

Russell, W.M.S. and Burch, R.L. (1959) *The Principles of Humane Experimental Technique*. Universities Federation for Animal Welfare, Potters Bar, England

Sams-Dodd, F. (2006) Strategies to optimize the validity of disease models in the drug discovery process. *Drug Discovery Today*, **11**, 355–363

Scharmann, W. (1999) Physiological and ethological aspects of the assessment of pain, distress and suffering. In: Humane Endpoints in Animal Experiments for Biomedical Research: Proceedings of the International Conference, 22–25 November 1998, Zeist, The Netherlands. Eds Hendriksen, C.F.M. and Morton, D.B., pp. 33–39. Royal Society of Medicine Press, London

Schnell, C.R. and Gerber, P. (1997) Training and remote monitoring of cardiovascular parameters in non-human primates. *Primate Report*, **49**, 61–70

Schwanig, M., Nagel, M., Duchow, K. and Kramer, B. (1997) Elimination of abnormal toxicity test for sera and certain vaccines in the European Pharmacopoeia. *Vaccine*, **15**, 1047–1048

Smyth, D. (1978) *Alternatives to Animal Experiments*. Scolar Press, London

Soothill, J.S., Morton, D. and Ahmad, A. (1992) The HID_{50} (hypothermia-inducing dose 50): an alternative to the LD_{50} for measurement of bacterial virulence. *International Journal of Experimental Pathology*, **73**, 95–98

Wells, D.J., Playle, L.C., Enser, W.E. *et al.* (2006) Assessing the welfare of genetically altered mice. *Laboratory Animals*, **40**, 111–114

Wolfensohn, S. and Honess, P. (2005) *Handbook of Primate Husbandry and Welfare*. Blackwell Publishing, Oxford

Wolfensohn, S. and Lloyd, M. (2003) *Handbook of Laboratory Animal Management and Welfare*, 3rd edn. Blackwell Publishing, Oxford

3 The design of animal experiments

Michael F.W. Festing

Introduction

This chapter is aimed at anyone involved in research using laboratory animals including: research workers, animal house staff and members of ethical review committees. It covers the main principles of experimental design, but deliberately does not cover the statistical analysis of the results. To some this may be strange because the design and statistical analysis of experiments are intimately linked. No experiment should ever be designed without a clear understanding of how the results will be statistically analysed. However, there are many good textbooks covering methods of analysing data once it has been collected as well as numerous statistical packages which will do the actual calculations. In contrast, there are few publications which deal specifically with the design of animal experiments. If an experiment has been well designed there should be no difficulty in getting the results analysed. The chapter contains no mathematics, which should endear it to the widest possible audience.

Experiments need to be well designed. Those which are biased or lack power (the ability to detect a response to a treatment) because they are too small may give the wrong answer and be totally wasted. Experiments which are excessively large may give the right results but with a waste of animals, money, time and other scientific resources. Unfortunately, surveys of published papers suggest that there is substantial room for improvement both in the design of experiments and in their statistical analysis. In many cases fundamental principles, such as the need to control random variation, randomisation and blinding (where possible), are either ignored or not reported. All too often methods of determining sample size depend more on tradition than clear scientific principles (Festing *et al.* 2002). Well designed experiments are not only more ethical, but they can also save money, time and effort and improve the chances of achieving the scientific objectives of the study.

Research strategy and the use of models in research

Most animal research is aimed directly or indirectly at curing or alleviating a specific human or animal disease. Careful thought needs to be given to developing a suitable research strategy, which may involve many experiments ranging from *in vitro* studies, through experiments on animals, possibly to clinical trials.

In vitro and animal studies usually involve modelling some aspect of animal or human disease. The models need to be relevant and capable of answering specific questions. It is highly unlikely that they exactly replicate the human condition, but they may lead to a better understanding of the disease process (Sams-Dodd 2006). There seems to be relatively little literature on the theory of models in biomedical research. Russell and Burch (1959) recognised that models have at least two dimensions which determine their use. They used the term 'fidelity' to describe the overall similarity of the model to the target (say humans). Thus non-human primates would normally be considered a high-fidelity model because they resemble humans in many ways. In contrast, a cell line would be a low-fidelity model because it is very unlike a human. Intuitively, scientists feel that they would like to work with high-fidelity models, yet they do not all work on primates. This is justified by considering another dimension; that is the ability of the model to distinguish between experimental treatments. A cell culture system which could distinguish between chemicals which are carcinogens and those which are not would be a preferred model in toxicity testing even though it is of low fidelity. Other attributes of models are also important (Festing 2000). They must resemble the target in ways relevant to the specific study, but must also be different from the target in other ways. For example, the mouse is widely used because it resembles humans in many ways, but also because it is different from humans in being small, economical to maintain easy to manipulate genetically, and because experiments can be done using the mouse which could not be done in humans. But the first step in using any model in research is to ensure, as far as possible, that the model is relevant. The second is to design experiments that are capable of detecting responses in the model. Models are not little humans, and attempts to make them seem more like humans, such as by using genetically heterogeneous animals so as to resemble the genetically heterogeneous human population, are often misguided. Research is a multistep process. The model is chosen because it is thought to be relevant to humans, but the experiment can only determine the response of the model, not the response of humans.

Steps in the design of an experiment

Defining the purpose of the experiment

There are three main types of experiment:

- Pilot experiments are small studies used mainly to examine the logistics of a proposed larger study, and to gather preliminary information, such as whether dose levels seem to be appropriate. They may involve a single animal or small groups if the aim is to gain some idea of inter-individual variation. In most cases the results will not be published, but will be used to design more definitive studies. Investigators are advised to make good use of pilot studies, which can often lead to substantial improvements in the design of larger scale studies.
- Exploratory experiments are used to study the pattern of response to some intervention, without necessarily having a clearly defined hypothesis which is being tested. They often involve measuring many outcomes or traits, and are used to generate hypotheses for further investigation. If many outcomes are measured, there can be serious problems with false positive results, so the results of the statistical analysis need to be treated with some caution.
- Confirmatory experiments are used to study a relatively simple hypothesis often concerning a single outcome, which is formulated before the experiment is started. However, many outcomes may be measured and the results may suggest other hypotheses which may need to be tested in further confirmatory experiments. Thus confirmatory experiments often have a dual confirmatory/exploratory role in testing hypotheses and suggesting new hypotheses which need testing.

An experiment which aims to explore a dose–response relationship will need to be designed differently from one which is designed to study, say, the effect of three diets on body weight in both males and females. So the purpose of each experiment needs to be clearly stated. However, in all cases the aim should be to design experiments which give the maximum amount of information using the minimum number of animals and other resources. Determining relevance to humans or other animals and deciding future action given the different possible outcomes, as noted above, is an entirely separate, non-statistical step which should be considered *before* starting the experiment.

In many cases the aim of the experiment is to compare the means of two or more groups of subjects which have had different treatments. Optimum group size depends mainly on the size of the differences between the group means and on inter-individual variability. If individuals are very variable, large differences between the group means could occur by chance. Great care therefore needs to be taken to choose uniform animals or to reduce variability using randomised block or crossover designs, discussed later in this chapter. Covariance analysis can also be used if some character related to the outcome variable can be measured before the experiment is started. Methods of estimating sample size are also discussed later in this chapter.

There are other types of experiment. In an uncontrolled experiment a treatment may be given to a single group of individuals to see whether, for example, the treatment has some immediately obvious effect on them such as hyperactivity. A control group is not required because animals do not normally become hyperactive within a short period of time without any treatment. An LD_{50} test is of this sort, but the outcome is so severe that for ethical reasons a more humane endpoint (Stokes 2000) should be used wherever possible. Experiments may also be done to estimate the mean or proportion of a group with some attribute such as a tumour, or to study the relationship between two variables such as time and growth rate. Occasionally an 'experiment' may either be successful or unsuccessful, such as in an attempt to develop a new strain of GM mice. This type of experiment is not considered here.

There is some confusion about what exactly constitutes an 'experiment'. Biologists will sometimes define an 'experiment' as something which was done to one or a group of animals at a particular time, with the statistical analysis combining data from several such 'experiments'. However, it is more appropriate to define an experiment as a planned strategy for collecting a set of data to answer a specific question. It is this whole set of data which is subject to the statistical analysis. Something which was done to the individual subject may more correctly be called a replicate or part of an experiment. A statistical analysis which combines the results of several independent experiments is called a meta-analysis. This is usually done by professional statisticians following well defined procedures. For example, in an attempt to determine how well animal experiments predict human responses, all papers which involved one of six different interventions in animals were combined using a meta-analysis to see whether they predicted known human responses to the same interventions (Perel *et al.* 2007). In three cases the conclusions of human and animal studies did not agree, although it was not clear whether this was because the animal model was not appropriate, or because the experiments were not sufficiently repeatable or because of methodological differences between the human and animal experiments. For example, some of the animal experiments may have been designed to study mechanisms rather than to predict the response in humans.

Identification of the experimental unit

A fundamental principle in designing an experiment is that there should be independent replication of the observations. The response of one subject should not be correlated with that of any other subjects. The 'experimental unit' (EU) is the individual subject in the experiment. It is also the unit of statistical analysis. Any two experimental units must be capable of receiving a different treatment. Very often it will be an animal, with animals being assigned to the treatments at random. However, if there are several animals in each cage, and they all receive the same treatment, then the cage, not the individual animal, is the experimental unit. Each cage will be assigned at random to one of the treatments and the statistical analysis will normally be done on the mean of all animals in the cage for whatever outcome(s) were being studied. In a teratology experiment a pregnant animal is treated with a test compound but measurements and counts of abnormalities are done on the foetuses. It is a common error to assume that each foetus is an experimental unit but in fact the mother is the experimental unit as it is the mother which was assigned to a treatment group. So in this case each mother will have a score based on the average number of abnormalities and measurements such as the mean weight of the pups in the litter. It may be necessary to take account of litter size in the statistical analysis as large litters will provide a better estimate of the susceptibility of the treated female than small litters, and females with large litters may respond differently from those with small ones.

Sometimes it is possible to do within-animal experiments. If the back of an animal can be shaved and treatments can be applied to individual patches of skin (eg, in testing for an allergic skin reaction), then the patch on the back of an animal is the experimental unit since any two patches can receive a different treatment. Similarly, if an animal can have a series of treatments done sequentially in random order, as is possible in an experiment to see if animals can taste certain solutions, and it can be assumed that each treatment does not alter the animal, then the animal for the period of treatment time will be the experimental unit.

Failure to identify the experimental unit correctly is not uncommon. One result is that 'n', the number of experimental subjects, is seriously over-estimated with the result that the statistical analysis and possibly the conclusions are incorrect.

Dependent and independent variables

There are two sorts of variables in an experiment. The independent variables include those factors which are being studied, and are deliberately varied as part of the experiment. This will usually include a factor called 'treatment' or it may have other names such as 'diet', 'strain' or 'sex' if these are the factors being deliberately varied. An independent variable may have several levels which may be quantitative (eg, dose 0, 2, 4, 8mg/kg) or qualitative (diets A, B, C, D). If the aim is to study a dose–response relationship, there may be many dose levels. If two or more variables are deliberately being varied simultaneously in the same experiment, then this is known as a 'factorial' experimental design. The variables may be of equal interest, or some may be included mainly in order to increase the generality of the result. For example, an experiment which shows that both sexes respond in the same way to an intervention provides a more general result than one done using only males. Occasionally, a fixed effect can be taken into account statistically. For example, outbred animals may be genotyped at some locus thought to be related to the outcome. In comparing treatment means, variation at this locus could be taken into account using covariance analysis (not discussed here).

Characters such as the sex and strain of the animals which can not be assigned to an animal at random are known as classification variables. Extra care needs to be taken to ensure that when strains, for example, are being compared that the animals are comparable in other ways. If the strains differ in age or the environment where they were bred, then these differences will be confounded with differences due to the strain and could be mistaken for such strain differences.

The independent variables can involve either fixed effects or random effects. A fixed effect is one over which the investigator has some control, and could include things like treatment, sex, strain, diet and housing conditions. Random effects are things like day-to-day variation, any remaining inter-individual variation, variation between rooms, cages (receiving the same treatment), or locations over which the investigator has little control. The strain of mouse is usually considered a fixed effect unless a group of strains used in an experiment is considered to be a random sample of all possible strains of mice and the aim of the experiment is to quantify the variation among strains. Thus in some cases whether a variable is considered fixed or random depends on the purpose of the experiment. Generally, random effects should be controlled as far as possible, and also taken account of by using an appropriate design. For example, a randomised block design will have one or more fixed effect factors such as treatment, and one random effect factor called 'block' which might be position in the animal house or a time variable. Uncontrolled variation either leads to more false-negative results, or sample size needs to be increased to average out the effect. This is discussed in more detail in the section on power analysis.

There are also many other factors which are not varied in the experiment, but which can still influence the outcome and need to be considered in interpreting the results. For example, if an experiment is done using only male animals on diet X using bedding type Y in plastic cages of size A × B × C, it is a matter of supposition as to whether similar results might have been obtained if the experiment had been done using females on diet A using bedding of type B in metal cages of size M × N × P. However, there is no way round this problem. All experiments are done under a particular set of conditions and it is never possible to be sure that they would be valid under a slightly different set of conditions.

The experimenter will usually measure one or more dependent variables which are used to measure the response to the treatments. Things like body and organ weights, haematology, clinical biochemistry, physiological variables such as heart rate and blood pressure, behaviour and measures of gene expression are examples of the sort of 'outcomes' or traits which may respond to the treatments, and which will be measured. Sometime there is a single outcome variable. At other times many variables may be measured. For example, in a microarray experiment there may be thousands of observations on each animal (or other experimental subject).

The randomised controlled experiment

The randomised controlled, double-blinded clinical trial, is the gold standard for the design of nearly all experiments, although with animal experiments it is much easier to control the many variables which can influence the outcome. Randomisation is of fundamental importance as it ensures that, provided it is maintained throughout the whole experiment, there will be no systematic difference between the treatment groups. Any differences must either be due to chance inter-individual variation or to the effect of the treatment. With proper randomisation the effect of the random variation can be estimated and taken into account in the statistical analysis. The aim of the statistical analysis is to quantify the part that chance may have played in determining group differences. If it is highly unlikely that the differences could be due to chance, then they are assumed to be due to the effect of the treatment. Of course, if the animals (it will be assumed from now on that the experimental subjects are animals, but they could equally well be cages of animals or tissue culture dishes) are very uniform, then chance differences between groups will be small and the experiment will have high probability of detecting any differences between treatments. So it is very important to control variation. This is discussed later in this chapter.

Randomisation in practice

Physical randomisation is very easy. For example, if the aim is to assign animals to five treatments (say a control and four dose levels), with six animals per treatment group, the numbers 1, 2, 3, 4 and 5 would each be written six times on separate pieces of paper or card. These would then be physically shaken in a suitable receptacle. The first animal is then taken, and a piece of paper is withdrawn from the receptacle (and not replaced) to show which group it should be assigned to, and so on.

Some statistical packages will take a column of numbers and re-arrange them in random order, so in this case a method very similar to physical randomisation could be used. Commonly used computer spreadsheets may have a function such as RAND() which generates a random number greater than or equal to 0 and less than one, evenly distributed. In the above example, the numbers 1, 2, 3, 4, 5 could each be put in a column six times. A column of 30 random numbers could then be put in the next column and both columns could be sorted by the random number column. This will put the numbers 1–5 (each six times) into random order. This could be done in the office, with the results being printed out and taken to the animal house for use. Many statistical texts also have tables of random numbers which can be used according to instructions.

With a randomised block design (discussed later in this chapter) the randomisation is done separately within each block, so it may be necessary to do several separate randomisations. But this presents few problems either with physical randomisation or using the computer.

Randomisation must be maintained throughout the whole experiment, with the animals housed in random position in the animal house and with the outcomes measured in random order, otherwise bias could be introduced. If the experiment involves surgery, the surgeon may improve his/her technique with practice. If all the controls are done first in order to gain practice, this will also introduce bias as the treated group will benefit from better surgery.

Blinding

Blinding or 'allocation concealment' is another important way of avoiding bias. Research workers are not unbiased observers of the results of their experiments. Very often they would like there to be a difference between the treatment groups. If there is any subjective element in assessing results, and the investigator knows the treatment group, then he/she may unconsciously bias the results by altering the scoring. This can be avoided by blinding. Of course, blinding is not always possible. There may be obvious differences between groups. Strains of mice being compared may differ in coat colour or groups may differ in body weight if diets are being compared. But if samples of tissue are taken from the animals, these should be coded so that any measurements can be done blind with respect to strain or treatment. Investigators should always mention whether or not they have used blinding in their experiments so that a reader will know whether the results are likely to be unbiased.

Any resulting publication should state whether randomisation and blinding were used, with the method of randomisation being stated. In one survey, animal experiments which were not blinded and/or randomised were significantly more likely to have a 'positive' outcome than those which were blinded and/or randomised (Bebarta *et al.* 2003), suggesting that these procedures really do reduce bias.

Controlling variability

Other things being equal, uniform material leads to high powered experiments, so control of variation is extremely important. Controlling genetic variation using inbred strains, for example, may mean that fewer animals need to be used in the experiment than if outbred stocks are used. However, if a single strain (inbred or outbred) is used, then strictly the results will be valid only for that strain. Crossover (within subject) designs in which each animal (or other subject) receives different treatments in random sequential order are particularly powerful because they automatically control the genetic and much of the environmental variation. Unfortunately, such designs cannot be used for long-term experiments or any experiment in which the treatment alters the animal.

Variation among the animals

Animals should, as far as possible, be the same weight, age and genotype and free of pathogens. Disease not only increases variability, it may also seriously interfere with the results. For example, diseased and disease-free animals may respond differently to a treatment. Most of the mice and rats supplied by reputable commercial breeders are now of SPF (specific pathogen free) quality and are routinely screened for the presence of pathogenic organisms. In-house bred animals should be similarly screened to ensure that they are pathogen-free.

Researchers using laboratory mice or rats should use isogenic (inbred or F1 hybrid) strains where all animals are genetically identical unless they can make a compelling case for using outbred stocks (Festing 1999). More details of the origin, maintenance and characteristics of isogenic strains are given in Chapter 4. The response to a treatment may be strain or genotype-dependent. More than one strain can be used in a factorial design (see later in this chapter) to see whether this is the case, usually without increasing the total number of animals needed.

Some people suggest that an outbred stock should be used on the grounds that humans are genetically heterogeneous, but this is false logic. Humans also vary in weight and age, but this does not mean that the animals used in an experiment should also be uncontrolled for weight and age. Uncontrolled genetic heterogeneity increases the phenotypic variability and reduces the power of the experiment leading to more false-negative results. Experiments may also be less repeatable because nothing is known about the genotypes of the individuals, which can therefore not be repeated. Even the degree of genetic variability within an outbred stock is unclear as it depends on the previous history of the stock. Certainly it is unlike the variability within human populations.

There is some evidence that stressed animals are also more variable. For example mice, which are social animals, are more variable in body weight when housed singly than when housed in groups (Chvedoff *et al.* 1980). Frequent sympathetic handling will tend to reduce stress associated with any procedures, another important source of variation. However, the effects of environmental enrichment are still unclear (see Chapter 10). In some cases it seems to increase variability, possibly because some 'enrichments' may increase aggression, but well designed and validated enrichments should decrease variability (Garner 2005).

Position in the animal house may also be important. Animals on the top shelf generally get more light and possibly a warmer temperature than those on lower shelves. Ideally, the animals should either be housed in random order on the shelves or a randomised block design (see later in this chapter) should be used in which each shelf has equal numbers of treated and control animals and any differences between shelves can then be eliminated in the statistical analysis. Certainly a randomised block design should be used if the animals need to be split into more than one location or treated at different times. If a power analysis (see later in this chapter) suggests that the experiment needs to be quite large, then it may be difficult to obtain large numbers of uniform animals all of similar weights and ages. Again, in this case a randomised block design should be considered.

Cage effects can be an important source of variation which may be difficult to deal with. Cages of identically treated animals may differ as a result of social interactions, unevenly distributed sub-clinical infection, cage position or other unknown factors. Moreover, individually housed animals may differ in their responses from those which are group housed. Possible ways of taking these effects into account in the design of the experiment are discussed in the section on factorial experimental designs.

Where some variation cannot be fully controlled, it is often useful to obtain individual measurements before starting applying the treatments. These can then be used to correct the observations using statistical methods such as the analysis of covariance. For example, final body or organ weights can be corrected for variation in initial body weight in this way. This does not obviate the need to choose animals of as uniform weight as possible and the use of randomised block designs, discussed later in this chapter, may be helpful.

Measurement error and variability in the procedures

Some outcomes, such as measuring the activities of enzymes or gene expression, may involve multiple steps. Tissues may need to be removed, extracted in some solution and assayed in various types of apparatus. There may be variation in the calibration of the instruments, in the composition of the reagents, incubation temperatures, pipetting errors etc, leading to considerable measurement errors. In such situations it may be advantageous to split the sample as soon as it is taken and run duplicate or triplicate determinations which are then averaged for the statistical analysis. This is sometimes called 'technical replication' compared with the 'biological replication' associated with differences between individuals. Note that technical replication does not increase the number of experimental units but it does increase the precision with which each experimental unit is measured so therefore contributes to a reduction in sample size or increase in power. The variation associated with the technical replication should not be used in assessing differences between treatments.

Behavioural observations provide another example. The animals may be observed and different types of behaviour recorded for relatively brief periods. Although such observations may be adequate, they may not fully reflect the behaviour. Modern apparatus is now available to record a wide range of behaviours automatically, sometimes with several animals per cage (Roughan & Flecknell 2003). This is likely to be more accurate than observing animals for only brief periods of time, although any technical limitations of such apparatus need to be taken into account. Also human observers may be more likely to identify interesting or anomalous events. Although automated behavioural recording systems are expensive they may still be cost effective when considering the total cost of a research project.

Experimental procedures themselves may introduce a considerable source of variability which reduces the power of the experiment (or requires larger sample sizes). Intraperitoneal injections are widely used in animal research, but the failure rate may be as high as 10–20%. This may result in statistical outliers which, if not taken into account, could have a serious effect on the power of the experiment (Das & North 2007). Other routes of injection may also have high failure rates, though these can usually be substantially reduced by training. Biophotonic methods appear to have many advantages as a training aid (Wiles *et al.* 2007). Skill should also improve with practice. As far as possible staff should be fully trained before participating in an experiment.

Sample size determination

Many scientists use sample sizes determined by tradition. In some disciplines, group sizes of eight are almost universal and some referees may go so far as to reject a paper which deviates from this norm. But traditional designs can be very inefficient leading to serious waste of animals and scientific resources. If there are several groups then the sample size of each group can usually be reduced, thereby saving animals. There are two methods discussed here which can be used to give a better estimate of the required sample size: 'power analysis' and the 'resource equation' method. Both of these methods have weaknesses, but are still substantially better than traditional methods of having a fixed number in each group.

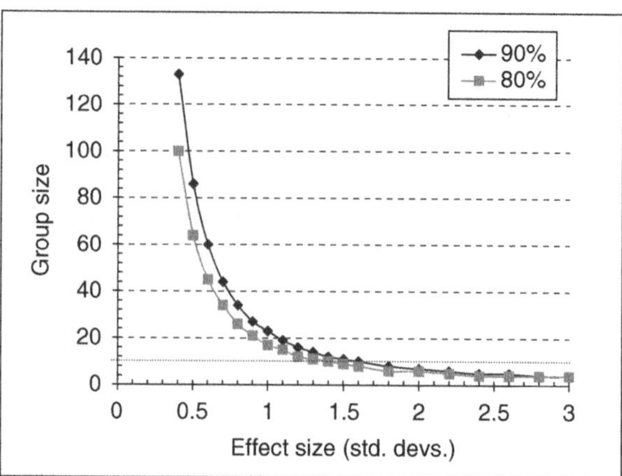

Figure 3.1 Power analysis estimates of sample size per group as a function of the effect size in standard deviations, assuming a two-sample t-test with a 5% significance level and an 80% or 90% power.

Power analysis

This method depends on a mathematical relationship between sample size and a number of other variables specified by the scientist. It is the method of choice for clinical trials or any other large, expensive but relatively simple experiment. In the situation where the aim is to compare the means of two groups (say treated and control) it requires the following specification:

- The type of statistical test which is to be used. This depends on the nature of the data. Quantitative data can normally be analysed using Student's t-test, the analysis of variance (which is mathematically identical in the special case of just two groups), or a non-parametric test, while qualitative data may be analysed using a chi-squared test, Fisher's exact test or a normal approximation of a binomial. In the example (below), it is assumed that a quantitative variable is measured and the means are to be compared using a two-sample Student's t-test.
- An estimate of the standard deviation, in the case of a quantitative variable. This has to come from a previous study, or a pilot experiment as the experiment has not yet been done. Unfortunately, pilot studies are usually small, so any estimate of variation will be imprecise. This may result in an under- or over-estimate of the numbers needed. This, and the fact that it cannot be used when the outcome has never before been measured, or where there is no good estimate of variability, is a potential drawback.
- The effect size. This is the minimum difference between the means of the two groups which would be of clinical or biological significance. Clearly, a very small difference would not be of great interest whereas it would be important to be able to detect a large difference. The effect size is the cut-off between these two.
- The required power. Somewhat arbitrarily the power is usually set at 80–90%. A power of 80% implies that if there is an effect as large as that specified, then there will be an 80% chance of detecting it. The power should be set taking account of the implications of failing to detect an effect. If this could be serious, say in toxicity testing where it might mean that a toxic effect was missed, then a higher power should be specified. However, it is not possible to specify a power of 100% as that would require an infinitely large experiment.
- The significance level. This is the probability of a false-positive result (ie, of claiming a treatment effect when in fact it is purely due to chance). This is usually set at 0.05 or 5% although this is entirely arbitrary and other levels may sometimes be set.
- The sidedness of the test. A two-sided test is used when it is not clear whether the mean of the treated group will be less than or greater than that of the control group. However, if the hypothesis is that the mean will move in a particular direction then a one-sided test should be specified.
- The sample size. This is usually what is being estimated. However, in some situations the sample size is fixed by the availability of animals. In this case the calculations can be used to determine the power of the experiment or the effect size likely to be detectable.

The formulae connecting these variables are not easy to use, but fortunately most good statistical packages will do the calculations and there are a number of web sites (eg, Biomath[1]) where the data can be entered and the results calculated. It is often useful to express the effect size in standard deviation units by dividing it by the standard deviation, as this puts everything into the same units and the required sample size can be read from a graph such as Figure 3.1. When there is more than one outcome variable, separate calculations are needed for each variable and the estimated sample sizes will differ depending on the variable of interest. It may be necessary to decide which outcome is most important, and base sample size on that variable.

Example: The mean body weight of a group of F344 male rats in a growth trial was 259 g with a standard deviation of 11.0 g (real data). Suppose a diet experiment is to be set up using these male F344 rats such that the experiment is able to detect a difference in mean body weight between the two

[1] http://www.biomath.info

diet groups of 10 g or more, assuming that the treatment does not alter the standard deviation. How many F344 rats will be needed?

Assume a two-sided t-test, a power of 90%, a significance level of 0.05 and an standard deviation of 11, then the aim is to be able to detect 10/11 = 0.91 standard deviations. From Figure 3.1 this would require about 25–30 rats per group. A more accurate estimate using the Biomath website suggests 27 rats per group.

If the mean body weight of the rats is 259 and the standard deviation 11, then among a group of 100 rats body weight could range from about 230 to 290 g. Suppose the rats were specified to range in weight from 250–270 g, then applying this to the real data, the standard deviation was found to be reduced to about 5 g. This would mean the experiment would only need to be able to detect an effect of 10/5 = 2 standard deviations, and from Figure 3.1 it would require only about 7–8 instead of 25–30 rats per group.

Some statistical packages also allow sample size calculations for qualitative (dead/alive, positive/negative) variables. In this case it is not necessary to specify the standard deviation as it is a function of the proportion affected. In general, many more animals are needed to compare two proportions than if a measurement variable can be used.

The resource equation method (for quantitative variables)

This method, described somewhat informally by Mead (Mead 1988) is the method that was used by most applied statisticians before power analysis became a practical possibility. It depends on the law of diminishing returns. Adding one more animal to a small experiment gives good returns in terms of increased power. However, doing the same to a large experiment will hardly increase power at all. The critical thing in most experiments is to have a good estimate of the variation, against which any differences in means are assessed. The 'error mean square' in an analysis of variance of the proposed experiment is an estimate of the population variance, and this needs to be estimated reasonably well. It depends on the size of the whole experiment and the number of treatment groups, not the individual group sizes. Mead suggests that if the error degrees of freedom (E) is between about 10 and 20, then the experiment will probably be of an appropriate size. However, these limits should not be applied too rigidly. A good case can be made for E being 25–30 or more to ensure equal group sizes, and it can go even higher when the experimental units are very cheap, such as when they are wells in a tissue culture dish. In a completely randomised design E is the total number of subjects minus the number of treatment groups.

$$E = \begin{pmatrix}\text{total number}\\ \text{of animals}\end{pmatrix} - \begin{pmatrix}\text{number of treatment}\\ \text{combinations}\end{pmatrix}, \text{ and } 10 < E < 20$$

For example, if a factorial experiment is planned with both sexes and three dose levels then there will be six treatment groups. If it is proposed that there should be eight animals in each treatment group (as is common), there will be 48 animals in total and E = 48 − 6 = 42. This experiment is unnecessarily large. Redesigning it with four animals per group, E = 24 −6 = 18, which is within the suggested limits of 10–20. Using the example of body weight of F344 rats discussed under power analysis, two groups of 10 rats per group gives E = 18, which is within the specified range. This is slightly more than the 7–8 rats per group needed to detect the 10 g or more treatment effect in the animals with a standard deviation of 5.0 g using power analysis.

A power analysis should be used in preference to the resource equation method wherever possible. Unfortunately, power analysis is not so easy to use when there are more than two groups because it is more difficult (but not impossible) to specify the effect size of interest. This difficulty is even greater when there are many outcomes (characters) being measured as separate calculations are necessary for each one with some sort of compromise being applied, unless the most important one can be identified. The resource equation method is useful when there is no previous estimate of the standard deviation. It is particularly suited to complex factorial experiments, and it is much better than relying on tradition.

Statistical analysis of planned experiments

Only a general description of the main methods used in the statistical analysis of experimental data is given here. Detailed accounts with numerical examples are given in many textbooks (Kvanli 1988; Altman 1991; Mead *et al.* 1993; Montgomery 1997; Petrie & Watson 1999; Festing *et al.* 2002). These days all the calculations will normally be done using a dedicated statistical package such as SPSS (SPSS Inc. 233 S. Wacker Drive, 11th floor, Chicago, Illinois 60606), MINITAB (Minitab Inc., Quality Plaza, 1829 Pine Hall Rd, State College PA 16801-3008, USA) or SAS (SAS UK, Wittington House, Henley Road, Medmenham, Marlow, Buckinghamshire, SL7 2EB). These are expensive commercial packages. The 'R' statistical software or 'language'[2] is widely used by professional statisticians and is free of charge, but it is command driven so initially may be difficult to learn. Some textbooks on the use of this language are now becoming available (Dalgaard 2003; Verzani 2005). Some free statistical software can be found on the Free Statistics[3] and StatPages[4] websites. The author does not recommend the use of spreadsheets as they are more difficult to use for this sort of analysis than dedicated statistical packages and may give non-standard output.

A large majority of experiments result in quantitative measurement data rather than discrete (eg, binary) data. These experiments can usually be analysed using Student's t-test or an analysis of variance (ANOVA), as long as the assumptions relevant to these tests are met (see next section). It may be necessary to transform a scale to reduce heterogeneity of variation and make the residuals (deviations from group means) have a more normal (bell-shaped) distribution. However, in cases where the data is very non-homogeneous so called 'non-parametric' methods may have

[2] http://www.r-project.org/
[3] http://www.freestatistics.altervista.org
[4] http://www.statpages.org

to be used. It is important to examine the data to get a feel for the type and distribution of the observations.

The first step should always be to screen the data for possible errors. This is usually best done graphically. Where outliers are detected the records should be traced back to ensure that they are not due to recording errors. Genuine outliers should not be discarded. A good way of dealing with them is to do the statistical analysis with and without them. If they make no difference to the conclusions, then they can be retained. However, if the aim is to obtain a good estimate of a mean or some other parameter such as the slope of a regression line, then there may be a case for deleting them provided that there are very few of them, there is a clear explanation as to why this is being done, and that analyses both with and without the outliers are presented (Das & North 2007).

The analysis of variance and the t-test

The aim of the analysis of variance and the t-test is to compare the means of two (in the case of the t-test) or two or more (in the case of the ANOVA) groups. The hypothesis to be tested is that there are no differences among the means (ie, that they could all be random samples from the same population). Where there are three or more means, the ANOVA does not indicate which means differ, only that it is unlikely that they could have come from the same population. Further tests such as *post hoc* comparisons or planned comparisons, described in most textbooks, are needed to determine which means differ. A 'one-way' ANOVA is used to compare means from a completely randomised single-factor design (see below). In this case unequal group sizes present no particular problem, although in most cases it is preferable to have equal group sizes. Randomised block designs are analysed using a 'two-way ANOVA *without* interaction' and factorial designs are analysed using a multi-way ANOVA *with* interaction. However, unequal group sizes cause problems with two-way designs and it is usually necessary to resort to a 'general linear model' ANOVA in such cases. This is available in all good statistical packages. Thus the ANOVA will deal with quite complex situations. Roberts and Russo (Roberts & Russo 1999) give an excellent introduction to the analysis of variance. The analysis of covariance (ANCOVAR) can sometimes be used to correct for other variables in order to further increase statistical power. For example, some of the variation associated with the initial body weight of the animals might be removed using this technique.

ANOVA and t-tests are mathematically identical when there are just two groups. However, the ANOVA is more versatile as it can be used to analyse complex experimental designs. Both depend on three assumptions:

1. the residuals (deviation of each observation from its group mean) have a normal distribution (note it is the residuals, not the 'data' that should have a normal distribution); a 'normal distribution' is a bell-shaped distribution;
2. the variation is the same in each group;
3. the observations are independent; this depends on correct identification of the experimental unit and appropriate randomisation.

The first two of these assumptions can be examined using graphical plots of the residuals, available in many good statistical software packages. For example, a normal probability plot of the residuals can be used to study assumption 1, above, and a plot of fits (group means) versus residuals can be used to investigate assumption 2, above. However, the ANOVA is said to be quite 'robust' to deviations from these assumptions. Only if they are seriously violated does the ANOVA give the wrong answer. Unfortunately, it is not easy to give clear guidance on exactly when parametric methods should be abandoned in favour of non-parametric methods. Robustness is a matter of degree. If the normality assumption is seriously violated, then the type I error (false positive) rate may be 0.1 rather than a nominal 0.05, but this would be an extreme case. Lack of homogeneity of variance should not be a serious problem if group sizes are equal with at least five subjects per group. However, with unequal group sizes serious errors in type I error rates may occur. Both parametric and non-parametric methods depend on the assumption of observations being independent. This depends on correct experimental design (Maxwell & Delaney 1989).

Where the assumptions are seriously violated, transformation to a different scale rather than the use of non-parametric methods may be the best approach as the power of non-parametric methods (see later in this chapter) is usually low. For example, biological data often have a log-normal distribution (ie, the logarithms of the actual values have a normal distribution). This is particularly the case when measuring the concentration of some substance in body fluids. It is not possible to have a concentration of less than zero, low concentrations may be common, but there may be a few very high values. Taking the logarithms of the observations will usually result in the residuals having a normal distribution. So in this case all the analyses will be done on the log-transformed data. Results can either be presented on this scale, or back-transformed to the original scale (although the standard deviation cannot be back-transformed).

The chi-squared and Fisher's exact tests for discrete data (counts)

Experiments which involve discrete (often binary) data which is summarised as the proportion or percentage of animals (say) having a particular attribute (eg, a tumour) in each group can usually be analysed using a chi-squared test. Note that all calculations are done using the actual numbers not the percentages. The null hypothesis is that there is no difference in the proportions in the two (or more) groups. All good statistical packages should be able to analyse such data. The main limitation of this test is that the expected numbers in all cells of the table should exceed five. If this is not the case, then it is necessary to use Fisher's exact test. There are numerous web sites which will do the calculations when there are just two groups (a web search on 'Fisher's exact test' will find them). For three or more groups more specialised software may be necessary.

Non-parametric methods

These methods are used when the data are very heterogeneous and no scale transformation can be found which would make it possible to use parametric methods. The methods tend to lack statistical power, so should not be used routinely. The main methods are the Mann-Whitney (also known as the two-sample rank sum, or the Wilcoxon two sample rank sum) test, the non-parametric equivalent of the t-test, which is used to compare the medians of two groups, the Kruskal-Wallis test, the non-parametric equivalent of the one-way ANOVA used to compare several medians, and the Friedman's test, which is the non-parametric equivalent of the two-way ANOVA without interaction, and can be used for randomised block designs (see later in this chapter). These tests are used to compare locations (eg, medians) of the groups, but problems may arise if the distributions are very different. Most textbooks include sections on these methods, they are available in all good statistical software packages, and there is a number of specialist textbooks explaining the methods (Sprent 1993).

Some experimental designs

The completely randomised (between subjects) design

This is the simplest design with a single factor, the treatment. There can be any number of levels and numbers of subjects on each treatment do not need to be equal, although it is usually most powerful if they are. One of the groups may be considered a 'control', or the aim may be to compare a set of qualitatively or quantitatively different treatments. The statistical analysis is relatively simple.

This design may be difficult to use for large-scale experiments as the larger the number of animals needed the more difficult it is to get a homogeneous group of animals all at the same time. The need to break the experiment down in time or space into more manageable bits also increases (this can be done with a randomised block design). Animals are assigned to treatment groups strictly at random, as shown in the example in Figure 3.2, and the positions within the animal house and the order in which the treatments are given and the outcome is measured should also be in random order. Wherever possible, the staff measuring the outcome should be blinded with respect to the treatment group as noted above.

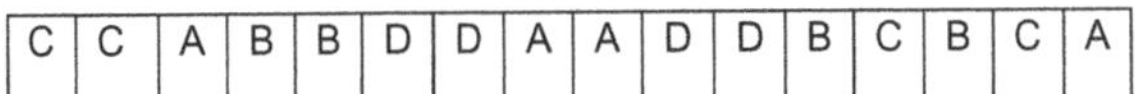

Figure 3.2 Example of the layout of a completely randomised design with four treatments (A, B, C, D) each with four animals. These are shown in random order. This could be maintained throughout the experiment or at least the recording of the observations should be in a re-randomised order. Thus, the first and second animals will be assigned to treatment C, the third to A etc. These should be housed on one shelf or split into two or more shelves in this random order, and all measurements of the outcome should be made in the same order. Note that using the Resource Equation method of sample size determination E = 16 – 4, which is 12, so the experiment is probably of an adequate size. Note also that the shelf level could be a source of variation which could be controlled not by randomisation, but by using a randomised block experimental design.

As with all the designs discussed here, there may be multiple outcomes. For example, a haematologist will look at the counts of a large number of blood cell types. In this case the statistical analysis either analyses each outcome separately, or some sort of 'multivariate' analysis is done which combines the different characters into a single composite character. However, this probably requires the advice of somebody with experience of these techniques. In some cases a character may be measured sequentially over a period of time. These samples will not be independent because if the animal has a high count on day 1 it is also likely to have a high count on day 2. Methods of analysing such data depend on individual circumstances. Suggested approaches include analysing the mean of the measurements, the slope of the line connecting them, the area under the curve or the time to reach a certain value. This should not be confused with a repeated measures design, discussed later in the chapter, where a single animal receives a series of different treatments.

The randomised block design

This design can be used to maximise statistical power in several situations. It is an extremely useful design widely used in agricultural research and it could be more widely used in research with laboratory animals. It involves splitting the experiment up into a number of 'mini-experiments', the results of which are then re-combined in the statistical analysis. Some of the reasons for using it include:

- If the animals are quite variable for weight or age or in some other identifiable characteristic such as batch or source. In this situation, animals which are similar should be grouped in a 'block' and then assigned at random to the treatments. Typically, a block will be the same size as the number of treatments. So if there are three treatments, then a block will consist of three animals as similar as possible which will be assigned at random to the three treatments. However, a block could consist of six animals with two assigned to each treatment although it is important that equal numbers are assigned to each treatment within each block.
- If sufficient animals of the required specification are not all available at the same time. In this case the experiment can be started with the first batch as block 1, then other blocks can be added as the animals become available.
- If there is some heterogeneity in the environment which may affect the outcome. For example, if the experiment needs to be split into two or more locations, or if account needs to be taken of a range of environments within a room. The top shelf in an animal house has a different environment from the bottom shelf, so each shelf might house a different block.
- To ensure that the results are repeatable over time. This is common with *in vitro* studies which are often repeated

two or more times on different days. The investigator often considers these to be separate 'experiments', and often is not clear how they can be combined. But if they are pre-planned, then they represent a single experiment split over a number of time periods and can be analysed as a randomised block experiment using a two-way ANOVA without interaction. Note that the animals assigned to a block should be as similar as possible, but there can be multiple differences between blocks. Thus block 1 might be uniformly heavy animals on the top shelf treated in week 1, with block 2 being light animals on a lower shelf treated in week 2 etc.

Randomisation is done separately within each block in this type of design, as shown diagrammatically in Figure 3.3. Note that a 'matched pairs' design is a randomised block with a block size of two, as is a study involving monozygous twins.

The repeated measures (within subject) and crossover design

In these designs the experimental unit is an animal (or cage of animals etc) for a period of time (the 'subject'). For example, if the aim is to compare the effects of four anaesthetics on blood pressure in, say, dogs, then the anaesthetics might be assigned to each dog sequentially in random order with blood pressure being monitored each time. It is assumed that the treatments make no permanent changes to the subjects, which will normally be rested between treatments. Where necessary this assumption can be tested by applying the same treatment a second time and comparing first versus second application. The experiment will usually involve several such subjects, depending on the required sample size, each receiving their four anaesthetics in random order. This is virtually the same design as the randomised block design with each dog being considered a 'block'. So, for example, Block 1 in Figure 3.3 might consist of a single animal given anaesthetics B, C, A, D in that random order.

Usually such a design will be extremely powerful because the variation within an animal over a period of time is much less than the variation between animals which may have both genetic and environmental components. The experiment is also analysed using a two-way ANOVA without interaction. Differences between subjects are assumed to be a random effect (like a block), with the treatments being a fixed effect.

A special case of the within animal experiment is a 'before and after' experiment where an animal is used as its own control. Thus, some outcome is measured in the untreated animal, then a treatment is applied and the same outcome is again measured to assess the effect of the treatment. While this is a useful design in many cases it suffers from the technical disadvantage that there is no randomisation. It is not possible to have an 'after' before the 'before'. The results therefore have to be interpreted with extra care.

Note that there can be some confusion in the name of the design because experiments where some outcome is measured several times following a treatment is *not* a repeated measures design because time is not a 'treatment'. It is a design with multiple outcomes. Methods of analysis of this type of data were discussed earlier in this chapter.

B	C	A	D	Block 1
D	A	B	C	Block 2
A	B	D	C	Block 3
A	C	B	D	Block 4
D	C	B	A	Block 5

Figure 3.3 Diagram of a randomised block design with four treatments (A, B, C, D) and five blocks. Note that animals are chosen for each block which are as similar as possible, and are then assigned to one of the four treatments at random. Blocks can be separated in time so, for example, block 1 can be started this week, block 2 next week etc. Blocks can also be separated in space, such as being on different shelves or in different rooms. The results should be measured in the same random order for each block. The results, assuming a quantitative outcome variable, are analysed using a two-way ANOVA without interaction.

The Latin square design

This design was developed for agricultural research where crop experiments are frequently laid out in fields and there may be a gradation in fertility from left to right (columns) and top to bottom (rows). It is rare in animal research. The design removes the rows and columns effects in order to increase statistical power. The number of treatments must be the same as the number of rows and the number of columns, hence it is 'square'. In animal research 'rows' might, for example, be represented by the shelf in a rack of cages and columns by position from left to right. Whether this would be worthwhile depends, of course, on whether there are important environmental effects of cage location. In Figure 3.4 every row and every column has all three of the treatments A, B and C. Thus the experiment is balanced in such a way that it is possible to remove the differences between both rows and columns so that the effects of the treatments can be assessed more accurately. The Latin

A	B	C
C	A	B
B	C	A

Figure 3.4 A 3 × 3 Latin square design. There are three treatments A, B and C, three rows and three columns. Every row and column has exactly one of each of the treatments. However, a 3 × 3 Latin square is too small for practical use. It can, however, be replicated with separate squares being combined in the statistical analysis.

square in Figure 3.4 was written with the three treatments A, B and C in this order in the first row, then displaced one column to the right in the second column etc. Randomisation is achieved by randomising whole rows and then whole columns.

With the 3 × 3 Latin square there will only be two degrees of freedom for the error term, which is far too few. In practice Latin squares are best with between five and seven different treatments involving 25–49 subjects in total. Any smaller and they will lack power, any larger and they become difficult to manage. However, it is possible to replicate small squares in order to increase their power.

The statistical analysis of a Latin square using a three-way ANOVA poses no problems. Data will normally be presented in the computer in four columns. The first will indicate the treatment, the second the row, the third the column and the fourth the observation or measurement. A three-way ANOVA will then be invoked with the column and row being random effects and the treatment being a fixed effect. However, complications will arise if there are missing values. Generally complex designs of this sort should not be used if missing values are likely to be common. A numerical example can be found in many statistical text books.

Factorial experimental designs

A factorial design is one in which two or more factors are varied in a single experiment. For example 'treatment' could be a factor with levels low, medium and high and strain may be another factor with levels C57BL/6, BALB/c. A factorial design based on these two factors would have all six combinations of treatment and strain. Where drugs or toxic agents are being studied one factor could be drug A (say at several dose levels) and another factor being drug B at several levels. The results will show whether the drugs potentiate or interact with each other. Similarly, it is often desirable to find out whether the response to some treatment depends on gender, strain, diet or any other factor which might influence the outcome.

Suppose an experiment is designed to compare a group of 12 C57BL/6 mice treated with a test chemical with 12 control C57BL/6 mice receiving the vehicle, but it would be desirable to know whether the response is the same in males and females. One way of doing this would be to do the experiment in males and then repeat it in females. This is known as the 'one variable at a time' approach, but it would mean using a further 24 mice and, because these are separate experiments, there is no way of testing whether males and females were responding in the same way. The alternative would be to use a factorial design with six male and six female mice receiving the test chemical and six male and six female mice receiving the vehicle control. This is a 2 × 2 factorial, with four treatments and would only involve 24 rather than 48 mice. It has the added advantage that it is possible to test whether the two sexes respond in the same way. Using the resource equation method of determining group size, E = 24 – 4 = 20, so the experiment seems to be of an appropriate size.

How should these animals be housed? This is not an easy question to answer.

- Housing one mouse per cage would ensure that each animal was independent, but mice are social animals and individual housing is stressful. It may be acceptable for a short period, but not for a long-term study.
- Housing them in four groups (by treatment and sex, six mice per cage) would be bad because the individuals would not be independent. Environmental or social effects may differ among cages. For example, males may fight in one cage but not in another one or one cage may get more light or be warmer than another.
- If the mice are individually treated, then it would be possible to house a treated and control mouse in each cage. This might be a problem if the treated mice become temporarily sick and get bullied by the control mice, or if the treated mice produce faeces or urine which affects the control mice. Assuming that these factors are not a problem, then this design is actually a split plot (discussed in the next section) rather than a factorial design. The comparison between the treated and control animals is more precise (because it is a within-cage comparison) than that between males and females (a between-cage comparison).
- The mice might be housed two per cage so that there were three cages of male treated, three of male control and the same for the females, giving a total of 12 cages. In this case the experimental unit is a cage with two mice. However, the statistical analysis could detect whether there are statistically significant cage effects. If not, then it might be acceptable to consider the individual mouse as the experimental unit.
- Another strategy would be to make the experimental unit a cage with two mice in it, but that would double the number of mice. Ethically, it is sometimes better to use more animals each of which suffers less, but each case needs to be considered on its merits.
- Another similar strategy would be to house the experimental animals one mouse per cage, and give each one a companion which is not part of the experiment and on which no observations are made.

Assuming that the individual mouse is the experimental unit (say it is housed with a companion) and the outcome variable is a quantitative measurement such as body weight or red blood cell count, the statistical analysis of this experiment will involve a two-way analysis of variance *with interaction*. This would indicate whether there was a statistically significant difference between the treated and control means averaged across the two sexes (known as the 'main effect' of the treatment), whether there was a significant difference between males and females averaged across the treatments (the main effect of gender), and whether the response in the males was the same as in the females (the interaction between treatment and gender). Of course, if the interaction is significant it implies that males and females respond differently. In this case it does not usually make sense to average across the sexes when looking at the response to the treatment. The four groups will need to be averaged separately.

Factorial designs can have any number of factors and any number of levels of each factor, although as complexity increases, the interpretation may become more difficult. In the above example it would be possible to have a third

Table 3.1 Layout of a 2 (treatments) × 2 (gender) × 2 (strain) factorial design with three mice in each treatment group. For discussion see text.

Strain	*Treated*		*Control*	
	Male	*Female*	*Male*	*Female*
C57BL/6	3	3	3	3
BALB/c	3	3	3	3

factor, strain, as shown in Table 3.1. This would make it a $2 \times 2 \times 2$, or 2^3 factorial design with eight treatment groups and would show whether the response to the treatment depended on both gender and strain. In this case E would be $24 - 8 = 16$, which is still of an adequate size.

Some scientists express concern about sample size in factorial experiments. In the above 2^3 example there will only be three mice in each of the eight treatment combinations, whereas in some fields of research there is a tradition of having eight animals per group. However, in this example when comparing the treated versus control mice there will be 12 animals in each group, as there will be for comparing males and females and the two strains. The concept of group size needs to be modified with this type of design. Moreover, in experiments of this type it is necessary to estimate the mean of a group, which can be done with quite small numbers, but it is also necessary to estimate the standard deviation which needs larger numbers. In the factorial design the sub-group means are estimated from three mice (in this example) which is perfectly adequate because the standard deviation is estimated from the whole experiment, and is based on 16 degrees of freedom. Statisticians sometimes call this 'hidden replication', and it accounts for the great efficiency of factorial designs.

Factorial designs provide extra information, when compared with a single factor design, at no extra cost in terms of animals and scientific resources. The value of factorial designs has been recognised by statisticians for many years. According to R.A. Fisher:

> *If the investigator … confines his attention to any single factor we may infer either that he is the unfortunate victim of a doctrinaire theory as to how experimentation should proceed, or that the time, material or equipment at his disposal is too limited to allow him to give attention to more than one aspect of his problem. … Indeed in a wide class of cases (by using factorial designs) an experimental investigation, at the same time as it is made more comprehensive, may also be made more efficient if by more efficient we mean that more knowledge and a higher degree of precision are obtainable by the same number of observations.* (Fisher 1960)

However, it is important for investigators to understand both the statistical analysis and interpretation of such experiments. One important limitation is that these designs should not be used where many missing numbers are expected, and group sizes should be equal otherwise the statistical analysis and interpretation is more complicated although still possible with good software.

As noted, factorial designs can have any number of factors and any number of levels of each factor. However, the 2^n series is of particular interest as it can be used to explore the relationships between many factors, each at two levels, without using excessive numbers of experimental units. Special methods are available for dealing with ten or more factors simultaneously. These depend on the assumption that high-level interactions are usually zero, so these interactions can be combined to give an estimate of error. This makes it possible to use as few as one animal per group in high-dimensional designs. More details are given by Montgomery (Montgomery 1997) and other specialised texts. These designs are common in industrial research when optimising output (say) from a chemical reaction which may involve many variables. In biomedical research they could play a useful role in optimising a screening programme for drug development (Shaw *et al.* 2002), and their more widespread use in toxicity testing using rats or mice of several inbred strains rather than an outbred stock has been advocated for many years (Russell & Burch 1959; Festing 1979, 1980, 1995).

The split-plot design

The split-plot design is somewhat similar to a factorial design although it is more complicated. Again it was developed from agricultural research involving field experiments on crops, but is often applicable to animal research. It is easiest to describe by an example.

Suppose several cages containing, say, two animals are assigned either as controls or to a treatment in the food or water. Within each cage it would be possible for some animals, chosen at random, to receive, say, a vitamin supplement by injection and the other one to receive a placebo. This design has two sorts of experimental units. So far as the treatments are concerned, the cage is the experimental unit, as it is the cage of animals which is assigned to one of the treatment groups. But so far as the vitamin supplement is concerned, the individual animal within a cage is the experimental unit since animals within a cage can have different vitamin treatments (or be of a different strain).

The split-plot design provides a relatively poor estimation of the main effect of treatments, depending on the number of cages, but a good estimate of the within-cage effect, eg, the effect of the vitamin supplement and also the interaction between vitamin supplement and treatment. The statistical analysis is done using a 'nested' ANOVA (the vitamin treatment is said to be nested within the cage) and probably requires expert statistical advice.

Other designs

There is a range of other experimental designs which can be used in particular circumstances. For example, incomplete block designs are used when there is a natural structure to the experimental units but the number of treatments is greater than the natural block size. This might occur, for example, if the aim is to compare the effects of, say, six micro-organisms on mice but only four isolators are available. These will need to be re-used in such a way as to ensure that each micro-organism is compared with every other one in a fair way. Sequential designs can be used in situations where a small number of units may be compared quickly, and the numbers can be extended if necessary in order to achieve a given level of statistical power. These can be useful designs to minimise animal use but, except in very simple cases, the statistical analysis can be complicated.

Concluding remarks

There are five criteria for a good experiment.

1. It should be unbiased with all treatment groups having the same environment unless environment is the subject of the study. This is achieved by ensuring that the animals (or other subjects) are randomised both in the allocation to a treatment, but also throughout the whole experiment. The investigator should also do the experiment blind with respect to the treatment groups so that no bias in introduced by inadvertently favouring one particular group.
2. All experiments should have adequate power so that if there is a scientifically or clinically important treatment effect there will be a high chance of detecting it and it will not be drowned out by 'noise' or random variation. The latter is achieved through two measures: First by controlling the variation. As far as possible animals should be the same age, weight, sex, health status, be housed in a controlled environment and have similar prior experience. Where there is detectable heterogeneity or where there is some natural structure to the experimental material, then a randomised block design may be appropriate. Similarly a within-subject crossover design is often very powerful because the variability within an animal is usually less that the variability between animals. Second, when the variability has been controlled, sample size can be determined using a power analysis or the resource equation methods. Although both have limitations, they are far better than traditional methods of having a fixed number per group in all experiments.
3. If it is important to know whether the results depend on the strain, sex, diet or other factor (and this is often the case) then a factorial design should be used in order to increase the range of applicability. Factorial designs should be used wherever possible, with the exception of studies where very unequal numbers in each group are unavoidable, because they provide extra information at no additional cost apart from a slight increase in the complexity of the statistical analysis. Using such designs it is possible to include both sexes or more than one strain in addition to a treatment without increasing the total number of animals which are used. However, if these designs are used it is essential to use the correct statistical analysis otherwise all the advantages are lost.
4. Experiments should be simple so that the chance of making a mistake is minimised. The experiment should always be pre-planned and additional treatment groups should not be added at a later date as randomisation will not be possible. The method of statistical analysis should be considered at the design stage, and not be left until after the experiment is finished.
5. Finally, the experiment should be amenable to statistical analysis. The most important criterion in this case is that there should be independent replication of the observations. This requires correct identification of the experimental unit, which may, for example, be a cage of animals if the treatment is given in the food or water, or a single animal if animals were individually treated.

References

Altman, D.G. (1991) *Practical Statistics for Medical Research.* Chapman and Hall, London

Bebarta, V., Luyten, D. and Heard, K. (2003) Emergency medicine animal research: does use of randomization and blinding affect the results? *Academic Emergency Medicine*, **10**, 684–687

Chvedoff, M., Clarke, M.R., Faccini, J.M. *et al.* (1980) Effects on mice of numbers of animal per cage: an 18-month study. (preliminary results). *Archives of Toxicology, Supplement*, **4**, 435–438

Dalgaard, P. (2003) *Introductory statistics with R.* Springer, New York

Das, R.G. and North, D. (2007) Implications of experimental technique for analysis and interpretation of data from animal experiments: outliers and increased variability resulting from failure of intraperitoneal injection procedures. *Laboratory Animals*, **41**, 312–320

Festing, M.F.W. (1979) Properties of inbred strains and outbred stocks with special reference to toxicity testing. *Journal of Toxicology and Environmental Health*, **5**, 53–68

Festing, M.F.W. (1980) The choice of animals in toxicological screening: inbred strains and the factorial design of experiment. *Acta Zoologica et Pathologica Antvipensia*, **75**, 117–131

Festing, M.F.W. (1995) Use of a multi-strain assay could improve the NTP carcinogenesis bioassay program. *Environmental Health Perspectives*, **103**, 44–52

Festing, M.F.W. (1999) Warning: the use of genetically heterogeneous mice may seriously damage your research. *Neurobiology of Aging*, **20**, 237–244

Festing, M.F.W. (2000) Reduction, model development and efficient experimental design. In: *Progress in the Reduction, Refinement and Replacement of Animal Experimentation.* Ed. Balls, M., pp. 721–727. Elsevier Sciences BV, Amsterdam

Festing, M.F.W., Overend, P., Gaines Das, R. *et al.* (2002) *The Design of Animal Experiments.* Laboratory Animals Ltd., London

Fisher, R.A. (1960) *The Design of Experiments.* Hafner Publishing Company, Inc, New York

Garner, J.P. (2005) Stereotypies and other abnormal repetitive behaviors: potential impact on validity, reliability, and replicability of scientific outcomes. *ILAR Journal*, **46**, 106–117

Kvanli, A.H. (1988) *Statistics: a Computer Integrated Approach.* West Publishing Company, St. Paul

Maxwell, S.E. and Delaney, H.D. (1989) *Designing Experiments and Analyzing Data.* Wadsworth Publishing Company, Belmont, California

Mead, R. (1988) *The Design of Experiments.* Cambridge University Press, Cambridge

Mead, R., Curnow, R.N. and Hasted, A.M. (1993) *Statistical Methods in Agriculture and Experimental Biology.* Chapman and Hall, London

Montgomery, D.C. (1997) *Design and Analysis of Experiments*, Wiley, New York

Perel, P., Roberts, I., Sena, E. *et al.* (2007) Comparison of treatment effects between animal experiments and clinical trials: systematic review. *British Medical Journal*, **334**, 197

Petrie, A. and Watson, P. (1999) *Statistics for Veterinary and Animal Science*. Blackwell Publications, Oxford

Roberts, M.J. and Russo, R. (1999) *A Student's Guide to the Analysis of Variance*. Routledge, London

Roughan, J.V. and Flecknell, P.A. (2003) Evaluation of a short duration behaviour-based post-operative pain scoring system in rats. *European Journal of Pain*, **7**, 397–406

Russell, W.M.S. and Burch, R.L. (1959) *The Principles of Humane Experimental Technique*. Special Edition, Universities Federation for Animal Welfare, Potters Bar, England

Sams-Dodd, F. (2006) Strategies to optimize the validity of disease models in the drug discovery process. *Drug Discovery Today*, **11**, 355–363

Shaw, R., Festing, M.F.W., Peers, I. *et al.* (2002) The use of factorial designs to optimise animal experiments and reduce animal use. *ILAR Journal*, **43**, 223–232

Sprent, P. (1993) *Applied Nonparametric Statistical Methods*. Chapman and Hall, London

Stokes, W.S. (2000) Reducing unrelieved pain and distress in laboratory animals using humane endpoints. *ILAR Journal*, **41**, 59–61

Verzani, J. (2005) *Using R for Introductory Statistics*. Chapman and Hall, London

Wiles, S., Crepin, V.F., Childs, G. *et al.* (2007) Use of biophotonic imaging as a training aid for administration of substances in laboratory rodents. *Laboratory Animals*, **41**, 321–328

4 Introduction to laboratory animal genetics

Michael F.W. Festing and Cathleen Lutz

Introduction

The aim of this chapter is to give an introduction to laboratory animal genetics both for the research worker wishing to use these animals and for the staff who will be required to breed and/or maintain them. Inevitably, most of the examples involve mice or rats. However the principles of genetics are universal, and one striking finding of recent years is the extent to which many genes and even genetic linkages have been conserved through evolution.

Research workers are now faced with a wide array of different species, stocks, inbred strains, mutants and transgenic strains from which to choose suitable experimental animals, assuming that the research cannot be done with some non-sentient alternative. However, only in mice is the full array of types available and even in the mouse there are no genetic 'models' for all diseases of interest. In rats there are many inbred strains, some mutants and a few transgenic strains, and in zebra fish there are many mutants, defined strains and transgenic strains but targeted mutagenesis is not yet possible. For larger and/or less widely used species, such as primates, cats, dogs, pigs and even rabbits and guinea pigs, the research worker usually has to be satisfied with the product of breeding colonies for which there is relatively little genetic information. However, knowledge of the genetic basis of susceptibility to disease and environmental agents is increasing exponentially at present so the demand for genetically defined animals of all species is likely to rise in the future. It is particularly important that people using rodents should make an informed choice of the type of animal for their particular project. Failure to do so could result in a waste of scientific resources and the unethical use of excessive numbers of animals.

Modes of inheritance

The characteristics of an individual, whether human, mouse or dog, are determined both by the composition and nature of the hereditary material that it receives from its parents, and by the environmental influences that it encounters during its growth and development.

The hereditary material consists of DNA (deoxyribonucleic acid) in the classical double-stranded helix made up of a sugar backbone and four bases: adenine (A), thymine (T), guanine (G) and cytosine (C). It is the sequence of these four bases which make up the genetic code which in turn determines the polypeptide synthesised by the gene. Genes are located on chromosomes (and some, in the mitochondria, not discussed here), one set of which is passed to an individual from each parent. Thus a mouse will normally have 40 chromosomes (20 pairs) 20 of which will have come from each parent. One pair of chromosomes varies between the sexes, with female mammals having a pair of X chromosomes of similar size and shape, while males are 'heterogametic' and have only one X chromosome and a smaller Y chromosome. In birds the females are heterogametic.

By April 2007 there were 22 188 known genes in the mouse which code for proteins and a further 3014 which code for RNA (ribonucleic acid)[1], but the genes in mammals constitute only about 2–3% of the total DNA, the rest consisting of various classes of repetitive sequences, non-functional genes (known as pseudogenes) and small amounts of DNA introduced by viruses. Each gene is situated at a particular position or 'locus' on the chromosome and usually consists of separated tracts that together code for polypeptides, known as 'exons' and non-coding sequences between the exons, known as 'introns'. There are also DNA sequences outside the gene known as the 'promoter' and 'enhancer' sequences that control the time and place in which it is expressed. The introns are eliminated and the set of exons that form a single gene are brought together during the complicated process of gene transcription and splicing to form messenger RNA which in turn codes for a specific polypeptide. Discussion of the genetic code and mechanism of gene transcription leading to the synthesis of polypeptides is beyond the scope of this chapter.

Mutations and polymorphisms

Sometimes a *mutation* occurs in a gene or larger segment of a chromosome either spontaneously or induced by radiation or a chemical. This can lead to a defective or abnormal gene product. It may also lead to a clearly visible abnormality in an animal such as albinism, obesity or hairlessness or it may have no obvious effect if, for example, it codes for resistance to a disease-causing organism which is not present in the colony. The mutant gene is known as an *allele* of the normal or so called *wild type* gene locus at which it occurs. Some of these mutations can occur in genes controlling biochemical pathways, and they may have a very slight effect on the

[1] http://www.ensembl.org

phenotype. These often continue to segregate within a population as *polymorphisms*.

Mammals are diploid, meaning that at each locus there are two copies of a gene, one from each parent. If these alleles are identical, then the animal is said to be homozygous at that locus. If they are different, then the animal is heterozygous at that locus. If a mutation is expressed only when the animal is homozygous for the mutation, then the mutation is said to be recessive. If it is expressed in the heterozygote it is said to be dominant or semi-dominant if it is intermediate between the homozygote and heterozygote.

Microscopic observation of the chromosomes has shown that a number of different chromosomal abnormalities may occur. Total loss or gain of one or more whole chromosomes (aneuploidy) is rare and is usually fatal at an early stage of development. However other types of abnormality are more common. These 'cytogenetic abnormalities' include the fusion of two chromosomes so that the total number of chromosomes is reduced, but one chromosome is much larger than normal. These are known as Robertsonian translocations, and they have been found in wild mice. Another type of translocation occurs when parts of two chromosomes break and join with one another. These 'reciprocal translocations' do not result in a reduction in the total number of chromosomes, but they may alter their relative sizes. Individuals carrying these are usually perfectly viable, though males may be sterile. There are also several other cytogenetic differences such as small deletions and inversions (where a bit of chromosome has broken in two places and re-joined the wrong way round) which can usually only be seen microscopically using stains which give a banding pattern to the chromosomes, or by using special breeding techniques.

Finally, certain characters may have a non-chromosomal mode of inheritance caused by the 'vertical' transmission of certain characteristics from parent to offspring via the cytoplasm, placenta, or the milk. The best known example of this is the vertical transmission of the Bittner mammary tumour virus which is passed from mother to offspring through the milk in certain susceptible strains of mice. Normally, the young will receive the virus, and this results in the development of mammary tumours in females of that strain. However, if the young are fostered to another strain which does not carry the virus, then the cycle will be disrupted and the young will not develop mammary tumours in subsequent generations. There are numerous other viruses which can be vertically transmitted from parents to offspring, though in most cases it is not possible to eliminate them by cross-fostering.

Nomenclature of simple mutants

The genetic nomenclature of mice and rats is controlled by the *International Committee on Standardised Genetic Nomenclature of the Mouse* and *The Rat Genome and Nomenclature Committee*[2]. The main purpose of standardised genetic nomenclature is to give each genetic locus and allele a unique name so that information about it can be accumulated in databases ranging from those involved with DNA sequences up to those which record the phenotypic consequences of the mutation. Clearly it would soon become chaotic if each investigator used a different name for the same gene or a name that has already been taken by a different gene.

There are detailed rules for different types of genes including spontaneous and induced mutations and various types of genetically modified animals as well as for inbred strains. However, only the nomenclature of gene mutations is discussed here. Nomenclature of inbred strains and genetically modified organisms is considered later.

When a mutation occurs, and it is shown to be inherited it is given a name which is usually descriptive such as 'obese'. In the case of a recessive gene this starts with a lower case letter and a gene symbol in italics (in this case '*ob*'). The normal unmutated allele is designated by a plus sign +, or as a superscript to the gene symbol ob^{+} if the context makes it necessary to indicate the locus. However, research on the obese locus has since shown that it codes for a protein which has been named leptin, so the name of the locus was changed to the leptin locus with the gene symbol *Lep*, and the allele is now indicated by a superscript Lep^{ob}. Note that the gene symbol now starts with an upper case letter as it is the allele not the locus which is recessive.

At a time of rapid research progress it is very common for gene names to change as more is known about them. Attempts are also made to use the same locus name and symbol across species. For example, the nude mutation in the mouse was found to be a homologue of a gene in *Drosophila* called forkhead 11 (a so-called homeobox gene which helps to determine body pattern, and a mutation of which causes a forked head in *Drosophila*) so the gene name is now forkhead box N1 with the gene symbol *Foxn1*. The nude mutation is therefore now designated $Foxn1^{nu}$. Human gene symbols are all given in upper case letters, which serves to indicate that a transgene (see later) is of human origin if shown in upper case letters. A complete list of previous names is maintained, at least for the mouse, and is available on the Jackson Laboratory website[3].

Table 4.1 lists some examples of relatively old mutations which are of biomedical interest. Note that in most cases the original name has been changed because the locus and DNA sequence are known.

Mendelian inheritance

The rules of Mendelian inheritance may be illustrated by reference to the albino locus which is about half way along chromosome 7 in the mouse. Alleles at this locus affect the activity of the enzyme tyrosinase, with the albino mutation now being designated Tyr^{c} (the c standing for colour). There are several different mutations or 'alleles' at this locus, including the chinchilla and Himalayan mutations, though there can only be two in an individual animal.

The monohybrid cross

Crosses involving mutants at a single locus (ie, a monohybrid cross) can be designated using the above symbols.

---

[2]http://www.informatics.jax.org/mgihome/nomen/index.shtml

[3]http://www.informatics.jax.org

Table 4.1 Example of some old mutants of interest in biomedical research. Note that most mutants are now listed as alleles of a renamed locus (eg, nu is now an allele of the *Foxn1* locus), but the function of the locus of others (eg, *qk*) has yet to be determined.

Gene symbol	*Locus (allele name)*	*Brief description*
A^y	Yellow	Yellow coat colour, obese, increased tumours
$Atp7a^{Mo\text{-}br}$	ATPase, Cu^{++} transporting, alpha polypeptide (brindled)	Sex-linked semi-dominant lethal, abnormal copper metabolism
Dh	Dominant hemimelia	Asplenic, skeletal abnormalities
Eda^{Ta}	Ectodysplasin-A (tabby)	Sex-linked, abnormalities of pelage
$Foxn1^{nu}$	Forkhead box N1 (nude)	Hairless, athymic, immunodeficient
Hr^{hr}	Hairless (hairless)	Hair loss, mild immunodeficiency
Kit^W	Kit oncogene (dominant spotting)	Anaemia, defective haematopoetic stem cells
$Kitl^{Sl}$	Kit ligand (steel)	Anaemia, deficiency of mast cells
$Lama2^{dy}$	Laminin, alpha 2 (Dystrophia muscularis)	Muscular dystrophy
Lep^{ob}	Leptin (obese)	Type II diabetes
$Lepr^{db}$	Leptin receptor (Diabetes)	Non-insulin dependent diabetes on a C57BL/Ks background, phenotype virtually identical to obese when on a C57BL/6 background
$Lyst^{bg\text{-}J}$	Lysosomal tracking regulator (Beige)	Dilute colour, lacks natural killer cells, immunodeficient
$Prkdc^{scid}$	Protein kinase, DNA activated, catalytic polypeptide (severe combined immune deficiency)	Immunoglobulin deficiency, severe immunological defects
$Ptpn6^{me}$	Protein tyrosine phosphatase non-receptor type 6 (motheaten)	Severe autoimmune disease
Qk	Quaking	Myelin deficiency, neurological abnormalities
T	Brachyury (brachyury)	Tailless, embryonic lethal, interesting genetics

Thus, crossing a mouse which is wild type at the albino locus and therefore is Tyr^+/Tyr^+ with one which is albino (Tyr^c/Tyr^c) is designated:

$$Tyr^+/Tyr^+ \times Tyr^c/Tyr^c.$$

The resulting 'F1' offspring will get one allele from each parent, so will have the genotype Tyr^+/Tyr^c. The appearance of an animal is referred to as its phenotype (in this case wild type), whereas its genetic make up is referred to as its genotype (in this case Tyr^+/Tyr^c).

If two of these F1 animals are crossed to produce an F2 generation:

$$Tyr^+/Tyr^c \times Tyr^+/Tyr^c$$

then each parent will produce gametes which are either Tyr^c or Tyr^+ and these will recombine at random to give the following types of mice in the statistical ratios 1:2:1:

$$Tyr^+/Tyr^+ \; Tyr^+/Tyr^c \; Tyr^c/Tyr^c$$

This results in a 3:1 ratio of animals with the wild-type phenotype and the albino phenotype. The phenotypically wild-type animals will either be homozygous for wild type or heterozygous.

The crossing of animals which differ at two loci is not considered here although in practice it is important as it is used to test whether the two loci are linked on the same chromosome, and if so how close they are to each other in terms of how frequently they re-combine. This is discussed briefly later in this chapter.

Sex linkage

Genes carried on the sex chromosomes are said to be sex linked, as their expression, and the frequencies of the different phenotypes differ between the sexes. The 'tabby' gene in the mouse has a sex-linked mode of inheritance. This dominant mutation was first designated *Ta* in 1953, but is now known to be an allele of a locus called ectodysplasin-A with the gene symbol Eda^{Ta}. In studying the mode of inheritance of such characters, the Y chromosome may be considered to be inert and devoid of hereditary material (though it does in fact carry some genes such as a Y-linked alloantigen and a sex-determining locus). Thus in the male with an X and a Y chromosome, all the genes on the X chromosome will be expressed (ie, will act as though they are dominant). Such a male is said to be *hemizygous* for the gene. So in the case of the *Eda* locus, the male will have the genotype $X^{Eda\text{-}Ta}/Y$ which is described as having a 'greasy coat' phenotype, while the female heterozygote has the genotype $X^{Eda\text{-}Ta}/X^{Eda\text{-}+}$ and is said to be have a tabby phenotype (a bit like a tabby cat). A cross between these two mice results in 25% greasy coat and 25% wild type males and 25% greasy coat and 25% tabby females. The female has two X chromosomes. However, one of these X chromosomes becomes inactive at an early stage of embryonic development. Either the maternally or the paternally derived chromosomes may be inactivated, and the choice seems to be random in any given cell. Once a chromosome has become inactive, in an embryonic cell, clones derived from that cell will have the genetic characteristics associated with the active X chromosome. If the female is heterozygous for a sex-linked gene such as tabby, the result is that the female becomes a mosaic of cells expressing the tabby gene *(Eda^{Ta})* and those expressing the wild-type gene (+). Tabby mice in fact have stripes which consist of patches of fur with the greasy-coat phenotype seen in males carrying tabby, and normal fur, hence their tabby appearance.

Linkage and linkage maps

Two loci will be linked (ie, they will not segregate independently) if they are close together on the same chromosome. Linkage will not be absolute, however, because during meiosis (the process of forming the gametes) the chromosomes twist together and often break, and rejoin. This leads to 'crossing over' or recombination, which will only be observable if both genetic loci are polymorphic. For example, one chromosome may carry the alleles designated by capital letters A and B while the other chromosome carries those designated by lower case letters a and b. After genetic recombination one chromosome will now carry A and b and the other a and B at these two loci. The frequency of such recombination will depend on how close the gene loci are on the chromosome. Linkage analysis measures this recombination involving at least three loci in order to obtain a 'linkage map' by observing the types of offspring from appropriate crosses. This has become increasingly easy in the last decade due to the development of large numbers of DNA-based genetic markers such as microsatellites (short stretches of repetitive DNA sequence, with the number of repetitions varying) and single nucleotide polymorphisms (a difference in the base at a particular locus in different animals).

Extensive linkage maps of the mouse and rat are now available. These may be used both for fundamental genetic studies such as in the identification and cloning of genes and also in a number of practical ways. It has been found that quite large parts of mouse chromosome have orthologous parts in humans, so if two mouse genes are linked, there is a good chance that the same genes will be linked in humans. As genetic mapping in the mouse is much easier than in humans, this is a substantial advantage. Physical maps showing the actual DNA sequences and the locations of individual genes and their components are also available now that rapid DNA sequencing methods have been developed.

Genes in populations of animals and the Hardy–Weinberg equilibrium

The examples of Mendelian inheritance given so far have been considered in relation to the mating of individuals of a designated genotype. Many research workers use outbred stocks of rats, mice, guinea pigs etc; stocks which are usually closed colonies, and still contain a considerable amount of genetic variation. The laws derived by Hardy and Weinberg independently in 1908 describe the distribution of genetic variants in such populations. The Hardy–Weinberg laws refer to a theoretically 'ideal' population which is infinitely large, which is maintained by random mating and which is closed to the introduction of new stock. The laws also assume that no selection of the offspring occurs, and that the gene locus has no effect on viability or reproductive performance. In practice, none of these conditions would hold with a real group of animals, but real populations may behave approximately as stated by the Hardy–Weinberg laws.

In the ideal population which is segregating at a locus with alleles *a* and *A* it would theoretically be possible to count or estimate the frequency of the *a* and *A* genes. For example, a sample of 500 animals (therefore having a total 1000 genes at each locus counting all animals) could be taken and the number of animals which were *AA*, *Aa* and *aa* determined. Suppose that it turned out that there were 405, 90 and 5 animals of each type respectively. Therefore, the frequency of the *a* allele is $(2 \times 5 + 90)/1000 = 0.10$, and the frequency of the *A* allele is $(2 \times 405 + 90)/1000 = 0.9$. The Hardy–Weinberg laws state that:

1. in the ideal population, gene frequency will remain constant, with no tendency to change from generation to generation;
2. the frequency of animals of genotypes *AA*, *Aa* and *aa* is determined solely by the gene frequencies and follows the binomial $(p + q)^2$ where p is the frequency of one allele and q $(= 1 - p)$ is the frequency of the other one.

The practical consequences of the Hardy–Weinberg laws are most commonly noticed in the maintenance of a coloured strain of animals such as hooded rats which carry wild-type at the albino locus although they are homozygous for the hooded gene *h* (ie, they are *hhCC* or *hhCc*). In one case, approximately 1% of all the rats produced in a hooded rat colony were albino. Such large numbers cannot arise as a result of new albino mutations, but are easily explained by references to the Hardy–Weinberg equilibrium.

If 1% of the animals are albino, the frequency of the albino allele, q, can be calculated as the square root of 0.01 which is 0.1, so p is 0.9 and the frequency of heterozygotes is $2pq = 2 \times 0.9 \times 0.1 = 0.18$ or 18%.

Although the effects of selection to eliminate a gene such as albinism in a hooded rat colony will not be considered in detail here, it is clear from the above that most of the albino genes are maintained in the heterozygous state, so that in the case of a recessive gene such as this one, culling of the 1% of albino animals will have relatively little effect on the future frequency of albino animals produced. The only practical way to eliminate a gene of this sort in an outbred population is to progeny test each breeding animal by crossing it to a homozygous recessive animal to see if any mutant offspring are observed. If not, and if sample size was reasonably large (say eight to ten offspring), then it is unlikely that the animal being tested carries the recessive mutation. This is a laborious process which has to be done on a large scale in order to reconstitute the outbred stock without the recessive mutation.

Directional selection

Selective breeding has been used to develop several rat models of spontaneous hypertension, a number of rat strains differing in behaviour and strains of mice which differ in their response to sheep red blood cell antigens, carcinogens and alcohol, to give just a few examples.

The usual method, known as 'mass selection by truncation', involves measuring the trait of interest in all animals. Only those animals which exceed a certain value (the point of truncation) are used for breeding. If the heritability of the character (briefly the extent to which any variation is inherited, as opposed to being due to environmental influences, usually designated h^2) is known, then the progress from this type of selection can be calculated from:

$$\text{Progress/generation} = h^2 \times \text{selection differential.}$$

The selection differential is the difference between the mean of the whole population, and the mean of the selected individuals. Thus, the greater the selection differential, the greater the progress.

Very small animals are often regarded as 'runts' and are not used for breeding in case they are genetically abnormal. As a result there has been mild selection over a long period for increased body weight in mice and rats. The 10-week body weight of the three outbred stocks of mice supplied by one commercial breeder all exceed the 10-week body weight of the 17 inbred strains supplied by the same breeder. Similar selection is practised with inbred strains, but as there is no genetic variation within an inbred strain the heritability is zero, and there has been no response to such selection. Breeders wishing to maintain the characteristics of their outbred stocks so that they do not become heavier over time should ensure that there is no selection for larger body weight.

Inbreeding

Inbreeding is the mating of related individuals. The more closely that they are related, the greater the degree of inbreeding. Thus the most intense inbreeding is self-fertilisation (in species where this is possible) as the closest possible relationship is that of an animal with itself. Next comes brother × sister and parent × offspring mating (which are of equal intensity), half-brother × sister mating and so on. At the other extreme, in large populations of animals maintained by random mating the average relationship between any two individuals will be slight, so the rate of inbreeding will be low (Figure 4.1). Inbreeding is measured in terms of the 'coefficient of inbreeding', which is usually given the symbol 'F' (not to he confused with Fl, F2 etc. which indicates filial generations from a given cross). Theoretically, F can range from 0.00 (ie, no inbreeding) to 1.00 (complete inbreeding).

The coefficient of inbreeding is a measure of the probability that two alleles at any given locus (one of which comes from each parent) are identical by descent (ie, that they are both copies of the identical piece of DNA in some ancestor). If the two genes are identical by descent the parents must have been related and the animal will, of course, be homozygous at that locus. Thus high levels of inbreeding are associated with high levels of homozygosity.

The calculation of the exact degree of inbreeding for any given animal will involve a study of the pedigree of the colony (if it is available) and will always be quoted relative to an arbitrary starting point at which the level of inbreeding

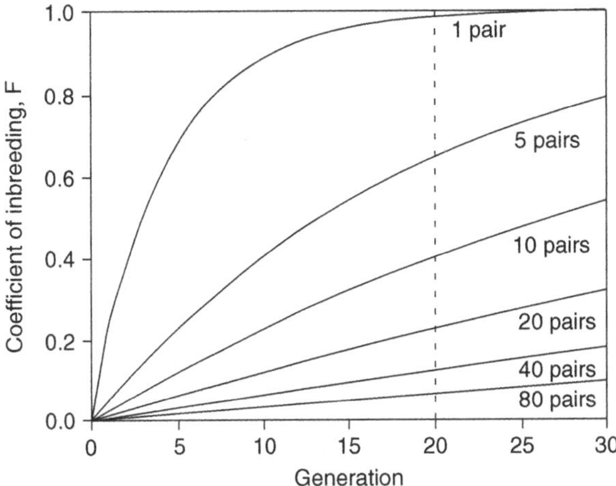

Figure 4.1 Coefficient of inbreeding as a function of the generation in colonies of various sizes. Note, it is assumed that at the start the coefficient of inbreeding is zero.

is assumed to be zero. The calculations also assume that at the locus in question heterozygotes do not survive any better than homozygotes.

Inbreeding usually leads to 'inbreeding depression', which is a general decline in reproductive performance, vigour and ability to survive. This is largely due to the 'uncovering' of mildly deleterious recessive genes as they become homozygous. Such depression will be most severe in the early stages of inbreeding because this is when the homozygosity is increasing rapidly (Figure 4.1). If a strain is already highly inbred further inbreeding will not significantly increase homozygosity, hence it should not result in further inbreeding depression.

Inbreeding also has the effect of increasing the total genetic variation provided all individuals are maintained, while at the same time decreasing the genetic variation within any one family. An 'inbred strain', as discussed later, consists of a single branch of a colony inbred by brother × sister mating. However, if the full set of all sublines has been retained (ie, a full set of independently inbred strains from the same initial colony), it would be found that the variation between these branches or strains would be very much greater than the variation present in the original colony. This means that, in general, a set of inbred strains will be more extreme in their phenotypic characteristics than would be found among individuals of an outbred stock. This point is of some importance in designing experiments based on a wide range of phenotypes, as it means that a collection of individuals of different inbred strains will cover a much wider range of phenotypes than will a collection of outbred individuals. A more detailed account of much of the material given so far is given by Green (1981) and Falconer (1981).

Effects of genetic background: variation in the expression of genes

The 'genetic background' is the rest of the genome apart from a specified gene or genes. The expression of many genes depends on this genetic background as well as on environmental influences. Chance effects during embryonic development may also play a part. In extreme cases, modifiers and environmental influences may prevent a gene from being expressed at all. Some genes may be lethal on some genetic backgrounds but perfectly viable on others. The viable yellow allele at the agouti locus in the mouse is one of the best examples of variable expression which is due both to environmental and genetic influences. Animals of the A^{vy}/a genotype can vary from pure yellow through a mottled yellow and agouti colour to a pseudo-agouti colour which closely resembles pure agouti. This variation occurs even when the genetic background is constant (ie, when the allele is in an inbred strain), showing that it is determined by unknown non-genetic or chance environmental influences. The frequency of the pseudo-agouti animals also varies according to the inbred strain in which the allele is maintained, showing that the variation is also dependent to some extent on genetic modifiers.

There is a powerful case for maintaining mutants and transgenes etc. on a standard inbred genetic background where the within-strain expression will be more uniform. Thus, in developing genetically modified animals it may be necessary to make crosses between strains largely because inbred strains do not always breed very well, but when studying the effects of the genetic modification it is good practice first to transfer the gene to an inbred background by backcrossing to produce a congenic strain (see below).

Polygenic characters and quantitative trait loci

Many characters such as body and organ weights, growth rate, litter size, behaviour, cancer incidence, metabolic rate, response to chemicals and certain immune responses have a polygenic mode of inheritance which depends on the simultaneous action of many genes. Many of these characters have a continuous distribution so that it is not possible to designate distinct classes and assign animals unambiguously to them. In other cases, there may be clearly distinct classes (eg, animals which develop a spontaneous tumour and those that do not) but when these animals are bred, it is not possible to show that the offspring are of the types and in the numbers that would be expected from Mendel's laws. Each quantitative trait locus (known as a QTL) has a Mendelian mode of inheritance but this is obscured by the simultaneous segregation of genes at many other loci and by environmental effects.

The development of substantial numbers of genetic markers such as microsatellites and single nucleotide polymorphisms (SNPs) has made it possible to map and in some cases identify individual QTLs. Typically, two inbred strains which differ in susceptibility to a disease or toxic agent are crossed to produce first an F1 hybrid and then either an F2 or a backcross generation. These will be genetically segregating for the susceptibility genes. Each individual is then phenotyped (ie, characterised) for susceptibility and genotyped at a large number of marker loci distributed across all chromosomes. Any association between susceptibility and one or more of the genetic markers implies linkage between the two.

Strains and stocks of laboratory animals

Outbred stocks

An outbred stock is a colony of genetically heterogeneous laboratory animals usually maintained as a closed colony. Such animals are available in all species. The most common outbred stocks are CD-1 and Swiss mice (Chia *et al.* 2005) and Sprague-Dawley and Wistar rats. The individuals are said to be 'genetically undefined' because the genotype of an animal at any given locus is usually unknown unless the animal is individually typed. Most outbred stocks of mice and rats are albino, some stocks of rats are hooded (white with a coloured head and front legs) and many breeds (ie, outbred stocks) of rabbits have a defined coat colour. Some colonies of dogs, primates and pigs may be typed at the major histocompatibility complex (MHC) or other loci of particular interest in a particular research project.

The characteristics of a particular stock can change as a result of directional selection, inbreeding and random genetic drift, resulting in departures from the ideal Hardy–Weinberg population. Daughter colonies in other locations will only have a sample of the genes present in the parental colony, depending on the size of the founding group of animals, hence even if colonies have the same name and come from the same stock, they will be genetically different. Commercial breeders overcome this problem to some extent by circulating stock among different breeding colonies, but this poses a health hazard because there is a danger that one of the colonies has become infected but this has not yet been recognised.

A high level of heterozygosity is usually associated with good reproductive performance. This usually also means that the animals are relatively cheap to buy. However, the cost of the animal is usually only a small fraction of the total cost of the experiment. Increased phenotypic variability means that either sample sizes will need to be increased or statistical power will be decreased in controlled experiments when compared with the use of inbred strains (see Chapter 3). Taking into account the many other advantages of inbred strains such as long-term stability, known genotype at many loci, easy genetic quality control and international distribution, the investigator needs to give serious consideration as to whether the use of outbred stocks can be justified in a particular research project. Basically, the default position should be to use inbred strains except in circumstances when the use of outbred stocks can be specifically justified.

Nomenclature

The International Committee on Laboratory Animals (now the International Council on Laboratory Animal Science, ICLAS) formulated rules for the nomenclature of outbred stocks in 1972[4]. Very briefly, to qualify for designation, an outbred stock should have been bred as a closed colony for at least four generations, and it should be maintained in such a way as to give less than 1% inbreeding per generation

[4]http://www.informatics.jax.org

(see next section). The stock code name should consist of two to four capital letters, eg, NMRI. A laboratory code for the breeder, consisting of a capital and one to four lower case letters should precede the stock name, and be separated by a colon, thus: Tif:NMRI. In alphabetised lists the prefix may be left off so that all stocks with the same name are listed together. It is the prefixed code and the colon which serve to distinguish between an outbred stock and in inbred strain. Further rules are given for the designation of mutant-bearing stocks and crosses between stocks. An appendix of the report also gives details of suitable breeding methods, discussed in the next section. There is no organisation which takes a particular interest in outbred stocks but a review of the origins and uses of outbred stocks of mice is given by Chia *et al.* (2005).

Maintenance of outbred stocks

The objective of maintaining an outbred stock is usually to minimise the rate of change over a period of time. Change can occur as a result of selection (either natural selection as a response to a changing environment or artificial selection imposed by those who control the colony), inbreeding, random drift, mutation and genetic contamination. Wherever possible deliberate selection should be avoided, except that abnormal or unhealthy animals should be culled. Inbreeding and random genetic drift can be controlled by maintaining as large a population as possible, and by careful choice of an appropriate breeding system. In a closed colony maintained by random mating, the rate of inbreeding per generation ΔF is:

$$\Delta F = 1/8N_m + 1/8N_f$$

where N_m and N_f are the numbers of breeding males and females, respectively. Note that the rate of inbreeding depends on the number of the least numerous sex. For example, if a colony is maintained with only four males the inbreeding will be at least 1/32 or 3.1% per generation however many females there are. Hence inbreeding is minimised by keeping equal numbers of each sex. This can be uneconomical with dogs and some other large species, where more males have to be kept than are really required to maintain the colony.

Inbreeding reduces heterozygosity by a certain percent each generation, so as heterozygosity decreases after each generation of inbreeding, it becomes less effective. The formula for calculating the inbreeding at generation t, designated F_t is

$$F_t = \Delta F + (1 - \Delta F) F_{t-1}$$

where F_{t-1} is the inbreeding from the previous generation. It is always assumed that the starting point is zero (ie, that the base population is not inbred). Table 4.2 shows the rate of inbreeding in random-mated groups of various sizes, according to these formulae. Random-mated colonies of 25 or more breeding pairs must be maintained in order to give less than 1% inbreeding per generation, which is the maximum recommended in the nomenclature rules.

A maximum avoidance of inbreeding system can halve the rate of inbreeding. Several such systems are available. The one shown in Table 4.3 is convenient as the mating schedule is the same each generation. Note that avoiding mating of close relatives does not reduce the overall rate because a high rate of inbreeding in one generation will be cancelled out in the next one. Where regular systems of this sort are not practicable, every attempt should be made to ensure that each breeding male contributes one male and each breeding female contributes one female to the next breeding generation.

Table 4.2 Inbreeding per generation for outbred colonies maintained with various numbers of males and females and random mating. Note that with random mating a minimum of 25 breeding pairs is needed to keep the inbreeding down to 1% per generation. Note also that the rate of inbreeding is halved with a maximum avoidance of inbreeding system if the numbers of the two sexes are equal.

Number of male breeders	*Number of female breeders*	*Inbreeding per generation*
4	4	6.3
4	40	3.4
13	13	1.9
10	20	1.9
25	25	1.0
80	80	0.3

Table 4.3 A maximum avoidance of inbreeding system for 12 breeding pairs. Note that such a system can be used for any number of breeding pairs, and it remains the same in each generation. This system with 12 pairs would result in approximately 1% inbreeding per generation. See text for further details.

New pair number	*Male from old pair munber*	*Female from old pair number*
1	1	2
2	3	4
3	5	6
4	7	8
5	9	10
6	11	12
7	2	1
8	4	3
9	6	5
10	8	7
11	10	9
12	12	11

Inbreeding and random genetic drift may be a problem in the maintenance of transgenic populations which are often maintained in small numbers. One result is that the expression of the transgene may change over a period of a few generations. Problems with inbreeding may also arise when maintaining some of the larger and more expensive animals such as primates where large breeding colonies may be extremely expensive to maintain and may produce more animals than are needed in research, but reducing population size may lead to inbreeding. Freezing of sperm and embryos may offer one possible solution to these problems.

Genetic contamination should be avoided by maintaining stocks with the same coat colour in different animal rooms where possible. Genetic monitoring methods may be used to ensure that rapid genetic change as a result of contamination or other cause does not occur. However, the genetic monitoring of outbred colonies is expensive and time consuming, and is rarely done. It is necessary to find some genetic markers which are segregating within the population, and then screen quite large numbers of animals to see if the gene frequency changes. These are statistical calculations rather than the all/nothing results obtained with inbred strains. In one case the gene frequency of a biochemical marker which was segregating within an outbred mouse colony, changed quite dramatically over a period of 2 or 3 years, suggesting genetic contamination (Papaioannou & Festing 1980). Methods of genetic quality control are discussed in more detail later.

Outbred stocks are sometimes found to be carrying deleterious recessive genes. These can usually only be eliminated by progeny testing each future breeder by mating it to an animal homozygous for the gene. If no mutant animals are produced among the first 10 offspring, the animal is probably not a carrier (Green 1981).

Research uses of outbred stocks

The use of outbred stocks of mice relative to inbred strains is declining because of their obvious limitations, though outbred rats are still widely used in some disciplines such as toxicology. They are rather a blunt research tool, but are still of value in some types of research, particularly when a good breeding performance is important. Thus their use may be justified in reproductive physiology, embryology and teratology. Being cheap, they may also be used when the cost of the animal is a significant proportion of the total cost of the experiment, such as in some types of biological assay. It may be necessary to use more outbred than inbred animals, but this may still work out more economical (though ethically less desirable) in some studies. Outbred stocks may also be used during the development of new techniques, in cases where the type of animal used is likely to be of little significance, and in teaching, where the uniformity and genetic stability found in inbred strains may have little value. Finally, outbred stocks will have to be used in cases where inbred strains are not available. This is usually the case for the larger species of laboratory mammals such a rabbits, dogs and primates.

There is a number of 'genetically heterogeneous' stocks which have been developed for genetic research. In the hands of genetically aware scientists such stocks are valuable for specific types of research. Chia *et al.* (2005) concluded that:

> *... outbred stocks (of mice) are a genetically ill-defined set of laboratory animals that are often erroneously used in toxicology, pharmacology and basic research. There is no system of genetic quality control for these stocks and even their names provide little help as to their genetic or phenotypic characteristics. These stocks should not be used in situations where smaller numbers of animals from a range of inbred strains would give optimal results, in terms of sensitivities to substances, for example, or for examining physiological parameters.*

They go on to say:

> *However, outbred stocks, especially the experimentally designed and carefully monitored heterogeneous stocks, are helpful in positional cloning of QTLs and as a phenotype and genotype pool from which to select specific traits of interest. Nevertheless we believe the vast majority of papers currently published that refer to the use of outbred stocks should in fact be using inbred lines, and any experimental plans, including grant applications and papers, using outbred stocks need to be fully justified to avoid the current waste of animals and funding.*

Inbred strains

An inbred strain is produced by 20 or more consecutive generations of brother × sister mating (younger parent × offspring mating is also permitted), with all individuals tracing back to a common ancestor in the 20th or a subsequent generation. This second requirement eliminates parallel branches which will differ genetically. The result is that the animals should be homozygous for at least 98.6% of loci (Figure 4.1). The animals should also be isogenic, that is, all animals should be genetically identical at every locus, although 100% homozygosity is never achieved.

The first inbred strain of mice was DBA, developed by C.C. Little in 1909, with the first inbred strains of rats and guinea pigs being developed at about the same time by Drs. Helen King and Sewell Wright, respectively (Festing 1979). Most of the strains used today can be traced back to the 1920s and 1930s, though some new strains continue to be developed. Over 450 independent inbred strains of mice have been described including many 'old' strains derived from laboratory and pet or fancy mice (Beck *et al.* 2000) as well as a few strains developed from wild mice and subspecies such as *Mus spretus*. The relationship between 102 inbred strains and major substrains based on 1636 informative SNP markers is shown in Figure 4.2 (Petkov *et al.* 2004). Strains could be classified into seven groups according to their genetic similarity. A later study involving 673 SNPs quantified the genetic distances between 55 common mouse strains (Tsang *et al.* 2005). Such data can be useful in the selection of strains of known genetic similarity for future studies. All the 'classical' inbred strains of mice have some admixture of genes from the mouse sub-species. For example, C57BL/6 has about 92% of genes from *Mus musculus domesticus*, 7% from *M. m musculus* and 1% from *M. castaneous* (Yang *et al.* 2007). There are also many 'derived' inbred strains of mice such as the congenic, coisogenic, recombinant inbred and chromosome substituted strains discussed in the next section.

Over 200 inbred strains of rats have also been described (Festing 1979), although some of these have subsequently died out. A list of rats strains with their history and information on their published characteristics is available at the Mouse Genome Informatics website[5]. There are also a few inbred strains of hamster, guinea pigs, rabbits and some other species (Festing 1979). Tables 4.4 and 4.5 show the inbred strains of mice and rats most commonly cited in

[5]http://www.informatics.jax.org

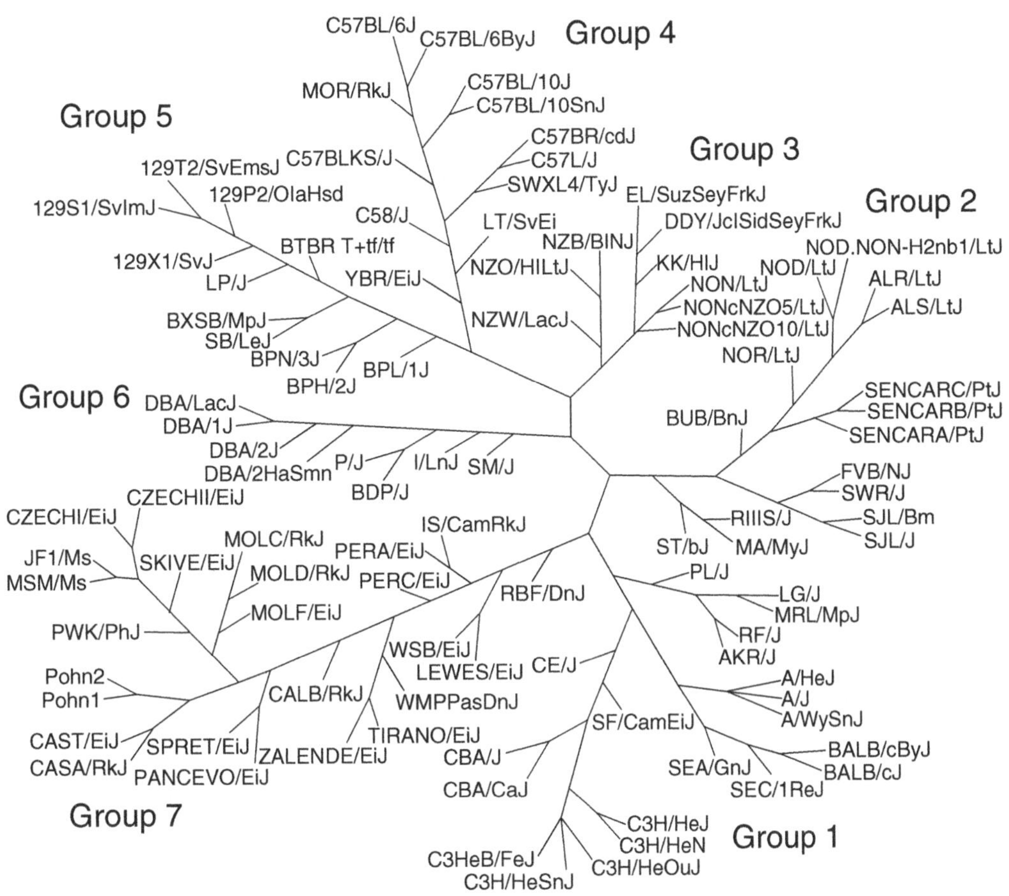

Figure 4.2 Mouse family tree. The 102 strains tested are organized into seven groups. Group 1, Bagg albino derivatives; Group 2, Swiss mice; Group 3, Japanese and New Zealand inbred strains; Group 4, C57/58 strains; Group 5, Castle's mice; Group 6, C.C. Little's DBA and related strains; Group 7, wild-derived strains. The length and angle of the branches have been optimised for printing and do not reflect the actual evolutionary distances between strains. Petko M. Petkov *et al.*, *Genome Research* 2004, **14**, 1806–1811, reprinted with permission.

PubMed over a 5-year period. Note that 66% of the mouse citations are for BALB/c and two sublines of C57BL and that the three most popular rat strains accounted for 69% of citations. These strains are probably being used largely because being inbred they represent standard, repeatable, experimental material and not for any particular characteristics that they may possess. Strain C57BL/6 is frequently used as a genetic background for genetic modifications.

The use of inbred strains is highly variable between disciplines. Virtually all critical experiments in immunology which use rodents now involve inbred strains. In contrast, those disciplines with a chemical orientation such as pharmacology and toxicology have not yet fully realised the potential value of such animals.

Nomenclature of inbred strains

Inbred strains are designated by a capital letter or letters or, less preferably, by a combination of letters and numbers, starting with a letter (eg, CBA, C57BL). Exceptions to this rule include strains, such as 129, which were already well established at the time the rules were formulated. Where it is necessary to indicate the level of inbreeding, this is given by an 'F' and the number of generations of brother × sister mating, eg, F100 indicates 100 generations of brother × sister mating. Care should be taken to ensure that the same strain designation is not used for both rat and mouse strains. Details of nomenclature are given at the Mouse Genome Informatics website.

Substrains are formed when a strain is split into two or more branches, and genetic differences between the branches are discovered or thought to be probable. Two branches of the same strain which have been separated between generations F20 and F40, or which have been separated after F40, but have been maintained separately for more than 20 generations should also be regarded as separate substrains, as in these circumstances it is highly probable that they will be genetically different at some loci. Substrains are indicated by a slash, followed by letters, which are laboratory codes, and/or numbers (eg, C57BL/6 and C57BL/10 are substrains 6 and 10 of strain C57BL which are known to differ at some loci). Substrain symbols may be accumulated (eg, C57BL/6J is a substrain of C57BL/6 developed at the Jackson Laboratory).

F1 hybrids between two inbred strains are indicated usually using abbreviated upper case strain names appending 'F1', for example B6D2F1, the F1 hybrid between strains C57BL/6 and DBA/2.

Table 4.4 Inbred strains of mice and frequency of citations in the PubMed bibliographic database, 2001–2005.

Strain*	Number of citations	Percent of total
BALB/c	20421	36.4
C57BL/6	10279	18.3
C57BL/10	6251	11.1
C3H	3764	6.7
ICR	3502	6.2
CBA	2167	3.9
A/J	1771	3.2
NOD	1722	3.1
DBA/1	1199	2.1
DBA/2	1178	2.1
MOLD	877	1.6
129/	619	1.1
HRS	479	0.9
MRL	411	0.7
NZB	294	0.5
NIH	291	0.5
AKR	290	0.5
SJL	200	0.4
NZW	112	0.2
CAST	76	0.1
KK	58	0.1
SENCAR	56	0.1
C57L	36	0.1
SAMR1	31	0.1
SAMP1	30	0.1
C57BR	11	0
NZO	10	0
	56135	100

*PubMed does not distinguish between sublines

Characteristics of inbred strains

An inbred strain is like an immortal clone of genetically identical individuals. Such strains have many useful characteristics, outlined below, but care should be taken in generalising results obtained with a single strain to the species as a whole. A more general result can usually be obtained by using more than one strain. This can usually be done without increasing the total number of animals using a 'factorial' experimental design (see Chapter 3). F1 hybrids, the first-generation cross between two inbred strains, have most of the useful features of inbred strains except that they are not homozygous so when mated the offspring will be genetically segregating for all those loci at which the parental strains differed. They are not, therefore, immortal. However, they tend to be much more vigorous than inbred strains so are more suitable for some research projects. The main disadvantage of inbred strains is that they do not usually breed as well as outbred stocks or F1 hybrids. Where this is critical, as in the development of genetically modified animals, research workers are often forced to use a genetically heterogeneous stock. However, once developed it is usually better to backcross the transgene to an inbred strain (see later in this chapter) in order to stabilise the strain/mutant characteristics.

Inbred strains have made a substantial contribution to biomedical research. More than 20 Nobel prizes have been awarded for work which would have been either impossible or much more difficult were such strains not available (Festing & Fisher 2000).

Table 4.5 Inbred strains of rats in order of the number of citations in PubMed 2001–2005 (data from www.isogenic.info).

Strain designation	Number of citations	Percentage
F344	4611	32.1
LEW	3227	22.5
SHR	2086	14.5
WKY	1821	12.7
BN	989	6.9
Dahl SS and SR	318	2.2
WF	309	2.2
ACI	224	1.6
BB	209	1.5
OLETF	171	1.2
WAG	95	0.7
BUF	90	0.6
PVG	79	0.6
LEC	66	0.5
OM	16	0.1
COP	15	0.1
BDIX	12	0.1
BDII	8	0.1
BH	7	0.0
Total inbred strains	14353	100.2

The main properties of inbred strains can be considered under the following headings.

Isogenicity

The individuals of an inbred strain are isogenic (all animals are identical at more than 99% of the genetic loci which were segregating in the original foundation colony). One consequence is that a single individual can be genotyped, and this will serve to genotype all animals of that strain. In fact the DNA of 16 inbred strains of mice has now been fully sequenced[6]. Two individuals of a strain will be histocompatible (ie, they will not reject skin grafts or other tissue from another member of the same inbred strain). F1 hybrids, the first-generation cross between two inbred strains, are also isogenic and will accept skin and tissue grafts from each other and from both parental strains without immunological rejection.

Homozygosity

Each inbred animal is homozygous at more than 99% of the loci which were segregating in the original population. They do not carry any hidden recessive genes (except for recent mutations) and will breed true. This is what makes the strains immortal as new generations of identical animals can be produced at will. When mutations do occur they will segregate briefly in the strain until they are fixed (with ¼ probability) or eliminated (with ¾ probability) by further inbreeding.

Long-term stability

An inbred strain will stay genetically constant for long periods of time. It cannot change as a result of selection, inbreeding, or random drift of polymorphic gene loci (the

[6] http://www.niehs.nih.gov/news/releases/2006/snp2.cfm

factors which cause change in outbred stocks). The only change that can occur is as a result of new, sometimes unnoticed, mutations becoming fixed. 'Quiet' mutations of this sort can sometimes remain undetected in a colony for many years (Stevens *et al.* 2007). Genetic drift occurs much more slowly than in an outbred stock because virtually all loci are homozygous so genetic drift can only occur as a result of new mutations, while in an outbred stock drift is a result of changes in gene frequency at many loci as well as being due to mutation at a few loci. It can also be prevented by maintaining banks of frozen embryos of inbred strains, which can be resuscitated periodically to replace colonies which may have fixed new undetected mutations. Investigators maintaining their own breeding colonies are advised to go back to the original source periodically (say every 20 generations) so as to minimise subline drift between the two colonies.

Phenotypic uniformity
The elimination of genetic variation generally leads to greater uniformity of most characteristics within an inbred strain. This is most obvious with a single polymorphic locus such as the major histocompatibility complex. However, it is also true for many polygenic characters, particularly those with a high heritability. Increased uniformity means that fewer inbred animals are needed relative to outbred animals to achieve a given level of statistical precision (Festing *et al.* 2002).

Individuality
Each inbred strain is a unique combination of alleles at approximately 25 000 loci, and therefore differs from every other strain. These differences can be of great interest in themselves. A study of why one strain develops a particular type of tumour, or a particular pattern of behaviour, while another strain does not, may throw considerable light on the development of tumours or behaviour patterns respectively.

Some examples of strain characteristics which are of biomedical interest in inbred strains are given in Table 4.6. Most mouse genes have human homologues so identification of the mouse genes associated with human disease can be an efficient and economical way of identifying human genetic disease susceptibility.

Identifiability
Once an inbred strain has been developed, and some of the polymorphic loci such as microsatellites and SNPs have been characterised to provide a 'genetic profile', the strain may then be identified by this genetic profile. Scientists using inbred strains would be advised to keep a sample of tissue or DNA so that if they obtain unexpected results the authenticity and integrity of the strains can be determined. There are commercial companies which will carry out the appropriate tests, given a sample of DNA or tissue.

Table 4.6 Examples of inbred mouse strains with characteristics of interest in biomedical research. Note that these conditions do not necessarily preclude the use of the strains in general research.

Strain	*Characters of interest*
129P1	One of several major substrains of the original strain 129. Pink-eyed chinchilla coat colour. Develops testicular teratomas. Used in the development of ES cells which are used in the production of targeted mutations ('knockouts')
A/J	Susceptible to the development of lung adenomas. High incidence of congenital cleft palate
AKR	High incidence of lymphatic leukaemia and short lifespan
BALB/c	Possibly the most widely used strain. Develops myelomas when treated with a carcinogen. Used in the development of monoclonal antibodies. Useful general purpose albino strain, but males may fight
C3H/HeJ	Unfostered strains (now rare) develop a high incidence of mammary tumours. General purpose strain. High incidence of hepatomas. Substrain resistant to bacterial lipopolysaccharide due to spontaneous mutation previously designated Lps^{d}, now $Tlr4^{Lps\text{-}d}$
CBA/Ca	General purpose strain with a high incidence of hepatomas
C57BL/6	Most widely used strain. Used as genetic background for many mutants and congenic strains. High preference for alcohol. Some micropthalmia and fur chewing on back
DBA/1	Susceptible to collagen-induced arthritis
DBA/2	Oldest strain. Susceptible to induction of audiogenic seizures
DDK	Semi-sterile when mated with C57BL males due to a defect of the F1 embryos
FVB	Relatively new strain. Breeds well. Large male pronucleus helpful in producing transgenic strains by microinjection
HRS	Carries hairless gene. Homozygotes for hr develop high incidence of leukaemia
I	Sex-linked phosphorylase kinase deficiency leading to 3–4-fold elevation of muscle glycogen
NOD	Developes insulin-dependent diabetes mellitus and associated pathology
NON	Obesity without diabetes
NZB	Develops autoimmune haemolytic anaemia
SJL	Develops reticulum-cell sarcoma (Hodgkin's disease). Males very aggressive
SWR	Polydipsia and polyurea on aging

Sensitivity
There is some evidence that inbred strains are more sensitive to environmental influences than are outbred stocks. This is an advantage to the extent that they may be more sensitive to an experimental treatment, but is a disadvantage in other respects. For example, a breeding colony may stop breeding as a result of some unknown environmental factor which may hardly influence an outbred stock. Their production and use requires more attention to details of husbandry and diet than is the case for outbred stocks. However, the actual breeding plan is much simpler. Very small populations can

be maintained, as an inbred strain will no longer be subject to further inbreeding depression, whereas the maintenance of outbred stocks requires large sample sizes and careful attention to methods of avoiding directional selection and genetic drift due to inbreeding.

International distribution
Inbred strains have an international distribution, so that work in the UK, USA, Germany and Australia, for example, can be carried out using virtually identical inbred mice or rats. This is possible due to the long-term stability of inbred strains, the fact that daughter colonies are genetically identical with the original colony and because genetic quality control is so much easier with inbred strains than with outbred stocks. Sublines separated for long periods will differ to some extent as a result of new mutations. This may affect the expression of mutations and transgenes. For example, the expression of the obese (Lep^{ob}) and diabetic ($Lepr^{db}$) mutations in mice differs between the sublines C57BL/6J and C57BL/6KsJ (Hummel *et al.* 1972). Such effects need to be taken into account in designing and interpreting such studies. Colonies may also differ as a result of environmental differences. There have been several examples of strain characteristics being seriously altered as a result of an infection, such as Tyzzer's disease or ectoparasites.

Background data
Inbred strains stay genetically constant for long periods so it is possible to build up reliable data on their phenotypic and genetic characteristics. The names of many of the most commonly used strains are included as key words in electronic bibliographical data bases, so it is possible to retrieve all papers in which a particular inbred strain was used provided authors have used correct nomenclature. The Mouse Phenome database[7] provides a substantial body of information on the comparative phenotypic characteristics of many strains. This gives tables and graphical displays of comparative strain characteristics for a wide range of phenotypes including appearance, behaviour, blood characteristics, reproductive performance, response to pathogens and many more characteristics. The Rat Phenome database[8], although less detailed, also provides a considerable amount of information about inbred strains and mutants of the rat.

Maintenance of inbred strains

Ideally, an inbred strain would remain genetically constant for an indefinite period. It should also be maintained as economically and efficiently as possible. Usually it is best to maintain a 'foundation stock' or 'stem-line' colony and a separate production colony as outlined in the next sections. Once a strain has been brother × sister mated for 20 or more generations, the main sources of change are from genetic contamination or as a result of the occurrence and fixation of new mutations, though some drift may occur due to 'residual heterozygosity', the small amount of heterozygosity remaining after 20 generations of inbreeding.

[7] http://www.informatics.jax.org
[8] http://rgd.mcw.edu/

The chance of genetic contamination can be minimised by keeping each strain physically separated as far as is practicable. If several strains must be kept in one room they should, ideally, have different coat colours. The cages should have clear colour labels, and the staff should be rigorously trained so as to be on their guard against genetic contamination. Staff should be assured that if a contamination occurs they will not get blamed otherwise they will tend to cover up any unusual behaviour in the colony. With mice and rats a monogamous breeding system with each pair staying together for the whole of their breeding life should he adopted, as this will minimise the chance of a mismating.

The best way of preventing genetic change due to new mutations would be to maintain a bank of frozen embryos of each strain, and thaw out samples to renew the colony at infrequent intervals (Hedrich & Reetz 1988).

Stem-line or foundation stock colony

This should be a small self-perpetuating colony of up to about 30 permanently mated monogamous pairs. Detailed pedigree and production records should be kept and care should be taken to ensure that no genetic contamination occurs. Ideally, this colony will be kept physically separate from all other colonies. Genetic quality control methods (see later in this chapter) should be used periodically to check genetic authenticity. Offspring from this colony will be used first to perpetuate the stem-line colony, and second as breeding stock for the production colony. All animals should trace back to a common ancestor about six to ten generations back. Sublines which breed poorly should be culled to try to eliminate quiet mutations which reduce breeding performance.

Production colony

Where large numbers of animals are to be bred (eg, by a commercial supplier) colonies of 100–1000 or more cages, possibly with several subdivisions such as an expansion colony (which may be pedigreed) and one or more generations of production stock, may be required. The production colony does not contribute to the long-term survival of the strain so animals may be mated as pairs or trios, or using some other system. Animals may be mated at random, rather than brother × sister, and detailed records of pedigrees need not be kept although they may be useful if problems arise. All animals in the production colony should trace back to stem-line ancestors within about four to six generations. In other words, up to about six generations may be used to multiply up the stem-line stock in the production colonies. Only in exceptional circumstances (eg, if the colony would otherwise be lost) should the random-mated production stock be used to perpetuate the inbred strain.

Research uses of inbred strains

Inbred strains may be used in many ways in research. The simplest case is when an inbred strain is chosen in preference to an outbred stock on the grounds that it is more uniform, genetically more stable, and better defined than the outbred stock even though either type could be used. There is a strong case for using, say, C57BL/6 or BALB/c mice and F344 rats as the universal standard in experiments where there is no *a priori* reason for choosing a particular strain. Such standard strains are widely used as a genetic background for mutants and transgenes, discussed later in this chapter.

An inbred strain may also be chosen because the experiment would otherwise be impossible. For example, a study may require the transfer of cells, tissues, or tumours from one animal to another without immunological rejection. This is only possible if the host is isogenic with the donor unless animals with a defective immune system are used. A considerable number of experiments in immunology and cancer research fall into this class.

An inbred strain may be chosen for a particular project because it develops a spontaneous disease or condition which is of intrinsic interest or may be considered to be a model of human disease. Many strains develop specific types of neoplasia either spontaneously or after the application of a carcinogen. These are often of value in research. For example, the myelomas which may be induced in BALB/c mice by mineral oil, were vital in developing monoclonal antibodies.

In some cases the research worker wishes to do experiments on a wide range of phenotypes within the species so as to be reasonably confident that the results are general and do not depend on some quirk of an individual strain. It is a fallacy to assume that testing on an outbred stock will achieve this objective. If the outbred stock is truly variable, then this will result on a considerable amount of background 'noise' which may obscure treatment effects. The use of several inbred strains using a 'multi-strain' experimental design without using excessive numbers of animals should, however, provide a wide range of phenotypes on which to test the treatment without any associated problems of experimental noise (Russell & Burch 1959; Heston 1968; Festing, 1995). Very often it is the unusual strain which is of greatest interest.

Several strains may also be used to explore the relationships between different characters. For example, if some response to a treatment is quantified in several strains, grouping the strains by their *H2* haplotype (using data taken from published literature) may show whether the response is *H2* related. Quantitative relationships between variables may also be explored in this way, to show, for example, the relationship between certain types of biochemical activity in the brain, and some types of behaviour (Gaitonde & Festing 1976). It is, of course, essential to use more than two strains in such experiments. Indeed, the use of several inbred strains in this way offers one of the most powerful methods of analysing the response to a treatment effect. The ultimate tool for research workers interested in this approach is a full set of recombinant inbred strains, discussed later in this chapter.

Derived inbred strains

Large numbers of new inbred strains have been developed from existing strains. The most common are the congenic strains where a mutation or genetic modification has been backcrossed to an inbred strain. However, there are many other types, discussed in the following paragraphs.

Coisogenic and segregating inbred strains

If a mutation (eg, for coat colour or other visible effect) occurs in an inbred strain, and is then bred separately, then it will differ from the inbred strain only at a single genetic locus, namely, the mutant locus. Two inbred strains which are genetically identical except at a single locus as a result of a mutation within the strain and subsequent separation of sublines are said to be *coisogenic*. A transgenic strain developed by micro-injection of DNA into a fertilised egg of an inbred strain will also be coisogenic with the parent strain. Targeted mutations developed within an inbred strain are also coisogenic with the background strain. Segregating inbred strains are developed by inbreeding with forced heterozygosity at a specific locus.

Nomenclature of coisogenic strains

Coisogenic and segregating inbred strains should be designated by the name of the inbred strain followed by a hyphen and the gene symbol so, C3H/N-$Kit^{W\text{-}v}$ is the N substrain of strain C3H carrying a mutation of the Kit oncogene with the allele designation *W-v* (viable dominant spotting, previously designated W^{v}) as a result of a mutation within the strain. 129-$Alox5^{tm1Fun}$ is a targeted mutation (the tm1 superscript shows it is the first one developed by 'Fun', a laboratory code) of the arachidonate 5-lipoxygenase locus coisogenic with strain 129. When a mutation is maintained in a heterozygous state, this may be indicated by including a + sign in the symbol (eg, C3H/N-$Kit^{W\text{-}v}$/+).

In the case of segregating inbred strains developed by inbreeding with forced heterozygosity, indication of the mutant locus is optional (eg, DW-+/$Pou1f1^{dw}$ an inbred strain DW carrying a dwarf mutation at the *Pou1f1* locus developed by inbreeding with forced segregation, could be designated simply as DW).

Maintenance of coisogenic and segregating inbred strains

Coisogenic strains are inbred strains and should be maintained in the same way as any other inbred strain. However, segregating inbred strains need to be maintained with continued segregation at the locus of interest. This usually involves mating animals with the mutant phenotype with those with a wild-type phenotype.

Congenic strains

These strains are an approximation of coisogenicity produced by backcrossing an allele from another strain or outbred stock into a specific inbred strain for 10 or more generations. The result is a pair of strains (the inbred partner and the congenic strain) which should be genetically identical at virtually all loci not linked to the differential locus. On average, the differential locus is accompanied by about 20 centiMorgans of associated chromosome which will contain some contaminating genes. In most cases these are of little importance, and can be ignored, though the possibility that they may interfere with research results should not be forgotten. The nomenclature also recognises partially congenic strains following five generations of backcrossing.

Congenic strains are developed when an investigator wants to determine the characteristics of a mutation or QTL on a different genetic background or to maintain it on a standard inbred background such as C57BL/6. For example, many targeted mutations (see later in this chapter) have been developed on one of the 129-background strains, but for comparative purposes it is convenient to have them on a C57BL/6 background, hence they are backcrossed to that strain.

Backcrossing for 10 generations takes a considerable time. It can be speeded up using marker-assisted or 'speed' backcrossing by simultaneously selecting for genetic markers on other chromosomes which differ between the donor and background strains, but resemble the background strain (Markel *et al.* 1997). This should approximately halve the time required.

Congenic strains were first developed systematically by Dr. George Snell at the Jackson Laboratory (for which he received the Nobel Prize in 1980) as a means of separating out the loci responsible for rejection of transplanted tumours. The strains which he developed were called 'congenic resistant' strains because they resisted a strain-specific transplantable tumour which would grow in the background strain. The resulting strains were mostly found to differ at the major histocompatibility locus.

Nomenclature of congenic strains

Congenic strains are designated by a full or abbreviated name of the background strain, followed by a period (full-stop) and the abbreviated name of the donor strain, followed by a hyphen and a gene symbol (eg, BlO.129-*H12*^{b}). Thus BlO (abbreviation for C57BL/10) is the background strain, 129 is the donor strain and *H12*^{b} is the allele of interest. When several strains are developed from the same donor strain they may be distinguished by a number and/or letter in parentheses (eg, B10.129(12M)-*H2*^{b}). Partially congenic strains have the same nomenclature except they have a semi-colon between the two strain designations, eg, B6;129S-*Inhba*^{tm1Zuk}, a partially congenic strain developed by backcrossing the first targeted mutation at the inhibin-beta-A locus developed by 'Zuk' (a laboratory code).

In other cases the full designation given above is not appropriate because the donor strain is not inbred, or because the congenic strain is already widely known. In such cases, a less complete symbol may be used (eg, A.SW, BlO.D2/n, the n in this case stands for 'new', C3H.SW+).

Maintenance

Congenic strains are inbred strains in their own right, and are maintained as such.

Research uses

The value of congenic, coisogenic and segregating inbred strains is that the differential locus and its effects may be studied on a chosen inbred genetic background, free of the noise associated with genetically determined variation in expression and penetrance found in a heterogeneous stock. For this reason many mutant genes such as obese (*Lep*^{ob}), dwarf (*Pou1f1*^{dw}), nude (*Foxn1*^{nu}) and yellow (*A*^{y}) have been placed on an inbred genetic background (usually C57BL/6).

Many congenic strains have also been developed which differ at the major histocompatibility complex (the *H2* complex in mice). A parasitologist or microbiologist may be interested in discovering whether the response to a parasite or bacterium depends on the *H2* genotype. All that is necessary in the first instance is to obtain, say, C57BL/10 (mice which are *H2*^{b}) and some strains congenic with this, but differing at the *H2* locus such as Bl0.D2 (which is *H2*^{d}), and BlO. BR (which is *H2*^{k}). The course of the infection would then be studied in the strains, and if they were found to differ, this would suggest that *H2* has some influence. Such a study does not depend on the research worker developing the highly specialised skills of tissue typing individual animals. The research worker would, however, be well advised to confirm his/her results using other pairs of congenic strains in order to rule out the possibility that the observed difference has some other cause (such as genetic contamination or mutation of one of the congenic lines).

Recombinant inbred (RI) strains

A set of recombinant inbred strains is developed by crossing two standard inbred strains followed by brother × sister inbreeding for 20 generations as a set of parallel strains (Bailey 1971). Ideally, at least 10–20 new inbred strains should be produced, though the more strains that are produced, the more useful the set will be. Each RI strain is an inbred strain in its own right, but its genotype will be composed of a recombination of the parental strain genes – hence the name recombinant inbred strain.

More recently a large collaborative study is developing a panel of 1000 RI strains from a cross involving eight diverse inbred mouse strains. Genetic analysis will involve comparisons of strains and crosses between them (Churchill *et al.* 2004).

Nomenclature

A set of recombinant inbred strains is designated by an abbreviation of the parental strain names separated by an X, with no intervening spaces. Thus CXB would be the designation of a set produced by crossing BALB/c (abbreviated C) with C57BL (abbreviated B). Different strains of the same series should be designated by a number or letter. Optionally, these may be separated by a hyphen thus: AXB5 or AXB-5. An exception is made in the case of strains already known by another designation. Thus Bailey's original seven strains are designated CXBD–CXBK (with CXBF missing).

Maintenance

Each recombinant inbred strain is an inbred strain in its own right, and should be maintained in exactly the same way as any other inbred strain.

Research uses

Recombinant inbred strains may be used for investigating the mode of inheritance of any character in which the parental strains differ. They are particularly valuable for studying characters requiring the destruction of the animal before it reaches breeding age, or discrete characters such as tumour incidence in which a good estimate of the phenotype of a strain can only be obtained by averaging across several individuals. They can also be useful in the analysis of polygenic characters and the identification of QTLs (Plomin *et al.* 1991). These strains have great potential for the study of genetic variation in response to toxic or pharmacologically active chemicals such as those which cause lung tumours in mice (Malkinson *et al.* 1985).

The characteristics of the parental strains to the treatment should be examined first. If these differ, then the response of the full set of recombinant inbred strains should be characterised, and the 'strain distribution pattern' (SDP) should be studied. If the recombinant inbred strains fall into two distinct groups with about half of them resembling one parent and the other half the other parent, then this is presumptive evidence that the response is governed by a single Mendelian locus. If some genetic marker agrees closely with the separation into two groups, then that is evidence for linkage between a gene near the marker and the phenotype. The development of microsatellite and other markers has made it possible to characterise some sets of RI strains at several hundred loci on all chromosomes. This makes it virtually certain that an approximate chromosomal location of a well behaved Mendelian gene could be identified just from the strain distribution pattern, provided a reasonably large set of RI strains was available.

However, if the strains grade continuously between the two parental strains, then this would be evidence that the response is controlled by more than one locus and/or environmental factors. When the thousand or so strains from the collaborative cross being developed by the Complex Trait Consortium[9] are available, they will be particularly useful for identifying and mapping QTLs.

Recombinant congenic strains

These strains have been developed largely for the study of complex traits. Two inbred strains are crossed and the offspring are backcrossed to one of the parental strains (the 'background' strain) usually for two (or sometimes more) generations before further generations of brother × sister mating to produce a set of 'recombinant congenic' or RC strains. They are regarded as fully inbred when the coefficient of inbreeding is the same as that used for inbred strains. With two backcrosses a further 14 generations of brother × sister mating are necessary. In use, the strains are individually phenotyped for a character of interest. Most of the RC strains will resemble the parental strain but some strains may carry a part of a chromosome from the donor strain carrying an allele which influences the trait of interest. Crosses between this strain and the parental strain can then be used to isolate and identify the gene responsible for the difference.

The set of strains is designated by BACKGROUND-STRAINcDONOR STRAIN-n, where n is a strain number. For example strain NONcNZO-1 is the first strain of a set of RC strains with strain NON being the background strain and NZO the donor strain.

[9] http://www.complextrait.org

Chromosome substitution (CSS) or 'consomic' strains

These strains are produced by substituting a chromosome from one strain into a background strain by backcrossing with selection for the whole donor chromosome. This provides a very powerful tool for finding out what QTLs there are on a given chromosome which are associated with strain differences between the two strains because segregation on all other chromosomes has been eliminated. In a study of 53 traits in the full set of 22 A/J into C57BL/6J mouse strains a total of 150 QTLs affecting levels of serum components, diet-induced obesity and anxiety were identified (Singer *et al.* 2004). Once a QTL has been identified on a whole chromosome it can be mapped by intercrossing the substituted strain with the background strain and looking for any association between the phenotype and a set of markers on that chromosome. Backcrossing can also be used to develop congenic strains for the QTL. Thus, once a set of CSS has been developed, it provides a powerful tool for complex trait analysis.

Nomenclature of CSS

The designation of these strains is HOST STRAIN-Chr $\#^{\mathrm{DONOR\ STRAIN}}$ where # is the chromosome number. So a consomic strain with a C57BL/6 genetic background with chromosome 1 from strain A/J is designated C57BL/6-Chr1$^{A/J}$.

Genetic quality control

Genetic contamination of inbred strains is not uncommon (Festing 1982), and can cause substantial disruption to the research programmes. Animals should only be obtained from a reliable source and, if they are to be bred on site, their authenticity should be checked as soon as possible. Breeding colonies of inbred strains should be kept physically separated as far as possible. If several strains must be kept in the same room, then they need clear labelling. Staff need to be well trained and alert to any changes in the colony. Changes in coat colour and/or breeding performance should certainly be investigated, but monitoring these is not sufficient to ensure authenticity.

In the past, use has been made of biochemical and immunological markers and bone morphology but modern methods depend on examination of microsatellite and SNP DNA markers.

Breeding performance

Inbred strains usually have a relatively poor breeding performance. F1 hybrids, in contrast, breed well due to hybrid vigour. Breeding performance is normally monitored routinely in order to detect any environmental influences which adversely affect output. However any breeding pair or group of related animals which breed exceptionally well should be regarded with some suspicion. It might be advisable either not to breed from such animals or to get them genetically typed using microsatellite or SNP markers.

Microsatellite and single nucleotide polymorphic markers

Microsatellites are short repetitive DNA sequences such as the dinucleotide sequence CA, commonly 50–200 bases in length, with unique sequence flanking DNA. There are several thousand microsatellites in vertebrate DNA and they are often highly polymorphic in the number of repeats. The microsatellite profile of a test animal is compared with the published microsatellite profile of the particular strain.

More recently, genome scanning using SNP markers has become both cheap and powerful. There are literally millions of SNPs in the mouse genome, where individuals or inbred strains differ. Individuals to be tested can be typed and compared with the known SNP profile of authentic strains. Where they differ, this can be quantified. This technique can also be used to examine the success of backcrossing in the development of congenic strains by getting both the congenic strain and the inbred partner scanned and compared. These techniques require expensive apparatus, but are commercially available. Samples of tissue or DNA can be sent by mail so there is no need to send live animals. Results might be available in 2–4 weeks.

Ovary transplants and embryo manipulation

A number of techniques which have been developed for studies of various aspects of reproductive biology and embryology have now assumed some importance in applied genetics.

Ovarian transplants

A technique for transplanting the ovaries between histocompatible hosts was developed some years ago, and has been used routinely to assist in the maintenance of some mutants which are difficult to breed, usually because the female dies young or is infertile.

Ovaries may be taken from donor females as young as 16 days of age. The ovaries may then be cut in half, with half being transplanted into each recipient. Thus a single mutant female provides sufficient material for four recipients.

The recipients must be histocompatible with the donor. Usually the donor is inbred and the recipient is an F1 hybrid (to obtain maximum breeding performance) in which the donor strain is one of the parents. For example, C57BL/6-*Lep*^{ob}/*Lep*^{ob} (obese) female mice are infertile, but their ovaries could be transplanted to B6D2F1 hybrid females without immunological rejection.

Once a phenotypically normal female has been given homozygous mutant (*m/m*) type ovaries, it can be mated with a normal +/+ male of the same strain to produce known heterozygotes, or with *m*/+ or *m/m* males to produce 50% or 100% homozygous mutant offspring, respectively.

Embryo transfers

The technique of embryo transfer may be used to study the effect of the material genotype on offspring characteristics, as an alternative to hysterectomy as a method of eliminating disease-causing organisms from a strain, provided suitable disease-free foster mothers are available, or to implant thawed frozen embryos.

Donor mice are (optionally) superovulated using an appropriate hormone regimen (eg, an injection of 2–10 IU of pregnant mare's serum gonadotrophin, PMSG, followed 44–48 h later with 2–10 IU of human chorionic gonadotrophin, hCG) and mated overnight. Vaginal plugs indicate successful mating. After about 3 days (depending exactly on the aims of the study), the mice are killed and the embryos flushed out of the oviduct and uterus. These embryos may be transferred directly to the oviduct or uterus of a pseudopregnant foster mother (ie, one that has been mated with a sterile male, usually 1 day after the donor females were mated), or they can be cultured in vitro for 24 h. The foster mother, which need not be histocompatible with the strain of the embryos, is anaesthetised and the embryos are transferred directly to the uterus via a dorsal abdominal incision. If sterile techniques are used, and the foster mother is pathogen-free, then this provides a method of eliminating pathogens from genetically valuable strains and stocks. Practical details are given by Papaioannou and Johnson (1993).

Freeze preservation of mouse embryos and sperm

Mouse embryos obtained as described above may also be frozen and maintained virtually indefinitely in liquid nitrogen before being thawed and placed in a foster mother. Various techniques and cryoperservatives are used. One of the most common methods is to use eight-cell embryos, which are flushed from the mother on day 3 of gestation. They are placed in vials or straws in a medium containing dimethyl-sulphoxide (DMSO) as a cryoprotective agent, and are frozen under carefully controlled conditions, using a slow cooling rate. Eventually, the vials are placed in liquid nitrogen. When the embryos are wanted, they are thawed in a controlled manner, and are usually cultured for 24h before being transferred to a foster mother. This makes a viability check possible, as the embryos should undergo some degree of development during this period. They are then transferred to pseudopregnant foster mothers as described above.

The main advantages of maintaining banks of frozen embryos are:

1. freeze preservation of embryos from inbred strains should prevent genetic drift due to new mutations;
2. it provides an economical method of maintaining strains and mutants which are not currently being used;
3. it provides an insurance against loss of valuable stocks and allows such stocks to be maintained in smaller, more economical numbers;
4. in some cases, frozen embryos may be transported more conveniently than live animals.

The freeze preservation of mouse sperm is relatively easy, compared with embryos (Nakagata 2000) and is now used in ENU mutagenesis programs (see below). Sperm may even be repeatedly frozen and thawed, and still be capable of producing viable offspring (Aoto *et al.* 2007, Ostermeier *et al.* 2008).

Genetically modified (transgenic and mutant) strains

Genetically modified strains of mice, and to a lesser extent other species, are now widely used in research. Initially, transgenic strains were developed by direct injection of DNA into early embryos. However, mutagenesis using ethyl-nitroso-urea (ENU), techniques for 'gene trapping', gene targeting using homologous recombination to produce 'knockout' and 'knockin' mice, the use of transposon-mediated mutagenesis and the use of RNAi (see later in this chapter) have transformed many areas of research. These techniques are described briefly in the following paragraphs.

Direct injection of DNA

Transgenic strains were first developed in the 1980s by direct injection of foreign DNA into the pro-nucleus of an early embryo in such a way that it became incorporated permanently into the host DNA. The transgene is incorporated at random (or at least in an unpredictable location) and very often consists of a tandem array of many genes end-to-end. Occasionally, if it gets incorporated into an existing gene it may cause an insertional mutation. The transgene needs a promoter and enhancer region as well as the coding region to allow it to be expressed. A dramatic demonstration of the method involved the transgenic insertion of the human growth hormone gene with a metallothionein promoter region into mice. When these mice were subsequently treated with zinc sulphate, which induced a high level of growth hormone, the mice grew extremely large (Palmiter *et al.* 1982). Unfortunately, the mice also developed a range of defects and had a short lifespan. Mouse strain inbred FVB is now widely used in the production of this type of transgenic strain because it breeds well and has a large male pro-nucleus into which it is relatively easy to inject the transgene (Taketo *et al.* 1991).

Hundreds of transgenic strains have now been produced using these techniques, and are listed in various electronic databases. Most have been developed to answer highly specific research questions, but a few have been produced for more general research purposes. For example, the 'immortomouse' was developed as an aid to the establishment of cell lines from different mouse tissues. It was developed by injecting a DNA construct containing a thermolabile version of the simian virus 40 (SV40) large T antigen fused with an *H2* (major histocompatibility complex) promotor region. *In vivo*, this transgene has little or no effect. However, when cells from these mice are grown *in vitro* at 33 °C (but not at 37 °C) in the presence of interferon (which induces SV40 T activity), they become immortal, due to the action of the SV40 T gene. Using this technique, it has been possible reliably to develop immortal cell lines from a range of tissues which have proved difficult to culture in the past (Jat *et al.* 1991).

'BigBlue' mice and rats and the 'Mutamouse' have also been developed as a means of assessing whether chemicals are mutagenic, and therefore potentially carcinogenic, *in vivo* (Gehlmann 1993). The animals carry a transgene in the form of a 'shuttle vector' with a reporter gene *lac Z* (and its suppressor locus *lac I* in the case of BigBlue), which codes for bacterial betagalactosidase. The reporter gene causes no ill effects in the animals. Animals are treated with the test chemical. If it is mutagenic, it will mutate some of the transgenes. The shuttle vector is then extracted from a target tissue such as the liver and the number of mutations is assessed and compared with a control.

Transgenic strains have also been developed with reporter genes such as the green fluorescent protein (GFP) and betagalactosidase controlled by specific promoters as an aid to understanding in which tissues or at which times a gene becomes active. For example damage to the adult neural cortex leads to loss of motor function. In a mouse model grafts of embryonic mouse cortical cells expressing GFP were grafted into the damaged area and it was observed that host and transplanted neurones formed synaptic contacts with the re-establishment of cortical circuitry suggesting that there is potential to use neural transplants in the reconstruction of brain injury (Gaillard *et al.* 2007).

Nomenclature of transgenic strains

Transgenic strains are designated by the background strain or background status followed by a hyphen then Tg(YYY)#Zzz, where YYY is the inserted gene, # is the serial number of the insert and Zzz is the laboratory code. For example STOCK Tg(GFPU)5Nagy is an outbred stock with a transgenic green fluorescent protein incorporated by microinjection into an early embryo. It is the fifth line that was developed by Nagy, a laboratory code. If the transgene should become inserted into a gene, then it will become an allele of that gene with the Tg(YYY)#Zzz being shown as a superscript of the gene designation. More details are given on the Jackson Laboratory website[10].

Chemical mutagenesis

One of the best ways of studying the function of a gene is to mutate it and see what happens. Chemical mutagenesis is now done almost exclusively using ENU because it gives a good yield of mutants and usually causes point mutations rather than deletions (Barbaric *et al.* 2007). Point mutations may not inactivate a gene, but may alter its function depending on exactly where in a given gene the mutation occurs. This is an advantage as a complete inactivation may be lethal and therefore more difficult to study. Chemical mutagenesis is a random process, so it is not normally possible to mutate a specified gene. Male mice are injected with ENU and after about 6 weeks, to allow the mutated sperm to develop and the males to become fertile again, are mated with normal females. The offspring are screened for abnormalities which might be caused by a dominant mutation. Techniques of screening have developed enormously in the last few years, with the EUMORPHIA Consortium developing many standardised methods[11] with clear standard oper-

[10] http://www.informatics.jax.org

[11] http://empress.har.mrc.ac.uk

ating procedures (Brown *et al.* 2005). Recessive mutations are detected with a further round of brother × sister breeding followed by further phenotypic testing. These screens involve the breeding of many mice, so care needs to be taken in optimising methods (Cordes 2005; Barbaric & Dear 2007).

With the automation of DNA sequencing techniques it is now also possible to screen samples of DNA from the offspring of mutagenised males for mutations in genes of specific interest (Michaud *et al.* 2005). Where phenotype can only be determined after killing the animal, such as those involving histology of internal organs, samples of sperm can be frozen before killing male mice. If a mutation is found, then it can be recovered from the frozen sperm.

Once an abnormal animal is detected further breeding is necessary to confirm that it is an inherited mutation and to map and identify the genetic locus. This can be time consuming as large numbers of mice may need to be bred and phenotypically typed.

Embryonic stem cells

Embryonic stem (ES) cells are cell lines derived from early embryos, which are said to be totipotent, being able to form any cell type in the body. ES cells are derived by culturing pre-implantation embryos in suitable culture medium which allows them to multiply but not to differentiate (Evans & Kaufman 1981). The cells can be manipulated and mutated *in vitro* using gene trapping or gene targeting (see later paragraph) and can then be injected into the blastocyst of an embryo where they are incorporated, so that the resulting mouse is a chimera. If cells from the ES cell line colonise the gonads of the chimeric mice then offspring of the ES cell genotype will be produced. Usually strains of different coat colour are used in making the chimeras so that mutant offspring can be easily recognised. The majority of ES cells used so far come from the 129 inbred mouse strain, substrains of which differ in many ways including coat colour (Simpson *et al.* 1997). When making targeted mutants (see below) it is important that the DNA in the targeting vector is from the same substrain as the ES cells. It has proved to be difficult to produce ES cells from other strains and it has so far been impossible to produce ES cell in the rat. More recently suitable media have been developed which allow the development of ES cells from other mouse strains such as C57BL/6, although some substrains seem to be more amenable than others. Some reports suggest, for example, that it is easier to establish ES cells from C57BL/6N than from C57BL/6J.

Mutagenesis using gene trapping

Gene trapping is used to randomly mutate genes which are expressed in ES cells. A DNA construct or vector is used which has a reporter gene such as green fluorescent protein or beta-galactosidase and a selectable marker such as *neo* (neomycin resistance) but no promoter region. ES cells are cultured with the DNA constructs, which are incorporated into the cells by electroporation (ie, subjecting the culture to an electric current) or by a modified virus. The DNA constructs are then randomly incorporated into the nuclear DNA. If one lands near or within an active ES cell gene then the reporter gene will become activated by the ES cell promoter. It will usually (but not always) also deactivate or mutate the ES cell gene. In order to obtain live mice the mutated ES cells are then injected into mouse blastocysts. The result is a chimeric mouse which, when bred, may produce mutant offspring. DNA surrounding the gene trap construct can be sequenced to map and identify the mutant gene.

The gene trap DNA construct can be made to include sequences such as *loxP* (see below) which allow it to be deleted in certain tissues and/or at certain times.

The advantage of gene trapping is that it can be done in ES cells in a standardised way on a large scale using the most appropriate constructs, but live mice do not need to be derived until such a time as there are facilities available to study them. The disadvantage is that it is a random process, so to begin with many of the mutated genes will be 'new', but eventually more mutations will occur in genes which have already been mutated. Thus diminishing returns will eventually make the process less efficient. International projects to knock out every mouse gene will eventually need to use gene targeting to knock out the remaining genes.

Transposon-mediated mutagenesis

Transposons or 'jumping genes' are sections of DNA which can move around in host DNA, sometimes causing insertional mutagenesis. They can also be used to insert genes into a host so may be of value in gene therapy. 'Sleeping Beauty' was a transposon found in fish which had been inactivated at least 10 million years ago, but was re-activated by genetic engineering (Wadman *et al.* 2005). It has been used for insertional and conditional gene trap mutagenesis in mice (Geurts *et al.* 2006) and also for the insertional mutagenesis of cancer genes where it can be made specific to particular tissues (Dupuy *et al.* 2006). It appears to be a promising new way of causing mutations in the mouse and possibly other species.

Gene targeting and the production of 'knockout' mice

Gene targeting is used to mutate a specific gene in ES cells whose sequence is already known (Mansour *et al.* 1988). The targeting vector consists of several thousand bases of DNA sequences identical to those of the gene of interest, a positive selectable marker such as a *neo* (neomycin resistance) gene complete with promoter sequences inserted into an exon and a negative selectable marker such as *tk* (thymidine kinase), again with promoter sequences, at one end. It may also include sequences such as *loxP* sites (see later in this chapter) which can be used to delete the construct in certain tissues or at certain times chosen by the investigator. The targeting vector is incorporated into ES cells, usually by electroporation or within a virus. Because the sequences exactly match the DNA sequences of the gene of interest, in a very small fraction of cells homologous recombination will occur and the targeting vector, excluding the *tk* gene (which does not match the sequence so is left out), will become incorporated into the DNA of the ES cell gene. Medium containing neomycin will ensure that cells where no targeting vector is incorporated do not survive and the inclusion of gancyclovir ensures that those cells which incorporate the targeting vector in a random location and still retain the *tk* gene do not survive, thereby enriching the culture in cells where homologous recombination has occurred. The *neo* disrupts the gene, thereby 'knocking' it out. Live 'knockout' mice are retrieved from chimeras formed by injecting the ES cells containing the contruct into blastocysts of a normal mouse strain. Many targeted mutants are now available and two large international consortia, KOMP and EUCOMM, are using gene targeting as well as gene trapping to knock out each of the mouse genes in order to find out their function.

Nomenclature

Targeted mutations result in new allele at the targeted locus. This is indicated by the gene symbol with a superscript tm#Lab code. For example B6;129-*Fshb*^{tm1Zuk} is the first targeted mutation of the follicle-stimulating hormone beta produced by Zuk (a laboratory code). It was produced on a 129 genetic background and has been partially backcrossed (between 5 and 10 generations) to strains B6 (an abbreviation for C57BL/6).

Gene targeting: 'knockin' mice

Knockin mice are being used to overcome some of the defects of transgenic strains produced by direct injection of DNA into early embryos. A non-critical gene is targeted with an insert consisting of the gene of interest flanked by DNA from the non-critical region. Homologous recombination is then used to insert the gene of interest into the site of the non-critical gene. In this way the investigator has complete control of the site of integration and avoids the problem of multiple copies being integrated. This ensures that the targeting construct is not interfering with an existing critical gene, so giving more reliable results. Nomenclature rules are given on the Jackson Laboratory website.

Conditional mutations

Techniques are now available to produce conditional knockouts either in a particular tissue or at a particular time. This is necessary because many genes are essential for development so that knocking them out altogether results in a lethal phenotype which is difficult to study. Cre and FLP are 'recombinases' or enzymes which recognise 34 base pair DNA sequences designated loxP in the case of Cre and FRT in the case of FLP. Cre acts to delete any DNA flanked by two loxP sites. Basically, two loxP sites are placed on either side of the essential functional gene of interest using homologous recombination techniques. These cause no problems, so the gene continues to be expressed. Many transgenic strains have been developed carrying the Cre recombinase under the control of tissue specific or inducible promoters. In the absence of loxP sites, this rarely has an effect on the mice. However, when the mouse strain carrying the loxP sites is crossed with a strain carrying the Cre recombinase the target gene of interest will be deleted in those tissues in which the Cre recombinase is being expressed. The use of both FLP/FRT and Cre/loxP gives even more flexibility to the system.

RNAi RNA interference

RNAi offers an additional way of studying the function of a gene by knocking it 'down' so that effectively it is not expressed. This can be done in a tissue- or time-specific manner using transgenic or gene targeting methods. So called small or short interfering RNA (siRNA) interferes with gene translation by interacting with messenger RNA (mRNA) from the targeted gene in a sequence-specific manner. A similar process occurs naturally when microRNA is produced both to control gene expression and to fight off a viral attack.

Very briefly, a construct containing a sequence that codes for a short hairpin RNA (shRNA) with a sequence specific for the gene of interest, is introduced either by direct injection into the male pro-nucleus of a one cell embryo, by viral transduction or using gene targeting with appropriate selectable markers to a specific non-critical locus. When the sequence is transcribed it forms a short hairpin RNA (shRNA) which is then cleaved by an enzyme called 'dicer' to produce siRNA. This is transported from the cell nucleus and interferes with mRNA of the gene of interest. By using the Cre-lox technique the gene of interest can be knocked down in a time- or tissue-specific manner (Gao & Zhang 2007; Kumar & Clarke 2007).

Concluding remarks

Mammalian genetics is developing rapidly at present as a result of new technology which, among other things, has made it possible to sequence the whole genomes of several species, including humans, the rat, mouse, dog and some species of non-human primate. Classical genetic techniques such as full-sib mating, backcrossing and selection have led to the development of many inbred, coisogenic, congenic and recombinant inbred strains of mice and rats and some other laboratory species. These have made a substantial contribution to biomedical research with several Nobel Prizes being awarded for work which would have been impossible without them. Mutations occurring spontaneously or as a result of irradiation of chemical mutagenesis have also been widely used in research. Some, such as the immune deficient nude and scid (severe combined immune deficiency) mutants, have not just been of interest in their own right but have also been used to grow grafts of tissue and tumours from humans and other species, making it possible to study aspects of biology which could not otherwise be studied. ENU mutagenesis is providing a steady stream of new mutants for further investigation.

The development of DNA-based techniques such as the polymerase chain reaction (PCR) resulted initially in the development of numerous genetic markers such as mini and microsatellites and single nucleotide polymorphisms. Linkage analysis, initially using phenotypic markers, but more recently using microsatellite and other DNA markers has led to the development of detailed genetic maps of most laboratory species. It is now possible to map quantitative trait loci and methods of identifying these loci are improving rapidly. Mutagenesis using gene trapping, and the development of embryonic stem cells followed by gene targeting using homologous recombination now makes it possible to knock out any gene and observe the consequences. The amount of data being generated is enormous, and the science of informatics has grown from almost nothing to assuming major importance in the last two decades. Powerful computers and the World Wide Web are also fundamental to these developments, enabling information to be shared immediately in a way which would be impossible with a paper-based science. Scientists need to understand the fundamentals of laboratory animal genetics if they are to use animals efficiently and humanely in the future.

Useful websites and collaborative genetics projects

The NIH Rat Genomics and Genetics Web site

http://www.nih.gov/science/models/rat/

This has pages on rat genomic and genetic resources, courses and meetings, funding opportunities, reports and publications, major resources and contacts.

RatMap

http://www.ratmap.org

RatMap is focused on presenting rat genes, DNA-markers and QTLs which are localised to chromosomes as well as rat gene nomenclature. It is maintained by the Department for Cell and Molecular Biology, Göteborg University, Sweden.

RGD (Rat Genotype Database)

http://rgd.mcw.edu

The aim of the RGD is the '..*establishment of a Rat Genome Database, to collect, consolidate, and integrate data generated from ongoing rat genetic and genomic research efforts and make these data widely available to the scientific community. A secondary, but critical goal is to provide curation of mapped positions for quantitative trait loci, known mutations and other phenotypic data.*'

The Complex Trait Consortium

http://www.complextrait.org

'*Quantitative genetics and QTL mapping have undergone a revolution in the last decade. Progress in the next decade promises to be even more rapid, and prospects for exploring the complex interplay between gene variants, disease, and the environment will be radically improved.*' The CTC organises meetings, publishes abstracts or full papers resulting from these meetings, provides some software for QTL research and generally keeps its members up to date with progress in complex trait analysis.

The International Mouse Strain Resource

http://www.findmice.org

The IMSR is a searchable online database of mouse strains and stocks available worldwide. It includes inbred, mutant, and genetically engineered mice. Note that the data found in the IMSR is as supplied by data provider sites.

International Gene Trap Consortium

http://www.genetrap.org

Gene trapping is a high-throughput approach that is used to introduce insertional mutations across the genome in mouse embryonic stem (ES) cells. In addition to generating standard loss-of-function alleles, newer gene trap vectors offer a variety of post-insertional modification strategies for the generation of other experimental alleles.

The International Gene Trap Consortium (IGTC) represents all publicly available gene trap cell lines, which are available on a non-collaborative basis for nominal handling fees. Researchers can search and browse the IGTC database for cell lines of interest using accession numbers or IDs, keywords, sequence data, tissue expression profiles and biological pathways.

It has four main components: Information, data access, tutorials and requests for the approximately 120000 cell lines which are available.

EUCOMM (European Conditional Mouse Mutagenesis Program)

http://www.eucomm.org/

This is a collaborative project set up under the European Union Framework 6 programme to develop a collection of 20000 conditional mouse mutations by gene trapping and homologous recombination on a C57BL/6 genetic background. The resulting mutants, made in a standardised way, will be made available to investigators world-wide. It includes participating laboratories in Germany, Italy, France and the UK. The gene trapping and the gene targeting vectors include both loxP and FRT sites, making future control and manipulation of the resulting mutants easier. It includes funds for training and databases. In addition it aims at the '*synergistic integration of EMMA, EUMODIC, EURExpress, FLPFLEX, EMAGE, FunGenES, PRIME and others and will collaborate with the Canadian NorCOMM, KOMP and members of the International Knockout Mouse Consortium (IKMC).*'

EUMODIC (The European Mouse Disease Clinic)

http://www.eumodic.org

This facility will undertake the primary phenotypic assessment of up to 650 lines of mice developed from ES cells produced by EUCOMM. Lines of particular interest will then be studied in more detail. It will make use of a sub-set of the comprehensive phenotyping protocols (EMPReSS) developed in the EUMORPHIA project.

EUMORPHIA

http://www.eumorphia.org

This was a project funded by the European Commission under FP5 from October 2002 until March 2006. The work created EMPReSS, a database of standard operating procedures (SOPs) for phenotyping mice, a database of mouse phenotyping information EUMODIC.

EMMA (The European Mouse Mutant Archive)

http://www.emmanet.org

This is a non-profit collaborative repository for mouse mutants and strains and for the cryopreservation of mouse mutants. The current membership includes the CNR Istituto di Biologia Cellulare in Monterotondo, Italy (core structure), the CNRS Centre de Distribution, de Typage et d'Archivage animal in Orleans, France, the MRC Mammalian Genetics Unit in Harwell, UK, the KI Karolinska Institutet in Stockholm, Sweden, the FCG Instituto Gulbenkian de Ciência in Oeiras, Portugal, the GSF Institute of Experimental Genetics in Munich, Germany and the EMBL European Bioinformatics Institute in Hinxton, UK. The EMMA network is directed by Professor Martin Hrabé de Angelis who also heads the GSF/IEG in Munich.

KOMP (The Knockout Mouse Project)

http://www.nih.gov/science/models/mouse/knockout/

This is an NIH-funded collaborative project, costing approximately $42 million, to produce a set of ES cells carrying null mutations with reporters at about 10000 loci, using gene targeting methods. A C57BL/6 genetic background is considered preferable and the programme includes grants for the further development of robust C57BL/6 ES cells. The programme will support a repository to house the collection and a 'repatriation' of about 1000 of existing knockouts and a centre to coordinate the data which will be generated. It is intended to be complementary with other projects around the world such as the EUCOMM, and all the resources generated will be made freely available to investigators. It is recognised that data on gene expression and phenotypic characterisation would increase the value of the project, but it would also substantially increase the costs, so are not included as part of the main project. It is noted that *'a complete catalog of mouse knockouts will totally alter the sociology of the mouse research community landscape'* which may be disruptive and will create the need for extensive education and re-training.

Mouse Genome Informatics at the Jackson Laboratory

http://www.informatics.jax.org

This is a comprehensive database of mouse genetics including lists of genes and markers, phenotypes, alleles, gene expression, gene sequences, linkage maps and mapping data, mammalian orthology, mouse tumour biology, probes and clones, nomenclature, inbred strains and their origins and characteristics and access to the mouse phenome database.

Glossary

Allele One of a pair of alternative, contrasting characters of which one is sometimes dominant and the other recessive. Each is determined by a gene occupying the same locus in a pair of homologous chromosomes.

Alloantigen An antigen which is capable of being recognised immunologically as foreign by another member of the same species.

Autosomes All chromosomes except the sex chromosomes.

Backcross A cross of an F1 hybrid to one of the parental strains or of a heterozygote to either of the parental homozygous types.

Coisogenic strains A pair of strains which are genetically identical apart from a single gene due to a mutation within an inbred strain followed by maintenance as two separate lines. Targeted mutagenesis also results in a pair of such strains.

Congenic strains A pair of strains which approximate a coisogenic status as a result of backcrossing a specified gene to an inbred strain. Usually 10 to 12 backcross generations are required. Partially congenic strains are recognised after five backcrosses.

Dibybrid cross A cross between two individuals which differ with respect to two specified pairs of genes.

DNA A macromolecule of genetic material which carries the genetic code specifying an individual.

Dominant The phenotypic expression of a character to the exclusion of its allelic (recessive) character.

Epistasis The dominant action of a gene over a non-allelic gene at a different locus, for example, the albino gene is epistatic to other coat colour genes.

Expressivity The degree of expression of a character controlled by a gene, in contrast with the frequency with which a gene produces its effect (penetrance).

F Coefficient of inbreeding. Probability (in the range 0.0 to 1.0) that two alleles at a locus are identical by descent.

F1, F2 etc. Indicates the filial generation following a specified cross between genetically dissimilar parents.

Forced heterozygosity Continuous matings of type Aa × aa, thereby ensuring that the locus is segregating among the progeny. In contrast a mating of type aa × aa would lead to the a allele becoming fixed in the progeny.

Gene A hereditary element comprising a specific location (locus) on a chromosome, and which either alone or in combination with other genes determines a heritable character.

Genetic monitoring Routine procedure for testing whether individuals are of the stated strain or genotype.

Genetic profile List of the alleles at certain specified loci which are present in a given inbred strain.

Genotype The genetic constitution of an individual.

Haplotype Composition of a specified group of closely linked genes which act as a functional unit (eg, the major histocompatibility complex).

Hemizygote An organism carrying a gene which is present on one chromosome, but absent on the homologous chromosome. In mammals it usually refers to males carrying an X-linked gene, there being no homologous locus on the Y chromosome. When a transgenic strain is crossed with a normal strain the progeny will also be hemizygous for the transgene.

Heritability Proportion of the total phenotypic variation which can be accounted for by heritable factors (H, in the broad sense) or by factors with an additive mode of inheritance (H, in the narrow sense).

Heterozygote An organism which has inherited from its parents different genes at a locus controlling a particular character. Adjective: heterozygous.

Histocompatible Ability to accept grafts of skin, tumours or other tissue from another individual without immunological rejection.

Homozygote An organism which has inherited from its parents identical genes controlling a particular character. Adjective: homozygous.

Hybrid In laboratory animal genetics, a hybrid is usually the F1 (first generation) offspring of a cross between two inbred strains. However, it can also be applied to the offspring of parents of unlike genetic composition such as animals known to differ at a single locus, or at several loci even though they are not fully inbred (eg, a cross between breeds of rabbits or outbred stocks of rats).

Inbreeding The mating of related individuals. In mammals brother × sister mating leads to the fastest inbreeding (see Strain (inbred)).

Intercross A cross between two hybrids.

Isogenic Genetically uniform. All individuals of identical genotype.

Knockout Strain developed by inactivation of a specific gene.

Linkage The non-random assortment of characters due to the genes for these characters being on the same chromosome. A series of linked gene pairs on the same chromosome is known as a linkage group.

Locus Position on a chromosome at which a gene is located. Each locus is given a name (eg, the 'agouti' locus) and a symbol usually consisting of one to three letters (eg, a).

Marker gene Gene which may be used to indicate the genotype at some other specified locus as a result of being closely linked to that locus. May also be applied to genes which are used to distinguish between different populations (eg, two inbred strains).

Mass selection Selection of the individuals which are in some sense 'best', without regard to their pedigree.

Mendelian inheritance Controlled by a pair of determinants (genes), which segregate during the formation of the gametes and recombine at random in the zygote.

Minisatellite Sequence of DNA of a few to several hundred bases in length, which is present at multiple locations in the chromosomes of an individual and which may differ between individuals in the number of repeats.

Microsatellite Simple sequence of bases often just two to four bases long (eg, CA), which is repeated up to a few tens or hundreds of times at each locus. These may be present at thousands of loci throughout the genome of an individual, but they very often have unique DNA flanking sequences which are used as the 'primers' in the polymerase chain reaction when used as genetic markers.

Modifiers Genes or non-genetic factors which alter the expression of a particular genotype.

Monohybrid cross A cross between two individuals which differ at one specified genetic locus.

Mutant Individual bearing a mutation.

Mutation A change in the nuclear substances (genes, chromosomes) of an organism. A mutation may arise from a change in the number of chromosomes, a change in part of a chromosome, or a change at a particular base in a gene. The latter is known as a 'point mutation'.

Outbred Usually refers to a genetically variable breeding group of animals maintained by random mating, maximum avoidance of inbreeding, or a haphazard mating scheme.

Penetrance Percentage frequency with which a particular gene produces its effect.

Phenotype The total expression of the genetic characteristics of an individual. Individuals of the same phenotype will look alike, but may differ genetically (ie, in genotype).

Polygenic Character whose mode of inheritance depends on many gene loci, whose individual effects are too small to be analysed individually without using special techniques. Polygenic characters are usually also dependent on non-genetic (ie, 'environmental') influences. See also QTL.

Population Group of organisms which potentially or actually may interbreed.

Primers Short, defined DNA sequences typically of about 20 bases which are used in the polymerase chain reaction to amplify a particular section of DNA.

Progeny test Evaluation of the genotype of an organism by a study of its offspring under controlled conditions.

QTL or Quantitative trait locus A genetic locus associated with a quantitative trait or character such as body weight, reproductive performance or susceptibility to the induction of tumours. Typically, such 'polygenic characters' (see above) will be controlled by many different loci and will also be influenced by environmental factors.

Random Occurring by chance.

Recessive Refers to a member of an allelic pair of genes which does not produce its effect in the presence of the other (dominant) gene.

Recombinant inbred strains A set of inbred strains produced by 20 generations of brother × sister mating of the offspring of a cross between two standard inbred strains.

Reporter gene A protein coding gene which encodes an enzyme or protein not normally present in the transgenic animal, and for which a sensitive assay procedure exists. For example the *lac Z* gene encodes bacterial beta-galactosidase which can be used to produce a blue-coloured stain in tissues in which it is expressed.

Segregating inbred strain An inbred strain produced by brother × sister mating in such a way as to maintain genetic segregation at a specified locus (eg, by mating m/m × +/m animals each generation). May also be produced by backcrossing the mutant to an inbred strain and subsequent matings as above.

Segregation The separation of the chromosomes and genes in the formation of the germ cells (ie, during meiosis). Each germ cell receives only one chromosome (and therefore gene) of each pair.

Sex-linked A character associated with one sex, due to the genes for the character being located on the sex chromosomes.

Shuttle vector A DNA construct which can be incorporated into a transgenic animal, but which can also be extracted again from the host DNA using defined restriction enzymes and packaged into a plasmid or bacteriophage so that it can be cloned into a bacteria again.

SNP or single nucleotide polymorphism Genetic variation among individuals due to a single DNA base change (or possibly a few close bases) which may or may not alter phenotype depending on where it occurs and the nature of the change.

Stem-line colony Small nucleus breeding colony of an inbred strain which reproduces itself specifically to perpetuate the strain, and which also produces surplus animals which may be used for further breeding in an 'expansion' or 'multiplication' (the terms are synonymous) colony.

Stock A closed colony of genetically heterogeneous laboratory animals maintained without deliberate inbreeding.

Strain (inbred) A group of laboratory animals produced as a result of at least 20 generations of brother × sister mating (or its genetic equivalent using other mating systems), with all individuals tracing back to a single breeding pair in the 20th or a subsequent generation.

X, Y chromosomes The sex chromosomes. In mammals the female has two X chromosomes, one of which becomes inactivated during early embryonic development. Males have an X and a Y chromosome. The latter has few genes, but determines sex. In birds the female has XY and the male XX chromosomes. The sex chromosomes in birds were once designated W and Z.

References

Aoto, T., Totsuka, Y., Takahashi, R. *et al.* (2007) Production of progeny mice by intracytoplasmic sperm injection of repeatedly frozen and thawed spermatozoa experimental technique. *Journal of the American Association of Laboratory Animal Science*, **46**, 41–46

Bailey, D.W. (1971) Recombinant inbred strains, an aid to finding identity, linkage, and function of histocompatibility and other genes. *Transplantation*, **11**, 325–327

Barbaric, I. and Dear, T.N. (2007) Optimizing screening and mating strategies for phenotype-driven recessive N-ethyl-N-nitrosourea screens in mice. *Journal of the American Association of Laboratory Animal Science*, **46**, 44–49

Barbaric, I., Wells, S., Russ, A. *et al.* (2007) Spectrum of ENU-induced mutations in phenotype-driven and gene-driven screens in the mouse. *Environmental and Molecular Mutagenesis*, **48**, 124–142

Beck, J.A., Lloyd, S., Hafezparast, M. *et al.* (2000) Genealogies of mouse inbred strains. *Nature Genetics*, **24**, 23–25

Brown, S.D., Chambon, P. and de Angelis, M.H. (2005) EMPReSS: standardized phenotype screens for functional annotation of the mouse genome. *Nature Genetics*, **37**, 1155

Chia, R., Achilli, F., Festing, M.F. *et al.* (2005) The origins and uses of mouse outbred stocks. *Nature Genetics*, **37**, 1181–1186

Churchill, G.A., Airey, D.C., Allayee, H. *et al.* (2004) The Collaborative Cross, a community resource for the genetic analysis of complex traits. *Nature Genetics*, **36**, 1133–1137

Cordes, S.P. (2005) N-ethyl-N-nitrosourea mutagenesis: boarding the mouse mutant express. *Microbiological and Molecular Biological Reviews*, **69**, 426–439

Dupuy, A.J., Jenkins, N.A. and Copeland, N.G. (2006) Sleeping beauty: a novel cancer gene discovery tool. *Human Molecular Genetics*, **15**, R75–R79

Evans, M.F. and Kaufman, M.H. (1981) Establishment in culture of pluripotential cells from mouse embryos. *Nature*, **292**, 154–156

Falconer, D.S. (1981) *Introduction to Quantitative Genetics*. Longman, London

Festing, M.F.W. (1979) *Inbred Strains in Biomedical Research*. Macmillan Press, Basingstoke

Festing, M.F.W. (1982) Genetic contamination of laboratory animal colonies: an increasingly serious problem. *ILAR News*, **25**, 6–10

Festing, M.F.W. (1995) Use of a multi-strain assay could improve the NTP carcinogenesis bioassay program. *Environmental Health Perspectives*, **103**, 44–52

Festing, M.F.W. and Fisher, E.M.C. (2000) Mighty mice. *Nature*, **404**, 815

Festing, M.F.W., Overend, P., Gaines Das, R. *et al.* (2002) *The Design of Animal Experiments*. Laboratory Animals Ltd, London

Gaillard, A., Prestoz, L., Dumartin, B. *et al.* (2007) Reestablishment of damaged adult motor pathways by grafted embryonic cortical neurons. *Nature Neuroscience*, **10**, 1294–1299

Gaitonde, M.K. and Festing, M.F.W. (1976) Brain glutamic acid decarboxylase and open field activity in ten inbred strains of mice. *Brain Research*, **103**, 617–621

Gao, X. and Zhang, P. (2007) Transgenic RNA interference in mice. *Physiology (Bethesda)*, **22**, 161–166

Gehlmann, R. (1993) Pros and cons of transgenic mouse mutagenesis test systems. *Journal of Experimental Animal Science*, **35**, 232–243

Geurts, A.M., Wilber, A., Carlson, C.M. *et al.* (2006) Conditional gene expression in the mouse using a Sleeping Beauty gene-trap transposon. *BMC Biotechnology*, **6**, 30

Green, E.L. (1981) *Genetics and Probability in Animal Breeding Experiments*. The Macmillan Press Ltd, Basingstoke

Hedrich, H.J. and Reetz, I.C. (1988) Strain preservation of rodent embryos: possibilities and limitations. In: *New Developments in Biosciences: Their Implications for Laboratory Animal Science*. Ed. Beynen, A.C., pp. 163–173. Martinus Nijhoff, Dordrecht

Heston, W.E. (1968) Genetic aspects of experimental animals in cancer research. *Japanese Cancer Association Gann Monograph*, **5**, 3–15

Hummel, K.P., Coleman, D.L. and Lane, P.W. (1972) Influence of genetic background on expression of mutations at the diabetes locus in the mouse.I. C57BL/KsJ and C57BL/6J strains. *Biochemical Genetics*, **7**, 1–13

Jat, P.S., Noble, M.D., Ataliotis, P. *et al.* (1991) Direct derivation of conditionally immortal cell lines from an H-2K{+b}-tsA58 transgenic mouse. *Proceedings of the National Academy of Sciences*, **88**, 5096–5100

Kumar, L.D. and Clarke, A.R. (2007) Gene manipulation through the use of small interfering RNA (siRNA): from in vitro to in vivo applications. *Advances in Drug Delivery Reviews*, **59**, 87–100

Malkinson, A.M., Nesbitt, M.N. and Skamene, E. (1985) Susceptibility to urethane-induced pulmonary adenomas between A/J and C57BL/6J mice: use of AXB and BXA recombinant inbred lines indicating a three-locus genetic model. *Journal of the National Cancer Institute*, **75**, 971–974

Mansour, S.L., Thomas, K.R. and Capecchi, R. (1988) Disruption of the protooncogene {Iint-2} in mouse embryo-derived stem cells: A general strategy for targeting mutations to non-selectable genes. *Nature*, **336**, 248–252

Markel, P., Shu, P., Ebeling, C. *et al.* (1997) Theoretical and empirical issues for marker-assisted breeding of congenic mouse strains. *Nature Genetics*, **17**, 280–284

Michaud, E.J., Culiat, C.T., Klebig, M.L. *et al.* (2005) Efficient gene-driven germ-line point mutagenesis of C57BL/6J mice. *BMC Genomics*, **6**, 164

Nakagata, N. (2000) Cryopreservation of mouse spermatozoa. *Mammalian Genome*, **11**, 572–576

Ostermeier, G.C., Wiles, M.V., Farley, J.S. *et al.* (2008) Conserving, distributing and managing genetically modified mouse lines by sperm cryopreservation. *PLoS One*, **3**, e2792

Palmiter, R.D., Brinster, R.L., Hammer, R.E. *et al.* (1982) Dramatic growth of mice that develop from eggs microinjected with metallothionein-growth hormone fusion genes. *Nature*, **300**, 611–615

Papaioannou, V. and Johnson, R. (1993) Production of chimeras and genetically defined offspring from targeted ES cells. In: *Gene Targeting*. Ed. Joyner, A.L., pp. 107–146. Oxford University Press, Oxford

Papaioannou, V.E. and Festing, M.F.W. (1980) Genetic drift in a stock of laboratory mice. *Laboratory Animals*, **14**, 11–13

Petkov, P.M., Ding, Y., Cassell, M.A. *et al.* (2004) An efficient SNP system for mouse genome scanning and elucidating strain relationships. *Genome Research*, **14**, 1806–1811

Plomin, R., McClearn, G.E., Gorer-Maslak, G. *et al.* (1991) An RI QTL cooperative data bank for recombinant inbred quantitative trait loci analysis. *Behavior Genetics*, **21**, 97–98

Russell, W.M.S. and Burch, R.L. (1959) *The Principles of Humane Experimental Technique*. Special Edition, Universities Federation for Animal Welfare, Potters Bar

Simpson, E.M., Linder, C.C., Sargent, E.E. *et al.* (1997) Genetic variation among 129 substrains and its importance for targeted mutagenesis in mice. *Nature Genetics*, **16**, 19–27

Singer, J.B., Hill, A.E., Burrage, L.C. *et al.* (2004) Genetic dissection of complex traits with chromosome substitution strains of mice. *Science*, **304**, 445–448

Stevens, J.C., Banks, G.T., Festing, M.F. *et al.* (2007) Quiet mutations in inbred strains of mice. *Trends in Molecular Medicine*, **13**, 512–519

Taketo, M., Schroeder, A.C., Mobraaten, L.E. *et al.* (1991) FVB/N: An inbred mouse strain preferable for transgenic analyses. *Proceedings of the National Academy of Sciences*, **88**, 2065–2069

Tsang, S., Sun, Z., Luke, B. *et al.* (2005) A comprehensive SNP-based genetic analysis of inbred mouse strains. *Mammalian Genome*, **16**, 476–480

Wadman, S.A., Clark, K.J. and Hackett, P.B. (2005) Fishing for answers with transposons. *Marine Biotechnology (NY)*, **7**, 135–141

Yang, H., Bell, T.A., Churchill, G.A. *et al.* (2007) On the subspecific origin of the laboratory mouse. *Nature Genetics*, **39**, 1100–1107

5 Phenotyping of genetically modified mice

Rikke Westh Thon, Merel Ritskes-Hoitinga, Hilary Gates and Jan-Bas Prins

Introduction

The development of techniques to create genetically modified mice has allowed tremendous progress in the fields of comparative medicine and genetics during the last decades. These animals have been used to provide a multitude of new disease models and their use has increased dramatically.

Each new genetically modified mouse generated is a potential new strain, which may or may not show altered characteristics (phenotypic changes) compared to the wild type. The phenotype of a genetically modified mouse is the sum of observable characteristics of an induced or spontaneous mutation.

The phenotypic consequences of a genetic modification cannot always be predicted and, consequently, it is necessary to characterise each new genetically modified animal's phenotype. Phenotypic characterisation, or phenotyping, is the discipline of identifying and describing new characteristics as compared to the non-mutated wild type. Ideally, phenotyping should uncover any new trait and a vast number of tests could be applied to the mouse in order to ensure that such traits are actually revealed. It is necessary to know the characteristics of an animal model so that decisions can be made as to whether the animal will be suitable for a particular line of research. The knowledge also helps with making welfare decisions for these animals.

Due to the tremendous increase in the number of newly generated genetically modified mice over the last decades, phenotyping has received considerable recent scientific attention and has become established as a discipline within laboratory animal science. Several journals have published special issues on phenotyping including Lab Animal Europe (Vol. 2, 2002), Laboratory Animals (vol. 37, Supplement 1, 2003) and the ILAR Journal (vol. 47, 2006). Even though much effort has been put into developing phenotyping protocols, the use of these protocols in practice lags behind, and the production of new strains far exceeds the number of strains that are characterised. Nonetheless, there are efforts to improve implementation (Hrabé de Angelis *et al.* 2006).

Welfare issues

The general situation

The current state of affairs regarding the welfare of genetically modified mice has been investigated in a survey of users, from a variety of different disciplines, of genetically modified mice in Denmark, UK, Sweden, Finland and the Netherlands (Thon *et al.* 2009). Despite publication of detailed protocols for phenotypic characterisation, the results indicated that very few genetically modified mice were systematically characterised. Only one of those interviewed had SOPs (standard operating procedures) for phenotypic characterisation. The importance of the role of animal care staff has been pointed out by others (Morton & Hau 2003), and in this survey many used daily observation/visual inspection of animals by animal technicians. Some scientists knew about published protocols, but very few had practical experience with the test methods, and general knowledge about phenotyping strategies and protocols was low. On the other hand, phenotyping as a concept was widely understood and it was clearly regarded as an advantage to the science.

During the interviews, it became clear that there was considerable doubt amongst users of genetically modified mice as to whether the published protocols would actually fulfil their particular needs. Furthermore, concern was expressed about the comprehensiveness of the protocols and lack of resources and time for phenotypic characterisation. The survey also demonstrated that the reason for characterizing genetically modified mice depended strongly on the scientific reason for creating or using the strain. The kind of phenotype information that was required differed between scientists. For example, some needed to identify characters relating to diseases, whereas other kinds of information were required for those producing and establishing a modified strain for commercial purposes.

At least four levels of, or types of, characterisation were identified:

1. welfare assessment;
2. one-trait assessment focused on the expected phenotypic effect of the genetic modification;
3. basic characterisation;
4. comprehensive characterisation.

The welfare of genetically modified animals

Genetic modification can give rise to unpredictable outcomes that may impact on animal well-being. Therefore, there is a need to pay special attention to the welfare of genetically modified mice. There has been a focus on animal welfare since the beginning of the era of genetic modification as demonstrated by the inception of an EU workshop in 1995 named Welfare Aspects of Transgenic Animals (Van Zutphen & van der Meer 1997). Since then, several articles and reports have addressed the issue (eg, Mepham *et al.* 1998; van der Meer *et al.* 1999; Van Hoosier 1999; Wood 2000; Dennis 2002; Brown *et al.* 2006). One study has shown that approximately one third of genetically modified mice, as reported to the Danish Animal Experiment Inspectorate, showed welfare consequences arising from the genetic modification (Thon *et al.* 2002). Animals generated with the purpose of serving as disease models are particularly likely to show impaired welfare.

Phenotyping is important for keeping and breeding genetically modified animals. It should provide information about any special problems of a particular strain, thereby allowing the animal care staff to take action and improve the conditions of the animals. Once an animal has been phenotyped for welfare, special measures can be taken to actually improve welfare, such as providing a special diet, special housing or medication. Ultimately, this will improve animal welfare and the loss of valuable strains can be prevented. In addition, a better ethical evaluation of the research can be carried out and humane endpoints can be defined.

Methods of welfare assessment

In the proceedings of the above-mentioned 1995 EU workshop, indices of good and bad welfare were defined (Broom 1995). Those relating to the former were listed as: changes to normal behaviours; changes to the ability of the animal to perform strongly preferred behaviours; and changes to physiological and behavioural indicators of pleasure. The list of indices reflecting poor welfare was much longer and included: reduced life expectancy; reduced ability to grow or breed; body damage; disease; immunosuppression; impairment of physiological and behavioural attempts to cope; behavioural pathology; self narcotisation when given the opportunity; changes to behavioural aversions; changes to normal behaviour; and changes to normal physiological processes and anatomical development.

The relevant tests for assessing the above mentioned indices can be roughly grouped into: (1) behavioural tests; (2) measurement of production parameters; and (3) physiological tests. The first two types of tests are performed relatively easily and require few resources. The last is more demanding. However, assessing animal well-being is always a laborious task and there are no 'easy' measures of welfare (Morton & Hau 2003).

van der Meer and co-workers have introduced a less comprehensive welfare test (van der Meer *et al.* 2001). It consists of non-invasive, mainly observational, easy-to-perform assessments based on three score sheets. One sheet is for scoring animals aged 0–6 days, one for animals 10–14 days and the last for animals around weaning. The indices used are: death in or out of the nest; milk spot; weight; fur growth; nipples; upper/lower incisors; and abnormalities. The most comprehensive (after weaning) test can be performed on an average litter of four to six pups by an animal technician within 15–20 minutes and requires a minimum of equipment. The score-sheet approach to measuring welfare in young pups has been further developed by Marques *et al.* (2007). The method has been improved by adding further individual tests to the screening from the day of birth. A training film has been produced to facilitate implementation.

A working group has published recommendations on welfare assessment of genetically altered mice (Wells *et al.* 2006). These authors recommend that any institution using genetically altered animals should have a standard welfare assessment in place. Newly generated strains should be checked, and because of the risk that a changed environment could cause welfare issues, so should well known strains that have just arrived in an animal unit. When the institute has become familiar with the strain there is no need for retesting unless adverse effects are observed during the daily routine handling. The group suggested that animals should be checked as neonates, at weaning and for the normal lifespan of the particular strain. The tests should preferably be non-invasive and easy to implement. The importance of accurate recording of test results was stressed. Parameters such as teeth eruption, walking, righting, ears/eyes opening, posture and reaction to cage opening/handling were suggested, and examples of assessment forms were provided. For pups, parameters to be recorded include colour, activity and milk spot. Furthermore, mortality rates, appearance, coat condition, posture/gait, clinical signs, relative size and other unexpected characteristics were suggested in the assessment of older animals.

The group also recommended that the information obtained by the welfare assessment should be used for a mouse passport or certificate which would always follow the animal in order to facilitate correct husbandry and treatment. The introduction of an animal certificate or passport has also been recommended by others (Mertens & Rülicke 2002; Jegstrup *et al.* 2003; Morton & Hau 2003). However, there has been some discussion within the phenotyping community as to whether the document should be both a physical paper certificate plus the corresponding information saved in a database, or just the information in a database. The first solution has the advantage of the information following the animal wherever it goes, but also includes the risk of paper documents disappearing or getting mixed up and the risk of circulation of outdated versions.

Morton and Hau (2003) present a very helpful guideline on how to establish a score sheet for assessment of animal welfare. They conclude that every welfare assessment is different depending on strain and experiment and, consequently, an individual score sheet should be designed for each new study covering the relevant welfare parameters.

Ironically, several of the tests suggested in phenotyping protocols may themselves impinge on the welfare of the tested animal. Hence, decisions on the potential adverse effect of chosen tests (eg, pain threshold and blood sampling) and on the number of mice tested should be made to avoid exposing mice to unnecessary suffering. The logical approach is to carry out a cost (harm)/benefit analysis (Richmond 2000) of the chosen test battery before phenotyping, and perform only the necessary tests based on these considerations.

Other advantages of phenotyping

The benefits of a better understanding of the welfare impacts of a genetic modification are also that the information contributes to a better description of the model, which is important for the science. Phenotyping is obviously necessary for geneticists working on the relationship between genes and phenotype to characterise a genetically modified animal. The success of an approach, such as induction of mutations by the use of ENU (N-ethyl-N-nitrosourea), is totally dependent on effective phenotyping. ENU mutagenesis is aimed at introducing random and mainly point mutations in the genes of premeiotic spermatogonia. After breeding, successful mutations are identified through thorough phenotyping of every animal. This way, any new trait that has arisen as a consequence of the ENU treatment can be discovered (phenotype-driven approach) (Brown *et al.* 2005). Animals carrying mutations created by other techniques should also be subject to phenotypic characterisation. Since the phenotype of any genetic modification is a complex interaction between gene allele and genetic background, among other factors, one cannot be sure that an expected phenotypic change has taken place even after successful targeted mutation and whether it is the only phenotypical change. The phenotyping strategy should, furthermore, optimise the chance of detecting unexpected effects of the mutation as well (Brown *et al.* 2006).

For decades, it has been accepted that microbiological and genetic characterisation of laboratory animals was a necessity in order to reduce variability and increase replicability of studies. The same argument is true for phenotypic characterisation of genetically modified animals. Lack of phenotyping increases the risk that unidentified traits could cause extraneous variability, as they are not taken into account when designing the experiment. This could increase the risk of systematic errors which might intervene and confound results leading to false conclusions. Phenotyping the mutant model before setting up the experiment will provide the user with scientifically important information about the animal and allow him/her to implement a better design of the experiment leading to more valid results. Therefore, a precise characterisation must be considered as an essential aid in designing a scientific experiment (Barthold 2004).

Furthermore, new and unexpected traits may be detected that could be of scientific interest in other areas of research, or might provide an important model for work in other fields and which may contribute to the Three Rs (replacement, refinement and reduction) as well.

Studies may suffer or be aborted as a consequence of surprises regarding unexpected phenotypes, which may only become apparent at a late stage. Unfortunately, this kind of negative outcome is very rarely published and the scale of the problem is hard to estimate. However, it is the experience of the authors that the event is not rare, and every time studies are aborted it will inevitably lead to waste of animals, time and effort. The risk of ending up in this kind of unfortunate situation could be minimised by phenotyping right at the start.

A critical evaluation through a cost (harm)/benefit assessment (Richmond 2000) of the justification of the use of genetically modified animals should precede their use in experiments. In order to assess the welfare 'cost', including the adverse effects of the genetic modification, it is crucial to characterise the animals. This can provide information about the potential suffering of the animal. Furthermore, phenotyping meets the needs of regulatory authorities as they increase their demands for information about genetically modified animals.

Early protocols for phenotyping

As long ago as 1968, Irvin introduced protocols for systematic identification of behavioural and physiological phenotypes of mice (Irwin 1968). These protocols were designed for the pharmacological and toxicological fields and were not aimed at genetically modified strains. However, they have served as an inspiration for more recent protocols such as the SHIRPA protocols (SmithKline Beecham, Harwell MRC, Imperial College School of Medicine at St Mary's, Royal London Hospital Phenotype Assessment) (Rogers *et al.* 1997). The SHIRPA protocols were initially developed for characterisation of neurological models and were based on the principle of a broad primary test battery followed by more specialised secondary and tertiary tests. The SHIRPA protocols have been in use for many years (sometimes in a modified form) and they have had a profound influence on more recent comprehensive phenotyping protocols. In 1997 Crawley and Paylor published a detailed description of a battery of tests for the investigation of behavioural phenotypes (Crawley & Paylor 1997).

The Mouse Phenome Project

The Mouse Phenome Project was initiated in 2000 by the Jackson Laboratories to develop a comprehensive database. The Mouse Phenome Database (MPD)[1] encompasses phenotypes from inbred mouse strains. It now also includes results of genetically modified mice. MPD aims at providing scientists with appropriate information about mice for: (1) physiological testing; (2) drug discovery; (3) toxicology studies; (4) mutagenesis; (5) modelling human diseases; (6) Quantitative Trait Locus (QTL) analyses and identification of new genes; and (7) unravelling the influence of environment on genotype (Bogue & Grubb 2004).

The data available at the MPD are the results of different research groups using different protocols and the database contains descriptions of how the data were generated. Due to their various origins, the protocols are of different designs, provide different levels of detail and vary in comprehensiveness. The protocols are organized in measurement categories in a hierarchical way starting with 15 top-level categories, such as anatomy, behaviour and heart/lung parameters, down to sub-levels of more detailed categories. The database provides several tools for downloading and viewing the phenome data. The tools can be used in combination to enable the scientist to mine the biological information for relevant patterns and correlations.

[1] http://phenome.jax.org/pub-cgi/phenome/mpdcgi?rtn=docs/home

The Eumorphia Project

Eumorphia (European Union Mouse Research for Public Health and Industrial Applications) was an integrated research programme funded by the European Commission. It was involved in the development of new approaches in phenotyping, mutagenesis and informatics leading to improved characterisation of mouse models for the understanding of human physiology and disease. Eighteen laboratories from eight European countries formed the consortium, which developed over 150 SOPs for phenotyping from 2002–2006[2]. The SOPs are standardised and validated on a cohort of inbred strains across a number of laboratories.

A primary screening protocol EMPReSS (European Mouse Phenotyping Resource for Standardised Screens) has been suggested for large-scale phenotyping (Brown *et al.* 2005). EMPReSS covers the major body systems and includes: clinical chemistry; hormonal and metabolic systems; cardiovascular system; allergy and infection; renal function; sensory function; neurological and behavioural function; cancer; bone/cartilage; and respiratory function; as well as generic approaches to pathology and gene expression. The Eumorphia project has established the EuroPhenome database to hold data on phenotypes obtained from the EMPReSS SOPs[3].

The project was geneticist driven and mainly aimed at serving programmes of large-scale generation of mutant mice with no *a priori* hypothesis about the function of mutated genes. The goal was to systematically mutate every gene in the genome thereby shedding light on the relationship between gene and phenotype (Brown *et al.* 2006). The tools developed for this purpose adopted a phenotype-driven approach of comprehensive testing in order to maximise the capture of new traits.

Unfortunately the EMPReSS protocols do not include welfare assessment and so this important aspect must be evaluated according to other protocols. However, they do include SOPs for a broad spectrum of phenotyping areas and employ a hierarchical approach. They are validated and standardised to a high degree making results comparable over laboratories and time; and since these protocols have been developed across Europe and are still being developed, eg with the Mouse Phenome Database and the Mouse Clinics adhering to these protocols, this approach appears to be the future of phenotyping in Europe.

The EUMODIC project

The European Mouse Disease Clinic EUMODIC[4] project started in 2007 and is funded by the European Commission. EUMODIC is undertaking a primary phenotype assessment of up to 650 mouse mutant lines, as a first step towards a comprehensive functional annotation of the mouse genome. In addition, a number of these mutant lines will be subject to more in depth secondary phenotype assessment. The EUMODIC consortium is of 18 laboratories across Europe, expert in the field of mouse functional genomics and phenotyping and with a track record of successful collaborative research in Eumorphia. EUMODIC has further developed a selection of the EMPReSS screens, and this selection is called EMPReSSslim, which is structured for comprehensive, primary, high throughput phenotyping of large numbers of mice. The EMPReSS tests are run in two 'pipelines' in order to minimise the number of tests that each animal undergoes and to allow the testing to take place over a 6 week period from 9–14 weeks of age. The sequence of tests in the two 'pipelines' is designed to allow the individual tests to be run at relevant ages so that earlier tests do not unacceptably influence the outcome of those that follow.

Mutant lines will be made available from another EU initiative, EUCOMM, the European Conditional Mouse Mutagenesis project[5]. The primary phenotype assessment using EMPReSSslim, will be undertaken in four large-scale phenotyping centres at the German Mouse Clinic (GMC), GSF (National Research Centre for Environment and Health), Germany; ICS (Institute Clinique de la Souris), France; MRC (Medical Research Council, Mammalian Genetics Unit), Harwell, UK; and the Wellcome Trust Sanger Institute, UK. A distributed network of centres with expertise in various phenotyping domains will undertake more complex, secondary phenotyping screens and apply them to mice that have shown interesting phenotypes in the primary screen.

Other protocols

The MuTrack[6] system was developed for the Tennessee Mouse Genome Consortium in connection with the National Institute of Health's neuromutagenesis programme (Baker *et al.* 2004). This is divided into ten primary screens covering aggression, aging, auditory, drug abuse, ethanol, epilepsy, eye, general behavioural, neurohistology and a social behaviour domain. Furthermore, it includes three secondary screens focusing on drug abuse, nociception and learning/memory. The protocols for screening are individually designed by different scientists and contain different details for screening purposes.

The protocols available at the PhenoSITE were developed in connection with the Japanese mouse mutagenesis program at RIKEN GSC (Genomic Sciences Centre)[7]. Their basic phenotype screen includes a modified SHIRPA and further tests, including: haematology and urine tests; radiography; seizure induction; home cage activity; open field and passive avoidance tests; and for late-onset phenotypes: fundus imaging, blood pressure, hearing and tumour development. The mice are tested between the ages of 8 and 12 weeks.

Mertens and Rülicke (1999, 2000, 2002) have developed a protocol with a slightly different and broader objective than that of the programmes above (Mertens & Rülicke 2000, 2002). It is based on two comprehensive standardised forms and covers registration of animals, recommendations for

[2]http://www.eumorphia.org
[3]http://www.europhenome.org
[4]http://www.eumodic.eu

[5]http://www.eucomm.org
[6]http://www2.tnmouse.org/neuromutagenesis
[7]http://www.gsc.riken.go.jp/mouse/aboutus/screening.htm

husbandry and breeding, phenotyping, welfare assessment and animal certificate/passport. The first form 'Data record form' includes score sheets for litters and individual health and development monitoring from birth until death or euthanasia. The tests are based on observation or other very simple tests. The second form 'Characterisation of genetically modified animal lines: Standard form' includes 'General information' which addresses the genetic modification, phenotype and clinical burden, ethical evaluation and information on breeding, husbandry and transportation, and 'Detailed information on genotype and phenotype' which goes into detail with new traits/observations that are specific for the particular strain.

Mouse clinics

The need for facilities and expertise for phenotyping is growing and, consequently, the concept of mouse clinics has emerged. However, there are still relatively few mouse genetics institutes around the world that have broad experience in phenotyping and which can be categorised as phenotyping centres or mouse clinics.

The German Mouse Clinic (GMC) at GSF, Munich[8] is an open platform for phenotyping and offers a service of examination of mouse mutants for external scientists, using a broad standardised phenotypic check-up with more than 300 parameters. The screens cover behaviour, bone and cartilage development, neurology, clinical chemistry, eye development, immunology, allergy, steroid metabolism, energy metabolism, lung function, vision, pain perception, molecular phenotyping, cardiovascular analyses and pathology. Mouse mutants accepted at the GMC are first examined in a primary screen. A standardised workflow for screening a mouse cohort of 40 animals (ten males and ten females of mutant and wildtype, respectively) has been developed according to EMPReSS protocols and takes about 10 weeks to complete. An application form and instructions for submission of a strain for free phenotyping can be found at the GMC website.

Commercial phenotyping

Another option is commercial phenotyping performed by companies offering this service to their customers. The following two are examples of such companies and the reader is encouraged to search the internet for others.

Charles River Laboratories[9] offer an extended range of tests, initially starting with a primary neurobehavioural observation based on a modified SHIRPA panel, which also includes basic pathology and clinical pathology. Necropsy is performed and tissues from 16 organs plus tissue from any identified abnormality are stained with haematoxylin and eosin and examined by a veterinary pathologist. Clinical pathology includes a complete blood count with differential and platelet count. Serum is submitted to a standard clinical chemistry profile and so is urine. Furthermore, the company offers a range of supplemental phenotyping panels relating to obesity, diabetes, oncology, embryonic lethality, osteoporosis and several other conditions.

Frimorfo[10] offers a diagnostic pathology-based characterisation. They also offer, through a network, screens relating to genetics, physiology and behavioural analysis. The histopathology includes immunohistochemistry, *in situ* hybridisation, standard and customised tissue microarrays and microscopy. Genetics includes zygosity, gene expression, reporter gene assay, apoptosis assays and cell proliferation assays. *In vivo* physiology includes respiratory and cardiovascular tests and *in vitro* blood chemistry and haematology. Behavioural analyses are divided into primary, secondary and tertiary test batteries much like the SHIRPA protocols. The tests are composed in packages focusing on different organ/tissue functions.

Before phenotyping – search for information

It is advisable to carry out a thorough literature/database search for existing information about a particular mouse strain before phenotyping. Results from animals with similar mutations and mutations in the same area of the genome also can be of great value when gathering information about the phenotype.

Regrettably, a comprehensive database of results from all genetically modified animals is not available; rather data are held in various forms at many sites worldwide and one has to carry out the laborious task of searching databases to retrieve information. Web addresses of screening protocols and databases of phenotypic characteristics can be found in the literature (Bolon 2006; Consortium (MPDIC) 2007). Furthermore, we have included a list of websites that we have found useful (see Useful websites at the end of this chapter). This list was made in 2008 and since web addresses frequently change, we urge the reader to make his/her own search as well.

The Mouse Phenome Database (MPD)[11] (Grubb *et al.* 2004; Blake *et al.* 2006) and the EuroPhenome resource[12] are central databases holding substantial information about phenotypes. The MPD contains information about both inbred and mutant strains. The EuroPhenome resource holds the results of the large-scale phenotyping projects from EMPReSS protocols. Both are annotated according to the Mammalian Phenotype (MP) Ontology (Gkoutos *et al.* 2005; Smith *et al.* 2005) and have tools for browsing and searching for phenotypes.

Phenomics data are fragmented and some are not publicly available. Various types have been generated (eg, detailed descriptions of mouse lines, first-line phenotyping data on new mutations and data on the normal features of inbred lines) depending on the groups presenting them. The issues arising as a result of there being several phenome databases using different systems is being addressed by the

[8] http://www.gsf.de/ieg/gmc
[9] http://www.criver.com
[10] http://www.frimorfo.com
[11] http://phenome.jax.org/pub-cgi/phenome/mpdcgi?rtn=docs/home
[12] http://www.europhenome.eu

InterPhenome project[13]. A working group, the Mouse Phenotype Database Integration Consortium (MPDIC), representing large parts of the phenotyping society has been formed and is striving to link these databases, set standards for data and to set up mechanisms to facilitate data exchange between and searches across the various databases (MPDIC, 2007).

Testing for new traits – the hierarchical approach

In principle any clinical test could be used to uncover phenotypic details about a specific genetically modified mouse and a variety of SOPs for these tests can be found in the published protocols. In view of the huge number of possible tests, it is worth prioritising these to obtain relevant results as quickly and efficiently as possible. A practical approach to gaining useful information about a mouse strain is to first apply a battery of relatively unsophisticated tests or primary screens such as those of the SHIRPA test (Rogers *et al.* 1997). These provide a superficial but broad assessment of a mouse phenotype. Various protocols have been proposed which employ this hierarchical approach, focusing either on specific functional domains such as behaviour (Crawley & Paylor 1997a; Crawley 2003) or employing a wider selection of screens (Rogers *et al.* 1997; Murray 2002). Results from these primary screens should point the way for following more detailed tests. For example, if a mouse shows a hearing deficiency in the auditory startle test during the primary phenotyping screen, a comprehensive examination of the auditory tract should follow. In this way, phenotypes of interest identified by the primary screen are followed up by more time-consuming, detailed secondary screens.

Delimiting the phenotyping process

When phenotyping a mouse strain, difficulties may be encountered in deciding how comprehensive the phenotyping project should be. How many and which tests should be included? Looking at the protocols for phenotyping published in the literature and on the internet, it is obvious that no working procedure is unanimously recommended. As pointed out earlier, genetically modified mice can be very different and are used in so many ways that specific phenotyping needs often arise. This is an area that needs further investigation to facilitate optimal choice of tests for the circumstances.

Therefore, before commencing the laborious task of phenotyping, some serious reflection on the level of characterisation is recommended. Firstly, consideration should be given to the particular need for information about a mouse strain. Some results are more relevant than others depending on what the strain is used for. Also, the resources (economy, time, expertise) available should be considered since there are limits in practice to how much can be investigated. Deciding how comprehensive the test battery should be is a difficult task, and this is usually made on the basis of common sense, experience and tradition. However, these approaches carry a risk of being non-systematic and subjectively biased, thereby influencing their validity. It is therefore advisable to carry out a systematic investigation into the need for phenotyping and the contribution that the individual protocols can yield in every case of phenotyping, before the project is started.

The question of how wide-ranging a basic phenotyping protocol should be – or what the minimum requirement for phenotyping is for relevant results – is still open and needs further investigation.

The dilemma of large-scale versus 'home' phenotyping

Huge efforts have been and are still being put into developing EMPReSS and the corresponding SOPs leading to better phenotyping tools. However, these developments will, in many cases, make the protocols more complex and demanding, and will require increased levels of expertise and further equipment.

The lack of phenotyping of mutants that are not part of large-scale projects, but have been locally produced and bred, is obvious. Scientists working with these animals are often more focused on their particular field of interest than on phenotyping, and protocols like EMPReSS are not easily implemented by people who are not phenotyping experts. It is probably unrealistic to expect many laboratories to develop the expertise, equipment, resources and infrastructure to carry out comprehensive phenotyping themselves. These two opposing tendencies raise the question as to whether, rather than 'home phenotyping', sophisticated phenotyping should be carried out at specialist centres. Phenotyping at specialist mouse clinics adhering to EMPReSS protocols has the advantage of a high professional standard, but might not always provide the user of a mutant with the specific information needed for their purpose and may not be affordable.

Capacity and need

As pointed out earlier, only a minority of genetically modified mice are phenotyped. This could be due to a lack of knowledge about the possibilities or the advantages of doing so. Nevertheless, a central problem in phenotyping today is the issue of current capacity versus need. There is still a huge mountain to climb to complete the phenotyping of every mutant. The capacity of existing mouse clinics is absolutely insufficient to phenotype all the mice generated and it would be of benefit to have several more of these facilities established. These clinics would accumulate expertise in phenotyping and could serve as consultants to users planning to phenotype their animals themselves.

New methods for phenotyping – speed and sophistication

The problem of capacity could be improved by developing new, inexpensive, rapid and reliable methods of phenotyp-

[13]http://www.interphenome.org

ing. This challenge is being met by the introduction of new technology which meets the above criteria. For example, a new technology named Luminex enables the detection and quantification of multiple RNA or protein targets simultaneously. It combines a flow cytometer, fluorescent-dyed microspheres (beads), lasers and digital signal processing to allow multiplexing of up to 100 assays within a single sample, and it is expected to revolutionise the rapidity and scale of assaying a wide spectrum of blood parameters. In the future we can expect micro technologies, remote monitoring and new imaging methods to have a large impact on the speed, price and quality of phenotyping (Johnson *et al.* 2006). Moreover, technologies that take welfare into consideration and can minimise trauma to animals, while still retaining sufficient sensitivity and replicability, will become an integrated component of the future phenotyping process (Pinkert 2003).

The environment – a challenge to phenotyping

The results of phenotyping not only depend on the genetic make-up of the mutant but can also be influenced by environmental factors, such as cage environment, diet and health status (Barthold 2004). Some phenotypes are not expressed by the animal until provoked by the environment; for example diabetes may not develop until the animals are fed a high-fat diet.

Another important environmental factor is the phenotyping test itself. One aspect of this is that different equipment may have different detection sensitivities and this must be considered. Also, many tests affect the animals in some way (eg, when taking a blood sample the animal is removed from its cage, immobilized and a vein is punctured). These procedures can significantly influence results obtained. Generally, when behavioural phenotyping results need to be comparable and replicable it is recommended that environmental conditions are standardised as much as possible and that the conditions under which the results are obtained are documented (Brown *et al.* 2006). Different environmental factors influence phenotyping results to different degrees and the results of behavioural tests are prone to being very sensitive to the environment. Research has shown that the environment of individual laboratories influenced behavioural results despite attempts to standardise between laboratories (Crabbe *et al.* 1999). On the other hand, some parameters seem rather resistant to environmental conditions. For example, caging and diet were found to have little effect on blood chemistry of a number of inbred strains (Arndt & Surjo 2001). It has been argued that when performing behavioural phenotyping, environmental background should be systematically varied instead of being standardised, because the parameters are so strongly modulated by the environment (Würbel 2002).

An open international network on behavioural phenotyping, the Mutant Mouse Behaviour Network (MMB) and the specific environmental challenges it offers has been established[14]. MMB was founded within the framework of the conference 'Behavioural Phenotyping of Mouse Mutants', February 2000, held in Cologne, Germany.

[14]http://www.medizin.uni-koeln.de/mmb-network/index.html

Further phenotyping issues to consider

The user of a genetically modified mouse should keep in mind that some phenotypic changes are subtle and can be compensated for by other mechanisms. Some may not be apparent in the young animal but are exposed at a later stage of life. Some phenotypes are seen only at a specific developmental stage and some in connection with specific physiological conditions such as pregnancy. For those reasons, animals should be characterised at different stages of their lives. It has been suggested that animals should be tested at three ages: young, adult and geriatric (Broom 1995; Morton & Hau 2003; Wells *et al.* 2006). Both homo- and heterozygous animals should be tested, and within every group they should be the same age as far as possible (age-matched). Also, one should be aware that a phenotype could vary between sexes and so both male and female animals should be tested.

Use of the pronuclear injection method can give rise to the formation of concatemers, head to tail, multicopy gene arrays of extrachromosomal DNA which might enter the genome, thereby generating a mutant carrying a transgene concatemer at one or more loci in the genome. Alternatively the result may be silencing of genes, transgene instability, low degree of transmission to offspring and somatic mosaicism of the F1 generation (Clark *et al.* 2007).

Some new traits have been shown not to reveal themselves until after a couple of generations (Van Hoosier 1999). Therefore, consideration should be given to phenotyping strains for several generations. Depending on the method of modification, new strains become genetically more 'stable' after breeding for some generations and characterisation of the strain at a 'stable' point will give the most reliable result (Mertens & Rülicke 2000). However, establishing this point by breeding several generations can be difficult and also contradictory to welfare considerations in case the strain has problems.

The order in which the individual tests are performed can influence the results. This has been investigated in behavioural tests and it has been reported that certain test variables are sensitive to the test order while others are resistant (McIlwain *et al.* 2001). Mice that have become experienced through their participation in some tests change their behaviour significantly in subsequent tests compared with naïve mice (Voikar *et al.* 2004). For this reason it is best to start with tests that assess anxiety and exploratory activity and to perform the cognitive tests at a later stage.

When phenotyping genetically modified animals, the question of controls needs to be dealt with. The most obvious choice is probably to use wild-type siblings as controls (Charsa *et al.* 2003). If the strain is kept by homozygous breeding and no wild-type siblings are available, the corresponding inbred strain should be used as a control. Wild-type siblings of a mixed genetic background are not ideal controls as one cannot be sure how much donor/recipient strain is represented in each animal and backcrossing to a congenic strain before phenotyping is therefore recommended.

Background of animals

Identical mutations might have different phenotypes because of their different genetic backgrounds, as when, for example, different inbred mouse strains carry the same mutation. The majority of phenotypic traits are of complex polygenic origin and their inheritance does not follow a simple single locus Mendelian pattern. In this case, the different phenotypes of mice with identical mutations in different strains can be attributed to independent modifier genes with allelic variations. In the end, it is not just the genes, but also other genetic modifiers that lead to the combined action of many genes and the differential patterns of transcription and translation that influence the development and phenotype of a genetic modification (Barbaric *et al.* 2007). Despite this, the phenotypic changes of genetically modified mice are still frequently attributed to just the induced mutation but, according to the above, it could be argued that testing the trait in different genetic backgrounds/strains would provide a clearer picture of the mutation.

Backcrossing of animals

Some mutant mice are kept of a 'mixed genetic background'. This means that the animals are not congenic, but a mixture of the strains used in the generation of the mutant (typically 129 and C57BL/6). With modifier genes in mind, there is no doubt that the 'mixed background' will give variations in the phenotype of these animals – even among siblings.

The Banbury Conference on Genetic Background in Mice (1997) recommended that backcrossing is carried out to obtain a congenic strain with the genetic background of an inbred strain. This is obtained by a minimum of ten generations of backcrosses to the recipient strain counting the first hybrid generation as F1 and the following backcrosses as N2–N10.

As backcrossing for ten generations is a very time-consuming exercise (2–3 years) an accelerated method for the production of a congenic strain has been developed which is based on background selection. This is called 'speed congenic' or 'marker-assisted selection'. The principle of this is to select breeders from each new generation with a genome as similar to the recipient strain as possible. This cuts the backcrossing time down to approximately 1 year (Wakeland *et al.* 1997; Wong 2002).

Furthermore, in order to prevent the mutant strain from accumulating genetic changes as a result of genetic drift over time it is recommended that the strain should be backcrossed to the parental inbred background every five to six generations (Banbury Conference on Genetic Background in Mice 1997).

Despite these recommendations, situations might occur where animals are not completely backcrossed to a congenic state before they are used. In that case, it is best to use a larger number of animals for the tests to compensate for the variation in the genetic background (Zeiss 2004). However, using more animals for the test has welfare aspects which should be considered beforehand.

Number of animals

The aim of phenotyping is to find new traits either for welfare assessment or scientific use. In order to optimize the chance of detecting these, a sufficient number of animals must be tested. As outlined earlier, traits might be subtle or only identifiable under certain conditions (eg, with age, stress or feeding a specific diet) (Fitzgerald *et al.* 2003; Davey & Maclean 2006). Furthermore, different test methods have different levels of sensitivity. Such factors make it difficult to estimate how many animals should be used for phenotyping a particular strain.

Mertens and Rülicke (2000) concluded that for animal welfare, time and expense reasons it is important to consider the number of animals thoroughly. They have stated that it is not feasible to make a clear-cut recommendation as many factors, such as genetic background, penetration and expression of the mutation and welfare implications, would influence the size of the group necessary. However, they recommended starting with approximately ten wild-type, ten hemi- or hetero- and ten homozygous animals (50% males and 50% females). This would allow statistical calculations and should be regarded as the minimal number of animals for testing. Depending on the results more animals could be included. This recommendation was supported by others (Bailey *et al.* 2006).

Some of the protocols mentioned earlier give recommendations on the number of mice that should be tested. The SHIRPA protocol does not *per se* give a recommendation regarding number of animals. However, Rogers *et al.* (1999) used two separate cohorts of ten males and ten females for the SHIRPA tests. One cohort was used for the elevated plus-maze and open field tests; the other cohort was used for the remaining tests. The order of testing was designed such that the procedures most likely to be affected by prior handling were carried out first (Rogers *et al.* 1999).

In the protocols of the Mouse Phenome Project some recommend a specific number of mice for the particular test, whereas others do not. The general recommendation is ten males and ten females at the age of 10–14 weeks (Bogue & Grubb 2004). The MuTrac system of the Tennessee Mouse Genome Consortium also recommends number of mice in some protocols varying from two to eight mice per test. To date, the EMPReSS protocols do not include recommendations for numbers of animals. However, at this moment ten males and ten females for each of the two 'pipelines' are used at MRC, Harwell, UK and at the German Mouse Clinic.

The issue of sample size has also been addressed by Meyer *et al.* (2007). The 'background noise' defined as the difference in response to the same test by mice of the same strain but from different laboratories/suppliers has been investigated. This intra-strain variability of response to a specific test will affect the number of mice recommended for each test, as the 'background noise' might mask potential phenotypic differences. Other parameters such as the variance of the trait in question (subtle/strong phenotype) will also influence this. A pilot study should be carried out in order to establish the values of the above parameters and calculate sample sizes accordingly (Meyer *et al.* 2007).

To conclude, several suggestions have been made regarding the optimal number of animals for phenotyping and the scientific rationale has not always been clear. This issue would benefit from further consideration.

A different, but often very troublesome issue that can affect the number of animals available for phenotyping is the breeding capability of genetically modified strains. Many mutants have reproduction problems making it difficult to get enough pups at approximately the same age (age-matched) for testing. This should be taken into consideration when planning the breeding of animals for phenotyping.

Summary of phenotyping issues to consider

In this paper we have tried to call attention to the many important aspects of phenotyping. Bearing in mind the many reasons for using genetically modified mice we shall not attempt to suggest which set of tests to use. Rather, we urge the scientist responsible for the characterisation of the animal to give the issue careful consideration based on the information in this chapter. We would, however, make the following outline as a guide to running a basic phenotyping project:

1. search for existing information;
2. conduct a welfare assessment;
3. investigate the basic functions of the animal, eg:
    - growth and development of the animal;
    - lifespan and age-specific mortality;
    - fertility;
    - physical examination;
    - clinical chemistry and haematology;
    - behaviour;
4. conduct necropsies.

In summary, we recommend testing every new strain at three stages: young, adult and geriatric. The mice in each group should be approximately the same age. Homo-, heterozygous and wild-type mice should be tested in both sexes. The strain should be backcrossed to congenezity for 10 generations or the number of backcrossings by marker assisted selection to obtain equivalent congenezity before phenotyping and the order of tests should be considered to minimise one test affecting the result of the next.

It is worth considering testing the strain for several generations and investigating the mutation in different inbred strains. Based on the literature, the number of animals in every test group should be at least 10 for the initial testing. Pilot studies for the identification of the optimal number of animals could be carried out.

Concluding remarks

Only very few genetically modified mice are systematically phenotyped – often the process involves no more than daily observation by animal technicians. The widespread use of such observation for the detection of welfare impingement and new phenotypic traits is in many cases regarded as sufficient. There is no doubt that a talented and experienced animal technician is likely to discover even subtle deviations in a genetically modified mouse. Nevertheless, there are traits that produce no immediately observable symptoms. Systematic testing using phenotyping protocols increases the chance of identifying traits, and should be carried out.

For welfare assessment, observation is an excellent tool, as much welfare assessment is based on behavioural studies. However, observation of behaviour alone is not sufficient to evaluate welfare. Observations should always be recorded for later reference.

Phenotyping takes time. Testing requires a certain number of age-matched pups. Producing these from a founder animal is a laborious and time-consuming task. Furthermore, carrying out the actual phenotyping tests can take months and if the mouse is tested at different ages, the time needed, of course, increases. However, the advantages of thoroughly phenotyping before using an animal for scientific purposes are obvious and the time for phenotyping should be allocated to any project including genetically modified rodents.

Phenotyping requires expertise. The tests that are used to identify new traits are often complicated and demanding to perform. Behavioural testing is the classic example of a task which requires special skills. Also laboratory animal histopathologists need many years of specialised education and training. The tendency of phenotyping protocols to grow both in size (by adding more tests) but also in complexity (by developing more sophisticated methods) is increasing the demand for specialised expertise and it cannot be expected that a research group or even a university animal facility, will possess all this know-how without the necessary investments.

Phenotyping costs money and a major issue may be the ability or willingness to meet the costs of detailed phenotypic characterisation. Today, many scientists are funded by time-limited grants and in order to obtain the next grant, they must provide satisfactory scientific results at the end of the previous period. Establishing the phenotype of a mouse model is, unfortunately, not yet regarded as a scientific result, and often the experimental work is initiated without previous phenotyping. The risk is that research may be carried out using animal models which later appear to be sub-optimal or may even be invalid.

In summary, the implementation of phenotyping will undoubtedly improve as new cheaper and faster high-quality methods are developed and the concept becomes further scientifically accepted.

Useful websites

British National Centre for Replacement, Refinement and Reduction of Animals in Research (NC3Rs)

http://www.nc3rs.org.uk

CF2 Mouse Phenotyping Platform

http://davinci.crg.es/mpc/cf2.php

Objectives are:

- to share common phenotyping protocols for large phenotypic analysis on mouse models;

- to share protocols and apparatus (EUMORPHIA-based protocols);
- to facilitate research/learning stages within the consortium;
- to define common strategies and/or establish different lines of phenotyping (eg, cardiovascular/general morphology and behaviour/neurology/imaging etc);
- to perform in depth studies of a limited number of aneuploid transgenics workshops.

Charles River Laboratories

http://www.criver.com

Consortium for Functional Glycomics – Mouse Line Phenotype Analysis

http://www.functionalglycomics.org/glycomics/publicdata/phenotyping.jsp

EUMODIC

http://www.eumodic.eu

EUMORPHIA

http://www.eumorphia.org

Europhenome Mouse Phenotyping Resource

http://www.europhenome.eu

The European Mouse Mutagenesis Consortium (EMMC)

http://www.eucomm.org

The EMMC is the European initiative contributing to the international effort on functional annotation of the mouse genome. Its objectives are to establish and integrate mutagenesis platforms, gene expression resources, phenotyping units, storage and distribution centres and bioinformatics resources. The combined efforts will accelerate the understanding of gene function and of human health and disease (Auwerx *et al.* 2004).

The European Mouse Mutant Archive (EMMA)

http://www.emma.rm.cnr.it

The European Mouse Phenotyping Resource for Standardised Screens, EMPReSS

http://www.empress.har.mrc.ac.uk

EMPReSS is a web-based resource for the visualisation, searching and downloading of standard operating procedures and other documents (Green *et al.* 2005).

Frimorfo

http://www.frimorfo.com

Functional Annotation of Mouse (FANTOM)

http://www.ddbj.nig.ac.jp/, http://fantom2.gsc.riken.jp, http://fantom3.gsc.riken.jp

The large mouse transcriptome project, Functional Annotation of Mouse (FANTOM), provides a wealth of data on novel genes, splice variants and non-coding RNA, and provides a unique opportunity to identify novel human disease genes. It will also facilitate the creation of transgenic mouse models to help elucidate the function of potential human disease genes (Hayashizaki & Kanamori 2004; Kiyosawa *et al.* 2004). After the development of original technologies (such as full-length cDNA libraries, CAGE, GSC) followed by massive application, the data have been analysed by the members of the Fantom-3 consortium ((Carninci *et al.* 2005; Katayama *et al.* 2005). The information is available to the public on the servers of DDBJ, National Institute of Genetics and RIKEN.

The Gene Expression Database (GXD)

http://www.informatics.jax.org or http://www.informatics.jax.org/menus/expression_menu.shtml

The GXD is a community resource for gene expression information in the laboratory mouse. By collecting and integrating different types of expression data, GXD provides information about expression profiles in different mouse strains and mutants (Hill *et al.* 2004).

GeneLynx Mouse

http://mouse.genelynx.org

Gene Lynx Mouse is a meta-database providing an extensive collection of hyperlinks to mouse gene-specific information in diverse databases available via the Internet. The GeneLynx project is based on the simple notion that given any gene-specific identifier (eg, accession number, gene name, text or sequence), scientists should be able to access a single location that provides a set of links to all the publicly available information pertinent to the specified gene. The recent climax in the mouse genome and RIKEN cDNA sequencing projects provided the data necessary for the development of a gene-centric mouse information portal based on the GeneLynx ideals. Clusters of RIKEN cDNA sequences were used to define the initial set of mouse genes. Like its human counterpart, GeneLynx Mouse is designed as an extensible relational database with an intuitive and user-friendly web interface. Data is automatically extracted from diverse resources, using appropriate approaches to maximise the coverage. To promote cross-database interoperability, an indexing utility is provided to facilitate the establishment of hyperlinks in external databases. As a result of the integration of the human and mouse systems, GeneLynx now serves as a powerful comparative genomics data mining resource (Lenhard *et al.* 2003).

The German Mouse Clinic

http://www.gsf.de/ieg/gmc

The German Mouse Clinic is an open access platform for standardised phenotyping (Gailus-Durner *et al.* 2005).

Institut Clinique de la Souris (ICS)

http://www-mci.u-strasbg.fr/service_intro.html

The Integrated Genomics Environment

http://rgd.mcw.edu/VCMAP

Integration of the large variety of genome maps from several organisms provides the mechanism by which physiological knowledge obtained in model systems such as the rat can be projected onto the human genome to further the research on human disease. Twigger *et al.* (2004) use new data and introduce the Integrated Genomics Environment, an extensive database of curated and integrated maps, markers and physiological results (Twigger *et al.* 2004).

The Jackson Laboratory

http://www.jax.org

LIFEdb

http://www.dkfz.de/LIFEdb

LIFEdb is implemented to link information regarding novel human full-length cDNAs generated and sequenced by the German cDNA Consortium with functional information on the encoded proteins produced in functional genomics and proteomics approaches. The database also serves as a sample-tracking system to manage the process from cDNA to experimental read-out and data interpretation. A web interface enables the scientific community to explore and visualise features of the annotated cDNAs and ORFs combined with experimental results, and thus helps to unravel new features of proteins with as yet unknown functions (Bannasch *et al.* 2004).

The Mouse Brain Library (MBL)

http://mbl.org

The MBL is comprised of four interrelated components: The Brain Library, iScope, Neurocartographer and WebQTL. The centerpiece of the MBL is an image database of histologically prepared museum-quality slides representing nearly 2000 mice from over 120 strains – a library suitable for stereologic analysis of regional volume. The iScope provides fast access to the entire slide collection using streaming video technology, enabling neuroscientists to acquire high-magnification images of any CNS region for any of the mice in the MBL. Neurocartographer provides automatic segmentation of images from the MBL by warping precisely delineated boundaries from a 3D atlas of the mouse brain. Finally, WebQTL provides statistical and graphical analysis of linkage between phenotypes and genotypes. This website provides universal access over the web to tools for the genetic dissection of complex traits of the CNS – tools that allow researchers to map genes that modulate phenotypes at a variety of levels ranging from the molecular all the way to the anatomy of the entire brain (Rosen *et al.* 2003).

The Mouse Genome Database (MGD)

http://www.informatics.jax.org

The MGD forms the core of the Mouse Genome Informatics (MGI) system: a model organism database resource for the laboratory mouse. MGD provides essential integration of experimental knowledge for the mouse system with information annotated from both literature and online sources. MGD curates and presents consensus and experimental data representations of genotype (sequence) through phenotype information, including highly detailed reports about genes and gene products. Primary foci of integration are through representations of relationships among genes, sequences and phenotypes (Eppig *et al.* 2005).

Mouse Genetic Resources – Shared Information of Genetic Resources (SHIGEN)

http://www.shigen.nig.ac.jp/mouse/mouse.default.html

Mouse Genome Resource (MGR)

http://www.ncbi.nlm.nih.gov/genome/guide/mouse

Mouse Models of Human Cancers Consortium (MMHCC)

http://web.ncifcrf.gov/researchresources/mmhcc/default/asp

The Mouse Phenome Database (MPD)

http://phenome.jax.org/pub-cgi/phenome/mpdcgi?rtn=docs/home

The Mouse Phenotype Database Integration Consortium (MPDIC)

http://interphenome.org

Multicentre Mouse Behavioural Trial

http://www.albany.edu/psy/obssr3

The Mutant Mouse Behaviour Network (MMB)

http://www.medizin.uni-koeln.de/mmb-network/index.html

The non-profit international MMB was founded within the framework of the conference 'Behavioural Phenotyping of Mouse Mutants', February 2000, held in Cologne, Germany. It intends to be a forum for presenting and discussing all topics dealing with the behavioural phenotyping of mice. The major aim of the MMB is to support the interdisciplinary finding of a consensus on the methods and techniques used for behavioural phenotyping of mouse mutants. That means that scientists involved in the development of mouse models have to consent to the fact that a consideration of all the parameters that might affect the behaviour is necessary. The network will provide a standardised database that includes detailed descriptions of test methods and of the relevant background parameters that might influence the behaviour of mice. Information will range from detailed descriptions of test methods, specifications of the equipment used, housing conditions and specifications of the animals used according to the international nomenclature. A mailing list has been established to provide a platform for the continuous exchange of information between the network members. Scientists from all research areas involved are free to provide detailed information about their experimental work. (Crabbe *et al.* 1999; Surjo & Arndt 2001).

My Mouse

http://mymouse.org/centers

NeuroMouse

http://www.mshri.on.ca/molec/henderson/neuromouse.htm

NIHR Health Technology Assessment Programme

http://www.hta.nhsweb.nhs.uk

PhenoSITE protocols

http://www.gsc.riken.go.jp/mouse/aboutus/screening.htm

The Pharmacogenetics Research Network and Knowledge Base (PharmGKB)

http://www.pharmgkb.org

The National Institutes of Health, recognizing: (1) the need for fully disclosable and publishable research in this domain; and (2) the need to store the results of this research in a public database, has funded PharmGKB. This will become a national resource containing high-quality structured data linking genomic information, molecular and cellular phenotype information and clinical phenotype information. For further information, please see http://www.nigms.nih.gov/funding/pharmacogenetics.html. The ultimate product of this project will be a knowledge base that will provide a public infrastructure for understanding how variations in the human genome lead to variations in clinical response to medications (Klein *et al.* 2001).

PRIME – Priorities for Mouse Functional Genomic Research Across Europe

http://www.prime-eu.org

The Rat Genome Database (RGD)

http://rgd.mcw.edu

The RGD aims to meet the needs of its community by providing genetic and genomic infrastructure while also annotating the strengths of rat research: biochemistry, nutrition, pharmacology and physiology. RGD works towards creating a phenome database. Recent developments can be categorised into three groups: (1) improved data collection and integration to match increased volume and biological scope of research; (2) knowledge representation augmented by the implementation of a new ontology and annotation system; (3) the addition of quantitative trait loci data, from rat, mouse and human to our advanced comparative genomics tools, as well as the creation of new, and enhancement of existing, tools to enable users to efficiently browse and survey research data. The emphasis is on helping researchers find genes responsible for disease through the use of rat models (De La Cruz *et al.* 2005).

RIKEN Mouse Encyclopedia Index

http://genome.rtc.riken.go.jp

Rodent Phenotyping

http://www.radil.missouri.edu/pheno

Sloan-Kettering Institute Mouse Project

http://mouse.ski.mskcc.org

The Structural Genomics Consortium

http://www.sgc.utoronto.ca

A group of multinational companies, together with the Wellcome Trust, is attempting to form a charitable organization, the Structural Genomics Consortium. The goal will be to obtain X-ray structures for a broad representation across families of human proteins and to place the structural coordinates in the public database (Williamson 2000).

TBASE

http://tbase.jax.org

Tennessee Mouse Genome Consortium

http://www.tnmouse.org/tmgc_public/mutant.php

TIGR Mouse Gene Index

http://www.tigr.org/tdb/mgi/index.html

University of California Genetically Engineered Mouse Research

http://ccm.ucdavis.edu/tgmouse

University of California Resource of Gene Trap Insertions

http://socrates.berkeley.edu/~skarnes/resource.html

University of Michigan Transgenic Animal Model Core Protocols

http://www.med.umich.edu/tamc/protocols.html

Whole Mouse Catalogue

http://www.rodentia.com/wmc

References

Arndt, S.S. and Surjo, D. (2001) Methods for the behavioural phenotyping of mouse mutants. How to keep the overview. *Behavioural Brain Research*, **125**, 39–42

Auwerx, J., Avner, P., Baldock, R. *et al.* (2004) The European dimension for the mouse genome mutagenesis program. *Nature Genetics*, **36**, 925–927

Bailey, K.R., Rustay, N.R. and Crawley, J.N. (2006) Behavioral phenotyping of transgenic and knockout mice: practical concerns and potential pitfalls. *Institute for Laboratory Animal Research Journal*, **47**, 124–131

Baker, E.J., Galloway, L., Jackson, B. *et al.* (2004) MuTrack: a genome analysis system for large-scale mutagenesis in the mouse. *BMC Bioinformatics*, **5**, 11

Banbury Conference on Genetic Background in Mice (1997) Mutant mice and neuroscience: recommendations concerning genetic background. *Neuron*, **19**, 755–759

Bannasch, D., Mehrle, A., Glatting, K.H. *et al.* (2004) LIFEdb: a database for functional genomics experiments integrating information from external sources, and serving as a sample tracking system. *Nucleic Acids Research*, **32** (Database issue), D505–D508

Barbaric, I., Miller, G. and Dear, T.N. (2007) Appearances can be deceiving: phenotypes of knockout mice. *Briefings in Functional Genomics and Proteomics*, **6**, 91–103

Barthold, S.W. (2004) Genetically altered mice: phenotypes, no phenotypes, and faux phenotypes. *Genetica*, **122**, 75–88

Blake, J.A., Eppig, J.T., Bult, C.J. *et al.* (2006) The Mouse Genome Database (MGD): updates and enhancements. *Nucleic Acids Research*, **34** (Database issue), D562–D567

Bogue, M.A. and Grubb, S.C. (2004) The Mouse Phenome Project. *Genetica*, **122**, 71–74.

Bolon, B. (2006) Internet resources for phenotyping engineered rodents. *Institute for Laboratory Animal Research Journal*, **47**, 163–171

Broom, D.M. (1995) Assessing the welfare of transgenic animals. In: *Welfare Aspects of Transgenic Animals. Proceedings EC-Workshop of October 30, 1995 Presented at EC-workshop*. Eds van Zutphen, L.F.M. and van der Meer, M., pp. 58–67. Springer, Berlin

Brown, S.D., Chambon, P. and de Angelis, M.H. (2005) EMPReSS: standardized phenotype screens for functional annotation of the mouse genome. *Nature Genetics.*, **37**, 1155 (http://www.empress.har.mrc.ac.uk, accessed 13 July 09)

Brown, S.D.M., Hancock, J.M. and Gates, H. (2006) Understanding mammalian genetic systems: the challenge of phenotyping in the mouse. *Public Library of Science Genetics*, **2**, e118

Carninci, P., Kasukawa, T., Katayama, S. *et al.* (2005) The transcriptional landscape of the mammalian genome. *Science*, **309**, 1559–1563

Charsa, R., Knoblaugh, S. and Ladiges, W. (2003) Phenotypic characterization of genetically engineered mice. In: *Handbook of Laboratory Animal Science*, Vol 1. Eds Hau, J. and Van Hoosier, G.L., pp. 205–230. CRC Press, New York

Clark, K.J., Carlson, D.F. and Fahrenkrug, S.C. (2007) Pigs taking wing with transposons and recombinases. *Genome Biology*, **8** (Suppl 1), S13

Crabbe, J.C., Wahlsten, D. and Dudek, B.C. (1999) Genetics of mouse behavior: interactions with laboratory environment. *Science*, **284**, 1670–1672

Crawley, J.N. (2003) Behavioral phenotyping of rodents. *Comparative Medicine*, **53**, 140–146

Crawley, J. N. and Paylor, R. (1997) A proposed test battery and constellations of specific behavioral paradigms to investigate the behavioral phenotypes of transgenic and knockout mice. *Hormones and Behavior*, **31**, 197–211

Crawley, J.N. and Paylor, R. (1997a) A proposed test battery and constellations of specific behavioral paradigms to investigate the behavioral phenotypes of transgenic and knockout mice. *Hormones and Behavior*, **31**, 197–211

Davey, R.A. and Maclean, H.E. (2006) Current and future approaches using genetically modified mice in endocrine research. *The American Journal of Physiology – Endocrinology and Metabolism*, **291**, E429–E438

De La Cruz, N., Bromberg, S., Pasko, D. *et al.* (2005) The rat genome database (RGD): developments towards a phenome database. *Nucleic Acids Research*, **33** (Database issue), D485–D491

Dennis, M.B., Jr. (2002) Welfare issues of genetically modified animals. *Institute for Laboratory Animal Research Journal*, **43**, 100–109

Eppig, J.T., Bult, C.J., Kadin, J.A. *et al.* (2005) The mouse genome database (MGD): from genes to mice – a community resource for mouse biology. *Nucleic Acids Research*, **33** (Database issue), D471–D475

Fitzgerald, S.M., Gan, L., Wickman, A. *et al.* (2003) Cardiovascular and renal phenotyping of genetically modified mice: a challenge for traditional physiology. *Clinical and Experimental Pharmacology and Physiology*, **30**, 207–216

Gailus-Durner, V., Fuchs, H., Becker, L. *et al.* (2005) Introducing the German Mouse Clinic: open access platform for standardized phenotyping. *Nature Methods*, **2**, 403–404

Gkoutos, G.V., Green, E.C., Mallon, A.M. *et al.* (2005) Using ontologies to describe mouse phenotypes. *Genome Biology*, **6**, R8

Green, E.C., Gkoutos, G.V., Lad, H.V. *et al.* (2005) EMPReSS: European mouse phenotyping resource for standardized screens. *Bioinformatics*, **21**, 2930–2931

Grubb, S.C., Churchill, G.A. and Bogue, M.A. (2004) A collaborative database of inbred mouse strain characteristics. *Bioinformatics*, **20**, 2857–2859

Hayashizaki, Y. and Kanamori, M. (2004) Dynamic transcriptome of mice. *Trends in Biotechnology*, **22**, 161–167

Hill, D.P., Begley, D.A., Finger, J.H. *et al.* (2004) The mouse Gene Expression Database (GXD): updates and enhancements. *Nucleic Acids Research*, **32** (Database issue), D568–D571

Hrabé de Angelis, M., Chambon, P. and Brown, S. (2006) *Standards of Mouse Model Phenotyping*. Wiley-VCH Verlag GmbH & Co. KGaA, Weinheim

Irwin, S. (1968) Comprehensive observational assessment: Ia. A systematic, quantitative procedure for assessing the behavioral and physiologic state of the mouse. *Psychopharmacologia Journal*, **13**, 222–257

Jegstrup, I., Thon, R., Hansen, A.K. *et al.* (2003) Characterization of transgenic mice – a comparison of protocols for welfare evaluation and phenotype characterization of mice with a suggestion on a future certificate of instruction. *Laboratory Animals*, **37**, 1–9

Johnson, J.T., Hansen, M.S., Wu, I. *et al.* (2006) Virtual histology of transgenic mouse embryos for high-throughput phenotyping. *Public Library of Science Genetics*, **2**, e61

Katayama, S., Tomaru, Y., Kasukawa, T. *et al.* (2005) Antisense transcription in the mammalian transcriptome. *Science*, **309**, 1564–1566

Kiyosawa, H., Kawashima, T., Silva, D. *et al.* (2004) Systematic genome-wide approach to positional candidate cloning for identification of novel human disease genes. *Internal Medicine Journal*, **34**, 79–90

Klein, T.E., Chang, J.T., Cho, M.K. *et al.* (2001) Integrating genotype and phenotype information: an overview of the PharmGKB project. Pharmacogenetics Research Network and Knowledge Base. *Pharmacogenomics Journal*, **1**, 167–170

Lenhard, B., Wahlestedt, C. and Wasserman, W.W. (2003) GeneLynx mouse: integrated portal to the mouse genome. *Genome Research*, **13**, 1501–1504

Marques, J.M., Augustsson, H., Ögren, S.O. *et al.* (2007) *A Characterization Routine for Improved Welfare in Pre-weaning Mice. Refinement of Mouse Husbandry for Improved Animal Welfare and Research Quality*. Doctoral thesis 2007:104. Uppsala, Sweden: Faculty of Veterinary Medicine and Animal Science, Swedish University of Agricultural Sciences

McIlwain, K.L., Merriweather, M.Y., Yuva-Paylor, L.A. *et al.* (2001) The use of behavioral test batteries: effects of training history. *Physiology and Behavior*, **73**, 705–717

Mepham, T.B., Combes, R.D., Balls, M. *et al.* (1998) The use of transgenic animals in the European Union: The report and recommendations of ECVAM Workshop 28. *Alternatives to Laboratory Animals*, **26**(1), 21–43

Mertens, C. and Rülicke, T. (1999) Score sheets for the monitoring of transgenic mice. *Animal Welfare* **8**, 433–438

Mertens, C. and Rülicke, T. (2000) Umfassendes Formular zur strukturierten Characterisierung gentechnich veränderter Tierlinien. *Altex*, **17**, 15–21

Mertens, C. and Rülicke, T. (2002) Phenotype characterisation and welfare assessment of transgenic mice. *3R-Info-Bulletin*, 3R Research Foundation, Switzerland. http://www.forschung3r.ch/en/publications/bu19_print.html

Meyer, C.W., Elvert, R., Scherag, A. *et al.* (2007) Power matters in closing the phenotyping gap. *Naturwissenschaften*, **94**, 401–406

Morton, D.B. and Hau, J. (2003) Phenotypic characterization of genetically engineered mice. In: *Handbook of Laboratory Animal Science*, Vol 1. Eds Hau, J. and Van Hoosier, G.L., pp. 457–481. CRC Press, New York

Mouse Phenotype Database Integration Consortium (2007) Integration of mouse phenome data resources. *Mammalian Genome*, **18**, 157–163

Murray, K.A. (2002) Issues to consider when phenotyping mutant mouse models. *Laboratory Animals*, **31**, 25–29

Pinkert, C.A. (2003) Transgenic animal technology: alternatives in genotyping and phenotyping. *Comparative Medicine*, **53**, 126–139

Richmond, J. (2000) Cost-benefit assessment: the United Kingdom experience. In: *Progress in the Reduction, Refinement and Replacement of Animal Experimentation*. Developments in Animal and Veterinary Sciences, 31. Eds Balls, M., Van Zeller, A.-M. and Halder, M., pp. 821–827. Elsevier, Amsterdam

Rogers, D.C., Fisher, E.M., Brown, S.D. *et al.* (1997) Behavioral and functional analysis of mouse phenotype: SHIRPA, a proposed protocol for comprehensive phenotype assessment. *Mammalian Genome*, **8**, 711–713

Rogers, D.C., Jones, D.N., Nelson, P.R. *et al.* (1999) Use of SHIRPA and discriminant analysis to characterise marked differences in the behavioural phenotype of six inbred mouse strains. *Behavioural Brain Research*, **105**, 207–217

Rosen, G.D., La Porte, N.T., Diechtiareff, B. *et al.* (2003) Informatics center for mouse genomics: the dissection of complex traits of the nervous system. *Neuroinformatics*, **1**, 327–342

Smith, C.L., Goldsmith, C.A. and Eppig, J.T. (2005) The Mammalian Phenotype Ontology as a tool for annotating, analyzing and comparing phenotypic information. *Genome Biology*, **6**, R7

Surjo, D. and Arndt, S.S. (2001) The Mutant Mouse Behaviour network, a medium to present and discuss methods for the behavioural phenotyping. *Physiology and Behavior*, **73**, 691–694

Thon, R., Lassen, J., Hansen, A.K. *et al.* (2002) Welfare evaluation of genetically modified mice – an inventory study of reports to the Danish Animal Experiments Inspectorate. *Scandinavian Journal of Laboratory Animal Science*, **29**, 45–53

Thon, R., Vondeling, H., Lassen, J. *et al.* (2009) An interview survey of phenotypic characterization of genetically modified mice. *Laboratory Animals*, **43**, 278–283

Twigger, S.N., Nie, J., Ruotti, V. *et al.* (2004) Integrative genomics: in silico coupling of rat physiology and complex traits with mouse and human data. *Genome Research*, **14**, 651–660

van der Meer, M., Costa, P., Baumans, V. *et al.* (1999) Welfare assessment of transgenic animals: behavioural responses and morphological development of newborn mice. *Alternatives to Laboratory Animals*, **27**, 857–868

van der Meer, M., Rolls, A., Baumans, V. *et al.* (2001) Use of score sheets for welfare assessment of transgenic mice. *Laboratory Animals*, **35**, 379–389

Van Hoosier, G.L. (1999) The age of biology: opportunities and challenges for laboratory animal medicine. *Scandinavian Journal of Laboratory Animal Science*, **26**, 181–192

Van Zutphen, L.F.M. and van der Meer, M. (1997) *Welfare Aspects of Transgenic Animals*. Springer Berlin, Germany

Voikar, V., Vasar, E. and Rauvala, H. (2004) Behavioral alterations induced by repeated testing in C57BL/6J and 129S2/Sv mice: implications for phenotyping screens. *Genes, Brain and Behavior*, **3**, 27–38

Wakeland, E., Morel, L., Achey, K. *et al.* (1997) Speed congenics: a classic technique in the fast lane (relatively speaking). *Immunology Today*, **18**, 472–477

Wells, D.J., Playle, L.C., Enser, W.E. *et al.* (2006) Assessing the welfare of genetically altered mice, laboratory environments and rodents' behavioural needs. *Laboratory Animals*, **40**, 111–114 (available at http://www.nc3rs.org.uk)

Williamson, A.R. (2000) Creating a structural genomics consortium. *Nature Structural and Molecular Biology*, **7**(Suppl), 953

Wong, G.T. (2002) Speed congenics: applications for transgenic and knock-out mouse strains. *Neuropeptides*, **36**, 230–236

Wood, P.A. (2000) Phenotype assessment: are you missing something? *Comparative Medicine*, **50**, 12–15

Würbel, H. (2002) Behavioral phenotyping enhanced – beyond (environmental) standardization. *Genes, Brain and Behavior*, **1**, 3–8

Zeiss, C.J. (2004) Phenotyping of genetically altered mice. In: *Laboratory Animal Medicine and Management*, document No B2518.0504. http://www.ivis.org/advances/Reuter/zeiss/chapter.asp?LA=1 (registration needed)

6 Brief introduction to welfare assessment: a 'toolbox' of techniques

Naomi Latham

Introduction

Animal research will often impact on the welfare of the animals: either, for example, because animals are deliberately exposed to, or genetically altered or manipulated to exhibit disease (eg, mouse models of Huntington's Disease, Mangiarini *et al.* 1996), or because animals are housed in 'standardised' laboratory environments which may not fully meet their natural adaptations and needs (Latham & Mason 2004). Methods of assessing welfare allow us to gauge the level of suffering in research (and indeed other) animals, and to find ways of refining research techniques and housing or husbandry practices so that we can minimise that suffering and increase positive feelings, such as pleasure. This chapter will start by identifying what is meant by welfare, why animal welfare is considered important and who is responsible for ensuring the welfare of research animals. It will then go on to discuss some of the commonly used welfare assessment methods (the welfare assessment 'toolbox').

What is animal welfare, and why is it important?

Over 200 years ago the barrister and philosopher Jeremy Bentham wrote of animals, '*The day may come, when the rest of the animal creation may acquire those rights which could have been withholden from them but by the hand of tyranny. … The question is not, Can they reason?, nor Can they talk?, but Can they suffer?*' (Bentham 1789). Since then, the question of what constitutes good animal welfare has been addressed in a number of ways, with some focusing on physical fitness and others on the ability of animals to 'live a natural life' (Duncan & Fraser 1997). However, Bentham's concerns about animal suffering continues to be at the core of animal welfare principles – most closely reflected by the so-called 'feelings-based' conception of welfare, whereby welfare is about the subjective feelings of animals (Dawkins 1988; Duncan 1993). Animal welfare is thus treated as analogous to human welfare – indeed, the term 'welfare' is sometimes used interchangeably with other terms commonly used to describe *human* welfare, such as 'quality of life' and 'well-being' (Christiansen & Forkman 2007). Like human welfare, current consensus is that good animal welfare is based upon good health and positive subjective states (also referred to as affective states or emotions, Rolls 1999); while poor welfare occurs when individuals experience negative subjective states, such as suffering, due to disease or injury, or as a result of aversive or frustrating environments (Dawkins 2006; Boissy *et al.* 2007; Yeates & Main 2008). However, unlike humans, the welfare of animals cannot be assessed by asking for a direct verbal indication of their subjective state (which is generally accepted as the 'gold standard' indicator of subjective experiences) (Paul *et al.* 2005). Instead, there is a range – a 'toolbox' – of indirect measures of the behavioural, physiological and neurophysiological/-chemical components of subjective states (measures that will be discussed later in the chapter). These tools can be used to ask two questions that, between them, capture both the physical and mental aspects of animal welfare: 'are animals healthy?' and 'do they have what they want?' (Dawkins 2004). Since these tools only provide an indirect indication of an animal's health or its subjective state it is usually considered good practice to base welfare assessments on a number of parameters rather than a single measure. There are several reasons why good laboratory animal welfare and appropriate, evidence-based assessment techniques are important.

The first of these reasons relates to the ethical obligations of researchers and animal facilities to ensure the welfare of sentient laboratory animals. For a general discussion about the ethical issues associated with animal research see Sandøe *et al.* (1995) and the 2005 report published by the Nuffield Council on Bioethics (Nuffield Council on Bioethics 2005). National regulation, eg, The Animals (Scientific Procedures) Act (1986) in the UK, may also place on researchers legal requirements to ensure the welfare of their animals. There is still debate about whether or not non-human animals are capable of consciously experiencing affective states (Dawkins 1993; MacPhail 1998; see also Mendl & Paul 2004). However, given that many vertebrates possess the brain structures associated with the initiation of emotional arousal (eg, the amygdala) some researchers suggest that we should '*remain open to the possibility that … primary-process forms of affective experience evolved long before human brain evolution allowed us to think and to talk about such things*' (Panksepp 2003; also, Burgdorf & Panksepp 2006; Kirkden & Pajor 2006). Concern about the ethics of animal research (particularly studies that involve suffering) also influences public support for animal research, and researchers and animal facilities need to be mindful of this. Thus, for example, polls of public opinion often reveal that the general public are in favour of animal research provided that the research is for serious medical purposes, that there are no alternatives and that animal suffering is minimised (Festing & Wilkinson 2007). However, while being mindful of ethical obligations and the public concern regarding animal research, animal welfare assessment must be rigorous and evidence-based. Moreover, welfare concerns must be assessed from the animals' viewpoint, not merely from an anthropomorphic view-point, which may be extremely inappropriate. Indeed, for a clear demonstration of the dangers of unfettered anthropomorphism see a recent article by Bekoff in New Scientist (Bekoff 2007) – in particular, the counter-argument by Dawkins in the same article.

A further reason for ensuring good welfare in research animals is the often mooted argument that '*good welfare* = *good science*' (Poole 1997). For example, one of the main behavioural welfare indicators used in research (and other captive) animals is highly repetitive stereotypic behaviour, eg, bar-chewing in mice. However, there is now a large body of evidence indicating that stereotypic behaviours not only stem from frustration (hence their use as a welfare indicator), but that they may also reflect underlying changes in CNS functioning which cause animals to become less able to inhibit responses even if they become inappropriate (termed 'perseverative' behaviour) (reviewed Garner 2006). Stereotypic behaviour has also been directly correlated with changes in neurotransmitter functioning in a variety of captive animals (McBride & Hemmings 2005; Lewis *et al.* 2006), and may reflect stress-induced sensitisation of the dopaminergic pathways (Cabib 2006). These changes then raise questions about whether research animals housed in stereotypy-inducing environments are valid models in ethological and biomedical research. This is just one example of ways in which 'standard' laboratory housing may produce subjects whose validity as models in ethological and biomedical research is questionable (see Sherwin 2004a for a review of numerous other potentially undesirable effects of 'standard' housing). Furthermore, it has been argued that impoverished environments (which are often used in the name of standardisation) may in fact reduce the reproducibility and external validity of results – the so-called '*standardisation fallacy*' (Würbel 2000). Indeed, a series of studies by Crabbe, Wahlsten and colleagues elegantly demonstrated that even when conditions were rigorously standardised conditions across three laboratories, there were significant strain differences in behaviour in a battery of standard tests (Crabbe 1999; Wahlsten 2001). Hence, refining environments and experimental procedures may be beneficial for both animal welfare and the quality of research (Sherwin 2004a; Würbel & Garner 2007; see also Ritskes-Hoitinga *et al.* 2006).

Who is responsible for animal welfare?

Responsibilities for animal welfare will differ according to local regulation, but it may be helpful to provide a specific example. In the UK, ultimate responsibility for the welfare of animals used in Home Office licensed research lies with each project licence holder – usually the primary researcher on the project (Home Office 1989). This researcher is responsible for checking the welfare of their animals both on a day-to-day basis and following any experimental procedures. Hence, he or she must not only be familiar with the normal physical appearance and behaviour of their animals, but also with the physiological and behavioural effects of any experimental treatments. This must be specific to their particular subject species, strain or even genotype. For example, researchers working with genetically altered animals must be aware of not only the 'normal' characteristics of the 'wild-type' (control) animals but also with the characteristics of animals with the 'modified' genotype (see Committee on Recognition and Alleviation of Distress in Laboratory Animals (CRADLA) 2008, p. 26). Furthermore, the 'normal' characteristics of animals may also depend upon their age and gender. For example, numerous age-related changes, including changes in pain sensitivity and emotional behaviour, have been documented in research animals; and there are many well documented gender differences in behaviour and physiological stress responses (reviewed CRADLA 2008, p. 27). Researchers should also ensure that they document any relevant information about the signs observed during disease progression or the after-effects of any experimental procedures so that changes in the condition of animals can be assessed and monitored accurately and efficiently (J. Rogers personal communication 2008). Finally, researchers should also try to ensure that they are familiar with the natural biology and behaviour of their subject animal, as this is often essential for understanding how the captive environment can influence welfare (Dawkins 1980), and identifying behaviours that indicate impaired welfare (discussed further later). Table 6.1 contains some key references for information about the natural ethology of the two most commonly used research animals, mice and rats.

However, as well as the main researcher there are various other people who can, and should, be involved in ensuring the welfare of research animals. These include animal care staff, NACWOs (Named Animal Care and Welfare Officers) – or comparable roles in non-UK facilities – and veterinarians (Home Office 1989). These members of staff can provide supplementary support, particularly where researchers are indisposed or unable to spend the time monitoring their animals' welfare, or if they are inexperienced at doing so. Animal care staff play a key role at the 'frontline' of animal husbandry. They may often notice small changes in the physical condition and behaviour of animals (eg, changes to the animal's coat, chromodacryorrhoea, lethargy etc) that may indicate welfare problems. These should be brought to the attention of the researcher or responsible person so that the cause(s) of the problem can be identified and, if possible, addressed. Veterinary staff can also become involved in order to advise animal care staff and researchers as to the best course of action. Indeed, input from animal care staff and veterinarians, who are impartial to the outcome of research, can be essential to avoid bias where the interests of the researcher may conflict with the welfare of the animals.

The 'welfare assessment toolbox'

There are several different reasons for assessing welfare, and these influence which tool may be right for the job.

Table 6.1 Key references providing information about the natural biology and behaviour of mice and rats (see also the species-specific chapters in this Handbook for information about these and other laboratory animals).

Species	*Relevant publications*
Mouse (*Mus musculus*)	• Latham and Mason (2004) From house mouse to mouse house: the behavioural biology of free-living *Mus musculus* and its implications in the laboratory. *Applied Animal Behaviour Science*, **86**, 261–289 • Olsson *et al.* (2003) Understanding behaviour: the relevance of ethological approaches in animal welfare science. *Applied Animal Behaviour Science*, **81**, 245–264
Rat (*Rattus norvegicus*)	• Burn (2008) What is it like to be a rat? Rat sensory perception and its implications for experimental design and animal welfare. *Applied Animal Behaviour Science*, **112**, 1–32 • Whishaw and Kolb, Eds (2004) *The Behavior of the Laboratory Rat*. Oxford University Press, New York • See also the website http://www.ratlife.org for a demonstration of how laboratory rats retain many 'natural' characteristics despite many generations of captivity

Thus, for example, the method will depend upon factors such as:

1. whether the day-to-day welfare of animals is being monitored;
2. whether welfare in particular environments is to be assessed, or how welfare changes following an environmental manipulation (eg, the provision of a potential environmental enrichment);
3. whether animals' preferences or strength of motivation for particular resources (ie, potential environmental enrichments) are being assessed; or
4. whether welfare (specifically pain) is being monitored following an experimental procedure.

The next sections describe the tools available to those wishing to assess welfare in relation to the conditions in which they might be useful. However, please note that this is only intended as a brief introduction to each of these methods. Many of the welfare assessment techniques described below could fill an entire chapter in themselves (and indeed do in other publications, eg, Appleby & Hughes 1995). Thus, those wishing to use any of the following methods are encouraged to familiarise themselves more fully with the literature about their chosen method(s) – particularly in relation to their subject animal of interest.

Table 6.2 Examples of routine observations of physical appearance (note some of these are specific to certain species).

Body area	*Observations*
Head	Is the head consistently being tilted to one side?
Eyes	Are the eyes sunken or bulging? Are the pupils constricted or dilated? Are there signs of opacity in the eyes? Are there abnormal secretions, crusting or signs of inflammation of the mucous membranes? Are there signs of chromodacryorrhoea[a]?
Nose	Are there abnormal secretions or crusting?
Teeth	Are the teeth overgrown or damaged?
Whiskers	Are there any signs of damage to the whiskers (possibly due to barbering) (Figure 6.1)?
Body	What is the body condition of the animal (eg, emaciated, obese etc)? Are there any obvious lumps? Is the body shape asymmetrical? Are there any wounds from fighting?
Fur	Is the fur dull? Are there signs of piloerection (raised fur)? Is there any hair loss?
Anogenital area	Are there signs of rectal or vaginal prolapse?
Breathing	Is the animal's breathing noisy or laboured?

[a] discussed in detail in Assessing welfare: physical and physiological measures section

Routine welfare monitoring

Physical condition

Monitoring the physical appearance of animals can be a quick and non-invasive method of assessing welfare, and one that can easily be incorporated into routine daily or weekly checks (Leach *et al.* 2008). Examples of some of the parameters that can be assessed are given in Table 6.2.

Physical condition measures such as these are often incorporated into distress scoring systems (see eg, the scoring sheets developed by Morton and Griffiths, originally published in 1985, and reproduced in CRADLA 2008 p. 109–110), body condition scoring assessments (Ullman-Cullere & Foltz 1999; Clingerman & Summers 2005) and guidelines for assessing health and physical condition in laboratory animals (eg, Foltz & Ullman-Cullere 1999). Many of these are general signs of an underlying problem and may not indicate the specific nature of that problem. Thus, animals exhibiting signs of poor physical condition (particularly multiple signs, or physical *and* behavioural signs (see later in this chapter)) should be assessed by a veterinarian. Assessment of such parameters is somewhat more qualitative (and hence can be more susceptible to between-observer variability, see eg, Beynen *et al.* 1987) than some other meas-

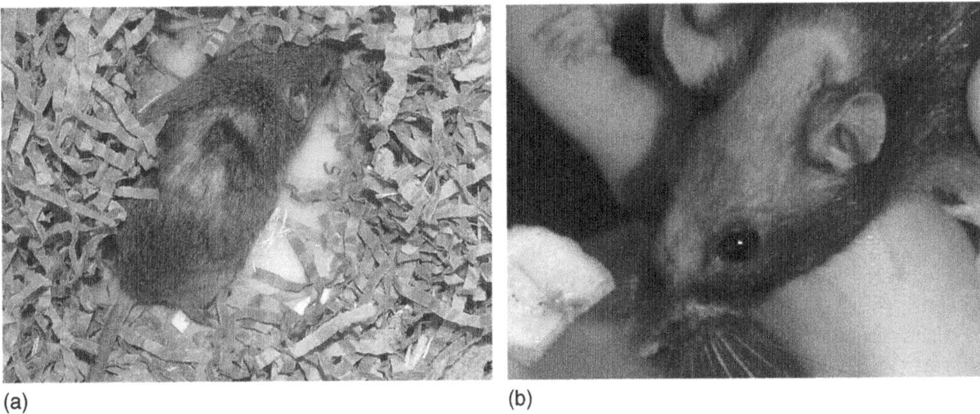

Figure 6.1 (a) A mouse that has been barbered on its head and whiskers and on its back respectively. (b) A rat that has been barbered on its head. (Pictures: N. Latham.)

ures of physical condition, eg, body weight (which will be discussed later on). However, assessment of physical appearance can have benefits over other more quantifiable measures in certain situations. For example, physical appearance can be assessed non-intrusively (ie, the animals can be assessed visually and do not need to be removed from the home cage); and body scoring systems may be useful in cases where weight loss may be counteracted by eg, tumour growth, organ enlargement or fluid accumulation (Ullman-Cullere and Foltz 1999). In certain situations, though, it may be beneficial to supplement visual examinations of an animal's condition with a physical examination. For example, Beynen *et al.* (1987) found that gallstone-bearing mice did not differ in physical appearance from non-gallstone-bearing individuals, but did differ by exhibiting signs of discomfort during abdominal palpitation.

Behaviour

Routine checks of home-cage behaviour can also be used to monitor welfare in laboratory animals (Leach *et al.* 2008) and, like physical parameters, behaviour is often incorporated into distress scoring systems (CRADLA 2008, p. 109–110) and guidelines on assessing health and welfare (Foltz and Ullman-Cullere 1999). Examples of home-cage behaviours that might indicate health and/or welfare problems are given in Table 6.3. (Note that this table deals primarily with those behaviours that might be observed in quick, routine checks on animals – it does not include those behaviours that must be assessed over longer time periods, such as stereotypic behaviour, as these will be addressed later in the chapter.) Observations of home-cage behaviour (eg, the frequency of twitching, writhing and rearing behaviour) can also be useful in assessing pain following experimental procedures (see section on Assessing pain).

Table 6.3 Examples of home cage behaviours that may indicate health and/or welfare problems in laboratory animals.

Inactivity or lethargy
Hyperactivity
Aggression
Abnormal gait
Reduced exploratory behaviour
Reduced use of resources, eg, nesting material and shelters
Social isolation
Hunched posture
Huddling
Ataxia (lack of coordination)
Signs of paresis or paralysis

Cage observations

Evidence of welfare problems may also come, indirectly, from observations of the cage. For example, evidence of unconsumed food or diarrhoea, blood or other secretions around the cage walls or bedding should lead to a closer examination of animals within the cage (and possibly also within neighbouring cages) to check for physical signs that may identify the affected individual(s), eg, matted fur around the anogenital area, signs of dehydration (eg, as assessed by the skin tent test) (Thurman *et al.* 1999). The resources provided within a cage may also stimulate questions about welfare, particularly if resources known to improve welfare are absent (eg, nesting material for mice). These types of measures have been termed *'resource input'* measures of welfare assessment (Leach *et al.* 2008).

Assessing welfare and changes in welfare: physical and physiological measures

Chromodacryorrhoea

Chromodacryorrhoea (also sometimes known as 'red tears' or 'bloody tears') is the name for red staining around the eyes and nose that occurs when the Harderian glands oversecrete porphyrin. This is commonly used as a welfare indicator in rats, with chromodacryorrhoea occurring (or becoming more severe) following 'stressors' such as cage-cleaning, handling or restraint (Harkness & Ridgway 1980; Mason *et al.* 2004; Abou-Ismail *et al.* 2008; Burn *et al.* 2008). Chromodacryorrhoea has also be used (in rats and other species) to assess the effects of certain pharmacological manipulations (Burgen 1949; Harkness & Ridgway 1980; Rupniak & Williams 1994), including the pharmacological induction of acute inflammation (Harper *et al.* 2001). Gender differences have been observed in studies assessing chromodacryorrhoea, but the differences are not consistent (Kerins *et al.* 2003; see also Harkness & Ridgway 1980; Martin *et al.* 1984). Chromodacryorrhoea has a number of advantages over other physiological measures of 'stress'. For example, it can be assessed non-invasively and relatively non-intrusively, and unlike other physiological stress responses (eg, hypothalamic–pituitary–adrenal (HPA) axis activity) it has not yet been reported to be increased by physical activity *per se* or 'excitement' (Burn *et al.* 2006). However, this measure has the disadvantage that it is of limited use in species other than rats (since many other laboratory species do not exhibit chromodacryorrhoea), and it is a product of parasympathetic activity, which is not well understood in terms of welfare.

The onset of chromodacryorrhoea is relatively quick. For example, chromodacryorrhoea has been reported to occur within 10 minutes of handling or 20 minutes of restraint (although onset can vary according to the size of the individual) and ceases after approximately 2h (Harkness and Ridgway 1980; Burn 2005). Since grooming (which can also be elicited by 'stressors') removes evidence of chromodacryorrhoea, observations must be made within the initial time period during which chromodacryorrhoea occurs (Burn *et al.* 2006). Numerical scoring systems are generally used to grade the severity of chromodacryorrhoea; for one example of a scoring system see Figure 6.2.

Body weight

Body weight is commonly used as an indicator of health and/or welfare in research animals. Body weight is often measured repeatedly during a study, in order to allow ongoing assessment of this measure as well as comparison between treatments (Spangenberg *et al.* 2006; Abou-Ismail *et al.* 2008; Simone *et al.* 2008). However, a number of other factors may also influence this measure, including age, activity levels and reproductive cycling (Spangenberg *et al.* 2005; CRADLA 2008, p. 34), as well as tumours and fluid accumulation (as discussed above). Thus assessments of body weight should ideally include comparisons with appropriate (eg, age- and sex-matched) controls. Body weight may also be used as a criterion for humane endpoints in studies, as the rapid loss of a certain percentage of weight can be considered one criterion for euthanasia, eg, 20% in rodents (Ullman-Cullere & Foltz 1999) or 20–25% of body weight in primates (Association of Primate Veterinarians 2008).

HPA axis activity

HPA axis activity culminates in the release of glucocorticoids – usually corticosterone in rodents and cortisol in other animals – from the adrenal cortex. This release of glucocorticoids functions to mobilise energy stores (CRADLA 2008, p. 37), and so HPA axis activity often increases in conditions where an increase in activity may be appropriate. For example, glucocorticoid levels exhibit circadian variation, with peak levels occurring prior to the onset of the active phase (Terlouw *et al.* 1995). Increases in HPA axis activity then additionally occur during flight/fight responses in aversive situations, but they also occur during other heightened states of arousal, including during coitus and hunting prey (Szechtman *et al.* 1974; Rushen 1991; Walker *et al.* 1992; Toates 1995). Thus, although HPA axis

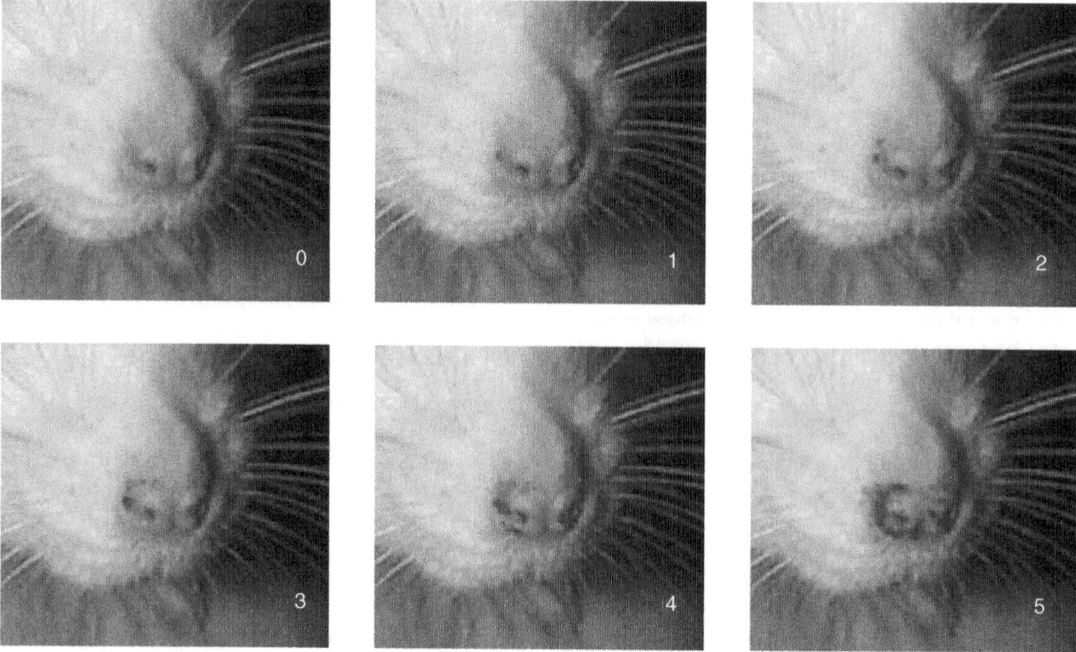

Figure 6.2 Scoring system for assessing severity of chromodacryorrhoea in rats. Note that the pictures are not actual photographs of chromodacryorrhoea of differing severities. The pictures have been digitally altered to illustrate the severity of chromodacryorrhoea required for each of the scoring grades. (Picture: Charlotte Burn.)

activity is commonly referred to as the 'physiological stress response', it is necessary to remember that increases in glucocorticoids are not restricted to aversive situations. Hence measures of HPA axis activation must be interpreted cautiously (and, preferably, in combination with other indices of welfare).

Glucocorticoids, or their metabolites, can be assessed in blood (Vahl *et al.* 2005), saliva (Lutz *et al.* 2000), urine (Touma *et al.* 2003), faeces (Lepschy *et al.* 2007) or even hair samples (Davenport *et al.* 2006), and the timescales differ for each of these sampling methods. Thus, glucocorticoids are released into the blood within a few minutes; they appear in the saliva a few minutes later (Kirschbaum & Hellhammer 2000); their metabolites appear in urine and faeces roughly 1–2 h and 9–10 h later respectively, although this varies according to species, sex, and the time of glucocorticoid release (Touma *et al.* 2003; Lepschy *et al.* 2007); and changes in glucocorticoid levels can be measured in hair samples some weeks later (Davenport *et al.* 2006). Due to the differences involved in sample collection and the timescales over which the responses appear there are pros and cons to each of the sampling techniques listed above, and these are detailed briefly in Table 6.4.

Other 'stress' hormones

Although HPA axis activity is the most commonly assessed hormonal 'stress' response, plasma levels of various other hormones are also sometimes monitored. These include catecholamines, such as adrenaline (epinephrine), prolactin, growth hormone, luteinising hormone and oxytocin (Manteca 1998; Paul *et al.* 2005; CRADLA 2008). Similar *caveats* to those that apply to HPA axis activity also apply to many of these measures in terms of the influence of circadian variation, invasive sampling techniques and the fact that these hormones are also released in response to neutral or even pleasurable stimuli. Indeed, oxytocin release (in contrast to many physiological measures) often occurs during bonding experiences, such as suckling and maternal care, and so tends to be interpreted as indicating positive affective responses (Carter 2001). Hence this may be a potential measure if we consider welfare to be not only about the reduction of negative feelings but the promotion of positive feelings (Paul *et al.* 2005; Boissy *et al.* 2007; Yeates & Main 2008).

Autonomic responses

Autonomic responses, such as heart rate (particularly 'stress-induced' elevations from baseline levels), heart rate variability, blood pressure and respiratory rate, are frequently used to assess welfare in farm animal and equine studies (Boissy *et al.* 2007; von Borell *et al.* 2007). Autonomic responses are also commonly used to monitor physiological functioning in biomedical research and to monitor general activity levels (Irvine *et al.* 1997; Gross *et al.* 2008). However, these measures seem to be less commonly used, at present at least, to assess welfare in research animals (although some examples include Beerda *et al.* 1998; Duke *et al.* 2001; Sharp *et al.* 2002; Arras *et al.* 2007). Autonomic responses may be less commonly used here because monitoring them often requires the use of telemetry devices that: (i) must be surgically implanted into the research subjects; and (ii) are still relatively large and heavy compared to the body size of most research animals (the vast majority of which are mice and rats). Thus, although some researchers report that telemetric

Table 6.4 Pros and cons of the different methods of glucocorticoid analysis.

Sample type	*Pros*	*Cons*
Blood	Allows accurate assessment of acute glucocorticoid responses	Sample collection is invasive Potential risk of sampling procedure influencing sample levels (if sample is not collected quickly enough) Provides information about levels at one moment in time ('point sample'[a]) Vulnerable to circadian variation[b]
Saliva	Allows accurate assessment of acute glucocorticoid responses Non-invasive sampling method	Only non-invasive in species that can be trained to provide samples or that readily chew the collection device Training may be lengthy and not always successful[c] Provides information about levels at one moment in time ('point sample'[a]) Vulnerable to circadian variation[b]
Urine/faeces	Non-invasive sampling method (unless urine is forcibly extracted at a particular time-point) Less vulnerable (but not invulnerable) to circadian variation Provides an assessment of glucocorticoid levels over several hours ('steady state' sample[a])	Assessment of acute responses may require repeated sampling during the time period at which responses typically appear in the urine/faeces
Hair	Non-invasive sampling method Not vulnerable to circadian variation	Provides only a chronic index of glucocorticoid responses

[a] CRADLA (2008)
[b] samples must be collected at the same time of day
[c] Lutz *et al.* (2000)

assessment of autonomic responses provides information about welfare that otherwise may not have been observed (Arras *et al.* 2007), the low popularity of this method may stem from the desire to avoid using a method that requires surgical implantation of a device that may cause discomfort once implanted. Nonetheless, where animals are telemeterised for the purposes of research, there is an opportunity to use the data for assessing welfare.

Assessing welfare and changes in welfare: behavioural measures

Behavioural signs associated with reduced welfare range from gross changes in the home cage behaviour of animals, to subtle (but significant) changes in cognitive testing paradigms. As alluded to earlier, the ability to identify changes, particularly in spontaneous home cage behaviour, that (are likely to) indicate reduced welfare requires an understanding of the species' natural behaviour and the animals' normal behaviour under captive conditions. Thus, researchers assessing behavioural measures of welfare should ensure that they are familiar with both of these aspects of their subject animals' behaviour.

Stereotypic behaviour

Stereotypic behaviours are highly repetitive behaviours caused by frustration or central nervous system dysfunction (Mason 2006). They are also often somewhat invariant, and they can appear to lack function; note that these descriptive characteristics also form the basis for more 'classical' definitions of stereotypic behaviour (Mason 1991). Common examples of stereotypic behaviour in laboratory rodents include bar-biting (Figure 6.3), somersaulting ('back-flipping') and jumping (Würbel 2006), while examples in research primates include pacing, rocking and digit-sucking (Novak *et al.* 2006). There is also an enormous diversity in the prevalence and severity of stereotypic behaviour observed in different laboratory species. For example, stereotypic behaviours have been estimated to develop in approximately 50% of mice in standard laboratory cages, but they appear to be much less common in rats and possibly even absent in guinea pigs (Würbel 2006, p. 88); lower prevalence of stereotypic behaviour has been reported more recently in mice, but behavioural observations were made during the light portion of the light cycle, when mice are typically less active (Leach & Main 2008). However, species differences may be due, in part, to inconsistencies in whether or not comparable behaviours are defined as stereotypic in different studies (see the example of bar-biting in rats cited by Würbel (2006) and discussed later in this section).

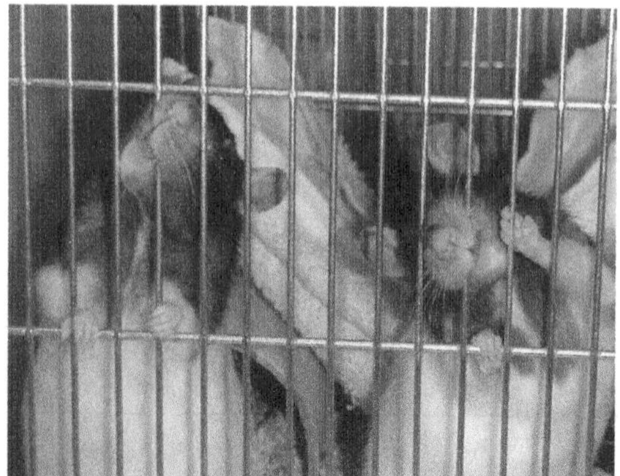

Figure 6.3 Bar-biting in rats. (Picture: Charlotte Burn.)

Stereotypic behaviour is the most commonly used behavioural measure of welfare, but the relationship between stereotypic behaviour and welfare is somewhat complex. The diversity of stereotypic behaviours performed by animals may reflect the diversity of underlying mechanisms that can cause their performance. Some stereotypic behaviours may indeed stem from repeated, frustrated attempts to perform motivated behaviours. Indeed, although stereotypic behaviours often superficially appear to be functionless, a number of studies have elegantly demonstrated the underlying motivation leading to the behaviour. For example, bar-biting in mice stems from attempts to escape from the cage (Nevison *et al.* 1999b) and stereotypic digging in gerbils stems from the desire for a naturalistic burrow (Wiedenmayer 1997). However, in some cases the performance of the stereotypic behaviour itself may be rewarding, acting as a substitute behaviour for motivated behaviours (termed 'DIY enrichments'). In other cases, the stereotypic behaviour may reflect environmentally induced changes in behavioural control processes that cause animals to be unable to inhibit behavioural responses to environmental stimuli ('perseverative' behaviour) (Mason & Latham 2004). Stereotypic behaviours may also, through frequent repetition, become performed out of habit (and shifted into an automatic form of processing known as 'central control'). As a result, different types of stereotypic behaviour (within the same species, and even within individuals) should not necessarily be considered directly comparable in their implications for welfare. Hence, while it is generally accepted that environments that increase stereotypic behaviour are associated with decreased welfare, those individuals exhibiting the most stereotypic behaviour within stereotypy-inducing environments may not have the worst welfare (as assessed by other welfare measures) – perhaps because they have found a stereotypic behaviour that helps them to 'cope' with their poor environment, or because their stereotypic behaviour reflects changes in behavioural control processes (Mason & Latham 2004).

The diversity of stereotypic behaviour, and the question of when the 'normal' performance of a behaviour becomes 'stereotypic' makes scoring the behaviours somewhat complex: and this is one method of welfare assessment that can be greatly enhanced by understanding the subject animals' natural behavioural repertoire (see references in Table 6.1 for information about the natural behaviour of mice and rats). Stereotypic behaviour can be scored from direct observations or video recordings of home-cage behaviour, and is often assessed by scan sampling (observing whether the behaviour occurs *at* specific time intervals, eg, every minute) or one-zero sampling (observing whether the behaviour occurs *during* specific time intervals) (Martin & Bateson 1993). Stereotypic behaviour is often used to compare different environments or treatments (Podberscek *et al.* 1991; Nevison *et al.* 1999a; Latham *et al.* 2008); or to assess the effects of adding environmental enrichments (Lidfors 1997); or even a rebound effect following the removal of enrichments (Bayne *et al.* 1992). However, one of the problems of using stereotypic behaviour is that scoring these behaviours is often somewhat subjective: researchers may make different decisions about when a behaviour is classed as stereotypic. For example, some authors score bar-biting as stereotypic after only 1 s of continuous bar-biting (Garner & Mason 2002), others score it as stereotypic after 10 s (Würbel & Stauffacher 1998). Furthermore, some researchers may not define behaviours as stereotypic if they are perceived as functional, or if they are not perceived as reflecting poor welfare. For example, Hurst *et al.* (1999, cited by Würbel 2006) did not classify bar-biting in rats as a stereotypic behaviour because it was considered to be 'functional' escape-related behaviour, yet bar-biting is commonly accepted as a stereotypic behaviour in mice (Würbel *et al.* 1996; Nevison *et al.* 1999a) even though it has also been shown to stem from escape behaviour (Nevison *et al.* 1999b). See also Mason (2006) and Latham and Würbel (2006) for discussions about whether wheel running, tail-chasing in dogs and the use of dummies (pacifiers) by human babies can or should be considered stereotypic behaviours. Thus, researchers/staff must ensure that they detail fully how they have scored stereotypic behaviour, and be careful about drawing comparisons between studies where stereotypic behaviour has been defined and scored in different ways.

Vocalisations

Vocalisations, including those outside the range audible to humans, have been well studied in research animals for many years, often in relation to reproductive behaviour (rats, McIntosh *et al.* 1984; gerbils, Holman 1980; hamsters, Cherry 1989; deer mice, Pomerantz & Clemens 1981; mice, Warburton *et al.* 1989). However, vocalisations are increasingly also being used as a tool to assess welfare. Much of this research has focused on vocalisations in rats (Brudzynski & Ociepa 1992; Burman *et al.* 2007; Mällo *et al.* 2007; Cloutier & Newberry 2008). However, vocalisations have also been used as a method of welfare assessment in a variety of other species (eg, olive baboons, Crowell Comuzzi 1993; dogs, Gazzano *et al.* 2008; marmosets, Cross & Rogers 2006). Most attention has been paid to vocalisations associated with negative subjective states, such as ultrasonic alarm calls (22 kHz) (Cuomo *et al.* 1992; Litvin *et al.* 2007; Wöhr & Schwarting, in press) or audible vocalisations (Burman *et al.* 2008) in rats. Indeed, questions concerning the welfare of animals within auditory range of conspecifics producing such vocalisations have also been raised (Burman *et al.* 2007). Since welfare researchers are increasingly acknowledging the importance of positive subjective states for good welfare (Boissy *et al.* 2007; Paul *et al.* 2005; Yeates & Main 2008), there is an increasing focus upon vocalisations that indicate positive feelings. The best known and most commonly studied of these is the 50 kHz call in rats – the so-called rat 'laughter', which can be elicited by tickling rats and mimicking play behaviour (Panksepp & Burgdorf 2000, 2003) or which increase during food consumption, mating, electrical self-stimulation of the brain or the use of addictive drugs (Wöhr *et al.* 2008). However, some researchers have recently suggested that experience, context and individual differences can influence 50 kHz calls, and that some caution is required when interpreting these calls with respect to their welfare implications (Wöhr *et al.* 2008).

Anticipatory behaviour

Anticipatory behaviour is the behavioural response that is *'elicited by rewarding stimuli that lead to and facilitate consummatory behaviour'* (Spruijt *et al.* 2001). Anticipatory behaviour is associated with feelings of 'wanting'; this is termed 'incentive salience' and is different to 'liking', which is the hedonic pleasure associated with consummatory behaviour (Berridge & Robinson 1998). Anticipatory behaviour has mainly been investigated in rats using classical Pavlovian training tasks, whereby a 'reward' (such as a sugary food, the opportunity to mate or interact with others) is announced by a 'conditioned stimulus', eg the sound of a bell. The amount of active behaviour performed by the animal(s) is then scored during the intervening period between the animal hearing the bell and the presentation of the reward (Van den Berg *et al.* 1999, 2000; Von Frijtag *et al.* 2000, 2001). This activity score is then compared with that of control animals that heard the bell but did not receive the reward. However, anticipatory activity is not expressed in the same way in different species. For example, rats exhibit an increase in anticipatory activity in the period between the conditioned stimulus and the arrival of the reward, while domestic cats exhibit a decrease in the number of behavioural transitions during this time. It has been suggested that this may reflect species differences in food-acquisition behaviour: for example, rats actively explore for food while cats often employ a 'sit-and-wait' strategy when close to prey (Van den Bos *et al.* 2003). Anticipatory behaviour can be used to assess sensitivity (incentive salience) to different types of rewarding stimuli (Van Der Harst *et al.* 2003b, 2005), or to assess (poor) housing-induced sensitisation of the mesolimbic dopaminergic system (Van Der Harst *et al.* 2003a).

Cognitive bias

Tasks assessing cognitive bias are one of the newest tools in the welfare assessor's toolbox. This method of animal welfare assessment was proposed by Mendl, Paul and colleagues (Mendl & Paul 2004; Harding *et al.* 2004; Paul *et al.* 2005), and is based on the wealth of evidence from the human literature that people who report negative feelings tend to make negative judgements about ambiguous stimuli or anticipated events, while those reporting positive feelings tend to make more optimistic judgements (Paul *et al.* 2005). In humans, cognitive biases are typically investigated using linguistic tasks (Mathews *et al.* 1989; Eysenck *et al.* 1991): for example, Mathews *et al.* (1989) found that clinically anxious subjects are more likely to interpret ambiguous words or phrases in a threatening sense (eg, die vs dye) than normal controls. Recently, these tasks have been modified for use in animals. Thus, Harding *et al.* (2004) trained rats to perform a lever press to one auditory stimulus (a tone) in order to receive a food reward and to refrain from pressing the lever following a different tone in order to avoid 30 s of loud white noise. The rats were then housed in different types of housing and subsequently tested with the training tones and three intermediate (ambiguous) tones. Harding and colleagues found that rats housed in 'unpredictable' housing made fewer and slower responses to the tone associated with food and the ambiguous tones that were closer to it – findings that are comparable with those in anxious or depressed humans. Similar techniques and results indicating 'pessimistic' and 'optimistic' behaviour have subsequently been published in further studies on rats and in European starlings (Bateson & Matheson 2007; Matheson *et al.* 2008; Burman *et al.* in press). Given the increased emphasis on positive subjective feelings in welfare research (Boissy *et al.* 2007; Yeates & Main 2008), tasks which enable us to assess positive feelings (such as optimism) are thus an important addition to the welfare assessment toolbox.

Assessing welfare and changes in welfare: brain measures

The processes that lead to affective states and the physiological and behavioural indicators of welfare that we assess are regulated by the brain. Thus, affective states are elicited by neural processing (eg, in the amygdala and limbic regions) of the rewarding and punishing properties of sensory stimuli (Rolls 1999; Panksepp 2003). Stimuli then elicit physiological responses by additional processing through regions including the hypothalamus, pituitary and brainstem; and behavioural responses by additional processing through the basal ganglia, ventral tegmental area, motor cortical areas and cerebellum (Sapolsky 1992; Toates 2004). Thus, welfare can be assessed by monitoring activity or changes in these regions: for example, by assessing glucocorticoid activity or receptor levels or neurotransmitter functioning (eg, dopaminergic functioning) (Broom & Zanella 2004). Indeed, a number of aspects of brain functioning have been correlated with physiological or behavioural indicators of welfare: for example, numerous studies have found a correlation between aspects of dopaminergic functioning (particularly dopamine receptor levels) and stereotypic behaviour (McBride & Hemmings 2005; Lewis *et al.* 2006). One disadvantage of assessing brain function is that it can be invasive, such as requiring surgical electrode implants or requiring *post-mortem* brain analysis, and in some cases the most humane killing methods cannot be used because they disrupt the brain regions of interest. However, technological advances mean that, with the right equipment, eg, functional magnetic resonance imaging (fMRI) or positron emission tomography (PET), it may be possible to assess brain activity during pleasant or unpleasant experiences non-invasively, although such methods are generally currently limited to the assessment of human emotional states (Phan *et al.* 2004).

Assessing animals' preferences and motivation for resources

In addition to assessing welfare itself, the welfare researchers' toolbox also includes tools for identifying potential methods of improving welfare. Thus, we can assess animals' preferences and motivation for resources by asking animals to 'vote with their feet' and tell us how they feel about their environment and choices that we offer them (Dawkins 1980; Kirkden & Pajor 2006). This is often used as a way of identifying potential refinements to laboratory housing (eg, environmental enrichments), and the two most commonly used methods (and hence those that will be discussed here) are preference tests and consumer demand studies. However, while these tools enable us to identify potential refinements, the long-term effects of these refinements should then be double-checked using the tools described in previous sections. This additional assessment is necessary because, for example, defendable resources may elicit undesirable behaviours such as territorial behaviour in group-housed animals; and animals (like humans) do not always make choices or behave in ways that maximise their long-term welfare (Silverman 1978; Rutherford 2002).

Preference tests

Preference tests (as their name implies) investigate the preference of animals for particular resources when given a choice, and they have been a popular tool in welfare research for many years (Fraser & Matthews 1995). Preference tests can be used to assess animals' preferences for different environmental characteristics such as: cage height and light intensity (Blom *et al.* 1992, 1995); different substrates (Van de Weerd *et al.* 1996); nesting material vs nest boxes (Van de Weerd *et al.* 1998); climbing structure orientation, eg, with marmosets (Pines *et al.* 2005); and social contact (Held *et al.* 1995). Preference for the resources is usually measured by time spent with (using) the resources (whereby most time = most preferred). However, there are a number of criticisms that have been levelled at preference tests and *caveats* that should be borne in mind when using them. These have been addressed in detail in a number of places (Duncan 1978; Fraser & Matthews 1995; Bateson 2004; Kirkden & Pajor 2006), so the main criticisms detailed in these other reviews will only be briefly discussed here. The first of these is that preference tests only tell you about the relative preference for different resources, not the absolute strength of motivation for any of the resources. Thus, a preferred resource may only be weakly more reinforcing – eg, a preference for strawberries over blackberries – or alternatively it may be much more reinforcing – eg, copulatory rather than exploratory behaviour.

Secondly, short-term and long-term welfare are not necessarily always compatible. Hence animals may exhibit preferences for resources that maximise their immediate welfare, but may adversely affect their longer-term welfare. For example, certain strains of rodents have long been used as models in studies of alcohol abuse (Green & Grahame 2008). A further interesting example is provided by Silverman (1978), who describes an inhalation toxicity study in which various rodent species were exposed to cigarette smoke. During the initial stages of the study a number of rats, mice and hamsters quickly developed a behaviour whereby they blocked the inlet tube with their faeces: thus apparently demonstrating an aversion to the cigarette smoke. However, later in the study some of the mice developed an apparent attraction to the cigarette smoke, persistently jamming their noses as far into the inlet pipe as possible.

Thirdly, behaviour in preference tests may be confounded by differential use of the resources, for example due to time of day effects (Van de Weerd *et al.* 1998), or strong but periodic motivation to use resources that provide opportunities for motivated behaviours (such as an enhanced motivation for nesting material in pre-parturient animals, or access to a potential mate when females are in oestrus). Fourthly, preferences can be influenced by the prior experience of the animals. Thus, for example, animals that are used to living in cages may initially show a preference for cages rather than an outdoor pen, a preference that may then change following exposure to the outdoor pens (eg, hens, Dawkins 1980; for some other interesting examples see, Fraser & Matthews 1995).

Finally, preference tests are designed to test preference between two substitutable resources (ie, two resources that satisfy the same motivation). Kirkden and Pajor (2006; see also Fraser & Matthews 1995) suggest that a preference test between non-substitutes (eg, food vs litter) would have little meaning from the animals' point of view since the comparison would not be between the resources but between the strengths of the different motivations. Thus, preference tests can provide useful information about environmental features that may enhance animals' welfare. However, preference tests must be carefully designed so that the link between an animal's preferences and their welfare is valid and reliable.

Consumer demand

Consumer demand tasks were introduced into animal welfare research in the 1980s, and they are based on ideas traditionally used by economists studying the spending patterns of humans faced with a choice of products and limited income (Dawkins 1983). The basic premise behind consumer demand tasks is that there is an inverse relationship between the price of a resource and the amount that a consumer will buy. By increasing the price of the resource the researcher can then quantify the value that the consumer places on the resource, measuring one or more of the following: (1) the top price that the consumer is willing to pay ('reservation price'); (2) the total amount of income spent on the resource ('consumer surplus'); and (3) the willingness of the consumer to keep on paying for the resource as the price increases ('elasticity of demand') (Varian 1993; Gwartney *et al.* 2005 pp. 56–82). The advantages and limitations of these methods in animal welfare research are addressed in detail by Kirkden and Pajor (2006; see also Jensen *et al.* 2004).

Consumer demand studies have an advantage over preference tests in that they can tell us about the strength of motivation for different resources; we can even determine the absolute strength of this motivation if we 'titrate' it against motivation for essential resources, such as food (termed *'yardstick'* resources, Dawkins 1983; see also Warburton & Mason 2003). In animal welfare studies, consumer demand tasks require animals to 'pay' to gain access to resources, either by performing an operant task (eg, lever pressing – termed fixed ratio (FR) schedules) (eg, Sherwin 2004b, 2007), or by increasing the effort required to acquire the resource (eg, pushing weighted doors or traversing water) (Sherwin & Nicol 1995, 1996; Seaman *et al.* 2008). Consumer demand tasks can thus be used to assess (quantitatively) motivation for different environmental characteristics in laboratory animals (Manser *et al.* 1996; Sherwin 1998; Seaman *et al.* 2008) and, indeed, farmed animals, where consumer demand techniques are probably even more extensively utilised (Gunnarsson *et al.* 2000; Mason *et al.* 2001; Jensen *et al.* 2004).

However, like preference tests, there is a number of factors that must be borne in mind when designing consumer demand tasks; these are also reviewed in more detail by Kirkden and Pajor (2006). For example, motivation for some resources may be influenced by whether or not the resource can be seen (ie, for some resources *'out of sight = out of mind'*) (Warburton & Mason 2003), and where the cost of accessing the resource must be *'paid'*, eg, whether the cost is paid on entry or exit from the resource (Warburton & Nicol 1998). Furthermore, many consumer demand tasks use animals that are individually housed, yet individual housing may affect motivation for resources (Sherwin 2003; Cooper 2004); see also the Anticipatory Behaviour section). Thus, finding methods of assessing motivation in group-housed animals (Sherwin 2004b, 2007) may be more complex, but ultimately more appropriate where animals are typically group housed (as most laboratory animals are).

Assessing pain

Animals' experience of pain has been the centre of as much debate as animals' experience of affective states ('emotions') such as pleasure or suffering. Pain in humans is defined as *'an unpleasant sensory and emotional experience associated with actual or potential tissue damage, or described in terms of such damage'* (International Association for the Study of Pain (IASP) 1979). However, this definition relies on verbal self-report and hence is not suitable for defining pain in animals (or indeed small children or mentally handicapped humans) (Rutherford 2002). Thus, a number of other definitions of animal pain have been proposed: for example, Rutherford (2002) cites a definition by Zimmerman that *'pain in animals is an aversive sensory experience caused by actual or potential injury that elicits protective motor and vegetative reactions, results in learned avoidance behaviour, and may modify species specific behaviour, including social behaviour.'* The relatively recent nature of this debate is perhaps not surprising given that it was less than 150 years ago that it was still commonly felt that people of some races, the poor and the uneducated were insensitive to pain: indeed, even within the last decade there has been discussion about whether very young human children experience pain (Weary *et al.* 2006). However, despite the debate about whether animals consciously experience pain, it is generally accepted that mammals and birds at least do have the underlying physiological and neurological structures necessary to experience pain, and exhibit physiological and behavioural responses comparable to human responses (Rutherford 2002).

As in general welfare assessment, the ability to assess pain is greatly enhanced by understanding animals' normal appearance and behaviour and species-typical pain responses (Flecknell & Molony 1997; American College of Laboratory Animal Medicine (ACLAM) 2007). Indeed, additional training in pain assessment techniques (particularly using visual examples of pain-related behaviour) may help researchers to identify and score pain more accurately and reliably (Flecknell & Roughan 2004); see Roughan and Flecknell (2006) for an example of a researcher training system. Like welfare, pain is often assessed by monitoring general measures of body functioning, such as changes in body weight, reduced feeding and drinking (Weary *et al.* 2006), physiological responses, including HPA axis activity (Wright-Williams *et al.* 2007) and behaviour, including pain-related behaviour and vocalisations (Cooper & Vierck 1986; Jourdan *et al.* 1998); see also ACLAM (2007) and Table 6.5.

In addition to the general observations in Table 6.5, pain assessment can measure the prevalence and severity of specific pain-related behaviours. Pain-related behaviour in laboratory animals has probably been most studied in rats, and four behaviours have been identified as likely reliable indicators of pain in rats: cat-like back arching, horizontal stretching followed by abdominal writhing, and twitching while inactive (Roughan & Flecknell 2001); the nature of the primary pain-related behaviour may, however, depend upon the nature and location of the pain (Flecknell and Roughan 2004). Four similar behaviours have also been identified as likely pain indicators in mice: flinching, writhing, rear leg lift and pressing the abdomen to the floor (Wright-Williams *et al.* 2007). These behaviours can be scored from direct observations or video recordings of animals in their home cages (or recovery cages), but observing and scoring these behaviours can be very time-consuming, and thus may not be practical in all situations (Flecknell and Roughan 2004). However, technological advances mean that such behaviours can now be scored in a fraction of the time by shape recognition software packages, such as HomeCageSys software (M. Leach, presentation at the inaugural symposium of the CIMPP, Sept 2007).

Concluding remarks

Animal welfare, like human welfare, is generally accepted to be about subjective feelings, such as pleasure and suffering. Despite ongoing debate about whether or not laboratory animals are capable of consciously experiencing subjective feelings, laboratory animal welfare is widely considered important, not only for ethical reasons but increasingly also because of its potential impact on scientific validity. Although animals cannot be asked about their feelings directly, there is a broad (and increasing) range of tools available which can be used to provide an indirect indication of animals' subjective states. Many of these tools have been described in this chapter. The diversity of tools in the welfare assessor's toolbox means that different methods are available for the different types of welfare assessment that might be necessary during the course of a research animal's life. Thus, the physical appearance and home-cage behaviour of animals can be used to monitor their welfare on a day-to-day basis; while longer-term or treatment effects on welfare can be assessed by measuring physiological responses (eg, HPA axis activity – the physiological 'stress response'), home-cage behaviour (eg, stereotypic behaviour), vocalisations and performance in behavioural paradigms that reveal sensitivity to rewarding stimuli and cognitive states, such as optimism.

Tools are also available (tasks designed to assess preference and motivation for resources) that enable potential refinements to laboratory housing to be identified – techniques that are regularly used in the growing field of refinement research. When used, and appropriately analysed, these techniques can help the identification and assessment of animals' negative and positive subjective states, and find techniques of refining housing and husbandry practices and experimental procedures that make a genuine and meaningful difference to the welfare of research animals. Thus, for example, such research has shown that laboratory mice prefer environments that contain nesting material and indeed will work to get nesting material (Roper 1975; Van de Weerd *et al.* 1998), and that providing nesting material can help to reduce behavioural problems such as aggression (Van Loo *et al.* 2002). Hence, the provision of nesting material is now widely recommended for laboratory mice (Jennings *et al.* 1998), and its presence in mouse cages is used as a 'resource input' measure of welfare by animal care staff and researchers (Leach *et al.* 2008).

Finally, for many years (even dating back to the thoughts of Jeremy Bentham) questions about welfare have focused upon animal suffering. Therefore, it is encouraging that the

Table 6.5 Observations for the clinical assessment of pain in mice, rats and rabbits (information from ACLAM 2007).

<table>
<tr><th>Mice</th><th>Rats</th><th>Rabbits</th></tr>
<tr><td colspan="3">• Squint-eyes
• Pale eyes (if albino)
• Reduced grooming
• Reduced level of spontaneous activity[a]
• Reduced food/water intake</td></tr>
<tr><td colspan="2">• Piloerection
• Increased aggressiveness when handled</td><td>• Changed posture, tucking of abdomen, tensing of muscles</td></tr>
<tr><td>• Hunched posture
• Distance themselves from cage mate</td><td>• Chromodacryorrhoea</td><td>• Guarding, attempt to hide, or aggressiveness
• Grinding of teeth</td></tr>
</table>

[a]citing Karas *et al.* 2001 and Goecke *et al.* 2005

increased interest in finding tools that enable us to assess positive subjective states reflects the increasing emphasis on the importance of ensuring that research animals not only do not suffer any more than is necessary, but that they experience positive subjective states, such as pleasure, and hence actually have good (and not just the absence of poor) welfare.

Acknowledgements

I would like to thank Charlotte Burn for the use of her pictures and chromodacryorrhoea scoring system, and Janet Rogers and Manuel Berdoy for helpful discussions about welfare assessment during the production of this chapter. I would also like to thank the two reviewers, whose constructive comments have helped to improve this review.

References

Abou-Ismail, U., Burman, O., Nicol, C. *et al.* (2008) Let sleeping rats lie: Does the timing of husbandry procedures affect laboratory rat behaviour, physiology and welfare? *Applied Animal Behaviour Science*, **111**, 329–341

American College of Laboratory Animal Medicine (2007) Guidelines for the assessment and management of pain in rodents and rabbits. *Journal for the American Association of Laboratory Animal Science*, **46**, 97–108

Animals (Scientific Procedures) Act (1986) Available online at: http://scienceandresearch.homeoffice.gov.uk/animal-research/legislation/

Appleby, M. and Hughes, B. (1995) *Animal Welfare*. CABI, Wallingford

Arras, M., Rettich, A., Cinelli, P. *et al.* (2007) Assessment of post-laparotomy pain in laboratory mice by telemetric recording of heart rate and heart rate variability. *BMC Veterinary Research*, **3**, 16

Association of Primate Veterinarians (2008) *APV position statement on humane endpoints of nonhuman primates in research*. Available online at: http://www.primatevets.org/Files/NHP_Endpoint_Guidelines-Final.doc

Bateson, M. (2004) Mechanisms of decision-making and the interpretation of choice tests. *Animal Welfare*, **13**, S115–120

Bateson, M. and Matheson, S. (2007) Performance on categorisation tasks suggests that removal of environmental enrichment induces 'pessimism' in captive European starlings (*Sturnus vulgaris*). *Animal Welfare*, **16**(S), 33–36

Bayne, K., Hurst, J. and Dexter, S. (1992) Evaluation of the preference to and behavioral effects of an enriched environment on male rhesus monkeys. *Laboratory Animal Science*, **42**, 38–45

Beerda, B., Schilder, M., van Hooff, J. *et al.* (1998) Behavioural, saliva cortisol and heart rate responses to different types of stimuli in dogs. *Applied Animal Behaviour Science*, **58**, 365–381

Bekoff, M. (2007) Do animals have emotions? *New Scientist*, **2605**, 42–47

Bentham, J. (1789) *Introduction to the Principles of Morals and Legislation*. Clarendon Press, Oxford

Berridge, K. and Robinson, T. (1998) What is the role of dopamine in reward: hedonic impact, reward learning or incentive salience? *Brain Research Reviews*, **28**, 309–369

Beynen, A., Baumans, V., Bertens, P. *et al.* (1987) Assessment of discomfort in gallstone-bearing mice: a practical example of the problems encountered in an attempt to recognize discomfort in laboratory animals. *Laboratory Animals*, **21**, 35–42

Blom, H., Van Vorstenbosch, C., Baumans, V. *et al.* (1992) Description and validation of a preference test system to evaluate housing conditions for laboratory mice. *Applied Animal Behaviour Science*, **35**, 67–82

Blom, H., Van Tintelen, G., Baumans, V. *et al.* (1995) Development and application of a preference test system to evaluate housing conditions for laboratory rats. *Applied Animal Behaviour Science*, **43**, 279–290

Boissy, A., Manteuffel, G., Jensen, M., *et al.* (2007) Assessment of positive emotions in animals to improve their welfare. *Physiology and Behavior*, **92**, 375–397

Broom, D. and Zanella, A. (2004) Brain measures which tell us about animal welfare. *Animal Welfare*, **13**, S41–45

Brudzynski, S. and Ociepa, D. (1992) Ultrasonic vocalization of laboratory rats in response to handling and touch. *Physiology and Behavior*, **52**, 655–660

Burgdorf, J. and Panksepp, J. (2006) The neurobiology of positive emotions. *Neuroscience and Biobehavioral Reviews*, **30**, 173–187

Burgen, A. (1949) The assay of anticholinesterase drugs by the chromodacryorrhoea response in rats. *British Journal of Pharmacology*, **4**, 185–189

Burman, O., Ilyat, A., Jones, G. *et al.* (2007) Ultrasonic vocalizations as indicators of welfare for laboratory rats (*Rattus norvegicus*). *Applied Animal Behaviour Science*, **104**, 116–129

Burman, O., Owen, D., Abou-Ismail, U. *et al.* (2008) Removing individual rats affects indicators of welfare in the remaining group members. *Physiology and Behavior*, **93**, 89–96

Burman, O., Parker, R., Paul, E. *et al.* (in press) A spatial judgement task to determine background emotional state in laboratory rats, *Rattus norvegicus*. *Animal Behaviour*

Burn, C. (2005) Effects of husbandry and the laboratory environment on rat welfare. In: *Zoology*. University of Oxford, Oxford

Burn, C. (2008) What is it like to be a rat? Rat sensory perception and its implications for experimental design and rat welfare. *Applied Animal Behaviour Science*, **112**, 1–32

Burn, C., Deacon, R. and Mason, G. (2008) Marked for life? Effects of early cage cleaning frequency, delivery batch and identification tail-marking on adult rat anxiety profiles. *Developmental Psychobiology*, **50**, 266–277

Burn, C., Peters, A. and Mason, G. (2006) Acute effects of cage-cleaning at different frequencies on laboratory rat behaviour and welfare. *Animal Welfare*, **15**, 161–172

Cabib, S. (2006) The neurophysiology of stereotypies II: The role of stress. In: *Stereotypic Behaviour: Fundamentals and Applications to Welfare*. Ed. Mason, G., pp. 227–255. CAB International, Wallingford

Carter, C. (2001) Is there a neurobiology of good welfare? In: *Coping with Challenge. Welfare in Animals Including Humans*. Ed. Broom, D., pp. 11–30. Dahlem University Press, Berlin

Cherry, J. (1989) Ultrasonic vocalizations by male hamsters: parameters of calling and effects of playbacks on female behaviour. *Animal Behaviour*, **38**, 138–153

Christiansen, S. and Forkman, B. (2007) Assessment of animal welfare in a veterinary context – a call for ethologists. *Applied Animal Behaviour Science*, **106**, 203–220

Clingerman, K. and Summers, L. (2005) Development of a body scoring system for nonhuman primates using *Macaca mulatta* as a model. *Laboratory Animal*, **34**, 31–36

Cloutier, S. and Newberry, R. (2008) Use of a conditioning technique to reduce stress associated with repeated intra-peritoneal injections in laboratory rats. *Applied Animal Behaviour Science*, **112**, 158–173

Cooper, B. and Vierck, C. (1986) Vocalizations as measures of pain in monkeys. *Pain*, **26**, 393–407

Cooper, J. (2004) Consumer demand under commercial husbandry conditions: practical advice on measuring behavioural priorities in captive animals. *Animal Welfare*, **13**, S47–56

Crabbe, J. (1999) Genetics of mouse behavior: interactions with laboratory environment. *Science*, **284**, 1670–1672

Committee on Recognition and Alleviation of Distress in Laboratory Animals (2008) *Recognition and Alleviation of Distress in Laboratory Animals*. National Academies Press, Washington

Cross, N. and Rogers, L. (2006) Mobbing vocalizations as a coping response in the common marmoset. *Hormones and Behavior*, **49**, 237–245

Crowell Comuzzi, D. (1993) Baboon vocalizations as measures of psychological well-being. *Laboratory Primate Newsletter*, **21**, 5–6

Cuomo, V., Cagiano, R., De Salvia, M. *et al.* (1992) Ultrasonic vocalization as an indicator of emotional state during active avoidance learning in rats. *Life Sciences*, **50**, 1049–1055

Davenport, M., Tiefenbacher, S., Lutz, C. *et al.* (2006) Analysis of endogenous cortisol concentrations in the hair of rhesus macaques. *General and Comparative Endocrinology*, **147**, 255–261

Dawkins, M. (1980) *Animal Suffering: The Science of Animal Welfare*. Chapman and Hall, London

Dawkins, M. (1983) Battery hens name their price: consumer demand theory and the measurement of ethological needs. *Animal Behaviour*, **31**, 1195–1205

Dawkins, M. (1988) Behavioural deprivation: a central problem in animal welfare. *Applied Animal Behaviour Science*, **20**, 209–225

Dawkins, M. (1993) *Through our Eyes Only? The Search for Animal Consciousness*. Spektrum/Freeman, Oxford

Dawkins, M. (2004) Using behaviour to assess animal welfare. *Animal Welfare*, **13**, S3–7

Dawkins, M. (2006) A user's guide to animal welfare science. *Trends in Ecology and Evolution*, **21**, 77–82

Duke, J., Zammit, T. and Lawson, D. (2001) The effects of routine cage-cleaning on cardiovascular and behavioral parameters in male Sprague-Dawley rats. *Contemporary Topics in Laboratory Animal Science*, **40**, 17–20

Duncan, I. (1978) The interpretation of preference tests in animal behaviour. *Applied Animal Ethology*, **4**, 197–200

Duncan, I. (1993) Welfare is to do with what animals feel. *Journal of Agricultural and Environmental Ethics*, **6**, 8–14

Duncan, I. and Fraser, D. (1997) Understanding animal welfare. In: *Animal Welfare*. Eds Appleby, M. and Hughes, B., pp. 19–31. CAB International, Wallingford

Eysenck, M., Mogg, K., May, J. *et al.* (1991) Bias in interpretation of ambiguous sentences related to threat and anxiety. *Journal of Abnormal Psychology*, **100**, 144–150

Festing, S. and Wilkinson, R. (2007) The ethics of animal research. Talking Point on the use of animals in scientific research. *EMBO Reports*, **8**, 526–530

Flecknell, P. and Molony, V. (1997) Pain and injury. In: *Animal Welfare*. Eds Appleby, M. and Hughes, B., pp. 63–73. CAB International, Wallingford

Flecknell, P. and Roughan, J. (2004) Assessing pain in animals – putting research into practice. *Animal Welfare*, **13**, S71–76

Foltz, C. and Ullman-Cullere, M. (1999) Guidelines for assessing the health and condition of mice. *Laboratory Animal*, **28**, 28–32

Fraser, D. and Matthews, L. (1995) Preference and motivation testing. In: *Animal Welfare*. Eds Appleby, M. and Hughes, B., pp. 159–174. CAB International, Wallingford

Garner, J. (2006) Perseveration and stereotypy – systems-level insights from clinical psychology. In: *Stereotypic Animal Behaviour: Fundamentals and Applications to Welfare*. Eds Rushen, J. and Mason, G., pp. 121–152. CAB International, Wallingford

Garner, J. and Mason, G. (2002) Evidence for a relationship between cage stereotypies and behavioural disinhibition in laboratory rodents. *Behavioural Brain Research*, **136**, 83–92

Gazzano, A., Mariti, C., Notari, L. *et al.* (2008) Effects of early gentling and early environment on emotional development of puppies. *Applied Animal Behaviour Science*, **110**, 294–304

Goecke, J., Awad, H., Lawson, J. *et al.* (2005) Evaluating postoperative analgesics in mice using telemetry. *Comparative Medicine*, **55**, 37–44

Green, A.S. and Grahame, N.J. (2008) Ethanol drinking in rodents: is free-choice related to the reinforcing effects of ethanol? *Alcohol*, **42**, 1–11

Gross, V., Tank, J., Partke, H.-J. *et al.* (2008) Cardiovascular autonomic regulation in non-obese diabetic (NOD) mice. *Autonomic Neuroscience: Basic and Clinical*, **138**, 108–113

Gunnarsson, S., Matthews, L., Foster, T. *et al.* (2000) The demand for straw and feathers as litter substrates by laying hens. *Applied Animal Behaviour Science*, **65**, 321–330

Gwartney, J., Stroup, R., Sobel, R. and Macpherson, D. (2005) *Economics. Private and Public Choice*. Thomson South-Western, Mason

Harding, E., Paul, E. and Mendl, M. (2004) Animal behaviour – cognitive bias and affective state. *Nature*, **427**, 312

Harkness, J. and Ridgway, M. (1980) Chromodacryorrhea in laboratory rats (*Rattus norvegicus*): etiologic considerations. *Laboratory Animal Science*, **30**, 841–844

Harper, R., Kerins, C., McIntosh, J. *et al.* (2001) Modulation of the inflammatory response in the rat TMJ with increasing doses of complete Freund's adjuvant. *Osteoarthritis and Cartilage*, **9**, 619–624

Held, S., Turner, R. and Wootton, R. (1995) Choices of laboratory rabbits for individual or group-housing. *Applied Animal Behaviour Science*, **46**, 81–91

Holman, S. (1980) Sexually dimorphic, ultrasonic vocalizations of Mongolian gerbils. *Behavioral and Neural Biology*, **28**, 183–192

Home Office (1989) *Code of practice for the housing and care of animals used in scientific procedures*. Available online at: http://www.homeoffice.gov.uk/docs/hcasp3.html

International Association for the Study of Pain (1979) Pain terms: a list with definitions and notes on usage. *Pain*, **6**, 249–252

Irvine, R., White, J. and Chan, R. (1997) The influence of restraint on blood pressure in the rat. *Journal of Pharmacological and Toxicological Methods*, **38**, 157–162

Jennings, M., Batchelor, G., Brain, P. *et al.* (1998) Refining rodent husbandry: the mouse. *Laboratory Animals*, **32**, 233–259

Jensen, M., Pedersen, L. and Ladewig, J. (2004) The use of demand functions to assess behavioural priorities in farm animals. *Animal Welfare*, **13**, S27–32

Jourdan, D., Ardid, D., Chapuy, E. *et al.* (1998) Effect of analgesics on audible and ultrasonic pain-induced vocalisation in the rat. *Life Sciences*, **63**, 1761–1768

Karas, A., Gostyla, K., Aronovitz, M. *et al.* (2001) Diminished body weight and activity patterns in mice following surgery: implications for control of post procedural pain/distress in laboratory animals. *Contemporary Topics in Laboratory Animal Science*, **40**, 83–87

Kerins, C., Carlson, D., McIntosh, J. *et al.* (2003) Meal pattern changes associated with temporomandibular joing inflammation pain in rats: analgesic effects. *Pharmacology Biochemistry and Behavior*, **75**, 181–189

Kirkden, R. and Pajor, E. (2006) Using preference, motivation and aversion tests to ask scientific questions about animals' feelings. *Applied Animal Behaviour Science*, **100**, 29–47

Kirschbaum, C. and Hellhammer, D. (2000) Salivary cortisol. In: *Encyclopedia of Stress*. Ed. Fink, G., pp. 379–383. Academic Press, Boston

Latham, N. and Mason, G. (2004) From house mouse to mouse house: the behavioural biology of free-living *Mus musculus* and its implications in the laboratory. *Applied Animal Behaviour Science*, **86**, 261–289

Latham, N., Mason, G. and Dawkins, M. (2008) Can we improve the welfare of laboratory cages by cleaning their cages less frequently? *Laboratory Animal*, **37**, 216–217

Latham, N. and Würbel, H. (2006) Wheel running: a common rodent stereotypy? In: *Stereotypic Animal Behaviour: Fundamentals and Applications to Welfare*, (eds G. Mason and J. Rushen). CAB International, Wallingford

Leach, M. and Main, D. (2008) An assessment of laboratory mouse welfare in UK animal units. *Animal Welfare*, **17**, 171–187

Leach, M., Thornton, P. and Main, D. (2008) Identification of appropriate measures for the assessment of laboratory mouse welfare. *Animal Welfare*, **17**, 161–170

Lepschy, M., Touma, C., Hruby, R. *et al.* (2007) Non-invasive measurement of adrenocortical activity in male and female rats. *Laboratory Animals*, **41**, 372–387

Lewis, M., Presti, M., Lewis, J. *et al.* (2006) The Neurobiology of Stereotypy 1: Environmental Complexity. In: *Stereotypic Animal Behaviour: Fundamentals and Applications to Welfare*. Eds Rushen, J. and Mason, G., pp. 190–226. CAB International, Wallingford

Lidfors, L. (1997) Behavioural effects of environmental enrichment for individually caged rabbits. *Applied Animal Behaviour Science*, **52**, 157–169

Litvin, Y., Blanchard, D. and Blanchard, R. (2007) Rat 22 kHz ultrasonic vocalizations as alarm cries. *Behavioural Brain Research*, **182**, 166–172

Lutz, C., Tiefenbacher, S., Jorgensen, M. *et al.* (2000) Techniques for collecting saliva from awake, unrestrained, adult monkeys for cortisol assay. *American Journal of Primatology*, **52**, 93–99

MacPhail, E. (1998) *The Evolution of Consciousness*. Oxford University Press, Oxford

Mällo, T., Matrov, D., Herm, L. *et al.* (2007) Tickling-induced 50 kHz ultrasonic vocalization is individually stable and predicts behaviour in tests of anxiety and depression in rats. *Behavioural Brain Research*, **184**, 57–71

Mangiarini, L., Sathasivam, K., Seller, M. *et al.* (1996) Exon 1 of the *HD* Gene with an expanded CAG repeat is sufficient to cause a progressive neurological phenotype in transgenic mice. *Cell*, **87**, 493–506

Manser, C., Elliott, H., Morris, T. *et al.* (1996) The use of a novel operant test to determine the strength of preference for flooring in laboratory rats. *Laboratory Animals*, **30**, 1–6

Manteca, X. (1998) Neurophysiology and assessment of welfare. *Meat Science*, **49**, S205–218

Martin, J., Driscoll, P. and Gentsch, C. (1984) Differential response to cholinergic stimulation in psychogenetically selected rat lines. *Psychopharmacology*, **83**, 262–267

Martin, P. and Bateson, P. (1993) *Measuring Behaviour: An Introductory Guide*. Cambridge University Press, Cambridge

Mason, G. (1991) Stereotypies: a critical review. *Animal Behaviour*, **41**, 1015–1037

Mason, G. (2006) Stereotypic behaviour in captive animals: fundamentals, and implications for welfare and beyond. In: *Stereotypic Animal Behaviour: Fundamentals and Applications to Welfare*. Eds Rushen, J. and Mason, G., pp. 325–326. CAB International, Wallingford

Mason, G., Cooper, J. and Clarebrough, C. (2001) Frustrations of fur-farmed mink. *Nature*, **410**, 35–36

Mason, G. and Latham, N. (2004) Can't stop, won't stop: is stereotypy a reliable animal welfare indicator? *Animal Welfare*, **13S**, S57–S69

Mason, G., Wilson, D., Hampton, C. *et al.* (2004) Non-invasively assessing disturbance and stress in laboratory rats by scoring chromodacryorrhoea. *ATLA, Alternatives to Laboratory Animals*, **32(1A)**, 153–159

Matheson, S., Asher, L. and Bateson, M. (2008) Larger, enriched cages are associated with 'optimistic' response biases in captive European starlings (*Sturnus vulgaris*). *Applied Animal Behaviour Science*, **109**, 374–383

Mathews, R., Richards, A. and Eysenck, M. (1989) Interpretation of homophones related to threat in anxiety states. *Journal of Abnormal Psychology*, **98**, 31–34

McBride, S. and Hemmings, A. (2005) Altered mesoaccumbens and nigro-striatal dopamine physiology is associated with stereotypy development in a non-rodent species. *Behavioural Brain Research*, **159**, 113–118

McIntosh, T.K., Barfield, R.J. and Thomas, D. (1984) Electrophysiological and ultrasonic correlates of reproductive behavior in the male rat. *Behavioral Neuroscience*, **98**, 1100–1103

Mendl, M. and Paul, E. (2004) Consciousness, emotion and animal welfare: insights from cognitive science. *Animal Welfare*, **13**, S17–25

Morton, D. and Griffiths, P. (1985) Guidelines on the recognition of pain, distress and discomfort in experimental animals and an hypothesis for assessment. *Veterinary Record*, **116**, 431–436

Nevison, C., Hurst, J. and Barnard, C. (1999a) Strain-specific effects of cage enrichment in male laboratory mice (*Mus musculus*). *Animal Welfare*, **8**, 361–379

Nevison, C., Hurst, J. and Barnard, C. (1999b) Why do male ICR(CD-1) mice perform bar-related (stereotypic) behaviour? *Behavioural Processes*, **47**, 95–111

Novak, M., Meyer, J., Lutz, C. *et al.* (2006) Deprived environments: developmental insights from primatology. In: *Stereotypic Animal Behaviour: Fundamentals and Applications to Welfare*. Eds Rushen, J. and Mason, G., pp. 86–120. CAB International, Wallingford

Nuffield Council on Bioethics. (2005) *The Ethics of Research Involving Animals*. Latimer Trend and Company Ltd, Plymouth

Olsson, I., Nevison, C., Patterson-Kane, E. *et al.* (2003) Understanding behaviour: the relevance of ethological approaches in laboratory animal science. *Applied Animal Behaviour Science*, **81**, 245–264

Panksepp, J. (2003) At the interface of the affective, behavioral, and cognitive neurosciences: decoding the emotional feelings of the brain. *Brain and Cognition*, **52**, 4–14

Panksepp, J. and Burgdorf, J. (2000) 50-kHz chirping (laughter?) in response to conditioned and unconditioned tickle-induced reward in rats: effects of social housing and genetic variables. *Behavioural Brain Research*, **115**, 25–38

Panksepp, J. and Burgdorf, J. (2003) 'Laughing' rats and the evolutionary antecedents of human joy? *Physiology and Behavior*, **79**, 533–547

Paul, E., Harding, E. and Mendl, M. (2005) Measuring emotional processes in animals: the utility of a cognitive approach. *Neuroscience and Biobehavioral Reviews*, **29**, 469–491

Phan, K., Wager, T., Taylor, S. *et al.* (2004) Functional neuroimaging studies of human emotions. *CNS Spectrums*, **9**, 258–266

Pines, M., Kaplan, G. and Rogers, L. (2005) Use of horizontal and vertical climbing structures by captive common marmosets (*Callithrix jacchus*). *Applied Animal Behaviour Science*, **91**, 311–319

Podberscek, A., Blackshaw, J. and Beattie, A. (1991) The behaviour of group penned and individually caged laboratory rabbits. *Applied Animal Behaviour Science*, **28**, 353–363

Pomerantz, S. and Clemens, L. (1981) Ultrasonic vocalizations in male deer mice (*Peromyscus maniculatus bairdi*): their role in male sexual behavior. *Physiology and Behavior*, **27**, 869–872

Poole, T. (1997) Happy animals make good science. *Laboratory Animals*, **31**, 116–124

Ritskes-Hoitinga, M., Gravesen, L. and Jegstrup, I. (2006) *Refinements benefits animal welfare and quality of science*. Available online at: http://www.nc3rs.org.uk/downloaddoc.asp?id=338&page=212&skin=0 (accessed 20 November 2009)

Rolls, E. (1999) *The Brain and Emotion*. Oxford University Press, Oxford

Roper, T. (1975) Self-sustaining activities and reinforcement in the nest building behaviour of mice. *Behaviour*, **59**, 40–57

Roughan, J. and Flecknell, P. (2001) Behavioural effects of laparotomy and analgesic effects of ketoprofen and carprofen in rats. *Pain*, **90**, 65–74

Roughan, J. and Flecknell, P. (2006) Training in behaviour-based post-operative pain scoring in rats – an evaluation based on improved recognition of analgesic requirements. *Applied Animal Behaviour Science*, **96**, 327–342

Rupniak, N. and Williams, A. (1994) Differential inhibition of foot tapping and chromodacryorrhoea in gerbils by CNS penetrant and non-penetrant tachykinin NK1 receptor antagonists. *European Journal of Pharmacology*, **265**, 179–183

Rushen, J. (1991) Problems associated with the interpretation of physiological data in the assessment of animal welfare. *Applied Animal Behaviour Science*, **28**, 381–386

Rutherford, K. (2002) Assessing pain in animals. *Animal Welfare*, **11**, 31–53

Sandøe, P., Crisp, R. and Holtug, N. (1995) Ethics. In: *Animal Welfare*. Eds Appleby, M. and Hughes, B., pp. 3–17. CAB International, Wallingford

Sapolsky, R. (1992) Neuroendocrinology of the stress-response. In: *Behavioral Endocrinology*. Eds Becker, J., Breedlove, S. and Crews, D., pp. 287–324. Massachusetts Institute of Technology, Cambridge, Massachusetts

Seaman, S., Waran, N., Mason, G. *et al.* (2008) Animal economics: assessing the motivation of female laboratory rabbits to reach a platform, social contact and food. *Animal Behaviour*, **75**, 31–42

Sharp, J., Zammit, T., Azar, T. *et al.* (2002) Does witnessing experimental procedures produce stress in male rats? *Contemporary Topics in Laboratory Animal Science*, **41**, 8–12

Sherwin, C. (1998) The use and perceived importance of three resources which provide caged laboratory mice the opportunity for extended locomotion. *Applied Animal Behaviour Science*, **55**, 353–367

Sherwin, C. (2003) Social context affects the motivation of laboratory mice, *Mus musculus*, to gain access to resources. *Animal Behaviour*, **66**, 649–655

Sherwin, C. (2004a) The influences of standard laboratory cages on rodents and the validity of research data. *Animal Welfare*, **13**, S9–15

Sherwin, C. (2004b) The motivation of group-housed laboratory mice, *Mus musculus*, for additional space. *Animal Behaviour*, **67**, 711–717

Sherwin, C. (2007) The motivation of group-housed laboratory mice to leave an enriched laboratory cage. *Animal Behaviour*, **72**, 29–35

Sherwin, C. and Nicol, C. (1995) Changes in meal patterning by mice measure the cost imposed by natural obstacles. *Applied Animal Behaviour Science*, **43**, 291–300

Sherwin, C. and Nicol, C. (1996) Reorganisation of behaviour in laboratory mice, *Mus musculus*, with varying cost of access to resources. *Animal Behaviour*, **51**, 1087–1093

Silverman, A. (1978) Rodents' defence against cigarette smoke. *Animal Behaviour*, **26**, 1279–1281

Simone, L., Bartolomucci, A., Palanza, P. *et al.* (2008) On-ground housing in 'Mice Drawer System' (MDS) cage affects locomotor behaviour but not anxiety in male mice. *Acta Astronautica*, **62**, 453–461

Spangenberg, E., Augustsson, H., Dahlborn, K. *et al.* (2005) Housing-related activity in rats: effects on body weight, urinary corticosterone levels, muscle properties and performance. *Laboratory Animals*, **39**, 45–57

Spangenberg, E., Bjorklund, L. and Dahlborn, K. (2006) Outdoor housing of laboratory dogs: effects on activity, behaviour and physiology. *Applied Animal Behaviour Science*, **98**, 260–276

Spruijt, B., van den Bos, R. and Pijlman, T. (2001) A concept of welfare based on reward evaluating mechanisms in the brain: anticipatory behaviour as an indicator for the state of reward systems. *Applied Animal Behaviour Science*, **72**, 145–171

Szechtman, H., Lambrou, P., Caggiula, A. *et al.* (1974) Plasma corticosterone levels during sexual behaviour in male rats. *Hormones and Behaviour*, **5**, 191–200

Terlouw, E., Schouten, W. and Ladewig, J. (1995) Physiology. In: *Animal Welfare*. Eds Appleby, M. and Hughes, B., pp. 143–158. CAB International, Wallingford

Thurman, J., Tranquilli, W. and Benson, G. (1999) *Essentials of Small Animal Anaesthesia and Analgesia: Small Animal Practice*. Blackwell Publishing, Oxford

Toates, F. (1995) *Stress: Conceptual and Biological Aspects*. John Wiley and Sons, Chichester

Toates, F. (2004) Cognition, motivation, emotion and action: a dynamic and vulnerable interdependence. *Applied Animal Behaviour Science*, **86**, 173–204

Touma, C., Sachser, N., Mostl, E. *et al.* (2003) Effects of sex and time of day on metabolism and excretion fo corticosterone in urine and feces of mice. *General and Comparative Endocrinology*, **130**, 267–278

Ullman-Cullere, M. and Foltz, C. (1999) Body condition scoring: a rapid and accurate method for assessing health status in mice. *Laboratory Animal Science*, **49**, 319–323

Vahl, T., Ulrich-Lai, Y., Ostrander, M. *et al.* (2005) Comparative analysis of ACTH and corticosterone sampling methods in rats. *American Journal of Physiology and Endocrinology Metabolism*, **289**, E823–828

Van de Weerd, H., Van Den Broek, F. and Baumans, V. (1996) Preference for different types of flooring in two rat strains. *Applied Animal Behaviour Science*, **46**, 251–261

Van de Weerd, H., Van Loo, P., Van Zutphen, L. *et al.* (1998) Strength of preference for nesting material as environmental enrichment for laboratory mice. *Applied Animal Behaviour Science*, **55**, 369–382

Van den Berg, C., Pijlman, T., Koning, H. *et al.* (1999) Isolation changes the incentive value of sucrose and social behaviour in juvenile and adult rats. *Behavioural Brain Research*, **106**, 133–142

Van den Berg, C., Van Ree, J. and Spruijt, B. (2000) Morphine attenuates the effects of juvenile isolation in rats. *Neuropharmacology*, **39**, 969–976

Van den Bos, R., Meijer, M., van Renselaar, J. *et al.* (2003) Anticipation is differently expressed in rats (*Rattus norvegicus*) and domestic cats (*Felis silvestris catus*) in the same Pavlovian conditioning paradigm. *Behavioural Brain Research*, **141**, 83–89

Van Der Harst, J., Baars, A. and Spruijt, B. (2003a) Standard housed rats are more sensitive to rewards than enriched housed rats as reflected by their anticipatory behaviour. *Behavioural Brain Research*, **142**, 151–156

Van Der Harst, J., Baars, A. and Spruijt, B. (2005) Announced rewards counteract the impairment of anticipatory behaviour in socially stressed rats. *Behavioural Brain Research*, **161**, 183–189

Van Der Harst, J., Fermont, P., Bilstra, A. *et al.* (2003b) Access to enriched housing is rewarding to rats as reflected by their anticipatory behaviour. *Animal Behaviour*, **66**, 493–504

Van Loo, P., Kruitwagen, C., Koolhaas, J. *et al.* (2002) Influence of cage enrichment on aggressive behaviour and physiological parameters in male mice. *Applied Animal Behaviour Science*, **76**, 65–81

Varian, H. (1993) *Intermediate Microeconomics: a Modern Approach*. WW Norton, London

von Borell, E., Langbein, J., Despres, G. *et al.* (2007) Heart rate variability as a measure of autonomic regulation of cardiac activity for assessing stress and welfare in farm animals – a review. *Physiology and Behavior*, **92**, 293–316

Von Frijtag, J., Reijmers, L., Van Der Harst, J. *et al.* (2000) Defeat followed by individual housing results in long-term impaired reward- and cognition-related behaviours in rats. *Behavioural Brain Research*, **117**, 137–146

Von Frijtag, J., Van den Bos, R. and Spruijt, B. (2001) Imipramine restores the long-term impairment of appetitive behaviour in socially stressed rats. *Psychopharmacology*, **162**, 232–238

Wahlsten, D. (2001) Standardizing tests of mouse behavior: reasons, recommendations, and reality. *Physiology and Behavior*, **73**, 695–704

Walker, C., Lightman, S., Steele, M. *et al.* (1992) Suckling is a persistent stimulus to the adreno-cortical system of the rat. *Endocrinology*, **130**, 115–125

Warburton, H. and Mason, G. (2003) Is out of sight out of mind? The effects of resource cues on motivation in mink, *Mustela vison*. *Animal Behaviour*, **65**, 755–762

Warburton, H. and Nicol, C. (1998) Position of operant costs affects visits to resources by laboratory mice, *Mus musculus*. *Animal Behaviour*, **55**, 1325–1333

Warburton, V., Sales, G. and Milligan, S. (1989) The emission and elicitation of mouse ultrasonic vocalizations: the effects of age, sex and gonadal status. *Physiology and Behavior*, **45**, 41–47

Weary, D., Niel, L., Flower, F. *et al.* (2006) Identifying and preventing pain in animals. *Applied Animal Behaviour Science*, **100**, 64–76

Whishaw, I. and Kolb, B. (2004) *The Behavior of the Laboratory Rat*. Oxford University Press, New York

Wiedenmayer, C. (1997) Causation of the ontogenic development of stereotypic digging in gerbils. *Animal Behaviour*, **53**, 461–470

Wöhr, M., Houx, B., Schwarting, R. *et al.* (2008) Effects of experience and context of 50-kHz vocalizations in rats. *Physiology and Behavior*, **93**, 766–776

Wöhr, M. and Schwarting, R. (in press) Ultrasonic calling during fear conditioning in the rat: no evidence for an audience effect. *Animal Behaviour*

Wright-Williams, S., Courade, J.-P., Richardson, C. *et al.* (2007) Effects of vasectomy surgery and meloxicam treatment on faecal corticosterone levels and behaviour in two strains of laboratory mouse. *Pain*, **130**, 108–118

Würbel, H. (2006) The motivational basis of caged rodents' stereotypies. In: *Stereotypic Animal Behaviour: Fundamentals and Applications to Welfare*. Eds Rushen, J. and Mason, G., pp. 86–120. CAB International, Wallingford

Würbel, H. (2000) Behaviour and the standardisation fallacy. *Nature Genetics*, **26**, 263

Würbel, H. and Garner, J. (2007) Refinement of rodent research through environmental enrichment and systematic randomization. *NC3Rs*, **9**, 1–9

Würbel, H. and Stauffacher, M. (1998) Physical condition at weaning affects exploratory behaviour and stereotypy development in laboratory mice. *Behavioural Processes*, **43**, 61–69

Würbel, H., Stauffacher, M. and Holst, D. V. (1996) Stereotypies in laboratory mice – quantative and qualitative description of the ontogeny of wire-gnawing and jumping in Zur:ICR and Zur:ICR nu. *Ethology*, **102**, 371–385

Yeates, J. and Main, D. (2008) Assessment of positive welfare: a review. *The Veterinary Journal*, **175**, 293–300

7 Welfare and 'best practice' in field studies of wildlife

Julie M. Lane and Robbie A. McDonald

Introduction

Wildlife research is exciting and is an appealing career for many aspiring scientists. The life of the wildlife biologist or vet and the thrill of capturing and handling wild animals are glamorised by the media, and the professions are often treated as being synonymous with working to promote animal welfare and conservation. However, field studies of wild animals carry with them multiple risks for the animal subjects. Unfortunately, these risks and problems are sometimes given scant consideration by practitioners, often because they are judged relative to natural processes or are incurred 'for the good of the species' or population. Whilst wild animals undoubtedly suffer a range of markedly inhumane fates in the wild, and while some are in grave need of intervention for conservation and management reasons, the ethical/moral absolute of the welfare of the individual animal and the corresponding deep concern felt by society, mean that field research on wild animals requires an approach to ethical issues and the implementation of the Three Rs (3 Rs, see Chapter 2) that is as rigorous as for other areas of research using animals.

For a range of historical and subjective reasons, 'wildlife' is most commonly construed as naturally free-living vertebrates, most commonly mammals and birds, and to a slightly lesser extent, reptiles, amphibians and 'fish'. The huge diversity within and among these taxa, means that there is little consistency in their physiology, let alone their behaviour. Even within species, individuals and populations are likely to be behaviourally distinct; indeed this fine-scale variation is itself often the focus of field investigation. Generalising the needs and responses of individuals of particular populations and species is, therefore, an ambitious and probably unrealistic endeavour. All investigators and regulators must view field studies on a case-by-case basis, bringing relevant experience to bear where possible, but being prepared for exception and novelty. Since much of the legislation dealing with scientific procedures on animals is restricted to vertebrates (see Chapter 8), invertebrates will not be considered in this chapter. *Octopus vulgaris*, for example, is covered by legislation in the UK and, at a European level, protection may be extended to all cephalopods and decapod crustaceans. Kept animals, such as companion animals and farm livestock, will also not be considered. However, cats (*Felis catus*), dogs (*Canis familiaris*), pigs/boar (*Sus scrofa*), goats (*Capra aegagrus hircus*), horses (*Equus caballus*) and other kept animals, such as ferrets (*Mustela furo*), mink (*Neovison vison*), often return to a free-living state, sometimes outside of their native range, where they can revert to wild-type appearance and behaviour. Such feral animals are, to all intents and purposes, wild and so they fall within the scope of this chapter.

The object of field studies is to examine how wild animals behave in the wild or in as natural a situation and habitat as possible. Observations in the field might require little direct intervention, and be as apparently straightforward as observing animals from a distance, comparable to a bird-watcher's hobby. However, other treatments, procedures and initial observations might take place in the laboratory, or in other situations where wild animals are held captive for periods of time. Interventions might carry forward into the field, obviously when animals are equipped with tags or telemetry devices and less conspicuously if they are treated with internal markers, drugs or if their social or physical environment is manipulated around them. Therefore, this review extends to any interaction with wild animals in the field, the taking of animals from the wild and includes making observations or applying treatments in captivity, where captivity is temporary and takes place in the field or requires holding animals for periods of between a few hours and a few days. We will not dwell on the use of wild-caught animals in prolonged or terminal laboratory work, but focus on cases where animals are subsequently released back to the wild.

When working with animals in the wild, the work and its potential effects on the animals are often subject to uncertainty and unpredictability. It is never certain, for example, how many animals might be caught in a trap round or cannon net or how individuals might behave or respond to capture or interventions. With experience, many of these risks can be identified and mitigated. Expecting the unexpected and building appropriate contingency plans and budgets carries financial costs, but these are usually minor relative to the cost of mistakes and misjudgement which may lead to the projects being abandoned because of failures to comply with legislation and/or public opposition.

Reasons for wildlife research

The management of wild animals is an intrinsic part of land management. Often these practices have developed over centuries of common practice and form part of routine pest management for disease control and crop protection, as well as for food and sport. More recently, as awareness of the threats to biodiversity conservation has increased, management is frequently undertaken to enhance the status of threatened species. As society and the environment change, it is becoming much more important that we understand how wild animals might respond to management actions. Regulatory authorities and private sector interests can also intervene in management, by requiring evidence of humane treatment, efficacy or cost-effectiveness.

Studies may be carried out to examine wild animal biology, including population dynamics and individual behaviour and welfare. Wild animals are also used as indicators of environmental health. For these studies, the benefits in terms of knowledge, understanding and the conservation of the species are usually clearly articulated, however, the costs incurred to the individual animals are often not as well understood.

One critical difference between wild animal studies and the use of laboratory animals in research is that the subject of interest and focus of investigation is usually the subject animal in its own right rather than it serving as a model for the human condition or as a model of any other living system. For this reason, total replacement of animals in wildlife research (unlike, for example, clinical studies) will never be a feasible option (see Cuthill (2007) and Barnard (2007) for fuller discussions on this topic) and for many wildlife studies captive or captive-bred animals will never be a substitute for free-living animals. Nonetheless, due consideration should always be given to seeking alternatives where possible.

Welfare implications of wildlife studies

Effects of stress

All interactions between humans and animals have the potential to cause stress and behavioural or physiological changes and this is particularly likely with wild animals, where any kind of direct interaction is usually perceived as a threat. Stress is an integral part of all animals' lives and the body has developed many mechanisms for coping with both psychological and physical stressors (Broom & Johnson 1993). However, acute or prolonged stress can have diverse, profound and deleterious effects on the psychological and physiological health of animals and it is usually in the latter case that animals are said to be 'suffering from distress'. In wildlife studies the onset of these stress-related effects is of particular importance as the effects are difficult if not impossible to determine. This is because animals are normally released into the wild before any symptoms become apparent and, unlike laboratory subjects, wild animals are not constantly provided with the essentials of life (such as food, water, shelter) and so their survival is routinely challenged on a range of fronts.

In severe cases, acute stress can cause death from cardiac failure, but in the majority of instances the effects of acute stress will be more long term and harder to define. Physiological indicators of stress that may be observed during capture include shortness of breath (panting) and tachycardia (racing heart). However, from a behavioural point of view stress reactions are more difficult to ascertain and very much rely on having detailed knowledge of the biology of the study animals. For example, some animals become motionless (eg, rabbits (*Oryctolagus cuniculus*)) or may appear relaxed (eg, badgers (*Meles meles*)) when confronted with a stressor, whereas other animals will be hyperactive and spend a great deal of time in escape behaviours (eg, rats (*Rattus* spp.)). In addition, variation in response to stressors can occur within a species, with differences apparent in the reactions of dominant and subordinate animals and between genders (Overli *et al.* 2006).

The long-term physiological components of stress can affect most aspects of an animal's biology. High levels of stress hormones (such as glucocorticoids) are linked to poor reproductive success in males and females (Rivier & Vale 1984; Sapolsky *et al.* 2000) and reduced immunity from disease (Munck *et al.* 1984), both of which have the potential for significant impact on a wild animal's life and fitness.

Injuries

Apart from physiological effects there are also adverse physical consequences of field studies, primarily arising from capture and captivity. These range from minor injuries such as skin abrasions and tooth and claw damage in animals attempting to escape from cage or box traps and abrasions from external devices (eg, radiocollars) up to more severe injuries such as broken limbs (eg, birds in mist nets, 'foul' captures in traps), adverse reactions to drugs, predator attacks or death (eg, fish in gill nets).

One particularly serious problem associated with capture of wild animals is myopathy. This can occur when an animal is subjected to stress and intense physical exertion. It is unusual with cage trapping but can be found with netting or prolonged pursuit and handling of large mammals, particularly deer (Haulton *et al.* 2001). The condition is caused by a build up of lactic acid in muscles leading to stiffness, paralysis and, in extreme cases, eventual death (Conner *et al.* 1987). Symptoms normally have a delayed onset (sometimes over 1 week) and hence are rarely identified during capture. It is imperative, therefore, that stress levels are kept low by ensuring confident and effective handling and brief periods of pursuit and capture.

Other welfare effects

If the welfare status of an animal is unduly compromised this has repercussions, not only in ethical terms, but also on the validity and rigour of the scientific study itself. The stress associated with capture (and particularly when associated with anaesthesia) can have wide-ranging effects on an animal's biology, behaviour and ecology, and allowances must be made for these. Poor welfare arising from studies can have effects on the areas discussed in the following paragraphs.

Social structure and behaviour

The establishment and maintenance of social status within animal groups is complex and varies greatly with taxonomy, environment and among individuals. Social rank in a group is determined by many factors, but higher rank is often gained through aggressive behaviour linked to levels of the male hormone testosterone (Abbott *et al.* 2003; Schaffner & French 2004). Stress can alter levels of testosterone and hence may have an impact on the dominance hierarchies of a population, particularly in group-living animals such as wolves (*Canis lupus*). In addition, even the temporary removal of an animal from its social group (especially the dominant male and female), may affect its position and the relative status of several others and be the cause of unrest and heightened aggression in the group. The effect of large-scale permanent removal of individuals on social structure has been well documented in badgers. Badger culling employed for the control of TB has resulted in disruption of territoriality, increased ranging behaviour and mixing between social groups (Carter *et al.* 2007).

Reproductive behaviour

The effect of stress on levels of sexual hormones is well documented and could have wide-ranging effects for males and females, with respect to their reproductive investment and success. Anaesthesia has the potential to cause abortion in the early part of gestation and premature birth in late pregnancy. It has also been shown that handling young can cause the mother to kill or abandon them. Therefore, where reproduction is not a focus of the research, studies might, where possible, avoid the sensitive parts of breeding seasons. There are also instances where the procedure itself can influence mating behaviour. This has been demonstrated in bird species that use 'badges of status', where ringing these birds can have an impact on mate choice (Burley 1986).

Foraging behaviour

Anaesthesia and stress can affect the metabolic condition and cognitive ability of an animal in the short term rendering it less able to forage. Alternatively, periods of captivity in the absence of preferred food may affect an animal's nutritional status and foraging choices upon release. This problem can be minimised if studies are conducted at times when there are fewer external pressures such as low food availability.

Spatial behaviour

Some animals have been shown to move away from an area from where they have experienced capture and anaesthesia presumably as the stress of this experience is associated with this geographical area (Teixeira *et al.* 2007). Others tend to be more sedentary than normal after capture and release. This has, potentially, wide-ranging effects on the population dynamics of group-living animals and also on the survival of individual animals that forsake their known home ranges and food sources.

While such changes may be temporary, resulting measures may give a misleading impression of typical ranging behaviour. Where observation periods are brief, these measures will be even more prone to bias.

Survival and mortality rates

Even the ringing of birds can have an effect on mortality in a population (Recher *et al.* 1985; Inglis *et al.* 1997). The procedure itself can directly affect the probability of survival and in addition, wild animals often carry underlying latent infections such as toxoplasmosis (eg, in sparrows) that may, as a result of lowered immunity due to stress, develop into clinical disease (Bermúdez *et al.* 2009).

Population dynamics

There is always the potential that the study itself might have a direct effect on the results. Increased mortality and disease are both possibilities but more subtle effects may be more difficult to determine. Moorhouse and Macdonald (2005) demonstrated that the sex ratio of a population of water voles was affected by the trapping and radio-tracking programme over a 3-year period. Over this time one discrete population of the water voles was regularly trapped and anaesthetised whereas a separate population was left undisturbed. After 3 years, both populations were trapped and the numbers estimated. It was found that the first population had a significantly higher ratio of males to females than the undisturbed voles. The conclusion being that the stress of capture and tracking had caused the mothers to produce higher levels of testosterone leading to an increase in male births.

Effects on others

One of the main differences in welfare terms between laboratory and wildlife studies is the fact that the latter have the potential to affect not only the study animals but also many other individuals in the surrounding area. Although this may not be avoidable it is always important to be aware of the consequences of any study and factor it into the ethical assessment.

Conspecifics

The effect of a study on an individual also has potential repercussions for conspecifics especially with respect to group living animals. This includes changes in dominance hierarchies and the onset of disease (see section on Survival and mortality rates).

Dependents

Removing parent animals from their dependents may cause malnutrition and, in severe cases, death of the young, particularly among animals with altricial young and those in the earliest stages of life. Treatment with drugs, including anaesthesia, has the potential to affect lactation (Yokoyama 1965), potentially exacerbating nutritional problems. Where breeding is not itself the focus of the study, trapping when young are dependent is a risk that should be avoided or mitigated. If there are obvious signs that the animals caught have dependent young (eg, lactation, brood patches), then it is advisable to release them as soon as possible, which may involve a judgement as to whether to carry out all of the intended procedures.

Non-targets
Capturing non-target species or individuals is almost unavoidable in wildlife studies, but the consequences can be more severe than those for the intended subject. For example, while the research might not be carried out during the breeding season of the subject it may be during that of non-target species; or the trap may not be appropriate (eg, weasels (*Mustela* spp.) caught in uncovered cage traps can die through hypothermia).

Three Rs and welfare

Exact numbers of wild animals used in regulated procedures are difficult to ascertain, and are not often collated specifically. In the UK, Home Office statistics[1] provide numbers of each species used in a range of subjects but it is not clear how many wild animals are studied in the field. For example 90 419 animals were used in the field of ecology in 2007. Of these 84 252 were fish, many of which were tagged and released as part of fisheries research though others were captive animals used in behavioural ecology research in the laboratory. The remaining individuals largely fell into the categories: Other rodent, Other carnivore, Other mammal (1405) and Other bird (3628) and Any amphibian (1027). Many of these studies of 'non-standard' species may have involved wild animals and will have been carried out at least partly in the field. In addition, wild species are also likely to have been used in other fields of study (eg, zoology, animal welfare). Many wildlife studies, including observational studies or minor interventions such as bird ringing, may not be regulated but nonetheless could affect the welfare of the subject animal.

Although the original definition of the Three Rs (replacement, reduction and refinement) was developed with laboratory studies in mind the principles and philosophy of this concept can be extended to many other areas in which there are human–animal interactions, as a means of ensuring the highest standards of welfare (Cuthill 2007). Unfortunately most of the information readily available with respect to the Three Rs tends to be aimed at their implementation in laboratory studies and many examples are not applicable to wildlife research (eg, cell culture, refinement of housing). This, however, should not lead to the conclusion that implementation of the Three Rs within wildlife research is not necessary or relevant. Here, a number of practical examples of how the Three Rs can be addressed in field studies is provided.

Replacement

Replacement is often not considered a viable option in studies of the behaviour and ecology of wildlife species, where the specific animals and their natural behaviour are intrinsic to the study (see section Reasons for wildlife research). However, there are alternative techniques that can give us a greater understanding of these topics without the use of animals themselves.

[1] http://www.homeoffice.gov.uk/rds

In silico studies (computer modelling)

This approach can be used to generate predictions of treatment effects, often taking into account uncertainty associated with observations and outcomes. In this way, the results of modelling can be more general than those of specific or localised observational studies. While such modelling requires understanding of the quality and representative nature of input data, modelling can also help evaluate the most important avenues of investigation allowing the field study to be refined. This approach has proven particularly effective in estimating population changes and for evaluating methods of management and disease control (Wilkinson *et al.* 2004).

Use of less sentient species

The substitution of a less sentient and/or non-protected species is usually classed as a form of replacement; this is not appropriate for the majority of wildlife studies, where the species itself is the subject of investigation. However, there is potential for using this type of replacement in ecotoxicology studies, where invertebrate models (eg, amphipods (*Gammarus pulex*)) can be used to assess levels of pollutants (Ashauer *et al.* 2007).

Read-across approach

This approach is more commonly associated with pharmaceutical and toxicity testing, usually in combination with computer modelling (Schultz *et al.* 2009). At a basic level it involves using data from one species to predict the outcome in others. Although this may not be appropriate for many field studies it may have uses, particularly in more heavily regulated areas such as ecotoxicology and developing population control methods. For example, if determining the effect of pesticides on non-target species data from wood mice (*Apodemus sylvaticus*) may be used to extrapolate to other small rodents such as harvest mice (*Micromys minutus*).

Reduction

Most of the principles and techniques of minimising animal use in the laboratory are also applicable to studies in the field.

Statistical design

The use of robust statistical approaches before, during and after the study can help ensure an efficient study where minimum numbers of animals are used and resources are deployed to best effect. Power analysis, where the project scale and sampling techniques are evaluated with respect to a range of probable effect sizes, is particularly important in planning investigations. It can now be applied to a range of complex analytical approaches, though this often requires repeated simulations of statistical outcomes rather than the off-the-peg power analyses available in standard packages (Dytham 2003).

As with laboratory studies, the precision and accuracy of observations in relation to the magnitude of any effect size are vital in considering the required sample size. Similarly variance in outcomes can be inflated by sampling across outwardly similar groups or environments, potentially masking treatment effects. Sampling design may need to be modified to account for, or avoid, these sources of potential variance. However, sample size and sampling design cannot be easily controlled in the field, and natural error variance and sampling error, if anything, tend to be more pronounced (Feinsinger 2001). The following factors often confound field investigations and should be taken into account in developing the study design:

- species, sex and age;
- weather conditions;
- presence and number of non-targets;
- interference by others (eg, members of the public).

The other factor to consider is that if the sample size is too small, repeating field studies to gain the data required is more difficult than in the laboratory, due to the inability to mimic the exact conditions used in previous trials.

Sequential testing

Sequential testing (or phasing) is where the sample size is not fixed in advance. Instead, data are evaluated as they are collected and further sampling is stopped in accordance with a predefined stopping rule as soon as significant results are observed. Thus a conclusion may sometimes be reached at a much earlier stage than would be possible with more classical hypothesis testing or estimation, with the potential to use fewer animals. With these techniques, as the study progresses, the design can be refined or the study halted as appropriate.

Using published or available data

Literature and other resources should be used to inform experimental design, perhaps in a power analysis, and hence reduce the number of animals or trials needed. It is important to note that the read-across approach works in this instance as well (ie, if no data are available for a particular species, searches should be made for data on related animals).

Sharing data

Data sharing is an important method for reducing animal use across the whole spectrum of animal-related studies. Data are normally shared within a scientific discipline via publications or presentations at conferences but this tends to focus only on positive results and finalised studies. It is as important, if not more so, that negative results and potential pitfalls of animal work are highlighted and a particularly good way of achieving this is by the use of specialist user groups on the web. These can provide an easily accessible and low-cost method to exchange data and ideas.

Samples can be shared as well as information. If different research teams (especially in the same geographical area) all require samples (eg, blood, hair, swabs) from the same species then it may be possible to work together so that the animals only need to be caught and sampled once. This needs to carry the caveat that the numbers, quantities and types of samples taken from an individual must remain within the best practice guidelines (see later in this chapter) and have the appropriate licensing authority.

Multi-use technique

This technique is particularly applicable to field use. It is a method of minimising the overall number of animals used by gaining data from one event that may be required for different parts of the study or for a completely separate study (eg, trapping animals for marking for ecological study and taking blood samples for a disease-monitoring programme). A good degree of forethought needs to be exercised when undertaking multi-use studies so that appropriate permissions are in place for all uses and any caveats observed before the studies are initiated.

Refinement

The main way of addressing refinement with respect to wildlife studies is through opting for the least invasive techniques and always to referring to 'best practice' guidelines and recent experience for capture, handling, marking and sampling appropriate for the species (see section Capture, handling, release). More specific, less-invasive methods are discussed in the following paragraphs.

Remote cameras

This method involves using remotely triggered cameras to gain information without any capture or manipulation of an animal. With digital technology, these cameras are more sophisticated and can create photographs in various formats, use time-lapse technology, can be motion-sensitive, and can operate at night using infra-red (Figure 7.1). Using video recording and/or still photographs has the advantage over direct observations in that there is less interference (and hence less stress imposed) on the animal and it requires less input from the investigator.

Non-invasive sampling methods

Many field studies involve taking samples to measure physiological parameters or pathological indicators. Although most of these factors have been traditionally measured in the blood, other less invasive approaches to sampling (eg, saliva and faeces) can be used in many instances to gain the same data. Faecal sampling is of particular interest as it can be used easily without disturbing the subject and without interfering with other welfare measures running in parallel, such as behavioural assessment (Lane 2006). Faecal sampling can be used to investigate hormone levels (eg, cortisol, testosterone), DNA analyses and for bait-marking purposes (Figure 7.2).

Identification

For some species natural markings can be used as a completely non-invasive method of identification (see Marking).

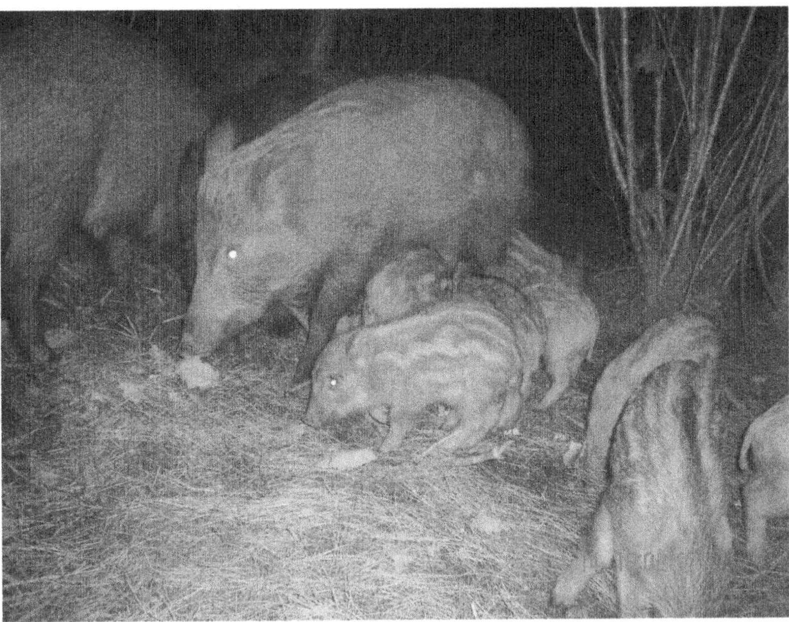

Figure 7.1 Image of wild boar using an infra-red camera trap.

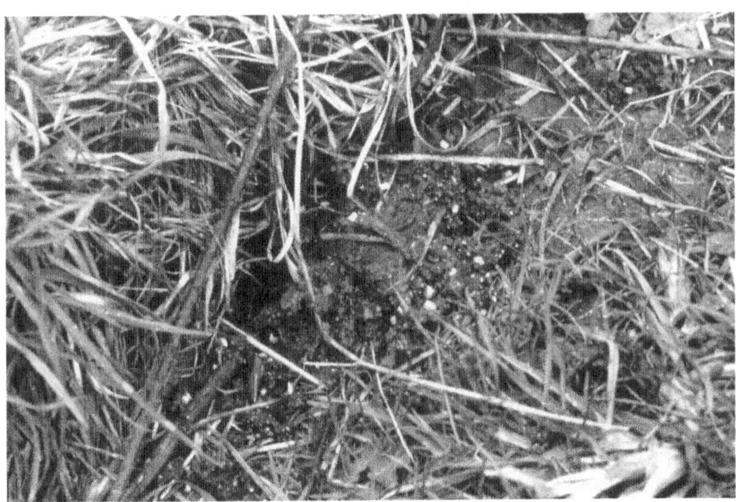

Figure 7.2 Coloured beads as bait markers in badger latrine. A non-invasive and effective method to monitor bait uptake and to determine territory structure is to add coloured beads to baits which can then be detected in the faeces negating the need for any procedure or capture of the animal.

It is also important to be aware of techniques that should not be used in most circumstances due to the availability of more refined alternatives. A good example of this is the use of toe-clipping to permanently mark small mammals and amphibians. This invasive technique causes tissue damage (Golay & Durrer 1994; Reaser 1995), affects survival (Clarke 1972) and has been demonstrated to cause pain and suffering (May 2004). For these reasons it should, wherever possible, be replaced by a non-invasive technique such as natural markings or, if this is not possible, a less damaging technique such as microchipping.

With respect to refinement it is always important to consider the fate of non-targets as well as study animals. Non-targets may encounter the same potential costs to welfare as the target animals such as stress and injury caused by cage trapping or mist netting. Hence, it is vitally important that best practice methods of capture are employed to reduce the incidence of non-target captures (see next section).

Capture, handling, release

Most wildlife studies in the field include the use of capture, mark and release programmes. The techniques adopted in these programmes can have far-reaching consequences, so it is important to be aware of, and where possible, minimise the potential adverse effects not only on the study animals but also the other animals in the environment.

General welfare issues

Time of year

Research may lead to disruption of normal animal activities, whether as part of the study procedure or incidental to it. Disturbance of breeding individuals and dependent juveniles is of particular concern. Investigators should be aware of the breeding seasons of the species that they propose to study and ensure that there are no significant welfare implications associated with the timing of their research.

Time of day

An awareness of an animal's circadian activities is essential for appropriate capture and handling. Nocturnal animals should be kept in darkness when held in traps, as being away from cover during daylight hours will cause them further stress. Animals that are caught without the use of food baits (eg, mist netting of birds and bats) should be released with enough time to forage. If this is not possible, consideration should be given to provision of supplementary food and water or a glucose solution before release.

Extreme weather conditions (heat or cold)

Checking weather forecasts should always be a priority when carrying out field work. In the UK, the Met Office provide a pay-for service in which detailed, tailored forecasts can be sent directly to an email account. Trapping should be avoided during extreme weather conditions to reduce the possibility of hyper- or hypothermia. Shelter and extra warmth should be considered especially when anaesthetising animals in cold conditions (eg, heat pads, blankets, bubble wrap).

Non-targets

The capture of non-targets is always a possibility with live trapping so, where possible, use methods which maximise capture of the intended target and reduce capture of other species (eg, set restraining traps on a run). However, always be prepared to deal with non-targets if the need arises. In some cases certain non-target species, usually invasive non-native species (eg, grey squirrel, mink in the UK) may not be released back to the wild under conservation legislation, hence provision for humane euthanasia of these species should be made.

Capture

The choice of capture method should be made according to the species involved and availability of technology and personnel, potentially including veterinary cover. Methods of capture may be physical, such as the use of traps and nets. Small–medium mammals and birds are often caught in live traps, and netting tends to be the most common method for catching small birds and bats. Larger mammals may be trapped by a variety of methods (live trapping, netting) and may also be chemically sedated using darts. Capture efficiency and capture-related mortality rates have been found to differ considerably between methods and operators and this should be considered before a decision is made.

Live trapping

It is vitally important that only as many animals as can be effectively and safely dealt with in the time period available are caught. The number of cage traps set, should be the number able to be checked and processed within the allocated time (usually a maximum of 24h, though note that traps checked once in a 24h period could in theory hold animals captive for nearly 48h). It is also beneficial to have a good idea of variation in trap efficiency in the study system (eg, number of captures/100 trap night) so that it can be checked that the plan is achievable. Traps should always be securely shut down or wired open if they cannot be checked with the required frequency.

Being caught and held in a trap can be a very stressful experience for an animal but the trauma can be minimised by:

- avoiding exposed areas (so they are less likely to be bothered by predators, noise, etc);
- providing shade/cover and bedding or similar material where applicable – apart from calming the animal this can also reducing biting and scratching (Figures 7.3, 7.4);
- ensuring traps (and animals) are clearly labelled, particularly if the animals are being moved for processing so that it is known exactly where to return them for release;
- checking frequently – especially with small animals such as shrews (preferably at least twice a day);
- with netting, being able to close down the nets as the handling capacity is approached in the specified time period; small animals have high metabolic rates and can quickly lose condition, so efficiency is of the essence.

Most cage traps rely on a baiting system so food is usually available but it is also recommended that water or food with high water content is provided. In addition, if using live traps for small mammals, food for shrews (eg, fly pupae) should be provided even if they are not the target.

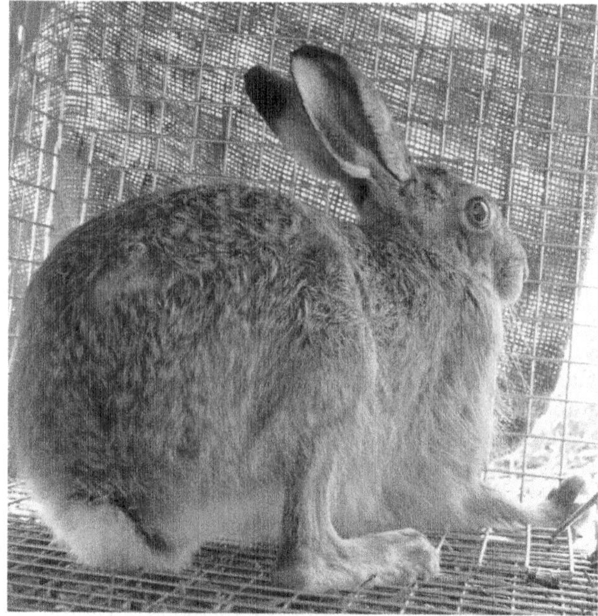

Figure 7.3 Brown hare (*Lepus europaeus*) in cage trap. Covering traps prevents exposure to the elements and predators and has a calming effect on most species.

Handling

Wild animals should not be handled unless necessary for the procedure. If handling is required the amount of contact should be kept to a minimum and the safety of the handler and of the animal needs to be considered (Figure 7.4). Wild animals are likely to bite or peck and scratch and are carriers of many zoonotic diseases (eg, *Leptospira*, *Cryptosporidium*) and so caution needs to be exercised at all times and risk assessments carried out before handling any wild animal. The method of handling will depend on the species of the animal and on the procedure to be carried out. However, there are key rules that should be followed:

- Handling should be kept to a minimum.
- Most animals like to be covered as it produces a calming effect. This is *not* the case for some species of deer (eg, muntjac (*Muntiacus* reevesi)), which find being covered more stressful.

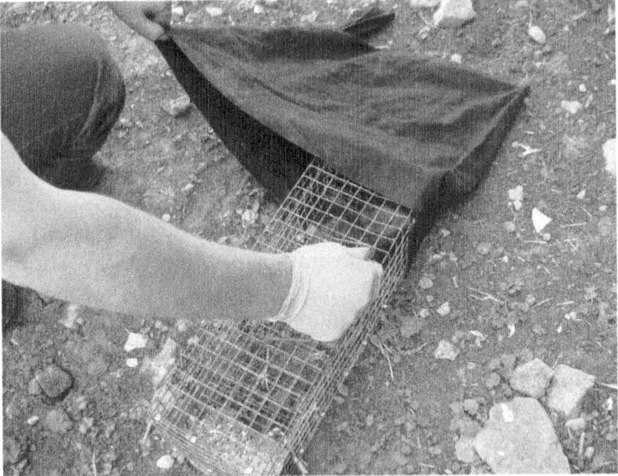

Figure 7.4 Transferring wild rat from cage trap. When dealing with wild animals it is always beneficial if they can be studied with minimal handling. A simple black bag provides a device to extricate wild rats simply and safely from a cage trap. The rats, seeking cover in the darkness, will run directly into the bag avoiding direct handling.

- Handlers need to be confident and competent at dealing with the appropriate species.
- Rodents should never be lifted by the end of tail.
- With birds the hold must include the wings and legs in order to prevent damage to these appendages. Certain species may have specific requirements for physical restraint, including those with long legs and necks (Figure 7.5). Birds breathe by a bellows-like action of the ribs and sternum. Therefore, care should be taken so that the method of restraint does not interfere with the ventilatory movements of the sternum or impede the respiratory air flow.

Anaesthesia

Under Schedule 2(A) of Animal Scientific Procedures Act, anaesthesia should be used for all regulated procedures unless the use of these compounds is likely to cause more harm and distress. For wild animals, it may be that some procedures that are not inherently painful (eg, fitting a radiocollar) may still require sedation and/or anaesthesia, even if brief, for the handler's safety and the animal's welfare.

With all wild animal anaesthesia, veterinary input and advice should be sought from the outset. Doses, routes and recovery should be discussed fully with a veterinary surgeon before embarking on anaesthetising any wild animal. The following information is for guidance only.

After administering an anaesthetic the animal must be monitored to check that they are at the required depth of anaesthesia and that their vital body functions have not become dangerously depressed. Respiratory and cardiac function must both be monitored closely. When anaesthetising wild animals in the field, inhalation or injectable anaesthetics may be used (see Hall *et al.* 2000 for overview, and see also Flecknell 2009).

Inhalation anaesthetics

These types of anaesthetics tend to be used for small mammals and birds. There are portable versions of gaseous

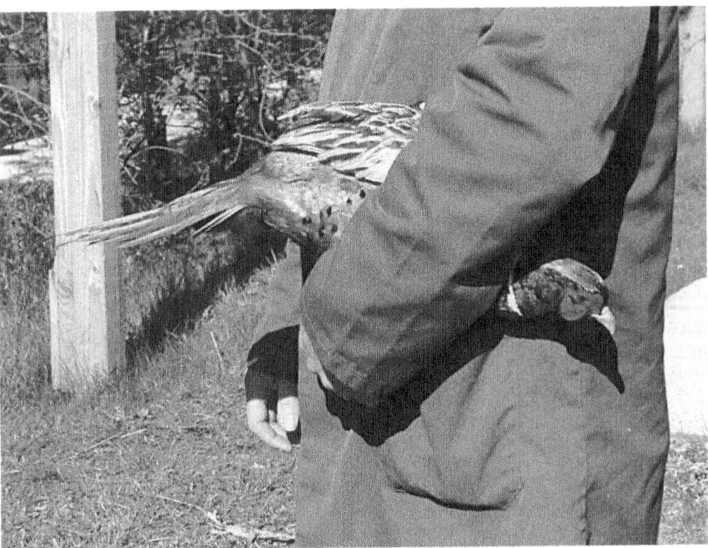

Figure 7.5 Correct handling of a pheasant. Wings and feet are safely secured so the bird cannot damage itself or the handler.

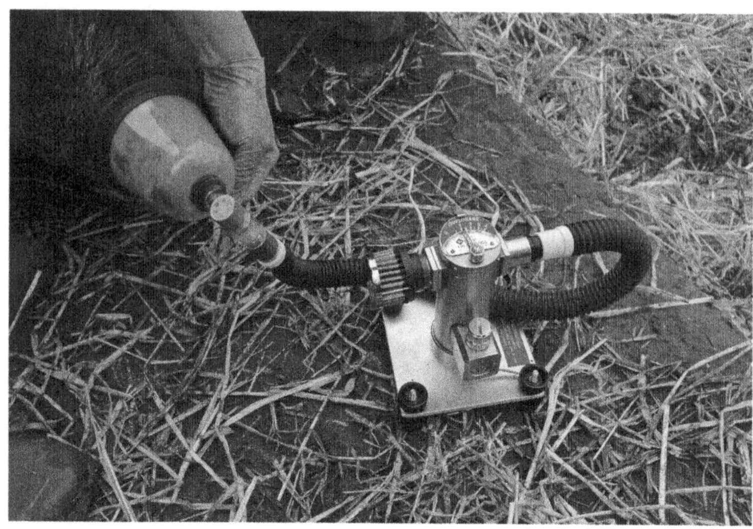

Figure 7.6 Anaesthesia of a wild boar. Portable gaseous anaesthetic machines are an effective and safe way of maintaining anaesthesia (after initial darting or injection) in medium- and large-sized mammals in field situations.

anaesthetic machines (Figure 7.6) or anaesthetics can be delivered in a chamber in which the liquid compound is poured onto a gauze or cotton wool pad. The former set-up is preferable is it allows much more control of the depth and recovery from anaesthesia and hence should be used whenever it is possible and practical to do so. In the latter device the gas concentration is dependent on the temperature, and in cold winter weather it may be difficult to ensure that the anaesthetic agent actually vaporises. All volatile anaesthetics are irritant when in their liquid state, so the chamber must be designed to separate the anaesthetic-soaked gauze or cotton wool from the animal.

It can be more difficult to safely judge the correct depth of anaesthesia for birds. The avian respiratory system, which consists of a pair of relatively fixed lungs and a group of mobile air sacs, is more efficient at gas exchange than that of mammals and, therefore, birds will often demonstrate a more rapid response to the effects of inhaled anaesthetics. In addition, due to the large volume of stored gases in air sacs, birds can be slow to eliminate the anaesthetics. Recovery from anaesthesia can be facilitated by maintaining the bird in lateral recumbency and turning it every few minutes.

Injectable anaesthetics

These are commonly used for larger mammals. They may be delivered through a hypodermic syringe to a trapped or caged animal (eg, badgers, wild boar), or from a distance via a dart (eg, wild boar, deer) and will usually be delivered intramuscularly.

Injectable anaesthetics may be used to induce anaesthesia, which is then maintained with a gaseous anaesthetic. In some instances, particularly with small animals that are highly active, such as weasels (*Mustela nivalis*) the opposite may apply, with short-term anaesthesia induced by inhalation and maintained by injection. It should also be noted that the injectable agent ketamine (when used in isolation) has been shown to cause psychosis in humans particularly with repeated use and hence should be avoided for wild animal anaesthesia unless used in a cocktail with other drugs (such as metomidine) (de Leeuw *et al.* 2004).

Darting

Use of a dart-gun to dart wild animals is a specialist skill and may be subject to a number of restrictions. In the UK, dart rifles and blow pipes are classified as Section 5 prohibited weapons under the Firearms Act and require both a permit from the Home Office and permission from the statutory authority before use. Furthermore, there are restrictions on the number of darts that may be held by one individual. Details may vary between authorities and advice should always be sought. When firing a dart, the aim is for the dart to hit the animal at right-angles, ensuring that the needle penetrates the subcutaneous fat and enters the muscle. The propellant pressure of the rifle should be adjusted depending upon the distance between the operator and the animal to ensure that the dart has sufficient velocity to penetrate to the muscle, but not so much that it enters the body cavity. It is essential to practise thoroughly and regularly before using this equipment on animals.

Sampling

Methods and volumes for blood sampling of wild species are similar in many instances to those for laboratory species (Joint Working Group on Refinement (JWGR), 1993), although sedation or anaesthesia may be needed for restraint. Due consideration should be given to the health and physiological status of the animal as this can affect the level of handling or the amount of blood withdrawal that can be safely undertaken without causing the animal to go into hypovolaemic shock. As with laboratory animals, no more blood should be taken than is necessary and where alternative less invasive methods are available (eg, use of saliva (Figure 7.7) or faeces) these should be chosen.

If hair and/or whiskers (vibrissae) are to be taken, cutting/shaving rather than plucking is preferable if the follicles are not required. Whiskers should be taken equally from both sides of the face and only a small percentage of the total number of whiskers should be removed at any one time. Feathers should be taken from less essential areas of birds (eg, from the back rather than the wings). For stable isotope

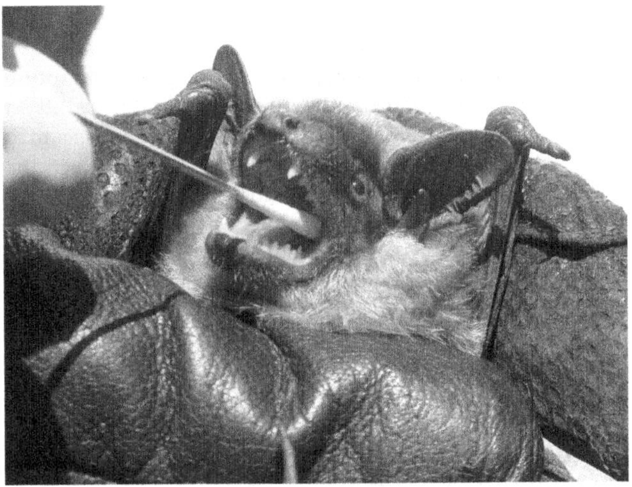

Figure 7.7 Salivary sampling of a serotine bat. Saliva can be collected without anaesthesia in many species and used instead of blood for a variety of physiological measures (eg, immunoglobulins, stress and reproductive hormones).

sampling of tissues it is important to consider the time at which tissues were formed.

Risk of infection is high in wild animals (perhaps particularly in fossorial species) and hence the use of antibacterial sprays and/or use of surgical glue, is recommended for skin protection following invasive sampling.

Marking

Recognition of individual animals plays an important part in most wildlife research. Marking can provide information about survival, site fidelity, population dynamics, social behaviour, feeding ecology and almost every facet of an animal's ecology. Several techniques are available (see also Chapter 18), such as:

- telemetry: external and internal, VHF, GPS and proximity transmitters;
- external ringing and tagging (bird and bat banding, mammal ear tags, wing tags);
- physical marking (tattooing, fur clipping, scale marking);
- internal marking (microchips, fish wire tags);
- natural markings.

Telemetric/GPS devices

A wide variety of attachment methods for both types of transmitters exists (collars, tags, implants). External devices should be as light in weight as possible and should not usually exceed 5% of the body mass of the animal (<3% is recommended). Devices that break away after sampling, at the end of the useful life of the transmitter or those with a remote release are preferable. Collars/harnesses should always be fitted to allow room for growth and natural variation in body mass, which can be pronounced in some species. For example, when fitting collars on small–medium mammals, insert fingers between the neck and the collar to judge the appropriate fit (Figure 7.8).

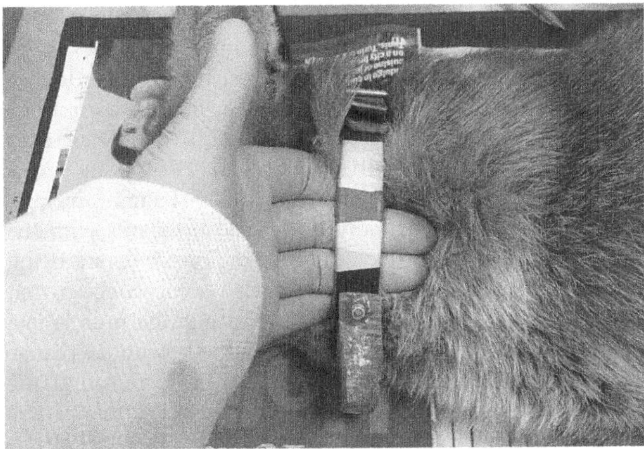

Figure 7.8 Fitting a radio collar to a red fox. It is essential that fitting of the collar is comfortable and allows for growth.

Ringing

This is the most accepted method of marking birds. In the UK, ringing is not regulated under legislation relating to animals used in research but attachment of any marks or tags to wild birds requires formal training and a permit from the British Trust for Ornithology[2]. Scientists can obtain scientific permits that are more restricted in their scope, but may require less diverse training and accreditation.

Tagging

When tagging animals, bright colours should be used with caution as they may affect camouflage and act as an attractant for predators – they also make the animals visible to members of the public. In addition, tags should be thoughtfully placed so that they are not likely to snag or get caught on vegetation, potentially leading to tissue damage, this is of particular relevance for animals that squeeze through crevices or holes (eg, bats, rats).

Physical marking

Fur clipping is a good non-invasive method of temporary marking an individual but its use is limited in most studies due to its short duration. In contrast, tattooing is a permanent mark and of great benefit in long-term population studies. However it should be noted that it always requires anaesthesia and does pose a risk of infection (especially for fossorial animals) and hence the use of antiseptic sprays or creams on the tattooed area is recommended.

Microchipping

Microchipping or the use of passive integrated transponders (PIT tags) represents a relatively recent advance in animal marking technologies (Camper & Dixon 1988) and has become the most popular method of choice for many small mammals and amphibia. The tag itself is a small cylinder (approximately 12 mm in length) and it is usually injected

[2] http://www.bto.org/ringing

subcutaneously in the scruff of the neck or can be implanted in the lymphatic cavity (particularly in amphibians or reptiles). Although available data suggest no strong evidence for lasting detrimental effects of these tags (Brown 1997) most studies concentrate on efficacy and cost rather than welfare, behaviour, growth and survival. There is anecdotal evidence suggesting that subcutaneous PIT tags can occasionally migrate, potentially leading to problems with the tag moving around the scapular region or even being expelled from the body. There is also some concern that implanting tags into the abdomen through the muscle is a relatively invasive procedure and has the potential to cause pain, necrosis of tissue and/or inflammation around the site. In addition, in some cases PIT tags are not retained as reliably as other marking techniques (Ott & Scott, 1999).

Natural marking

Individual identification based upon natural markings is an under-utilised refinement method. The theory behind individual identification involves the use of physical markings, patterns or coloration to distinguish between conspecifics. The advantage of this method is that it enables identification without extended periods of handling, therefore minimising disturbance to the animal. It also has low cost compared to other methods (Doody 1995). The age of digital photography has also provided a method of storing a large number of pictures, which can be viewed easily and transferred between facilities. The method has now been used for range of different species including many types of amphibian (Doody 1995; Loafman, 1991), cetaceans (Rugh *et al.* 1992; Neumann *et al.* 2002), birds (Bretagnolle *et al.* 1994), cheetahs (Kelly 2001) and whalesharks (Arzoumanian *et al.* 2005).

Invasive tissue marking

Marking techniques that cause significant tissue injury, such as branding and toe, ear and tail clipping, should be avoided. If no alternative methods can achieve the desired results then researchers need to ensure that the marking process does not cause unnecessary tissue damage, pain, and/or severe blood loss. Adequate pain control is a necessity when undertaking such procedures.

The method used will depend on the species and type of study. When choosing a marking technique, primary consideration should be given to methodologies that are the least invasive, do not require recapture for identification, and will remain visible for the duration of the study. In addition, marks should:

- be quick and easy to apply;
- be readily visible and distinguishable;
- persist on animals until all research objectives are fulfilled;
- not introduce bias by having variable tag retention rates;
- not cause long-term adverse effects on health, behaviour, longevity or social life;
- comply with any legal restrictions or regulations;
- allow for seasonal changes in mass and growth of juvenile animals.

Release

Animals should be released back to the point of capture when fully recovered from the procedures performed. If an animal is injured or showing signs of illness euthanasia may be required. The most humane method of dispatch in the field will depend on the species and the experience of the investigator. Table 7.1 lists some suggested methods but see also Chapter 17 and AAZV (2006). The investigator should always have the necessary equipment to euthanase target or non-target animals where appropriate (eg, anaesthetics for overdose) or, in the case of larger animals where veterinary advice may need to be sought, contact numbers for 24-hour cover.

To treat or not to treat?

There are often ethical and moral dilemmas to be faced in the treatment of wild animals. Interference with a natural process could lead to perturbation of the ecological balance and this must be considered when deciding whether or not to treat a wild animal. As a general guideline, it is accepted that injuries and illnesses that have anthropogenic causes should be treated (see Figure 7.9 for an example flow chart). In many other cases, the researcher must make an informed choice based upon his/her knowledge of the animal, the injury (or illness) and the situation. The final decision should be one that the researcher has the ability and confidence to defend.

Legislation appropriate to wildlife studies

Anyone proposing to conduct research on, study, capture, hold or release wildlife should be familiar with, and comply

Table 7.1 Methods of dispatch. Please note that these methods are not the only, or necessarily the most appropriate methods to be used in all situations. The method of dispatch used should always be decided depending on the health status of the individual, the situation, the setting, the competence of the personnel and local regulations.

Animal	*Suggested method of dispatch*
Small rodents Rats Birds	Dislocation of neck or overdose of gaseous anaesthesia
Rabbit	Dislocation of neck (requires highly skilled operator)
Hedgehog	Overdose of gaseous anaesthesia
Badger	Overdose of anaesthesia (injectable)
Bats	Overdose of gaseous anaesthesia
Fox Deer Wild boar	Overdose of anaesthesia (injectable) or shooting

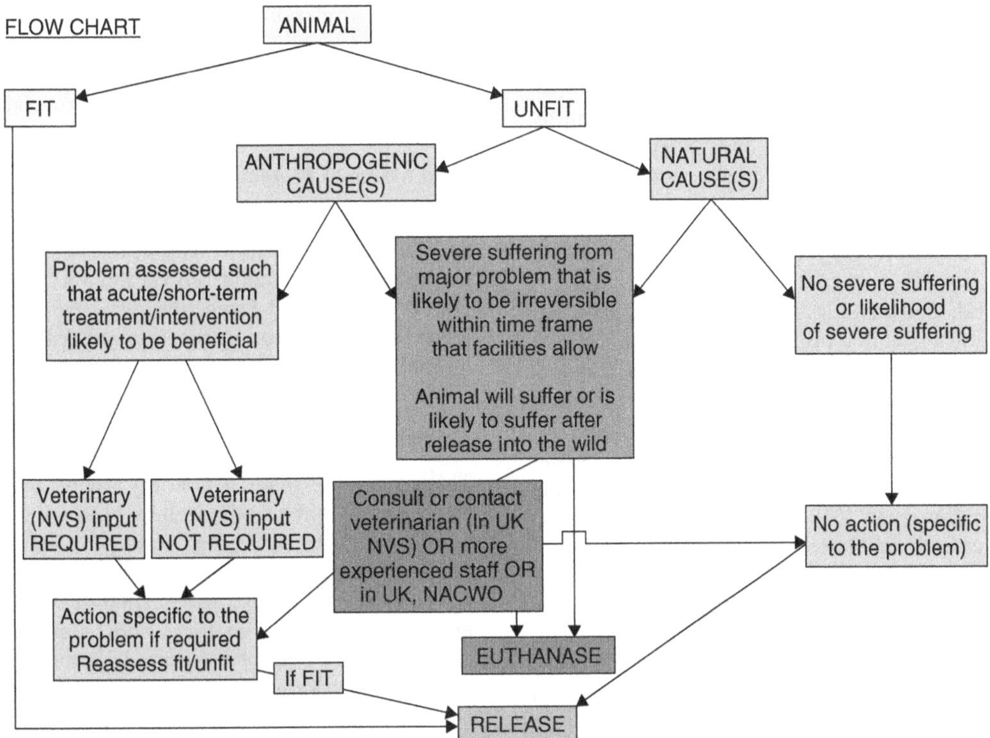

Figure 7.9 Example flow chart on dealing with injured animals in the field. It is vital that all field workers are aware of how to deal with injured target and non-target animals. This flow chart shows an example of strategies for dealing with injuries that are due to the procedure (iatrogenic) or for which the animal sustained prior to capture. In the UK veterinary advice is likely to come from the named veterinary surgeon (NVS). NACWO stands for named animal care and welfare officer, who in the UK is responsible for the day-to-day care of protected animals used in research.

with, the relevant legislation governing their use. In many cases, licences or permits are required to conduct work with wildlife. As an example, the paragraphs below list some of the provisions pertaining to wildlife research in the UK.

Legislation relating to the use of animals in research

In the UK, the Animals (Scientific procedures) Act 1986 (A(SP)A) states that all regulated work must be carried out a designated establishment (DE) unless the work requires:

- wild animals or farm species at sites that could not be reasonably part of a DE;
- studies that depend upon access to the wild environment or commercial husbandry standards.

When regulated work under A(SP)A is carried out at field sites these are classed as PODEs (places other than designated establishments). At PODEs procedures must be conducted and welfare standards maintained as near as practicable to those achievable in DEs. Additional conditions also apply to PODEs to enable appropriate controls to be applied, such as notification conditions (ie, usually the inspector is required to be notified of all PODE sites at least 72h before the onset of a regulated study). Land-owner's consent, where appropriate, must be obtained prior to applying for a licence under A(SP)A and provision must be made to allow inspectors onto all PODE sites.

Wildlife studies and/or techniques that are not regulated under A(SP)A include:

- the ringing, tagging or marking of an animal or the use of any other humane procedure for the sole purpose of enabling an animal to be identified is not a regulated procedure under A(SP)A if it causes only momentary pain or distress and no lasting harm;
- humane killing by a recognised method;
- procedures applied in the course of recognised veterinary practice;
- capture and release of wild animals unless the method of capture itself is being studied.

However, it should be noted that any of the above do become regulated if anaesthesia is used. Advice should always be sought from the local Home Office inspector in case of any doubt as to whether a procedure is regulated or not.

Certain species to be used in research may be obtained only from a designated breeding establishment, unless an official exemption is granted. Therefore, it is also illegal to trap these animals in the wild without an exemption granted by the Home Office. The animals on this list include mouse, rat, rabbit, ferret and quail. Moreover release of animals back to the wild will only be authorised if:

- the maximum possible care has been taken to safeguard the animal's well-being;
- the animal's state of health allows it to be set free;

- setting the animal free poses no danger to public health and the environment.

A(SP)A licences do not absolve the licensee from their duties under other wildlife legislation. Hence all work must comply with other appropriate legislation and other applicable licences must be in place before any studies commence.

Wildlife and Countryside Act

The Wildlife and Countryside Act 1981 is the principle mechanism for the legislative protection of wildlife in Great Britain but does not extend to Northern Ireland, the Channel Islands or the Isle of Man; the Wildlife (Northern Ireland) Order is equivalent in many respects. Most countries have similar legislation, particularly in the EU. This legislation is the means by which the Convention on the Conservation of European Wildlife and Natural Habitats (the 'Bern Convention') and latterly the Council Directive on the Conservation of Wild Birds (79/409/EEC) are implemented in Great Britain. Similar legislation is enacted to fulfil these obligations elsewhere in the United Kingdom. The Wildlife and Countryside Act (WCA) is divided into four parts with Part I being concerned with the protection of wildlife.

Part I of WCA protects all wild birds and protected animals (includes some mammals, all species of bat; species of dolphin; porpoise; otter; amphibians; reptiles; and many species of insects). A wild bird is defined as any bird of a species that is resident in or is a visitor to the European Territory of any member state in a wild state. Under the WCA it is an offence to:

- take, injure, kill or sell a protected species;
- disturb a protected species in its nest or place of shelter;
- possess a protected species.

There are additional clauses and various additional forms of protection.

However, many activities prohibited under the WCA can be carried out after acquiring a licence issued by the appropriate authority to avoid committing an offence. For example scientific study that requires capturing protected animals can be allowed by obtaining a licence.

Other wildlife legislation

The Conservation (Natural Habitats, etc) Regulations 1994

These implement the Council Directive 92/43/EEC in Great Britain under which it is an offence, with certain exceptions, to:

- deliberately capture or kill any wild animal of a European protected species;
- deliberately disturb any such animal;
- deliberately take or destroy eggs of any such wild animal;
- damage or destroy a breeding site or resting place of such a wild animal;
- deliberately pick, collect, cut, uproot or destroy a wild plant of a European protected species;
- keep, transport, sell or exchange, or offer for sale or exchange, any live or dead wild animal or plant of a European protected species, or any part of, or anything derived from such a wild animal or plant.

Wild Mammal Protection Act 1996

This act covers unprotected mammals to prevent unnecessary suffering by certain methods such as self-locking snares, explosives, drowning, asphyxiation and use of live decoys. The Wild Mammal Protection Act 1996 does not apply in legal pest control or in the humane killing of an injured animal.

Animal Welfare Act 2006

This act ensures that it is not only against the law to be cruel to an animal, but also the welfare needs of the animals must be met. A 'protected animal' under this act is domesticated, not living in a wild state, or under control of man (either permanently or temporarily). The latter does include wild animals captured even for a short period. An offence is caused when an '*act of a responsible person causes an animal to suffer ... and suffering is unnecessary*'. '*Suffering for a legitimate purpose*', eg, research is permissible but only if suffering is proportionate to purpose of the conduct, and it could not have been avoided or reduced, and the conduct concerned was that of a reasonably competent and humane person.

CITES

The Convention on International Trade of Endangered Species provides protection to specified endangered species and on the taking, handling and transport of samples taken or collected from them[3]. This can constrain the international movement of samples collected for scientific purposes so advice should always be sought about the application of CITES regulations in research on CITES listed species.

Other examples of legislation include acts that are designed for the protection of specific groups of wildlife. In the UK this includes acts such as:

- The Protection of Badgers Act 1992;
- The Deer Act 1991;
- The Ground Game Act 1880;
- The Whaling Industry (Regulation) Act 1934;
- The Conservation of Seals Act 1970;
- The Salmon and Freshwater Fisheries Act 1975;
- The Dangerous Wild Animals Act 1976;

Some of these acts have parallel legislation in Scotland and Northern Ireland.

Licences

Natural England (the Countryside Council for Wales, Scottish Natural Heritage and Northern Ireland Environ-

[3] http://www.defra.gov.uk/animalhealth/CITES/

ment Agency have similar arrangements) is responsible for issuing licences and permits through their Wildlife Management and Licensing Service under a range of wildlife legislation for activities that would otherwise be illegal but where a valid justification exists.

International legislation

Many countries have their own guidance and legislation regarding the use of animals in research and the protection of animals in the wild. It is important that researchers are aware of the local regulations in different countries and abide by these and the best practice guidelines (see below). Links and information are available regarding animal research and welfare legislation for many areas in the world, including USA, New Zealand, Canada and Europe[4].

Best practice guidelines

The key to carrying out wildlife studies in the field to the highest standards is to follow best practice guidelines wherever possible. Below is a selection of relevant websites, most of which have links to further resources.

UK

National Centre for the Replacement, Refinement and Reduction of Animals in Research (NC3Rs)

http://www.nc3rs.org.uk

Microsites on a number of topics with relevance to field studies; of particular interest is their site on Three Rs and wildlife research, but also there are sites on dosing and sampling and anaesthesia that include information appropriate to studying animals in the field.

Association for the Study of Animal Behaviour (ASAB)

http://asab.nottingham.ac.uk/ethics/guidelines.php

Guidelines relating to conducting animal research with some areas particularly associated with field studies (eg, marking) and also has links with other websites that contain information with respect to welfare and ethical treatment of animals.

British Association for Shooting and Conservation (BASC)

http://www.basc.org.uk/

Although not a welfare organisation, BASC has codes of practice on trapping of pest mammals and pest birds which include information on the different legislations, and practical tips on topics, such as how to reduce non-targets and the appropriate setting and positioning of traps which may be of help in conducting field studies of these species.

[4] http://www.animalethics.org.au/legislation/international

Worldwide

Norwegian Consensus-platform for Replacement, Reduction and Refinement of Animal Experiments (norecopa)

http://www.norecopa.no

Guidelines for wildlife research particularly relating to the Three Rs.

Canadian Council for Animal Care (CCAC)

http://www.ccac.ca

Three Rs microsite with a special section on its implementation on wildlife research and refinement alternatives for marking and tagging.

Concluding remarks

This chapter is intended as a signpost to the issues that a potential researcher should be considering but does not cover all outcomes that are possible in an ever-changing environment. Before embarking on a field study, preparation is key. A checklist of considerations can be of great benefit, an example of which is given below:

- Do you need to use animals to achieve your aims?
- Are you using the lowest number of animals to achieve your aims?
- Are you using the least invasive but effective methods?
- Have you checked best practice guidelines?
- Have you got the appropriate legal authorities (eg, licences)?
- Have you sought advice from others (eg, veterinary surgeon)?
- Have you checked the weather forecast?
- Have you checked breeding seasons?
- Have you checked your field equipment is the most appropriate for your target species and is fully functional?
- Have you minimised non-target risk?
- Do you know how to treat/dispatch injured animals?
- Do you know how to check and ensure the welfare of the animals before discharging them from your care?

The wildlife researcher has to be prepared for any eventuality and ensure the welfare of the animals within their care is maintained at the highest possible level. This is best achieved by always considering the Three Rs, being aware of best practice guidelines and taking advice from colleagues and other experts in the relevant scientific fields.

References

AAZV (2006) *Guidelines for Euthanasia of Nondomestic Animals*. American Association of Zoo Veterinarians. http://www.aazv.org (accessed 21 July 09)

Abbott, D.H., Keverne, E.B., Bercovitch, F.B. *et al*. (2003) Are subordinates always stressed? A comparative analysis of rank differences in cortisol levels among primates. *Hormones and Behavior*, **43**, 67–82

Ashauer, R., Boxall, A.B. and Brown, C.D. (2007) New ecotoxicological model to simulate survival of aquatic invertebrates after exposure to fluctuations and sequential pulses of pesticides. *Environmental Science and Technology*, **41**, 1480–1486

Arzoumanian, Z., Holmberg, J. and Norman, B. (2005) An astronomical pattern matching algorithm for computer-aided identification of whalesharks Rhincondon type. *Journal of Applied Ecology*, **42**, 999–1011

Barnard, C. (2007) Ethical regulation and animal science: why animal behaviour is special. *Animal Behaviour*, **74**, 5–13

Bermúdez, R., Faílde, L.D., Losadab, A.P. *et al.* (2009) Toxoplasmosis in Bennett's wallabies (*Macropus rufogriseus*) in Spain. *Veterinary Parasitology*, **160**, 155–158

Bretagnolle, V., Thibault, J. and Dominici, J. (1994) Field identification of individual osprey using head marking pattern. *Journal of Wildlife Management*, **58**, 175–178

Broom, D.M. and Johnson, K. (1993) *Stress and Animal Welfare*. Blackwell Publishing, Oxford

Brown, L.J. (1997) An evaluation of some marking and trapping techniques currently used in the study of anuran population dynamics. *Journal of Herpetology*, **31**, 410–419

Burley, N. (1986) Sexual selection for aesthetic traits in species with biparental care. *American Naturalist*, **127**, 415–445

Camper, J.D. and Dixon, J.R. (1988) Evaluation of a microchip marking system for amphibians and reptiles. *Journal of Herpetology*, **22**, 425–433

Carter, S.P., Delahay, R.J., Smith, G.C. *et al.* (2007) Culling-induced social perturbation in Eurasian badger *Meles meles* and management of TB in cattle: an analysis of a critical problem in applied ecology. *Proceedings of The Royal Society of London B*, **274**, 2769–2777

Clarke, R.D. (1972) The effect of toe clipping on survival in fowlers toad (*Bufo woodhousei fowleri*). *Copeia*, **1**, 182–185

Conner, M.C., Soutiere, E.C. and Lancia, R.A. (1987) Drop-netting deer: costs and incidence of capture myopathy. *Wildlife Society Bulletin*, **15**, 434–438

Cuthill, I.C. (2007) Ethical regulation and animal science: why animal behaviour is not so special. *Animal Behaviour*, **74**, 15–22

Doody, J.S. (1995) A photographic mark-recapture method for patterned amphibians. *Herpetological Review*, **26**, 19–21

Dytham, C. (2003) *Choosing and Using Statistics. A Biologists Guide*. Blackwell Publishing, Oxford

Feinsinger, P. (2001) *Designing Field Studies for Biodiversity and Conservation*. Island Press, Washington, DC

Flecknell, P.A. (2009) *Laboratory Animal Anaesthesia*, 3rd edn. Academic Press, London

Golay, N. and Durrer, H. (1994). Inflamation due to toe clipping in natterjack toads (*Bufo calamita*). *Amphibia–Reptilia*, **15**, 81–83

Hall, L.W., Clarke, K.W. and Trim, C.M. (2000) Anaesthesia of birds, laboratory animals and wild animals. In: *Veterinary Anaesthesia*, 10th edn., pp. 463–478. Elsevier Press Ltd, London

Haulton, S.M., Porter, W.F. and Rudolph, B.A. (2001) Evaluating 4 methods to capture white-tailed deer. *Wildlife Society Bulletin*, **29**, 255–264

Inglis, I.R., Isaacson, A.J., Smith, G.C. *et al.* (1997) The effect on the woodpigeon (*Columba palumbus*) of the introduction of oilseed rape into Britain. *Agriculture Ecosystems & Environment*, **61**, 113–121

Joint Working Group on Refinement (1993) Removal of blood from laboratory mammals and birds. First Report of the BVA/FRAME/RSPCA/UFAW Joint Working Group on Refinement. *Laboratory Animals*, **27**, 1–22

Kelly, M.J. (2001) Computer-aided photograph matching in studies using individual identification: and example from Serengeti cheetahs. *Journal of Mammalogy*, **82**, 440–449

Lane, J. (2006) Can non-invasive glucocorticoid measures be used as reliable indicators of stress in animals? *Animal Welfare*, **15**, 331–342

de Leeuw, A.N.S., Forrester, G.J. and Spyvee, P.D. (2004) Experimental comparison of ketamine with a combination of ketamine, butorphanol and medetomidine for general anaesthesia of the Eurasian badger (*Meles meles L.*). *Veterinary Journal*, **167**, 186–193

Loafman, R. (1991) Identifying individual spotted salamanders by spot pattern. *Herpetological Review*, **22**, 91–92

May, R. (2004) Ecology: ethics and amphibians. *Nature*, **431**, 403

Moorhouse, T.P. and Macdonald, D.W. (2005) Indirect negative impacts of radio-collaring: sex ratio variation in water voles. *Journal of Applied Ecology*, **42**, 91–98

Munck, A., Guyre, P.M. and Holbrook, N.J. (1984) Physioloigical functions of glucocrticoids in stress and their relation to pharmacological actions. *Endocrine Review*, **5**, 25–41

Neumann, D.R., Leitenberger, A. and Orams, M.B. (2002) Photo identification of short beaked common dolphins (*Delphinus delphis*) in north east New Zealand: a photo catalogue of recognisable individuals. *New Zealand Journal of Marine and Freshwater Research*, **36**, 593–604

Ott, J.A. and Scott, D.E. (1999) Effects of toe clipping and PIT-tagging on growth and survival in metamorphic Ambystomaopacum. *Journal of Herpetology*, **33**, 344–348

Overli, O., Sorensen, C. and Nilsson, G.E. (2006) Behavioral indicators of stress-coping style in rainbow trout: Do males and females react differently to novelty? *Physiology & Behavior*, **87**, 506–512

Reaser, J. (1995) Marking amphibians by toe-clipping; a response to Halliday. *FROGLOG*, **12**, 1–2

Recher, H., Gowing, G. and Armstrong, T. (1985) Causes and frequency of deaths among birds mist-netted for banding studies at 2 localities. *Australian Wildlife Research*, **12**, 321–326

Rivier, C. and Vale, W. (1984) Influence of CRF on reproductive functions in the rat. *Endocrinology*, **114**, 914–921

Rugh, D.J., Braham, H.W. and Miller, G.L. (1992) Method of photographic identification of bowhead whales, *Balaena mysticetus*. *Canadian Journal of Zoology*, **70**, 617–624

Sapolsky, R.M., Romero, L.M. and Munck, A.U. (2000) How do glucocorticoids influence stress responses? Integrating permissive, suppressive, stimulatory and preparative actions. *Endocrine Reviews*, **21**, 55–89

Schaffner, C.M. and French, J.A. (2004) Behavioral and endocrine responses in male marmosets to the establishment of multi-male breeding groups: Evidence for non-monopolizing facultative polyandry. *International Journal of Primatology*, **25**, 709–732

Schultz, T.W., Rogers, K. and Aptula, A.O. (2009) Read-across to rank skin sensitization potential: subcategories for the Michael acceptor domain. *Contact Dermatitis*, **60**, 21–31

Teixeira, C.P., De Azevedo, C.S. and Mendl, M. (2007) Revisiting translocation and reintroduction programmes: the importance of considering stress. *Animal Behaviour*, **73**, 1–13

Wilkinson, D., Smith, G.C. and Delahay, R.J. (2004) A model of bovine tuberculosis in the badger *Meles meles*: an evaluation of different vaccination strategies. *Journal of Applied Ecology*, **41**, 492–501

Yokoyama, A.K. (1965) The effect of anaesthesia on milk yield and maintenance of lactation in the goat and rat. *Journal of Endocrinology*, **33**, 341–351

8 Legislation and oversight of the conduct of research using animals: a global overview

Kathryn Bayne, Timothy H. Morris and Malcolm P. France

Introduction

This chapter serves to highlight key aspects of laws, regulations, policies and/or codes that apply to the use of animals in biomedical research and testing. An exhaustive review of all relevant, but adjunct regulations (eg, pertaining to animal transportation both domestically and internationally; occupational health and safety; importation/exportation; etc) is beyond the scope of this chapter. In addition, in some jurisdictions the conduct of veterinary clinical research and veterinary clinical trials of new devices, vaccines and pharmaceuticals may be covered by separate mechanisms of oversight. However, as these subjects can have a significant role in the operation of an animal facility, readers are encouraged to review applicable standards in these areas.

Many, but not all, countries and jurisdictions around the world have laws, regulations, policies and other systems of oversight relating to the use of animals in science. There are variations in scope, scale, approach; in legal basis; in social and cultural perspectives; and in implementation. Variability in regulatory delivery and application of such oversight is likely to continue, but there is increasing convergence of the outputs of this oversight. In particular, there is increased emphasis on a wider scope of oversight to include all facets of animal use, in particular on ethical aspects, and on standards and approaches to animal care and welfare.

The regulatory environment for animals in biomedical research and testing is, therefore, both variable across countries, and also in many parts of the world is in a state of evolution. Different approaches have been taken by various countries to improve the welfare of animals used in research, to develop and maintain high-quality science and to address ethical issues. In some countries, the individual scientist is licensed to conduct research, while elsewhere the institution (eg, university or pharmaceutical company) may hold the licence to do animal-based research. In some countries, a wide range of animals (vertebrate and invertebrate, warm and cold blooded) is covered by government standards, while in other countries there are no government regulations, or government standards cover select species of animals. Some countries require ethical review of proposed research, while in others no institutional or governmental review of the proposed study is necessary before work can begin. Similarly, some countries require researchers to have appropriate training and qualifications while others do not. Voluntary oversight schemes are of importance in several countries. This chapter describes some of the similarities and distinctions between countries/regions where biomedical research is conducted by describing the regulatory climate and systems of oversight in several countries. Its purpose is to provide an introduction to the range of legislative approaches, and it is neither a summary of all national regulations nor a critical review.

The increasing availability of laws and regulations in an electronic format has enhanced access to this information by countries that are in the process of developing their own standards. Some countries (eg, Singapore) have assessed the regulations of many different countries and selected those that apply best for their cultural and scientific environment. Such action can lead to a convergence of approaches in providing animal research oversight, as oversight systems viewed as useful are used as resources for developing a customised regulatory framework. In general, such increased availability of information has increased harmonisation in approaches to assuring research animal welfare.

The increasing internationalisation of research has led to greater interest in systems of accreditation, both for institutions in emerging scientific locations to demonstrate their standards and for institutions in established scientific areas to assure standards. Non-governmental oversight bodies (eg, the Association for Assessment and Accreditation of Laboratory Animal Care International) have a key role, and in some cases the primary role, in harmonising standards for animal care and use around the world, for example by requiring committee review of proposed research at institutions in countries where there is no such requirement. Thus, while approaches may differ among countries, the goals of good animal welfare, attention to ethics and high-quality science are the same. Nonetheless, differences remain in the standards required by different nations. Therefore, there is an ongoing imperative, both for animal welfare reasons and to ensure a level playing field, that regulations and other means of oversight should reflect current knowledge of animal welfare science.

History

Animals have been used in science for centuries (Dunlop & Williams 1996), but formal oversight of such animal use developed from the eighteenth century. This was the period when study of animals was revived on a larger scale in European and North American universities, having fallen into disuse after earlier extensive use by Greek and Arab societies. As this use grew, so too did concern, both for the animals themselves, and also about how lack of respect for animals and how they were used would *'corrupt'* humans. Even before laws were proposed in the nineteenth century in the United Kingdom (UK), to regulate research using animals, the tensions between the need for such research and animal welfare were present. There was both support for animal use as well as concern for their *'pain and suffering'* (Dunlop & Williams 1996). It is interesting that one prescient set of principles for research laid out at that time was that there should be: (1) no alternative; (2) a clear objective; (3) avoidance of repetition of work; (4) minimisation of suffering; and (5) full and detailed publication (Rupke 1987). See also the discussion of early proposals similar to the Three Rs (3 Rs) in Chapter 2.

A general trend in oversight has been to move the focus from avoiding 'cruelty' and on sanitary aspects, to a wider perspective on experimental animal health, welfare and ethics. Early laws and guidelines gave fellow scientists control over other scientists' specified use of animals (Select Committee on Animals in Scientific Procedures 2002) and were aimed at controlling and excluding diseases that clearly confounded early animal experimentation (Walker & Poppleton 1967).

It is important to reiterate that oversight can include voluntary as well as legally required activities, and both approaches may be useful mechanisms to address broader animal welfare and ethical issues (Orlans 2001). For example, the basic Russian law on animal experimentation (Russian Ministry of Health 1973) focuses on hygiene, husbandry and facilities but, in practice, establishments are becoming increasingly aware of broader issues. Key guidance documents have been translated into many languages, including Russian (eg, National Research Council 1996). A recent example of new regulatory requirements is the Japanese Guidelines on animal experimentation which now include aspects such as replacement, reduction and refinement (Science Council of Japan 2006).

Principles

The Three Rs

The principles of the Three Rs, consisting of replacement, reduction and refinement (see Chapter 2) were developed by the UFAW Scholars, Professors William MS Russell and Rex Burch. The Three Rs were first presented at a UFAW symposium in 1957 entitled *'Humane Techniques in the Laboratory'* and published as *'The Principles of Humane Experimental Technique'* in 1959 (Russell & Burch 1959). The term alternatives, while sometimes confused with replacement is commonly used to refer to all Three Rs. Definitions of the Three Rs have evolved over the last half century (Buchanan-Smith *et al.* 2005), but the original text (Russell & Burch1959) remains valid and important:

> We shall use the term 'replacement technique' for any scientific method employing non-sentient material which may in the history of experimentation replace methods which use conscious living vertebrates.
>
> Reduction means reduction in the numbers of animals used to obtain information of a given amount and precision.
>
> Suppose, for a particular purpose, we cannot use replacing techniques. Suppose it is agreed that we shall be using every device of theory and practice to reduce to a minimum the number of animals we have to employ. It is at this point that refinement starts, and its object is simply to reduce to an absolute minimum the amount of distress imposed on those animals that are still used.

Since 1957, and in particular over the last 20 years, the Three Rs have increasingly become, either explicitly (eg, Science Council of Japan 2006) or implicitly (eg, Interagency Research Animal Committee (IRAC) 1985), a key, if not the leading, ethical principle for the care and use of animals used in science.

International Guiding Principles for Biomedical Research Involving Animals

The International Guiding Principles for Biomedical Research Involving Animals were developed by the Council for International Organizations of Medical Sciences (CIOMS 1985). CIOMS is an international, non-governmental, non-profit organization established jointly by the World Health Organization and the United Nations in 1949 and is representative of a substantial proportion of the biomedical scientific community. These principles for animal experimentation were, in part, created because national and international ethical codes and laws for human experimentation mandate that new substances or devices should not be used for the first time on human beings unless previous tests on animals have provided a reasonable presumption of their safety. The principles provide a framework for ethical animal use (Box 8.1). Other areas covered include animal acquisition, transportation, housing, environmental conditions, nutrition, the provision of veterinary care, the maintenance of records, euthanasia, the monitoring of animal care and use, the implementation of the Three Rs, and the training of investigators and others in animal care and use.

The World Organisation for Animal Health (OIE)

Recently the OIE have taken an interest in the use of animals in research. Proposals have been published for OIE members to follow when formulating regulatory requirements for the use of live animals in research, testing or teaching (World Organisation for Animal Health 2009). The proposed standards give prominence to the Three Rs, protocol and programme review, training of those involved in veterinary care, the animal facilities, as well as animal health control.

Engineering versus performance standards

Standards can be performance based, specifying the outcomes but not the methods to achieve outcomes, or engineering based, specifying measurements, activities or

Box 8.1 CIOMS International Guiding Principles for Biomedical Research Involving Animals

I. The advancement of biological knowledge and the development of improved means for the protection of the health and well-being both of man and of animals require recourse to experimentation on intact live animals of a wide variety of species.

II. Methods such as mathematical models, computer simulation and *in vitro* biological systems should be used wherever appropriate.

III. Animal experiments should be undertaken only after due consideration of their relevance for human or animal health and the advancement of biological knowledge.

IV. The animals selected for an experiment should be of an appropriate species and quality, and the minimum number required to obtain scientifically valid results.

V. Investigators and other personnel should never fail to treat animals as sentient, and should regard their proper care and use and the avoidance or minimisation of discomfort, distress, or pain as ethical imperatives.

VI. Investigators should assume that procedures that would cause pain in human beings cause pain in other vertebrate species, although more needs to be known about the perception of pain in animals.

VII. Procedures with animals that may cause more than momentary or minimal pain or distress should be performed with appropriate sedation, analgesia, or anaesthesia in accordance with accepted veterinary practice. Surgical or other painful procedures should not be performed on unanaesthetised animals paralysed by chemical agents.

VIII. Where waivers are required in relation to the provisions of article VII, the decisions should not rest solely with the investigators directly concerned but should be made, with due regard to the provisions of articles IV, V, and VI, by a suitably constituted review body. Such waivers should not be made solely for the purposes of teaching or demonstration.

IX. At the end of, or, when appropriate, during an experiment, animals that would otherwise suffer severe or chronic pain, distress, discomfort, or disablement that cannot be relieved should be painlessly killed.

X. The best possible living conditions should be maintained for animals kept for biomedical purposes. Normally the care of animals should be under the supervision of veterinarians having experience in laboratory animal science. In any case, veterinary care should be available as required.

XI. It is the responsibility of the director of an institute or department using animals to ensure that investigators and personnel have appropriate qualifications or experience for conducting procedures on animals. Adequate opportunities shall be provided for in-service training, including the proper and humane concern for the animals under their care.

processes (National Research Council 1996). Performance standards have the advantage of flexibility, which may be useful where species, previous history of the animals, facilities, expertise of the people and research goals need to be taken into account, but are open to more variability. The performance approach requires professional input and judgement to achieve outcome goals. Engineering standards are useful to establish a baseline, but are not as useful when a goal or outcome, such as well-being, sanitation, or personnel safety, needs to be specified. Moreover, they may not encourage the development of higher standards. Optimally, engineering and performance standards should be used in tandem, thereby providing baseline standards while allowing flexibility and the application of informed professional judgement.

Adequate veterinary care

Veterinary care by trained and experienced specialists is fundamentally important to the delivery of a programme of humane and scientifically valid animal care and use. This is reflected in many countries' provisions for regulation or oversight.

The United States Department of Agriculture's (USDA) Animal Welfare Regulations (US Department of Agriculture 1991) and the Public Health Service (PHS) Policy on Humane Care and Use of Laboratory Animals (Policy) (Office of Laboratory Animal Welfare (OLAW) 2002) stipulate that the veterinarian has the authority to oversee several key components of the animal care and use programme, including: animal procurement and transportation; quarantine, stabilisation and separation of animals; surveillance, diagnosis, treatment and control of disease; surgery; the selection of analgesic and anaesthetic agents; method of euthanasia; animal husbandry and nutrition; sanitation practices; zoonosis control; and hazard containment. The veterinarian must be qualified through either experience or training in laboratory animal medicine or in the species being used. The veterinarian brings a specific perspective to the deliberations of the Institutional Animal Care and Use Committee (IACUC), and is a voting member of the IACUC. The Animal Welfare Regulations describe the programme of adequate veterinary care as including:

- the availability of appropriate facilities, personnel, equipment and services;
- the use of appropriate methods to prevent, control, diagnose and treat diseases and injuries, inclusive of the availability of emergency, weekend and holiday care;
- daily observation of all animals to assess their health and well-being;
- guidance to researchers regarding handling, immobilisation, anaesthesia, analgesia, tranquillisation and euthanasia;
- nutrition;
- pest and parasite control;
- adequate pre-procedural and post-procedural care in accordance with current professional standards (see also Animal and Plant Health Inspection Service

(APHIS) Tech Note March 1999, Animal Care Policy #3[1], and APHIS Form 7002 (APHIS 1992)).

The Report of the American College of Laboratory Animal Medicine on Adequate Veterinary Care in Research, Testing and Teaching (1996) describes a programme of adequate veterinary care as including:

- disease detection and surveillance, prevention, diagnosis, treatment and resolution;
- provision of guidance on anaesthetics, analgesics, tranquilliser drugs and methods of euthanasia;
- the review and approval of all pre-operative, surgical and post-operative procedures;
- the promotion and monitoring of an animal's well-being before, during and after its use;
- involvement in the review and approval of all animal care and use at the institution.

This report is used by the Association for Assessment and Accreditation of Laboratory Animal Care (AAALAC International, see later in this chapter) as a reference standard in its assessments of animal care and use programmes.

More recently, the Federation of European Laboratory Animal Science Associations (FELASA), the European Society of Laboratory Animal Veterinarians (ESLAV) and the European College of Laboratory Animal Medicine (ECLAM) have produced European Guidelines for the Veterinary Care of Laboratory Animals (Joint Working Group on Veterinary Care 2008) These are designed to inform the general requirement for veterinary care and advise in the European Directive controlling animal experimentation (European Council 1986). Core veterinary roles include:

- all activities directly related to the animals to promote their welfare, such as during transportation, health monitoring and health management, husbandry, selection of environmental enrichment, surgery, anaesthesia, analgesia and euthanasia;
- scientific activities, often as a scientific collaborator and adviser in laboratory animal science;
- activities related to regulatory and administrative compliance; the veterinarian must be knowledgeable about relevant legislation, including any appropriate ethical review process;
- education and training of personnel and guidance of administrative staff, animal care staff and scientists to the benefit of the animals, the science and the institution.

The guidelines also emphasise the need for appropriate training and continuing professional development to ensure competence is established and maintained.

Training

The importance of adequate training for all those involved in the animal care and use programme is underscored by the emphasis it receives in regulation and policy such as the US Animal Welfare Regulations, PHS Policy, the *Guide for the Care and Use of Laboratory Animals* (*Guide*) (NRC 1996), and the Council of Europe Convention for the Protection of Vertebrate Animals used for Experimental and other Scientific Purposes Resolution on education and training of persons working with laboratory animals (Council of Europe 1993). This emphasis is also reflected in other jurisdictions.

The US Animal Welfare Regulations and PHS Policy require institutions to ensure that people caring for or using animals are qualified to do so. The Animal Welfare Regulations stipulate that several key topics be included in the institution's training programme. They are:

- humane methods of animal maintenance and experimentation, including the basic needs of each species of animal, proper handling and care for the various species of animals used by the institution, proper pre-procedural and post-procedural care of animals, and aseptic surgical methods and procedures;
- the concept, availability and use of research or testing methods that limit the use of animals or minimise animal distress;
- proper use of anaesthetics, analgesics and tranquillisers for any species of animal at the institution;
- methods to report any deficiencies in animal care and treatment;
- use of the services at the National Agricultural Library, such as appropriate methods of animal care and use, alternatives to the use of live animals in research, prevention of unintended and unnecessary duplication of research involving animals, information regarding the intent and requirements of the Animal Welfare Act.

The *Guide* urges that adequate training should be provided to members serving on the IACUC so that they can appropriately discharge their responsibilities. In addition, the *Guide* recommends that the professional and technical personnel caring for animals should be trained, as should investigators, research technicians, trainees (including students) and visiting scientists. The *Guide* also endorses training in occupational health and safety, in procedures that are specific to an employee's job and in procedures specific to research (eg, anaesthesia, surgery, euthanasia, recognition of the signs of pain and/or distress, etc).

Over the last decade, there has been regionalisation and internationalisation of training standards. A particularly strong example is the development of training guidelines across Europe. These are based on a resolution adopted out of the Council of Europe Convention for the Protection of Vertebrate Animals used for Experimental and other Scientific Purposes (Council of Europe (COE) 1986). This resolution on education and training of persons working with laboratory animals (COE 1993) defined four categories of persons working with laboratory animals and their training needs:

- Category A: persons taking care of animals;
- Category B: persons carrying out procedures;
- Category C: persons responsible for directing or designing procedures;
- Category D: laboratory animal science specialists.

[1]http://www.aphis.usda.gov/animal_welfare/downloads/policy/policy3.pdf

FELASA has elaborated these training requirements for each of these categories into training guidelines (FELASA 1995, 1999, 2000) and an accreditation scheme for provision of this training (FELASA 2002). These guidelines have become the *de facto* requirement for training and education across Europe, and are also being used elsewhere in the world.

This trend to wider application of guidelines is seen in other areas. Animal technology certification is heavily influenced by the certification programmes of the American Association for Laboratory Animal Science across the Americas, whilst in Europe and beyond, the European Federation of Animal Technicians is increasingly influenced by the programmes from the UK Institute of Animal Technology. More recently, there have been moves to share standards for certification of specialists in Laboratory Animal Medicine by the formation of an International Association of Colleges of Laboratory Animal Medicine[2].

Institutional and governmental authorisation

Institution-based review is the commonest method of authorisation around the world. Whilst there may be oversight of these activities by a national authority, often this is the single layer of authorisation.

The committee or process that is designated to review proposed uses of animals has been variously called the Animal Care Committee (Canada), Ethics Committee (Europe) and the IACUC (US). This group of individuals, operating as a committee or process, representing institutional and public interests, has the responsibility for oversight and evaluation of the entire animal care and use programme and facilities. Because they act on behalf of the institution, their role is pivotal to engendering a humane and progressive animal care and use programme. The term programme is used to describe all aspects of animal care and use. The successful programme is overseen by a committee that is engaged, knowledgeable and receives strong administrative support. Because the committee is responsible for investigating reports of concern regarding animal welfare, the committee's functions must be well known throughout the institution and there must be ready (and confidential) access to the committee.

Previously, where there was central authorisation by a national or regional authority, an approach common in Europe, this was often the sole process. The trend is now to include local institutional or regional 'ethical' review, in conjunction with governmental authorisation procedures. These two approaches can be complementary or additive, depending on the detailed requirements.

Special procedures often operate for approval of the use of certain species, such as non-human primates, dogs, cats, and equidae (eg, Council of Europe 1986; US Department of Agriculture 1991).

The ethical component of this review activity may be explicit or implicit, depending on regulatory requirements, but especially on the cultural norms in each jurisdiction. For example, in Europe, at present, it is commonly explicit but not always legally mandated (FELASA Working Group on Ethical Evaluation of Animal Experiments 2007). In Asia it may be less explicit in terms of 'ethical review'; but ethics is implicit in approaches such as memorials to animals used in research which encourage reflection on ethical aspects of such animal use (Slaughter 2002).

Inspection and compliance

Systems of inspection, with consequences for non-compliance, are operated in some jurisdictions, although they may or may not be perceived as fully or effectively implemented (European Parliament 2002). The inspection system is usually government controlled but there may also be other means of oversight, such as the peer-review system used by AAALAC International. Sanctions for non-compliance are highly varied and may include fines, imprisonment, denial of authority to conduct research or withdrawal of accreditation.

International accreditation of animal care and use programmes

There are two systems currently in place that accredit programmes that use animals in research, testing or teaching. One is the accreditation offered by the Canadian Council on Animal Care (CCAC), which is generally limited to institutions located in Canada (see below). The other is AAALAC International's global accreditation system. AAALAC International is a non-profit organization that was formed in 1965. AAALAC's mission is to promote the humane treatment of animals in science through confidential, voluntary accreditation of animal care and use programmes. The Association is comprised of a Board of Trustees from 69 scientific organizations, patient advocacy groups, laboratory animal medical and science organizations and research lobby groups; a Council on Accreditation made up of veterinarians, animal researchers, research administrators and facility managers who are experts in the field of laboratory animal science and medicine; a roster of consultants who assist Council with the on-site evaluations and an office staff. The Board of Trustees sets the vision and general direction of the Association, the Council on Accreditation is responsible for the conduct of site visits and for determining the accreditation status of institutions, and the office staff (US, Europe and Pacific Rim regional offices) serves as a point of coordination of these activities and as an information resource to the laboratory animal using community.

AAALAC does not establish policies to which institutions must conform. Rather, AAALAC International relies principally on the *Guide*, as well as national laws, regulations and policies, and numerous scientifically based standards, referred to as '*reference resources*', which address specific subject areas (eg, recombinant DNA, surgery, euthanasia), for evaluation of animal care and use programmes around the world (Bayne & Martin 1998; Bayne & Miller 2000). The accreditation process includes an extensive internal review conducted by the institution, which is summarised in an animal care and use programme description. On-site visits are announced and conducted every 3 years. There is also

[2] http://www.iaclam.org

an annual report requirement. The standards and process for accreditation are described in the Association's Rules of Accreditation. Non-conformance with AAALAC International standards results in formal notification that full accreditation has not been granted and provision of a timeline for correcting identified deficiencies. Sustained or serious non-conformance can result in revocation of accreditation.

Regional and international harmonisation of guidelines

Regionally or internationally, some organisations promote greater harmonisation of standards. As examples, FELASA has also issued guidelines that include health monitoring, control of pain and distress and use of transgenic animals, and the International Council for Laboratory Animal Science (ICLAS) has a programme of producing harmonised guidance that includes euthanasia and humane endpoints.

Western Europe

After much public debate the UK passed the first legislation in the world to regulate animal research. The 1876 UK Cruelty to Animals Act made provision to permit certain experiments on live animals subject to support from eminent scientists (Nuffield Council on Bioethics 2005). This law was replaced in 1986 with the UK Animals (Scientific Procedures) Act. This introduced formal controls on sources of animals, re-use of animals and euthanasia. It also set out requirements to consider alternatives, to ensure training, to set up an advisory committee and to publish wide-ranging codes of practice on health, refinement, husbandry and care (Her Majesty's Stationery Office 1985). Previously, these wider aspects had developed as voluntary guidelines (Biological Council 1984). Such broadening of the scope was part of the trend for more comprehensive laws, such as the European Directive for the protection of animals used for experimental and other scientific purposes (European Council 1986) and the International Guiding Principles for Biomedical Research Involving Animals (Council for International Organizations of Medical Sciences 1985).

The use of animals in scientific procedures in Europe is covered by two overlapping legal instruments that are currently very similar. The first is the Council of Europe Convention for the Protection of Vertebrate Animals used for Experimental and other Scientific Purposes (Council of Europe 1986), and the second is the European Union's Council Directive on the approximation of laws, regulations and administrative provisions of the member states regarding the protection of animals used for experimental and other scientific purposes (European Council 1986).

The 47 member states of the Council of Europe can choose whether to participate in developing a convention, and can choose whether to ratify it. In 2007 less than half the member States of the Council of Europe had ratified the Convention for the Protection of Vertebrate Animals used for Experimental and other Scientific Purposes. In contrast, European Union directives must be implemented by member states (through national law as, for example, with the Animals (Scientific Procedures) Act 1986 in the UK), and must be adopted by any new state which joins the Union. Both the European Convention and Directive provide a framework which member states may choose to develop into more detailed regulations and guidance in the implementation of their provisions. Box 8.2 gives an overview of the provisions of the Convention and Directive.

The methods of implementing the Directive and Convention vary among European states (Nuffield Council on Bioethics 2005) and they are permitted to adopt stricter measures. Some states have centralised national authorisation, some have regional authorisation. Some require authorisation for all procedures, some allow minor procedures to start after notification. Commonly among the states a two-licence system is operated: one for the establishment, one for the project. A few states also require individuals to be licensed. National inspection regimes vary, with inspection visits ranging from frequent to occasional. Increasingly, a formalised process of ethical review is used, either mandated by law or voluntarily (FELASA Working Group on Ethical Evaluation of Animal Experiments 2007). Further restrictions on animal species (eg, apes), purposes (eg, safety testing of cosmetics) or procedures (eg, the LD_{50} test) have been implemented in one or more European states.

Two complementary changes are underway in Europe. The standards in animal care and husbandry listed in Appendix A of the Convention have been reviewed over several years as part of the Multilateral Consultation of Parties to the Convention. Discussions on this were informed by working parties comprising representatives of science, industry and animal welfare groups. The parties to the Convention ratified an updated Appendix A in June 2006 (Council of Europe 2006). The changes from the previous versions were considerable, with much greater emphasis on the quality of the environment and accommodation because of its potential to affect animal well-being. For some species, particularly birds, dogs and non-human primates, enclosure sizes were increased considerably (Federation of European Laboratory Animal Science Associations 2007). In June 2007, a Commission Recommendation (2007 526 EC) replaced the existing Annex II guidance, with new guidelines aligned to the revised Council of Europe guidelines (Appendix A of Convention ETS 123), on accommodation and care of laboratory animals.

In 2001, the European Commission proposed revision of the European Directive because of its concerns about variation in its implementation across Europe, changes in scientific practice and advances in science, and because of its concern for more explicit reference to the use and development of alternatives to animal use. Since then, various reports and assessments have been undertaken, including a report by the European Parliament's Environment & Public Health Committee; a Commission-sponsored technical review; input from the European Food Safety Authority; an impact assessment by the Commission; and a public consultation (European Commission 2007a). The Commission's proposal on the new Directive was published in November 2008 and is now subject to dynamic revision between the Commission, the European Parliament and the European Council of Ministers. Areas for revision include:

Box 8.2 Overview of the provisions of the European Convention and 1986 Directive (C – unique to Convention; D – unique to Directive).

Animals protected:

- Live non-human vertebrates, including free-living and/or reproducing larval forms, but excluding other foetal or embryonic forms.
- Use of stray animals prohibited.
- Restrictions on the use of wild or endangered species (D).

Activities regulated:

- Experimental or other scientific use of an animal which may cause it pain, suffering, distress or lasting harm. Includes the birth of an animal in any such conditions.
- Excludes the least painful methods accepted in modern practice of killing or marking an animal.
- Non-experimental, veterinary and agricultural activities excluded.

Reasons allowed for one or more of the following purposes only:

- Avoidance or prevention of disease or abnormality in man, vertebrate or invertebrate animals or plants. Includes production and quality, efficacy and safety testing of drugs, substances or products.
- Diagnosis or treatment of disease in man, vertebrate or invertebrate animals or plants.
- Detection, assessment, regulation or modification of physiological conditions in man, vertebrate and invertebrate animals or plants.
- Protection of the environment.
- Scientific research (C).
- Education and training, and forensic inquiries (C).

Animal environment, care and husbandry:

- Standards for this in an Appendix (A) (C) or an Annex (II) (D).
- Environment checked each day and action taken if required.

Three Rs:

- Cannot use an animal if another scientifically satisfactory method is reasonably and practicably available.
- Choice of species to be carefully considered.
- Procedures selected which use the minimum number of animals, cause the least pain, suffering, distress or lasting harm, and which are most likely to provide satisfactory results.
- General or local anaesthesia or analgesia or other methods to eliminate as far as practicable pain, suffering, distress or lasting harm must be applied throughout the procedure unless they confound experiment or themselves cause more harm.
- The development of the Three Rs is encouraged.
- States to recognise the results of procedures carried out in other states.

Notification and authorisation:

- Procedures in which an animal will or may experience severe pain which is likely to endure must be specifically declared and justified to, or specifically authorised by, state authorities.
- Authorisation for any procedure shall be granted only to persons deemed to be competent by the state authorities, and if the experimental or other scientific project concerned is authorised in accordance with the provisions of national legislation.

Actions at the end of experiments:

- Animal to be killed and this is required during the course of the experiment if the animal is in unrelieved severe pain or distress.
- Animals may be re-used, under certain conditions, or released, but not if not previously used in an experiment causing severe pain or distress.
- Animal may, under certain conditions, be released.
- There must be veterinary involvement in decisions made at the end of the experiment if the animal is not killed.

User establishments:

- Registered and comply with standards for animal environment, care and husbandry.
- Design, construction and functioning of facilities and equipment to ensure that the procedures obtain consistent results with the minimum number of animals and the minimum degree of pain, suffering, distress or lasting harm.
- Persons who are administratively responsible for the care of the animals and the functioning of the equipment to be identified.
- Sufficient trained staff.
- Adequate arrangements for the provision of veterinary advice and treatment.
- Veterinarian or other competent person charged with advisory duties in relation to the well-being of the animals.
- Persons who carry out procedures, or take part in procedures, or take care of animals used in procedures to have appropriate education and training.
- Records kept of animal acquisition and use.
- Periodic inspection by the state (D).

Breeding and supply establishments:

- Registered and comply with standards for animal environment, care and husbandry.
- Person in charge of the establishment competent to administer for suitable care for animals.
- Requirements for records, with special provision for records identification of dogs and cats
- Some species must be purpose bred unless specific exemption: mouse, rat, guinea pig, golden hamster, rabbit, dog, cat and quail.
- Periodic inspection by the state (D).

Statistical information made available to the public for each state:

- The numbers and kinds of animals used in procedures.
- The numbers of animals in selected categories used in procedures directly concerned with medicine and in education and training (C).
- The numbers of animals in selected categories used in procedures for the protection of man and the environment.
- The numbers of animals in selected categories used in procedures required by law.
- Commercial information protected (D).

- regulation of individuals, places and projects with prior authorisation of procedures;
- establishment of an inspection system in each member state and EU audit of inspection;
- requirement for member states to promote the Three Rs;
- establishment of institutional ethical review to advise on the Three Rs and review certain projects annually;
- classification of projects by severity;
- restrictions on the use, breeding and acquisition of non-human primates;
- prescribed minimum standards for animal care and accommodation;
- extension of the scope to some invertebrates, animals bred for tissues and immature forms;
- further restrictions on the re-use of animals;
- requirement for a national animal welfare and ethics committee and a national reference laboratory to validate alternatives;
- requirement for public non-technical summaries of projects;
- measures to promote the avoidance of duplication in regulatory testing.

The revised Appendix A of the Convention has therefore become the current standard for animal use in the European Union (European Commission 2007b), as well as in countries which have ratified the Council of Europe Convention, and it is now being implemented over a period of several years.

In addition, for the European Union states, the revised Directive will become the current regulation for standards for animal use, once the revision process is complete.

North America

Canada

The Canadian constitution precludes federal legislation pertaining to the use of animals in research, testing or education because such use is under provincial jurisdiction. Six provinces have established legislation regarding animal research, five of which reference the CCAC guidelines and policies. In addition, although there is no federal requirement to participate in the CCAC assessment programme, the two principal funding agencies require grantee institutions to have a Certificate of Good Animal Practice® and to comply with CCAC guidelines and policies for continued funding. Contractors performing work for the federal government are required to adhere to CCAC guidelines, as specified in the Public Works and Government Services Canada, Standard Acquisition Clauses and Conditions Manual, Section 5, Subsection A, Clause A9015C: Experimental Animals.

The CCAC, founded in 1968, places responsibility for humane animal care and use with the animal care committee (ACC) at each institution. The ACCs are granted specific authority and provided with terms of reference under which they operate (eg, membership, authority, responsibilities and functioning). The CCAC's mission is:

> *to act in the interests of the people of Canada to ensure through programs of education, assessment and persuasion that the use of animals, where necessary, for research, teaching and testing employs optimal physical and psychological care according to acceptable scientific standards, and to promote an increased level of knowledge, awareness and sensitivity to relevant ethical principles.*

Thus, the CCAC has two principal functions: (1) the development of guidelines and policies to govern experimental animal care and use; and (2) to monitor compliance with those guidelines and policies. The CCAC is an independent organisation and receives funding from the Medical Research Council (MRC) and the Natural Sciences and Engineering Research Council (NSERC).

The CCAC establishes guidelines for its certified institutions to follow, currently contained in the two-volume *Guide to the Care and Use of Experimental Animals* (CCAC 1984; Olfert *et al.* 1993). Adjunct guidelines address topics such as animal use protocol review, transgenic animals, selecting appropriate endpoints and developing an animal user training programme. The CCAC also has established several policies, including the ethics of animal research, review of scientific merit, social and behavioural requirements of experimental animals, acceptable immunological procedures and categories of invasiveness.

On-site assessments using panels of experts from the animal care and use community and a representative nominated by the Canadian Federation of Humane Societies are conducted triennially. An institution is deemed to be in compliance if the CCAC report prepared by the assessment panel and approved by the Assessment Committee, a standing committee composed of at least four Council members, contains only regular, minor and/or commendatory recommendations, and the institution submits an implementation report for any regular recommendations that is judged to be satisfactory. Institutions which have been found to be in compliance or conditional compliance will receive a CCAC Certificate of Good Animal Practice®. If the CCAC report contains major and/or serious recommendations whose correction does not require verification by an on-site reassessment, but rather can be verified through documentation and the institution provides to the CCAC an implementation report that is judged to be satisfactory, then compliance is maintained. An assessment report containing major or serious recommendations may place the institution in a status of conditional compliance, probation or non-compliance. All relevant funding agencies and government ministries and departments are notified of an institution's non-compliance with CCAC guidelines (Canadian Council on Animal Care 2000). Sustained non-compliance with CCAC guidelines and policies can ultimately result in withdrawal of all animal-based research funding to the institution.

The United States

In the US, oversight of animal care and use for research, testing and teaching is achieved by numerous laws, regulations, policies and guidelines from two principal government organisations: the USDA and the PHS. Other guidance may be derived from scientific panels and endorsed by the government as required standards. Federal laws are annually compiled and categorised into their respective subjects (eg, agriculture) and published as the United States Code (USC). The USC includes a discussion of the intent of Congress for establishing the law and any interpretations from the courts. Regulations are promulgated to enforce the corresponding law. Proposed regulations are published in the Federal Register for public comment. After the responsible agency reviews and addresses the public comments, the regulations are again published in the Federal Register in final format and then incorporated into the Code of Federal Regulations (eg, 9 CFR) (Johnson & Morin 1983; Johnson *et al.* 1995). In general, laws address two specific areas: animal welfare and procurement, and animal importation and shipment.

US Department of Agriculture

Federal laws for the humane treatment of animals have been in place since 1873. The first federal law to protect non-farm animals was not passed until 1966 and was called the Laboratory Animal Welfare Act, administered by APHIS, USDA. The Laboratory Animal Welfare Act of 1966 was amended in 1970, 1976, 1985, 1990, 2000 and 2008 to broaden coverage of the law. Public Law 91-579, Animal Welfare Act of 1970, increased the species of animals covered under the law to include all warm-blooded animals and increased the scope of applicability of the law to include the time animals were held in the facility. Specifically exempted were horses not used in research and agricultural animals used in food and fibre research, retail pet stores, state and county fairs, rodeos, purebred cat and dog shows, and agricultural exhibitions. Public Law 94-279, Animal Welfare Act Amendments of 1976, included common commercial carriers, such as airlines, and this subsequently led to standards being developed for shipping containers and conditions of shipment. Public Law 99-198, Improved Standards for Laboratory Animals Act, added several new provisions to the law including: minimisation of animal pain and distress and consideration of alternatives to painful procedures; consultation with a doctor of veterinary medicine for any practice which could cause pain to animals; limitation on conducting more than one major survival surgery on an animal (ie, multiple major survival surgical procedures may be permitted if they are interrelated to the scientific goal of the study); establishment of an IACUC to provide oversight of the animal care and use programme and facilities; provision of specific training to personnel; provision of exercise to dogs; and a stipulation to promote the psychological well-being of non-human primates. The 1990 amendment to the Animal Welfare Act, Public Law 101-624, Food, Agriculture, Conservation, and Trade Act of 1990, Section 2503, Protection of Pets, established a holding period for dogs and cats at shelters and other holding facilities prior to sale to dealers supplying animals for research. The law also requires dealers to provide written certification to the recipient regarding the background of each animal.

The 1970 amendment to the Animal Welfare Act defined an animal as: *'any live or dead dog, cat, monkey (nonhuman primate animal), guinea pig, hamster, rabbit, or other such warm-blooded animal as the Secretary may determine is being used, or is intended for use, for research, testing, experimentation, or exhibition purposes, or as a pet.'* In this way, the Secretary of the Department of Agriculture was provided the authority to determine which animals would be covered by the Act. In 1977 the USDA promulgated regulations that specifically excluded rats, mice and birds from the definition of 'animal'. The Helms amendment to the 2002 Farm Bill explicitly excluded rats, mice and birds used for research from the Act. Because the USDA regulates only those species covered by the Animal Welfare Act, the passage of this bill into law removed USDA oversight of these species. Rationale for Congress to accept their exclusion from the Act was based in large part on the fact that these species are covered by other federal (eg, PHS Policy) and private (eg, AAALAC International) systems of oversight, and there are reports that approximately 95% of research using rats and mice is funded by the National Institutes of Health and thus are covered by the Health Research Extension Act/Public Health Service Policy (Federation of American Societies for Experimental Biology 2002).

Since the 1966 Act, the USDA has been vested by Congress with both promulgation and enforcement authority. The USDA is required to conduct unannounced annual inspections of research facilities, with follow-up inspections until any cited deficiency has been corrected. Exempt from this provision are federal research facilities. Research institutions, intermediate handlers and common carriers are required to register with the USDA, while animal dealers and exhibitors must be licensed. Research facilities and US government agencies are required to purchase animals only from licensed sources, unless the source is exempted from obtaining a license. Failure to comply with regulatory requirements, despite formal notification of an item(s) of non-compliance and an opportunity to effect a correction, can result in fines levied on the facility, suspension of authority to operate and even permanent revocation of the facility's license to operate. Thus, the enforcement arm of the USDA's oversight responsibility is strong, and has been used over the years to improve animal welfare at dealers, exhibits and research facilities.

Public Health Service Policy

The other federal agency charged with oversight of research animal care and use is the PHS. The PHS Policy was implemented in 1973 and was revised in 1979. The PHS Policy covers all vertebrate animals used in research, testing or teaching. Today, the PHS authority is derived from Public Law 99-158, the Health Research Extension Act of 1985, Section 495, Animals in Research. Under this Act, institutions conducting animal research using PHS funding, such as through the National Institutes of Health (NIH), must comply with the PHS Policy on Humane Care and Use of Laboratory Animals (Office of Laboratory Animal Welfare 2002). The PHS Policy requires submission by the funding recipient (referred to as an *'awardee institution'*) of an Animal Welfare Assurance Statement, and which must be approved by the PHS's Office of Laboratory Animal Welfare (OLAW), a component of the NIH, and commits the institution to following the US Government Principles for the Utilization and Care of Vertebrate Animals Used in Testing, Research, and Training (IRAC 1985) which are largely based on the CIOMS Principles, and the *Guide*. In addition to stating a commitment to animal welfare, the Assurance Statement must designate clear lines of authority and responsibility for institutional oversight of the work, inclusive of a designated *'Institutional Official'* who is ultimately responsible for the animal care and use programme; identify a qualified veterinarian who is involved in the programme; provide a description of the occupational health and safety programme for relevant personnel in the programme; describe mandated training; and describe the facility. The assurance is re-negotiated with OLAW every 5 years. OLAW can approve, disapprove, restrict or withdraw approval of the Assurance.

PHS awarding agencies, such as the NIH, may not make an award for an activity involving live vertebrate animals unless the prospective awardee institution and all other institutions participating in the animal activity have an approved Assurance with OLAW and provide verification that the IACUC has reviewed and approved those sections of the grant application that involve the use of animals. Applications from organisations with approved Assurances must address five specific points pertaining to the use of animals:

- a detailed description of the proposed work, including species, strain, sex, age and number of animals to be used in the proposed work;
- a justification of the use of animals, species and number of animals;
- information regarding the veterinary care for the animals;
- a description of the procedures for ensuring that discomfort, distress, pain and injury will be minimised;
- a description of the method of euthanasia and the reason for the selection of that method, including a justification for any method that does not conform with the American Veterinary Medical Association's (AVMA) Euthanasia Guidelines (2007).

Awardee institutions that do not comply with the standards of the *Guide*, the USDA Animal Welfare Regulations and other standards referenced in the PHS Policy (eg, the AVMA's Euthanasia Guidelines (American Veterinary Medical Association 2007)), may have their Assurance Statement restricted, which in turn can limit access to PHS funding for research. Sustained non-compliance with the PHS Policy can result in withdrawing the approval of the assurance and cessation of all PHS funding for animal-based activities.

The awardee institution must also submit an annual report. Institutions that are reviewed by an outside accrediting body, such as AAALAC International (Category 1 institutions), must indicate in the annual report if that accreditation status has been removed. Institutions that are not accredited by an external review group (Category 2) must provide the most recent copy of their IACUC's semiannual programme review and facility inspection with the Assurance. The role of the IACUC in providing local oversight of animal care and use is a key element of the PHS Policy. Although the required composition of the IACUC for the PHS differs slightly from USDA requirements, due to a Memorandum of Understanding concerning laboratory animal welfare among APHIS/USDA, the Food and Drug Administration (FDA) and the NIH that sets forth procedures for co-operation among the three agencies in their oversight of animal care and use programmes, the general functions and responsibilities of the IACUC are similar.

OLAW conducts site visits of awardee institutions both *'for cause'* and *'not for cause'*. In addition, an ongoing significant mission of OLAW is the educational outreach it performs in collaboration with awardee institutions. Jointly sponsored workshops focus on information of value to Institutional Officials and IACUCs to provide appropriate oversight of animal care and use. OLAW also provides guidance through articles in journals, commentary on other articles, NIH Guide Notices and a listserve.

Other laws, regulations and policies

In 1978 the FDA initially promulgated regulations for the conduct of animal research on new or existing pharmaceutical agents, food additives or other chemicals. These regulations, known as the Good Laboratory Practice (GLP) regulations (which have been subsequently revised), specify appropriate diagnosis, treatment and control of Disease in animals used in the work (see 21 CFR Part 58[3] (Code of Federal Regulation 1998)). The Environmental Protection Agency (EPA) has issued companion regulations (Code of Federal Regulation 1997) for conducting research pertaining to health effects, environmental effects and chemical fate testing in a separate set of GLP regulations[4]. Both the FDA and EPA GLP regulations rely heavily on adequate and detailed record keeping. Records must include standard operating procedures, animal identification, food and water analysis, documentation that any pesticides or chemicals used near the animals do not interfere with the study, and documentation of any disease and treatments animals experience. On-site inspections are conducted to ensure compliance with GLP standards.

The Department of Defense (DoD) developed a 'Policy on Experimental Animals' in 1961 to ensure that all research at DoD facilities involving animals was conducted in accord with certain principles of animal care (Rozmiarek 2007). Later versions of this policy included overseas sites. Subsequently a joint regulation, entitled 'The Use of Animals in DoD Program', from the Army, Navy, Air Force, Defense Nuclear Agency and Uniformed Services University required all DoD facilities to *'seek accreditation by AAALAC'* and to establish local institutional animal care and use committees (Department of Defense 1995).

State laws to protect animals have a long history, with the first anti-cruelty law passed in 1641 in the Massachusetts Bay Colony to prevent riding or driving farm animals beyond established limits (US Congress Office of Technology Assessment 1986). All 50 states and the District of Columbia have enacted anti-cruelty laws. The overarching goals of these laws are to protect animals from cruel treatment, require that animals have access to suitable food and water and require that animals have shelter from extreme weather. Some state laws define 'animal' and some do not. In common

[3]http://edocket.access.gpo.gov/cfr_2004/aprqtr/pdf/21cfr58.1.pdf

[4]http://ecfr.gpoaccess.gov/cgi/t/text/text-idx?c=ecfr&sid=cd55b9ce1e35880245e76f6ba16ab76d&rgn=div5&view=text&node=40:23.0.1.1.11&idno=40

among the state laws is the diversity of approaches to providing protection to animals. Some states have additional provisions for animals used in research, and many states prohibit the sale of pound animals into the research stream. In general, criminal penalties are imposed for offences. On occasion, state anti-cruelty laws have been used against research facilities. In recent years, state and federal laws have been used by private citizens or citizen groups claiming 'standing to sue' on behalf of animals. The issue of 'standing' has undergone a long litigation process and a chronology of court decisions on this issue has been compiled by the National Association for Biomedical Research (1999).

Because animal research can involve a variety of different species, several other federal acts, laws and treaties have bearing on animal use. These include the US Endangered Species Act, which restricts the research conducted on these animals to those studies that would directly benefit the species under investigation; the Marine Mammal Protection Act, which provides authority for scientific research on marine mammals by special permit; the Convention on International Trade in Endangered Species of Wild Fauna and Flora (CITES), which requires signatory countries to obtain a permit for the import or export of certain species; the Lacey Act, which governs import, export and interstate commerce of foreign wildlife; and the Migratory Bird Treaty Act, which makes it unlawful to take or possess any protected bird except by permit.

Asia

Japan

Effective 1st June 2006, the Science Council of Japan (SCJ) issued 'Guidelines for Proper Conduct of Animal Experiments' as a result of the amended Law for the Humane Treatment and Management of Animals (amended 2005) and at the request of the Ministry of Education, Culture, Sports, Science and Technology (MEXT) and the Ministry of Health, Labour and Welfare (MHLW). Of particular note, the amended law and SCJ Guidelines requires attention to the Three Rs in the planning and conduct of research, though in practice, particular emphasis is placed on refinement. The detailed guidelines promulgated by the SCJ build upon the more basic guidelines, 'Fundamental guidelines for proper conduct of animal experiment and related activities in academic research institutions under the jurisdiction of the Ministry of Education, Culture, Sports, Science and Technology', 'Basic policies for the conduct of animal experimentation in the Ministry of Health, Labour and Welfare' and 'Standards Relating to the Care and Management of Laboratory Animals and Relief of Pain (Ministry of Environment, 2006)'.

The SCJ Guidelines encourage each institution to develop and implement its own policies for the conduct of animal-based research. The SCJ guidelines place ultimate responsibility for all experiments with the director of the institution, but also encourage the formation of an IACUC. Therefore, the IACUC's role is to provide the institutional director with a report on the committee's deliberations regarding a proposed study, and then the director approves or disapproves the protocol. The number of IACUC members may vary with the size and complexity of the institution, but the committee should include researchers who conduct animal experiments, laboratory animal specialists and *'other persons of knowledge and experience'* (Science Council of Japan 2006). The primary role of the IACUC is to evaluate the scientific merit of the proposed study, taking into consideration the aforementioned law, standards and policies. The IACUC is also charged with reviewing the education and training of the investigator and to make recommendations to the director of the institution as necessary.

The SCJ Guidelines provide general recommendations regarding items for the IACUC to consider when reviewing a protocol, items that should be contained on the protocol form, facility and equipment considerations, animal restraint, food and water restriction, surgical procedures, analgesics and anaesthetics, humane endpoints, euthanasia, safety considerations and reporting of experimental results. This latter item suggests that the investigator report to the director of the institution the number of animals used, whether any changes were made to the protocol and the results of the experiment. Other topics covered include laboratory animal selection and receipt, the care and management of laboratory animals, laboratory animal health management, as well as education and training. Under the topic of laboratory animal care and management, cage space is discussed. The Guidelines recommend considering the animal's characteristics (species, age, etc) and its behaviour when determining appropriate cage size, or alternatively to use the *Guide* (NRC 1996). The Standards provide additional guidance on environmental conditions and other related animal care and use programme information. Although a government inspection system does not validate conformity with these standards and guidelines, a third party audit system is encouraged, which may be met by a relatively new national audit system or through assessments and accreditation provided by AAALAC International.

Korea

The first Korean Animal Protection Law was passed in 1991 that formally permitted the use of animals for teaching, research, *'or other scientific study'*. The law was amended in January 2007 with a 1-year period for institutions to come into compliance (Korean Animal Protection Law 2007). The amended law addresses several key principles, including consideration of harm/benefit, alternatives, using the minimum number of animals necessary to achieve the scientific goal, ensuring appropriate training and experience of the investigator, pain mitigation and euthanasia. Importantly, the amended law requires the establishment of an Animal Experimentation Ethics Committee to *'oversee the protection and ethical treatment'* of research animals. The composition of the committee is specified as a chair and 3–15 members, one third of whom must be independent of the institution. The committee must have a veterinarian; a person who represents animal welfare and is recommended by a private organization; a lawyer; and a professor that is in charge of animal protection and welfare at an institution of *'higher education'*. The committee is appointed by the head of the facility and the chair is elected from among the committee members. A fine may be levied against the head of an animal facility who has not appointed an Animal Experimentation Ethics Committee. Under the terms of the amended law, an annual report must be submitted to the Minister of Agriculture and Forestry regarding animal experimentation activities.

People's Republic of China

The 'Regulations for Administration of Laboratory Animals' was approved by the State Council in 1988 (State Science and Technology Commission 1988). The Ministry of Health subsequently published Implementing Detailed Rules of Medical Laboratory Animal Administration. In general, these regulations are designed to ensure high-quality animals for research. The standards, 'Laboratory animal – Requirements of environment and housing facilities' (GB 14925-2001) were revised in 2001. Standards are described regarding construction of the animal housing areas; separation of animals by source, species, strain, experiment and pathogen status; quality of food, water and bedding provided to the animals; quarantine procedures; preventive medicine; and animal transportation. In 2006, the Ministry of Science and Technology (MOST) issued guidelines for the humane treatment of laboratory animals. This was the first state policy-related document which directs administrators and technicians to attend to the welfare of laboratory animals. In this manner, concepts such as the Three Rs and scientific merit have begun to be included in Chinese regulations.

The Beijing Municipality has additional regulations regarding the Administration of Laboratory Animals (Beijing Municipal Science and Technology Commission 1997). These regulations are specific to '*artificially raised and bred animals with control of microbes and parasites carried by them and definite genetic background and clear sources that are used for scientific researches, teaching, production, examinations and other scientific experiments*'. The Beijing regulations require a license be obtained from the Beijing Municipal Science and Technology Commission for the use of laboratory animals in breeding, research or testing. The municipal regulations require personnel training, and technical staff must complete a technical competency assessment. Proper care, handling and treatment of the animals are emphasised throughout the regulations. Similar approaches are established in other cities where scientific research is important, such as Shanghai.

Taiwan, ROC

In Taiwan, the Animal Protection Law (Taiwan Animal Protection Law 1998), under the auspices of the Council of Agriculture (COA), has provisions that address animals used for commercial purposes (eg, meat, milk, fur, etc), science (teaching and research) and animals kept as pets. Chapter II, Article 12 of the Animal Protection Law precludes the killing of animals, with certain exceptions such as killing for scientific purposes. Chapter III, Articles 15–18 specify the conditions for the '*scientific utilization of animals*'. Included in this chapter is the mandate that the minimum number of animals necessary will be used in ways that cause the minimum amount of pain or injury. Article 16 requires that the institution that is using animals form an '*animal experimentation management unit*' to oversee the scientific utilization of the laboratory animals. In addition, the institution must establish an ethics committee, which must include a veterinarian and one representative of a private '*animal protection group*'. Under this law, the institution is entitled to employ an '*animal protection inspector*' or use voluntary '*animal protectors*' to assist with the supervision of animal use, including inspection of locations where animals are housed and used. In 2001 the COA announced regulations for establishing Laboratory Animal Care and Use Panels for institutions using vertebrate animals. Training sessions were provided for the panel members and the COA developed a Guideline for the Care and Use of Laboratory Animals for use by the panels.

India

The Animal Welfare Board of India was set up in accordance with Section 4 of the Prevention of Cruelty to Animals Act 1960 (No. 59 of 1960). The Ministry of Food and Agriculture constituted the Animal Welfare Board of India in 1962. Since 1998, oversight of the Animal Welfare Board is the purview of the Ministry of Social Justice and Empowerment. Among the functions of the Board are: to advise the government on promulgating rules with a view to preventing unnecessary pain or suffering of captive animals and on potential amendments to the law. Chapter 4 of the Prevention of Cruelty to Animals Act addresses experimentation on animals. Included in the act is the authority for the government to appoint a Committee for the Purpose of Control and Supervision of Experiments on Animals (CPCSEA). The committee must ensure that animals are not subjected to unnecessary pain or suffering before, during or after the performance of experiments on them. To achieve this, the committee may, subsequent to notification in the Gazette of India, develop rules regarding the conduct of experiments. In general, the rules for animal experimentation pertain to appropriate qualifications of individuals conducting the experiment, minimisation of animal pain by the use of anaesthetics, euthanasia, consideration of alternatives to animal experimentation, that pre- and post-procedural care be provided to the animal, and that suitable records are maintained. The committee can authorise inspection of the location of the experiment and can suspend animal work by an individual or an institution.

The Indian National Science Academy is responsible for the development of guidelines for the operation of Institutional Animal Ethics Committees (IAEC). For example, protocols must be provided to the IAEC 30 days in advance of the committee meeting. The IAEC's principal responsibility is the review and authorisation of proposed animal experimentation. Each IAEC includes a member of the Committee for the Purpose of Control and Supervision of Experiments on Animals. Most experimentation is conducted on small laboratory animals (eg, mice, rats, guinea pigs, rabbits); permission must be obtained from a subcommittee of the CPCSEA to conduct research on larger animals.

Singapore

Singapore recently established Guidelines on the Care and Use of Animals for Scientific Purposes (National Advisory Committee for Laboratory Animal Research 2004). These cover animal care and use for scientific purposes based on ethical, legal and scientific considerations, Institutional Animal Care and Use Committees and training of personnel involved in the care and use of animals for scientific purposes. Implementation is institution based, and they draw heavily on US, Australian and Canadian standards for husbandry, care and protocol authorisation, and on European standards for training guidelines.

Australia and New Zealand

Australia

The Australian Code of Practice for the Care and Use of Animals for Scientific Purposes (National Health and Medical Research Council 2004) provides a national standard for the use of animals in research, testing and teaching and since it is integrated into state-based animal welfare legislation, it is legally binding in each jurisdiction. Now in its seventh edition, the Code of Practice began in 1969 as an initiative of the scientific community aimed at establishing ethical and welfare standards for animal research. It is published by the National Health and Medical Research Council (NHMRC) which is Australia's peak statutory health body and whose responsibilities include the promotion of ethical behaviour in the conduct of research. Periodic revisions to the code are conducted with public consultation through a Code Liaison Group which includes representation from animal welfare groups in addition to government research bodies and academia. This process of periodic revision and the legally binding status of the code means that the regulatory framework can respond to changes in the biological sciences and community attitudes more readily than is usually possible through the formal legislative process. The NHMRC supports the enhancement of laboratory animal welfare in other ways too including through its Animal Welfare Committee, which provides advice to the Council on the conduct and ethics of animal experimentation. The Animal Welfare Committee participates in the revision of the Code of Practice and has developed numerous policies, guidelines and publications on topics such as advice for independent members of AECs, the care of genetically modified animals, monoclonal antibody production and the training of surgeons using animals.

The Code of Practice covers all live non-human vertebrates and also cephalopods. It emphasises the responsibilities of investigators, teachers and institutions to:

- *ensure that the use of animals is justified, taking into consideration the scientific or educational benefits and the potential effects on the welfare of animals;*
- *ensure that the welfare of animals is always considered;*
- *promote the development and use of techniques that replace the use of animals in scientific and teaching activities;*
- *minimize the number of animals used in projects; and*
- *refine methods and procedures to avoid pain or distress in animals used in scientific and teaching activities*

The Code of Practice endorses the principles of the Three Rs and also provides practical guidance by setting out general principles for the care, housing and humane use of animals. Importantly, it also requires the establishment of AECs for each research institution. Membership of an AEC must include a veterinarian, a scientist, a person with a demonstrable commitment to animal welfare but who is not employed by the institution, and a person viewed by the wider community as bringing a completely independent view and who is both independent of the institution and who has never been involved with the scientific use of animals. In addition, the AEC should appoint to its membership a person responsible for the routine care of animals from within the institution. AECs must have terms of reference that are publicly available and must include provision for oversight of all aspects of the animal care and use programme, assessment of animal use proposals, withdrawing approval of a project, authorising emergency treatment or euthanasia of animals and making recommendations to the institution to ensure compliance with the Code of Practice.

To assist with regulatory oversight, the Code of Practice provides guidance for the external review of animal research institutions and their AECs although details of the implementation varies between states according to legislation. In the state of New South Wales, for example, the legislation requires the establishment of a 12-member panel constituted by representatives from animal welfare organisations, the research sector and government. The panel has broad responsibilities that include serving as a conduit for community input to policy development, advising on the resolution of complaints and oversight of institutional self-regulation through on-site inspections and audits in collaboration with government veterinary inspectors. It has also published guidelines on practical aspects of laboratory animal care with an emphasis on evidence-based approaches.

In addition to state and territory laws dealing specifically with animal welfare, other laws at both the state and federal levels extend into the regulatory environment of animal research in Australia. These include laws relating to quarantine, wildlife management, genetic manipulation and occupational health and safety.

Recently, the Federal Government released the Australian Animal Welfare Strategy (Commonwealth of Australia 2005). This comprehensive strategy covers not only laboratory animals but all use of animals in Australia. In common with the Code of Practice, however, broad consultation was prominent in its development with input being sought from animal welfare groups, government, industry and the general public. The goals of the Strategy include the enhancement of existing animal welfare arrangements and development of nationally consistent policies which will, among other things, take into account scientific evidence and social considerations. At present, the prospect of federal legislation governing animal research seems unlikely since the Australian Constitution is usually interpreted as delegating animal welfare matters to the state governments. However, the integration of the Code of Practice into state animal research legislation, does, in effect, achieve the Strategy's goal of a consistent national policy in this area.

Another recent publication has been the NHMRC's 'Guidelines to promote the wellbeing of animals used for scientific purposes: The assessment and alleviation of pain and distress in research animals' (National Health and Medical Research Council 2008). The guidelines offer definitions of animal welfare and well-being and contain *'Factsheets'* addressing a diversity of topics relevant to research proposal review, including food and water restriction, tumour induction, polyclonal antibody production and several others.

New Zealand

Animal use in New Zealand was initially regulated by the Animals Protection Act 1960 and, in particular, its 1983 amendment which stipulated conformance with a code of ethical practices when using animals for research or testing. The Act covered all vertebrate animals kept in captivity or which are dependent upon humans for care. The 1983 amendment also established a National Animal Ethics Advisory Committee (NAEAC).

The Animal Welfare Act of 1999 (Ministry of Agriculture and Forestry (MAF) 1999) replaced the Animals Protection Act of 1960 to meet changing societal views toward the use of animals. It also expanded the types of animals covered under law to include most of those that can feel pain, excluding shellfish and insects due to the lack of evidence that would support their ability to feel pain. Part 6 of the Animal Welfare Act requires that an institution hold a Code of Ethical Conduct (CEC) approved by the Director-General of the MAF before research, testing or teaching with animals can be done. Organisations and individuals who wish to engage in research, testing or teaching may, however, use another organisation's code and animal ethics committee. The goal of the CEC is to ensure that the applicant's staff have the *'appropriate qualifications and expertise'* to carry out the proposed procedures on animals (Ministry of Agriculture and Forestry 2006). The CEC describes the policies and procedures implemented by the code holder to ensure that the use of animals in research, testing and teaching complies with the Animal Welfare Act. Specifically, a system of record keeping and monitoring of all animal activities is required. Subsequent to the CEC's initial approval, it must be reviewed and renewed after a maximum of 5 years. This role has been assumed by NAEAC. The 1999 Animal Welfare Act also calls for an independent, periodic review of the programme to ensure it conforms to the CEC, the Act, and other relevant regulations.

As noted, the holder of a CEC must form an animal ethics committee (AEC). The committee is appointed by the code holder who may be the chief executive of the institution or his/her nominee. The AEC must be comprised of at least four members and have a minimum of three external members, including a senior member of the organisation; an outside veterinarian; a person representing animal welfare groups who is not affiliated with the institution and is not involved with animal research, testing or teaching; and a person to represent the public (lay member). The NAEAC has published a guide to assist the lay member in his/her role on the AEC (National Animal Ethics Advisory Committee 2007). The AEC is responsible for overseeing conduct of research at the institution, including reviewing proposed projects, monitoring the conduct of the project, reviewing project renewals, monitoring management practices and facilities to ensure conformance with the CEC, suspending or revoking project approval and recommending to the code holder changes to the CEC. Each proposed project must include a harm/benefit analysis and must address reduction, replacement and refinement (the Three Rs) of animal use. If the animal(s) is euthanased at the end of a manipulation, Part 6 does not require that the AEC consider the ethical question of killing the animals. Rather, the harm/benefit analysis that must be considered with each proposal is limited to the pain and/or distress that the animal may experience. Part 6 of the Animal Welfare Act provides for circumstances where pain, distress, and *'compromised care'* of the animals may be allowed such that the researcher cannot be prosecuted for not conforming with Parts 1 or 2 of the Act.

The Animal Welfare Act stipulates that the physical, health and behavioural needs of animals used in research, testing and teaching are met in a manner that conforms with good practice and available scientific knowledge. To that end, the NAEAC and MAF published a 'Good practice guide for the use of animals in research, testing and teaching' (National Animal Ethics Advisory Committee 2002) with the stated purpose of promoting *'the humane and responsible use of animals for scientific purposes'* by describing guidelines for good practice. The guide addresses the acquisition of animals, facility construction and operation, management of animals in breeding and holding areas, responsibilities of investigators and responsibilities of teachers. Of particular note is the Animal Welfare Score Sheet provided as an appendix.

Finally, the Animal Welfare Act requires that all code holders submit to MAF annual animal use statistics. These data are made available to the general public. These reports contain data regarding animal source, the purpose of the experiment, a grading of the animal procedure severity and other related information.

Examples of oversight elsewhere in the world

Mexico

Technical specifications for the production, care, and use of laboratory animals (Norma Oficial Mexicana para la Producción, Cuidado y Uso de los Animales de Laboratorio) are contained in the federal Mexican law, NOM-062-ZOO-1999. The law covers dogs, cats, pigs and non-human primates. In addition, Mexico City has enacted a law in 1981 for the prevention of cruelty to animals (Ley del Distristito Federal para la Prevención de la Crueldad a los Animales).

Russia

Russian regulations (Sanitary Regulations for the Organization, Equipment and Maintenance of Animal Facilities for Experimental Biology (Vivaria) 1973), describe the location and design of animal facilities; sanitation requirements of animal facilities; housing and husbandry requirements; acquisition and quarantine of animals; standards for personal hygiene; and standards for the humane treatment of animals. Included in the latter section is the requirement to minimise pain experienced by the animal through the use of anaesthetics and analgesics.

Israel

The Israeli Animal Welfare Law (Experiments with Animals) 1994 establishes a review system and standards that are very similar to the US institutional based system. However, oversight of contentious procedures is performed directly by a National Council for Experiments in Animals, whose composition includes scientists, animal welfare representatives and non-affiliated members. The Council may withhold permission to conduct animal research if a reasonable alternative is available. The Council also visits animal facilities.

South America

In Brazil, animal welfare is encompassed in the Constitution (Article 225) and the Federal Decree on Anti-Cruelty (1934). The Brazilian Environmental Crimes Law (1998) supplements the Constitution to include cruelty crimes against animals. Article 32 of the Environmental Crimes Law specifically addresses the use of animals in research. This Article encourages the use of alternatives and requires the use of anaesthesia for painful procedures. Various states and municipalities have additional animal laws in place. In Peru, the protection of Domestic Animals Law (2000) covers the use of cats and dogs used in research.

South Africa

The South African National Standard, 'The care and use of animals for scientific purposes' (SANS 10386:2008 (South African Bureau of Standards 2008)) encompasses all aspects of the care and use of animals for medicine, biology, agriculture, veterinary and other animal science, as well as industry and teaching. These standards define an animal as *'live, sentient non-human vertebrate, including eggs, foetuses and embryos, that is fish, amphibians, reptiles, birds and mammals … and higher invertebrates such as the advanced members from the Cephalopoda and Decapoda'*.

Acknowledgements

The authors wish to express their gratitude to Dr. Gilly Griffin, Guidelines Program Director, Canadian Council on Animal Care and for her contribution to ensuring the accuracy of some of the information presented in this chapter.

References

American College of Laboratory Animal Medicine (1996) *Report of the American College of Laboratory Animal Medicine on Adequate Veterinary Care in Research, Testing and Teaching*. Cary, NC. http://www.aclam.org/education/guidelines/position_adequatecare.html (accessed 3 June 2008)

American Veterinary Medical Association (2007) *AVMA Guidelines on Euthanasia*. Schaumburg, IL. http://www.avma.org/issues/animal_welfare/euthanasia.pdf (accessed 27 April 2008)

Animal Plant Health Inspection Service (1999) *Ensuring adequate veterinary care: roles and responsibilities of facility owners and attending veterinarians*. Tech Note, March 1999. http://www.aphis.usda.gov/lpa/pubs/tneavc.pdf (accessed 27 April 2008

Animal Plant Health Inspection Service (1992) *Form 7002. Program of Veterinary Care for Research Facilities or Exhibitors/Dealers*. June 1992. http://www.aphis.usda.gov/animal_welfare/downloads/policy/policy3.pdf (accessed 27 April 2008)

Bayne, K. and Martin, D. (1998) AAALAC International: Using performance standards to evaluate an animal care and use program. *Laboratory Animals*, **27**, 32–35

Bayne, K. and Miller, J. (2000) Assessing animal care and use programs internationally. *Lab Animal*, **29**, 27–29

Beijing Municipal Science and Technology Commission (1997) *Regulations of Beijing Municipality for Administration of Laboratory Animals*. People's Republic of China. http://www.baola.org/ENGLISH/default.htm# (accessed 27 April 2008)

Biological Council (1984) *Guidelines of the Use of Living Animals in Scientific Investigations*. Biological Council, London

Buchanan-Smith, H.M., Rennie, A.E., Vitale, A., Pollo, S., Prescott, M.J. and Morton, D.B. (2005) Harmonising the definition of refinement. *Animal Welfare*, **14**, 379–384

Canadian Council on Animal Care (1984) *Guide to the Care and Use of Experimental Animals, Volume 2*. Ottawa, Canada. http://www.ccac.ca/en/CCAC_Programs/Guidelines_Policies/GUIDES/ENGLISH/toc_v1.htm (accessed 27 April 2008)

Canadian Council on Animal Care (2000) *CCAC Policy on Compliance and Noncompliance*. http://www.ccac.ca/en/CCAC_Programs/Guidelines_Policies/POLICIES/COMPLI.HTM. (accessed 27 April 2008)

Code of Federal Regulations (1998) *Title 21: Food and Drugs*; Chapter 1: Feed and Drug Administration, Department of Health and Human Services; Subchapter A: General; Part 58: Good Laboratory Practice for Nonclinical Laboratory Studies, Office of the Federal Register, Washington, DC

Code of Federal Regulations (1997) *Title 40: Protection of the Environment*; Chapter 1: Environmental Protection Agency; Subchapter E: Pesticide Programs; Part 160: Good Laboratory Practice Standard, Office of the Federal Register, Washington, DC

Commonwealth of Australia (2005) *Australian Animal Welfare Strategy*. Department of Agriculture, Fisheries and Forestry. Canberra, Australia. http://www.daff.gov.au/animal-plant-health/welfare/aaws (accessed 27 April 2008)

Council for International Organizations of Medical Sciences (1985) *International Guiding Principles for Biomedical Research Involving Animals*. Geneva. http://www.cioms.ch/1985_texts_of_guidelines.htm (accessed 27 April 2008)

Council of Europe (1986) *Convention for the Protection of Vertebrate Animals used for Experimental and other Scientific Purposes* (ETS 123). Strasbourg. http://conventions.coe.int/treaty/en/Treaties/Html/123.htm (accessed 27 April 2008)

Council of Europe (1993) *Convention for the Protection of Vertebrate Animals used for Experimental and other Scientific Purposes* (ETS 123) Resolution on education and training of persons working with laboratory animals adopted by the Multilateral Consultation on 3 December 1993. Council of Europe, Strasbourg. http://www.coe.int/t/e/legal_affairs/legal_co-operation/biological_safety,_use_of_animals/laboratory_animals/Res%20training.asp#TopOfPage (accessed 27 April 2008)

Council of Europe (2006) *Multilateral Consultation of Parties to the European Convention for the Protection of Vertebrate Animals used for Experimental and other Scientific Purposes* (ETS 123) Appendix A. *Cons 123 (2006) 3*. http://www.coe.int/t/e/legal_affairs/legal_co-operation/biological_safety,_use_of_animals/laboratory_animals/2006/Cons123(2006)3AppendixA_en.pdf (accessed 27 April 2008)

Department of Defense (1995) *The Use of Laboratory Animals in DoD Programs*, Directive Number 3216.1. http://www.army.mil/usapa/epubs/pdf/r40_33.pdf (accessed 27 April 2008)

Dunlop, R. and Williams, D. (1996) Bioethics, Animal Experimentation and Sentience. In: *Veterinary Medicine: An Illustrated History*. pp. 619–642. Mosby, Philadelphia

European Commission (2007a) *Review of Directive 86/609*. http://ec.europa.eu/environment/chemicals/lab_animals/nextsteps_en.htm (accessed 27 April 2008)

European Commission (2007b) Commission recommendations of 18 June 2007 on guidelines for the accommodation and care of animals used for experimental and other scientific purposes. Annex II to European Council Directive 86/609. See 2007/526/EC. http://eurlex.europa.eu/LexUriServ/site/en/oj/2007/l_197/l_19720070730en00010089.pdf (accessed 13 May 2008)

European Council (1986) Council Directive 86/609/EEC of 24 November 1986 on the approximation of laws, regulations and administrative provisions of the Member States regarding the protection of animals used for experimental and other scientific purposes. *Off J Eur Comm L* **358**, 1–29. http://eur-lex.europa.eu/LexUriServ/LexUriServ.do?uri=CELEX:31986L0609:EN:NOT (accessed 27 April 2008)

European Parliament (2002) *Report on Directive 86/609 on the protection of animals used for experimental and other scientific purposes* (2001/2259(INI)). Committee on the Environment, Public Health and Consumer Policy. http://ec.europa.eu/environment/chemicals/lab_animals/pdf/evans_report.pdf (accessed 27 April 2008)

Federation of American Societies for Experimental Biology (2002) *FASEB letter to the Office of Management and Budget on rats, mice and birds*. 8th January 2002. http://opa.faseb.org/pdf/ltr1x8x02.pdf (accessed 18 July 2008)

Federation of European Laboratory Animal Science Associations (1995) FELASA recommendations for the education and training of persons working with laboratory animals: Categories A and C. *Laboratory Animals*, **26**, 121–131. http://www.felasa.eu/recommendations.htm (accessed 27 April 2008)

Federation of European Laboratory Animal Science Associations (1999) FELASA recommendations for the education of specialists in laboratory animal science: Categories A and C. *Laboratory Animals*, **33**, 1–15. http://www.felasa.eu/recommendations.htm (accessed 27 April 2008)

Federation of European Laboratory Animal Science Associations (2000) FELASA recommendations for the education and training of persons carrying out animal experiments (Category B). *Laboratory Animals*, **34**, 229–235. http://www.felasa.eu/recommendations.htm (accessed 27 April 2008)

Federation of European Laboratory Animal Science Associations (2002) FELASA recommendations for the accreditation of laboratory animal science education and training. *Laboratory Animals* **36**, 373–377. http://www.felasa.eu/recommendations.htm (accessed 27 April 2008)

Federation of European Laboratory Animal Science Associations (2007) *Euroguide: On the accommodation and care of animals used for experimental and other scientific purposes*. Royal Society of Medicine Press, London. http://www.rsmpress.co.uk/bkfelasa.htm (accessed 27 April 2008)

Federation of European Laboratory Animal Science Associations (FELASA) Working Group on Ethical Evaluation of Animal Experiments (2007) Principles and practice in ethical review of animal experiments across Europe: summary of the report of a FELASA working group on ethical evaluation of animal experiments. *Laboratory Animals*, **41**, 143–160. http://www.felasa.eu/recommendations.htm (accessed 27 April 2008)

Her Majesty's Stationery Office (1985) *Scientific Procedures on Living Animals* (Cmnd.9521). London. http://www.archive.official-documents.co.uk/document/hoc/321/321-xa.htm (accessed 27 April 2008)

Interagency Research Advisory Committee (1985) US Government Principles for the Utilization and Care of Vertebrate Animals Used in Testing, Research, and Training. *Federal Register*, May 20, **50**. http://grants.nih.gov/grants/olaw/references/phspol.htm#USGovPrinciples (accessed 27 April 2008)

Johnson, D. and Morin, M. (1983) U.S. laws, regulations, and policies important to managers of nonhuman primate colonies. *Journal of Medical Primatology*, **12**, 223–238

Johnson, D., Morin, M., Bayne, K. *et al.* (1995) Laws, regulations, and policies. In: *Nonhuman Primates in Biomedical Research: Biology and Management*. Eds Bennett B.T., Abee C.R. and Henrickson R., pp. 15–31. Academic Press, Inc., New York

Joint Working Group on Veterinary Care: Voipio, H-M., Baneux, P., Gomez de Segura, I. A. *et al.* (2008) Guidelines for the veterinary care of laboratory animals: report of the FELASA/ECLAM/ESLAV Joint Working Group on Veterinary Care. *Laboratory Animals*, **42**, 1–11

Korean Animal Protection Law. 26 January 2007. http://www.aapn.org/koreanlaw.html (accessed 27 April 2008)

Ministry of Agriculture and Forestry, New Zealand (2006) *Guide to the preparation of codes of ethical conduct*. http://www.biosecurity.govt.nz/files/regs/animal-welfare/pubs/naeac/naeaccec.pdf (accessed 18 July 2008)

Ministry of Agriculture and Forestry, New Zealand (1999) Animal Welfare Act 1999. Public Act 1999, Number 142. http://newzealand.govt.nz/record?recordid=2367 (accessed 27 April 2008)

Ministry of Environment, Japan (2006) *Standards relating to the care and management of laboratory animals and relief of pain* (Notice No. 88). http://www.env.go.jp/nature/dobutsu/aigo/anim_guide/index.html (accessed 27/04/2008)

National Advisory Committee for Laboratory Animal Research (2004) *Guidelines on the Care and Use of Animals for Scientific Purposes*. Singapore. http://www.ava.gov.sg/NR/rdonlyres/C64255C0-3933-4EBC-B869-84621A9BF682/8338/Attach3_AnimalsforScientificPurposes.PDF (accessed 27 April 2008)

National Animal Ethics Advisory Committee (2002) *Guide for the Use of Animals in Research, Testing and Teaching*. Ministry of Agriculture and Forestry, Wellington, New Zealand. http://www.biosecurity.govt.nz/files/animal-welfare/naeac/papers/guide-for-animals-use.pdf (accessed 18 July 2008)

National Animal Ethics Advisory Committee (2007) *A guide for lay members of Animal Ethics Committees*. http://www.biosecurity.govt.nz/files/regs/animal-welfare/pubs/naeac/2007-lay-members.pdf (accessed 18 July 2008)

National Association for Biomedical Research (1999) Animal Legal Defense Fund (ALDF), *et al.* v. Glickman, *et al.* and NABR. U.S. District Court for the District of Columbia, Civil Action No. 96-408 (CRR), U.S. Court of Appeals No. 97-5009 consolidated with 97-5031 and 97-5074. Summary as of 8 June 1999. Washington, DC

National Health and Medical Research Council (2004) *Australian Code of Practice for the Care and Use of Animals for Scientific Purposes*. Australian Government. http://www.nhmrc.gov.au/ethics/animal/issues/index.htm (accessed 27 April 2008)

National Health and Medical Research Council (2008) *Guidelines to promote the wellbeing of animals used for scientific purposes: The assessment and alleviation of pain and distress in research animals*. http://www.nhmrc.gov.au/publications/synopses/ea18syn.htm (accessed 18 July 2008)

National Research Council (1996) *Guide for the Care and Use of Laboratory Animals*. National Academies Press, Washington DC. http://www.nap.edu/readingroom/books/labrats/ (accessed 27 April 2008)

Nuffield Council on Bioethics (2005) *The Ethics of Research using Animals*. London. http://www.nuffieldbioethics.org/go/ourwork/animalresearch/introduction (accessed 27 April 2008)

Office of Laboratory Animal Welfare, National Institutes of Health (2002) *Public Health Service Policy on Humane Care and Use of Laboratory Animals*. Bethesda, MD

Olfert, E., Cross, B. and McWilliam, A. (1993) *Guide to the Care and Use of Experimental Animals, Volume 1*, 2nd edn. Canadian Council on Animal Care, Ottawa

Orlans, B. (2001) Ethical themes of national regulations governing animal experiments: An international perspective. In: *Applied Ethics in Animal Research. Philosophy, Regulation, and Laboratory Applications*. Eds Gluck, J., DiPasquale, T. and Orlans, B., pp. 131–147. Purdue University Press, West Lafayette

Rozmiarek, H. (2007) Origins of the IACUC. In: *The IACUC Handbook*, 2nd edn. Eds Silverman, J., Suckow, M. and Murthy, S., pp. 1–9. CRC Press LLC, New York

Rupke, N. (1987) *Vivisection in Historical Perspective*. Croon-Helm, London

Russell, W. and Burch, R. (1959) *The Principles of Humane Experimental Technique*. Methuen, London (2nd Edn 1992, UFAW). http://altweb.jhsph.edu/publications/humane_exp/het-toc.htm (accessed 27 April 2008)

Russian Ministry of Health (1973) *Guidelines for Animal Experiments* (1045-73 and 52-F3-24.04.95). Moscow

Sanitary regulations for the organization, equipment and maintenance of animal facilities for experimental biology (vivaria) (1973) No. 1045-73. Russia.

Science Council of Japan (2006) *Guidelines for Proper Conduct of Animal Experiments*. Tokyo, Japan. http://www.scj.go.jp/ja/info/kohyo/pdf/kohyo-20-k16-2e.pdf (accessed 27 April 2008)

Select Committee on Animals in Scientific Procedures (2002) *Memorandum by the Chief Inspector*, **III** 179, (HL paper 150-III). House of Lords, London

Slaughter, B. (2002) Animal use in biomedicine: an annotated bibliography of Buddhist and related perspectives. *Journal of Buddhist Ethics*, **9**, 149–158. http://www.buddhistethics.org/9/slaug021.html (accessed 27 April 2008)

South African Bureau of Standards (2008) *Standards Bulletin*, September 2008. https://www.sabs.co.za/pdf/Business_Units/Standards_SA/09-08.pdf (accessed 24 June 2009)

State Science and Technology Commission (1988) *Regulations of People's Republic of China for Administration of Laboratory Animals*. Beijing

Taiwan Animal Protection Law. 4 November 1998. http://www.animallaw.info/nonus/statutes/sttaapl1998.htm (accessed 27 April 2008)

The Prevention of Cruelty to Animals Act 1960 (59 of 1960), Amended by Central Act 26 of 1962, Republic of India. http://envfor.nic.in/legis/awbi/awbi01.pdf (accessed 18 July 2008)

US Department of Agriculture (1991) Code of Federal Regulations, Title 9, Part 3, Animal Welfare; Standards; Final Rule. *Federal Register*, **56**, 1–109

US Congress, Office of Technology Assessment (1986) State regulation of animal use. In: *Alternatives to Animal Use in Research, Testing, and Education*. pp. 305–331. US Government Printing Office, Washington, DC

Walker, A. and Poppleton, W. (1967) The establishment of a specific pathogen-free (SPF) rat and mouse breeding unit. *Laboratory Animals*, **1**, 1–5

World Organisation for Animal Health (2009) *Use of Animals in Research, Testing and Teaching: Proposals for Terrestrial Animal Health Standards*. http://www.aphis.usda.gov/import_export/animals/oie/downloads/tahc_mar09/tahc_use_ani_res_test_teaching_mar09.pdf (accessed 23 June 2009)

9 Planning, design and construction of efficient animal facilities

Barbara Holgate

Introduction

Research animal facilities are complex and highly technical buildings which need to be planned to address the need to provide for the health and welfare of the animals, as well as the health and safety of the people working within the facility. In view of this, the planning and design process for a new or refurbished facility needs to be carefully thought through and to involve all those with an interest in the final functioning of the facility.

The key groups to involve at the planning stage include:

- the scientists who will plan and conduct studies within the facility;
- the animal technicians who will service the facility and care for animals within it;
- the engineering and other support staff who maintain the fabric of the building;
- health and safety advisors;
- regulators.

This is also the point at which to consider how the animals' needs can best be met.

The objectives and critical success factors for the new facility need to be specified very clearly. These are likely to include:

- capacity to meet research objectives by reducing environmental variability in animal studies and maximising the capacity to capture data;
- maximising animal welfare;
- providing a pleasant and safe environment for people to work in;
- maximising the future flexibility and adaptability of the facility;
- minimising the total lifetime cost of the facility;
- completing the project on time and within budget;
- building a state-of-the-art facility in order to attract and retain talented researchers.

Establishing the detailed objectives may not be easy: reviewing past and current volumes and types of research and scientific procedures involving animals is necessary, but may not give a clear indication of future needs. Departmental plans, including recruitment patterns and future plans, are important to consider in establishing trends. There is a clear benefit in trying to make facilities as future-proof as possible, by designing with flexibility and adaptability in mind and, if possible, allowing for expansion. One or two examples of recent shifts in trends may help illustrate the need for flexibility. In many countries, total animal usage was fairly steady or declining until the rapid expansion in recent years of the use and breeding of genetically altered animals (especially mice). An even more recent trend is the expansion in use of zebrafish. UK Home Office statistics for 2008 (Home Office 2009) summarise recent trends for the UK, and may be useful in helping to predict trends elsewhere also. Over many years, the use of mice has increased, and the use of rats has decreased. The number of animals used in breeding has increased steadily, as has the proportion of those animals which are genetically altered – this had reached 37% in 2008. The overall percentages for different species used in the UK in 2008 are shown in Table 9.1.

The design process and design team

For a successful project, a large amount of thorough preparation is needed before the first pile is driven. This should start many years before the facility is required, and one of the first steps is gaining recognition and acceptance of the fact that a new or refurbished facility is required. This may require collation of large amounts of data on occupancy of existing facilities, and predictions of future work, both in terms of volume and type.

A useful activity at this early stage is process mapping (Bicheno 2004). This is a formal way of capturing existing activities, and also allows the opportunity to identify scope for improvement, either within the existing facility or in the future facility that is to be designed. In some cases, the additional efficiencies that may be identified might postpone the need to build or extend facilities; if not, then the results of the exercise are useful confirmation that a new facility is indeed necessary.

Once there is some commitment to build a new facility, a design team should be assembled. In the early stages, this should include, at minimum, representatives of the future users of the facility (typically researchers, animal technicians and laboratory animal veterinarians), a project manager, an architect and engineering representatives. Although a small design team can usually make progress more rapidly, it is essential that the user population is adequately represented. Failure to consult widely and appropriately may well result in a design which is at worst unsuitable for the proposed

Table 9.1 UK Home Office statistics for species used in scientific procedures in 2008.

Species	*Percentage of total*
Mice	66%
Rats	10%
Fish	17%
Birds	3%
Other mammals	3%
Reptiles and amphibians	1%

use, or at best very unpopular, leading to multiple complaints and dissatisfaction.

There is a significant advantage in engaging architects and engineers that have prior experience of the design and construction of animal facilities. This shortens the education process that otherwise is required to inform these individuals about the detailed requirements of such facilities. It also allows visits to existing facilities where they have been engaged previously, to learn from the relative successes and failures (Association for Assessment and Accreditation of Laboratory Animal Care (AAALAC) 1998). If possible, several such visits should be arranged and discussions should take place with the current users of those facilities to seek their views.

Traditionally, the design goes through several iterations, from initial concept, to the development of a brief, and then of the detailed tender documents which are used to engage contractors to build the building. More recently, an approach known as 'alliance contracting' has gained popularity, where contractors are engaged at an early stage, involved in development of the design, and then share in the risks and benefits that develop through the project. This approach has arisen mainly because of cases in the past, in which contractors have taken on too much risk in accepting contracts and have either gone out of business or ended up in lengthy legal disputes with the contracting parties (Egan 1998).

Key information required in early planning

Species

While the full range of species that may be kept in a facility can be difficult to predict, a facility designed to house rodents can generally be adapted to house the majority of small species that might be considered. This could even be extended to include some aquatic or amphibious species such as fish and toads. Among the points to consider here are to ensure that the load-bearing capacity of the floor of the facility will cope with the additional weight of containers filled with water, that there is a means of dealing with water from spillage or leaks, either through drainage or vacuuming, and that the ventilation system can deal with high relative humidity within the area.

Facilities intended for large animals (eg, dogs, farm animals, macaques) are rather different, and it can be very difficult to adapt the functions of a facility designed for large animals to suit smaller ones, and *vice versa*. Larger animals such as dogs, pigs and primates will normally be kept in large enclosures rather than in racks of cages within a room, and these animals are much more capable of causing damage to fixtures and finishes, therefore the choice of materials must be much more durable than is necessary with rodents and other small animals. Large-animal facilities also require more extensive consideration of noise reduction and the means of dealing with the larger volumes of bedding and other waste. Again, flexibility is desirable, and several establishments have designed accommodation that is adaptable to the needs of both pigs and dogs.

Capacity

Calculating the required capacity for a new facility is often a process of educated guesswork. Information that may be available to help the calculations will include historical data and future estimates of the number of animals used annually, the duration of typical studies or, most usefully, the number of each type of animal that may be held at any given time. Another critical factor is whether or not animals are held individually, or group housed, and what provisions are made for environmental enrichment. Space allowances must, of course, at minimum, comply with local legislation for a particular type of animals involved (Home Office 1989, 1995; Institute of Laboratory Animal Resources (ILAR) 1996; Council of Europe 2006), but more generous provision allows for a wider range of enrichment approaches.

Capacity for breeding and supply of animals

The majority of research facilities now source many of the animals that they use from commercial suppliers and breeders. In general, these suppliers can provide animals more efficiently than on-site breeding facilities. There may be exceptions, such as the creation and breeding of genetically altered animals, where the breeding is in essence an experiment in its own right, and the researcher may wish to keep the various steps of the breeding programme under their direct control. There can also be exceptions where, because of long transport routes, or concerns over security, the decision may be taken to undertake in-house breeding of key species and strains. However, it can usually be assumed that space should be provided for the holding, acclimatisation and conduct of procedures on animals, but not for their breeding and supply.

Holding capacity

The information required to inform estimation of the necessary holding capacity includes:

- The number of each animal to be housed at any time. If possible, it is useful to have an estimate of the average population, the minimum and the maximum, as, depending on the urgency of the work, it may be possible to smooth out the peaks and troughs in population rather than provide capacity for the worst-case scenario.
- The range of ages and weights of animals to be kept, and the effect this may have on stocking density.

- Whether any animals will need to be housed singly, or whether they can be group housed, taking into account legislation on stocking densities.
- It is also helpful to find out whether animals awaiting procedures can be housed in accommodation with those of other investigators, or whether they need to be segregated from other groups. This may be affected by factors such as health and immune status, and susceptibility to disturbance.
- Cage and rack design. There is considerable variation in the stocking densities that can be accommodated within a given footprint, depending on the style of caging that is chosen. Many of the cage manufacturers have developed higher stocking density systems, by reducing the space between cages in a rack, increasing the height of racks or introducing so-called 'library' systems, where racks are rolled to and fro to open up working space when required, rather than providing a permanent space between racks. Increasing stocking density in these ways will have a significant effect on ventilation needs. It is also wise to consider the impact on ergonomics; placing and managing cages on the top and/or bottom row of racks can involve uncomfortable stretching and may be injurious to staff over time.

Capacity for procedures

It is important to try to gain estimates from the researchers that will be using the facility on the number of animals they foresee undergoing experimental procedures at any given time, and the duration of those procedures. In general, it can be difficult for research groups to share either procedure rooms or rooms for holding animals under study. However, in order to achieve efficient use of space, such sharing should be encouraged whenever possible.

There is a trend to gather more information from each animal than was possible in the past (which, as a general principle, is to be encouraged). This means that more measuring and observational equipment is required, and hence the proportion of procedure to holding space is increasing. As a rule of thumb, 10 years ago, the proportion of procedure space to holding space was around one third to two thirds. However, that is changing and many newer facilities are designed to provide two thirds procedure space and one third holding space. If one includes some of the highly complex imaging facilities that are now being built, that proportion seems set to shift even further. It is essential to obtain as much information as possible about the experimental procedures that are planned and to build in flexibility to accommodate those which may not yet have been anticipated.

Health status and barrier requirements

The health status of most research animals has improved considerably over the last 10–15 years, and suppliers can generally provide common rodent strains to a reliable specific pathogen free (SPF) status. Hence some of the historical concerns over segregation, containment and quarantine of groups of animals have diminished. This may not apply to genetically altered animals (GAA) obtained from other research establishments rather than commercial suppliers. In addition, many GAA strains have altered immune status and are more susceptible to infections. Research may involve the use of infectious agents (including those that have been genetically modified), and an understanding will be required of the hazard categories to which they belong and the necessary containment requirements. For many reasons, then, it is very important to develop an understanding of the health and immune status of the animals to be used, and the work to be conducted, in defining the required barrier structures, systems and procedures. In a multi-user research facility, it is usual to have to provide for groups of animals with different health or immune status, and so a single, facility-level barrier system is unlikely to be satisfactory. It is more likely that a local barrier system that allows protection or containment at room, isolator or cage level will be required. Components of barrier systems are outlined in Table 9.2.

Site

Ideally, the chosen site would be large enough to allow an ideal footprint size and to minimise disturbance to neighbouring facilities, would have good access to utilities, be accessible for the researchers and be secure. Very often, there is little choice of site, where the proposed new animal facility is to be located within an existing research establishment; and this will mean that conflicts and compromises will need to be carefully managed.

Points to consider in selecting a suitable site include:

- Access – both during construction and operation of the building. Management of the construction issues is a specific engineering discipline (construction design and management – CDM) and will require an early study to confirm that the building can indeed be constructed on the site proposed.
- Planning restrictions. These can often include restrictions on the height of the building and on visual appearance. Early consultation with planning authorities is advisable, in order to identify and address potential concerns.
- Scope for future expansion. This is an ideal – often the site is only just large enough for the current requirement. But if extension at a later date is a possibility, then care must be taken not to 'sterilise' the site for further expansion by the positioning of the current development.
- Access to utilities. It must be possible to supply all the required utilities and services to the site, and not to disrupt existing services.
- Access to outside space for large-animal enclosures. This may introduce security concerns and can also mean noise disturbance to nearby buildings.
- Relationship with other nearby buildings. This can include a range of issues, from ensuring researchers can access the animal facility without undue travel time from other laboratories, to assessing the prevailing wind direction, as occupants of buildings downwind of the facility may be affected by smells.

- Geographical and physical hazards (such as the likelihood of floods or major storms).

Costs

Animal facilities have always been relatively expensive and the situation is only likely to worsen, as the work becomes more equipment-intensive. As the rate of change in scientific procedures increases, it becomes harder to prevent obsolescence of facility designs, and therefore the lifespan of buildings (ie, time before their refurbishment, modification or replacement) is tending to decrease. Quoting sample costs here is of little value, as they are not comparable between countries, nor will they remain static over time. However, it may be useful to make some brief comparisons with other types of buildings. A modern, well equipped, rodent research facility (eg, with automated cage-wash and imaging facilities) would be at the top end of building costs, comparable with highly automated laboratory buildings. On the other hand, in the design and construction of a recently completed dog breeding facility, using simple but robust materials, final costs were comparable with those for standard office accommodation on a per square metre basis. Another worthwhile comparison is to benchmark areas of usable space versus circulation space and plant room space (Clough 1999).

The lifetime costs of the facility should also be considered. One issue that can arise in the design and construction of new facilities is that the project capital costs are considered separately from the revenue costs of running a building. Project managers are often under extreme pressure to ensure that their building project is completed within or below budget. To this end, they may be tempted to cut costs in construction and fit-out that would actually result in reduced running costs. Examples of finishing and equipping that may impact on running costs include:

- Quality of finishes. High-quality floor finishes can be extremely expensive per square metre. However, economising in this area can result in a poor finish which wears badly, is hard to clean and maintain, and needs replacing within a short space of time. This increases the total running costs and is also very disruptive.
- Automation. Automated cage wash areas require a very high capital investment. However, fewer staff are required to carry out the cage cleaning operation, so over the lifetime of the building the initial investment

Table 9.2 Components of barrier systems.

Item	*Comment*
Separation of building from hazards (other research facilities, wild rodents)	Although this is a good method of preventing spread of infections, the cost of constructing multiple small facilities makes it difficult to achieve
Exclusion of wild rodents and insects from facility	Rodent-proof doors, or rodent barriers, are recommended at all entrances into the facility. Insecto-cutors are required inside all external doorways
Staff changing routines, protective clothing	Not essential if the barrier is at cage or isolator level, but important if at facility or similar level. May require shower and full change to be really effective. Common sources of infection include hands and respiratory system
Air pressure regimes	Keeping animal holding rooms at positive pressure can help exclude pathogens, but also pushes allergens out of the animal rooms into staff areas, which can increase the risk of development of laboratory animal allergy (LAA)
Air filtration	High-efficiency particulate air (HEPA) filtration is required for maximum protection. This can be at facility level or below (isolator, cage). Lower levels of filtration may be appropriate in conventional facilities. HEPA filtration of extract may also be required if containment of infections is required
Sterilisation and disinfection	All items entering a fully barriered area require treatment (eg, autoclaving, irradiation and/or surface disinfection by spraying, fogging or immersion) to minimise the potential of carrying infections into the area
Isolators	Isolators (usually flexible film isolators) represent the maximum barrier possible, as all items entering the isolator are sterilised or disinfected, and people do not enter the working area
Individually ventilated cages (IVCs)	IVCs can represent an effective barrier, if air is HEPA filtered into the cages, other materials are sterilised before use and all operations requiring opening of the IVC are carried out in a biological safety cabinet. Strict compliance with operating procedures is essential to maintain these systems effectively
Quarantine	An important procedure when adding animals from a less trusted source to animals of a known health status, allowing time for health screening of the new population before they are added to the existing animals
'Clean to dirty' flow of operations	Theoretically, people and materials moving from a 'dirty' area may carry pathogens with them, so ensuring work flows in the opposite direction should reduce the risks
Restricted access	Restricting access to the minimum number of staff, and ensuring they are all trained in correct procedures, should minimise the risks of introduction of new infections

can result in significant savings. As an additional benefit, automation can also minimise the exposure of staff to laboratory animal allergens.

- Ventilation of safety cabinets. Once-through, non-recirculating Class II cabinets can be more expensive to install than other systems, because of the ductwork required. However, because fewer fans and filters are required in the immediate working area, there may be efficiency gains because staff can adopt a more ergonomic working position, and maintenance may be easier and cheaper.

Design considerations

Structure

Modern buildings are commonly constructed with a steel frame. It is important to be aware at an early stage of the spacing between components of the steel frame and to attempt to lay out a grid which is both structurally strong but also reduces interference with room layouts (for example, avoid positioning columns in the centre of rooms). Larger grid spacing requires bigger steel columns and beams, which can add costs and reduce ceiling headroom for distribution of services. Typical grid spacing is around 6–8 m, which allows for room widths of 3–4 m. This is in line with typical animal room widths.

Single or multi-storey?

Single storey facilities are undoubtedly easier to construct and operate. Typically, they would involve a single storey of animal facility, with plant room above. However, the size of site available may often dictate that a multi-storey facility is constructed, or there may be a requirement to build an animal facility as a single floor within a multi-storey research facility. The issues that can arise with multi-storey facilities include:

- movement of people, animals and materials around the facility and, in particular, the need for lifts;
- floor loading by heavy equipment (eg, autoclaves, MRI and PET scanners);
- potential leakage from cage wash facilities or other 'wet' facilities if these are not placed on the lowest floor;
- distribution routes for ventilation, access for maintenance.

Services

Animal facilities will typically need good supplies of electricity, steam, water (including chilled water for cooling) and drainage. Often these will be taken from existing site supplies, but it is essential to ensure that there is adequate supply capacity, and that there are backup systems in case of any interruption. Enquiries should be made about the quality of steam – wet or 'dirty' steam can cause problems with autoclaves and cage washers, as can a lack of steam pressure. Table 9.3 outlines some of the service requirements.

Table 9.3 Checklist of typical service requirements.

Service	*Comment*
Electricity	Required for the majority of equipment, and for lighting. Back-up supply likely to be required for some equipment, especially IVCs and isolators, where failure to supply fresh air to the animals can result in mortality after short periods of time. Electrical power requirements need to be carefully planned in relation to the equipment to be run
Water	Required for hygiene procedures, animal drinking water, staff facilities and cooling
Heat	May be locally generated (in which case fuel such as gas or oil is required) or site supply (eg, hot water, steam)
Laboratory gases	Commonly oxygen, carbon dioxide. Other specialist gases may be needed. Scavenging of waste anaesthetic gases is likely also to require consideration
Drainage	Drainage from sinks and toilets definitely required. Floor drains only essential for large species. Where installed in large animal facilities, floor drains must be designed to prevent blocking with bedding and similar materials

Functional relationships

The layout of an animal facility is critical to its success. Animals, people and materials will need to enter the facility and be moved around within it, then people and waste materials will need to exit (see Figure 9.1). All these different categories of inputs and outputs will need to be handled safely and efficiently, with the minimum of crossing of movement routes (especially for 'clean' versus 'dirty' items). In addition, movement into or near animal holding areas should be minimised to avoid disturbance. Single-corridor versus dual-corridor systems need to be considered: dual-corridor systems make segregation of clean and dirty materials much easier, but are costly in terms of space. Clough (1999) outlines common functions and their relationships and a range of single- or dual-corridor layouts.

Storage

Most facility managers claim that they do not have enough storage space, and this is generally a commodity that is under pressure during the design of a building. To a degree, this is inevitable, as space in animal facilities is expensive and priority tends to be given to the absolutely essential functions such as animal holding, procedures and plant. Some potential solutions to solve the issue include:

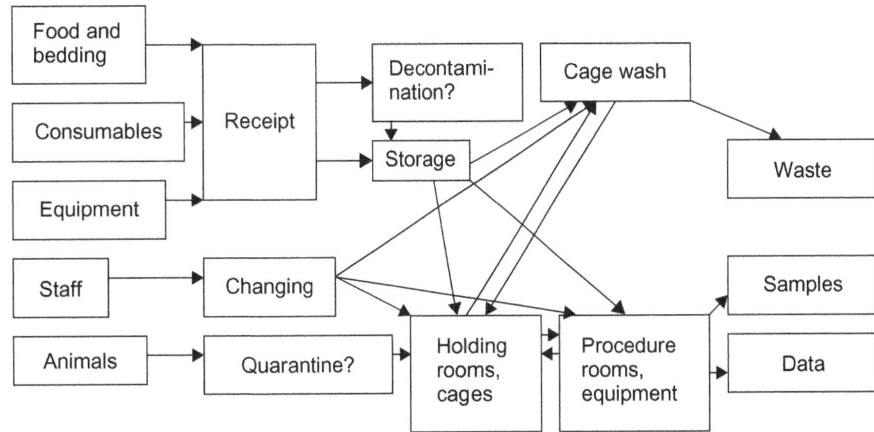

Figure 9.1 Simple process map for planning purposes.

- Working with suppliers to develop 'just-in-time' methods.
- Use of lower specification, cheaper storage space outside the main facility, in conjunction with smaller storage spaces within the facility for immediate use. Several facilities have adopted this approach for bulky items (such as food and bedding), or for equipment that is used infrequently.
- Use of efficient storage and retrieval methods, such as automated 'Kardex'-type systems. Even if not used for automatic re-stocking, these systems make good use of vertical space and reduce corridor space needed to access all parts of the storage system.

Corridors

Corridors are essential but take up a lot of space. They need to be wide enough to allow easy flow of people and materials around the building. The NIH recommendation for single-corridor buildings is 2.1 m clear width (National Institutes of Health (NIH), 1999). In dual-corridor systems, corridors can be narrower as there is less two-way traffic.

Doors

Doors will generally need to be 1.1–1.2 m wide to enable movement of people and materials into rooms. Vision panels can be very useful, but on doors into animal holding rooms these should be provided with a light tight cover or blind.

For safety reasons, doors should normally open into rooms (not out of them into corridors). Alternatively, sliding doors may be used (though these are usually more expensive). Doors should be constructed in such a way as to resist the ingress of moisture into the structure or fabric. Doorways may need to be designed to contain or exclude rodents. This can be achieved with rodent-proof doors or by the use of rodent barriers. Where rodent barriers are used, they can potentially pose a trip hazard: this may be reduced by ensuring either the barrier or the slots which hold it are flexible and safely collapse if a person knocks into the barrier.

Lifts

Animal facilities on a single floor are undoubtedly easier to design and manage than multi-floor facilities. However, limited land space may drive the need for multi-floor facilities. In these cases, dual lifts are strongly recommended, with separation of clean and dirty functions. The shaft of the dirty lift should generally be at negative pressure to the rest of the facility (NIH 1999).

Windows

Traditionally, few if any windows have been built into animal facilities, for two main reasons. Firstly, there have been concerns that windows are a weak point in security, and secondly, they can make controlling photoperiods more difficult. However, more recently, there has been a desire to make the working conditions for people inside animal facilities more pleasant, and it seems that access to daylight can be very positive in this respect. It can also create the impression of a more open facility. Careful placement of windows in administrative areas, or on outside corridor walls, can achieve these positive gains without significant adverse impact. Skylights and light tubes can be useful alternatives. In large-animal facilities (for example, housing dogs or primates), access to daylight can be seen as a positive enrichment and recommendations to this effect are now starting to appear in some national and international guidelines (Council of Europe 2006).

Floors and floor drains

Floors should be made from robust and durable materials, capable of physical cleaning and disinfection.

Drains are essential for large-animal facilities, where large volumes of water may be used in cleaning. However, difficulties are commonly experienced in achieving an adequate floor fall towards floor drains, resulting in pooling of fluids. For this reason, where drains are not essential, it is suggested they may be best avoided.

As well as choosing an appropriate flooring material, it is essential to make sure that the contractors laying the floor are skilled and experienced. Poor-quality workmanship is a frequent cause of problems in this area.

Where drains are provided, the drain traps should be kept filled with water and additional means of preventing the ingress of wild rodents may be necessary. If floor drains are used in rodent facilities, the design should also prevent the escape of the animals housed. Drains in large-animal facilities will need to be of adequate diameter and it is highly likely that stainless steel mesh baskets will need to be provided in the drains to catch sawdust bedding and prevent clogging further down.

The load-bearing capacity of floors will need to be taken into account; especially as very large items of equipment are increasingly being used. For example, MRI and PET facilities involve very heavy equipment and may be best placed on ground or basement floors.

Walls

Walls need to have smooth, moisture resistant finishes, capable of withstanding regular fogging or disinfection. It is not always necessary to have heavy-duty construction (eg, plastered block walls). Lightweight construction of stud and plasterboard, with an appropriate finish (eg, Vinyl sheet), can be satisfactory in small animal facilities. The advantage of this type of construction is that it is relatively flexible, and removal of a wall, or creation of a new one, can be done with the minimum of disruption. Prefabricated panel systems may also be appropriate – there are several systems in use in hospitals which may be worthy of consideration. The key point to be covered in the building brief is that the walls, along with the floors, must be capable of regular cleaning and disinfection. Attention to sealing joints and coving angles, where appropriate, is very important.

Bumpers and guards

Due to the relatively heavy traffic within animal facilities, walls, doors and lifts will require bump rails and corner protection to avoid damage. These must be positioned at the correct height to prevent sharp corners on trolleys and cage racks from making contact with the finishes to be protected, and should be robust and firmly fixed. Bump rails must be deep enough to protect surface-mounted items such as electrical sockets.

Ceilings

Ceilings should be smooth, to avoid the creation of dust-traps. Depending on the function of the particular room, they should be moisture resistant and capable of cleaning. However, where ceilings are not going to be subject to contact with a lot of water or disinfectants, there may be an opportunity to use sound-absorptive materials to reduce sound levels within the room. As far as possible, the design of the facility should avoid the need to access above ceilings to conduct maintenance on, for example, ventilation and lights.

Drinking water for animals

Animals should be supplied with uncontaminated drinking water. The precise quality of water, and the treatment required to achieve this quality, will usually depend on the health and immune status of the animals concerned. For example, in a barriered breeding unit, it might be appropriate to filter, chlorinate and irradiate the water with UV light. On the other hand, water supplies to a conventional dog unit could be taken straight from the municipal supply. Water supplied to immunocompromised animals within isolators may well need to be completely sterile. Acidification may need to be considered – it has been used as a means of controlling infection with organisms such as *Pseudomonas aeruginosa*. Hard water may need to be treated to avoid deposits within delivery systems. Reverse osmosis appears to be the method of choice for this purpose, as it requires no addition of chemicals.

The water delivery systems for animals need to be considered. Traditionally there have been two choices: either automatic water systems or bottles. More recently, suppliers have been offering the option of supplying water in plastic pouches (similar to pouches used for sterile intravenous fluids). Attributes of different water delivery systems are summarised in Table 9.4.

Procedure rooms

General procedure space will be required in research facilities, in which to conduct routine and common activities such as dosing animals, collecting samples and making observations. This space can be suitable for diverse activities – typical requirements are that it is quiet, close to the holding area, well lit and sufficiently spacious to allow for equipment. Typically, such rooms will contain laboratory benching and cupboards, a sink, plentiful electrical sockets and data sockets, and little else in the way of fixed equipment; researchers will bring equipment to the room as and when required. Cantilever benching is often favoured, as it allows easy floor cleaning.

More specialised space is required for surgical procedures and for *post-mortem* examinations.

Increasingly, in all procedure areas, provision is required for engineering controls to reduce exposure to laboratory animal allergens. Options include Class II cabinets, downflow tables and laminar air flow (LAF) booths. Operator protection and ease of use varies, with Class II cabinets being hardest to use from an ergonomic perspective, but offering best protection, while downflow tables and LAF booths offer less protection but greater ease of use.

Cage wash facilities

It has been recognised in recent years that cage changing and cleaning is one of the activities that may lead to the highest exposure to laboratory animal allergens. Various approaches have been taken in order to try to reduce this exposure. Mobile bedding disposal stations are available, which draw air from the front of the cabinet to the back,

Table 9.4 Attributes of different animal drinking water systems.

Automatic system	*Bottles*	*Pouches*
Expensive initial outlay	Bottles relatively cheap. Bottle washing equipment can be expensive (especially if largely automated)	Capital outlay depends on system: pouch-making machine can be expensive; ready-made pouches require no machine but increase revenue costs
Low labour requirement	Can be labour intensive, especially if washing process not automated	Low labour requirement
Constant supply of water (but system still needs regular checking to detect failures)	Water levels require frequent checking	Water levels need checking, but, depending on volume of pouch, less often than with bottles
Failures may not be obvious	Failures generally obvious	Failures generally obvious
Difficult to avoid flooding in conjunction with solid-floored cages	Flooding limited to volume within bottle	Flooding limited to volume within pouch
Impossible to measure water consumption	Easy to measure water consumption	Easy to measure water consumption
Difficult to administer treatments in water to small groups of animals	Easy to administer treatments in water to animals within an individual cage	Easy to administer treatments in water to animals within an individual cage

filter and recirculate it, thus protecting the operator from the allergen-laden dust which would otherwise enter their breathing zone during cage changing. However, these stations tend to be somewhat restricted in size, and can lead to ergonomic issues whilst handling cages within them. This has led to the development of large, walk-in, down-flow booths, where there is much greater access to the actual point of bedding disposal. These are much better ergonomically, but still rely on much repetitive manual work. The most sophisticated cage change and cage wash facilities now incorporate robots to empty cages of waste material and place them on the conveyor of tunnel washers. When the cleaned and dried cages have reached the far side of the tunnel wash, further robots take them off the conveyor, and add clean sawdust and stack them ready for use. These systems are very expensive to install, but capable of high throughput and almost continuous operation, and clearly offer the maximum protection from exposure to laboratory animal allergens. They are, however, only likely to provide an appropriate economic pay-back in large facilities.

Another recent development in cage washing equipment has been the possibility of using cage washers for fumigation, when connected to vaporised hydrogen peroxide (VHP) generators. VHP is an effective surface sterilant and is becoming popular for room and building fumigation. Connected to a cage washer in this way, it can be used to sterilise large items of equipment or bagged consumables.

Autoclaves

If the barrier requirements necessitate an autoclave for sterilisation, then key considerations include:

- ensuring the chamber is large enough to take the largest item requiring sterilisation;
- ensuring the different cycles available are suitable for all the types of materials to be sterilised;
- ensuring the cycle time is short enough to avoid bottlenecks in the operation of the facility; the barrier system will break down if the capacity of the autoclave is insufficient to supply enough sterile materials.

It is also wise to plan how maintenance, repairs and replacement will be carried out without having to cease operation of the facility.

Data handling

Research is a data-intensive process, and it is important to provide sufficient capacity in the facility for collection and transfer of data. High-speed network links and multiple computers allow data to be collected directly, without transcription. Many recording devices (weighing balances, measuring callipers, for example) can be directly linked to computers. Wireless networks may allow the computer to be taken cage-side for immediate recording of observations.

Environmental specifications

This is a key area in the design and construction of an animal facility, and generally represents a high percentage of the overall building cost. National guidelines usually specify performance requirements and may require proof that these are met before the building can be used, hence achieving compliance is a critical success factor for a building project. It must be noted that the majority of guidelines specify the *macro* environment for keeping various species (ie, the room environment), and were probably, partly, empirically derived from environmental parameters that were found to provide comfortable working conditions for staff. The immediate environment around the animals (ie, the micro environment within the cage) can be significantly different. From a functional perspective, as well as meeting compliance requirements for the macro environment, the building design should also ensure the micro environment will support the satisfactory health and welfare of the animals.

Temperature

Theoretically, it seems logical to keep animals within their thermo-neutral zone (TNZ); coping with more extreme ranges may be physiologically possible, but requires considerable energy expenditure and adaptation, and there is evidence of altered experimental results at different temperature ranges (Romanovsky *et al.* 2002). However, Romanovsky and colleagues also explain that the TNZ can vary across different experimental set-ups, even for the same animal. They describe TNZ values from the literature that vary widely, including values for the rat that vary from 18–34 °C. Much of this variation may be a result of the micro environment and the behavioural responses of the animals. Gordon *et al.* (1998) describe the concept of the 'operative' ambient temperature by modelling heat loss in different circumstances. In an acrylic cage with a wire top and no bedding, the 'operative' temperature was more than 10 °C cooler than a similar cage with wood shavings and a filter top. This probably explains why rodents which 'choose' an ambient temperature of up to 30 °C do not appear to suffer cold stress when kept in cages with bedding within a room where the ambient temperature is around 22 °C. One can envisage a future where the performance criteria for the animal facility will be to prove that animals are within their TNZ in whatever caging system is provided. In the current circumstances, while it is necessary to achieve compliance with guidelines and codes of practice, it is also wise to be aware of the potential effects of temperature variations and instability on the research to be conducted in the facility.

In designing a facility, decisions will need to be taken on the range of temperatures which can be set for animal rooms, and whether they are controlled at the level of the individual room, at the level of the whole facility or somewhere in between. Individual room control will add significantly to the costs, while increasing the flexibility to hold species with different temperature ranges, as set out in legislation or codes of practice.

Relative humidity (RH)

Published guidelines recommend RH ranges which avoid extremes (Home Office 1989; ILAR 1996). Low humidity can cause increased heat loss, and 'ringtail' in some strains of rats. High humidity can reduce the ability to lose heat, and has been associated with rapidly increasing levels of ammonia within cages. A set point of 50%, with variation of 15% around the set point, is achievable and avoids likely problems. The ventilation system must be designed to meet these limits within the range of external relative humidity experienced at the location of the facility.

Sound, noise and vibration

There are some circumstances where it is possible that noise within an animal facility will cause physical damage to an animal – loud barking by dogs has been raised as a concern in terms of damage to their own and their handlers' hearing (Sales *et al.* 1997). However, there is a growing body of evidence that noise and vibration can disrupt studies in animals through disturbance and stress effects (Faith 2007). Sudden impact noises may be more of a concern than high but constant background noise levels, as they are more likely to induce a startle response in the animals. It is thus difficult to define acceptable noise levels, but experience suggests that noise levels quoted in the UK Home Office Codes of Practice appear to avoid major disruption (Home Office 1989). Where it is known that planned research is particularly susceptible to noise disruption (such as telemetry or behaviour studies), additional measures, such as sound insulation between rooms or the use of subdivisions within rooms (eg, mobile cabinets with built-in ventilation), may be necessary. The use of such cabinets has been reported to reduce noise levels within the containers by 30dB in comparison with the surrounding room (Mayers 2007).

It is well understood that rodents have a different hearing range to humans, and so sources of ultrasound as a cause of disturbance to the animals must also be considered (Sales *et al.* 1988).

Light

The aim of the lighting system should be to meet the following functions:

- to provide sufficient light to inspect animals and ensure they are healthy;
- to provide sufficient light to conduct procedures (which might include surgery);
- to ensure light levels in the animal's immediate environment are low enough to avoid retinal degeneration or aversiveness;
- to provide a means of controlling photoperiod (including reverse light cycles, which allow the study of animals during their active phase);
- to assist in the provision of a pleasant working environment.

The first two requirements can be contradictory, as high light levels may be aversive to albino rats (Blom *et al.* 1995) but are required to allow intricate work by people. This contradiction can be resolved by positioning of lights, use of tinted or opaque cage material and switching off 'task' lights when not required. Modern building regulations in many countries also require that thought is given to the energy efficiency of lighting. This can include tactics such as linking lights in administrative areas to passive infrared detectors, so that the lights only switch on when people enter the rooms. Energy-efficient light bulbs may be used and these have the added benefit that they last longer and require less maintenance. Light emitting diode (LED) technology is showing significant promise in this area. Energy-efficiency requirements may drive the need to consider the use of daylight where possible: this can also make for a more pleasant working environment, but it is important to ensure animal holding areas can be made lightproof, so as not to interfere with photoperiods.

A wide variety of research programmes may require the use of reverse light cycles. Traditionally, this has been achieved by the use of red sleeves around fluorescent strip lights. However the colour density of these sleeves can be variable, and there has been some interest in looking at sodium lights, as a more reliable means of providing a wavelength that is not visible to rodents (McLennan & Taylor-Jeffs 2004). Aside from this, there is little strong evidence about the effects of different light colours, and standard fluorescent or incandescent lights have been used for many years without apparent issues (Clough 1999).

Heating, ventilation and air conditioning systems

The main objectives of a ventilation system should be to supply adequate oxygen, to remove excess heat generated by animals, people and equipment, to extract waste gases and particulates, and to maintain an appropriate relative humidity. Additionally, the ventilation system may be designed to maintain pressure differences between different parts of the facility. The ventilation system should do all this without creating draughts which may be uncomfortable for the occupants. AAALAC reports that inadequacies of ventilation systems are one of the commonest reasons for failing inspections (AAALAC 2007), and that this was, typically, because specifications for temperature, humidity or air change rates were not being met. Given that these performance data are specified at an early stage in most projects, and have been relatively constant for many years, it is somewhat surprising that such failures are so common.

The key driver for designing the system is usually the removal of heat generated by animals, humans and equipment. Hence a good estimate of stocking density is an important starting point in calculations. Air change rates sufficient to achieve this aim will also deal successfully with waste gases and smells in most cases.

Distribution of the air in the rooms is critical in achieving appropriate delivery of fresh air and removal of waste gases. Clough (1999) describes common positions for supply and extract vents to achieve good distribution of air, and the design of systems can now also be informed by computer modelling. Prior to this, physical mock-ups were often used, either using live animals, or simulations with small heat-generating objects such as light bulbs.

A very useful summary of details from guidelines, and data such as heat production from different species, is provided at the Phoenix website (Phoenix 2003).

There is a number of approaches that can be taken to the distribution of HVAC (heating, ventilation and air conditioning) ducting within a building. Broadly, these are either horizontal (walk-on ceilings or parallel interstitial space) or vertical (vertical risers). Vertical distribution takes up horizontal space within rooms, but allows the overall building height to be lower. It can be more energy efficient than horizontal distribution. Horizontal distribution generally provides better access for maintenance.

The HVAC system should be designed to provide some degree of surplus capacity or redundancy. For example, it may be possible to supply the facility from two air handling units, both sized to run at 60% capacity during normal operation. In case of failure of one unit, the other can be ramped up to deliver around 80% of the normal requirements of the facility.

The HVAC system must be designed to help achieve the target noise levels for the facility. Air flow velocity, duct and diffuser size, turbulence due to changes of duct direction and vibrating fans are just some examples of sources of noise in these systems, which need to be minimised if the recommended levels are to be achieved.

Individually ventilated cage systems and integration with HVAC

The IVC system has become a common means of keeping rodents in recent years. The technology evolved from the simple filter cage (Kraft 1958) to systems which have delivery and extraction of air from each cage, and in which HEPA filtration can be provided on both supply and extract if required. Supply and extract can be balanced to provide positive or negative pressure with respect to the surrounding room. If combined with an appropriate transfer station (eg, microbiological safety cabinet or similar) for all manipulations involving opening of the cage, good containment of or protection from pathogens can be provided, as well as good micro-environmental conditions (Lipman 1999). Details of specific systems are best discussed with the various manufacturers, who can provide details and performance features of their current models. However, some general points on whether and how to integrate IVC systems with HVAC systems are provided here. Early IVC systems were self-contained, with fan units for supply and extract normally standing next to, or fixed on top of, the cage rack. More recently, manufacturers and ventilation engineers have considered integration of the cage ventilation with the building HVAC systems. The pros and cons of the various options have been reviewed (Stakutis 2003) and can be briefly summarised as follows:

- Independent supply and exhaust fans. These are easy to fit into existing facilities, but can be noisy, cause vibrations and generate extra heat, which is retained in the room as the extracted air is recirculated. The space requirements are larger. Control systems are simpler and only small numbers of racks are affected by any failures.
- Independent supply and exhaust fans with thimble or capture hood for exhaust. In theory, this has the advantage that exhaust gas is extracted from the room, rather than recirculated within it. However, it is expensive (all the costs of the first system, plus the cost of thimbles) and can be very difficult to balance satisfactorily.
- Independent supply fan, exhaust ducted into building ventilation system. Here the supply fan is as in the previous two options, but the exhaust gas is extracted purely by the building ventilation system. This approach removes heat and waste gases more reliably, and is potentially less expensive than individual extract fans on each cage rack. Valves connecting into the ventilation extract need to be flow-independent, which can add cost and complexity. Consideration also needs to be given to whether the extract needs to be HEPA filtered, and if so, at what level (at cage level, or more centrally within the building extract ventilation ducting, for example).

- Supply and extract provided by building ventilation system. Here the rack has no independent fans, but relies on the building system for all air movement. In theory, this system will give least noise and vibration locally, and generate no extra heat within the room. No independent power supply is needed within the room. However, there are disadvantages – the valves connecting to the ventilation system all need to be variable flow, which adds cost to the HVAC system. The positioning of the racks within the rooms becomes somewhat less flexible, as the connections to the ventilation system have to be fixed during construction.

As indicated by some of these considerations, integration of an IVC system with the HVAC system is not a trivial undertaking, and if felt desirable, it should be planned at a very early stage of the building design, with close co-operation between the IVC manufacturers and the HVAC designers.

Sustainability

Concerns about global warming and carbon footprints mean that new and refurbished buildings need to take account of energy efficiency and sustainability. Local regulations may require individual electricity metering of different areas of the animal facility in order to record consumption.

HVAC systems are major consumers of energy, and a critical consideration is whether or not air can be recirculated. Recirculation may involve the risk of cross-contamination with pathogens. Whilst in some cases this may be overcome with filtration of air, in others the risk might be considered too great (for example, biohazard areas or areas where non-human primates are housed (ILAR 1996)).

While windows may make the facility more pleasant to work in, and reduce the amount of artificial lighting required, they can also increase solar gain in the facility and increase the need for cooling (which can add significantly to the energy consumption).

More radical approaches might include use of solar panels or wind production of electricity, or novel approaches to insulation (such as the use of grass or moss roof coverings).

Commissioning

Snagging and commissioning are important phases at the end of a project, before the building is handed over for operation. Clear performance targets should have been set during design, and it is essential to make sure these have been met before accepting handover of the building. Sufficient time must be left for commissioning – a period of several months to complete this and get the building running fully is not unusual.

Concluding remarks

Animal facilities are complex, costly and time consuming to build. Such projects require a multidisciplinary team approach, with a strong supportive but challenging team ethos in order to make good progress and deliver a satisfactory result which will meet the objectives. As time progresses, the technical solutions available for tackling the various challenges of maintaining the animal house environment increase but, at the same time, the standards to be met also advance (whether they are standards for animal welfare, human safety or environmental impact). Recent trends (eg, increasing use of imaging, genetically modified animals and fish) show how rapidly requirements can change – this is likely to remain the case, and hence the key challenge for those planning future facilities is likely to be how to build in the maximum flexibility and adaptability.

References

Association for Assessment and Accreditation of Laboratory Animal Care (1998) *Connection* Newsletter, Fall 1998. http://www.aaalac.org/publications/Connection/Fall_1998.pdf (accessed 31 July 2008)

Association for Assessment and Accreditation of Laboratory Animal Care (2007) *Facilities and Operations*, Resources webpage: presentations. http://www.aaalac.org/resources/available.cfm (accessed 31 July 2008)

Bicheno, J. (2004) *The New Lean Toolbox*. PICSIE Books, Buckingham, UK

Blom, H.J.M., Van Tintelen, G., Baumans, V. *et al.* (1995) Development and application of a preference test system to evaluate housing conditions for laboratory rats. *Applied Animal Behaviour Science*, **43**, 279–290

Clough, G. (1999) The animal house: design, equipment and environmental control. In: *UFAW Handbook on the Care and Management of Laboratory Animals*, 7th edn. Ed. T. Poole, pp. 97–134. Blackwell Publishing, Oxford

Council of Europe (2006) *European Convention for the Protection of Vertebrate Animals used for Experimental and other Scientific Purposes, Revised Appendix A, Guidelines on Accommodation and Care (ETS 123).* Strasbourg. http://conventions.coe.int/Treaty/EN/Treaties/PDF/123-Arev.pdf (accessed 31 July 2008)

Egan, Sir J. (1998) *Rethinking Construction*. HMSO, London

Faith, R. (2007) *The Need for Sound and Vibration Standards in US Research Animal Rooms*. ALN Magazine, July/August. http://www.animallab.com/articles.asp?pid=265 (accessed 31 July 2008)

Gordon, C.J., Becker, P. and Ali, J.S. (1998) Behavioural thermoregulatory responses of single- and group-housed mice. *Physiology & Behaviour*, **65**, 255–262

Home Office (1989) *Code of Practice for the Housing and Care of Animals Used in Scientific Procedures*. HMSO, London. http://scienceandresearch.homeoffice.gov.uk/animal-research/publications-and-reference/publications/code-of-practice/code-of-practice-housing-care/?view=Standard&pubID=428573 (accessed 31 July 2008)

Home Office (1995) *Code of Practice for the Housing and Care of Animals in Designated Breeding and Supplying Establishments*. HMSO, London. http://scienceandresearch.homeoffice.gov.uk/animal-research/publications-and-reference/publications/code-of-practice/housing-of-animals-breeding/?view=Standard&pubID=428587 (accessed 31 July 2008)

Home Office (2009) *Statistics of Scientific Procedures on Living Animals, Great Britain 2008*. The Stationery Office, London

Institute of Laboratory Animal Resources (1996) *Guide for the Care and Use of Laboratory Animals*. ILAR, Commission on Life Sciences,

National Research Council. National Academy Press, Washington, DC

Kraft, L.M. (1958) Observations on the control and natural history of epidemic diarrhea of infant mice (EDIM). *Yale Journal of Biology & Medicine*, **31**, 121–137

Lipman, N.S. (1999) Isolator rodent caging systems (state of the art): a critical view. *Contemporary Topics*, **38**, 9–17

Mayers, R. (2007) Personal communication.

McLennan, I.S. and Taylor-Jeffs, J. (2004) The use of sodium lights to brightly illuminate mouse houses during their dark phases. *Laboratory Animals*, **38**, 384–392

National Institutes of Health (1999) *Vivarium Design Policy and Guidelines*. http://orf.od.nih.gov/PoliciesandGuidelines/DesignPolicy/vivtoc.htm (accessed 31 July 2008)

Phoenix (2003) *Standards and Guidelines*. www.phoenixcontrols.com/documents/ch6englishAR.pdf (accessed 31 July 2008)

Romanovsky, A.A., Ivanov, A.I. and Shimansky, Y.P. (2002) Ambient temperature for experiments in rats: a new method for determining the zone of thermal neutrality. *Journal of Applied Physiology*, **92**, 2667–2679

Sales, G.D., Wilson, K.J. and Milligan, S.R. (1988) Environmental ultrasound in laboratories and animal houses: a possible cause for concern in the welfare and use of laboratory animals. *Lab Animal*, **22**, 369–375

Sales, G.D., Hubrecht, R., Peyvandi, A., Milligan, S. and Shield, B. (1997) Noise in dog kennelling: is barking a welfare problem for dogs? *Applied Animal Behaviour Science*, **52**, 321–329

Stakutis, R.E. (2003) Cage rack ventilation options for laboratory animal facilities. *Lab Animal Europe*, **3**, 31–38

10 Enrichment: animal welfare and experimental outcomes

Robert Hubrecht

'The need for designing animal facilities that provide the basic needs of shelter, food, water and a degree of environmental stability has long been appreciated. Currently, however, it is recognized that science also has an ethical responsibility to house animals according to their species specific needs, and that responsibility invokes the concept of behavioural and environmental enrichment.' (Wolfle 2005)

Introduction

It is now almost 50 years since Russell and Burch pointed to the need to refine animal experiments by reducing *'to an absolute minimum the amount of stress imposed on those animals that are still used'* (Russell & Burch 1959, reprinted 1992, p. 134). More recently Buchanan-Smith *et al.* (2005) clarified the definition of refinement as: *'any approach which avoids or minimises the actual or potential pain, distress and other adverse effects experienced at any time during the life of the animals involved, and which enhances their well-being'*. Enrichment having any of these effects is a refinement, which should be implemented wherever possible.

For many years unenriched housing was the norm, but over the last 20 years or so, there has been remarkable growth in the provision of enriched housing conditions for animals used in research. There is a number of factors that are likely to have contributed to this change, not least the development of enrichment in other areas of animal husbandry. Zoos were relatively early adopters of enrichment in the 1970s (Markowitz 1982); included: concerns about the occurrence of abnormal behaviour (eg, Hediger 1950); a better understanding of natural animal behaviour and of the effect of environmental variables on the behaviour, better understanding and physiology of captive animals (Shepherdson 1998, 2003). Within agricultural practice, the Brambell report on farm animal welfare of 1965 stimulated welfare research, calling for studies in the fields of veterinary medicine, stress physiology, animal science and animal behaviour (Fraser 2008). Moreover, a prominent member of the Brambell Committee Dr. Thorpe, suggested that animal welfare might be advanced by studies of motivation and preference: an early call for studies that have since become a major component of enrichment research. Animal welfare science has, since then, developed rapidly; its research influencing current practice with respect to enrichment provision in laboratory animal housing, as well as the newer regulations and codes of practice governing laboratory animals (see Chapter 8). However, it is important to recognise that the impetus for improvements in housing and husbandry has not just come from legislators and animal welfare researchers but also from those directly involved in using and caring for animals in research. Many institutions, even facilities carrying out regulatory work, have developed innovative enrichment strategies as a means to achieving high welfare standards (Dean 1999; Johnson *et al.* 2003).

Nonetheless, experience shows that implementation of enrichment varies between institutions and countries and that some species are either more likely to be provided with enrichment, or are provided with more varied enrichment than others. Moreover, on some occasions researchers or others may resist the use of enrichment. Reasons for these differences in implementation may include concerns about: cost; standardisation; bias of experiments; increase in variation; potential risk to the animal; or a lack of understanding of the welfare impact of enrichment. In order to assess, and perhaps be able to address these concerns, it is important that animal care staff understand the implications of enrichment for welfare and experimental outcomes. The aim of this chapter is to provide a short introduction to the subject by discussing: what enrichment is; why and when it is needed; how it might interact with research requirements; and the practicalities of providing environments that meet animals' needs.

Terminology

As others have noted, enrichment is not a term that has always been used consistently (Bayne 2005; Benefiel *et al.* 2005; Würbel & Garner 2007). As a paradigm in neurobiological research, where it is used to investigate the plasticity of the neural system, it has been defined as *'a combination of complex inanimate and social stimulation'* (Rosenzweig *et al.* 1978, cited in Praag *et al.* 2000). In these neurobiological studies, various modifications are made to standard housing and husbandry practices. Standard unenriched conditions for rodents used in such studies typically comprise socially housed animals in a relatively small enclosure fitted either with a grid floor, or a solid floor with a substrate to absorb waste. Enriched conditions have included: social housing in large groups; larger than normal enclosure sizes; and the provision of various physical items such as tunnels, nesting material, running wheels, etc. Food locations are often also frequently changed (Praag *et al.* 2000).

The purpose of such studies is not to inform animal husbandry decisions, although in some cases the enrichment used in these studies might incidentally have improved welfare. However, for those concerned about animal husbandry, the purpose of enrichment is that it should be beneficial to the animals. Hence, Shepherdson (1998) defines enrichment as *'an husbandry principle that seeks to enhance the quality of captive animal care by identifying and providing the environmental stimuli necessary for optimal psychological and physiological well-being'*. Newberry (1995) defined environmental enrichment as *'an improvement in the biological functioning of captive animals resulting from modifications in their environment'*, and Olsson and Dahlborn (2002) suggest that changes to the environment should only be considered as enrichment when their use results in an improvement in animal welfare.

Not surprisingly, welfare legislation and codes of practice for animals used in research also link enrichment with welfare. So, for example, the Library of Congress defines enrichment as *'enhancing the environment of confined animals in order to encourage natural behaviors and improve their quality of life'* (Kreger 1999). Similarly, a US report on the psychological well being of non-human primates, says that environmental enrichment *'is an independent variable that refers to manipulations to improve the environments of captive primates to enhance psychological well-being'* where *'enrichment is used in the sense of providing for species-appropriate activities in an otherwise restricted and limited environment'* (National Research Council (NRC) 1998, p. 10). In Europe, an amendment to *The European Convention for the Protection of Vertebrate Animals used for Experimental and other Scientific Purposes* (ETS 123) states that *'special relevance should be given to the enrichment of the environment of the respective species according to their needs'*[1] and the recently revised Appendix A to the Convention (Council of Europe 2006) refers to environmental enrichment as being *'an important factor for the welfare of the animals'*. Although the ultimate aim of enrichment in these documents is to have a beneficial impact on the animals, there are differences between them regarding the specific outcome expected (eg, to encourage natural behaviour, enhance psychological well-being, etc). This probably reflects different underlying assumptions regarding the nature of animal welfare. Various definitions of welfare have included concepts such as the ability to perform natural or normal behaviour, evolutionary fitness, feelings, etc (Fraser *et al.* 1997); see also Chapter 6.

The terms behavioural enrichment and environmental enrichment have sometimes been used in rather different ways. Behavioural enrichment has been used to refer to strategies likely to elicit certain species-specific behaviours, whilst environmental enrichment referred to attempts to provide a sufficiently complex environment that would stimulate a wide range of species-typical behaviours (Markowitz 1998). These days, environmental enrichment is more often used in animal welfare science to refer to all attempts to provide a more suitable social and physical environment for captive animals. Approaches to achieve this have included: modifications of the enclosure structure or its surrounds; changes to social structure or opportunities for social interaction; the provision of objects within the enclosure to increase complexity and choice; increased opportunities for sensory stimulation; changes to feeding methods; and strategies to occupy the animals (Bloomsmith *et al.* 1991; Young 2003). To help focus attention on the diversity of enrichment needed, some authors have subdivided the term into subcategories For example, Bloomsmith *et al.* (1991) lists five subcategories: social, occupational, physical, sensory and nutritional. Divisions such as these should be used with care as the categories can overlap. A cage mate (social enrichment) might also be thought to be a form of occupational or sensory enrichment.

The use of the term enrichment to describe a wide variety of changes to a range of husbandry conditions leads to difficulties in using the term in a way that is generally understood. Because enrichment is used by some branches of science in a welfare-neutral way, and because not all attempts at welfare-based enrichment are successful or biologically relevant, Würbel and Garner (2007) have proposed using sub-categories. This subdivision into: pseudo-enrichment (enrichment that does not benefit the animal), conditionally beneficial enrichment (enrichment that is beneficial for some animals or under some circumstances) and beneficial enrichment, seems a very useful way forward.

Why is enrichment needed?

Enrichment and evolutionary niches

Traditional standard laboratory housing provides a very limited environment compared to the natural environments in which animals evolved, which are usually complex and rich in stimuli. Therefore, enrichment has been described as more of a reversal of the impoverishment normally found in the laboratory setting than an enrichment over a natural setting (Praag *et al.* 2000). There is, as will be discussed in the following sections, a considerable body of evidence from both deprivation studies and studies of environmental enrichment (which are fundamentally similar except for the reversal of the experimental and control groups (Fuller 1967)), that barren environments, or housing designed without taking into account the natural history of the animal, can result in abnormal development, physiology and behaviour.

Animals are complex organisms with behaviour and physiology adapted towards their natural ecosystems. The evolutionary process works so that organisms tend to behave and function in ways that maximise their chances of reproduction and reduce their chances of dying before achieving their reproductive potential. This does not, of course, mean that animals in natural environments always experience good welfare. All environments, including natural ones, are likely to include some stressors (defined as

[1] http://www.coe.int/t/e/legal_affairs/legal_co%Doperation/biological_safety%2C_use_of_animals/laboratory_animals/Res%20accommodation.asp#TopOfPage

real or perceived perturbations to an organism's physiological homeostasis or psychological well-being (NRC 2008, p. 2)). However, animals have evolved to respond to a range of natural stressors with coping mechanisms that may include behavioural, hormonal or immune function changes. In captivity, problems can arise if the environment does not allow an appropriate coping response or if the coping response is overloaded, leading to a breakdown of homeostasis and a state of distress.

It is generally accepted that some degree of predictability and control are important in reducing the likelihood that stress will tip into distress, and that control over the environment requires that the environment possesses a certain degree of complexity (Wiepkema & Koolhaas 1993; Rennie & Buchanan-Smith 2006; NRC 2008). There is, however, a balance to be struck between too much and too little predictability (Sambrook & Buchanan-Smith 1997).

Enrichment can allow more opportunities for animals to make choices that allow them to maintain homeostasis or to control social interactions. Mice are commonly housed at 20–24 °C which is outside their thermoneutral zone of 26–34 °C, and given the choice prefer warmer temperatures (Gaskill *et al.* 2009). Nesting material can allow them to create an area with a microclimate and express such choice. Similarly, visual barriers, that allow animals to move out of sight of other animals, may allow them to cope with the ups and downs of social life and to maintain harmonious social groupings.

While the proximate aims of providing enrichment for welfare reasons may be to reduce abnormal behaviour, stimulate normal behaviour, allow the animal to exercise choices etc; for many, the ultimate goal is to improve the animal's affective state. This, sometimes referred to as the animal's emotions or feelings, is part of the mechanism by which animals make choices so as to maximise their chances of survival and reproduction. Hence, environments that frustrate strongly motivated behaviour or that tip the balance of adverse stimuli towards the negative result in poor welfare. It is becoming increasingly accepted that we should not simply be concerned about animals' negative experiences but should also try to promote positive ones (Yeates & Main 2008). To paraphrase Fraser (2008, p. 69), for animals' welfare to be satisfactory, they should experience a minimum of suffering and they should be allowed the normal pleasures of life. As discussed in the sections below, there is a growing body of research indicating that animals' affective states can be adversely affected by traditional standard housing and that they are motivated to attain certain enriched environments.

Motivation for enrichment

If it can be shown that animals really value a particular enrichment, that is, that they are strongly motivated to use it, then that provides a powerful, although not compelling, argument, for its implementation to improve the animals' welfare. Conversely, it is likely that an animal's welfare will be poor if it is strongly motivated to do something but cannot do so because of an inadequate environment. Animal welfare scientists have developed a range of study techniques that provide different types of information on animals' motivation for various resources (see also Chapter 6). The simplest of these are observational studies that report on the animals' use of various enrichment options when they are added to an existing enclosure. Such studies have shown that primates, for example, will use various types of enrichment including foraging devices, toys/manipulanda and mirrors (Lutz & Novak 2005). Dogs make extensive use of platforms and chews when given the opportunity (Hubrecht 1993, 1995a; Joint Working Group on Refinement (JWGR) 2004), and if not provided with chews may chew inappropriate pen materials such as plaster or steel cord. A somewhat more complicated type of study which allows the researcher to rank animals' motivation for resources is the choice or preference test. Such studies have shown that mice, for example, prefer nesting material to a nest box and prefer effective nesting materials to less easily used materials (Olsson & Dahlborn 2002); there are many other examples.

However, neither observational studies nor choice tests provide much indication regarding the extent to which an animal wants a resource. To address this issue, operant studies have been used to assess the strength of animals' motivation for resources (Patterson-Kane *et al.* 2008). In these studies, sometimes known as demand studies, the animals may have to push a lever a number of times in order to obtain a resource, or might have to travel or cross an aversive substrate. By changing the cost that the animal has to pay to access the resource, the experimenter can gain an estimate of the value of that resource to the animal. Such studies have shown that mice are strongly motivated to explore and patrol all accessible areas of their environment (Sherwin & Nicol 1996) and will work for access to resources such as a larger cage and running wheels, enrichment items and deep sawdust (Sherwin 1996). Moreover, the mice worked as hard to maintain access to these resources as for food, giving some idea of the importance of these resources to these animals. Other studies have shown that rats work harder for social contact than for an empty home cage (Patterson-Kane *et al.* 2002), and will lift substantial weights to gain access to a novel environment or a resting place with a solid floor (Manser *et al.* 1996).

These studies have an obvious appeal and have provided extremely useful data on the features that should be provided for various species. However, their interpretation is not always straightforward, demand studies have their limitations (Kirkden & Pajor 2006) and there is ongoing scientific debate on these studies regarding appropriate experimental design and choice of measures. Animals' preferences and choices may be affected by context, experience, time of presentation and the options that are offered to the animal. Moreover, animals' short-term choices may not always be in their best long-term interests; for example, an animal might work hard for a high-calorie treat but eating too many might have long-term health consequences. It is also the case that demand studies on larger species used in research such as dogs and primates are lacking, probably because of the practical and financial difficulties involved in constructing large test apparatus. Despite the difficulties outlined above there is a need to extend demand-study research to these species.

Abnormal behaviour in unenriched or standard housing

Abnormal behaviour is a sign that, at some point, conditions for the animal have not been adequate, and seems to be relatively common in some species used in research. It has been estimated that around 50% of mice, the animals most commonly used in research, stereotype, performing repetitive behaviours such as bar biting, jumping and looping around the cage (Würbel & Stauffacher 1994, reported in Würbel 2006). The prevalence of the behaviour may come as a surprise to some animal care staff, but this is because much of the behaviour is performed at night. Extrapolating from the figures above, Mason and Latham (2004) estimated that the numbers of laboratory housed mice exhibiting abnormal behaviour may amount to a total of 7.5 million worldwide. Gerbils are also prone to develop stereotypies in standard laboratory housing (Wiedenmayer 1997). Similarly for primates, 89% of individually housed rhesus monkeys at a research centre showed abnormal behaviour, with pacing occurring in 78% and self-injurious behaviour occurring in 11% (Novak *et al.* 2006). In carnivores, home range size is linked to their propensity to develop stereotypies (Clubb & Mason 2003). As dogs can range over substantial areas (Hubrecht 1995b) it is, perhaps, not surprising that they also develop stereotypies when kept in restricted social or environmental conditions. In one study, 13% of single-housed laboratory dogs spent more than 10% of their time in repetitive behaviour patterns (Hubrecht *et al.* 1992), and some dogs spent up to 51% of their time performing these behaviours.

It is well known that inadequate social environments during development can lead to abnormal behaviour in the adult. Harlow and his followers in the 1960s demonstrated the importance of a normal social environment for macaques during their development (Novak *et al.* 2006; NRC 2008, Chapter 3). Similarly, Fuller (1967) showed that dogs reared under a partial social isolation regimen became less social and interacted less with their environment; early weaning of mice can lead to increased anxiety, as tested in an elevated plus maze, and poorer maternal behaviour (Kikusui *et al.* 2005). Separation of animals after they have developed social ties can also cause problems. Self-injurious behaviour is much more common in individually housed than socially housed rhesus macaques (Novak *et al.* 2006) while Fox and Stelzner (1966, 1967) found that isolating dogs from conspecifics led to later deficits even if human social contact was provided.

Stimulation of normal behaviour and reduction of abnormal behaviour in enriched environments

Enrichment of barren environments can stimulate an increase in behaviours that are deemed to be normal within the caged environment, typical of behaviour in the wild or simply thought of as desirable behaviour. Young (2003) reviews the literature for this on farm, zoo and laboratory animals. Lutz and Novak (2005) and Honess and Marin (2006) provide extensive reviews of the effects of various types of enrichment on non-human primate behaviour. Enrichment can be used to stimulate desirable behaviours, such as chewing of toy items, as an alternative to the cage or walls by dogs (Hubrecht 1993), and play (marmosets, Ventura & Buchanan-Smith 2003). It may also be used to reduce undesirable behaviours such as aggression in rodents (mice, van Loo *et al.* 2002; rats, Johnson *et al.* 2004) or primates (Honess & Marin 2006).

However, it is important to consider what is meant by normal and to interpret these studies with care. Normal behaviour, as seen in the wild, is not necessarily closely linked with good welfare (see Chapter 6). Behaviour such as aggression is normal, although it may be undesirable in the research environment depending on the context, level and duration of aggression. Similarly, anti-predator behaviour is undoubtedly normal behaviour but its expression is unlikely to be linked to a state of good welfare. When considering how much time is spent in various behaviours, there can be difficulties in determining what would be a normal time-budget for the behavioural repertoire for a species (Veasey *et al.* 1996). It is also necessary to take into account the full spectrum of behaviour elicited by a particular enrichment. For example, Marashi *et al.* (2003) found that enriching male mouse cages increased play (an indicator of good welfare) but also found that aggression, possibly linked to territoriality, was increased.

Enrichment can not only promote normal behaviour, but also reduce abnormal behaviour. Shyne (2006) carried out a meta-analysis of zoo animal enrichment studies, showing that attempts to enrich housing have generally been effective in reducing stereotypies, but to have their best effect, animals should be exposed to an enriched social and physical environment throughout their development. Enrichment later in the animal's life can still be beneficial, but may not undo the damage caused by an inadequate environment during development (squirrel monkeys, Fekete *et al.* 2000; deermice, Hadley *et al.* 2006). Social enrichment, rather than physical items such as toys or foraging devices, seems to be more likely to result in improvements for non-human primates (Lutz & Novak 2005). Nonetheless, some improvement can occur; for example, mealworm feeders decreased marmoset stereotyped pacing (Vignes *et al.* 2001), and Würbel *et al.* (1998) showed that the provision of a tube for mice reduced wire-gnawing by 40%. It has been asserted that because that there is little evidence that enrichment of rodents' cage environments reverses abnormal behaviour, it has no effect on their well-being (Benefiel & Greenough 1998). However, stereotypies resulting from chronic exposure to a sub-optimal environment can be thought of as a behavioural scar (Mason 1991). Hence, stereotypies are not necessarily a good indicator of current welfare status (see Chapter 6) and they can be resistant to improvements in housing condition. Failure to eradicate established stereotypies, therefore, does not necessarily indicate that the enrichment is a failure.

Enrichment and stress

Animals used in research are inevitably exposed to stressors, both during husbandry and during experimental procedures. Enrichment that improves their ability to cope and reduces fear and stress will improve their welfare.

There is evidence for a range of species that enrichment can produce less fearful, more confident and adaptable animals than those kept in barren conditions (Chamove 1989; Prior & Sachser 1994; Larsson *et al.* 2002; van de Weerd *et al.* 2002; Young 2003, p. 34; van Loo *et al.* 2004). A study carried out by Sherwin and Olsson (2004) in which mice were allowed to self dose with an anxiolytic, indicated that mice housed in enriched cages may be less anxious than those housed in standard cages. Environmental complexity can decrease stress reactivity as shown by behaviour in the elevated plus maze, defaecation in a novel environment, defensive responses to a predator and open-field exploration (Lewis 2004). Young (2003, p. 40) cites evidence for the beneficial effects of certain enriched environments on a range of physiological indicators of stress on a variety of species. More recent studies include those by: Benaroya-Milshtein *et al.* (2004) in which enrichment such as ladders, tunnels and running wheels attenuated behavioural and physiological responses to an electrical shock; and van Loo *et al.* (2004) who showed that provision of nesting material reduced corticosterone levels in male Balb/c and CD-1 mice. Changes in stress responses can lead to different disease outcomes, most of which are beneficial (Praag *et al.* 2000); and it has been suggested that the beneficial effects of enrichment observed in mouse models of Huntington's disease and Alzheimer's disease could lead to new avenues of research for effective treatment of humans (Hockly *et al.* 2002; Jankowsky *et al.* 2005).

Reductions in stress responses such as these suggest that enrichment not only has the potential to improve the animals' welfare during husbandry but could also help to refine procedures. For example, Meijer *et al.* (2006) found that enrichment and frequent handling of mice reduced their temperature and heart rate following procedures such as injection or restraint.

Those implementing enrichment programmes should be aware that some common forms of enrichment may not work for a specific gender or strain, resulting in increased stress rather than a reduction. For instance, it can be counter-productive to provide shelters for some strains of male mice, as the enrichment is associated with increases in testosterone, aggression and corticosterone that are probably linked to increases in territoriality (Haemisch *et al.* 1994; Haemisch & Gartner 1994; Nevison *et al.* 1999; van Loo *et al.* 2002).

Enrichment and quality of science

Researchers may be concerned that enrichment could affect their results (Benefiel *et al.* 2005). There is a number of potential issues wrapped up in this concern. These are: that enrichment might affect validity by biasing results by producing abnormal animals; that it might decrease reliability by increasing between-subject variation thus reducing test sensitivity; or it might decrease replicability by increasing between-laboratory variation (Garner 2005; Würbel & Garner 2007). These issues are addressed in the following sections.

Bias

Enrichment (as defined by Rosenzweig *et al.* 1978) certainly has the potential to affect experimental outcomes (Federation of European Laboratory Animal Science Associations (FELASA) 2006). Enrichment can result in: increased neurogenesis; increased capilliary development; the formation and changes to the efficiency of synapses; and changes to neurotransmitter activity (reviewed in Healy & Tovée 1999; Praag *et al.* 2000; Lewis 2004). Rats kept in an enriched environment (ie, with a selection of toys/chews and conspecifics) increase brain size by about 5% with the largest changes occurring in the cortex. Similar effects have been found for other mammalian and avian species, including cats, monkeys and even humans (Healy & Tovée 1999).

Animals kept in enriched environments often show improved memory, learning and behavioural plasticity (Lewis 2004) which may well be related to changes to structures such as the cortex, hippocampus and thalamus (Nithianantharajah *et al.* 2004). It is interesting to note here that, while enrichment does promote neurogenesis, the changes produced by enrichment on spatial learning and habituation are not dependent on this but may result from synaptic changes (Meshi *et al.* 2006).

Enrichment can affect the senses and their development as visual acuity of enriched mice was 18% greater than those of mice kept in standard conditions (Prusky *et al.* 2000). Cortical sensory maps can also be affected. When rats are kept in a naturalistic environment, complete with conspecifics, subterranean tunnels and opportunities for foraging, the cortical representations of the rats' sensory whiskers become refined and more focused, contracting by up to 46% compared to rats housed in standard cages (Polley *et al.* 2004).

So, can enrichment bias experimental outcomes? Benefiel *et al.* (2005) list a range of effects of various types of enrichment on experimental variables that include a range of ameliorative, and sometimes negative, effects on animals used as disease models. Olsson and Dahlborn (2002) provide a detailed review of the effects of enrichment on mice (see also FELASA 2006) and Bayne (2005) lists effects on primates, rabbits and rodents. Some of these effects may be modulated by stress responses, which, as we have seen, can be affected by enrichment. Moreover, changes in anxiety and stress responses can persist for some time after the enrichment is ended (Larsson *et al.* 2002).

At first glance this literature might suggest that, at least for studies where stress responses are measured or might influence the variable in question, enrichment should be avoided. However, it is important to note that the reviews included studies where the aim was not always to improve welfare and the enrichment was more elaborate than would normally be used for animals under study (Olsson & Dahlborn 2002; Benefiel *et al.* 2005). Moreover, the enrichment used in studies where negative effects occurred was clearly not beneficial and thus these studies are irrelevant to considerations of the impact of beneficial enrichment. It is also important to consider whether animals kept in a beneficially enriched environment are more likely to deliver externally valid data. As described earlier, enriched environments are closer to the environments in which animals evolved. It seems likely, therefore, that standard laboratory conditions lead to reductions in size and capabilities of the brains of laboratory animals, which raises questions about the validity of learning and memory research carried out on animals housed in these conditions (Healy & Tovée 1999). Moreover, mismatches between evolved behaviours and the captive environment provided by standard housing (Würbel 2001) are, as already discussed, likely to lead to stressed animals and increased incidence of abnormal behaviour, which could affect the quality of science (see review by Sherwin 2004). Conversely, as Garner (2005) suggests, beneficial enrichment should result in animals that are more like the natural animal in terms of their neural development, physiology and behaviour; and in most cases these should be better experimental models with improved external validity. To summarise, beneficial enrichment should help to avoid bias caused by housing conditions rather than create it.

Despite the arguments outlined above, the situation might arise where there are data indicating that beneficial enrichment has an effect on the experimental variable in question, and the researcher is unconvinced that there is a scientific need for a more normal animal. To answer this, the ethical imperative is to provide, if possible, an environment that meets the animals' needs and it is worth considering the following discussion points: It may be that, as enrichment would be provided to both treatment and control groups, there would be no effect on any difference between the groups. Consider whether the magnitude of any effect produced by enrichment would be trivial compared to the experimental effect. The importance of an enrichment effect should also be judged in context with other factors such as: strain differences (Kim *et al.* 2002); normal husbandry routines (Duke *et al.* 2001); site differences, etc.

Finally, while there is a growing body of literature on the value of many types of enrichment and this has helped to inform guidance given in this volume and elsewhere, it remains true, as pointed out by Würbel and Garner (2007), that further work is needed to clarify the relationship between housing conditions, external validity and welfare, and work of this sort would help inform decisions regarding optimal enrichment.

Replicability and variation

Researchers may be concerned that variable implementation of enrichment will reduce standardisation between sites leading to reduced replicability. However, so-called standard housing is, itself, not particularly standardised, with variation between sites and between countries in cage design, materials and husbandry. Some sites use grid floor cages whilst others use solid-bottomed cages; cages may be made from different materials or ventilated in different ways. Moreover, even when conditions between laboratories are rigorously standardised, systematic differences between the laboratories still remain (Crabbe *et al.* 1999). Further, Würbel (2000) and Würbel and Garner (2007) have argued that institutional standardisation leads to poor external validity, and that it can actually reduce between-laboratory replicability as different laboratories adopt different standards. They suggest that a better approach would be to design factorial experiments with subject animals exposed to a variety of husbandry and environmental conditions including various types of enriched environments.

A related issue is replicability over time. Researchers may be concerned that the introduction of enrichment will impair comparison of current results with those from previous studies (historical data). However, this problem should only be a temporary one; as once an enrichment programme is in place new historical data will rapidly be generated.

With respect to within-study variation, there have been a number of studies reporting variously that enrichment increases variation (Eskola *et al.* 1999; Mering *et al.* 2001; Tsai *et al.* 2002, 2003), reduces it (Eskola *et al.* 1999; van de Weerd *et al.* 2002) or has no effect (Eskola *et al.* 1999; Augustsson *et al.* 2003). Taken together, these studies seem to indicate that there is no obvious effect on variation. Moreover, the enrichments used in these studies were not always those that are commonly used in laboratory facilities to improve welfare and not all may have been beneficial. Only one study, published in the journal *Nature*, has explicitly tested the effects of enrichment on variation and replicability (Wolfer *et al.* 2004). In this study, three laboratories raised three batches of female mice of two strains and their hybrids. The mice were housed in small standard cages or large enriched cages, and the results indicated that enrichment neither increased individual variability in behavioural tests nor the risk of obtaining conflicting data in replicate studies. The authors conclude that, at least for female mice, environmental enrichment should '*improve the animals well-being without reducing the precision and reproducibility of the data derived from them, while attenuating abnormal brain function and anxiety – both of which are possible confounds in animal experiments*'.

Factors to consider when choosing enrichment

What are the benefits of the proposed enrichment?

The aim of enrichment in laboratory animal husbandry is to improve welfare. However, what does this mean in practice? Young (2003, p. 2) provides the following list of goals, which should help to focus planning and to assess success:

Goals of enrichment are to:

1. increase behavioural diversity;
2. reduce the frequencies of abnormal behaviour;
3. increase the range or number of normal behaviour patterns;
4. increase positive utilisation of the environment;
5. increase the ability to cope with challenges in a more normal way.

As discussed earlier, some so-called enrichments may turn out to have no or negative effects on the animals' welfare. Therefore, it is important to avoid filling the animals' enclosure with a random selection of items in the hope that the animal will make use of them. Instead, enrichment choices should be based on a sound understanding of the animal's biology and preferably on experimental research. A good example of enrichment that combines these features is the provision of refuges with tunnels for gerbils.

Gerbils commonly develop stereotyped behaviour in the laboratory. The reason for this was not understood until Wiedenmayer (1997) showed that gerbils not only need a refuge, but also a tunnel of a certain length leading to that refuge to avoid the development of stereotyped digging behaviour. It is likely that this is because gerbils, in the wild, dig burrows that are connected to the surface by tunnels of a sufficient length to reduce the risk of predation and to protect them from other hazards (Chapter 23). As a result, it seems that they are strongly motivated to keep digging if they are not able achieve this goal in captivity. Those implementing behavioural strategies should therefore review the literature to familiarise themselves with the natural history of the species and to identify any proven beneficial enrichments.

While enrichment should be biologically relevant (Garner 2005) it need not be naturalistic (ie, designed to mimic features of the wild environment). However, non-naturalistic objects such as bells, marbles, metal manipulanda, etc, should be evaluated to ensure that they really are a beneficial enrichment and that they are not harmful or distressing to the animals. Even if animals do make use of, or manipulate, enrichment items, it is important to consider whether they are doing so for positive reasons and not, perhaps just trying to remove them from their living areas. The answers to these questions lie in carefully designed behavioural experiments, which, if the enrichment is a commercially marketed one, should be the responsibility of the manufacturer. To help encourage manufacturers to carry out this research, customers of companies selling enrichment should ask to see the scientific data that supports their claims.

Enrichment and animal safety

As the aim of enrichment in laboratory animal husbandry is to improve animal welfare only beneficial, or conditionally beneficial, enrichments should be used. However, the addition of any novel item to an animal's environment carries some risks. It is therefore necessary to attempt to identify these and to weigh them against the likely benefits arising from the enrichment before using a new enrichment. This assessment is likely to require considerable input from care staff, which includes veterinary care staff (Nelson & Mandrell 2005). A good example of the costs and benefits of enrichment is social housing. It is increasingly accepted that social animals should be housed in harmonious social groups (eg, European Commission 2007). Social housing allows animals to interact with each other, thus permitting the expression of species-specific behaviours and keeping them occupied. It may also have other less obvious benefits. For example, Schapiro and Bushong (1994) found that incidences of diarrhoea and dehydration were reduced in socially housed macaques. On the other hand, it is not possible to guarantee that groups will continue to be socially harmonious and social housing carries risks. Bayne (2005) reviews literature for non-human primates where social housing resulted in deaths or increases in self-injurious behaviour. Dogs housed socially also may fight, and in some cases the injuries may be severe, perhaps even resulting in death. For animals at the losing end of these encounters, social housing as enrichment will have failed. Generally, however, although some animals may need to be housed singly, experience shows that aggression can be minimised with good management practices. This is an ethical issue where the consensus is that the benefits to the majority outweigh the risks to the few (Hubrecht & Buckwell 2004; Joint Working Group on Refinement (JWGR) 2004, 2009).

Physical items can also result in injury, either directly, or by increasing aggression. Bayne (2005) reviews harms (as well as benefits) arising from attempts to provide enrichment for non-human primates as well as rodents and rabbits. Animals can become entangled in objects. Murchison (1993), for example, described a case of a pig-tailed macaque becoming entangled in a ring toy. Items placed into a cage may be ingested, even if that is not the specific aim of the enrichment, so there may be risks of choking or obstruction. It is possible that certain types of food enrichment, if not properly controlled, may lead to obesity or tooth decay. Moreover, commonly used enrichments may result in problems for particular strains, eg, nesting material for nude mice (Bazille *et al.* 2001). Enrichment may result in increased aggression either because the items may be desirable resources in themselves, or because they allow the animals to divide the enclosure into territorial units as previously described for male mice. Enrichment within the animals' environment can make cleaning more difficult, and the enrichment items themselves could act as fomites (Bayne *et al.* 1993). To help put these risks into context it is worth considering that no environment is entirely safe, that incidences of disease related to enrichment items seem to be very rare, that enrichment can also reduce aggression (Honess & Marin 2006) and that injuries can occur even in an unenriched environment. Marmosets have been known to entangle their arms in the mesh of their cages; dogs without chews may chew through the steel cable holding up pop holes or even at the walls, with consequent tooth damage. The increased risk of injury from most physical enrichment options is likely to be small, and there are few published reports of enrichment devices resulting in injury (Young 2003; Nelson & Mandrell 2005). This lack of data may not be surprising, given its sensitive nature, but there are obvious benefits that could arise if both failures and successes were published. While the increased risk of injury or disease when using well established enrichment items is small, it is best to avoid problems. The checklist of safety considerations provided by Young (2003) is a useful starting point in carrying out a risk assessment. As Young points out, safety assessment should be an ongoing process, as animals may use enrichment in new and unexpected ways.

Enrichment and human safety

Enrichment strategies must meet the needs of staff and researchers as well as the animals. Clearly any enrichment must be practical and cost effective, and any health and safety issues for the staff must also be addressed. Concerns may include trip hazards, increased weight of enclosures, increased exposure to allergens, exposure to sharp objects (eg, after animals have gnawed or broken them). Some species such as primates or apes may cause injury by throwing enrichment items. Excessive enrichment might also compromise the ability of staff to avoid potentially dangerous animals. Again, an attempt should be made to identify risks to human safety before introducing the enrichment and to find ways of ameliorating these by reconsidering housing and management regimens.

Enrichment and the experiment

Previous sections have discussed the issues of enrichment and experimental outcomes, but it goes without saying that before introducing enrichment both scientists and care staff must be content that it will not adversely affect the outcomes of experiments in which the animals or their offspring might be used. Where there are concerns that a proposed enrichment might have such effects, it is important to carefully assess the validity of these concerns, bearing in mind that enrichment programmes have been successfully adopted in many experimental protocols. It is also important to consider whether the procedures carried out on the animals might impact on the way in which they interact with the enrichment. If, for example, the research involves damage to the animals' motor or sensory function, then this might necessitate changes to enrichment regimens to avoid safety issues.

Validating new enrichment

Ensuring that enrichment is beneficial is an important component of any programme. This issue is discussed in detail in a FELASA working group document (FELASA 2006), which points out that the techniques used to demonstrate a welfare benefit (eg, preference/choice tests, demand studies, physiological measurements) can be difficult to use and to interpret. As previously discussed, choice tests, for example, can provide some indication of the relative value that an animal attaches to a resource, but they do not tell how much an animal either likes or dislikes a resource, or why the animal has made the choice. The test might therefore reflect the animal's motivation to minimise deprivation, maximise pleasure or monitor unwanted problems; and the value of the enrichment in question would be very dependent on which of these was the underlying motivation. Past experience of the animal can also strongly affect preference test outcomes, and in some cases animals may make short-term choices that result in a long-term reduction in welfare or health, such as through diet choices that ultimately result in obesity or dental caries. Finally, the enrichment needs of animals can vary between strain, by gender and with age.

The requirement for validation of enrichment will depend to a great extent on the novelty of the enrichment being introduced. For the reasons outlined above, the initial determination of the types of enrichment required by a species will normally best be carried out either by, or in collaboration with, specialist animal welfare scientists who will be aware of the pitfalls of these studies and will have the necessary experience to choose appropriate measures and study designs.

Once an enrichment has been validated as beneficial it would normally be a waste of time and resources for individual laboratories to repeat this process. For example, it is well known that foraging enrichment is beneficial for primates and further research to corroborate this is unnecessary. Nonetheless, there may be local variations in the implementation of categories of enrichment, and these details may need to be evaluated to ensure that they function as expected, there are no safety concerns and that the enrichment will not compromise the study.

Managing an enrichment programme

Successful enrichment strategies depend on good communication and management. Research institutions should be committed from top management down to providing a high quality of housing for their animals; and animal care staff, veterinarians and research scientists should have bought into this concept. Enrichment should not be introduced piece-meal, but should be properly planned and discussed, particularly with the scientists who will be using the animals.

It may be helpful to have a committee charged with implementing the programme; even if this is not the case, enrichment should be the subject of regular review to ensure that it is being implemented, that there are no problems and to assess its efficacy against current knowledge. For some research programmes, the normal enrichment and housing conditions may not be compatible with the aims of the research, but requests to keep animals without enrichment should always be carefully examined to determine whether an alternative enrichment programme, perhaps using different materials, is possible.

Management should ensure that there is a reasonable and sufficient budget to meet enrichment needs and to fund any research necessary to validate the programme. However, simple enrichments can be as effective as more complex and expensive options (Schapiro *et al.* 1997). Enrichment items need not be expensive, and have been made from everyday items such as old water bottles, cardboard rolls, etc. Nonetheless, such items should be used with care as they may contain undesirable substances, and their composition may not remain consistent. Commercial enrichment products have the advantage that they can often be obtained with a certificate of analysis, which is necessary for regulatory studies. Further advice on implementing enrichment within a GLP framework is available from FELASA (2006).

The extra costs arising from an enrichment programme should not impact adversely on research. For commercial establishments, the costs of enrichment are usually trivial compared to overall budgets. Moreover, as enrichment becomes more widely accepted, competitive disadvantages between commercial organisations adopting enrichment should decrease. For academic establishments it may be harder to find the extra funds but, at least within the UK, the major funding bodies emphasise the importance of the Three Rs, and of housing animals in a complex and varied physical environment in appropriate social groupings, with the aim of promoting exercise and performance of species-typical behaviours (Medical Research Council (MRC) 2008). Moreover, funding bodies have indicated that they would consider offering funding to enable establishments to achieve high standards (Animal Procedures Committee (APC) 2005).

Within the animal house, records should be kept of the enrichment used and of any rotation of enrichment items. As part of continuing professional development, staff should keep up-to-date with the literature on enrichment, should visit other research sites and attend conferences at which enrichment is discussed. It is also useful to invite experts on various species to visit and comment on the enrichment programmes in place. When animals are bought in from outside institutions, it is important to determine the husbandry and enrichment systems of the supplying institution. This is partly to minimise adverse effects resulting from a change of husbandry, and also to encourage the worldwide spread of high standards (APC 2007). Finally, institutions should make efforts to disseminate information on the successes or failures of their enrichment programmes.

References

Animal Procedures Committee (2005) *Report of the Animal Procedures Committee for 2005*. The Stationery Office, London. http://www.apc.gov.uk/reference/apc_ann_rep_2005.pdf (accessed 23 April 2009)

Animal Procedures Committee (2007) *Consideration of Policy Concerning Standards of Animal Housing and Husbandry for Animals from Overseas Non-designated Sources*. http://www.apc.gov.uk/reference/2007%2004%2004%20web%20version%20standards.pdf (accessed 23 April 2009)

Augustsson, H., van de Weerd, H.A., Kruitwagen, C.L.J.J. and Baumans, V. (2003) Effect of enrichment on variation and results in the light/dark test. *Laboratory Animals*, **37**, 328–340

Bayne, K. (2005) Potential for unintended consequences of environmental enrichment for laboratory animals and research results. *ILAR Journal*, **46**, 129–139

Bayne, K.A.L., Dexter, S.L., Hurst, J.K. *et al.* (1993) Kong® Toys for laboratory primates: are they really an enrichment or just fomites? *Laboratory Animal Science*, **43**, 78–85

Bazille, P.G., Walden, S.D., Koniar, B.L. *et al.* (2001) Commercial cotton nesting material as a predisposing factor for conjunctivitis in athymic nude mice. *Lab Animal*, **30**, 40–42

Benaroya-Milshtein, N., Hollander, N., Apter, A. *et al.* (2004) Environmental enrichment in mice decreases anxiety, attenuates stress responses and enhances natural killer cell activity. *European Journal of Neuroscience*, **20**, 1341–1347

Benefiel, A.C., Dong, W.K. and Greenough, W.T. (2005) Mandatory 'enriched' housing of laboratory animals: the need for evidence based evaluation. *ILAR Journal*, **46**, 95–105

Benefiel, A.C. and Greenough, W.T. (1998) Effects of experience and environment on the developing and mature brain: implications for laboratory animal housing. *ILAR Journal*, **39**, 5–11

Bloomsmith, M.A., Brent, L.Y. and Schapiro, S.J. (1991) Guidelines for developing and managing an environmental enrichment program for nonhuman primates. *Laboratory Animal Science*, **41**, 372–377

Buchanan-Smith, H.M., Rennie, A.E., Vitale, A. *et al.* (2005) Harmonising the definition of refinement. *Animal Welfare*, **14**, 379–384

Chamove, A.S. (1989) Cage design reduces emotionality in mice. *Lab Animal*, **23**, 215–219

Clubb, R. and Mason, G. (2003) Animal welfare: captivity effects on wide-ranging carnivores. *Nature*, **425**, 473–474

Council of Europe (2006) *Multilateral Consultation of Parties to the European Convention for the Protection of Vertebrate Animals used for Experimental and other Scientific Purposes (ETS 123) Appendix A. Cons 123 (2006) 3*. Available from URL: http://www.coe.int/t/e/legal_affairs/legal_co-operation/biological_safety,_use_of_animals/laboratory_animals/2006/Cons123(2006)3AppendixA_en.pdf (accessed 17 March 2009)

Crabbe, J.C., Wahlsten, D. and Dudek, B.C. (1999) Genetics of mouse behavior: interactions with laboratory environment. *Science*, **284**, 1670–1672

Dean, S.W. (1999) Environmental enrichment of laboratory animals used in regulatory toxicology studies. *Laboratory Animals*, **33**, 309–327

Duke, J.L., Zammit, T.G. and Lawson, D.M. (2001) The effects of routine cage-changing on cardiovascular and behavioral parameters in male Sprague-Dawley rats. *Contemporary Topics in Laboratory Animal Science*, **40**, 17–20

Eskola, S., Lauhikari, M., Voipio, H.M. *et al.* (1999) Environmental enrichment may alter the number of rats needed to achieve statistical significance. *Scandinavian Journal of Laboratory Animal Science*, **26**, 134–144

European Commission (2007) Commission recommendations of 18 June 2007 on guidelines for the accommodation and care of animals used for experimental and other scientific purposes. Annex II to European Council Directive 86/609. See 2007/526/EC. http://eurlex.europa.eu/LexUriServ/site/en/oj/2007/l_197/l_19720070730en00010089.pdf (accessed 13 May 2008)

Federation of European Laboratory Animal Science Associations (2006) *FELASA Working Group Standardization of Enrichment Working Group Report*. http://www.lal.org.uk/pdffiles/FELASA_Enrichment_2006.pdf (accessed 27 March 2009)

Fekete, J.M., Norcross, J.L. and Newman, J.D. (2000) Artificial turf foraging boards as environmental enrichment for pair-housed female squirrel monkeys. *Contemporary Topics in Laboratory Animal Science*, **39**, 22–26

Fox, M.W. and Stelzner, D. (1966) Behavioural effects of differential early experience in the dog. *Animal Behaviour*, **14**, 273–281

Fox, M.W. and Stelzner, D. (1967) The effects of early experience on the development of inter and intraspecies social relationships in the dog. *Animal Behaviour*, **15**, 377–386

Fraser, D. (2008) *Understanding Animal Welfare: The Science in its Cultural Context*. John Wiley & Sons, Chichester, UK

Fraser, D., Weary, D.M., Pajor, E.A. *et al.* (1997) A scientific conception of animal welfare that reflects ethical concerns. *Animal Welfare*, **6**, 187–205

Fuller, J.L. (1967) Experiential deprivation and later behaviour. *Science*, **158**, 1645–1652

Garner, J.P. (2005) Stereotypies and other abnormal repetitive behaviors: potential impact on validity, reliability, and replicability of scientific outcomes. *ILAR Journal*, **46**, 106–117

Gaskill, B.N., Rohr, S.A., Pajor, E.A. *et al.* (2009) Some like it hot: mouse temperature preferences in laboratory housing. *Applied Animal Behaviour Science*, **116**, 279–285

Hadley, C., Hadley, B., Ephraim, S. *et al.* (2006) Spontaneous stereotypy and environmental enrichment in deer mice (*Peromyscus maniculatus*): reversibility of experience. *Applied Animal Behaviour Science*, **97**, 312–322

Haemisch, A. and Gärtner, K. (1994) The cage design affects intermale aggression in small groups of male laboratory mice: strain specific consequences on social organization, and endocrine activations in two inbred strains (DBA/2J and CBA/J). *Journal of Experimental Animal Science*, **36**, 101–116

Haemisch, A., Voss, T. and Gärtner, K. (1994) Effects of environmental enrichment on aggressive behavior, dominance hierachies, and endocrine states in male DBA/2J Mice. *Physiology and Behavior*, **56**, 1041–1048

Healy, S.D. and Tovée, M.J. (1999) Environmental enrichment and impoverishment: neurophysiological effects. In: *Attitudes to Animals Views in Animal Welfare*. Ed Dolins, F.L., pp. 54–76. Cambridge University Press, Cambridge

Hediger, H. (1950) *Wild Animals in Captivity*. Butterworths, London

Hockly, E., Cordery, P.M., Woodman, B. *et al*. (2002) Environmental enrichment slows disease progression in R6/2 Huntington's disease mice. *Annals of Neurology*, **51**, 235–242

Honess, P.E. and Marin, C.M. (2006) Enrichment and aggression in primates. *Neuroscience and Biobehavioral Reviews*, **30**, 413–436

Hubrecht, R.C. (1993) A comparison of social and environmental enrichment methods for laboratory housed dogs. *Applied Animal Behaviour Science*, **37**, 345–361

Hubrecht, R.C. (1995a) Enrichment in puppyhood and its effects on later behavior of dogs. *Laboratory Animal Science*, **45**, 70–75

Hubrecht, R.C. (1995b) Dog welfare. In: *The Domestic dog: Evolution, Behaviour, and Interactions with People*. Ed Serpell, J., pp. 179–198. Cambridge University Press, Cambridge

Hubrecht, R. and Buckwell, A.C. (2004) The welfare of laboratory dogs. In: *Welfare of Laboratory Animals*. Ed Kaliste, E., pp. 245–273. Kluwer Academic Publishers, Dordrecht

Hubrecht, R.C., Serpell, J.A. and Poole, T.B. (1992). Correlates of pen size and housing conditions on the behaviour of kennelled dogs. *Applied Animal Behaviour Science*, **34**, 365–383

Johnson, C.A., Pallozzi, W.A., Geiger, L. *et al*. (2003) The effect of an environmental enrichment device on individually caged rabbits in a safety assessment facility. *Contemporary Topics in Laboratory Animal Science*, **42**, 27–30

Jankowsky, J.L., Melnikova, T., Fadale, D.J. *et al*. (2005) Environmental enrichment mitigates cognitive deficits in a mouse model of Alzheimer's disease. *Journal of Neuroscience*, **25**, 5217–5224

Johnson, C.A., Pallozzi, W.A., Geiger, L. *et al*. (2003) The effect of an environmental enrichment device on individually caged rabbits in a safety assessment facility. *Contemporary Topics in Laboratory Animal Science*, **42**, 27–30

Johnson, S.R., Patterson Kane, E.G. and Niel, L. (2004) Foraging enrichment for laboratory rats. *Animal Welfare*, **13**, 305–312

Joint Working Group on Refinement (2004) Refining dog husbandry and care – eighth report of the BVAAWF/FRAME/RSPCA/UFAW Joint Working Group on Refinement. *Laboratory Animals*, **38**, S1–S94

Joint Working Group on Refinement (2009) Refinements in husbandry, care and common procedures for non-human primates. Ninth report of the BVAAWF/FRAME/RSPCA/UFAW Joint Working Group on Refinement. *Laboratory Animals*, **43**, S1:1–S1:47

Kikusui, T., Isaka, Y. and Mori, Y. (2005) Early weaning deprives mouse pups of maternal care and decreases their maternal behavior in adulthood. *Behavioural Brain Research*, **162**, 200–206

Kim, S., Lee, S., Ryu, S. *et al*. (2002) Comparative analysis of the anxiety-related behaviors in four inbred mice. *Behavioural Processes*, **60**, 181–190

Kirkden, R. and Pajor, E. (2006) Using preference, motivation and aversion tests to ask scientific questions about animals' feelings. *Applied Animal Behaviour Science*, **100**, 29–47

Kreger, M. (1999) *Environmental Enrichment for Nonhuman Primates Resource Guide*. Animal Welfare Information Center, Beltsville, Maryland

Larsson, F., Winblad, B. and Mohammed, A.H. (2002) Psychological stress and environmental adaptation in enriched vs. impoverished housed rats. *Pharmacology, Biochemistry and Behavior*, **73**, 193–207

Lewis, M.H. (2004) Environmental complexity and central nervous system development and function. *Mental Retardation and Developmental Disabilities Research Reviews*, **10**, 91–95

Lutz, C.K. and Novak, M.A. (2005) Environmental enrichment for non-human primates: theory and application. *ILAR*, **46**, 178–191

Manser, C.E., Elliott, H., Morris, T.H. *et al*. (1996) The use of a novel operant test to determine the strength of preference for flooring in laboratory rats. *Laboratory Animals*, **30**, 1–6

Marashi, V., Barnekow, A., Ossendorf, E. *et al*. (2003) Effects of different forms of environmental enrichment on behavioral, endocrinological, and immunological parameters in male mice. *Hormones and Behavior*, **43**, 281–292

Markowitz, H. (1982) *Behavioural Enrichment in the Zoo*. Van Nostran Reinhold, New York

Markowitz, H. (1998) Enrichment for animals. In: *Encyclopedia of Animal Right and Animal Welfare*. Ed Bekoff, M., pp. 156–157. Fitzroy Dearborn, Illinois

Mason, G.J. (1991) Stereotypies: a critical review. *Animal Behaviour*, **41**, 1015–1037

Mason, G.J. and Latham, N.R. (2004) Can't stop, won't stop: is stereotypy a reliable animal welfare indicator? *Animal Welfare*, **13**, S57–S69

Medical Research Council (2008) *Responsibility in the Use of Animals in Bioscience Research: Expectations of the Major Research Council and Charitable Funding Bodies*. http://www.mrc.ac.uk/Utilities/Documentrecord/index.htm?d=MRC001897 (accessed 23 April 2009)

Meijer, M.K., Kramer, K., Remie, R. *et al*. (2006) The effect of routine experimental procedures on physiological parameters in mice kept under different husbandry conditions. *Animal Welfare*, **15**, 31–38

Mering, S., Kaliste Korhonen, E. and Nevalainen, T. (2001) Estimates of appropriate number of rats: interaction with housing environment. *Laboratory Animals*, **35**, 80–90

Meshi, D., Drew, M.R., Saxe, M. *et al*. (2006) Hippocampal neurogenesis is not required for behavioral effects of environmental enrichment. *Nature Neuroscience*, **9**, 729–731

Murchison, M.A. (1993) Potential animal hazard with ring toys. *Laboratory Primate Newsletter*, **32**, 7

Nelson, R.J. and Mandrell, T.D. (2005) Enrichment and nonhuman primates: 'First, Do No Harm'. *ILAR*, **46**, 171–177

Nevison, C.M., Hurst, J.L. and Barnard, C.J. (1999) Strain-specific effects of cage enrichment in male laboratory mice (*Mus musculus*). *Animal Welfare*, **8**, 361–379

Newberry, R.C. (1995) Environmental enrichment: increasing the biological relevance of captive environments. *Applied Animal Behaviour Science*, **44**, 229–243

Nithianantharajah, J., Levis, H. and Murphy, M. (2004) Environmental enrichment results in cortical and subcortical changes in levels of synaptophysin and PSD-95 proteins. *Neurobiology of Learning and Memory*, **81**, 200–210

Novak, M.A., Meyer, J.S., Lutz, C. *et al*. (2006) Deprived environments: developmental insights from primatology. In: *Stereoptypic Animal behaviour: Fundamentals and Applications to Welfare*. Eds. Mason, G. and Rushen, J., pp. 19–57. CAB International, Wallingford

National Research Council (1998) *The Psychological Well-Being of Nonhuman Primates: A Report of the Committee on the Well-Being of Nonhuman Primates*. Institute for Laboratory Animal Research, National Research Council, National Academy Press, Washington, DC

National Research Council (2008) *Recognition and Alleviation of Distress in Laboratory Animals*. Committee on Recognition and Alleviation of Distress in Laboratory Animals. National Research Council, National Academy Press, Washington, DC. http://grants.nih.gov/grants/olaw/NAS_distress_report.pdf (accessed 23 March 2009)

Olsson, I.A.S. and Dahlborn, K. (2002) Improving housing conditions for laboratory mice: a review of environmental enrichment. *Laboratory Animals*, **36**, 243–270

Patterson-Kane, E.G., Hunt, M. and Harper, D. (2002) Rats demand social contact. *Animal Welfare*, **11**, 327–332

Patterson-Kane, E.G., Pittman, M. and Pajor, E.A. (2008) Operant animal welfare: productive approaches and persistent difficulties. *Animal Welfare*, **17**, 139–148

Polley, D.B., Kvasnák, E. and Frostig, R.D. (2004) Naturalistic experience transforms sensory maps in the adult cortex of caged animals. *Nature*, **429**, 67–71

Praag, H.V., Kempermann, G. and Gage, F.H. (2000) Neural consequences of environmental enrichment. *Nature Reviews: Neuroscience*, **1**, 191–198

Prior, H. and Sachser, N. (1994) Effects of enriched housing environment on the behaviour of young male and female mice in four exploratory tasks. *Journal of Experimental Animal Science*, **37**, 57–68

Prusky, G.T., Reidel, C. and Douglas, R.M. (2000) Environmental enrichment from birth enhances visual acuity but not place learning in mice. *Behavioural Brain Research*, **114**, 11–15

Rennie, A.E. and Buchanan-Smith, H.M. (2006) Refinement of the use of non-human primates in scientific research. Part II: housing, husbandry and acquisition. *Animal Welfare*, **15**, 215–238

Rosenzweig, M.R., Bennett, E.L., Hebert, M. *et al.* (1978) Social grouping cannot account for cerebral effects of enriched environments. *Brain Research*, **153**, 563–576

Russell, W.M.S. and Burch, R.L. (1959) *The Principles of Humane Experimental Technique*. Methuen & Co Ltd, London, reprinted UFAW 1992, Potters Bar

Sambrook, T.D. and Buchanan-Smith, H.M. (1997) Control and complexity in novel object enrichment. *Animal Welfare*, **6**, 207–216

Schapiro, S.J., Bloomsmith, M.A., Suarez, S.A. *et al.* (1997) A comparison of the effects of simple versus complex environmental enrichment on the behaviour of group-housed, subadult rhesus macaques. *Animal Welfare*, **6**, 17–28

Schapiro, S.J. and Bushong, D. (1994) Effects of enrichment on veterinary treatment of laboratory rhesus macaques (*Macaca mulatta*). *Animal Welfare*, **3**, 25–36

Shepherdson, D.J. (1998) Tracing the path of environmental enrichment in zoos. In: *Second Nature: Environmental Enrichment for Captive Animals*. Eds. Shepherdson, D.J., Mellen, J.D. and Hutchins, M., pp. 1–12. Smithsonian Institution, Washington, DC

Shepherdson, D.J. (2003) Environmental enrichment: past, present and future. *International Zoo Yearbook*, **38**, 118–124

Sherwin, C.M. (1996) Laboratory mice persist in gaining access to resources: a method of assessing the importance of environmental features. *Applied Animal Behaviour Science*, **48**, 203–213

Sherwin, C.M. (2004) The influences of standard laboratory cages on rodents and the validity of research data. *Animal Welfare*, **13**(S), 9–15

Sherwin, C.M. and Nicol, C.J. (1996) Reorganization of behaviour in laboratory mice, *Mus musculus*, with varying cost of access to resources. *Animal Behaviour*, **51**, 1087–1093

Sherwin, C.M. and Olsson, I.A.S. (2004) Housing conditions affect self-administration of anxiolytic by laboratory mice. *Animal Welfare*, **13**, 33–38

Shyne, A. (2006) Meta-analytic review of the effects of enrichment on stereotypic behavior in zoo mammals. *Zoo Biology*, **25**, 317–337

Tsai, P.P., Pachowsky, U., Stelzer, H.D. *et al.* (2002) Impact of environmental enrichment in mice. 1: effect of housing conditions on body weight, organ weights and haematology in different strains. *Laboratory Animals*, **36**, 411–419

Tsai, P.P., Stelzer, H.D., Hedrich, H.J. *et al.* (2003) Are the effects of different enrichment designs on the physiology and behaviour of DBA/2 mice consistent? *Laboratory Animals*, **37**, 314–327

van de Weerd, H.A., Aarsen, E.L., Mulder, A. *et al.* (2002) Effects of environmental enrichment for mice: variation in experimental results. *Journal of Applied Animal Welfare Science*, **5**, 87–109

van Loo, P.L.P., Kruitwagen, C.L.J.J., Koolhaas, J.M. *et al.* (2002) Influence of cage enrichment on aggressive behaviour and physiological parameters in male mice. *Applied Animal Behaviour Science*, **76**, 65–81

van Loo, P.L.P., van der Meer, E., Kruitwagen, C.L.J.J. *et al.* (2004) Long-term effects of husbandry procedures on stress-related parameters in male mice of two strains. *Laboratory Animals*, **38**, 169–177

Veasey, J.S., Waran, N.K. and Young, R.J. (1996) On comparing the behaviour of zoo housed animals with wild conspecifics as a welfare indicator. *Animal Welfare*, **5**, 13–24

Ventura, R. and Buchanan-Smith, H.M. (2003) Physical environmental effects on infant care and development in captive *Callithrix jacchus*. *International Journal of Primatology*, **24**, 399–413

Vignes, S., Newman, J.D. and Roberts, R.L. (2001) Mealworm feeders as environmental enrichment for common marmosets. *Contemporary Topics in Laboratory Animal Science*, **40**, 26–29

Wiedenmayer, C. (1997) Causation of the ontogenetic development of stereotypic digging in gerbils. *Animal Behaviour*, **53**, 461–470

Wiepkema, P.R. and Koolhaas, J.M. (1993) Stress and animal welfare. *Animal Welfare*, **2**, 195–218

Wolfer, D.P., Litvin, O., Morf, S. *et al.* (2004) Laboratory animal welfare. Cage enrichment and mouse behaviour. *Nature*, **432**, 821–822

Wolfle, T.L. (2005) Environmental enrichment. *ILAR Journal*, **46**, 79–82

Würbel, H. (2000) Behaviour and the standardization fallacy. *Nature Genetics*, **26**, 263

Würbel, H. (2001) Ideal homes? Housing effects on rodent brain and behaviour. *Trends in Neurosciences*, **24**, 207–211

Würbel, H. (2006) The motivational basis of caged rodents' stereotypies. In: *Stereoptypic Animal Behaviour: Fundamentals and Applications to Welfare*. Eds. Mason, G. and Rushen, J., pp. 19–57. CABI, Wallingford

Würbel, H., Chapman, R. and Rutland, C. (1998) Effect of feed and environmental enrichment on development of stereotypic wire-gnawing in laboratory mice. *Applied Animal Behaviour Science*, **60**, 69–81

Würbel, H. and Stauffacher M. (1994) Standard-haltung für labormäuse – probleme und lösungsasätze. *Tierlaboratorium*, **17**, 109–118

Würbel, H. and Garner, J.P. (2007) Refinement of rodent research through environmental enrichment and systematic randomization NC3Rs #9 Environmental enrichment and systematic randomization. Jan 2007 http://www.nc3rs.org.uk (accessed 13 July 2007)

Yeates, J.W. and Main, D.C.J. (2008) Assessment of positive welfare: a review. *Veterinary Journal*, **175**, 293–300

Young, R.J. (2003) *Environmental Enrichment for Captive Animals*. Blackwell Publishing, Oxford

11 Special housing arrangements

Mike Dennis

Introduction

Whilst it is desirable to maintain laboratory animals in accommodation that is as close as possible (excluding harmful aspects) to their natural habitats, there are several reasons why special housing arrangements are required in some cases in order to meet more exacting experimental requirements than are provided by conventional caging or penning systems.

Special housing arrangements may be required to achieve any of the following:

- to prevent contamination of germ-free animals;
- to protect animals that are particularly sensitive to infection, for example genetically immunocompromised animals such as severe combined immunodeficient (SCID) or nude (athymic) mice;
- to protect animal handlers from allergens or infections that are deemed to be a potential risk (eg, from animals of unknown health provenance or that have been administered an infectious agent).

Many approaches and systems have been developed over the years to address these issues but the main principles involve a physical barrier, a directional/laminar airflow or a combination of both.

Physical barriers may be provided by:

- protective clothing;
- animal rooms;
- plastic film isolators;
- filter-top boxes;
- independently ventilated cages;
- laminar flow hoods;
- isolation booths;
- rigid cabinets.

All barriers, even one as simple as protective clothing, can have an impact upon the welfare of the animals This chapter will first describe the types of containment systems currently in use and then address their use with individual species. It will not cover highly specialised housing situations such as tethering or metabolic cages as their use is generally short term and the welfare issues associated with their use are generally covered by a project licence or other equivalent experimental permission/justification.

Types of containment

Protective clothing

This is probably the most common physical barrier used in animal facilities. Personal protective equipment (PPE) may be as simple as a gown over normal clothing and a pair of gloves, but may also include hats and masks. For higher levels of operator protection it may be necessary for a complete change of clothes and the use of respiratory protective equipment (RPE) (Figure 11.1). Other protection strategies may require the use of powered respirators or suits with their own integral air supplies, depending on the danger presented by the infectious agent is that is being used (Figures 11.2, 11.3).

Welfare considerations

Protective clothing may impact on animal welfare in a number of ways. This impact may be accentuated if a sudden change in regime is adopted, for example after an experimental challenge (ie, a sudden change in appearance and practices may well have an influence on the dynamics of the relationship between the animal, its handler and even its cage mates). Animals that have become habituated to their care staff may be affected by any of the following changes:

- Odours: the use of PPE may remove smells that have become familiar to the animals; or PPE equipment may have a distinctive odour of its own that is not pleasant to the animals.
- Colours: a change in the colour of protective apparel from the previous everyday laboratory gown may affect some species.
- Noise from powered air supplies: these may disturb animals and even if they may seem quiet to the wearer, there may be sub- or super-sonic noise that can be disturbing to certain species.
- Visibility: the profile of an individual may be changed by protective wear such that they can no longer be recognised. Face masks or other RPE hide usual visual signals that may be used by some species.
- Startling sudden appearance without the usual clues of approach (eg, if emerging from a changing room, rather than directly from a corridor.

- Gloves: the wearing of gloves has been shown to affect dexterity and this may result in clumsier, more stressful handling of smaller species.

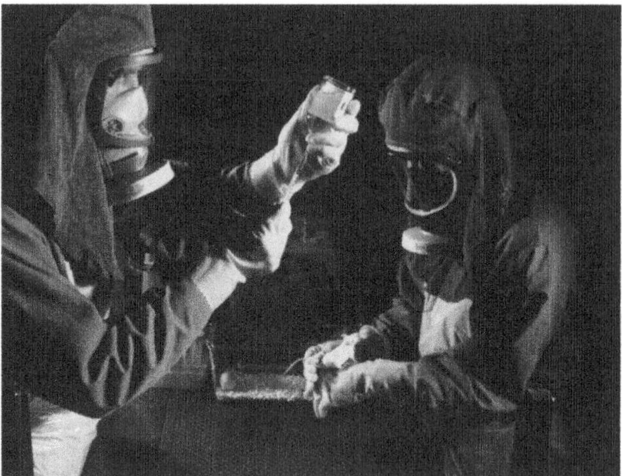

Figure 11.1 The use of RPE plus down-draught table to protect the operators during procedures on infected animals. (Courtesy of Health Protection Agency.)

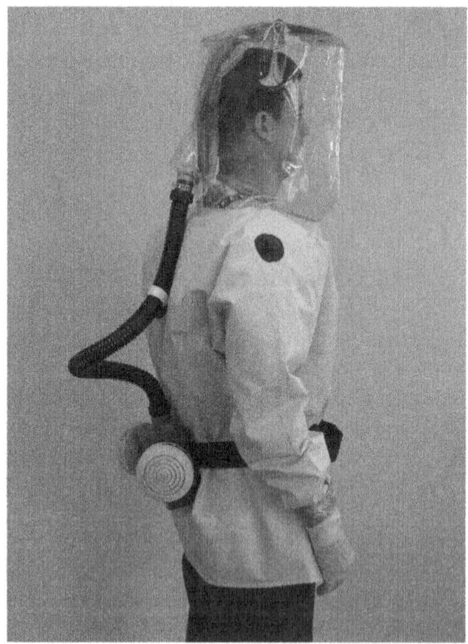

Figure 11.2 A Martindale-type suit with a filtered, powered air supply. (Courtesy of Health Protection Agency.)

Welfare aspects of higher levels of PPE (eg, suits, half suits, powered RPE with full clothing change)

The use of specialised apparel with higher levels of PPE usually involves strict changing and showering regimes that are time consuming and reduce the number of visits that can be made per day. In addition, protective equipment can restrict movement, hearing and dexterity, and its use has an inherent level of discomfort that reduces the amount of time that can be safely spent on any one visit. A further problem

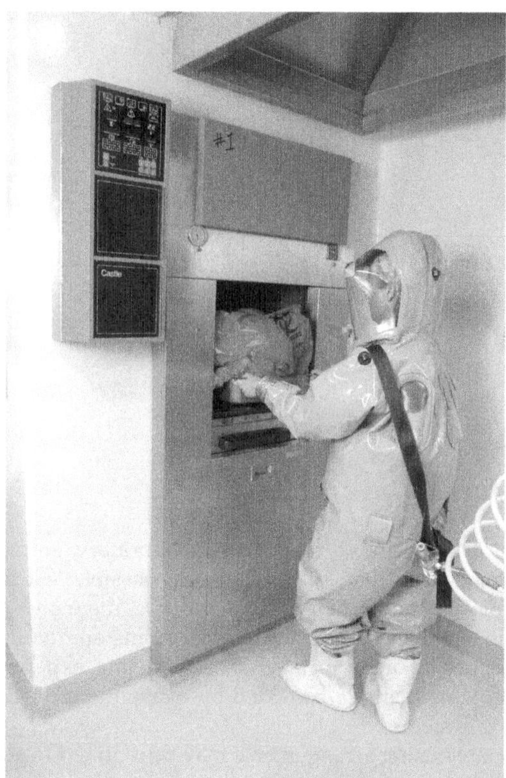

Figure 11.3 A one-piece full suit that might be required for work with dangerous pathogens. (Courtesy of the Canadian Science Centre for Human & Animal Health.)

with this equipment is the lack of facial signals to animals because of reduced clarity or reflectivity of visors or other head-gear.

The animal room

In some cases the boundaries of the animal room itself may be considered as the primary barrier between the animals and the rest of the facility. This type of barrier system is likely to be required where the work involves species that cannot be housed with any degree of practicability in other containment systems. Examples may include adult farm animals such as cattle, pigs or sheep. In such cases and where high-level containment is required, the room might need to be modified and this may impact upon animal welfare in ways that are not immediately obvious. Containment of pathogens dangerous to humans or to other animals may require the provision of *en suite* changing rooms, showers, fumigation chambers and autoclaves. The supply air, extracted air, or both may require high-efficiency particulate air (HEPA) filtration and the room may need to be maintained at negative pressure, depending on the defined biosafety level.

Welfare considerations

Practices within the room may be affected by the containment level specified for the room: for example if effluent treatment is part of the containment strategy, then the use of water for cleaning down may be restricted. In addition, the type of bedding that can be used may be restricted to avoid blocking the drains that lead to the treatment plant. Due consideration needs to be given to where procedures and necropsies are to be performed, bearing in mind both the welfare of other animals and any safety requirement to prevent release of any pathogens. It is highly likely where the confines of the room itself are used as the primary barrier, that protocols will also prescribe some level of protective clothing for animal care and scientific staff, as described in the section on clothing above. The needs of high-level biocontainment may dictate the use of sealable submarine-type doors to prevent escape of pathogens, to enhance air pressure cascades and to allow regular fumigation. Current biosecurity requirements often demand that facilities using certain agents should have robust physical security, such as coded locks or swipe access, to limit access. As layers of mechanical or procedural strategies are built up to address safety issues or to ensure the integrity of the experiment, then more attention needs to be paid to the impact upon the welfare of the animals as they become more isolated from the rest of the facility and its day-to-day activities. Table 11.1 provides a summary of potential welfare issues and solutions relating to using rooms as a barrier.

Flexible film isolators

Flexible film isolators are used extensively for the microbial isolation of experimental animals. The original flexible film isolators were developed by Trexler and Reynolds (1957), and designed specifically to maintain germ-free (animals with no detectable microbial flora) or gnotobiotic animals (derived germ-free but having a defined, given microbial agent) and to prevent contamination of these animals by environmental microbes. Germ-free animals are derived free of microbial contamination by removal directly from the uterus under sterile conditions either by hysterotomy or hysterectomy in the case of mammals (decontamination of newborn has also been reported) or by decontamination of eggs in the case of birds.

Flexible film technology has proved to be extremely effective and adaptable as a microbiological barrier and a wide range of species, from rodents to farm animals such as pigs, sheep and calves, have been maintained under gnotobiotic conditions (Tavernor *et al.* 1971; Alexander *et al* 1973; Dennis *et al.* 1976). Microbial isolation is achieved by the physical barrier of the flexible film canopy, enhanced by positive pressure and HEPA filtration of both incoming and outgoing air.

Germ-free or gnotobiotic animals are used in research for various reasons: to investigate the role of commensal bacteria in development of the immune system (Butler *et al.* 2005; Hope *et al.* 2005); in studies of gene expression (Chowdhury *et al.* 2007); or to provide an insight into diseases of unknown aetiology (Wyatt *et al.* 1979; Bridger *et al.* 1984).

Welfare and handling considerations

The use of isolators can impact upon animal handling with potential knock-on welfare consequences in various ways:

- If the operator's vision is reduced or restricted this may impact upon animal observations and checks on well-

Table 11.1 Potential welfare issues of the room as a containment barrier.

Parameter	*Potential welfare issue*	*Solution*
HEPA filtration	Room reliant on air handling system for adequate ventilation/environmental control. Failure of fans could lead to inability to control temperature, humidity and build-up of waste gases	Build in redundancy on air handling equipment and have reliable emergency power with automatic cut in
Negative (or positive) air pressure	Needs to be well controlled. Sudden changes in pressure can be distressing	Have feedback between supply and extract, build in a delay in variable fan speed to allow for door opening
Limited access due to time-consuming changing and showering regimes	Reduced time and frequency of observation and interaction with animals	Consider CCTV and environmental enrichment appropriate for species. Consider practices that reduce the time taken to enter/exit (eg, is showering necessary? Could air showers be used?)
En-suite autoclave/ fumigation chamber	Exposure to noise, heat, noxious fumes	Ensure good sound and heat insulati on, use an ante-room if possible, have local ventilation that will cope with steam or leakage of fumigant
Procedures and necropsies	Requirement for biocontainment may preclude separate procedures room or use of a shared postmortem room	Have, as a minimum, a screened-off area that is well ventilated. Use a cascade pressure regime away from the animal accommodation to the procedures area
Effluent treatment	Capacity issues or fear of blockage may restrict use of water and certain types of bedding. This may impact on natural behaviours such as foraging for food	Consider using a system of screen filters for the drains and have separated areas where deep litter can be used and then bagged for disposal
Use of PPE/RPE	Stress may be caused by unfamiliar suits/respirators and lack of usual facial and olfactory signals	Acclimatise animals by wearing apparel on occasions before study start or by hanging suits in room

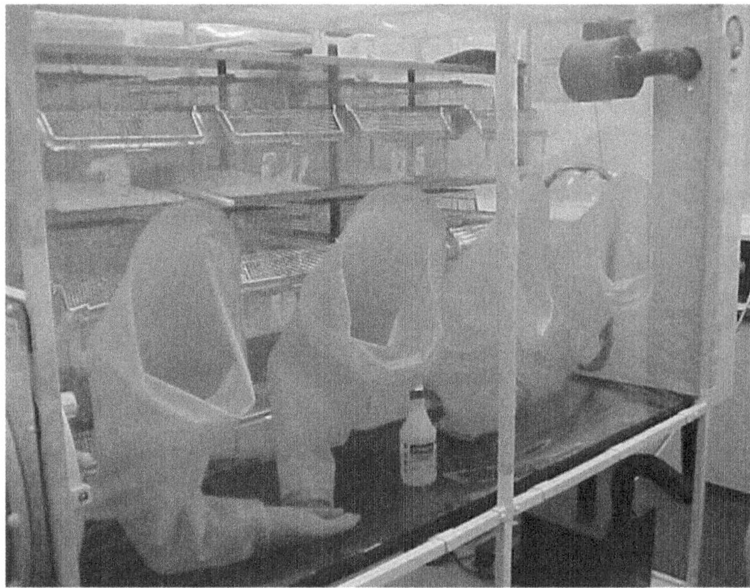

Figure 11.4 A flexible film isolator used to house infected mice or guinea pigs. (Courtesy of Health Protection Agency.)

being. Plastic canopies, even if of clear PVC, will reduce optical clarity, although clearer panels can be introduced to enhance visibility in key areas of the canopy.

- Reduced dexterity may affect the handling of smaller species and hinder sampling or administration procedures. Access to cages and to the animals will be via glove sleeves built into the walls of the isolator (Figure 11.4) or by the use of integral half suits (Figure 11.5). These gloves will normally be fixed in place and will thus have to be of a size to accommodate all users.
- The length and position of glove sleeves may mean that there are certain areas within the isolator that cannot be reached. There needs to be a contingency plan in place to deal with animals that have escaped from cages within the isolator so that this will not compromise the experiment (eg, by chewing through the isolator wall or a glove) or stress the animals during attempts at recapture.
- The reduced or absent gut microflora of gnotobiotic animals may affect their digestion or utilisation of nutrients that are usually made available by commensal organisms. In addition, the normal microflora may act as a barrier to pathogenic or opportunist organisms, and animals in which this flora is absent or restricted may be more susceptible to infection.
- Some species may be colostrum-deprived in order to maintain germ-free status and so be deficient in protective maternal antibodies, resulting in greater susceptibility to disease by opportunist organisms, or to any pathogens given experimentally.

The environment within isolators is dependent upon a constant adequate airflow through the isolator to prevent high temperature, high humidity or build up of ammonia and welfare will be at risk if these systems should fail. The removal of waste is time consuming and is a risk to the integrity of the system.

The introduction of food, water, bedding and other materials into isolators requires strict decontamination protocols. Usually, these materials are pre-sterilised by autoclaving, filtration or irradiation and sealed into plastic bags or other containers that can then be introduced to the isolator via a transfer port after surface decontamination. The use of chemical disinfection may potentially expose animals to unpleasant or toxic fumes. It is important to select non-toxic disinfectants, those that break down rapidly to non-toxic components (eg, peracetic acid breaks down to water, carbon dioxide and oxygen) or to design isolators to have some sort of ventilation system to remove unpleasant or toxic fumes.

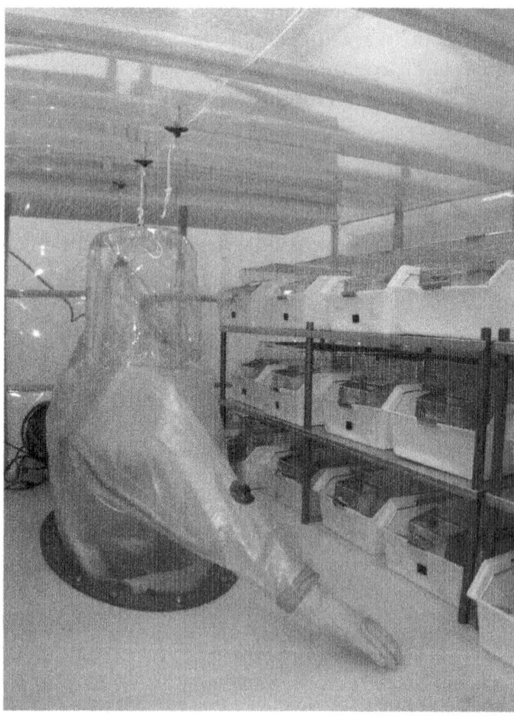

Figure 11.5 The interior of a half-suit isolator used to house infected guinea pigs. (Courtesy of Health Protection Agency.)

It is important to check that treating food by autoclaving or irradiation will not result in loss of essential trace elements or nutritional value.

Table 11.2 Potential welfare issues of isolators.

Parameter	*Potential welfare issue*	*Solution*
Air supply	Restricted space requires constant airflow to be maintained to avoid build up of humidity, temperature or waste gases (eg, ammonia). Failure of power or fans will rapidly cause problems	Have over-capacity for fans. Have reserve fan or twin-motored fan. Emergency generator is essential and battery back-up to power fans is recommended
Use of supply ports	Potential route for contamination. Potential for exposure to chemical disinfectants	Minimise frequency of use of entry ports by use of supply isolators and/or extended waste bags. Choose disinfectants that will decompose into non-toxic components or ventilate the port
Sterilisation of food	This may affect nutritional value	Select least drastic sterilisation technique. When specifying diet composition allow for decay of essential vitamins or trace elements
Interaction with staff	Reduced visibility, dexterity and ergonomics may limit observation of animals, precision for handling or procedures and may reduce the time staff can spend at one session	Consider lighting levels, glove positions, number of cages per isolator and positioning. Consider half suits for improved ergonomics. Environmental enrichment and group housing can be the same as for conventional rooms
Procedures and necropsies	Confined space and biosafety requirements may lead to procedures and necropsies being performed in close proximity to other animals	Where possible have a separate isolator or cabinet attached for conduct of procedures/necropsies. For more intricate procedures removal to a downdraught table may be required
Natural microflora	May affect ability to utilise food	Consider supplementation of diet or possibility of introducing a balanced microflora
Escape from cage	Escaped animals may damage canopy or sleeves and this may compromise the experiment There may be areas in the isolator that cannot be reached due to restrictions of glove sleeves	A strict regime of checking cage security is required. Caps can be used to prevent access to glove sleeves Design out any dead spaces or ensure that some form of humane capture such as netting can be used successfully

More recently, isolator technology has been adapted as a strategy for primary containment of infected animals and, in this scenario, the isolator is maintained under negative pressure to enhance operator protection. The same points listed apply regarding potential impact on animal welfare. Flexible canopies need robust support to prevent collapse on to the animals' cages due to the negative pressure (UK Health and Safety Executive guidelines (Guidance on the use, testing and maintenance of laboratory and animal isolators for the containment of biological agents[1]) recommend a minimum operating pressure of 30 Pa below laboratory pressure). In order to safeguard animals' welfare, isolators need to be equipped with alarms that indicate out-of-range pressure changes and air supply failure. They also need to be linked to standby generators and to emergency battery back-up that will cut in to maintain the air supply, allowing sufficient operating time to allow any remedial action to be completed.

Rigid isolators

Rigid isolators operate in the same way as flexible film isolators, but their walls are made of rigid plastic. This makes them more resistant to physical damage, but the rigid nature of the walls limits the access reach of glove sleeves: this normally necessitates the use of integral half suits to improve access and user ergonomics. The other disadvantage of these isolators is that they are less able to absorb sudden pressure fluctuations such as those that occur when entering the glove sleeves or half suit and this could potentially compromise the protective efficacy of a negative- or positive-pressure regime unless carefully managed. Rigid isolators have been used where a more robust structure is required such as for housing infected marmosets (Brown & Hearson 2008) or poultry (Timms *et al.* 1979). Table 11.2 provides a summary of potential welfare issues and solutions relating to using isolators.

Individually ventilated cages

The principle of the individually ventilated cage (IVC) is for each to be a mini containment system (Figure 11.6). Each cage has a removable lid that, for effective containment purposes, is clamped and sealed to the top rim of the cage. Ventilation for the occupants is provided by plugging each cage into a dedicated rack system that has either an integrated air supply/extract or which, less frequently, plumbs into the room air-handling system in some way. The supply and extract air can be balanced to provide either positive or negative pressure within the cage, depending upon the experimental requirements. For effective high-level biocontainment the integrity of these air penetrations is managed by the use of small in-line HEPA filters or by snap-shut valve systems or a combination of both. IVCs are often used as the preferred option for protecting staff from exposure to animal allergens (Renström *et al.* 2001) or, in older facilities, as a less expensive method of meeting recommended air change rates, in place of total refurbishment.

[1] http://www.hse.gov.uk

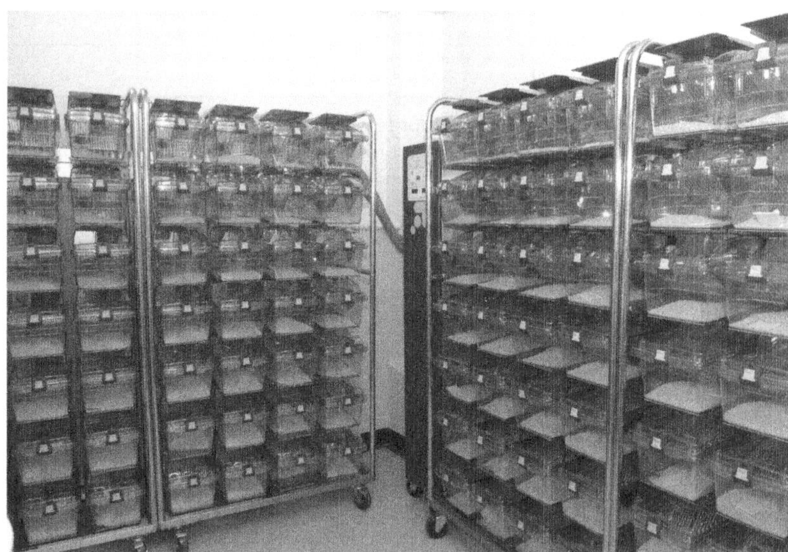

Figure 11.6 A rack of IVCs used to house mice. (Courtesy of Arrowmight.)

Welfare considerations in the use of IVCs

Individually ventilated cages are capable of providing good air change rates and environmental conditions when working well (Clough *et al* 1995; Höglund & Renström 2001). However, dust clogging of filters may affect performance (Höglund & Renström 2001). They can provide protection from external disease or cross-contamination from experimental infection (Lipman *et al.* 1993; Morrell 1997), but there is reduced visibility of the occupants. Kallnik *et al.* (2007) found that for some inbred mouse strains, housing in IVCs reduced activity and increased anxiety-related behaviour. To improve visibility, the food hopper can be moved to the rear of the cage.

These cages are labour-intensive to service: a change of bedding requires transfer of each cage to cabinet prior to removal of lid and strict disinfection regimes to prevent cross-contamination (Figure 11.7) (Höglund & Renström 2001). There is a risk of uneven distribution of air throughout cages depending on their position on the rack. Other potential disadvantages or problems include:

- There is a risk of suffocation if the air supply fails (therefore, they need good back-up support and visible evidence of airflows for each cage on the rack, plus good alarm systems) (Krohn & Hansen 2002). An uninterruptible power supply (UPS) is essential to guarantee the well-being of the occupants.
- Care must be taken that the noise and vibration of air handling units is not transferred to the cages. This should include any frequencies beyond the normal human range. Noise level considerations should also extend to the cabinet where cage changes or procedures may be conducted.
- Disturbance during cage changes may affect breeding performance (Reeb-Whitaker *et al.* 2001). In the most recent systems, the improved level of ventilation means that cages need cleaning out at fortnightly rather than weekly intervals.
- Reduced frequency of cleaning may mean that welfare problems may go unnoticed unless a strict discipline of observation by animal care staff is enforced. This practice may also require the use of large food hoppers and drinking bottles that may intrude upon and reduce the amount of three-dimensional cage space available to the occupants.
- A drive towards more efficient use of room space may lead to the deployment of cage racks that are too tall for direct observation of all animals. Similarly, library racking systems may present a tempting economy of room usage, but working practices must be in place to ensure that cages are observed at least once per day by a competent individual.

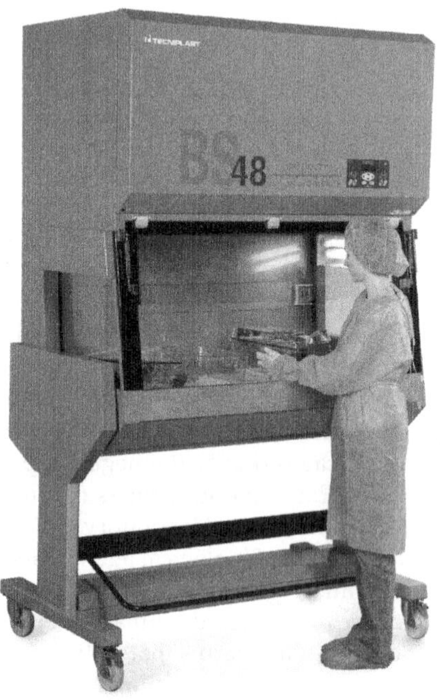

Figure 11.7 An IVC being serviced in a Class II type cabinet. (Courtesy of Tecniplast UK.)

Table 11.3 provides a summary of potential welfare issues and solutions relating to using IVCs.

Table 11.3 Potential welfare issues of IVCs.

Parameter	*Potential welfare issue*	*Solution*
Air supply	Sealed lids and small volume of airspace requires constant airflow to be maintained to avoid build up of humidity, temperature or waste gases (eg, ammonia) Failure of power or fans will rapidly cause problems and may lead to suffocation if prolonged	Have a system that ensures even distribution of air to all cages. Have reserve fan or twin-motored fan. Emergency generator is essential and battery back-up to power fans is recommended (UPS). A schedule of regular servicing should be in place to ensure optimum performance
Filtration	Effective biocontainment will involve filtration of air. Filters will become clogged with dust and dander and this will affect performance	Either change filters frequently (expensive) or have a disposable pre-filter that can be discarded Have a monitoring system that will warn of reduction in performance (preferably for each cage)
Cage cleaning/changing	Every event such as addition of food and water, changing bedding, close inspection of animals, will require removal to a cabinet	Reduce change requirements to a minimum by optimising air change rates
Interaction with staff	Reduced visibility and ergonomics may limit observation of animals Requirement to move to cabinet before removing lid may reduce the time staff can spend at one session	Organise cages to allow maximum visibility of occupants (eg, move food hopper from front of cage) Have strict daily observation regime in place Mobile transportation units are available to move batches of cages whilst maintaining air supply
Procedures	Cages need to be transferred to a cabinet or downdraught table to conduct experimental procedures. This will be time-consuming and may lead to fatigue	Design experiments so that groups of animals can be dealt with in a tolerable time period. Do not be over-ambitious with the types of procedures that can be conducted, bearing in mind group sizes and the limitations of cabinet work
Cross-contamination	The use of a cabinet for husbandry or procedures means that there is a risk of cross-contamination between groups of animals	Strict operating procedures are required to schedule the order in which groups of cages are opened and to define disinfection regimes for exposed surfaces

Filter-top cages

Filter-top cages provide a simple method of preventing cross-contamination between cages by providing a physical barrier to larger particles (Figure 11.8). Typically they consist of a shoebox-type cage with a lid consisting of a polycarbonate frame fitted with a piece of filter media. Such systems have been shown to protect the cage occupants from exposure to pathogens in adjacent cages (Lipman *et al.* 1993). Whilst they can be used successfully to prevent cross-contamination between groups of infected animals such as hamsters infected with *Clostridium difficile* (Shone personal communication), they are not recommended for use with pathogens dangerous to humans without the additional use of some other, more robust form of containment.

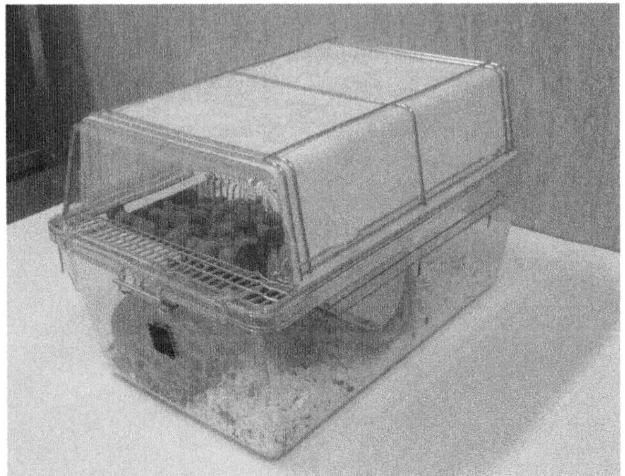

Figure 11.8 A filter-top box housing hamsters infected with *Clostridium difficile*. (Courtesy of Health Protection Agency.)

Welfare considerations in the use of filter-top cages

The presence of a filter lid reduces visibility of the occupants and of food and water levels. Also, the presence of a filter without a forced air supply reduces ventilation and can lead to a build up of waste gases. Reviews of the environmental conditions within such cages indicate that the reduced airflow observed within these cages could lead to a build-up of gaseous pollutants that may adversely affect the animals' health (Keller *et al.* 1989) and that the high relative humidity, ammonia and carbon dioxide levels result in lower body weight gain and lower water consumption (Corning & Lipman 1991; Memarzadeh *et al.* 2004).

However, if due consideration is given to the number of animals housed per cage, the provision of bedding that will absorb waste effectively and to the frequency of bedding change (Reeb *et al.* 1998), then these cages provide a simple and effective means of preventing cross-contamination.

The filter lid should only be removed in a contained environment such as a safety cabinet, otherwise the benefits of using the lid will be lost and the resultant cross-contamination may invalidate the experiment. A strict working practice regime, including disinfection, placing only similarly infected groups of cages in the cabinet at the same time, and working from the lowest dose upward, is required for this system to work effectively.

Ventilated cabinets

Ventilated cabinets are cabinets with sets of shelves on which the animal cages are placed. They can provide low-grade protection or isolation (Figure 11.9). There are usually one or two doors at the front to allow access to the cages, and air is supplied either by an integral air-handling system or by plumbing into the room air system. The air handling can usually be switched between supply or extraction so that the cabinet can be operated at either negative or positive pressure. The shelves may be perforated to allow better distribution of air. Ventilated cabinets are frequently used in combination with filter-top cages, as any protective efficacy is lost as soon as a cabinet door is opened. Ventilated cabinets can be fitted with a range of optional extras to suit user requirements, such as building in a variable circadian rhythm with light/dark time control or fitting temperature control to allow post-operative recovery.

Welfare considerations in the use of ventilated cabinets

Ventilated cabinets limit the observation of occupants, especially if used in combination with filter-top boxes. Ventilation is limited in the event of a power failure. As with other ventilated systems due consideration should be given to the transfer of noise and vibration from air handling systems. There may be a temptation to conduct more than one experiment in a room as the cabinets appear very self-contained. For such a strategy to succeed there need to be strict protocols in place for removal of cages for husbandry or experimental procedures.

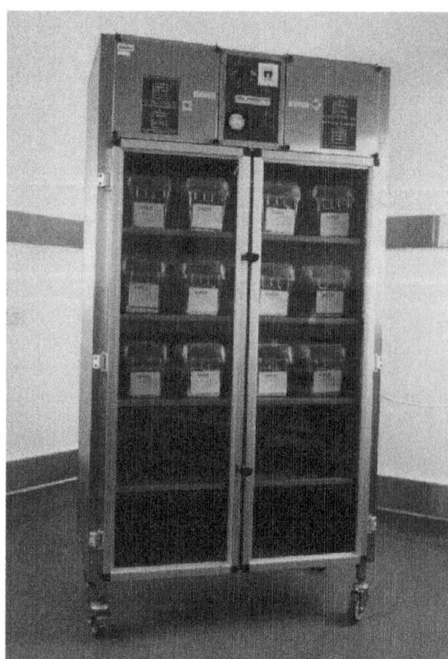

Figure 11.9 A typical ventilated cabinet containing mouse cages. (Courtesy of Tecniplast UK.)

Laminar flow booths or cubicles

Laminar flow booths are essentially miniature rooms with their own air handling systems and they are used to subdivide an animal room into several independent units. Their main advantage is that this subdivision of a room can enable more efficient use of space where this is at a premium by allowing several different experiments to be conducted simultaneously (Figure 11.10).

Typical isolation booths include: a wall system, a ceiling containing controls and an air handling system and a vertically telescoping front access door with transparent windows. They can be operated at either positive pressure, to protect the occupants, or at negative pressure, to protect staff. They can be custom built to fit any particular space and are usually accessed from the front by upward-opening sectioned doors. As with ventilated cabinets, any protective efficacy afforded by the pressure differential or direction of airflow is considerably reduced when the doors are opened to access the occupants of the booth. The use of upwardly telescoping, rather than outward-opening doors reduces this effect and allows the air handling system to cope more efficiently with the breach in the barrier that is created. The vulnerability of the occupants of such systems to power or fan failure is very much dependent on the size of the booth.

For smaller booths, animals will need to be removed to a separate area or cabinet to perform daily husbandry or procedures, but larger booths can incorporate a section to allow such functions.

Welfare considerations in the use of laminar flow booths

These booths can provide a degree of microbiological separation but they permit only poor observation of occu-

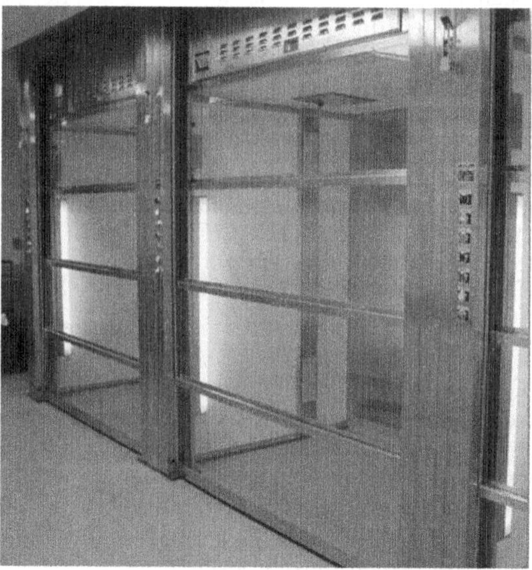

Figure 11.10 A typical containment booth with upwardly telescoping sectioned doors. (Courtesy of Britz & Co., USA.)

pants from outside the booth. Other potential problems include:

- limited ventilation in the event of power failure;
- as with other ventilated systems, there is the potential for transfer of noise from air handling equipment or generated by the flow of air.

The environment of a booth can be easier to control in terms of air changes, temperature and humidity than that of an entire room. A controlled light–dark system can also be incorporated if required. A strict regime of daily practice is required for staff to prevent cross-contamination between booths and where smaller booths are sharing an area or cabinet for procedures, robust protocols must be in place to prevent cross-contamination between separate experiments. As with any enclosed system a reliable UPS is essential.

Bespoke systems

For some species, no systems that offer acceptable levels of operator protection are commercially available and bespoke systems have to be developed according to need. An example of this is the directional flow containment system developed at the UK Centre for Emergency Preparedness and Response (CEPR) to enable group housing of macaques that have been challenged with infectious agents (Figure 11.11a,b). Here, operator protection depends upon a directional flow of air that is maintained to a minimum velocity of 0.7 m/s at all times, even when accessing the animals. The room air-handling system is used to provide the ventilation for the system. The primates are physically isolated from the general room area by a solid transparent plastic barrier fixed to the front of the cage system. This barrier serves to enhance the directional airflow and to provide a physical barrier to potentially contaminated material generated by coughing, urination or defecation.

The risks associated with the husbandry of infected primates are controlled by strict discipline with regard to feeding, watering and waste removal regimes. The risks associated with handling of the primates are controlled by a strict regime whereby animals are sedated by injection before any handling or removal from the cage. Injection for sedation is accomplished by the use of a winding mechanism that gently brings the animal to the front of the cage and a strategically placed access door to allow injection. Sedated animals are removed from the cage into a carrying box that will be used at all times for transportation to and from a separate procedures area. All procedures are conducted on validated downdraught tables.

Welfare considerations of bespoke systems

Access to the animals is restricted compared to the situation when using an open cage system. It is essential that all systems are designed so that animals can be accessed and isolated without causing undue stress for sedation or for remedial treatment in case of injury. In these systems, observations of animals can be limited by reflection of the plastic barrier. Overhead lighting needs to be positioned carefully to avoid this. Observation periods are also limited due to the demanding entry and exit procedures that require the use of protective clothing and strict disinfection regimes. Solid barriers inevitably alter the relationship between the care staff and the animals. This is no great problem if the animals are housed in social groups. Such systems can change the ergonomics of husbandry procedures and consideration needs to be given at the design stage to the potential for fatigue or strain in staff conducting day-to-day husbandry procedures.

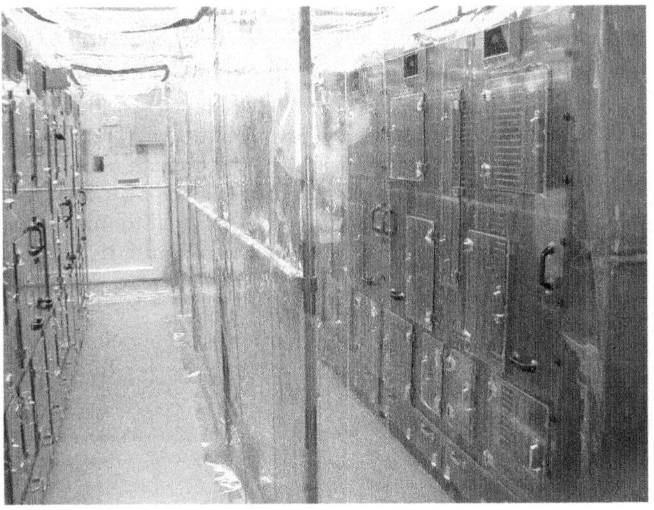
(a)

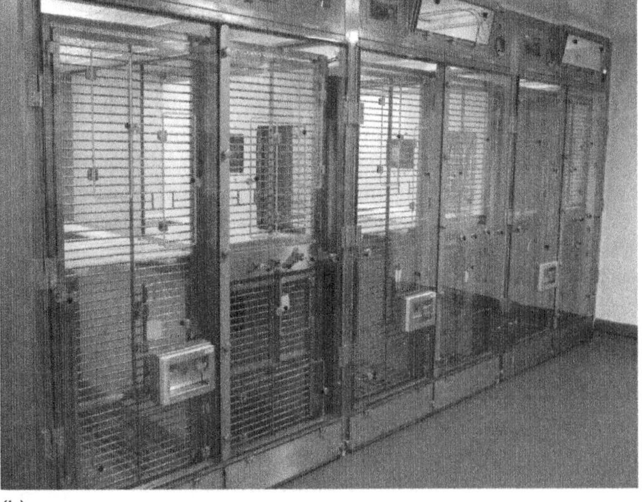
(b)

Figure 11.11 Two versions of a directional flow containment system that can house social groups of macaques infected with level 3 pathogens. (a) Flexible film technology is used to form an additional barrier and to subdivide areas for different functions. (Courtesy of Bell Isolation Systems Ltd.) (b) There is a directional flow unit only, with separate rooms for other functions such as procedures. Note the increased cage size, meeting ETS 123 housing standards. (Courtesy of Health Protection Agency.)

Species

Mice

IVCs are now in common usage for mice for containment of infection, for reduction of animal allergens or to protect susceptible animals from outside contamination. The ability to 'quarantine' animals of unknown health status in such systems has led to increased usage linked to the increasing traffic of transgenic strains of mice between research groups in different countries.

The other obvious attraction of these systems is that more efficient use can be made of animal accommodation, whilst not compromising health status (increases in stocking density of up to 50% are claimed). Thus, IVC systems are seen as a preferred option to improve standards of environmental health for both staff (allergen containment) and animals (cross-contamination, environmental control) without investing heavily in facility refurbishment or in new facilities.

Ventilation is provided by plugging individual cages into an air-handling system that is either integral to the cage rack or is plumbed in to the room air supply. Protection is afforded by maintaining either a positive or negative pressure within each cage. This works well whilst the cages are attached within the rack but the challenge to bio-containment status comes when the cages have to be removed in order to change bedding, food and water, or to handle the animals. Containment integrity after removal from the rack can be maintained, to some extent, by an airtight seal between the lid and the box. This airtight seal presents a potential threat to the welfare of the occupants should the air system fail or should the box not be replaced accurately on the rack. Manufacturers have overcome this problem by placing an additional filter on the lid of the box that will allow passive exchange of gases and by adding pressure alarms and emergency battery power that will allow continued operation for a finite time until power is restored and by engineering in accurate locating systems. The effect of various ventilation rates from 30–100 air changes per hour (ACH) has been evaluated (Reeb *et al.* 1998) and whilst all rates kept ammonia levels below 3 parts per million (ppm), carbon dioxide levels, relative humidity and temperature were found to vary according to air change rate. The authors concluded that ventilation rates of 30ACH were adequate if bedding was changed weekly, but this needed to be increased to 60ACH in case of a fortnightly change frequency.

Removal of the lid for any husbandry or procedural functions is generally performed within a safety cabinet (usually Class II) but strict working protocols must be put in place to prevent cross-contamination between groups of animals. Any assessment of working practice should include the likelihood of contamination when handling the animals for operations such as cage changing or procedures: this is usually addressed either by changing gloves between each cage (very time consuming) or using disposable forceps to pick up the mice (this requires careful choice of implement and of experienced staff to avoid injury to the animals).

Other containment systems used for mice include:

- isolators;
- filter-top cages;
- ventilated cabinets;
- ventilated booths;
- suited laboratories.

Welfare considerations with the use of containment systems for mice

Mice should be kept in groups wherever possible. Bedding and nesting materials should be provided; this includes the consideration of the importance of location of nest boxes as described by Kostomitsopoulos *et al.* (2007). Plastic, autoclavable nest boxes are available specifically for containment systems and treats, disposable tunnels and mouse refuges are readily available.

Containment strategies should be selected that allow maximum observation of animals but minimise laborious clothing change procedures. Where ventilated containment systems are used due consideration must be given to avoid exposing mice to excessive air change rates or air velocities (see also Chapter 21). All aspects of ergonomics should be considered so that staff are not reluctant to observe and care for animals. The preventative maintenance implications to keep containment systems running efficiently and safely for animal welfare should be considered.

Rats

IVCs are now manufactured at an appropriate size to maintain rats. Other suitable containment systems for rats include:

- isolators;
- ventilated cabinets;
- ventilated booths;
- suited laboratories.

Welfare issues with the use of containment systems for rats

As with mice, rats should be housed in social groups of three to five (Patterson-Kane *et al.* 2001) wherever possible. Cage height may be important to allow rats to stand erect. It has been noted that rats prefer a lower air change rate, below 80ACH (Krohn *et al.* 2003). Rats are also affected by ammonia build-up (Gamble & Clough 1976) compared to mice, who are thought to be more ammonia tolerant (Smith *et al.* 2004), so an optimal ventilation rate needs to be established. Provision of refuge and shredded nesting materials are thought to provide the best environmental enrichment for rats but they do not show any preference for tunnels or pipes (Bradshaw & Poling 1991).

Hamsters

Suitable containment systems for hamsters include:

- filter-top boxes;
- isolators;
- ventilated cabinets;

- ventilated booths;
- suited laboratories.

Welfare considerations with the use of containment systems for hamsters

Hamsters are more solitary than rats and mice and care is needed when housing them in social groups unless they are put together at an early age. They have a need to burrow or hide in shelters, so deep litter and appropriate nesting materials are of great benefit. It should be borne in mind that hamsters are very adept at chewing through cages.

Guinea pigs

Suitable containment systems for guinea pigs include:

- isolators;
- ventilated cabinets;
- ventilated booths;
- suited laboratories.

Welfare considerations with the use of containment systems for guinea pigs

Animals should be housed in groups or pairs with deep litter if possible. Sudden noises or movements should be avoided during husbandry or experimental procedures. Guinea pigs do well with a set routine and adapt poorly to changes, especially more mature animals. They may be upset by changes in the type of food hopper, water bottle or the type of food (Wolfensohn & Lloyd 1998) and they may be upset by a sudden move from conventional to contained housing.

Rabbits

Suitable containment systems for rabbits include:

- isolators;
- ventilated cabinets;
- ventilated booths;
- directional flow systems;
- suited laboratories.

Welfare considerations with the use of containment systems for rabbits

The use of senses such as smell or hearing may be impeded by the enclosure, by directional airflow or the use of protective clothing. A risk assessment taking into account the infectious agent may allow group housing in floor pens or large cages with deep litter if this results in no increased biological risk to handlers. This type of housing may be accommodated in a bespoke directional-flow system and will have the potential benefit of reducing stereotypic behaviours. Boxes or tubes should be provided as refuges from aggression. Cages should be of a size to allow the animals to stand on their hindlegs, or climb on ledges to get a better view. The housing should allow animals to get an early warning rather than be startled by the sudden appearance of an operator (as might happen if they were housed in an isolator system similar to those shown in Figures 11.12 or 11.13).

Ferrets

Ferrets are considered to be good models for several human respiratory infections, including influenza, to which they are

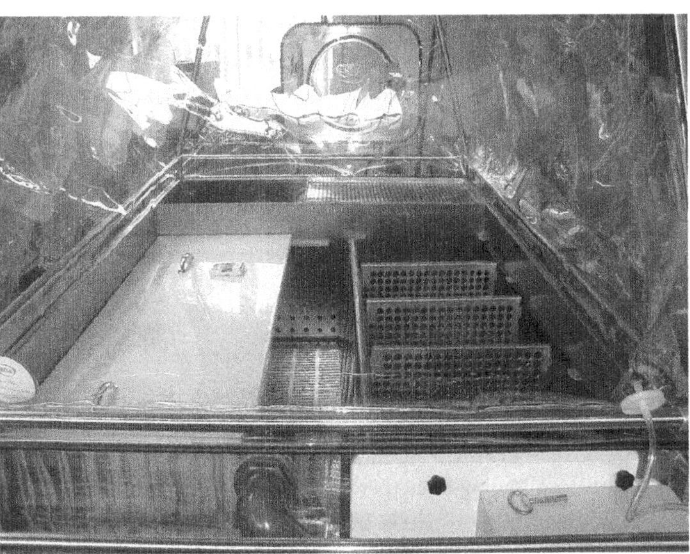

Figure 11.12 The interior of a containment isolator for piglets. (Courtesy of Bell Isolation Systems Ltd.)

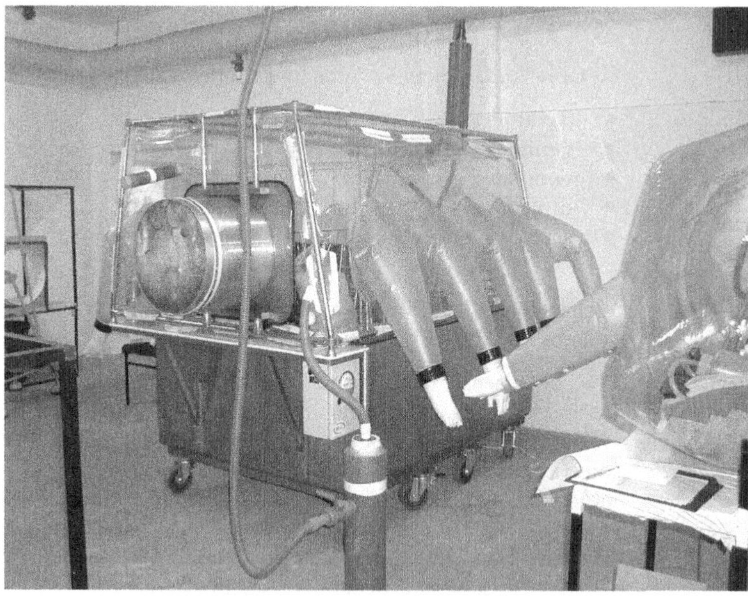

Figure 11.13 An isolator for gnotobiotic calves. (Courtesy of Bell Isolation Systems Ltd.)

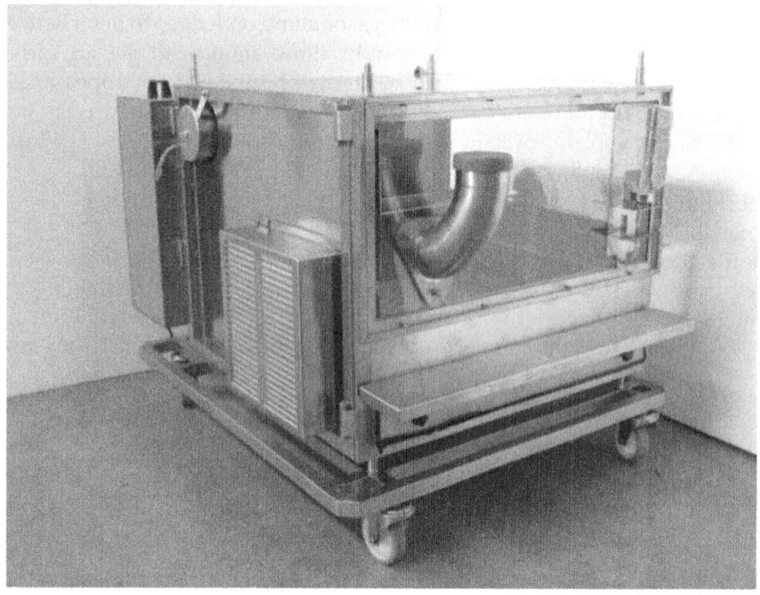

Figure 11.14 A ventilated unit for use with ferrets infected with a high-level pathogen. (Courtesy of Tecniplast UK.)

naturally susceptible; they have been shown to respond to infection in the same way as humans.

Suitable containment systems for ferrets include:

- ventilated cages (Figure 11.14);
- ventilated booths;
- directional flow systems;
- suited laboratories.

Welfare considerations with the use of containment systems for ferrets

Ferrets should be housed in social groups or pairs where possible. Risk assessment should be undertaken to give consideration to allowing floor pens with deep litter, tunnels and disposable boxes if there is no increased risk to handlers. Consideration should be given to a bespoke system that will allow this whilst satisfying the experimental requirements for safe access to the animals for husbandry and procedures. Sullivan and Reardon (2008) report that ferrets used as a model for H5N1 influenza, requiring high-level containment, can be given the same level of enrichment as that provided prior to infection.

Non-human primates

Suitable containment systems for non-human primates include:

- rigid isolators (New World only);
- directional flow systems: see Figure 11.11;
- negative pressure rooms plus RPE;
- suited laboratories.

Welfare considerations with the use of containment systems for non-human primates

Primates should be housed in social groups wherever possible. Marmosets are usually pair-housed for experimental work as a vasectomised male and female, whereas tamarins and Old World primates such as macaques can be successfully housed in single-sex social groups. After social groups have been established, sufficient time should be allowed before the start of a study to ensure that the groupings are compatible and stable.

Provide foraging in deep litter or foraging tray/box if not possible, vary the diet, add toys, puzzle feeders, mirrors, etc, and alternate these to maintain interest. The author has found that providing a TV can be useful enrichment. The TV should be visible for all individuals, with a range of DVDs. Duration and content should be varied to avoid losing the novelty value.

CCTV with a view of all animals and a zoom facility can be used to study abnormal behaviour or overt clinical signs without disturbing the animals. Far more subtle information about well-being can be acquired if the animals are not reacting to human presence. CCTV can also be used to record, so that any missed time periods can be reviewed (Figure 11.15).

Staff familiar with individual animals should be those that assess clinical or behavioural signs. Humane endpoints with clear definition of criteria that are unambiguous and easy to evaluate should be used.

Animals should be acclimatised to the containment system or to protective clothing, using staff who are familiar to the animals. Where possible, train the animals to come to the front of cage or to the area where sedation will be given. Train them to take oral dose, use target training for groups, and use positive reinforcement. Train animals to allow them to be weighed by, for example, entering a detachable weighing box.

In addition to the above:

- Provide a nest box or bucket for marmosets or tamarins to sleep in and hammocks for macaques.
- Maintain the same social groups throughout and plan experimental groups to allow same partners. Plan for eventuality of when humane endpoints are met. Plan necropsy schedules so that animals are not left alone, if at all possible.
- Remote telemetry allows continuous data capture (temperature, blood pressure, ECG, respiration rate, mobility), without repeated sedation. It provides improved experimental data and may assist in establishing early humane endpoints; but choose a system that allows group housing where possible and balance the harms to the animals in terms of surgical implantation, against the benefits (Figure 11.16).
- Ensure that staff are fully trained to understand animals' behaviour and the impact of their own behaviour so as to minimise aggression.
- Design cages so that animals can be separated if aggressive, or isolated for sedation or veterinary treatment if injured. It is of little value having vast cages if animals cannot be captured/sedated without prolonged stress to the animals and staff. Brown and Hearson (2008) describe a humane way of restraining marmosets without stress or injury, using a netting cassette.
- Make cages as complex as possible, using partitions and shelves, or perches for smaller species. This makes the environment more interesting and allows refuge from peers or more dominant animals.
- Feed in an appropriate manner, so that all members of the group can access adequate food: this avoids disrupting groups by minimising aggressive incidents at feeding.

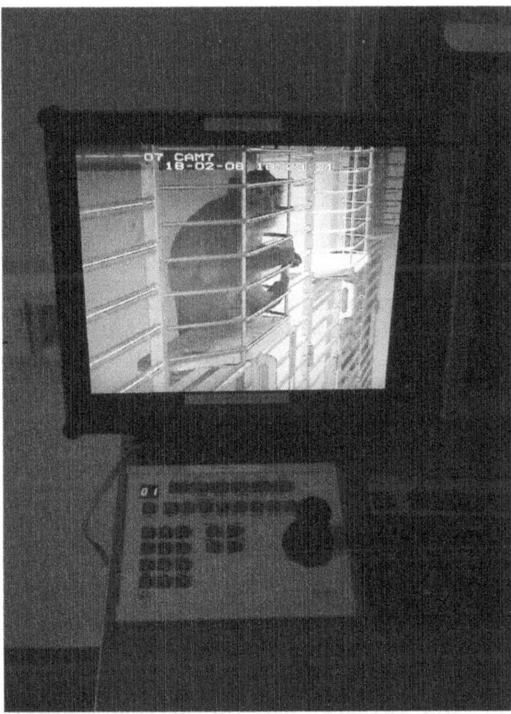

Figure 11.15 Animals being observed by CCTV. (Courtesy of Health Protection Agency.)

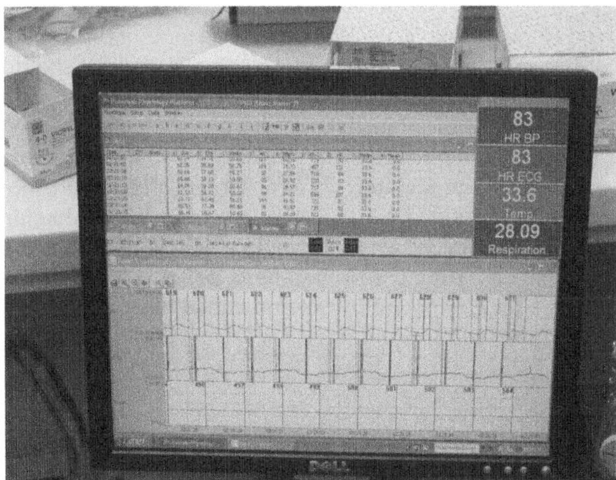

Figure 11.16 Real-time display of cardiac and respiratory data from a telemetry implant. (Courtesy of Health Protection Agency.)

Pigs

Young piglets can be housed in flexible film isolators, but will outgrow such limited accommodation within a few months (Figure 11.12). Other suitable containment systems for pigs include:

- directional flow systems;
- negative pressure rooms plus RPE, or suited laboratories.

Welfare considerations with the use of containment systems for pigs

A deep substrate should be provided to permit natural behaviours such as rooting for food. Enrichment, such as toys, plastic bottles, boxes and play chains, should also be provided. Interactions with handlers are important, so consider how high-quality interaction can be achieved. It is important that there is a system to enable restraint for examination or sampling without causing stress.

Ruminants

Young calves and lambs have been reared in modified flexible film isolators either as germ-free animals or to contain an experimental infection (Figure 11.13). However, like piglets, they will outgrow this type of accommodation within a few months. Adult animals require negative pressure rooms plus RPE, or suited laboratories.

Welfare considerations with the use of containment systems for ruminants

From a welfare point it is preferable to house animals in isolators in pairs rather than as individuals as this type of containment gives a high degree of isolation from outside stimuli. The plastic canopy insulates from noise and the height of the base container limits vision of the external environment.

For containment of larger juveniles and adult ruminants, the most practicable alternative is the use of negative pressure rooms with staff wearing PPE (and RPE if necessary). In such accommodation, it is essential that consideration is given to providing more than just a concrete floor. Rubber matting, or straw or other bedding if at all possible, should be provided. It is important to ensure that systems are in place that allow the animals to be restrained for examination or sampling without stress. It is important also to ensure that a diet containing suitable fibre to prevent digestive problems can be provided without compromising any drainage/effluent treatment systems. In most cases these problems can be addressed by the use of high-fibre, pelleted rations supplemented with mineral blocks and cubed hay.

Birds

Suitable containment systems for birds include:

- isolators (Figure 11.17);
- negative pressure rooms plus RPE or suited laboratories.

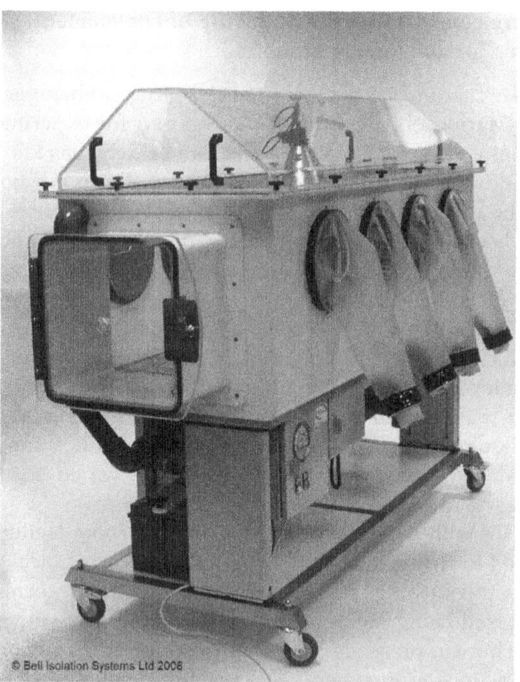

Figure 11.17 An isolator designed for use with poultry. (Courtesy of Bell Isolation Systems Ltd.)

Welfare considerations with the use of containment systems for birds

Environmental enrichment, such as sand baths, artificial turf, provision of perches, has been shown to improve the condition of domestic hens (Abrahamsson *et al.* 1996). Enrichment objects reduce aggression between birds (Gvaryahu *et al.* 1994). Ventilation systems will be required in enclosed systems to prevent ammonia build-up. The filters can be affected by rapid clogging with dust.

Check list for containment

The check list below is designed to help avoid overlooking any important aspects when planning to use containment facilities.

- Is a containment system really necessary? Is its use going to decrease the risks associated with your experiment (are the animals shedding infectious particles, are they infectious by aerosol or by direct contact) or could you actually be increasing risks (eg, needle-stick or bites due to decreased dexterity)?
- Does it do what it is supposed to do (contain or protect)?
- Does it still contain/protect during associated practices (eg, feeding, watering, cage changing, experimental procedures) and does any ancillary equipment offer the same level of protection?
- Can you demonstrate/quantify the effectiveness of operator protection?
- Is it practical to use (ergonomics, dexterity)?
- Can you actually perform all the experimental requirements?
- Can the animals be housed in social groups?

- Can they be accessed easily for food, water, health checks or handling?
- Can the animals be restrained or sedated without undue stress?
- Can they be readily observed for abnormal clinical signs, behaviour?
- Is rapid intervention practicable (eg, humane killing at endpoint, separation if aggression observed, remedial veterinary care)?
- Can they escape and if so can they be retrieved?
- Is air supply optimised for air changes, temperature and humidity?
- Can these conditions be sustained over an extended period?
- Are noise levels acceptable at all times?
- What measures are necessary against power failures?

Legislative requirements

Each country will have its own legislative requirements but there is general consistency especially in assigning containment levels to specific pathogens. In general, biological agents are assigned to a hierarchical grouping according to the perceived threat to human health. These are normally called biocontainment or biosafety levels or the hierarchy may be named after the national body that assigns these 'risk' or 'hazard' groups. Thus for a particular infectious agent you will encounter a number of risk assessment phrases such as biocontainment level (eg, BCL3), biosafety level (eg, BSL3) in the US (Centers for Disease Control and Prevention and National Institutes for Health 2007) or, in the UK, Advisory Committee on Dangerous Pathogens level (eg, ACDP3; Advisory Committee on Dangerous Pathogens (1995)). Criteria that affect this categorisation include: the ability of the pathogen to infect humans; the seriousness of disease; the ability to spread from person to person; and whether prophylaxis (eg, a vaccine) or therapy is readily available. A good general outline of guidance on biohazard categories and the equipment and facilities required to operate safely is given in World Health Organization (2004).

To further complicate matters, many countries have assigned a similar hierarchical system to pathogens that may threaten the environment or agricultural species of economic importance. In this case the hierarchy is based more upon the potential to infect farm animals, the likelihood of escape into the environment and the consequences of infection, rather than the risk to human health. Here you will encounter categorisation of microbes under regulations such as Specified Animal Pathogen Order (eg, SAPO3) or BSL-3 Ag in the US (USDA Agricultural Research Service, Heckert & Kozlovac 2007). In some cases, eg, anthrax, the pathogen may come under both human and animal pathogen legislation and the containment strategy will need to take both into account.

Yet more legislation applies to genetically modified organisms and yet another hierarchy is applied based on the nature of the genetic alteration, whether this has enhanced or diminished the ability to infect or cause disease, whether the altered organism can survive outside the laboratory and whether the altered genes can be passed on to organisms in the outside environment. Be aware that this legislation will apply to genetically altered animals as well as microbes, so containment protocols and risk assessments will need to address the issue of escaped animals and how these might interact genetically with the wild population.

The future

As long as there is a requirement for animal models of infectious diseases there will be a need to use containment strategies to protect the operators. The principles underpinning current containment systems have changed little over the years, relying on some sort of physical barrier supplemented by a differential pressure regime: the main changes that have been seen relate mainly to improving the engineering associated with filtration, pressure and temperature control, alarm systems and emergency back-up capabilities. Thus, the use of isolators, IVCs and cabinets will continue to expand as the expectations of health and safety regulators increase. Furthermore, there is currently an explosion of investment worldwide in high-containment laboratories, driven in part by the perceived threats of bioterrorism, emerging diseases (eg, H5N1 influenza, severe acute respiratory syndrome (SARS)) and changing patterns in disease prevalence due to climate change and population mobility (eg, vector-borne diseases). The main driver for improving these systems is always going to be minimising risk to the operators and will thus be focused on ergonomics and infection hazards. Many of these agents cause serious disease or death and there are some that have an infectious dose for humans of one organism. Thus, potentially lethal needlestick injuries, bites or scratches must be prevented at all costs. Inevitably, any disease-containment strategy will add to the time taken to perform a given task. Copps (2005) gives an example of a single blood sample from one pig that will take 15 minutes at BCL-2, 30 minutes at BCL-3 and 60 minutes at BCL-4, taking into account the time taken to don and doff protective clothing, check all systems, restrain the animal, disinfect and shower out. The challenge will be to optimise animals' welfare within these parameters.

The value of giving animals the ability to manipulate their environment and express preferences, even in a small way, should not be underestimated as it allows them to cope better with the housing conditions necessitated by the procedures.

Given the range of materials available for the construction of cages and enrichment equipment there is little excuse for not addressing the welfare needs of all species of laboratory animals even under the most stringent biocontainment regimes. If animal-friendly materials are not sterilisable for re-use then they should considered as disposable and destroyed or made safe in the most appropriate manner. Several laboratories that specialise in high containment have demonstrated that cage sizes can be maximised, that materials such as plastics and wood can replace stainless steel and that group housing is possible. Biotelemetry can be especially useful in the context of biocontainment, where human presence is kept to a minimum, as it allows continuous monitoring of physiological parameters that can be used to inform on humane endpoints or to indicate a point in the disease progression when extra monitoring or care will be required. Telemetric systems are now being developed that allow concurrent monitoring from multiple animals within group housing (Williamson *et al.* 2007) and it is hoped that these will evolve to be applicable to more species and to be minimally invasive, whilst still providing meaningful physiological data. In addition, the creative use of CCTV can enable continuous monitoring of animals and can even be advantageous in observing natural behaviour that cannot be seen during human presence.

References

Advisory Committee on Dangerous Pathogens (1995) *Categorisation of Biological Agents According to Hazard and Categories of Containment*, 4th edn. HSE books, Sudbury, UK

Abrahamsson, P., Tauson, R. and Appleby, M.C. (1996) Behaviour, health and integument of four hybrids of laying hens in modified and conventional cages. *British Poultry Science*, **37**, 521–540

Alexander, T.J.L., Lysons, R.J., Elliott, L.M. *et al.* (1973) Techniques for rearing gnotobiotic lambs. *Laboratory Animals*, **7**, 239–254

Bradshaw, A.L. and Poling, A. (1991) Choice by rats for enriched versus standard home cages: plastic pipes, wooden platforms, wood chips and paper towels as enrichment items. *Journal of the Experimental Analysis of Behaviour*, **55**, 245–250

Bridger, J.C., Hall, G.A. and Brown, J.F. (1984) Characterization of a calici-like virus (Newbury agent) found in association with astrovirus in bovine diarrhea. *Infection & Immunity*, **43**, 133–138

Brown, M. and Hearson, S. (2008) Refining handling for marmosets in high levels of biocontainment. *Animal Technology and Welfare*, **7**, 39–41

Butler, J.E., Francis, D.H., Freeling, J. *et al.* (2005) Antibody repertoire development in fetal and neonatal piglets. IX. Three pathogen-associated molecular patterns act synergistically to allow germ-free piglets to respond to type 2 thymus-independent and thymus-dependent antigens. *Journal of Immunology*, **175**, 6772–6785

Centers for Disease Control and Prevention and National Institutes of Health (2007) *Biosafety in Microbiological and Biomedical Laboratories (BMBL)*, 5th edn. US Government Printing Office, Washington, DC

Chowdhury, S.R., King, D.E., Willing, B.P. *et al.* (2007) Transcriptome profiling of the small intestinal epithelium in germ-free versus conventional piglets. *BMC Genomics*, **8**, 215–230

Corning, B.F. and Lipman, N.S. (1991) A comparison of rodent caging systems based on microenvironmental parameters. *Laboratory Animal Science*, **41**, 498–503

Clough, G., Wallace, J., Gamble, M.R. *et al.* (1995) A positive, individually ventilated cage system: a local barrier system to protect both animals and personnel. *Laboratory Animals*, **29**, 139–151

Copps, J. (2005) Issues related to the use of animals in biocontainment research facilities. *ILAR Journal*, **46**, 34–43

Dennis, M.J., Davies, D.C. and Hoare, M. (1976) A simplified apparatus for the microbiological isolation of calves. *British Veterinary Journal*, **132**, 642–646

Gamble, M.R. and Clough, G. (1976) Ammonia build-up in animal boxes and its effect on rat tracheal epithelium. *Laboratory Animals*, **10**, 93–104

Gvaryahu, G., Ararat, E., Asaf, E. *et al.* (1994) An enrichment object that reduces aggressiveness and mortality in caged laying hens. *Physiology & Behaviour*, **55**, 313–316

Heckert, R.A. and Kozlovac, J.P. (2007) Biosafety levels for animal agricultural pathogens. *Applied Biosafety*, **12**, 168–174

Höglund, A.U. and Renström, A. (2001) Evaluation of individually ventilated cage systems for laboratory rodents: cage environment and animal health aspects. *Laboratory Animals*, **35**, 51–57

Hope, J.C., Thom, M.L., Villarreal-Ramos, B. *et al.* (2005) Vaccination of neonatal calves with *Mycobacterium bovis* BCG induces protection against intranasal challenge with virulent *M. bovis*. *Clinical Experimental Immunology*, **139**, 48–56

Kallnik, M., Elvert, R., Erhardt, N. *et al.* (2007) Impact of IVC housing on emotionality and fear learning in male C3HeB/FeJ and C57BL/6J mice. *Mammalian Genome*, **18**, 173–186

Keller, L.S., White, W.J., Snider, M.T. *et al.* (1989) An evaluation of intra-cage ventilation in three animal caging systems. *Laboratory Animal Science*, **39**, 237–242

Kostomitsopoulos, N.G., Paronis, E., Alexakos, P. *et al.* (2007) The influence of the location of a nest box in an individually ventilated cage on the preference of mice to use it. *Journal of Applied Animal Welfare Science*, **10**, 111–121

Krohn, T.C. and Hansen, A.K. (2002) Carbon dioxide concentrations in unventilated IVC cages. *Laboratory Animals*, **36**, 209–212

Krohn, T.C., Hansen, A.K. and Dragsted, N. (2003) The impact of cage ventilation on rats housed in IVC systems. *Laboratory Animals*, **37**, 85–93

Lipman, N.S., Corning, B.F. and Saifuddin, M.D. (1993) Evaluation of isolator caging systems for protection of mice against challenge with mouse hepatitis virus. *Laboratory Animals*, **27**, 134–140

Memarzadeh, F., Harrison, P.C., Riskowski, G.L. *et al.* (2004) Comparison of environment and mice in static and mechanically ventilated isolator cages with different air velocities and ventilation designs. *Contemporary Topics in Laboratory Animal Science*, **43**, 14–20

Morrell, J.M. (1997) Efficacy of mini-containment units in isolating mice from micro-organisms. *Scandinavian Journal of Laboratory Animal Science*, **24**, 191–199

Patterson-Kane, E.G., Harper, D.N. and Hunt, M. (2001) The cage preferences of laboratory rats. *Laboratory Animals*, **35**, 74–79

Reeb, C., Jones, R., Bedigan, H. *et al.* (1998) Microenvironment in ventilated animal cages with differing ventilation rates, mice populations and frequency of bedding changes. *Contemporary Topics in Laboratory Animal Science*, **37**, 43–49

Reeb-Whitaker, C.K., Paigen, B., Beamer, W.G. *et al.* (2001) The impact of reduced frequency of cage changes on the health of mice housed in ventilated cages. *Laboratory Animals*, **35**, 58–73

Renström, A., Björing, G. and Höglund, A.U. (2001) Evaluation of individually ventilated cage systems for laboratory rodents: occupational health aspects. *Laboratory Animals*, **35**, 42–50

Smith, A.L., Mabus, S.L., Stockwell, J.D. *et al.* (2004) Effects of housing density and cage floor space on C57BL/6J mice. *Comparative Medicine*, **54**, 656–663

Sullivan, A. and Reardon, H. (2008) The use of multiple species and models at MRC NIMR: care and welfare implications. *Animal Technology & Welfare*, **7**, 35–38

Timms, J.R., Cooper, D.M., Millard, B.J. *et al.* (1979) An isolator for avian disease research. *Laboratory Animals*, **13**, 101–105

Trexler, P.C. and Reynolds, L.I. (1957) Flexible film apparatus for the rearing and use of Germfree Animals. *Applied Microbiology*, **5**, 406–412

Tavernor, W.D., Trexler, P.C., Vaughan, L.C. *et al.* (1971) The production of gnotobiotic piglets and calves by hysterotomy under general anaesthesia. *Veterinary Record*, **88**, 10–14

Williamson, E.D., Savage, V.L., Lingard, B. *et al.* (2007) A biocompatible microdevice for core body temperature monitoring in the early diagnosis of infectious disease. *Biomedical Microdevices*, **9**, 51–60

World Health Organization (2004) *Laboratory Biosafety Manual*, 3rd edn. WHO, Geneva

Wolfensohn, S. and Lloyd, M. (1998) *Handbook of Laboratory Animal Management and Welfare*, 2nd edn. Blackwell Publishing, Oxford

Wyatt, R.G., Mebus, C.A., Yolken, R.H. *et al.* (1979) Rotaviral immunity in gnotobiotic calves: heterologous resistance to human virus induced by bovine virus. *Science*, **203**, 548–550

12 Refinements in in-house animal production and breeding

Roger Francis

Introduction

From time to time all animal house managers, whether in academic institutes or research laboratories, are likely to be asked to breed animals in-house rather than obtaining them from commercial breeders. Scientists often consider that it would be far easier and cheaper for them to have their own colonies of animals, bred in-house and under their control. While this chapter is aimed primarily at the scientist who wishes to have animals bred in-house, and it does not apply directly to commercial breeding establishments, many of the issues raised may also apply when purchasing from commercial breeders. For example, it is just as important for users to provide the commercial breeder with precise information on numbers required and when they are required so as to minimise wastage.

The resource implications of breeding in-house should not be under-estimated. Laboratory animal housing is expensive to provide and maintain. The requirements necessary to protect both the animals (eg, in the UK, Home Office 1989, 1995) and the personnel working within the animal unit (eg, Health and Safety Executive 2002; European Agency for Safety and Health at Work[1]) have led to the development of very specialised environmental needs. The maintenance of laboratory animals within specialist animal units requires: regulated relative humidity; precise temperature ranges; controlled rates of change of high-quality air (HEPA-filtered); dual lighting systems (a normal lower level for the animals and a higher level for humans to work in); dawn and dusk lighting and photoperiod control etc. Depending upon the nature of the work undertaken, specialist drainage systems with catchment containment systems for sterilisation of effluent prior to discharge may be required. In addition to these specialist environmental controls, animal accommodation must also have high-quality, easily cleaned finishes. Infrastructure and running costs make animal accommodation extremely expensive per square metre to maintain, and users have to judge the costs and benefits of using available space for breeding or for research animals.

It is just as important to have the resources to maintain high-quality breeding animals as it is to have adequate infrastructure. Questions to consider before breeding in-house include: Are there adequate trained staff for the species to be bred? Are staff familiar with the species, and with the type of housing required? Will they need specific training in order to work with new housing systems such as containment systems? Is veterinary advice available to develop and run the necessary programmes for screening, routine treatments, vaccinations etc? Are the animal care technicians fully conversant with the information technology required to maintain and monitor the breeding colonies and to facilitate regular communication between the animal unit and the scientist?

The Three Rs in animal production

The topic of animal breeding and production, as opposed to the use of animals in research, may not be one that immediately springs to mind when considering the Three Rs (Russell & Burch 1959, see also Chapter 2). However, two of the Three Rs, reduction and refinement, are very relevant to the ethical production of laboratory animals.

Proper planning of production and usage should be undertaken in pursuit of reduction, to minimise the chances of any overproduction. Centralising animal production within multiple-user establishments can lead to reductions by reducing the replication of strains within the same establishment. Challenging assumptions about the need to use only one sex of animal, or animals at very precise weights or ages may also help to reduce the size of the colony required.

When establishing new colonies, the user groups and animal technicians should meet prior to starting the colony to discuss special needs and how these can be addressed. They should meet regularly to review progress and discuss whether the initial discussions were appropriate and effective. Senior technicians should produce reports on production, usage and wastage at regular intervals for users and the animal house committee, to enable trends to be monitored.

Where several animal units are spread across a campus or site there should be a central register of strains kept, their usage and surpluses or tissue availability.

Refinement is very important in the management of breeding colonies. Well trained animal technicians, who are specifically aware of the care and needs of breeding stock, are integral to keeping healthy animals to good welfare

[1] http://osha.europa.eu/en/legislation/directives/index_html/@@legislation_overview

standards. The maintenance of high health status is essential but has considerable cost implications.

Refinement includes reducing suffering due to disease or morbidity. Good record systems (see the section on communication) can be used to monitor the efficiency of the colony, and can provide early indicators of problems, such as an increase in, or high levels of, pre-weaning mortality. Any problems must be investigated. For example, is an elevated incidence of pre-weaning mortality because nervous or stressed dams are killing their offspring? Would giving more nesting material reduce the loss? Or could it be caused by an underlying disease problem? If the latter is suspected, then health screening should take place and veterinary advice should be sought. For genetically altered (GA) animals, does a passport (a description of the animal the way in which it has been altered and the consequences of the alteration (Figure 12.1, see also RSPCA booklet GA Passports: *The key to consistent animal care*, In Press)) exist for the line? If so get a copy and continue to update it with your own findings. For all species research the literature for up-to-date advice on enclosure design and enrichment (see species-specific chapters).

Making the decision

Despite all the disadvantages, there is a number of reasons why it may be necessary to produce animals in-house. It may be that the species, strain or animals of an appropriate health status are not readily available from commercial establishments within the same country. The animals may be required at a stage that is not readily available from commercial suppliers or which would might result in, for example, undue stress during transport, eg, timed pregnancy, timed lactation, animals prior to normal weaning age, aged animals.

Establishing user requirements

When a research worker or a research group asks for animals to be bred in-house, the first question has to be what species/strains are required? If these are readily available commercially, the next question is what is the case for producing the animal in-house? If the requirement is for a commonly available species or strain after the normal weaning age then this it is likely to be more efficient and cost-effective to purchase the animals from a commercial animal producer. However, if the requirement is for species, strains or developmental/life cycle stages that are not readily available then in-house breeding will need to be explored and discussed.

Before establishing in-house breeding colonies, animal unit managers should insist on written confirmation of what is required: species, strain, numbers, age, sex, special requirements, dates or times when required, and including details of endpoints, financial arrangements, start and finish dates, and legal requirements (legal authority may be needed for production of some strains). It should be made clear that only the principle investigator can make changes to these specifications and that any changes must be in writing. This is so that requirements are carefully planned and costly changes avoided. Much of this information is relevant also when sourcing animals from commercial suppliers. Do not forget to agree a contingency plan (see later in this chapter).

Nomenclature	
Originator	
Source	
Contact details	
Email address/ Telephone	
Detail of modification	
Background strain	
Number of backcrosses	
Website/references	
Health and welfare	
Coat colour	
Eye colour	
Any physical abnormalities	
If yes describe coping strategies	
Immune status	
Housing system	
Current health status	
Date of last health screen (attach report)	
Behavioural traits	
Coping strategies	
Phenotypic tests used	
Breeding and general care	
Husbandry recommendations	
Cage changing frequency	
Substrate used	
Current food type and manufacturer	
Refuge/shelters used	
Nesting material	
Environmental enrichments used	
BREEDING DATA	
Breeding system used	
Age at first pairing ♂ ♀	
Breeding longevity	
Average litter size	
Pre-weaning mortality	
Average weight at weaning ♂ ♀	
Growth curves Attach if available	
Longevity	

Figure 12.1 Examples of a genetically altered animal passport.

Breeding facilities and health status

Having decided on species and/or strain, there are many issues to address relating to health status. For example: Is the unit able to maintain the required animals at an appropriate health status? Does the animal unit have barrier systems, equipment and sufficient trained staff to maintain the animals appropriately? Can regular health screening be carried out (Laboratory Animal Breeders Association (LABA) 2002)? Are there legal constraints on transporting animals that are part of a scientific study? The method of housing must also be considered in conjunction with the users' needs. Are the users prepared to comply with the biosecurity arrangements (barriers etc) required to maintain the health status of their animals, and do they understand the terminology relating to this (see below)? In establishments with multiple user groups, it may be that some groups (eg, immunologists) require animals of different status than other users. Nonetheless, unless the research topic is the animal disease there can be no justification for keeping animals with compromised health status.

Because of modern requirements for high health status animals, the breeding of animals using conventional methods has become much rarer. As a minimum, most will need to be maintained in a barrier system producing specific pathogen free (SPF) animals. This places restrictions on the amount of access that user groups will have to their animals and may necessitate the scientist handing over the daily running of the colony to the animal house technicians, who then issue the animals as required. It may be necessary to maintain animals within individually ventilated cages, racks, or container systems, or negative- or positive-pressure isolators, all of which require highly developed standard operating procedures (SOPs) and place considerable restrictions on access and usage. One option may be to house nucleus or pedigree lines separately in higher containment systems while expansion colonies could be housed in simpler containment systems. Considerable care must always be taken when buying in animals to establish new colonies, and a period of quarantine and health screening is necessary to ensure that the new animals are of the appropriate health status.

Predicting usage

Users must appreciate that the supply of animals cannot be simply switched on or off. Depending on the stage of development/life cycle that is required, it may be several months before an in-house colony is in a position to supply animals on a regular basis. For some species (primates, cats and dogs), it could be several years before a breeding colony could supply animals. Even when colonies of animals are in full production, users must appreciate the need to communicate their requirements. For instance, if the user requires 8-week-old mice then the production of those mice needs to be set up some 11–12 weeks before the user's required date.

If animals must be produced in-house then, wherever possible, the user should be required to provide a reasonable usage plan. There will be peaks and troughs in usage, for instance there is normally a drop in use around and

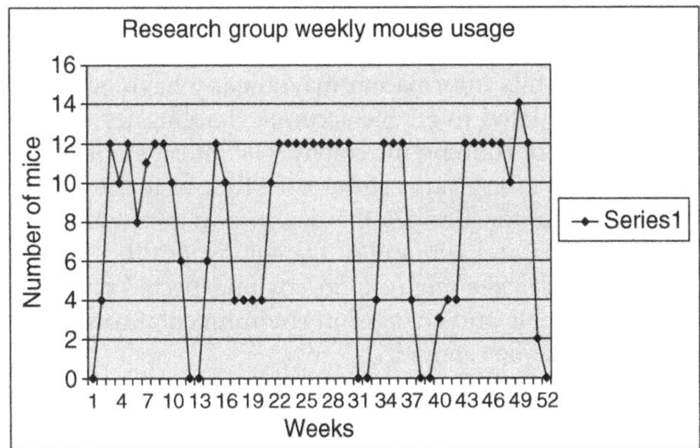

Figure 12.2 Weekly usage of mouse pups by a research group.

during holidays. Experience in academia shows that there may be a surge in use at the start of each academic term and then again when students have departed in early summer. Therefore, to minimise wastage, it is important to know when the research groups are planning to take annual holidays, or when they are attending conferences. Figure 12.2 shows the usage by a research group of 10–12-day-old mouse pups each week, with zero use in weeks 52 and 1 coinciding with the Christmas/New Year holiday, another break at weeks 13–14 (the Easter holiday), a drop to only 4 animals per week for a 4-week period, 2 weeks' annual holiday with no usage during weeks 30–31 followed by no usage in weeks 38–39 when the research group was away at a conference. Such changes should be predicted and planned for so as to minimise wastage.

Research workers may not appreciate the size of colonies needed to produce the numbers of animals that they require each week. The smaller the numbers required the more difficult it is to keep the colony viable. Colonies consist of current breeders, replacement breeders, growing stock and within most colonies there will be animals that may already have already been used, unless there are clear instructions regarding culling. A colony to supply six male mice a week at 8 weeks of age could consist of between 60–80 animals.

If a colony is to successfully produce the required animals over a number of years it will need to be robust, and the management required to achieve this will depend on colony type. If the colony is to have an inbred status, then there will have to be sufficient animals to maintain pedigree lines and, where appropriate, to maintain expansion colonies. If the colony is outbred, then the population must be large enough to maintain a gene pool so as to allow unrelated pairings and to prevent inbreeding (see also Chapter 4).

Communicating with the users

Good communications between the animal producer and the user are essential and with the use of electronic transfer of information, records can be regularly updated, on a weekly basis or more frequently if desired. Indeed, if the animal technicians update computer records of animal production and usage on a daily basis, then this information can also be sent daily to users. Simple spreadsheets can be used to report on the number of animals produced, used, culled etc. Much of this information may already have been collected and collated to enable accurate charging for the full cost recovery of running the colony. The information can be distributed to user groups at the same time as to the animal unit administrator. Besides the day-to-day information on the production and running of the colony, health information (eg, health screening results), any unexpected problems with the animals and changes in environmental conditions etc should also be reported.

The communication needs to be two way. The principle investigator should provide details of the planned usage, as discussed above, and should also give feedback on how the work is progressing and if there is likely to be change in usage. User groups will often get a better service from the animal unit if they take the trouble to explain what they are doing and hoping to achieve. If the research group gives the animal care staff a presentation on the area of research and explains the needs of the group, this can frequently result in better utilisation of the animals.

Contingency plans

Having agreed to production of animals in-house, in an appropriate housing system and to a predetermined health status, the next stage is to develop, in discussion with users, a contingency plan to address arrangements if things go wrong. This might cover: What happens when things break down (as they inevitably will)? Or what will happen if a problem emerges during health screening. Dependent upon the nature of the problem and the veterinary advice, will it be necessary to cull the entire colony? Would the use of a firebreak (stopping breeding for a period of time) allow a disease 'to burn itself out'? Could the colony be treated? Would the treatment conflict with the research programme? Whatever course of action is taken in such circumstances there would be a considerable impact, not only on the breeding colony, but also in terms of delay to research programmes. This will have further serious cost implications for the user groups, in terms of lost time, inability to meet deadlines, staff time and deciding who pays for the health treatments and the colony while it is non-productive and being rebuilt? Potential knock-on consequences for other user groups and their animals held within the unit should also be considered.

Transport

Another important consideration is transport and the effect it has upon animals (see Chapter 13). Animals are regularly transported around the world for laboratory use. Generally these will be normal healthy animals, but there are times when it may be necessary to transport surgically prepared or GA animals. Special care and coping strategies must be put in place to ensure that such animals do not suffer during transport. In the case of surgically prepared animals, veterinary advice should be sought before the animals undergo transportation. With GA animals, referral to the passport for the genotype should show if the animals need specialist care during transportation. Animals that have been transported for more than a short distance should be allowed at least a week to acclimatise, and some species can take much longer. When transporting laboratory animals, due consideration must be given to the legislation and codes of practice on animal transportation within each area or country the animals will be travelling through (eg, Council of Europe 1986, 2006; European Council (1986)); National Institutes of Health 2004; Laboratory Animal Science Association 2005; HMSO 2006). Given the potential stressors of transport and re-housing, it may be possible to make an ethical argument for in-house breeding, especially if the animals are required in a compromised state or at some stages of development/life cycle.

Financial costs

Historically, users in academia have not paid the full costs of their animal colonies, often paying only for consumables, such as food, bedding and possibly caging. Recently, within the UK, there has been a move to full economic costing (FEC) with the result that that research animals are now very expensive for users to maintain. FEC means that the user pays for food and bedding as well as a footprint charge for the space taken up by the colony. This will cover fuel, maintenance, replacement build costs, all labour charges for the animal unit including ancillary staff and administrative staff, and consumables including clothing, laundry, environmental enrichment, equipment depreciation, quarantine, health screening etc. The result is that buying animals in has become a more attractive option; a researcher who uses six male mice bought in from a commercial supplier each week, finds that he or she is will only be paying for 12 animals per week (six housed for a week acclimatisation, plus the six they are about to use) instead of meeting the costs of maintaining a breeding colony of 60–80 animals. FEC results in the more efficient use of animals and space and, through this, the more ethical use of animals. Purchase from commercial companies may often offer ethical advantages. Commercial companies, through economies of scale, are able to minimise wastage, and are well placed to use, for other scientific purposes, those animals that have to be killed or to supply them as food for zoo animals.

Partial in-house production

There may be good reasons for partial in-house production. Although timed-mated animals can be bought in, the stress of transportation and the legal constraints are considerable and the failure rates can be quite high. In-house production might also be necessary if there is a need for lactating females or specific age pups pre-weaning. Obtaining aged animals presents different sets of problems as these are not generally available from commercial suppliers (most of their rats and mice are used or killed by 12 weeks of age) although some companies will keep animals to specific ages at a cost. If the animals required are not commercially available then there is no choice but to produce in-house. On the other hand, if the animals are commercially available, then it might be possible, in the case of timed pregnant or lactating animals, to buy in animals of breeding age and to time mate the animals in-house. If the dams are not used (ie, where it is the pups that are used for the research) they could be remated if necessary. In the case of aged animals, these should be bought in as old as possible and kept until the appropriate age. When maintaining groups of aged animals there is always the risk of animals being lost to natural causes. Good communication is essential to ensure that users are aware of the health status of aged animals.

Calculating colony size

Once the principle investigator has provided information on animals, and stage of development required it is possible to calculate the required colony size. For this, it is important to know whether the animals will breed throughout the year or if they are seasonal breeders. If the latter, can the animal be induced to produce outside the normal season by manipulation of the environment, especially photoperiod and possibly temperature? Where seasonal manipulation is practised, care must be taken to ensure that the animals, especially birds, where necessary, get appropriate rest periods enabling them to complete physiological changes, such as moulting. In intensive breeding programmes, the duration of the breeding life of both male and females should be taken into account, especially if the females are producing and rearing very large litters; the calculations must reflect this and allow for adequate replacements.

Information required to calculate the size of breeding colonies

In order to calculate breeding colony size, the following information is needed:

- Number of animals required to supply scientific needs (if a single sex is required, colony size will need to be doubled) and for replacement breeding stock.
- Reproduction data for the species, or more specifically the strain, including: type of oestrous cycle, length of cycle, breeding season, age at first breeding, gestation period, average litter size, litter interval, weaning age, age at first breeding, if seasonal breeders, then number of young per season, and economic breeding life. Obtain a growth curve for the strain so that all concerned are aware of the age/weight relationship.
- Shelf life. How long will the animal remain usable? Check the growth curve to see how long an animal remains within the required weight range.
- Breeding system: inbred, outbred, permanent pairs, temporary pairs, harems, hand mated (for timed pregnancy etc).
- Variance allowance. When calculating the size of the colony required to produce a given number of animals, it is not possible to state exact litter sizes, so a small number of extra animals (a variance allowance) has to be included to ensure that adequate animals are produced. *The Manual of Animal Technology* (Barnett 2006) recommends adding variance allowances of 5% for colonies of 1000 pairs, 10% between 1000 and 100 pairs and 15% for less than 100 pairs.

Having ascertained the above and calculated the size of the breeding colony, it is then necessary to calculate the number of animals needed to get the stock to the stage required. This will be the numbers of animals required each week from the time of weaning to the age at which they will be issued, plus the number of animals required to be kept on as replacement breeders.

Preservation of colonies

As mentioned earlier, it may be possible to maintain a smaller pedigree colony under higher health status housing with restricted personnel access (such colonies not only provide greater accuracy and control of production but also act as a safeguard should the expansion colony become infected), to supply an expansion colony for providing animals for the user. In the case of an outbred colony there must be a breeding system in place to maintain the gene pool as large as possible. Whatever system is used, there is always a possibility of genetic drift, incorrect matings or the risk of genetic loss if the colony becomes infected by disease. This can be safeguarded against by cryopreservation of gametes or embryos at the earliest possible stage in the development of a colony. Colonies should also be genetically monitored from time to time to ensure that the strains are still the authentic strain.

References

Barnett, S.W. (2006) *Manual of Animal Technology*. Blackwell Publishing, Oxford

Council of Europe (1986) Convention for the Protection of Vertebrate Animals used for Experimental and other Scientific Purposes (ETS 123). Strasbourg. http://conventions.coe.int/treaty/en/Treaties/Html/123.htm (accessed 27 April 2008)

European Council (1986) Council Directive 86/609/EEC of 24 November 1986 on the approximation of laws, regulations and administrative provisions of the Member States regarding the protection of animals used for experimental and other scientific purposes. *Off J Eur Comm L*, **358**, 1–29. http://eur-lex.europa.eu/LexUriServ/LexUriServ.do?uri=CELEX:31986L0609:EN:NOT (accessed 27 April 2008)

Council of Europe (2006) *Multilateral Consultation of Parties to the European Convention for the Protection of Vertebrate Animals used for Experimental and other Scientific Purposes (ETS 123) Appendix A*. Cons 123 (2006) 3. Available from URL: http://www.coe.int/t/e/legal_affairs/legal_co-operation/biological_safety,_use_of_animals/laboratory_animals/2006/Cons123(2006)3AppendixA_en.pdf

Health and Safety Executive (2002) *Control of Laboratory Animal Allergy EH76*. HSE Books, Suffolk

HMSO (2006) *The Welfare of Animals (Transport) (England) Order 2006*. HMSO, London. http://www.opsi.gov.uk/si/si2006/uksi_20063260_en.pdf (accessed 1 June 2008)

Home Office (1989) *Home Office Code of Practice for the Housing and Care of Animals in Designated Scientific Procedure Establishments.* HMSO, London. http://scienceandresearch.homeoffice.gov.uk/animal-research/publications/publications/code-of-practice/ (accessed 1 June 2008)

Home Office (1995) *Home Office Code of Practice for the Housing and Care of Animals in Designated Breeding and Supplying Establishments.* HMSO, London. http://scienceandresearch.homeoffice.gov.uk/animal-research/publications/publications/code-of-practice/ (accessed 1 June 2008)

Laboratory Animal Breeders Association (2002) Recommendation for health monitoring of rodent and rabbit colonies in breeding and experimental units. *Lab Animals*, **36**, 20–42

Laboratory Animal Science Association (2005) Guidance on the transport of laboratory animals. Report of the Transport Working Group established by LASA. *Lab Animals*, **39**, 1–39

National Institutes of Health (2004) *Animal Transportation Guidelines.* National Institute of Health, USA. http://oacu.od.nih.gov/ARAC/animaltransport.pdf (accessed 1 June 2008)

Russell, W. and Burch, R. (1959) *The Principles of Humane Experimental Technique.* Methuen, London

13 Transportation of laboratory animals

William J. White, Sonja T. Chou, Carl B. Kole and Roy Sutcliffe

Introduction

Laboratory animals represent only a small fraction of animals moved in commerce and they differ from many in usually having a more defined health status. A wide range of purpose-bred or wild-caught animals could be used in research, but, in practice, only a small number of species are used. Animals used, and transported for research purposes, include rats, mice, guinea pigs, gerbils, hamsters, rabbits, cats, dogs, swine, non-human primates (only a few species), fish (principally zebra fish), and rarely frogs, sheep, goats, cattle and poultry (mostly chickens). The greatest numbers of shipped containers holding laboratory animals, as well as the greatest number of shipments, are of rats and mice. This chapter focuses on the transport of common laboratory animals although the principles can be applied across many species destined for research use. Species-specific information for less commonly used species can be found in other more comprehensive sources (International Air Transport Association (IATA) 2008a).

General principles

When transporting laboratory animals, the objective is to move them in a manner that does not jeopardise their well-being or health status, minimises controllable sources of stress and ensures their safe arrival at their destination. Part of the stewardship of animal care and use is to understand, and provide for, needs and eventualities arising during transport.

There are various reasons for transporting laboratory animals. Animals are commonly produced in commercial facilities, using specialised housing and handling systems that can reliably exclude disease-causing and unwanted micro-organisms. These animals must be transported to the institutions that use them in research, testing or other activities. In the past, this traffic between commercial breeders and users comprised most of the transportation of laboratory animals. However, over the last few decades, the development of genetic manipulation techniques has led to increasing numbers of animals, with unique genotypes and phenotypes, being bred in small research colonies. These colonies have increasingly become a source of supply for other institutions, either as a small commercial enterprise, or for use on a collaborative basis. Collaborative studies between two or more institutions may require that animals are transported more than once in larger multi-institutional studies. The number of institutionally produced animals that must be transported may be relatively small for any given institution, when compared to commercial producers, but across institutions the aggregate may represent a substantial number of journeys.

Research institutions often have a limited number of options regarding methods for transporting animals between institutions. In the UK and continental Europe, ground transportation by contracted carriers is more common than air transport because of the relatively short distances within and between countries. The majority of ground shipments involve journey times of less than 24h. Carriage by air still remains the most rapid means of transport over long distances and represents the only practical option for transporting animals between continents.

The type of journey, its duration, the physical environment during carriage, the design of the container, along with other factors influences the animals' safety and well-being during the journey. Transportation involves removal of animals from a controlled home environment and their placement in a varying and less controlled environment in which they may be transported with other animals from other locations or with non-animal freight. Even if proper arrangements and procedures are followed, it is, unfortunately, often likely that some animals will experience some discomfort or stress; adverse events may occur, albeit very rarely. In order to minimise adverse events and stress, it is essential to: understand the biological and behavioural requirements of the species; properly plan the journey; and provide adequate contingency provisions prior to commencing the journey. In practice, this means that the consignor should clearly understand all aspects of the procedures involved in transporting their animals as well as the variables that may be encountered during the journey. Since transporting animals between research institutions is not a daily or even a weekly event for most institutions, a detailed written set of procedures and a check list can be very useful in assuring that all steps in the journey have been carefully considered and that appropriate actions have been taken.

General requirements

Animal transportation includes the entire period from packing, through dispatch, carriage and receipt by the consignee to the unpacking of the animals at their final destination. It is important during the transportation process:

- that appropriate containers be used, constructed of strong, durable materials which meet or exceed all national and international guidelines;
- that the animals and their shipping containers be protected from adverse weather conditions such as precipitation, direct sunlight and high winds which can affect the ambient conditions within the container or the security of the container;
- that the animals be provided with an adequate supply of fresh or conditioned air that provides for their thermoregulatory, respiratory and metabolic needs;
- that the animals be protected from exposure to extremes in environmental conditions, especially high temperatures;
- that the animals be prevented from escaping, or from falling out of the container, or extending appendages outside the container, or from experiencing other conditions that result in physical harm, including illness, injury or death;
- that factors that may cause animal discomfort or stress during the journey are recognised and, where possible, minimised.

The health and welfare of animals

Animals to be shipped should be in good clinical health. Prior to packing, each animal should be examined by an appropriately trained animal care provider, experienced in recognising signs associated with illness in that species. Animals should be excluded from shipment if there is behavioural or other clinical evidence of abnormalities that would make them unsuitable for transportation. In some cases, transport may involve animals with inherited abnormalities due either to spontaneous mutations or genetic manipulation. If animals have adapted to these abnormalities so that there are no apparent functional deficits or if the phenotypic expression of these abnormalities, in the judgment of the health care provider, does not present a risk to their well-being in transit, then these animals may be considered for transport. This is subject, however, to appropriate documentation of their abnormalities and the granting of any necessary regulatory permission for their transport. Similarly, diseased or injured animals may be considered for transport only when the purpose of such transport is for the diagnosis or treatment of the condition.

Shipment of pregnant animals should be avoided when possible. Shipment during the last 20% of gestation is risky, as it may be associated with stress-induced abortion. If the pregnancy is not the result of a carefully timed mating, shipment during this period could result in the animal delivering during shipment with risk to both the foetus and the mother. The risk of adverse events occurring during transport increases with the increasing body size of the mother and the size of the foetal mass being carried and also varies with the species. Time-mated rodents can be successfully shipped during the first two thirds of pregnancy and with caution during the first portion of the last third.

There is some variation in guidance on shipment of pregnant animals. Article 9 of The European Convention for the Protection of Animals during International Transport (Council of Europe 2003) states that pregnant female mammals shall not be transported either during the last tenth of the gestation period or for at least 1 week after they have given birth. However, the Laboratory Animal Science Association (LASA) recommends that pregnant animals should not normally be transported during the last fifth of gestation to minimise the risk of abortion or parturition in transit (LASA 2005). Larger species, such as dogs and non-human primates, can be transported nearer the time of parturition provided that the journey is direct, of relatively short duration and can be undertaken under appropriate veterinary direction and supervision. Guidance on this varies with different codes of practice, regulatory bodies and by species. However, as a general rule, shipment during the last 5–10% of gestation is considered more risky particularly for larger species. Nursing animals with their young may be transported when the young are a minimum of 7 days of age and with additional bedding and nesting material (LASA 2005).

Transport of unweaned animals presents a considerable risk to their safety and well-being. Unweaned animals may, depending upon their age, have difficulty in regulating body temperature, be incapable of eating solid food and may be unfamiliar with, or unable to access, water sources within the container. Some species such as guinea pigs can be weaned at a very early age since they are precocious at birth and capable of regulating body temperature and consuming solid food within a few days of birth. While there is no universal minimum age for shipment, animals must be capable of functioning independently from their mothers, consuming solid food and water as well as maintaining normal physiological and metabolic functions. Shipping a lactating female with her young, especially over long distances, may result in her failing to care for her young and their death. The risk of this varies somewhat between species and with the age of the young but, as a general rule, shipping lactating females and young constitutes an unacceptable risk to their health and well-being and is not recommended.

Immunologically deficient, or immunocompromised animals, are commonly transported for research purposes. Some genetically modified animals can possess unrecognised immune defects that may alter their susceptibility to disease. These animals may, as a result of acquiring human or environmental commensal organisms, develop illness that would not be experienced by animals that did not have immune dysfunction. Whenever immunologically deficient or immunologically compromised animals are transported, great care must be taken with all packing and handling and disinfection processes, to ensure that the animals will not be exposed to infectious agents. Other than these considerations, the requirements for successful transport of these animals are the same as for immunocompetent animals of the same species.

A number of anatomical conditions, such as genetic hairlessness or obesity, may impact upon the metabolism and physiology of laboratory animals during transportation and provisions should be made to account for these anatomical differences.

The greater insulation provided by body fat in obese animals compromises their ability to dissipate heat and to adapt to elevated environmental temperatures. Reducing the number of animals placed in a shipping container will help lessen the risk of excess heat by decreasing the total amount of heat generated within the container. Consideration should also be given to postponing shipments of such animals during abnormally warm weather if there is a possibility that the ambient environmental conditions could exceed acceptable ranges even for brief periods of time.

Certain strains of laboratory rodents lack a protective hair coat and this compromises their ability to thermoregulate at lower environmental temperatures and also makes them more susceptible to cuts and abrasions from rough surfaces within their shipping containers. When hairless animals are transported, extra care must be taken to select a container that does not have exposed or rough edges that could injure unprotected skin. In addition, when hairless animals are shipped during periods of cold weather, the provision of extra bedding and nesting materials will help to provide insulation within the shipping container during transport. In some instances, when hairless animals are produced as a result of breeding homozygous and heterozygous animals for the desired genotype, haired cage mates of the same microbiological status are also produced. Inclusion of some of these haired colony animals can also be used to provide additional thermal protection, as they huddle with the hairless animals.

Some laboratory animals can have metabolic or physiological conditions that may predispose them to challenges during transport. Diabetic animals, for example, require greater water intake than non-diabetic animals in order to maintain homeostasis. They also produce, as a result, large volumes of urine, which can result in unacceptably wet bedding in the transport container. In order to provide an appropriate environment, more bedding material or the addition of absorbent pads may be required. Consideration should also be given to decreasing the number of animals per container to help address this problem.

Health

As previously discussed, health is an important concern in the transport of laboratory animals. In general, we can place infections into three groups as they relate to transportation: (1) infections that pose a risk to domestic animals or humans; (2) infections that pose a risk to the transported animals themselves; and (3) infections that may produce no clinical disease but make the animals unsuitable for some types of research. The health certifications for transport of animals, required to allow them to move in commerce and between countries, usually focus on infections that have human or agricultural/domestic animal significance. A health certificate issued by a competent veterinary authority prior to a journey or by virtue of customs inspection directed at assessing health during the journey, is the principle safeguard for assuring that the clinical health of the animal(s) is appropriate for them to make or continue a journey.

Infections that may not be harmful to the carrier animals, and which may not be regulated in transport may, nevertheless, make the animal unsuitable for its intended research purposes. The risk that animals can carry such infections, either as a result of infection at the source colony or during transportation, is a potential reason to hold newly received animals in quarantine housing until their health status can be verified.

Institutions transporting animals often provide health screening information for the source colony. While commercial suppliers of laboratory animals often perform extensive and frequent health screening of closed colonies, the health screening of animals may vary considerably between research institutions. A thorough description of the health monitoring programme for the colony should be sought in order to determine what, if any, additional testing should be done upon the receipt of the animals by the consignee. Verifying health status on arrival is recommended as a reasonable precaution when receiving animals from unfamiliar sources.

IATA has defined two health status categories for laboratory animals. They are (1) Conventional, and (2) Specific Pathogen Free (SPF) (International Air Transport Association 2008a). IATA defines Conventional animals as *'those for which the presence or absence of specific micro-organisms and parasites is unknown due to the absence of testing, treatment or vaccination. ... Usually, no physical precautions, such as specialised housing, are undertaken prior to or during shipment to prevent introduction of infection.'* IATA defines Specific Pathogen Free animals as *'being free of one or more parasites or infectious micro-organisms'* (IATA 2008a). They further classify SPF animals into two subcategories: (1) Conditioned SPF, and (2) Barrier-raised SPF. Conditioned SPF animals are defined as *'those that have undergone testing, treatment and/or vaccination to ensure the absence of one or more parasites or microbial agents. Conditioned SPF animals are often not maintained in specialised housing to prevent introduction of infectious agents, and are usually shipped in unfiltered containers'* (IATA 2008a). IATA cites as examples, non-human primates, dogs and cats as conditioned SPF animals (IATA 2008a). Barrier-raised SPF animals are *'animals that have been raised in the absence of one or more parasites or microbial agents in specialised facilities to exclude these agents as well as agents of agricultural and human significance. Their microbial status has been established either by testing each individual animal or by sampling representative animals from the colony. Filtered SPF shipping containers are required for transport of these animals, as are special procedures and equipment for packing, unpacking and handing them'* (IATA 2008a).

During transport, animals of differing health status and of different species might be shipped together in the same cargo area of the aircraft (Figures 13.1 and 13.2). Similarly, depending upon whether dedicated ground transportation or a common carrier is used, animals from more than one source, and hence potentially of different health statuses, could be shipped in the same vehicle. Commercial suppliers of SPF animals generally produce and ship only barrier-raised SPF animals (although the pathogens from which they are free can vary considerably between suppliers). Since the cargo compartment, whether it is in a ground transport vehicle or an aircraft, is one microbiological space, it is up to the shipping institution ('consignor/shipper') to select an appropriate container to maintain the microbio-

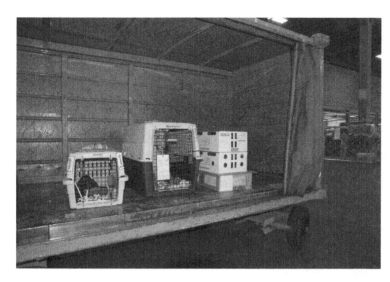

Figure 13.1 Example of multiple species being held together in a ramp cart in the same airport staging area prior to loading on an aircraft.

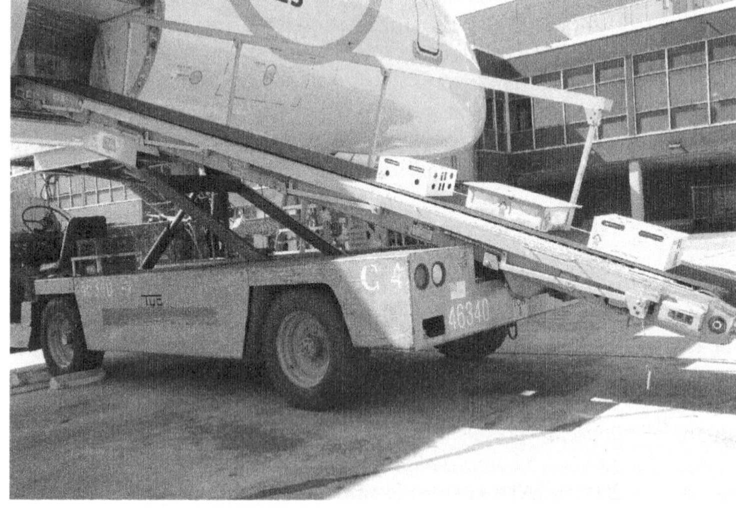

Figure 13.2 Containers of mice and rats being loaded into the climate-controlled hold of an aeroplane that contains other perishable goods.

logical status of the animals that are being shipped. No assumption should be made regarding the microbiological status of the outside of the shipping container when received at the consignee's institution: containers may have been exposed to unwanted micro-organisms during transit. In the case of SPF animals, surface disinfection of the container before unpacking is an important precaution to take in preventing unwanted introduction of contaminants. Aqueous halogen-based disinfectants are very useful for this purpose.

Laboratory animals, which have been infected with agents that pose a threat to humans, animals of agricultural importance, or other domestic animals or wildlife, always provide a challenge for the shipper. An infectious substance is defined as any substance which is known or can be reasonably expected to contain pathogens which can cause disease in humans or animals.

Infectious substances can be divided into two categories: Category A – an infectious substance transported in a form that, if exposure to it occurs, is capable of causing permanent disability, life-threatening or fatal disease in otherwise healthy humans or animals; and Category B - an infectious substance that does not meet the criteria of Category A. The International Civil Aviation Organization (ICAO) Technical Instructions for the Transport of Dangerous Goods (ICAO 2007–2008) and the IATA's Dangerous Goods Regulations (IATA 2008b) provide additional detail on the transportation of these substances.

Live animals that have been intentionally infected or are suspected to contain an infectious substance must not be transported unless the substance cannot be consigned by any other means. Under such circumstances, infected animals may only be transported under terms and conditions approved by the appropriate national authorities and the carrier.

Genetically modified animals are frequently submitted for transportation. Their transport is regulated under IATA's Dangerous Goods Regulations (IATA 2008b) for genetically modified organisms. IATA defines genetically modified organisms (GMOs) as organisms in which genetic material has been purposely altered through genetic engineering in a way that does not occur naturally. GMOs, including laboratory animals which do not meet the definition of infectious substances as defined previously, but are capable of genetically altering natural populations of animals as a result of natural reproduction, are not subject to the IATA Dangerous Goods Regulations when authorised for transport or use by the appropriate national authorities of the states of origin transit and destination. Thus, such animals do not have to be packaged and labelled as dangerous goods or meet transport standards that differ from other animals of the same species. However, shipments of such animals could be required by the countries of origin, transit or destination to have authorisation (and perhaps additional labelling) to leave, transit through or enter these countries. It is the responsibility of the consignor (shipper) to ensure that the animals to be transported comply with regulations regarding genetic modification, including local regulations in the countries of origin and destination. In most countries, transport of genetically engineered laboratory animals is allowed. In some parts of the world, misunderstanding of the terms transgenic, genetically modified (GM), engineered or manipulated can cause delays in transportation. Shippers should ensure they have secured in advance the appropriate documentation and authorisation for the movement of their shipments. Animals that are genetically modified, but which do not harbour or express pathogens or toxins are not considered to be 'dangerous goods' by the IATA, and may be shipped provided this is done in compliance with other live animal shipping requirements. However, unforeseen welfare problems associated with their phenotypic expression may arise and this risk can be avoided by transporting GM animals as cryopreserved embryos or cryopreserved gametes. Such options should be considered when planning shipment of GM stock.

Bedding, food and water

Bedding is commonly provided for laboratory animals in shipping containers. It serves several functions, the most important of which is the absorption of moisture from urine, water released from hydration sources such as water bottles or gelled water, as well as from animal sources such as condensation from insensible water loss on internal container surfaces. Bedding also provides a means to dilute and dry out faeces produced by the animals during transport. In the case of small mammals, bedding provides a source of insulation. Due to positional changes of the container during various stages of the transportation process, as well as due to the disturbances caused by the transportation environment, nest building may not always occur. The efficacy of the bedding material, as insulation and for absorbency, varies with the nature of the bedding material itself.

Sufficient bedding materials must be provided to maintain a dry and sanitary environment during shipping. Care must be taken, however, not to place so much bedding within a shipping container that it occludes ventilation openings. In the case of SPF animals, it may be necessary to provide suitably disinfected bedding that matches their microbiological status.

Recently, concerns have been raised over wood products used for bedding, as well as in shipping container construction and in pallets used to support and secure shipping containers during transit, with respect to their potential to carry plant diseases and agricultural pests across borders. Additional requirements for the treatment of such materials to eliminate these risks, as well as other measures imposed by countries and carriers, may eventually affect the use of untreated wood products in transportation.

Animals in transit should be provided with access to food and water during the journey. Ideally, the food provided to the animals during shipment should be of the same type and microbiological status as that they were fed at the institution of origin. Barrier-raised SPF small mammals that are shipped in filtered containers in order to preserve their microbiological status must be provided with food and water of a compatible microbiological status. In such instances, since there will be no opportunity during the course of the journey to replenish the food and water without opening the container (and thus potentially altering their microbiological status), sufficient quantities must be placed within the container at the time of packing. Larger animals, such as non-human primates and dogs, are almost always shipped in non-filtered containers, which allow for food and water to be replenished at scheduled stops during shipment. The design of these shipping containers for larger animals usually includes devices built into the container for addition of feed and water during the course of the journey. When large domestic animals undergo ground transportation, regulatory bodies require provision of feed and water, observation of the animals and specified rest periods at prescribed intervals. In the case of air transport of larger laboratory animals, there is usually no access to the cargo hold by personnel for the purposes of feeding and watering during flight and this has to be done following landing.

In their home environments, common laboratory animals are usually fed a dry pelleted or extruded diet. For non-human primates this is often supplemented by fruits and vegetables. Such foods, with high water content, can serve as an additional source of water during shipment. Unfortunately, these can spoil easily and may require some level of preparation prior to being introduced into the container. Opening the shipping container during the journey for purposes of introducing or removing materials carries with it the risk of escape. Food and water containers that are built into the shipping container but accessible from the outside may provide a route for escape or entrapment and great care must be taken when re-feeding or replenishing water supplies during the journey. It is a good practice to provide sufficient food and water not only to allow for the anticipated length of the journey but also for at least an additional 24h of transportation in case of any unforeseen delays.

Presentation of food and water should be done using a method that is appropriate to the past experience of the animals and to the behaviour patterns of the species. Purpose-bred dogs, for example, are accustomed to eating and drinking out of bowls in a lighted environment. Many common laboratory rodents, by contrast, feed principally at night; and despite the use of feeders in a laboratory environment, some rodents such as hamsters and gerbils will remove all feed from the feeder and hoard them in piles. Feeders or feed bowls are unnecessary for rodent transport since these animals forage for feed in the wild and do so quite readily when it is placed in with the bedding material.

Food consumption while in transit will often be less than when the animals are in their home environment. Commonly, this is reflected in weight loss, which will be rapidly regained during the first few days in their new home environment. The use of novel food items during transit may also contribute to reduced intake and weight loss.

Access to drinking water during transit is important to help animals maintain hydration and thermoregulate. Water in liquid form can be provided in refillable water bowls in the case of certain large animals (eg, non-human primates) or through the use of water kits in the case of small animals (eg, rodents). A water kit (Figure 13.3) consists of a sealed flexible pouch of water of the appropriate microbiological quality that is placed in a holder affixed to the wall of the container. Animals access water through a disposable drinking valve that is inserted into the pouch by puncturing the wall of the pouch. When water bowls are used, substantial amounts of water can be spilled out of the bowl either through the course of drinking or by movements of the container or movements of the animal. Similarly, with a water kit much of the water can be spilled if there is leakage around the insertion point of the drinking valve or by animals brushing against the valve thereby releasing water. This can result in the bedding within the container becoming wet. If a water kit is to be used, the animals should be conditioned to the use of a drinking valve as compared to the use of water bottles or other means of providing water in their home environment.

Alternatively, a gelled water source can be provided. Gelled water is a hydrocolloid-stabilised material containing between 70 and 98% water by weight. Various sources of calories in the form of carbohydrates can also be added to the gelled water as well as flavouring and stabilising ingredients to prevent spoilage. Animals have taste preferences and hence the presence or absence of certain nutrients may affect the consumption of gelled water during transit. A number of commercially available sources of this material have been shown to be accepted by various species. When a large amount of gelled water is placed in a container in order to provide for extended journeys, it is important to assure that it is suitably affixed within the container as movement of this material within the container during transit could result in injury to small animals.

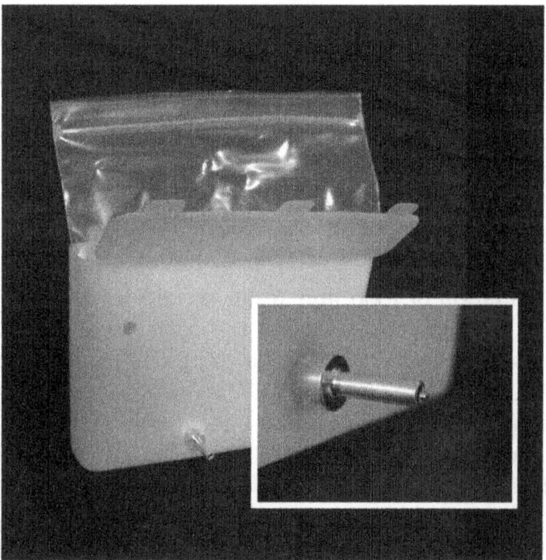

Figure 13.3 A drinking water kit consisting of a plastic holder, a sealable plastic bag for holding the water and a drinking valve for dispensing water (the inset is a close-up view of the disposable drinking valve).

Stress during transportation

Transient periods of stress will occur during transportation. This may be reflected in changes in heart rate, respiratory rate, behaviour, food and water consumption, and in changes in the cellular and chemical composition of blood. Changes in one of these parameters are not necessarily diagnostic of stress nor is it practical to routinely assess these parameters during the transportation process. Moreover, there are species differences in what constitutes an environmental stress and the magnitude of its effects as well as the manifestation of those effects. Given these limitations coupled with the limited number of species-specific studies on transportation stress, it is difficult to provide specific and widely applicable recommendations aimed at minimising stress in transport. Obviously, one should prepare carefully so as to avoid extreme situations wherein environmental control is lost.

The length of the journey is an important variable affecting stress in shipment. Avoidance of delays in shipment and transfers by good journey planning is important to minimise the overall level of stress associated with the journey. From an animal welfare point of view, transport distance and time should be kept to a minimum, and an uninterrupted journey is preferable.

Research on domestic farm animals suggests that the process of loading and unloading animals from shipping containers is more stressful than are other components of the journey (Knowles *et al.* 1995; Warriss *et al.* 1995). For this reason, acclimatisation of larger laboratory animals, such as domestic farm animals, to the container as well as to the loading and the unloading process may mitigate some of the stress encountered during the journey. For larger species, their efforts in counteracting the movements of the transport vehicle whilst in motion (Warriss *et al.* 1995) may cause additional stress. This may be less of a concern for smaller species that do not have to balance a large body mass at a substantial height above the floor. It is possible that species with more advanced cognitive abilities, such as non-human primates, may be more aware of their change in circumstances and be more predisposed to fear during transport, resulting in additional stress. Changes in presumptive measures of stress should be interpreted in context. For example, simply moving mice from one room or floor of a building to another can alter plasma cortisol levels (Tuli *et al.* 1995). Sheep undergoing a 24h journey showed increases in heart rate, plasma cortisol and glucose during loading and the initial stages of the journey but after 9h of travel, these had returned to normal levels (Knowles *et al.* 1995).

Experience has shown that there is considerable risk in sedating laboratory animals prior to transport in order to counteract stress and destructive behaviours. Tranquillisers and other psychoactive drugs can reduce the ability of animals to respond to stresses during transport, affect their ability to thermoregulate and have unpredictable cardiovascular effects. In addition, the reaction of various species to these drugs cannot always be foreseen. For these reasons, the routine use of psychoactive medication is not recommended.

In order to enable animals to recover adequately from stress experienced during transport, it is very important that they are given a recovery period at their final destination prior to use in a research programme. This period of acclimatisation allows for recovery from the effects of stress during shipment and also allows the animals to adapt to changes in housing and husbandry. In the case of group-housed animals whose groups have changed prior to shipment or which have a disrupted social structure, this period of acclimatisation permits the re-establishment of social order and resumption of natural behaviours. During this period, some presumptive measures of stress such as changes in electrolyte concentrations, haematological parameters, blood corticosteroid levels and a variety of physiological parameters can return to normal levels. Transportation-induced changes in the immune system may take longer to recover than fluid balance, electrolytes, plasma cortisol or glucose (Wallace 1976). The longer and more stressful the journey, the longer it may take for this stabilisation to occur.

During transport, animals can lose varying amounts of body weight, often of the order of 10% or sometimes even a little more. Most of this loss occurs early in the transport process, much of which is attributable to the voiding of faeces and urine as well as decreased food and water intake. Most, if not all, of this weight is recovered within a few days upon return to a more stable environment in the acclimatisation period post shipping. Grooming and exploratory behaviour in rats and mice are restored early in the acclimatisation period as are plasma cortisol concentrations, which may have been elevated upon receipt (Landi 1982); full acclimatisation may require up to 4 days (Tuli *et al.* 1995). There are species as well as strain and stock variations in the time required to fully acclimate. Various components of immune function may take longer to recover to pre-transport capability, as may certain other metabolic functions (Damon *et al.* 1986; Bean-Kundsen & Wagner 1987; Olubadeno *et al.* 1994).

Laws, regulations and standards

The current European regulations on animal welfare in transport (European Council 2004) came into force on 5 January 2007. While EU regulation is directly applicable, some national legislation is needed to provide for enforcement and penalty provisions, derogations from the rules and to levy the charges for authorisations. In the UK, this is done through separate enforcement legislation in England, Scotland, Wales and Northern Ireland. For example, the legislation which implemented the previous Directives in Northern Ireland (the Welfare of Animals (Transport) Order (Northern Ireland) 1997 (WATO)) has been replaced by The Welfare of Animals (Transport) Regulations (Northern Ireland) 2006, as amended by the Welfare of Animals (Transport) (Amendment) Regulations (Northern Ireland) 2007. Some useful guidance on the EU regulation has been published on the web. For example, see the DARDNI (Department of Agriculture and Rural Development Northern Ireland) website[1].

The current EU regulation aims to improve animal welfare through raising transportation standards. In particular, it provides significant improvements in enforcement capability for all species transported. The EU regulation covers the transport within the EU Community, in connection with an economic activity, of all live vertebrate animals (excluding man). The regulation does not apply to the transport of non-vertebrates such as insects, worms, crustaceans (eg, crab, lobster), cephalopods (eg, octopus, squid) and molluscs (eg, shellfish, snails). However, general welfare in transport provisions protecting non-vertebrates from injury or unnecessary suffering are contained in regulations for devolved administrations in the UK.

The Convention on International Trade in Endangered Species of wild flora and fauna (CITES) and the World Health Organization through OIE (World Organization for Animal Health) have agreed that the IATA Live Animals Regulations (LAR) be employed as guidelines for the air transportation of animals. The LAR set standards concerning the transport of animals by air which include advice on general care and loading, the design and construction of containers together with appropriate packing, feeding and watering arrangements (IATA 2008a). The LAR have been adopted by the European Union as minimum standards for transporting animals, and, globally, most airlines and countries will only accept animals packed and transported according to the LAR standards. The Animal Air Transportation Association *Manual for the Transportation of Live Animals*[2] also contains useful information, especially concerning European legal requirements for transport of large animals (Animal Transportation Association 2000). Other useful guidance is available; see for example the publications by Elmore (2008) and Institute for Laboratory Animal Research (2006).

Transport containers

The specifications of animal transport containers (also termed shipping containers) can vary substantially depending upon the source (ie, commercial or locally constructed) and the local, national, or international guidance upon which their design is based. The most detailed specifications for shipping containers are found in the LAR published annually by IATA. This guidance is organised by species and container type. Given its international acceptance, this guidance forms the basis for the minimum standards for container design. These may need to be modified to meet the requirements of some countries of origin and, if applicable, the countries of transit and destination. For some species such as non-human primates, dogs and cats, and farm animals (as mentioned above), it may be necessary to acclimatise them to the shipping containers prior to loading.

[1] http://www.dardni.gov.uk/guidance-welfare-of-animals-transport-08-08.doc

[2] http://www.aata-animaltransport.org

Container design and construction

The most common design of animal transport container is in the form of a rectangular box, the dimensions and shape of which are largely dictated by the species for which it is intended. Various types of containers have been developed commercially for transporting laboratory animals, some of which are illustrated in this text.

Adequate ventilation is essential and the shipping container should be designed so that it can incorporate filtered or non-filtered ventilation apertures according to the microbiological status of the animals. The container and air vents should be designed so that vents cannot be occluded, even when stacked (Figure 13.4). Many containers have additional built-in features such as spacers or stand-offs to aid in ventilation (Figure 13.5). Air vents should be sited on at least two opposite sides of the container. The combined area of the ventilation apertures should be determined according to the species, dimensions of the container, intended stocking density, whether filter material covers the ventilation apertures and the range of ambient conditions expected to prevail during transport. Ventilation apertures should be covered with wire mesh of such a gauge that no part of the animal can protrude, and be designed such that the animal cannot damage the mesh with its teeth or feet.

While non-filtered transport containers are available for rodents and rabbits (Figure 13.6), animals with restricted microbial status destined for research use should be transported under SPF conditions using microbiologically secure containers (Figures 13.5, 13.7 and 13.8) to protect them from infectious agents. SPF transport containers have ventilation apertures that are covered with some form of filter material of a pore size and filtration efficiency selected according to the degree of filtration and airflow required. Since most infectious agents are carried on particulates of larger diameter than the mean pore diameter of standard filters and since air velocity across the filters is low, small pore-size filters are not usually required. It is important to remember that filter material can decrease the ventilation rate within a container by 70% or more depending on thickness and pore size. Other factors such as stocking density within the container should be adjusted accordingly to compensate for decreased ventilation imposed by the addition of filters.

Filtered containers require a viewing port (viewing window) to allow assessment of animals whilst in transit (Figure 13.9). This is particularly important for journeys that cross national borders where some form of official inspection may be required.

A variety of materials is available for container construction. For rodents and rabbits, the most commonly used

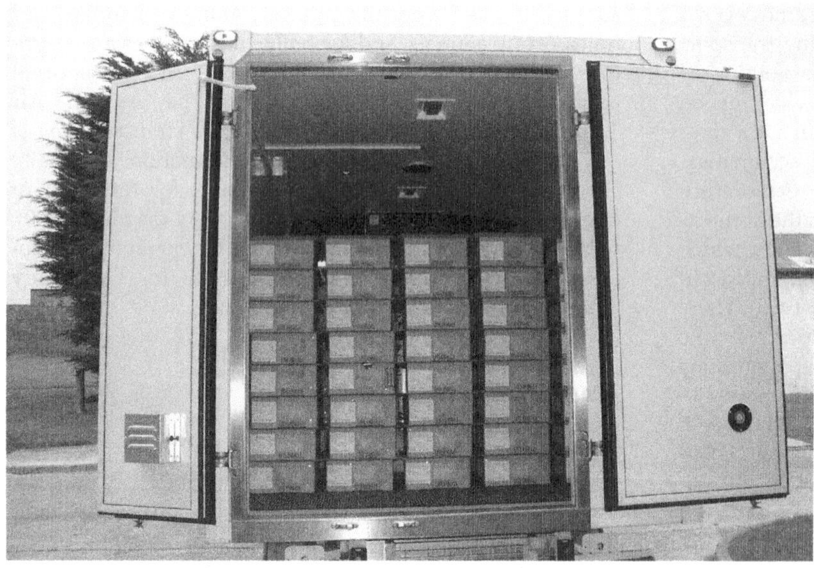

Figure 13.4 The back of a partially loaded, climate-controlled truck containing rodent shipping containers with integral ventilation stand-offs. The air channels between the containers allow circulation of air across the filtered openings.

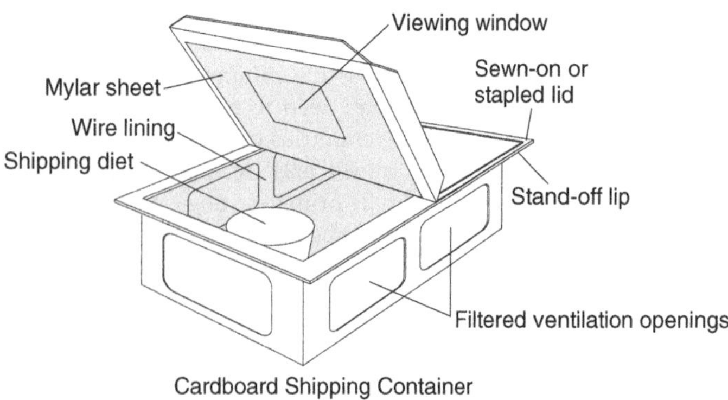

Figure 13.5 Diagram of a cardboard shipping container used for transport of mice and rats. The principle features of this design of container are noted on the illustration.

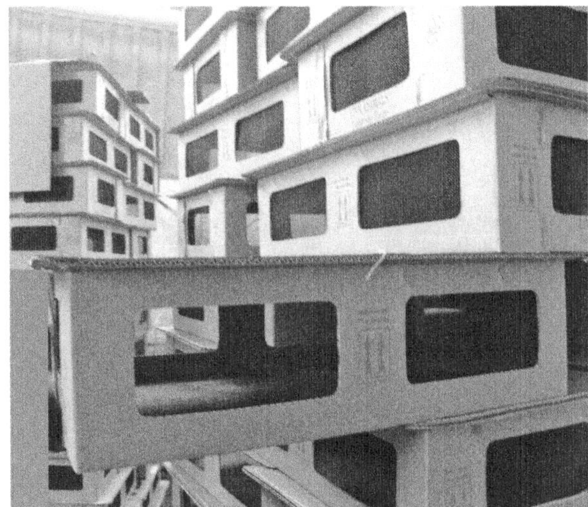

Figure 13.6 Unfiltered rodent shipping containers.

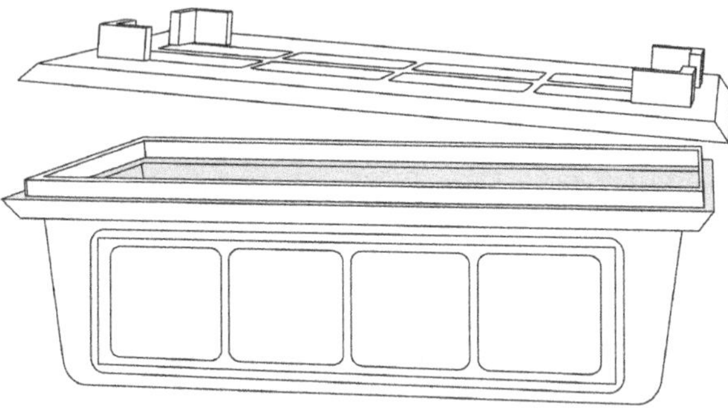

Figure 13.7 A drawing of a plastic shipping container used for transporting rodents. Ventilation openings (four) are visible along the side with similar ventilation openings located on the lid of the container. Plastic stand-offs are located on the top and a continuous stand-off runs around the top of the base of the container providing a channel for ventilation along the sides of the container.

materials are plastic or varying strengths of corrugated cardboard or corrugated polypropylene. Each container may be partitioned into separate compartments, or two or more separate, primary containers may be placed into an overshipper for transport (Figure 13.8). Corrugated cardboard and corrugated polypropylene are relatively cheap and easy to dispose of, or recycle, and therefore are commonly used in non-reusable containers. For transporting larger species, materials used to construct containers include wood, plastic, metal or fibreglass. Such containers when made of plastic can be injection or vacuum moulded or, in the case of wood or metal, constructed with a strong framework and joints sheathed with solid panels with reinforced ventilation openings (Figure 13.10). Care must be taken to avoid using materials which adversely affect the health or welfare of the animal(s) to be transported, such as wood that has been treated with preservatives.

The container should be durable, non-toxic and able to withstand stacking without causing damage or crushing. Wooden containers should be constructed so that the animal cannot bore, claw or bite them open at the seams or joints. Nails, bolts, staples, sharp edges or other protrusions, on which animals could injure themselves, should be avoided; all slats and uprights should have rounded edges and be installed so that the animals cannot entrap their extremities.

The interior surface of the container must be of solid construction and can be protected to some extent from the effects of damp seepage due to urine by coating the inner surface with plastic or wax. For rodents that chew and gnaw, a wire mesh lining may be applied over all internal surfaces, including the floor and filtered ventilation openings, of disposable cardboard shipping containers to prevent escape. The wire should be applied so that the animals do not have access to loose or sharp edges. Some animals such as hamsters that aggressively dig and chew at surfaces must be shipped in containers with a double layer of wire lining covering all internal surfaces to prevent escape. Moulded plastic containers that provide a rugged smooth surface constructed such that corners and ventilation openings are not within the animals bite radius, do not require a wire lining

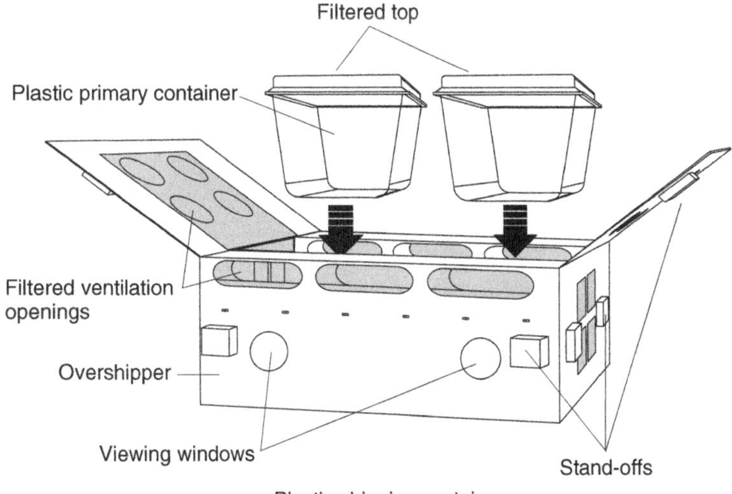

Figure 13.8 Two plastic filtered shipping containers are placed within a cardboard overshipper with filtered openings. The overshipper contains two viewing windows as well as rigid foam stand-offs to allow for unobstructed ventilation.

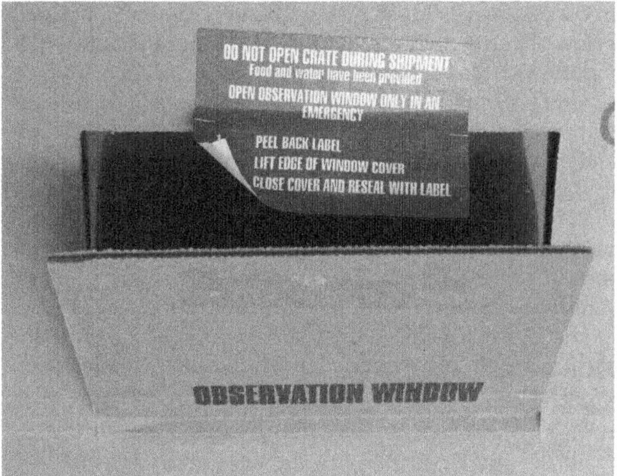

Figure 13.9 A disposable cardboard shipping container with a viewing window that can be accessed by peeling back an instruction label and lifting up a cut-out in the cardboard. The viewing window is constructed of Mylar™.

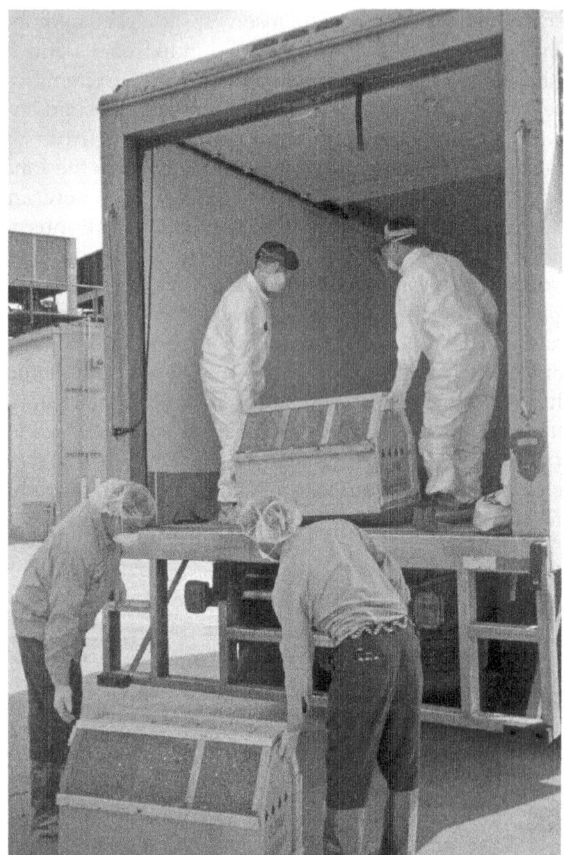

Figure 13.10 Wooden non-human primate shipping containers being loaded into a climate-controlled truck. The containers are designed to hold up to three non-human primates each with separate ventilation openings.

when used with certain species. These are designed for specific species and may not work for others. Similarly, the lids of some shipping containers can be lined with a thick sheet of Mylar that, by its smooth surface design, does not fall within the animal's bite radius.

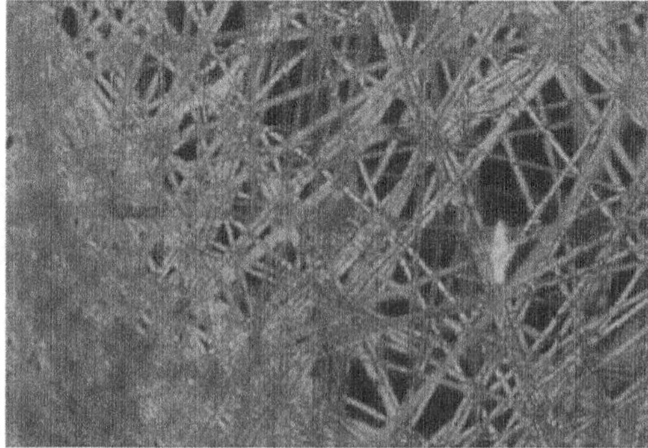

(a)

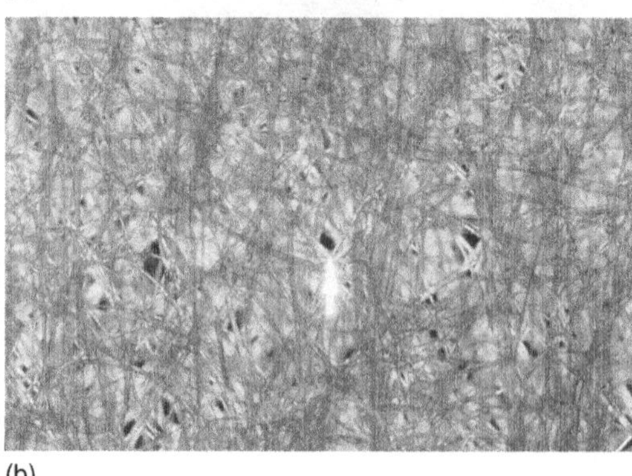

(b)

Figure 13.11 Top is a 10x magnification of a spun-bound polyester filter typically used to cover ventilation openings in shipping containers used for certain SPF laboratory animals. Note the varying pore size openings. Bottom is the same filter material after being used to ship animals and subsequently autoclaved. Note that the remaining pores are very small in diameter. The use of moist heat has caramelised food particles and adhering dust has occluded most of the pores in the material. Effective ventilation is substantially reduced.

The lid or door of the container must fit the container securely to prevent accidental opening. Containers should have adequate hand holds or other lifting devices to enable them to be lifted without undue tilting or bringing the handlers in close contact with the animals.

If containers are to be used on more than one journey, it must be possible to adequately clean and sterilise them. Although some shipping containers for laboratory rodents may be sanitisable, the integrity of cardboard and plastic containers may change after autoclaving, irradiation or chemical disinfection. The protective plastic or wax, for example, that lines corrugated cardboard is destroyed by heat sterilisation within an autoclave. After transport, the pores of the air filters covering the vents may be obstructed by debris such as food dust, bedding, animal fur and dander, or be compromised due to autoclaving, thereby reducing airflow into the container (Figure 13.11). Therefore, whenever possible, use new shipping crates which are commonly available through commercial sources to ensure safe animal transport and biosecurity.

Transport container stocking density

Animals should have adequate space to provide for normal postures and postural adjustments within a transport container, including the ability to stand quadrupedally, stretch, turn around and lie down. Recommendations for transport container height and stocking density are based on species and body weight, as well as ambient temperature control and overall heat output of animals within in a given area with ventilation apertures. The calculation of animal heat output is based in part on the work by Kleiber (1975) and Besch and Woods (1977), which is outlined by Swallow (1999). The results of these and other engineering studies, modified by experience using various stocking densities, have formed the basis for the current recommendations. Stocking density guidelines for shipping laboratory animals in filtered containers to maintain their SPF status as well shipment using non-filtered containers are found in the LAR.

Compatible animals are best transported in a socially harmonious group within the same shipping container or container compartment. Species should never be mixed within the same transport container. Rodents shipped within a container should come from the same colony, be of similar age, of the same sex as appropriate, and when possible be from the same weaning or social group. Similarly, when it is necessary to transport breeding adults and their offspring, they should travel in the same container, if possible. The maximum number of animals per compartment should be reduced when the ambient temperature at ground level exceeds 24 °C. Rabbits are usually transported singly or in divided boxes with or without filtered air vents.

In the UK and continental Europe, dogs may travel in a loose housing system in small single-sex groups using the cargo area of a suitably equipped ground vehicle. However, this arrangement is forbidden in certain other countries when transporting dogs by air and by ground. In these cases, each dog must have its own container, except when specifically permitted by the competent authority. These containers can be used to transport two compatible animals of comparable size (up to 14kg each) or up to three animals not exceeding 6 months of age, from the same litter. To ensure compliance with current regulations, it is important to verify exceptions with the local competent authority (European Council 2004).

Same-sex adult macaques that have been maintained in an established compatible cohort should travel as pairs. Juveniles should be transported in pre-established single-sex pairs. Animals under 3kg can be shipped using three-compartment containers (Figure 13.10), while those over 3kg should be shipped in two-compartment containers. If co-housing is not feasible, then the animals should be shipped either in the company of compatible conspecifics in partitioned containers, or in separate containers loaded adjacent to each other. Pregnant females and females with suckling young are generally not accepted for air transport.

Labelling and marking

Each shipping container should be marked durably and legibly on the outside with the following information:

- Marked 'LIVE ANIMALS' or 'LABORATORY ANIMALS' for filtered containers containing SPF animals (Figures 13.12 and 13.13).
- Marked 'THIS WAY UP', including orientation arrows.
- Specifications of the animals within the container and ID, if applicable (usually found on the shipping label).
- The full name, address and 24h contact information for consigner and consignee.
- Any special feeding and watering instructions.

Journey planning

Mode of transport

Laboratory animals can be transported either by ground or by air. In some instances, short water-borne voyages are also required (usually in a vessel designed to carry vehicles), for example when transporting animals from the UK to conti-

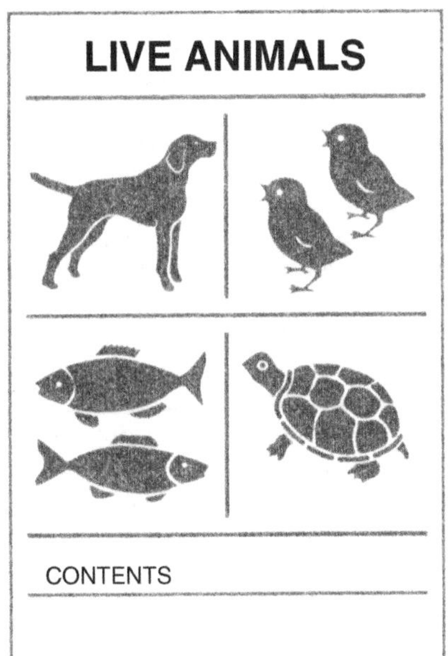
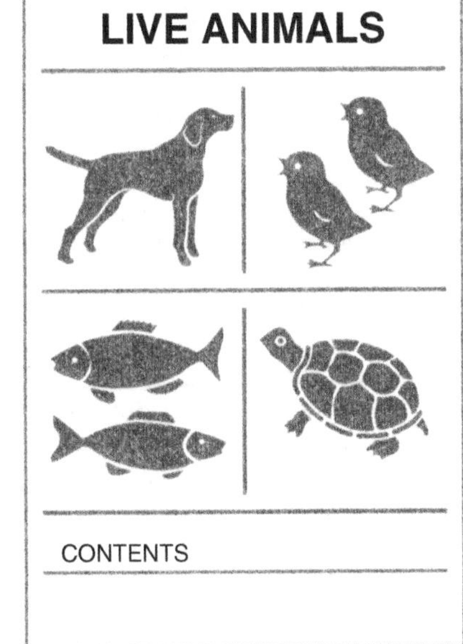

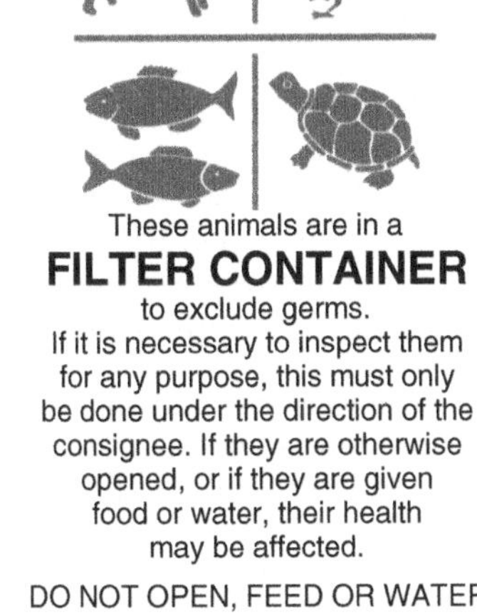

Figure 13.12 Illustrations of IATA-approved shipping labels. The 'LIVE ANIMALS' label is used when shipping any live animal or the 'LABORATORY ANIMALS' label can be used instead when shipping SPF laboratory animals.

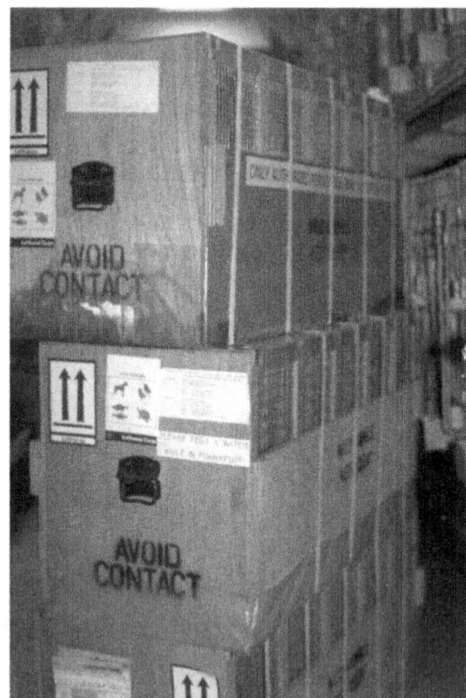

Figure 13.13 Wooden non-human primate shipping containers with directional arrow labelling, live animals labelling and transportation documents attached to the outside of the container. Other labelling imprinted on the container is used to advise personnel that only authorised individuals should handle these containers.

nental Europe. The majority of laboratory animals required for research travel relatively short distances by road. Many laboratories make use of the services of specialised laboratory transport companies. Such transporters (including some commercial laboratory breeders) operate their own fleets of environmentally controlled vehicles in accordance with national and European laws. These animal transporters can also be a helpful source of information on the ground transportation process and on the required documentation and other shipping requirements.

Ground transport

Purpose-bred laboratory animals such as rodents and rabbits must be transported in an environmentally controlled vehicle that can be easily sanitised and which provides ventilation rates and can maintain temperature parameters as set forth in EU regulations (eg, 1/2005/EC which requires that temperature within the cargo area be monitored and recorded throughout the journey). Among the new safeguards for ground transportation of animals that were introduced in the EU by regulation 1/2005/EC were higher standards for vehicles and equipment, and stricter requirements for those dealing with animals 'in transit' including training and certification. This regulation also provides measures to ensure better enforcement of EU rules for transport. Article 3 and Article 27 of this regulation detail general conditions for the transport of animals, as well as requirements for inspections and for annual reports by the competent national authority. Authorisation is generally required for journeys but transporters undertaking journeys of less than 65km from place of departure to place of destination do not require authorisation nor are they required to use drivers/attendants who have been trained and who hold a certificate of competency (Article 6.7). A journey log or appropriate satellite navigation record must be kept for each journey.

Regulation 1/2005/EU requires that all transported animals must be fit for travel. This applies to the transport of all laboratory animals including those undergoing regulated procedures under the authority of the Animals (Scientific Procedures) Act (A(SP)A 1986). Exceptions may be authorised under A(SP)A where there might be a compelling scientific need to move ill or injured animals. However, in such cases an appropriately certified veterinarian is required to confirm that such animals are fit for the intended journey. There are additional specific requirements regarding feeding and watering intervals and certain general loading requirements for cats, dogs, poultry, domestic birds and rabbits.

The journey log required by European regulation is the official record of the ground transportation journey. It includes sections on planning, place of departure, place of destination, a declaration by the transporter and an anomaly report. As envisioned, it would serve as a mechanism for approval by the competent authority of the journey prior to the journey beginning and would contain specifics of the actual journey as it occurred. This record would remain within the EU and be available for inspection for a period of 3 years.

Air transport

The air transport process also has a ground transportation component which must meet applicable ground transport regulations. Air transport begins when the animal shipment arrives at the air cargo facility and is accepted by the carrier. Where international shipments are made outside the European Union, a customs broker or freight forwarder will need to be engaged to assist in the export process. The air waybill is the official acceptance document used by the carrier for air transport wherein liability is accepted by the carrier. This liability is limited by international convention and should be supplemented by additional coverage if the animals are very valuable. The waybill is also the document that the shipper uses to describe the contents of the shipment. Since the carrier and its personnel are not experts in animal biology and care or in taxonomy, they depend upon the shipper to provide the necessary information on the waybill to indicate the required conditions for carriage. It is the duty of the shipper to provide adequate amounts of food, bedding and water to sustain the animals during travel. The shipper must also supply the appropriate documents for export, carriage and import to satisfy existing laws and regulations in the countries of export and import.

Animals are classified as perishable cargo and are provided a climate-controlled environment in the aircraft. The consignor should provide the carrier with any specific environmental requirements for the animals being shipped. If there are no specific requirements given, general guidance for the species as found in the IATA's Live Animals Regulations will be used. If very tight temperature or other environmental restrictions are required the shipment may not be able to be accommodated. Air cargo personnel are provided training in handling animal containers as well as basic information on animals in transport. Typically, carrier personnel use a checklist to ensure that all the appropriate steps and paperwork have been completed. They are not responsible, however, for making judgments on whether documentation has been completed correctly.

Once the appropriate paperwork is completed, the shipment will be moved to a section of the cargo facility where it can be held in a well ventilated and quiet area. Not all airports, however, have dedicated areas for this purpose. Hence, animals may share space with other perishable cargo, live animals or personnel.

After holding in the cargo facility (typically 4–6h in advance of flight departure), the shipment will be transported to the flight line for loading on to the aircraft. Typically, animals are loaded on to the aircraft last, for a first-off unloading at the final destination. Once on the aircraft, the animals are kept in a darkened environment. Even though space has been reserved for animal shipments, circumstances can arise resulting in their being kept off a particular flight for a variety of reasons including incompatibility with other priority cargo (eg, mail, human remains) and temperature embargos.

Upon arrival, the unloading process is a mirror image of the loading process. Arrangements should be made by the consignee (person receiving the shipment at the final destination), either directly or preferably through the use of a broker or customs agent, for pick up once the animals have cleared customs. The vehicle used for this should be capable of providing a conditioned environment.

Due to the complexity of air transportation and the potential for intermediate stops and delays in flight schedules, it is important that contingency plans be made during the journey planning process. The carrier should be made aware of special requirements of the animals and should be given contact information for both the shipper and the consignee, in case of unforeseen delays or adverse events.

Documentation

Depending on the animals to be transported, their health status, the mode of transportation and the final destination of the animals, a number of documents need to be prepared and authorised and should accompany the shipment. Some certifications are time sensitive and must be submitted as originals, not copies. It is a good idea to keep copies of all documents required for shipment in case of loss during shipment – an event that could strand animals at boarder crossings or airports. A list of documents for transport of animals within Europe is provided by the EU[3].

One of the documents necessary for the shipment of laboratory animals is the Export Health Certificate (EHC). This is needed for the shipment of animals between countries. Guidance in relation to this requirement is generally given by the competent authority (eg, in the UK, this is The Department for Environment, Food and Rural Affairs (DEFRA)). An EHC is an official veterinary document used to confirm that a consignment of animals or animal products meets certain health criteria. Shippers wanting to export live animals, animal products or germ plasm to an EU member state will need the health certificate signed by a government-approved 'official veterinarian'. Further information on EHCs can be obtained by contacting DEFRA in the UK or similar competent authorities in exporting or receiving countries.

Other documents that may be required include: import licences issued by the state veterinary service; CITES permits where necessary; invoices for custom purposes; fitness to travel documents, including records of certain laboratory tests, vaccinations or treatments; quarantine labels, if applicable; transfer authorisations from specific bodies that regulate the use of laboratory animals; an animal transport certificate or group plan; and, in the case of ground transportation, vehicle registration details and insurance.

Information specific to the animals being transported, including species, strain, scientific name, number, sex, age, weight, individual identification and any special care requirements related to phenotype should accompany each shipment. Some of this information is required on other documents, but placing it in one location can prove helpful. In addition, the name, address, and 24h telephone contact numbers for the consignor (person with ultimate responsibility for the shipment), intermediaries, consignee and the shipper's attending veterinarian can also be helpful in case of difficulties during shipment.

All the required documents should be collated and attached to the first container of each consignment. It is advisable to make sure that the necessary documents have been aligned with the United Nations (UN) layout key for trade documents. These are internationally agreed standards that are easily translated because common information appears in standard positions on all forms. Many countries have trade facilitation organisations, for example, SITPRO[4] in the UK, that can provide advice on UN aligned documents.

Correct and complete documentation is essential to avoid delays in transit. Animal shipments are often delayed in customs due to failure to provide correct documents containing the appropriate wording, signatures and authorisations. Accompanying documents can be lost in transit, highlighting the need to keep copies of all necessary documents. There is currently an air freight industry initiative to make many documents electronic so that they can be sent in advance of shipment to the competent authorities at the point of entry (POE). Basic documentation requirements for international shipment for various countries can be found in The Air Cargo Tariff (TACT) Manuals (IATA 2008c) and the LAR (IATA 2008a), both published by IATA. If a customs

[3]http://eur-lex.europa.eu/LexUriServ/LexUriServ.do?uri=OJ:L:2005:003:0001:0044:EN:PDF

[4]http://www.sitpro.org.uk

broker is employed to facilitate the shipment, they can also provide guidance on the required documents. Individual country embassies are also a source of information. It is also helpful to have the consignee at the destination assist in determining what documentation is required and for an electronic copy of all shipment documents to be sent in advance of the shipment to the consignee.

Points of entry

Most countries have a limited number of designated locations (border inspection posts (BIPs)) where animals can enter the country. For example, the EU and the US, operate a system of BIPs or points of entry (POE) which are approved for the importation of different species such as farm livestock, equidae, rabies-susceptible animals, birds, fish, or any combination of the above, including laboratory animals. Animal consignments may be inspected by officials upon arrival. Authorities often require advance notification of the import or export of live animals (especially in the case of larger animals) so that the appropriate inspection personnel can be available. Recipients of animals should note that such inspections take time and journey plans should allow for delays at BIPs.

Both consignor and consignee should agree in advance of any shipment the conditions of transportation, including the departure and arrival times so that, at their destination, the animals can be placed in previously prepared cages, fed, watered and rested as quickly as possible. On arrival, animals should be removed from their transport container and examined by a responsible person with the least possible delay.

Journey time

Most laboratory animals travel within containers with food, water and bedding sufficient in quantity for the journey. Under these conditions, there is not usually a maximum permitted journey time. However for some animals, particularly larger species, there can be specific restrictions regarding journey time and rest stops (European Council 2004). Given the broad definition of animal in this regulation, guidance might be included in future revisions to cover more traditional laboratory species.

Acknowledgements

Mr. Gregg Pittelkow of Northwest Airlines for donating air transport illustrations. Dr. David Elmore of Charles River for donating illustrations of non-human primate transport. Dr. Jeremy Swallow of Pfizer for his original text in the 7th edition of the UFAW Handbook.

References

Animal Transportation Association (2000) *AATA Manual for the Transportation of Live Animals*, 2nd edn. AATA, Redhill, Surrey

Bean-Knudsen, D.E. and Wagner, J. E. (1987) Effect of shipping stress on clinicopathologic indications in F344/N Rats. *American Journal of Veterinary Research*, **48**, 306–308

Besch, B.E.L. and Woods, J.E. (1977) Heat dissipation biorhythms of laboratory animals. *Laboratory Animal Science*, **27**, 54–59.

Council of Europe (2003) *European Convention for the Protection of Animals During International Transport*. European Treaty Series No. 193. Council of Europe, Strasburg

Damon, E.G., Eidson, A.F., Hobbs, C.H. *et al.* (1986) Effect of acclimation on nephrotoxic response of rats to uranium. *Laboratory Animal Science*, **36**, 24–27

Elmore, D.B. (2008) Quality management for the international transportation of nonhuman primates. *Veterinaria Italiana*, **44(1)**, 141–147

European Council (2004) *The Welfare of Animals During Transport*. Council Directive 1/2005/EC. (available at http://ec.europa.eu/food/animal/welfare/transport/index_en.htm accessed 11 March 2009)

International Air Transportation Association (2008a) Live Animals Regulations, 35th edn. IATA, Montreal. (available at http://www.iata.org accessed 11 March 2009)

International Air Transportation Association (2008b) *Dangerous Goods Regulations*, 49th edn. IATA, Montreal

International Air Transportation Association (2008c) *The Air Cargo Tariff (TACT) Manuals*. IATA Netherlands Data Publications, The Netherlands

International Civil Aviation Organization (2007–2008) *Technical Instructions for the Safe Transport of Dangerous Goods by Air* (including Addendum/Corrigendum 1/8/07). ICAO, Montreal

Institute for Laboratory Animal Research (2006) *Guidelines for the Humane Transportation of Research Animals*. National Academies Press, Washington, DC

Kleiber, M. (1975) *The Fire of Life: an Introduction to Animal Energetics*. Robert E. Kreiger, Huntingdon

Knowles, T.G., Brown, S.N., Warriss, P.D. *et al.* (1995) Effects on sheep of transport by road for up to 24 hours. *Veterinary Record*, **136**, 431–488

Laboratory Animal Science Association (2005) Guidance on the transport of laboratory animals. Report of the Transport Working Group established by LASA. *Laboratory Animals*, **39**, 1–39

Landi, M.S. (1982) Effects on shipping on the immune function in mice. *American Journal of Veterinary Research*, **43**, 1654–1657

Olubadeno, J.O. (1994) The effects of stress on lipoproteins and catecholamines in rats. *Cellular Immunology and Molecular Biology*, **40**, 1201–1206

Swallow, J.J. (1999) Transporting Animals. In: *The UFAW Handbook on The Care and Management of Laboratory Animals, Vol 1 Terrestrial Vertebrates*, 7th edn. Ed Poole, T., pp. 171–187. Blackwell Publishing, London

Tuli, J.S., Smith, J.A. and Morton, D.B. (1995) Stress measurements after transportation. *Laboratory Animals*, **29**, 132–138

Wallace, M.E. (1976) Effects of stress due to deprivation and transport in different genotypes of house mouse. *Laboratory Animals*, **10**, 335–347

Warriss, P.D., Brown, S.N., Knowles, T.G. *et al.* (1995) Effects on cattle of transport by road for up to 15 hours. *Veterinary Record*, **136**, 319

14 Nutrition, feeding and animal welfare

Bart Savenije, Jan Strubbe and Merel Ritskes-Hoitinga

Introduction

It is essential for the welfare of animals that adequate food, containing essential nutrients, is provided and ingested (National Research Council (NRC) 1995; Beynen & Coates 2001; Ritskes-Hoitinga 2004). Physical and mental processes are dependent on and influenced both by what is ingested, and when and how food is eaten (Ritskes-Hoitinga & Chwalibog 2003). Food ingestion is essential for homeostasis, a regulated state of internal balance (Strubbe 2003; Ritskes-Hoitinga & Strubbe 2004), although it always leads to some homeostatic disturbance, for example through the thermogenic effect. As many bodily functions naturally show biological rhythms, fluctuations due to food intake may result in good animal welfare, as long as the animal is able to return to the homeostatic state. Introducing species-specific fluctuations into the laboratory feeding process may, therefore, contribute positively to the welfare of laboratory animals.

This chapter provides some key concepts in nutrition, with the aim of helping animal care staff to prevent the occurrence of nutrition-based pathological and behavioural disorders in animals in their care. Using and implementing this basic knowledge will not only support good animal health and welfare, but will also contribute to standardisation and replicability of experiments. In the second part of the chapter, aspects related to feeding, rhythmicity and environmental factors and procedures are discussed. A range of examples is provided to illustrate how nutrition and feeding can influence animal welfare and experimental results. The authors suggest that better animal welfare can be achieved when nutrition is better adapted to the species-specific adaptive capabilities for returning to homeostasis (Ritskes-Hoitinga & Strubbe 2004). Thus, refining the feeding process by providing correct nutrition, together with appropriate foraging and feeding opportunities, should contribute to the animals' welfare as well as improve the quality of the science by reducing variation resulting from stress.

Proper study design

Minimum nutrient requirements

Animals' needs for macronutrients (lipid, carbohydrates, proteins) and the micronutrients (minerals, vitamins, trace elements) and water differ between species. For example, vitamin C is an essential nutrient for guinea pigs and primates, whereas rats and mice do not need to ingest it. For each animal species extensive scientific documentation on (essential) nutrient requirements has been assembled in the documents of the NRC (1977–2003). Estimated nutrient requirements for each species and stage of life are presented by the NRC (1977–2003). These recommendations are usually higher than the minimum requirements, as they are often based on the intention of obtaining maximum growth. Maximum growth is, however, probably not optimal for the health of laboratory animals. For example, *ad libitum* feeding can result in kidney degeneration in rodents, whereas food restriction prevents kidney degeneration completely (Hart *et al.* 1995). As these guidelines are currently the best available and are based on scientific evidence, it is advisable to use them until new scientific evidence comes available. However, it is important to be aware that there can be strain differences in nutritional requirements, and that this may also apply to genetically modified strains (Ritskes-Hoitinga 2004). For example, in phosphatidylethanolamine N-methyltransferase (PEMT) knockout mice, the *de novo* synthesis of choline is disrupted, so the NRC's minimum dietary choline recommendation for mice is likely to be insufficient for this strain (Zhu *et al.* 2003). In such cases it is necessary to establish the nutritional requirements of the strain, in order to provide a special diet fulfilling those particular needs.

It is also essential to provide for animals' differing needs during their various life stages (ie, growth, maintenance, reproduction, lactation or work). Failure to do this can lead to incorrect interpretation of experimental results as in the report that genetically modified potatoes could compromise the immune system of young rats (Ewen & Pusztai 1999). In this study, the diet only provided 6% protein; it was later concluded that the results were invalid, as young growing rats need 15% dietary protein (Horton 1999).

Manufacture of diet, chow versus purified diets, pellet hardness

Chow diets are the standard diets in most laboratory animal facilities, and are usually produced from natural ingredients. Manufacturers provide a whole range of diets adapted to particular animal species and their stage of life. Because natural ingredients differ, the commercially available chow diets not only vary in composition between various companies, but can vary also between batches from the same company (Ritskes-Hoitinga & Chwalibog 2003; Ritskes-Hoitinga 2004).

Where natural-ingredient chows are used, it is advisable to obtain a batch analysis certificate with each batch used, to provide exact information on nutrient and contaminant levels. If a batch analysis certificate is not available, researchers will not be able to reject batches that may interfere with the results of their study (Nygaard Jensen & Ritskes-Hoitinga 2007). Moreover, unexpected outcomes where dietary composition may have been the cause would not be able to be explained. Some dietary chows are produced that are intended for use in several species, eg, rat, mouse and hamster. In these cases one has to be aware that individuals could ingest toxic levels of certain nutrients if they eat more than the intended amount of food where the concentration of the nutrient has been determined at the highest minimum concentration needed for one of the species, eg, iron in a diet for rat, mouse and hamster (Beynen & Coates 2001).

Purified or semi-purified diets are formulated with a combination of natural ingredients, pure nutrients and ingredients of varying degrees of refinement, resulting in far more standardised compositions than natural-ingredient diets. For rodents the American Institute of Nutrition, AIN-93 diet (Reeves *et al.* 1993) is recommended, as the composition is such that (with slight modifications) it fulfils nutrient requirements (NRC 1995; Ritskes-Hoitinga 2004). Often, with these diets the composition is such that pelletting is not possible so that alternative types of presentation become necessary (Ritskes-Hoitinga & Chwalibog 2003). Because purified diets are constituted with a better control of dietary composition, more reliable and reproducible results are obtained (compare Ritskes-Hoitinga *et al.* 1989 and 1991). From the point of view of good science, purified diets ought to be used much more frequently than is currently the case. However, depending on composition, there can be problems with palatability and variation in intake: the choice of diets has to be made on a case-by-case basis. Pilot studies are advisable where the effect of the dietary composition is unknown and uncertain.

The hardness of pellets and blocks is measured as the amount of pressure that is required for crushing a pellet. If pellets are too hard (over 20 kp/cm^3), the growth of preweaned mice is reduced significantly (Koopman *et al.* 1989). This is partly because the young mice have to work hard to eat the pellets, and partly because the lactating females are not able to eat enough to satisfy the needs of both themselves and their young (Koopman *et al.* 1989).

About 30% of genetically modified mice have been reported to show signs of weakness and to have reproduction difficulties (FELASA Working Group *et al.* 2007), and this has led to the marketing of special high-fat diets for breeding transgenic mice. The eating problems may be the result of a 'general weakness' of genetically modified strains, but dental problems, muscular weakness, neurodegenerative disorders etc, could all contribute to a reduced food intake. The higher-fat diets marketed for these animals are not as hard, so mice do not need to work as much and can ingest food more easily. The disadvantage of a higher fat content is an increased risk that the mice will develop atherosclerosis. In addition to the various kinds of pelleted diets, manufacturers also produce so-called extruded diets, which have a softer composition and which provide greater availability of nutrients. The reader should consult the manufacturers for detailed information.

Contaminants and trace elements

Contaminants are defined as undesirable substances (usually foreign) which, when present at sufficiently high concentration in the food, can affect the animal and therefore the outcome of experiments (British Association of Research Quality Assurance (BARQA) 1992). Maximum permitted levels of dietary contaminants have been published by the United States' EPA (Environmental Protection Agency 1979); BARQA (1992); GV-Solas (2002). For certain contaminants like selenium, an essential trace element with a narrow safety margin, information on maximum safe levels is provided by the NRC (1995). A table comparing the maximum contaminant levels specified in the three guidelines listed above can be found in Ritskes-Hoitinga (2004). Which guidelines are followed will depend on the goal of the scientific procedure and on the necessity to protect welfare (Ritskes-Hoitinga 2004; Ritskes-Hoitinga & Strubbe 2004). The researcher should decide and choose maximum contaminant levels permissible in order to avoid compromising the results. When working under Good Laboratory Practice (GLP) guidelines the maximum levels must always be defined before the start of the study.

Avoiding toxic nutrient levels: quality assurance, diet and experimental outcomes

Quality control

Manufacturers design diets to contain (much) more than the required minimum nutrient densities. This helps to prevent nutrient deficiencies, even taking into account periods of storage during which some nutrients (eg, some vitamins) may be lost. Moreover, variation in nutrient concentrations in so-called standard chows can be quite considerable, due to the use of natural ingredients that vary in composition (Beynen & Coates 2001; Nygaard Jensen & Ritskes-Hoitinga 2007). This variation can affect results (Wainwright 2001; Ritskes-Hoitinga 2004) and sometimes nutrient concentrations may get close to toxic levels. It is therefore important to have an analysis certificate for each batch of diet used, so that experiments can be planned correctly and unwanted effects prevented. Diet can also be used in environmental enrichment strategies where the animals are provided with choice of diet or allowed to work for food. However, this approach complicates matters with respect to standardisation and quality control and can have adverse consequences. This topic is dealt with more extensively in a later section.

The NRC reports (NRC 1977–2003) provide information on the minimum nutrient requirements for each species, and on known toxic levels of these nutrients. Unless the goal of the experiment is to examine toxicity, nutrient levels that might cause toxic effects should obviously not be used, as this would both compromise animal well-being and experimental results. Even when the goal is to examine nutrient toxicity, very high concentrations are not advisable as they may result in reduced growth and early death. From an animal welfare point of view, testing the dose–response relationship of several subtoxic concentrations is preferable to testing one or two high toxic concentrations (Ritskes-Hoitinga *et al.* 1998). Moreover, such a strategy will provide more detailed information on the metabolic effects of the nutrient, and this approach is therefore an important refinement.

Safety margins

Methionine is an example of a nutrient with a narrow safety margin. The minimum recommended level for mice during growth is 0.3% (NRC 1995). When studying the influence of higher dietary methionine levels on atherothrombosis in ApoE deficient mice, dietary methionine levels of 2.2% and 4.4% (W/W) proved to be toxic, resulting in reduced growth and premature death (Zhou *et al.* 2001; Ritskes-Hoitinga 2004). In a follow-up study, a dietary methionine level of 1.4% (W/W) did not give any obvious signs of toxicity, thereby resulting in better mouse health and welfare and a more reliable interpretation of study results (Zhou *et al.* 2003).

Toxic effects

The recommended nutrient levels for good health and those that cause toxicity vary between species. For sheep, the copper density of the diet is critical, as the difference between that for good health and that causing toxicity is very narrow. Errors in feed mixing can easily lead to mortality in this species (NRC 1995-Sheep 1985). Sheep are able to store sufficient reserves of copper to tide them over periods of up to 4–6 months when grazing copper-deficient forage (NRC 1985). When used in research, sheep are often fed pelleted chow as well as hay and grass on a daily basis, in order to avoid mineral and vitamin deficiencies. In these cases total copper intake must be kept below toxic levels. Moreover, because sheep are usually group-housed, a chow diet can lead to copper intoxication in some individuals, if the food intake is not distributed evenly among the individuals in the group. Characteristic symptoms copper intoxication are haemolysis, icterus (easily detected directly around the eyes) and haemoglobinuria (NRC 1985).

Dietary phosphorus (P) levels are critical in mice, rats and rabbits, as excessive concentrations lead to soft tissue calcification (NRC 1995; van der Broek 1998; Ritskes-Hoitinga *et al.* 2004a). This typically affects the kidneys in rabbits and (female) rats, whereas in mice more widespread calcification involving kidney, tongue and heart is seen. Kidney calcification can negatively affect kidney function (Ritskes-Hoitinga *et al.* 2004a, 2004b). Not all dietary P is available to mice and rats as they cannot access that bound to phytates, whereas rabbits can access all dietary P because of the role of their intestinal microflora (NRC 1995-Rabbits 1977). The recommended dietary P level (at a calcium level of 0.5%) for growing mice and rats is 0.3 % (NRC 1995), and for rabbits 0.2% (NRC 1977). This minimum recommended dietary (available) P level for rabbits is also the maximum recommended level (Ritskes-Hoitinga *et al.* 2004a).

Deficiencies

Usually manufacturers ensure that the nutrient densities of diets exceed the minimum requirements, which helps to prevent nutrient deficiencies following storage. Providing animals with the opportunity to forage and/or select what they want to eat in addition to a complete chow diet, means that intake needs to be carefully monitored. For example, it is well known that providing sunflower seeds to parrots *ad libitum*, in addition to a complete diet, can lead to vitamin A deficiency, as the parrots prefer to eat sunflower seeds. Similarly, scattering corn and wheat in the substrate provides rodents with foraging opportunities, and is thought to be enrichment. However, the amount that is provided needs to be calculated and monitored. Rodents eat according to energy need, so it is important to ensure that most of the energy intake is not from the corn and wheat, as this will suppress intake of the complete diet, potentially leading to mineral and vitamin deficiencies. In summary, it is important to calculate the amount of treats that can be provided without disturbing the balance of nutrients required for health.

Foraging is an important activity of primates in the wild, and can be profoundly affected by captivity (Wolfensohn & Honess 2005). Collecting and eating food is necessary to satisfy physiological, behavioural and social needs, and it is therefore important to consider both forage and eating time when feeding primates. Small portions should be provided unpredictably rather than providing large portions in a predictable schedule (Wolfensohn & Honess 2005). Tables listing the nutrient densities of foods commonly used for primates are presented in the *Nutrient Requirements of Non-Human Primates* (NRC 1995-Nonhuman primates 2003). The size of the food pieces should be such that the primates can hold them, as primates like to manipulate their food. It is important to keep track of the nutrient balance of the total ration presented, as commercial diets are formulated to have a balanced composition according to the animals' needs and this balance may be disturbed if inappropriately large amounts of additional items that do not have a balanced composition are consumed. It is often recommended that a varied diet should be provided (eg, fruit supplements with the chow diet), and care is needed to ensure that the balanced composition of the total diet is maintained (Wolfensohn & Honess 2005). As dietary supplements are also given for environmental enrichment or as part of positive reinforcement training, the selection of these treats and the amounts given are crucial. Treats that are nutritionally complete or high in moisture and low in calories, such as fresh fruit and vegetables, are better choices than nuts and raisins, as these are energy dense and nutritionally incomplete. Data on the nutrient composition of commonly used food supplements are provided by Wolfensohn and Honess (2005) and the Foods Standards Agency and Institute of Food Research (2002). Age-related disorders in primates are often related to nutrition. Dietary restriction that does not lead to essential nutrient deficiencies may tend to increase longevity and to decrease the incidence and age of onset of age-related degenerative conditions. Dominant animals may become obese (Kemnitz 1984) as they may dominate access to food. This can be modified by changing spatial distribution and mix of food types.

Isocaloric exchange

When a standard complete food is offered *ad libitum*, animals ingest according to their energy need. Energy need depends on the life stage, and is generally defined in MJ metabolisable energy per metabolic weight ($kg^{0.75}$): for growth the need is typically recommended as $1.2\,MJ/kg^{0.75}/day$ (but this depends upon rate of growth in relation to adult body mass and species that grow very rapidly, eg altricial birds, have greater daily requirements per metabolic weight than more slowly growing ones such as primates), for maintenance the need is typically about $0.45\,MJ/kg^{0.75}/day$, for gestation, about $0.60\,MJ/kg^{0.75}/day$ (depending on species and litter size) and for lactation, about $1.3\,MJ/kg^{0.75}/day$ (depending on species and other factors). Metabolic weight is used to make proper comparisons between species, correcting for size-related variation in metabolic rates. Because fat in the diet has an energy density 2.25 times higher than that of carbohydrate and protein, changing the fat concentration will result in a change in energy concentration of the diet and thus on amount of food ingested. If the fat content of the diet is changed, compensation is necessary by changing carbohydrates (or proteins) on the basis of calories (isocaloric exchange) not weight, This is the only way to ensure that the intake of all nutrients, except for fat and carbohydrate (or protein), remains similar in test and control group. Only isocaloric exchange isolates the effect of a change in fat (and carbohydrate) content in the diet and makes it possible to reliably interpret study results. Examples of how this is done can be found in Beynen and Coates (2001), Ritskes-Hoitinga and Chwalibog (2003) and Ritskes-Hoitinga (2004).

Aspects of feeding

Rhythms of feeding in nature versus the laboratory situation

Living organisms in nature are continuously influenced by external stimuli, many of them having regular or rhythmic patterns. These include lunar/tidal, solar/daily and seasonal/yearly patterns of light, temperature, food availability, and so on. Because these environmental rhythms are usually quite predictable, animals can usually adapt their physiology to cope with them. The ability to anticipate critical environmental events has clear advantages and survival value in nature, and may be related to the fact that predictability and controllability often have a stress-reducing effect on animals. Species have evolved adaptive anticipatory strategies through the process of natural selection with the result that many species have innate behaviours that are environmentally and temporally appropriate, such as hibernation, migration and seasonal reproduction. Other behaviours that maximise reproductive success include eating patterns that minimise exposure to predators or harsh environments while maximising food consumption. Learning can modify the timing of innate feeding behaviours based upon whether past behaviours were successful in providing adequate nutrients or not. Hence, animals are able to adjust their patterns of ingestive behaviour to adapt to a wide spectrum of environmental conditions, as long as these conditions are predictable (Strubbe 1994b).

These evolved characteristics and strategies are still present in animals in the laboratory today, although domestication has led to changes (Strubbe 1999); chickens housed in battery cages spend less time voluntarily foraging for food than wild jungle fowl (Ritskes-Hoitinga & Strubbe 2004). It is necessary to know what these genetically determined characteristics are and whether and how one must to adapt to them in the laboratory, because they can impact on the animals' well-being and the experimental results. For instance, for practical reasons most scientific tests on animals in the laboratory are performed during the light phase. However, for nocturnal animals this seriously interferes with sleeping behaviour. Regular and predictable changes found in nature are usually absent in the laboratory. The very important light–dark cycle is normally replicated artificially in the laboratory and kept constant throughout the year, in order to synchronise daily rhythms. However, it is not necessary to mimic all natural conditions to produce better welfare for the laboratory animals. Reducing or eradicating infectious diseases in the laboratory clearly improves animal welfare and experimental results.

One of the best-understood rhythmic patterns is the 24h circadian cycle that underlies many physiological processes and behaviour. The rat is the species that has been most extensively investigated with regard to rhythms and their links to feeding, because this animal exhibits most of the general characteristics of mammalian timing systems. Rats are nocturnal and this remains the case when they are maintained under experimentally controlled light–dark rhythms in the laboratory. Under undisturbed *ad libitum* feeding conditions in the laboratory, rats maintained on a 12h dark and 12h light schedule eat most of their total daily food during the dark hours, with peaks at the beginning (dusk) and end (dawn) of the dark period (Kersten *et al.* 1980).

Whereas the dusk peak is needed to compensate for the lower energy stores in the body following the resting phase, the dawn peak has a more anticipatory function to maintain adequate energy over the forthcoming resting phase (Strubbe *et al.* 1986a). Even before the dawn peak the stomach is hard packed (Armstrong *et al.* 1978) and rats do not reduce feeding when liquid food is infused into the stomach (Strubbe *et al.* 1986a). This indicates that satiety signals are neglected during this period in order to allow preparatory 'over-consumption'.

While each rat may have its own characteristic feeding pattern, such patterns usually do not deviate much from the common pattern in free-feeding animals in the laboratory and from animals in nature. This pattern represents a conserved, probably genetically determined, natural behaviour that, in the wild, would reduce the risk of predation.

Light aversiveness

Nocturnal feeding in rats could, at least in part, be a product of light avoidance. Light is known to be aversive to some nocturnal species and in particular to albino species. When rats are provided with smaller and darker nest boxes inside their cages, they spend most of their time during the light phase inside these nest boxes. This remains true when the food hopper and water bottle are placed at a location remote from the nest box (Strubbe *et al.* 1986b; Brinkhof *et al.* 1998). During the dark phase, rats eat in close proximity to the food hopper, whereas when they eat during the light phase, they make rapid excursions from the nest box to the food hopper, take a morsel of food and quickly return to the nest box to consume it. Consumption of food in the nest box increases with light intensity and can therefore be used as a measure of the light's aversiveness (Brinkhof *et al.* 1998; Strubbe & Woods 2004). Aversion to light should, therefore, be taken into account when assessing feeding activity in rats during the light phase. In commonly used rat and mouse cages, the layer of food pellets in the food tray offers some protection from the light. Extremely bright light is, however, never advisable since it may induce retinal damage (Schlingmann *et al.* 1993, 1995). The message here is that the presence of a burrow will certainly increase animal welfare for nocturnal animals, and for rats large burrows are recommended (Jegstrup *et al.* 2005).

Circadian rhythms

When an animal lives in an environment in which it is exposed to predictable light cycles every 24 h, its behavioural patterns entrain on (or synchronise with) the light cycle of the environment. Important patterns can be revealed when the normal light–dark cycle is absent. Thus, when light is kept constant (either with continuous light or continuous dark), animals are no longer able to synchronise with the environment. The result is that many behavioural patterns, including feeding patterns, are governed by a, now unentrained, endogenous oscillator. This operates at a 'free running' rhythm with a daily period that is near, but not identical, to that of one rotation of the earth. From this the term, circadian has been derived (circa = approximately, dies = day). The free running period (tau) is dependent on the individual and is genetically determined, so that in the absence of a light–dark change, or other effective cue, animals' rhythms will be at different phases, which could increase experimental variance. For this reason, a constant light–dark cycle is usually maintained in the laboratory. It is therefore important always to control and check the lighting conditions in the experiment rooms and when experiments are performed in the laboratory, it is extremely important to do this under entrained conditions, unless specific chronobiological experiments require a 'free run' design.

The anatomical site of the light-entrainable oscillator or clock that controls circadian rhythms has been the subject of considerable investigation. The hypothalamic suprachiasmatic nucleus (SCN), which lies just dorsal to the optic chiasm, has been identified as the site of the clock that generates circadian rhythms in mammals. When the SCN is lesioned in mammals, there is immediate and permanent disruption of the circadian rhythm of food intake and the animal's feeding pattern becomes arrhythmic (Strubbe *et al.* 1987).

Importantly, a SCN lesion does not induce blindness, and during the dark phase rats will still eat in the vicinity of the food hopper and in the light they will still take each food pellet back to the nest box. SCN lesions also disrupt many other behavioural and physiological circadian rhythms. For example, in restriction experiments where rats are forced to eat and drink during the light phase, there are strong interacting influences between food intake and sleep (Spiteri *et al.* 1982; Strubbe *et al.* 1986b; Brinkhof *et al.* 1998; Ritskes-Hoitinga & Strubbe 2004). As soon as the *ad libitum* food intake is reinstated, rats revert to their original pattern of food intake (Spiteri 1982). Rats forced to eat during the light phase suffer gastrointestinal problems, comparable to the problems associated with jetlag and shift work in humans (Ritskes-Hoitinga & Strubbe 2004). Interacting effects between circadian clock influences and behaviour and physiology are abolished in rats with SCN lesions (Strubbe *et al.* 1987; Strubbe & van Dijk 2002). This suggests that circadian pacemaker activity in the SCN normally dominates the temporal patterning of food intake, water intake and sleeping behaviour and is not shifted permanently by long-term shifts in food or water availability. As humans work mostly during the light phase, researchers must carefully consider in the implications of their choices as to how and when they feed and treat nocturnal animals in the laboratory.

Memory for feeding time and feeding schedules

In the laboratory, feeding schedules can be part of the experimental design. Rats are quick learners and will readily adapt to these feeding schedules, however, in other rodent species, such as the mouse and hamster, this can be much more difficult, if not impossible. Hamsters on a schedule of one meal of 2 h/day experienced a very rapid drop in body weight (20% in 1 week), making it necessary to stop this experiment (Ritskes-Hoitinga, unpublished observations). It is essential to know and adapt to the characteristics of the species in feeding studies, and where there is uncertainty, pilot studies are recommended. If food restriction is a scientific necessity, feeding meals at certain times can be used to achieve the restriction. Sometimes exact coupling of food intake between test and control groups is necessary in order to promote standardisation, so-called 'pair feeding' (see below).

Meal feeding

Although feeding schedules are used to increase standardisation of experiments, they are, mostly, quite unnatural and artificial. Such schedules interfere with the natural rhythms of drinking, eating and sleeping as dictated by the circadian oscillators. Interference will also occur with the rhythms of many (food-related) physiological processes. When food is consumed, especially large meals, the food itself perturbs many ongoing physiological processes that are closely regulated by the body. As obvious examples, blood glucose concentration and metabolic rate both increase during and after meals, and the effects are greater when larger meals are eaten. In order to minimise the impact of these challenges, the well prepared individual can make meal-anticipatory responses that lessen the magnitude of the meal-induced perturbations. This has obvious advantages for an individual who, due to environmental constraints, is forced to consume all of its daily food in one or two very large meals. Rats can easily be trained to ingest the required amount of food in a limited amount of time. Within a week's time, rats can be trained to ingest their daily food intake in two meals of 0.5 h each during the light phase (Ritskes-Hoitinga *et al.* 1995). One meal of 2 h/day can be sufficient for an (adult) rat to obtain the necessary energy and nutrients but this does depend on the physiological state of the animal. Although rats can be trained to adapt to eating one or two meals per day, the internal rhythm of the circadian clock is maintained. Therefore, in these scheduled feeding designs, there is a strong interference with the circadian feeding behaviour and concomitant gastrointestinal physiology. The time of day when the food is offered is critical to physiology and welfare. Meal-feeding during the dark phase as compared to during the light phase, resulted in bile flow and physical activity being comparable to *ad libitum* feeding (Ritskes-Hoitinga & Strubbe 2004) and resulted in more normal physiological responses.

Animals can eventually adapt to feeding schedules in which fewer, larger meals are eaten, and this is usually associated with more efficient handling of the diet, including a slower gastrointestinal passage time and hypertrophy of the gastrointestinal wall. These changes help the animal to cope with the situation, despite the fact that the feeding schedule can be unsuited to its physiology and uncomfortable.

Virtually every digestive or metabolic variable that has been investigated changes in anticipation of meals. These meal-related changes are often called cephalic responses, because many of them are initiated by signals from the brain. When six equal meals are spread over the daily cycle with equal inter-meal intervals, these anticipatory responses are not seen (Strubbe 1992; Kalsbeek & Strubbe 1998). However, where rodents are used and the study requires a schedule of one to two meals per day, these anticipatory responses do occur. Generally it is preferable to feed more often as rats normally eat eight to ten meals per day. Welfare is certainly affected when forced artificial schedules are used.

Restricted feeding

Severe obesity and diabetes mellitus are becoming increasingly prevalent in Western societies, and reducing body weight by adequate control of food intake is one of the best therapies. However, it is also one of the most difficult treatments in humans, since it usually induces a feeling of a permanent state of hunger and as a consequence stress and mood problems, such as depression, occur. This is also the case in several husbandry systems, for instance in broiler breeders, where severe long-term food restriction is applied during rearing to prevent health and reproduction problems at a later age (De Jong *et al.* 2003).

In food restriction studies, instead of food being provided *ad libitum*, the energy supply is restricted, while still ensuring nutritional adequacy, ie, that all essential nutrients are supplied in the required amounts (Hart *et al.* 1995). For dogs, pigs, cats, monkeys and many other animals it is considered bad veterinary practice to feed *ad libitum*, as the animals will become obese (Hart *et al.* 1995).

Long-term food restriction

Rodents are fed *ad libitum* in the majority of experimental studies. Feeding rodents *ad libitum* may be attractive from a practical point of view because no special feeding system or special care is required. However, on the basis of results from long-term toxicological studies, it is questionable whether this is a sound scientific or welfare approach.

Ad libitum feeding leads to long-term negative health effects compared with restricted feeding (75% of *ad libitum* intake). These include shorter survival time, increased rates of obesity, degenerative kidney and heart disease, and cancer at an earlier age (Hart *et al.* 1995). Food restriction can have other positive effects on health. For instance, the relative body weight reduction 48 h after surgery (jugular cannulation) is smaller in food-restricted animals as compared to *ad libitum* fed rats (both at 3–4 and 17–18 months of age) (Hart *et al.* 1995). It is claimed that animals become more 'robust' when food intake is restricted, that is, that they can cope better with experimental stressors and related procedures (Keenan *et al.* 1999). Diluting the diet, for example, by including a higher fibre content under *ad libitum* conditions, does not give the same positive health effects as compared to food restriction (Hart *et al.* 1995).

In most instances, health problems due to being overweight are not considered a problem, because laboratory animals do not live to an age at which problems occur. However, for research into aging and kidney physiology, there are clear reasons to use food restriction instead of *ad libitum* feeding. Long-term food restriction is also very useful when long-term reductions of body weight are required, such as in obesity and type 2 diabetes research.

Keenan *et al.* (1999) have demonstrated that *ad libitum* feeding is the least controlled experimental factor in the laboratory. Considerable variation in experimental results from rodents on *ad libitum* feeding schedules was seen during the 1980s to 1990s in toxicology (Keenan *et al.* 1999). One possible explanation could be the continuous selection of faster growing individuals in outbred strains (Keenan *et al.* 1999). As rapid growth has often been considered an indicator of good health, robustness and leading to better reproduction, heavier individuals may have been selected for the breeding process. However, faster growth tends also to be associated with a shorter lifespan. By selecting within outbred colonies on the basis of fast growth, subpopulations may arise, leading to more variation within outbred populations. Feeding rodents at approximately 75% of the *ad libitum* food intake is recommended for long-term toxicity studies in order to make certain that a sufficient number of animals survive the required 2-year period (Hart *et al.* 1995). Under *ad libitum* feeding conditions, body fat content can be more than 25% (Toates & Rowland 1987). By restricting food intake to 85% of *ad libitum* intake, body fat content will be less than 10%, which is similar to that found in wild-caught animals (Toates & Rowland 1987). In order to make sure that all individuals eat the same amount of food, it is advised to house them individually (Keenan *et al.* 1999). However, this may have a negative welfare impact because of social isolation, as rodents are social animals. In order to solve this, one possibility is to feed group-housed animals individually. In line with current agricultural practice, microchips, computer technology and automated feeding devices have been used for feeding individual rats restrictedly under permanent group housing conditions. This strategy needs to be further developed.

An aspect of food restriction that deserves much more attention is the issue of standardisation and reduction. Under *ad libitum* feeding conditions, animals can freely choose the amount of food eaten. By definition, animals are fed a standardised amount of food under restricted feeding conditions, which automatically improves standardisation of experiments. Upon testing chloral hydrate in rats under *ad libitum* versus food-restricted conditions, it was found that a significant difference in the liver enzyme activity of LA (lauric acid) between control and test group occurred at a dose of 100 mg/kg (Leaky *et al.* 2003; Ritskes-Hoitinga 2006; Ritskes-Hoitinga *et al.* 2006). Under *ad libitum* conditions 86 animals per group were necessary, whereas only 7 animals were needed under food-restricted conditions to prove that this difference was statistically significant (Figure 14.1). This indicates that a reduction of 92% in the number of animals used was possible under these conditions because the magnitude of the effect was much greater under restricted feeding conditions than under *ad libitum* feeding, which is a well known effect of food restriction (Hart *et al.* 1995).

However, it is not only from the point of view of the numbers of animals used, that welfare issues associated to food restriction need to be addressed. Long-term food restriction may (temporarily) cause feelings of hunger. This can be a strong stressor leading to abnormal behaviour such as stereotypies and will affect animal's welfare by causing mood problems (Dixon *et al.* 2003). One study with rabbits showed that a lower frequency of stereotypical behaviour occurred when rabbits were offered a restricted amount of food at their natural time of the day compared with restricted feeding at an unnatural time of day and as compared to *ad libitum* feeding (Krohn *et al.* 1999). This indicates that feeding a restricted amount of food at the 'proper' time is beneficial for welfare, even when compared to *ad libitum* feeding. When a restricted feeding schedule is used, it should be remembered that as soon as food becomes available again, the animal will ingest a large meal in order to compensate for energy deficits from the fasting period.

Short-term food deprivation

Short-term food deprivation, such as overnight fasting or other food deprivation schedules, is often used in research. For example, fasting may be necessary when blood samples need to be lipid-free for certain analyses. These short-term food restriction periods (ie, hours) are needed for certain experiments and can also improve standardisation and reproducibility of experiments. However, food deprivation for a period of 24 h results in a different metabolic state than under *ad libitum* feeding conditions (Strubbe & Alingh Prins 1986). After rats have been deprived of food for a period of 24 h or more, all glycogen deposits have been used. Food deprivation in rats for a period of 12 h leads to a shift from carbohydrate to fat metabolism (Strubbe & Alingh Prins 1986). An excellent overview of how food restriction influ-

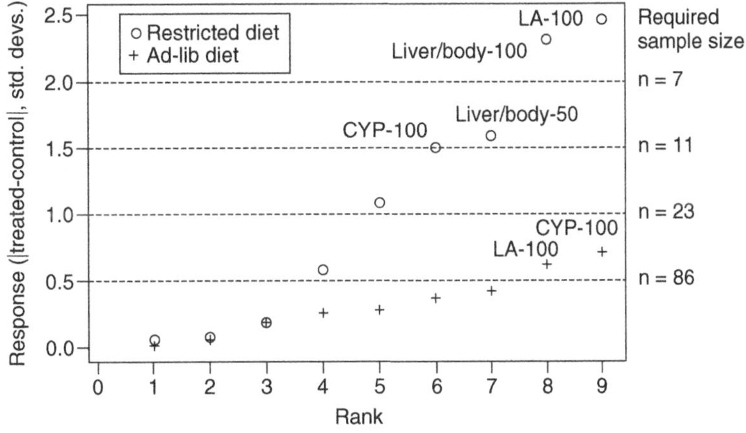

Figure 14.1 Chloral hydrate caused a significant increase in the liver enzyme activity LA-100 (LA is lauric acid, 100 refers to a dose of 100 mg/kg). Under *ad libitum* conditions, 86 animals were needed in order to show a statistically significant difference, whereas under food restriction conditions, only seven animals were necessary to find a significant difference between the treatment and control group (ie, a 92% reduction). Food restriction also leads to an increase in effect size as compared to *ad libitum* conditions (Leaky *et al.* 2003; Ritskes-Hoitinga 2006). 'Effect size' is the magnitude of the difference between the treated and control group, calculated by taking the absolute differences between the treated and control means and dividing this difference by the standard deviation for each group; 'rank' indicates the numerical position of a certain parameter in the magnitude of the effect size; crosses refer to *ad libitum* fed groups, circles refer to restrictedly fed groups; CYP-100 refers to liver enzyme activity measurement of the enzyme CYP at a dose of 100 mg/kg; liver/body is the liver/body weight ratio at the dose of 50 and 100 mg/kg. (Dr. Michael Festing is greatly acknowledged for these calculations.)

ences the physiology and well-being of various species has been published by Rowland (2007).

Pair feeding

If a test group's voluntary food intake differs from that of the controls, it is advisable to take steps to equalise the intake between the groups. Such differences can occur when the palatability of the test diet is negatively influenced, or where the substance has a negative effect on appetite or health, resulting in reduced food intake. For standardisation, test and control animals must ingest a similar amount of food at a similar time of day, otherwise it will be impossible to judge the effects of the test substance and/or procedure independently of its effects on food intake. Because NRC requirements are based on obtaining maximum growth rate, a level of 75% of the NRC recommendations is still considered sufficient to fulfil all needs.

There are four possible methods for achieving pair feeding and these are: (1) weighing; (2) coupling of food dispensers; (3) gavage/permanent stomach cannula; and (4) feeding machine. In the first method the amount of food eaten by the test group is weighed, and the control group is fed the same amount of food the next day. A disadvantage of this method can be that the total daily food supply is provided at once to the control animals, perhaps at an unnatural time point of the day (eg, perhaps during the resting phase in rodents). This may induce quite a different eating pattern and overloading of gastrointestinal processes in the controls as compared to the test animals, thereby preventing proper comparison between test and control animals. In the second method, using food dispensers, rats can be trained to obtain a pellet by pressing a lever. By coupling food dispensers for test and control animals, the dispenser of the control rat provides a pellet at exactly the same time as the test animal 'asks for' and eats a pellet. This system standardises amounts eaten and ingesting patterns. In the third method, permanent stomach cannulation and gavage make it possible to provide all animals with exactly the same amount of food at the same time points (Balkan *et al.* 1991). However, inserting a permanent stomach cannula requires a surgical procedure and both the stomach cannula and gavage method omit the oral digestive process. In the fourth method, feeding machines with regulated opening of valves make it possible to open and close food hoppers at the same times during the day for test and control animals. Meal training is another possible solution for a pair-feeding schedule.

Gavage feeding

In research on pharmaceutical agents or nutrients, it can be important to avoid any negative influence of taste on food intake. In such cases, gavage is used to introduce substances directly into the stomach. Gavage may also be required for radioactive isotopes or immunosuppressants, where exact dosing is required and health-damaging substances must not be spilled into the environment. However, the application of a meal directly in the stomach as compared to voluntary eating of a similar meal, can affect experimental results (Vachon *et al.* 1988). In this study by Vachon *et al.* (1988), voluntary consumption yielded results more comparable to those from from human studies. A disadvantage of stomach tubing is that it bypasses all the oropharyngeal processes, including the physical effects of chewing and the addition of salivary enzymes that initiate the digestive process. Gavage can also cause stress to the animals, resulting in suppression of gastrointestinal activity. By training the animals to become accustomed to the procedure and giving them positive rewards, the use of the stomach tubes becomes gradually less stressful.

Another possibility is to insert permanent cannulas in the stomach (or small intestine), which makes it possible to apply substances directly into the stomach or small intestine without stress (Strubbe *et al.* 1986a) and without risk of contamination of the environment and the person executing it. These permanent cannulas are used, for example, to measure the satiety effects of filling the gastrointestinal system with purified nutrients at different anatomical locations. After the initial surgical procedure, rats can walk freely in their home cage. Due to the presence of the cannula attachment to the skull, individual housing is often used, however, this will impact on the animals' welfare. Social housing is possible if the cannula attachments are protected from bites by a metal cap.

Working for food

When food is always available, but not 'free', animals readily change their feeding patterns based upon other kinds of constraints. When an energy cost is placed on gaining access to food, rats change their strategy to minimise total daily work while maintaining a constant body weight (Collier *et al.* 2007). Specifically, as the cost of gaining access to food increases (eg, the number of responses an animal must make to gain access to food; or some other aspect of physical effort), two changes occur: the rats eat larger meals, and they eat fewer meals (Figure 14.2).

It is difficult to determine how much time/energy ought to be spent on working for food. The choice the animals make does not necessarily optimise long-term welfare. Sometimes, the animals are inclined to eat a large amount of easily available food fast, in order to make energy deposits. This in turn, may have a negative impact on the animals' health and welfare in the long term. As a result of domestication and selection, animals may change in ways that impact on their needs for optimal welfare. Comparing the behaviour of the white leghorn chicken and its ancestor, the wild jungle fowl, a remarkable difference has occurred in food searching behaviour. When given the choice between freely available food from a plate and food that was hidden in the bedding in a semi-natural environment, the white leghorn chose to search for food in the bedding and consumed 30% of their feed from this source, whereas wild jungle fowl consumed 70% of the total diet from the hidden food (Ritskes-Hoitinga & Strubbe 2004). This indicates that there may be a behavioural adaptation as a result of domestication and selecting strains for increased production.

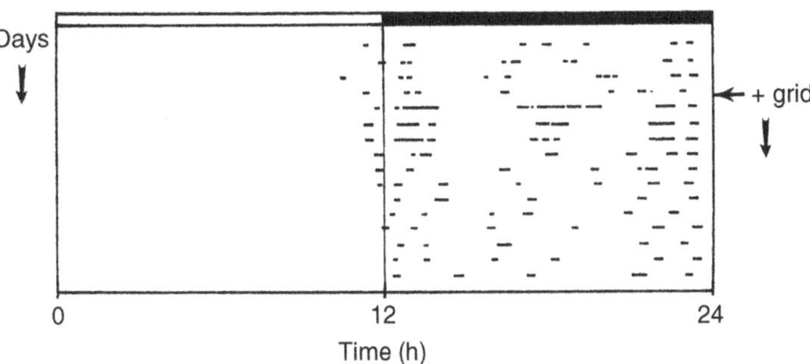

Figure 14.2 Daily pattern of food intake of a rat on consecutive days. The black lines represent bouts of feeding activity. On day 5, the distance between the food hopper bars was reduced, requiring increased effort to obtain food through the bars. Notice the large meals of extremely long duration in the beginning. After a few days, the animals could work their way through the narrowed food hopper bars just as fast as before. Reproduced from Ritskes-Hoitinga, M. and Strubbe, J.H. (2004) Nutrition and animal welfare. In: *The Welfare of Laboratory Animals*. Ed. Kaliste, E., pp. 51–80. With kind permission of Springer Science and Business Media.

Diets

A change is likely in the animal's feeding strategy if diet and palatability are changed. However, after a few days the free-feeding pattern will return to the original state with the same meal frequency (Strubbe & van Dijk 2002; Ruffin *et al.* 2004).

A regular chow diet can be used for animal maintenance and during numerous types of scientific procedures but, in nature, a greater variety of ingredients is often available and consumed. So, is greater variety and the opportunity to choose and select better for the welfare of the animals? When rats were given the choice between various diets providing energy from different sources, the rats chose carbohydrate-rich diets in the evening hours, and fat-rich diets just before the start of the resting period (Strubbe 1994a, 1994b). The same time-dependent pattern of macronutrient selection was also seen in humans (van het Hof *et al.* 1997). The evolutionary explanation may be that carbohydrate-rich diets will quickly provide the animal with a source of readily available energy, necessary to supply the energy deficits that have arisen during the resting phase. The selection of macronutrients is governed by several neurotransmitters in the central nervous system such as galanin, neuropeptide Y (NPY) and serotonin (Strubbe 1994a; Kyrkouli *et al.* 2006). At present, in the authors' laboratory, the animals are often only offered one standard diet throughout the day but varying the diets offered can improve their welfare. It has been reported that monkeys that had access to a herb garden in the Zoo 'Apenheul' at Apeldoorn in the Netherlands, made a selection of specific herbs according to their health state[1]. Food selection is individually determined, and it may be better for welfare to permit individual selection of foods. At first glance, this may appear to conflict with attempts to standardise experiments, however, if individual needs are properly met, standardisation of experiments can be improved by adopting this approach. It will be a challenge to define how this should be achieved in practice.

Normal feeding patterns in rats also vary with their physiological and metabolic state. When energy demands are increased, such as during lactation or during forced daily exercise, rats first increase the size of meals up to their normal maximal meal size and later increase the number of such meals as energy demands increase further (Strubbe & Gorissen 1980).

Group housing

Although restricted feeding schemes and solitary housing have advantages for the standardisation and execution of experiments, restricted feeding schedules and solitary housing may have welfare consequences. Animals of social species ought to be housed socially, unless there are clear reasons for doing otherwise. When harmonious social housing is not possible, then all possible efforts should be made to improve animal welfare in other ways.

Housing and husbandry conditions can influence both the amount of food animals ingest, and the animals' feeding patterns. Whether an animal is group or individually housed has implications for food intake and results of scientific procedures. Individually housed mice of both sexes were found to have higher food intake than mice housed in groups of two, four or eight per cage (Chvedoff *et al.* 1980; Beynen & Coates 2001). Mice housed individually or at two per cage had a higher body weight and body weight variability than the other groups. When the mice were housed at eight per cage, gastritis occurred more frequently compared with individually housed mice (Chvedoff *et al.* 1980). These results indicated that four mice per cage was the optimum group size in this particular study. Peters and Festing (1990) showed that maximum body weight gain at different cage densities depended on the cage size and the mouse strain chosen: the inbred Balb/c thrived best in a high-density housing, whereas the outbred MF1 had a higher body weight gain in low-density housing. If mice are housed in a group, they usually lie together, reducing their total surface area. Reduced heat loss per animal in the group is the result and, due to this 'behavioural thermoregulation', food intake is reduced (De Vries *et al.* 1993; Woods & Strubbe 1994). If test compounds are incorporated in the food, the investigator should be aware of the phenomenon that group size influences intake and, therefore, the intake of the compound.

Behavioural and ingestion patterns can also be influenced by the social structure in the group. A dominant animal may prevent others from eating at certain times. Food intake patterns of socially compatible groups of S3 rats showed the normal feeding pattern with a clear dawn peak for all individuals. In contrast in a group that was socially incompatible, the dominant animal prevented the rats lower in

[1]http://www.kennislink.nl/publicaties/wat-kunnen-wolapen-ons-leren-over-gezondheidsbevorderend-gedrag

hierarchy from having a dawn peak at the natural time. Some had to shift to an earlier time during the dark phase, and some even shifted to the beginning of the light phase (Ritskes-Hoitinga & Strubbe 2004). It is unclear whether the phase of circadian rhythm had shifted permanently.

Thus, group housing can influence experimental outcome, either by influencing food intake and feeding patterns or by other factors. In one case, incompatibility between individuals in a group of dogs led to stress and vomiting of food until 8 h after the meal. Ingestion of this vomited food caused a disturbance of the experimental results. Upon changing the treatment and handling of the group of dogs in many ways, a social compatible group of individuals led to more reliable and reproducible results (Ritskes-Hoitinga *et al.* 2006).

Concluding remarks

When carrying out research using animals, it is a challenge to feed them in such a way that their health and welfare is maintained and results are reliable and reproducible. To do this requires knowledge of nutritional and behavioural requirements. This chapter provides an overview of factors that must be taken into account when feeding animals in the laboratory. Much more research is needed into how different feeding methods can be used as enrichment in order to improve laboratory animal welfare.

References

Armstrong, S., Clarke, J. and Coleman, G. (1978) Light-dark variation in laboratory rat stomach and small intestine content. *Physiology and Behavior*, **21**, 785–788

Balkan, B., Steffens, A.B., Bruggink, J.E. *et al.* (1991) Hyperinsulinemia and glucose tolerance in obese rats with lesions of the ventromedial hypothalamus: dependence on food intake and route of administration. *Metabolism: Clinical and Experimental*, **40**, 1092–1100

Beynen, A.C. and Coates, M.E. (2001) Nutrition and experimental results. In: *Principles of Laboratory Animal Science*. Eds van Zutphen, L.F.M., Baumans V. and Beynen, A.C., pp. 111–128. Elsevier Scientific Publishers, Amsterdam

Brinkhof, M.W., Daan, S. and Strubbe, J.H. (1998) Forced dissociation of food- and light-entrainable circadian rhythms of rats in a skeleton photoperiod. *Physiology and Behavior*, **65**, 225–231

British Association of Research Quality Assurance (BARQA) (1992) *Guidelines for the Manufacture and Supply of GLP Animal Diets*. BARQA, Ipswich

Chvedoff, M., Clarke, M.R., Faccini, J.M. *et al.* (1980) Effects on mice of number of animals per cage: an 18-month study (preliminary results). *Archives in Toxicology*, **4** (Suppl.), 435–438

Collier, G., Johnson, D. and Mathis, C. (2007) The currency of procurement cost. *Journal of the Experimental Analysis of Behavior*, **78**, 31–61

De Jong, I.C., Van Voorst, A.S. and Blokhuis, H.J. (2003) Parameters for quantification of hunger in broiler breeders. *Physiology and Behavior*, **78**, 773–783

De Vries, J., Strubbe, J.H., Wildering, W.C. *et al.* (1993) Patterns of body temperature during feeding in rats under varying ambient temperatures. *Physiology and Behavior*, **53**, 229–235

Dixon, D.P., Ackert, A.M. and Eckel, L.A. (2003) Development of, and recovery from, activity-based anorexia in female rats. *Physiology and Behavior*, **80**, 273–279

Environmental Protection Agency (1979) Proposed health effects test standards for toxic substances control act test rules. Good laboratory standards for health effects. *Federal Register*, **44**(91), 27362–27375

Ewen, S.W.B. and Pusztai, A. (1999) Effect of diets containing genetically modified potatoes expressing *Galanthus nivalis* lectin on rat small intestine. *The Lancet*, **354**, 1353–1354

FELASA Working Group: Rülicke, T., Montagutelli, X., Pintado, B. *et al.* (2007) FELASA guidelines for the production and nomenclature of transgenic rodents. *Laboratory Animals*, **41**, 301–311

Foods Standard Agency and Institute of Food Research (2002) *McCane and Widdowson's The Composition of Foods*, 6th edn. Royal Society of Chemistry, London

GV-Solas (2002) *Guidelines for the Quality-Assured Production of Laboratory Animal Diets*. Gesellschaft für Versuchstierkunde – German Society for Laboratory Animal Science, Berlin

Hart, R.W., Neumann, D.A. and Robertson, R.T.E. (1995) *Dietary Restriction: Implications for the Design and Interpretation of Toxicity and Carcinogenicity Studies*. ILSI Press, Washington

Horton, R. (1999) Genetically modified foods: 'absurd' concern or welcome dialogue? *The Lancet*, **354**, 1314–1315

Jegstrup, I.M., Vestergaard, R. and Ritskes-Hoitinga, M. (2005) Nest building behaviour in male rats in three inbred strains: BDIX/Orl Ico, BN/HsdCpb and Lewis/Mol. *Animal Welfare*, **14**, 149–156

Kalsbeek, A. and Strubbe, J.H. (1998) Circadian control of insulin secretion is independent of the temporal distribution of feeding. *Physiology and Behavior*, **63**, 553–558

Keenan, K., Ballam, G., Soper, K. *et al.* (1999) Diet, caloric restriction, and the rodent bioassay. *Toxicological Sciences*, **52** (Suppl), 24–34

Kemnitz, J.W. (1984) Obesity in macaques: spontaneous and induced. *Advances in Veterinary Science and Comparative Medicine*, **28**, 81–114

Kersten, A., Strubbe, J.H. and Spiteri, N.J. (1980) Meal patterning of rats with changes in day length and food availability. *Physiology and Behavior*, **25**, 953–958

Koopman, J., Scholten, P., Roeleveld, P. *et al.* (1989) Hardness of diet pellets and its influence on growth of pre-weaned and weaned mice. *Zeitschrift für Versuchstierkunde*, **32**, 71–75

Krohn, T., Ritskes-Hoitinga, J. and Svendsen, P. (1999) The effects of feeding and housing on the behaviour of the laboratory rabbit. *Laboratory Animals*, **33**, 101–107

Kyrkouli, S.E., Strubbe, J.H. and Scheurink, A.J.W. (2006) Galanin in the PVN increases nutrient intake and changes peripheral hormone levels in the rat. *Physiology and Behavior*, **89**, 103–109

Leaky, J.E.A., Seng, J.E., Latendresse, J.R. *et al.* (2003) Dietary controlled carcinogenicity study of chloral hydrate in male B6C3F1 mice. *Toxicology and Applied Pharmacology*, **193**, 266–280

National Research Council (1977–2003) Nutrient Requirements of Sheep 1985; of Dogs 1985; of Beef Cattle 1984; of Mink and Foxes, 1982; of Laboratory Animals (Rat, Mouse, Guinea pig, Hamster, Gerbil, Vole), 1977 and 1995; of Poultry 1994; of Fish 1993; of Horses 1989; of Dairy Cattle 1989; of Swine 1998; of Cats 1986; of Goats 1981; of Nonhuman Primates 2003, 2nd edn; of Rabbits 1977. National Academy Press, Washington, DC

Nygaard Jensen, M.N. and Ritskes-Hoitinga, M. (2007) How isoflavone levels in common rodent diets can interfere with the value of animal models and with experimental results. *Laboratory Animals*, **41**, 1–18

Peters, A. and Festing, M. (1990) Population density and growth rate in laboratory mice. *Laboratory Animals*, **24**, 273–279

Reeves, P.G., Nielsen, F.H. and Fahey, G.C. Jr. (1993) AIN-93 purified diets for laboratory rodents: final report of the American Institute of Nutrition ad hoc writing committee on the reformulation of the AIN-76A rodent diet. *Journal of Nutrition*, **11**, 1939–1951

Ritskes-Hoitinga, M. (2004) Nutrition of laboratory mice. In: *The Laboratory Mouse, Handbook of Experimental Animals Series*. Ed. Hedrich, H., pp. 463–479. Elsevier Academic Press, Amsterdam

Ritskes-Hoitinga, M. (2006) Heeft een rat Boeddhanatuur? http://www.ru.nl/aspx/download.aspx?File=/contents/pages/11712/070406ritskeshelemaal.pdf (accessed 15 April 2009)

Ritskes-Hoitinga, M., Bjoerndal Gravesen, L. and Jegstrup, I.M. (2006) Refinement benefits animal welfare and quality of science. http://www.nc3rs.org.uk/news.asp?id=212 (accessed 15 April 2009)

Ritskes-Hoitinga, J. and Chwalibog, A. (2003) Nutrients requirements, experimental design and feeding schedules in animal experimentation. In: *Handbook of Laboratory Animal Science, Vol. 1.*, 2nd edn. Eds Hau, J. and van Hoosier, G., pp. 281–310. CRC Press, London

Ritskes-Hoitinga, J., Grooten, H.N., Wienk, K.J. *et al.* (2004a) Lowering dietary phosphorus concentrations reduces kidney calcification, but does not adversely affect growth, mineral metabolism, and bone development in growing rabbits. *British Journal of Nutrition*, **91**, 367–376

Ritskes-Hoitinga, J., Lemmens, A.G., Danse, L.H.J.C. *et al.* (1989) Phosphorus-induced nephrocalcinosis and kidney function in female rats. *Journal of Nutrition*, **119**, 1423–1431

Ritskes-Hoitinga, J., van het Hof, K.H., Kloots, W.J., *et al.* (1995) Rat as a model to study postprandial effects in man. In: *Proceedings of The World Congress on Alternatives and Animal Use in the Life Sciences: Education, Research, Testing*. Eds Goldberg, A.M. and van Zutphen, L.F.M., pp. 403–410. Alternative Methods in Toxicology and the Life Sciences

Ritskes-Hoitinga, J., Mathot, J.N.J.J., Danse, L.H.J.C. *et al.* (1991) Commercial rodent diets and nephrocalcinosis in weanling female rats. *Laboratory Animals*, **25**, 126–132

Ritskes-Hoitinga, M., Skott, O., Uhrenholt, T.R. *et al.* (2004b) Nephrocalcinosis in rabbits – a case study. *Scandinavian Journal for Laboratory Animal Science*, **31**, 143–148

Ritskes-Hoitinga, M. and Strubbe, J.H. (2004) Nutrition and animal welfare. In: *The Welfare of Laboratory Animals*. Ed. Kaliste, E., pp. 51–80. Kluwer Academic Publishers, Dordrecht

Ritskes-Hoitinga, J., Verschuren, P.M., Meijer, G.W. *et al.* (1998) The association of increasing dietary concentrations of fish oil with hepatotoxic effects and a higher degree of aorta atherosclerosis in the ad lib-fed rabbit. *Food and Chemical Toxicology*, **36**, 663–672

Rowland, N.E. (2007) Food or fluid restriction in common laboratory animals: balancing welfare considerations with scientific inquiry. *Comparative Medicine*, **57**, 149–160

Ruffin, M., Adage, T., Kuipers, F. *et al.* (2004) Feeding and temperature responses to intravenous leptin infusion are differential predictors of obesity in rats. *American Journal of Physiology. Regulatory, Integrative and Comparative Physiology*, **286**, 756–763

Schlingmann, F., Pereboom, W.J. and Rémie, R. (1993) The sensitivity of albino and pigmented rats to light. *Animal Technology*, **44**, 71–84

Schlingmann, F., de Rijk, S.H.L., Pereboom, W.J. *et al.* (1995) Light intensity in animal rooms and cages in relation to the care and management of albino rats. *Animal Technology*, **44**, 97–107

Spiteri, N., Prins, A., Keyser, J. *et al.* (1982) Circadian pacemaker control of feeding in the rat, at dawn. *Physiology and Behavior*, **29**, 1141–1145

Spiteri, N.J. (1982) Circadian patterning of feeding, drinking and activity during diurnal food access in rats. *Physiology and Behavior*, **28**, 139–147

Strubbe, J.H. (1992) Parasympathetic involvement in rapid meal-associated conditioned insulin secretion in the rat. *American Journal of Physiology*, **263**, R615–R618

Strubbe, J.H. (1994a) Neuro-endocrine factors. In: *Food Intake and Energy Expenditure*. Eds Westerterp-Plantenga, M.S., Fredrix, E.W.H.M. and Steffens, A.B., pp. 175–182. CRC Press, London

Strubbe, J.H. (1994b) Circadian rhythms of food intake. In: *Food Intake and Energy Expenditure*. Eds Westerterp-Plantenga, M.S., Fredrix, E.W.H.M. and Steffens, A.B., pp. 155–174. CRC Press, London

Strubbe, J.H. (1999) Circadian organization of feeding behaviour. In: *Regulation of Food Intake and Energy Expenditure*. Eds Westerterp-Plantenga, M.S. and Steffens, A.B., pp. 135–157. Edra, Milan

Strubbe, J.H. (2003) Hunger, meals and obesity. In: *Encyclopedia of Cognitive Science*, Vol **2**. Ed. Nadel, L., pp. 432–437. Nature Publishing Group, London

Strubbe, J.H. and Alingh Prins, A.J. (1986) Reduced insulin secretion after short-term food deprivation in rats plays a key role in the adaptive interaction of glucose and free fatty acid utilization. *Physiology and Behavior*, **37**, 441–445

Strubbe, J.H. and Gorissen, J. (1980) Meal patterning in the lactating rat. *Physiology and Behavior*, **25**, 775–777

Strubbe, J.H., Keyser, J., Dijkstra, T. *et al.* (1986a) Interaction between circadian and caloric control of feeding behavior in the rat. *Physiology and Behavior*, **36**, 489–493

Strubbe, J., Prins, A., Bruggink, J. *et al.* (1987) Daily variation of food-induced changes in blood glucose and insulin in the rat and the control by the suprachiasmatic nucleus and the vagus nerve. *Journal of the Autonomic Nervous System*, **20**, 113–119

Strubbe, J.H., Spiteri, N.J. and Alingh Prins, A.J. (1986b) Effect of skeleton photoperiod and food availability on the circadian pattern of feeding and drinking in rats. *Physiology and Behaviour*, **36**, 647–651

Strubbe, J.H. and van Dijk, G. (2002) The temporal organization of ingestive behaviour and its interaction with regulation of energy balance. *Neuroscience Biobehaviour Reviews*, **26**, 485–498

Strubbe, J.H. and Woods, S.C. (2004) The timing of meals. *Psychological Reviews*, **111**, 128–141

Toates, F.M. and Rowland, N.E.E. (1987) *Feeding and Drinking*. Elsevier, Amsterdam

Vachon, C., Jones, J., Wood, P. *et al.* (1988) Concentration effect of soluble dietary fibers on postprandial glucose and insulin in the rat. *Canadian Journal of Physiology and Pharmacology Links*, **66**, 801–806

van der Broek, F. (1998) *Dystrophic Cardiac Calcifications in Laboratory Mice*. PhD thesis, Utrecht University, The Netherlands

van het Hof, K., Weststrate, J., van den Berg, H. *et al.* (1997) A long-term study on the effect of spontaneous consumption of reduced fat products as part of a normal diet on indicators of health. *International Journal of Food Sciences and Nutrition*, **48**, 19–29

Wainwright, P.E. (2001) The role of nutritional factors in behavioural development in laboratory mice. *Behavioral Brain Research*, **125**, 75–80

Wolfensohn, S. and Honess, P. (2005) *Handbook of Primate Husbandry and Welfare*. Blackwell Publishing, Oxford

Woods, S.C. and Strubbe, J.H. (1994) The psychobiology of meals. *Psychonomic Bulletin and Review*, **1**, 141–155

Zhou, J., Møller, J., Danielsen, C.C. *et al.* (2001) Dietary supplementation with methionine and homocysteine promotes early atherosclerosis but not plaque rupture in ApoE-deficient mice. *Arteriosclerosis, Thrombosis, and Vascular Biology*, **21**, 1470–1476

Zhou, J., Møller, J., Ritskes-Hoitinga, M. *et al.* (2003) Effects of vitamin supplementation and hyperhomocysteinemia on atherosclerosis in apoE-deficient mice. *Atherosclerosis*, **168**, 255–262

Zhu, X., Song, J., Mar, M.H. *et al.* (2003) Phosphatidylethanolamine N-methyltransferase (PEMT) knockout mice have hepatic steatosis and abnormal hepatic choline metabolite concentrations despite ingesting a recommended dietary intake of choline. *Biochemical Journal*, **15**, 987–993

15 Attaining competence in the care of animals used in research

Bryan Howard and Timo Nevalainen

Introduction

During the last two decades, there has been very considerable improvement in our understanding of the needs of animals, although there is much still to learn, and many of the measures implemented to improve husbandry have been empirically formulated. There is an urgent need for more investigative work into the most appropriate husbandry conditions of many laboratory species and those who are routinely engaged in animal care may often be well placed to carry out or assist in such research.

In addition to animal welfare-based changes to the way animals are housed and cared for, there have been other developments that have brought science into the animal facility and technology into the day-to-day routines of staff working there. New ways of keeping animals include: the group housing of rabbits, primates and dogs; ventilated racks and other biocontainment facilities; high-intensity aquatic environments; computerised systems for monitoring the environment and maintaining animal records; and high-performance room ventilation systems, which minimise carbon costs whilst maintaining rigorously defined air quality within rooms with a low burden of aeroallergens. Changes such as these have coincided with the emergence of new experimental methods and models, including transgenics, high health status, chronic studies on animals with instrumentation, radiotelemetry and indwelling catheters.

The importance of ensuring competence of those who care for and use animals has never been higher. Training programmes should be designed and delivered with a view to developing the knowledge and skills appropriate to the duties of individuals, whilst promoting the diversity and flexibility necessary for career development. All staff must commit to their own development, so it is important that at the outset they explicitly agree what constitutes satisfactory performance in relation to the outcomes required and that the reasons for training and the ways in which both staff and the organisation will benefit are made clear (Silverman 2002). Training helps staff to develop basic competencies and, in the case of ongoing training, to use new equipment and procedures. Training is important for maintaining and updating knowledge about legislative and regulatory developments, and for the renewal of competencies, particularly in areas not frequently addressed (Pritt & Duffee 2007). The amount and nature of training required by individuals is likely to differ, which, with variation in preferred learning styles, resource allocation and conflicting work demands puts considerable pressure on those responsible for delivering training in the workplace. Training without follow-up is ineffective and a clear, transparent means of measuring progress should be set in place that allows both staff and their supervisors to monitor and recognise success as the learning objectives are achieved.

Legal and ethical considerations

All those working with animals need to be made aware of their obligations under national and regional legislation, and this is an essential part of the training process (see also Chapter 8). In most instances, legislation adopts the ethical framework of the Three Rs of Russell and Burch (Russell & Burch 1959). In general terms, this states that animals should only be used when no non-sentient alternatives exist, that then as few as possible should be used, and that the experiments should be conducted so as to minimise the adverse impact on each animal concerned (see Chapter 2).

Everyone involved in the care and use of laboratory animals is partially responsible for an activity which requires legislation to make it legal, and consequently must make ethical decisions and accept the consequences of those on an ongoing basis. The people who have most influence on the well-being of laboratory animals are those who care for them on a regular basis. Although the conduct of scientific procedures almost invariably impacts on their well-being, that impact is usually transient or of relatively short duration. On the other hand, animals must be bred, transported and cared for before the study starts and during its progress; and at the end of the investigation they must usually be humanely killed. Animal care staff and their supervisors are in the frontline of this process and it is important that they should clearly understand the ethical principles involved and the concerns which society expresses. Appreciation of this can be particularly difficult when some individuals, albeit only a tiny minority, threaten violence or intimidation against those involved. While it may not always be appropriate to focus on the theoretical background of ethical decision making, all persons involved in animal experimentation should be able to apply ethical principles to clarify and feel confident about their role and the activities of the institution and regulatory systems within which they work. Moreover, a common ethical appreciation of those caring for and conducting experiments on animals within a particular establishment results in the development of shared values, which underpin a pervasive culture of care. Such an institutional culture is intolerant of acts which unnecessarily impair animal welfare, thereby supporting legal compliance, establishing ethical sustainability and ultimately enhancing the robustness of scientific studies.

Because of the underlying importance of these ethical principles in relation to the day-to-day activities of animal care staff and others, it is important that staff are made aware of the ethical framework and the law as soon as they commence work. These are important topics in formal training courses, but should also be promoted by ethical review processes within establishments and by supervisors and colleagues. This is one of several topics in which formal teaching, by lectures, seminars or study of online materials, is less effective than interactive teaching, in which learners are encouraged to ask questions and to solve problems that address ethical issues. Good communication is central to developing shared ethical values, and both care staff and scientists should be able to talk freely with each other using a common understanding focused on high-quality care routines, welfare issues and science and based on acceptance of individual responsibility and accountability.

Other purposes of education and training

Consideration of the needs for education and training should not be restricted to regulatory requirements, but should use them as a starting point. Regulatory requirements tend to be broadly drafted and include general statements such as the need for 'appropriate education'. Details of curriculum content, the minimum length of initial training and maintenance of up-to-date knowledge and skills are not addressed in detail (see for example European Directive 86/609, European Council 1986). A similar situation applies in the United States (see Duffee *et al.* 2003). Although the objectives of national laws and regulations on education and training are similar, the means by which they are achieved and implemented can differ considerably.

Training is also necessary to achieve high-quality science and good animal welfare (Nevalainen 2004). University science curricula do not usually specifically address issues relating to animal welfare, good scientific practice or associated ethical subjects. A strong case can be made for referring to these topics within the curriculum. Many undergraduates who are taking biology-based courses will not progress to carry out research involving animals, and therefore do not need to gain competences in these areas, but it is important that all of those who acquire or use information in a scientific or technical way should appreciate how that information has been obtained. The value of including such information in undergraduate degree courses has been explored by assessing student opinions (Carlsson *et al.* 2001) but more needs to be done to determine the most appropriate level and time of presentation.

Sources of information

Various courses and training opportunities are available, such as those organised by major laboratory animal breeders, which deal with general laboratory animal care, as well as the research techniques used by particular establishments or research groups. In addition, national/regional laboratory animal science associations frequently hold symposia or conferences, at which specific aspects of animal use are discussed and placed within context. Ideally, completion of such courses should be recognised formally, so that credit can be given to individuals who take the time and effort to keep their skills up to date.

Efforts have been made in some areas to harmonise training, but this may be easier for general courses than for specific research techniques, because of the greater number of organised training opportunities, the much greater size of the target group and the development of national and international guidelines. Specialist knowledge, for example in the husbandry and care of genetically altered animals, can be gained at an individual level by reading texts and visiting specialist websites, for example that of the International Society for Transgenic Technologies[1] etc.

Harmonisation of general courses within countries has been achieved in some cases, but to achieve the same within a continent or globally is much more of a challenge. None the less, efforts in that direction have been initiated by the International Council for Laboratory Animal Science (ICLAS)[2]. In contrast, the quality and volume of specific training offered by research groups is highly variable, and it is difficult to conceive a mechanism for ensuring sufficient training for the variety of specific procedures conducted.

What is competency?

Competency has been incorporated into European legislation for over two decades (European Council 1986), and remains central to current proposals to revise the European Directive 86/609[3], although this identifies a competent person only as someone '*who is considered by a member state to be competent to perform the relevant function described in the Directive*'. Beyond this the proposed Directive provides no guidance as to what might be expected from a competent person, although it recognises that quality and professional competence is required for assuring the welfare of animals, both for overseeing the care of animals on a daily basis and during the conduct of procedures. Reference is made to some duties which must be carried out only by competent persons, including performance of euthanasia and confirming the well-being and health of animals at least once daily. Those conducting scientific procedures must have appropriate veterinary or scientific education and training and have evidence of the requisite competence (Article 20, paragraph 2, sub-paragraph 1). Authorisation to carry out such investigations is valid only for a strictly limited period (5 years)

[1] http://www.transtechsociety.org/.
[2] www.iclas.org/harmonization.htm.
[3] http://www.europarl.europa.eu/sides/getDoc.do?pubRef=-//EP//TEXT+TA+P6-TA-2009-0343+0+DOC+XML+V0//EN&language=EN

and at the end of that time extensions shall be granted only on the basis of evidence of continuing competency.

There is very little agreement about the meaning of the word 'competence', although most people agree that it refers to the ability to perform a task or perhaps the skill with which it is performed. However, the word is more frequently used in a broader way, to refer to a person's overall ability to carry out a role satisfactorily, rather than just certain elements of it. It is also sometimes used to describe the detailed aspects of an individual's job performance, for example; '*this technician had demonstrated competency in sexing day-old mice*'. The EU Knowledge System for Lifelong Learning defines competence as '*an ability that extends beyond the possession of knowledge and skills. It includes cognitive competence, functional competence, personal competence and ethical competence*'[4].

For the purpose of this chapter, competence will be regarded as the ability of an individual to properly perform specific tasks that fall within their job remit. The term encompasses a combination of knowledge, skills and attitudes, which are applied to tasks being undertaken and which ensure that these are carried out efficiently and effectively. In the case of laboratory animal science, the relevant attitudes encompass recognition and application of the Three Rs at every opportunity, a high level of skill and empathy with animals for which the individual is responsible, openness and willingness to seek assistance and guidance whenever appropriate, and the ability to effectively communicate concerns if issues relating to animal welfare arise.

In the case of animal care staff, the range of skills that a competent person should possess would include the following:

- appreciation of the ethical issues associated with the scientific use of animals and the application of the Three Rs;
- working knowledge of national and local legislation and regulations; insofar as these relate to the sourcing, care and use of the species concerned, including any requirements of local ethical or care and use committees;
- ability to recognise departures from good health and knowledge of actions to take where this is detected;
- knowledge and skill in the handling and caring of animals including breeding stock and animals undergoing experiments;
- awareness of normal behaviour, and ability to recognise the causes and signs of pain, discomfort or distress and awareness of how to minimise these;
- skill in the administration of medicines (where prescribed by a veterinarian), basic husbandry procedures such as identification methods, breeding and checking for physical signs of good health;
- dexterity in animal handling, skill in selecting a suitable method and carrying out euthanasia if necessary and awareness of how to dispose of carcases;
- ability to communicate effectively with other care staff, including supervisors, and with scientists who may be carrying out experiments on animals being cared for;
- appreciation of the importance of good hygiene and biosecurity, and awareness of the procedures necessary to maintain these;
- appreciation of health and safety issues which may arise in the animal facility and awareness of how these should be addressed;
- understanding the importance of maintaining accurate records and aptitude in record maintenance.

Additionally, specific competencies may be developed relating to the ability to administer compounds, withdraw biological samples, carry out specific observations or make measurements using validated equipment, as directed by a scientist or other person, appropriately authorised and subject to compliance with local and legal requirements. Those with aptitude may develop competencies such as managing staff, overseeing facilities or the provision of specialist services.

A distinction can be made between basic competences relating to the ability to perform relatively routine tasks efficiently and effectively, following detailed instructions, where relevant, and more advanced competences in which individuals vary their behaviour when necessary, but always in an appropriate way. Highly competent people react almost intuitively by assessing the situation in its context, drawing from a repertoire of possible actions, determining which of these is most appropriate, monitoring the consequences of that action and adjusting their actions as appropriate. Highly competent people require experience and the ability to monitor outcomes and adapt actions according to the consequences. Such behaviour involves a continuous process of acting and reflecting. Basic and advanced competence can be developed by training. Both require an understanding of regulatory and other constraints on actions, and the ability to ensure that appropriate authority is obtained where necessary.

Development of competency involves a complex mix of education and teaching. Education is the process by which knowledge is accumulated, whereas teaching can be defined as the promotion and facilitation of learning. Of itself, teaching imparts neither knowledge nor skill – it simply helps the learner to acquire, understand and interpret information efficiently and effectively. The term training has been used to describe the facilitation of skills development. From the perspective of competence, teaching involves instruction and practice, which develop and enhance performance so as to help learners to carry out their responsibilities. The development of appropriate attitudes is a much more complicated issue, and depends partly upon the previous experience of the learner, organisational attitudes within the workplace and the professionalism and enthusiasm of those responsible for delivering training and education. The extent to which inherent attitudes can be modified by training is the subject of considerable debate, but there is no doubt that both the attitude of teachers and relationships with peers have an important influence.

Oversight of training

As noted earlier competence is '*the ability of an individual to properly perform specific tasks*'. This ability requires possession

[4]http://www.gramlinger.net/f_arbeit/LLL/glossary.pdf.

of appropriate manual skills, but without an appreciation of the principles that underlie the task, performance becomes automatic and unresponsive to any variation in demands, such as might arise from an unexpected event or a significant observation, this should not be regarded as competence.

A distinction also needs to be made between knowledge and understanding (Foshay & Tinkey 2007). The former refers to information which can be recalled to mind, but the latter requires that the facts can be assembled and used to enable concepts and principles to be developed and assessed and so contributes to flexibility of actions. Whilst knowledge of facts may be necessary to underpin understanding, additional processing is necessary to use them in a meaningful way.

Basic technical procedures can be learnt by following a series of steps without understanding why they are taken or the consequences of performing them; this is knowledge without understanding and an example might be close adherence to a standard operating procedure (SOP). However, when something is meaningfully understood, it is remembered much longer, provides the basis for developing further understanding and can be adapted to deal with emergencies or novel and perhaps more complex situations. For factual knowledge to become meaningful knowledge, it needs to be linked to a broader, previously learned, closely related context; a process known as assimilation. The weaker the association with that context, the less coherent is the resultant understanding and it may become necessary to substantially revise that context in order to enable conflicts to be resolved. The education, training and development of persons working with laboratory animals requires the learning of skills, the presentation and assimilation of knowledge and the incorporation of all these into a framework of understanding and responsiveness.

Although all individuals are ultimately responsible for developing their own knowledge and competence, legislation usually places additional responsibilities on those overseeing animal facilities. This responsibility often resides in a committee, such as an institutional animal care and use committee (IACUC) or ethical review committee, or an individual who has been granted a licence authorising specific animal experimentation at the establishment. Whatever the details of the arrangement, it is important that management should provide opportunities for individuals to acquire knowledge and skills, and establish mechanisms to ensure satisfactory standards of performance. Each establishment should establish a flexible framework to identify training needs and provide a mechanism for the promotion of learning, for example by delivering formal or informal training. The remit should include both primary training and lifelong learning, also known as continuing professional development (CPD). There are three key stages in such a framework:

1. planning and developing strategies to meet shortfalls and improve performance of the research programme;
2. taking action to maximise the performance of staff in the workplace;
3. evaluating the impact of training and development on the performance of individuals and the research output of establishment.

Many practical benefits result from a logically structured training programme including:

- Increased productivity in terms of scientific output and the quality of publications generated by skilled and motivated people who work more effectively.
- Improved motivation and greater understanding of the role of staff within the workplace. Improved personal development and recognition of achievements. This enhances morale, reduces staff turnover and absenteeism, and creates a climate in which change is more readily embraced. Motivation also encourages teamwork in the conduct of scientific investigations, with closer liaison between animal care staff scientists and those overseeing projects.
- Reduced costs and wastage, because skilled and motivated people work more effectively and consistently, delivering higher-quality scientific outputs.
- Recognition that the facility is comprised of effective and well trained individuals. This together with improved quality of programmes makes it easier to attract grants or commissions, or to identify promising research leads and lines. At academic establishments in many European countries, there is increased emphasis on the consistency and quality of scientific work.

The development of a training programme provides an opportunity to review current policies and practices and to identify areas where improvement is possible. It also provides a framework for planning future strategy and developing actions, and enables the creation of a structured system to enhance the effectiveness of training and development activities. Critical to this stage is the identification of priorities for education and training (Conarello & Shepherd 2007). The programme should take account of the size and type of establishment, the current knowledge and skills of staff, the complexity of the work, the rate of staff turnover and the level of support and advice available within the workplace. The framework provided by the four Federation of European Laboratory Animal Science Associations (FELASA) categories is often a convenient starting point. One strategy is to benchmark the provision of education and training against that of similar establishments undertaking similar work, and to adopt similar performance standards. Alternatively, views may be sought of key individuals such as line managers, veterinarians, senior scientists or their representatives, a member of the ethical review process and perhaps other key individuals such as client representatives or officials concerned with regulatory compliance. Often such a body already exists in the form of an animal care and use committee or similar, and in such cases this is likely to be the most effective tool. The training plan must identify clear targets based on the Three Rs, quality of science and the business or academic objectives of the organisation. The process should take account of perceived future skills requirements resulting from the introduction of new equipment or new technologies. While the training programme is being developed, there must be wide consultation with staff, particularly in large organisations or where staff work in distinct teams in different parts of a single organisation, for example where biosecurity arrangements preclude frequent mixing.

Mention has been made earlier of the importance of developing a culture of care within the establishment. Staff involved in animal experimentation should be trained to understand and appreciate what is required of them and to know how to perform effectively (Romick *et al.* 2006). Staff should be equipped with the necessary training, information tools and materials to perform effectively alongside others, and should be well acquainted with actions to be taken when problems arise. This information can be communicated by a variety of means, including: team briefings, focused seminars dealing with the technical and scientific progress of specific projects, circulation of newsletters, staff meetings and performance reviews. Whichever method is used, regular flow of information is important to ensure that all staff are acquainted with the activities of the organisation.

Job categories

Within Europe, appropriate education and training of all those engaged in the use of live vertebrate animals for scientific purposes are required by both the Council of Europe (Convention ETS 123, Article 26, Council of Europe 1986) and the European Union (Council Directive 86/609/EEC, Article 14, European Council 1986). In 1993, the parties of the European Convention ETS 123, issued a resolution to promote the development and uptake of training and educational programmes to meet the competency requirements set out in the Convention. The resolution acknowledged FELASA proposals, which identified four different categories of persons working with experimental animals:

- Category A: persons taking care of animals;
- Category B: persons carrying out experimental procedures;
- Category C: persons responsible for directing or designing experiments;
- Category D: laboratory animal science specialists.

FELASA subsequently published further clarification of these requirements basing its recommendations on functions common to the different categories, rather than on nomenclature, which may vary from country to country (FELASA 1995, FELASA 1999, FELASA 2000). Recommendations for practical, theoretical and ethical aspects were applicable for all categories and included implementation of the Three Rs, and the teaching syllabus for Category C persons is coming to be accepted more widely as providing a basis for training staff working in a range of different areas.

FELASA Category A Persons

These are sometimes known as animal care staff or, when their duties are principally related to routine animal husbandry and care, as animal caretakers. Four levels of complexity of job function are identified within this category.

Level 1 relates to persons who provide basic laboratory animal care, working in accordance with verbal or written instructions and under close supervision by an experienced member of staff. Such staff should appreciate the needs of the animals they work with and understand the legal and ethical principles associated with their care and use. Amongst other things, Level 1 staff may carry out routine cleaning, feeding and watering, check animals for their well-being, operate and maintain cleaning and sterilisation equipment and monitor and record animal environmental conditions.

Level 2 persons have more experience and are able to work more independently. They are expected to have greater knowledge and practical skills than Level 1 staff and may work within specialised animal facilities involving special biocontainment measures or complex care routines and may assist in training Level 1 animal care staff. They are likely to be responsible for daily routines, breeding programmes and specialist husbandry procedures such as post-surgical care and monitoring.

Level 3 persons may hold supervisory or managerial posts and be regularly involved in training and developing animal care staff and overseeing their activities. They are also responsible for more complex activities such as allocation of resources, oversight of breeding programmes, monitoring heath and safety issues, preparing reports and liaising with researchers.

Level 4 persons are familiar with theoretical and practical aspects of laboratory animal science and may occupy senior managerial positions within complex animal facilities or possess other specialised skills relevant to their organisation. Some personnel at this level may have responsibilities resembling those of FELASA Category D laboratory animal specialists. Category A Level 4 staff may not be present in small-scale animal facilities.

At the time of writing, FELASA is revising its Category A training guidelines and is likely to recommend fewer levels.

FELASA Category B persons

These are scientists who carry out experiments on animals (FELASA 2000). Article 26 of the Council of Europe Convention (Council of Europe 1986) requires that such persons shall be appropriately educated and trained. The competencies identified by FELASA for those working at Category B level include awareness of the ethical framework within which animal experiments are conducted and national and European legislation and regulations which have arisen from these. They should be skilled in performing the techniques they will use, be able to handle animals of the relevant species without stressing them, be able to recognise departures from good welfare and to take appropriate action to avoid or at least minimise these when they occur. Within Europe, there remain considerable differences between national requirements for training and development, although there is a proposal in the draft new Directive, to urge member states to work towards common standards. Similarly, the European Science Foundation has called on member organisations to develop and organise accredited courses on laboratory animal science, including information on animal alternatives, welfare and ethics with a view to establishing more uniform standards[5].

---

[5]European Science Foundation Policy Briefing 15 (August 2001 – second edition). Use of animals in research http://www.esf.org/publications/policy-briefings.html

FELASA Category C persons

These persons design and oversee experiments on living animals (FELASA 1995). They should possess a university degree or equivalent in a biomedical discipline at the level of Bachelor or Master, and have completed a basic training programme equivalent to 80h. In addition, where it is intended to use specialised techniques, such as surgery, or to work with different species, such as non-human primates, dogs or cats, additional expertise should be obtained by collaborating with experienced investigators and animal care staff, or by attending specialised courses. Category C persons must: appreciate the basic needs and care of animals and the importance of maintaining them in good health; have familiarity with methods of alleviating pain, including correct use of anaesthetic and analgesic regimes; and understand the need for safe working practices. Because they may be involved in designing experiments, they must also be aware of the importance of implementing the Three Rs.

FELASA Category D Persons

These are specialists in laboratory animal science (FELASA 1999). The category may include veterinarians, some Category A staff at Level 4, nutritionists, geneticists, architects designing and supervising construction of facilities, pathologists working in diagnostic laboratories etc. Most specialists are university graduates who have acquired particular expertise and experience relevant to laboratory animal science. In addition, they should be aware of all key aspects of the care and uses of laboratory animals. Category D persons should be capable of managing animal, human and physical resources in a laboratory animal facility, securing the health and welfare of animals, providing support to investigators, ensuring compliance with all relevant laws, regulations and guidelines, ensuring the availability of education and training in the humane care and use of laboratory animals and making personal contributions to the humane care and use of laboratory animals by carrying out research in laboratory animal science.

FELASA recommendations for the syllabus for Category A persons

FELASA proposed that Category A persons preparing for a career in animal care, should initially study for Level 1 examinations (FELASA 1995). These involve learning to handle the commoner species of laboratory animals – the rat, mouse, guinea pig, hamster and rabbit. They should also learn the different techniques and demonstrate competence in handling them and carrying out euthanasia. Trainees are also expected to understand relevant legislation and ethics, and to know how to meet the basic needs of animals including their care and husbandry, as well as learning about routines in animal houses, including health checks, etc.

After a period of approximately 2 years gaining relevant experience by working in animal facilities, FELASA envisaged Category A persons commencing studies towards Level 2. They are expected to develop a deeper appreciation of legislation relating to the care and uses of laboratory animals and an awareness of safety issues in the animal facility, including safe working practices. During this period, care staff should acquire an understanding of the biology and husbandry requirements of a range of different species, including their nutritional requirements and relevant feeding practices, and the principles and practices underlying management of breeding colonies. They should understand the impact of ill-health on animal colonies and be competent to assess, record and report the health status of species for which they are responsible. Care staff are expected to develop competence in handling a range of less common species of animals, to understand the different methods of euthanasia and know how to choose between them. The syllabus also requires an understanding of the commoner scientific and technical procedures that might be carried out on laboratory animals.

Level 3 builds on the experience gained at Level 2 and at least 3 years of relevant work experience at Level 2 is recommended. Level 3 training prepares personnel for management responsibilities, and includes study of theoretical and practical aspects of managing an animal facility, including budgetary controls, resources allocation and oversight of staffing. Staff at this level are expected to have a good working knowledge of legislation. They should understand the principles of designing animal facilities and the practicalities of environmental monitoring (including the need for and the use of measuring equipment). The syllabus includes more detailed study of the care requirements of a range of different species, a working knowledge of how to recognise and alleviate pain, suffering and distress. It also requires an understanding of the management of conventional and specialised breeding and non-breeding colonies, including a more detailed understanding of their nutritional requirements and the way these should be met. It is also expected that personnel at this level should understand the principles of study design and the conduct of experimental procedures, including anaesthesia, surgery, post-operative care, etc.

Implementation of training schemes for animal care staff training schemes

Several national training schemes have been established for animal care staff and some of these are recognised worldwide. Three of these will be considered in outline here: those organised by the American Association for Laboratory Animal Science (AALAS), the Institute of Animal Technology (IAT) and the Canadian Association for Laboratory Animal Science (CALAS). In general, the syllabus does not differ greatly from that recommended by FELASA.

Each scheme recognises three levels of competence, summarised in Table 15.1. The lowest level in each case is appropriate for trainee technicians who have relatively recently entered the field and the experience required is relatively basic. AALAS requires those seeking this qualification to have at least 6 months' experience of laboratory animal science, depending upon their academic qualifications at the time the work commences. IAT does not lay down specific requirements; CALAS expects applicants to have a high

Table 15.1 Levels of competence recognised by three major care-staff associations.

Organisation	*Qualification*		
	Basic	*Intermediate*	*Advanced*
AALAS	Assistant laboratory animal technician	Laboratory animal technician	Laboratory animal technologist
IAT	First Certificate in Animal Husbandry	First Diploma in Animal Technology	National Certificate in Animal Technology
CALAS	Associate registered laboratory animal technician	Registered laboratory animal technician	Registered master laboratory animal technician

school diploma or have worked in animal facility full-time for at least 3 years and to have already successfully completed three basic study modules. In each case, assessment is based on written examinations. IAT and CALAS also stipulate an oral examination and, in the case of the latter, a formal practical examination.

For all three organisations the intermediate level qualification is the basic qualification for experienced laboratory animal technicians. Entry requirements are rather more diverse. The stipulation by AALAS is similar to that for the entry level – at least 6 months work-experience, possibly extending up to 3 years, depending on previous formal educational experience. In the case of the IAT, a candidate would normally hold the First Certificate in Animal Husbandry, although this is not mandatory and some exemptions are available for previous educational experience. CALAS is more prescriptive and requires 5 years of experience after successful completion of the basic qualification.

The most advanced level of qualification is intended for individuals entering senior management positions within animal care facilities. Entry requirements are generally more rigorous, and in the case of CALAS include completion of the intermediate qualification and 5 years of additional continued employment in the field of laboratory animal science.

All organisations encourage involvement with continuing educational programmes, and contribute to the provision of these, but CALAS is the only one requiring all persons holding registered qualifications to meet annual requirements in order to maintain their status.

By contrast, in Australia a national scheme for training animal care staff has been established by the National Training Information Service, and is delivered by a number of local providers at Certificate and Diploma levels over a period of 2 years. The process is competency-based and recognises three levels, corresponding to those who perform care tasks, those who manage them and persons who evaluate and revise practices[6].

Orientating the new employee

Recruitment of new employees is often regarded as a means of addressing a particular task within the department, but it should also be seen in the context of developing future talent and contributing to the overall culture of care within the establishment (Pritt & Duffee 2007). The first few days are important in setting ground rules for the new position, but also in shaping the attitude of a new colleague and integrating him or her into the workforce. Orientation is best done by the immediate line manager, who understands the role of the new employee but is not so senior as to appear remote from the work to be done; although it is helpful to briefly introduce the recruit to senior management at an early stage (Silverman 2002). Make sure that sufficient time is made available for the person to fully understand the key aspects of their role. If it is not the immediate supervisor who is providing the orientation, new employees should be introduced to that person as soon as possible.

Right at the beginning of employment, the line manager should ensure that immediate work details such as the employment contract, pay roll, medical tests etc are dealt with; it may also be necessary for recruits to attend courses or be briefed about responses to emergencies, such as fire procedures and what to do in case of accidents. On a new employee's first day it makes good managerial sense also to sit down and discuss the function of the organisation and the facility within which the employee will be working, the staffing structure and the organisational culture, including responsibilities, humane treatment of animals, sources of advice, whistle-blowing policies, etc. A clear, alternative channel of communication should be established wherever possible, although not for regular use. Where the organisation has a clear mission statement this should be presented and placed in context. Inform the new person about the management style of the organisation and the department, how the role of each individual relates to the organisation and what is expected of them. This personal touch demonstrates the manager's awareness of the activities of the department and informs the recruit about the context of the role so that it is easier for them to come back with questions subsequently should that be necessary. The training expectations and opportunities and the routes for promotion should also be explained. Where it is anticipated that close supervision will be needed for some time this should be indicated clearly.

It is a good idea to accompany new employees to the first rest break of the day, and at this to introduce him or her or to other staff. This provides a relatively stress-free way of introducing the employee to colleagues and vice versa.

If possible, a check list should be developed for orientating new employees. This should identify what information needs to be given up front, and what new arrivals should work out for themselves. Examples of the former may

[6] http://www.ntis.gov.au

include matters bearing on health and safety, current working routines (such as working hours, lunch and rest breaks), holiday entitlements etc and key contacts both for gaining advice and seeking assistance when necessary; it is a good idea to have this laid out in a staff handbook or similar so that misunderstandings can be avoided. The nature of material which new employees should work out for themselves depends upon the level of employment, and may be relatively basic, or may relate to much more complex issues, for example staffing roles, workloads and procedures and practices. It is also helpful to have available written briefing materials appropriate to the role of the employee. Such materials may include information about staffing numbers, grades and competences, animal health records, SOPs, minutes of committee meetings etc; again, a check list is helpful.

Developing practical skills

The most effective method of delivering training depends upon the topic to be addressed, the learner's background and preferred way of learning, the trainer's skills and preferences and the facilities available. Wherever possible, a mix of teachers and teaching styles is preferable to a continuous series of lectures, practical classes or seminars. Formal lectures should be restricted to between 45 minutes and an hour, followed by a short break (or a question and answer session) during which students can assimilate what they have been told. Whatever method of training is adopted, students should be encouraged to actively use the information by encouraging participative learning, which is a powerful way of reinforcing learning and relating it to real-life issues.

Competence in the care of animals depends crucially on practical skills, the development of which is an essential part of training in laboratory animal science and requires careful consideration. Hands-on exercises provide a means of relating theoretical understanding (taught alongside or previously) to hands-on skills. Despite this, the teaching of practical skills often receives less attention than that given to knowledge and understanding, probably because it involves a more demanding learning environment and it is more difficult to assess and record levels of performance. These obstacles are easier to overcome than is often assumed.

No course can teach all of the practical skills required by someone working in laboratory animal science, so the objective is to equip students with sufficient theoretical understanding and practical skill to enable them to address practical issues in a safe, ethical and systematic way and to know when to seek help and from whom. Practical skills may be developed as part of formal training courses, subsequently under supervision or, ideally, both. Whichever route is chosen, learning should be supported by enthusiastic, experienced staff. This helps to develop a commitment to achieving and sustaining practical competence in preparation for working independently. In order to ensure the quality of the process, it is important that learning takes place within a structured framework, is overtly linked to underlying theoretical principles, is formally documented and is properly assessed. However, it must also be made clear that this basic training is only the first stage of a lifelong process of learning and development, during which time practices and procedures are likely to change.

Animal care staff can generally devote considerable time to developing expertise and competence, but throughout this process they should be supported and mentored by experienced colleagues. It is particularly important that new employees are made to feel part of a team and that the contribution of their work to the team and the animals for which they care is acknowledged. It is during this early period of training that a good working relationship with more experienced care staff is developed.

If it is proposed to use live animals, the instructor should judge whether this is essential for development of the relevant skills, students must be made aware of their ethical and legal responsibilities and it may be necessary to consult with the ethical review process before commencing. Animals should never be subjected to unnecessary pain, suffering or harm, although the use of animals to teach techniques such as handling, restraint, sexing and basic technical procedures, can cause distress to naïve animals. One way of dealing with this difficulty is to maintain a small stock of animals that have been accustomed to being handled, and are used principally for training purposes. Such animals become compliant, their behaviour is more predictable and they are less likely to be perceived as threatening. Animals used for teaching practical skills should be in good health.

If possible, lessons should be organised to be species- or technique-specific, and learner groups kept as small as possible; one-to-one training is best. In addition, only the smallest number of animals necessary to develop appropriate skills should be used and there must be adequate technical oversight so that each student can be closely supervised during the learning period, and given assistance if necessary. Learners should be allowed to progress at their own pace, to ask questions, receive accurate and supportive feedback and helped promptly to rectify faults. If a formal lesson is involved, it must allow sufficient time for a concluding question and answer session. This allows learners and teacher to critically assess progress and performance. In addition tutors should subsequently assess how well the session went.

Before initiating lessons involving the handling of animals, it is a good idea to explain the techniques with the help of video presentations, practise with surrogate models and then to progress to non-sentient models, which are made as realistic as possible. Sometimes it may be appropriate to carry out a technique on a recently killed animal or possibly one that has been anaesthetised or sedated. These techniques allow tasks to be paused during their performance thereby allowing discussion of key aspects, which would not be possible using conscious animals. When this stage has been completed, or where sentient animals are not involved, teaching usually proceeds with the demonstrator carrying out the practical task, with a commentary explaining its purpose and importance, indicating possible health and safety issues and emphasising possible refinement and reduction methods, safe working practices etc. Skilled performance of a task is characterised by speed and dexterity. Indeed some tasks are difficult to conduct at slow speed;

examples include: capturing an animal in a large cage, opening the mouth of a rabbit or rat to examine its teeth or performing euthanasia.

After demonstrating the task, each student should be asked to repeat it several times, and whilst doing so to provide a commentary. Putting the process into words helps learners to remember the different stages or steps involved. In addition, requiring students to demonstrate a technique immediately after it has been shown to them is a useful way of identifying deficiencies or problems that exist in the completion of that skill and enabling these to be corrected before they become assimilated.

As with teaching theoretical knowledge, a list of practical skills, which a student is required to learn, should be shown to students at the beginning of their training. Also, each class should be logically structured, and one way of achieving this is to prepare a worksheet, which lists the stages and competencies expected. An assessment schedule should be prepared, based on those key points and the assessment process itself should be clearly separated from the process of learning. It is good practice to ask whether the trainee is ready for the assessment to begin or whether he or she would prefer to defer it to later. The proficiency with which the task is performed should be judged using a formal check sheet which lists the key elements which make it up; for example such a list might include having minimal impact on the animal's well-being, successfully achieving the required effect, speed, precision, safe working practices, understanding the underlying rationale etc. Wherever possible a means should also be found of allowing the trainee to comment on the learning process and difficulties which he or she may have experienced, so that future learning sessions can take account of these perceptions.

When training personnel who are already working with laboratory animals at a different establishment, learning may be enhanced by adopting a bidirectional process, in which the instructor asks how the procedure is done at the learner's home institution followed by a discussion about the strengths and weaknesses of various aspects of the method.

Evaluating competence

It is important that supervisors should be able to assess the competence of those for whom they are responsible. This presupposes that competency can be demonstrated by measurable actions and that the effectiveness with which these are performed can be assessed. Competence cannot easily be measured by setting written examinations or formally structured practical examinations. In particular, it is difficult to assess the attitudes of individuals or their ability to respond promptly and effectively to the unexpected, and in such matters the quality of supervision and workplace support is paramount. Fortunately, in the case of animal care staff, basic competence can usually be judged by observing the performance of individuals in the workplace, the way they handle and respond to the needs of animals, their ability to identify signs of distress or disturbance and their appreciation of the biological requirements of an animal.

Records of competence

In order for an establishment to provide evidence that measures have been taken to ensure that staff working with laboratory animals are competent, it is important that appropriate records are maintained (Pritt *et al.* 2004). Records should include all staff, including researchers, animal care staff, long-term visitors and students, maintenance, quality assurance and other technical staff whose work may have a direct or indirect effect on the well-being of laboratory animals. At regular intervals line managers should review progress with each employee to ensure that appropriate competences are either proven, or being addressed; this can take place at periodic staff appraisals or performance reviews.

An induction checklist similar to that recommended for the orientation of new employees, can be used for those whose work involves only a very limited range of issues.

Records of training and competence have a number of functions:

- They enable each staff member to be able to demonstrate that they have taken measures to develop appropriate competences.
- They provide staff members with an overall training structure, which over time they will expect to complete. They also demonstrate progress.
- They enable supervisors and managers to gain an overview of the training and development currently undertaken, the resources required to meet this and future demands.
- They demonstrate compliance with the requirements of the Directive and national legislation.
- They save time by ensuring that staff and their supervisors can find relevant information easily.
- They provide a means of analysing areas where a particular focus on training is appropriate, in order to ensure that all staff are bought up to a satisfactory level of competence.
- They may be useful in allocating scientific and technical staff to particular projects, for which they have demonstrated competence.

A distinction should be made between records of competence and records of training, which are less immediate measures of performance. The record should establish when employees started to learn about each task which they are expected to perform, when and by whom competence was deemed to have been achieved, evidence of periodic updating and, where appropriate, the level of that competence. For example, an employee may be deemed competent to perform a task under supervision, unsupervised or to train others to do it. As competences progress, the trainer or line manager should sign off each task for each student. Personnel who attend external training sessions should maintain certificates of attendance with the remainder of the file, in a scanned electronic format when this is necessary.

Records may be kept as a hard copy files such as a looseleaf folder. This is a relatively simple process, is easily understood, robust, in so far as only one copy exists and it therefore contains all relevant documents and can be made the responsibility of each employee. The disadvantage is that they are available only to the person who holds them,

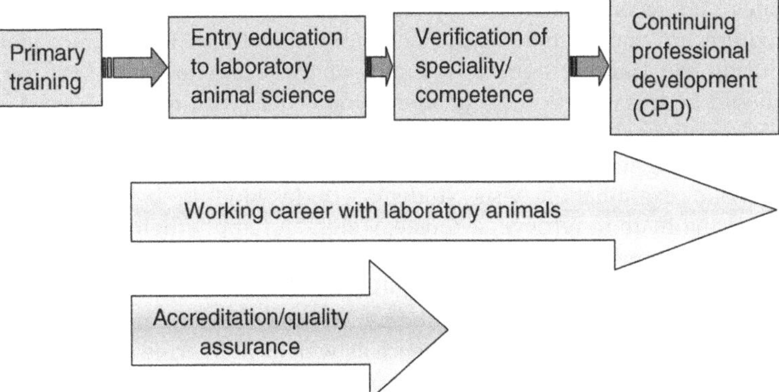

Figure 15.1 Schematic representation of life-long education in laboratory animal science.

they could be misplaced, it is time consuming to compare training and competencies of a number of employees and they are geographically restricted to one area of the organisation and therefore unavailable to others who may wish to make use of them.

There are several benefits to maintaining records of competence on relational databases. They can be set up to actively notify staff, supervisors and managers of the current status of training and additional requirements; they may also facilitate evaluation of courses attended by summarising assessment outcomes, course or course provider evaluations and assessments and comments. Electronic records are easily backed up and retrieved and may be distributed by e-mail or printed out when necessary. However, it is important to ensure that electronic records are filed securely, that they are accurate and kept up to date and can only be accessed by authorised personnel.

Life-long learning or continuing professional development

The necessity of life-long learning, also called continuing professional development (CPD), cannot be overemphasised. Training and education in laboratory animal science must be seen as a continuum starting immediately after completion of entry or formal training and proceeding throughout an individual's career; this is illustrated in Figure 15.1. During this process, there are various quality assurance elements (eg, accreditation of entry education programmes, certification of individuals, speciality examinations and assessment of competence).

It is anticipated that in Europe revision of the Directive (86/609/EEC) will extend the requirement for education and training to include maintenance of competence in all categories. In Europe, the speciality board for veterinarians – ECLAM (European College of Laboratory Animal Veterinarians) – and in the US, ACLAM (American College of Laboratory Animal Medicine), have both introduced systems of life-long learning[7,8]. In the US, AALAS also has a Registry Program for all levels of animal care technicians where documented CPD is required. There is an urgent and compelling need to establish additional systematic frameworks for life-long learning for all the categories of individuals working with laboratory animals, and at the time of writing FELASA has engaged with this task by setting up a working group to consider a number of proposals.

The existing and future systems of life-long learning rely on: supplementary courses, such as those described for experimental design (Howard *et al.* 2009); seminars which are organised by several commercial companies; scientific meetings; workshops; and electronic course offerings. It is also likely that more training and education opportunities suitable for life-long learning will appear in the near future. The importance of supervision and CPD training in achieving and maintaining competence and in contributing to good science and welfare needs to be more widely recognised within the research community, both locally within research establishments and by those funding research[9].

In all training and education there are some items which one is required to master, some with which one should be familiar and finally those which may be nice to know. Allocation of learning should be weighted accordingly with required items filling a majority (about 80%) of the allocated time, while the 'nice to know' pieces may only need a 5% timeslot.

Quality schemes

The delivery of training is a long-term process usually involving inputs from a number of different individuals. In view of this, it is most important that there is a mechanism in place to ensure high-quality delivery at an appropriate level and time, and that it is effective and within budget. Wherever possible, the assurance of quality should involve a mechanism quite independent of the training process, so as to avoid any conflict of interest. At its simplest, this may involve scrutiny of the results of assessment but a more thorough approach is to also consider the experience of those who have been trained, the quality of their work before and after training and their productivity.

People need to be competent in all aspects of animal care and use with which they will be involved. There are various ways of assessing competence and various problems that need to be overcome in order to do so. Practical skills cannot usually be taught in a short course so there need to be ways of assessing people over the requisite period. Most guide-

[7]http://www.eclam.org/index.php?id=3
[8]http://www.aclam.org/education/training/index.html.

[9]http://www.apc.gov.uk/reference/2006%2012%2013%20Home%20Office%20response%20on%20Mod%20training.pdf.

lines and recommendations in laboratory animal science require an examination at the end, and sometimes also during the training period. The aim of the examination should be to assess how the student would deal with real-life situations. It is good practice for instructors to combine various taught elements in order to check comprehension. A good examination tests students' understanding by requiring them to retrieve, evaluate, weigh and apply their knowledge and to demonstrate learnt skills.

Irrespective of the training method, feedback from the trainees is a crucial part of the process. This may be done at the end of the educational experience as well as at intermediate time points. Common approaches are by use of an anonymous form or by verbal communication. Questionnaires are increasingly being used on the internet, and quite often a standard format is adopted within an institution, which allows comparisons with other courses.

In addition to training period evaluation, participants can be asked to carry out a self-evaluation (ie, do they feel that they truly learned and did the final outcome genuinely match expectations they had prior to the course). This can be anonymous if in a written form.

The way in which feedback is used for planning future training depends on several factors. Sometimes teachers have difficulties in finding proper ways to make improvements because the feedback may be conflicting. Usually feedback which has active elements proves the most useful and rewarding.

As indicated above, some countries have established schemes to certify the education and training of both animal technicians and veterinary specialists in laboratory animal science or medicine. For example, in UK the Home Office requires that Named Veterinary Surgeons have received appropriate post-graduate specialist training. At present, there are few schemes with similar aims for research technicians and scientists, and attendance at a course of verified quality is often considered to be sufficient. Unfortunately, there are limited opportunities for research technicians to achieve specialist competence certification. There is an example of such a system in a related professional area. The Federation of European Toxicologists & European Societies of Toxicology (EUROTOX) administers a programme based on theoretical training in toxicology and associated practical working, completion of which allows use of the title 'European registered toxicologist'[10].

Within Europe, the most widely based accreditation scheme is that established by FELASA in 2002. This offers assurance about course quality and is intended to promote wider harmonisation of education and training provision in laboratory animal science (FELASA 2002). The scheme is operated by an accreditation board and is open to courses which develop full competence in any of the FELASA categories. It also provides for the recognition of other well established, non-European courses in laboratory animal science, provided they lead to the development of comparable competences. Currently, the scheme does not extend to CPD, although this may be added in the future. Course organisers wishing to apply for accreditation submit details of the curriculum, describe the methodology and materials used in teaching and course frequency and size. The board also requests sight of assessment results, evaluations of the course by students and information about the background of teaching staff; clarification or further information may be requested if necessary. Members of the board visit each course and prepare a report which is considered by the full board and also sent to the course organiser. Courses organisers submit an annual, or for courses lasting more than 1 year, biennial report. The accreditation process is conducted and maintained in strict confidence.

[10]http://www.sciencedirect.com/science?_ob=ArticleURL&_udi=B7GJ4-4S9NG6T-3&_user=10&_rdoc=1&_fmt=&_orig=search&_sort=d&view=c&_acct=C000050221&_version=1&_urlVersion=0&_userid=10&md5=4bc1b154ca5a32720e84b38bc119b635.

References

Conarello, S.L. and Shepherd, M.J. (2007) Training strategies for research investigators and technicians. *ILAR Journal*, **48**, 120–130

Council of Europe (1986) *Convention for the Protection of Vertebrate Animals used for Experimental and other Scientific Purposes* (ETS 123). Strasbourg. http://conventions.coe.int/treaty/en/Treaties/Html/123.htm (accessed 27 April 2008)

Duffee, N., Nevalainen, T. and Hau, J. (2003) Education and training. In: *Handbook of Laboratory Animal Science, Vol I. Essential Principles and Practice*, 2nd edn. Eds Hau J. and van Hoosier, G.L. Jr, pp. 63–75. CRC Press, Boca Raton

Carlsson, H.E., Hagelin, J., Höglund, A.U. *et al.* (2001) Undergraduate and postgraduate students' responses to mandatory courses (FELASA category C) in Laboratory Animal Science. *Laboratory Animals*, **35**, 188–193

European Council (1986) Council Directive 86/609/EEC of 24 November 1986 on the approximation of laws, regulations and administrative provisions of the Member States regarding the protection of animals used for experimental and other scientific purposes. *Off J Eur Comm L*, **358**, 1–29. Brussels. http://eur-lex.europa.eu/LexUriServ/LexUriServ.do?uri=CELEX:31986L0609:EN:NOT (accessed 27 April 2008)

Federation of European Laboratory Animal Science Associations (1995) FELASA recommendations on the education and training of persons working with laboratory animals: Categories A and C. *Laboratory Animals*, **29**, 121–131

Federation of European Laboratory Animal Science Associations (1999) FELASA guidelines for education of specialists in laboratory animal science (Category D). *Laboratory Animals*, **29**, 1–15

Federation of European Laboratory Animal Science Associations (2000) FELASA recommendations for the education and training of persons carrying out animal experiments (Category B). *Laboratory Animals*, **34**, 229–235

Federation of European Laboratory Animal Science Associations (2002) FELASA recommendations for the accreditation of laboratory animal science education and training. *Laboratory Animals*, **36**, 373–377

Foshay, W.R. and Tinkey, P.R. (2007) Evaluating the effectiveness of training strategies: performance goals and testing. *ILAR Journal*, **48**, 156–162

Howard, B., Hudson, M. and Preziosi, R. (2009) More is less: reducing animal use by raising awareness of the principles of efficient study design and analysis. *ATLA*, **37**, 33–42

Nevalainen, T. (2004) Training for reduction in laboratory animal use. *ATLA*, **32** (Suppl 2), 65–67

Pritt, S., Samalonis, P., Bindley, L. *et al.* (2004) Creating a comprehensive training documentation program. *Lab Animal*, **33**, 38–41

Pritt, S. and Duffee, N. (2007) Training strategies for animal care technicians and veterinary technical staff. *ILAR Journal*, **48**, 109–119

Romick, M.L., Chavez, J. and Bishop, B. (2006) An interdisciplinary performance-based approach to training laboratory animal technicians. *Lab Animal*, **35**, 35–39

Russell, W. and Burch, R. (1959) *The Principles of Humane Experimental Technique*. Methuen, London. (2nd edn 1992 UFAW) http://altweb.jhsph.edu/publications/humane_exp/het-toc.htm accessed September 2007 (accessed 27 April 2008)

Silverman, J. (2002) *Managing the Laboratory Animal Facility*. CRC Press, Boca Raton

16 Positive reinforcement training for laboratory animals

Gail Laule

Introduction

Every animal kept in captivity deserves high standards of animal care. Laboratory animals are no exception; nonetheless, animals housed and managed in a laboratory setting do provide unique challenges. Issues of particular welfare importance, and of relevance to this chapter, are that they may be handled more frequently and subjected to a wider range of more invasive husbandry and medical procedures than most other captive animals.

To maximise the welfare of laboratory animals, it is most desirable to perform these procedures with as little stress for the animals as possible. Less stressed animals make better research models and produce the most reliable research results (Bloomsmith 1992; Reinhardt 1997a, 1997b; Lambeth *et al.* 2006). There are, therefore, dual incentives to protect and enhance the well-being of the animals and mitigate the special conditions of the laboratory setting.

In day-to-day management activities, animals are being trained all the time, whether the staff realise it or not. Every time anyone interacts with an animal, there is some training/communication occurring. The more frequent the interaction, the more established the resultant behaviours become. Animal care staff such as veterinarians, researchers and technicians can produce changes in the animals' behaviour even though they may be unaware that they are effectively training the animal. When a member of animal care staff places a desirable food item in a cage, opens the door and the animal moves into that cage, training has occurred because behaviour has been impacted which can be explained in operant conditioning terms. Nonetheless, much better results can be attained by consciously and deliberately implementing the training process.

The specific terms and techniques of operant conditioning have changed little since B.F. Skinner conducted his original research and presented his results in his book, *The Behavior of Organisms,* in 1938. What has evolved, however, has been the increasing use of these techniques in the care and management of captive animals. There has also been a corresponding development of interest in measuring the effects of training through objective and scientific studies. Therefore, this chapter provides a review of basic training methods, practical suggestions for integrating a positive reinforcement training approach into the management of animals in the laboratory setting, as well as examples of new applications and assessments of training.

Most of the applications of training for management, husbandry and medical purposes in the biomedical field have focused on non-human primates and dogs. As a domestic species and common household pet, laboratory dogs are usually managed differently to other animals, with direct contact in the form of petting, playing, walking on a leash and manual restraint for simple procedures. Training is used to augment an inherently positive human–animal relationship where simple verbal praise has significant value to many individual animals. There are many good resources on the training of dogs within the laboratory setting (Joint Working Group on Refinement (JWGR) 2004; Lindsay 2005; Meunier 2006) and many others on general dog training that present positive training techniques that can be applied to the laboratory setting (Donaldson 1996; Pryor 1999; McConnell 2002; Colflesh 2004) so this area will not be covered in depth in this chapter.

On the other hand, non-human primates are wild animals and do not have an inherent affiliation to humans, in fact, often quite the opposite. The variety of species and numbers of individual animals in laboratories make them prime subjects for a detailed discussion on methods to most effectively and humanely manage and maintain primates in the laboratory setting. The use of training techniques with primates is focused on developing a positive human–animal relationship, gaining safe access to individuals whether singly housed or in a group setting, and gaining an animal's voluntary co-operation in husbandry and medical procedures so that more negative forms of restraint and coercion can be reduced or eliminated.

Farm animals used in research are also prime candidates for training, especially swine. As another group of domesticated animals, the emphasis is on developing a positive human–animal relationship and using positive handling techniques to minimise stress during restraint and to gain voluntary co-operation to the extent of their cognitive abilities, with swine being more amenable to more complex training objectives.

Finally, rodents, rabbits and birds, which make up the vast majority of animals used in research, raise different issues, as they are small enough to be easily handled and restrained for most procedures. Although rodents are capable of learning a wide range of tasks as evidenced by numerous experiments by Skinner and others (Skinner 1938; Ferster 1953; Skinner & Ferster 1970; Hernstein 1997), in most cases training will be fairly basic, with a focus primarily on developing a positive human–animal context based on patience and empathy, and a calm, gentle handling style. A culture of training animals to cooperate also encourages a proactive approach to finding the most positive, least invasive method of achieving research objectives.

Despite the differences in training objectives between species, the techniques discussed in this chapter are universal and applicable to all species and individuals to varying degrees. An array of benefits is possible for all laboratory animals, and therefore these techniques should be considered and applied whenever it is reasonable and feasible to do so.

Positive reinforcement training

Operant conditioning offers two basic options for managing behaviour: positive reinforcement and negative reinforcement or escape/avoidance. The training discussed and recommended in this chapter is based on the use of positive reinforcement. In a positive reinforcement-based system, animals are rewarded with something they like for responding appropriately to the animal care staff's cues or commands (Pryor 1999). Animals gain the opportunity to voluntarily co-operate in procedures, rather than being forced to do so. Positive reinforcement training does not require food or water deprivation. Animals are always provided their daily allotment of food and water and training rewards are often the more preferred diet items, or special treats reserved for training alone.

This differs from negative reinforcement training, where the animal performs the correct behaviour in order to escape or avoid something it does not like. This 'something' can be as simple as being physically handled or lightly restrained. Operationally, it may not be feasible to use positive reinforcement exclusively; however, the positive alternatives should be exhausted before any kind of negative reinforcement is employed. If an escape/avoidance technique is necessary, its use should be kept to a minimum and balanced by positive reinforcement. For example, restraining an animal in a squeeze cage can be immediately followed by offering the animal a preferred food treat.

Negative reinforcement

The use of negative reinforcement to modify and control behaviour is achieved by pairing pain, discomfort or an unpleasant experience with a particular object or behaviour (Pryor 1999). Fear of the discomfort triggers an escape/avoidance response, which leads to performance of the desired behaviour. Unfortunately, captive animal management practices have traditionally included a large measure of negative reinforcement. The most commonly used negative reinforcers in the laboratory include equipment like nets, gloves or crowding boards used to coerce animals into squeeze cages and other restraint devices. In most facilities, devices like squeeze backs are used as a routine means of encouraging and/or forcing animals to the front of the cage for access and manipulation. Unfortunately, the use of tactics like these is sometimes accompanied by other unpleasant stimuli like authoritative or loud voices and physical threats, up to and including chasing of animals (ie, primates in large corral situations, livestock in pens) by animal care staff.

Although negative reinforcement works, it could be argued that there is an inherent cost to the animal's overall welfare by being forced to co-operate through the threat of a negative event or experience that elicits fear or anxiety (Reinhardt 1992; Laule & Desmond 1997; Pryor 1999). Studies with farm animals have shown a high degree of fear response associated with negative handling methods, which is surprising since these are domesticated species. In one study on the handling of heifers, using negative methods that included hits and slaps, remote blood sampling through indwelling jugular catheters showed both acute and chronic stress responses in fearful animals (Breuer *et al.* 1998). Negative handling methods with chickens often lead to escape reactions with associated injury, decreased breeding behaviour and greater inter-flock aggression (Jones 1997).

A study on dog training methods found that dogs trained exclusively using reward-based methods were reported to be significantly more obedient and to exhibit fewer problem behaviours, such as food stealing and over-excitement, than dogs trained using negative methods (including punishment), or even a combination of positive and negative methods (Hiby *et al.* 2004).

Smith and Swindle (2006, p. 62) note that swine are highly intelligent and have excellent memories. Therefore, much more effort is necessary to overcome the effects of negative handling experiences compared with the effort expended in using positive reinforcement for training (Smith & Swindle 2006).

Benefits of positive reinforcement training

In contrast to the costs to animal welfare associated with the use of negative reinforcement, positive reinforcement can achieve similar results with minimal costs and significant benefits. Positive reinforcement training (PRT) can be used to enhance the care, management and welfare of laboratory animals in a number of ways (Kirkwood *et al.* 1989; Reinhardt 1997b; Laule *et al.* 2003). From an animal welfare perspective, PRT may provide animals with greater choice and control and a chance to work for their food (Neuringer 1969; Anderson & Chamove 1984; Sackett 1991; Laule & Desmond 1997), both factors that have been associated with enhanced psychological well-being (Hanson *et al.* 1976; Markowitz 1982; Mineka *et al.* 1986).

For example, consider the animal receiving an injection for a research protocol. Without training, the animal has no choice as to how that event occurs. If escape/avoidance training is used, the threat of a negative stimulus is necessary to achieve the desired behaviour in which the animal presents a leg for the injection, thus exposing the animal to stress from both the injection and the threat. Using a positive reinforcement approach, the animal is trained through shaping and rewards to voluntarily present a leg for an injection, and concurrently desensitised to the procedure to reduce the associated fear or anxiety. (The processes of shaping and desensitisation are described in detail later in this chapter.) It would seem logical to argue that having a clearer choice as to how events such as injections happen, and being less fearful of them, will contribute to an animal's psychological well-being.

PRT provides the tools to improve husbandry and veterinary care (Reichard & Shellabarger 1992; Laule & Desmond 1994; Bassett *et al.* 2003; Schapiro *et al.* 2005; Coleman *et al.* 2008), enhance co-operation in collection of urine, semen and blood samples (Phillipi-Falkenstein & Clarke 1992; VandeVoort *et al.* 1993; Stone *et al.* 1994; Laule *et al.* 1996; Reinhardt 1997b; McKinley *et al.* 2003; Smith *et al.* 2004), reduce abnormal and/or stereotypic behaviour (Laule 1993; Bloomsmith *et al.* 2007; Bourgeois *et al.* 2007), reduce aggression (Bloomsmith *et al.* 1994), improve socialisation (Desmond *et al.* 1987; Desmond and Laule 1994; Bloomsmith *et al.* 1997; Baker 2004), enhance enrichment programmes (Bloomsmith *et al.* 1997; Laule & Desmond 1997) and increase the safety of the attending personnel (Bloomsmith 1994). A summary of literature on training primates is provided by Prescott *et al.* (2005), together with a clear step-by-step guide for a transport box training protocol.

PRT provides the opportunity for subjects to be desensitised to frightening or painful events, so the events become less frightening and less stressful (Reinhardt *et al.* 1990; Turkkan *et al.* 1990; Perlman *et al.* 2004; Videan *et al.* 2005; Lambeth *et al.* 2006). Many husbandry and veterinary procedures can be implemented with less disruption to all animals, by reducing the need to separate animals from their social groups for many procedures (Schapiro *et al.* 2003; Laule & Whittaker 2007). With greater accessibility to more co-operative animals comes a reduction in the use of restraint and anaesthesia (Bloomsmith 1992; Reinhardt *et al.* 1995; McKinley *et al.* 2003).

Experience has shown that trained animals maintain a high degree of reliability in participating in these procedures and are less stressed while doing so (Reinhardt *et al.* 1990; Turkkan *et al.* 1990; Lambeth *et al.* 2006). Evidence for this includes reports from a number of investigators of reductions in cortisol levels, stress-related abortions, physical resistance to handling and fear responses such as fear-grinning, screaming and acute diarrhoea in a variety of primate species (Moseley & Davis 1989; Vertein & Reinhardt 1989; Reinhardt *et al.* 1990).

One area of great interest and concern is the reduction of self-injurious behaviours (SIBs) in captive primates. Bloomsmith *et al.* (2007, p. 211) reviewed a number of recent studies that, '... *although preliminarily in nature, indicate that stereotyped behaviour and SIB in nonhuman primates can be modified through the use of operant conditioning.*' No studies achieved complete elimination of the problematic behaviour, but significant reductions were documented.

Training objectives

The following are examples of training objectives relevant to the laboratory setting:

- achieve voluntary co-operation by animals in husbandry, medical and research procedures (ie, blood draw, injections, urine collection, enter restraint cage, blood pressure measurement, topical treatment, oral dosing, etc);
- reduce fear and discomfort;
- decrease abnormal or stereotypic behaviour;
- reduce or eliminate aggressive behaviour toward conspecifics and/or animal care staff;
- facilitate introductions and socialisation with conspecifics.

Training methods

To achieve all the benefits that PRT offers requires skilful and effective implementation. It is beyond the scope of this manual to provide a step-by-step guide to the training of laboratory animals. However, throughout this chapter some sample training protocols for specific behaviours have been provided. The following is a brief discussion of the basic tools and techniques of PRT, and suggested steps to be taken in the training process. Although these are used most often with primates, the basics of PRT, i.e. giving an animal something they like for responding correctly, applies to the management of any animal.

Positive reinforcer

A positive reinforcer is anything that the animal likes. Food, tactile contact, verbal praise, a favoured enrichment item, access to conspecifics and play are all potential reinforcers. Food, which is the most often used reinforcer, can be part of the normal diet, enrichment allotment or an extra treat. It is always desirable to have a variety of reinforcers to choose from.

Conditioned reinforcer (bridge)

A conditioned reinforcer is an initially meaningless signal that, when repeatedly associated with primary reinforcers such as food, becomes a reinforcer, in and of itself. The animal learns that every time it hears the signal, a reward will follow. The most commonly used conditioned reinforcers in animal training are a spoken word, such as 'good', a hand-held clicker or a dog whistle. The use of a conditioned reinforcer, particularly a clicker, is highly recommended for training laboratory animals. It is a way of saying, 'Good, that is what I want!' It provides precise information that tells the animal exactly what you're looking for. Immediately following the response, the actual reward or positive reinforcement is delivered. The whistle or clicker is called a 'bridge' because it bridges the gap between the behaviour occurring and the food reward being delivered.

Stationing

In order to train any behaviour, you must have the animal's attention. This requires reinforcing the animal for remaining in one place and looking at you. Stationing requires periodic reinforcement on an ongoing basis.

Target

A target is an object the animal is trained to move towards and to touch. Commonly used targets include a ball on the end of a stick, a plastic bottle, a wooden dowel or any object that can be easily held by the trainer or attached to the enclosure. Primates are normally trained to touch their hand to the target. With other species, such as dogs, cats, rodents, cattle and pigs, the animal is taught to touch the target with the nose. This usually occurs spontaneously as most animals are curious to touch or sniff something new. However, if necessary, the behaviour can be taught by moving the object towards the animal's hand or nose a little bit at a time and reinforcing each time it gets closer. At the same time, the trainer should reinforce any forward movement the animal makes towards the target, until contact is made.

A target is useful in several ways. First, the trainer can control gross movement, by rewarding the animal for coming to the target when presented or for going to a target pre-placed elsewhere in the cage. Second, the animal can be trained to stay at the target to achieve or extend stationing. Once this behaviour is established, socially housed animals can be trained to each remain at their own individual target, allowing the trainer to access individual animals within the group. Finally, the target can be used to more safely access body parts, by training the animal to move a foot, paw, arm, leg, chest, back, side, etc to the target.

Shaping or successive approximation

The primary method for training behaviour is shaping, which is the process of breaking a behaviour into small, individual steps that build upon each other, eventually leading to the completed behaviour. Teaching an animal to touch a target by moving it incrementally closer and closer and reinforcing any movement the animal makes towards it, no matter how small or tentative, is a simple example of shaping. In most cases, shaping starts with reinforcing a naturally occurring behaviour. For example, to train a dog to open its mouth, the first step may be to hold a food treat up for it to see. When the mouth opens in anticipation, a quick 'Good' followed by the delivery of the treat is the first step in the shaping process. The following training protocol illustrates the potential approximations in training a pig to enter a squeeze cage which might be necessary for certain procedures.

- Choose a verbal and/or hand cue for the behaviour, such as 'inside'; use a hand-held clicker as a bridge.
- Place the squeeze cage in the enclosure, or attach to the door of the home cage, and bridge and reinforce when pig looks at the squeeze cage.
- Bridge and reinforce any movement towards the squeeze cage.
- A target can be used to direct the animal to the squeeze cage.
- Bridge and reinforce any exploratory behaviour such as sniffing the squeeze cage, looking inside, touching it with nose or foot.
- Bridge and reinforce any forward movement into the squeeze cage; a target can be attached to the inside back of the squeeze cage and the animal reinforced for moving towards it.
- Use verbal cue 'inside' whenever the animal initiates movement towards the squeeze cage or trainer encourages movement towards or into the squeeze cage.
- Once the animal is entering the squeeze cage, send the animal in and out of the squeeze cage (reinforcing movement in both directions) to firmly establish the cue and strengthen the desired behaviour.
- Reinforce the animal for remaining in the squeeze cage for progressively longer periods of time.
- Begin to move the door, a small amount at a time for short periods of time, bridging and reinforcing each approximation, and slowly increase both until the pig will remain inside while the door closes.
- Slowly increase the amount of time the door is closed.
- When the pig is comfortable in the squeeze cage with the door closed, begin to repeat the last two steps with the squeeze back until the pig will stand calmly when completely restrained by the squeeze back.

The key to successful shaping is the ability to identify appropriate-sized steps. Steps that are too big can create confusion and frustration in the animal. Too small steps can lead to loss of motivation and boredom. Generally speaking, the most common mistake made by new trainers is to expect too much from the animal and attempt steps that are too big. The aim should always be to end each training session on a positive note, no matter how small the step achieved.

Time out

Punishment, by definition, is designed to eliminate behaviour and occurs after the behavioural response. (Note: The term 'punishment' is often confused with 'negative reinforcement' which has the opposite effect and significantly different timing. Negative reinforcement is designed to increase the likelihood of a behaviour occurring and is used at the same time the behaviour occurs.) In positive reinforcement training, the only acceptable punisher is a time out. Physical punishment is not appropriate except in a life-threatening situation for person or animal. A time out is a very mild form of punishment in which reinforcement is withheld for a brief period of time immediately following an inappropriate response. A time out can vary in quality and length, from the trainer breaking eye contact for several seconds, to walking away for a couple of moments at the most. A time out is a very simple, powerful response to misbehaviour, with two basic rules:

- Do not use a time out too often, or it will lose its effectiveness.
- Always follow a time out by giving the animal another chance. Even if you leave the area altogether, come back and start fresh with no grudges.

Extinction

Extinction is a very useful method of reducing or eliminating a problem behaviour by no longer reinforcing it. The trainer must determine what exactly the reinforcement is (food, attention, etc) and then ensure that it is consistently withheld whenever the behaviour occurs. Extinction is most effective when paired with reinforcement of a more desirable alternative behaviour. For example, a macaque has been inadvertently reinforced with attention for reaching out to grab people with her hand. The remedy is to ensure that all staff stop giving her attention whenever she reaches out and, simultaneously, that the animal is given attention every time she keeps her hand inside the cage.

Regression

Training and learning are complex processes and progress is not linear. In fact, it occurs in steps forwards and backwards. Progress the animal makes one day, seems to be forgotten by the next. Then suddenly learning accelerates, and the animal moves two steps forwards. Each of those steps backwards is called regression, and it is a normal part of training.

Addressing fear

Animals in laboratory environments are faced with a wide array of fearful stimuli and experiences. Hediger (1950) warned of the potential of an enemy–prey relationship developing between humans and captive animals. Animal care staff are in the position of power – controlling food, water, access to physical spaces, choice of conspecifics, movement patterns, daily routines, implementation of research protocols and so on (Caine 1992; Laule 2003). The more negative events the animal experiences in relation to humans, the stronger the link between the stimuli (humans) and the fear response (Hemsworth & Coleman 1998). Studies have shown repeatedly that routine procedures by familiar personnel may result in persistent stress responses (Malinow *et al.* 1974; Manuck *et al.* 1983; Line *et al.* 1989). Increased fighting and wounding in chimpanzees is seen at times of greater human activity (Maki *et al.* 1987; Lambeth *et al.* 1997).

The first strategy employed by animals when feeling threatened and/or fearful is normally escape or flight. However, laboratory animals often cannot escape the fearful stimuli (humans) nor, in most cases, can they even get out of visual range of humans. When an animal cannot escape from a threat, this tends to lead to either the fight response, which we label as aggression (Hediger 1950), or an avoidance behaviour (Boissy 1995). Avoidance is often seen as the rodent who runs from the human hand, the dog that cowers in the corner of the kennel, the pig who emits a loud vocalisation or squeal when approached, or the primate who is pressed against the back of the cage and refuses to approach, even for a food treat.

Laboratory animals will show fearful responses when subjected to a wide array of medical procedures, particularly invasive ones such as blood draws, dosing of medications, injections and administration of topical drugs. Similarly, restraint procedures such as the use of a squeeze cage, tether, gloves, pole and collar, restraint chair, sling and restraint board trigger varying degrees of fear, discomfort and stress in most animals.

More and more studies have shown that routine procedures traditionally viewed as neutral events can be quite stressful to a laboratory animal. Studies on primates in laboratories, conducted nearly 20 years ago by Line and Markowitz and their colleagues (Line *et al.* 1987, 1989) found prolonged alterations in heart rates and cortisol levels after routine procedures such as cage cleaning. Increases in glucocorticoid concentrations, weight loss and suppressed immune system response have been reported in rodents (Obernier & Baldwin 2006), rabbits (Toth & January 1990) and dogs (Bergeron *et al.* 2002) when they are moved, even if it is just to a new cage in the same facility. Whary and colleagues (1993, p. 331) report that in rodent stress studies '*... the most important stress-inducing factor is a sudden change in housing method rather than the method itself*'. Other common procedures that can elicit fear or anxiety in laboratory dogs include change in routine, separation from a stable social group, wearing equipment such as jackets and introduction to new people or conspecifics (Beerda *et al.* 1999).

When ongoing fear is unresolved, the animal can remain in a chronic stress response or state of distress (Moberg 1985; Toates 1995). This state has significant and detrimental physiological effects including slower growth, lower reproductive success and immunosupression (Selye 1976; Broom & Johnson 1993; Wielebnowski 2002). It can also lead to an array of abnormal behaviors (Meyer-Holzapfel 1968; Erwin & Deni 1979; Anderson & Chamove 1980).

Non-human primates are particularly prone to stereotyped behaviours when housed currently (or previously) in sub-optimal or inappropriate environments. These include pacing and repetitive somersaulting, headnodding, self clasping and rocking (Bellanca & Crockett 2002; Lutz *et al.* 2003; Bourgeois & Brent 2005); abnormal appetitive behaviours such as coprophagy and regurgitation and reingestion (Bellanca & Crockett 2002; Struck *et al.* 2007); over-grooming and resultant alopecia (Honess *et al.* 2005); and self-injurious behaviours with and without wounding (Tiefenbacher *et al.* 2004; Bloomsmith *et al.* 2007; Bourgeois *et al.* 2007). Rodents display repetitive backflipping (Callard *et al.* 2000), stereotypic digging (Wiedenmayer 1997), barbering (DeLuca 1997) and bar- and wire-biting (Orok-Edem & Key 1994; Würbel *et al.* 1998). Rabbits exhibit excessive grooming and bar-gnawing (Hansen & Berthelsen 2000). Dogs and cats engage in self-injurious biting (Laboratory Animal Refinement and Enrichment Forum (LAREF) 2007); and pigs engage in bar-biting and excessive rooting and rubbing (Smith & Swindle 2006).

From a practical perspective, it will be difficult to gain the voluntary co-operation of an animal in any husbandry or research procedure if that animal is overwhelmed by fear. The animal must be able to tolerate the stimulus to the degree that a food reward is accepted and learning is possible. Therefore, it is important to:

1. recognize fear;
2. acknowledge its effects;
3. adjust behavioural criteria and expectations accordingly;
4. develop and implement strategies to reduce fear.

Positive reinforcement training provides animal care staff with the techniques to adopt a proactive approach to diminish the level of fear and thus the accompanying stress that an animal experiences. Doing so can directly enhance welfare, reduce resultant abnormal behaviour and increase the likelihood of achieving a greater degree of co-operation by the animal in behavioural objectives.

Improving the human–animal relationship

An appreciation of the human–animal relationship is important. A patient, empathetic handler will contribute much towards the well-being of an animal, no matter what the circumstance or the species. Whether handling a rat, restraining a dog or reassuring a primate, a gentle hand, quiet voice and measured approach can create a more positive experience for the animal.

Smith and Swindle (2006) emphasise the importance of the influence of animal care staff on pig behaviour in the laboratory. With gentle handling and positive reinforcement techniques pigs can be readily trained to tolerate a simple physical examination, to walk out of their cages to another location and to accept restraint, including manual, mechanical (i.e. a sling) and chemical.

One of the most effective ways to establish a positive relationship with captive animals is to have some positive interaction with them on a daily basis. Bayne *et al.* (1993) found that 3–5 minutes of daily positive interactions and treat provisioning for singly housed rhesus macaques (Macaca mulatta) resulted in decreased abnormal behaviour and overall fear. Similarly, Baker *et al.* (2003) found that PRT, used as an enrichment strategy for primates, resulted in reduction of abnormal behaviour and anxiety-related behaviour. Studies have shown that petting a dog can have a calming effect and decrease heart and respiratory rates (Gantt *et al.* 1966) and may be effective in reducing cortisol responses to aversive situations, such as physical examinations, injections and blood sampling (Hennessy *et al.* 1998). Ferrets that are handled regularly become less troublesome to handle and less fearful (Ball 2006). Numerous studies demonstrate the beneficial effects of frequently handling research animals in a patient and calm manner before initiation of study protocols (Meaney *et al.* 1991; Chapillon *et al.* 2002; Conour *et al.* 2006).

Tuli *et al.* (1995, p. 132) suggest that 'animals habituated to a handler or animals that are gentled in early life show less handling stress in later life'. Davis (2002) documented the ability of a variety of species to discriminate between handlers that were either simply familiar or those that had been associated with a positive experience. Finally, Wolfle (1985, p. 450) argues, *'It is not an overstatement to say that the right animal technician instils qualities in the animals that make them better and more reliable research subjects.'*

PRT is a powerful vehicle for creating a positive bond between human and animal. The very nature of the process – gaining the voluntary co-operation of the animal and rewarding behavioural performance with something the animal likes – enhances both the behaviour and the motivation to perform it, and all within the context of a positive interaction. Furthermore, specific training techniques that are directed at reducing fear can serve the dual purpose of achieving a positive human–animal relationship while reducing stress on the animal.

Desensitisation

Desensitisation is a process designed to 'train out', or overcome, fear. By pairing positive rewards with any action, object or event that causes fear, that fearful entity slowly becomes less negative, less frightening and less stressful. The effectiveness of desensitisation can be assessed in two ways. Is there a positive change in the animal's willingness to voluntarily co-operate in the event? And are there changes in the animal's behaviour in relation to the fearful entity that indicate reduced stress or fear? Through desensitisation, animals learn to tolerate and eventually accept a wide array of frightening or uncomfortable stimuli. Effective desensitisation relies on two elements: precise reinforcement and good judgement in determining where the process should start and how fast to move through the steps to the completed behaviour.

Precise reinforcement means catching the exact moment the animal experiences the stimulus. For example, when training an animal to accept an injection, or to tolerate a blood draw, the feeling of a needle piercing the skin is a potentially frightening and painful experience. Effective desensitisation requires pairing many positive rewards directly with that experience, or with a similar experience. Training may include pairing positive rewards with the experience of being touched with a progression of items, starting with the trainer's finger or a wooden dowel, then a capped syringe, then a needle with the end cut off so it is blunted and finally the real needle. In each case, the bridge (such as verbal 'good' or clicking sound) must occur at the exact moment the animal feels the object touch the skin. The bridge is then immediately followed by a reward. The animal must experience this over and over again, with the touch slowly moving from very light to the final experience of actually piercing the skin. If desensitization is done well, the animal will voluntarily accept the injection, or allow the blood draw, and recognisable signs of stress and fear will be diminished or absent.

The second key to effective desensitisation is determining the starting point and how fast to progress. If fear of the syringe is so great that the animal cannot accept a food reward in its presence, then learning cannot occur. In that case, the first step may be to offer the animal a brief glimpse of the syringe, or increase the distance between the syringe and the animal, pairing these experiences with the bridge and food reward. The next step may be moving the syringe towards the animal in small increments, each one paired with the bridge and reward. How quickly progress occurs and how big each step is depend on how the animal reacts to each approximation.

Desensitisation can be used in many situations. Animals can be desensitised to husbandry and research procedures, new enclosures, unfamiliar people, specific people like the veterinarian, novel objects, strange noises and other possible aversive stimuli.

Habituation or acclimatision

Habituation refers to the process of gradually getting an animal used to a situation which it normally avoids, by prolonged exposure. It differs from desensitisation in that there is no direct pairing of a positive reinforcer with the stimulus, or with the experience of fear or anxiety in relation to the stimulus. The animal simply experiences the event repeatedly until it no longer displays the behavioural signs of fear or stress. At that point it is assumed to have habituated to it. This is a widely accepted approach to managing laboratory animals and their fearful, painful or stressful experiences (Ruys *et al.* 2004). The reliance on habituation, rather than desensitisation, is one of practicality. Time constraints and limited staff place pressures on animal care staff to get the necessary behaviour in the easiest and quickest way possible.

For example, habituation is often used to accustom primates to chair restraint. It is readily acknowledged that forced restraint is stressful for an animal. Behavioural signs include physical resistance and struggling, heightened agitation, alarm vocalisations and facial expressions of fear and defensive threats (Reinhardt *et al.* 1995). Physiological changes include increased respiration and heart rate, activation of the hypothalamic–pituitary–adrenal (HPA) axis and the secretion of glucocorticoids in proportion to the intensity of the perceived threat.

With repeated exposure to the restraint, behavioural and physiological responses diminish, which is cited as evidence that the animal has become habituated to the experience. However, as one study by Ruys *et al.* (2004) showed, this may not be indicative of actual habituation to the event. Changes in behaviour may be simply an effective coping strategy as the animal learns that attempts to escape are futile and therefore submits. Study results showed that after repeated chairing of rhesus macaques (Macaca mulatta), although expected behavioural changes occurred, there was still an HPA response, albeit diminished, and increased cortisol levels, especially in the initial period of restraint. Their conclusion was that '*... the pattern of results that we found suggests that rhesus macaques habituate behaviourally but not physiologically to their chair restraint*' (Ruys *et al.* 2004, p. 212).

This study is referenced because it is a good reminder that compliance on the part of the animal may not be indicative of the level of stress the individual is experiencing. The handling and training methods used should increase behavioural compliance and at the same time reduce stress and fear. Simply providing repeated exposure to an uncomfortable event may not be enough. A better approach is to reverse the process through the use of desensitisation techniques. As the animal becomes less fearful, behavioural compliance increases.

This was demonstrated in a study by Lambeth *et al.* (2006) where researchers examined records of 575 anaesthesia events for 128 chimpanzees. Animals either voluntarily presented an arm or leg for the injection, or were given the injection involuntarily, through coercion or the use of a dart gun. The training process used a combination of shaping and desensitisation. Haematological and serum chemistry values indicative of acute stress in chimpanzees (ie, total white blood cell (WBC) counts, absolute segmented neutrophils (SEG), glucose (GLU) levels and haematocrit (HCT) levels) were analysed in both conditions. Results showed that total WBC counts, blood GLU levels and SEG levels were significantly lower in animals that voluntarily presented than in animals that received an injection involuntarily. Perhaps the most noteworthy results came from within-subject conditions showing that individuals had significantly lower WBC and GLU levels when they voluntarily presented for the injection than when they did not.

Therefore, whenever possible, it is worth the time and effort to desensitise animals to uncomfortable or frightening events, rather than by simply habituating them to it. However, habituation can be quite useful as a preliminary step before formal desensitisation. For, example, in the sample training protocol for training a pig to enter a squeeze cage, the first step might be to attach the squeeze cage to the pig's enclosure and allow free access to it for a couple days. Adding some food inside may make exploration of the cage more likely. This process of habituation, implemented before actual PRT begins, may shorten the time required for training and desensitisation. Furthermore, if habituation is the only method employed, animal care staff should at the very least provide some positive reinforcements, i.e. food rewards, in conjunction with the experience as frequently and as generously as possible.

Socialisation training

With the growing requirement to house social primates in pairs or small groups, it is necessary to have the ability to facilitate introductions and increase the likelihood of maintaining stable groupings of animals. One PRT method has been used successfully with a wide range of species to address these objectives (Desmond & Laule 1994; Laule & Whittaker 2007).

Co-operative feeding

Co-operative feeding is a technique used to enhance positive social behaviour and reduce agonistic behaviour (Bloomsmith 1992; Bloomsmith *et al.* 1994; Cox 1987; Desmond *et al.* 1987; Laule & Whittaker 2007). It is of particular value in managing socially housed primates in laboratories. Many staff caring for captive animals have used subterfuge and distraction when attempting to provide subordinate animals with food, enrichment or other desirable resources. However, these techniques actually exacerbate aggression, causing dominant animals to become more vigilant in order to maintain control of the desirable resources. In captivity, aggressive interactions can have serious consequences if group members or cage mates are unable to escape the aggressors.

Co-operative feeding conforms to operant conditioning theory, which states that the consequences of a behaviour determine whether or not it will recur (Pryor 1999). During co-operative feeding, the dominant animal receives reinforcement, in the form of desirable foods, whenever the subordinate animal receives these resources. This technique reinforces the dominant animal for behaviour that is co-operative rather than aggressive, thus strengthening co-operative behaviours. When consistently and skilfully applied, co-operative feeding has two positive outcomes: (1) the dominant animal becomes less aggressive and more tolerant, and (2) the subordinate animal becomes less fearful and more willing to accept rewards in the presence of the dominant animal.

Co-operative feeding can be used to enhance introductions of animals, prior to and after they are given physical access to each other. Initial training can be done with animals separated in adjacent cages. However, they must have visual access to each other so the dominant animal can see what s/he is being reinforced for. A housing situation with multiple animals may require more than one trainer in the initial stages. If so, one trainer should control the dominant animal and the other trainer feed the rest of the animals, following the protocol so the dominant animal is being reinforced specifically for the other animals being fed. The training should progress so that eventually one person feeds the animals.

The following is a sample protocol for applying co-operative feeding to two pair-housed primates. Tools include a clicker and food, including some special food items for the dominant (target) animal.

- Cue the target animal to sit, then reinforce.
- Give the second animal a piece of food and as he takes it, bridge and reinforce the target animal with two to three pieces of food for sitting and staying without interfering (if necessary, cut the food smaller to keep volume down).
- Provide verbal and visual information to the target animal – look at him and say 'Good!' as you feed the other animal, say 'No' if he breaks position and immediately ask him to sit again.
- Ignore minor interferences (head bob, reaching for food, etc) as long as the second animal is successful in taking food.
- If the target animal is aggressive towards or intimidates the second animal so he won't take food, bring the target animal back to sit/stay, then resume the feed.
- Use a high rate of continuous reinforcement at first (one piece for second animal, two to three pieces for the target animal) then as progress is made, the amount and frequency of reinforcement for the target animal can be slowly reduced.
- Give the target animal a special treat at the end of every successful session.

Training programme development

The success of a positive reinforcement-based animal training programme in the laboratory environment depends on many factors. Primary among them is the ability of the personnel to understand the principles of operant conditioning and effectively apply PRT techniques. Training is a skill that takes time and practice to develop. Poorly planned and implemented training will yield minimal benefits at best. Second, the commitment and motivation of personnel will have an enormous impact on the quality of the training experience and the results achieved. Third, consistency in handling and training techniques between all staff who work with the animals is critical. Positive reinforcement methods should be applied to the daily husbandry and cleaning routine as well as to the training of specific behaviours for research protocols. Fourth, learning occurs through repetition. Therefore, the more opportunity the animal has to practise the behaviour, the quicker results will be realised.

It is important that every institution recognises the need to invest resources in training staff in PRT techniques. By developing staff that are familiar with these techniques and have some degree of competence in using them, the quality of care of laboratory animals can be greatly improved. Although it may not be feasible to develop equal training skills in all animal care personnel, one approach that is effective is to develop multiple levels of skills in staff. For example, everyone who works with the animals should have a basic understanding of operant conditioning techniques and be capable of using and maintaining trained behaviour once it is complete. They should also be capable of implementing simple training protocols, for example, incorporating reinforcement into interactions with animals when they comply with husbandry and medical procedures. A smaller subset of staff should have training skills that allow them to design training protocols and train new behaviour. These individuals can then plan and implement PRT to improve daily handling and husbandry procedures and better prepare animals for research protocols. Finally, at least one individual on site should have sufficient training skills to resolve difficult situations as they arise, as well as coordinate and oversee PRT activities.

Despite the complexity of this process, if viewed in the long term, the apparent costs of implementing a positive reinforcement training programme can be turned into real benefits for the staff, animals and the institution. Training sessions provide a context where person and animal can have a mutually positive interaction and positive interactions ultimately strengthen the human–animal bond, enhancing the quality of life for laboratory animals. Finally, in a pragmatic sense, training success can reduce the use of restraint and anaesthesia and save time, labour and money over the long term (Bloomsmith 1992; Luttrell *et al.* 1994; McKinley *et al.* 2003).

Practical approach to training laboratory animals

The reality of life in the laboratory may not always be ideally suited to a formal PRT programme. For example, care staff are normally responsible for large numbers of animals, limiting the amount of time they can spend with individual animals. Housing conditions vary from small caging, that severely restricts the animal's range of physical movement, to big corrals with large numbers of animals, that are difficult to access on an individual basis. Research protocols often dictate or restrict the amount and type of food animals can receive, the type of physical activity they can engage in and acceptable enrichment options. Finally, staff are often given only short periods of time to prepare animals for research procedures.

In many cases, PRT, in its purest form, may not be feasible in this setting. Limitations in the training skills of staff and time constraints may not allow for the step-by-step shaping process of a behaviour using totally positive reinforcement. The cognitive abilities of different animals, as well as the complexity of the behavioural requirements, will also vary. Although the techniques of PRT are universal, species and individuals within species will have their own unique temperament. A significant element of skilful training is the ability to be sensitive and responsive to these often subtle differences, and to adapt and respond appropriately. However, even with basic skills, it is feasible to integrate positive reinforcement techniques into existing management procedures for most species. In order to develop such a system, the following actions are recommended and ideally should be integrated into existing operational procedures.

1. Use the basic principles of positive reinforcement training to improve the human–animal relationship. For example, in a primate colony, moving through a room with multiple cages and stopping for even a few seconds to say some kind words and deliver a food treat to each animal can contribute greatly to a positive human–animal relationship. It may reduce the animal's fear of humans and create the context for more co-operation on the part of the animal in future procedures. Therefore, it is most beneficial to incorporate this simple conditioning into care routines at breeding centres and import/quarantine facilities. Whenever possible, hand feeding and rewarding can evolve into training of simple cues and responses such as coming to the front of the cage and remaining there, sitting, climbing on the cage front, presenting a hand or arm and so on. This is also a great opportunity to start the training process with young animals, which are generally quite responsive to PRT. The sooner this process is begun, the greater the benefits in the long term.
2. Provide animals with the opportunity and motivation to co-operate voluntarily in activities and procedures by incorporating two basic positive reinforcement training techniques into interactions. First, provide a cue or a signal that clearly tells the animal what he is being asked to do. If the animal can perceive and understand the signal, it can then respond with the correct behaviour. Second, if the animal responds appropriately, provide a reward. Even if the animal care staff must resort to negative reinforcement (ie, moving a cage back to restrict space, or showing the animal a net) to gain compliance, when the behaviour occurs, the treat is given. Over time, the use of negative reinforcement is steadily decreased until it is no longer necessary. With a clear signal and regular reinforcement, the animal now has the information necessary to co-operate and the motivation to do so. It is surprising how often those two elements are overlooked.
3. Always give the animal a reasonable opportunity to co-operate in the desired behaviour. Time constraints may be an issue, and numbers of animals that require training may be high, but every animal deserves a measure of patience on the part of the human. For example, if a primate must be restrained in a squeeze cage, rather than immediately moving the cage wall all the way forward, the wall should be moved in increments, offering the animal the chance to co-operate by moving to the front of the cage after each increment. When it complies, a reward is given. Total co-operation will not be immediate, but over time the animal will learn what is expected and will probably co-operate without having to be fully restrained. In the same way, when it is necessary to handle or restrain a rodent or rabbit, a patient, gentle hand and a treat following the procedure is the most humane and positive way to carry out the task and gain greater co-operation.
4. Always look for and employ the least invasive methods to achieve objectives. Research protocols put great demands on animals and animal care staff. Results are dependent upon consistent means of collecting samples, administering oral medications, applying topical applications and so on. However, it is often possible to meet the specific study requirements in a less invasive or stressful way. For example, collecting urine samples from group-housed callitrichids through training animals to urinate quickly and reliably into a vial (McKinley *et al.* 2003) or on a clean platform inside the cage (Smith *et al.* 2004) yields the same results, ie, the individual urine sample, as separating animals for extended periods of time until they urinate. In two studies, one with rats (Huang-Brown & Guhad 2002) and another with rabbits (Marr *et al.* 1993), animals were trained to take their oral doses of medication in chocolate and a sucrose solution respectively. In both cases, drug absorption and serum levels were appropriate. This allowed the animals to avoid a very stressful experience of gastric gavage, while meeting the study needs.
5. Plan ahead: prepare for research protocols by identifying which animals will be involved, what behaviours are needed, what equipment will be used, how long the procedure will take, how often it will occur and other relevant factors. Then focus some effort on a daily basis towards preparing the animals for the protocol. There are two fundamental objectives of this work. First, to desensitise each animal to components of the process that may be new, frightening or uncomfortable such as medical equipment, the feel of a needle prick, the experience of being restrained and so on. The second is to gain the voluntary co-operation of the animal in as much of the research protocol as possible.
6. Find ways to train regularly and frequently – animals, like humans, learn through repetition. Ideally, PRT sessions should be conducted on a daily basis with each of the animals. For best results, it is advisable to limit the number of individuals conducting new training. During this phase, consistency between sessions is a critical factor in the effectiveness of the training and how quickly new behaviours are completed. Consistency

can be achieved in a couple of ways. Individual animal care staff can be assigned to individual animals, training them for all new behaviours related to the protocol. It is also possible to assign a back-up trainer to work on the behaviours during the primary trainer's days off, as long as good communication is maintained between those individuals. This allows for a 7 days a week training regimen, providing opportunities for daily practice and repetition. Another option is to divide up responsibility for training new behaviour so that several individuals work with each animal, but each person only works on his or her assigned behaviour.

7. Incorporate PRT into the daily routine. If regular training sessions are not possible, then training should be incorporated into the daily routine. For example, every time animal care staff interact with the animals during cleaning, feeding, visual inspections etc, they carry with them an instrument or apparatus that will be used in the procedure and give each of the animals a treat. If possible, when some large piece of equipment is to be used, it should be brought into the room and the animals given a treat while it is present. A simple process like this, done regularly, can dramatically reduce the fear response to the item. Similarly, training for voluntary co-operation in the research procedure can be initiated and implemented. Even a couple of behavioural responses each day can have a beneficial impact. For example, a member of animal care staff can introduce a target to teach stationing and each day ask the animal to come to the target for his enrichment. Or he or she can: carry a syringe and just show it to each animal prior to giving the enrichment; or hold the dog or cat's paw for a couple of seconds; pick up the rat or rabbit; rub the pig's belly with the sling, and then reinforce or enrich. By identifying individual components of the final behaviour and working on these relatively small units on a daily basis, the animal is slowly conditioned to accept and co-operate with the process. Even if the final behaviour is not trained in its entirety, there is a greater likelihood that the animal will be more co-operative and less fearful when the actual procedure is implemented.
8. If habituation is used to provide repeated exposure of the animal to a procedure, add reinforcement to the process. As discussed earlier, habituation may only eliminate the behavioural responses to the situation, but not actually reduce the associated stress. By adding at least a cursory element of desensitisation to the process, ie, pairing this repeated exposure with positive rewards, the animal has the opportunity to comply and feel less fearful while doing so.

Concluding remarks

The use of positive reinforcement training as an animal care and management tool offers many benefits to biomedical facilities and to their animals, staff and researchers. Primary among these is the ability to gain the voluntary co-operation of animals in husbandry and research procedures. Through techniques like desensitisation, the fear and stress associated with these procedures can be significantly reduced. PRT can be applied in a wide array of situations with a wide variety of species. When appropriately and skilfully applied, positive reinforcement techniques represent a viable option to the traditional approach to the management of laboratory animals. By making the shift to a more positive reinforcement-based system, the welfare of the animals is significantly enhanced while providing better research models for the biomedical community.

References

Anderson, J.R. and Chamove, A.S. (1980) Self-aggression and social aggression in laboratory-reared macaques. *Journal of Abnormal Psychology*, **89**, 539–550

Anderson, J.R. and Chamove, A.S. (1984) Allowing captive primates to forage. In: *Standards in Laboratory Animal Management*, Vol. 2. pp. 253–256. Universities Federation for Animal Welfare, Potters Bar, UK

Baker, K.C. (2004) Benefits of positive human interaction for socially housed chimpanzees. *Animal Welfare*, **13**, 239–245

Baker, K., Bloomsmith, M., Griffis, C. *et al.* (2003) Self-injurious behavior and response to human interaction as enrichment in rhesus macaques. *American Journal of Primatology*, **60**, 94–95

Ball, R.S. (2006) Issues to consider for preparing ferrets as research subjects in the laboratory. *ILAR Journal*, **47**, 348–357

Bassett, L., Buchanan-Smith, H., McKinley, J. *et al.* (2003) Effects of training on stress-related behavior of the common marmoset (*Callithrix jacchus*) in relation to coping with routine husbandry procedures. *Journal of Applied Animal Welfare Science*, **6**, 221–233

Bayne, K., Dexter, S. and Strange, D. (1993) The effects of food provisioning and human interaction on the behavioral well-being of rhesus monkeys (*Macaca mulatta*). *Contemporary Topics (AALAS)*, **32**, 6–9

Beerda, B., Schilder, M.B., Bernadina, W. *et al.* (1999) Chronic stress in dogs subjected to social and spatial restriction. Hormonal and immunological responses. *Physiology and Behavior*, **66**, 243–254

Bellanca, R.U. and Crockett, C.M. (2002) Factors predicting increased incidence of abnormal behavior in male pigtailed macaques. *American Journal of Primatology*, **58**, 57–69

Bergeron, R., Scott, S.L., Edmond, J.P. *et al.* (2002) Physiology and behavior of dogs during air transport. *Canadian Journal of Veterinary Research*, **66**, 211–216

Bloomsmith, M.A. (1992) Chimpanzee training and behavioural research: a symbiotic relationship. In: *Proceedings of the American Association of Zoological Parks and Aquariums Annual Conference*, pp. 403–410. AAZPA, Maryland

Bloomsmith, M.A. (1994) Evolving a behavioral management program in a breeding/research setting. In: *Proceedings of American Association of Zoological Parks and Aquariums Annual Conference*, pp. 8–13. AAZPA, Maryland

Bloomsmith, M., Lambeth, S., Stone, A. *et al.* (1997) Comparing two types of human interaction as enrichment for chimpanzees. *(Abstract) American Journal of Primatology*, **42**, 96

Bloomsmith, M., Laule, G., Thurston, R. *et al.* (1994) Using training to modify chimpanzee aggression during feeding. *Zoo Biology*, **13**, 557–566

Bloomsmith, M.A., Marr, J.M. and Maple, T.L. (2007) Addressing nonhuman primate behavioral problems through the application of operant conditioning: is the human treatment approach a useful model? *Applied Animal Behaviour Science*, **102**, 205–222

Boissy, A. (1995) Fear and fearfulness in animals. *Quarterly Review of Biology*, **70**, 165–191

Bourgeois, S.R. and Brent, L. (2005) Modifying the behaviour of singly caged baboons: evaluating the effectiveness of four enrichment techniques. *Animal Welfare*, **14**, 71–81

Bourgeois, S.R., Vazquez, M. and Brasky, K. (2007) Combination therapy reduces self-injurious behavior in a chimpanzee (*Pan troglodytes troglodytes*): a case report. *Journal of Applied Animal Welfare Science*, **10**, 123–140

Breuer, K., Coleman, G. and Hemsworth P. (1998) The effect of handling on the stress physiology and behaviour of nonlactating heifers. In: *Proceedings of Australian Society for the Study of Animal Behaviour, 29th Annual Conference*. pp. 8–9, Institute of Natural Resources, Massey University, Palmerston North, New Zealand

Broom, D.M. and Johnson, K.G. (1993) *Stress and Animal Welfare*. Chapman & Hall, London

Caine, N.G. (1992) Humans as predators: observational studies and the risk of pseudohabituation. In: *The Inevitable Bond: Examining Scientist-Animal Interactions*. Eds Davis, H. and Balfour, D., pp. 357–364. Cambridge University Press, New York

Callard, M.D., Bursten, S.N. and Price, E.O. (2000) Repetitive backflipping behaviour in captive roof rats *(Rattus rattus)* and the effect of cage enrichment. *Animal Welfare*, **9**, 139–152

Chapillon, P., Patin, V., Roy, B. *et al.* (2002) Effects of pre-and post natal stimulation on developmental, emotional, and cognitive aspects in rodents: a review. *Developmental Psychobiology*, **41**, 373–387

Coleman, K., Pranger. L., Maier, A. et al. (2008) Training rhesus macaques for venipuncture using positive reinforcement techniques: a comparison with chimpanzees. *Journal of the American Association for Laboratory Animal Science*, **47**, 37–41

Colflesh, L. (2004) *Making Friends: Training Your Dog Positively*. Howell Book House, Hoboken NJ

Conour, L.A., Murray, K.A. and Brown, M.J. (2006) Preparation of animals for research – issues to consider for rodents and rabbits. *ILAR Journal*, **47**, 283–293

Cox, C. (1987) Increase in the frequency of social interactions and the likelihood of reproduction among drills. In: *Proceedings of the American Association of Zoological Parks and Aquariums Western Regional Conference*, pp. 321–328. AAZPA, Maryland

Davis, H. (2002) Prediction and preparation: Pavlovian implications of research animals discriminating among humans. *ILAR Journal*, **43**, 19–26

DeLuca, A.M. (1997) Environmental enrichment: does it reduce barbering in mice? *Animal Welfare Information Center Newsletter*, **8**, 7–8

Desmond, T. and Laule, G. (1994) Use of positive reinforcement training in the management of species for reproduction. *Zoo Biology*, **13**, 471–477

Desmond, T., Laule, G. and McNary, J. (1987) Training for socialization and reproduction with drills. In: *Proceedings of the American Association of Zoological Parks and Aquariums Annual Conference*, pp. 435–441. AAZPA, Maryland

Donaldson, J. (1996) *The Culture Clash*. James and Kenneth, Berkley, CA

Erwin, J. and Deni, R. (1979) Strangers in a strange land: abnormal behaviors or abnormal environments? In: *Captivity and Behavior: Primates in Breeding Colonies, Laboratories, and Zoos*. Eds Erwin, J., Maple, T.L. and Mitchell, G., pp. 1–28. Nostrand Reinhold Co., New York

Ferster, C.B. (1953) The use of the free operant in the analysis of behavior. *Psychological Bulletin*, **50**, 263–274

Gantt, W.H., Newton, J.E., Royer, F.L. *et al.* (1966) Effect of person. *Conditioned Reflex*, **1**, 18–35

Hansen, L.T. and Berthelsen, H. (2000) The effect of environmental enrichment on the behaviour of caged rabbits *(Oryctolagus cuniculus). Applied Animal Behaviour Science*, **68**, 163–178

Hanson, J., Larson, M. and Snowdon, C. (1976) The effects of control over high intensity noise on plasma cortisol levels in rhesus monkeys. *Behavioural Biology*, **16**, 333–340

Hediger, H. (1950) *Wild Animals in Captivity*. Butterworth, London

Hemsworth, P.H. and Coleman, G.J. (1998) *Human-Livestock Interactions: The Stockperson and the Productivity and Welfare of Intensively-Farmed Animals*. CAB International, Wallingford, UK

Hennessy, M.B., Williams, M.T., Miller D.D. *et al.* (1998) Influence of male and female petters on plasma cortisol and behaviour: Can human interaction reduce the stress of dogs in a public animal shelter? *Applied Animal Behavior Science*, **61**, 63–77

Hernstein, R.J. (1997) *The Matching Law: Papers in Psychology and Economics*. Eds Rachlin, H. and Laibson, D.I. Harvard University Press, Cambridge MA

Hiby, E.F., Rooney, N.J. and Bradshaw, J.W. (2004) Dog training methods: their use, effectiveness and interaction with behaviour and welfare. *Animal Welfare*, **13**, 63–69

Honess, P.E., Gimpel, J.L., Wolfensohn, S.E. *et al.* (2005) Alopecia scoring: the quantitative assessment of hair loss in captive macaques. *Alternatives to Laboratory Animals*, **33**, 193–206

Huang-Brown, K.M. and Guhad, F.A. (2002) Chocolate, an effective means of oral drug delivery in rats. *Lab Animal*, **31**, 34–36

Joint Working Group on Refinement (2004) Refining dog husbandry and care: Eighth report of the BVAAWF/FRAME/RSPCA/UFAW Joint Working Group on Refinement. *Laboratory Animals*, **38** (Suppl. 1), 1–94

Jones, R.B. (1997) Fear and distress. In: *Animal Welfare*. Eds Appleby, M.C and Hughes, B.O., pp. 75–87. CAB International, UK

Kirkwood, J., Kichenside, C. and James, W. (1989) Training zoo animals. In: *Proceedings of Animal Training Symposium: A Review and Commentary on Current Practices*, pp. 93–99. Universities Federation for Animal Welfare, Potters Bar

Laboratory Animal Refinement and Enrichment Forum (2007) Maladaptive behaviors: stereotypical behavior; hair pulling-and-eating and alopecia (hair loss); self-injurious biting. In: *Making Lives Easier for Animals in Research Labs: Discussions by the Laboratory Animal Refinement and Enrichment Forum*. Eds Baumans, V., Coke, C., Green, J. *et al.*, pp. 39–45. Animal Welfare Institute, Washington, DC

Lambeth, S.P., Bloomsmith, M.A. and Alford, P.L. (1997) Effects of human activity on chimpanzee wounding. *Zoo Biology*, **16**, 327–333

Lambeth, S.P., Hau, J., Perlman, J.E. *et al.* (2006) Positive reinforcement training affects hematologic and serum chemistry values in captive chimpanzees (*Pan troglodytes*). *American Journal of Primatology*, **68**, 245–256

Laule, G.E. (1993) The use of behavioural management techniques to reduce or eliminate abnormal behaviour. *Animal Welfare Information Center Newsletter*, **4**, 1–11

Laule, G.E. (2003) Positive reinforcement training and environmental enrichment, enhancing animal well-being. *Journal of the Veterinary Medical Association*, **223**, 969–973

Laule, G.E., Bloomsmith, M.A. and Schapiro, S.J. (2003) The use of positive reinforcement training techniques to enhance the care, management, and welfare of primates in the laboratory. *Journal of Applied Animal Welfare Science*, **10**, 31–38

Laule, G.E. and Desmond, T.J. (1994) Use of positive reinforcement techniques to enhance animal care, research, and well-being. In: *Proceedings of Wildlife Mammals as Research Models: in the Laboratory and Field*. A seminar sponsored by the Scientists Center for Animal Welfare at the American Veterinary Medical Association Annual Meeting, pp. 53–59. SCAW, Maryland

Laule, G.E. and Desmond, T.J. (1997) Positive reinforcement training as an enrichment strategy. In: *Second Nature: Environmental Enrichment for Captive Animals*. Eds Sheperdson, D., Mellen, J. and Hutchins, M., pp. 302–312. Smithsonian Institution Press, Virginia

Laule, G.E., Thurston, R.H., Alford, P.A. *et al.* (1996) Training to reliably obtain blood and urine samples from a diabetic chimpanzee (*Pan Troglodytes*). *Zoo Biology*, **15**, 587–591

Laule, G.E. and Whittaker, M.A. (2007) Enhancing nonhuman primate care and welfare through the use of positive reinforcement training. *Journal of Applied Animal Welfare Science*, **10**, 31–38

Lindsay, S.R. (2005) *Handbook of Applied Dog Behavior and Training. Vol III. Procedures and Protocols*. Blackwell Publishing, Oxford

Line, S., Clarke, A.D. and Markowitz, H. (1987) Plasma cortisol of female rhesus monkeys in response to acute restraint. *Laboratory Primate Newsletter*, **26**, 1–4

Line, S., Morgan, K.N., Markowitz, H. *et al.* (1989) Heart rate and activity of rhesus monkeys in response to routine events. *Laboratory Primate Newsletter*, **28**, 9–12

Luttrell, L., Acker, L., Urben, M. *et al.* (1994) Training a large troop of rhesus macaques to co-operate during catching: analysis of the time investment. *Animal Welfare*, **3**, 135–140

Lutz, C., Well, A. and Novak, M. (2003) Stereotypic and self-injurious behavior in rhesus macaques: a survey and retrospective analysis of environment and early experience. *American Journal of Primatology*, **60**, 1–15

Maki, S., Alford, P.L. and Branmblett, C. (1987) The effects of unfamiliar humans on aggression in captive chimpanzee groups. *(Abstract) American Journal of Primatology*, **12**, 358

Malinow, M.R., Hill, J.D. and Ochsner, A.J. (1974) Heart rate in caged rhesus monkeys (*Macaca mulatta*). *Laboratory Animal Science*, **24**, 537–540

Manuck, S.B., Kaplan, J.R. and Clarkson, T.B. (1983) Behavioural induced heart rate reactivity and artherosclerosis in cynomolgus monkeys. *Psychosomatic Medicine*, **45**, 95–108

Markowitz, H. (1982) *Behavioral Enrichment in the Zoo*. Van Nostrand Reinhold Co., New York

Marr, J.M., Gnam, E.C., Calhoun, J. *et al.* (1993) A non-stressful alternative to gastric gavage for oral administration of antibiotics in rabbits. *Lab Animal*, **22**, 47–49

McConnell, P. (2002) *The Other End of the Leash. Why We Do What We Do Around Dogs*. Valentine Books, New York

McKinley, J., Buchanan-Smith, H.M., Bassett, L. *et al.* (2003) Training common marmosets (*Callithrix jacchus*) to cooperate during routine laboratory procedures: ease of training and time investment. *Journal of Applied Animal Welfare Science*, **6**, 209–220

Meaney, M.J., Mitchell, J.B., Aitken, D.H. *et al.* (1991) The effects of neonatal handling on the development of the adrenocortical response to stress: Implications for neuropathology and cognitive deficits in later life. *Psychoneuroendocrinology*, **16**, 85–103

Meunier, L.D. (2006) Selection, acclimation, training, and preparation of dogs for the research setting. *ILAR Journal*, **47**, 326–247

Meyer-Holzapfel, M. (1968) Abnormal behaviour in zoo animals. In: *Abnormal Behaviour in Animals*. Ed. Fox, M.W., pp. 476–503. Saunders, London

Mineka, S., Gunnar, M. and Champoux, M. (1986) The effects of control in the early social and emotional development of rhesus monkeys. *Child Development*, **57**, 1241–1256

Moberg, G.P. (1985) Influence of stress on reproduction: a measure of well-being. In: *Animal Stress*. Ed Moberg G.P., pp. 245–267. American Physiological Society, Bethesda, MD

Moseley, J. and Davis, J. (1989) Psychological enrichment techniques and New World monkey restraint device reduce colony management time. *Laboratory Animal Science*, **39**, 31–33

Neuringer, A. (1969) Animals respond for food in the presence of free food. *Science*, **166**, 339–341

Obernier, J.A. and Baldwin, R.L. (2006) Establishing an appropriate period of acclimatization following transportation of laboratory animals. *ILAR Journal*, **47**, 364–369

Orok-Edem, E. and Key, D. (1994) Responses of rats (*Rattus norvegicus*) to enrichment objects. *Animal Technology*, **45**, 25–30

Perlman, J.E., Thiele, E., Whittaker, M.A. *et al.* (2004) Training chimpanzees to accept subcutaneous injections using positive reinforcement training techniques. *American Journal of Primatology*, **62**(Suppl. 1), 96

Phillipi-Falkenstein, K. and Clarke, M. (1992) Procedure for training corral-living rhesus monkeys for fecal and blood sample collection. *Laboratory Animal Science*, **42**, 83–85

Prescott, M.J., Bowell, V.A. and Buchanan-Smith, H.M. (2005) Training laboratory-housed non-human primates, Part 2: Resources for developing and implementing training programmes. *Animal Technology and Welfare*, **4**, 133–148

Pryor, K. (1999) *Don't Shoot the Dog. The New Art of Teaching and Training*. Bantom Books, New York

Reichard, T. and Shellabarger, W. (1992) Training for husbandry and medical purposes. In: *Proceedings of the American Association of Zoological Parks and Aquariums Annual Conference*, pp. 396–402. AAZPA, Maryland

Reinhardt, V. (1992) Improved handling of experimental rhesus monkeys. In: *The Inevitable Bond: Examining Scientist-Animal Interactions*. Eds Davis, H. and Balfour, A., pp. 171–177. Cambridge University Press, Cambridge

Reinhardt, V. (1997a) Training nonhuman primates to cooperate during blood collection: a review. *Laboratory Primate Newsletter*, **36**, 1–4

Reinhardt, V. (1997b) Training nonhuman primates to cooperate during handling procedures: a review. *Animal Technology*, **48**, 55–73

Reinhardt, V., Cowley, D., Scheffler, J. *et al.* (1990) Cortisol response of female rhesus monkeys to venipuncture in homecage versus venipuncture in restraint apparatus. *Journal of Medical Primatology*, **19**, 601–606

Reinhardt, V., Liss, C. and Stevens, C. (1995) Restraint methods of laboratory nonhuman primates: a critical review. *Animal Welfare*, **4**, 221–238

Ruys, J.D., Mendoza, S.P., Capitanio, J.P. *et al.* (2004) Behavioral and physiological adaptation to repeated chair restraint in rhesus macaques. *Physiology and Behavior*, **82**, 205–213

Sackett, G. (1991) The human model of psychological well-being in primates. In: *Through the Looking Glass*. Eds Novak, M. and Petto, A., pp. 35–42. American Psychological Association, Washington, DC

Schapiro, S.J., Bloomsmith, M.A. and Laule, G.E. (2003) Positive reinforcement training as a technique to alter nonhuman primate behavior: quantitative assessments of effectiveness. *Journal of Applied Animal Welfare*, **6**, 175–187

Schapiro, S.J., Perlman, J.E., Thiele, E. *et al.* (2005) Training nonhuman primates to perform behaviors useful in biomedical research. *Lab Animal*, **34**, 37–42

Selye, H. (1976) *Stress in Health and Disease*. Butterworth, Boston

Skinner, B.F. (1938) *The Behavior of Organisms*. Appleton-Century-Crofts, New York

Skinner, B.F. and Ferster, C.B. (1970) Schedules of reinforcement. In: *Festschrift for B. F. Skinner*. Ed. Dews, P.B., pp. 37–46. Irvington, New York

Smith, T.E., McCallister, J.M., Gordon, S.J. *et al.* (2004) Quantitative data on training New World primates to urinate. *American Journal of Primatology*, **64**, 83–93

Smith, A.C. and Swindle, M.M. (2006) Preparation of swine for the laboratory. *ILAR Journal*, **47**, 358–363

Stone, A.M., Bloomsmith, M.A., Laule, G.E. *et al.* (1994) Documenting positive reinforcement training for chimpanzee urine collection. *(Abstract) American Journal of Primatology*, **33**, 242

Struck, K., Videan, E.N., Fritz, J. and Murphy, J. (2007) Attempting to reduce regurgitation and reingestion in a captive chimpanzee through increased feeding opportunities: a case study. *Lab Animal*, **36**, 35–38

Tiefenbacher, S., Fahey, M.A., Pouliot, A.L. *et al.* (2004) Effects of diazepam treatment on the incidence of self-injurious behavior in individually housed male rhesus monkeys. *American Journal of Primatology*, **62**, 112

Toates, F. (1995) *Stress. Conceptual and Biological Aspects*. John Wiley and Sons, Chichester

Toth, L.A. and January, B. (1990) Physiological stabilization of rabbits after shipping. *Laboratory Animal Science*, **40**, 384–387

Tuli, J.S., Smith, J.A. and Morton, D.B. (1995) Stress measurements in mice after transportation. *Lab Animal*, **29**, 132–138

Turkkan, J., Ator, N., Brady, J. *et al.* (1990) Beyond chronic catheterization in laboratory primates. In: *Housing, Care and Psychological Well-being of Captive and Laboratory Primates*. Ed. Segal, E., pp. 305–322. Noyes Publishing, New York

VandeVoort, C., Neville, L., Tollner, T. and Field, L. (1993) Noninvasive semen collection from an adult orangutan. *Zoo Biology*, **12**, 257–265

Vertein, R. and Reinhardt, V. (1989) Training female rhesus monkeys to cooperate during in-homecage venipuncture. *Laboratory Primate Newsletter*, **28**, 1–3

Videan, E.N., Fritz, J., Murphy, J. *et al.* (2005) Training captive chimpanzees to cooperate for an anesthetic injection. *Lab Animal*, **34**, 43–48

Wiedenmayer, C. (1997) Stereotypies resulting from a deviation in the ontogenetic development of gerbils. *Behavioural Processes*, **39**, 215–221

Wielebnowski, N.C., Fletchall, N., Carlstead, K. *et al.* (2002) Noninvasive assessment of adrenal activity associated with husbandry and behavioral factors in the North American clouded leopard population. *Zoo Biology*, **21**, 77–98

Wolfle, T. (1985) Laboratory animal technicians: their role in stress reduction and human–companion animal bonding. *Veterinary Clinics of North America: Small Animal Practice*, **15**, 449–454

Würbel. H., Chapman, R. and Rutland, C. (1998) Effect of feed and environmental enrichment on development of stereotypic wire-gnawing in laboratory mice. *Applied Animal Behaviour Science*, **60**, 69–81

17 Euthanasia and other fates for laboratory animals

Sarah Wolfensohn

To be or not to be: that is the question:
Whether 'tis nobler in the mind to suffer
The slings and arrows of outrageous fortune,
Or to take arms against a sea of troubles,
And by opposing end them? To die. ...
Shakespeare: Hamlet (1601) Act 3 Scene 1

Is it is better to be dead, or better to be alive and suffering? Does being a laboratory animal count as an 'outrageous fortune'? Is that any worse or better than being a farm animal or a pet or a wild animal (Wolfensohn & Honess 2007)? These are difficult questions with no simple answers, as ethicists, philosophers and even great playwrights have found. Many hours, days or even careers have been spent debating this question down the centuries. But endless debate does not help the welfare of a laboratory animal whose fate a scientist, a vet, an animal care technician or an ethical review committee is trying to decide. Decisions on euthanasia must be reached swiftly and appropriate actions taken promptly if suffering is to be prevented. Euthanasia is defined as the bringing about of a gentle and easy death (Oxford English Dictionary); so should not, itself, cause pain or suffering.

The optimum time at which to kill an animal in the laboratory will be affected by a range of parameters, and the combination of the factors that lead to a decision as to precisely when to carry out euthanasia has evolved into the concept of the humane endpoint (Hendriksen & Morton 1998). The idea behind the humane endpoint is to define a set intervention point which allows the collection of quality scientific data but limits the amount of suffering, either contingent or direct (Russell & Burch 1959), to which the animal may be subjected. The endpoint may be purely temporal; for example, the animal will be killed x hours/days/weeks after a particular technique is carried out when the adverse effects are not expected to increase but a time limit is set nonetheless, thus reducing the potential for contingent suffering. Or there may be a defined measurable point relating to a physiological parameter; for example, when the blood glucose level reaches x mmol/l which indicates that the animal is in the required physiological state to gather the data, but not yet experiencing deteriorating clinical signs. Or, in some cases, the defined intervention point may be based on a collection of scores cumulatively measured, sometimes with weightings for more challenging clinical conditions, to ensure that any potential suffering is limited to the minimum consistent with obtaining satisfactory data. The collection of usable data is essential since, without that, any suffering caused would be pointless and unethical, as the animal would have been used without purpose or scientific output. Well designed experiments detect early signs of distress, allowing the definition of a point at which adequate data can be obtained, but the suffering of the animals is kept to a minimum. The precise time at which to kill the animal must be based on appropriate and accurate clinical judgement, assessing the degree of suffering and the potential loss of data. Ideally, the maximum achievable information should be obtained from each animal while keeping suffering and distress to the minimum. Using this concept of the humane endpoint will refine the procedure and reduce the costs to the animals, improving the justification and the cost–benefit equation for the experiment. It is unusual for laboratory animals to reach death in a laboratory as an expected consequence of a procedure without the intervention of euthanasia. For further detail on humane endpoints see Chapter 2.

Someone in the laboratory will have to carry out the procedure of euthanasia and actively kill the animal rather than leaving it to die, and this in itself generates a particular set of problems. Euthanasia is not necessarily the most difficult part of the procedure for the animal, indeed if carried out competently it may be easier for the animal than those parts of the procedure that may have caused pain, suffering or distress. On the other hand, the carrying out of euthanasia can be the most difficult part for the researcher.

For a doctor, euthanasia is illegal in most countries. For medical practitioners, treatment is aimed at palliative care, analgesia and supportive therapy, a quality death, but one that occurs naturally and is not actively brought about. Conversely, for veterinary practitioners, euthanasia is part of everyday life in the surgery. The majority of domesticated animals end their lives at the hand of man: millions of food animals are slaughtered in the UK each year (see Table 17.1), production animals are killed once they cease to be viable economic units and pet animals are often subjected to euthanasia once a decline to inevitable death begins to be apparent. The reasons for requesting pet animal euthanasia are many, some of which reflect concern for the animal's well-being; but some are a mixture of concern for the animal and concern for the owner's feelings and their own ability to cope with death, and some are a reflection of the brutal financial facts of animal care and death. Phrases such as 'I

Table 17.1 Number of agricultural animals slaughtered in the UK in 2006 (MLC 2007).

Species	*Number of animals slaughtered*
Cattle	2 643 000
Sheep	16 414 000
Pigs	9 096 000
Broilers	807 200 000
Turkeys	17 300 000

wouldn't want him to suffer', 'I don't want to see him suffer', 'I want to be able to remember him as happy', 'I don't want the children to see him die', 'I don't want to pay for treatment' are regularly heard in veterinary consulting rooms and reflect the complex interactions of factors that lead to the decision of when, or if, to carry out euthanasia.

For the veterinary surgeons themselves, carrying out euthanasia can give rise to a mixture of emotions depending on the individual circumstances. They are in a unique position of being able to offer a quiet and painless death to animals under their care (Bowlt 2007), but in some cases it may be interpreted by the pet owner or by the veterinary surgeon himself, as a failure on the part of the veterinary surgeon to effect a satisfactory cure (BVA Ethics and Welfare Group 2007). Depression is common among veterinary surgeons and as a demographic group they have one of the highest suicide rates, possibly due to stigmatism of mental health disorders and a reluctance to seek medical help, professional and social isolation and ease of access to lethal drugs. Combined with the acceptance of killing as an act, a proven ability to carry it out efficiently and a high level of stress in the working environment, the proportional mortality ratio for veterinarians is significantly higher than for medical or dental practitioners, farmers or pharmacists (Mellanby 2005; Bartram & Boniwell 2007). Coping with death of research animals can also take its toll on the emotions of those involved (Pekow 1994; Halpern-Lewis 1996).

All of these factors play their part in the way that euthanasia is viewed in the context of a laboratory animal environment; sometimes making the researcher more and sometimes less willing to carry out euthanasia. Individual psychological state is important and must be handled carefully by all those involved, but must not be allowed to affect the welfare of the animal under study.

Experimental animals may need to be killed for a variety of reasons but virtually all will be killed long before their natural life expectancy comes to an end. It may simply be that the end of the experiment has been reached and all the necessary data have been collected. Animals may also be killed if their health gives cause for concern, if they have reached the end of their breeding life, if they are unwanted stock, or if tissues and blood are required for *in vitro* studies. Article 8 of Council Directive no. 86/609/EEC states that the animal should not be subjected to severe pain, distress or suffering and that if it is not possible to treat it with pain-relieving means it shall be immediately killed by a humane method. Killing an animal is never a pleasant task for the person carrying it out; but it does not have to be unpleasant for the animal, provided it is carried out competently, swiftly and humanely.

An animal is regarded as continuing to live until the permanent cessation of the circulation or the destruction of the brain, therefore any method of killing used must ensure that one or both of these criteria is met. As with any scientific procedure, humane killing requires a certain amount of preparation. Points that should be considered include:

- **Training.** The person carrying out the killing must be able to do so without causing distress to the animals involved. Any method of killing can cause distress if badly performed, so staff must be suitably trained and competent in the methods and with the equipment they will be using.
- **Handling.** Animals must be handled carefully and competently without causing them distress. Animals will often be calmer if held by a person with whom they are familiar. Staff must be competent to hold animals properly and securely. Some methods of killing may require two or more people to hold the animal; there must be sufficient trained people available to do the job properly.
- **Location.** If an animal is frightened but conscious it may show behavioural responses such as vocalisation, struggling, urination and defecation. Any fear or distress experienced can be communicated by sound or smell to other animals causing further distress. Some of these responses may be exhibited by unconscious animals before death occurs. When killing entire cages of animals it is advantageous to kill them in the home cage as this causes much less stress (Hackbarth *et al.* 2000) than removing them to an unfamiliar location. In the case of rodents, the reactions of conspecifics may not be apparent when an animal is killed in the same room; although for other species it is considered preferable to remove them to another area away from the group before they are killed. In any event, in an emergency, it is better to euthanase the animal immediately rather than to move it.
- **Equipment.** Some methods of killing require equipment such as anaesthetic induction chambers, carbon dioxide cylinders, bottles of anaesthetic agents, needles and syringes, or firearms. It is essential to make sure that any equipment is clean, prepared and ready for use at the start, cleaned again before subsequent use with another animal, and that the operator is fully competent to use it.

There are several different methods of euthanasia available. There is a variety of guidelines that can provide assistance with the considerations relating to the carrying out of euthanasia (Canadian Council on Animal Care (CCAC) 1980; Close *et al.* 1996, 1997; American Veterinary Medical Association (AVMA) 2001, 2007; Reilly 2001; American Association of Zoo Veterinarians (AAZV) 2006; Office International des Epizooties (OIE) 2007). The following points should be considered when choosing a method of humane killing (Wolfensohn & Lloyd 2003; Carbone *et al.* 2004):

- death must occur without producing pain;
- the time required to produce loss of consciousness must be as short as possible;

- the time required to produce death must be as short as possible;
- the method must be reliable and non-reversible;
- there must be minimal psychological stress on the animal;
- there must be minimal psychological stress to the operators and any observers;
- it must be safe for personnel carrying out the procedure;
- it must be compatible with the requirements of the experiment;
- it must be compatible with any requirement to carry out histology on the tissues;
- any drugs used should be readily available and have minimum abuse potential;
- the method should be economically acceptable;
- the method should be simple to carry out with little room for error.

The different methods are often divided into those using physical methods and those using chemicals administered by various routes.

Chemical methods of euthanasia

Overdose of injectable anaesthetic agent

The aim is to cause respiratory depression, leading to hypoxia and death. With modern injectable agents used in combination to achieve balanced anaesthesia, there is generally a fairly wide safety margin, and indeed with some anaesthetics it is actually quite difficult to kill an animal using a reasonable injection volume. The drug of choice to carry out euthanasia is therefore pentobarbital, which does not have a wide safety margin and so has been superseded as an agent to provide quality anaesthesia. It is preferable to give it intravenously for the most rapid action but in the smaller species it is generally administered intraperitoneally, using a suitably sized needle. The smaller the needle, the better, as it will cause less pain on insertion. Pentobarbital causes pain on injection and combination with a local anaesthetic agent will help to reduce this (Ambrose *et al.* 2000). In larger animals, if it is not possible to locate a vein, the animal should be sedated first with an agent administered by an easier route. When the sedative has taken effect and the animal can be handled more easily, the pentobarbital can be administered intravenously to kill it quickly and humanely. Pentobarbital must not be given intramuscularly as it is very irritant to the tissue and this will cause pain. Intrathoracic injections in the conscious animal are also painful, and an intracardiac injection of pentobarbital should only be attempted after the animal has been rendered unconscious.

Exposure to carbon dioxide and overdose of anaesthetic by inhalation

The use of carbon dioxide for euthanasia, while very common, is controversial, leading to much debate over the most humane method of euthanasia (Conlee *et al.* 2005; Hawkins *et al.* 2006). One of the principal advantages is that it can be carried out leaving the animal in its home cage and placing the entire cage in a carbon dioxide cabinet. The animal is not handled and the operator is able to remain detached from the process of killing. A controllable source of carbon dioxide should be used, it is not acceptable to use dry ice; preferably there should be a thermostatic mechanism to ensure that the gas reaching the animal from the cylinder is not uncomfortably cold.

Neonatal animals and cold-blooded vertebrates are resistant to hypoxia, and diving birds and mammals can hold their breath for long periods, so the use of carbon dioxide is not recommended in these animals. It is now established that rats and mice find carbon dioxide aversive (Leach *et al.* 2002a) and its use as a euthanasia agent is considered unacceptable by many (Leach *et al.* 2004). Carbon dioxide exposure causes immediate bradycardia due to nasal nociception activation and pain, although Hackbarth *et al.* (2000) found that when rats were exposed to carbon dioxide in the home cage without disturbance there were no such aversive signs. For humans, carbon dioxide inhalation is painful at 50–100% exposure concentrations (Danneman *et al.* 1997). If rodents are exposed to a high concentration (>50%) of carbon dioxide, the time to unconsciousness and therefore the time for which the pain has to be endured is at least 10–15 s (Hawkins *et al.* 2006). Many guidelines for euthanasia state that the concentration of carbon dioxide should be *rising*. However, if the chamber is filled slowly it can take around 2 minutes to reach unconsciousness at 35% carbon dioxide (Golledge *et al.* 2005). While this avoids the acute pain seen with 100% carbon dioxide, there is significant dyspnoea and tachypnoea which may be very distressing to the animal even if it is not actually painful. In Hawkins *et al.* (2006) it is stated that carbon dioxide aversion in rats starts at 10–15% concentration and that this aversion is very high, not even being overcome by motivation of 24 h of food deprivation. In humans, dyspnoea occurs at 7% carbon dioxide, is severe at 15–20% and said to be very unpleasant. Rats will show escape behaviour at 15–20% carbon dioxide. The choice with carbon dioxide would therefore appear to be between a high concentration initially, resulting in a faster more painful death; or a lower rising concentration of carbon dioxide, resulting in a slower death with less pain but more distress from dyspnoea. Neither of these is satisfactory.

The question is therefore whether there are any better methods that combine the advantages of not having to handle the animal and the aesthetic acceptability of being remote from the animal at the point of death, but which does not cause the animal respiratory distress or pain.

The use of carbon dioxide for stunning or for euthanasia in farm animals has also been shown to be aversive, whereas combination of the carbon dioxide with argon is less so (Gregory *et al.* 1987; Raj 1999 (pigs); Raj & Whittington 2003 (chicks)). The use of argon raises health and safety concerns since it is difficult to detect and when used in rats and mice they still show some aversive behaviour even though this is less than with carbon dioxide (Leach *et al.* 2002b).

Euthanasia can be carried out by administering an overdose of inhalation anaesthetic. The animal is placed in a suitable induction chamber with the vapour. It is important that the animal is physically separated from the liquid agent since volatile anaesthetics are very irritant to mucous membranes. While inhalation anaesthetics are less aversive than carbon dioxide, they are still not particularly pleasant. Halothane has been found to be least aversive for rats and enflurane for mice (Leach *et al.* 2002b), although such agents should be used with appropriate scavenging systems to ensure compliance with health and safety regulations. It is important to ensure that the animal is left in the chamber with the inhalation anaesthetic for long enough, and to confirm that it is dead, since it may recover if it is removed too soon and allowed to breathe room air.

Rodents communicate by pheromones in urine and faeces and placing the animals on disposable paper which can be replaced each time, is a simple way of controlling this potential stress factor. Chambers of this type should always be used in an extraction cabinet or with a suitable ducting system to reduce exposure of staff to the volatile agent. Similarly, as for injectable agents, modern inhalational anaesthetic agents are developed to have a wide safety margin so it can be quite difficult to kill an animal with such agents. It may therefore be preferable to use them to induce unconsciousness and then kill the animal using carbon dioxide at 100%. This way the detection of pain from nociception will be avoided and death from hypoxia is rapid. It has therefore been suggested to use halothane (but this agent is shortly to be withdrawn from some markets) to induce loss of consciousness, then to infuse carbon dioxide to cause death. However the change from use of a single agent is not currently acceptable in some jurisdictions (Home Office 1997) and it is not so simple or convenient for the user. It also may give rise to a training issue, but these considerations should not be used as an excuse not to change if multiple agents would be more humane. No doubt the use of carbon dioxide versus other methods will be subject to further debate in the future. Inhalation methods may be less suitable for large animals since they are more difficult to restrain.

Overdose of anaesthetic by immersion

For fishes and small amphibia, euthanasia can be achieved by percutaneous administration of tricaine methane sulphonate (MS 222), administered by immersion. As for inhalation euthanasia in the rodent, care must be taken to ensure that the animal is left in the solution for an adequate length of time and that death has occurred when it is removed.

Physical methods of euthanasia

Physical methods of euthanasia can be distasteful to have to carry out, and this can lead to a tendency to be hesitant. However, if carried out properly these methods are often less distressing to the animal, since unconsciousness is very quickly achieved. Death should be confirmed by exsanguination by severing major vessels or by destruction of the brain. Manual dexterity and an ability to handle the animal confidently are essential to minimise any apprehension. They should be practised first on dead animals, after careful observation of the method carried out by a competent and experienced person. Physical methods are appropriate for small rodents, rabbits and birds and also for amphibians, reptiles and fishes. Dislocation of the neck causes extensive damage to the brainstem and instantaneous unconsciousness. Dislocation must be carried out quickly and with confidence, otherwise there might not be complete separation of the cervical vertebrae and the animal may experience distress or pain. It may be preferable to sedate or anaesthetise animals prior to cervical dislocation. It may be necessary to wrap birds to prevent involuntary flapping of the wings.

Concussing the animal by striking the back of the head renders the animal unconscious, following which death must be ensured by dislocation of the neck or by exsanguination. As with dislocation of the neck, confidence in handling the animal and manual dexterity are required to carry out this method without causing distress to the animal. Support the animal by the hindquarters and swing the body downwards such that the back of the head comes sharply into contact with a hard surface such as a work bench. Considerable training and practice on dead animals is required to ensure competence with this method, and it is difficult to ensure that animals are stunned consistently. For amphibia, reptiles and fishes the brain must be destroyed immediately following concussion, as in these species the brain is very tolerant to hypoxia, and it cannot otherwise be guaranteed that concussion is irreversible or that unconsciousness will last until death.

For ungulates the animal may be killed by one of the standard methods of slaughter, such as use of a free bullet, a captive bolt, or electrical stunning followed by destruction of the brain or exsanguination. However these methods are controlled by other legislation including control of firearms and will therefore only be available to those who have been appropriately trained and issued with the relevant licences.

For foetal, larval and embryonic forms there are other methods that can be used which take into account the degree of development of the nervous system in the various animals. Overdose of injectable anaesthetic may be used as for adult animals of all species. Refrigeration, disruption of membranes or maceration can be used for birds and reptiles, but the death of the reptile embryo must be ensured by overdose of anaesthetic, maceration or immersion in tissue fixative. Cooling of foetuses until movement has stopped followed by immersion in cold tissue fixative is appropriate for mouse, rat and rabbit foetuses. Decapitation can be used for foetal mammals and birds up to 50 g weight, using a pair of sharp scissors. In some jurisdictions decapitation for neonatal rodents is considered an appropriate method of euthanasia.

Other methods of euthanasia

Other methods of killing may be employed occasionally if there is a scientific need. Microwaves can be used to fix brain metabolites without losing anatomical integrity (Ikarashi *et al.* 1984; Stavinoha *et al.* 1978). Specialist apparatus and careful technique are required. The microwaves are focused on particular areas of the brain, producing death very rapidly. Electrical stunning may be used as in routine preslaughter stunning for ungulates and also for other species such as poultry or rabbits. It requires specialist equipment, and death must be confirmed using another method. Pithing may be carried out in unconscious fish, amphibia or reptiles. A sharp needle is inserted through the foramen magnum and agitated to destroy the brain. This requires technical skill in order to ensure rapid death, and must not be carried out in conscious animals. Rapid freezing using liquid nitrogen can be used *in situ* or following decapitation to freeze the brain. The animal must be rendered unconscious first, as it can take up to 90s to freeze deep structures. Decapitation may not be humane in conscious animals, because of the length of time it takes for the decapitated head to lose consciousness, particularly in cold-blooded vertebrates. If this method is required for scientific reasons, there must be particular justification, and consideration given to sedating or anaesthetising the animal first.

Confirmation of death and disposal of carcases

After carrying out any method of euthanasia it is vital to check that the animal is really dead before disposing of the carcase. Thus the process of killing must be completed by one of the following six methods:

- confirm permanent cessation of the circulation, if possible by severing the major vessels;
- destruction of the brain with a permanent loss of brain function; all signs of reflex activity must have ceased;
- dislocation of the neck, following concussion or overdose of anaesthetic;
- exsanguination;
- onset of rigor mortis;
- mechanical disruption by destruction of the body in a macerator.

All animal carcases are classed as clinical waste and as such must be disposed of correctly either by maceration or in clinical waste bags that are then incinerated. There should be local rules relating to the method of disposal in each animal unit.

Alternatives to euthanasia

For most laboratory animals the carrying out of euthanasia is an integral part of the experimental procedure, as tissues are collected for examination and generation of critical data. However there are some procedures that can be completed and all necessary scientific data collected without necessitating the death of the animal. At the end of these procedures, some animals are then used as breeders, some are returned to stock for use in further procedures, some are moved out of being laboratory animals into other sectors such as agriculture as farm animals or rehomed as pets. The first critical decision is to ensure that the maximum amount of data has been generated from each individual, without causing additional harm, and thus prevent more animals having to be used. In the case of surplus ex-breeding or stock animals, it may be possible to harvest blood or tissue at euthanasia which can then be used in *in vitro* experiments which are increasingly being developed as replacement alternatives to the use of live animals in research. However a number of laboratory species including dogs, rabbits and species of primates, such as common marmosets, squirrel monkeys, capuchins, stump-tailed macaques and chimpanzees, have been successfully retired to private homes, zoos, sanctuaries or professional collections in the UK, Europe and USA. This is reported to be beneficial for staff morale as well as the animals (Laboratory Animal Science Association (LASA) 2004) and can help further develop a culture of care.

Re-homing ex-laboratory animals must be considered very carefully since the re-homing facility must be able to accommodate the animals properly and there must be adequate resources to care for them in the longer term. Whoever will be caring for the animals must have suitable training and experience. Depending on the animal's age, state of health, previous experiences and the physical and social conditions in which they are to be kept, there are potentially significant welfare costs to laboratory animals that are re-homed. Re-homing should only be considered if it is clear that the process will be truly in the best interests of the individual animal, that it will not harm its welfare, and that the new home offers it a good quality of life. The factors that must be considered when re-homing dogs have been described in detail in the LASA (2004) guidance on re-homing and in the Joint Working Group on Refinement (JWGR) report (2004).

Re-use of animals in further experimental procedures in order to avoid euthanasia may result in a decrease in the total number of animals used thus applying the principle of reduction. However it also presents the specific ethical question of animal numbers versus animal suffering. The suffering (both contingent and direct) of an individual animal must be weighed against the welfare impact of obtaining, housing and preparing (surgically in some cases, or by training) a different animal. In the European Union re-use is subject to legal constraints defined in Council Directive no. 86/609/EEC and it is considered that a reduction in total number of animals used does not justify causing a significant increase in suffering for the individual animals involved.

Intuitively, longevity is an aim of most humans, provided that one remains in good health. However, for a laboratory animal, longevity may not be in its welfare interests. For a start, the laboratory environment may not be the ideal one in which to keep some species (Berdoy 2002). Limits should therefore be set on the length of time for which animals are maintained. It is not necessarily easy to define a set of temporal criteria and decisions may have to be made on a case-by-case basis. The points that should be considered include:

- The health of the animal. This should include both physical and psychological health and welfare and should be regularly reviewed by the animal care staff, veterinary staff and ethologist (as appropriate). Any abnormal behaviours should be noted as well as physiological indicators of poor well-being.
- The adequacy of animal's environment. Whatever the housing system there must be good quality and quantity of space, with attention to all three dimensions, and provision for social interactions, if appropriate for the species.

There should be a good reason for maintaining animals kept in the laboratory long term other than as subjects in experiments or as breeders. For example, they may be kept as a companion for an experimental animal when using species such as sheep, dogs or primates. Additional resources such as enrichment, training and exercise will be necessary and there should be a written plan for such animals as well as for experimental ones.

As an example, ex-breeder primates are a particular case where there can be a tendency to allow animals to live out their natural lifespan but where arguments may be put forward for euthanasia once an animal reaches a specific age or has given birth a specified number of times. Again, decisions should be made on a case-by-case basis. In wild primate populations, as in most species, the cessation of breeding is frequently determined by the death of the individual (from disease, parasites, predation, fighting or a basic inability to feed sufficiently) and is quite likely to occur before any biological reproductive senescence occurs. In harem, or multimale systems, males may breed for as long as they retain the required social status to maintain reproductive access to females, and females may breed for as long as they are able to achieve the necessary breeding condition.

There is no evidence for the existence of a menopause in New World primates and they appear to continue breeding, albeit with reduced frequency as they get older, well into old age with lifespans of typically 10–20 years (higher in some species: 40–45 in *Cebus* sp. and 30–35 in *Ateles* sp.) (Hendrickx & Dukelow 1995). In macaques, the menopause, including stopping of the menstrual cycle and ovulation, has been determined to be at about 25–30 years of age; and it may be accompanied by appearance changes, such as changes in face colouration and a greying and thinning of the hair. In addition to changes in the reproductive physiology and anatomy, post-menopausal changes may occur, for example to the skeletal and cardiac system (Hendrickx & Dukelow 1995). Although an aging individual may have ceased to breed frequently, and there may be an increase in the number of stillbirths in older females, this does not mean that this animal does not perform an extremely valuable social role within the group in which it lives. In captive populations removing older animals ranging from social perturbation (and hence stress) caused by removing a socially influential older animal to loss of any role they might have played in educating younger members of the group in parenting skills. This is particularly true of the removal of older, high-ranking females in matrilineal macaque societies.

The periodic change of the resident breeding male occurs naturally in macque harem and multimale groups and this helps to maintain breeding production; avoiding female boredom with their partner. However, the removal (either culling or individual housing) of older females from their group should be avoided unless there are over-riding animal health concerns. In the interests of the animal's health and welfare it may be appropriate to embark upon a course of contraception for older females that are experiencing problems such as repeated stillbirths, but it is important for their welfare that they be allowed to remain with their social group.

The use of a welfare assessment grid can be helpful in balancing some of the difficult decisions about the future of an animal. The axis can be use to give a schematic representation of parameters including clinical condition, psychological well-being, behaviour and environmental conditions (Wolfensohn & Honess 2007).

Concluding remarks

There is no doubt that the purposeful killing of animals by people, when done badly, can cause extreme suffering and it matters not whether the animal is being killed for food, for population management or as part of a research project. Its capacity to suffer is the same, whatever the purpose. There is an ethical obligation and a practical opportunity to minimise any associated suffering when animals are killed and this should be done each and every time (Mellor 2000). Whatever the answers to these questions might be, it is both worthwhile and ethically imperative to find scientifically based refinements to minimise suffering at euthanasia.

An animal's quality of life has been defined as being made up of three components: its value to itself, its value to science and its value to its peer group (Sandoe & Christensen 2007). Alternative views are that the animal has no value at all, has a value for that individual only, or that its value exceeds what is 'in it' for the animal in question. Any domestic species, whether farmstock, companion animal or laboratory animal is man's product, arguably for man's use and would not exist if man had not organised for it to do so (Allen 2007). The same author continues that since a post-weaning animal does not have grieving relatives, the most sensible, pragmatic, economic and humane solution whether it is sick and suffering, old and debilitated or simply no longer wanted for its intended use, is to kill it. However, animals, both domestic and wild have varied roles in society and their value can be economic, cultural, political, emotional or religious (Gardiner 2007). They are also attributed an inherent 'animal value' that exists by virtue of them being sentient beings. Antonites (2001) argues that while sentience is important it is not a sufficient condition and it is the demonstration of rational consciousness in animals that leads to the ethical and welfare implications. Kirkwood and Hubrecht (2001) expand on the meaning of consciousness and cognition and conclude that despite the diversity of opinion it is of great relevance to animal welfare. For further discussion on the ethics of killing animals which have an inherent value either to themselves or to others see Nuffield Council on Bioethics (2005).

Each individual's view of this will affect their attitude to choices made about treatment, endpoints and euthanasia method. Ethically driven scientific evaluations are used to improve the humaneness of livestock slaughter through such organisations as the Humane Slaughter Association[1]. Killing used in vertebrate pest control is also under discussion since many of the current methods of rodent control fall short of a humane ideal (Universities Federation for Animal Welfare (UFAW) 2006), but questions remain between the objective scientific evaluations and their interpretation as to how much suffering an animal experiences and the relativi-

[1]http://www.hsa.org.uk

ties of different types of suffering. Specifically, how does one compare the intensity of suffering versus its duration? Or how can two different types of suffering be compared; for example Mellor and Litten (2004) give the example: is severe breathlessness a greater welfare insult than severe and unquenchable thirst? Moreover, there is the question of quality of life versus quantity of life. It is perhaps inevitable that a veterinary surgeon will have a different perspective on the value of an animal's life compared to the view of the pure scientist. The former has committed his/her professional life to the welfare of animals committed to his/her care, whereas for the latter the animal is a tool to formally investigate a hypothesis. But while we may not all agree on the value of an animal's life we should all agree on the significance of animal welfare and strive to maximise it.

References

American Association of Zoo Veterinarians (2006) *Guidelines for Euthanasia of Non-domestic Animals.* AAZV, Yulee, FL

Allen, T. (2007) Views on euthanasia. *Veterinary Record*, **162**, 72

Ambrose, N., Wadham, J. and Morton, D. (2000) *Refinement of Euthanasia. Progress in the Reduction, Refinement and Replacement of Animal Experimentation.* Elsevier Science, Oxford

Antonites, A. (2001) Animals – more than sentience: ethical and welfare implications. *Animal Welfare*, **10**, S236

American Veterinary Medical Association (2001) 2000 Report of the AMVA panel on euthanasia. *Journal of the American Veterinary Medical Association*, **218(5)**, 669–696

American Veterinary Medical Association (2007) AVMA Guidelines on Euthanasia June 2007 (formerly Report of the AMVA Panel on Euthanasia). http://www.avma.org/issues/animal_welfare/euthanasia.pdf (accessed 16 April 2009)

Bartram, D. and Boniwell, I.B. (2007) The science of happiness: achieving sustained psychological well being. *In Practice*, **29**, 478–482

Berdoy, M. (2002) *The Laboratory Rat: A Natural History Film.* http://www.ratlife.org/ (accessed 16 April 2008)

Bowlt, K. (2007) Views on euthanasia. *Veterinary Record*, **160**, 915–916

British Veterinary Association Ethics and Welfare Group (2007) Report of meeting with Lord Joffe. *Veterinary Record*, **160**, 780

Carbone, L., Baumans, V. and Morton, D.B. (2004) Report of the Workshop on Euthanasia Guidelines and Practices. *Alternatives to Laboratory Animals*, **32** (Suppl. 1), 445–446

Canadian Council on Animal Care (1980) *Guide to the Care and Use of Experimental Animals*, Vol **1**. CCAC, Ottawa

Close, B., Banister, K., Baumans, V. *et al.* (1996) Recommendations for euthanasia of experimental animals. Part 1: report of a working party. *Laboratory Animals*, **30**, 293–316

Close, B., Banister, K., Baumans, V. *et al.* (1997) Recommendations for euthanasia of experimental animals. Part 2: report of a working party. *Laboratory Animals*, **31**, 1–32

Conlee, K.M., Stephens, M.L., Rowan, A.N. and King, L.A. (2005) Carbon dioxide for euthanasia: concerns regarding pain and distress, with special reference to mice and rats. *Laboratory Animals*, **39**, 137–161

Danneman, P.J., Stein, S. and Walshaw S.O. (1997) Humane and practical implications of using carbon dioxide mixed with oxygen for anaesthesia and euthanasia of rats. *Laboratory Animal Science*, **47**, 376–385

Gardiner, A. (2007) Views on euthanasia. *Veterinary Record*, **161**, 144

Golledge, H., Roughan, J., Niel, L., Richardson, C., Wright-Williamson, S. and Flecknell, P. (2005) Carbon dioxide euthanasia in rats – behavioural and autonomic system responses to exposure. Abstract, SECAL-ESLAV 2005 International Congress, Elche, Spain

Gregory, N.G., Moss, B.W. and Leeson, R.H. (1987) An assessment of carbon dioxide stunning in pigs. *Veterinary Record*, **121**, 517–518

Hackbarth, H., Küppers, N. and Bohnet, W. (2000) Euthanasia of rats with carbon dioxide – animal welfare aspects. *Laboratory Animals*, **34**, 91–96

Halpern-Lewis, J.G. (1996) Understanding the emotional experiences of animal research personnel. *Contemporary Topics*, **35**, 58–60

Hawkins, P., Playle, L., Golledge, H. *et al.* (2006) *Newcastle Consensus Meeting on Carbon Dioxide Euthanasia of Laboratory Animals.* 27 and 28 February 2006 Newcastle upon Tyne UK. http://www.lal.org.uk/workp.html (accessed 14 May 2009)

Hendriksen, C.F.M. and Morton, D.B. (1998) Humane end points in animal experiments for biomedical research. In: Proceedings of the International Conference 22–25 November 1998 Zeist, The Netherlands.

Hendrickx, A.G. and Dukelow, W.R. (1995) Reproductive Biology. In: *Nonhuman Primates in Biomedical Research: Biology and Management.* Eds Bennett, T.B., Abee, C.R. and Hendrickson, R., pp. 365–374. American College of Laboratory Animal Medicine Series. Academic Press, San Diego

Home Office (1997) *Code of Practice: The humane killing of animals under Schedule 1 to the Animals (Scientific Procedures) Act 1986.* ISBN 0102653976. HMSO, London

Ikarashi, Y., Maruyama, Y. and Stavinoha, W.B. (1984) Study of the use of the microwave magnetic field inactivation for the rapid inactivation of brain enzymes. *Japanese Journal of Pharmacology*, **35**, 371–387

Joint Working Group on Refinement (2004) Refining dog husbandry and care. Eighth report of the BVAAWF/FRAME/RSPCA/UFAW Joint Working Group on Refinement. *Laboratory Animals*, **38** (Suppl. 1), S1:1–S1:94

Kirkwood, J.K. and Hubrecht, R. (2001) Animal Consciousness, cognition and welfare. *Animal Welfare*, **10**, S5–17

Laboratory Animal Science Association (2004) *Guidance on the Rehoming of Laboratory Dogs.* www.lasa.co.uk/position_papers/publications.asp (accessed 2 June 2008)

Leach, M.C., Bowell, V.A., Allan, T.F. *et al.* (2002a) Aversion to gaseous euthanasia agents in rats and mice. *Comparative Medicine*, **52**, 249–257

Leach, M.C., Bowell, V.A., Allan, T.F. *et al.* (2002b) Degrees of aversion shown by rats and mice to different concentrations of inhalational anaesthetics. *Veterinary Record*, **150**, 808–815

Leach, M.C., Bowell, V.A., Allan, T.F. *et al.* (2004) Measurement of aversion to determine humane methods of anaesthesia and euthanasia. *Animal Welfare*, **13**, S77–86

Mellanby, R.J. (2005) Incidence of suicide in the veterinary profession in England and Wales. *Veterinary Record*, **157**, 415–417

Mellor, D. (2000) Learning from refinement strategies applied at low and high levels of noxiousness. In: *Progress in the Reduction, Refinement and Replacement of Animal Experimentation.* Eds Balls, M., van Zeller, A-M. and Halder, M.E., pp. 65–77. Elsevier Science, Amsterdam

Mellor, D.J. and Litten, K.E. (2004) Using science to support ethical decisions promoting humane livestock slaughter and vertebrate pest control. *Animal Welfare*, **13**, S127–132

Meat and Livestock Commission (2007) *A Pocketful of Meat Facts 2007.* MLC, Milton Keynes

Nuffield Council on Bioethics (2005) The ethics of research involving animals. http://www.nuffieldbioethics.org (accessed 2 June 2008)

Office International des Epizooties (2007) Guidelines for the slaughter of animals. In: *Terrestrial Animal Health Code 2007 16th edition:*

Appendix 3.7.5. OIE World Organisation for Animal Health. http://www.oie.int/ (accessed 2 June 2008)

Pekow, C.A. (1994) Suggestions from research workers for coping with research animal death. *Lab Animal*, **23**, 28–29

Raj, A.B.M. and Whittington, P.E. (2003) Euthanasia of day old chicks with carbon dioxide and argon. *Veterinary Record*, **136**, 292

Raj, A.B.M. (1999) Behaviour of pigs exposed to mixtures of gases and the time required to stun and kill them: welfare implications. *Veterinary Record*, **144**, 165

Reilly, J.S. (2001) Euthanasia of animals used for scientific purposes. *Australian and New Zealand Council for the Care of Animals in Research and Teaching*. Adelaide University, Adelaide, South Australia

Russell, W.M.S. and Burch, R.L. (1959) *The Principles of Humane Experimental Technique*. Special Edition, UFAW 1992

Sandoe, P. and Christensen, S.B. (2007) The value of animal life: how should we balance quality against quantity. *Animal Welfare*, **16**, S109–115

Stavinoha, W.B., Frazer, J.W. and Modak, A.T. (1978) Microwave fixation for the study of acetylcholine metabolism. In: *Cholinergic Mechanisms and Psychopharmacology*. Ed. Jenden, D.J., pp. 169–179. Plenum Publishing Corp, New York

Wolfensohn, S. and Honess, P. (2007) Laboratory animal, pet animal, farm animal, wild animal: Who gets the best deal? UFAW Symposium: Quality of Life: The Heart of the Matter. *Animal Welfare*, **16** (Suppl), 117–123

Wolfensohn, S.E. and Lloyd, M.H. (2003) *Handbook of Laboratory Animal Management and Welfare*, 3rd edn. Blackwell Publishing, Oxford

Universities Federation for Animal Welfare (2006) *UFAW Workshop on Rodent Control Methods.* http://www.ufaw.org.uk/

PART 2
SPECIES KEPT IN THE LABORATORY

Mammals

18 Wild mammals

Ian R. Inglis, Fiona Mathews and Anne Hudson

Introduction

A range of wild mammal species is studied in the laboratory or other captive conditions. Many of the principles for keeping wild animals (eg, nutrition, climatic requirements) are similar to those for domesticated animals of the same species but, as emphasised below, it is very important to take careful account of behavioural and other differences to avoid stress or ill-health. This chapter touches on special requirements for a small selection of species kept for research in Europe but cannot provide detail on the very wide range of species kept worldwide.

As noted above, although some wild animals used in research are closely related to common laboratory animals, for example, the Norway rat (*Rattus norvegicus*), the house mouse (*Mus musculus*) and the European wild rabbit (*Orytolagus cuniculus*), their requirements can be profoundly different (see also Chapter 25). Applying the standard protocols and housing conditions developed for laboratory strains is likely not only to compromise their welfare, but also adversely affect the quality of the data collected. The process of domestication in laboratory strains has selected, both deliberately and accidentally, for traits such as docility and inquisitiveness. In addition, inbreeding has reduced the inter-individual variability that characterises natural populations. This means that laboratory animals are generally easier to handle than their wild counterparts, are less stressed by standard procedures and the close proximity of humans and are more predictable in their responses.

Many other wild animals studied in the laboratory have no domesticated relatives. Examples include Daubenton's bats (*Myotis daubentoni*), red fox (*Vulpes vulpes*), badger (*Meles meles*) or wild boar (*Sus scrofa*). The lack of relevant baseline information on 'normal' physiological profiles, such as haematological reference ranges, for most species presents significant challenges. Similarly, baseline data on 'normal' behaviour are frequently lacking. It can therefore be difficult to apply the conventional methods for scoring well-being familiar to researchers working with laboratory animals, or to define thresholds at which interventions to alleviate suffering should be implemented. The onus is therefore on researchers to familiarise themselves with relevant literature from a range of sources – for example from zoo medicine and conservation biology – and also to apply the precautionary principle when judging whether welfare is compromised.

It is useful to consider the evolutionary context of an animal's response in captivity: for example, for a mouse, sleeping in the open would be maladaptive in the wild, and this behaviour in the laboratory is more likely to indicate exhaustion than relaxation (Mathews *et al.* 2004). Taking evasive action to the threat of predation (such as a human entering the room) is an appropriate response, and does not, in itself, indicate compromised welfare. However, if efforts to escape are thwarted (for example if no hiding places are provided); if there is repeated exposure to the stressor; or several stressors are experienced simultaneously (such as exposure to humans and the provision of new food types) then psychological and physiological distress are likely (Moberg 2000).

Wild mammals are usually kept for applied research into: (1) methods of population control (eg, Shepherd & Inglis 1987, 1993; Smith *et al.* 1994); (2) the transmission of diseases and parasites (eg, Tesh & Arat 1967; Crouch *et al.* 1995); (3) environmental protection, where the animals are used to test for possible contamination (eg, Beardsley *et al.* 1978; Barber *et al.* 2003; Thompson 2007); and (4) for studies relating to conservation or breeding. However, wild mammals have also been used for more academic reasons, such as to investigate various forms of learning (eg, Shumake *et al.* 1971; Powell 1974; Cowan 1977; Inglis & Shepherd 1994) and behaviour (eg, Odberg 1987; Hurst 1990; Wurbel *et al.* 1998; Hendrie *et al.* 2001).

For many types of work, there can be good justification – from the perspective of animal welfare as well as research output – to undertake it in the laboratory rather than the field. In the UK, special dispensation is needed to release wild animals back into the wild after a procedure. This requires competent and authorised persons to judge that the animal is fit for release and that no long-term adverse implications are expected from the procedure. In many cases, research in the field or re-release to the wild would not be appropriate. For example, when testing new rodenticides, all subjects need to be monitored and humane endpoints applied. However, this is not always the case and, historically, work has often been conducted in the laboratory for reasons of convenience. Advances in methods of tracking, remote monitoring, non-invasive sampling (for example, using hormone profiles in faecal samples to judge reproductive status) and field anaesthesia mean that there is now much more scope to conduct research on wild animals in their natural environment. It is therefore important to carefully evaluate the welfare costs of conducting the research in the laboratory versus the field. In some cases, the quality of the research may also be improved by working with wild mammals *in situ*: for example, captivity is likely to influence disease dynamics due to the effects of stress, alteration of population processes etc, and so field research may be preferred (eg, Mathews *et al.* 2006; Amengual *et al.* 2007; Vaz 2007; Beldomenico *et al.* 2008; see also Chapter 7).

This chapter discusses only those aspects of maintenance, care and handling of wild mammals that differ from the techniques usually employed with laboratory strains.

Potential health hazards to humans

Working with wild mammals is hazardous. They frequently show aggressive behaviour when approached or handled. In addition, allergy to laboratory animals (ALA) is common particularly when, to avoid disturbance, cages and pens of wild mammals are less frequently cleaned than those of laboratory strains. The most common symptoms are blocked sinuses, sneezing and watering eyes. Particular attention must be paid to the potential transmission of zoonotic parasites and pathogens from wild animals to humans. It is important to recognise that screening of natural populations for parasites and pathogens is often somewhat haphazard. Screening is largely driven by concern for disease outbreaks important to the health of humans or their livestock. There has tended to be little proactive screening, and baseline information on the prevalence of most pathogens is scant or non-existent for many species (Mathews 2009). This chapter, therefore, is only able to highlight some of the better known parasites and pathogens that occur in European wildlife. Researchers must be alert to the possibility that other zoonoses are likely to be present, and the implications of these agents for human health may not be known; for example, most emerging infectious diseases appear to be zoonotic in origin (Taylor *et al.* 2001). Parasites and pathogens not only threaten the health of staff and of other animals in the facility, but they may also influence the animals' responses to experimental interventions. Recent evidence suggests that animals need not even be in direct contact with infected individuals in order to mount immune responses (eg, Curno *et al.* 2009). Particular care should, therefore, be taken whenever a new cohort of animals is brought to the laboratory.

One of the most serious diseases likely to be carried by wild rodents is Weil's disease or leptospirosis, caused by the spirochaete *Leptospira icterohaemorrhagiae*. Wild rats are the most common host but the house mouse (Twigg *et al.* 1969), water vole (pers. obs.) and other mammals including rabbit (Chalmers *et al.* 2009) and hedgehog (Dyachenko *et al.* In press) can also carry the organism. Once the spirochaete is contracted, a rat passes through a brief bacteraemic period of acute infection, which is not accompanied by obvious symptoms of disease. This is then followed by a chronic stage when the organism is harboured in the kidneys and is excreted in the urine throughout the remaining lifetime of the host without clinically affecting its health. *Leptospira icterohaemorrhagiae* enters the human body through abrasion in the skin, or via the mucous membranes of the eyes, nose, throat or lungs. It is uncertain whether the spirochaete can also be transmitted through unabraded skin. There have been reports of mouse colonies infected with *Leptospira ballum* causing illness in personnel (eg, Stoenner & Maclean 1958). The early stages of Weil's disease produce general flu-like symptoms and it is, therefore, important that staff inform their doctors that they have contact with wild rodents.

Rat-bite fever in man is caused by two organisms that naturally inhabit the bucconasal cavities of wild rats (Somerville 1961). *Streptobacillus moniliformis* is pathogenic to mice, whereas both rats and mice are the normal host to *Spirillum minus*. The human diseases lead to local irritation followed by generalised febrile illness with a macular rash. As its name implies, rat-bite fever is usually contracted from a rodent bite.

Pasteurella pestis, the plague bacillus (Hudson *et al.* 1964), is transmitted through several species of fleas that parasitise wild mammals. As it is easy to control these insect vectors, the danger of human infection from a sanitised colony of wild rodents is small. *Pasteurella septica* may be of more practical importance. It is found in the respiratory tracts of many mammals and is transmitted to humans by bites.

Salmonellae are a common cause of food poisoning. *Salmonella typhimurium* and *Salmonella enteriditis* are the two types most frequently associated with colonies of wild mammals. Newly infected colonies can suffer high losses. Chronic infection leads to a prolonged carrier state in which the carriers show no symptoms but shed infective agents from the alimentary tract. Human infection occurs via the oral route and results, within hours or days, in fever and gastrointestinal distress.

Lymphocytic choriomeningitis is a viral disease of humans that in its rarest form may cause a fatal encephalitis. The virus is commonly found in house mice but rarely in other wild rodents (Maurer 1964). Laboratory personnel are thought to acquire the virus by ingestion.

Toxoplasma gondii, a parasitic protozoan, can be carried by many mammal species, (including humans who are 'dead end' hosts). This causative agent of the disease toxoplasmosis is usually minor and self-limiting but it can have serious, or even fatal, effects on a foetus whose mother contacts the disease during pregnancy. The life cycle of *T. gondii* has two phases. The sexual part of the life cycle takes place only in the members of the felidae family, whilst the asexual part of the life cycle can take place in any mammal. The early stages of toxoplasmosis can produce no symptoms, or mild fever, enlarged lymph nodes in the neck and muscle pains.

Cryptosporidiosis and giardiasis are protozoan diseases affecting the intestines of mammals. The parasites are spread by faecal–oral route. Symptoms appear from 2–10 days after infection and can last for up to 2 weeks. As well as watery diarrhoea there are often stomach pains or cramps and a low fever but not all individuals have symptoms. Infection can be life-threatening in immunocompromised people and animals.

Rabies is a very dangerous viral disease but one that is unlikely to pose a hazard in a well managed animal unit in Europe. The virus is geographically distributed in endemic pockets, which periodically erupt into neighbouring regions. Although carnivores and bats are the usual carriers, all mammals are susceptible. The virus enters through skin wounds usually caused by bites inflicted by infected animals in the virulent stage of the disease. Where wild mammals have to be imported from regions with endemic rabies, vaccination in conjunction with quarantine should prove effective against carriers of the virus. European bat lyssavirus II (EBL 11) is endemic in Daubenton's bats in the UK (Brookes *et al.* 2005). Although passive surveillance has failed to identify bat rabies in other British bats caution should still be exercised, as a range of European bats is known to be naturally infected with EBL 1 and EBL 11 (Harris *et al.* 2006). It is important to note that infected bats may not exhibit symptoms of rabies for a considerable period. All staff working with bats must therefore be vaccinated against rabies, and appropriate gloves should be worn whenever handling the animals.

Dermatomycoses are frequently acquired by wild mammals. The affected regions on the animal develop bald circular patches, which gives the condition its vernacular name 'ringworm'. The causative agent is usually *Trichophyton mentagrophytes* and there can be a much higher proportion of carriers than of clinically infected animals, particularly in wild mice.

Cestode infection is an important hazard (eg, Gibson 1967). The tapeworm *Hymenolepis nana* is common in wild rodents and can infect humans via the oral route. *Hymenolepis diminuta* is also found in wild rodents but only rarely in humans.

Arthropod parasites are usually restricted to a few closely related hosts. Some, especially fleas and *Sarcoptes* mites, do attempt to invade humans but the infections are usually self-eliminating irritations of a duration that varies with the physiological sensitivity of the persons involved, and they are easy to control. However, in addition to being a nuisance, ectoparasites are potential vectors of disease; as discussed above, several flea species transmit *Pasteurella pestits*, the plague bacillus.

Precautions

When working with any wild mammals, as with laboratory animals, scrupulous personal hygiene and adherence to all safety codes are essential. The following precautions reflect specific hazards associated with working with wild mammals.

1. Adequate protective clothing should be worn at all times (ie, a minimum of laboratory coat or overalls, overshoes or boots, masks and gloves) in the animal unit and removed before entering non-infective areas. If disposable clothing is not worn, provision must be made to isolate soiled garments from other laundry.
2. All clothing worn in the animal unit must be dealt with as a potential hazard. Even if clothing has not come into direct contact with wild mammals there could still be allergens present and hence it should not be taken out of the unit. Wherever possible, the laundering of protective clothing should be done within the animal unit.
3. All equipment should be thoroughly washed and disinfected or sterilised after use. Disinfectants with low odour, which are biodegradable, and are effective against a wide range of pathogens and parasites should be used. Note that some agents that infect wild animals are particularly resistant to disinfection (such as *Cryptosporidium parvum* and *Mycobacterium bovis*). Care should be taken to ensure that appropriate disinfectants are used; many virucides are NOT effective against a sufficient range of pathogens.
4. Non-standard housing such as floor pens should be vacuumed rather than swept, or doused with water first, to reduce the risk of allergy.
5. All cuts, scratches and abrasions, particularly on the hands and forearms, must be covered with waterproof dressings before entering the animal unit.
6. Hands and forearms need to be thoroughly washed with adequate soap before entering areas outside the animal room.
7. Gloves should always be worn when cleaning out and washing cages, and when handling wild mammals.
8. When conducting experimental procedures with, or sexing, wild rodents, safety glasses should be worn in order to minimise the risk of urine passing through the mucous membranes of the eye.
9. Particularly when working with wild rodents, staff must report animal bites; it is essential that medical attention is given within 24 h.
10. Risk assessments should be carried out laying down basic information on relevant zoonontic diseases (eg, Weil's disease). Staff should inform their doctor that they work with wild mammals.
11. Staff should undergo a course of anti-tetanus injections and regularly receive booster injections.
12. Staff should have annual checks carried out to make sure they are not developing symptoms of animal allergies.

Capture of wild animals

Information on welfare issues relating to the capture and use of wild animals is given in Chapter 7. An important additional consideration when conducting laboratory research is that the animals are removed from the site of capture. Wild animals are parts of communities and ecosystems, and the removal of individuals therefore has consequences for the remaining animals. The effects may range from starvation of dependent young, to the removal of a predator or preybase. The Three Rs principles can be applied to help minimise these effects. Reduction in the numbers of animals used may be possible through improved study design. Alternatively, impacts on the population may be reduced if smaller numbers of animals are caught at a greater number of sites (this strategy may also help avoid problems of pseudoreplication in the study design). Refinement to the protocol might include avoidance of capture during the breeding season and possibly (depending on the type of research) conducting the work in the field. Replacement could be achieved through the use of a related laboratory animal or a captive-bred wild-type animal; or, where there are conservation concerns, the use of a more common, related species.

Transport of wild animals to the animal unit

Detailed information on the transport of laboratory animals is given in Chapter 13. Animals being transported in the UK are protected under the Animal Health Act 1981 (including the Welfare of Animals During Transport Order 1997) and the Protection of Animals Acts 1911–2000.

Specific reference is made under the Animal Health Act 1981 Transit of Animals (General) Order 1973 to the transport of those wild species listed under CITES. Article 11 (2) states that: *'No person shall transport an animal to which the Convention on International Trade in Endangered Species refers except in compliance with the CITES guidelines for transport and preparation for shipment of live wild animals or in compliance with the standards set by the International Air Transport Association'*. Specific reference is also made in the Animal Health Act to the transportation of deer in velvet. Article (6) states that: *'No person shall transport a deer in velvet unless the journey is of 50 km or less and special precautions are taken to protect it from injury or unnecessary suffering.'*

Every effort should be made to minimise transport times: as a general rule, the amount of stress experienced increases with journey length. Because the animals need to be captured prior to transport, a considerable time may have elapsed before arrival at the laboratory, even if the transport distance is short (for example, if some animals were trapped early in the night): the total amount of time for which the animal has lacked control over its environment must therefore be evaluated. The cumulative effects of several stressors (capture, transport, introduction to laboratory, etc) may result in high levels of stress or even distress, with consequences for the animal's psychological state and physiological function (Moberg 2000). Interventions such as the provision of high-energy foods to help prevent exhaustion, or the use of chemical sedatives may be necessary.

Wild rodents can be transported in the cage traps in which they were captured providing that these are covered to give the animals darkness and security. Preferably, cages with nest boxes should be used. Sufficient pelleted diet should be added to the traps together with a few cut potatoes or apples to provide moisture. Small groups of mice captured in the same locality may be transported together within large bins; as well as food, these bins should contain ample hay or straw to reduce the chance of fighting during transit. Some species that are caught in nets will need to be placed in suitable transport cages/bags, eg, bats can be placed in cloth bags. To transport some large mammals for very short distances it may be possible simply to securely fasten a hessian sack over the head. The transportation of several species requires expert assistance; for example, it is difficult to transport deer safely although they may be quietened and restrained if their heads and limbs are covered.

Arrival of wild mammals at the animal unit

Wild animals are likely to have suffered considerable stress as a result of capture and transport, even under optimal conditions. For example, even short transport distances in badgers have important effects on innate immune responses, and a period of undisturbed recovery is required for the animals to return to normal profiles (McLaren *et al.* 2003).

The introduction of wild mammals into an animal unit poses the severe risk of spreading diseases and parasites to laboratory stocks. Ideally wild mammals should be housed in a separate building from laboratory stocks. If this is not possible they must be removed as far as possible from laboratory strains; for example, in a separate isolated corridor. There are several key husbandry duties that are essential to prevent the spread of disease and parasites:

1. separate and complete sets of equipment must be kept for wild and laboratory stocks;
2. wild mammals should never be moved through areas containing laboratory strains;
3. it is essential that different personnel care for wild and laboratory animals;
4. experimental procedures that involve both laboratory and wild animals must be carried out first in the rooms containing the laboratory strains;
5. laboratory breeding stock must be health screened at least once per year.

Upon arrival at the animal facility, it may be necessary to treat the animals for ectoparasites and/or endoparasites (Tuffery & Innes 1963). Veterinary advice should be sought to develop appropriate preventative medicine programmes and procedures for each species kept. Some care should be taken in extrapolating treatments from related domesticated species as what can be safe for one species may not be for another (especially, for example, in the use of live vaccines). Whether the removal of the natural parasite burdens is required depends on the research question. For example, if the work is intended to study dominance or mating behaviour and extrapolate to wild populations, then removal of parasites could interfere with data interpretation since parasite loads influence social status and mate selection. Where parasite removal is desirable, care should be taken to choose an agent and method of application that does not harm the animal or interfere with experimental results. For example, a reliable method to rid wild rodents of ectoparasites is to immerse the animal, still inside the cage trap, in a solution of Amitraz 251 for a few seconds. The animals will need to be dipped again 14 days later. For bats, permethrin-based powders should be used and systemic spot-on treatments avoided due to their potential toxicity. Alternatively, the majority of mites can be removed without chemical treatment by placing the animals on light-coloured cotton cloths and changing these daily. In addition, several species will require inoculation; for example, wild rabbits should be vaccinated against myxomatosis and rabbit viral haemorrhagic disease, whilst red foxes in the UK need vaccination procedures against canine distemper, hepatitis, parvovirus, parainfluenza and canine leptospirosis. As noted above, vaccination of wild animals should be considered carefully as live vaccine strains safe for use in some species may cause severe disease in others.

Monitoring the health and welfare of the animals

Health monitoring is a legal requirement in several countries, including the UK. Monitoring can be carried out in three ways: (1) the daily checking of each animal for signs of clinical disease; (2) the regular screening of a predetermined number of animals to determine what microorganisms are present and/or to which they have previously been exposed; and (3) *post-mortem* examination of any animal that dies. Routine health screening is rarely carried out for wild mammals but should be conducted if health concerns arise or if it is important to assess the subclinical disease burden. A predetermined number of representative animals (preferably a mixture of sexes and ages) is selected for a detailed study of the micro-organisms and antibodies present. Larger species can be sampled at the institution and the resulting samples sent to the analytical laboratory; whilst for smaller species the whole body can be sent away for analysis. The samples that may be collected for analysis include: fresh faeces (or gut contents in small species) for signs of protozoa and parasite eggs/segments/larvae; hair and skin scrapes for signs of ectoparasites; ear swabs for signs of mites; and throat and nasal swabs for signs of bacteria and viruses. A clotted blood sample is taken for antibodies to listed micro-organisms and for serum biochemistry. It is important to recognise that the parasites and pathogens included in routine screening of standard laboratory species may not be those of most relevance to wild animals, and specific tests may therefore need to be requested.

There may be interactions between the health status of the animal and some aspects of the research work. Some of these interactions are obvious; for example, respiratory infection may result in high mortality when the animals are anaesthetised. Other interactions are subtler; for example, Sendai virus in rats causes immunosuppression and then permanently modulates the animal's immune response, and in mice the hepatitis virus also has major effects on immune responses.

Staff should be able to spot signs of illness, pain and distress in those wild mammals for which they are responsible. However, this is not always easy because it may be difficult to see or interpret signs of chronic pain, and indicators of chronic pain or distress are usually more insidious in the early stages. Although fundamental uncertainty exists when assessing subjective experiences such as pain and suffering in animals, nevertheless there are some reliable signs. For example, an animal may show protective behaviour towards an injured part, such as limping after an injury to a leg, going off feed because of abdominal injury, or actively seeking relief from pain by ingesting both opiate and non-opiate analgesics. Careful observation is often required to detect those changes in an animal's appearance and behaviour which indicate that deterioration has occurred. It must also be remembered that, particularly for wild animals in captivity, distress caused by fear should be considered as important as suffering induced by pain.

Although it is clear that animals can experience and suffer pain and stress, measuring the intensities of these states is very difficult. The UK National Centre for the Replacement, Refinement and Reduction of Animals in Research has suggested the following strategy, which is applicable to wild animals:

- If methods of pain assessment have been developed for the species used, then these should be adapted to the requirements of the particular research procedure being undertaken.
- If methods of pain assessment are not available, consider devoting resources to developing some form of scoring system.
- If pain scoring is not possible, determine the analgesic protocol based on clinical experience with other surgical procedures in that, or related, species.
- If possible, use dose rates that have been established using studies that have employed pain-scoring systems.
- When data on pain scoring is not available, estimate doses from results of analgesiometric studies using tonic (longer lasting) nociceptive stimuli (eg, late phase formalin test).
- Use pre-emptive analgesia and consider using multi-modal strategies.
- Attempt to evaluate the efficacy of the analgesic regimen selected, if only by clinical assessment.

Housing and handling

General considerations

In the UK, wild mammals are not included within Schedule 2 of the Animals (Scientific Procedures) Act 1986 as far as the provision of light, heat etc is concerned. The housing and the animal unit environment for wild mammals should be appropriate for each species and, in the UK, professional help and advice must be sought from the Named Veterinary Officer (NVO) and the Named Animal Care and Welfare Officer (NACWO) of the animal unit.

Wild mammals should be kept in conditions that conform as far as is possible to their natural habitat. Whilst many of the larger mammals (eg, fox, deer) should be held only in outdoor facilities (see below), several of the smaller mammals can be successfully housed within indoor laboratory facilities (see below). Whilst housing requirements vary widely between wild species nevertheless there are some general guidelines.

The wild animals' exposure to humans should be minimised. Refuges should be provided that allow the animals to hide from view. 'Look out' places where animals can rest and spot the approach of humans are also environmental features that help to reduce stress. The animals should be provided with the materials required to perform natural behaviours such as nesting materials and substrates suitable for digging. For example, when given the opportunity, captive-bred bank voles will build straw nests and dig burrows in peat substrate.

Environmental enrichment must be provided (see Chapter 10). The form of such enrichment will depend on the species but should include not only objects that animals can manipulate but also static features that increase the complexity of movement throughout the cage/pen/enclosure. Hiding some of the animal's food helps to maintain more normal exploratory and foraging behaviour patterns and to prevent stereotypic behaviour. Species that are incompatible (for example, predator and prey, animals requiring different environmental conditions, animals of different health status) should not be housed in the same room nor, in some cases, within smell or earshot.

Standard housing and care regimes established for the commonly used laboratory animals are not necessarily suitable for wild mammals or for individuals of wild species born in captivity. For example, olfactory cues are extremely important in communication in wild animals, and frequent removal of scent marks by cleaning of pens and cages will adversely affect the animals' welfare. Frequent cleaning will also entail the stress of exposure to humans and unfamiliar objects such as a holding cage and new bedding. A compromise between the need to prevent disease and the need to minimise stress is therefore required.

Many wild animals are unable to operate water bottles or other dispensing equipment, or require time to acquire the skill. Shallow drinking bowls should always be provided in the first instance, and removed only if there is evidence that the animals are able to use dispensers. Note that some species, such as the water vole or beaver, prefer to defecate in water, and so the resource should be provided for this purpose and refreshed regularly. Wild mammals can have difficulty recognising unfamiliar food (eg, laboratory chow). In addition, digestive problems can be produced by sudden changes in diet when the animals arrive in the laboratory (eg, the change from a grass-based diet to pelleted food in rabbits). Mortality can be markedly decreased by initially providing familiar foods and introducing novel foods slowly.

The temperature and humidity of indoor rooms housing wild mammals should be as carefully controlled as is the practice for laboratory strains of the same species. The control of such variables for wild mammals housed in outdoor facilities is not possible and it is essential that suitable shelter/refuge areas are provided.

Avoid high light levels; an intensity of 350–400 lux at bench level is adequate for routine experimental and laboratory activities. When nocturnal mammals are housed indoors, light-induced retinal damage can occur if the periods of darkness are too short to allow recovery. A daily cycle of 12:12h is suitable for the majority of mammals housed in indoor rooms. For observation and experimental purposes nocturnal animals may be housed under 'reverse photoperiod' conditions (ie, the light and dark periods are switched over and a dim red light is substituted for the dark period). Red light can also be used to provide appropriate 'twilight' periods for crepuscular animals. Changes in the lighting regime should always be conducted gradually, giving the animals time to habituate.

The control of noise is important in the care of all animals but particularly so for wild mammals. Loud, unexpected and unfamiliar sounds are more disruptive than constant sounds, regardless of whether the animal is housed inside or outside. There is no indication that constant background noise, such as that generated by air-conditioning and similar equipment, is harmful providing it is not too loud; indeed, having a radio playing at low volume for a few hours a day may assist the acclimatisation of wild mammals. The general background sound level in an empty indoor animal room should be kept below about 50dB. Some wild animals, particularly bats but also shrews and mice, hear and make use of ultrasound. Ultrasound is generated by a range of equipment (notably computers, but also burglar alarms, sensors, washing machines etc) and is not apparent to humans. It is therefore recommended that the range of ultrasound heard by the species in question is identified and compared with the ultrasound present in the laboratory (which can be cheaply monitored using a heterodyne bat detector). For example, Daubenton's bats echolocate at 30–90 kHz and are therefore particularly likely to be disturbed by sounds within this range.

Specific examples

Wild mice and voles (*Mus musculus, Apodemus sylvaticus, Apodemus flavicollus, Clethrionomys glareolus, Microtus agrestis*)

Wild mice and voles can be kept and will breed in most types of cage but, as a general rule, the larger the cage area the more likely they are to breed. Males show high levels of aggression if housed together, unless they were litter mates and have been housed together continuously, but females provided they have been kept with other females during adolescence, are highly social and prefer to nest together. Wild adult females brought into the laboratory are highly likely to be pregnant, and need careful monitoring. Mice can breed extremely rapidly, and therefore need to be separated as soon as possible after weaning in order to avoid unwanted litters. Adjustment of photoperiod can be used as a method of bringing female bank voles into oestrus.

A range of bedding material can be used (eg, hay, paperwool, shredded paper) and it is important to provide an ample supply of bedding because mice like to burrow and to cover their young. If possible, opportunities to burrow should be provided, for example through the use of peat substrate. The authors have successfully used deep polypropylene storage boxes (50 cm × 50 cm) filled with peat and covered with a lid made of wire mesh within a square wooden frame. A nest box should also be provided in the cage. The cages should not be frequently changed or washed because this removes the mouse pheromones that enable the animals to recognise their familiar environment, and as a result the animals become more stressed. Depending on the number of mice housed together, cleaning out should occur about once a fortnight, and certainly not more than once a week. Environmental enrichment (eg, toilet rolls, sputum cups, sticks, blocks of wood) should be provided. Wild mice, particularly when stressed, may gnaw continually at the diet in the hopper thereby forming a large pile of chewed food in the base of their cage. To help stop wastage of diet the food hoppers may only be filled half way.

Wild mice can also be housed in groups within indoor arenas that provide free movement within a large area. The mouse arenas used by the authors each consist of a wooden floor, 2 m × 3 m, with 1 m high sheet metal walls. The floors and walls slot together enabling several arenas to be joined together to form a larger unit. The wooden floor is covered with a layer of shavings and/or hay. Food bowls, water fonts, nest boxes and enrichment objects are provided. A breeding colony is started with one male and two females and the authors have found that mice breed freely in such arenas. New mice cannot be introduced into an established colony, as the group members will kill them.

Wild mice are far less tractable than their laboratory relatives and, unfortunately, their small size means that it is not practicable to handle them wearing gloves that are strong enough to withstand the frequent bites that occur. Although rubber gloves covered with cotton gloves are not thick enough to withstand a bite they do provide some protection since the slight gap between the glove and finger means that bites do not normally penetrate the skin, and they do provide protection against excreta, etc. A house mouse may be picked up by the base of its tail (although there is evidence that this is a stressful procedure) but the tip of the tail should not be held because the outer skin can be sloughed off as an anti-predator strategy. Make small circular movements whilst holding the mouse; this prevents it from climbing up its tail to bite you. Wood mice and yellow-necked mice have delicate tails, and these should be picked up by scruffing (holding a large pinch of loose skin from across the shoulder blades) which prevents the animal turning around and biting the handler, gently cupped in the palms of the hand rather than lifted by their tails (Figure 18.1). It is preferable to transport a wild mammal indirectly if at all possible, and short, 5 cm diameter tunnels made of plastic with a removable cap at one end can be used to transport wild mice (J.L. Hurst, personal communication). Mice will readily run into such tunnels and their tails can then be grasped easily and the animal transferred within the tunnel. Mice in arenas take shelter in nest boxes when disturbed and, if these boxes are fitted with doors that can be firmly closed, they can be transported within the boxes.

Wild rat (*Rattus norvegicus*)

Wild rats are best kept in groups of related individuals within large arenas; they will readily breed under such conditions. Each group of rats is started using a male and female that have been trapped on the same local farm and then kept in quarantine for at least a month. Figure 18.2 shows one of the wild rat arenas used by the authors. These are housed within a large, bird-proofed agricultural building with roof lights to provide daylight. Each arena measures 10 m 5 m with 1.5 m high walls made of zinc-coated steel. For the housing of small groups (ie, less than 10) it is possible to insert a partition down the centre of each arena, as shown in Figure 18.2. The tops of the walls are angled inwards to

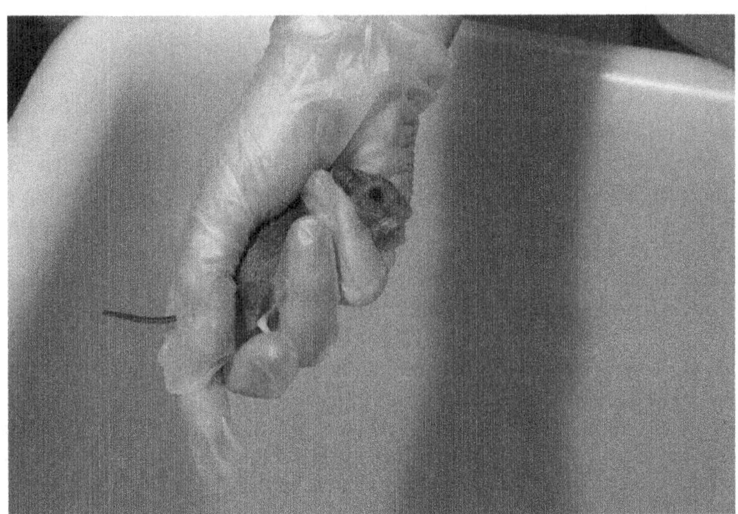

Figure 18.1 Handling wood mice. Courtesy of The Food and Environment Research Agency, British Crown Copyright, 2009.

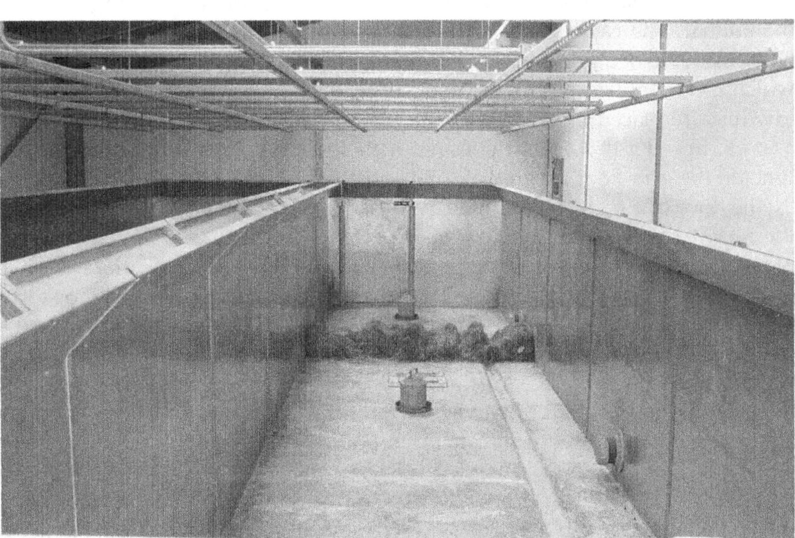

Figure 18.2 Wild rat arena. Courtesy of The Food and Environment Research Agency, British Crown Copyright, 2009.

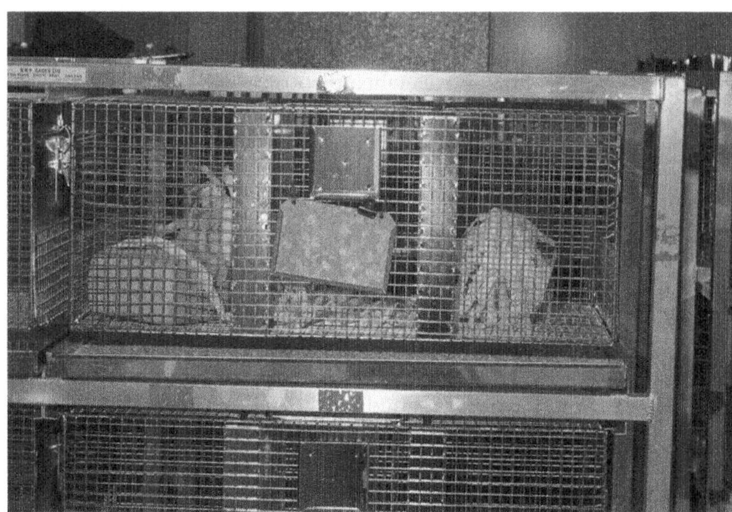

Figure 18.3 Wild rat cage showing the vertical runners down which metal partitions can be slid. Courtesy of The Food and Environment Research Agency, British Crown Copyright, 2009.

prevent escapes. Wild rats climb extremely well and it is crucial that all joins between metal sheeting and wall surfaces do not leave vertical gaps. The floors are made of concrete and a drainage system is required. As well as food and water bowls, hay bales containing nest boxes are placed in the middle of the arena to provide nesting and harbourage. The food bowls can be placed upon the pans of balances set into the arena floors. A computer program has been developed that analyses the changes in weight of the various balances such that the amounts of food removed during feeding bouts can be measured in real time and assigned to individual rats, providing the animals differ sufficiently in their initial body weights. In this manner experimental studies have been conducted on undisturbed groups of wild rats (eg, Shepherd & Inglis 1987). As only healthy individuals are used to start colonies, the arenas can also be used a source of animals for laboratory work. Baited cage traps are used to remove animals from the arenas.

Wild rats are able to chew through polypropylene and wood and it is therefore better if they are to be kept in the laboratory that they are housed in metal cages. It is difficult to clean cages of wild rats, as removing the animal from the cage is both hazardous to the operator and very stressful to the animal. The cages used by the authors therefore have bottoms made of a grid of thick bars with trays underneath which can be pulled out for cleaning. The trays lined with sawdust are placed under the cages and are changed twice a week. In order that the rat does not have to spend all the time on the grid floor, an area of solid substrate is provided by the floor of a metal box or hideaway that is clipped onto the back of the cage; this hideaway is open towards the back of the cage to allow observation. It is also helpful to be able to place a metal partition into the cage; for example this can be inserted vertically down a slot midway along the top of the cage. Thus when placing anything into the cage, such as a food pot, the rat can be confined in another part of the cage by inserting the partition. Shelters need to be provided, such as the inners from toilet rolls, or urine bottles, and paper strips.

If arenas are not available, wild rats can be successfully bred in the animal unit. Stainless steel mesh cages (each 60 cm × 35 cm × 25 cm) are used (Figure 18.3). These cages have doors at either end and allow two metal partitions to be inserted; the cage can thus be divided into three sections should it be necessary to separate the members of the pair. Two nest boxes are provided, one at either end of the cage, so that male and female can have their own space. As there must be minimal human disturbance the male is not removed during the breeding programme. The second nest box provides him with shelter when the female is pregnant, or rearing young. Having two nest boxes is also essential when the pair are first placed together because there will inevitably be some fighting during the first 2 days. The animals must be observed closely during this period to ensure that they can, if necessary, be separated to prevent serious injury. Noises coming from the female's nest box indicates that a litter has been born, and after a further 10 days it is possible to inspect the inside of the nest box without risking death to the litter.

Wild rats should never be handled directly without first having been anaesthetised. They can bite viciously without warning and can carry a number of serious diseases (see earlier in this chapter). A safe, indirect way method to handle a wild rat involves the use of a strong, black, cloth bag which should be large enough to fit over the end of a cage and long enough to allow the rat to move well into the bag (at least 75 cm × 45 cm). The partition is placed into the cage to confine the rat to the end opposite the door that will be opened. The mouth of a black cloth bag is secured tightly over the opening end of the cage so that when the cage door is opened it is completely enveloped by the bag (Figure 18.4). The partition is then removed and the rat will normally enter the darkness of the bag with little delay. Once the rat is well inside the bag one hand is placed across the bag to stop the rat moving back towards the cage whilst the other hand removes the mouth of the bag from the cage and ties it securely. The rat will normally remain sufficiently quiet for a number of tasks, such as weighing, to be carried out. To place the rat back into the cage, the bag is placed in the cage, the neck of the bag is untied and the door of the cage firmly held closed. The bag is then carefully pulled through a small gap between door and cage (Figure 18.5). This will force the rat towards the mouth of the bag and into the cage. The cage door is then made secure. Cardboard and

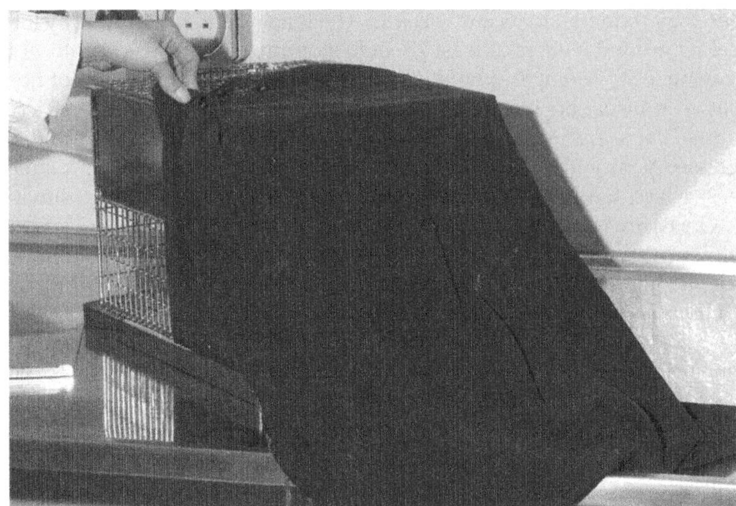

Figure 18.4 Demonstration of how a wild rat is moved from the cage into a strong, black, cloth bag. Courtesy of The Food and Environment Research Agency, British Crown Copyright, 2009.

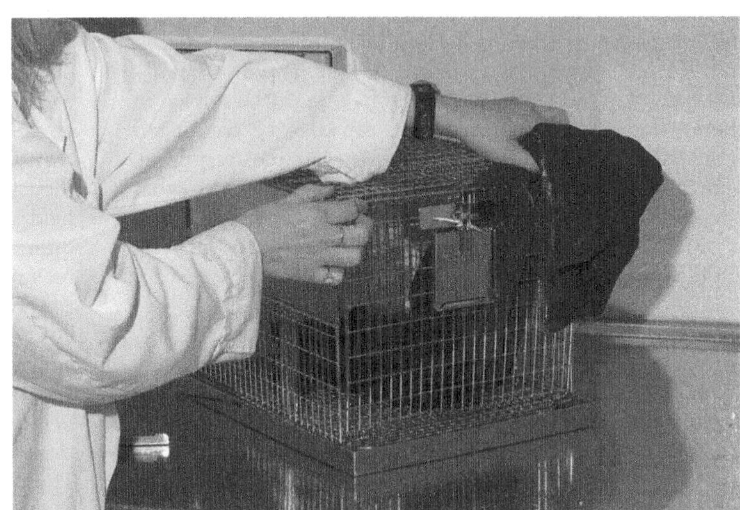

Figure 18.5 Demonstration of how a wild rat is moved from the cloth bag into the cage. Courtesy of The Food and Environment Research Agency, British Crown Copyright, 2009.

plastic tubes with one blind end have also been successfully used by the authors for rats and water voles. The animals readily enter the tube, the end of which can be rapidly covered. This method is particularly useful if the animal needs to be anaesthetised, as the tube can serve as an induction chamber.

Wild rabbit (*Oryctolagus cuniculus*)

Wild rabbits should not be housed in plastic/metal cages indoors as they tend to injure themselves. Weak backs also become a serious problem when wild rabbits are housed in cages; this is thought to be due to lack of exercise. If it is necessary to keep wild rabbits indoors, they can be housed in floor pens (eg, the authors keep individual rabbits floor pens measuring 1.1 m × 1.3 m × 1.1 m). The floor of the pen should be covered with sand or straw; if the floor is just a hard substrate like concrete the animals will become stressed. Raised platforms or boxes that can be used as 'lookout posts' should be provided. Environmental enrichment in the form of tubes and large cardboard boxes filled with paper or straw for burrowing and nesting, should also be provided because, without environmental enrichment, rabbits tend not to use empty floor space and fail to get sufficient exercise.

Rabbits can be housed in groups/pair/singles. However they are social animals, and much better standards of welfare are achieved by group housing. This can be achieved easily if youngsters, between 4 and 8 weeks of age, or female littermates are housed together. Neutering of male rabbits is likely to be required if they are to be group-housed successfully. Otherwise they will need to be separated at puberty in order to avoid fighting. It can be difficult to introduce older unfamiliar rabbits to each other. The introduction needs to be very carefully monitored, and adequate shelter and refuges must be provided (see Chapter 28). The use of a new pen (rather than introducing one animal to another's 'home' enclosure), prior familiarisation with the scent of the new individuals by introducing soiled bedding, and neutering, can all help to improve the success rate.

Rabbits held in outside accommodation require wooden boxes that provide refuge from hot sunshine and protection from small predators like stoats and weasels. Groups of rabbits can be held outside in grassed paddocks enclosed with heavy gauge, small mesh, wire netting fences to prevent entry by rodents, stoats and weasels. The fencing should go below ground level to at least 75 cm to stop the rabbits burrowing out. A single strand electric wire can be strung between insulators just above the fence to prevent entry by foxes. Pairs and single rabbits can be housed in smaller grassed pens with a concrete area at one end where wooden nest boxes, food and water bowls are placed.

Great care is required when handling a wild rabbit because violent struggling can result in not only in deep scratches for the handler but also the animal breaking its back. The technique of handling a wild rabbit is basically the same as that used for a laboratory rabbit (see Chapter 28). The animal must be well supported or it will begin to thrash its hindlegs thereby causing serious back injuries. When disturbed, wild rabbits will usually retreat to their wooden nest boxes and the handler can then close the entrance door of the box and gain access to the animal by removing the roof of the box. The rabbit should be lifted by grasping over the flattened ears and nape of the neck with one hand whilst the other hand is placed around the hindquarters and the animal is drawn against the handler's body. The rabbit is then placed into a large, cotton, drawstring bag. Rabbits will normally rest quietly in these bags and can conveniently be carried in them. Many common procedures can also be conducted whilst the animal is in the bag (for example, weighing, extracting blood from the marginal ear veins) providing that care is taken to ensure that only the body part in question is out of the bag; the rest of the body, in particular the eyes, should remain inside the bag.

Grey squirrel (*Sciurus carolinensis*)

In the UK, a licence is required to hold grey squirrels in captivity because they are classed as a non-native species. In order to obtain the licence you will need to demonstrate that the squirrels are unable to escape from captivity. A licence is also required if the intention is to release the animal back into the wild, as might, for example, be needed by an ecological study. This exemplifies the need to consider local biosecurity laws and regulations for the containment of non-native species. Where containment requirements are strict, this may impose constraints on husbandry methods that may be in conflict with health and welfare interests and plans will need to be developed to deal with or mitigate this situation.

Squirrels are less stressed if housed in groups but, if required, can be kept singly. A large space with plenty of foliage and branches is required to provide the animals with shelter and environment enrichment. Figure 18.6 shows the enclosures used by the authors. Each enclosure is 2.5 m × 9.8 m × 2.8 m, with a substrate of part grass and part concrete upon which the food and water bowls are placed. Ideally the floor should provide some opportunity for digging; if not then containers filled with soil or shavings must be provided. Even though squirrels can share nest boxes there should be at least one nest box per squirrel fixed high on the walls of the enclosure.

Grey squirrels can give serious bites and the handler should wear thick, protective gloves. Upon entering the enclosure all the squirrels are likely to retreat into their nest boxes. The roof of a nest box is removed and the squirrel is gently pinned down with a gloved hand. The handler must then feel around the animal's body until he or she can put their finger and thumb round its neck; the squirrel must be held securely above its shoulders in order to prevent it biting. Once the handler has a firm hold around the squirrel's neck with one hand and the other hand is supporting the animal's rump, the squirrel can be lifted out of the nest box. As well as supporting the rump it is a good idea to gently grip the back legs to prevent the squirrel from kicking. The squirrel can now be placed into a large cotton bag. Before letting go of the squirrel ensure that the bag is closed closely around the arm that is gripping the animal's neck. The neck can then be released and the arm slowly pulled out of the bag whilst ensuring that the squirrel can not escape before the bag can be closed.

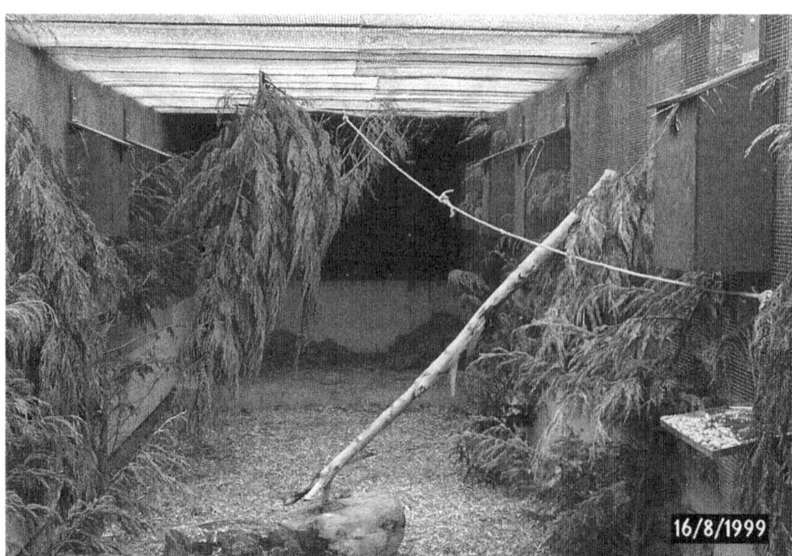

Figure 18.6 Squirrel enclosure. Courtesy of The Food and Environment Research Agency, British Crown Copyright, 2009.

Stoat (*Mustela erminea*) and weasel (*Mustela nivalis*)

Weasels and stoats should be housed singly to avoid fighting. A wooden and wire mesh cage approximately 75 cm × 105 cm × 45 cm is suitable. The authors use a cage that has a door at the side to enable cleaning out and a metal chute used when feeding the animal. The metal chute is placed through the mesh of the top of the cage with approximately 8 cm protruding above the cage. The chute has a shutter at both ends; the bottom shutter (ie, the one inside the cage) can be operated from outside the cage by using a wire. With the bottom shutter closed, the top shutter is opened and food placed within the chute. The top shutter is then closed and the bottom shutter opened, thereby allowing the food to drop onto the floor of the cage. A nest box is also provided with a door that can be operated remotely from outside the cage. In this way the stoat or weasel may be confined within the nest box when the cage is cleaned, and the animal can be transported within the nest box if required.

Thick protective gloves must be worn for handling these animals. The live trap or nest box containing the stoat or weasel is placed in a deep trough and the animal is released into the bottom of the trough. The animal is firmly held down by placing fingers and thumb round its neck; it must be held above the shoulders or it will be able to turn and bite the handler. The animal is then lifted out of the trough by supporting its rump/hindquarters with the other hand.

Fox (*Vulpes vulpes*)

The authors house foxes within enclosures approximately 4.5 m × 6.0 m (Figure 18.7). The animals are usually housed singly; although foxes from the same litter that were captured as cubs can be kept together. Each pen has a concrete floor and 1 m high concrete walls supporting thick wire mesh walls and a wire mesh roof. A wooden outer roof above the wire mesh roof provides shelter and protection from the elements. The concrete floor is sloped providing good drainage and the drains lead to a separate septic tank that is emptied periodically. Shelves are placed on the top of the concrete walls to enable the fox to lie out (Figure 18.7). Nest boxes, foliage and other objects are provided for environmental enrichment. The pen has a door leading into a grassed paddock (completely enclosed by wire mesh) measuring approximately 4.5 m × 10 m that also contains foliage and enrichment objects.

Handling a fox normally requires two people. The animal is encouraged into a nest box, the roof of the box removed, and the noose from a dog-catcher placed over its head and around its neck; the slack in the noose is then gently taken up and the noose locked. This will enable the fox to be inspected within the nest box or moved.

Wild boar (*Sus scrofa*)

Wild boar are secretive and largely nocturnal animals that will shy away from humans. However, when the sows are defending their young they can attack and can be very dangerous due to their size (150+ kg), speed, agility and aggressive defence of their young. In the UK wild boar are listed as dangerous animals under the Dangerous Wild Animals Act 1976. Although in captivity boar will, over time, become habituated to the presence of people it must be remembered that they will never become as docile as the domestic pig. The UK Farm Animal Welfare Council (FAWC) describes them as '*highly strung nervous animals, which can be easily excited or frightened and thus become highly aggressive*'.

The authors keep wild boar within two grassed paddock areas, each 27 m × 80 m in size, enclosed by a double fence consisting of an external 2 m high galvanised wire mesh fencing and an internal 8500 V three-tier electric fence (Figure 18.8). A metal race is used to move boar from one paddock to the other, or to restrain one or more boar when required. Pig arcs and basic sun shelters are provided. The pig arcs need to be capable of housing a sow and the many piglets she can have. The arcs have solid sides and provide good shelter from the weather but afford little visibility into

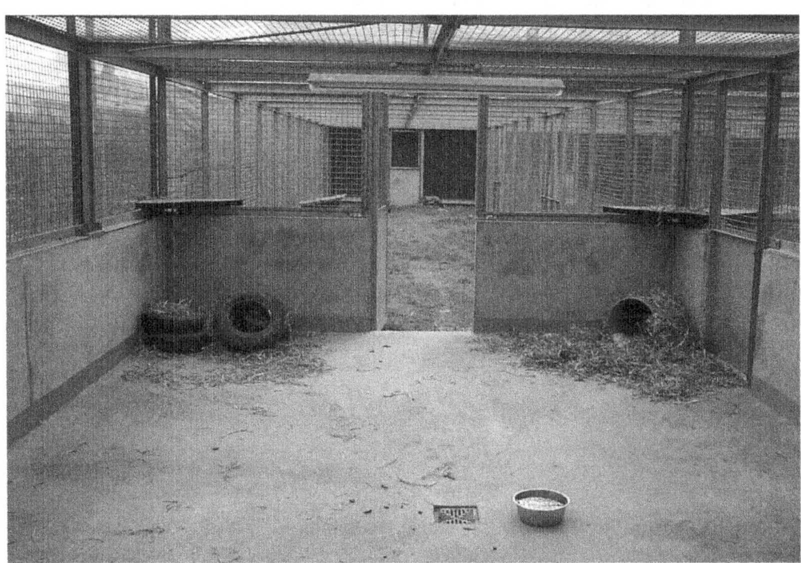

Figure 18.7 Fox enclosure. Courtesy of The Food and Environment Research Agency, British Crown Copyright, 2009.

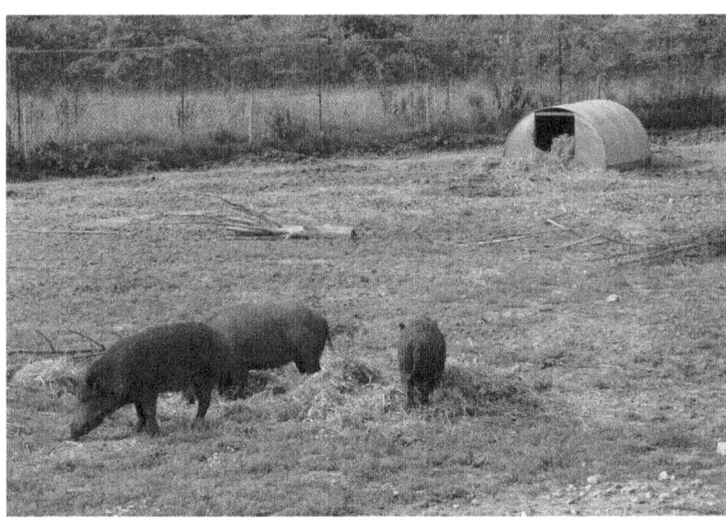

Figure 18.8 Wild boar enclosure showing a pig arc and the surrounding double fence consisting of a wire mesh fence and a three-tier electric fence. Courtesy of The Food and Environment Research Agency, British Crown Copyright, 2009.

the rest of the paddock. The sun shelters give the boar both a place to rest and a good view of the paddocks and the other sows and piglets, whilst reducing their exposure to the sun. Foliage is also provided within each paddock to enable the wild boar to build nests, to lie in or to chew. It is essential that an area of the paddock is designated as a wallow; the animals lie in the wet mud to protect themselves from sunburn and external parasites, and to cool down on hot days. Rubbing posts are also placed in various locations around the paddock. The only safe way to handle wild boar is to sedate and then anaesthetise them.

Laboratory procedures

Procedures and principles are generally the same for wild and conventional laboratory animals, but it is necessary to take note of special handling requirements, of the often unknown disease and reproductive history, and of specific differences that there may be in physiology, behaviour and responses to drug doses. In the UK, the majority of procedures must be conducted under a Home Office Project Licence by suitably qualified staff who hold the necessary Personal Licence. Most wild animals of conservation concern, for example bats and otters are also covered by additional regulations such as, in the UK, The Wildlife and Countryside Act 1981 and The Conservation (Natural Habitats, &C) Regulations 1994. This means that all procedures, as well as the removal of animals from the wild, must be licensed by the appropriate authority (in England this is Natural England), and this procedure is independent of the Home Office Licensing system. Because changes in wildlife law occur quite frequently, researchers are advised to consult the appropriate licensing authorities in their countries for species-specific advice.

Marking

In general, the range of marking techniques that are available for laboratory strains, such as implantation of transponders or 'smart tags', can also be used on wild species (eg, Ball *et al.* 1991). Short-term marks such as clipping the guard hairs (fur clipping) may also be used if an enduring mark is not necessary. Helpful information is provided by Beausoleil *et al.* (2004) and Mellor *et al.* (2004).

Anaesthesia

Small wild mammals are most easily anaesthetised using gaseous anaesthetics, especially isoflurane or sevoflurane. These must be delivered through a metered system, being much too volatile to be used safely with other techniques. Larger mammals can be anaesthetised using injectable anaesthetics and, since with wild species intravenous injection is usually not practical, the drugs are delivered intramuscularly. To allow maximum control over the depth and duration of anaesthesia, anaesthesia induced by an injectable agent can be maintained by gaseous anaesthetics. If the animal is free-ranging, then remote delivery of the sedative by dart-gun will be necessary and this, in the UK, requires a prohibited weapon licence, which specifies that the gun and ammunition are only to be used for the treatment of animals. There are similar arrangements for people who need pistols or revolvers to kill animals humanely. Darting is a skilled and dangerous business. The size of needle, volume and viscosity of the fluid and the amount of power used to project the dart need to be appropriate to the size of the muscle mass and thickness of the skin of the target species. Obviously, the use of inappropriate equipment and materials can cause serious damage to the animal. Darting usually requires a drug mixture containing various proportions of medetomidine, butorphanol and ketamine. In larger mammals such a drug cocktail may result in too large a volume of liquid, and in such cases alternative drugs like Tiletamine or Immobilon may have to be used. Specialist veterinary advice is needed in the development of protocols for chemical capture, sedation and anaesthesia. Information on latest methods for such procedures are available from specialist veterinary texts and series such as Fowler and Miller (2008).

Collection of blood

General advice on blood sampling is provided in the reoprt by the Joint Working Group on Refinement (JWGR 1993). Blood is taken from wild small mammals, rats and water voles from the coccygeal or tail vein of the anaesthetised animal. Although the scales on the tails make it difficult to see the vein, this technique can be perfected with little difficulty. A temporary tourniquet and the use a vasodilator help to raise the vein. Disposable plastic hypodermic syringes with 0.50 mm needles are used for wild rats and with 0.25 mm for wild mice. These can be flushed with sodium citrate solution to prevent clotting. The needle is inserted pointing towards the anterior end of the animal. With small animals, the suction from a syringe will tend to make the vein collapse and so better success may be achieved by allowing the blood to drip out into a collecting pot. Alternatively, heparinised capillary tubes can be used to gather sample volumes of up to 100 µl. The authors have also successfully gathered high-quality samples from water voles using the Multivette 600 capillary blood collecting system (Sartsedt Inc.), which not only maximises sample volumes but reduces the risk of contamination. Sampling from the orbital sinus should be avoided because of the high risk of adverse sequelae. Similarly, sequential sampling from the tail tip (by cutting off the tip of the tail) is contraindicated, and should never be used in rats because the vertebrae extend to the tail tip.

Anaesthetised squirrels can be bled from the jugular vein. However, if the animal is held in a squeeze tube it is possible, by restraining it on its back and holding its hindlimbs apart, to take blood from the medial femoral vein of conscious squirrels. Stoats and weasels are difficult to blood sample and so blood has to be taken from the jugular vein under general anaesthetic. Sedated foxes can be blood sampled like a dog; the cephalic, jugular and lateral saphenous veins are all easily accessible. Badgers can be bled from the jugular vein under anaesthetic. Anaesthetised wild boar should have blood samples removed from a superficial vein of the medial branch of the saphenous vein that is located on the medial surface of the leg just proximal and anterior to the hock.

No anaesthesia is required to collect blood from the marginal ear vein of the wild rabbit. The rabbit is held in a cotton bag with one ear protruding. A patch of fur above the ear vein is shaved with a scapel blade and the area wiped with cotton wool soaked in 70% ethanol. A small nick is made in the peripheral ear vein with the point of a sterile surgical blade (no. 11 size) and the drops of blood are collected in a hand-held tube. It is rarely necessary but if required, light pressure applied to the area with a cotton wool pad will stop the bleeding at the end of the procedure. Alternatively, blood can be withdrawn from the vein using a needle and hypodermic syringe.

Blood can be drawn from the veins that run semi-parallel to the tail in the interfemoral (tail) membrane of bats. The brachial vein near the elbow may also be used, but this carries greater risk of muscle damage. Note that the handling of wild-caught bats in the UK requires special authorisation from the statutory licensing authority. The vein should be raised using light pressure, and an incision made with a small needle (25 mm). Blood drops can then be collected using a heparinised capillary tube. Haemostasis is achieved by applying light pressure, and if necessary by the application of a clotting agent. The small body size of bats places a significant constraint on the volume of blood that may be collected. The total volume sampled should not exceed 1% of the body weight. For most European species, volumes of 50–100 µl are recommended.

Collection of urine

Urine can be a useful biological sample in which to measure a range of metabolites as well as some infectious agents (eg, *Leptospira*). In most larger mammals (>100 g), samples can be obtained from anaesthetised animals by using external manual palpation of the bladder. Samples can also be collected from small to medium-sized animals by placing the animal in a cage with a mesh floor. The mesh should be small enough to prevent faeces from falling into the collecting chamber below. To minimise the risk of contamination, the urine should be removed as soon as possible after it has been voided.

Euthanasia

The primary aim of all methods of euthanasia is to bring about death in a rapid and painless manner (see Chapter 17). Guidelines for euthanasia of non-domesticated animals are provided by the American Association of Zoo Veterinarians (2006). Methods that are inherently humane may nevertheless cause suffering if practised by nervous or unskilled individuals and not performed with deliberation and purpose. Developing the required skill in methods of euthanasia should be obtained by practice on dead animals, where possible, after observation of the technique by trained personnel.

A frequently used method of euthanasia for laboratory strains is the administration of an overdose of a general anaesthetic, leading to cardiac and respiratory arrest and the death of the animal. Intravenous or intraperitoneal injection of pentobarbital (100–150 mg/kg) is commonly used because it is rapidly acting, easy to administer and relatively inexpensive. However, in wild animals both of these routes may be difficult and inhalation anaesthesia is frequently used instead.

Carbon dioxide is commonly used as an inhalation agent for euthanasia. However, the sudden exposure of animals to 100% carbon dioxide can induce severe dyspnoea and cause distress, and the technique is therefore not recommended (Conlee *et al.* 2005). Whenever practicable, the animal should be exsanguinated, or have its neck dislocated, before disposal of the body.

When dispatching a large wild animal it is usually necessary to first administer a sedative, often by darting (see earlier in this chapter), and then to give a follow-up injection of the anaesthetic overdose. (It is important to remember that in the UK if an animal is to be sedated before overdosing with an anaesthetic this requires specific permission on the relevant Project and Personal Licences of the operative.)

References

Amengual, B., Bourhy, H., López-Roig, M. *et al.* (2007) Temporal dynamics of European Bat Lyssavirus Type 1 and survival of Myotis myotis bats in natural colonies. *PLoS ONE*, **2**, e566

American Association of Zoo Veterinarians (2006) Guidelines for euthanasia of non-domestic animals. http://www.aazv.org

Ball, D.J., Argentieri, G., Krause, R., *et al.* (1991) Evaluation of a microchip implant system used for animal identification in rats. *Laboratory Animal Science*, **41**, 185–186

Barber, I., Tarrant, K.A. and Thompson, H.M. (2003) Exposure of small mammals, in particular the wood mouse *Apodemus sylvaticus*, to pesticide seed treatments. *Environmental Toxicology and Chemistry*, **22**, 1134–1139

Beausoleil, N.J., Mellor, D.J. and Stafford, K.J. (2004) Methods for marking New Zealand wildlife: amphibians, reptiles and marine mammals. Department of Conservation, New Zealand. http://www.doc.govt.nz/upload/documents/science-and-technical/MarkingMethods.pdf. (accessed 06 July 2009)

Beardsley, A., Vagg, M.J., Beckett, P.H.T. *et al.* (1978) Use of the field vole (*M. agrestis*) for monitoring potentially harmful elements in the environment. *Environmental Pollution*, **16**, 65–71

Beldomenico, P.M., Telfer, S., Gebert, S. *et al.* (2008) The dynamics of health in wild field vole populations: a haematological perspective. *Journal of Animal Ecology*, **77**, 984–997

Brookes, S.M., Aegerter, J.N., Smith, G.C. *et al.* (2005) Europea bat lyssavirus in Scottish bats. *Emerging Infectious Diseases*, **11**, 572–578

Chalmers, R.M., Robinson, G., Elwin, K. *et al.* (2009) Cryptosporidium sp. Rabbit Genotype, a newly identified human pathogen. *Emerging Infectious Diseases*, **15**, 829–830

Conlee, K.M., Stephens, M.L., Rowan, A.N. *et al.* (2005) Carbon dioxide for euthanasia: concerns regarding pain and distress, with special reference to mice and rats. *Laboratory Animals*, **39**, 137–161

Cowan, P.E. (1977) Neophobia and neophilia: new object and new place reactions of three *Rattus* species. *Journal of Comparative and Physiological Psychology*, **91**, 63–71

Crouch, A.C., Baxby, D., McCracken, C.M. *et al.* (1995) Serological evidence for the reservoir hosts of cowpox virus in British wildlife. *Epidemiology of Infection*, **115**, 185–191

Curno, O., Behnke, J.M., McElligott, A.G. *et al.* (2009) Mothers produce less aggressive sons with altered immunity when there is a threat of disease during pregnancy. *Proceedings of the Royal Society, London (B)*, **276**, 1047–1054

Dyachenko, V., Kuhnert, Y., Schmaeschke, R. *et al.* (in press) Occurrence and molecular characterization of Cryptosporidium spp. Genotypes in European hedgehogs (*Erinaceus europaeus* L.) in Germany. *Parasitology*.

Fowler, M.E. and Miller, R.E. (Eds) (2008) *Zoo and Wild Animal Medicine: Current Therapy*, Vol 6. Saunders Elsevier, St Louis, Missouri

Gibson, T.E. (1967) Parasites of laboratory animals transmissible to man. *Laboratory Animals*, **1**, 17–24

Harris, S.L., Brookes, S.M., Jones, G. *et al.* (2006) Passive surveillance (1987 to 2004) of United Kingdom bats for European bat lyssaviruses. *Veterinary Record*, **159**, 439–446

Hendrie, C.A., Van Driel, K.S., Talling, J.C. *et al.* (2001) PBI Creams: a spontaneously mutated mouse strain showing wild animal-type reactivity. *Physiology & Behavior*, **74**, 621–628

Hudson, B.W., Quan, F.F. and Goldenberg, M.I. (1964) Serum antibody responses in a population of *Microtus californicus* and associated species during and after *Pasteurella pestis* epizootics in the San Francisco Bay area. *Zoonoses Research*, **3**, 15

Hurst, J.L. (1990) Urine marking in populations of wild house mice. Communication between males. *Animal Behaviour*, **40**, 209–222

Inglis, I.R. and Shepherd, D.S. (1994) Rats work for food they then reject: support for the information-primacy approach to learned industriousness. *Ethology*, **98**, 154–164

Joint Working Group on Refinement (1993) Removal of blood from laboratory mammals and birds. First Report of the BVA/FRAME/RSPCA/UFAW Joint Working Group on Refinement. *Laboratory Animals*, **27**, 1–22

Mathews, F. (2009) Zoonoses in wildlife: integrating ecology into management. In: *Advances in Parasitology, Vol. 68*. Ed. Webster, J.P., pp. 185–209. Academic Press, Burlington

Mathews, F., Macdonald, D.W., Taylor, G.M. *et al.* (2006b) Bovine tuberculosis (*Mycobacterium bovis*) in British farmland wildlife: importance to agriculture. *Proceedings of the Royal Society, London (B)*, **273**, 357–365

Mathews, F., McLaren, G.W., Gelling, M. *et al.* (2004) Keeping fit on the ark: assessing the suitability of captive-bred animals for release. *Biological Conservation*, **121**, 569–577

Maurer, F.D. (1964) Lymphocytic choriomeningitis. *Laboratory Animal Care*, **14**, 415

McLaren, G.W., Macdonald, D.W., Georgiou, C. *et al.* (2003) Leukocyte coping capacity: a novel technique for measuring the stress response in vertebrates. *Experimental Physiology*, **88**, 541–546

Mellor, D.J., Beausoleil, N.J. and Stafford, K.J. (2004) Marking amphibians, reptiles and marine mammals: animal welfare, practicalities and public perception in New Zealand. Department of Conservation, New Zealand. http://www.doc.govt.nz/upload/documents/science-and-technical/MarkingPre.pdf (accessed 27 August 2009)

Moberg, G.P. (2000) Biological responses to stress: implications for animal welfare. In: *The Biology of Animal Stress: Basic Principles and Implications for Animal Welfare*. Ed. Moberg, G.P. and Mench, J.A., pp. 1–21. CAB International, Wallingford

Odberg, F.O. (1987) The influence of cage size and environmental enrichment on the development of stereotypies in bank voles (*Clethrionomys glareolus*). *Behavioural Processes*, **14**, 155–173

Powell, R.L. (1974) Comparative studies of the preference for free vs response-produced reinforcers. *Animal Learning and Behaviour*, **2**, 185–188

Shepherd, D.S. and Inglis, I.R. (1987) Feeding behaviour, social interactions, and poison bait consumption by family groups of wild rats living in semi-natural conditions. In: *Stored Products Pest Control*. Ed. Lawson, D., pp. 97–105. British Crop Protection Council, London

Shepherd, D.S. and Inglis, I.R. (1993) The development of toxic bait aversions in wild and domesticated rats following brief exposure to food containing an acute rodenticide. *Journal of Wildlife Managment*, **57**, 640–647

Shumake, S.A., Thompson, A.R.D. and Caudil, C.J. (1971) Taste preference behaviour of laboratory versus wild Norway rats. *Journal of Comparative and Physiological Psychology*, **77**, 498–494

Smith, P., Inglis, I.R., Cowan, D.P. *et al.* (1994) A symptom-dependent taste aversion induced by an anticoagulant rodenticide in the brown rat (*Rattus norvegicus*). *Journal of Comparative Psychology*, **108**, 282–290

Somerville, R.G. (1961) Human viral and bacterial infections acquired from laboratory rats and mice. *Laboratory Animal Centre Collected Papers*, **10**, 21–32

Stoenner, H.G. and Maclean, T.D. (1958) *Leptospirosis ballum* contracted from Swiss albino mice. *American Medical Association Archives of International Medicine*, **101**, 606

Taylor, L.H., Latham, S.M. and Woolhouse, M.E.J. (2001) Risk factors for human disease emergence. *Philosophical Transactions of the Royal Society of London Series B – Biological Sciences*, **356**, 983–989

Tesh, R.B. and Arat, A.A. (1967) Bats as laboratory animals. *Health Laboratory Science*, **4**, 106–112

Thompson, H.M. (2007) Addressing issues in pesticide risk assessment for birds and mammals. *Outlooks in Pest Management*, **18**, 23–27

Tuffery, A.A. and Innes, J.R.M. (1963) Diseases of laboratory rats and mice. In: *Animals for Research*. Ed. Lane Petter, W., pp. 57–69. Academic Press, London

Twigg, G.I., Cuerden, C.M., Hughes, D.M. *et al*. (1969) The leptospirosis reservoir in British wild mammals. *Veterinary Record*, **84**, 424–426

Vaz, V.C., D'Andrea, P.S. and Jansen, A.M. (2007) Effects of habitat fragmentation on wild mammal infection by *Trypanosoma cruzii*. *Parasitology*, **134**, 1785–1793

Wurbel, H., Chapman, R. and Rutland, C. (1998) Effect of feed and environmental enrichment on development of stereotypic wire-gnawing in laboratory mice. *Applied Animal Behaviour Science*, **60**, 69–81

19 The laboratory opossum

John L. VandeBerg and Sarah Williams-Blangero

Biological overview

General biology of marsupials

The term marsupial derives from the Latin word *marsupium*, meaning little pouch. However, the word is somewhat deceptive because males of most species and even females of some species, including *Monodelphis* species, have no pouch.

Fossil evidence suggests that marsupials originated in North America, and dispersed to South America and then Australia. However, it has been argued that marsupials may have arisen on the ancient Southern continent of Gondwana (O'Brien & Graves 1990). In any case, it is generally accepted that the Australian forms were separated from the South American forms well before Australia split off from Antarctica 45 million years ago.

Marsupial lineages had disappeared from North America by 25 million years ago, as had the single species that reached Europe. The Virginia opossum (*Didelphis virginiana*), which is the only indigenous marsupial in North America today, is a recent arrival, having come from South America only about 4 million years ago. Of the other 291 extant marsupial species recognised by Nowak (1999), 73 are indigenous to South and Central America, 217 are indigenous to Australia and New Guinea and one (the Tasmanian tiger, *Thylacinus cynocephalus*) is probably extinct.

The most important feature of marsupials from the standpoint of unique research opportunities is the early developmental stage at which all marsupials are born. The gross anatomy of a neonate resembles that of a mouse at 12.5 days of gestation and that of a human at 6 weeks of gestation. Each neonate quickly attaches to a teat which swells in the mouth. The neonate is unable to release the teat until considerable further development has occurred. This early developmental stage at birth is common to all marsupials and renders the newborn marsupial, in essence, an extrauterine foetus that can be manipulated and observed in ways not possible with eutherian mammals.

In addition, marsupials have a variety of unique anatomical characteristics of the jaw, skull, teeth and reproductive system (Tyndale-Biscoe 1973). The early developmental stage of marsupials at birth and their distinctive anatomy are interpreted not as reflecting a more primitive stage in evolutionary development than eutherians, but rather as alternative strategies for achieving an equally adaptive endpoint. Thus, marsupials are useful for comparative research designed to improve understanding of the evolution of genetic and physiological mechanisms in mammals. *Monodelphis domestica* is a marsupial species that is well suited to research and the laboratory environment.

There are three orders of American marsupials: Didelphimorphia (American opossums) with 15 genera and 66 species; Paucituberculata (shrew opossums) with two genera and seven species; and Microbiotheria with one species (the monito del monte) (Nowak 1999). Only four species, all American opossums, have been used extensively as laboratory animals, although the adaptability of many others to laboratory conditions has never been explored. Two of the four species are large pouched opossums (family Didelphidae), and two are small pouchless opossums (family Marmosidae).

Marsupials in the laboratory

Didelphis virginiana has been used extensively as a laboratory animal in North America, and its close relative *Didelphis marsupialis* has been used in South America. The care, experimental manipulation and use of these species in laboratory research were reviewed in detail by Jurgelski (1987). However, *Didelphis* have limited utility because they are relatively large (1.0–5.5 kg), are aggressive towards one another and are seasonal breeders. Furthermore, reproductive success is low among captive-born animals, particularly males (VandeBerg 1990). No one has developed a long-term, self-propagating breeding colony of *Didelphis*. Therefore, experimental animals or breeders needed to produce first-generation captive progeny are usually captured from the wild. These animals have additional disadvantages in that they are of unknown age and health status, and generally carry a heavy parasite load. Furthermore, they are a potential source of pathogens that are causal agents of a variety of serious human diseases (Jurgelski 1987). Despite the shortcomings of these two species, they are likely to continue to be used as experimental animals for research that requires a relatively large marsupial or depends on the unique characteristics of these species.

Marmosa robinsoni, a small American opossum (40–70 g for females and 60–130 g for males) that appeared to have promise as a laboratory marsupial, was bred in captivity for several generations during the 1960s and 1970s (Barnes & Barthold 1969; Barnes 1977). However, fecundity decreased with each successive generation, and satisfactory conditions for long-term propagation of this species were never identified.

Monodelphis domestica

The grey short-tailed opossum (*Monodelphis domestica*) is the only American marsupial species that has proven to be successful as a self-perpetuating population in captivity. It has many characteristics that render it ideally suited as a laboratory animal, and it is widely used in North America and Europe. Breeding colonies have also been established in Australia and Brazil for specific experimental applications. Some stocks of this species have been produced in captivity for as many as 43 generations with no apparent detrimental effects on fertility, fecundity or health status. Because of the selection that has undoubtedly taken place over these generations, *Monodelphis domestica* presently in captive colonies may be quite different from their wild counterparts. For these reasons, laboratory stocks of this species are now referred to as the laboratory opossum. Figure 19.1 shows an adult female laboratory opossum.

Monodelphis domestica has been inappropriately described as the Brazilian opossum or grey opossum in the literature. The term Brazilian opossum is incorrect because many opossum species are native to Brazil, and *Monodelphis domestica* is also found in Bolivia and Paraguay. The grey opossum is also not an appropriate designation for *Monodelphis domestica* because some other opossum species also have grey pelage. Appropriate common names for this species are grey short-tailed opossum, laboratory opossum (when used in reference to laboratory stocks rather than wild animals) and *Monodelphis domestica*. However, the confusion demonstrates the importance of using scientific names where appropriate. The genus name *Monodelphis* may be used as an abbreviation without the species name when it is clear that *Monodelphis domestica* is implied, much as *Drosophila* is often used in reference to *Drosophila melanogaster*.

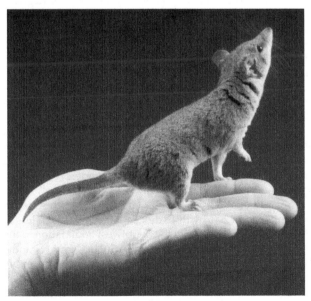

Figure 19.1 An adult female laboratory opossum.

The 15 species of the genus *Monodelphis* (short-tailed opossums) are distributed from Panama to Argentina. Linnaeus in 1758 coined the term *Didelphis* meaning two wombs, because it was known that the females of this species have an internal uterus like other mammals, as well as a pouch in which much of early ('foetal') development takes place (Tyndale-Biscoe 1973). The short-tailed opossums were named *Monodelphis* by Burnett in 1830 (Pine & Handley 2008) who recognised them as being closely related to *Didelphis* but lacking a pouch.

The omnivorous *Monodelphis domestica* is nocturnal and individuals are most active during the first few hours of the evening (Streilein 1982). Under natural conditions, they consume insects and other invertebrates, small vertebrates and various fruits. They are efficient predators, particularly adept at killing scorpions and cockroaches. They reproduce throughout the year in their natural habitat.

Size range and lifespan

Monodelphis domestica is among the largest of the short-tailed opossums. Adult laboratory-reared females typically weigh 60–100g and males 90–150g, although individuals of some stocks tend to be larger, and individuals within many stocks may exceed these ranges (VandeBerg 1990). Laboratory opossums begin to show physical signs of aging at approximately 3 years of age and generally die during the fourth year of life. The oldest individual in the colony maintained at the Southwest Foundation for Biomedical Research (San Antonio, Texas) reached the age of 4 years and 7.5 months (unpublished data). Reproductive and developmental data are summarised in Table 19.1.

Social organisation

Little is known about the natural social organisation of *Monodelphis domestica*. Individuals are difficult to capture because they are solitary and nomadic, and the estimated population density is less than four per hectare (2.47 acres) in areas where the animals are most common (Streilein 1982). Furthermore, they are terrestrial and do not congregate at isolated trees where species of semi-arboreal marsupials are more easily found.

Fully enclosed nests with an opening just large enough to allow entry are built by both males and females in hollow logs, fallen tree trunks or among rocks (Nowak 1999). Both males and females use their slightly prehensile tails to carry nesting material to the nest.

It has been stated in the literature that the species was named *domestica* because it frequently inhabits human households and plays a welcome role in controlling insect and rodent populations. However, human dwellings are not considered to be a frequent habitation site for these animals (I. Santos, personal communication).

Reproduction

In both the wild and captivity, *Monodelphis domestica* is a non-seasonal breeder. Female laboratory opossums reach

Table 19.1 Laboratory opossum: reproductive and developmental data.

Parameter	*Normal value*
Weight at birth (mg)	~100
Weight at 2 weeks (mg)	~840
Weight at 8 weeks (g)	~20
Weight of adult female (g)	60–100
Weight of adult male (g)	90–150
Dental formula	$I^5_4C^1_1Pm^3_3M^4_4$
Range of litter size	4–13
Typical litter size	7–8
Age at weaning (weeks)	8
First oestrus (in presence of a male) (days)	140
Full sexual maturity (months)	6
Time of ovulation after exposure to male (days)	5–10
Time of copulation to fertilisation (days)	1
Gestation (days)	13.5
Minimum interbirth interval (with successful weaning) (weeks)	11
Typical age of reproductive failure, females (months)	18–24
Typical age of reproductive failure, males (months)	24–30
Typical lifespan (months)	36–42

sexual maturity by 5 months of age (Stonebrook & Harder 1992) and males achieve sexual maturity 2–3 weeks later. The youngest female reported to have given birth was 141 days old, but few females conceive prior to 140 days of age. For most females, the prime reproductive period is prior to 18 months. Not all successful breeders continue to reproduce that long, and most females cease to reproduce by 24 months of age. Males are frequently successful breeders until 24–30 months of age and sometimes for several months more.

Standard biological data

The body temperature of *Monodelphis domestica* is 32.6 °C (Dawson & Olson 1988), respiratory rate at rest is approximately 54 breaths per minute, systolic blood pressure is approximately 188 mmHg and heart rate is approximately 345 beats per minute (Kraus & Fadem 1987). Maximal hearing sensitivity is from 8–64 kHz (Frost & Masterton 1994). The dental formula for *Monodelphis domestica* follows the standard opossum pattern of $I^5_4C^1_1Pm^3_3M^4_4$ (Reig *et al.* 1987; Macrini 2004; van Nievelt and Smith 2005).

Genetics

The karyotype of *Monodelphis domestica* contains 2n = 18 chromosomes. The autosomes are large and easily distinguished from one another. Two hundred and thirty-three bands can be observed in the G-banded karyotype (Pathak *et al.* 1993). The X chromosome is much smaller than the autosomes, and the Y is much smaller than the X. The karyotype is ideally suited for cytogenetic investigations.

Early surveys of genetic variants among laboratory opossums revealed 13 polymorphic proteins and two polymorphisms at the DNA level (Perelygin *et al.* 1996; reviewed by VandeBerg and Robinson 1997). The laboratory populations derived from the four founding sites in Brazil had significantly different gene frequencies for these early markers, and some alleles are specific to one population or another (van Oorschot *et al.* 1992a).

Breeds and strains

The laboratory opossum, like the Syrian hamster, differs from other laboratory animals in that the details of its origins are precisely known and well documented (Table 19.2) (VandeBerg & Robinson 1997). The first captive animals ancestral to the present laboratory population were four males and five females captured in 1978 near the town of Exu in the state of Pernambuco, Brazil. They were shipped to the National Zoological Park in Washington DC, where all of them reproduced. Twenty pedigreed first- and second-generation descendants were provided to one of the authors (JLV) in 1979. These animals were used to establish the initial breeding colony of laboratory opossums at the Southwest Foundation for Biomedical Research. Genetic material from all nine of the original wild-caught founders from Exu is present in the laboratory stock known as Purebred Population 1.

Table 19.2 summarises the populations present in the Southwest Foundation laboratory opossum colony. These populations are the source of most, if not all, the other laboratory colonies of *M. domestica* in the world.

A single shipment of 40 fully pedigreed laboratory opossums, all derived from the nine original founders from Exu (Purebred Population 1), was sent from the Southwest Foundation to the Zoological Society of London, Regent's Park, London, in 1983. A successful breeding colony was established there and became a source of animals for European investigators. Several shipments totalling 56 descendents of the founders of Populations 1 and 2 were also made from the Southwest Foundation to German institutions during the 1980s. It is believed that all populations of *Monodelphis domestica* in Europe are derived from these shipments to London and Germany.

More recently, laboratory opossums were exported from the UK to Australia. The Australian animals were descended from the 40 individuals sent to London in 1983, and thus all trace their ancestry to the original nine founders of Purebred Population 1.

An additional colony established outside North America was initiated in 2007 with 16 descendants of the founders of Population 1 shipped from the Southwest Foundation to the Federal University of Mato Grosso do Sul in Campo Grande, Brazil. Previously, there had been no self-sustaining captive colonies of this species in Brazil.

Because the number of founders is limited, most laboratory opossums are partially inbred. However, several stocks

Table 19.2 Laboratory stocks of Monodelphis domestica.

Laboratory code for wild populations	*Year of importation to the USA*	*Town of origin*	*Number of founders*	*Purebred laboratory population (no. of founders)*	*Admixed populations*	
					Laboratory designation	*Proportionate genetic contribution to each individual*
1	1978	Exu	9	Yes (9)	–	–
2	1984–1988	Piraua	14	Yes (7)	Admixed Population 2	≥78% Pop. 2, ≤22% Pop. 1
3	1990	Joaima	2	No (0)	Admixed Population 3	≥64% Pop. 3, ≤36% Pop. 1
4	1992	Conselheiro Mota	1	No (0)	Admixed Population 4	50% Pop. 4, 50% Pop. 1
5	1993	Brecha (Bolivia)	2	No (0)	Admixed Population 5	≥54% Pop. 5, ≤46% Pop. 1

exist that have no shared relatives with Purebred Population 2 (Table 19.2). Therefore, animals with an inbreeding coefficient of zero can be produced by matings between animals from Purebred Population 2 and any animals of Purebred Population 1, Admixed Population 3, Admixed Population 4 or Admixed Population 5.

Sources of supply (conservation status)

The species *Monodelphis domestica* is broadly distributed in much of eastern and central Brazil and in Bolivia and Paraguay. The natural habitat of *Monodelphis domestica* encompasses the relatively dry Chaco, Cerrado and Caatinga biomes, where they are most frequently found among rock outcrops (Streilein 1982). The species is not endangered or threatened. However, wild-caught animals are difficult to obtain because their population densities are low, making them somewhat difficult to trap.

The laboratory opossum colony at the Southwest Foundation for Biomedical Research is the source population for all of the captive colonies of *Monodelphis domestica* in the world, although a limited number of descendants of the nine founders from Exu (Population 1) were distributed directly by the National Zoological Park in the late 1970s and early 1980s.

Uses in the laboratory

The continuous availability and non-seasonal reproduction of laboratory opossums have made possible, for the first time in history, the large-scale experimental use of a marsupial species. Consequently, the laboratory opossum has become by far the most extensively used marsupial in research. A total of 895 publications citing *Monodelphis domestica* were indexed in BIOSIS Previews (all life science subjects) between 1978, the year in which the first *Monodelphis domestica* arrived in the USA, and 2006 (two in 1978 and 50 in 2006). In comparison, the numbers of publications citing other marsupial species have remained approximately constant and at a much lower level for any one species (VandeBerg & Robinson 1997). The diversity of research topics is too great to allow a detailed summary in this chapter, but several major areas of research are summarised below.

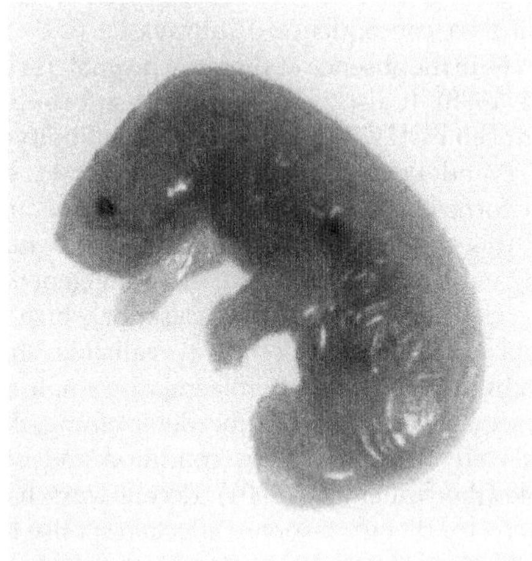

Figure 19.2 A newborn laboratory opossum.

The most obvious distinctive feature of marsupials, the birth at such an early stage of development, was a major driving force for establishing a laboratory marsupial. The features of the newborn laboratory opossum (Figure 19.2) have been exploited in research on function of the embryonic nervous system in long-term cell culture (Stewart *et al.* 1991), healing of the neonatal spinal cord after complete transection or crushing (Fry & Saunders 2000; Mladinic *et al.* 2005; Lane *et al.* 2007), effects of oestrogen on testicular development (Fadem & Tesoriero 1986), ontogeny of skin healing and development of capacity for scarring (Armstrong & Ferguson 1995), and development of neuropeptides, steroid receptors, and the visual system (reviewed by Kuehl-Kovarik *et al.* 1995).

Research in immunobiology provides an example of the use of laboratory opossums in a comparative approach to answer questions about function and evolution (Stone *et al.* 1996). Both the cellular (Stone *et al.* 1997) and humoral (Croix *et al.* 1989; Shearer *et al.* 1995) immune responses have been investigated. Evidence from those early studies suggested that the immunobiological characteristics of *Monodelphis* are similar in many respects to those of eutherian mammals. For example, skin graft responses are similar to those of eutherian mammals, suggesting considerable polymorphism of the MHC class I locus. However, *Monodelphis* exhibits a limited mixed lymphocyte culture (MLC) response, suggesting that class II loci may be highly restricted in extent of variability (Stone *et al.* 1998). An additional difference between *Monodelphis* and eutherian mammals is that the primary humoral response is mediated equally by IgM and IgG, as compared with predominantly IgM in eutherian mammals. It had been suggested that marsupials may have a less complex immune system than eutherian mammals, but recent findings have established that the genomic regions that specify key elements of the immune system are highly similar in the marsupial and eutherian lineages (Wong *et al.* 2006; Belov *et al.* 2007).

The laboratory opossum is also uniquely suited as a model for some human diseases. It is the only mammal other than humans known to be susceptible to malignant melanoma as a consequence of ultraviolet (UV) radiation alone; that is, in the absence of chemical promoters (Robinson *et al.* 1994, 1998). It also is susceptible to a form of corneal cancer induced by UV radiation, and susceptibility is highly heritable (VandeBerg *et al.* 1994; Kusewitt *et al.* 2000). Although corneal cancer is rare in humans, the high heritability of this disease in laboratory opossums makes it a potentially valuable model for investigating genetic mechanisms in carcinogenesis. A third disease for which the laboratory opossum has become a valuable model is dietary-induced hypercholesterolaemia. A single recessive gene is primarily responsible for determining that some individuals are resistant to this condition and others are susceptible (Rainwater *et al.* 2001). Recent work has shown that the gene for dietary response affects response to dietary cholesterol but not to saturated fat (Kushwaha *et al.* 2004a), and that factors associated with different dietary responses are absorption of dietary cholesterol, production of apolipoprotein B and expression of hepatic genes involved in cholesterol homeostasis (Kushwaha *et al.* 2004b, 2005; Chan *et al.* in press).

Monodelphis domestica displays considerable promise for research on allografting and xenografting, the interactions between graft and host and the development of tolerance. Allogeneic grafts of melanoma cells into opossum pups lead to tumour growth and systemic metastasis (Robinson & Dooley 1995). Remarkably, even mouse and human cancer cells can cause tumours to develop, some of which metastasise when implanted into pups (Fadem *et al.* 1988; Wang *et al.* 2003). Immunotolerance of xenografts can be induced by injecting multiple desensitising doses of cancer cells (Wang & VandeBerg 2005). These findings establish a foundation for exploiting *Monodelphis domestica* in research on the cascade of interactions between host and tumour cells, and the immunobiological mechanisms that are involved.

A xenograft model has also been developed for investigating cell transplant strategies to repair diseased or injured retinas (Sakaguchi *et al.* 2004). This model involves transplanting murine brain progenitor cells and retinal progenitor cells into the eyes of 5–10-day-old *Monodelphis* pups.

One of the primary reasons for developing *Monodelphis domestica* as a laboratory animal was the need for a small marsupial that could be produced in large numbers for research on the marsupial system of sex chromosome dosage compensation: paternal X-chromosome inactivation in somatic cells of females (VandeBerg 1983; VandeBerg *et al.* 1983). It took more than two decades for molecular technologies to advance to the state where they could be brought to bear on understanding the reasons for the difference between paternal X inactivation in the opossum model and the random inactivation that is characteristic of eutherian mammals. However, a flurry of recently published manuscripts has established that marsupials lack the inactivation centre that is present on eutherian X chromosomes; these reports have provided details about inactivation of the X-chromosome in X-bearing spermatozoa prior to fertilisation (Davidow *et al.* 2007; Hornecker *et al.* 2007; Mikkelsen *et al.* 2007; Namekawa *et al.* 2007; Shevchenko *et al.* 2007). However, since the mechanism by which paternal X inactivation occurs is still not understood, this field of research is likely to continue providing new insights into this unusual form of regulation of gene expression at the level of the whole chromosome.

Monodelphis domestica exhibits a variety of interesting genetic and physiological characteristics. For example, females exhibit greatly reduced rates of recombination in comparison with males (and with eutherian females) (van Oorschot *et al.* 1992b, 1993; Samollow *et al.* 2007); *Monodelphis* has a photolyase capable of repairing UV-induced DNA damage (cyclobutane pyrimidine dimers) (reviewed by Ley *et al.* 2000), whereas eutherian mammals do not; and the sperm heads of *Monodelphis* precisely align in pairs during passage through the epididymis and possibly achieve maximal progressive motility via this adaptation (Taggart *et al.* 1993). Some other marsupial species are known to share one or more of these characteristics with *Monodelphis*, but none provides such a convenient and economical opportunity for further investigation.

Cells from *Monodelphis* have been cultured for a variety of research purposes under conditions suitable for culture of cells from eutherians, but the optimal temperature for cell culture is less than 37 °C. Cell types that have been cultured include lymphocytes (Robinson *et al.* 1996), fibroblasts (Merry *et al.* 1983; Robinson *et al.* 1994), melanocytes (Dooley *et al.* 1995) and melanoma cells (Robinson *et al.* 1994).

Procedures for long-term (10-day) culture of the intact central nervous system of 2-day-old pups have been developed and used to investigate the actions of amines and transmitters, and the activation and inactivation of gamma-aminobutyric acid (GABA) receptors (Stewart *et al.* 1991; Mollgard *et al.* 1994).

Embryos have been cultured by several groups (Moore & Taggart 1993; Johnston *et al.* 1994; Selwood *et al.* 1997). Embryos cultured at 32.6 °C, the body temperature of *Monodelphis domestica*, progress further than those cultured at 37 °C (Selwood & VandeBerg 1992). Parthenogenic development to the two-cell stage occurred in 8% of oocytes cultured at 32.6 °C.

The recent development of high-quality genomic tools specific to *Monodelphis domestica* (Samollow 2006) is certain to stimulate an acceleration of research with this species in many biological disciplines. These tools include a physically anchored genetic linkage map with 150 highly polymorphic loci (Samollow *et al.* 2007), a cytogenetic BAC map (Duke *et al.* 2007) and a high-quality draft of the genome sequence (Mikkelsen *et al.* 2007). The laboratory opossum was the first marsupial selected for genome sequencing by the National Human Genome Research Institute. This first marsupial gene sequence has been instrumental in revealing the complexities of the marsupial immune system, and a prominent role for the evolution non-protein-coding sequences in mammalian diversification (Mikkelsen *et al.* 2007; Lemos 2007). A genomic tool that is not yet available for *Monodelphis domestica* is a species-specific microarray. However, cross-species applications of mouse and human microarrays have been successfully used to profile gene expression changes during melanomagenesis and spinal cord development (Wang *et al.* 2004; Lane *et al.* 2007).

Laboratory management and breeding

General husbandry

Housing

Polypropylene and polycarbonate cages (mouse shoebox cages) of two standard sizes are generally used: a 'large cage' sized 43 cm × 22 cm × 13 cm (l × w × h); and a 'small cage' sized 27 cm × 17 cm × 12 cm. Each cage is fitted with a standard stainless steel top used for rodents. However, the tops used in breeding colonies must fit within 0.75 cm of the cage edges, and the space between the bars on the top must not exceed 0.75 cm. Pre-weanlings can escape through openings as small as 1.0 cm, which is a standard distance between bars on some tops sold for use with rodents. Filter covers may be used to protect against airborne pathogens, but they are not essential in a well managed colony. Multiple cages are kept in racks (Figure 19.3). There have been no recent studies on housing requirements for this species.

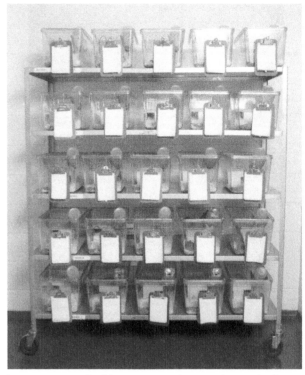

Figure 19.3 A rack of large cages, each containing a pair of animals and a nest box. The life history record of each animal is kept in a spiral notebook affixed to a clipboard on the front of each cage.

Environmental provisions and enrichment

The cage bottom is covered with aspen or pine shavings to a depth of approximately 2.5 cm. The animals are hygienic and generally choose a single corner of their cage as a toilet area. In addition to bedding, each cage is provided with paper towelling, cut into 5 mm × 18 cm strips by a paper shredder, for nesting material. The amount of nesting material provided is about 3 g for a single animal, 5–6 g for a pair or a female with a litter and 10–12 g for a group of weanlings caged together. The early stage of development at birth, incapability of thermoregulation at birth and lack of a maternal pouch make nesting material especially important for neonatal survival.

Nest boxes are provided in cages that contain breeding pairs, a female with a litter or a group of weanlings. Nest boxes can be constructed of any material that can be easily cleaned and permit a female to be checked for the presence of a litter with minimal disruption. Polypropylene or plastic food storage boxes with removable lids and an entrance hole cut from one side will suffice. In the authors' colony, aluminium nest boxes (18 cm × 13 cm × 10 cm) are generally used which are constructed locally. Each box has a removable 'shoe box' type lid and an entrance measuring 5 cm × 4.5 cm (w × h). A convenient alternative to a nest box is a round glass jar 16.5 cm long, 8.9 cm in diameter, with an opening 8.3 cm in diameter. However, it is easier to check females for the presence of litters if a nest box with a removable lid is used (Figure 19.4).

From the perspectives of psychological well-being and environmental enrichment, ample nesting material is essential for all animals whether they are single- or pair-housed, and at least one nest box is essential for pair-housed animals. Both males and females may spend many hours per day assembling bundles of nesting material, curling their semi-prehensile tails around a bundle and carrying it around the cage. In some instances, bundles of nesting material are woven into elaborate nests, even by animals that are not in breeding situations. A nest box is essential for paired animals in order to provide a haven in which one member of the pair may be able to protect itself from an aggressive mate, and for providing seclusion for mothers with litters. There have been no recent publications on enrichment for this species.

Social grouping

Litters are weaned at 8 weeks of age and under optimal conditions the animals are caged individually (a small cage is sufficient). Littermates may be caged communally in a large cage containing a nest box, but there is risk of aggression. If caged communally beyond 4 months of age, many animals become aggressive towards one another and severe

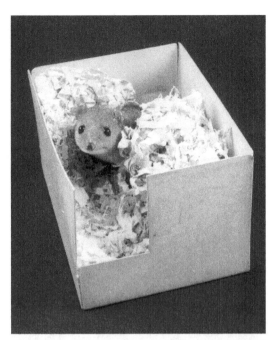

Figure 19.4 A female with a 4-week-old litter in a nest box from which the lid has been removed. The nest is well formed except across the top where the lid contacted the sides of the nest itself.

injuries or death are likely outcomes. Therefore, individual caging is mandatory after 4 months of age.

Presentation of food and water

Feeders designed for rodents are unsatisfactory for laboratory opossums; Rather, food pellets are placed directly on the bedding in a clean area of the cage. To ensure *ad libitum* feeding, a sufficient quantity of pellets is added three times a week.

Water is provided in glass, polycarbonate or polypropylene bottles fitted with rubber stoppers and stainless steel sipper tubes. Automatic waterers are not recommended because *Monodelphis* are unable to adapt to any of several designs that have been tested.

Identification and sexing

Littermates are separated into individual cages by 4 months of age and the only contact between animals after that age occurs during pairing of females and males. Therefore, after the separation of littermates, each individual can be tracked by an ID number that is recorded in a record booklet or on a cage card that is maintained with each animal as it is moved from cage to cage.

Ear punching and the shearing of identification patterns on the back are practical methods of identifying individuals if there is a need to do so with group-housed littermates, provided the identification patterns are monitored and renewed as needed. Subcutaneous transponders may also provide an efficient means for identification of individual *Monodelphis*.

Monodelphis can be easily sexed long before weaning because the testicles are contained in a pendulous scrotum attached to the body by a thin stalk.

Physical environment and hygiene

Room temperature is maintained at 23.5–26.5 °C, slightly higher than that recommended for rodents. Although no controlled experiments have been reported, the neonatal survival rate is suspected to be higher at this slightly elevated temperature.

Fluorescent lighting is used in a cycle of 14 h light and 10 h dark, and humidity is maintained at 55–60%. Humidity levels below 35% lead to desiccation and necrosis of the ears and tails of some individuals.

The animal rooms should be kept as quiet as practicable. Loud noises such as those that occur during construction cause stress that may lead to increased levels of aggression and cannibalism. Additionally, *Monodelphis domestica* can hear at ultrasound frequencies inaudible to humans and sources of high-frequency noise should be minimised.

Once a week, all animals are moved to clean cages with fresh bedding. Nest boxes and well constructed nests are moved to the new cage if they are not soiled. Care is taken to disturb as little as possible the nests of mothers with litters less than 3 weeks old in order to discourage cannibalism. Nest boxes are generally washed in a cage washer every 2 weeks when litters are not present.

Health monitoring and quarantine

Monodelphis is an exceptionally healthy laboratory animal and has required no health monitoring procedures other than routine daily observation.

Animals captured from wild populations typically carry endoparasites and should be kept in quarantine while the bedding is changed three times per week to break the life cycle of these parasites. Endoparasites are generally eliminated within a few weeks by this procedure. Ectoparasites have not been documented on newly captured animals.

Transport

For general advice on transport see Chapter 13. Local transportation in a climate-controlled vehicle suited for animal transport is safely conducted with the animals in their standard cages. Temperature should be maintained as constant as is practical. For trips during which the temperature might drop below the normal laboratory range for this species (23.5–26.5 °C), the animals should be transported in cages with nest boxes and several days after the addition of nesting material so that ample nests will have been constructed.

For shipping by air, animals can be placed in standard mouse shipping boxes purchased from commercial mouse suppliers, into which plywood partitions have been placed (International Air Transport Association 2008). Each animal must be placed singly within a partitioned enclosure to prevent fighting en route. Even littermates that have been caged together since weaning are likely to be aggressive during transport. Care must be taken in constructing partitions to ensure that a portion of each compartment has open access to at least one ventilation opening.

The authors typically partition each box into six compartments (Figure 19.5), the dimensions of which are 18cm × 13cm × 18cm (l × w × h). The box is divided into four compartments if fewer than five animals are to be transported.

The floor of each compartment is covered with about 2.5cm of shavings and about 15g of nesting material is provided for each animal. Two quarters of one orange are usually provided at one end of each compartment, and apple quarters or pieces of watermelon have also been used successfully. Alternatively, water gel packs can be used, especially for trips of extended duration.

Attempts to ship females with suckling pups have had limited success because of cannibalism. However, no problems have been encountered in shipping pregnant females, even in the late stages of pregnancy.

Animals should be acclimatised to a new environment in solitary cages. Pairings of breeders should not occur less than 1 week after arrival to minimise the risk of aggressive behaviour.

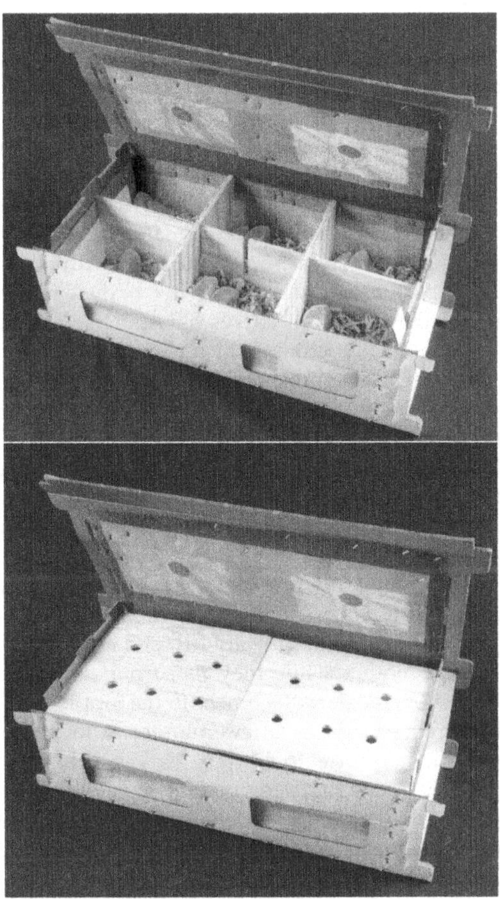

Figure 19.5 Top: a shipping box ready for six animals to be placed inside. Note the nesting material on top of the wood shavings and the two orange quarters in each. Bottom: a plywood cover with holes for air exchange is placed inside the box before closing the cardboard top to ensure that animals cannot gain access to an adjacent compartment and to facilitate putting individual animals into, and retrieving them from, the compartments.

Breeding

Condition of adults

Females are biologically capable of rearing up to four litters per year, although this level of success is rare. More than four litters can be produced by a single female in a year if the pups are removed for experimental purposes prior to weaning and the female is returned immediately to breeding. One female subjected to this protocol produced 67 progeny in 1 year. The largest number of progeny weaned by a female in the Southwest Foundation colony is 49.

A single male can be paired with a different female every 2 weeks, and could in theory sire up to 26 litters per year. The largest number of weaned progeny sired by a male in the Southwest Foundation colony is 105.

Female laboratory opossums reach sexual maturity by 5 months of age (Stonebrook & Harder 1992), 2–3 weeks earlier than males. Oestrus is induced at any time of the year by the presence of a strange male, generally 5–10 days after the animals are caged together. The induction of oestrus occurs even immediately after a litter dies or is removed prior to weaning, if a female is provided with a male. This characteristic is highly advantageous in comparison to many marsupial species that are seasonal breeders. This characteristic also facilitates timed pregnancies and the collection of staged embryos.

The only practical strategy for determining if an animal is fertile is to pair it with a member of the opposite sex which has a recent history of fertility. If an animal does not reproduce after four such opportunities, it is judged to be infertile.

Pairing

Monogamous pairings are made to minimise aggressive behaviour and to prevent interference with mating. Under normal conditions, a mature male and female are placed together in a large cage (with a nest box and nesting material). Pairing should be done early in the day so that animal care staff can be alert for undue aggression for at least a few hours after pairing. A low level of aggression is common and does not pose a high risk, but occasionally the animals must be separated due to aggressive fighting.

Conceptions are not likely to occur more than 10–12 days after pairing, so males are typically removed after 2 weeks, at which time they may be paired with another female. After removal of the male from the cage, the female is kept solitary for at least 2 weeks (the gestation period), usually in a small cage. If a litter has not been born (or has died or been removed), the female may be paired again with the same or a different male. If a litter is born, the mother and her nest are carefully transferred to a large cage and the nest is placed in the nest box if it was not constructed inside the box.

The day of mating cannot be precisely ascertained by techniques that are used for rodents. There is no vaginal plug and sperm are rarely detected in vaginal smears. Furthermore, the time of ovulation is difficult to predict from vaginal smears because cornified cells from the lateral vaginae may infiltrate the posterior vaginal sinus, masking changes in the cytology of the cells that line the posterior vaginal sinus

(Fadem & Rayve 1985). Therefore, several laboratories have adapted video systems to determine the precise timing of mating (Baggott & Moore 1990; Mate *et al.* 1994; Kuehl-Kovarik *et al.* 1995). Generally, a group of cages is filmed under red light during the dark phase when most matings occur. The film can be fast forwarded for examination each day to identify the exact time of copulations. Another strategy has been to keep the paired animals separated by a perforated plexiglass partition except for 1–2 h at the end of the light period and at 12 h intervals after that until mating occurs (Kuehl-Kovarik *et al.* 1995). Mating usually takes place within 20 minutes of removal of the partition.

Generally, no harm arises from leaving a male paired with a female longer than 2 weeks, provided he is removed within the first 2 weeks after a litter is born to prevent him from eating the pups when they are left alone by the mother. However, there is little chance of conception from a prolonged pairing and there is always risk of aggression.

Fertility decline and aggression

Risk of aggression is especially high among older animals, particularly females. For most females, the prime reproductive age is up to 18 months, and most cease to reproduce by 24 months of age. Cessation of reproductive success is often accompanied by aggressive behaviour toward prospective mates. Females in the authors' colony are routinely removed from the breeding programme at between 18 and 24 months of age depending on their reproductive history, history of aggression towards potential mates and importance of the particular animal to its breeding programme. However, the oldest female that produced a litter in the authors' colony was 34 months old at the time of conception and she succeeded in rearing the litter to weaning.

Some elderly males become aggressive to their potential mates, so a judgement is made as to which males are allowed to continue as studs beyond 2 years of age. The oldest male that sired a litter in the authors' colony was 40 months old at the time the litter was conceived.

Embryonic development

The embryonic development of *Monodelphis* has been described in detail (Baggott & Moore 1990; Mate *et al.* 1994; Selwood *et al.* 1997). According to Mate *et al.* (1994), ovulation and fertilisation occur about 24 h after mating. Between 2 and 3 days later (days 3 and 4 after mating), most embryos are at the four-cell stage, and on day 5 most are at the 16–32-cell stage. Complete unilaminar blastocysts are present on day 7 and bilaminar blastocysts on day 8. The first somites are formed in the primitive streak by day 10, the heart and blood vessels by day 11 and paddle-shaped forelimbs by day 12. By day 14, the forearm is well developed with claws on the digits, and birth occurs on day 15. Thus, development from the bilaminar blastocyst stage to birth takes place in a mere 7 days.

Production

At the time of pairing, a male and a female are placed together in a large cage containing bedding, nesting material, a nest box and fresh feed and water (Figure 19.6). Both males and females build nests.

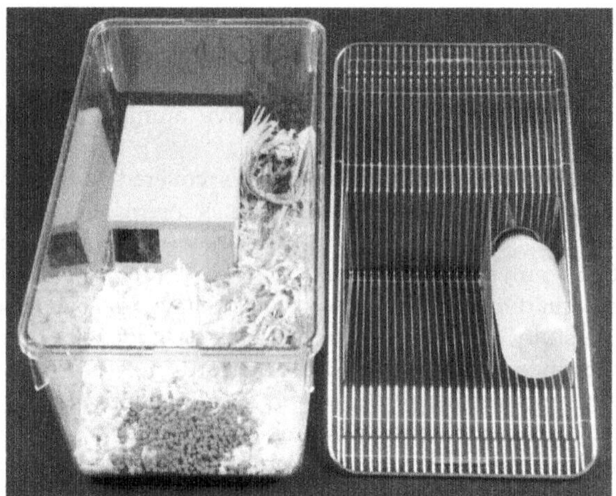

Figure 19.6 A large cage ready for a pair of animals. Fox chow is placed on the bedding near the front of the cage. Nesting material is divided into two portions to limit competition for it. Typically, one animal builds a nest inside the nesting box and the other builds a nest outside.

Birth occurs approximately 14.5 days after copulation and 13.5 days after ovulation and fertilisation (Mate *et al.* 1994). Under normal circumstances, birth probably occurs in the seclusion of the nest and nesting material should be provided to allow for this behaviour. Pregnant females may be observed or filmed giving birth if deprived of nests.

Females may become more active for a few minutes before birth. At the moment of birth, the female places one side of the dorsal surface of her rump on the floor, with hindfeet in the air; props the anterior part of her body by placing a forepaw on the floor; and curves her spine so her head is near the urogenital opening, which is raised to extrude the neonates on to the mammary area.

As many as 15 neonates have been observed in a newborn litter. However, the maximum number of newborns that are capable of surviving is equal to the number of teats of the mother; that number is 13 in most individuals, but may be only 11 or 12 (Robinson *et al.* 1991). Typical litter size (determined after attachment to the nipples) varies among stocks, but 7–8 is common for many stocks, and 9–12 is not unusual. Occasionally, a litter of 13 is reared to weaning.

The neonates are light grey at birth and are licked vigorously by the mother while they flail from side to side in worm-like movements. Attachment to the nipples generally occurs within seconds, or a few minutes at most, and the colour of the skin turns to a bright pink shortly thereafter. Neonates that do not find a teat continue crawling, generally in an upward direction and remain light grey. After the unattached neonates reach the dorsal side of the mother, they are cannibalised.

The young

Litter survival is highly variable, depending on the breeding stock, the age and reproductive experience of the dam and the size of the litter. In general it exceeds 50%, but survival is reduced in highly inbred litters and in litters born to older females (approaching 2 years of age and beyond). Small litters tend to be lost more frequently than large litters; litters of three or less rarely survive to weaning, so, if it is necessary to return the female immediately to breeding, the litter has to be euthanased. It is important that extraneous noise be kept to a minimum in breeding colonies to reduce the risk of cannibalism of litters by their mothers.

The newborn marsupial has an embryonic two-layered forebrain, no cerebellum, embryonic eyes, no ears and hindlimbs at the paddle stage of development. Anatomically, it resembles a mouse at 12.5 days of gestation. The newborn *Monodelphis* weights about 100 mg and is approximately 1 cm in length. It attaches to a teat within seconds or minutes of birth. Each newborn remains attached to the same nipple for at least the first week of life. At 2 weeks of age, each pup weighs about 840 mg (VandeBerg 1990) and may be left alone in the nest, although pups are frequently present on the nipples during the third week of life both when the mother is resting and when she is active. The pups begin to grow fur during the third week of life and their eyes open about 1 month postnatally.

Laboratory opossums are routinely weaned at 8 weeks of age, when they weigh about 20 g. Occasionally, when the size of the young is judged to be smaller than normal at that age, they are left with the mother until 9–11 weeks postpartum, when lactation usually ceases. Weaning is accomplished simply by placing littermates in a large cage by themselves or by placing each one in a small cage. The weanlings continue to grow rapidly for 200–250 days, after which growth plateaus (see growth curves in Cothran *et al.* 1985). Growth of females and onset of puberty may be stimulated if they are paired with males prior to 6 months of age (Stonebrook & Harder 1992). Conversely, females exhibit pronounced growth retardation if they are deprived of mates after about 6 months of age (Cothran *et al.* 1985; VandeBerg 1990).

Breeding systems

Most aspects of breeding systems are similar to those for mice and rats, with the exception of inbreeding.

For stocks where the number of animals and reproductive success are especially limited, a useful practice is to pair proven breeders with animals that are virgin or have failed to reproduce. This practice helps to ensure that animals capable of reproduction are provided the best opportunity for success before they are culled on the basis of reproductive performance.

At the Southwest Foundation for Biomedical Research, more than 95 000 laboratory opossums have been produced and weaned. Pedigree data are maintained for each individual in a computerised database, and the inbreeding coefficient of each individual is calculated using software developed at the institution (Dyke 1989). Because the number of founders was small, all individuals are partially inbred except those that can be produced by intercrosses between several stocks (as discussed under Breeds, strains and genetics).

Initial attempts were made to develop inbred strains by full sibling matings, but all lines were eventually lost as a consequence of reduced fecundity, as well as high mortality of litters within the first 2 weeks of life. One line achieved an inbreeding coefficient (F) of 0.911 (equivalent to just over 11 generations of full sibling matings) before it was lost (VandeBerg & Robinson 1997).

More recently, a series of partially inbred stocks has been developed by matings involving full siblings interspersed with matings between relatives less closely related than full siblings (VandeBerg & Robinson 1997). Six of these stocks currently have inbreeding coefficients in excess of 0.90. Selective breeding practices are being employed to increase the inbreeding coefficients gradually while maintaining satisfactory levels of fecundity and litter survival rates, and two stocks have inbreeding coefficients in the range of 0.95–0.96 (equivalent to 14–15 generations of full sibling matings).

The partially inbred stocks have been derived from Purebred Population 1 and Admixed Population 2. Despite not having achieved the status of fully inbred strains (F = 0.986, equivalent to 20 generations of full sibling matings), these partially inbred stocks are useful for research where uniform experimental subjects are desired, for research on histocompatibility and for intercross and backcross mating strategies for gene mapping and other genetic objectives.

Feeding

Natural and laboratory diets

In captivity, *Monodelphis* will consume virtually any small animal, such as cockroaches, crickets, earth worms, scorpions, mice, lizards, snakes and *Tenebrio* larvae. They will also eat most fruits. However, the recommended diet is a reproduction grade of dried pelleted fox chow (reviewed by VandeBerg 1990) for which no supplements are required.

Dietary requirements

Dietary experiments have been conducted with commercially prepared foods for cats, dogs, marmosets, mink and foxes, as well as more natural diets containing meat, insects, eggs, milk, infant mice and fruit. The optimal diet of those that have been rigorously tested experimentally was found to be the reproductive grade of fox chow as noted above (VandeBerg 1990). The diet currently used at Southwest Foundation for Biomedical Research contains not less than 35% crude protein 13% crude fat and 4.5% crude fibre (dry weight). Specific dietary requirements have not been defined.

Water

All animals should have access to fresh water *ad libitum*. At the authors' facility, tap water is provided in bottles that were sanitised on the same day. A freshly sanitised bottle of water is provided weekly when the cage is changed.

Laboratory procedures

Handling

Monodelphis domestica is a most gentle and docile wild mammal in response to human handling. Even individuals captured from wild populations can be picked up by experienced handlers with little risk of being bitten. At the Southwest Foundation facility, the only hand coverings used are latex disposable gloves. Under most circumstances the animal is picked up by the tail, as is typically done with laboratory mice (Figure 19.7). Animals may also be picked up by placing the fingers under the midsection and the thumb over the back, just behind the front legs of the animal, as shown in Figure 19.8.

If a *Monodelphis* is not handled properly, it is likely to bite. The animals have sharp, needle-like teeth, and most adults, particularly the larger males, are capable of puncturing human skin. Inexperienced or careless handlers are generally bitten under either of two circumstances. One is when they move their hand too fast in attempting to capture an animal. *Monodelphis* has an extremely fast reflex to bite anything that moves rapidly, whether it be prey (presumably a hunting adaptation) or a human hand. The biting reflex is often quicker than the initial movement of the human hand to grab the tail (or animal). In contrast, moving the hand slowly to the animal and picking the animal up slowly will almost never elicit a bite, even though some animals back into the corner of the cage hissing with an open mouth and displaying their teeth. The second circumstance in which an inexperienced or careless handler is likely to be bitten is when an attempt is made to restrain any part of the body of the animal. If the body of an unanaesthetised animal must be restrained, light leather gloves, such as golf gloves, should be used.

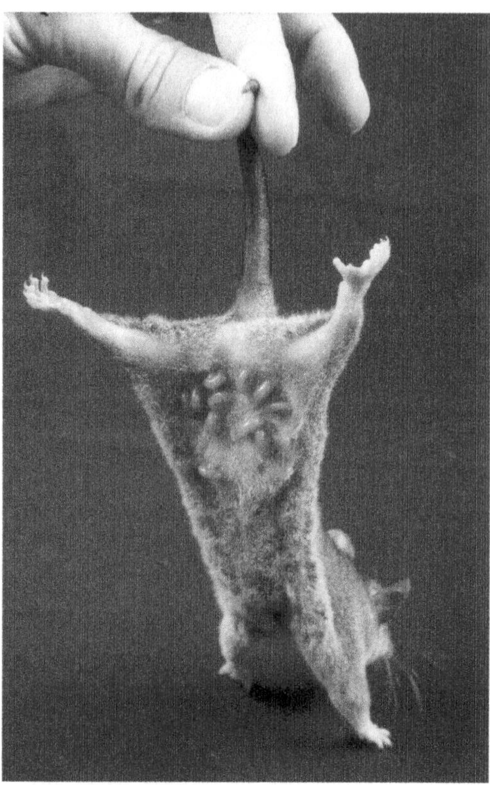

Figure 19.7 Picking up an animal by the tail. This female has a newborn litter.

Physiological monitoring

Body temperature can be assessed by thermocouples as a deep colonic measure at an insertion depth of 3–4 cm (Dawson & Olson 1988). A temperature-sensitive microchip transponder also could be used.

General advice on refinement of blood collection, within the Three Rs framework, is provided by the Joint Working Group on Refinement (JWGR) (1993). Blood can be collected easily and routinely by cardiac puncture of animals anaesthetised with isoflurane. A 1.27 cm, 27G (0.406 mm nominal outside diameter) needle on a 1 ml tuberculin syringe is typically used, although a larger syringe may be used for collecting larger volumes of blood. Experienced technical staff collecting blood routinely are able to obtain 0.8–1.0 ml of blood in 95% of attempts, with no obvious adverse impact on health (Robinson & VandeBerg 1994).

Cardiac puncture, under anaesthetic, has been conducted repeatedly over time on an animal without apparent ill effects. In an investigation of the effects of chronic blood loss, 2 ml of blood was removed weekly from each of 20 animals for 13 weeks (Manis *et al.* 1992). No apparent changes in health status occurred, although haematopoietic characteristics were altered.

Another procedure for collecting blood is to make an incision through the ventral tail artery of an anaesthetised animal after a heat lamp has been placed above it to dilate the blood vessels (Kraus & Fadem 1987). This procedure can yield 1–2 ml of blood. The wound is cauterised upon completion of the procedure and sealed with flexible collodion.

Large volumes of blood can be collected by exsanguination using the cardiac puncture method. Experienced personnel can routinely collect at least 5 ml and often as much as 6–7 ml from each animal that weighs 100 g or more (Robinson & VandeBerg 1994).

Urine may be collected by putting individual animals in cages with wire mesh bottoms placed over collection pans

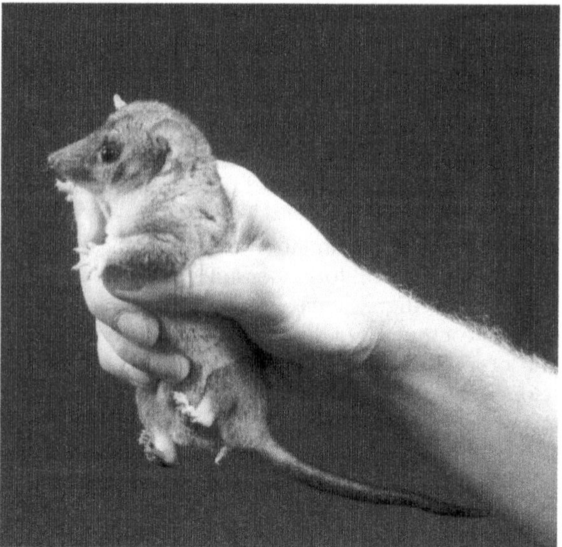

Figure 19.8 Picking up an animal by placing the fingers under the midsection with thumb and index finger just behind the front legs of the animals.

as described by Christian (1983). The collection pans should contain a layer of mineral oil to prevent evaporation of urine and faeces.

For milk collection within 2 weeks postpartum, the sucklings must be pulled off the teats and euthanased. For older litters, the mothers can simply be separated from their litters temporarily. Two hours after the separation of mothers from their litters, dams are anaesthetised with isoflurane and injected intramuscularly with 0.75 ml oxytocin (Samples *et al.* 1986). Milk droplets are exuded by manually squeezing the mammary glands, and they are collected in capillary tubes. Between 5 and 10 µl of milk can be collected during the first few days of lactation, and up to 80 µl during the later stages (Crisp *et al.* 1989).

Administration of medicines

General advice on refinement of the administration of medicines or test substances can be found in JWGR (2001).

Anaesthesia and analgesia

Light anaesthesia by inhalation is recommended for all injections because it is difficult to restrain *Monodelphis*. The procedures for injections of *Monodelphis* are the same as those for rodents. Subcutaneous injections are generally given in the shoulder area, intramuscular injections in the hindleg area and intraperitoneal injections in the caudal abdomen.

Detailed procedures for anaesthesia were described by Robinson and VandeBerg (1994). However, procedures for anaesthesia by inhalation have been further optimised in recent years.

The most satisfactory inhaled anaesthetic in the authors' experience is isoflurane. Although considerable care must be taken to maintain depth of anaesthesia without killing the animal, isoflurane is relatively safe in the hands of experienced personnel for short-term anaesthesia (up to 1 h). Animals are provided with water but no food overnight prior to anaesthesia, in order to minimise the risk of vomiting and aspirating stomach contents during or after sedation. In the authors' laboratory, animals are placed in a chamber with six individual compartments lined with paper towels. The chamber is flooded with a mixture of isoflurane/oxygen delivered from an anaesthesia machine. The oxygen flow rate is set at 0.8 l/min and the isoflurane level is set at 4% V/V. The animals can be monitored through the clear acrylic sides of the chamber. The length of time required to sedate the animals is variable, but most animals are thoroughly sedated within 5 minutes. Animals are removed from the chamber based on their appearance.

Depth of anaesthesia can best be judged by toe pinching and respiratory rate. Deep anaesthesia sufficient for cardiac puncture or surgical procedures is indicated by failure to withdraw a foot in response to a pinch. Respiratory rate should be watched continuously during the procedure and during the recovery period; a sudden reduction in rate of breathing or sporadic breathing indicates that an animal is at high risk of death. If respiration ceases, an animal can often be resuscitated by placing one or two drops of doxapram hydrochloride (20 mg/ml) on the tongue of the animal. If respiration does not commence within a few seconds, one end of a 20 cm length of plastic tubing is placed over the animal's nostrils and snout, firmly against the skin, and the person conducting the procedure blows into the other end at intervals of 1–2 s so that that the animal's lungs inflate on each occasion. The tubing has an external diameter of 15 mm and an inside diameter of 11 mm.

For recovery from anaesthesia, an animal is placed into an acrylic chamber on its ventral surface on a heating pad covered with absorbent paper and maintained at 30 °C. If there is any sign of respiratory distress, the procedures for resuscitation are immediately performed. Most animals are fully recovered and able to walk without losing balance within 10–30 minutes, when they are returned to their cages.

For inducing deep anaesthesia for a prolonged period of time, a combination of inhalation and injection anaesthesia was developed in the early 1990s (Robinson & VandeBerg 1994). In this protocol, the animal was lightly anaesthetised with isoflurane and then injected subcutaneously with 0.0025 ml (= 50 µg) per gram of body weight of sodium pentobarbitone (pentobarbital) (20 mg/ml) followed by an intramuscular injection of 0.0054 ml (= 2 µg atropine and 40 µg ketamine) per gram of body weight of an atropine/ketamine mixture (1.25 ml atropine (0.4 mg/ml) + 0.1 ml ketamine HCl (100 mg/ml)). Occasionally during prolonged anaesthesia, one or two additional injections of sodium pentobarbitone (pentobarbital) were required to maintain deep anaesthesia. The authors have not used this protocol in their laboratory for many years, but would recommend now that isoflurane replace halothane, and that a more advanced injectable anaesthetic be considered as a replacement for sodium pentobarbital. Telazol (30 mg/kg) or a mixture of medetomidine (100 µg/kg), butorphanol (0.2 mg/kg) and ketamine HCl (10 mg/kg) have been used to immobilise Virginia opossums (*Didelphis virginiana*) for short periods of time (Stoskopf *et al.* 1999), suggesting possible replacements of sodium pentobarbital. More research is required to establish an up-to-date protocol for long-term anaesthesia of laboratory opossums.

Light anaesthesia of dams and litters with halothane or isoflurane has been used for procedures that can be completed quickly. However, litter loss is unacceptably high when dams with litters are subjected to deep anaesthesia with isoflurane. Deep and prolonged anaesthesia with the combination inhalation and injection anaesthesia protocol causes minimal loss of litters (E.S. Robinson, personal communication). Halothane/nitrous oxide anaesthesia has also been used successfully to anaesthetise dams and pups for the conduct of neonatal surgery (Armstrong & Ferguson 1995). It has been reported that feeding a mother mealworms immediately after recovery from anaesthesia may reduce the incidence of cannibalism (Saunders *et al.* 1995).

Another approach to anaesthesia of a mother with attached pups is to anaesthetise it lightly using a 50 ml conical tube delivering the regulated anaesthetic mixture over the head of the mother (Wang & VandeBerg 2003). This procedure enables anaesthesia of the dam without affecting the pups, greatly reducing the risk of losing the litter.

Anaesthesia of sucklings within the first 2 weeks of life has been accomplished by cooling them with ice (Morykwas *et al.* 1991; Stewart *et al.* 1991) or by using a series of puffs of dry ice dust (Taylor & Guillery 1995). The methods are effective because the neonates are not capable of thermoregulation; furthermore, the nervous system is poorly developed with an embryonic forebrain and no cerebellum. Because neurones in mammals cease to function when body temperature is reduced to 20 °C, as compared with 0–4 °C in poikilotherms, cooling is an effective form of anaesthesia for altricial mammalian neonates which are incapable of thermoregulation. Hypothermia is recommended for surgical procedures on altricial neonates by the Institute of Laboratory Animal Research (ILAR) (1992) and the Canadian Council on Animal Care (1993), and the subject was reviewed by Martin in 1995.

Procedures for ovariectomy, castration, partial hepatectomy, unilateral hysterectomy, vasectomy and embryo transfer have been described in detail (Kraus & Fadem 1987; Robinson & VandeBerg 1994). In addition, procedures have been developed for tail amputations and eye removals, which are sometimes necessary following trauma (usually fighting) or infection (Robinson *et al.* 1994). The procedure for anaesthesia by inhalation and injection is generally used for major surgery, but simple procedures can be conducted under isoflurane anaesthesia alone. Techniques are similar to those used for rodent surgery. However, incisions must be closed with sutures rather than surgical clips, because the animals are adept at removing the clips.

Buprenorphine is used as a post-surgical analgesic. Immediately after surgery, 0.1 mg/kg is injected subcutaneously along the lateral abdomen. For the next 2 days, buprenorphine is administered orally at 0.18 mg/kg twice a day. If the animal appears to be experiencing discomfort, the dose is increased to 0.25 mg/kg.

Euthanasia

Euthanasia is most easily accomplished by inhalation because the animals are difficult to restrain for physical methods of euthanasia. Carbon dioxide or isoflurane are suitable inhalants for the purpose of euthanasia (see also Chapter 17). After the animal has ceased to breathe, cervical dislocation is performed to ensure that it is dead. Alternatively, after induction of anaesthesia using injectable agents (eg, tiletamine/zolazepam mixture), animals can be euthanased with an overdose of intravenous or intracardiac barbiturates (Pye 2006).

Young animals within the first 2 weeks of life are resistant to carbon dioxide and isoflurane, and are easy to restrain. Therefore, decapitation is an appropriate form of euthanasia for this age group.

Common welfare problems

Disease

Laboratory opossums are relatively free of infectious disease so little is known about appropriate treatments or medicines. As is standard procedure with other small readily available laboratory animals, a colony can be protected from transmissible diseases by euthanasing animals suspected of being infected, and conducting a complete pathological and microbiological evaluation. Appropriate prevention measures can be implemented on the basis of the results. Comprehensive texts on wild animal medicine are available (eg, Holz 2003).

Prophylaxis

Infectious diseases are virtually non-existent in animals that are properly managed and fed a nutritionally adequate diet. However, some of the animals involved in early dietary trials were prone to opportunistic respiratory infections. The affected animals were restricted to groups receiving diets that turned out to be nutritionally suboptimal.

Signs of disease

Common clinical signs of disease include rapid breathing, poor coat condition and loss of body weight. If an animal suspected of having an infectious disease is discovered in a colony, it should be necropsied by a veterinary pathologist, and all husbandry procedures and conditions, including nutritional adequacy of the diet, should be carefully assessed.

Loss of hair near the tail on the rump occurs commonly in females, especially when they are lactating, and rarely in males. There is no apparent detriment to health from hair loss which is thought to be due to hormonal changes.

Haematological and serum chemical values have been determined for healthy laboratory opossums maintained under standard conditions (VandeBerg *et al.* 1986; Cothran *et al.* 1990). These values may be useful as reference values in instances where health problems are suspected.

Common diseases

Wild-caught animals may harbour a variety of endoparasites, including *Capillaria*, *Trichuris*, *Cruzia*, *Strongylus* and fluke-like and *Hymenolepis*-like species, although no disease states induced by these parasites have been observed (Hubbard *et al.* 1997). There have been no reports of ectoparasites in wild or captive populations of *Monodelphis domestica*.

Based on 150 necropsies of *Monodelphis* that became ill or died spontaneously at the Southwest Foundation for Biomedical Research, the most prevalent pathological changes were in the digestive (38%), urogenital (19%), cardiovascular (12%) and respiratory (19%) systems (Hubbard *et al.* 1997). The primary disease problems were rectal prolapse, congestive heart failure and dermatitis. Rectal prolapse was a common problem in laboratory opossum females in earlier years (Cothran *et al.* 1985), but for unknown reasons this condition has become rare. It is likely that animals resistant to this condition under laboratory conditions have been highly favoured by selection.

The most common neoplasia is pituitary adenoma, followed by uterine lesions and cutaneous lipomas (Kuehl-Kovarik *et al.* 1994; Hubbard *et al.* 1997).

No zoonoses have been identified and, as far as the authors are aware, abnormal behaviours related to housing conditions have not been reported.

Reproductive problems

In addition to those animals that fail to reproduce (see Breeding), some females that readily produce litters routinely lose them during the first 2 weeks after parturition. In the authors' colony, females that fail to wean three consecutive litters are generally culled.

When the mother of a valuable litter dies, fostering can be employed to rear the litter to weaning if the pups are old enough to release the teat. However, milk production may not be sufficient for survival of members of an existing litter in addition to foster pups. Therefore, fostering is generally practised only when the mother of an especially valuable litter dies. In that case, a foster mother is required whose pups are at the same age as the orphaned litter, and whose litter size is at least as large as the litter to be fostered. The foster mother's pups are euthanased and replaced in the nest by the foster pups.

Fostering has been successful for litters between 2 and 4 weeks of age. Beyond that age, orphaned litters can be reared by feeding fox chow liquefied with tap water; it is fed via an eye dropper three to four times per day. In addition, half-and-half cow's milk is provided in a shallow dish, such as a Petri dish. As the animals mature, the amount of water added to the fox chow is gradually reduced until it has a pasty consistency by the time the animals are 6 weeks old. By 6–7 weeks of age, the animals can eat moistened fox chow in a shallow dish. By 7–8 weeks, they are able to consume fox chow pellets.

References

Armstrong, J.R. and Ferguson, M.W.J. (1995) Ontogeny of the skin and the transition from scar-free to scarring phenotype during wound healing in the pouch young of a marsupial, *Monodelphis domestica. Developmental Biology*, **169**, 242–260

Baggott, L.M. and Moore, H.D.M. (1990) Early embryonic development of the grey short-tailed opossum, *Monodelphis domestica, in vivo* and *in vitro. Journal of Zoology*, **222**, 623–639

Barnes, R.D. (1977) The special anatomy of *Marmosa robinsoni*. In: *The Biology of Marsupials*. Ed. Hunsaker, D., **II**, pp. 387–413. Academic Press, New York

Barnes, R.D. and Barthold, S.W. (1969) Reproduction and breeding behaviour in an experimental colony of *Marmosa mitis* Bangs (Didelphidea). *Journal of Reproduction and Fertility*, **6 S**, 477–482

Belov, K., Sanderson, C.E., Deakin, J.E. *et al.* (2007) Characterization of the opossum immune genome provides insights into the evolution of the mammalian immune system. *Genome Research*, **17**, 982–991

Canadian Council on Animal Care (1993) Euthanasia. In: *Guide to the Care and Use of Experimental Animals*, 2nd edn. Vol. 2. pp. 141–153. Canadian Council on Animal Care, Ottawa

Chan, J., Donalson, L.M., Kushwaha, R.S. *et al.* (in press) *Differential expression of hepatic genes involved in cholesterol homeostasis in high and low responding strains of laboratory opossums. Metabolism*

Christian, D.P. (1983) Water balance in *Monodelphis domestica* (Didelphidae) from the semiarid caatinga of Brazil. *Comparative Biochemistry and Physiology*, **74**(A), 665–669

Cothran, E.G., Aivaliotis, M.J. and VandeBerg, J.L. (1985) The effects of diet on growth and reproduction in the gray short-tailed opossum (*Monodelphis domestica*). *Journal of Experimental Zoology*, **236**, 103–114

Cothran, E.G., Haines, C.K. and VandeBerg, J.L. (1990) Age effects on hematologic and serum chemical values in gray short-tailed opossums (*Monodelphis domestica*). *Laboratory Animal Science*, **40**, 192–197

Crisp, E.A., Messer, M. and VandeBerg, J.L. (1989) Changes in milk carbohydrates during lactation in a didelphid marsupial, *Monodelphis domestica. Physiological Zoology*, **62**, 1117–1125

Croix, D.A., Samples, N.K., VandeBerg, J.L. *et al.* (1989) Immune response of a marsupial (*Monodelphis domestica*) to sheep red blood cells. *Developmental and Comparative Immunology*, **13**, 73–78

Davidow, L.S., Breen, M., Duke, S.E. *et al.* (2007) The search for a marsupial XIC reveals a break with vertebrate synteny. Chromosome *Research*, **15**, 137–146

Dawson, T.J. and Olson J.M. (1988) Thermogenic capabilities of the opossum *Monodelphis domestica* when warm and cold acclimated: similarities between American and Australian marsupials. *Comparative Biochemistry and Physiology*, **89**(A), 85–91

Dooley, T.P., Mattern, V.L., Moore, C.M. *et al.* (1995) UV-induced melanoma: a karyotype with a single translocation is stable after allografting and metastasis. *Cancer Genetics and Cytogenetics*, **83**, 155–159

Duke, S.E., Samollow, P.B., Mauceli, E. *et al.* (2007) Integrated cytogenetic BAC map of the genome of the gray, short-tailed opossum, *Monodelphis domestica. Chromosome Research*, **15**, 361–370

Dyke, B. (1989) *PEDSYS. A Pedigree Data Management System. Users Manual*. PGL Technical Report No. 2. Southwest Foundation for Biomedical Research, San Antonio, Texas

Fadem, B.H., Hill, H.Z., Huselton, C.A. *et al.* (1988) Transplantation, growth, and regression of mouse melanoma xenografts in neonatal marsupials. *Cancer Investigations*, **6**, 403–408

Fadem, B.H. and Rayve, R.S. (1985) Characteristics of the oestrous cycle and influence of social factors in gray short-tailed opossums (*Monodelphis domestica*). *Journal of Reproduction and Fertility*, **73**, 337–342

Fadem, B.H. and Tesoriero, J.V. (1986) Inhibition of testicular development and feminization of the male genitalia by neonatal estrogen treatment in a marsupial. *Biology of Reproduction*, **34**, 771–776

Frost, S.B. and Masterton, R.B. (1994) Hearing in primitive mammals: *Monodelphis domestica* and *Marmosa elegans. Hearing Research*, **76**, 67–72

Fry, E.J. and Saunders, N.R. (2000) Spinal repair in mammals, a novel approach using the South American opossum *Monodelphis domestica. Clinical and Experimental Pharmacology and Physiology*, **27**, 542–547

Holz, P. (2003) Marsupials. In: *Zoo and Wild Animal Medicine*, 5th edn. Eds Fowler, M.E. and Miller, R.E., pp. 288–303. WB Saunders, Philadelphia

Hornecker, J.L., Samollow, P.B., Robinson, E.S. *et al.* (2007) Meiotic sex chromosome inactivation in the marsupial *Monodelphis domestica. Genesis*, **45**, 696–708

Hubbard, G.B., Mahaney, M.C., Gleiser, C.A. *et al.* (1997) Spontaneous pathology of the laboratory opossum (*Monodelphis domestica*). *Laboratory Animal Science*, **47**, 19–26

Institute of Laboratory Animal Resources (1992) *Recognition and Alleviation of Pain and Distress in Laboratory Animals*. National Academy Press, Washington, DC

International Air Transport Association (2008) *Live Animals Regulations*, 35th edn. International Air Transport Association, Montreal

Johnston, P.G., Dean, A., VandeBerg, J.L. *et al.* (1994) HPRT activity in embryos of a South American opossum *Monodelphis domestica. Reproduction, Fertility and Development*, **6**, 529–532

Jurgelski, W. (1987) American marsupials. In: *The UFAW Handbook on the Care and Management of Laboratory Animals*, 6th edn. Ed. Poole T.B., pp. 189–206. Longman Scientific and Technical, Harlow

Joint Working Group on Refinement (1993) Removal of blood from laboratory mammals and birds. First Report of the BVA/FRAME/RSPCA/UFAW Joint Working Group on Refinement. *Laboratory Animals*, **27**, 1–22. http://www.lal.org.uk/pdffiles/BLOOD.PDF (accessed 19 January 2009)

Joint Working Group on Refinement (2001) Refining procedures for the administration of substances. Report of the BVAAWF/FRAME/RSPCA/UFAW Joint Working Group on Refinement. *Laboratory Animals*, **35**, 1–41. http://www.lal.org.uk/pdffiles/refinement.pdf (accessed 19 January 2009)

Kraus, D.B. and Fadem, B.H. (1987) Reproduction, development and physiology of the gray short-tailed opossum (*Monodelphis domestica*). *Laboratory Animal Science*, **37**, 478–482

Kuehl-Kovarik, C., Sakaguchi, D.S., Iqbal, J. *et al.* (1995) The gray short-tailed opossum: a novel model for mammalian development. *Lab Animal*, **24**, 24–29

Kuehl-Kovarik, M.C., Ackermann, M.R., Hanson, D.L. *et al.* (1994) Spontaneous pituitary adenomas in the Brazilian gray short-tailed opossum (*Monodelphis domestica*). *Veterinary Pathology*, **31**, 377–379

Kusewitt, D.F., Hubbard, G.B., Warbritton, A.R., *et al.* (2000) Cellular origins of ultraviolet radiation-induced corneal tumours in the grey, short-tailed South American opossum (*Monodelphis domestica*). *Journal of Comparative Pathology*, **123**, 88–95

Kushwaha, R.S., VandeBerg, J.F., Rodriguez, R. *et al.* (2005) Low-density lipoprotein apolipoprotein B production differs between laboratory opossums exhibiting high and low lipemic responses to dietary cholesterol and fat. *Metabolism Clinical and Experimental*, **54**, 1075–1081

Kushwaha, R.S., VandeBerg, J.F., Rodriguez, R. *et al.* (2004a) Cholesterol absorption and hepatic acyl-coenzyme A: cholesterol acyltransferase activity play major roles in lipemic response to dietary cholesterol and fat in laboratory opossums. *Metabolism*, **53**, 817–822

Kushwaha, R.S., VandeBerg, J.F. and VandeBerg, J.L. (2004b) Effect of dietary cholesterol with or without saturate fat on plasma lipoprotein cholesterol levels in the laboratory opossum (*Monodelphis domestica*) model for diet-induced hyperlipidaemia. *British Journal of Nutrition*, **92**, 63–70

Lane, M.A., Truettner, J.S., Brunschwig, J.P. *et al.* (2007) Age-related differences in the local and molecular responses to injury in developing spinal cord of the opossum, *Monodelphis domestica*. *European Journal of Neuroscience*, **25**, 1725–1742

Lemos, B. (2007) The opossum genome reveals further evidence for regulatory evolution in mammalian diversification. *Genome Biology*, **8**, 223

Ley, R.D., Reeve, V.E. and Kusewitt, D.F. (2000) Photobiology of *Monodelphis domestica*. *Developmental and Comparative Immunology*, **24**, 503–516

Macrini, T.E. (2004) *Monodelphis domestica*. *Mammalian Species*, **760**, 1–8

Manis, G.S., Hubbard, G.B., Hainsey, B.M. *et al.* (1992) Effects of chronic blood loss in a marsupial (*Monodelphis domestica*). *Laboratory Animal Science*, **42**, 567–571

Martin, B.J. (1995) Evaluation of hypothermia for anesthesia in reptiles and amphibians. *ILAR Journal*, **37**, 186–190

Mate, K.E., Robinson, E.S., VandeBerg, J.L. *et al.* (1994) Timetable of *in vivo* embryonic development in the grey short-tailed opossum (*Monodelphis domestica*). *Molecular Reproduction and Development*, **39**, 365–374

Merry, D.E., Pathak, S. and VandeBerg, J.L. (1983) Differential NOR activities in somatic and germ cells of *Monodelphis domestica* (Marsupialia, Mammalia). *Cytogenetics and Cell Genetics*, **35**, 244–251

Mikkelsen, T.S., Wakefiled, M.J., Aken, B. *et al.* (2007) Genome of the marsupial *Monodelphis domestica* reveals innovation in non-coding sequences. *Nature*, **447**, 167–177

Mladinic, M., Wintzer, M., Del Bel, E. *et al.* (2005) Differential expression of genes at stages when regeneration can and cannot occur after injury to immature mammalian spinal cord. *Cellular and Molecular Neurobiology*, **25**, 407–426

Mollgard, K., Blaslev, Y., Stagaard, J. *et al.* (1994) Development of spinal cord in the isolated CNS of a neonatal mammal (the opossum *Monodelphis domestica*) maintained in longterm culture. *Journal of Neurocytology*, **23**, 151–165

Moore, H.D.M. and Taggart, D.A. (1993) *In vitro* fertilization and embryo culture in the grey short-tailed opossum *Monodelphis domestica*. *Journal of Reproduction and Fertility*, **98**, 267–274

Morykwas, M.J., Ditesheim, J.A., Ledbetter, M.S. *et al.* (1991) *Monodelphis domesticus*: a model for early developmental wound healing. *Annals of Plastic Surgery*, **27**, 327–331

Namekawa, S.H., VandeBerg, J.L., McCarrey, J.R. *et al.* (2007) Sex chromosome silencing in the marsupial male germ line. *Proceedings of the National Academy of Sciences*, **104**, 9730–9735

Nowak, R.M. (1999) *Walker's Mammals of the World*, 6th edn. The Johns Hopkins University Press, Baltimore

O'Brien, S.J. and Graves, J.A.M. (1990) Geneticists converge on divergent mammals: an overview of comparative mammalian genetics. *Australian Journal of Zoology*, **37**, 147–154

Pathak, S., Ronne, M., Brown, C.L. *et al.* (1993) A high-resolution banding ideogram of *Monodelphis domestica* chromosomes (Marsupialia, Mammalia). *Cytogenetics and Cell Genetics*, **63**, 181–184

Perelygin, A.A., Samollow, P.B., Perelygina, L.M. *et al.* (1996) A new DNA marker *U1557* is linked to protease inhibitor (*PI*) and adenylate kinase-1 (*AK-1*) in the laboratory opossum, *Monodelphis domestica*. *Animal Genetics*, **27**, 113–116

Pine R.H., Handley, C.O. Jr. (2008) Genus *Monodelphis* Burnett, 1830. In: *Mammals of South America, Volume 1: Marsupials, Xenarthrans, Shrews, and Bats*. Ed. Gardner, A.L., pp. 82–85. University of Chicago Press, Chicago

Pye, G.W. (2006) *Marsupials*. In: *Guidelines for Euthanasia of Nondomestic Animals*. Ed. Kirk-Baer, C., pp. 52–56. American Association of Zoo Veterinarians (AAZV) http://www.aazv.org

Rainwater D.L., Kammerer, C.M., Singh, A.T.K. *et al.* (2001) Genetic control of lipoprotein phenotypes in the laboratory opossum, *Monodelphis domestica*. *GeneScreen*, **1**, 117–124

Reig, O.A., Kirsch, J.A.W. and Marshall, L.G. (1987) Systematic relationships of the living and Neocenozoic American 'opossum-like' marsupials (suborder Didelphimorphia), with comment on the classification of these and of the Cretaceous and Paleogene New World and European metatherians. In: *Possums and Opossums: Studies in Evolution*. Ed. Archer, M., pp. 1–89. Surrey Beatty and Sons and the Royal Zoological Society of New South Wales, Sydney

Robinson, E.S. and Dooley, T.P. (1995) A new allogeneic model for metastatic melanoma. *European Journal of Cancer*, **31**(A), 2302–2308

Robinson, E.S., Hubbard, G.B., Colon, G. *et al.* (1998) Low-dose ultraviolet exposure early in development can lead to widespread melanoma in the opossum model. *International Journal of Experimental Pathology*, **79**, 235–244

Robinson, E.S., Renfree, M.B., Short, R.V. *et al.* (1991) Mammary glands in male marsupials. 2. Development of teat primordia in *Didelphis virginiana* and *Monodelphis domestica*. *Reproduction, Fertility, and Development*, **3**, 295–301

Robinson, E.S. and VandeBerg, J.L. (1994) Blood collection and surgical procedures for the laboratory opossum (*Monodelphis domestica*). *Laboratory Animal Science*, **44**, 63–68

Robinson, E.S., VandeBerg, J.L, Hubbard, G.B. *et al.* (1994) Malignant melanoma in ultraviolet-irradiated laboratory opossums: initiation in suckling young, metastasis in adults, and xenograft behavior in nude mice. *Cancer Research*, **54**, 5986–5991

Robinson, E.S., VandeBerg, J.L., Watson, C.M. *et al.* (1996) Intersexual phenotypes and sex chromosome complements of five gray short-tailed opossums. *Laboratory Animal Science*, **46**, 555–560

Sakaguchi, D.S., Van Hoffelen, S.J., Theusch, E. *et al.* (2004) Transplantation of neural progenitor cells into the developing retina of the Brazilian opossum: An *in vivo* system for studying stem/progenitor cell plasticity. *Developmental Neuroscience*, **26**, 336–345

Samollow, P.B. (2006) Status and applications of genomic resources for the gray, short-tailed opossum, *Monodelphis domestica*, an American marsupial model for comparative biology. *Australian Journal of Zoology*, **54**, 173–196

Samollow, P.B., Gouin, N., Miethke, P. *et al.* (2007) A microsatellite-based, physically anchored linkage map for the gray, short-tailed opossum (*Monodelphis domestica*). *Chromosome Research*, **15**, 269–281

Samples, N.K., VandeBerg, J.L. and Stone, W.H. (1986) Passively acquired immunity in the newborn of a marsupial (*Monodelphis domestica*). *American Journal of Reproductive Immunology and Microbiology*, **11**, 94–97

Saunders, N.R., Deal, A., Knott, G.W. *et al.* (1995) Repair and recovery following spinal cord injury in a neonatal marsupial (*Monodelphis domestica*). *Clinical and Experimental Pharmacology and Physiology*, **22**, 518–526

Selwood, L., Robinson, E.S., Pedersen, R.A. *et al.* (1997) Development *in vitro* in marsupials: a comparative review of species and a timetable of cleavage and early blastocyst stages of development in *Monodelphis domestica*. *International Journal of Developmental Biology*, **41**, 397–410

Selwood, L. and VandeBerg, J.L. (1992) The influence of incubation temperature on oocyte maturation, parthenogenetic and embryonic development *in vitro* of the marsupial *Monodelphis domestica*. *Animal Reproduction Science*, **29**, 99–116

Shearer, M.H., Robinson, E.S., VandeBerg, J.L. *et al.* (1995) Humoral immune response in a marsupial *Monodelphis domestica*: anti-isotypic and anti-idiotypic responses detected by species specific monoclonal antiimmunoglobulin reagents. *Developmental and Comparative Immunology*, **19**, 237–246

Shevchenko, A.I., Zakharova, I.S., Elisaphenko, E.A. *et al.* (2007) Genes flanking *Xist* in mouse and human are separated on the X chromosome in American marsupials. *Chromosome Research*, **15**, 127–136

Stewart, R.R., Zou, D.-J., Treherne, J.M. *et al.* (1991) The intact central nervous system of the newborn opossum in long-term culture: fine structure and GABA-mediated inhibition of electrical activity. *Journal of Experimental Biology*, **161**, 25–41

Stone, W.H., Bruun, D.A., Foster, E.B. *et al.* (1998) Absence of a significant mixed lymphocyte reaction in a marsupial (*Monodelphis domestica*). *Laboratory Animal Science*, **48**, 184–189

Stone, W.H., Bruun, D.A., Manis, G.S. *et al.* (1996) The immunobiology of the marsupial, *Monodelphis domestica*. In: *Modulators of Immune Responses. The Evolutionary Trail*. Eds Stolen J.S., Fletcher, T.C., Bayne, C.J., Secombes, C.J., Zelikoff, J.T., Twerdok, L.E. and Anderson, D.P., pp. 149–165. SOS Publications, Brackenridge Series, Fair Haven, NJ

Stone, W.H., Manis, G.S., Hoffman, E.S. *et al.* (1997) Fate of allogenic skin transplantations in a marsupial (*Monodelphis domestica*). *Laboratory Animal Science*, **47**, 283–287

Stonebrook, M.J. and Harder, J.D. (1992) Sexual maturation in female gray short-tailed opossums, *Monodelphis domestica*, is dependent upon male stimuli. *Biology of Reproduction*, **46**, 290–294

Stoskopf, M.K., Meyer, R.E., Jones, M. *et al.* (1999) Field immobilization and euthanasia of American opossum. *Journal of Wildlife Diseases*, **35**, 145–149

Streilein, K.E. (1982) Behavior, ecology, and distribution of South American marsupials. In: *Mammalian Biology in South America*. Eds Mares, M.A. and Genoways, H.H., pp. 231–250. Pymatuning Symposia in Ecology. Special Publications Series. Linesville, PA: Pymatuning Laboratory of Ecology, University of Pittsburgh

Taggart, D.A., Johnson, J.L., O'Brien, H.P. *et al.* (1993) Why do spermatozoa of American marsupials form pairs? A clue from the analysis of sperm-pairing in the epididymis of the grey short-tailed opossum, *Monodelphis domestica*. *Anatomical Record*, **236**, 465–478

Taylor, J.S.H. and Guillery, R.W. (1995) Does early monocular enucleation in a marsupial effect the surviving uncrossed retinofugal pathway? *Journal of Anatomy*, **186**, 335–342

Tyndale-Biscoe, C.H. (1973) *Life of Marsupials*. Edward Arnold, London

van Nievelt, A.F.H. and Smith, K.K. (2005) Tooth eruption in *Monodelphis domestica* and its significance for phylogeny and natural history. *Journal of Mammalogy*, **86**, 333–341.

van Oorschot, R.A.H., Birmingham, V., Porter, P.A. *et al.* (1993) Linkage between complement components 6 and 7 and glutamic pyruvate transaminase in the marsupial *Monodelphis domestica*. *Biochemical Genetics*, **31**, 215–222

van Oorschot, R.A.H., Porter, P.A., Kammerer, C.M. *et al.* (1992b) Severely reduced recombination in females of the South American marsupial *Monodelphis domestica*. *Cytogenetics and Cell Genetics*, **60**, 64–67

van Oorschot, R.A.H., Williams-Blangero, S. and VandeBerg, J.L. (1992a) Genetic diversity of laboratory gray short-tailed opossums (*Monodelphis domestica*): effect of newly introduced wild-caught animals. *Laboratory Animal Science*, **42**, 255–260

VandeBerg, J.L. (1990) The gray short-tailed opossum (*Monodelphis domestica*) as a model didelphid species for genetic research. *Australian Journal of Zoology*, **37**, 235–247

VandeBerg, J.L. (1983) Developmental aspects of X chromosome inactivation in eutherian and metatherian mammals. *Journal of Experimental Zoology*, **228**, 271–286

VandeBerg, J.L., Cothran, E.G. and Kelly, C.A. (1986) Dietary effects on hematologic and serum chemical values in gray short-tailed opossums (*Monodelphis domestica*). *Laboratory Animal Science*, **36**, 32–36

VandeBerg, J.L., Johnston, P.G., Cooper, D.W. *et al.* (1983) X-chromosome inactivation and evolution in marsupials and other mammals. *Isozymes. Current Topics in Biology and Medical Research*, **9**, 201–218

VandeBerg, J.L. and Robinson, E.S. (1997) The laboratory opossum (*Monodelphis domestica*) in biomedical research. In: *Recent Advances in Marsupial Biology*. Eds Saunders, N. and Hinds, L., pp. 238–263. University of New South Wales Press, Syndey

VandeBerg, J.L., Williams-Blangero, S. Hubbard, G.B. *et al.* (1994) Susceptibility to ultraviolet-induced corneal sarcomas is highly heritable in a laboratory opossum model. *International Journal of Cancer*, **56**, 119–123

Wang, Z., Dooley, T.P., Curto, E.V. *et al.* (2004) Cross-species application of cDNA microarrays to profile gene expression using UV-induced melanoma in *Monodelphis domestica* as the model system. *Genomics*, **83**, 588–599

Wang, Z., Hubbard, G.B., Pathak, S. *et al.* (2003) *In vivo* opossum xenograft model for cancer research. *Cancer Research*, **63**, 6121–6124

Wang, Z. and VandeBerg, J.L. (2003) Survival anesthetic and injection procedures for neonatal opossums. *Contemporary Topics in Laboratory Animal Science*, **42**, 41–43

Wang, Z. and VandeBerg, J.L. (2005) Immunotolerance in the laboratory opossum (*Monodelphis domestica*) to xenografted mouse melanoma. *Contemporary Topics in Laboratory Animal Medicine*, **44**, 39–42

Wong, E.S., Young, L.J., Papenfuss, A.T. *et al.* (2006) In silico identification of opossum cytokine genes suggests the complexity of the marsupial immune system rivals that of eutherian mammals. *Immunome Research*, **2**, 4

20 Tree shrews

Eberhard Fuchs and Silke Corbach-Söhle

Biological overview

General biology

The first report of tree shrews dates back to 1780. The description and an accompanying sketch were from William Ellis who maintained a naturalist's journal during Captain's Cook's third Pacific voyage of the ship *Discovery*. Uncertainties concerning the taxonomic affinities of tree shrews originated with this description in which tree shrews were designated 'squirrels', a confusion that still occasionally persists today. About 80 years ago, a variety of reports described similarities between tree shrews and primates, and the conclusion that there was a direct phylogenetic relationship between modern tree shrews and primates was predominantly made by Le Gros Clark (1924), largely on the basis of brain anatomy. His view was endorsed in G.G. Simpson's classification of the mammals (Simpson 1945). In the following years, several authorities (see eg, Luckett 1980) had doubts about this phylogenetic link and, as a result, excluded tree shrews from primates. An intensive discussion of tree shrews and their phylogenetic relationships is provided in Luckett (1980), Martin (1990) and Emmons (2000). Today, tree shrews are placed in their own order, Scandentia, and according to very recent molecular phylogenetic studies they are placed together with primates and dermoptera within the clade Euarchonta (Kriegs *et al.* 2007). Currently the tree shrew genome is being cloned as part of the Mammalian Genome Project, funded by the National Institutes of Health (NIH).

Tree shrews (family Tupaiidae) are subdivided in two subfamilies: the diurnal subfamily Tupaiinae containing five genera (*Tupaia*, *Anathana*, *Dendrogale*, *Lyonogale*, *Urogale*) and the nocturnal subfamily Ptilocercinae, with a single genus, the pen-tailed tree shrew *Ptilocercus*. The geographic distribution of the Tupaiidae extends from India to the Philippines, and from Southern China to Java, Borneo, Sumatra and Bali. Natural habitats are tropical forests and plantation areas (Table 20.1).

In general, tree shrews are similar to squirrels in their external appearance and habits and the Malay word 'tupai' (from which the name *Tupaia* is derived) is used for both tree shrews and squirrels, whereas the Malay word 'tana' (found in the species *Lyonogale tana*) is used only for tree shrews. Despite their name, tree shrews have nothing to do with real shrews and most species of tree shrews are much more active on the ground than in trees. Although there are clear differences between tree shrew species, they share a basic common pattern that can be described with reference to the relatively well known Belanger's tree shrew *Tupaia belangeri* (Figure 20.1). All are relatively small, agile and, in general, omnivorous with a preference for small fruits and invertebrates, especially arthropods. Tree shrews range from the predominantly arboreal (*Dendrogale*, *Tupaia minor*, *Ptilocercus*) to the predominantly terrestrial (*Lyonogale*, *Urogale*), but most tree shrew species are semi-arboreal and usually forage on the ground. The terrestrial tree shrews have a long snout and sharp claws both of which are used to obtain food by rooting through the leaf litter on the forest floor. Species which are more arboreal are smaller than the terrestrial species. They have shorter snouts, smaller or poorly developed claws, long tails and more forward-facing eyes. When eating, all species will hold food between the front paws. In general, tree shrews have a well developed visual system and, for some species, colour vision has been documented. The vocal repertoire of *Tupaia belangeri* consists of eight distinct sounds. Within this repertoire, four basic acoustic structures can be distinguished which can be associated with functional categories such as alarm, attention contact and defence (Binz & Zimmermann 1989). No ultrasonic vocalisations could be found in *Tupaia belangeri* (Kirchhof *et al.* 2001). The same authors report that during agonistic encounters, adult males elicit five distinct call types, partially with graded variants. The calls show harmonic or noisy spectra ranging from 0.4–20 kHz. The call structure depends on the dominant status and the motivation of the individuals. Increasing pitch indicates increasing fear, while decreasing pitch and larger frequency range indicate increasing aggression (Kirchhof *et al.* 2001).

All tree shrews seem to use nests both for sleeping and rearing of offspring. Nests may be located in trees or on the ground level. Even tree shrews, which spend most of their time in trees, avoid climbing on fine branches and do not leap within or between trees. Typically, they use broad branches as support and trees as a vertical extension of the terrestrial substrate (Martin 1990).

Size range and lifespan

Depending on the species, the body weight of tree shrews ranges between 45 and 350 g (see Table 20.1) with adult

Table 20.1 Tree shrews, Scandentia, their biological data and distribution (with modifications from von Holst (1988)) (BW, body weight; HBL, head–body length; TL, tail length; NN, number of nipples; GP, gestation period; LS, litter size; BIW, birth weight; W, weaning; P, puberty; L, longevity in captivity).

	Body	*Reproduction*	*Life history*	*Distribution*
Subfamily Tupaiinae *Tupaia* (tree shrews) *T. belangeri, T. glis, T. gracilis, T. javanica, T. longipes, T. minor, T. montana, T. nicobaria, T. palawanensis, T. picta, T. splendidula*	BW: 50–270 g HBL: 12–21 cm TL: 14–20 cm NN: 1–3 pairs	GP: 41–55 days LS: 1–5 BIW: 6–10 g	W: around 30 days P: around 2 months L: 9–12 years	Tropical forests, semi-terrestrial
Lyonogale (Malaysian tree shrews) *L. tana, L. dorsalis*	BW: approx. 300 g HBL: approx. 22 cm TL: approx. 17 cm NN: 2 pairs	GT: 45–55 days LS: 1–4 BIW: approx. 10 g	W: around 30 days P: around 2 months L: Unknown	Mainly terrestrial, primary and secondary forests
Urogale (Philippine tree shrew) *U. everetti*	BW: 220–350 g HBL: approx. 20 cm TL: approx. 15 cm NN: 2 pairs	GP: approx. 55 days LS: 1–4 BIW: approx. 10 g	W: around 30 days P: probably 2 months L: 6 years	Terrestrial
Anathana (Indian tree shrew) *A. ellioti ellioti, A. ellioti pallida, A. ellioti wroughtoni*	BW: approx. 180 g HBL: approx. 19 cm TL: approx. 18 cm NN: 3 pairs	Unkown	Unkown	Tropical forests, semi-terrestrial
Dendrogale (smooth-tailed tree shrew) *D. melanura, D. murina*	BW: approx. 60 g HBL: approx. 13 cm TL: approx. 13 cm NN: 1 pair	Probably like *Tupaia*	Probably like *Tupaia*	Mainly arboreal
Subfamily Ptilocercinae *Ptilocercus lowii* (pen-tailed tree shrew)	BW: approx. 15 g HBL: approx. 14 cm TL: approx. 17 cm NN: 2 pairs	GP: unknown LS: probably 1–4 BIW: unknown	Unknown	Nocturnal, arboreal, tropical forests

males being usually heavier than adult females (own observation). Their lifespan in the wild is still unknown but in captivity, *Tupaia glis* (Bever & Sprankel 1986) and *Tupaia belangeri* (own observations) can live 10 years or more.

Social organisation

Despite extensive morphological description and behavioural studies in the laboratory, remarkably little is known about the behaviour and the ecological roles of tree shrews in the wild (Emmons 1991, 2000; Emmons & Biun 1991). Based on observations of Kawamichi and Kawamichi (1979), males of the common tree shrew *Tupaia glis*, which are close relatives to the Belanger's tree shrew, have relatively stable home ranges of about 2 acres. The territory of an adult male overlaps to a certain extent with the home range of one adult female and also includes the ranges of a small number of juveniles. This suggests that common tree shrews are basically monogamous in the wild, which is in agreement with observations made in the laboratory where tree shrews can be effectively maintained in pairs. The same authors also reported territorial marking behaviour using the chest gland, and territorial fights between adults of the same sex. Chemical signals play an important role in territorial behaviour of male tree shrews. Scent substances are found in glandular secretions, urine, faeces and saliva, and contain information concerning the identity and physiological state of the individual. Laboratory experiments have shown that in males, both the production of the scent substances and the marking behaviour are controlled by androgens (von Holst & Buergel-Goodwin 1975; von Holst & Eichmann 1998; Eichmann & von Holst 1999).

Standard biological data

The dental formula of the Tupaiidae is: $I^2_3C^1_1Pm^3_3M^3_3$ (Butler 1980). Core body temperature and its circadian rhythm have been studied by telemetry in *Tupaia belangeri*. Minimal body temperature during the night was about 35 °C while during day time the core temperature increased to a maximum of about 40 °C (Refinetti & Menaker 1992 and own observations). This day/night difference of about 5 °C is much larger than that of most endotherms. Since body temperature rhythm is synchronised with the rhythm of locomotor activity, the diurnal temperature curve shows a bimodal shape which clearly differs from the cosine waveform that characterises the temperature rhythms of other species (Figure 20.2).

Systolic blood pressure recorded using the tail-cuff method similar to that often used in rats yielded a mean systolic blood pressure of 125 mmHg (Fuchs *et al.* 1993). When using this technique it is not necessary, as is the case with rats, to warm the tree shrew's tail before measurement.

Heart rates in tree shrews show a surprising pattern of variance. Telemetric analysis has revealed that heart rate is strictly correlated with the behaviour and the emotional status of the animals. A heart rate between 240 and 300 beats/min (own observations) is characteristic of resting periods, while during physical activity, heart rate is in the range of 250–350 beats/min and can increase up to 650 beats/min in emotionally exciting situations (Stohr 1988; Muller & Hub 1992). *Tupaia belangeri* shows a high locomotor activity revealing a clear bimodal pattern with a clear trough in the early afternoon (Kurre & Fuchs 1988) (Figure 20.2).

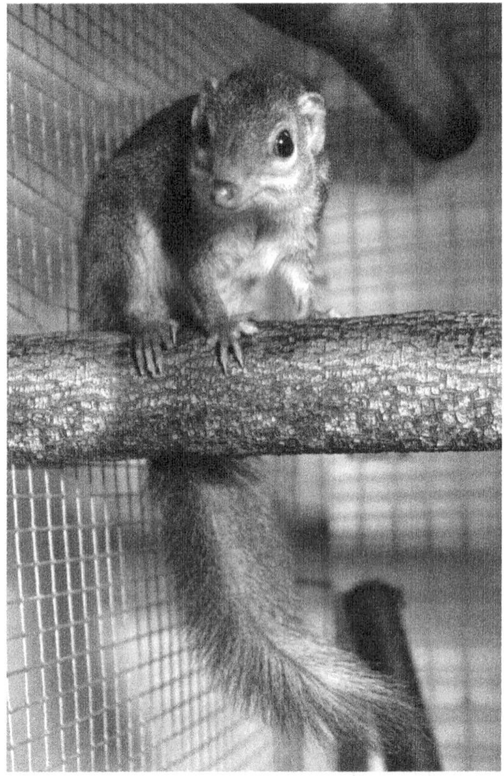

Figure 20.1 Adult male *Tupaia belangeri* from the German Primate Center.

Reliable data on serum constitutents are only available for *Tupaia belangeri*. Table 20.2 summarises serum values reported by Schwaier (1975). An overview of serum and endocrine data is given by von Holst (1977). Erythrocyte numbers are in the range of $8 \times 10^6/\text{mm}^3$, leucocytes in the range of $3 \times 10^3/\text{mm}^3$ and mean thrombocyte numbers in the range of $170 \times 10^3/\text{mm}^3$ (Zou *et al.* 1983). Basal concentrations for plasma norepinephrine (noradrenaline) range from 2.8–36.3 ng/ml and for epinephrine (adrenaline) from 1.3–19.1 ng/ml (Fuchs 1984). Corticosterone is the principal corticosteroid (mean 9 ng/ml) in the peripheral plasma and in unstressed animals the corticosterone : cortisol ratio is 4.5 : 1 (Collins *et al.* 1984). Values of urinary hormones for *Tupaia belangeri* are summarised in Table 20.2.

Breeds, strains and genetics

When selecting a breeding stock for tree shrews, it is important to know the exact origin of the animals. Sometimes, it can be extremely difficult to distinguish between closely related species since traditional classifications do not provide substantial help. Based on their external morphology alone, *Tupaia glis* and *Tupaia belangeri* are very difficult to distinguish from one another. The exact taxonomic classification could be ascertained by means of geographical origin, morphological criteria, cytogenetic analysis and analysis of acoustic signals (Toder *et al.* 1992).

Sources of supply

The Three Rs are a fundamental ethical requirement in laboratory animal science (see Chapter 2). To refine animal experiments and to reduce the number of animal subjects to a minimum, full control over the genetic background and lifespan of the subjects is required. Therefore, it is strongly recommended that animals should only be purchased from laboratory breeding colonies. Information on sources of

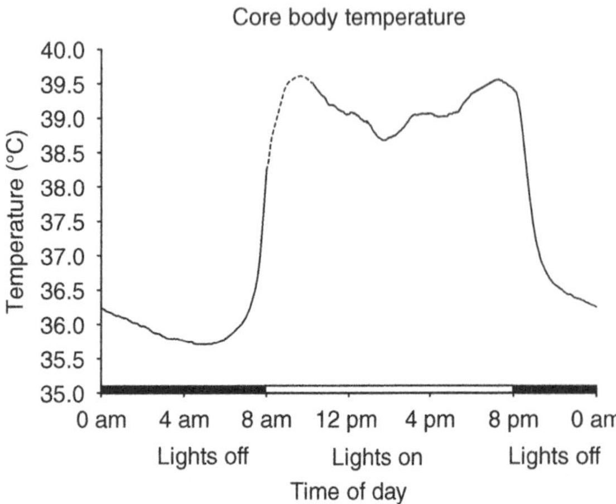

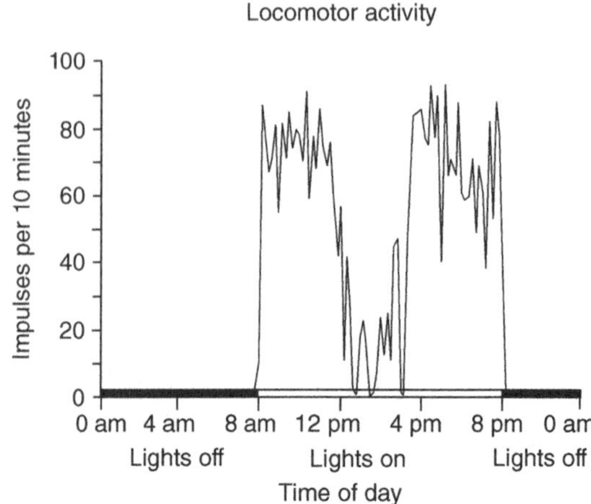

Figure 20.2 Circadian pattern of core body temperature and locomotor activity.

Table 20.2 Physiological data of adult Tupaia belangeri. Blood serum values from Schwaier (1975) and morning urine values from Fuchs (1988).

Parameter	*Serum/plasma*			*Urine*			
	Unit	*mean*	*SD*	*Gender*	*Unit*	*mean*	*SD*
Na^+	mmol/l	141	2.7	M	µmol/ml	95	34
				F	µmol/ml	120	48
K^+	mmol/l	5.2	0.75	M	µmol/ml	85	65
				F	µmol/ml	152	43
Na^+/K^+				M		1.05	0.5
				F		0.82	0.3
Mg^{2+}	mmol/l	2.12	0.24	M	µmol/ml	3.5	2
				F	µmol/ml	4.3	2.2
Ca^{2+}	mmol/l	5.58	0.88	M	µmol/ml	1.25	0.6
				F	µmol/ml	1.35	0.5
Fe^{2+}	µmol/l	95					
Cl^-	mmol/l	105	3.3				
Osmolarity	mOsmol/l	318	7.8	M	mOsmol/kg H_2O	2000	750
				F	mOsmol/kg H_2O	1950	350
pH				M		6.75	0.6
				F		6.75	0.4
Creatinine	µmol/l	62		M	µmol/ml	10.5	4.4
				F	µmol/ml	11.2	3.8
Urea		25.8	7.8	M	µmol/µmol Crea	0.9	0.8
				F	µmol/µmol Crea	0.9	0.2
Uric acid	mol/l	48		M	µg/µmol Crea	16	14
				F	µg/µmol Crea	15	8
Cholesterol	mmol/l	2					
Triglycerides	mol/l	1					
Glucose	mg/100 ml	115.9	16.3	M	mg/µmol Crea	0.1	0
				F	mg/µmol Crea	0.08	0
Protein	g/100 ml	6.5		M	mg/ml	2.65	1.1
				F	mg/ml	0.3	0.2
Protein/Crea				M	mg/µmol Crea	0.25	0.1
				F	mg/µmol Crea	0.27	0.1
Prolactin	ng/ml	12					
Cortisol	µg/ml	8.8		M	pg/µmol Crea	180	
Corticosterone				M	pg/µmol Crea	335	130
Gastrin	pg/ml	55					
GPT	U/l	10.9	6.2				
GOT	U/l	58	16.8				
LDH	U/l	1872	802				
AP (age 14–27 months)	U/l	90.8	48.2				
GH	ng Eq/ml	>50					
Epinephrine (adrenaline)	ng/l	7.5–11		M	pg/µmol Crea	47	39
Norepinephrine (noradrenaline)	ng/l	5–6.9		M	pg/µmol Crea	103	75
ACTH	pg/ml	65					
TSH	pg/ml	3.5					
FSH	pg/mg	89					
LH	ng/ml	24					

supply can be obtained from the German Primate Center, Göttingen, Germany[1].

Uses in the laboratory

Evidence derived from studies on the brain of *Tupaia* by Sir Wilfred Le Gros Clark played a major role in the acceptance of the classification of Tupaiids as primates. Their popularity as experimental subjects in neurobiology, in particular neuroanatomy, has been a direct consequence of their former phylogenetic status in which they were classified as primitive primates (Campbell 1980). The vast majority of experimental work with *Tupaia* has been on the visual system since they were considered ideal subjects to gain insight into the organisation of the early primate visual system. However, it became clear from comparative studies that *Tupaia* possesses none of the features characteristic of primate visual systems (Campbell 1980).

[1] http://www.dpz.eu

Tree shrews have proved to be useful animal models in many instances where a small omnivorous non-rodent species is required (Cao *et al.* 2003). Of course, they should only be used where it is appropriate and necessary for the study. They can be used in many fields of preclinical research such as toxicology and virology, in particular in studies investigating herpes and hepatitis viruses (Hunt 1993; Xu *et al.* 2007). Further, various aspects of behaviour, infant development, communication and social structures can be studied in tree shrews (Martin 1968a, 1968b; Hertenstein *et al.* 1987). Based on a study by von Holst (1972), psychosocially stressed male tree shrews were thought to be a suitable model to study the mechanisms of acute renal failure. However, the authors and others (Steinhausen *et al.* 1978) were unable to replicate these results.

Tree Shrews' pronounced territoriality, especially that of males, can be used to establish natural challenging situations under experimental control in the laboratory. When living in visual and olfactory contact with a male conspecific by which it has been defeated, the subordinate Belanger's tree shrew shows dramatic behavioural, physiological and neuroendocrine changes. As we know today, these stress-induced alterations result entirely from the continuous visual presence of the dominant conspecific. In contrast, dominant tree shrews show no noticeable biobehavioural alterations. It is an interesting aspect of preclinical research that many of the alterations in subordinate tree shrews are similar to the symptoms observed in depressed patients and can be counteracted by several classes of antidepressant drugs (Fuchs 2005).

There is a high degree of genetic homology between tree shrews and primates for several receptor proteins of neuromodulators (Fuchs & Flugge 2002) and the amyloid-beta precursor protein (Pawlik *et al.* 1999); this and the three to four times longer lifespan of tree shrews than that of rodents (Keuker *et al.* 2005), suggest that this species may possibly come to be used in future studies focusing on aging-related brain changes in socially homogeneous and stable cohorts.

Laboratory management and breeding

General husbandry

Housing

Tree shrews have been housed in enclosures of various sizes. Cages and cage equipment should be adapted to the natural behaviour patterns of the animals, providing enough space for their locomotor activities. The cage equipment thus should include substrates for climbing, such as suitable branches and wire mesh. A broad branch (diameter approximately 7 cm), board or tube should be fixed near the top of the cage where the animals can rest during their siestas. Objects for scent marking such as branches, and pasteboard tubes for hiding and marking should also be offered. Outside the cages, wooden sleeping boxes and, for breeding pairs, a separate nest box and nesting material should be provided. Schwaier (1973) recommended the installation of tunnels made out of flexible plastic tubing, of suitable diameter, which can be fixed outside the cages allowing opportunities for greater travel. When cages are side by side they must be separated by opaque screens, which prevent interactions other than the exchange of calls and dispersed odours. Cages face to face separated by a corridor are quite satisfactory because they allow visual interactions without the threat of an immediate attack. Below the cages are waste trays with sawdust or paper to catch excrement and food. In general, the caging conditions should allow control and observation of the animals during the active period by the animal care staff. Construction of the animal facilities should allow each room to be emptied of animals from time to time to allow for cleaning, disinfection and repairs. In the rooms all possible routes of escape must be screened with small diameter wire mesh. To avoid startling the animals, it is recommended that staff should give a sign to the animals before entering an animal room, for example, by knocking on the door.

Tree shrews are best housed at a temperature of approximately 25 °C. Temperatures less than 20 °C can be dangerous for the offspring. Humidity is also critical. Experience suggests that minimal levels required are in the range of 45–50%.

Little systematic research has been carried out on housing of tree shrews; a description of a successful facility is provided here. In the German Primate Center, Göttingen, *Tupaia belangeri* are housed in steel cages (size 50 cm × 80 cm × 130 cm (w × d × h) (Figure 20.3), or 65 cm × 85 cm × 85 cm (w × d × h)). Outside the cages are wooden nest boxes with removable covers (18 cm × 15 cm × 15 cm (w × d × h); entrance 6 cm diameter). These boxes are made from waterproof plywood, which is highly resistant to water and heat and can be effectively cleaned. As the animals stay in the box all night, moisture arises and the animals become damp unless open-pored material is used for the nest box. Therefore, boxes made of plastic or metal are inappropriate. The animals can be locked in the box by a shutter and the box can be removed from the cage. Breeding pairs are housed in modular units (two units with nest boxes) which can be separated by a wire mesh frame.

The animal quarters are air-conditioned with a relative humidity of 60 ± 7%, a temperature of 27 ± 1 °C, and a 10-fold air-exchange per hour. The animal rooms are illuminated (L : D = 12 : 12) from 8:00 am to 8:00 pm with six neon lamps (58 W each, light intensity about 900 lux). After lights are on and before lights are shut down a 30 minute 'sun rise' and a 30 minute 'sun set' with reduced light intensity are programmed. In addition to the neon lamps, each room is equipped with two ultraviolet lamps, which are regulated by a separate timer. The total UV exposure time per day is 2 h (four intervals of 30 minutes each). During the night there is no natural or artificial illumination of the rooms. Each animal room is equipped with one loudspeaker, which is active from 8:30 am to 7:30 pm broadcasting news, reports and some music at low volume. Cages are cleaned once a week with water, the paper under the cages is changed daily, and the waste trays with sawdust are cleaned once a week. No detergents are used in the animal rooms.

Presentation of food and water

Food is supplied in glazed stoneware or stainless steel dishes (diameter about 8 cm, height about 3 cm) which are

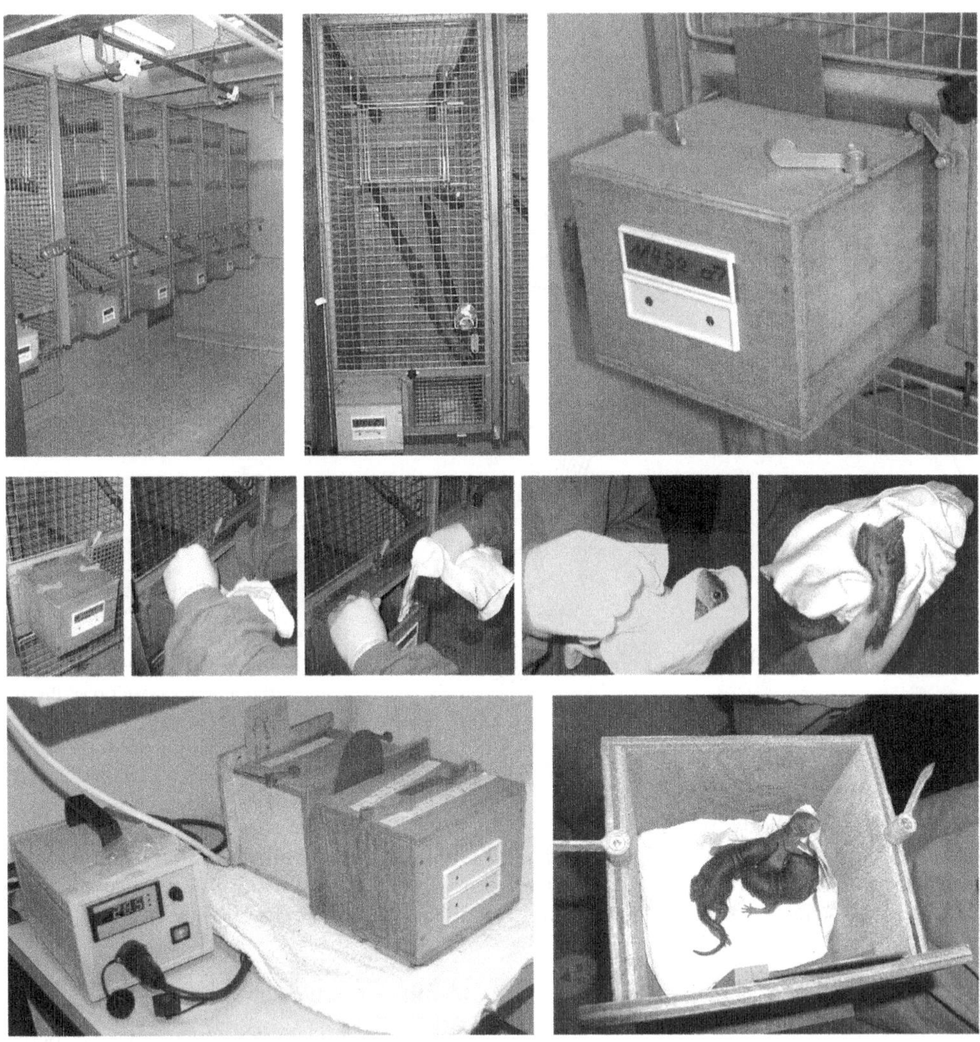

Figure 20.3 Housing and rearing *Tupaia belangeri* in the German Primate Center. Upper row: Animal room, a single cage and a nest box closed with a slider. Middle row: Catching a tree shrew from its nest box with a cloth. Lower row: Housing for newborn tree shrews.

changed and cleaned daily. Tap water is provided in bottles or in dishes.

Identification and sexing

Animals should be individually marked, which can be achieved by subcutaneous implantation of transponders or by cutting patterns into the tail hair. Tattooing is hard to perform and the marks often do not last long. Other methods such as notching the inside of the ear or even amputation of claws are prohibited by law in most countries.

The external genitalia of adult male tree shrews consist of a slender and elongate penis, which is posterior to scrotal testes. Retraction of the testes into the abdominal cavity can occur under experimental conditions of stress. In female *Tupaia*, *Lyonogale*, *Urogale* and *Dendrogale*, the clitoris is greatly elongated and grooved on its ventral surface. In neonatal *Tupaia*, the urethra enters the clitoris and extends throughout its length as the clitoral urethra, whereas in the adult the urethra opens together with the vagina as a urogenital sinus at the base of the clitoris. Therefore, infant and juvenile females and males might sometimes be mixed up because the vaginal orifice at the base of the clitoris is sealed. In contrast to the penis, the clitoris does not have a tubular sheath (Figure 20.4).

Health monitoring, quarantine and barrier systems

From the information available to date, the maintenance of tree shrews involves very little risk to human health but, nevertheless, they should be handled with caution. Routine colony health-screening procedures should be carried out and veterinary assistance must be available. Newly acquired animals must be kept in quarantine and require veterinary treatment for external and internal parasites. As pointed out earlier, environmental and social stressors may be a cause of health problems in tree shrews. They may induce sudden and dramatic weight loss or even wounds. Therefore, animal care staff should routinely monitor the animals for signs of illness, such as no food and water intake,

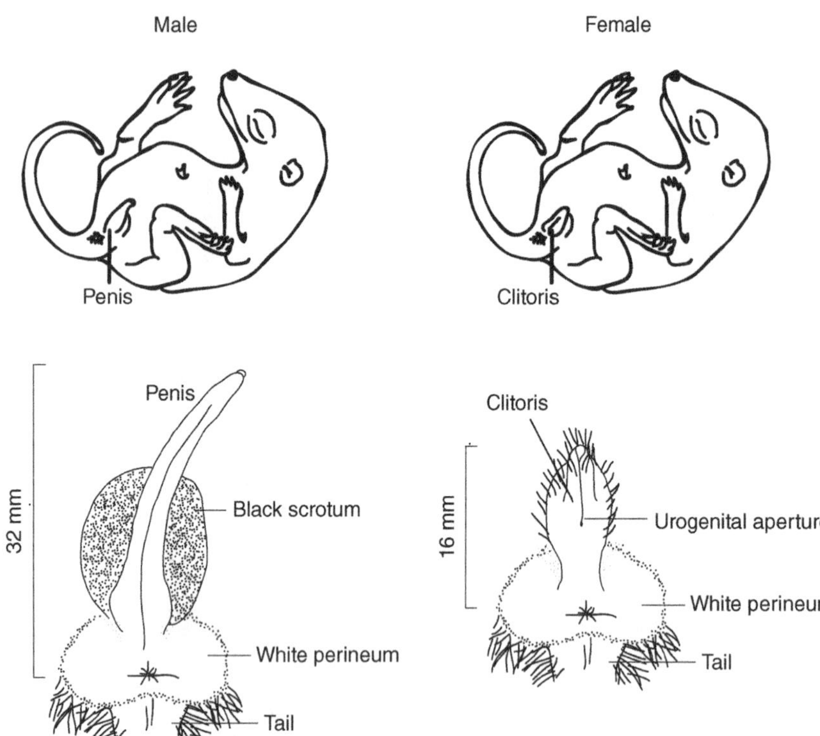

Figure 20.4 Ventral view of the external genitalia of infant and adult tree shrews (*Tupaia belangeri*). Note the penis of the infant tree shrew is twice as long as the clitoris and the anterior position of the scrotum in the adult male tree shrew (Bearder & Pitts 1987, adapted from Martin 1968a).

diarrhoea, weight loss, aberrant body posture or movements, rough fur and lethargy or apathy. When the animals are handled for the routine weighing procedure (at least once a month), they should also be checked for signs of cataracts or tumours.

Transport

For shipment, each individual should be confined to a small dark wooden compartment or its nest box. The size of the compartment is determined by the body weight of the animal and both national and international regulations. It must have openings for sufficient ventilation and should be lined with nesting material. Moist fruits, cooked moist rice and water in a gel form (available commercially) should be provided. Before shipping, animals should be habituated to water provided in gel form. See also Chapter 13.

Due to the high metabolic rate and the sensitivity of tree shrews to disturbances, newly arrived animals are often quite exhausted. For recovery, they should be supplied with sugar water or apple juice and a high-calorie diet. The sleeping boxes should be warmed with an electric cushion (30 °C), lights in the room should be dimmed and disturbances should be avoided.

Breeding

Adults

Females can give birth to their first litter at an age of about 4 months. Males become fertile between 4 and 5 months. The best age for first pregnancy seems to be between 6 and 9 months. If the animal is older, problems such as infertility, stillbirth, cannibalism or abortion occur more often. In males, stress can result in testicular inactivity (Fischer *et al.* 1985; Brack & Fuchs 2000).

Identifying fertile state

Based on the length of the intervals between copulation periods observed in captivity, several authors have suggested an 8–12 day (anovulatory) oestrous cycle in various species of *Tupaia* and ovulation is supposed to be induced by copulation (Martin 1990). However, it is still a matter of discussion whether ovulation is triggered by copulation (induced ovulation) and/or whether an oestrus cycle exists. No cyclic changes in vaginal smears have been detected by the authors or others. In addition, the authors could not find any cyclic alterations in urinary excretion of sex hormones. According to Cao *et al.* (2001) ovulation can be induced by combined injections of pregnant mare serum gonadotrophin and human chorionic gonadotrophin.

Mating systems

In tree shrews, mating is one of the critical and in many cases most difficult part of breeding. If a female accepts a male, copulation may be observed within a few hours. In many cases, however, placing an adult male and an adult female together in one cage will result in aggressive interactions. There are two main reasons for these fights. One is that the individuals just do not like each other; 'love at first sight' and its cardiovascular consequences have been described by von Holst (1987). Another reason is territoriality. If the mating cage is the territory of one partner, this animal –

male or female – defends its area against the intruder. In many cases the animals become gradually familiar with another and amicable physical attractions can be observed at the 'border' between the cages so that the partition can be removed after some days. However, if aggressive interactions or fights do not cease, other partners have to be tested. When a well matched couple is found and stable pair-bonding is established, constant reproductive success is guaranteed. Under natural and laboratory conditions, breeding may occur at any time of the year and no seasonal breeding peaks have been described.

When the female leaves the nest after giving birth and having suckled the young, copulation with the male usually occurs within a few hours. Therefore, leaving a couple together is convenient and ensures regular births. Repeated pregnancy cycles are typical of a highly successful breeding colony of *Tupaia belangeri*, and female receptivity and copulation are often confined to the post-partum oestrus (Martin 1968a, 1968b).

Conception and pregnancy

In *Tupaia belangeri*, pregnancy can be detected by palpation from the second week of gestation onwards. Significant weight gain (30–50 g) and marked swelling of the abdomen are observed within 2 weeks before term. Duration of pregnancy in regular breeding pairs is in the range of 41–45 days. Breeding success is a good indicator of the general condition of the colony. Even with harmonious, healthy and well nourished breeders, successful breeding can be disrupted by a variety of disturbances. Tree shrews are highly susceptible to stress and many of the problems in housing them are related to this. Loud noises, strange persons and unfamiliar care staff, overcleaning, inadequate furnishing of the cages and crowding have all been shown to be the reasons for abortion, shortened pregnancies, cannibalism or reduced amounts of milk resulting in starvation of the offspring.

Nesting

About 1 week before term, the female starts to carry nesting material into one of the two nesting boxes. For nesting material, we offer shredded paper, wood-wool or dry leaves. If no nesting material is available, the females will use pellets.

Parturition

After a relatively short gestation period, tree shrews give birth to naked and altritical pups. In most cases births occur in the morning hours, but sometimes they also occur in the afternoon.

Early development

The infants are born without fur; their ears open at around 10 days and their eyes after 20 days. The development strongly depends on the milk supply and health condition. The nipple count for all species of tupaiids falls within the range of one to three pairs. Field and laboratory studies indicate that the number of pups per litter is one to four (in some cases in the authors' colony there were five young per litter which were successfully raised). The birth weight is about 10 g.

Immediately after birth, the young are nursed and the weight of optimally fed babies is in the range of 14–20 g. Females tend to be a little heavier than males. Schwaier (1973) reports a litter size of 2.23 and sex ratio of 0.82 (males: females). For another colony of *Tupaia belangeri*, a sex ratio of 1.8 and a litter size of 2.4 was reported (Hertenstein *et al.* 1987). A survey of the *Tupaia belangeri* colony at the German Primate Center, Göttingen (1984–2007, total 2962 animals) revealed a sex ratio of 0.95 (m : f) and the following litter sizes: singletons: 158; twins: 462; triplets: 461; quadruplets: 113; quintuplets: 9.

A detailed description of growth and reproductive development in *Tupaia belangeri* from birth to sexual maturity is given by Collins and Tsang (1987) and Hertenstein *et al.* (1987).

The maternal behaviour in *Tupaia* is unusual among mammals and has been described in detail by Martin (1968a, 1968b). The tree shrew species that have been investigated (*Tupaia belangeri, Tupaia minor, Lyonogale tana*) all show an unusual nursing schedule with the infants kept in separate nests and visited by the mother for suckling only once every 48 h.

The pups receive about 5–10 ml milk. Due to the thin skin the dilated stomach appears as a light patch in the abdomen (Figure 20.5). The fat content in tree shrew milk is very high (about 25%) while the sugar concentration is low. The energy content of the tree shrew milk lies within the range of other mammals which is in general related to body size (Martin 1990). Since any suckling visit takes only 5–10 minutes, a tree shrew infant will be in contact with its mother less than 2 h during the 30 day nest phase, following which the infant is independent of its mother for milk supply. Thus, tree shrews have the lowest mother–infant contact and parental investment yet described for viviparous mammals (Martin 1990). The pattern of minimal mother–infant contact is strikingly different from the characteristic primate pattern of elaborated maternal care, juvenile dependence and enhanced social organisation (Martin 1990). In a recent field study, Emmons and Biun (1991) investigated the maternal behaviour of the Malaysian tree shrew *Tupaia* (*Lyonogale*) *tana*. Their observations confirmed the peculiar 'absentee' system previously demonstrated only in the laboratory. For the first month of life, the pups stay in a nest apart from the mother, who visits them every other day to nurse them for about 2 minutes. After they leave the nest, the mother spends a lot of time with them daily for at least 3 weeks. The male that shared the mother's territory frequently interacted with the mother during the nestling phase of the pups, but had no contact with them.

Death of young is due to premature birth (non-inflated lungs, interstitial pneumonia), cannibalism or starvation. Cannibalism of the new-born young by the mother or other adults occurs under stressful laboratory conditions which contribute to high mortality and also leads to modifications of maternal suckling behaviour. It has been observed by von Holst (1969) that increasing stress in the group modifies the suckling intervals and led to increased cannibalism of young *Tupaia belangeri* under experimental conditions.

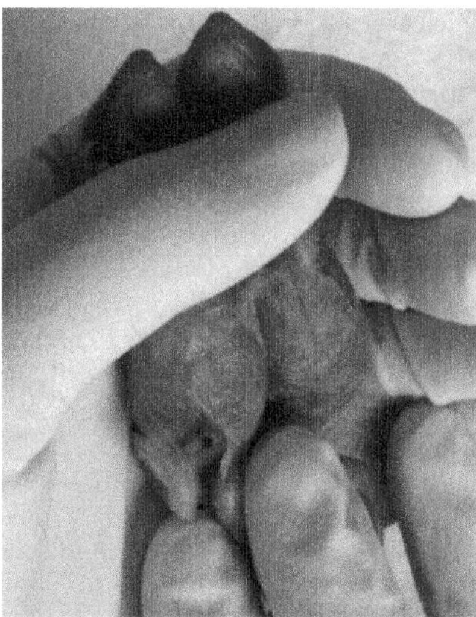

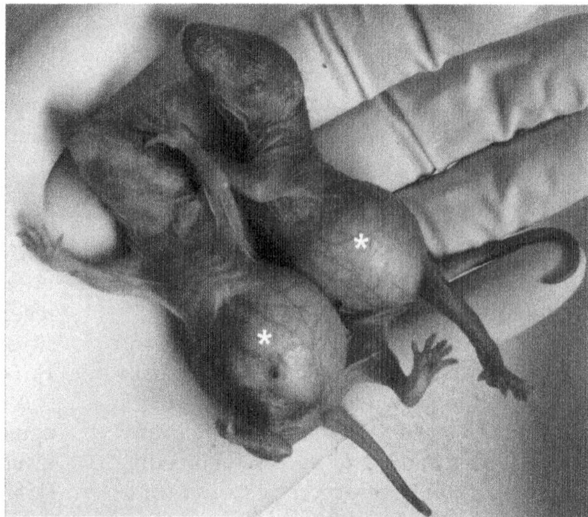

Figure 20.5 Newborn *Tupaia belangeri* before (left) and after suckling (right). Due to the thin skin the dilated stomachs appear as light patches (*) in the abdomen.

According to reports in the literature, newborn *Tupaia belangeri* are marked by a maternal scent substance which protects against cannibalism (von Stralendorff 1982). In contrast to these observations, the authors were successful with cross-fostering strategies in cases where the mothers were unable to suckle and raise their offspring.

In order to avoid cannibalism and to control suckling success the authors separate the neonates from the parents immediately after birth. For the next 3 weeks they are kept in a nest box elsewhere in the animal facility (Figure 20.3). Since temperature regulation is immature in newborn tree shrews the floor of the nest box is warmed by a temperature-controlled heating cushion (eye heating cushion, temperature about 27 °C) during the first 10 days (Figure 20.3). If they are kept too warm, they will develop a lighter fur colour; as they get older, the animals turn to their normal colour. Mothers are transferred to their litter every day for a maximum of 30 minutes. It is important to note that some females suckle their young only every second day; others have very clear daily time windows within which suckling will take place. The best suckling rhythm for each breeder can only be found by careful observation of individual animals.

Hand rearing

The extremely high fat content of the tree shrew milk is probably one reason why hand rearing is regarded as being very difficult. For successful hand rearing Tsang and Collins (1985) developed a liquid formula and a protocol which conforms to the natural weaning pattern of *Tupaia belangeri*.

Weaning and rearing

Tupaia belangeri can be weaned around day 35. In the authors' colony the young are separated from the parents at 50–60 days of age. Weaned *Tupaia* of the same sex and about equal age can be housed in peer groups (up to 10 animals depending on the size of the cage and the number of nest boxes). At 8–10 weeks of age, females and males gradually become fertile and consequently aggressive interactions increase. It is then time to separate the animals. In many cases smaller all-female groups (three animals) are stable. Males are housed singly or together with a female.

Feeding

Natural and laboratory diets

Tree shrews of the genus *Tupaia* are predominantly insectivorous. Besides insects they use fruit to add extra calories or nutrients such as calcium to a high-protein diet.

At the authors' colony, as basic food *Tupaia belangeri* are provided with a specially developed pelleted *Tupaia* diet. In addition, the animals get small pieces of fruit (such as apples, oranges, bananas, grapes, kiwi) and vegetables twice a week. Once a week, they get fruit juice and vitamins, cooked eggs or baby food and on weekends, small pieces of crisp bread. As rewards they get meal-worms, raisins, pieces of banana, dates and figs. Breeding pairs or recovering animals get, in addition to the standard food, cat chow or mashed bananas.

In the laboratory, tree shrews are reported to eat almost anything. Therefore, when pellets are not available they can be fed with steamed rice and chopped beef heart; they especially prefer soft, fat and sweet food, and all kinds of fruits and vegetables. There are, however, indications for allergic mechanisms against soybean products and oat flakes (Brack *et al.* 1990).

Water

As judged from the water content of their faeces, tree shrews absorb little water from their ingesta and they cannot stay without water for more than 1 day without serious problems. Consequently, water bottles must be controlled daily and water must always be present *ad libitum*; the mean water intake is 350 ml/kg. Tap water should be changed at least once a week. Bottles and nipples should be washed with hot water or sterilised between changes. No detergents should be used.

Laboratory procedures

Handling and training

For quick and easy catching tree shrews can be locked in their nesting boxes as the animals usually slip into the boxes as soon as somebody enters the room. When removing the animals and to protect the experimenter's hands, the animal is gently wrapped in a cloth (40 cm × 40 cm) (Figure 20.3). Since their teeth are small, bites are not dangerous but can be painful. Using this technique, no difficulties occur with the usual procedures such as daily external body inspection, weighing, urine and blood collection, temperature and blood pressure recording, and application of substances by different routes. Tree shrews can be easily trained for memory tests, for example, by positive reinforcement techniques (Ohl *et al.* 1998; Bartolomucci *et al.* 2001; see also Chapter 16).

Physiological monitoring

Rectal temperature can easily be measured by thermometers of the type used in humans. Transmitters can be implanted for long-term studies.

Collection of specimens – blood, urine

Blood withdrawal (about 500 µl) by puncturing the venous plexus at the lower side of the tail with a small scalpel is recommended by some authors. Prior to puncture, the tail should be shaved and rubbed with a silicon paste which improves the blood collection. Blood flow can be enhanced by holding the tail under a heating lamp. This technique, however, requires experience and is therefore often unsatisfactory. Another approach is described by Schwaier (1974), taking blood from the saphenous vein. Following the recommendations of GV-SOLAS for small laboratory animals, not more than 0.7 ml blood per 100 g body weight at a time should be collected. In cases of repeated blood sampling (eg, over 2 weeks) not more than 0.07 ml/100 g body weight should be collected within 24 h. Despite being completely relaxed during blood sampling, the procedure *per se* seems to be stressful for the animals as documented by increased basal heart rate over several days after one blood sampling procedure (Stohr 1988).

Morning urine can easily be collected from animals that have been confined to their nest box shortly before the lights turn on in the animal rooms. A slight massage of the hypogastrium gives between 1 and 7 ml of urine. Another approach is to place plastic mats with wells under the cages and to collect the urine later with a pipette out of the wells.

Urine analysis has proved to be a stress-free and reliable procedure for long-term monitoring of the physiological status of *Tupaia belangeri*. Among these are parameters for metabolic activity (Johren *et al.* 1991), various bioactive compounds (Collins *et al.* 1989; Fuchs & Schumacher 1990; Fuchs *et al.* 1992) and urinary proteins which play a crucial role in olfactory communication (Weber & Fuchs 1988). Age and time of the day may have an impact on the values (Fuchs 1988; van Kampen & Fuchs 1998). For urinary data see Table 20.2.

Administration of medicines

Most routes of applications, such as subcutaneous, intramuscular, intraperitoneal or oral, are easy to perform. For intravenous injections it is recommended to use the saphenous vein (Schwaier 1974).

Anaesthesia

Adequate anaesthesia is a prerequisite for using an animal species in the laboratory for a wide range of experiments. Early studies used pentobarbital in a comparatively high dose of 75 mg/kg.

A quick and safe injection anaesthetic is the so called Goettinger Mixture II (GM II) consisting of ketamine (50 mg/ml), xylazine (10 mg/ml) and atropine (0.1 mg/ml). The dosage is 0.1 ml/100 g body weight. Anaesthesia usually occurs within 5 minutes of the intramuscular injection, and general anaesthesia lasts about 20–45 minutes. For longer general anaesthesia, inhalation anaesthesia is recommended. For inhalation anaesthesia, animals had to be artificially ventilated through an endotracheal tube (home-made from high-med-PE-micro-tube, inner diameter 1.75 mm, outer diameter 2.08 mm). Our experiences with a respirator for small animals show that 0.5–2% isoflurane in a mixture of 30% oxygen and 70% N_2O, with a respiration rate of 35 per minute with an inspiratory phase of 35% and plateau phase of 5% work fine for *Tupaia belangeri*.

Inhalation anaesthesia is used following induction by injection anaesthesia (eg, GMII). The jaw bone is placed on the fingers and the head is fixed by placing the thumbs behind the skull. The mouth is opened by introducing the laryngoscope. Sometimes the epiglottis can be held down with the tip. After inserting the endotracheal tube, correct placement must be checked by auscultation; once corrrect placement is confirmed, the tube can be held in place with a strip of adhesive tape (Figure 20.6).

Euthanasia

The use of animals in research, including euthanasia, is a sensitive issue. Because of differences in national regulations, each researcher will be required to obtain clearance from the local or national ethical committee for research prior to conducting euthanasia. In our opinion, cervical dislocation is not an appropriate method of euthanasia for tree shrews. We recommend either an overdose of sodium

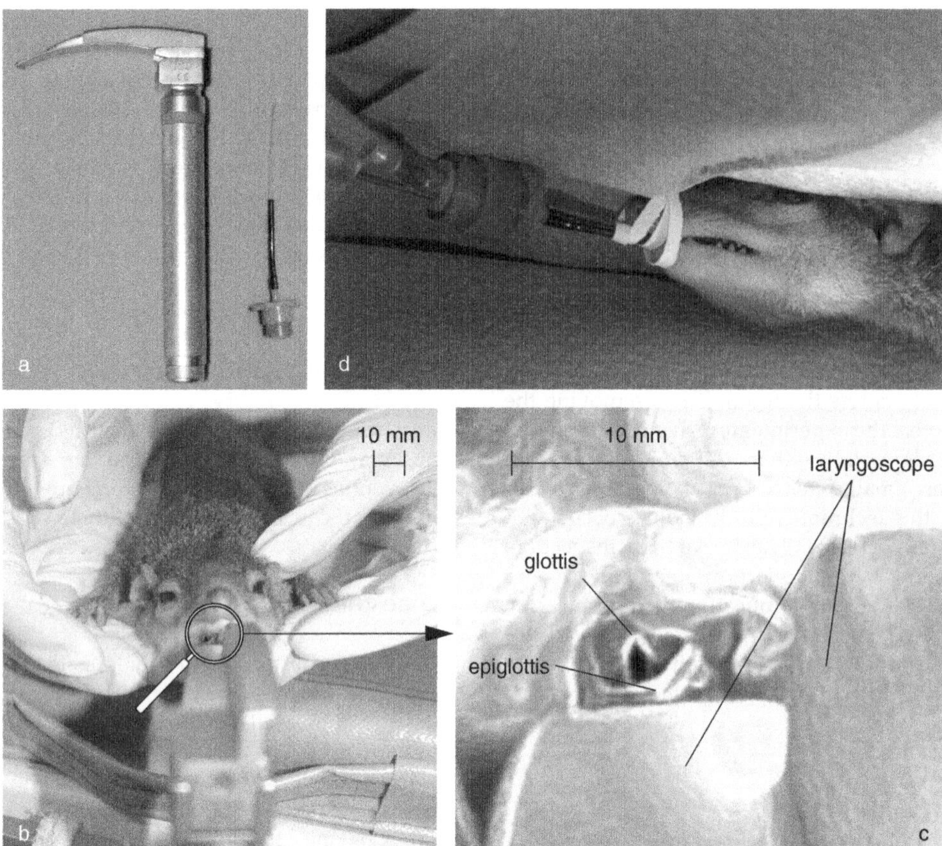

Figure 20.6 Intubation of a tree shrew (*Tupaia belangeri*) for inhalation anaesthesia. (a) Laryngoscope and homemade micro-tube (for details see text). (b) Fixation of the head and position of the laryngoscope. (c) Enlarged view of (b) showing glottis and epiglottis. (d) After successful intubation, the tube is held in place with a strip of adhesive tape.

pentobarbital, for example, or decapitation. Carbon dioxide has been used on tree shrews and has proven to be an appropriate means of euthanasia. In any case, after exposing animals to an overdose of anaesthetics it is always mandatory to confirm death by, for example, cervical dislocation, as an appropriate secondary means of euthanasia.

Common welfare problems

Health problems

Tree shrews experience relatively few health problems. However, our experience shows that gastritis can be a frequent problem. In this case, animals stop eating and a lack of faeces can also be observed. Gastritis can be effectively treated with cimetidine (10 mg/kg body weight, twice daily orally).

Diarrhoea is another symptom often seen in a colony. Mostly *Escherichia coli variatio haemolytica*, *Klebsiella pneumonia* or protozoa (*Giardia*, *Trichomonas*, *Entamoeba*) are the cause of this symptom. Before antibiotic treatment of diarrhoea, appropriate diagnostic and resistance tests are strongly recommended.

Infection with the cestode *Tupaiataenia quentini* was successfully treated with praziquantel (Brack *et al.* 1987). Intestinal trichomoniasis with *Tiritrichomonas mobilensis* (mostly in the caecum) has also been described as well (Brack *et al.* 1995). Enteropathy of the upper digestive tract was due to a foodstuff allergy against oat flakes and soybean products (Brack *et al.* 1990).

Penis prolapse is another possible health problem. We found this in several males of different ages with unknown cause. The prolapse is not lethal by itself, but since there is no effective treatment and the penis becomes irritated and swollen, in most cases, the animal has to be euthanased.

Automutilation can often occur if the cages are too small, overcrowed or the animals are disturbed too much. Moving the animal to a bigger or quieter area in the facility is the first step in treatment. In some cases, standard antibiotic treatment and amputation of the affected body part (eg, a toe or the distal part of the tail) is necessary.

Tupaia seem to be prone to the spontaneous development of gallstones with fatty and cholesterol-rich diets (Schwaier 1979). In two reports mite infestations were described (Bever 1985; Brack *et al.* 1989).

Most tumours of the genital system of male animals have a Leydig cell origin and occur unilaterally. Tumours of the female genital system are predominantly mammary tumours or sometimes ovarian tumours. Tumours of the haematopoietic system are malignant lymphomas; tumours of the integument occur mostly in the jugulo-sternal gland. Similar to humans, the incidence of tumours increases with age (Brack

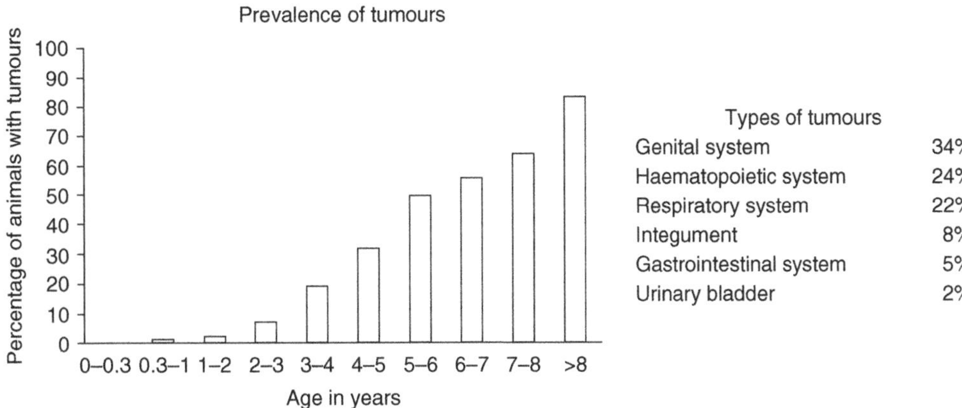

Figure 20.7 Common spontaneous tumours and incidence of tumours, which rises with age (with modifications from Brack 1998).

1998). The most common spontaneous tumours are summarised in Figure 20.7.

Two tree shrew specific viruses are known and reported in the literature so far: the Tupaia herpes virus (THV) (five different types), which might be a cause for tumours (Darai *et al.* 1982), and the potentially non-pathogenic Tupaia paramyxovirus (TPMV) (Tidona *et al.* 1999).

Concluding remarks

Despite their obvious attractiveness there are limitations to the use of tree shrews in research. Major limitations are housing and breeding, both of which are time consuming and expensive. Obviously, this constraint explains why many laboratories are not capable of using these animals for their study programmes. Further research is required to collect basic data on tree shrews to inform their housing and care.

References

Bearder, S. and Pitts, R.S. (1987) Prosimians and tree shrews. In: *The UFAW Handbook on the Care and Management of Laboratory Animals.* Ed Poole, T.B., pp. 551–567. Longman Scientific & Technical, Harlow

Bever, K. (1985) Mite infestation of *Tupaia glis* DIARD, 1820. *Primate Report*, **13**, 69–70

Bever, K. and Sprankel, H. (1986) A contribution to the longevity of Tupaia glis DIARD, 1820 in captivity. *Zeitschrift für Versuchstierkunde*, **28**, 3–5

Binz, H. and Zimmermann, E. (1989) The vocal repertoire of adult tree shrews (*Tupaia belangeri*). *Behavior*, **109**, 142–162

Brack, M. (1998) Spontaneous tumours in tree shrews (*Tupaia belangeri*): population studies. *Journal of Comparative Pathology*, **118**, 301–316

Brack, M., Fooke, M., Wirth, H. *et al.* (1990) Futtermittelallergie bei Spitzhörnchen (*Tupaia belangeri*). In: *Verhandlungsbericht des 32. Internationalen Symposiums über die Erkrankungen der Zoo- und Wildtiere Eskilstuna*, pp. 99–105. Akademie-Verlag, Berlin

Brack, M. and Fuchs, E. (2000) Incidence of testicular lesions in a population of tree shrews (*Tupaia belangeri*). *Comparative Medicine*, **50**, 212–217

Brack, M., Gatesman, T.J. and Fuchs E. (1989) Otacariasis in tree shrews (*Tupaia belangeri*) caused by *Criokeron quintus*. *Laboratory Animal Science*, **39**, 79–80

Brack, M., Kaup, F.J. and Fuchs, E. (1995) Intestinal trichomoniasis due to *Tritrichomonas mobilensis* in tree shrews (*Tupaia belangeri*). *Laboratory Animal Science*, **45**, 533–537

Brack, M., Naberhaus F. and Heyman E. (1987) *Tupaia taenia quentini* (Schmidt and File, 1977) in *Tupaia belangeri* (Wagner, 1841): transmission experiments and Praziquantel treatment. *Laboratory Animals*, **21**, 18–19

Bartolomucci, A., de Biurrun, G. and Fuchs, E. (2001) How tree shrews perform in a searching task: evidences for strategy use? *Journal of Comperative Psychology*, **115**, 344–350

Butler, P.M. (1980) The Tupaiid dentation. In: *Comparative Biology and Evolutionary Relationships of Tree Shrews.* Ed. Luckett, W.P., pp. 171–204. Plenum Press, New York

Campbell, C.B.G. (1980) The nervous system of the Tupaiidae: Its bearing on phyletic relationships. In: *Comparative Biology and Evolutionary Relationships of Tree Shrews.* Ed. Luckett, W.P., pp. 219–242. Plenum Press, New York

Cao, X., Ben, K. and Wang, X. (2001) Ovulation in the tree shrew (*Tupaia belangeri*) induced by gonadotrophins. *Reproduction, Fertility and Development*, **13**, 377–382

Cao, J., Yang, E.B., Su, J.J., Li, Y. and Chow, P. (2003) The tree shrews: adjuncts and alternatives to primates as models for biomedical research. *Journal of Medical Primatology*, **32**, 123–130

Collins, P.M., Dobyns, R.J. and Tsang W.N. (1989) Urinary immunoreactive androgen levels during sexual development in the male tree-shrew (*Tupaia belangeri*). *Comparative Biochemistry and Physiology*, **92A**, 489–494

Collins, P.M. and Tsang, W.N. (1987) Growth and reproductive development in the male tree shrew (*Tupaia belangeri*) from birth to sexual maturity. *Biology of Reproduction*, **37**, 261–267

Collins, P.M., Tsang, W.N. and Metzger J.M. (1984) Influence of stress on adrenocortical function in male tree shrew (*Tupaia belangeri*). *General and Comparative Endocrinology*, **55**, 450–457

Darai, G, Koch, H.G., Flugel, R.M. *et al.* (1982) Tree shrew (*Tupaia*) herpesviruses. *Developments in Biological Standardization*, **52**, 39–51

Eichmann, F. and von Holst, D.V. (1999) Organization of territorial marking behavior by testosterone during puberty in male tree shrews. *Physiology and Behavior*, **65**, 785–791

Emmons, L.H. (1991) Frugivory in treeshrews (*Tupaia*). *The American Naturalist*, **138**, 642–649

Emmons, L.H. (2000) *Tupai: A Field Study of Bornean Treeshrews.* University of California Press, Berkeley

Emmons, L.H. and Biun, A. (1991) Malaysian treeshrews. Maternal Behavior of a wild treeshrew, *Tupaia tana*, in Sabah. *National Geographic Research & Exploration*, **7**, 70–81

Fischer, H.D., Heinzeller, T. and Raab, A. (1985) Gonadal response to psychosocial stress in male tree shrews (*Tupaia belangeri*) morphometry of testis, epididymis and prostate. *Andrologia*, **17**, 262–275

Fuchs, E. (1984) Activity of the sympatho-adrenomedullary system in male *Tupaia belangeri* under control and stress situations. In: *Stress – The Role of Catecholamines and Other Neurotransmitters*. Eds Usdin, E., Kvetnansky, R. and Axelrod, J., pp. 595–602. Gordon and Breach, Langhorne

Fuchs, E. (1988) *Physiologische Charakterisierung von Spitzhörnchen (Tupaia belangeri) unter besonderer Berücksichtigung nichtinvasiver Untersuchungsmethoden*. Habilitationsschrift, Universität Karlsruhe

Fuchs, E. (2005) Social stress in tree shrews as an animal model of depression: an example of a behavioral model of a CNS disorder. *CNS Spectrum*, **10**, 182–189

Fuchs, E. and Flugge, G. (2002) Social stress in tree shrews: effects on physiology, brain function, and behavior of subordinate individuals. *Pharmacology Biochemistry Behavior*, **73**, 247–258

Fuchs, E., Johren, O. and Flügge, G. (1993) Psychosocial conflict in the tree shrew: effects on sympathoadrenal activity and blood pressure. *Psychoneuroendocrinology*, **18**, 557–565

Fuchs, E., Johren, O. and Goldberg, M. (1992) Psychosocial stress affects urinary pteridines in tree shrews. *Naturwissenschaften*, **79**, 379–381

Fuchs, E. and Schumacher, M. (1990) Psychosocial stress affects pineal function in the tree shrew (*Tupaia belangeri*). *Physiology and Behavior*, **47**, 713–717

Hertenstein, B., Zimmermann, E. and Rahmann, H. (1987) Zur Reproduktion und onogenetischen Entwicklung von Spitzhörnchen. *Zeitschrift des Kölner Zoo*, **30**, 119–133

Hunt, R.D. (1993) Herpesviruses of primates: an introduction. In: *Nonhuman Primates*. Eds Jones, T.C., Mohr, T.U., Hunt, R.D., pp. 74–78. Springer-Verlag, Berlin

Johren, O., Topp, H., Sander, G. *et al.* (1991) Social stress in tree shrews increases the whole-body RNA degradation rates. *Naturwissenschaften*, **78**, 36–38

Kawamichi, T. and Kawamichi, M. (1979) Spatial organization and territory of tree shrews (*Tupaia glis*). *Animal Behavior*, **27**, 381–393

Keuker, J.I.H., Keijser, J.N., Nyakas, C. *et al.* (2005) Aging is accompanied by a subfield-specific reduction of serotonergic fibers in the tree shrew hippocampal formation. *Journal of Chemical Neuroanatomy*, **30**, 221–229

Kirchhof, J., Hammerschmidt, K. and Fuchs E. (2001) Aggression and dominance in tree shrews (*Tupaia belangeri*). Agonistic pattern is reflected in vocal patterns. In: *Prevention and Control of Aggression and the Impact on its Victims*. Ed. Martinez, M., pp. 409–414. Kluwer Academic/Plenum Publishers, New York

Kriegs, J.O., Churakov, G., Jurka, J. *et al.* (2007) Evolutionary history of 7SL RNA-derived SINEs in Supraprimates. *Trends in Genetics*, **23**, 158–161

Kurre, J. and Fuchs, E. (1988) Messung der Spontanaktivität von Spitzhörnchen (*Tupaia belangeri*) mit Passiv-Infrarot-Detektoren. *Zeitschrift für Versuchstierkunde*, **31**, 105–110

Le Gros Clark, W.E. (1924) On the brain of the tree shrew (*Tupaia minor*). In: Proceedings of the Zoological Society of London, pp. 1053–1074

Luckett, W.P. (1980) *Comparative Biology and Evolutionary Relationships of Tree Shrews*. Plenum Press, New York and London

Martin, R.D. (1968a) Reproduction and ontogeny of tree-shrews (*Tupaia belangeri*), with reference to their general behaviour and taxomonic relationships. *Zeitschrift für Tierpsychologie*, **25**, 409–495

Martin, R.D. (1968b) Reproduction and ontogeny in tree-shrews (*Tupaia belangeri*), with reference to their general behaviour and taxonomic relationships. *Zeitschrift für Tierpsychologie*, **25**, 505–532

Martin, R.D. (1990) *Primate Origins and Evolution*. Chapman & Hall, London

Muller, E.F. and Hub, T. (1992) O_2-uptake and heart rate in tree shrews. In: IPS Congress Strasbourg, abstract 370

Ohl, F., Oitzl, M.S. and Fuchs, E. (1998) Assessing cognitive functions in tree shrews: Visuo-spatial and spatial learning in the home cage. *Journal of Neuroscience Methods*, **81**, 35–40

Pawlik, M., Fuchs, E., Walker, L.C. *et al.* (1999) Primate sequence of amyloid-b protein in tree shrew that do not develop cerebral amyloid deposition. *Neurobiology of Aging*, **20**, 47–51

Refinetti, R. and Menaker, M. (1992) Body temperature rhythm of the tree shrew, *Tupaia belangeri*. *The Journal of Experimental Zoology*, **263**, 453–457

Schwaier, A. (1973) Breeding Tupaias (*Tupaia belangeri*) in captivity. *Zeitschrift für Versuchstierkunde*, **15**, 255–271

Schwaier, A. (1974) Method of blood sampling and intraveneous injection in Tupaias (tree shrews). *Zeitschrift für Versuchstierkunde*, **16**, 35–36

Schwaier, A. (1975) *Die Verwendung von Tupaias (Praeprimaten) als neues biologisches Testobjekt in der Präventivmedizin und angewandten medizinischen Forschung*. Bericht für das Bundesministerium für Forschung und Technologie, Bonn

Schwaier, A. (1979) Tupaias (tree shrews) a new animal model for gall stone research. 1st observation of gall stones. *Research in Experimental Medicine*, **176**, 15–24

Simpson, G.C. (1945) The principles of classification and a classification of mammals. *Bulletin of the American Museum of Natural History*, **85**, 1–350

Steinhausen, M., Thederan, H., Nolinski, D. *et al.* (1978) Further evidence of tubular blockage after acute ischemic renal failure in *Tupaia belangeri* and rats. Virchows Archiv Part A. *Pathological Anatomy and Histology*, **381**, 13–34

Stohr, W. (1988) Longterm heartrate telemetry in small mammals: a comprehensive approach as a prerequisite for valid results. *Physiology and Behavior*, **43**, 567–576

Tidona, C.A., Kurz, H.W., Gelderblom, H.R. *et al.* (1999) Isolation and molecular characterization of a novel cytopathogenic paramyxovirus from tree shrews. *Virology*, **258**, 425–434

Toder, D, von Holst, D. and Schempp, W. (1992) Comparative cytogenetic studies in tree shrews (*Tupaia*). *Cytogenetic and Cell Genetics*, **60**, 55–59

Tsang, W.N. and Collins, P.M. (1985) Techniques for hand-rearing tree-shrews (*Tupaia belangeri*) from birth. *Zoo Biology*, **4**, 23–31

van Kampen, M. and Fuchs, E. (1998) Age-related levels of urinary free cortisol in the tree shrew. *Neurobiology of Aging*, **19**, 363–366

von Holst, D. (1969) Sozialer Stress bei Tupajas (*Tupaia belangeri*). Die Aktivierung des sympathischen Nervensystems und ihre Beziehung zu hormonal ausgelösten ethologischen und physiologischen Veränderungen. *Zeitschrift für vergleichende Physiologie*, **63**, 1–58

von Holst, D. (1972) Renal failure as the cause of death in *Tupaia belangeri* exposed to persistent social stress. *Journal of Comparative Physiology*, **78**, 236–273

von Holst, D. (1977) Social stress in tree shrews: problems, results, and goals. *Journal of Comparative Physiology*, **120**, 71–86

von Holst, D. (1987) Physiologie sozialer Interaktionen – Sozialkontakte und ihre Auswirkungen auf Verhalten sowie Fertilität und Vitalität von Tupaias. *Physiologie aktuell*, **3**, 189–208

von Holst, D. (1988) Heutige Spitzhörnchen. In: *Grzimeks Enzyklopädie Säugetiere*, Vol. 2, pp. 5–12. Kindler, München von Holst, D. and Buergel-Goodwin, U. (1975) Chinning by male *Tupaia belangeri*: the effects of scent marks of conspecifics and other species. *Journal of Comparative Physiology*, **103**, 153–171

von Holst, D.V. and Eichmann, F. (1998) Sex-specific regulation of marking behavior by sex hormones and conspecifics scent in tree shrews (*Tupaia belangeri*). *Physiology and Behavior*, **63**, 157–164

von Stralendorff, F. (1982) Maternal odor substances protect newborn tree shrews from cannibalism. *Naturwissenschaften*, **69**, 553

Weber, M.H. and Fuchs, E. (1988) 1D-micro-slab-PAGE of urinary proteins of tree shrews (*Tupaia belangeri*). A tool for non-invasive physioloiccal studies. *Zeitschrift für Versuchstierkunde*, **31**, 55–63

Xu, X., Chen, H., Cao, X. *et al.* (2007) Efficient infection of tree shrew (*Tupaia belangeri*) with hepatitis C virus grown in cell culture or from patient plasma. *Journal of General Virology*, **88**, 2504–2512

Zou, R., Dai, W., Ben, K. *et al.* (1983) Blood picture of the tree shrew *Tupaia belangeri*. *Zoological Research*, **4**, 291–294

21 The laboratory mouse

Vera Baumans

Biological overview

General biology

The house mouse is a cosmopolitan species, which is commensal with man and is capable of adapting to a wide variety of environmental conditions. Its laboratory counterpart originated from wild mice caught and bred by mouse fanciers for their behaviour or coat colours. During the early twentieth century, they were also increasingly bred for scientific purposes. The increase of biomedical research at this time, the interest in Mendelian genetics and the advantage of a small, inexpensive mammal that could be easily housed and bred were crucial to the development of the laboratory mouse.

Like most rodents, the mouse is a nocturnal burrowing and climbing animal, which shows a clear circadian rhythm with peaks of activity during the dark period (Figure 21.1). Maintenance behaviour, such as eating and drinking, occurs mostly during the night (Schlingmann *et al.* 1998).

Mice have acute hearing and respond to a range of ultrasonic frequencies; for example, the retrieval response of the female is elicited by ultrasonic calls from pups that are out of the nest. The sense of smell is also highly developed in mice, and is not only used to detect food and predators. Mice have a wide repertoire of olfactory social signals that include pheromones and the creation of patterns of urine marks on the substrates of their environments. Mice normally excrete large amounts of protein in the urine. In contrast to their olfactory and auditory acuity, vision is poor in mice, especially in albinos (see section on Environmental provisions section).

Selected physiological data for mice are summarised in Table 21.1. Sex, strain, age, reproductive phase and environment can have a dramatic influence on physiological and behavioural data. Body weight and growth curves are also influenced by these factors. Body weights of both sexes increase rapidly during the first 6–8 weeks, but they grow more slowly after this until 6 months of age, when a plateau is reached for a few months, followed by a decline. As small animals, mice have a relatively large surface area per gram of body weight. This results in dramatic physiological changes in their response to fluctuations in the ambient temperature (Fox *et al.* 2002). In general, they cannot regulate body temperature as well as other mammals and do not tolerate heat well; they have no sweat glands, they cannot pant and their ability to salivate is limited (Fallon 1996; Fox *et al.* 2002). There is some evidence that the tail has a thermoregulatory function in small rodents (Joint Working Group on Refinement (JWGR) 1993).

The mouse is an omnivorous animal. Each half of the jaw contains one incisor and three molars (dental formula: $I^1{}_1C^0{}_0Pm^0{}_0M^3{}_3$). Canine teeth and premolars are absent, resulting in an open space, the diastema. The incisors and molars grow continuously and are worn down by mastication.

The proximal part of the stomach is squamous and non-glandular, whereas the distal part is glandular (Fox *et al.* 2002; Havenaar *et al.* 2001). In females the urethra ends in the ventral wall of the vagina. She has three pairs of mammary glands in the cervicothoracic region and two pairs in the inguinoabdominal region (Figure 21.2).

Size range and lifespan

Adult mice are 12–15 cm long from the nose to the tip of the tail, with the length of the tail approximately equalling that of the body. The newborn mouse weighs between 1 g and 2 g, and gains weight very rapidly during the 3 week suckling period. Intrinsic variables such as genotype, sex, strain and age of the mouse and extrinsic variables such as diet, number of mice per cage and environmental temperature account for the variation in adult body size (Cunliffe-Beamer & Les 1987).

Many environmental and genetic factors influence the lifespan of the mouse. These include diet, number of animals per cage, subclinical infections, husbandry procedures, genetic predisposition to tumours, strain, gender and the presence or absence of deleterious mutant genes (Cunliffe-Beamer & Les 1987). Mice from short-lived strains (eg, CBA) have a life expectancy of between 5 and 16 months, while mice from long-lived strains (eg, C57BL6) often survive to 24 or even 36 months of age.

Social organisation

Mice are social animals, which live in compatible, single male dominated groups that are mostly family based. The organisation of a mouse colony tends to be a dominance hierarchy under confined or crowded conditions but is

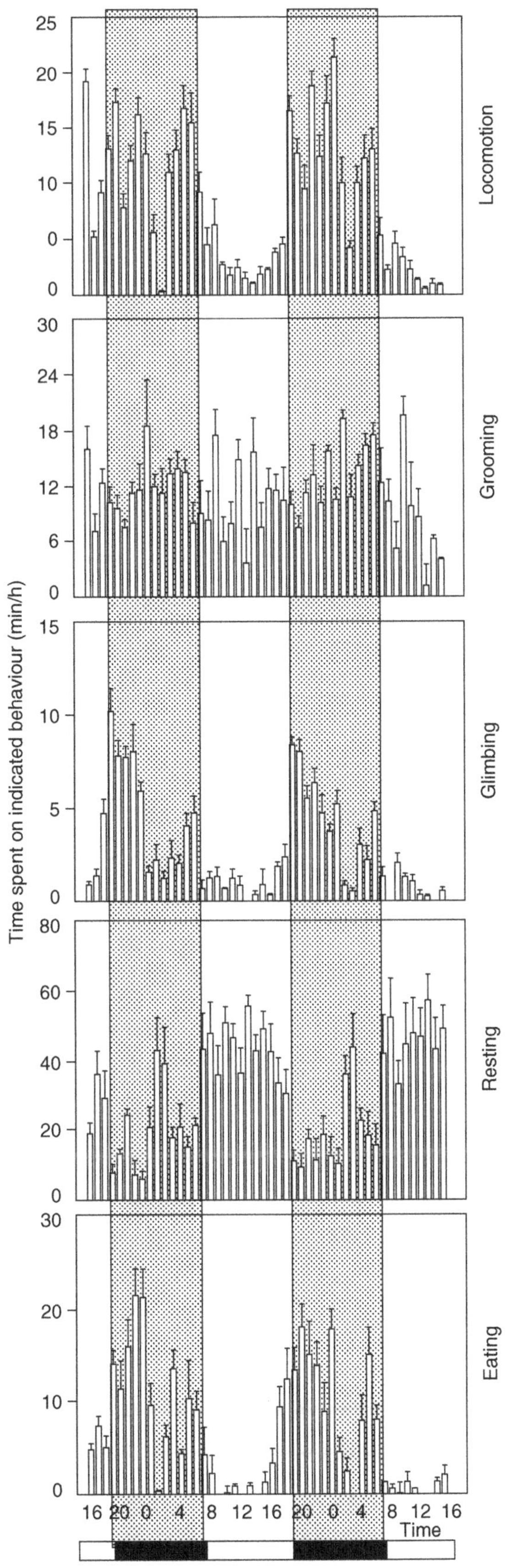

Figure 21.1 Circadian rhythm in the mouse. Black bars indicate the dark period (Schlingmann *et al.* 1988).

territorial under less restricted ones (Mackintosh 1981; van Loo *et al.* 2003; Latham & Mason 2004; Barnett 2007). Differences in behaviour between inbred strains may reflect behavioural adaptations to different habitats of the feral populations from which the ancestors of the inbred strain originated; for example, BALB/c mice appear to be well adapted to surface living, making superficial nests and showing territorial behaviour, while C57BL mice are more adapted to living in holes and do not show clear territorial behaviour (van Oortmerssen 1971; Busser *et al.* 1974).

Pheromones serve as a principal mechanism for communication and affect developmental and reproductive processes (Fox *et al.* 2002; Latham & Mason 2004). Mice use a variety of specialised scent glands, together with urine, faeces and vaginal secretions for olfactory communication. Urine is a particularly important source of odour (Hurst *et al.* 1993).

Reproduction

Sexual maturity in mice occurs very early in life. Oestrogen-dependent cornification of the epithelium at the vaginal opening may occur as early as 24–28 days (Fox *et al.* 2002), but sexual maturation varies with strain and environmental influences. Ovarian follicle development begins at 3 weeks of age and matures by 30 days. Puberty in males occurs up to 2 weeks later.

Female mice are polyoestrous, spontaneous ovulators and they cycle every 4–5 days. Factors such as season, diet, genetic background and environmental factors influence the oestrous cycle. The cyclicity of oestrus and ovulation are controlled by the diurnal rhythm of the photoperiod, and oestrus and ovulation most often occur during the dark phase (Fox *et al.* 2002). Light cycles of 12–14 h light and 10–12 h dark are necessary to maintain regular oestrous cycles. Light intensities in the range commonly encountered in animal rooms can affect the oestrous cycle (Clough 1984), eg, too much light or a too long period of dark will cause irregularities in the oestrous cycle. Pheromones and the social environment also affect the oestrous cycle. Female mice housed in groups become dioestrous, anoestrous or pseudopregnant (the Lee-Boot effect), while the introduction of a male into such a group synchronises their oestrous cycles (the Whitten effect). If the female is housed with a second male within 24 h after a successful mating, implantation of fertile egg cells will be prevented and the female will return to oestrus in 4–5 days (the Bruce effect). These effects are mediated by pheromones in the urine of the males (Cunliffe-Beamer & Les 1987).

Mating also often occurs during the dark phase (Fox *et al.* 2002), and can be detected within 24 h after copulation by the formation of a waxy vaginal plug (a mixture of sperm and secretions from the seminal vesicles and the coagulating glands of the male). As this detection method is not always reliable it is often combined with detection of spermatozoa in the vaginal fluid after flushing. Elevated environmental temperatures (>28 °C) and high noise levels can reduce female fertility (Cunliffe-Beamer & Les 1987).

The gestation period of non-lactating females is 19–21 days, depending on the strain. Pregnancy can be diagnosed

Table 21.1 Standard biological data environmental requirements and physiological parameters of mice (partly from Scott 1991; Wolfensohn & Lloyd 2003; Fox *et al.* 2002; Havenaar *et al.* 2001).

Environmental requirements[a]	
Temperature (°C)	20–24
Relative humidity (%)	55 ± 10
Ventilation (changes/hour)	15
Light–dark (hours)	12–12 or 14–10[a]
Minimum cage floor size	
One individually housed adult (cm^2)	330
Breeding animal with pups (cm^2)	330
Group (cm^2/adult)	80
Minimum cage height (cm)	12
General physiological parameters	
Adult weight (g)	
Male	25–40
Female	18–35
Lifespan (years)	1–3
Heart rate (/min)	300–800
Blood pressure	
Systolic (mmHg)	133–160
Diastolic (mmHg)	102–110
Blood volume	
Plasma (ml/100 g)	3.15
Whole blood (ml/100 g)	5.85
Tidal volume (ml)	0.18 (0.09–0.38)
Minute volume (ml/min)	24 (11–36)
Stroke volume (ml/beat)	1.3–2.0
Respiration rate (/min)	100–200
Body temperature (°C)	36.5–38.0
Number of chromosomes (2 n)	40
Body surface for a 20 g animal (cm^2)	36
Water intake (ml/100 g/day)	15
Food intake (g/100 g/day)	15
Reproductive and developmental data	
Puberty (weeks)	
Female	4–5
Male	5–7
Breeding age (weeks)	
Female	8–10
Male	8–10
Fertilisation	2 h after mating
Segmentation of ovum to:	
Formation of blastocele (days)	2–4
Implantation (days)	4–5
Usual end to breeding life (months)	6–12
Female fecundity	6–10 litters
Male breeding life	1 year
Oestrous cycle (days)	4 (2–9)
Duration of oestrus (hours)	12–14
First oestrus (days)	25–28
Duration of pregnancy (days)	19 (18–21)
Pseudopregnancy (days)	10–13
Interbirth interval (weeks)	3.5–6
Litter size	6–12
Dental formula	$I^1{}_1C^0{}_0Pm^0{}_0M^3{}_3$
First solid food intake (days)	11–12
Weight at birth (g)	0.5–1.5
Weight at weaning (g)	10
Weight of adult (g)	30–40
Weaning age (days)	21–28
Nipples show (days)	9
Eyes open (days)	12–13
Vagina opens (weeks)	5
Pairs of nipples	5
Ano-genital distance – male (mm)	10–15
Ano-genital distance – female (mm)	5–6
Blood parameters	
Blood volume (ml/kg)	76–80
Plasma volume (ml/100 g)	3.15
Whole blood (ml/100 g)	5.85
Blood urea nitrogen (mg/100 ml)	12–30
Haematocrit (vol. %)	39–49
Plasma	
pH	7.2–7.4
CO_2 (mmol/l)	21.9
CO_2 pressure (mmHg)	40 + 5.4
Leucocyte count	
Total (per µl)	8.4(5.1–11.6) × 10^3
Neutrophils (%)	17.9(6.7–37.2)
Lymphocytes (%)	69(63–75)
Monocytes (%)	1.2(0.7–2.6)
Eosinophils (%)	2.1(0.9–3.8)
Basophils (%)	0.5(0–1.5)
Platelets (per µl)	600(100–1000) × 10^3
Packed cell volume (%)	44(42–44)
Red blood cells (per µl)	8.7–10.5 × 10^6
Haemoglobin (g/dl)	13.4(12.2–16.2)
Maximum single bleeding (ml/kg per 2 wks)	8
Average volume obtained when bleeding out (ml/kg)	30
Recommended volume replacement after surgery (ml/mouse)	approx. 1
Clotting time (min)	2–10
PTT (s)	55–110
Prothrombin time (s)	7–19
Glucose (mg/100 ml)	124–262
Under stress conditions this value may rise up to 2× normal	
Serum protein (g/100 ml)	4–6
Creatinine (mg/100 ml)	0.3–1
Total bilirubin (mg/100 ml)	0.1–0.9
Albumin (g/100 ml)	2.5–4.8
Globulin (g/100 ml)	0.6
Cholesterol (mg/100 ml)	26–82
Urine (ml/day)	1–1.5
Specific gravity	1.030–1.070
pH	5.011
Osmolality (Osm/kg)	1.06–2.63
Creatinine (mg/100 g/24 h)	2.6 ± 0.91
Glucose (mg/24 h)	0.53 ± 0.19
Protein (mg/24 h)	0.7 ± 0.33
Albumin (mg/ml)	11.9 ± 0.2

[a] European Directive 86/609/EEC Annex II revised L197/1

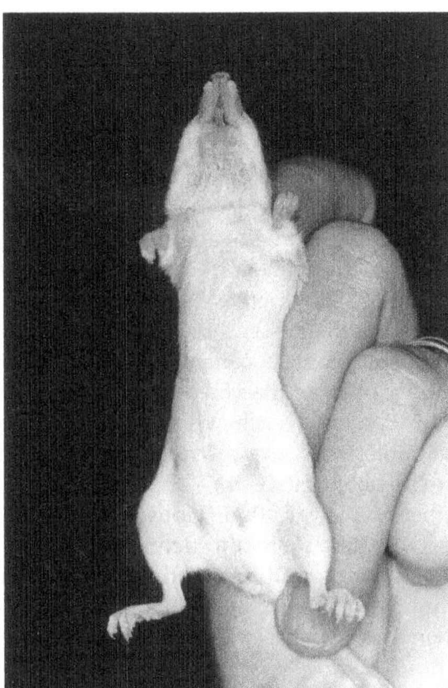

Figure 21.2 Mammary glands in the female mouse. (Photo: T.P. Rooymans.)

early by abdominal palpation between the 7th and 10th day of gestation, when the uterus feels like a string with knots in it. At days 15 and 16 the uterus feels uniformly enlarged. At the end of pregnancy, the skulls of the foetuses become firm and can be palpated. Towards parturition, pregnant females also build nests for giving birth (see later).

Litter size commonly ranges from 1–14 pups, depending on the strain. During parturition, pups and placentas are delivered simultaneously. Nursing females usually lactate for 3 weeks. Post-partum oestrus occurs within 24 h of parturition, but results less frequently in fertile matings, possibly because lactation delays implantation and prolongs gestation after post-partum oestrus for up to 12 days (Havenaar *et al.* 2001; Fox *et al.* 2002; Hedrich & Bullock 2004). Cannibalism (which is strain-dependent) can be minimised in most cases by providing a quiet place with reduced light intensity and nesting material.

The effective reproductive life of a female mouse approaches 2 years but, as litter size decreases with aging, females are usually retired by 1 year of age.

Uses in the laboratory

The mouse is the most widely used vertebrate species in biomedical research. Their short reproductive cycle, short lifespan, small size and low cost of maintenance make them suitable models for humans and animals in many aspects of biomedical research, including cancer and drug research, vaccine and monoclonal antibody preparation and evaluation of the safety and effectiveness of pharmaceutical products. As a result of the rapid advances in biotechnology, new strains expressing novel genetic characteristics are being created at a remarkable rate, so that there are now more than 1000 genetically defined inbred strains of laboratory mice.

Genetics, strains and stocks

See also Chapter 4.

Laboratory mice have 40 chromosomes that are differentiated by the size and pattern of transverse bands. Genetic mapping in mice began in the early 1900s, and the first linkage in the mouse was discovered by Haldane *et al.* (1915). Extensive linkage maps and an impressive array of inbred strains are now available to expedite sophisticated genetic research.

The most thoroughly studied genetic systems of the mouse are the histocompatibility loci. Histocompatibility (H) loci control expression of cell surface molecules that modulate major immunological phenomena, such as as the recognition of foreign tissue. For example, the time, onset and speed of skin graft rejection are controlled by two groups of H loci. The group of major H loci is called H2 and is located on chromosome 17. These genes cause rapid rejection (10–20 days) of grafts that display foreign H2 antigens. The group of minor H loci consists of genes scattered throughout the genome. These genes are responsible for delayed graft rejection. Genes associated with the H2 complex also control other immunological functions, such as cell–cell interactions in primary immune responses and the level of response to a given antigen. Immune-mediated responses to infectious agents such as viruses and complement activity are influenced directly or indirectly by the H2 complex (Fox *et al.* 2002; Hedrich & Bullock 2004).

Inbred mice are widely used for research in fields such as immunology, oncology, microbiology, biochemistry, pharmacology, physiology, anatomy and radiobiology and offer a high degree of genetic uniformity. Clarence C. Little developed the first inbred mouse strain, DBA, in 1909. Animals of an inbred strain are homozygous and genetically very similar to other mice of the same strain and sex. They are produced by brother × sister matings for at least 20 generations (Fox *et al.* 2002; van Zutphen *et al.* 2001). At this stage, the inbreeding coefficient should be ~ 0.99 (ie, residual heterozygosity approximately 1%). The assumption that all sources of the same inbred strain provide genetically identical mice is not valid, as animals maintained at different institutions for many generations may show genetic drift, even though they originate from the same source. Therefore, genetic monitoring of colonies is a prerequisite for standardisation of laboratory animals resulting in a reduction in the number of animals used.

Inbred strains can be created with very specific characteristics, enabling researchers to develop very specific animal models for biomedical research. Thus, they might be highly sensitive to, for example, tumour development or be immunodeficient (the athymic nude or the severe combined immunodeficient (SCID) mouse). It is obvious that the welfare of these strains might be easily compromised as they might be more sensitive to bacterial, viral and fungal infections than outbred mice or they might suffer from their induced diseases (Baumans 2004).

By contrast, outbred mice are genetically heterogeneous and are often produced by breeding systems that minimise inbreeding. Random pairing is best planned with the aid of tables of randomised numbers or a randomising device (see Chapter 4). However, a small colony may become inbred, or at least not that genetically heterogeneous, as eventually all animals will become genetically related. In a population of 25 breeding pairs, for example, heterozygosity will decrease by 1% per generation with standard randomisation techniques. A stock is regarded as outbred when it has been maintained as a closed colony for at least four generations. To minimise changes caused by inbreeding and genetic drift, the population should be maintained in such numbers as to give less than 1% inbreeding per generation.

Symbols

Rules for the nomenclature of different 'breeds' of mice are well defined. The term 'stock' is used to denote an outbred population of mice while the term 'strain' is used to denote an inbred population. The outbred stock designation consists of a symbol indicating the current breeder/holder of the stock, followed by a colon and the stock symbol consisting of two to four capital letters (eg, Crl:NMRI).

Inbred strains should be designated according to the rules for the nomenclature by one to four capital letters (eg, A; DBA) or for some old strains by a combination of capital letters and numbers (eg, C57BL; 129). Inbred strains can be divided into substrains. The strain designation is followed by a slash and the substrain designation which may consist of a combination of numbers and letters. The letters usually represent the laboratory code. For example, C57BL/6J means that this strain originated from female 57 at the Cold Spring Harbor Laboratory (C) and was the black line (BL). The 6 indicates subline number 6 and bred at the Jackson laboratory (J).

F1 hybrids are animals resulting from a cross between two inbred strains. They are genetically uniform and heterozygous for those genes for which the two parental strains differ. A coisogenic strain is a subline which differs from the original inbred strain by only one gene which is the result of a mutation. The symbol for a coisogenic strain must consist of the full strain and substrain designation, followed by a hyphen and the symbol of the mutant gene (eg, C3H/HeJ-Lps, a mutant substrain of C3H with a gene causing resistance to bacterial lipopolysaccharide).

A congenic strain is an inbred strain where a genetic trait has been introduced by repeated backcrossing with an inbred strain. The designation of congenic strains is similar to that of coisogenic strains. However, if congenic strains differ at the major histocompatibility locus, it is acceptable to give an abbreviated strain name, followed by a full stop and the abbreviation of the name of the donor strain (eg, B10.D2, which refers to a C57BL/10 carrying the H2 haplotype of the DBA/2 inbred strain) (van Zutphen *et al.* 2001).

Recombinant inbred (RI) strains are produced by brother × sister mating of individuals from the F2 generation of a cross between two (unrelated) inbred strains which are termed progenitor strains. The RI strains can be regarded as established after a minimum of 20 generations of brother × sister matings and will then form a set or series of RI strains. They are designated by combining abbreviated names of both the parental strains which are separated by a capital X. The parallel lines are given numbers (eg B6XH-1 which is the first recombinant inbred strain derived from the progenitor strains C57BL/6J and C3H/HeJ). RI strains represent a fixed set of randomly assorted genes of both progenitors. These strains are very valuable for genetic research, in particular for studies on linkage analysis and for the identification and genetic analysis of complex genetic traits (van Zutphen *et al.* 2001; Hedrich & Bullock 2004).

The sequence of the mouse genome is a key informational tool for understanding the contents of the human genome. The availability of more than 50 commonly used laboratory inbred strains of mice, each with its own phenotype for multiple variable traits, has provided an important opportunity to map quantitative trait loci (QTLs) that underlie heritable phenotypic variation (Mouse Genome Sequencing Consortium, 2002). A system to define parameters as body weight, behavioural patterns and disease susceptibility among a number of inbred lines is under construction in the Mouse Phenome Database[1] (Mouse Genome Sequencing Consortium, 2002).

Transgenic animals

See also Chapter 4.

Genetically engineered or modified mice are those with induced mutations, including mice with transgenes, with targeted mutations (knockouts) and with retroviral, proviral or chemically induced mutations[2]). Transgenic technology focuses on the introduction or exclusion (knockouts) of functional genetic material in the germ line of an animal, thus changing the genetic characteristics of an organism and its progeny. The most frequently used methods for genetic transformation of the germ line are microinjection of DNA into the pronucleus of fertilised oocytes and the injection of transfected embryonic stem (ES) cells into normal mouse blastocysts, resulting in a subsequent generation of chimeras. These techniques have led to the rapid development of a variety of animal models, designed for the study of gene regulation, gene expression, pathogenesis and the treatment of human and animal diseases (eg, Alzheimer's disease, growth hormone disturbances, poliovirus vaccine testing in humans or mastitis in cows).

Although there may be numerous benefits of producing transgenic lines, this development does raise some ethical and welfare issues. For example, the increase in the use of genetically modified animals has caused an increase in numbers of mice used of more than 23% per year; this is not only due to growth in the numbers of these animals in research but also to the large number of mice necessary to create each genetically modified line, such as breeding males, donor females, vasectomised males and pseudopregnant recipient females. Furthermore, non-transgenic and wild-type littermates may be produced that are not suitable for research or further breeding (Dennis 2002).

---

[1] http://www.jax.org/

[2] http://www.jax.org/jaxmice

Moreover, the process of transgenesis by microinjection may compromise welfare through the experimental procedures used during the process of transgenesis. The donor animals, vasectomised males and foster mothers which are needed for the production of the transgenic offspring may experience discomfort from procedures, such as early mating (from 3 weeks onwards), anaesthesia, surgery and injections (JWGR 2003).

At the level of integration of the microinjected DNA into the genome, unintentional insertional mutations may occur, potentially also resulting in welfare problems. At the level of expression of the introduced gene detrimental side effects may occur. For example, the giant mouse that over-produced growth hormone suffered from chronic kidney and liver dysfunction (Poole 1995; Crawley 2000). In this mouse the presence of a both functional and non-functional microinjected DNA construct increased mortality and body weight of the pups in the first 2–3 days after birth, whereas no significant differences in behaviour and morphological development were observed later on (van der Meer *et al.* 2001a).

From an ethical point of view it might be argued that the integrity of the animal is compromised as the genome is modified (van der Meer *et al.* 1996, 2001b). Furthermore, concern has been expressed with respect to the patentability of transgenic animals, such as the oncomouse. Finally, it has been suggested that the escape of transgenic animals could impose a risk for animal populations in the wild. However, escapes from modern, well built laboratories are unlikely and it appears that laboratory animals are not very viable in the wild (van der Meer *et al.* 1996, 2001).

In conclusion, transgenic technology has a great potential for increasing the understanding of the role of genes and may provide suitable animal models for human and animal disease, but the welfare of transgenic animals has to be carefully monitored, at least until the second generation of offspring. A surveillance system including score sheets can be helpful in identifying welfare problems, and can be used together with humane endpoints, in order to prevent unnecessary suffering through euthanasia of severely affected animals (Mertens & Rulicke 1999; van der Meer *et al.* 2001). Data banks from existing genetically modified animals will be useful to help predict potential impairments in new genetically modified lines yet to be created (Baumans 2005a). See also Chapter 5 for further information on phenotyping.

Sources of supply

Laboratory mice can be obtained in several ways (see also Chapter 12). Commercial laboratory animal breeders can supply a vast array of well defined, high-quality animals of outbred, inbred, hybrid or mutant bearing strains or stocks. In-house breeding is now mostly limited to strains or stocks which are not commercially available and/or to the maintenance of colonies associated with studies of reproduction and genetics, such as the production of transgenic animals (see also see Chapter 4). In-house breeding may often seem cheaper, but many costs may be hidden, such as those of husbandry, quality control and overheads, including maintenance costs and salaries of the animal staff. In-house breeding may result in less efficient use of animals as large-scale breeders can even out fluctuations in demand. However, in-house breeding may be necessary for developmental studies.

The assumption that all sources of the same strain provide genetically identical mice is not valid, as animals maintained at different institutions for many generations may show genetic drift, although they originate from the same source (Cunliffe-Beamer & Les 1987). Therefore, genetic monitoring of colonies is a prerequisite for standardisation of laboratory animals.

Also, it should not be assumed that clinically normal mice from different sources are comparable with respect to their health status, as there may be the potential for even clinically 'healthy' mice to introduce unwanted pathogens such as mouse hepatitis virus and Sendai, which could jeopardise research results (Cunliffe-Beamer & Les 1987).

Laboratory management and breeding

General husbandry

Housing

The laboratory mouse has partially adapted to captive life, but still shows similarities to its wild counterparts. Mice are active, highly explorative animals, which, in the wild, spend considerable time foraging, seeking a wide variety of food. They construct elaborate nests and burrows and form complex social structures. All these behaviours, which they remain strongly motivated to perform, are still present in the laboratory mouse. Housing systems for laboratory animals have often been designed on the basis of economic and ergonomic aspects (such as equipment, costs, space, work load, ability to observe the animals and to maintain a certain degree of hygiene) with little or no consideration for animal welfare.

Such conditions deprive animals of the possibility of performing a full repertoire of normal behaviour, such as exploring, resting, climbing, grooming, foraging, nesting and social behaviour. This may then lead to frustration and suffering (Dawkins 1990; Sherwin 2000) expressed in abnormal behaviour such as stereotypies, due to lack of stimulation (van de Weerd & Baumans 1995; Würbel 2001). The environment of a mouse should consist of a wide range of stimuli, including the social environment of conspecifics and humans and the physical environment, such as the cage and its contents (Figure 21.3).

Laboratory mice are usually bred and housed in shoe-box shaped cages made of polycarbonate, polypropylene or stainless steel with solid or wire-mesh floors (Figure 21.4). Wire-mesh floors are used if experiments require continuous collection of faeces and/or urine or elimination of contact between the animal and bedding material. However, since mice are nesting animals, in a choice test they prefer solid floors with sawdust for digging, nesting and resting rather than grid floors (Blom *et al.* 1996); solid bottom cages containing bedding and nesting materials should therefore be used whenever possible (Council of Europe 2006; European Commission 2007).

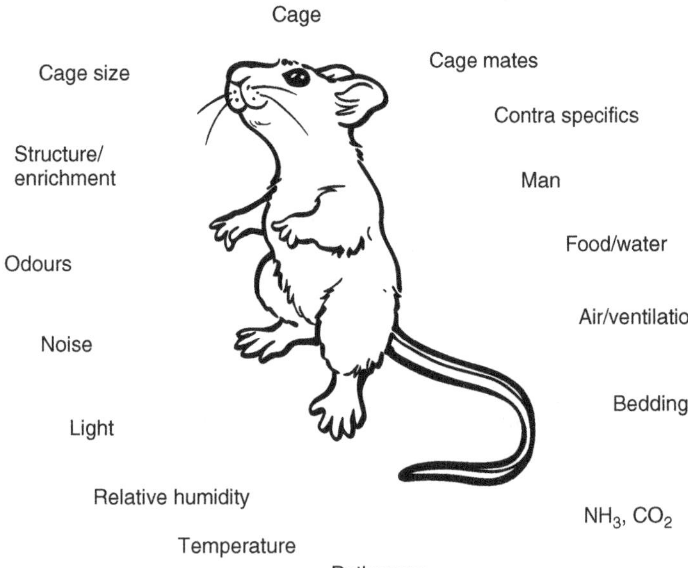

Figure 21.3 Stimuli in the environment of laboratory animals.

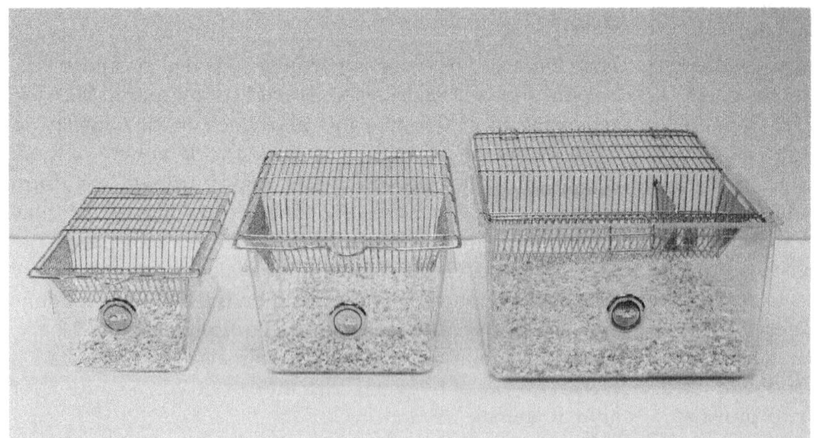

Figure 21.4 Polycarbonate cages for mice with sawdust-covered solid floors. (Photo: T.P. Rooymans.)

Boxes made of plastics may have varying degrees of translucency and also different abilities to withstand steam sterilisation. Cage lids are usually made of stainless steel and have an indentation forming a food hopper. Mice eat directly from the hopper through spaces about 3–5 mm wide. It is important to appreciate that small mice can escape through spaces more than 6 mm in width. Water can be provided from a bottle attached to each cage or by an automatic watering system (see Presentation of food and water).

Bedding should be provided that is comfortable for resting, that absorbs urine and is used by the animals for depositing odour patterns. There should be a balance in terms of cleaning, between increasing the anxiety of the animals by removing familiar odour patterns on the one hand, and minimising the build-up of harmful ammonia on the other (Eveleigh 1993). It has been shown that olfactory cues from nesting and bedding material affect aggression in a different way: transfer of nesting material reduces aggression, whereas sawdust containing urine/faeces intensifies aggression (Hurst *et al.* 1993; van Loo *et al.* 2000). All laboratory rodents spend considerable time manipulating bedding, often creating tunnels (where the depth and consistency is sufficient) as well as building nests to provide shelter and warmth.

Sawdust is widely used as bedding material, but fine particles can cause preputial and respiratory problems. The type of wood can affect physiological parameters in the animal such as hepatic microsomal enzyme function (Vesell 1967; Haataja *et al.* 1989). Hygroscopic material like cat litter should be avoided as it may cause dehydration in the newborn. Nesting material, such as paper towels, tissues and wood wool, can provide shade from lighting, the opportunity to regulate their microclimate, such as temperature, and a shelter to hide from conspecifics and the ability to control the environment (van de Weerd & Baumans 1995) (Figure 21.5). Therefore, nesting material should be provided not only for breeding female mice, but for all laboratory mice.

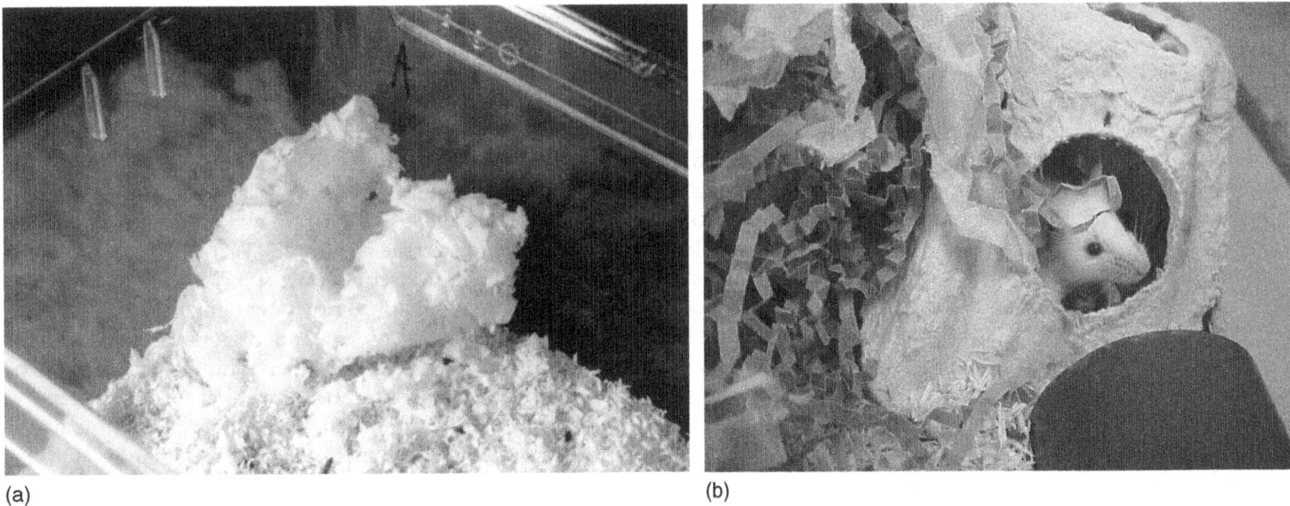

(a) (b)

Figure 21.5 (a) Bowl-shaped nest of BALB/c mice. (b) Environmental enrichment for mice. (Photos: T.P. Rooymans.)

Bedding and nesting material should:

- be in accordance with the mouse's needs;
- not be toxic or harmful to the animal;
- be absorbent, but not dehydrating for neonates;
- not be excessively dusty;
- be economical to use and dispose of;
- be inedible, to avoid interference with experiments.

Housing and husbandry have a major impact on the laboratory animal throughout its life, not only during, but also before and after scientific procedures. It is important to consider the species-specific needs in relation to housing and feeding regimes; and also to take into account within-species variation associated with genetic background. While laboratory animals have partially adapted to captive life, they still show similarities to their wild counterparts. The environment of captive animals should cater for physiological and behavioural needs such as resting, nest building, hiding, exploring, foraging, gnawing and compatible social contacts (Olsson & Dahlborn 2002; Baumans 2004).

Many laboratory animal species such as rodents and rabbits are highly susceptible to predators, and are thus likely to show strong fear responses in unfamiliar situations if they cannot shelter. This is shown by attempts to flee, biting when handled, or sudden immobility to avoid being detected. For this reason, cages should be provided with shelter or hiding places. Careful handling from a young age, together with conditioning to experimental and husbandry procedures, will probably reduce these stress responses considerably (Hurst 1999). Ideally, the animal should feel secure in a complex, challenging environment that it can control (Poole 1998). A sense of security can be achieved by providing nestable and manipulable and effective nesting material, hiding places and compatible cage mates.

In practice, however, laboratory animals are usually housed throughout their lives in relatively barren cages and given unrestricted access to food. This frequently results in adverse effects on the behaviour and physiology of the animals, and in a shortened lifespan due to overfeeding and inactivity (van de Weerd *et al.* 1997b; Mattson *et al.* 2001). Standardisation of environmental conditions has been designed to reduce individual differences within animal groups (intra-experimental variation), ultimately facilitating the detection of treatment effects, and to reduce differences between studies (inter-experiment variation), ultimately increasing the reproducibility of results across laboratories (Olsson *et al.* 2003; van Zutphen 2001). Nevertheless, despite rigorous attempts to equalise conditions among sites, tests with different inbred mouse strains, simultaneously carried out in three recommended laboratories, revealed significant effects from their respective sites for nearly all variables tested (Crabbe *et al.* 1999; Wahlsten *et al.* 2003). It seems that barren, restrictive and socially deprived housing conditions interfere with the development and function of brain and behaviour (Renner & Rosenzweig 1987; Würbel 2001; Benefiel *et al.* 2005), and restrictions such as those imposed by the standard rodent cage are potentially stressful (Mench 1998; Ladewig 2000). In other words, the barren environment that has been devised to minimise uncontrolled environmental effects on the animals may ironically be a primary source of pathological artefacts.

Current thinking (Council of Europe 2006) is that appropriate structuring of the cage/pen environment may be more beneficial than provision of a large floor area, although a certain area is necessary to provide a structured space. Except for locomotor activity (eg, playing), mice do not actually use open space as they are thigmotaxic, meaning that they use barriers and walls rather than the open space. Instead they use resources and structures within the area for specific behaviours.

Environmental enrichment

One way of improving the living conditions of laboratory animals is to give animals opportunities to perform more species-specific behavioural repertoires through enrichment of their environment. Enrichment can be defined as any modification in the environment of captive animals that seeks to enhance their physical and psychological well-being by providing stimuli that meet their species-specific needs (Newberry 1995; Baumans 2005b). This approach has been increasingly introduced into laboratory animal research facilities (Olsson & Dahlborn 2002). From a welfare point of view, it seems to be a good development, as there is general agreement that the well-being of the animals improves with the provision of environmental enrichment (see also Chapter 10). For example, beneficial effects of environmental enrichment have been described in animals with brain damage and disturbed motor function; an increased arborisation of dendrites has been found in the brains of these animals (Mohammed *et al.* 2002). The effects of environmental enrichment are dependent on the type of enrichment used. In the field of neuroscience, enrichment mainly refers to social housing in a large, complex cage containing different toys that are changed frequently in order to induce changes in the brain and behaviour (see Chapter 10). In animal welfare research, enrichment focuses on specific needs such as nest building, hiding and gnawing, in order to improve the well-being of the animals without major changes in physiology and behaviour (Zhu *et al.* 2006).

Enrichment of the animal's environment can be focused on both the social environment and the physical environment, consisting of sensory stimuli (auditory, visual, olfactory and tactile) and nutritional aspects (supply and type of food). The animal's psychological appraisal of its environment in terms of controllability and predictability can be improved by structuring the cage with nest boxes, tubes, partitions and nesting material (van de Weerd & Baumans 1995; Baumans *et al.* 2007). van de Weerd *et al.* (1997b) and van Loo *et al.* (2005) showed that paper tissue, for example, was strongly preferred by mice as a component of their cage (Figure 21.5). Enrichment items need to be designed and evaluated on the basis of knowledge gained in enrichment studies (van Loo *et al.* 2005) and knowledge of biology and behaviour of the animal. Furthermore it is important to know which type of housing and enrichment the animals were provided with at the breeder's facility, as differences may also have an impact on the animal and consequently on the scientific outcome. Besides meeting the needs of the animal, enrichment items should be practical and inexpensive, and pose no risk to humans, the animals used or the experiment. There is some concern, however, as to whether environmental enrichment conflicts with the standardisation of experiments. The question is: 'Do enriched animals show more variability in their response to experimental procedures because they show more diverse behaviours?' Some researchers think they do. In complex environments, for example, animals are not just responding to one stimulus but to many variable stimuli at once, and this can result in increased variation among subjects (Eskola *et al.* 1999; Tsai *et al.* 2003).

The counter-argument is that because an animal can perform more of its species-specific behaviour in enriched environments, it may be able to cope better with novel and unexpected changes and thus in fact show a more uniform response. If animals from enriched housing conditions are likely to be physiologically and psychologically more stable, it follows that they may be considered as more refined models that ensure better scientific results. In practice, however, results from different studies seem to indicate that the effects of enrichment on the variability in results depend on the parameter being measured, the strain of animal and the type of enrichment (van de Weerd *et al.* 2002; Wolfer *et al.* 2004).

It seems clear, therefore, that environmental enrichment should comprise a well designed and critically evaluated programme that benefits the animals as well as the experimental outcome; it should not be a process of randomly supplying objects that staff consider attractive for the animals. Enrichment needs to be regarded as an essential component of the overall animal care programme, and just as important as nutrition and veterinary care. The key component of the enrichment programme is the animal care staff, who must be motivated and educated (Stewart & Bayne 2004).

In summary, evaluating enrichment in terms of the animal (ie, by assessing the use of and preference for a certain enrichment, and the effect on behaviour, the performance of species-typical behaviour and physiological parameters) is essential. Equally important is evaluating the impact of enrichment on the scientific outcome (see Chapter 10) (van de Weerd *et al.* 2002; Baumans 2005b).

Space recommendations

It is difficult scientifically to specify the minimum cage sizes for maintaining laboratory animals; much depends on the strain, group size and age of the animals, their familiarity with each other and their reproductive condition. Cage sizes recommended in current European guidelines on accommodation for laboratory animals are generally based on scientific evidence; where such evidence is lacking or insufficient, they are based on what is described as best practice (Council of Europe 2006), which has been agreed upon by researchers, veterinarians and animal staff.

Specifications for laboratory housing of mice are expressed in two documents issued in 1986. One is the Council of Europe's (1986) European Convention for the protection of vertebrate animals used for experimental and other scientific purposes (Convention ETS 123) with its Appendix A, Guidelines for the accommodation and care of animals, revised in 2006. The other is the very similar European Union's (1986) Council Directive on the approximation of laws, regulations and administrative provisions of the Member States regarding the protection of animals used for experimental and other scientific purposes (Directive 86/609/EEC) with its Annex II, Guidelines for accommodation and care of animals (revised in 2007). Article 5.1 of the Convention requires that '*Any restriction on the extent to which an animal can satisfy its physiological and ethological needs shall be limited as far as practicable*', while Article 5.b of the Directive requires them to '*be limited to the absolute minimum*'. In the USA, guidelines on accommodation and care of laboratory animals are included in the National Research Council's (1996) Guide for the Care and Use of Laboratory Animals of the National Research Council, although mice, rats and birds do not come under the official legislation in the USA. Space recommendations should allow housing of mice in harmonious groups. Increasing the complexity of the cage is more important than increasing floor area as such, as the inclusion of structures will provide more opportunities for activity and will increase the usable space. Furthermore, mice partition their space into sleeping, defecating, urinating and feeding areas, so the available space and structure in the cage should be sufficient and should also cater for play behaviour in young animals. Incentives for activity should be provided in the cage, such as nesting material and climbing possibilities (Council of Europe 2006; European Commission 2007).

The use of environmental enrichment to improve the well-being of laboratory animals is widely promoted and is currently incorporated in European legislation (Kornerup Hansen & Baumans 2004; Council of Europe 2006; EU European Commission 2007). Many other countries have similar legislation and regulations on this matter, eg Australia (National Health and Medical Research Council (NHMRC) 2004; Animal Research Review Panel (ARRP) draft).

Other organisations besides governments are involved in developing guidelines and regulations on animal use. In Europe, the 2001 position paper of the European Science Foundation, an association of the major science-funding organisations, endorsed the principles of the Three Rs and the need for laboratory animal welfare research (European Science Foundation 2001).

Environmental provisions

Although environmental measurements are taken at the room level (macro-environment), the conditions in the cage actually affect the animal's micro-environment. Mice 'engineer' their own micro-environments by huddling and building nests and in this way they are able to exert some control over temperature, humidity and light conditions. Furthermore, the micro-environment will vary, depending on the position of the cage on the rack, crowding of the rack, cage type, stocking density in the cage, type and amount of bedding and cleaning frequency. Also the use of filter caps and individually ventilated cages (IVCs) will affect the rate of air exchange, build up of ammonia, temperature and humidity (Serrano 1971; Baumans *et al.* 2002). IVC systems are designed to reduce infection risks, ammonia and carbon dioxide concentrations, cleaning frequency, workload and allergens. However, the high ventilation rate and reduced handling of animals in IVC systems are potential drawbacks. To protect the animals from draught due to the forced ventilation, nesting material or a hiding place should be provided (Baumans *et al.* 2002, 2007).

When the environmental temperature falls below the thermoneutral zone (where body temperature is regulated by conduction and convection of heat), body temperature is maintained by behavioural adaptation, such as nest building and/or increased metabolic rate. Environmental temperature has been shown to influence reproduction, organ weight, food and water intake and haematological parameters. These data indicate that the optimal temperature range for mouse rooms is 20–26 °C (Yamauchi *et al.* 1983). According to the European Directive, the environmental temperature requirements range between 20 and 24 °C. The upper end of this range (22–24 °C) should be considered if the mice have to be housed in wire-bottom cages because of greater air exchange between the cage and the room, or if hairless or nude mice are being housed in cages with limited amounts of bedding (see also Chapter 10, which discusses evidence that the thermoneutral zone of mice is 26–34 °C). Blom *et al.* (1993) studied preferences of mice for temperature and found that individual BALB/c mice preferred a cage temperature of 28 °C, whereas C57BL/6 preferred 24 °C and that preference depended upon the type of cage flooring.

Ventilation rates should be based on the heat production of the animals. Air changes are less important than creating an efficient flow in the room to keep ammonia levels within the animal's immediate environment at an acceptable level. The health of staff also needs consideration with respect to exposure to animal allergens, such as dander and urine. To reduce the possibility of airborne introduction of infectious diseases into an animal room, high-efficiency particulate air (HEPA) or similar filtration of incoming air should be considered and is mandatory for maintaining specified pathogen free or gnotobiotic mice.

It is important to avoid extremely high or low humidities and rapid changes in humidity. At low humidity levels, mice may suffer from respiratory problems due to excessive dustiness of bedding and feed, and drying of mucous membranes. At high humidity levels, bedding may become damp and fail to evaporate moisture leading to rapid soiling of cages and increased production of ammonia by urease-producing bacteria. Furthermore, infections of the upper airways may occur more easily.

Cage cleaning regimes should be a compromise between maintaining hygiene and keeping odour patterns left by the animals (van Loo *et al.* 2000). Normally, cages are cleaned once a week. Water bottles should also be changed at least once a week.

Lighting conditions for the essentially nocturnal mouse are very important. Lighting must be controlled to avoid external lighting fluctuations. Mice exposed to too high an intensity of light may show retinal atrophy in the long term (Clough 1984). Animals should be subjected to a regular light–dark cycle, generally 12 h light: 12 h dark, but there is some debate concerning the effect on animal behaviour of creating artificial 'dawn' and 'dusk' periods (Latham & Mason 2004). In some cases, a reversed lighting schedule, with lights on at night, can be useful for observing activity of rodents during the working day; red light can be used to facilitate daytime husbandry as most rodents are less sensitive to red light (Spalding *et al.* 1969). Mice show a preference for a low light intensity. Maximum light intensity in the room should not exceed 350 lux and the intensity levels within the cage should be lower, or the animal should be given the opportunity to withdraw to shaded areas, such as a shelter or nest (Council of Europe 2006; European Commission 2007).

Many noises audible to the human ear and ultrasound (frequencies higher than the human range, >20 kHz) are important for rodents. Mice are more likely to be disturbed by high-pitched sounds and ultrasounds than they are by lower frequencies; care must be taken not to use equipment which emits these ultrasounds, such as electronic devices and computer screens (Clough 1984; Sales *et al.* 1999; Latham & Mason 2004; Voipio *et al.* 2006). It has been suggested that a constant background noise, such as radio music, has some benefits in facilitating breeding and making animals less excited, although it could also stress some animals. However it may benefit the staff more, which could have beneficial consequences for the animals in turn (Sherwin 2002); it certainly should not exceed 55 dB. Alarm systems, telephones and door bells within rodent facilities should sound outside the animals' hearing range where this does not conflict with their audibility to humans (Council of Europe 2006;

Federation of European Laboratory Animal Science Associations (FELASA) 2007).

Social housing

As mice are gregarious animals, it is preferable to keep them in groups rather than in individual housing, but the groups must be stable and harmonious in order to avoid or minimise aggression within groups (Council of Europe 2006; European Commission 2007). Allocating animals to new, unfamiliar groups may be a source of intense, stressful conflicts (Brain 1990). The evidence suggesting that individual housing in mice can be deleterious is not convincing (Brain & Benton 1983; Krohn *et al.* 2006) but strain differences have been found (Haemisch & Gärtner 1994). Individually housed mice are still provided with olfactory, auditory and (probably less importantly) visual cues from conspecifics in the room, whereas isolated animals are also deprived of this input. However, 'living apart together' (two mice in a cage, separated by a grid partition), did not appear to be beneficial to mice submitted to abdominal surgery. Increased heart rate levels and differences in behaviour as compared with both socially housed and individually housed animals indicate that 'living apart together' may even be the most stressful of the three housing conditions, whereas social housing appeared to be the best (van Loo *et al.* 2007). It is natural for many rodents to live in mixed sex groups but breeding frequently increases agonistic behaviour and laboratory mice are usually kept in single sex groups, which is unnatural in itself. Excessive agonistic behaviour depends on the animal's familiarity with its cagemates as well as its sex and age at the time of grouping (Council of Europe 2006; European Commission 2007; FELASA 2007).

Adult males from specific strains, eg BALB/c, may fight excessively when kept in single sex groups. Male mice of all ages tested so far have a preference for social contact during rest periods. During activity periods, the preference for social contact increases with age. Aggression can be reduced by: transferring used nesting material to the clean cage, at the time of cage cleaning (but not the soiled bedding material as the urine pheromones increase fighting); keeping no more than three males per cage; and minimising disturbances such as removing a group member temporarily (van Loo *et al.* 2003; Baumans *et al.* 2007).

'Barbering' or 'trimming' (hair nibbling and whisker chewing) occur frequently in both sexes of some strains of mice (Figure 21.6). Usually one of the mice retains its whiskers and it is assumed that this is the dominant animal within the cage, but this is not conclusive (van de Weerd *et al.* 1992; Garner *et al.* 2004). Removal of the barber mouse may lead to another mouse taking over the barbering role. Barbering may not be restricted to whiskers: head and body fur may also be involved, as can occur in the C57BL6 strain. The aetiology of barbering is not clear. Genetic factors may play a role as well as boredom of the animals (van den Broek *et al.* 1993). In caged mice, barbering is another example of an abnormal behaviour that has become a normative behaviour pattern within the context of inadequate living conditions (Garner *et al.* 2004; Baumans *et al.* 2007). Interestingly, mice will allow themselves to be barbered, even if they are given the opportunity to withdraw from the barber (van den Broek *et al.* 1993). However, Garner *et al.* (2004) point to a number of welfare issues that arise from barbering, including referring to a reference on degenerative alterations in somatosensory cortical areas corresponding to the whiskers.

Presentation of food and water

The mouse is an omnivorous animal. The incisors and molars grow continuously and are worn down by mastication. Attention should be paid to malocclusion leading to under-nutrition.

Feeding behaviour in rodents shows a diurnal pattern with the majority of food consumed during the dark period. Fasting overnight, sometimes part of an experiment, might lead to an increase of activity, resulting in unwanted variation in experimental results (Baumans 1999).

Food is usually presented *ad libitum* as pellets in the food hopper on the cage, which prevents soiling of food by the

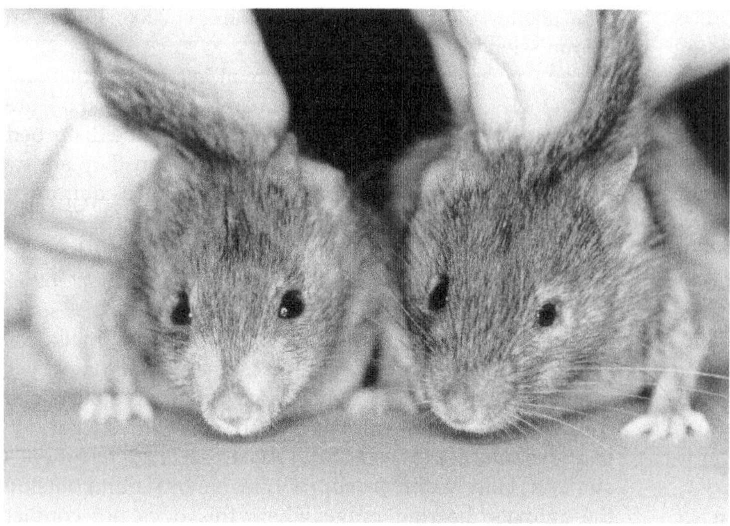

Figure 21.6 Whisker chewing ('barbering') in mice: barbering mouse (right); barbered mouse (left). (Photo: T.P. Rooymans.)

animals. The food rack should be kept sufficiently full, as it is difficult for the animals to gnaw the food when there are only a few pellets left. Restricted feeding has been shown to be beneficial in the long run in terms of reduced morbidity and mortality in the earlier stages of life (Mattson *et al.* 2001).

Enrichment related to food, such as grain scattered through the bedding, will meet the animal's need for foraging and will prevent boredom due to the gap in the animal's natural time budget usually filled with foraging (Baumans 2005b), although it might interfere with experiments, eg, certain nutritional research. BALB/c and C57BL/6 mice kept in enriched environments with nesting material have been found to weigh more than mice housed under standard conditions, although the latter consumed more food, probably due to the insulating effect of the nest or to reduced boredom (van de Weerd *et al.* 1997a).

Water can be provided in a bottle attached to each cage, and this should be changed at least once a week; an alternative is an automatic watering system, which supplies water through a valve connected to a piping system and serves a rack of cages from a central reservoir. The water valve can be located either outside or inside the cage. There is always some risk that the valve may become obstructed, resulting in dehydration of the animals or flooding in the cage. For this reason, automatic watering systems must be closely monitored to be certain that the water pressure is adequate and must be regularly cleaned and checked for contamination with bacteria and fungi.

Identification and sexing

Many permanent or temporary methods of identifying individual mice have been developed. Permanent methods include tattooing (on the tail or toe), toe clipping and ear punching. However, toe clipping is not recommended for welfare reasons (Baumans 2005a), and ear punching may be obliterated and damaged by fighting. Subcutaneous implantation of a microchip is a safe and long lasting, but expensive way of identification and might not be suitable for newborn mice. Temporary methods of identification include pen marks on the tail (Figure 21.7), clipping or plucking unique patterns in the fur, which may be visible for about 14 days, or dyeing the fur with a harmless dye, such as food dyes. Tail clipping is commonly used in genetically modified mice in order to take tissue samples from the offspring for identifying their genetic makeup. Concerns have, however, been raised about this procedure on the grounds that it may cause lasting harm in terms of pain, and disturbance of the thermoregulatory function of the tail.

The sex of the animal can be determined by comparing the anogenital distance, which is larger in males than in females. In females, a hairless strip is visible between anus and genital papilla (Figure 21.8). In males, testes can be present in the scrotum, but they can also be retracted through the inguinal canal into the abdomen, especially when the animal is scared or stressed.

Health monitoring, quarantine and barrier systems

Scientific data obtained from animal experiments should be reproducible and reliable and therefore the health status of the animals should be defined. Microbiological quality control aims at control of the barrier system and the animal itself. Only careful monitoring of animal facilities will provide useful information about the microbiological quality of the animals. Most infections in rodents are subclinical and modifications of research results due to natural infections often occur in the absence of clinical disease. For instance, Sendai virus infection, which is associated with a decreased B-cell and T-cell response after antigenic stimulation, enhances the production of interferon and decreases the serum level of the 3rd complement factor (C3) (Boot *et al.* 2001; FELASA 2002).

Laboratory animals can be classified according to their microbiological status (conventional, specific pathogen free (SPF) or gnotobiotic). Conventional animals can harbour a whole range of infectious micro-organisms, since they are kept without the application of preventive hygienic measures. Conventional animals are still widely used in biomedical research. Mice should be considered as conventional animals if their microbiological status is unknown. As a rule,

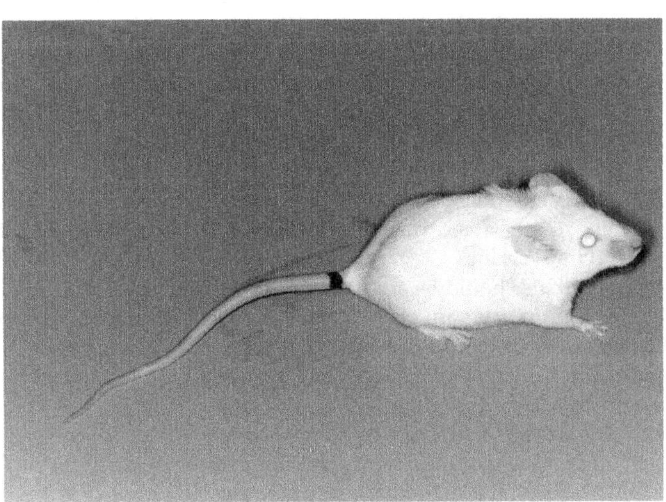

Figure 21.7 Identification by pen mark on the tail. (Photo: T.P. Rooymans.)

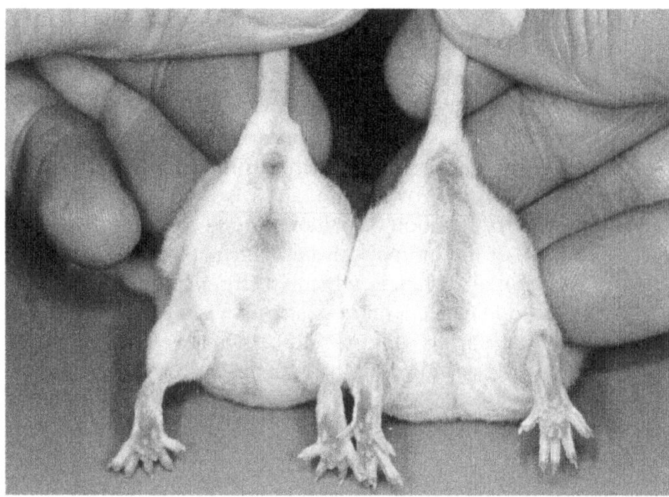

Figure 21.8 Sex differences in the mouse: male (right) and female (left). (Photo: T.P. Rooymans.)

these animals are 'quarantined' for a period of time before use. The length of this period is based upon the longest incubation time required for excluding infections. This implies the expectation that the 'quarantine' period would reveal certain clinical symptoms in the animals. However, most infections in laboratory animals are latent and can only be detected with specific screening programmes, which may be too costly to use as a routine.

SPF animals are free from a number of potentially pathogenic micro-organisms. SPF only designates which micro-organisms are known not to be in the colony at the time of the last testing. There are various reasons why SPF animals are used; for example, testing the safety of products and the performance of animal experiments with no interference from infections. The duration of experiments partly determines the likelihood of contamination. Long-term experiments are at greater risk than short-term ones.

Gnotobiotic animals are animals with a defined microflora and can be divided into germ-free (GF) and colonisation-resistant flora (CRF) animals. GF animals can be obtained from conventional counterparts by performing a hysterectomy (rederivation) and are kept under sterile conditions within isolators. GF animals are very susceptible to infections by micro-organisms that only rarely cause disease in conventional animals. To provide GF animals with some resistance to opportunistic infections, they can be deliberately given flora, which provide the formerly GF animal with a general resistance to the growth of other bacteria (colonisation resistance). CRF animals are housed as GF animals within isolators. Frequently, CRF animals are used to start SPF breeding colonies (Boot *et al.* 2001). Gnotobiotic animals are used for various purposes, such as the production of viral vaccines.

The animals should be screened periodically. The screening programme may involve serological tests, bacterial cultures, parasitic examinations and regular histopathological examination of major organs. The frequency of screening should be every 3 months with a minimal sample size of eight individual sera from mice randomly sampled from each unit for the most frequently occurring micro-organisms (FELASA 2002). If a particular agent is present in about 25% of the population, a sample size of 10 animals would be required in order for a 95% probability of detecting an infected animal. When an insufficient number of animals is present in an experiment to carry out the health-monitoring programme, sentinel animals can be used, which are obtained from a colony with a known microbiological status and introduced into the experiment animal unit.

Barrier systems

To maintain the microbiological status of gnotobiotic animals, including CRF animals, these animals should be kept separated from the environment in isolators made of steel or plastic (Figure 21.9). All equipment, including food and bedding, is sterilised and introduced through a lock which can be sterilised by, for example, peracetic acid vapour.

For short-term experiments, animals can be housed in cages with a protective hood (filter top) (Figure 21.10), which are only opened within laminar air flow cabinets. IVC systems are now widely used in combination with laminar air flow cabinets as work stations in order to create a bio-containment zone at cage level. As the airflow within the cage may be quite high (up to 100 air changes per hour) the animals may suffer from the high ventilation rate inside the cage. This might be reduced by providing nesting material or a shelter where the animals can hide from draughts (Baumans *et al.* 2002).

Animal rooms are cleaned with hot water, preferably with high-pressure equipment. Cleaning of cages and drinking bottles makes disinfection and sterilisation more effective. Physical and chemical methods exist for disinfection and sterilisation and depend upon the material to be treated and the micro-organisms likely to be present.

The effect of cleaning and disinfection can be monitored using agar plates, on which the number of bacterial colonies is counted and strips, which show colour changes, may monitor the autoclaving process or formaldehyde treatment. Modern autoclaves have inbuilt registration and control systems.

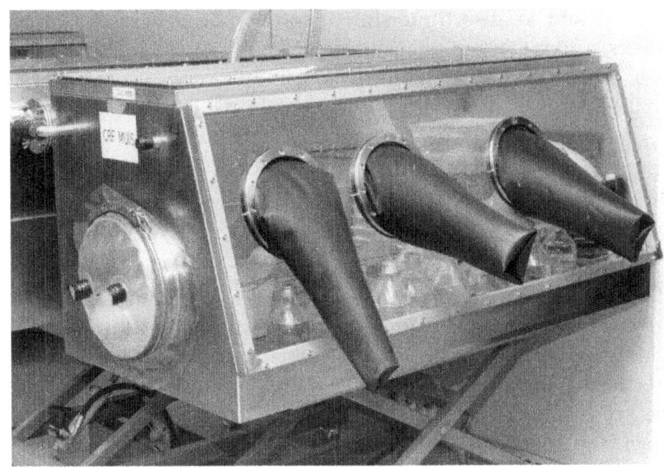

Figure 21.9 Steel isolator with lock and gloves. (Photo: T.P. Rooymans.)

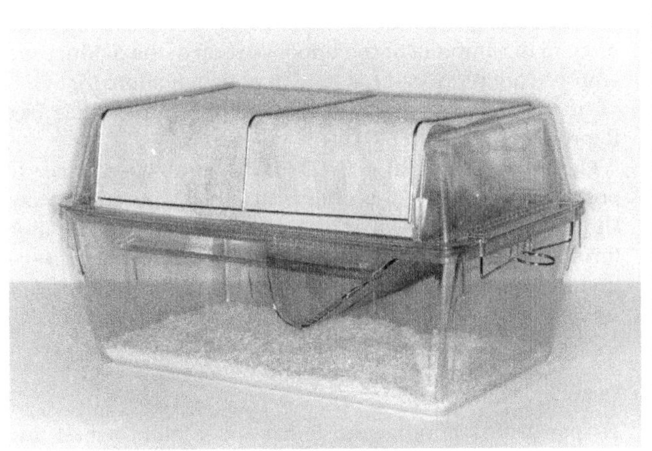

(a)

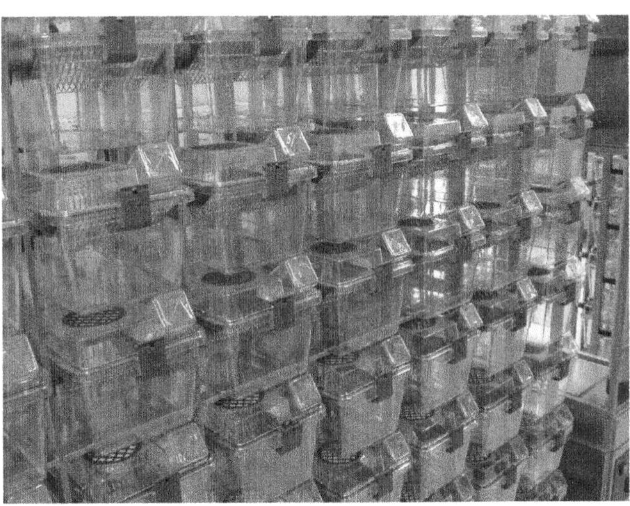

(b)

Figure 21.10 (a) Filter-top cage. (b) Individually ventilated cage (IVC) rack. (Photos: T.P. Rooymans.)

Transport

Transport of mice, even over short distances and/or under optimal conditions, is a stressful event for the animal. For example, immune functions are altered by shipment, and require at least 2–5 days to return to normal, and reproductive performance can be decreased (Cunliffe-Beamer & Les 1987). The extent to which the well-being of the animal is compromised depends upon its health status, age (old and very young animals are more susceptible), density of animals in the cage, conditions in transport vehicle and cage, such as temperature, ventilation, food and water supply, and the acclimatisation period (5–7 days) in the new environment.

Mice that are being moved over a short distance within the same facility can be transported in a clean cage or cardboard carton. For longer journeys, the cardboard container should be coated with moisture-impervious material. Ventilation openings should be present on at least the two opposite sides. The openings should be provided with steel wire mesh and filters to prevent escape or contamination en route (Figure 21.11). Bedding should always be supplied for

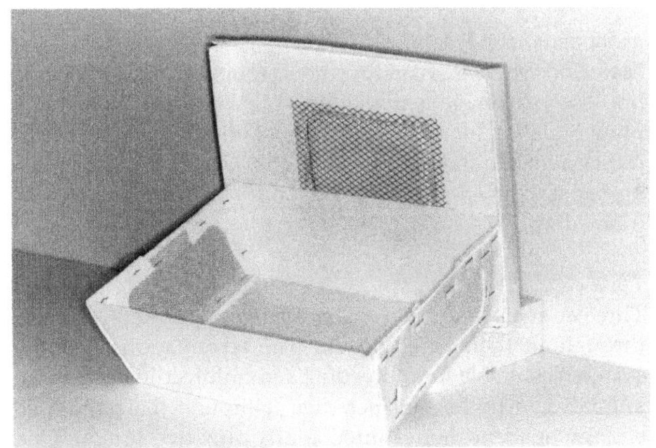

Figure 21.11 Disposable transport cage of cardboard, the inside covered with plastic, provided with wire mesh and filters. (Photo: T.P. Rooymans.)

comfort and to absorb moisture. Food can be provided as pellets, and water as 'solid' water, eg, agar, apples or potatoes or commercially available gel in the cage (see also Chapter 13).

Breeding

Selection of breeding stock

The primary objective of a good breeding programme is to produce the maximum number of quality mice at the lowest cost. Selecting breeding stock is important for the consistent production of healthy and fertile animals. The criteria for the selection of breeding stock may include the following (Buckland *et al.* 1981):

- The female parent should have a good overall breeding record and should not be prone to killing her young.
- The animals should be in good health and show no deformities.
- If possible, animals should not be selected from the first or second litters as they are usually small and do not reflect the size and standard of future litters.
- Animals should be selected from litters showing an average litter size for the strain, average weaning weight for the strain and equal sex ratio within litters.
- The parent animals should not be aggressive when handled.

Condition of adults

Ovarian follicle development begins at 3 weeks of age and matures by 30 days (see Reproduction section). Vaginal opening and the first oestrus may occur at 24 days of age, but complete sexual maturity is usually delayed until 7–9 weeks of age. For reproductive and developmental data see Table 21.1. The stages of the oestrous cycle can be identified by external appearance of the vaginal orifice or by examination of vaginal smears using a moistened cotton wool swab.

Mating systems

Monogamous pairs

Male and female remain together throughout their breeding life. The advantage is that the post-partum oestrus (oestrus immediately after the birth of the young) can be used, but the system requires more space and labour (one cage per breeding pair). It is, however, the system of choice for inbreeding.

Trios

Three animals (one male and two females) are kept together throughout their breeding life. The advantage is that the system is suitable for inbreeding and outbreeding and more animals can be housed per cage (although there must be enough space to house three adults plus two litters). One potential disadvantage is that, when both females produce offspring simultaneously, it may be unclear which female produced which young.

Harem

Groups of animals are housed together usually one male and four females, which is space and labour saving. More males may cause increased fighting, resulting in poor welfare and reproduction. When the females are pregnant they can be moved to a littering cage or stay in the harem. The latter may be less successful due to more disturbance and less tolerance when more than two females are present and it may be unclear which mother is fostering which pups.

Conception and pregnancy

When the cervix and vagina are stimulated physically during oestrus, prolactin is released from the anterior pituitary, which stimulates the corpus luteum to secrete progesterone, a process that continues for about 13 days. If fertilisation occurs, the placenta takes over progesterone production. If fertilisation does not take place, a pseudopregnant period starts, during which oestrus and ovulation do not occur for about 20 days. Fertilisation usually takes place in the ampulla or the upper portion of the oviduct and embryos are produced for 10–12 h post-ovulation. Mating is normally detected by formation of a vaginal plug (see Reproduction).

Gestation is normally 19–21 days. As a consequence of post-partum oestrus, lactation and gestation may occur simultaneously. However, lactation can delay gestation through delayed implantation, and this may prolong gestation for up to 12–13 days in certain inbred strains (Fox *et al.* 2002).

Nesting

As parturition approaches, female mice build a nest and spend time huddled in it. Thus, pregnant female mice should be provided with nesting material, such as soft paper (see housing section), which does not dehydrate the neonates.

Parturition

During the last 2 days of gestation, the female's nipples become prominent, mammary glands become distended and a slight mucus discharge from the vagina may be observed. Foetal movement that is obvious through the abdominal wall of the dam and foetal descent into the pelvic inlet are usually indicative of parturition within 12 h. The majority of births occur during the dark period.

Mice are born in either an anterior or posterior presentation. The female mouse normally walks around the cage during labour and delivery. After the pup is born, the female retrieves it, cleans it and places it in the nest. Pups and placentas are delivered simultaneously. Several minutes may elapse between the delivery of successive pups. Some females do not retrieve pups when they are born, but wait and retrieve them in groups. Primiparous females are more likely to reject litters than multiparous females.

Cannibalism of handled newborn mice can be minimised by ensuring that neonates are warm and free of blood and rubbed with bedding material from the home cage when they are returned to the nest; sedation of the dam may also be considered.

The young

The newborn mouse is relatively immature with closed eyes and ears and no fur (Figure 21.12). The development of external characteristics can be used to estimate the age of young mice (Table 21.2).

Maternal care can account for about 70% of the variation in body weight of neonatal mice. Milk production increases up to 12 days post-partum, and then declines until weaning at about 21 days. Transmission of passive immunity after birth by colostral antibodies has been demonstrated to a wide variety of antigens, including viruses, bacteria and parasites. Antibodies continue to be secreted in the milk throughout lactation (Fox *et al.* 2002). Milk uptake in newborn mice can be checked by looking at the 'milk spot', the milk-filled stomach of the young, showing through the furless skin of the belly.

Hand rearing of orphan or rejected newborn mice is not easy because of their small size, 4 h feeding schedule and susceptibility to temperature fluctuation. If the dam dies or lactation fails when the litter is about 14 days of age, placing a moistened or soft diet and water in the cage may improve survival of the pups. A powdered diet can be made by grinding pelleted mouse food and a soft diet can be made by soaking the pelleted feed in water. Small petri dishes make good disposable food or water containers. By 18–19 days of age, small pieces of pelleted food should replace part of the powdered or soft diet. By 21–24 days of age, normal pelleted food can be provided if the mice are able to reach the feeder.

Fostering newborn mice to other lactating females may be used for hysterectomy-derived neonates, when the dam has died or in certain teratological studies. The foster mother should deliver her litter 1–4 days before the anticipated birth of the litter that will be fostered. The foster mother is removed from her nest and placed in a separate cage. Her litter and the litter to be fostered are mingled together. The litter to be fostered is placed in the nest after being rubbed with soiled bedding material and the foster mother's litter removed. The foster mother is then returned to her cage but a few of the mother's pups may be left in the nest if the litter to be fostered contains only two or three pups and if each litter can be identified by, for example, coat colour. This procedure ensures that the litter size is adequate to maintain lactation. Research protocols may require partial exchange of litters between lactating female mice (cross-fostering). Age differences between litters to be cross-fostered should not exceed 4 days, and preferably should be only 1–2 days,

Table 21.2 Characteristics of mice from birth to 4 weeks of age.

Age	*Characteristics*
Birth	Blood-red skin colour
1 day	Lighter red skin colour. Milk visible in stomach (Figure 21.13)
2 days	Lighter skin colour. Ears flat against head
3 days	Ear elevated about 45° away from head, ears open
4 days	Ears elevated 90° away from head
5 days	Skin thicker. Milk no longer visible in stomach
6 days	Fur starts as a fine stubble over back (Figure 21.14)
7 days	Complete coat of fine fuzzy fur is visible
8 days	Lower incisors visible, but not erupted
9 days	Inguinal nipples visible in female
10 days	Lower incisors erupted
11 days	Upper incisors erupted
11–12 days	First solid food intake
11–14 days	Eyelids open. Slit-like palpebral opening
3 weeks	Oval palpebral opening, fine soft fur
4 weeks	Round palpebral opening, smooth fur
4–5 weeks	Vagina opens

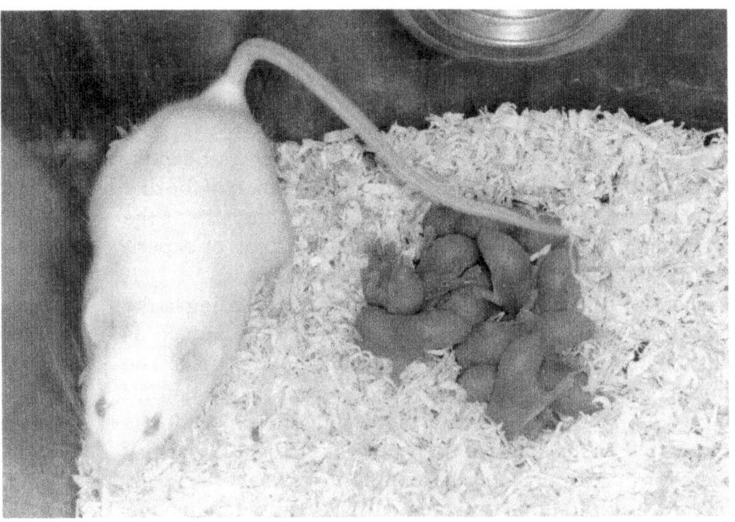

Figure 21.12 Mother with newborn mice. (Photo: T.P. Rooymans.)

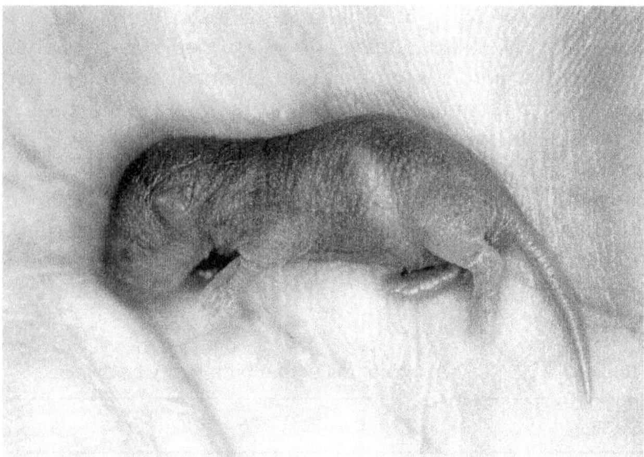

Figure 21.13 Young mouse, age 5 days. Note the milk spot. (Photo: T.P. Rooymans.)

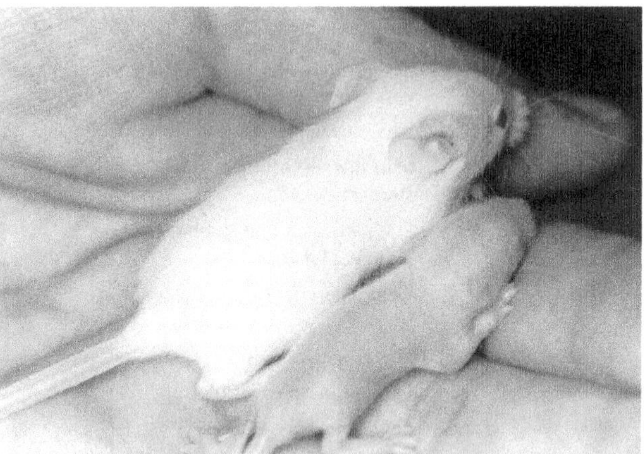

Figure 21.14 Young mice, aged 14 days and 6 days. (Photo: T.P. Rooymans.)

because larger, older pups will crowd out smaller younger pups as they compete for milk.

Mice are normally weaned at 3 weeks, when they start to eat pelleted food.

Feeding

Laboratory diets

The health status, performance and metabolism of experimental animals are influenced by the composition of the diet and the feeding practice. Thus, nutrition not only affects the well-being of the animals but also the outcome of experiments (see Beynen *et al.* 2001 and Chapter 14).

Diets for laboratory animals are classified according to the degree of refinement of the ingredients and are known as natural ingredient, purified or chemically defined diets. The most commonly used diets for laboratory mice are natural ingredient diets. In these diets, a minimum of processing is performed on the ingredients. Natural ingredient laboratory diets for mice are usually based upon one or more cereals or cereal by-products to which fats, protein, vitamins and minerals are added. The source of fat is usually vegetable oil, while protein sources include fish meal, milk solids and soybean meal. Nutrient concentration can vary considerably as a consequence of changes in the source of ingredients used in the manufacturing of the diet, as nutrient concentrations of natural ingredients are not fixed.

Chemically defined diets are often used in nutritional or toxicology studies. Chemically defined diets are formulated with pure chemicals, eg, individual amino acids replace whole proteins, which make the diets expensive. Purified diets are formulated with a combination of natural ingredients, pure chemicals and ingredients of varying degrees of refinement, for example, protein may be supplied as casein.

Mouse diets can be provided in pellet (compressed or expanded), meal and semi-moist or gel form. Pelleted diets are easy to feed and have minimal waste compared to the other forms of diets. Meal diets are used when test compounds must be added to the diet. The animals may waste large amounts and the diet has to be fed in the cage. Meal diets may be pelleted after the test compound is added if the compound is not heat- or moisture-sensitive. Gel-form diets are made by mixing equal parts agar and meal. These diets are often used in toxicological studies where it is important to incorporate dusty or highly toxic test compounds. Gel diets are easily contaminated by bacteria and should be stored under refrigeration.

Standard laboratory diets for mice are usually formulated either for maintenance of adult mice or for growth and reproduction. Maintenance diets are usually lower in fat (4–5%) compared to growth and reproduction diets (7–11%). Minimum protein levels range from 12–14% for maintenance and 17–19% for reproduction. Breeding female mice may be undernourished if fed on a maintenance diet, while adult mice that are not breeding may become overweight if maintained on growth and reproduction diets.

Different inbred strains of mice vary in their dietary requirements of protein, vitamins and minerals. Rapidly growing young mice and pregnant or lactating female mice have higher energy requirements than adult mice. Mice reared under germ-free or gnotobiotic conditions require higher dietary levels of B_{12} and K vitamins in order to compensate for losses during sterilisation of the diet and for the absence of B and K vitamin synthesis by intestinal microflora. SPF mice have additional requirements for vitamin K. The efficiency of feed utilisation can be altered by the number of mice per cage. Mice caged in groups of six to eight use food more efficiently than mice caged in smaller groups or caged individually (Cunliffe-Beamer & Les 1987).

The diet is a potential source of micro-organisms that can be pathogenic to laboratory animals. Food for gnotobiotic animals must be sterilised by either autoclaving or by gamma-radiation; food for SPF animals is also usually sterilised. Autoclaving causes some destruction of most of the vitamins and may denature proteins and cause the pellets to stick together (this situation can be improved by treating the pellets with talc powder). Irradiation is less damaging, although it causes some loss of vitamins, particularly vitamin K. Losses on irradiation are much greater in the presence of water, therefore moist diets or aqueous solutions should not be sterilised by gamma-radiation (Beynen *et al.* 2001).

Water

Drinking water is a potential source of pathogenic organisms, metals and organic chemicals. The type and amount of contamination will depend on the source of the drinking water. Tap water is not sterile and quickly becomes contaminated with even more bacteria after the bottle is placed on the cage. Water bottles may be contaminated if they are improperly washed or drinking tubes or bottles are in contact with saliva and faeces. Some mice push faeces and bedding into the drinking tube.

Water bottles and drinking tubes can be sources of *Pseudomonas aeruginosa* and other coliform bacteria. *P. aeruginosa* kills mice that have been immunosuppressed (by irradiation or other means) and has been associated with otitis media and encephalitis in recently shipped mice. Autoclaving filled water bottles and drinking tubes eliminates bacterial contamination arising from the source of the water or from ineffectively washed bottles or tubes; however, autoclaving does not prevent in-use contamination of the water. Bacterial contamination can be controlled by acidification (pH 2–3) or chlorination (15–20 parts per million active chloride).

The concentration of metals and organic chemicals in drinking water will vary with the source and type of pipe used to transport the water. Trace elements and heavy metals and organic chemicals can be sources of contamination or confounding variables in nutritional or toxicological experiments. Chemical contaminants can be removed by reverse osmosis, deionisation or microfiltration.

Laboratory procedures

Handling and restraint

Mice can be caught inside the cage by grasping the base of the tail with the thumb and index finger; they can be picked up by the tail and transferred to, for example, a clean cage (Figure 21.15). When holding a mouse by the tail, its weight should be supported on a surface such as the opposite arm or cage lid rather than allowing it to dangle. The tail must not be held by the tip as this may cause the skin to be sloughed off. However, J.L. Hurst and colleagues (data in preparation) have recently reported that mice picked up and held by the tail (while supporting their weight on the arm or hand) subsequently attempt to avoid contact with the handler and show much stronger anxiety in standard tests than those picked up and held by one of three alternative methods for routine handling: cupped directly on the open hand, handled indirectly in a home cage tunnel or picked up in a tunnel and transferred to the open hand. They report that mice handled using these alternative methods rapidly become tame to human contact, spending much time voluntarily interacting with the handler after only a few handling experiences as well as showing low anxiety in standard tests. If the animal needs to be restrained, it should be placed on a rough surface, such as the cage lid. The loose skin of the neck between the ears can be held between thumb and index finger of the other hand (Figure 21.16). The mouse is lifted and the tail is secured between the fourth or fifth finger and the palm of the hand. This technique leaves one hand free for injections or other procedures (Figure 21.17).

One should be careful not to pull the skin too tightly, as the mouse may be choked. One should always watch the colour of the mucous membranes of the nose and mouth for that reason. Neonatal mice (less than 2 weeks of age) are picked up by grasping the loose skin over neck and shoulders with thumb and index finger.

Strains of mice differ in temperament. Some strains are very calm and rarely try to bite or escape, for example BALB/c, while others are 'nervous' and can jump 'like popcorn', such as C57BL. All mice go through a 'jumpy' stage at about 3 weeks of age. Working with mice should always be done quickly, quietly and gently.

Plastic or metal devices to restrain mice for procedures such as tail vein injections, blood pressure measurements or irradiation can be manufactured (Figure 21.18). Training mice to be handled might reduce stress, by using alternative handling techniques that avoid picking up mice by the tail and encourage voluntary interaction with the handler (see earlier in this section). However, restraint will always cause more or less stress (Meijer 2006).

Unnecessary disturbance or manipulation of a post-parturient female and her litter should be avoided for the

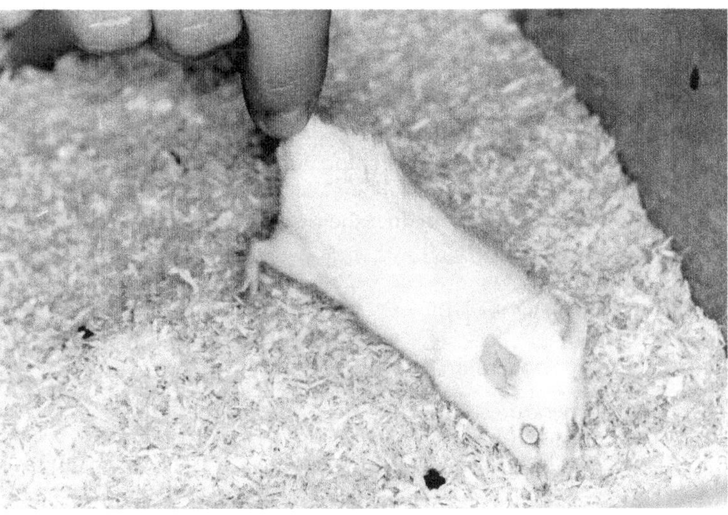

Figure 21.15 Lifting a mouse from the cage. (Photo: T.P. Rooymans.)

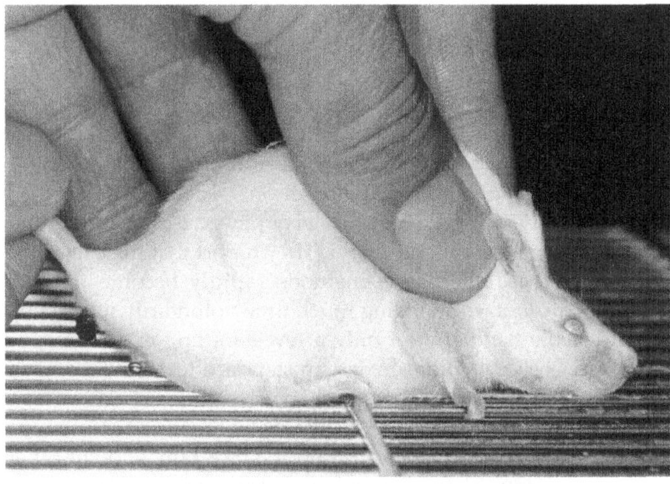

Figure 21.16 Restraint of a mouse. (Photo: T.P. Rooymans.)

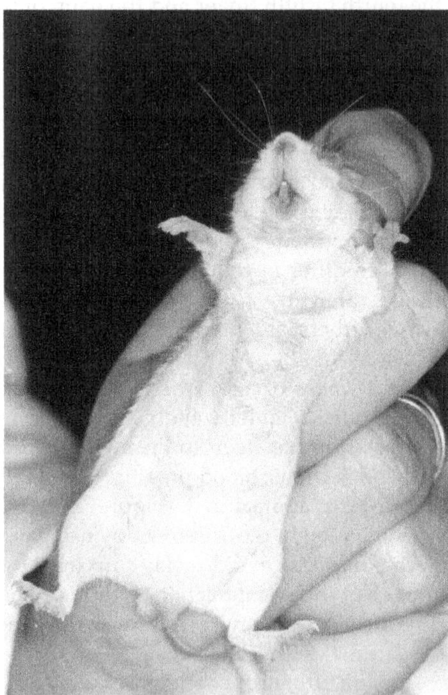

Figure 21.17 Restraint of a mouse. (Photo: T.P. Rooymans.)

first few days following birth. If handling of neonates cannot be avoided, the risk of cannibalism or rejection of the litter can be reduced by gentle handling of the dam and offspring, placing the dam in a separate cage while the litter is being handled, and wearing plastic gloves in order to prevent the neonates from acquiring human scent. Rubbing the pups with bedding material from the home cage when they are returned to the nest can also reduce the risk of cannibalism.

Physiological monitoring

Recording body temperature

The rectal temperatures of healthy mice vary in the range 36.5–38 °C and can be measured by inserting a thermocouple into the rectum. Rectal temperature is influenced by environmental temperature, age, strain and stress (eg, restraint).

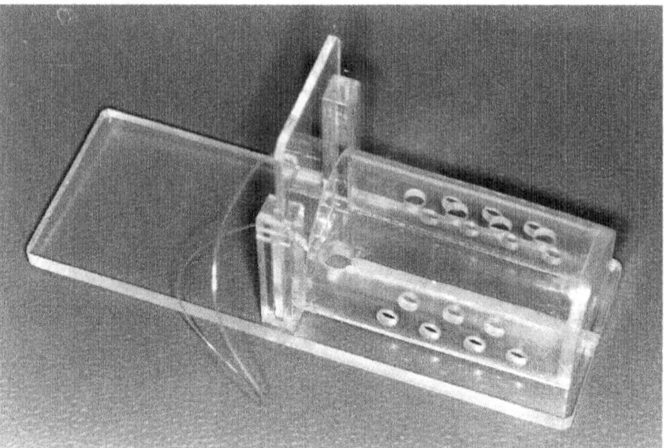

Figure 21.18 Plastic device for restraining mice. (Photo: T.P. Rooymans.)

Core temperature can also be measured by using telemetry. Although the transmitter, which has to be placed in the abdominal cavity, is still rather big for a mouse, it has been shown that behaviour and bodyweight return to normal within 10 days after implantation (Baumans *et al.* 2001a). This method has already been used to record mouse core temperature, heart rate and activity. Once the device has been implanted, measuring seems to be a stress-free method in the freely moving animal (Kramer *et al.* 1993; Meijer *et al.* 2006).

Collection of specimens

Collection of blood

General advice on blood sampling can be found in JWGR (1993). The total volume of blood in a living mouse is rather constant and is about 8% of its body weight. If the volume of a sample withdrawn exceeds 10% of the total blood volume, hypovolaemia and cardiovascular failure ('shock') may occur. As a general rule, a maximum of approximately 8 ml/kg bodyweight of blood can be removed from a live mouse every 2 weeks (Baumans *et al.* 2001b; Pekow & Baumans 2002). Blood samples can be obtained from various sites of the body, using a variety of methods. The choice of the method will depend upon several factors, such as the purpose of blood collection (arterial, venous or a mixture of the two), the duration and frequency of sampling and whether or not it concerns a terminal experiment. Samples obtained from various methods will not be identical with respect to cellular or other constituents. Anaesthesia may be required for some methods.

Blood samples can be collected from various sites:

- Small volumes of blood (for example for a smear) may be obtained by snipping off the very tip of the tail, which will result in a mixture of venous and arterial blood, together with tissue fluid. This method is suitable when small samples are required every few hours. The scab on the tail wound can easily be removed.
- The lateral tail vein can be punctured with a 0.6–1.0 mm needle after warming of the tail in warm water, under a heating lamp or in a climatic chamber (Figure 21.19). The mouse can be anaesthetised or placed in a restraining device. The ventral tail artery can be used in the same way. Using razor blades to cut the vein may prolong bleeding and create scar tissue, but the yield may be higher.
- The lateral saphenous vein can be punctured in the restrained mouse in the same way (Figure 21.20).
- Blood can be aspirated from the jugular vein, mostly by surgical exposure of the vein under anaesthesia, which provides a sterile blood sample.

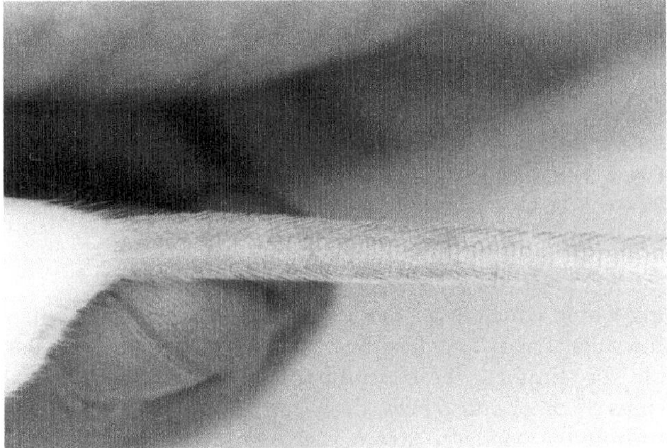

Figure 21.19 Lateral tail vein. (Photo: T.P. Rooymans.)

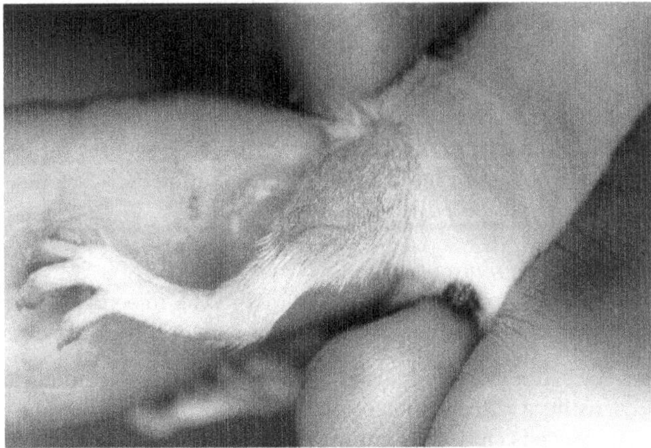

Figure 21.20 Lateral saphenous vein. (Photo: T.P. Rooymans.)

- Arterial blood can be obtained from the abdominal aorta, brachial artery or carotid artery under anaesthesia.
- Puncture of the orbital blood vessels. For this procedure the anaesthetised animal is firmly held by the skin at the nape of the neck, which causes distension of the jugular vein. A fine glass tube or a Pasteur's pipette is then placed at the inner canthus of the eye and gently advanced alongside the globe into the vessels. The tube ruptures the vessels and blood can be withdrawn by capillary action. Contamination with tissue fluids and porphyrins from the Harderian gland can occur. It is not possible to take sterile blood samples using this method. Also complications, such as haemorrhage, inflammation and blindness, may occur, especially when the same eye is used repeatedly. Moreover, this technique may be aesthetically unpleasant for the operator to perform. For these reasons, this method is not considered acceptable in some countries (Baumans *et al.* 2001b) and is generally not recommended. However, the extent of trauma is proportional to the skill of the technician.
- Submandibular bleeding from the facial vein (Golde *et al.* 2005). This technique is now getting more popular; however, it should be performed under anaesthesia and haemorrhage or damage of the facial nerve and artery may occur.
- Cardiac puncture. In this method, blood is collected directly from the ventricle of the heart of the anaesthetised animal. Puncturing the atrium can be dangerous, due to the risk of leakage into the pericardium, resulting in cardiac arrest and death. When the animal has to survive the procedure, these risks must be taken into account.
- Implantation of indwelling cannulae can be used when repeated blood sampling is required. The indwelling catheter can be implanted via the jugular vein into the cranial vena cava and exteriorised at the top of the head, where it is secured with screws and acrylic glue or between the shoulders. The catheter's dead space is usually filled with with a substance containing heparin.
- Exsanguination. To obtain the maximum amount of blood, decapitation can be performed using a guillotine or scissors, or by puncturing the aorta under anaesthesia. In this way about 30 ml/kg body weight or up to 50% of the total blood volume can be obtained. Exsanguination is also possible by removing the eyeball under anaesthesia and collecting blood from the eye artery.

Collection of faeces and urine

Mice often urinate and/or defecate purely as a result of being handled, which may provide the opportunity for collecting small samples of urine and faeces. Placing the animal in a plastic bucket will result in urination and urine can be collected with a syringe (van Loo *et al.* 2003; Meijer *et al.* 2006). Metabolic cages must be used for the quantitative collection of urine and faeces. The animals are housed on a grid above a funnel in which the urine and/or faeces are collected and separated (Figure 21.21).

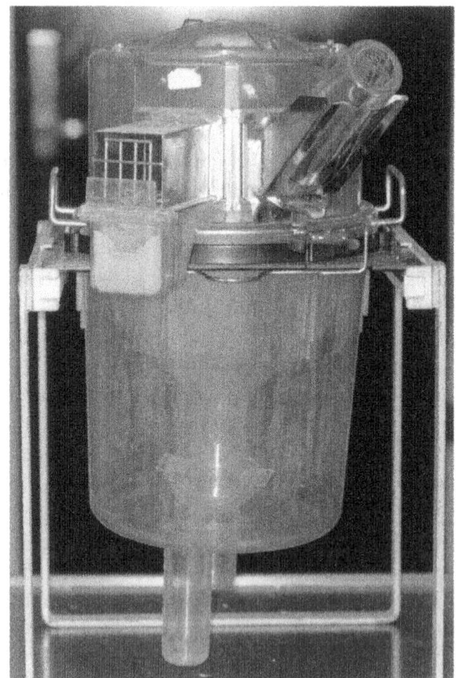

Figure 21.21 Metabolism cage with food hopper, water bottle and funnel. (Photo: T.P. Rooymans.)

Collection of milk
Mouse milk can be collected using milking 'machines' with single or multiple teat cups. Prior to milking, the lactating female is separated from her litter for 8–12h. Then, the mammary glands are washed with warm water and the mouse may be injected subcutaneously with oxytocin to stimulate milk flow.

Collection of sperm
Sperm for artificial insemination is usually obtained from the epididymides of a recently killed male mouse. However, electroejaculation of male mice has been described. A balanced salt solution with glucose should be used to dilute mouse semen (Cunliffe-Beamer & Les 1987; Hedrich & Bullock 2004).

Administration of substances

Dosing and injection procedures

General advice on the administration of substances can be found in JWGR (2001). Three methods for the administration of substances can be distinguished: via skin, enteral and parenteral (Baumans *et al.* 2001b).

Application to skin or mucous membranes
The substance is applied in solution or as ointment on shaven skin or mucous membranes. This method is inaccurate and may cause discomfort to the mouse if the substance is irritating.

Enteral administration
Enteral administration means that the substance is brought into the gastrointestinal tract orally through food or drinking water, which is not very accurate and impossible when the substance is unpalatable, insoluble or chemically unstable. To stimulate the consumption of, for example, medicines or other substances, these can be administered in fat drippings, raspberry cream, yoghurt sweets or chocolate which are highly appreciated by mice.

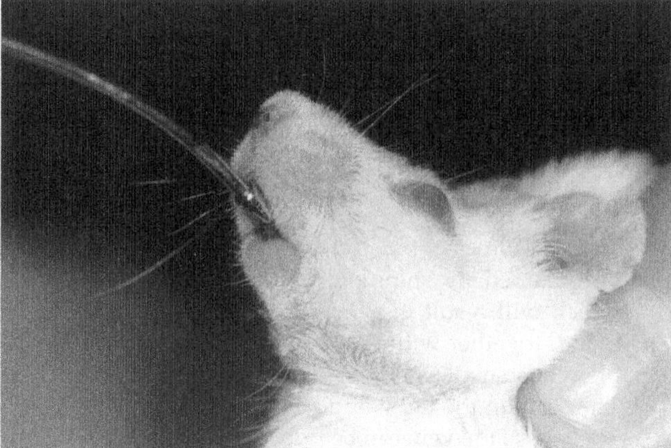

Figure 21.22 Administration of substances via stomach/oesophageal tube. (Photo: T.P. Rooymans.)

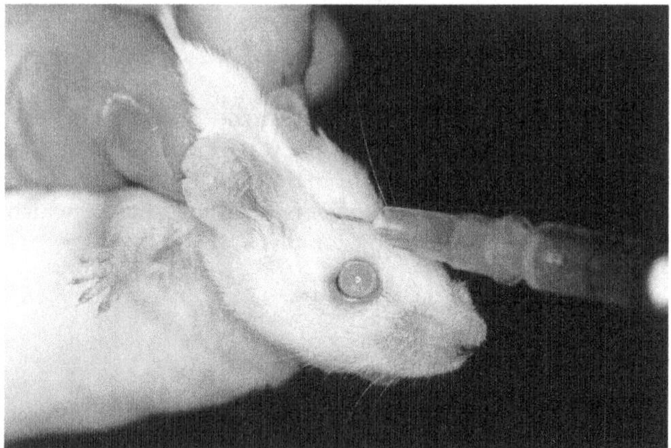

Figure 21.23 Subcutaneous injection under the skin of the neck. (Photo: T.P. Rooymans.)

Administration via a stomach/oesophageal tube is more accurate and can be performed by a curved needle with a blunt end (external diameter 0.8mm), such as an infant lacrimal sac canula (Figure 21.22). The mouse is held firmly by the scruff whilst passing the needle along the palate into the oesophagus. The animal should be allowed to 'swallow' the needle. As the head is directed upwards, the risk of entering the trachea is minimal. The maximum volume to be administered should be 0.25–0.5ml.

Parenteral administration
Parenteral administration refers mainly to injections. The most frequently used injection techniques in the mouse are:

- Subcutaneous (sc): usually under the skin of the neck using a 0.45mm needle (26G). Resorption of the substance is slow. Maximum volume to be administered is 0.25–0.5ml (Figure 21.23).

- Intramuscular (im) injections are usually avoided in the mouse because of its small muscle mass. If necessary, intramuscular injections of 0.05 ml or less may be made into the lateral thigh muscles using a 0.40 mm needle (27G). The tip of the needle should be directed away from the femur and sciatic nerve.
- Intraperitoneal (ip) injections may cause damage to the internal organs. To avoid the urinary bladder the injection should be given slightly off the midline. The needle should neither be inserted horizontally (between the skin and the abdominal wall) nor vertically (risking damage to the kidney). The injection should be given in the lower left or right quadrant of the abdomen. There is a slight risk of causing damage to the intestines (mainly due to their mobility) (Figure 21.24). To be sure the procedure has been carried out properly, the plunger must be retracted to determine whether any urine, intestinal contents or blood have been aspirated. The maximum volume to administer is 0.5–1.0 ml with a 0.45 mm needle (26G) (Baumans *et al.* 2001b; Pekow & Baumans 2002).
- Intravenous (iv) injection into the tail vein is usually the fastest and most accurate method, but requires more technical skill. The maximum volume to administer as bolus is 0.125 ml with a 0.45 mm (26G) or 0.50 mm (25G) needle. For preparation of the vein see section Collection of blood.

Points of special attention when carrying out these procedures are:

- Use clean, sharp, short and sterile needles.
- Use an appropriate needle size. A thin needle causes less pain and prevents the fluid from flowing back. The required thickness of the needle (gauge) will depend upon the viscosity of the fluid. When using very thin needles, there is a risk of cracking. On the other hand larger needle sizes for viscous injections require shorter injection time and because of shorter restraint time appear to be less distressing to the animal (Barclay *et al.* 1988).
- Never inject more fluid than the recommended maximum volume.
- Avoid air bubbles in the injection fluid (which can cause embolism).
- The injection fluid must be brought to room or body temperature prior to use.
- Some injection fluids can cause tissue irritation, for example, high or low pH, and should therefore be administered after having been diluted with saline. These substances should, preferably, be given intravenously, as they quickly become diluted in the blood. When using the ip route, dilution also occurs, but there is a risk of peritonitis (Baumans *et al.* 2001b).

Anaesthesia and analgesia

The principles of anaesthesia/analgesia and an overview of substances and dosages are described by Flecknell (1996, 2009). Pain occurring during surgical procedures can be prevented by the use of appropriate anaesthetic techniques. Most anaesthetics affect many body systems, and so may interact with experiments. To minimise such interactions, anaesthetic regimens should be selected with care, by considering the pharmacology of the drugs involved. Uncontrolled pain may interact with the experimental procedures.

A variety of anaesthetics can be used, depending on the type, duration and purpose of the experiment, strain and age of the mouse and the skill of the personnel. An ideal anaesthetic should induce a stable anaesthesia, be easy to administer, not influence physiology, be reversible and be safe for the animal and personnel.

General anaesthesia can be produced by inhalational agents such as halothane, isoflurane and ether. (The latter is generally not recommended and banned in some countries for the irritant properties to mucous membranes and the induced excitation which is unpleasant for the animal. Its explosive properties also make it a safety hazard.) Anaesthesia can also be produced by injectable agents such as pentobarbitone, ketamine and fentanyl/fluanisone plus midazolam.

Personnel anaesthetising mice with volatile anaesthetics should be aware of the hazards associated with prolonged exposure to these agents. The facemasks that are used to

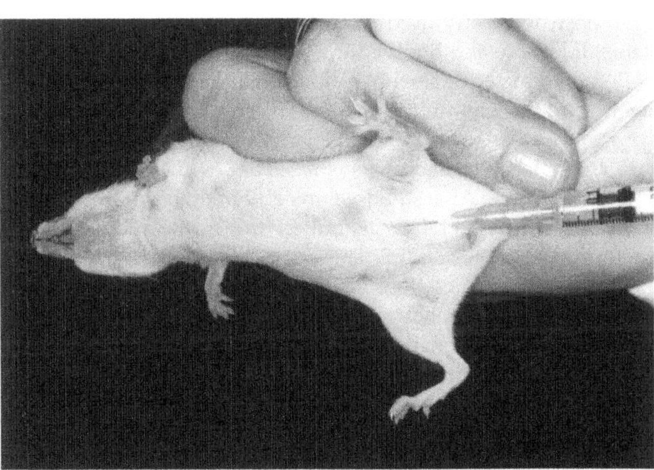

Figure 21.24 Intraperitoneal injection. (Photo: T.P. Rooymans.)

administer inhalant anaesthetics to mice usually leak the anaesthetic agent into the surrounding environment. The exposure to personnel can be reduced by placing the anaesthetic apparatus inside a fume hood or preferably by ducting the vapours to the outside using a suitable scavenging system.

The following are recommended for anaesthetising mice (see also Flecknell (2009)):

- Fentanyl/fluanisone (Hypnorm, Janssen) (0.4 ml/kg ip) with midazolam or diazepam (5 mg/kg ip). When using midazolam the components are mixed with water for injection. This anaesthetic mixture provides anaesthesia for 30–40 minutes and can be reversed partially by nalbuphine (4 mg/kg ip or sc).
- Ketamine (75 mg/kg ip) can also be used in a mixture with medetomidine (1.0 mg/kg ip), mixed in one syringe. This combination can be partially reversed by atipamezole (1 mg/kg sc). Another combination is ketamine (80–100 mg/kg ip) and xylazine (10 mg/kg ip) administered together as a single ip injection and reversed by atipamezole (1 mg/kg sc). Both of these mixtures provide moderate anaesthesia for 20–30 minutes, but are often insufficient for major surgery (Flecknell 1996).
- Pentobarbital is not a drug of choice in major surgery on account of its inadequate analgesic properties. When it is used, it should be administered at a dosage of 40–50 mg/kg ip. Overdosage or underdosage occur frequently (Flecknell 1996) and dilution may be useful to prevent peritoneal irritation.
- Inhalation anaesthesia can be achieved with halothane, isoflurane or enflurane using an anaesthetic chamber. Atropine (0.04 mg/kg sc, ip) can be administered to reduce salivation.

Local anaesthetics are used for anaesthesia of specific parts of the body, while the animal remains conscious. Local anaesthesia in the mouse is usually restricted to:

- surface anaesthesia, where the local anaesthetic is applied to the skin or mucous membranes as a gel, spray or cream;
- local infiltration of a local anaesthetic into the deeper layers of tissue, which can be used for procedures such as skin biopsies.

The most frequently used local anaesthetic agents are procaine, lidocaine and bupivacaine.

Before inducing anaesthesia, the animal should be in good health and sufficiently acclimatised to an experimental environment. Pre-anaesthetic fasting is unnecessary and undesirable in mice (Hellebrekers *et al.* 2001) as they show no vomit response. Anaesthetised mice should be placed in their cages in a lateral or ventral recumbent position with the head slightly extended. This position minimises aspiration of salivary secretions and reduces the intrathoracic pressure caused by abdominal viscera pressing against the diaphragm. If prolonged surgical procedures or recovery periods are anticipated, sterile physiological saline or balanced salt solutions should be administered sc or ip (0.5–1 ml per 15–25 g body weight).

The depth of anaesthesia can be estimated by:

- the righting reflex: the animal turns over to a position on its feet after being placed on its back;
- the pedal withdrawal reflex, when a digit or interdigital skin is pinched;
- movement of whiskers and ears in response to a puff of air.

Opthalmic ointment or artificial tears should be used to prevent drying of the cornea during anaesthesia.

Post-operative pain, and pain occurring as a result of non-surgical experimental procedures, can be alleviated by the administration of analgesics. In order to control pain effectively, it is essential to be able to assess the degree of pain that is being experienced by the animal. Post-operative care should be provided. This is likely to include: analgesics and fluids; a quiet, warm place, such as an incubator, intensive care unit or a cage provided with a heating pad or lamp to maintain body temperature; and observation and attention by skilled personnel. Monitoring of urine output and defecation gives an indication of the hydration status and condition of the gastrointestinal tract, respectively. Behavioural scoring systems and food and water intake can be used in the assessment of pain in the animal post-operatively. Twitching, flinching, stretching, reduced climbing and locomotion can be seen (Baumans *et al.* 1994; Baumans & Brain 2001; Roughan & Flecknell 2003; van Loo *et al.* 2007; National Research Council 2008) and reduced nest building can be observed (Arras *et al.* 2007; van Loo *et al.* 2007). It has been demonstrated in humans that effective analgesia reduces the time needed for post-operative recovery (Flecknell 1996; Hellebrekers *et al.* 2001, see also Flecknell 2009)).

The following analgesics can be used in the mouse (Flecknell 1996; Hellebrekers *et al.* 2001):

- non-steroidal anti-inflammatory drugs (NSAIDs), such as carprofen (5 mg/kg sc, 12 hourly), aspirin (120 mg/kg per os 4 hourly) and flunixin (2.5 mg/kg sc, im, 12 hourly);
- opioid analgesics, such as buprenorphine (0.05–0.1 mg/kg sc, 12 hourly).

Surgical procedures in mice require aseptic conditions (sterile instruments, cap, mask, gown and gloves). The mouse's hair can be removed by shaving and the skin decontaminated with 70% alcohol or povidone–iodine. Tissues should be handled using a 'no touch' technique. This means that only the tips of the surgical instruments touch the mouse and surgical instruments are returned to a sterile surface between successive procedures.

Endpoints

It is important to determine humane endpoints (the humane killing of animals at a stage that the first signs of approaching death are recognised). The animal would benefit, as unnecessary suffering is avoided or reduced, and also researchers would benefit as the scientific results would be more valid, data being less variable and timely collection of samples being scheduled. Clinical signs that can help to determine humane endpoints are rapid weight loss (15–20%), prolonged diarrhoea, nasal discharge, coughing, neoplasia accounting for 10–20% bodyweight, self-mutilation, central nervous system signs, severe ulceration or bleeding, drop in body temperature >4 °C, inability to ambulate, laboured breathing and cyanosis. A pilot study may help specify humane endpoints in particular experiments (Baumans *et al.* 1994; Hendriksen & Morton 1999; Morton & Hau 2003).

Euthanasia

Mice are killed in the laboratory at the end of an experiment, to provide blood and other tissues, to counter suffering when it exceeds an acceptable level, when they are no longer suitable for breeding or when there is surplus stock.

The 1986 Council Directive of the EEC on the protection of animals used for experimental and other scientific purposes (86/609/EEC) requires humane killing of experimental animals, with a minimum of physical and mental suffering. Methods of euthanasia should be painless, achieve rapid unconsciousness and death, require minimum restraint, avoid excitement, be appropriate for the age, species and health of the animal, must minimise fear and psychological stress in the animal, be reliable, reproducible, irreversible, simple to administer and safe for the personnel and (if possible) aesthetically acceptable. It is important that personnel are trained and experienced in recognising and confirming death in the animals (EC Working Party reports on euthanasia of experimental animals 1996, 1997).

Acceptable methods of euthanasia in mice are:

- Stunning by a blow on the head, followed by exsanguination.
- Cervical dislocation, in which the cervical vertebrae are separated from the skull using a pencil or similar placed in the neck and followed by a pull on the tail base.
- Decapitation, by guillotine or scissors although this method is still under discussion with regard to the onset of unconsciousness.
- Inhalational anaesthetics such as halothane, enflurane and isoflurane in overdose.
- Carbon dioxide >70%, which may cause excitation and stress, due to irritation of the mucous membranes and the induced hypoxia. The animal is placed in a chamber either prefilled with the gas, which will cause a short-lasting distress, but seems to result in a rapid loss of consciousness, or exposed to rising concentrations which seem to cause less distress but prolong consciousness. The optimal filling rate is still uncertain and prefill and rising concentrations both can cause welfare problems. However, rats exposed to carbon dioxide in their home cage instead of in a gas chamber did not show signs of distress (Hackbarth *et al.* 2000). There is still some discussion as to whether the addition of oxygen to high carbon dioxide concentrations contributes to the animal's welfare; it may reduce but not overcome welfare problems. It is also possible that high oxygen would prolong consciousness. It is clear that further studies are needed in this respect (Newcastle Consensus meeting on Carbon Dioxide Euthanasia of Laboratory Animals 2006).
- Sodium pentobarbital, iv or ip. The agent should be diluted for ip injection to prevent irritation and pain to the peritoneum.

Killing methods acceptable for use in unconscious mice include rapid freezing, exsanguination or potassium chloride injection.

If a foetus is removed from the anaesthetised mother, it may be killed by decapitation. Foetuses not anaesthetised prior to removal from the mother may be killed by rapid cooling in liquid nitrogen. Newborn mice can be killed by stunning or decapitation (EC Working Party reports on euthanasia of experimental animals 1996, 1997).

Common welfare problems

Disease

Signs of disease

Signs associated with disease include withdrawal from the group, hunched-up position, ruffled fur, sunken eyes, reduced growth rate, emaciation, diarrhoea, 'chattering' (a clicking sound associated with severe respiratory infections), laboured breathing, cyanotic or pale extremities, reduction in the number of offspring born or weaned, reduction in the number of breeding pairs producing offspring or increased mortality (Figure 21.25). However, many infectious diseases of mice cause few, if any, obvious signs of disease. These latent infections can have a significant impact on experiment results, as they do not cause clinical signs in infected mice, but they can alter histology or immune responses. *Pseudomonas aeruginosa* can be present in the intestine of mice without any apparent ill effects. However, if these same mice are irradiated or subjected to other immunosuppressive procedures, *P. aeruginosa* can cause a fatal septicaemia.

The signs associated with an infection, especially viral infections, vary depending upon strain, age and microflora of the mouse, previous exposure of the mouse to the infectious agent and the strain of the infectious agent.

To make a correct diagnosis of a disease, specific skills and experience in pathology and related disciplines including microbiology are needed. A complete diagnostic examination should include the history of the disease (sex, age, strain, microbiological status, source, use, performed procedures), environment, clinical signs, such as general condition, respiratory system, circulatory system and locomotion; also additional information from blood samples, urine, skin scrapings etc, *post-mortem* and microbiological examination (eg, histology, detection of antibodies) (van Dijk *et al.* 2001).

Common diseases

Tables 21.3, 21.4 and 21.5 contain lists of the major viral, bacterial and parasitic infections of mice. Specialists in laboratory animal medicine should be consulted to develop a disease-control programme.

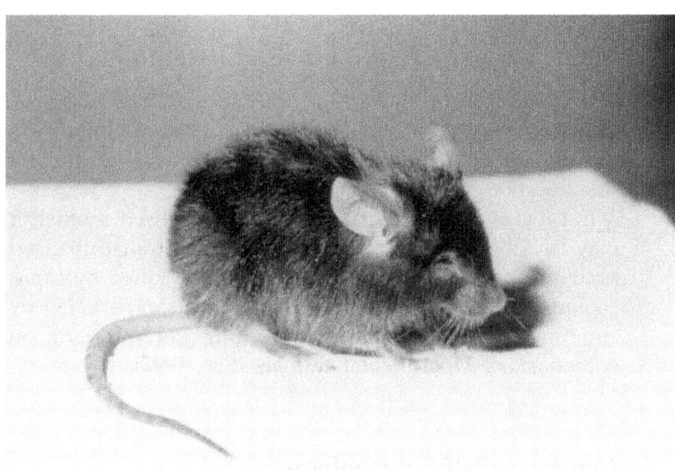

Figure 21.25 A sick mouse with sunken eyes, ruffled fur and a hunched up position. (Photo: T.P. Rooymans.)

Prophylaxis

Genetic and environmental factors play an important role in the causation of disease. Genetic factors are involved in disease susceptibility, eg, differences between mouse strains in tumour incidence (BALB/c, CBA, DBA/2) and myocardial calcification (C57BL/6). Environmental factors, eg, nutrition, husbandry, infections and other noxious agents can contribute to the causes of disease. Hygiene and improvement of the microbiological status will reduce the incidence of infections dramatically. Good management with health-monitoring programmes, knowledge of the biology of animals and epidemiology of diseases is a prerequisite (see Health monitoring, quarantine and barrier systems).

Key elements in an effective disease-control programme for mouse colonies are:

- microbiological assessment of breeding colonies;
- microbiological assessment of cell lines, transplantable tumours or other biological materials;
- development of standardised husbandry procedures that minimise transmission of infections between cages and between rooms;
- microbiological and mechanical monitoring of cage washing equipment, autoclaves and environmental conditions;
- understanding and controlling personnel (see Health monitoring, quarantine and barrier systems).

Abnormal behaviour

An important concept in the well-being of animals is homeostasis, which implies that the animal is in harmony with its internal and external environment and is able to keep that environment controllable and predictable. When homeostasis cannot be maintained, discomfort or stress may occur, which can become manifest as a disease or abnormal behaviour, such as the development of stereotypies.

Stereotypies can be defined as repeated, simple behavioural patterns, which seem to be meaningless and are typical of the individual animal, such as circling movements or constant jumping in the cage (Baumans 2005a). Whether stereotypy is a sign of abnormal brain function, or whether it is 'merely' a sign of chronic frustration, which is still a serious welfare problem, stereotypy is likely to be associated with differing stress responses between individuals (Garner & Mason 2002). Minimal responses or lack of reaction to stimuli (apathy) can also be considered as abnormal behaviour. Together with clinical and physiological parameters, abnormal behaviour may indicate that the well-being of the animal is compromised.

Reproductive problems

Reproductive problems may be caused by internal factors, such as: diseases and infections, eg pyometra in female mice or inflammation of the seminal vesicles in the male; chemicals, oestrogenic stimulation by oestrogen-like substances in the diet; immaturity or senescence; nutritional restriction; disturbances of maternal care, such as cannibalism, neglect of the young, insufficient milk production; or environmental factors, such as high (>28 °C) or low (<10 °C) temperatures in the cage, bedding containing fine particles (which may cause preputial inflammation in the male, preventing mating), deprivation of nesting material, noise and disturbance in the animal room (which may prevent mating or cause cannibalism or neglect of the newborn young) and overcrowding (Harkness & Wagner 1995). During the process of inbreeding a decline in reproductive performance may occur.

Acknowledgement

All photographs in this chapter are by T.P. Rooymans.

Table 21.3 Viral diseases of mice (Cunliffe-Beamer & Les 1987; O'Brien & Holmer 1993; Boot *et al.* 2001; FELASA 2002; Fox *et al.* 2002) (ELISA, enzyme-linked immunosorbent assay; HAR, haemagglutination reaction; IB, immunoblot; IFA, indirect immunofluorescence assay; LDH, lactate dehydrogenase; PCR, polymerase chain reaction; VN, virus neutralisation).

Name (synonyms: virus family)	*Incidence*	*Clinical signs*	*Pathological lesions*	*Diagnosis (suitable tests methods)**	*Control*	*Transmission of infection*	*Comments*
Mouse coronavirus							
Mouse hepatitis virus (MHV)	Frequent	Acute, inapparent infection, wasting disease in nude or thymectomised mice, diarrhoea (often fatal) in suckling mice or immunodeficient mice, ruffled fur, inactivity, dehydration, immunomodulatory effects	1. Respiratory pattern: replication in upper respiratory mucosa with dissemination to multiple organs in susceptible hosts including liver leading to multifocal necrotising hepatitis 2. Enteric pattern: bowel infection with the formation of multinucleate syncytial giant cells pathognomonic	ELISA, IFA	Self-limiting in immune competent mice; hysterectomy derivation; cessation of breeding	Air-borne, direct contact. Biological products	Chronic intestinal carriers, neurotrophic, hepatotrophic and enterotrophic strains of virus, alters immune responses
Parvovirus							
Minute virus of mice (MVM)	Frequent	Inapparent infection, infection of neonates retards growth, diarrhoea. Neuropathogenic in suckling mice	None, mild hypoplasia of external germinal layer of cerebellum, renal infarcts. Foetal resorption	ELISA, IFA, IB, VN	Hysterectomy derivation	Chronic carriers. Contact with infected mouse, urine, faeces	Chronic renal carriers, alters immunological responses and tumour development
Mouse parvovirus (MPV)	Frequent	Inapparent infection	Lymphocytotropism	ELISA, IFA, IB, VN	Hysterectomy derivation	Chronic carriers. Contact with infected mouse, urine, faeces	Chronic renal carriers, alters immunological responses and tumour development
Paramyxovirus							
Sendai (SV)	Frequent	No pathology in natural infections. Inapparent infection, ruffled fur, sometimes catarrhal bronchitis, dyspnoea, death in young mice. 129/J and DBA/2 strain more sensitive. Often complicated by secondary infections (*Pasteurella*)	Interstitial pneumonia with necrosis followed by marked squamous metaplasia of bronchial epithelium	ELISA, IFA	Vaccination for small numbers of animals, select breeders with antibody, hysterectomy derivation	Extremely contagious. Direct contact, aerosols biological products. Cessation of breeding and no introduction of new stock may be effective in elimination	Acute self-limiting infection in immunocompetent mice, post-infection alteration of immune responses. Influence on foetal development
Pneumonia virus of mice (PVM)	Moderate	Inapparent infection	Interstitial pneumonia, mild bronchial reactions compared to Sendai virus infection	ELISA, IFA, PCR	Select breeders with antibody, improve ventilation, hysterectomy derivation	Aerosols, direct contact	Acute self-limiting infection (pneumonia) in immunocompetent mice

Table 21.3 *Continued*

Name (synonyms: virus family)	*Incidence*	*Clinical signs*	*Pathological lesions*	*Diagnosis (suitable tests methods)**	*Control*	*Transmission of infection*	*Comments*
Rotavirus							
Epizootic diarrhoea of infant mice (EDIM); mouse rotavirus enteritis	Moderate	Acute, mild to severe watery yellow diarrhoea with constipation in 7–16-day-old mice, no signs in adult mice	Colon and caecum distended, mucoid yellow or grey–green content, vacuolated epithelium, no inflammation	ELISA, IFA	Hysterectomy derivation, filter covers on cages combined with culling of infected litters	Air-borne. Cessation of breeding and no introduction of new stock may be effective in elimination	Self-limiting infection
Arenavirus							
Lymphocytic choriomeningitis virus[*] (LCMV)	Moderate	Congenital or neonatal infection: inapparent infection with late onset immune complex disease, runting, some mortality. Infection in adult: clonic convulsion, tremors, die or recover within 3–6 days	Lymphoid infiltrate in choroid plexus, proliferation of lymphoid cells and lymphocytolysis, in spleen and lymph nodes, vacuolar degeneration of neurones. Necrosis of lymphoid and hepatic tissue	ELISA, IFA	Prevent wild mice from entering premises, select non-viraemic breeders, destroy carriers	Vertical transmission. Zoonosis	Clinical signs vary with age, genotype, viral strain and route of inoculation, lifelong viraemia in persistently infected mice, alters immunological responses. Infects endocrine glands
Herpesvirus							
Mouse cytomegalovirus (MCMV)	Moderate	Inapparent infection, suppression of immune system	Intranuclear inclusion in salivary gland duct epithelium and spleen, experimental disease produces a variety of lesions	ELISA, IFA	Filter covers on cages, prevent wild mice from entering premises	Close contact; may be vertical	Natural infection of laboratory mice is infrequent, virus excreted in saliva
Mouse thymic virus (MTV)	Rare	None in natural or experimental infection	Thymic necrosis if inoculated into mice less than 10 days old	ELISA, IFA	Prevent wild mice from entering premises	Chronic infection	Virus can be isolated from salivary glands and saliva of adult mice, susceptibility of inbred strains varies
Picornavirus							
Theiler's mouse encephalomyelitis virus (TMEV), mouse polio	Moderate	Inapparent infection, flaccid paralysis of hindlegs may occur	No macroscopic lesions, acute necrosis of ganglion cells in anterior horn	ELISA, IFA	Foster nursing, hysterectomy derivation	Faecal–oral route	Virus shed in faeces, experimental infections result in encephalitis or demyelination
Orthopox virus							
Ectromelia, mouse pox	Rare	Acute, inapparent infection; skin lesions on feet, tail, nose; found dead	Hepatic, splenic, lymph node, thymic necrosis, intestine engorged, dermal oedema and lymphocytic infiltrate, epidermal necrosis	ELISA, IFA	Culling and disinfection	Through skin abrasions. Biological products. Vertical transmission	Clinical signs influenced by gnotpye, virus resistant to many disinfectants

Hantaviruses*	Rare	Subclinical infection	Virus detectable in lung tissue	ELISA, IFA	Prevent wild mice from entering premises culling of infected animals. Hysterectomy derivation	Excreta/secreta, air-borne, biological products, zoonosis	Lifelong excretion in urine and faeces
Papovavirus K papova virus, (KPV), mouse pneumonitis virus	Rare	Inapparent infection unless inoculated into neonates, then laboured respiration and death	Consolidated lungs, thickened alveoli, endothelial cells swollen, hepatocyte vacuolation	ELISA, IFA, PCR	Hysterectomy derivation		Low incidence and low antibody titres
Polyoma virus (MPV)	Rare	Inapparent infection, experimental infection of neonates produces tumours in a variety of organs	Tumours rare in natural infection, demyelination reported in nude mice	ELISA, HAR, IFA	Hysterectomy derivation, prevent wild mice from entering premises	Urine, faeces, saliva	Virus shed in urine, saliva, faeces
Lactate dehydrogenase elevating virus (LDV)	Rare	Inapparent infection, paralysis of immunosuppressed C58 or AKR mice	Elevation of serum LDH, neuronal degeneration with mononuclear infiltrate in AKR, C58 mice	LDH plasma test, PCR	Eliminate infected animals. Pass tumours in another rodent species	Mouse biological products most likely source	Lifetime high-titre viraemia, not readily transmitted by natural means, alters immunological responses of infected mice, associated with transplantable tumours and mixed cell lines
Adenovirus Mouse adenovirus, (MadV): MAd-1, MAd-2	Rare	Inapparent infection. In infant and athymic mice fatal wasting disease	MAd-1: necrosis brown fat, myocarditis, adrenocortical changes, intranuclear inclusions in kidney tubulus MAd-2: enterotropic infection with inclusion bodies in enterocytes	ELISA, IFA	Hysterectomy derivation, improve sanitation procedures	MAd-1: urine MAd-2: faecal–oral route	Antibody present in 15–45% of older mice in an infected colony, transmits readily between cage mates (via urine?), less transmission between cages
Reovirus Reovirus 3 (Reo 3)	Rare	Often subclinical. Experimental infection leads to encephalitis, pulmonary oedema, emaciation, oil-matted hair, steatorrhoea, runting in suckling mice, jaundice	Necrosis in liver, exocrine pancreas, salivary gland, heart and brain, pancreas	ELISA, IFA, HAR, VN	Hysterectomy derivation	Faecal–oral route	Influences DNA replication, monoclonal antibody production. Clinical signs rarely reported

*also zoonotic disease

Table 21.4 Bacterial and other diseases of laboratory mice (Cunliffe-Beamer & Les 1987; O'Brien & Holmer 1993; Boot *et al.* 2001; FELASA 2002; Fox *et al.* 2002) (ELISA, enzyme-linked immunosorbent assay; IFA, indirect immunofluorescence assay; MA, microagglutination; PCR, polymerase chain reaction).

Genus and species	*Incidence*	*Clinical signs*	*Pathological lesions*	*Diagnosis*	*Control*	*Comments*
BACTERIA						
Pasteurella pneumotropica	Frequent	Inapparent infection, abscesses, pyometra, pneumonia, conjunctivitis	Abscesses	ELISA, IFA, MA. Isolate organism from upper respiratory tract, vagina or lesions	Culling of animals. Hysterectomy derivation	Viable foetuses may be derived from infected uteri
Staphylococcus aureus	Frequent	Inapparent infection, dermatitis, abscesses head/neck, conjunctivitis	Acute ulcerative dermatitis	Isolate organism from lesions	Eliminate affected mice, improve sanitation, monitor personnel. Hysterectomy derivation	Athymic mice especially susceptible
Citrobacter rodentium (freundii 4280)	Moderate	Transmissible colon hyperplasia. Soft faeces, ruffled fur, occasional rectal prolapse	Mucosal hyperplasia in descending colon ('pipe-like colon')	PCR. Isolate organism from faeces, pathognomonic lesion	Eliminate sick animals. Filter-top cages. Neomycin sulphate (2 mg/ml) or tetracycline (0.5–1 mg/ml). Temporary cessation of breeding	Not all *C. freundii* isolates are pathogenic
Clostridium piliforme (Tyzzer's disease)	Moderate	Inapparent infection, sudden death	Focal necrosis of liver, hyperaemic large intestine	ELISA, IFA. Identify organisms in liver or intestinal mucosa (special stains required), serological tests	Hysterectomy derivation. Sterilisation of rooms, materials	Activated by immunosuppression. Resistent to desinfectants
Mycoplasma pulmonis	Moderate	Inapparent infection, chattering, dyspnoea, ruffled coat, rhinitis, bronchopneumonia, otitis, reproductive failure	Suppurative rhinitis, chronic bronchopneumonia with syncytial giant cells	ELISA, PCR. Isolate organism from upper respiratory or genital tracts, serological tests	Hysterectomy derivation, tetracycline suppresses clinical signs	Can be isolated from uterus with viable foetuses. Synergistic effect with other infections
Pseudomonas aeruginosa	Moderate	Inapparent infection, mice found dead, occasional otitis media	Multiple areas of necrosis and haemorrhage	Isolate organism from intestinal tract or lesions	Acidification or chlorination of water	Activated by stress or immunosuppression
Corynebacterium kutscheri	Rare	Murine pseudotuberculosis. Inapparent infection, abscesses in liver, lung, kidney	Septic emboli and abscesses in many organ, pneumonia	Isolate organism from lung, liver or spleen	Hysterectomy derivation	Activated by stress or immunosuppression
Corynebacterium bovis	Rare	Scaly skin disease in nude mice, mortality in newborns	Skin lesions	Isolate organism from skin and mouth of nudes	Hysterectomy derivation	Activated by stress or immunosuppression
Klebsiella pneumoniae	Rare	Rough fur, hunched posture, anorexia, dyspnoea. Opportunistic pathogen	Pneumonia, empyema, abscesses	ELISA, IFA. Isolate organism from lung or abscesses	Hysterectomy derivation. Antibiotics only in single cases	Can be part of normal intestinal flora
*Salmonella enteritidis**	Rare	Inapparent infection, septicaemia, anorexia, lethargy, weight loss, soft faeces	Acute: hyperaemic viscera, catarrhal enteritis. Subacute: hyperaemic intestinal mucosa, necrotic foci in liver and spleen, lymph nodes enlarged	Isolate organism from intestinal tract, liver, spleen, lymph nodes	Hysterectomy derivation, repeated faecal cultures and elimination of state carriers, such as wild rodents	Antibiotics do not eliminate carrier

*Salmonella typhimurium**	Rare					
*Streptobacillus moniliformis**	Rare	Sudden death, acute sepsis, polyarthritis, paralysis, stillbirth, abortion, abscess, keratoconjunctivitis, chronic skin ulceration	Septicaemia with focal necrosis in spleen, liver and lymphe nodes, chronic infection causes arthritis	ELISA, IFA, PCR. Isolate organism from joint fluid	Exclusion of wild rodents or carrier animals	Spontaneous disease rare in mice, inapparent infection in rat. Disabling – lethal infection
CAR bacillus (cilia-associated respiratory bacillus)	Rare	Chronic respiratory disease, loss of body weight	Large numbers of bacilli present between cilia on respiratory epithelium	ELISA, IFA, PCR	Quarantine diseased animals	Insufficient information on importance of infection
Helicobacter sp.		Chronic hepatitis, gastritis	Focal non-suppurative inflammation liver, hepatocytomegaly, bile duct hyperplasia	PCR. Isolate organism from bile canaliculi	Hysterectomy derivation, antibiotics intensively (Fox *et al*. 2002)	Chronic inflammation liver and/or gastrointestinal tract. Elevated liver enzymes
Streptococcus sp. α-haemolytic β-haemolytic		Respiratory infection, haemorrhagic discharge from body orifices, especially in immunodeficient mice	Pneumonia, pleuritis, abscesses in cervical and submandibular lymph nodes	Isolate organism from lesions	Kill infected mice. Hysterectomy derivation	Transmission of infection via faeces
CHLAMYDIA						
Chlamydia trachomatis		Rough fur, dyspnoea, cyanosis, chattering	Patchy to diffuse interstitial pneumonitis	Elementary bodies in macrophages or bronchial epithelium (special stains required)	Hysterectomy derivation	Not reported since 1950s
MYCOTIC DISEASES						
Pneumocystis carinii		Pneumonia in immunodeficient mice	Interstitial alveolitis, cysts	ELISA, PCR, silver staining lung	Hysterectomy derivation	Mainly in immunodeficient mice
DERMATOPHYTES						
*Microsporum gypseum**		Inapparent infection		Isolate fungi from hair and skin cultures, microscopic examination of hairs for hyphae and spores	Difficult, kill infected mice	Rare in mice
Trichophyton spp.*		Inapparent infection, sparse hair coat		Isolate fungi from hair and skin cultures, microscopic examination of hairs for hyphae and spores	Difficult, kill infected mice	Rare in mice
RICKETTSIA						
Eperythrozoon coccoides		Inapparent infection, anaemia	Anaemia, splenomegaly	Ring-shaped organisms attached to red blood cells	Eliminate lice, hysterectomy derivation, tetracycline	Splenectomy activates inapparent infections, potentiates certain viral infections, antagonises experimental plasmodium infections

* also zoonotic disease

Table 21.5 Parasitic infections of mice (Cunliffe-Beamer & Les 1987; O'Brien & Holmer 1993; Boot *et al.* 2001; FELASA; 2002; Fox *et al.* 2002).

Common name	*Genus and species*	*Incidence*	*Clinical signs*	*Diagnosis and control*	*Potential effects on research results*
Lice	*Polyplax serrata*	Rare	Pruritis, anaemia	Identify the parasite in hair samples	Transmits *Eperythrozoon coccoides*
Mites	*Myobia musculi*	Frequent	Inapparent infection; pruritis; alopecia; dermatitis	The most efficient treatment is ivermectin spray solution (ivermectin 1% diluted 1:100 with a mixture of propylene glycol and water 1:1)	Serum protein alterations, elevated serum IgE
	Myocoptes musculinus	Frequent	Inapparent infection; pruritis; alopecia; dermatitis		
	Radfordia affinis	Rare	Inapparent infection; pruritis; alopecia; dermatitis		
	*Ornithonyssus bacoti**		Anaemia		Transits rickettsial diseases
Nematodes (pinworm)	*Aspicularis tetraptera*	Frequent	Inapparent infection (reduced growth rate?)	Seen with naked eye in gut, particularly caecum	Perturbation of host immune system
	Syphacia obvelata	Moderate	Inapparent infection (reduced growth rate)	Sticky tape test on perineum to see banana-shaped eggs of *Syphacia* sp. Fenbendazole 50ppm in feed to control	Perturbation of host immune system. May influence intestinal physiology
	Syphacia muris	Moderate	Sometimes enteritis	Ivermectin treatment, 2 mg/kg per os twice at 10-day intervals	Perturbation of host immune system
Protozoa	*Giardia muris*	Moderate	Inapparent infection → enteritis, weight loss, abdominal distention may occur	See organism on wet mount of faecal material or H&E section; Ttrophozoites in intestinal tract. 0.1% dimetridazole in drinking water for 14 days may control clinical disease; sanitation, disinfection	
	Spironucleus muris	Moderate	Inapparent infection. Diarrhoa; weight loss; occasional mortality seen in young post-weanling mice		Alter macrophage and other immunological responses
	Tritrichomonas spp.	Frequent	Inapparent infection; no known pathological significance	Commensal organism, no treatment warranted	None known
Cestodes (tapeworms)	*Hymenolepsis nana**	Moderate	Inapparent infection → local enteritis	Diagnosis by observation of parasite in gut. Praziquantel (0.05% in diet for 5 days)	
	Taenia taeniaeformis (*Cysticercus fasciolaris*)	Rare	Asymptomatic (rodents are intermediate host)	Observation of cysts in liver on *post-mortem*	

* zoonotic disease

Further reading

Foster *et al.* (1981) provide an overview of the history of the mouse in biomedical research. General advice on enrichment can be found in *Enrichment Strategies for Laboratory Animals* by the Institute for Laboratory Animal Research (ILAR 2005)

References

Arras, M., Rettich, A., Cinelli, P., Kaisermann, H.P. and Burki, K. (2007) Assessment of post-laparotomy pain in laboratory mice by telemetric recording of heart rate and heart rate variability. *BMC Veterinary Research*, **3**, 16

Animal Research Review Panel (in preparation) *Guideline 21: Guidelines for the Housing of Mice in Scientific Institutions*. Animal Welfare Branch, NSW Dept of Primary Industries, Orange, Australia

Barclay, R.J., Herbert, W.J. and Poole, T.B. (1988) *The Disturbance Index: a Behavioural Method of Assessing the Severity of Common Laboratory Procedures on Rodents*. Universities Federation for Animal Welfare, Potters Bar

Barnett, S.W. (2007) *Manual of Animal Technology*. Blackwell Publishing, Oxford

Baumans, V., Brain, P.F., Brugére, H. *et al.* (1994) Pain and distress in laboratory rodents and lagomorphs. *Laboratory Animals*, **28**, 97–112

Baumans, V. (1999) The Laboratory Mouse. In: *UFAW Handbook on the Care and Management of Laboratory Animals*, Vol. 1, 7th edn. Ed. Poole, T., pp. 282–312. Blackwell Publishing, Oxford

Baumans, V. (2004) The welfare of the laboratory mouse. In: *The Welfare of Laboratory Animals*. Ed. Kaliste, E., pp. 119–152. Animal welfare and nutrition series. Kluwer Academic Publishers, Dordrecht

Baumans, V. (2005a) Science-based assessment of animal welfare: *laboratory animals. Revue Scientifique et Technique (International Office of Epizootics)*, **24**, 503–514

Baumans, V. (2005b) Environmental enrichment for laboratory rodents and rabbits: requirements of rodents, rabbits and research. In: *Enrichment Strategies for Laboratory Animals. ILAR Journal*, **46**, 162–170

Baumans, V., Bouwknecht, J.A., Boere, H.A.G. *et al.* (2001a) Intra-abdominal transmitter implantation in mice: effects on behaviour and body weight. *Animal Welfare*, **10**, 291

Baumans, V. and Brain, P.F. (2001) Recognition of pain and distress. In: *Principles of Laboratory Animal Science*, revised edn. Eds van Zutphen, L.F.M., Baumans, V. and Beynen, A.C., pp. 265–276. Elsevier, Amsterdam

Baumans, V., Coke, C., Green, J. *et al.* (2007) Making lives easier for animals in research labs. Discussions by the Laboratory Animal Refinement & Enrichment Forum. Animal Welfare Institute, Washington. http://www.awionline.org

Baumans, V., Remie, R., Hackbarth, H.J. and Timmerman, A. (2001b) Experimental procedures. In: *Principles of Laboratory Animal Science*, revised edn. Eds van Zutphen, L.F.M., Baumans, V. and Beynen, A.C., pp. 313–333. Elsevier, Amsterdam

Baumans, V., Schlingmann, F., Vonck, M. and van Lith, H.A. (2002) Individually ventilated cages: beneficial for mice and men? *Contemporary Topics in Laboratory Animal Science*, **41**, 13

Benefiel, A.C., Dong, W.K. and Greenough, W.T. (2005) Mandatory 'enriched' housing of laboratory animals: the need for evidence-based evaluation. In: *Enrichment Strategies for Laboratory Animals. ILAR Journal*, **46**, 95–105

Beynen, A.C. and Coates, M.E. (2001) Nutrition and experimental results. In: *Principles of Laboratory Animal Science*, revised edn. Eds van Zutphen, L.F.M., Baumans, V. and Beynen, A.C., pp. 111–127. Elsevier, Amsterdam

Blom, H.J.M., van de Weerd, H.A., Hoogervorst, M.J.C. *et al.* (1993) *Preference for Cage Temperature in Laboratory Mice as Influenced by the Type of Cage Flooring*. Thesis Utrecht University, The Netherlands

Blom, H.J.M., van Tintelen, G., van Vorstenbosch, C.J.A.H.V., Baumans, V. and Beynen A.C. (1996) Preferences of mice and rats for type of bedding material. *Laboratory Animals*, **30**, 234–244

Boot, R., Koopman J.P. and Kunstý, I. (2001) Microbiological standardization. In: *Principles of Laboratory Animal Science*, revised edn. Eds van Zutphen, L.F.M., Baumans, V. and Beynen, A.C., pp. 149–171. Elsevier, Amsterdam

Brain, P.F. (1990) Stress in agonistic contexts in rodents. In: *Social Stress in Domestic Animals*. Eds Zayan, R. and Dantzer, R., pp. 73–85. Kluwer, Dordrecht

Brain, P.F. and Benton, D. (1983) Conditions of housing, hormones and aggressive behavior. In: *Hormones and Aggressive Behavior*. Ed. Svare, B.B., pp. 349–372. Plenum, New York

Buckland, M.D., Hall, L., Mowlem, A. and Whatley, B.F. (1981) *A Guide to Laboratory Animal Technology*. William Heinemann Medical Books Ltd, London

Busser, J., Zweep, A. and van Oortmerssen, G.A. (1974) *The Genetics of Behaviour*. Ed. van Abeelen, J.H.F. American Elsevier Publishing Company, New York

Clough, G. (1984) Environmental factors in relation to the comfort and well-being of laboratory rats and mice. In: *Standards in Laboratory Animal Management*, pp. 7–24. UFAW, Potters Bar

Council of Europe (1986) European Convention for the Protection of Vertebrate Animals used for Experimental and other Scientific Purposes (ETS 123). Council of Europe, Strasbourg Revised 2006 http://www.coe.int/t/e/legal_affairs/legal_cooperation/biological_safety,_use_of_animals/laboratory_animals/2006/Cons123(2006)3AppendixA_en.pdf (accessed 10th November 2009)

Council of Europe (2006) Multilateral Consultation of Parties to the European Convention for the Protection of Vertebrate Animals used for Experimental and other Scientific Purposes (ETS 123) Appendix A. *Cons 123 (2006) 3*. Available from URL: http://www.coe.int/t/e/legal_affairs/legal_co-operation/biological_safety,_use_of_animals/laboratory_animals/2006/Cons123(2006)3AppendixA_en.pdf (accessed 10th November 2009)

Crabbe, J.C., Wahlsten D. and Dudek, B.C. (1999) Genetics of mouse behavior: interactions with laboratory environment. *Science*, **284**, 1670–1672

Crawley, J. (2000) *What is Wrong with My Mouse? Behavioural Phenotyping of Transgenic and Knock out Mice*. John Wiley & Sons, Chichester

Cunliffe-Beamer, T.L. and Les, E.P. (1987) The laboratory mouse. The laboratory mouse. In: *The UFAW Handbook on the Care and Management of Laboratory Animals*. Ed. Poole, T., pp. 275–308 UFAW, Potters Bar

Dawkins, M.S. (1990) From an animal's point of view: Motivation, fitness and animal welfare. *Behavioural and Brain Sciences*, **13**, 1–9

Dennis, Jr M.B. (2002) Welfare issues of genetically modified animals. *ILAR Journal*, **43**, 100–109

European Commission (2007) Commission recommendations of 18 June 2007 on guidelines for the accommodation and care of animals used for experimental and other scientific purposes. Annex II to European Council Directive 86/609 See 2007/526/EC http://eurlex.europa.eu/LexUriServ/site/en/oj/2007/l_197/l_19720070730en00010089.pdf (accessed 13 May 2008)

European Council Directive (1986) *Directive on the approximation of laws, regulations and administrative provisions of the member states regarding the Protection of vertebrate animals used for Experimental and other Scientific Purposes (86/609/EEC).* Annex II revised L197/1 (2007)

European Science Foundation (2001) Use of animals in research. *ESF Policy Briefing*, **15**, 1–6

EC Working Party report on euthanasia of experimental animals (1996) Recommendations for euthanasia of experimental animals part 1. *Laboratory Animals*, **30**, 293–316

EC Working Party report on euthanasia of experimental animals (1997) Recommendations for euthanasia of experimental animals part 2. *Laboratory Animals*, **31**, 1–32

Eskola, S., Lauhikari, M., Voipio, H.M. *et al.* (1999) Environmental enrichment may alter the number of rats needed to achieve statistical significance. *Scandinavian Journal Laboratory Animal Science*, **26**, 134–144

Eveleigh, J.R. (1993) Murine cage density: cage ammonia levels during reproductive performance of an inbred strain and two outbred stocks of monogamous breeding pairs of mice. *Laboratory Animals*, **27**, 156–160

Fallon, M.T. (1996) Rats and mice. In: *Handbook of Rodent and Rabbit Medicine*. Eds Laber-Laird, K., Swindle, M.M. and Flecknell, P., pp. 1–38. Pergamon Veterinary Handbook Series, Elsevier Science Ltd, Oxford

Federation of European Laboratory Animal Science Associations (2002) FELASA recommendations for the health monitoring of rodent and rabbit colonies in breeding and experimental units. *Laboratory Animals*, **36**, 20–42

Federation of European Laboratory Animal Science Associations (2007) *Euroguide on the Accommodation and Care of Animals Used for Experimental and Other Scientific Purposes*. Royal Society of Medicine Press Limited, London

Flecknell, P.A. (1996) *Laboratory Animal Anaesthesia*. Academic Press, London

Flecknell, P.A. (2009) *Laboratory Animal Anaesthesia*, 3rd edn. Academic Press, London

Foster, H.L., Small, J.D. and Fox, J.G. (eds) (1981) *The Mouse in Biomedical Research*. Academic Press, New York

Fox, J.G., Anderson L.C., Loew F.M. *et al.* (2002) *Laboratory Animal Medicine*, 2nd edn. Academic Press, New York

Garner, J.P., Dufour, B., Gregg, L.E. *et al.* (2004) Social and husbandry factors affecting the prevalence and severity of barbering ('whisker trimming') by laboratory mice. *Applied Animal Behaviour Science*, **89**, 263–282

Garner, J.P. and Mason, G.J. (2002) Evidence for a relationship between cage stereotypies and behavioural disinhibition in laboratory rodents. *Behavioural Brain Research*, **136**, 83–92

Golde, W.T., Gollobin, P. and Rodriguez, L.L. (2005) A rapid, simple and humane method for submandibular bleeding of mice using a lancet. *Lab Animal Europe*, **5**, 29–34

Haataja, H., Voipio, H.M., Nevalainen, A., Jantunen, M.J. and Nevalainen, T. (1989) Deciduous wood chips as bedding material: estimation of dust yield, water absorption and micro-biological comparison. *Scandinavian Journal Laboratory Animal Science*, **16**, 105–111

Hackbarth, H., Küppers, N. and Bohnet, W. (2000) Euthanasia of rats with carbon-dioxide – animal welfare aspects. *Laboratory Animals*, **34**, 91

Haemisch, A. and Gärtner, J. (1994) The cage design affects intermale aggression in small groups of male laboratory mice: strain specific consequences on social organization and endocrine activations in two inbred strains (DBA/2J and CBA/J). *Journal of Experimental Animal Science*, **36**, 101–116

Haldane, J.B.S., Sprunt, A.D. and Haldane, N.M. (1915) Reproduction in mice. *Journal of Genetics*, **5**, 133–135

Harkness, J.E. and Wagner, J.E. (1995) *The Biology and Medicine of Rabbits and Rodents*, 4th edn. Williams and Wilkins, Baltimore

Havenaar, R., Meijer, J.C., Morton, D.B. *et al.* (2001) Biology and husbandry of laboratory animals. In: *Principles of Laboratory Animal Science*, revised edn. Eds van Zutphen, L.F.M., Baumans, V. and Beynen, A.C., pp. 19–28. Elsevier, Amsterdam

Hedrich, H.J. and Bullock, G. (2004) *The Laboratory Mouse*. Elsevier Academic Press, Boston

Hellebrekers, L.J., Booij, L.H.D.J. and Flecknell, P.A. (2001) Anaesthesia, analgesia and euthanasia. In: *Principles of Laboratory Animal Science*, revised edn. Eds van Zutphen, L.F.M., Baumans, V. and Beynen, A.C., pp. 277–311. Elsevier, Amsterdam

Hendriksen, C.F.M. and Morton, D. (1999) *Humane endpoints in animal experiments for biomedical research*. In: Proceedings International Conference 22–25 Nov 1998, Zeist, The Netherlands. The Royal Society of Medicine Press Limited, London

Hurst, J.L., Fang, J. and Barnard, C.J. (1993) The role of substrate odours in maintaining social tolerance between male house mice, *Mus musculus domesticus*. *Animal Behaviour*, **45**, 997–1006

Hurst, J.L. (1999) Introduction to rodents. In: *UFAW Handbook on the Care and Management of Laboratory Animals*, Vol. 1, 7th edn. Ed. Poole, T., pp. 262–273. Blackwell Publishing, Oxford

Institute for Laboratory Animal Research (2005) *Enrichment Strategies for Laboratory Animals*. ILAR Journal **46**. National Research Council, Washington, US

Joint Working Group on Refinement (1993) Removal of blood from laboratory mammals and birds. First Report of the BVA/FRAME/RSPCA/UFAW Joint Working Group on Refinement. *Laboratory Animals*, **27**, 1–22

Joint Working Group on Refinement (2001) Refining procedures for the administration of substances. Report of the BVAAWF/FRAME/RSPCA/UFAW Joint Working Group on Refinement. *Laboratory Animals*, **35**, 1–41

Joint Working Group on Refinement (2003) Refinement and reduction in production of genetically modified mice. Sixth Report of the BVAAWF/FRAME/RSPCA/UFAW Joint Working Group on Refinement. *Laboratory Animals*, **37** (Suppl. 1), S1–S49

Kornerup Hansen, A. and Baumans, V. (2004) Housing, care and environmental factors. In: *The Welfare of Laboratory Animals*. Ed. Kaliste, E., pp. 37–50. Kluwer Academic Publishers, Dordrecht

Kramer, K., van Acker, S.A.B.E., Voss, H.P. *et al.* (1993) Use of telemetry to record ECG and Heart rate in freely moving mice. *Journal of Pharmacological and Toxicological Methods*, **30**, 209–215

Krohn, T.C., Sörensen, D.B., Ottesen, J.L. *et al.* (2006) The effects of individual housing on mice and rats. A review. *Animal Welfare*, **15**, 343–352

Ladewig, J. (2000) Chronic intermittent stress: a model for the study of long-term stressors. In: *The Biology of Animal Stress*. Eds Moberg, G.P. and Mench, J.A., pp.159–169. CAB International, Wallingford

Latham, N. and Mason, G. (2004) From house mouse to mouse house: the behavioural biology of free-living *Mus musculus* and its implications in the laboratory. *Applied Animal Behaviour Science*, **86**, 261–289

Mackintosh, J.H. (1981) Behaviour of the house mouse. *Symposium of the Zoological Society London*, **47**, 337–365

Mattson, M.P., Duan, W., Lee J. *et al.* (2001) Suppression of brain aging and neurodegenerative disorders by dietary restriction and environmental enrichment: molecular mechanisms. *Mechanisms of Ageing and Development*, **122**, 757–778

Meijer, M.K. (2006) *Neglected Impact of Routine: Refinement of Experimental Procedures in Laboratory Mice*. Thesis, Utrecht University

Meijer, M.K., Spruijt, B.M., van Zutphen, L.F.M. *et al.* (2006) Effect of restraint and injection methods on heart rate and body temperature in mice. *Laboratory Animals*, **40**, 382–391

Mench, J.A. (1998) Why it is important to understand animal behaviour. *ILAR Journal*, **39**, 20–26

Mertens, C. and Rulicke, T. (2000) A comprehensive form for the standardized characterization of transgenic rodents: genotype, phenotype, welfare assessment, recommendations for refinement (in German). *ALTEX : Alternativen zu Tierexperimenten*, **17**, 15–21

Mohammed, A.H., Zhu, S.W., Darmopil, S. *et al.* (2002) Environmental enrichment and the brain. In: *Progress in Brain Research*, Vol **138**. Eds Hofman, M.A., Boer, G.J., Holtmaat, A.J.G.D. *et al.*, pp. 109–133. Elsevier Science BV, Amsterdam

Morton, D. and Hau, J. (2003) Welfare assessment and humane endpoints. In: *Handbook of Laboratory Animal Science*, Vol 1, 2nd edn. Eds Hau J. and Van Hoosier G.L., pp. 457–486. CRC Press, Boca Raton

Mouse Genome Sequencing Consortium (2002) Initial sequencing and analysis of the mouse genome. *Nature*, **420**, 520–562

National Health and Medical Research Council (2004) *Australian Code of Practice for the Care and Use of Animals for Scientific Purposes*, 7th edn. NHMRC, Canberra

National Research Council (1996) *Guide for the Care and Use of Laboratory Animals*, 7th edn. National Academy Press, Washington, DC. http://www.nap.edu/readingroom/books/

National Research Council (2008) *Recognition and Alleviation of Distress in Laboratory Animals*. National Academy Press, Washington, DC http://books.nap.edu/openbook.php?record_id=11931

Newberry, R.C. (1995) Environmental enrichment: increasing the biological relevance of captive environments. *Applied Animal Behaviour Science*, **44**, 229–243

Newcastle Consensus meeting on Carbon Dioxide Euthanasia of Laboratory Animals (2006) http://www.nc3rs.org.uk/downloaddoc.asp?id=416&page=292&skin=0 (accessed 10th November 2009)

O'Brien, C. and Holmer, M. (1993) The mouse, part two. *Anzccart News*, **6**, 4–6

Olsson, A.S. and Dahlborn, K. (2002) Improving housing conditions for laboratory mice: a review of environmental enrichment. *Laboratory Animals*, **36**, 243–270

Olsson, A.S., Nevison, C.M., Patterson-Kane, E.G. *et al.* (2003) Understanding behaviour: the relevance of ethological approaches in laboratory animal science. *Applied Animal Behaviour Science*, **81**, 245–264

Pekow, C.A. and Baumans, V. (2002) Common non surgical techniques and procedures. In: *Handbook of Laboratory Animal Science*, Vol **1**, 2nd edn. Eds Hau J. and Van Hoosier G.L., pp. 351–390. CRC Press, Boca Raton

Poole, T.B. (1995) Welfare considerations with regard to transgenic animals. *Animal Welfare*, **4**, 81–85

Poole, T.B. (1998) Meeting a mammal's psychological needs: basic principles. In: *Second Nature: Environmental Enrichment for Captive Animals*. Eds Shepherdson, D.J., Mellen, J.D. and Hutchins, M., pp. 83–96. Smithsonian Institution Press, Washington

Renner, M.J. and Rosenzweig, M.R. (1987) *Enriched and Impoverished Environments*. Springer-Verlag, New York

Roughan, J.V. and Flecknell, P.A. (2003) Pain assessment and control in laboratory animals. *Laboratory Animals*, **37**, 172

Sales, G.D., Milligan, S.R. and Khirnykh, K. (1999) Sources of sound in the laboratory animal environment: a survey of the sounds produced by procedures and equipment. *Animal Welfare*, **8**, 97

Schlingmann, F., van de Weerd, H.A., Baumans, V. *et al.* (1988) A balance device for the analysis of behavioural patterns of the mouse. *Animal Welfare*, **7**, 177–188

Scott, L. (1991) *Mouse Management*. University of Melbourne, Australia

Serrano, L.J. (1971) Carbon dioxide and ammonia in mouse cages: effect of cage covers, population and activity. *Laboratory Animals*, **21**, 75–85

Sherwin, C.M. (2000) Frustration in laboratory mice. *Scientists Centre for Animal Welfare Newsletter*, **22**, 7–12

Sherwin, C.M. (2002) Comfortable quarters for mice in research institutions. In: *Comfortable Quarters for Laboratory Animals*, 9th edn. Eds Reinhardt V. and Reinhardt A., pp. 6–17. Animal Welfare Institute, Washington http://www.awionline.org/www.awionline.org/pubs/cq02/Cq-mice.html (accessed 10th November 2009)

Spalding, J.F., Holland, I.M. and Tietjen, G.L. (1969) Influence of the visible color spectrum on activity in mice. *Laboratory Animal Care*, **19**, 209–213

Stewart, K.L. and Bayne, K. (2004) Environmental enrichment for laboratory animals. In: *Laboratory Animal Medicine and Management, International Veterinary Information Service, B2520.0404*. Eds Reuter, J.D. and Suckow, M.A., p. 10. International Veterinary Information Service, Ithaca, New York

Tsai, P.P., Stelzer, H.D., Hedrich, H.J. *et al.* (2003) Are the effects of different enrichment designs on the physiology and behaviour of DBA/2 mice consistent? *Laboratory Animals*, **37**, 314–327

van den Broek, F.A.R., Omtzigt, C.M. and Beynen A.C. (1993) Whisker trimming behaviour in A2G mice is not prevented by offering means of withdrawal from it. *Laboratory Animals*, **27**, 270–272

van der Meer, M., Baumans, V., Olivier, B. *et al.* (2001a) Behavioral and physiological effects of biotechnology procedures used for gene targeting in mice. *Physiology and Behavior*, **73**, 719–730

van der Meer, M., Baumans, V. and van Zutphen, L.F.M. (1996) Transgenic animals: what about their well-being. *Scandinavian Journal of Laboratory Animal Science*, **23**, 287–290

van der Meer, M., Rolls, A., Baumans, V. *et al.* (2001b) Use of score sheets for welfare assessment of transgenic mice. *Laboratory Animals*, **35**, 379–389

van de Weerd, H.A., van den Broek, F.A.R. and Beynen, A.C. (1992) Removal of vibrissae in male does not influence social dominance. *Behavioural Processes*, **27**, 205–208

van de Weerd, H.A. and Baumans, V. (1995) Environmental enrichment in rodents. In: *Environmental Enrichment Information Recources for Laboratory Animals 1965–1995*. AWIC Resource Series no 2. AWIC, USA, UFAW, England

van de Weerd, H.A., van Loo, P.L.P., van Zutphen, L.F.M. *et al.* (1997a) Nesting material as environmental enrichment has no adverse effects on behavior and physiology of laboratory mice. *Physiology & Behavior*, **62**, 1019–1028

van de Weerd, H.A., van Loo, P.L.P., van Zutphen, L.F.M. *et al.* (1997b) Preferences for nesting material as environmental enrichment for laboratory mice. *Laboratory Animals*, **31**, 133–143

van de Weerd, H.A., Aarsen, E.L., Mulder, A. *et al.* (2002) Effects of environmental enrichment for mice: variation in experimental results. *Journal Applied Animal Welfare Science*, **5**, 87–109

van Dijk, J.E., van Herck, H. and Bosland, M.C. (2001) Diseases in laboratory animals. In: *Principles of Laboratory Animal Science*, revised edn. Eds van Zutphen, L.F.M., Baumans, V. and Beynen, A.C., pp. 173–195. Elsevier, Amsterdam

van Loo, P.L.P., Blom, H.J.M., Meijer, M.K. *et al.* (2005) Assessment of the use of two commercially available enrichments by laboratory mice by preference testing. *Laboratory Animals*, **39**, 58–67

van Loo, P.L.P., Kuin, N., Sommer, R. *et al.* (2007) Impact of 'living apart together' on postoperative recovery of mice compared with social and individual housing. *Laboratory Animals*, **41**, 441–455

van Loo, P.L.P., Kruitwagen, C.L.J.J., van Zutphen, L.F.M. *et al.* (2000) Modulation of aggression in male mice: influence of cage cleaning regime and scent marks. *Animal Welfare*, **9**, 281–295

van Loo, P.L.P., van Zutphen, L.F.M. and Baumans, V. (2003) Male management: coping with aggression problems in male laboratory mice. *Laboratory Animals*, **37**, 300–313

van Oortmerssen, G.A. (1971) Biological significance, genetics and evolutionary origin of variability in behaviour within and between inbred strains of mice. *Behaviour*, **38**, 1–92 van Zutphen, L.F.M. (2001) History of animal use. In: *Principles of Laboratory Animal Science*, revised edn. Eds van Zutphen, L.F.M., Baumans, V. and Beynen, A.C., pp. 2–5. Elsevier, Amsterdam

van Zutphen, L.F.M., Hedrich, H.J., Van Lith, H.A. *et al.* (2001) Genetic standardization. In: *Principles of Laboratory Animal Science*, revised edn. Eds van Zutphen, L.F.M., Baumans, V. and Beynen, A.C., pp. 129–147. Elsevier, Amsterdam

Vesell, E.S. (1967) Induction of drug-metabolizing enzymes in liver microsomes of mice and rats by softwood bedding. *Science*, **157**, 1057–1058

Voipio, H.M., Nevalainen, T., Halonen, P. et al. (2006) Role of cage material, working style and hearing sensitivity in perception of animal care noise. *Laboratory Animals*, **40**, 400–409

Wahlsten, D., Metten, P., Phillips, T.J. *et al.* (2003) Different data from different labs: lessons from studies in gene–environment interaction. *Journal of Neurobiology*, **54**, 283–311

Wolfensohn, S. and Lloyd, M. (2003) *Handbook of Laboratory Animal Management and Welfare*, 3rd edn. Blackwell Publishing, Oxford

Wolfer, D.P., Litvin, O., Morf, S. *et al.* (2004) Cage enrichment and mouse behaviour. *Nature*, **432**, 821–822

Würbel, H. (2001) Ideal homes? Housing effects on rodent brain and behaviour. *Trends in Neuroscience*, **24**, 207–210

Yamauchi, C., Fujita, S., Obara, T. *et al.* (1983) Effect of room temperature on reproduction body and organ weights, food and water intakes and hematology in mice. *Experimental Animals*, **32**, 1–12

Zhu, S., Pham, T.M., Åberg, E. *et al.* (2006) Neurotrophin levels and behaviour in BALB/c mice: impact of intermittent exposure to individual housing and wheel running. *Behavioural Brain Research*, **167**, 1–8

22 The laboratory rat

Jaap M. Koolhaas

Biological overview

General biology

The laboratory rat is the domesticated form of the species *Rattus norvegicus* or brown Norway rat. Although the genus *Rattus* contains 66 species, the most commonly known other rattus species is *Rattus rattus* or black rat. The genus belongs to the family of the Muridea and the order of Rodentia. The two species differ considerably in their habitats, behaviour and ecology. The wild *Rattus norvegicus* has agouti-coloured fur, meaning that it has the agouti gene which produces hairs with colour bands varying between brown–black and red–yellow. *Rattus rattus* may have a more variable coat colour, but is mainly dark brown or black. The most conspicuous difference between the two species concerns the relatively large, mouse-like ears of *R. rattus*. The two species share more or less the same habitat, but *R. norvegicus* lives mainly in burrow systems at ground level, whereas *R. rattus* tend to occupy higher areas in trees and roofs.

Whereas most species of *Rattus* are indigenous in subtropical and tropical areas, both *R. norvegicus* and *R. rattus* are cosmopolitan and can be found on all continents. The Norway rat has a rather interesting recent evolutionary history. The species seems to have originated in central Asia, and has spread over almost all of the world during the last two or three centuries (Hedrich 2000). This spread was strongly facilitated by the increase in long-distance trading in the early eighteenth century. Early *R. norvegicus* colonies were established by Russian ships and wrecks in the Baltic region; meanwhile, they dispersed overland, reaching Paris by about 1750 and Switzerland by 1809. *R. norvegicus* reached Greenland about 1780, the eastern part of the United States in 1775 and the Pacific coast in 1851. In all of these areas they rapidly displaced *R. rattus*, and often became a major pest.

The Norway rat is a generalist which is able to survive in a wide variety of habitats and climatic conditions. The species greatly benefits from the presence of human beings and may live in buildings, harvest stores, sewer systems and on rubbish dumps. In nature, however, it prefers to live in burrow systems usually located near water. The burrow system occupies 2–4 m^2 and consists of tunnels 5–7 cm in diameter and 0.25–1.5 m long (Pisano & Storer 1948). The tunnels usually end in small chambers used for nesting and storage of food. The area around the burrow system can be considered as the territory and will be defended against unfamiliar conspecifics. However, the home range of the animals (ie, the range in which they search for food) may be about 100 m^2. The rat is a nocturnal animal and generally has three activity periods, one at the beginning, one in the middle and one at the end of the night. It feeds during these activity periods taking three to five separate meals. The worldwide success of the Norway rat is partially due to the fact that the species is omnivorous, having a remarkable capacity to balance its nutrient intake in a broad range of dietary conditions.

The senses of smell, hearing and touch are highly developed. Behaviour is strongly determined by olfactory signals. In a social setting, male rats are able to recognise social status of other males, reproductive status of females and kinship solely on the basis of olfactory cues (Beynon & Hurst 2004). Moreover, rats are very sensitive to olfactory signals from predators such as cats and alarm pheromones from other rats (Dielenberg & McGregor 2001). Rats emit a large repertoire of ultrasonic vocalisations: 22 kHz sounds occur in aversive stressful situations; pups emit 40 kHz sounds when left alone by the nursing mother and have a clear function in eliciting pup retrieval by the mother. Recent evidence suggests that the 50 kHz sound, in particular the frequency modulated form, reflects a state of positive affect (a positive emotional state), since it is emitted by adults during sexual and aggressive behaviour and in response to rewarding conditions (Panksepp 2007; Portfors 2007), although see also Chapter 6, Vocalisations. Although the function of these vocalisations is still not fully clear, the rat can hear frequencies up to 80 kHz. Tactile receptors are particularly well developed on the head, around the whiskers, on the paws and on the tail. Studies indicate that the rat whisker system has a sensitivity of less than 90 μm, which is comparable to that of primate fingertips (Carvell & Simons 1990).

Rats have dichromatic colour vision. One type of cone in the retina has a photo pigment with a maximal sensitivity at a wavelength of 510 nm (green) (Neitz & Jacobs 1986), which declines rapidly at wavelengths above 560 nm (red–infrared). A second type of cone has its maximal sensitivity in the near ultraviolet range (360 nm) (Jacobs *et al.* 1991). Visual acuity is generally low, albino strains being more variable and often lower in visual acuity than pigmented strains (Prusky *et al.* 2002).

Size range and lifespan

The size of a rat is usually expressed in terms of body weight. Growth rate depends not only on strain, but also on quality and availability of food, as well as environmental factors such as temperature and social situation. Male laboratory rats are particularly prone to develop obesity and may reach a weight of about 800 g.

Size can also be determined using morphological parameters such as body and tail length. Body length is measured from the tip of the nose to the middle of the anus and tail length from the middle of the anus to the tip of the tail. Although the body length to tail length ratio is rather constant in adult rats, the absolute values, particularly the length of the tail, may be influenced by the environmental temperature during rearing.

The maximum lifespan of wild rats kept in a semi-natural enclosure is about 600 days for males and 700 days for females, whereas the median lifespan (50% survival) is 300 days for males and 550 days for females (Calhoun 1962). Notice that the maximum and median lifespan are different measures of longevity, which cannot be compared directly. In laboratory strains longevity may vary considerably depending on the strain and diet. The maximum lifespan of the Wistar strain, for example, is about 1200 days (3.2 years) for males and 1400 days (3.8 years) for females. Median lifespan for the Wistar rat is 850 days for males and 900 days for females (Ghirardi *et al.* 1995).

Social organisation

The fact that the Norway rat is a social species by nature has often been under-emphasised, if not ignored, in the design and interpretation of laboratory experiments. Although much remains unknown about the rat's social system, it is clear that the species is gregarious and that social hierarchies easily develop in groups of rats. Generally, in groups of wild rats, one dominant male can be distinguished which lives together with a number of females and often younger males. In this latter group of males, two social layers may be distinguished: a group of socially active subdominant males and subordinate males. Dominant males that are replaced by a former subdominant male tend to be relegated to the position of a social outcast, being chased by most of the other colony members and having a peripheral existence at the outskirts of the colony. The group size of populations of feral rats may vary considerably, depending on environmental conditions such as food availability and nesting conditions. However, in larger colonies, smaller subgroups will emerge, which usually consist of family members (Calhoun 1962).

Reproduction

The rat has an exceptionally high reproductive capacity. Both males and females are, on average, sexually mature at the age of 2–3 months. The oestrous cycle is 4–5 days. At the time of oestrus, receptivity occurs in the second half of the dark period (Barbacka-Surowiak *et al.* 2003). In the wild, a receptive female will be followed and mounted by the dominant male and often by a number of other male colony members as well (McClintock & Adler 1978). After several successful copulations, the female's willingness starts to decline; this is indicated by aggressive actions and escape behaviour by the female. Gestation is 20–21 days, and during the few days prior to delivery of the pups, the pregnant female starts to build a nest and will defend her nest against both male and female colony members. This maternal aggression will continue throughout the first week of nursing, after which it gradually declines and another reproductive cycle may start (Rosenblatt *et al.* 1994). In temperate regions, wild rats have a clear seasonal variation in reproduction governed by day length and food availability. Some studies of laboratory rats indicate the presence of an intrinsic annual cycle (Claassen 1994; De Boer *et al.* 2003). The average litter size is approximately 10 and in the wild, sex ratio depends on season, population density and food availability (Bacon & McClintock 1994; Parshad 1997).

Standard biological data

Some of the basic physiological and morphological data of the Wistar rat are presented in Table 22.1, but see Krinke *et al.* (2000) for more extensive information. These data should, however, be used with some caution, as many of the parameters are not static but highly dynamic in time, varying both diurnally and throughout life. Moreover, there are significant strain differences, and within strains there may be differences between suppliers, in particular where outbred or random-bred strains are concerned.

Most physiological parameters show a strong circadian variation and are highly responsive to environmental stressors. Figure 22.1 shows the circadian variation in some neuroendocrine and physiological parameters measured in 4-month-old male Wistar rats, measured using stress-free

Table 22.1 Basic biological data of Wistar rats.

Parameter	*Normal value*
Chromosome number	42
Lifespan (years)	2–4
Body weight at birth (g)	4.5–6
Daily food intake (g/100 g BW)	10
Daily water intake (ml/100 g BW)	10–15
Defecation (g/24 h)	9–13
Urine production (ml/24 h)	10–15
Weight of organs (in % BW)	
Adrenal (single)	0.02
Blood	5–7
Brain	1
Heart	0.5
Kidney (single)	0.5
Liver	3
Lung	1
Ovary (single)	0.05
Spleen	0.2
Testis (single)	0.5
Thymus	0.07
Thyroid	0.005

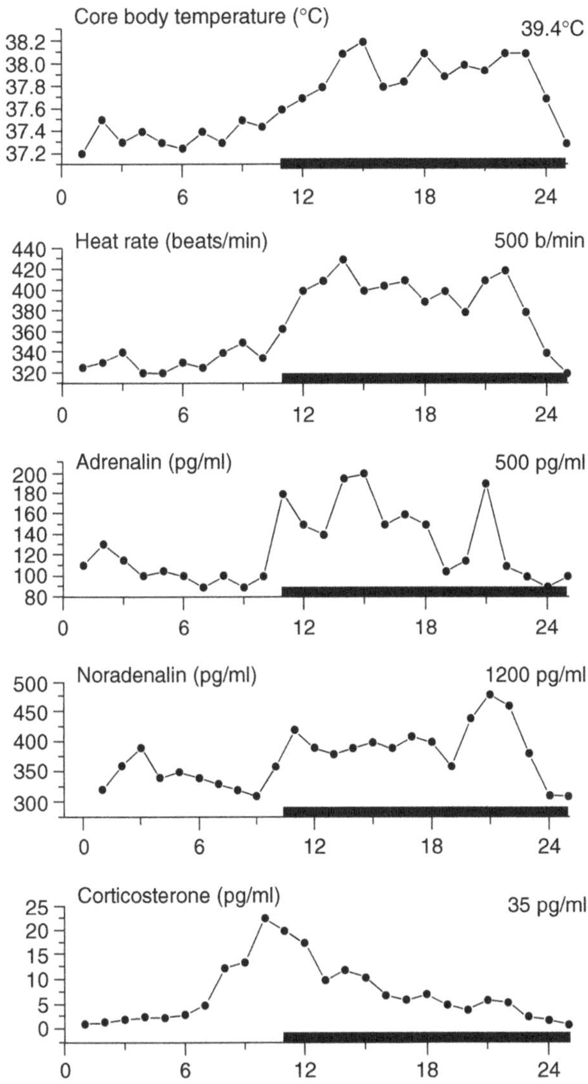

Figure 22.1 Circadian variation in plasma corticosterone, noradrenalin and adrenalin levels, heart rate and core body temperature in adult male Wistar rats. The black bar indicates the dark period of the light–dark cycle. The data on the right-hand side of each graph indicate the maximum response levels obtained during 15 minutes restraint stress (unpublished data from the author).

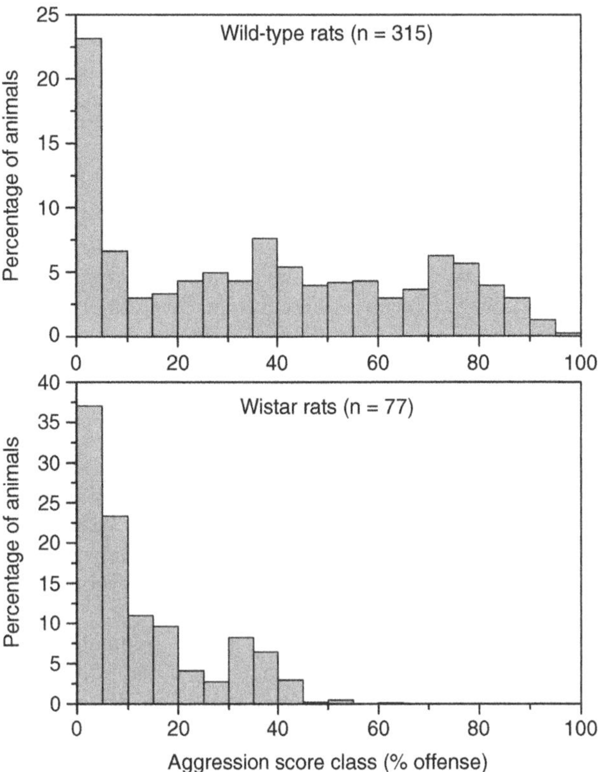

Figure 22.2 Frequency distribution of the individual levels of aggressive behaviour in the Wistar rat (Harlan) and the wild-type Groningen rat.

methods (permanent jugular vein cannulation, radiotelemetry). The figure in the right-hand part of each graph shows the maximum value of these parameters obtained during 15 minutes' restraint (data collected by the author).

Breeds, strains and genetics

Most of the laboratory rat strains are albino or derived from an albino form. Although the precise origin of the albino rat is unknown, it is very likely that the first laboratory albinos came from collections kept for breeding and show purposes. The use of rats for research in the laboratory started at the end of the nineteenth century, by a number of French and English scientists. More systematic breeding started in the early twentieth century in the United States by King and Donaldson at the Wistar Institute. They extensively compared up to 25 generations of laboratory-bred wild rats with the same generations of albino rats. The initial differences were considerable. More recent studies confirm the general idea that laboratory strains of rats must be considered as a very special selection from the original wild species *Rattus norvegicus* (De Boer *et al.* 2003). Figure 22.2 shows the frequency distribution of the individual level of aggressive behaviour in a population of Wistar rats and a population of a laboratory-bred wild-type rats (De Boer *et al.* 2003). Compared to this semi-wild population, even the use of the outbred Wistar strain shows a strong selection bias. Currently, more than 400 inbred strains are available and about 50 outbred or random-bred strains. A list of available inbred strains is presented in the International Index of Laboratory Animals (Festing 1993), and a more recent overview can be found at the MGI website[1]. A more extensive description of the origin and stockholders of these strains is given by Hedrich (1990). Provided a constant monitoring of the genetic stability of an inbred strain is carried out, they have the advantage that they remain genetically stable over a long period of time. However, it is important to be aware that the use of inbred strains depends on the nature of the experiments. The main disadvantage of inbred strains is that each of them represents a very narrow selection of the wide and functional genetic variation observed in a wild population. Consequently, one may question the general validity

[1] http://www.informatics.jax.org/external/festing/rat/STRAINS.shtml

of the results. Therefore, if the results of the experiments are to be extrapolated to the human population, as for example in toxicity testing, the use of at least two inbred strains is often preferable (see Chapters 3 and 4). An analysis, using DNA markers, of the genetic relationships or genetic distance between 60 inbred rat strains has been published by Otsen *et al.* (1995).

The disadvantage of outbred strains is that each breeding colony may be different due to genetic drift. Hence, a Wistar or Sprague-Dawley rat from one breeder may be genotypically and phenotypically different from those obtained from a different source. Considerable differences in neuroanatomy, behaviour and pharmacology have been reported, for example, in Sprague-Dawley rats obtained from different commercial breeders (Rex *et al.* 2007).

Examples of frequently used strains:

- Wistar albino. This strain was developed at the Wistar Institute in 1906. The animals are easy to handle and male aggressive behaviour develops relatively late. It is an outbred or random-bred strain and a large number of varieties exist worldwide.
- Sprague-Dawley albino. This strain originates from R.W. Dawley from Wisconsin in 1925. Originally female Wistar rats were crossed with males from an unknown origin. The animals are gentle and may grow to a large size. This random- or outbred strain may vary considerably across breeders.
- Long-Evans hooded. This strain was originally developed at Berkeley, California in 1910 by crossing Wistar females with wild male rats. The head and extremities are black, and the rest of the body is white. It has pigmented eyes, and, although this strain can be easily handled, the level of aggressive behaviour is generally high.

Apart from the traditional inbred and outbred strains, a wide variety of genetic selection lines are available. These lines are genetically selected for the presence or absence of certain behavioural or physiological characteristics. For example, the Roman High Avoidance (RHA) and the Roman Low Avoidance (RLA) lines are selected for their behavioural performance in an active shock avoidance paradigm, using the Roman Wistar as the parental population. The Kyoto Wistar was used to select the Spontaneous Hypertensive Rat (SHR) line, using high sympathetic reactivity as a selection criterion. Most of these genetic selection lines are not commercially available, and can only be obtained via the specific research institutes that breed and select these lines.

Genomics

The analysis of the full rat genome is an important recent development. This project was a joint effort by 13 research institutes, coordinated by the American National Institute of Health to produce the Rat Genome Database[2]. Recently, a genome wide analysis of single nucleotide polymorphisms (SNPs) has also became available for 35 different rat strains including wild rats (Nijman *et al.* 2008).

[2]http://www.nih.gov/science/models/rat/

Laboratory management and breeding.

General husbandry

Housing

In the past, laboratory rats have been housed under a wide variety of conditions and in cages of all sorts of materials. Most countries have formal rules and guidelines for accommodation and care of laboratory animals, for example: the European *Directive for the Protection of Animals used for Experimental and Scientific Purposes 1986*, for which the guidelines were recently updated (European Commission 2007), or the American *Guide for the Care and Use of Laboratory Animals* (National Research Council 1996). These guidelines specify floor area required per animal in relation to weight and number of cage mates, and the minimum cage height. Although these guidelines may differ between countries, they have led to a considerable degree of standardisation of housing conditions and improvement of welfare. However, it is difficult to scientifically specify the minimum sizes of pens and cages for maintaining laboratory rats as much depends on the strain, group size and age of the animals, their familiarity with each other and their reproductive status. For example, increasing the available floor area per animal does not necessarily improve housing conditions, because in some more socially active strains, well defined dominance relationships may develop. This in turn may lead to a larger variation between individuals and even the development of stress pathologies (Tamashiro *et al.* 2005).

In view of the importance of play in the development of adult social behaviour and adaptive capacity it is recommended that animals are provided with sufficient space during the first 3–4 weeks after weaning, with a maximum of seven or eight animals on a floor space of about $0.2\,m^2$ (Yildiz *et al.* 2007). For most strains, this density will be adequate until the animals reach a body weight of around 300 g. As the animals grow older and become larger, the number of animals may be reduced to three per $0.2\,m^2$ cage. There is general agreement on stocking densities in the various European, American and Australian regulations and codes of practice. When changing to a different housing system or different rat strains, it is generally recommended that all animals are carefully monitored in terms of their behaviour, breeding performance and general condition.

Most modern cages have their walls and floor made from solid macrolon with a stainless steel mesh lid. These cages are available in different sizes and are relatively cheap and easy to clean. Although stainless steel cages with a wire mesh floor may be easier to clean, the rats have no opportunity for behavioural thermoregulation; consequently, they should only be used when temperature, humidity and ventilation (draught) are well controlled. Indeed, when given a choice, rats prefer solid floors for resting (Manser *et al.* 1995). Within the ambient temperature range of 20–28 °C no thermoregulatory differences have been observed between animals housed on acrylic floors or metal floors. Below this range, however, animals housed on metal floors show a significant increase in metabolism, whereas above 28 °C animals housed on acrylic floors have problems controlling their body temperature (Gordon & Fogelson 1994).

Environmental provisions

In general, cages should be provided with adequate bedding material. The main function of bedding is to absorb urine and faeces. However, bedding material seems to be essential for certain biological needs as well. It provides insulation and with some materials the opportunity for nest building. Therefore, using appropriate bedding material may be an easy way to improve the well-being of laboratory rats. A variety of bedding materials is commercially available, ranging from wood chips, wood shavings and sawdust to absorbent paper. Experiments using preference tests have shown that male rats generally prefer bedding which consists of large fibrous particles (Blom *et al.* 1996). This preference may be due to several factors. Experimental evidence suggests that rats prefer bedding material which they can manipulate. Certain types of bedding material should be avoided if they contain irritating dust, or produce high levels of ultrasound in a frequency range for which rats are extremely sensitive when the animal moves (Blom *et al.* 1996).

Certain experimental conditions preclude the use of bedding material, for example in experiments where diet is critical and where the ingestion of bedding could affect the experimental results. In these conditions, it may be necessary to use a wire mesh floor and carefully controlled environmental conditions.

Several studies show that environmental enrichment may be another important provision for the animals. Animals raised from weaning in an environment enriched with objects such as ladders, balls, tubes and boxes are better in several learning tasks, are less defensive, show more exploration, and have a thicker cerebral cortex and a higher synaptic density than rats raised under standard conditions (Smith & Corrow 2005). Although environmental enrichment is generally considered to improve animal welfare and is advised in most of the codes of practice, the scientific evidence in support of this conclusion is still rather limited, and the value very much depends on the enrichment used (see reviews by Benefiel *et al.* (2005), Gonder and Laber (2007) and Chapter 10 this volume). Moreover, it may have unexpected and unintended consequences as well. Minor changes in the cage may alter the animal's behaviour and physiology considerably and often in an unexpected direction. In view of the wide range of supplies available for enrichment, and hence the lack of standardisation, this will reduce the reproducibility of experimental data (Bayne 2005; Benefiel *et al.* 2005). The bottom line is that environmental conditions and provisions are reflected in the physiology, neurobiology and behaviour of the animal. More fundamental research is required to determine whether, and in which direction, this altered state affects the capacity of the animal to cope with the laboratory environment and the conditions of animal experimentation.

Social grouping

Rats are social animals by nature, and an extensive literature shows that they are very sensitive to social isolation (Hall 1998). Although isolation at any age can have permanent effects on behaviour and physiology, some periods seem to exist throughout which rats are particularly vulnerable to social isolation. In particular, pre-weaning maternal separation and handling affects a wide variety of adult behavioural and neurobiological processes. Another sensitive period is the one when juveniles spend much time playing, particularly post-natal weeks 5 and 6. Even brief social isolation during these 2 weeks has a significant effect on subsequent adult social behaviour and stress reactivity (Gutman & Nemeroff 2002). In adulthood, long-term social isolation is well known to induce a number of behavioural disturbances such as increased locomotor activity, learning deficits, anxiety and aggression (Arakawa 2005; Malkesman *et al.* 2006). Some experiments have indicated that isolation at adulthood may induce a state of anxiety or depression which is presumably due to changes in central serotonergic neurotransmission, and which are difficult to restore with resocialisation (Maisonnette *et al.* 1993; Silva *et al.* 2003). Although these data indicate that the social environment has a strong and often lasting impact on behaviour and physiology, the consequences for animal welfare are not always clear and have not been studied very well (Krohn *et al.* 2006). Great care should be taken in standardising the social environment and, wherever possible, rats should be housed in a social group to ensure that they are normal both behaviourally and physiologically. In the author's experience, a reliable standardised method of avoiding the effects of social isolation, without encountering problems with dominance relationships, is to house individual male rats with a female sterilised by ligation of her fallopian ducts.

In the breeding colony, rats are usually housed in all male and all female groups. These groups should be of a standard size and composed of littermates. Mixing litters may affect the social relations between group members and may induce social stress. Mixing groups of adult male rats should be avoided, as it can result in serious dominance fights, and consequently in injury and social stress. In some experiments, regular mixing of social groups has been used as a procedure to study the adverse effects of social stress (Mormede 1997).

Presentation of food and water

Food is generally presented in food trays forming part of the lid of the cage and standard procedure is to provide food *ad libitum*. However, a large number of experiments show that longevity is increased when food availability and/or caloric intake is restricted (for a recent review see Goto *et al.* 2007). In a well controlled study, Roe *et al.* (1995) found that a restriction of food intake to 80% of the *ad libitum* intake increased the 30 months survival from 42% to 68%. Moreover, under such food restriction regimes, the incidence of neoplasms is significantly reduced, in particular in the aging animal. This suggests that welfare may be improved with a restricted diet if the animal is to be kept into its old age.

Water should always be given *ad libitum*. However, in a recent review, Rowland (2007) argued that 12–24 h of water deprivation falls well within the regulatory range of physiological and behavioural adaptive mechanisms of the rat. The behavioural and physiological adjustments to these periods of water deprivation seem to minimise the additional physiological and psychological stress of deprivation. Water is usually given in containers with a stainless steel nipple. This allows the water intake in individual cages to be monitored and controlled. Several sizes of water bottles for rats are available commercially. In large animal facilities, automatic watering systems may be used. However, these systems must be checked regularly to ensure that the water valves are functioning properly to avoid the possibility of the animals becoming dehydrated or the cage flooding.

Identification and sexing

Many experimental procedures require individual marking of animals for which several methods can be used. Due consideration should be given to using the least invasive method that is compatible with the study. The easiest way is to write a number at the base of the tail with a permanent marker. However, as a result of tail skin growth and renewal, these marks have to be renewed every 2 weeks. This is also the case with coloured dyes applied to the fur. Tattooing numbers or codes on the tail ears or toes is a more permanent way of marking. Another method of individual marking is to use an ear notch or ear-punch code, or to use numbered metal ear tags. However, because of the important role of auditory information in the social communication of rats, and because ears can be damaged by fighting, and the markings obliterated, these methods are often unsuitable. Rats can also be identified by means of injectable microchips or transponders. These chips are commercially available and sufficiently miniaturised. Each chip is provided with a unique code, and in some systems an additional code for the experiment can be added. The chip can be read without handling the animal using a portable reader provided with a display. Data from the reader can also be downloaded on to a computer. These electronic identification systems are reliable, and further developments are to be expected. For example some systems include the facility to measure body temperature or heart rate in association with the individual code of the animal.

The sexes can readily be distinguished on the basis of the anogenital distance (Figure 22.3). In males, the distance between the urethra and the anus is greater than in females. Moreover, males can be distinguished by the wrinkled, sparsely haired scrotum at the root of the tail. In a cool environment, the testes may be retracted. The vagina of the female is an orifice at some distance caudal to the urethra.

Physical environment and hygiene

Rats are normally housed in well ventilated rooms in which temperature, light and humidity are controlled. They can be bred and maintained in a wide range of environmental temperatures, provided that a sufficient degree of behavioural thermoregulation such as nest building is possible (Gordon 1990). Most codes of practice specify a room temperature of 20–22 °C mainly for the purpose of standardising laboratory experiments. Temperature should be measured in the cage because this may deviate strongly from room temperature, depending on the ventilation, the density of animals per cage and the location of the cage with respect to the heating system of the room. When rats are kept in wire mesh cages, the environmental temperature should not drop below 22 °C, and there should be no draughts.

The animal room should be well ventilated without creating draughts. It is difficult to give a standard recommendation on the number of air changes per hour, as it depends on: the number of animals kept in the room, their size, the humidity of the air and the cage cleaning routine. However, a few general guidelines can be provided. The main purpose of ventilation is to provide the animals with air of good quality. Apart from the obvious requirements of sufficient oxygen and low levels of carbon dioxide, the concentration of ammonia should be kept as low as possible. Ammonia is a breakdown product of urea and is harmful to the animals because it may facilitate bacterial infections of *Mycoplasma pulmonis* in the mucous membranes of the eyes, nose and the respiratory tract (Schoeb *et al.* 1982). As long as the bedding remains dry, ammonia will not be formed. This, in turn, depends on the number of animals per cage, the humidity, the ventilation and the frequency of cleaning. A smell of ammonia in the animal room, however, is a good indication that the animals are overcrowded or the cages need clean-

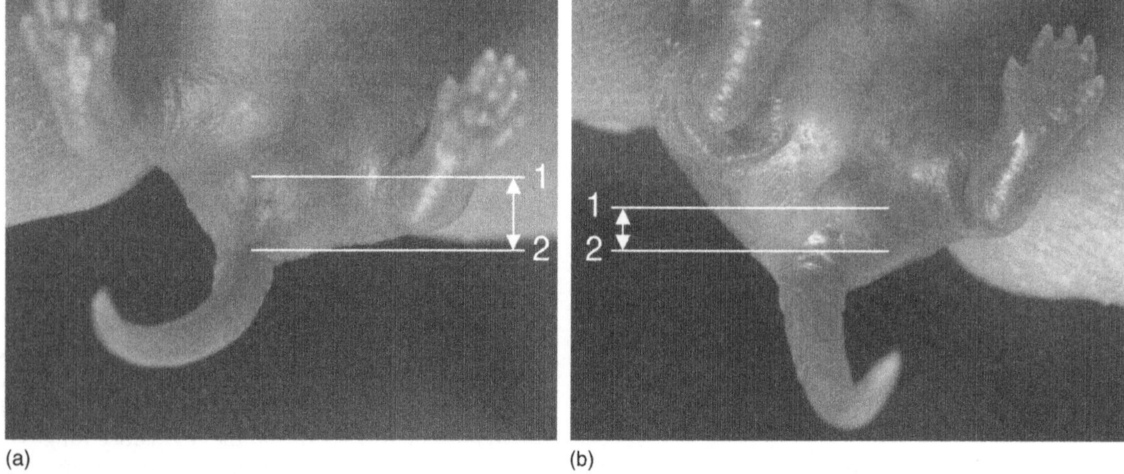

Figure 22.3 Sexing newborn rats (male on left, female on right). Note the greater distance between urethra (1) and anus (2) in the male.

ing. Humidity should be around 50%. When it drops below 30%, young animals tend to develop ring tail (Njaa *et al.* 1957). Cages should not be cleaned more often than once a week, because cleaning in itself is a considerable stressor and may disrupt the social structure in the cage. However, any increase in ventilation should not result in draught. On average 8–20 air changes per hour should suffice for a normally populated animal room (Clough 1984).

The use of individually ventilated cages (IVC) is increasingly common. A wide variety of systems is commercially available. Ventilated caging strongly improves the working conditions of animal care staff in terms of exposure to allergens. However, few studies have addressed the question of rat welfare in these housing systems. Depending on the system, ventilation rate may range between 40 and 50 air changes per hour, but 120 air changes per hour can also be found. In a study on the impact of cage ventilation on rats, Krohn *et al.* (2003) concluded that the number of air changes should be kept below 80 changes per hour according to preference tests and telemetric measurements of heart rate and blood pressure. It is not clear why the ventilation rate of IVC systems differ so strongly from the recommended ventilation rate of animal rooms. Most likely, this discrepancy is due to the fact that the ventilation rate of small cages is technically easier to increase than that of a whole animal room. Nevertheless, from a biological point of view, the currently used ventilation rates of individual ventilated cages might be considered as a rather artificial laboratory condition, since feral rats live in burrow systems with hardly any ventilation in the nesting chambers.

Rats are generally kept in light-controlled rooms with a photoperiod of 12 h light and 12 h dark. Different photoperiods such as 16 h light and 8 h dark are sometimes to improve for example breeding results. However, it is important to realise that the photoperiod may strongly affect experimental results (Prendergast *et al.* 2007; Prendergast & Kay 2008).

Rats are extremely sensitive to light, in particular albino strains. Retinal damage in albino rats due to light exposure is frequently reported (Perez & Perentes 1994). On the basis of the analysis of retinal damage it is recommended that the light intensity as measured at the level of the bedding of the cage should not exceed 50 lux (Perez & Perentes 1994; Semple-Rowland & Dawson 1987). However, when behavioural measures are also considered, such as activity and light avoidance, welfare of the animal seems to be optimised at levels below 25 lux. As a result of their sensitivity to light, rats may differ in the degree of retinal damage depending on the distance between the cage and the light source. A more uniform light intensity may be obtained by putting shelves at some distance above the cages.

Health monitoring, quarantine and barrier systems

Infections of laboratory animals can severely influence the outcome of experiments. Therefore, a health monitoring programme is essential to ensure reliability and reproducibility of research data. The Federation of European Laboratory Animal Science Associations (FELASA) advises that breeding units of laboratory rats should be screened every 3 months with respect to serology, bacteriology, parasitology and pathology with a sample size of at least four animals (FELASA 1994). Table 22.2 summarises the recommended viral, bacterial and parasitic infections to be monitored. It is recommended that positive serological results should be confirmed using another method or a repeated investigation. Bacterial and fungal infections should be investigated in samples from nasal turbinates/nasopharynx, trachea, prepuce/vagina and caecum. In addition, serum samples should be tested for mycoplasmas and *Leptospira* spp. Parasitology should be based on a microscopic examination of the skin, and of fresh wet samples of the ceacal contents, the inner lining of the ileum and of faecal flotation.

Depending on the requirements of the experiments, rats can be housed under different regimes with respect to microbiological control. In many experiments, it is sufficient to keep the animals under conventional clean conditions. This means that there are no special barrier systems and that the microbiological status of the animals is not guaranteed. However, with regular health monitoring and some precautions with respect to cleaning regime, quarantine, and traffic of animal care staff, healthy and highly standardised animals can usually be obtained.

Other experiments require a more strict microbial status. To guarantee the microbiological status of the animals, a strict barrier system is required. These systems usually

Table 22.2 Recommended list of viral and bacterial infections to be monitored every 3 months in rat breeding colonies (FELASA 2002).

Viral infections	*Test frequency*
Kilham rats virus	3 months
Rat parvovirus	3 months
Toolan's H-1 virus virus	3 months
Pneumonia virus of mice	3 months
Sendai virus	3 months
Sialodacryoadenitis/rat coronavirus	3 months
Hantaviruses	Annually
Mouse adenovirus type 1 (FL)	Annually
Mouse adenovirus type 2 (K87)	Annually
Reovirus type 3	Annually
Bacterial, mycoplasmal and fungal infections	
Bordetella bronchiseptica	3 months
Clostridium piliforme	3 months
Corynebacterium kutscheri	3 months
Mycoplasma spp.	3 months
Pasteurella spp.	3 months
Salmonella spp.	3 months
Streptobacillus moniliformis	3 months
Streptococci β-haemolytic	3 months
Streptococcus pneumoniae	3 months
Helicobacter spp.	Annually
Parasitology	
Ecotoparasites	3 months
Endoparasites	3 months

consist of physical barriers, combined with strict rules regarding disinfection of cages, utensils and personnel. A microbiologically defined breeding colony is started with animals obtained by caesarean section and fostered with microbiologically defined or germ-free mothers kept in isolators, according to standard procedures.

In some highly controlled experiments, it is necessary to keep rats in germ-free conditions. Special isolators are required to prevent contamination. These animals are. however. highly abnormal, because they lack the natural micro-organisms involved in essential processes such as digestion and heat production.

Transport

Long-distance transportation of rats should be avoided wherever possible because of the long-lasting effects of stress on behaviour and physiology (Koolhaas *et al.* 1997). When rats are obtained from a commercial breeder, they should be allowed a recovery period of at least 1 week, but preferably 2–3 weeks. Although the animals can be transported in cages used for standard laboratory housing, special disposable transport cages are available as well. When the rats are shipped by air, the transport cage should meet the criteria of the International Air Transport Association *Dangerous Goods Regulations Manual* (IATA 2010). Although it is unlikely that animals will drink or eat, owing to the stress involved in transportation, if the journey is expected to last longer than 24 h, they must be provided with food and water. For a general discussion of transport issues see Chapter 13.

Breeding

The adults

Rats are sexually mature at around 2 months of age. The fertile state of the female is most easily recognised by her behaviour in the presence of a male rat. Females in oestrus perform a highly characteristic soliciting behaviour, consisting of hopping and ear-wiggling and presenting the anogenital region to the male (Erskine 1989). When the male attempts to mount her, a receptive female adopts the lordosis position. Experienced animal care staff can induce lordosis in the female rat by gently palpating her flanks. A more elaborate way of determining the fertility state of the female is by monitoring the oestrous cycle by means of daily vaginal smears. These smears are taken by flushing the vagina with a drop of saline using a small drip pipette, or by taking a sample with a small flexible spatula. The sample is subsequently put on a glass slide, dried and stained with cresyl violet. The phase of the oestrous cycle can be determined under the microscope on the basis of the presence and quantity of cornified epithelial cells and leucocytes. Table 22.3 summarises some of the basic data on reproduction in the rat.

The male will frequently mount an oestrous female and, after several intromissions, an ejaculation occurs. This sequence of events may be repeated two or three times with

Table 22.3 Reproductive parameters.

Female	*Normal value*
Mammary glands	6 pairs
Vaginal opening (day)	28–60
First oestrus (day)	40–65
Oestrous cycle	Polyoestrus
Length of oestrous cycle (days)	4–6
Stage 1 dioestrus	6 h
Stage 2 pro-oestrus (early)	60 h
Stage 3 pro-oestrus (late)	12 h
Stage 4 oestrus	10–20 h
Stage 5 metoestrus	8 h
Age at first mating (day)	50–100
Gestation period	21–23
Size of litter	3–18
Male	*Normal value*
Descent of testes (day)	15–50
Age at sexual maturity (day)	40–50
Age at aggressive maturity (day)	90–120
Age at end of mating (months)	9–24
Minimum number of intromissions	3–10
Length of ejaculation (s)	10–20

a post-ejaculatory interval of 5–10 minutes. After a while, the female ceases courtship behaviour and defends herself from the male. Simultaneously, the vaginal fluid and the ejaculate coagulate and form a plug. The presence of such a plug is often used as evidence of mating. When the time of conception has to be determined accurately, either the behaviour of the male and female can be observed directly, or a series of vaginal smears can be taken and monitored for the presence of sperm.

Sperm cells can be detected microscopically in the vaginal smear up to 12 h after conception. It is difficult to detect pregnancy before the 15th day post conception. After day 15, foetuses can be detected by palpation, body weight rapidly increases, the female starts to perform nest-building behaviour and maternal aggression towards males gradually develops.

On the day of delivery, the pregnant rat becomes restless, and nest-building behaviour reaches its maximum. Pups are delivered at intervals of 5–10 minutes, usually during the last hours of the dark period and the beginning of the light phase. After delivery of a pup, the mother bites the umbilical cord, eats the placenta and cleans the neonate. A weak or stillborn neonate will usually be eaten immediately.

The young

A healthy rat neonate is pink coloured and begins to suckle within the first few hours after birth. Disturbance of the delivery process should be avoided, because this may lead to infanticide by the mother. From the second day onwards, a beige spot shining through the abdominal wall of the pup indicates the amount of milk it has consumed. Normally, mothers nurse their pups for about 1 h, after which she leaves the nest for several hours to rest and eat. The mother keeps the pups together in the nest, and when one escapes from the nest, she rapidly retrieves it. Pup retrieval is facilitated by ultrasonic vocalisations emitted by pups which have become separated from their mother and littermates (see Stern and Lonstein (2001) for a review on maternal behaviour). A healthy neonate has a pink colour and a well filled abdomen. Pups with a dark pink, violet or cyanotic, often wrinkled skin are indicative of a mother with insufficient milk supply. A somewhat disturbed nest and the absence of pup retrieval is indicative of a mother who is not nursing her pups properly.

Pups are extremely sensitive to rearing conditions. A large amount of literature shows that the adult behavioural, neurobiological, immunological and neuroendocrine reactivity (Tang *et al.* 2006) is affected by quality of nursing, neonatal handling, maternal separation, environmental enrichment and social isolation. Increasing evidence shows that these effects are mediated by the epigenetic process of DNA methylation resulting in permanent blockade of the expression of specific genes (Meaney & Szyf 2005; Szyf *et al.* 2008). Some of these influences seem to become more prominent in the aging rat, indicating that neonatal environmental factors affect the speed of aging (Meaney *et al.* 1991). In view of these influences of rearing conditions, it is recommended that neonates are raised with as little disturbance as possible, and that the cleaning regime, number of pups and sex ratio per nest are standardised. Any manipulation of the litter, such as reducing size or mixing with others, should be done on the first day after birth.

At birth, the pups are hairless, toothless and blind. The newborn is essentially poikilothermic and must rely upon the maternally maintained microenvironment and huddling of the litter to achieve thermal homeostasis. Within 2 weeks, thermoregulation matures, the coat develops and the eyes open. By day 9 the incisor teeth are sufficiently developed to gnaw and by day 11 the first solid food is usually taken.

The young are generally weaned at the age of 21 days, and subsequently housed in groups of the same gender. The period immediately after weaning till the age of about 60 days is characterised by intense play fighting. This is essential for the development of normal adult social behaviour (Pellis & Pellis 1998).

Breeding systems

Several systems can be used for breeding rats depending on whether inbred or outbred strains are used. The main purpose of any breeding system is to maintain a standard genetic quality of animals over generations. Inbreeding requires the crossing of closely related animals, usually brother × sister mating. To maintain adequate control over the genetic quality of the foundation stock, monogamous mating is recommended. In random-bred colonies, inbreeding is inevitable, but the degree of inbreeding depends on the breeding system used. When a monogamous mating system is used, the inbreeding coefficient, which represents the loss of genetic variation in the colony (ΔF) will be $1/(2N)$, where N is the total number of breeding animals. This means that the smaller the breeding colony, the greater will be the degree of inbreeding. Polygamous mating can be used for the expansion or production stock. However, using one male with several females for foundation stock, increases not only the risk of inbreeding, but also the likelihood of uncontrolled selection, and selection based on breeding performance. It is therefore better to use a monogamous rotation mating scheme. Rotation schemes are designed to reduce the degree of inbreeding by 50%. If a random-bred colony is maintained as a closed colony for at least four generations, and the number of breeding animals is sufficiently large for a $\Delta F < 1\%$, the colony may be designated as an outbred stock (Willis & Dalton 1998; Zimmermann *et al.* 2000).

Random-bred and outbred strains have a certain degree of genetic heterogeneity. In some experiments, this heterogeneity may be desirable, for example when results should have some degree of general validity in a population. It has the advantage that the results are based upon a broad spectrum of genotypes. In other experiments, genetically homogeneous inbred strains are required. This has the advantage that the individual variation is reduced and hence the number of animals required per experiment. However, it is important to realise that the results may only be valid for the particular genotype in question. To minimise this problem, F1 hybrids of two inbred strains can be used; they are still genetically homogeneous, but share the genetic characteristics of two different genotypes.

Feeding

The Norway rat is omnivorous by nature, and has a remarkable capacity to adjust its diet and food intake for specific dietary deficiencies (Markison 2001). The rat is widely used to study the mechanisms of food intake and body weight regulation (Schwartz *et al.* 2000). Feeding occurs in a specific daily pattern (Figure 22.4). Most of the food intake takes place during the dark period with a higher incidence of feeding in the first and last 2h of the dark period (Strubbe & Woods 2004). Rats exhibit a clear preference for certain diets and, in the laboratory, they show preferences for specific nutrients, which vary across the light–dark cycle (Tempel *et al.* 1989; Shor-Posner *et al.* 1994). Figure 22.4 also shows the daily variation in preference for carbohydrate, fat and protein-enriched lab chow. Nutrient balance and in particular amino acid intake is also maintained by coprophagia. Depending on the nutritional balance of their food, rats may eat 10–50% of their own faeces (Fajardo & Hornicke 1989). Moreover, recent studies show a strong influence of the social environment on food preference, ie, individual rats rapidly adopt the food preference of their cage-mates (Galef 2003). Finally, the rat is well known for its conditioned taste aversion, namely its capacity to associate a certain type of food or taste with sickness (Mediavilla *et al.* 2005).

Food is generally supplied *ad libitum*. However, it is now well established that food restriction will increase life expectancy and reduce tumour development in aging rats (Roe *et al.* 1995; Goto *et al.* 2007). Despite these studies, rats are still bred with *ad libitum* food availability. Commercially available diets are generally made from natural ingredients. Although most manufacturers specify the formula of their diets, the exact concentration of dietary components, nutrients and contaminants may vary considerably. This variation may either be due to different brands or to the use of different natural ingredients within the same brand. If such

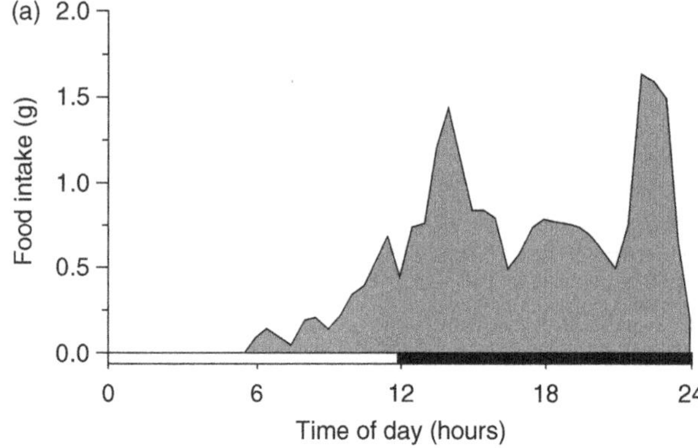

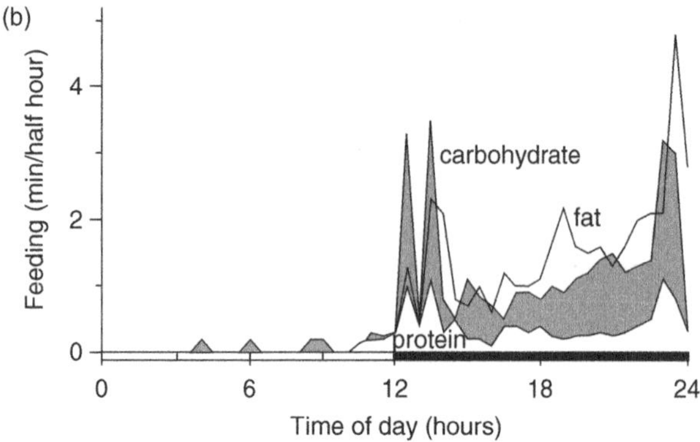

Figure 22.4 Circadian variation in food intake (a) and nutrient preference (b) in male Wistar rats. The black bar indicates the dark period of the light–dark cycle.

variations are likely to have an adverse or unpredictable effect on the experimental results it may be necessary to use a chemically defined or purified diet.

Laboratory procedures

Handling and training

Rats can usually be handled easily without the use of gloves or forceps. Before handling a rat, it is important to ensure that the animal is awake and alert. Rats which are not used to handling should be picked up by the base of the tail and immediately put on the arm of the handler (Figure 22.5). To comfort the animal, one may gently stroke the back of the animal and the neck region. They like being petted and tickled, during which they emit ultrasonic vocalisations as a sign of positive affect (Panksepp 2007). After a few minutes, the animal is usually willing to be picked up with the hand around its body (Figure 22.6). Rats recognise humans as individuals, so that it is always best if they are handled by a familiar person, usually the animal care staff. If rats are routinely gently handled and petted they are much less likely to be stressed by routine experimental procedures such as injections. A good relationship with a handler makes an important contribution to the welfare of these animals. Force should not be necessary and avoided as much as possible, because it will result in stress to the rat and elicit defensive responses. However, some strains of rats may be aggressive or nervous and difficult to handle. In this situation, it will be

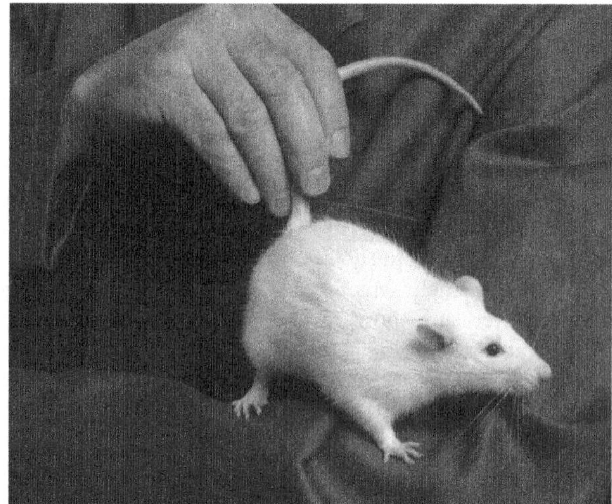

Figure 22.5 Method of holding a rat which has not been handled previously.

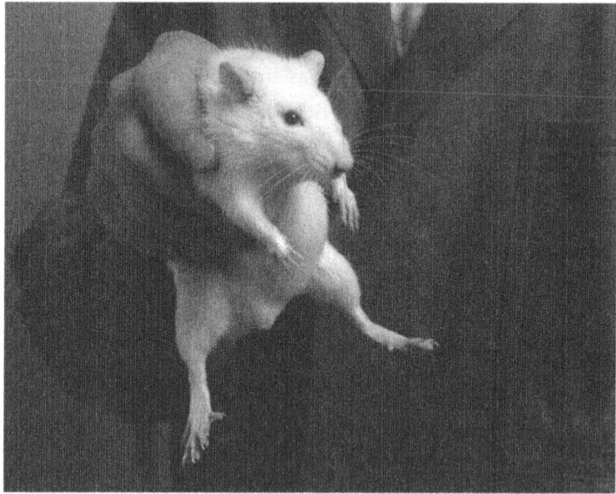

Figure 22.6 Holding a friendly rat or one used to handling.

necessary to handle the rat more firmly to avoid biting and escape. The best way of holding a defensive rat is presented in Figure 22.7. The animal should be approached from the back, with one hand grasping the base of the tail and the other hand should be laid on the back of the animal. The thumb and forefinger should form a circle around the neck of the animal, with one forepaw included in the ring. The other forepaw can be fixed between the forefinger and the middle finger. In general, rats are very easily trained to co-operate. It is recommended, therefore, to adapt the animals to the handling procedure several days before the animal will be used for experimentation. See also Chapter 16.

Physiological monitoring

A wide variety of techniques is available to monitor physiological processes in rats. A summary of the most common experimental and surgical techniques is presented by Waynforth and Flecknell (1992), whereas a more advanced manual of microsurgical techniques is presented by Dongen *et al.* (1990). However, many of these techniques are too

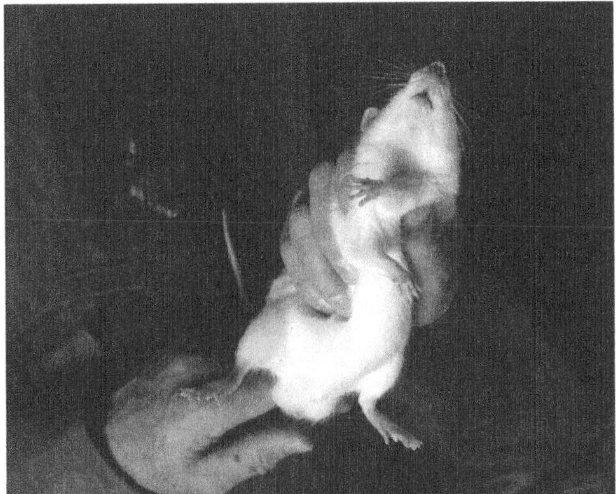

Figure 22.7 Restraining a rat.

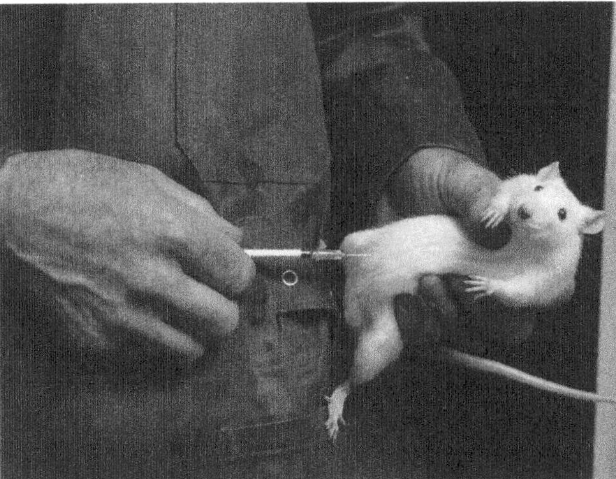

Figure 22.8 Giving an intraperitoneal injection to a well handled rat.

complex to be suitable as a standard daily laboratory procedure. Because stress from handling significantly affects their physiology, data should be obtained from undisturbed animals. Body temperature, for example, is often recorded using a thermistor inserted into the rectum to a depth of 3–5 cm. However, handling is unavoidable for this procedure; so in fact it measures stress-induced hyperthermia. Recent developments in chip technology using implanted transponders combine the identification of the individual with a body temperature measurement in the freely moving animal. More detailed and permanent recordings of body temperature can be obtained using permanently implanted transmitters. Transmitter systems are also suitable for monitoring heart rate, blood pressure, electroencephalograms (EEG) and electrocardiograms (ECG) in freely moving animals.

Blood samples can be collected in several ways. A decision tree for the choice of the best method can be found on the website of the National Centre for the Replacement, Refinement and Reduction of Animals in Research[3]. Generally, for the assay of stress-sensitive and rapidly changing substances in the blood, a permanently implanted jugular vein canula is recommended (Waynforth & Flecknell 1992). This technique allows repeated sampling over a period of several weeks. Another method of sampling to obtain reliable baseline values of stress-sensitive substances is to collect trunk blood from decapitated animals. This method, of course, has the disadvantages that it is fatal for the animal and does not allow repeated measures from the same individual. Moreover, great care should be taken that the whole procedure from catching, handling and decapitation of one animal does not affect stress levels in the subsequently sampled animals (Zethof *et al.* 1995). For the assay of less reactive substances, blood may be collected with a syringe from the tail vein. When a large volume of blood is required, a cardiac puncture can be used with the animal under deep anaesthesia (Joint Working Group on Refinement (JWGR) 1993).

Urine and faeces can be collected by housing the animals in commercially available metabolism cages. Faeces can be used to measure baseline concentrations of steroid hormones (Lepschy *et al.* 2007).

Administration of medicines

Most of the commonly used techniques to administer substances to rats are extensively described in Waynforth and Flecknell (1992) and by the JWGR (2001). As some of these procedures can be rather stressful to the animal and may, therefore, interfere with the experiment, alternative stress-free methods will be indicated here.

Intravenous (iv) injections can be given via the sublingual vein or the lateral vein at the root of the tail in an anesthetised rat (needle size: 0.5–0.6 mm). When frequent iv injections are required or the injection is to be combined with subsequent blood sampling, the implantation of a permanent jugular vein catheter is recommended. This method allows a stress-free iv injection to be given in freely moving animals.

Intraperitoneal (ip) injections are given in the lower left quadrant of the abdomen, to avoid damage to vital organs such as liver, stomach and spleen (needle size: maximum 0.9 mm). It is not usually necessary to restrain the animal so that an animal which is used to handling can be given an ip injection as depicted in Figure 22.8. More nervous, defensive animals will need to be held more firmly, including their hindquarters, and a second person may be needed to give the injection.

Subcutaneous (sc) injections can be given by placing the animal on top of the cage or on a table and raising a fold of the skin of the neck (needle size: 0.5–0.6 mm). The needle should be slid into the fold with its tip parallel to the body surface. When a more chronic administration of substances is required, it may be better to use osmotic mini pumps, the implantation of pellets or silicon capsules, in preference to a frequent injection schedule. Osmotic mini pumps are commercially available in a range of infusion rates and durations.

Intragastric administration of fluids can be performed by gavage of the oesophagus using a curved needle with a small bulb at the tip. Different sized rats need different sizes

[3]http://www.nc3rs.org.uk/bloodsamplingmicrosite/

of gavage needle (Waynforth & Flecknell 1992). For per oral administration the rat is held firmly by the skin of the neck and the back so that the head is kept immobile and in line with the back. Great care should be taken that the injection fluid does not enter the trachea. When frequent intragastric administrations are required, a permanent intragastric catheter may be implanted.

Anaesthesia and analgesia

General anaesthesia can be induced either by inhalation or by injection of anaesthetics by intraperitoneal, intramuscular or intravenous route. There are excellent standard works available with all the detailed information on anaesthesia and pain management (Flecknell & Waterman-Pearson 2000; Flecknell 2009). Reference to these books is strongly recommended. Table 22.4 summarises the inhalation and injection anaesthetics recommended for use in rats.

Inhalational anaesthetics are generally preferable because they have the advantage of easy adjustment of the depth of anaesthesia and rapid recovery. Induction of anaesthesia with volatile anaesthetics can be achieved using an induction chamber connected to a vaporiser. After induction of anaesthesia, gas can be delivered through a face mask or via an endotracheal tube; a calibrated vaporiser should be used. The volatile anaesthetic is mixed with air or a mixture of N_2O and O_2 (1:1).

Several types of injectable anaesthetics are suitable for rats. The selection of these anaesthetics depends on a variety of factors such as: the duration of the surgery; the preferred degree of muscle relaxation; and the appropriate level of analgesia. In rats, the anaesthetic is generally given as a single intraperitoneal injection. However, it is important to appreciate that the response to these injectable anaesthetics may vary strongly between individual animals and between sexes and strains. Therefore, when using a new anaesthesia regimen for the first time, the dosage required should be carefully assessed.

It is sometimes useful to reduce possible side effects of the anaesthetic compound by administering certain drugs as premedication. Sedatives or tranquillisers can be used to reduce the stress associated with the induction of anaesthesia and to promote a smooth recovery. However, most of these compounds have little or no analgesic properties and cannot be used to reduce post-operative pain. Anticholinergic agents may be used to reduce the production of saliva and to reduce undesirable autonomic responses.

During surgery, the depth of the anaesthesia should be monitored frequently. This can be assessed easily by checking some reflexes of the animal. A correctly anaesthetised rat shows a regular deep respiration and an absence of the righting reflex when being placed on its back. Pinching the tail with the finger nails does not induce a flick of the tail or vocalisations and a puff of air on the eyes does not induce an eye blink reflex. In view of the sensitivity of the rat's eyes for bright light, they should be protected from the surgical light, and a drop of saline in the eye will prevent the eye from dehydration during long surgical procedures.

Table 22.4 Inhalation and injection anaesthetics recommended for use in rats.

Drug and indication	*Dose and route of administration*	
Premedication (anticholinergics)		
Atropine	0.05 mg/kg sc	
Premedication (sedatives)		
Diazepam	2.5 mg/kg ip	
Acepromazine	2.5 mg/kg sc	
Hypnorm (fentanyl/ fluanisone)	0.4 ml/kg ip	
Xylazine	10 mg/kg sc	
Medetomidine	0.5 mg/kg sc	
Anaesthesia (short duration, 5–10 minutes)		
Alphaxalone	10–12 mg/kg iv	
Propofol	10 mg/kg iv	
Methohexitone	7–10 mg/kg iv	
Anaesthesia (medium duration, 20–60 minutes)		
Hypnorm/ midazolam	2 ml/kg ip (1 part Hypnorm, 1 part midazolam and 2 parts water for injection)	
Ketamine/ xylazine	90 mg/kg ip 10 mg/kg ip	
Ketamine/ medetomidine	75 mg/kg ip 0.5 mg/kg ip	
Pentobarbital	40–55 mg/kg ip	
Anaesthesia (long duration, non-recovery)		
Chloralose	130 mg/kg ip	
Urethane	1–2 g/kg ip	
Anaesthesia (inhalation agents, short/medium/long duration)		
Halothane	Induction concentration 4–5%	Maintenance concentration 1–2%
Isoflurane	Induction concentration 4%	Maintenance concentration 1.5–3%
Methoxyflurane	Induction concentration 4%	Maintenance concentration 0.5–1%

Many anaesthetics interfere with the thermoregulation of the animal. Therefore, body temperature should be carefully monitored during anaesthesia. An electric blanket controlled by a thermostat and integrated with a rectal temperature probe should be used.

Generally, rats recover rapidly from major surgery. However, a post-operative recovery period of at least 1 week is recommended. Moreover, pain should be relieved using analgesic treatment. The most common analgesics for rats are summarised in Table 22.5 (Bertens *et al.* 1993; Flecknell & Waterman-Pearson 2000; Flecknell 2009).

Analgesics administered systemically may have side effects which interfere with the experiment. In these situations, the use of local analgesic ointment to treat surgical

Table 22.5 Alphabetical list of analgesics for postoperative pain relief.

Drug	Dose
Aspirin	100 mg/kg per os, 4 hourly
Buprenorphine	0.01–0.05 mg/kg sc, iv 8–12 hourly
Butophanol	2 mg/kg sc, 4 hourly
Codeine	60 mg/kg sc, 4 hourly
Flunixin	2.5 mg/kg sc, im, 12 hourly
Morphine	2.5 mg/kg sc, 2-4 hourly
Nalbuphine	1–2 mg/kg im, 3 hourly
Paracetamol	100–300 mg/kg per os, 4 hourly
Pentazocine	10 mg/kg sc, 4 hourly
Phenacitin	100 mg/kg per os, 4 hourly
Pethidine	10–20 mg/kg sc or im, 2–3 hourly

wounds should be considered. This will also prevent the animal from biting surgical wounds and stitches. Recovery is improved after a few days when group housing can be re-established.

Euthanasia

The most appropriate way of killing rats is, to some degree, determined by the type of experiment involved. When the body will not be used for further experimental purposes, the best way of killing the animal is using a rising concentration of carbon dioxide and oxygen (6:4). After the animal has lost consciousness, the concentration of carbon dioxide is raised to 100% and kept at this level for at least 10 minutes. Although this method is widely used throughout the world, there is a significant debate on the stressful nature of this technique (Conlee *et al.* 2005). The immediate use of 100% carbon dioxide should be avoided, because it induces severe dyspnoea and signs of stress. Alternative methods include pre-euthanasia anaesthesia and the use of argon rather than carbon dioxide. Carbon dioxide should not be used to kill neonatal rats because they are relatively resistant to it. When specimens have to be obtained, administering a lethal dose of anaesthetic is usually an appropriate method. However, if the anaesthetic agents could interfere with the experimental results, physical methods of euthanasia are inevitable. Methods include concussion of the brain, cervical dislocation and decapitation (using a special guillotine or sharp scissors). The choice of method will depend on the size of the animal and local regulations. See also Chapter 17.

Common welfare problems

Disease

Rats can be kept free of disease relatively easily under conventional husbandry conditions, provided that these conditions meet certain criteria. For example, it is essential to avoid overcrowding not only in the breeding cages, but also in the whole animal room. Moreover, proper ventilation, humidity control, a cleaning regime using dust-free bedding material, and the use of filter caps are the best prophylactic precautions that can be taken. Reports in the literature suggest that a restricted feeding regime may be the best way to reduce the incidence of neoplasm in aging rats (Roe *et al.* 1995).

The most important indicators of disease and/or lack of well-being in rats are summarised below.

- Appearance. Piloerection and a rough greasy or matted pelage, sometimes with loss of hair, a loose skin, signs of muscle wastage on the back, dehydration and reduced body weight may all be observed. Eyelids are half or fully closed and the eyes have the appearance of being sunken. Red secretion from the lacrimal glands accumulates around the eyes (chromodacryorrhoea).
- Faeces. Soft faeces, or diarrhoea, a dirty tail and an unpleasant smell are indicative of an intestinal infection.
- Behaviour. Initially, animals may be more alert and aggressive, but will become progressively more passive; they stop eating and drinking and reduce exploratory behaviour (Roughan & Flecknell 2003). Sometimes rats gnaw affected parts of the body.
- Posture. The animal frequently lies down, initially curled up with the head touching the abdomen, later stretched with the tail extended. A hard belly indicates abdominal pain. A tilted head is indicative of an infected middle ear.
- Locomotion. A diseased rat moves slowly with a stiff-legged gait and arched back.
- Vocalisation. Squeaking when handled.
- Physiology. Sneezing may be the first sign of a respiratory infection. When the condition of the animal worsens, breathing is audible and laboured and the respiratory frequency increases. Hypothermia indicates a serious condition and a pale appearance is indicative of anaemia or loss of blood.

Sick animals must always be examined by a veterinarian for a complete clinical and *post-mortem* diagnosis. However, many diseases may take a subclinical course with no apparent signs of illness. It is important to be aware of such subclinical diseases, such as latent viral infections, because they may interfere with the standardisation of the experiments. Regular microbiological monitoring of the rat population is therefore essential.

The most common infectious diseases of rats involve infections of the respiratory tract by *Mycoplasma pulmonalis*, *Pasteurella* spp. and *Pneumococcus* spp. Under proper husbandry conditions, the disease will only be apparent in some animals. However, the disease may become a serious problem under less optimal husbandry conditions, or when experimental procedures compromise the physical condition of the animals. If the disease cannot be controlled by chemotherapy or by antibiotics, sick animals must be removed from the colony as soon as possible. Respiratory diseases are transmitted by air or by contact between the animals. Reducing the pH of drinking water is sometimes used to reduce the spread of the infection in a colony through contaminated drinking spouts. See Fox *et al.* (2002) for more extensive information on diseases and their treatment and control.

Abnormal behaviour

Rats rarely show obvious signs of abnormal behaviour. The incidence of stereotypies is very low under standard housing conditions. Abnormal behaviour is usually expressed as an increase in reactivity to environmental stimuli leading to panic reactions, or as increased passivity or state of depression. Occasionally, abnormal aggressive behaviour may occur in group-housed males. One male may continuously attack one of his cage mates, leading to serious wounding or death of the victim, and sometimes to cannibalism. There are no known solutions to this problem, other than killing the particular group of animals.

Another type of abnormal behaviour is chewing the fur of cage mates. The cause of this problem and its solution are unknown.

Reproductive problems

Rats, in particular the outbred strains, generally reproduce without any problems. After giving birth, the mothers of some strains may be infanticidal. This usually results from disturbance to the nest and the nursing mother caused by cage cleaning or other activities in the animal unit. Sensitive strains should be bred in separate, quiet breeding facilities, and pregnant females should be provided with nest boxes and nesting material.

References

Arakawa, H. (2005) Interaction between isolation rearing and social development on exploratory behavior in male rats. *Behavioral Processes*, **70**, 223–234

Bacon, S.J. and McClintock, M.K. (1994) Multiple factors determine the sex ratio of postpartum-conceived Norway rat litters. *Physiology & Behavior*, **56**, 359–366

Barbacka-Surowiak, G., Surowiak, J. and Stoklosowa, S. (2003) The involvement of suprachiasmatic nuclei in the regulation of estrous cycles in rodents. *Reproductive Biology*, **3**, 99–129

Bayne, K. (2005) Potential for unintended consequences of environmental enrichment for laboratory animals and research results. *ILAR Journal*, **46**, 129–139

Benefiel, A.C., Dong, W.K. and Greenough, W.T. (2005) Mandatory "enriched" housing of laboratory animals: the need for evidence-based evaluation. *ILAR Journal*, **46**, 95–105

Bertens, A.P.M.G., Booij, L.H.D.J., Flecknell, P.A. *et al.* (1993) Anaesthesia, analgesia and euthanasia. In: *Principles of Laboratory Animal Sciences*. Eds Zutphen, L.F.M., Baumans, V. and Beynen, A.C., pp. 267–298. Elsevier, Amsterdam

Beynon, R.J. and Hurst, J.L. (2004) Urinary proteins and the modulation of chemical scents in mice and rats. *Peptides*, **25**, 1553–1563

Blom, H.J.M., Van Tintelen, G., Van Vorstenbosch, C.J.A.H.V. *et al.* (1996) Preferences of mice and rats for types of bedding material. *Laboratory Animals*, **30**, 234–244

Calhoun, J.B. (1962) *The Ecology and Sociology of the Norway Rat*. Government Printing Office, Washington, DC

Carvell, G.E. and Simons, D.J. (1990) Biometric analyses of vibrissal tactile discrimination in the rat. *Journal of Neuroscience*, **10**, 2638–2648

Claassen, V. (1994) *Neglected Factors in Pharmacology and Neuroscience Research*. Elsevier, Amsterdam

Clough, G. (1984) Environmental factors in relation to the comfort and well-being of laboratory rats and mice. In: *Standards in Laboratory Animal Management*, Vol. **1**. pp. 7–24. UFAW, Potters Bar

Conlee, K.M., Stephens, M.L., Rowan, A.N. *et al.* (2005) Carbon dioxide for euthanasia: concerns regarding pain and distress, with special reference to mice and rats. *Laboratory Animals*, **39**, 137–161

De Boer, S.F., Van Der Vegt, B.J. and Koolhaas J.M. (2003) Individual variation in aggression of feral rodent strains: a standard for the genetics of aggression and violence? *Behavior Genetics*, **33**, 485–501

Dielenberg, R.A. and McGregor, I.S. (2001) Defensive behavior in rats towards predatory odors: a review. *Neuroscience and Biobehavioral Reviews*, **25**, 597–609

Dongen, J.J.V., Remie, R., Rensema, J.W. *et al.* (1990) *Manual of Microsurgery on the Laboratory Rat*. Elsevier, Amsterdam

Erskine, M.S. (1989) Solicitation behavior in the estrous female rat: a review. *Hormones and Behavior*, **23**, 473–502

European Commission (2007) Commission recommendations of 18 June 2007 on guidelines for the accommodation and care of animals used for experimental and other scientific purposes. Annex II to European Council Directive 86/609. See 2007/526/EC. http://eurlex.europa.eu/LexUriServ/site/en/oj/2007/l_197/l_19720070730en00010089.pdf (accessed 13 May 2008)

Fajardo, G. and Hornicke, H. (1989) Problems in estimating the extent of coprophagy in the rat. *British Journal of Nutrition*, **62**, 551–561

Federation of European Laboratory Animal Science Associations (1994) Recommendations for the health monitoring of mouse, rat, hamster, guineapig and rabbit breeding colonies. *Laboratory Animals*, **28**, 1–12

Federation of European Laboratory Animal Science Associations (2002) FELASA recommendations for the health monitoring of rodent and rabbit colonies in breeding and experimental units. *Laboratory Animals*, **36**, 20–42

Festing, M.F.W. (1993) *International Index of Laboratory Animals*, 6th edn. Festing, Leicester

Flecknell, P.A. (2009) *Laboratory Animal Anaesthesia*, 3rd edn. Academic Press, London

Flecknell, P.A. and Waterman-Pearson, A. (2000) *Pain Management in Animals*. W.B. Saunders, London

Fox, J.G., Anderson, L.C., Loew, F.M. *et al.* (Eds.) (2002) *Laboratory Animal Medicine*. American College of Laboratory Animal Medicine, Academic Press, New York

Galef, B.G. Jr. (2003) Social learning of food preferences in rodents: rapid appetitive learning. *Current Protocols in Neuroscience*, **8**, 5

Ghirardi, O., Cozzolino, R., Guaraldi, D. *et al.* (1995) Within- and between-strain variability in longevity of inbred and outbred rats under the same environmental conditions. *Experimental Gerontology*, **30**, 485–494

Gonder, J.C. and Laber, K. (2007) A renewed look at laboratory rodent housing and management. *ILAR Journal*, **48**, 29–36

Gordon, C.J. (1990) Thermal biology of the laboratory rat. *Physiology & Behavior*, **47**, 963–991

Gordon, C.J. and Fogelson, L. (1994) Metabolic and thermoregulatory responses of the rat maintained in acrylic or wire-screen cages: implications for pharmacological studies. *Physiology & Behavior*, **56**, 73–79

Goto, S., Takahashi, R., Radak, Z. *et al.* (2007) Beneficial biochemical outcomes of late-onset dietary restriction in rodents. *Annals of the New York Academy of Sciences*, **1100**, 431–441

Gutman, D.A. and Nemeroff, C.B. (2002) Neurobiology of early life stress: rodent studies. *Seminars in Clinical Neuropsychiatry*, **7**, 89–95

Hall, F.S. (1998) Social deprivation of neonatal, adolescent, and adult rats has distinct neurochemical and behavioral consequences. *Critical Reviews in Neurobiology*, **12**, 129–162

Hedrich, H.J. (1990) Inbred strains in biomedical research. In: *Genetic Monitoring of Inbred Strains of Rats*. Ed. Hedrich, H.J., pp. 1–7. Gustav Fisher Verlag, Stuttgart

Hedrich, H.J. (2000) History, strains and models. In: *The Laboratory Rat*. Eds Krinke, G., Bullock, G. and Bunton, T., pp. 3–16. Academic Press, New York

International Air Transport Association (2010) *Dangerous Goods Regulations*. http://www.iata.org/ps/publications/dangerous-goods-regulations-dgr

Jacobs, G.H., Neitz, J. and Deegan, J.F. (1991) Retinal receptors in rodents maximally sensitive to ultraviolet light. *Nature*, **353**, 655–656

Joint Working Group on Refinement (1993) Removal of blood from laboratory mammals and birds. First Report of the BVA/FRAME/RSPCA/UFAW Joint Working Group on Refinement. *Laboratory Animals*, **27**, 1–22

Joint Working Group on Refinement (2001) Refining procedures for the administration of substances. Report of the BVAAWF/FRAME/RSPCA/UFAW Joint Working Group on Refinement. *Laboratory Animals*, **35**, 1–41

Koolhaas J.M., Meerlo, P., Boer, S.F. d. *et al.* (1997) The temporal dynamics of the stress response. *Neuroscience & Biobehavioral Reviews*, **21**, 775–782

Krinke, G., Bunton, T. and Bullock, G. (Eds) (2000) *The Laboratory Rat*. Academic Press, New York

Krohn, T.C., Hansen, A.K. and Dragsted, N. (2003) The impact of cage ventilation on rats housed in IVC systems. *Laboratory Animals*, **37**, 85–93

Krohn, T.C., Sorensen, D.B., Ottesen, J.L. *et al.* (2006) The effects of individual housing on mice and rats: a review. *Animal Welfare*, **15**, 343–352

Lepschy, M., Touma, C., Hruby, R. *et al.* (2007) Non-invasive measurement of adrenocortical activity in male and female rats. *Laboratory Animals*, **41**, 372–387

Maisonnette, S., Morato, S. and Brandao, M.L. (1993) Role of resocialization and of 5-HT1A receptor activation on the anxiogenic effects induced by isolation in the elevated plus-maze test. *Physiology & Behavior*, **54**, 753–758

Malkesman, O., Maayan, R., Weizman, A. *et al.* (2006) Aggressive behavior and HPA axis hormones after social isolation in adult rats of two different genetic animal models for depression. *Behavioral Brain Research*, **175**, 408–414

Manser, C.E., Morris, T.H. and Broom D.M. (1995) An investigation into the effects of solid or grid cage flooring on the welfare of laboratory rats. *Laboratory Animals* **29**, 353–363

Markison, S. (2001) The role of taste in the recovery from specific nutrient deficiencies in rats. *Nutritional Neuroscience*, **4**, 1–14

McClintock, M.K. and Adler, N.T. (1978) The role of the female during copulation in wild and domesticated Norway rats *(Rattus norvegicus)*. *Behaviour*, **67**, 67–96

Meaney, M.J., Aitken, D.H., Bhatnagar, S. *et al.* (1991) Postnatal handling attenuates certain neuroendocrine, anatomocal and cognitive dysfunctions associated with aging in female rats. *Neurobiology of Aging*, **12**, 31–38

Meaney, M.J. and Szyf, M. (2005) Environmental programming of stress responses through DNA methylation: life at the interface between a dynamic environment and a fixed genome. *Dialogues in Clinical Neuroscience*, **7**, 103–123

Mediavilla, C., Molina, F. and Puerto, A. (2005) Concurrent conditioned taste aversion: a learning mechanism based on rapid neural versus flexible humoral processing of visceral noxious substances. *Neuroscience & Biobehavioral Reviews*, **29**, 1107–1118

Mormede, P. (1997) Genetic influences on the responses to psychosocial challenges in rats. *Acta Physiologica Scandinavica. Suppl*, **640**, 65–68

National Research Council (1996) *Guide for the Care and Use of Laboratory Animals*. National Academies Press, Washington, DC. Available from URL: http://www.nap.edu/readingroom/books/labrats/

Neitz, J. and Jacobs, G.H. (1986) Reexamination of spectral mechanisms in the rat (*Rattus norvegicus*). *Journal of Comparative Psychology*, **100**, 21–29

Nijman, I.J., Kuipers, S., Verheul, M. *et al.* (2008) A genome-wide SNP panel for mapping and association studies in the rat. *BMC Genomics*, **9**, 95

Njaa, L.R., Utne, F. and Braekkan, O.R. (1957) Effect of relative humidity on rat breeding and ringtail. *Nature*, **180**, 290–291

Otsen, M., Bieman, M.-D., Winer, E.-S. *et al.* (1995) Use of simple sequence length polymorphisms for genetic characterization of rat inbred strains. *Mammalian Genome*, **6**, 595–601

Panksepp, J. (2007) Neuroevolutionary sources of laughter and social joy: modeling primal human laughter in laboratory rats. *Behavioural Brain Research*, **182**, 231–244

Parshad R.K. (1997) Effect of restricted feeding of prepubertal and adult male rats on fertility and sex ratio. *Indian Journal of Experimental Biology*, **31**, 991–992

Pellis, S.M. and Pellis, V.C. (1998) Play fighting of rats in comparative perspective: a schema for neurobehavioral analyses. *Neuroscience & Biobehavioral Reviews*, **23**, 87–101

Perez, J. and Perentes, E. (1994) Light-induced retinopathy in the albino rat in long-term studies. An immunohistochemical and quantitative approach. *Experimental and Toxicologic Patholology*, **46**, 229–235

Pisano, R.G. and Storer, T.I. (1948) Burrows and feeding of the Norway rat. *Journal of Mammalogy*, **29**, 374–383

Portfors, C.V. (2007) Types and functions of ultrasonic vocalizations in laboratory rats and mice. *Journal of the American Association of Laboratory Animal Sciences*, **46**, 28–34

Prendergast, B.J., Kampf-Lassin, A., Yee, J.R. *et al.* (2007) Winter day lengths enhance T lymphocyte phenotypes, inhibit cytokine responses, and attenuate behavioral symptoms of infection in laboratory rats. *Brain Behavior and Immunity*, **21**, 1096–1108

Prendergast, B.J. and Kay, L.M. (2008) Affective and adrenocorticotrophic responses to photoperiod in Wistar rats. *Journal of Neuroendocrinology*, **20**, 261–267

Prusky, G.T., Harker, K.T., Douglas, R.M. *et al.* (2002) Variation in visual acuity within pigmented, and between pigmented and albino rat strains. *Behavioural Brain Research*, **136**, 339–348

Rex, A., Kolbasenko, A., Bert, B. *et al.* (2007) Choosing the right wild type: behavioral and neurochemical differences between 2 populations of Sprague-Dawley rats from the same source but maintained at different sites. *Journal of the American Association of Laboratory Animal Sciences*, **46**, 13–20

Roe, F.J.C., Lee, P.N., Conybeare, G. *et al.* (1995) The Biosure Study: Influence of composition of diet and food consumption on longevity, degenerative diseases and neoplasia in wistar rats studied for up to 30 months post weaning. *Food and Chemical Toxicology*, **33**, 1S–100S

Rosenblatt, J.S., Factor, E.M. and Mayer, A.D. (1994) Relationship between maternal aggression and maternal care in the rat. *Aggressive Behavior*, **20**, 243–255

Roughan, J.V. and Flecknell, P.A. (2003) Evaluation of a short duration behaviour-based post-operative pain scoring system in rats. *European Journal of Pain*, **7**, 397–406

Rowland, N.E. (2007) Food or fluid restriction in common laboratory animals: balancing welfare considerations with scientific inquiry. *Comparative Medicine*, **57**, 149–160

Schoeb, T.R., Davidson, M.K. and Lindsey, J.R. (1982) Intracage ammonia promotes growth of *Mycoplasma pulmonis* in the respiratory tract of rats. *Infection and Immunity*, **38**, 212–217

Schwartz, M.W., Woods, S.C., Porte, D., Jr. *et al.* (2000) Central nervous system control of food intake. *Nature*, **404**, 661–671

Semple-Rowland, S.L. and Dawson, W.W. (1987) Cyclic light intensity threshold for retinal damage in albino rats raised under 6 lux. *Experimental Eye Research*, **44**, 643–661

Shor-Posner, G., Brennan, G., Ian, C. *et al.* (1994) Meal patterns of macronutrient intake in rats with particular dietary preferences. *American Journal of Physiology*, **266**, R1395–402

Silva, R.C., Santos, N.R. and Brandao, M.L. (2003) Influence of housing conditions on the effects of serotonergic drugs on feeding behavior in non-deprived rats. *Neuropsychobiology*, **47**, 98–101

Smith, A.L. and Corrow, D.J. (2005) Modifications to husbandry and housing conditions of laboratory rodents for improved well-being. *ILAR Journal*, **46**, 140–147

Stern, J.M. and Lonstein, J.S. (2001) Neural mediation of nursing and related maternal behaviors. *Progress in Brain Research*, **133**, 263–278

Strubbe, J.H. and Woods, S.C. (2004) The timing of meals. *Psychological Review*, **111**, 28–141

Szyf, M., McGowan, P. and Meaney, M.J. (2008) The social environment and the epigenome. *Environmental and Molecular Mutagenesis*, **49**, 46–60

Tamashiro, K.L., Nguyen, M.M. and Sakai, R.R. (2005) Social stress: from rodents to primates. *Frontiers in Neuroendocrinology*, **26**, 27–40

Tang, A.C., Akers, K.G., Reeb, B.C. *et al.* (2006) Programming social, cognitive, and neuroendocrine development by early exposure to novelty. *Proceedings of the National Academy of Sciences, USA*, **103**, 15716–15721

Tempel, D.L., Shor-Posner, G., Dwyer, D. *et al.* (1989) Nocturnal patterns of macronutrient intake in freely feeding and food deprived rats. *American Journal of Physiology*, **256**, R541–R548

Waynforth, H.B. and Flecknell, P.A. (1992) *Experimental and Surgical Technique in the Rat*, 2nd edn. Academic Press, London

Willis, M.B. and Dalton, C. (1998) *Dalton"s Introduction to Practical Breeding*. Blackwell Publishing, Oxford

Yildiz, A., Hayirli, A., Okumus, Z. *et al.* (2007) Physiological profile of juvenile rats: effects of cage size and cage density. *Laboratory Animals*, **36**, 28–38

Zethof, T.J.J., Van der Heyden, J.A.M., Tolboom, J.T.B.M. *et al.* (1995) Stress-induced hyperthermia as a putative anxiety model. *European Journal of Pharmacology*, **294**, 125–135

Zimmermann, F., Weiss, J. and Reifenberg, K. (2000) Breeding and assisted reproduction techniques. In: *The Laboratory Rat*. Eds Krinke, G., Bullock, G. and Bunton, T., pp. 177–198. Academic Press, New York

23 The laboratory gerbil

Eva Waiblinger

Biological overview

Taxonomy

The Mongolian gerbil (*Meriones unguiculatus*) is the most widely used species of gerbil, and gerbil-like rodents, in the laboratory. There are several other species in the genera *Gerbillus* (gerbils, between 54 and 62 species) and *Meriones* (sand rats, 14 species). Gerbil taxonomy and phylogeny have recently been discussed by various authors (Michaux *et al.* 2001; Palinov 2001; Jansa & Weksler 2003; Steppan *et al.* 2004; Chevret & Dobigny 2005). This chapter will be limited to the Mongolian gerbil, or jird. The gerbil's scientific name *Meriones unguiculatus* means 'little clawed warrior' after Meriones, a marshal and relative of the Cretan king Idomeneus in the Trojan War. Meriones is said to have been one of the warriors in the Trojan Horse.

Standard biological data

Basic biological data on the gerbil have been described by McManus (1972b), Thiessen and Yahr (1977), Tumblebrook Farm (1979), and by Field and Sibold (1999). Gerbils have 44 chromosomes, four pairs of mammary glands, and have a typically rodent dental formula (one incisivus, a diastema and three molars in each half mandible). The body temperature is 38.1–38.4°C (measured by rectal probe), heart rate is 360 bpm (range 260–600 bpm) and the respiration rate is 90 per min with a range of 70–160 per min. Gerbils drink 9.63 +/− 1.95% of body weight per day, which corresponds to 4–7 ml per day per 100 g body weight. Caloric uptake is 40.32 +/− 4.92 kcal per day per 100 g body weight, corresponding to 5–8 g per day per 100 g body weight. Urine volume is 3–4 ml per day and the urine is highly concentrated.

Size range and lifespan

Gerbils are of intermediate size between a rat and a mouse (body length 11–13.5 cm). The fur-covered tail is slightly shorter than the body (9.5–12 cm), with a small tuft of black hair at the tip. An erect adult gerbil is about 15 cm high. At birth pups weigh about 3–4 g, at 20 days around 16 g, at 30 days 25 g, at 40 days 40 g, at 3 months 65 g, at 6 months 70–90 g; adult males weigh between 80 and 130 g, and females between 60 and 100 g. Gerbils can live up to 6 years, however, 3–4 years is more usual (Thiessen & Yahr 1977).

External features

The external features of a typical laboratory gerbil are shown in Figure 23.1. The wild type has an agouti-brown coat and a cream-coloured belly. Males are generally heavier than females (Agren *et al.* 1989a, 1989b). The hindlegs are relatively long compared to the forelegs. The animals often sit on their haunches to look around, feed or groom themselves, and the long hindpaws are used extensively during digging behaviour to vigorously kick out and remove loose substrate from under the belly. Hopping locomotion can only be observed if the gerbils have a large area of several square metres with rough flooring available, but their locomotion is never comparable to kangaroo-type hopping which can be seen in *Jaculus jaculus*, the giant jumping rat. Gerbils perform rapid foot-thumping with the hindfeet during alarming situations, and the males foot-thump after copulation (Roper & Polioudakis 1977; Holman & Seale 1991). In erect, attentive posture, gerbils stand up on the toes, and the tail acts as extra support. In the laboratory, gerbils do not readily climb, at least not upside down at the cage top as mice do (Lerwill 1974; Roper & Polioudakis 1977). This is due to their fur-covered soles of the hindpaws, and lack of friction pads and opposable toes. If startled, however, gerbils can readily jump over a 30 cm high barrier (wild gerbils can jump up to 60 cm; I.W. Stuermer, personal communication). Adult animals can comfortably crawl through tubes or tunnels of a diameter of 5 cm.

Senses and communication

Sound production

Gerbils are able to produce sounds of between 20 and 150 kHz with peak intensities up to 106 dB (Thiessen *et al.* 1978). Ultrasonic calling rate in gerbil pups increases from birth until day 4, then decreases, and from day 20 onwards, no vocalisations were detected by De Ghett (1974). Broom *et al.* (1977) and Lerwill (1978) have also described the ontogeny of sound production in gerbils. Male gerbils' pre-, within- and post-copulatory vocalisations differ, with

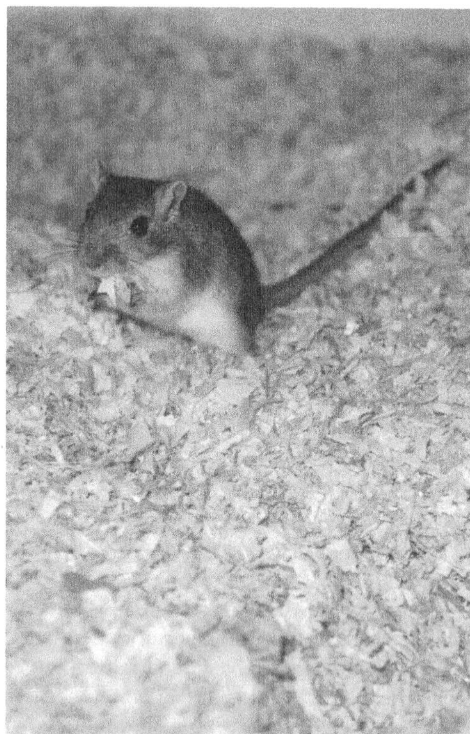

Figure 23.1 A typical inquisitive laboratory gerbil.

upsweep (28–35 kHz), unmodulated (26 kHz) and modulated (28–38 kHz) calls; females vocalise much less during copulation (Holman 1980; Holman & Seale 1991).

Hearing capacities

Gerbil ears are not mature at birth. The sound-conducting apparatus and inner-ear structures develop between day 16 and 20 (Finck *et al.* 1969). Woolf and Ryan (1984) however found the first cochlear microphonic potentials at day 12, with a very high 103 dB threshold. Juvenile gerbils first approach an auditory stimulus (low-intensity tape-recorded gerbil social call compared to broad-band white noise or lacking stimulus) at 16 days of age (Kelly & Potash 1986). Hearing sensitivity increases up to the age of 9 months. Adult gerbils respond to frequencies from 100 Hz to 60 kHz (Ryan 1976), with maximum sensitivity (<10 dB) between 4 and 44 kHz. In older gerbils (between 12 and 28 months), sensitivity is reduced at the range of 8–24 kHz, however this is only the case in domesticated, not wild gerbils (Stuermer & Wetzel 2006; Eckrich *et al.* 2008). Minimum resolvable angles (MRAs) for sound localisation in azimuth for broad-band noise is 23° (if the animal is stimulated from the front) and 45° (stimulated from the back) (Maier & Klump 2006). Gerbils use both phase and intensity differences to localise sounds (Heffner & Heffner 1988).

Vision

Jacobs and Deegan II (1994) described gerbils as 'visually alert rodents'. Visual performance in gerbils (spatial and temporal resolution, size constancy, pattern discrimination) was analysed by Ingle (1981), using gerbils trained in behavioural tasks. The retinas have rods (peak sensitivity at 499–501 nm (Jacobs & Nietz 1989), about 87% of receptor population) and cones (12–14% of total receptor population). There seem to be two types of cones: 95–97.5% of the cone population is green sensitive (peak sensitivity at 493 nm, very close to the rod sensitivity, but at high illumination levels), only 2.5–5% of the cones are blue sensitive (sensitivity possibly between 420 and 430 nm). Therefore gerbils can be said to have dichromatic, blue–green colour discrimination abilities (Jacobs & Nietz 1989; Govardovskii *et al.* 1992; Bytyqi & Layer 2005). Gerbils are also sensitive to ultraviolet (UV) light. Jacobs and Deegan II (1994) found indications for another UV sensitive pigment having a peak sensitivity at 360 nm. Receptor density was found to be 314 000–332 000/mm^2 for rods and 45 000–50 000/mm^2 for cones (Govardovskii *et al.* 1992). Visual acuity was found to be 1.8–2 cycles/degree at 70 cd/m^2 (Baker & Emerson 1983; Wilkinson 1983), the acuity for horizontal gratings being better than for vertical gratings. Gerbils have a good stereopsis, depth perception and cliff response (Collins *et al.* 1969). The gerbil visual system seems to be well adapted to diurnal life. It is not known whether albino-eyed gerbils have reduced acuity and are more susceptible to bright light than dark-eyed ones, as is the case in rats (Birch & Jacobs 1980).

Olfaction and scent marking

Gerbils are macrosmates with high densities of olfactory receptors and a well developed bulbus olfactorius (Loskota *et al.* 1974b; Thiessen & Yahr 1977). Gerbil pups show responses to odours from as early as day 4, and strongly prefer home cage odour between day 8 and 14 (Cornwell-Jones & Azar 1982). Gerbils also show pronounced scent-marking behaviour, smearing sebum of their ventral gland, which is present in both sexes, on objects in their territory and also on group members (for a detailed description of scent gland functions, see Thiessen and Yahr (1977)). Marking behaviour is characterised by the animal stretching out, lowering the abdomen and then crawling forward, dragging the gland over the substrate (Roper & Polioudakis 1977). In the wild, gerbils predominantly mark along the border of their territory, with the dominant breeding male marking most, followed by the breeding female and adult male offspring (Agren *et al.* 1989a, 1989b). Since scent-marking is controlled by androgens, males scent-mark more frequently than females (Thiessen & Yahr 1977). Gerbils of black coat colour mark more frequently than agouti animals (Dizinno & Clancy 1978). In isosexual groups of males, scent-mark frequency can be used as an indicator of rank (Shimozuru *et al.* 2006a), whereas body weight is usually taken as correlate of rank in mixed-sex groups (Weinandy 1995). Females scent-mark their pups, which might help the mother to recognise her own offspring (Wallace *et al.* 1973), and the pups recognise maternal nest odours and are attracted to them (Yahr & Anderson-Mitchell 1983). According to Roper and Polioudakis (1977), scent-marking is used to mark and identify group and family members. Gerbils can discriminate between odours of familiar and unfamiliar conspecifics (Tang Halpin 1975; Yahr 1977). Age, social stress and social defeat decrease scent-marking behaviour in male gerbils (Yamaguchi *et al.* 2005; Shimozuru *et al.* 2006b).

Activity patterns

Gerbils are polyphasic, diurnal and crepuscular. They exhibit two major peaks of activity after dawn and around dusk, but are also active during the day (Susic & Masirevic 1986; Weinandy 1995; Weinert *et al.* 2007). Daily activity patterns are temperature dependent in the wild (Leont'ev 1954) and in seminatural conditions (Randall & Thiessen 1980). When activity is measured using a running wheel, activity shifts mostly to the night; however, this seems to be an artefact induced by the running wheel (Refinetti 2006).

Social organisation

Extended family groups and sexual suppression

In the wild, gerbils live in extended families with one breeding pair and its offspring of several generations, in group sizes of 2–17 animals (Agren *et al.* 1989a, 1989b). Leont'ev (1954) even captured up to 26 animals in one burrow. As a rule, only the dominant pair reproduces, whilst adult offspring of both sexes remain with the parents and usually do not reproduce (Roper & Polioudakis 1977; Swanson & Lockley 1977; Agren *et al.* 1989a, 1989b; Solomon & Getz 1996). It is unclear whether gerbils really are monogamous. Agren *et al.* (1989a) found that females in oestrus actively solicit copulations of neighbouring males. So far, no paternity analyses have been performed in wild gerbil groups or in naturally grown families in semi-natural housing, therefore information on extra-pair reproduction is lacking. Adult sons often exhibit well developed ventral glands and testes; adult daughters' ventral glands, uteri and ovaries are undeveloped. Payman and Swanson (1980) and Swanson and Lockley (1977) suggested that suppression of sexual maturation in daughters is caused by the presence of the mother and her next litter. Clark and Galef found that sisters, but also other familiar animals, inhibit each other's reproductive development, with this inhibition being even more pronounced in the presence of the mother. In contrast, exposing suppressed females to unfamiliar males speeds up their maturation (Clark & Galef 2001a, 2002; Clark *et al.* 2002). Sexually suppressed adult group members participate in digging the communal burrow, hoarding food, territorial defence and co-operative breeding (Agren *et al.* 1989a, 1989b). Animals of a group also coordinate their actions according to the behaviour of group members, especially in predator avoidance (Ellard & Byers 2005).

Reasons for philopatry

In wild gerbils, adult offspring remain with the family and parents (ie, 'philopatry') long after weaning. Apparently, the presence of older offspring was not found to enhance reproductive success of the parents in the laboratory (Ostermeyer & Elwood 1984). French (1994) suggested that remaining with the parents offers opportunities for reproduction during prolonged interbirth intervals of the dominant female. According to French (1994), seven of 49 (14.3%) female offspring managed to produce offspring in the presence of the mother, albeit with lower pup weight and higher mortality; Scheibler *et al.* (2004) observed only two of 56 (3.8%) daughters giving birth while still with the family. Salo and French (1989) consecutively showed that adult offspring remaining with the family and helping at the nest can acquire essential parental skills which later improve their own reproductive performance, irrespective of sex. Since extended residence in the parental group by non-breeders can enhance their reproductive performance, it is advisable to leave future breeding animals longer with their parents.

Sudden intra-group aggression and expulsion of group members

One problem often encountered is a sudden outbreak of aggression in hitherto peaceful groups of animals, followed by expulsion of group members. If these animals are not removed, they will be killed. The problem is quite severe in pet gerbils, but its frequency in the laboratory is unknown. The author's experience is that such periods of aggression can also occur in same-sex groups, without increasing animal numbers, even in groups of only two same-sex animals. Researchers at the University of Halle have analysed this problem in naturally grown family groups of laboratory gerbils in semi-natural enclosures (Scheibler *et al.* 2004). Aggression originated from the founder female in 60% of the cases, who was either pregnant or lactating, or the founder male (13%). Pup mortality was very high during these periods of aggression (70%). Increased reproductive competition, especially for the female breeding position, seems to trigger such periods of aggression in reproducing families (Scheibler *et al.* 2005a, 2005b, 2006a). However, there is no explanation so far for such periods of sudden aggression occurring in hitherto stable same-sex groups.

Reproduction

Under laboratory conditions gerbils reproduce all year round, whereas in the wild, the main reproductive season is from late winter to summer, with only two to three litters per year (Naumov & Lobachev 1975). During a lifetime, females produce eight litters, on average, but there have been females with 17 and more. The young are altricial (naked, blind and highly dependent on the parents) and are kept in the nest or nest chamber and retrieved by the parents if they crawl out of the nest.

Lack of inbreeding avoidance

Gerbils are able to recognise kin independent of familiarity (Valsecchi *et al.* 2002). Valsecchi's findings did not undermine Agren's suggestion (Agren 1984a) that there is a particular period of time (60–70 days of age) during which prolonged social contacts between males or females result in the establishment of a sibling bond between these animals, inhibiting reproduction. Despite female gerbils' ability to recognise kin, they do not avoid reproduction with close relatives such as siblings.

Role of the male in rearing young

In gerbils, the male actively participates in raising the pups. They collect nesting material, help build the nest, warm and clean the pups, and might occasionally also retrieve a pup back to the nest (Clark *et al.* 2001; Clark & Galef 2001b; Weinandy *et al.* 2001). Males and females coordinate their activities at the nest in a manner that ensures constant supervision and care of the pups, so that if the female leaves the nest, the male guards the pups and *vice versa* (Waring & Perper 1980). The presence of the father increases pup activity and physical contact between pups and parents. Pups with the father present open their eyes earlier (Salo & French 1989; French 1994; Piovanotti Arua & Vieira 2004).

Bruce effect

There are contradictory results on the Bruce effect in gerbils (disruption of pregnancy or failure of implantation following exposure of the female to a strange male). Norris and Adams (1979a) failed to find evidence of the Bruce effect in gerbils, except when newly mated pairs were separated (Norris 1985). However, Rohrbach (1982) found that both the presence of a strange male or female, as well as changes in the housing conditions (cold, change to smaller or new cage) can block implantation in mated female gerbils. The presence of strange males reduces maternal care in lactating females, resulting in high pup losses.

'Stud' males and 'dud' males

Mertice Clark and Bennett Galef have demonstrated in a series of experiments that gerbil males differ strongly in their reproductive performance depending on their position in their mothers' wombs (Clark *et al.* 1992, 1998; Clark & Galef 1994, 1999, 2000). Males ('dud' males) situated between two sisters in the uterus will have much lower adult circulating testosterone levels, low territorial and sexual activity levels, but very high nest-bound activity levels (nest building and caring for pups), whereas males gestated between two brothers ('stud' males) will develop into sexually and territorially very active adults, but with less interest in pup care. According to these authors, this phenomenon leads to a testosterone-mediated trade-off between parental and sexual efforts, but its function and adaptive quality is yet unclear (Vandenberg 1993). Some males gestated between sisters have testosterone levels as low as those of females and are unable to mate and impregnate females. Generally, the serum level of testosterone in male gerbils determines whether these animals exhibit sexual or pup care behaviour. 'Dud' males have about half the testosterone levels of their 'stud' conspecifics, and wild gerbil males have much lower testosterone levels than laboratory gerbils (Blottner & Stuermer 2006; Stuermer *et al.* 2006). Circulating levels of testosterone in male laboratory gerbils ranges from 0.35–3.72 ng/ml, with temporal variation. At the age of around 10 weeks (70–80 days), testosterone levels are highest (up to and even over 4 ng/ml), then again drop to 1–2 ng/ml thereafter (Clark & Galef 2001b; Clark *et al.* 2004).

Uses in the laboratory

To assess the most common uses of gerbils in the laboratory, a quick search on ISI Web of Science yielded at least 711 published English papers on *Meriones unguiculatus* between January 2000 and October 2007. Most papers dealt with ischaemia (ie, stroke research) (336 papers, 47.2%). Due to the lack of carotid arterial anastomoses (incomplete circle of Willis) in the majority of gerbils the effect of vascular clamping of the carotids is more reproducible from animal to animal than in other species (Tumblebrook Farm 1980, 1985; and personal communication, C. Nitsch, Functional Neuroanatomy, University of Basel). However, Laidley *et al.* (2005) demonstrated that 23–39% of laboratory gerbils had a complete or unilateral complete circle of Willis, therefore the role of gerbils in stroke research is questionable. A large part of the references dealt with research into parasitic and other infectious diseases (110 papers). Gerbils are used in filariasis research as hosts for *Brugia pahangi* and *B. malayi*, as and are used also in echinococcosis, amoebiasis, babesiosis, giardiasis, trypanosomiasis, and schistosomiasis research. They are also occasionally used as hosts for ascarids, *Taenia* sp., *Trichostrongylus* sp. and *Neospora caninum*, and have been used as 'feeding stations' for ticks (*Ixodes ricinus*), and are also used in research into *Helicobacter pylori* infection.

Gerbils are frequently used in neurology research (98 references in total), which centres on the auditory system (53 out of 98 references). Gerbil behaviour and behaviour associated with reproduction were the subject of 61 references, followed by epilepsy and seizure research (49 references). Gerbils seem to be especially seizure-prone, seizures occur in response to sensory stimulation or forced exploratory behaviour and it seems the propensity for seizures is partly hereditary. In the 1970s, Loskota first established non-inbred seizure-prone and seizure-resistant strains of gerbils by selective breeding. As a result, gerbils became a model for spontaneous or conditioned seizures (Loskota *et al.* 1972; Loskota & Lomax 1974, 1975). Today there are several seizure-prone inbred strains of gerbils available. However, the propensity for seizures might present a problem in the general husbandry of these animals, wherever epilepsy is not the subject of research.

Questions on nutrition, in particular bioavailability of beta-carotene, were addressed in 17 studies. Five addressed new methods for biomedical procedures (blood collection, intravenous (iv) injections, anaesthesia and total body electrical conductivity (TOBEC) measurements), and some tentatively suggested gerbils as models for schizophrenia (Bagorda *et al.* 2006), psychosis (Brummelte *et al.* 2007) and depression (Hendrie & Pickles 2000; Starkey & Hendrie 1997; Jaworska *et al.* 2008). The remaining 26 references covered a variety of subjects including cancer, genetics, general anatomy, toxicology, circadian rhythms and thermoregulation. Only six studies dealt with behaviour or reproduction of gerbils in the wild or the behaviour of recently caught wild gerbils in the laboratory.

Breeds, strains and genetics

Provenance and breeding history

Wild Mongolian gerbils originate from the central Asian semi-deserts and steppes and can be found in Mongolia, Inner Mongolia (China) and southern Siberia. In the wild, they live in extended, territorial family groups (Agren *et al.* 1989a, 1989b), which inhabit self-dug burrows, that are widely branched and up to 60–80 cm deep (Bannikov 1954; Naumov & Lobachev 1975; Scheibler *et al.* 2006b). Gerbils prefer habitats with short, sparse vegetation and dry, loose and sandy soil (Bannikov 1954; Liu *et al.* 2007).

The Mongolian gerbil was discovered in 1866 by the French missionary Abbé Armand David. Travelling from Bejing to north-west China he found three '*yellow rats with long, hair-covered tails*'. He sent these animals to the director of the Paris Natural History Museum, Monsieur Milne-Edwards, who named the species *Meriones unguiculatus* (Milne-Edwards 1867). In 1935, 20 pairs of gerbils were caught by C. Kasuga in the Amur river valley in Manchuria and exported to Japan, where the Kitasato Institute established a closed breeding colony (Rich 1968). In 1949 another breeding colony was established at the Central Laboratories for Experimental Animals, Tokyo, by M. Nomura. From this breeding stock, in 1954, 11 pairs were sent to V. Schwentker who had founded the West Foundation/Tumblebrook Farm in 1940 at Brant Lake (USA) to introduce new laboratory animal species to the USA. Only four males and five females bred, so all animals of the Tumblebrook Farm colony descended from these animals. From Tumblebrook Farm, gerbils reached various laboratories and research groups at universities and pharmaceutical companies, for example the Worcester Foundation for Experimental Biology, Shrewsbury, Massachussetts, where a sub-colony was established in 1962.

In the 1960s, the gerbil was established as a laboratory animal in Europe (Rich 1968). In 1964 J.H. Marston imported 12 pairs from Massachussetts to Birmingham (Norris 1987). With the exception of 12 pairs imported by the Laboratory Animal Centre, Carshalton, in 1966 direct from Schwendtkers foundation colony, this random-bred colony at Birmingham has been used to generate the breeding stock for laboratories thoughout the UK and Europe, and has also established the gerbil as a pet animal. In 1995, Ingo W. Stuermer's German–Mongolian expedition caught wild Mongolian gerbils in Mongolia, and 60 of these animals were used for breeding in Germany (Strain Ugoe:MU95) to analyse domestication-induced changes in gerbil morphology, behaviour, reproduction, endocrinology and neurobiology (Stuermer 1998; Stuermer *et al.* 1998, 2003; Blottner *et al.* 2000; Neumann *et al.* 2001). Most animals used today are descendants of the colonies mentioned above. Currently, only a few studies are conducted with wild gerbils in their natural habitat (Wang & Zhong 2006; Liu *et al.* 2007; Zhang & Wang 2007). In the wild, *Meriones unguiculatus* is not endangered and is often viewed as an agricultural pest (Prof. R.Samjaa, personal communication), and also as a reservoir for bubonic plague-carrying fleas (Jun *et al.* 1993; Davis *et al.* 2004).

Domestication

Nowadays, more than 50 generations and several bottlenecks separate laboratory gerbils from their wild ancestors caught in 1935 (Rich 1968). There are pronounced differences between wild and laboratory gerbils. In 1995, a German–Mongolian research team caught about 170 wild gerbils in Mongolia, then housed and bred them in the lab and compared these F0, F1 and F2 animals with laboratory gerbils (Stuermer 1998; Blottner *et al.* 2000; Neumann *et al.* 2001; Stuermer *et al.* 2003, 2006). The latter show typical signs of domestication: higher body weight with higher variability, higher testes, liver and total fat weight, lower brain weight (17.7% lower), lower heart, lung, kidney and stomach weights, shorter intestinal tract length, higher testicular activity, greater litter size (mean 5.6 pups in laboratory gerbils compared with 4 in first generation wild gerbils bred in the laboratory), but also faster auditory discrimination learning in laboratory gerbils compared to wild gerbils. Microsatellite variability, and probably also genetic variability in general, is reduced in laboratory gerbils. Wild gerbils develop less stereotypic digging, but since this abnormal behaviour develops during ontogeny, and is caused by housing conditions in the laboratory, it is not surprising that adult wild gerbils did not develop this behaviour. Epileptic seizures do not occur in wild gerbils, but started to appear in their offspring. Stuermer observed rapid changes towards domestication characteristics with only a few generations of breeding wild gerbils in the laboratory. Despite these obvious changes, basic behavioural needs are still the same in all gerbils, as is demonstrated by their intensive digging behaviour, need for a burrow, social contact, gnawing and hoarding activities.

Colour mutations

Since the occurrence of the first coat colour mutations, black and spotted, a wide variety of coat colours has emerged (Waring *et al.* 1978; Swanson 1980; Waring & Poole 1980; Henley & Robinson 1981; Leiper & Robinson 1984, 1985, 1986; Matsuzaki *et al.* 1989). To date, there are at least seven loci coding for gerbil coat colour known, some of them with up to four alleles. However, agouti, black and spotted are still the most frequent colours in laboratory gerbils; other colours are rarely used. Colour varieties and breeding for colour is more common in pet gerbils. There are differences in behaviour and physiology between the agouti and black (Dizinno & Clancy 1978), and females seem to prefer males of their own fur colour (Wong *et al.* 1990). Also, there seems to be a connection between coat colour and seizure propensity in gerbils (Gray-Allan & Wong 1990; Fujisawa *et al.* 2003). When breeding the gerbil in the laboratory it is important to note that 'spotted' is a homozygously lethal, dominant gene (Waring *et al.* 1978). Therefore, if two spotted gerbils are mated, about a quarter of their offspring will die *in utero*. To improve reproductive output, spotted gerbils should always be mated to non-spotted ones.

Strains and supplies

A number of strains are available from the major breeders. Most of these gerbils are inbred due to several bottlenecks and founder effects in the history of laboratory gerbil breeding. Several authors have described and bred seizure-prone animals (Gray-Allan & Wong 1990; Buckmaster & Wong 2002; Fujisawa *et al.* 2003). However, these animals are not currently available from the major laboratory animal breeding companies. The original authors would have to be contacted for these strains.

Laboratory management and breeding

General housing and husbandry

Temperature and humidity range

Originating from arid steppes with continental climate (a dry climate with temperature extremes), gerbils can tolerate a wide range of temperatures. In the wild, they would escape these extremes by going underground into their borrows. Without a burrow, but with the opportunity to build an isolating nest and with deep substrate, they can tolerate between 0 and 35°C provided that that humidity is low and food is available *ad libitum*. Juvenile gerbils are unable to thermoregulate before the age of 12 days. Endothermic capacity then increases until the age of 21 days (McManus 1972b). Adults are more temperature tolerant (18–29°C) than juveniles (19–24°C) in the laboratory, therefore gerbils should be kept at temperatures between 20 and 24°C and humidities between 35 and 55% (ie, at lower humidities than suggested for other laboratory rodents) (Council of Europe 2006). At higher humidities, gerbils develop a matted, ruffled fur due to activation of the harderian gland. The secreted substances of this gland are distributed all over the fur by the animals grooming themselves, then evaporate and help cool the body. If humidity is too high, no evaporation occurs and harderian secretions remain in the fur, rendering it matted (Thiessen & Yahr 1977; Grant & Thiessen 1989).

Burrow/shelter

In the wild, gerbils dig their own extended burrow systems. Bannikov (1954) recorded 14–504 burrows per hectare; the author observed regions in Mongolia with gerbil burrows every 10–15 m. Gerbil burrows contain several of metres of tunnels, food and nest chambers (Naumov & Lobachev 1975; Thiessen & Maxwell 1979; Brunner 1993; Scheibler *et al.* 2006b). The burrow is one of the most important resources for gerbils in the wild: it offers protection from climatic extremes and from predators, allows for raising pups in relative safety and for storage of food (Naumov & Lobachev 1975; Thiessen & Yahr 1977, p. 64). Captive and domesticated gerbils show pronounced burrow digging behaviour. Raising gerbils without a burrow or burrow-like structure in the laboratory has a profound effect on their behaviour. Wiedenmayer found that lack of an adequate burrow structure consisting of at least a nest chamber and access tunnel leads to stereotypic digging in the corner of the cage, an abnormal behaviour exhibited for up to 21% of active time, with bout lengths from 12 s up to several minutes at a time (Wiedenmayer 1995, 1996, 1997a, 1997b). Gerbils reared in a burrow structure (Figure 23.2), however, do not develop stereotypic digging. Laboratory gerbils should, whenever possible, be provided with an artificial burrow system that consists of a dark nest chamber of at least 13 cm × 13 cm × 13 cm, accessible via a dark tunnel (length about 15–20 cm, diameter about 5 cm). Wiedenmayer's findings were independently confirmed by Schmook (2004) and the author of this chapter (Waiblinger & König 2004). Schmook even found that established stereotypic digging in adult gerbils can be reduced if an artificial burrow is added. In Switzerland, these findings led to an adjustment of the minimum housing requirements of gerbils in the laboratory. According to the revised Swiss Animal Protection Ordinance, laboratory gerbils need to be provided with an artificial burrow structure or the opportunity to dig in deep substrate. Also, The Council of Europe ETS No. 123 recommends either a thick layer of substrate for digging or a burrow substitute for gerbils. Unfortunately, no such artificial burrow system is commercially available to date. One prototype example can be seen in Figure 23.3.

The presence or absence of a shelter also affects other behaviour. Upon presentation of a startling visual stimulus, shelter-reared gerbils respond by fleeing, foot-thumping and concealment, whereas open-reared gerbils approach the stimulus. After 24 h of access to a shelter, open-reared gerbils also start to flee into the shelter (Clark & Galef 1977, 1979; Cheal & Foley 1985; Cheal *et al.* 1986). In the author's experience, gerbils reared with a burrow are shyer and more difficult to handle. Offering gerbils an artificial burrow increases costs and animal care workload. Depending on the research project for which the animals are intended, rearing with shelter may or may not be advisable. See also Chapter 10 regarding enrichment.

Minimum cage requirements

Gerbils should be kept in solid-bottomed cages with a thick layer of substrate (at least 5 cm) to allow for digging. It must be gnaw-resistant, for example made from polycarbonate. Cage height should be at least 15 cm but 18 cm is better to allow the animals to rear on their hindlegs. The EU Council's Group of Experts on Rodents and Rabbits suggested a minimum cage floor area of 1200 cm^2 and a height of 18 cm for gerbils, with 150 cm^2 per animal weighing less than 40 g, and 250 cm^2 per animal weighing more than 40 g, either for same-sex groups or breeding pairs and their offspring (Council of Europe 2006). If an artificial burrow (nest box and 20 cm access tube) has to be fitted in a cage, the minimum floor area for breeding pairs should be 1500–1800 cm^2, otherwise these structures are difficult to fit in conveniently (author's own experience).

Environmental provisions

Digging and chewing opportunities

Since gerbils are proficient diggers and gnawers, they should be provided with digging and gnawing opportunities: digging substrate such as wood chip bedding, and chewable

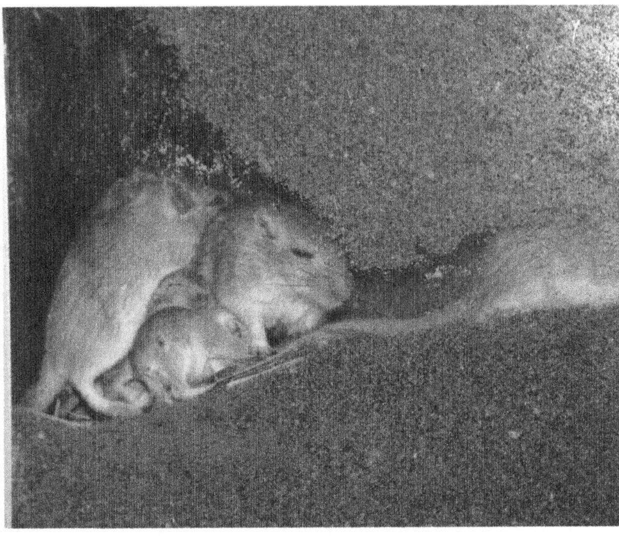

(a)

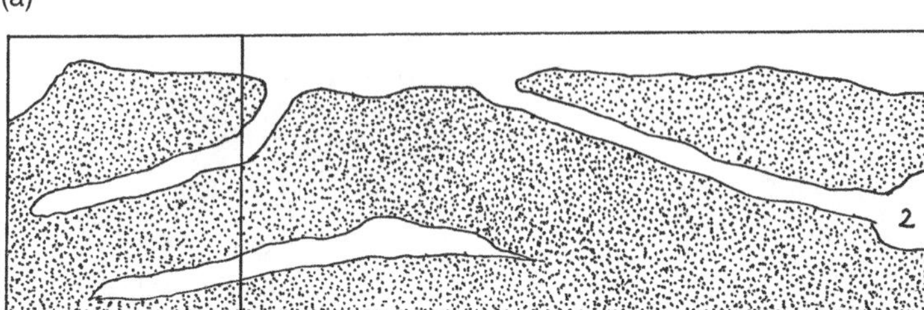

(b)

Figure 23.2 Laboratory gerbils in a self-dug burrow in moist sand (a) and layout of such a burrow (b), dug in terrarium measuring 0.5 m × 1.5 m × 0.6 m, side views. The big terrarium contained a smaller one, placed upside down into the bigger one, inaccessible to the animals. The gerbils were only able to dig tunnels in a 10 cm thick layer of moist sand between the two terrarium walls, therefore practically all tunnel and nest structures were visible from the outside (system described by Hauzenberger *et al.* 2006). 1: litter nest, 2: sleeping nest (Waiblinger, Ramer & Riva, unpublished).

materials such as hay, straw, tissues, paper, cardboard, branches and wood sticks. All this material is autoclaveable, and if the gerbils are not used for nutritional studies, there is no reason for not providing them with gnawing material. As substrate, wood chips and wood shavings are generally used, for example aspen shavings.

Sand bath

In pet gerbil housing, offering a sand bath (bird or chinchilla sand) has proved very successful for fur cleanness and fur shine, and Pendergrass and Thiessen (1983) have shown that sandbathing helps thermoregulation in gerbils. In the author's experience gerbils regularly use the sand bath, first to wallow and roll in it, then as a latrine.

Running wheels

Running wheels are not a necessary provision; Sherwin (1998) either found no or negative effects on gerbils. At the University of Halle, it was found that wheel running and bar gnawing are mutually replaceable abnormal behaviours (Master thesis B. Hünemörder, personal communication), and that activity patterns of gerbils differ significantly between those with running wheels and those without. The latter exhibit the typical biphasic crepuscular activity pattern, the former only one activity peak during night-time (Refinetti 2006; Weinert *et al.* 2007). If running wheels are used, they should be 30 cm in diameter, and not have rails or spokes, but a solid running surface.

Social grouping

Gerbils should not be housed alone whenever possible. Neonatal maternal separation leads to behavioural and neurochemical depression-like changes that differ in males and females, with more pronounced effects in males (Jaworska *et al.* 2008). If adult pair-bonded gerbils are separated, fatness and transient depression- and anxiety-like symptoms can be observed (Starkey & Hendrie 1997, 1998a, 1998b; Hendrie & Pickles 2000; Starkey *et al.* 2007), as well as pregnancy failure (Norris 1985). Singly housed gerbils show pathological changes in the dopamine innervation of their prefrontal cortex that impair learning and working memory (Winterfeld *et al.* 1998), and increased activity and heart rate (Weinandy 1995). If separated for too long, they may react with aggres-

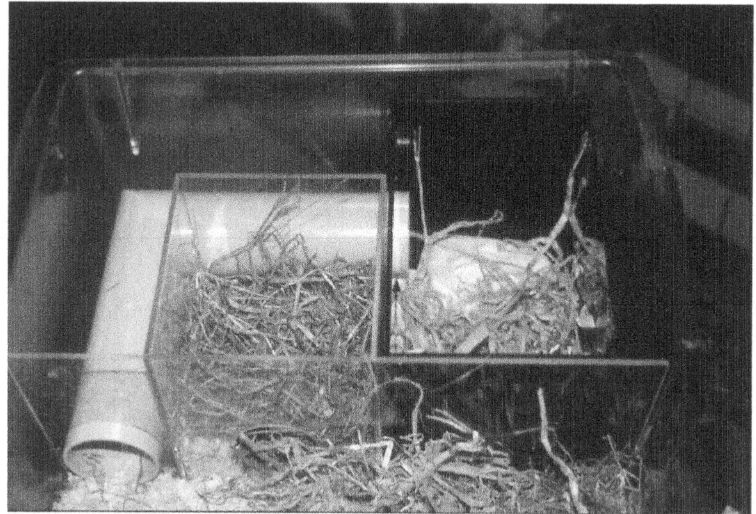

(a)

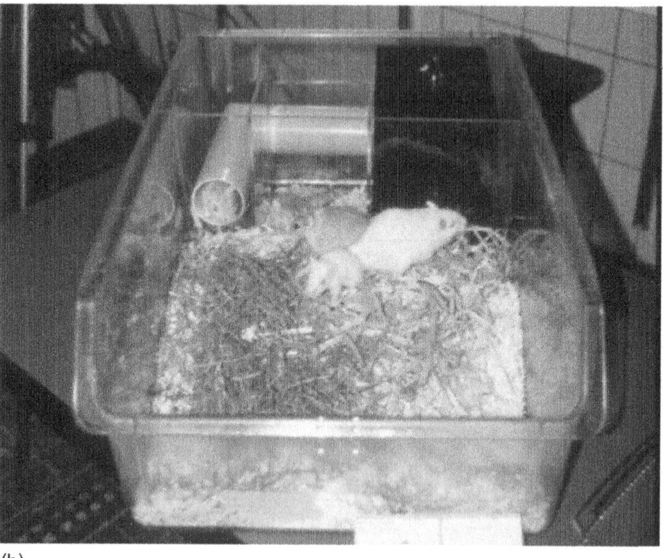

(b)

Figure 23.3 (a) Artificial burrow system which can be inserted into a laboratory cage type IV. (b) It consists of a dark nest box, access tube and an additional transparent box.

sion upon regrouping with their old group-mates. The author observed aggression occurring after just 2 days of separation.

Gerbils can be kept in breeding pairs of one female and male with their offspring. The offspring can remain for some time after the birth of the next litter (see sections on extended family groups and sexual suppression, and on abnormal behaviour). Some authors also suggested polygynous breeding pairs with one male and two females (Marston & Chang 1965). On the other hand, gerbils can be satisfactorily kept in same-sex groups of two or more animals. It is the experience of the author, and of thousands of pet gerbil owners, that in contrast to male mice and to recommendations made by the Council of Europe (2006 p. 19), male gerbils can easily be kept in same-sex groups. Same-sex male groups are usually more harmonious than same-sex female groups.

The following suggestions reflect the author's experience in grouping gerbils since there are no systematic studies on the success of the various grouping methods. Creating new adult gerbil groups is difficult because of aggression exhibited towards strange animals and should be avoided, except when forming opposite-sex breeding pairs (Clark *et al.* 1986). In this case, grouping during oestrus is advisable. Preferably, same-sex groups should be formed before the age of 7–8 weeks. Unfamiliar animals should always be brought together in an unfamiliar enclosure, such as a freshly prepared cage, and be observed for at least 2 h. The animals can alternatively be separated by a screen or wire mesh partition for 5–7 days before allowing direct contact (Clark *et al.* 2002). Intensive ano-genital sniffing, chasing, slashing tail and grinding teeth are signs of high arousal and gerbils displaying such behaviours should be distracted by food, sound or short blasts of air. If fighting starts, the animals should immediately be separated (wearing thick gloves is advisable) and they should not be reintroduced to each other. On the other hand, the author's experience is that, if a gerbil pokes its head under the snout of another, performs high, but audible cheeps, and is groomed on the back or belly, grouping was successful. Animals sleeping huddled together can be left alone.

Identification and sexing

Gerbils can easily be marked by clipping their fur in defined patterns. If only the upper parts of the hairs are shaved, the darker underfur will show. Colour dyes can also be used, however clipping fur is much easier and will last for 5–6 weeks in adults. Placing subcutaneous transponders for identification between the shoulder blades needs a short anaesthesia, but will mark the animals permanently. The newest transponders are only 4 mm long and less than 1 mm in diameter. Toe-clipping should not be used, except as a last resort for neonates where the other marking methods are not applicable. However, Leclercq and Rozenfeld (2001) have suggested plantar tattooing of neonates as an alternative to toe-clipping.

For sexing, the animals should be placed on a smooth surface and lifted at their tail-base since they should not be placed on their back. Sexing is easy in adult gerbils: the distance between genital papilla and anus is double in males, the connecting line is thin and covered with fur. Scrotal sacs are darkly coloured in agouti males. In females, the anogenital distance is much shorter, and there is a triangular naked area between genital papilla and anus (Figure 23.4). In juvenile animals, anogenital distance is the only distinguishable feature. In female neonates, the teats are visible, in males, the genital papilla is more prominent and has a roundish opening.

Physical environment and hygiene

Because of low urine quantities, gerbil cages do not have to be cleaned as often as mouse cages. Depending on stocking density and cage size, they might only be cleaned every 1–2 weeks. Cleaning is stressful to these animals, since they leave scent marks all over their territory. Weinandy measured stress responses in gerbils subjected to different stressors, using implanted heart-rate transmitters and found that cage change is less stressful than group recomposition, but more so than handling, confrontation with an intruder or confrontation with a resident animal, and that gerbils needed about 30 minutes for their heart rate to return to baseline after cage cleaning if this was done in their active time, and 120 minutes if cages were cleaned during their inactive time (Weinandy 1995; Weinandy & Gattermann 1997). Cages can also be partially cleaned, for example to avoid disturbing lactating or pregnant females.

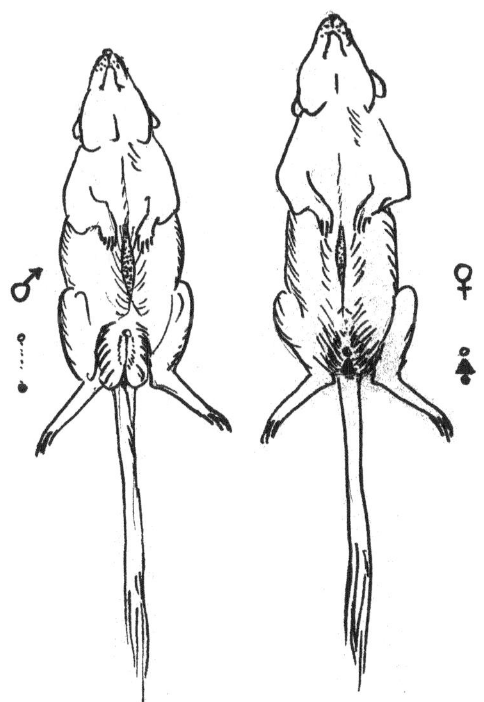

Figure 23.4 Sexing adult gerbils. In males (left), the distance between genital papilla and anus is much greater than in females (right). The latter exhibit a triangular naked area between papilla and anus.

Health monitoring and quarantine

Health monitoring involves close observation of appearance (eg shiny, smooth fur vs. matted, ruffled fur), body weight (ie, weight loss as an indicator of poor health) and behaviour on a regular basis. Gerbils should be inquisitive and active, and should eat and drink normally. Implanted heart rate transmitters or temperature-sensitive transponders can give additional information, but since these methods are, to some degree invasive, they are not suitable for all cases. Gerbils purchased from outside should be quarantined and screened for infectious agents as appropriate.

Transport

Only healthy animals should be transported. Special care has to be taken if pregnant or lactating females are transported. Only animals compatible with each other should be transported together; groups should not be mixed for transport. Transport boxes should allow sufficient air circulation, but also protect the animals from adverse environmental influences. Gnaw-proof boxes of non-toxic material must be used to prevent animals from escaping. Transport time must be minimised. Food and water should be provided on both short and long transports, since delays can always occur. Water can be offered in the form of gel packs ('solid drink'), moistened food and/or vegetables of high water content such as cucumbers, apple or lettuce. See also Chapter 13 and Laboratory Animal Science Association (LASA) (2005).

Breeding

Condition of adults

Gerbils are less prolific breeders than mice or rats, due to longer interbirth intervals, smaller litter sizes and higher pre- and post-natal pup mortality. Future breeding animals should remain with their parents as long as possible. This is advantageous for future breeding performance since the animals thus gain experience in pup care, resulting in measurable benefits of their own future reproductive performance (Salo & French 1989; French 1994). Norris and Adams (1972) found that the shortest interval (40 days) from pairing to parturition was achieved if mature, sexually experienced males were paired with inexperienced or experienced females, and longest (up to 90 days) if inexperienced males of 60 days were used. Clark *et al.* (2002) introduced females of various ages (35, 70, 90, 100 days) to experienced males and found latency to parturition being 34, 36, 45, and 78 days, respectively. The probability of younger females getting impregnated by the first male they were paired with was much higher. Older females tended to have smaller litters than younger females, and longer interbirth intervals, but they were more likely to retrieve removed pups to the nest, spent more time in contact with and nursing the pups, and their pups also grew more rapidly. Older mothers gave birth to more male-biased litters, as predicted by parental investment theory. It is therefore difficult to suggest an optimal age for pairing female gerbils. Future breeding animals should be introduced to each other between the ages of 60 and 90 days. Gerbils should not be paired too early, since familiarity resulting from growing up together can inhibit or delay reproduction in females (Clark & Galef 2001a, 2002; Clark *et al.* 2002).

Identifying fertile state

In laboratory males, testes descend at 30–45 days of age. Roughly 40 days later, active spermatogenesis and mating behaviour begin (70–84 days). Suggested breeding age for males is 75–85 days (Field & Sibold 1999). Without serum testosterone analyses, it is impossible to distinguish so-called 'stud' or 'dud' males (ie, those that will be able to father many offspring or not, see Reproduction section). However, since males with low circulating testosterone levels and lower litter sizes care better for their young, the effect of a low testosterone level is somewhat compensated.

Vaginal opening is at 40–76 days of age, depending on the animal's social surroundings (Norris & Adams 1979b). Sexual maturity is reached at 63–84 days of age if the female is separated from her mother and sisters after weaning. Females are able to breed from 3 months to about 3 years and longer (Field & Sibold 1999; I.W. Stuermer, personal communication). The mean age of wild gerbil females first giving birth was 199 days (F0, wild-caught); for the offspring (F1) of wild-caught gerbils this figure was 71 days (Blottner & Stuermer 2006; Stuermer *et al.* 2006). If paired at 60 days, earliest age at first conception lies around day 75, but Clark and colleagues (2002) observed the first litter being born to a female aged 69.7 days, if paired at the age of 35 days.

Breeding systems

The social system of gerbils indicates monogamous pairing as the optimal breeding system (Agren 1984b; Clark *et al.* 1986; Solomon & Getz 1996; Saltzman *et al.* 2006). Polygynous systems can result in aggression between the females, but some authors prefer this mating system (Marston & Chang 1965; Scheibler *et al.* 2005a, 2005b).

Fostering is possible in gerbils and is most successful within 24 h after parturition. For artificial insemination the same techniques are used as in rats and mice. After PMSG and hCG treatment, sperm is injected into both uterine horns. Artificial insemination has a success rate of about 50%. Reasons for infertility in females are often neoplasia of the ovaries and uterus, or ovarian cysts. Ovarian cysts have a prevalence of 4.3–50% in gerbils.

Conception and pregnancy

Basic reproductive data are taken from Burley (1979), Marston and Chang (1965), Norris (1987), Norris and Adams (1972, 1974, 1981a, 1981b, 1982) and Tumblebrook Farm (1979).

Mating occurs when females are in oestrus during normal oestrous cycles, during post-partum oestrus (13 h after parturition, 80% fertility) and after weaning, if the female was not impregnated during post-partum oestrus. The cycle length is 4–6 days. Peak activity of mating is 2–3 h before the onset of the dark phase in the late afternoon, duration of oestrus is between 12 and 18 h. The onset of post-partum oestrus is about 13.5 h after parturition, ie, the delivery of the last pup. This duration of this oestrus is somewhat shorter: 7–9 h (Prates & Guerra 2005). Mean ovulation range is 6.6 ova (range 4–9). During post-partum oestrus, females spend more time in pup-related behaviours, such as crouching over the pups, licking them, staying in the nest with them or nest building, than males. Males exhibited more female-directed behaviour such as allogrooming and sniffing, and engaged in intense copulatory behaviour (593 mounts or one mount every 47 s). Even during delivery, males attempted to mount, but were rejected at all times by the female. Gerbil males do not help females during parturition as occurs with dwarf hamsters. Paternal behaviour is suppressed by sexual motivation on the day of their mate's parturition and post-partum oestrus. Parental behaviour by males is pronounced before and after this day (Clark *et al.* 2004).

Oestrus can either be identified by female behaviour (Weinandy *et al.* 2002), or determined using vaginal smears (Marston & Chang 1965), which, however, is not very reliable, and further confused by the vaginal plug after mating. Leucocytes, epithelial cells with nucleus and cornified cells indicate phase I (also seen during pregnancy and pseudopregnancy); few leucocytes, many epithelial cells, early stages of cells with nucleus and cornified cells indicate phase II; and the lack of leucocytes plus many cornified cells indicate phase III, ie, oestrus. After mating, the vaginal smear is sperm-positive. During pregnancy, erythrocytes can also be seen in the vaginal smear from day 12 onwards and the vaginal opening is narrowed. During lactation a vaginal membrane develops which persists until weaning.

Copulatory behaviour patterns of females on the day of oestrus were described by Burley (1979). These included piloerection, present posture, darting and foot stamping, as well as an increase of female-initiated allogrooming and sniffing of the male's head and anogenital region. During oestrus, the male shows piloerection posture, presenting posture, intensive sniffing and chasing of the female before mounting the female, who responds with lordosis. Mounting occurs many times over a period of about 6 h. Mating is accompanied by the male regularly foot stamping. Duration of a mount is about 2 s. After mounting, both male and female lick their genitalia. A concealed vaginal plug develops in the upper part of the reproductive tract, but only remains in place for a day.

Implantation usually occurs 7–8 days after fertilisation. Pregnancy duration is between 24 and 28 days. However, if fertilisation occurred during post-partum oestrus, implantation of the blastocyst is retarded even further. According to Norris and Adams (1981a, 1981b), pregnancy duration is then increased by 1.9 days per neonate, if three or more pups of the previous litter are suckled. Pregnancy duration can increase to a maximum of 48 days. Pregnancy has a strong impact on maternal resources, especially if females are both pregnant and nurse the last litter. Females whose dams were both nursing while gestating them and were pregnant while suckling them are less fecund (smaller, more female-based litters) and show lower attachment to their mates (Clark *et al.* 2006). Pregnancy can be palpated from day 15 onwards, the teats are clearly visible from day 14. The female gains 10–30 g during pregnancy. Mating with unfertile males can lead to a pseudopregnancy of 13–23 days. Embryo-transfer has been described by Norris and Adams (1986).

Mean number of litters per reproductive lifespan in females is 7.6 ± 3.8, with a maximum of 17 (author's breeding colony), with litter size decreasing after the tenth litter. Life reproductive success is 33–48 young born per female (maximum 54).

Nesting

The female builds the pup nest, but the male is also involved in nest building. Both males and females shred material (tissues, straw, hay, textiles) into small pieces, collect these in their mouth and carry bundles of them to their nest. If a nest box or shelter is available, gerbils also pad it out with nesting material. A nest is either globular or more frequently hemispherical, with a depression in the centre. Globular nests are constructed if the gerbils are kept at low ambient temperatures and if the female is caring for offspring. Nest-building serves both thermoregulatory and reproductive functions. One needs to be aware that the nest is located underground in wild gerbils, so depth underground adds additional insulation.

Parturition

Parturition occurs usually during the night, its duration depends of the number of pups. The birth of one pup lasts 10–15 minutes; the whole parturition is somewhat longer than 1 h. The female eats placentae and stillbirths. The number of pups depends on the age and condition of the female, with very young and older females delivering smaller litters. The pups are altricial. Except for the first day post-partum the male is involved in pup care. experienced males, either through prolonged residence with their own parents or through having raised their own young, are beneficial for the pups' development. Males are active in nest building, huddle over, clean and occasionally retrieve pups.

The young

Basic developmental data are taken from Marston and Chang (1965), Norris (1987), Norris and Adams (1972, 1974, 1982) and Tumblebrook Farm (1979).

Litter size and development

The litter size of wild gerbils averages 4.5. In laboratory gerbils, the litter size is 5.5, with a range of 1–12. Depending on whether the female is both pregnant with the next litter and suckling pups of the present one, inter-litter interval varies between 25 and 49 days. Mean inter-litter interval is 29–35 days (colony dependant). Neonatal mortality is around 20%, with most mortality in the first 5 days. Exceptionally large litters may show mortality up to 57%, and, likewise, single-pup litters may have high mortality (eg, 75%). Sex ratio is 1.03 at birth, but decreases to 1.0 at weaning age due to higher mortality in males (Field & Sibold 1999). Causes of pup mortality are lack of care, insufficient milk, suffocation, or failure of older pups to reach food or water due to poor cage layout.

Ear opening occurs between days 12 and 14, the first hair appears at 5–7 days, incisors erupt at 10–16 days, and the eyes open between days 16 and 20 (14 days earliest eye opening). Upon eye opening and eruption of the incisors, pups start to venture out of the nest box, digging and eating solid food. Birth weight is inversely correlated with litter size. Singletons might weigh up to 3.3 g, compared with about 2.6 g in pups from large litters (over 10 pups). Males are about 5% heavier than females, a sexual dimorphism that is increased to 10% at older ages. Adult weight is reached at the age of 3 months.

Weaning age

Gerbil pups are artificially weaned at between 20 and 30 days, however, 21 days should be the earliest, and weaning at 28–35 days is recommended. The time between 3 and 4 weeks is critical, since the pups switch from milk to solid food only during this week and change to being completely homeothermic. Food and water should be placed within the cages from day 14 since such small pups cannot reach up to the food hopper and nipple of water bottle. Pups take their first solid food (vegetables or salad) from day 16, and dry pelleted food from day 18 onwards. Weaning weight should be at least 12–18 g, preferably 20 g, and pups should be checked for regular eating and lack of diarrhoea before separating them. Several aspects of behaviour suggest that an even later separation of pups and family would be advantageous: if gerbils are separated before the next litter of younger siblings is born, a significant increase of bar-gnawing is noted after the separation. Additionally, remaining with the family for the duration of the raising of another litter provides future breeding animals with relevant experience.

Infanticide

Infanticide is very rare, but does occur in both males and females. It occurs spontaneously (Saltzman *et al.* 2006) or under poor husbandry conditions, for example if the female is undernourished during lactation. The author observed one female eating her 7-day-old pups after the animal care staff forgot to replenish the food. In contrast to house mice, infanticidal gerbil females do not first kill the pups, but might start to eat them from the tail region. If male gerbils are food-deprived, they might also become infanticidal (Elwood & Ostermeyer 1984).

Feeding

Water

Gerbils exhibit several adaptations to dry climate: they excrete relatively low amounts of urine (3–4 ml per day compared to 6 ml in the golden hamster, also an animal of arid habitats) and quite dry faecal pellets (McManus 1972a). They tolerate quite high salt concentrations (McManus 1972a). Mongolian gerbils are able to survive without drinking water or consuming green foodstuffs by the use of metabolic water, arising, for example via the oxidation of lipids (Wang *et al.* 2003). If provided with *ad libitum* water, gerbils consume 4–10 ml of water per day (McManus 1972a; Field & Sibold 1999). Experiments summarised by Thiessen and Yahr (1977) show that depending on the composition of the food (its fat content), water-deprived gerbils die after losing 30% of their body weight. Water deprivation also results in a halt of reproduction in breeding pairs. Pregnant and lactating females are especially susceptible to water under-supply. In the laboratory, with dry food pellets and low humidity, *ad libitum* water supply should be provided in any case. This is in accordance with recently revised European guidance (Council of Europe 2006): '*Uncontaminated drinking water should always be available to all animals.*'

In general it is easier to provide water *ad libitum* via bottles or an automated drinking system than by regular supply with greens and vegetables. However, salad, dandelion leaves, cucumber, carrots, pumpkin (seeds and flesh), zucchini, fennel, etc are well liked by gerbils, as are fruit such as apples, pears, melon, etc. In contrast to the situation in the degu (*Octodon degus*), gerbils have not been found to be susceptible to type 2 diabetes (Besselmann & Hatt 2004), therefore sweet fruit and vegetables can be offered occasionally.

Food

In the wild, gerbils are granivorous–herbivorous animals (Wang *et al.* 2003). Their diet consists of green parts of plants and seeds, for example of grasses, wormwood (*Artemisia* sp.), and various other, locally available plants with the occasional insect or larva as a supplement (Bannikov 1954; Naumov & Lobachev 1975; Scheibler *et al.* 2006b).

Gerbils hoard food extensively, both in the wild and in the laboratory (Naumov & Lobachev 1975; Agren *et al.* 1989b; Tsurim & Abramsky 2004). The author has seen laboratory gerbils stuffing food pellets in one corner of their cage, if loose food is available. In the wild, gerbils hoard up to 20 kg of food for winter (Naumov & Lobachev 1975), and pet gerbils sometimes hoard several kilograms of food despite the relatively constant temperatures of their surroundings. Gerbils have been used to analyse food-searching strategies and patch-choice theory in the laboratory (Forkman 1991, 1993a, 1993b). Food preferences are socially transferred in gerbils. Mothers pass on their food preferences to their pups (Valsecchi *et al.* 1996, 2002), but gerbils also learn food preferences from familiar or related conspecifics (Galef *et al.* 1998). Hunger also influences the acquisition of food preferences (Forkman 1995).

In the laboratory, gerbils can be fed standard mouse, rat or hamster breeding chow; however, the protein content needs to be 22% and fat content only 4% to prevent the development of obesity. This pellet diet can be supplemented with grains and seed mixtures. Gerbils can be easily trained for various laboratory routines by rewarding them with sunflower seeds or pumpkin seeds. These seeds have a very high fat content and should be used with restraint.

Food and water should be provided in a way that allows all animals, including pups, to access them. One way of presenting food is scatter it on the bedding. In the author's opinion, this has several advantages over presenting it only in the food hopper: it is accessible for all animals, it is hoardable, and the animals are occupied searching for food in the bedding. Since gerbils produce very few drops of urine, their bedding stays clean for a longer time than that of mice or rats, therefore food in the bedding will not be contaminated by urine so quickly. Gerbils eat about 18 times during the day at random times, therefore their stomachs contain a little food all the time (Kanarek *et al.* 1977). As a rule, food should be presented *ad libitum* and should not be time restricted.

Laboratory procedures

Handling

If carefully habituated, gerbils can be caught with cupped hands. An easy way to catch them is to use tubes since they will readily enter any tube provided. Usually they are caught at the base of their tail, with the body being immediately supported by the other hand. If gerbils are caught at the tip of their tail, they tend to struggle and kick vigorously, resulting in shedding of the skin of the tail (degloving). Gerbils can be restrained by a neck-grip, also securing them at the base of the tail. However, they often struggle very much when placed on their back. In small animal practice, a soft towel is often used to restrain adult gerbils. They are tightly wrapped in a towel from behind and will often remain still as long as some pressure, but not too much, is applied around their body (Figure 23.5). Gerbil pups can

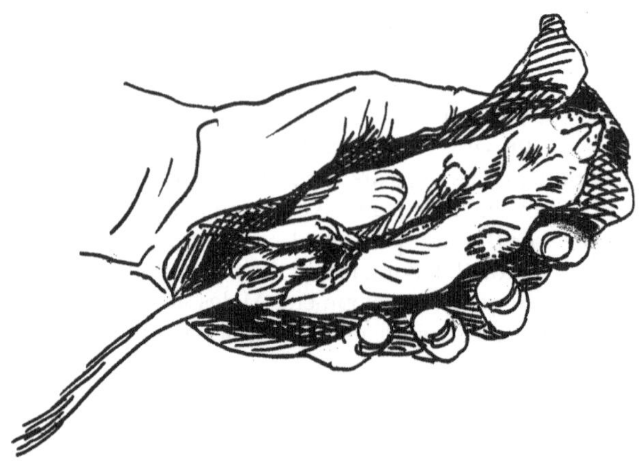

Figure 23.5 Gerbil restrained by wrapping the animal in a towel, a method often used in small animal practices.

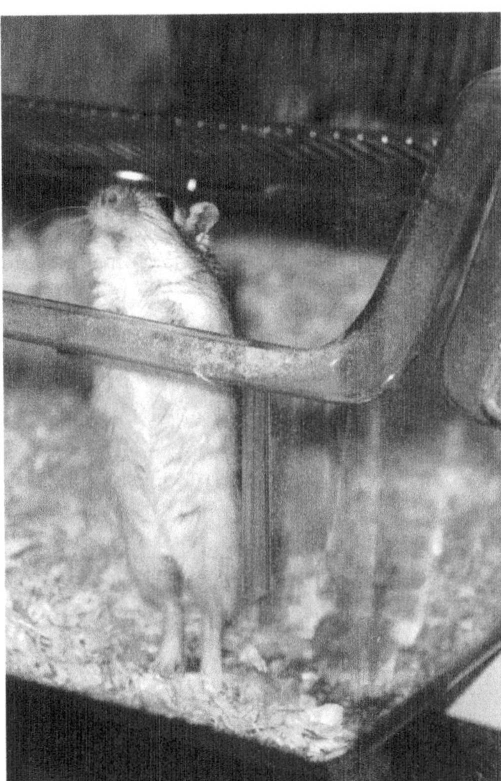

Figure 23.6 Gerbil habituated to coming forward in the laboratory cage, using positive reinforcement.

comfortably snuggle in a slightly closed fist. Gerbils can be habituated very well to handling procedures by offering them a treat if they come forward in the cage voluntarily and climb on a hand, and by rewarding them after replacing them in the cage and after procedures (Figure 23.6).

Physiological monitoring

Recording body temperatures

As noted earlier, gerbils have a body temperature of around 37.4–38.4°C. Body temperature can be measured by using a rectal probe, but this needs handling and manipulation, which itself could induce stress and temperature changes. For regular temperature readings, a subcutaneous temperature-sensitive passive transponder, injected (under isoflurane anaesthesia) between the shoulder blades, is recommended (Kort *et al.* 1998; Newsom *et al.* 2004). Infrared laser scanners can also be used to measure body surface temperature in slightly restrained animals. If gerbils are implanted with heart rate transmitters, core temperature can be measured (Weinandy 1995; Moons *et al.* 2007), but this needs major surgery.

Collection of specimens

Blood

Haematological and clinical chemistry data are provided by Field and Sibold (1999 p. 10–11). Blood volume is 6.7% of body weight or 66–78 ml/kg (van Zutphen *et al.* 2001). To be on the safe side, maximal blood volume to be collected should not be more than 10% of the purported maximal blood volume. The Swiss Laboratory Animal guidelines allow collection of a maximum of 1 ml in a gerbil weighing 80 g, or a maximum of 20% of the total blood volume within 2 weeks[1]. See also Joint Working Group on Refinement (JWGR) (1993) for general guidance on blood collection.

Blood collection routes have been summarised by Field and Sibold (1999). Blood can be collected from the lateral tail vein after warming the tail, either by placing it in warm water, by setting the animal under a infrared lamp or in a warmed chamber (30–35°C for 10–15 minutes) to allow for vasodilation. Another accepted method is the puncture of the saphenous vein (Hem *et al.* 1998). Small amounts of blood (0.1–0.2 ml) can also be attained by cutting the tip of the tail, a procedure that is usually only allowed once per animal in animal welfare guidelines. Retro-orbital sinus blood collection is also possible in gerbils, but it needs to be performed under anaesthesia, and, according to many animal welfare laws and guidelines, must be performed not more frequently than 2 weeks apart at the same eye. Unfortunately, puncture of the sublingual vein under inhalation anaesthesia has not been described in gerbils so far, despite its advantages over retro-orbital puncture in rats (safe, quick, improved healing) (Zeller *et al.* 1998). Cardiac puncture should be reserved for terminal blood collection and must only be performed under anaesthesia.

Urine

To collect urine, gerbils can be placed individually in metabolic cages. A much simpler method is to place filter paper in bedding-free cages. However, there is a danger of the gerbils shredding the paper within hours. Gerbils can also be placed in wire mesh bottom cages with a sheet of metal below to collect urine over 24 h (Fenske 1990, 1996; Waiblinger & König 2004). Handling can also be used to induce urination.

Faecal samples

Faecal samples can easily be collected, since they are dry and do not stick to the bedding. Gerbils produce about 15–20 dry pellets or 1.5–2.5 g faeces per day (author's own experience) Collecting these from the bedding is more tedious than using a metabolic cage, but probably less stressful for the animal, since it can be left in its own cage and bedding. Cortisol extraction from faeces has been done, however, Fenske (1996) found a dissociation of plasma and faecal/urinary cortisol after application of stressors (see above). However, faecal cortisol measurements might be used to assess long-term stressors.

Vaginal smears

To take vaginal smears, the same methods can be used as with mice: using a pasteur pipette with a rubber teat and irrigating the vagina with a small volume of sterile, warmed physiological saline. However, vaginal smears are not very well suited for determining oestrous state in gerbils.

[1] http://www.bvet.admin.ch/themen/tierschutz/00777/00778/index.html?lang=de>Richtlinie/Guideline No. 800.116-3.02

Milk

Collection of milk in gerbils has been described by Rassin *et al.* (1978). For the exact method of collecting milk from small rodents, see Feller and Boretos (1967) and Raffel and König (1999).

Administration of medicines

Dosing and injection procedures

Routine application procedures used for mice and rats can generally also be used for gerbils. Since gerbils should neither be held by their tails nor turned on their back, the procedure for intraperitoneal injection should be modified. The gerbil is placed on the wire top of a cage, where it will try to walk away. First the base of the tail is picked up with one hand, and the hindquarters of the animal lifted slightly off the grid. With the same hand, thumb and forefinger, the loose skin at the neck is picked up and the animal can be raised to an upright, vertical position (head up), at which time the injection can be made with the free hand or by an assistant. Intravenous injection in the femoral vein and the external jugular vein, both under anaesthesia, have been described since the lateral tail vein is not as easily accessible for injections in gerbils as in mice or rats due to their furry tail (Pérez-García *et al.* 2003; Kakol Palm & Hollaender 2007). Subcutaneous injections are usually given in the loose skin between the shoulder blades. In general 23–25 G needles are used. Details on dosing various common substances can be found in Field and Sibold (1999), pp. 73–75.

Anaesthesia and analgesia

In commercial small animal veterinary practice, isoflurane inhalation anaesthesia via precision vaporiser is generally used as the method of choice for small mammals such as gerbils. It is used at 2–5% for induction, and 1.2–2.3% for maintenance. Recovery from isoflurane anaesthesia is usually very quick. Methoxyflurane has also been used in gerbils (Norris 1981). It is to be noted that these gaseous anaesthesia agents do not have analgesic properties, and therefore pre- and post-surgery analgesia must be used where appropriate. Field and Sibold (1999) present a list of commonly used, injectable anaesthetics and their combinations (p. 77). Some common intraperitoneally injectable anaesthesias for gerbils are: 50 mg/kg ketamine and 2 mg/kg climazolam; 50 mg/kg ketamine and 2 mg/kg xylazine; or pentobarbital 60–80 mg/kg (duration 30–45 minutes). See also Flecknell (2009).

Post-operative pain should be relieved in gerbils using appropriate analgesia (this is required by most countries' animal welfare guidelines). A suitable analgesia regimen for gerbils might be 0.05–0.2 mg/kg buprenorphine sc or 0.003 mg/kg fentanyl sc (1 : 10 in NaCl; 1/3 of dose every 20 minutes) before surgery, and 5 mg/kg carprofen sc or 1 drop of meloxicam solution (5 mg meloxicam/ml) every 12–24 h after surgery, as required. Field and Sibold (1999) again list suitable analgesia agents for gerbils (p. 97), however, they centre on the opioids and do not give information about non-steroidal anti-inflammatory drugs (NSAIDs) such as paracetamol or diclofenac. A list of suitable NSAIDs can be found in Flecknell (2007).

Humane endpoints

If an animal shows signs of morbidity (disease or illness) for some days or is moribund (dying), then its condition should immediately be evaluated and a decision made as to treatment or euthanasia. In general, signs of morbidity are similar to those seen in hamsters and mice. Common signs, according to Field and Sibold (1999) include:

- hunched posture;
- ruffled fur;
- rapid weight loss (10–15% in a week);
- hypothermia or hyperthermia (depends on the experiment, ie, studies on infectious diseases differ from cancer studies);
- increased respiration rate;
- diarrhoea or constipation;
- changes in activity and behaviour;
- paralysis or other CNS signs.

For most of these signs, score sheets can be used. Body temperature can be measured non-invasively using subcutaneous, temperature-sensitive passive transponders (Kort et al 1998; Toth 1997, 2000). Frequent monitoring for signs of morbidity is paramount if humane endpoints are to be applied.

Euthanasia

Methods used for euthanasia must be painless, safe to apply and ensure a quick loss of consciousness. In the recommendations for euthanasia of experimental animals, the EU Commission working party suggests the following methods of euthanasia for rodents in general, not specifically for gerbils (Close *et al.* 1996, 1997), although national regulations may vary. See also Chapter 17.

Physical methods

Physical methods suitable for gerbils are: stunning (only by well trained personnel), cervical dislocation or decapitation (only with specialised apparatus). If microwaves are used for euthanasia, only specialised apparatus adapted to the size of the animal and the species must be used to focus the irradiation exactly on the brain (Close *et al.* 1996, 1997).

Chemical methods, injectable agents

Generally, if venepuncture and intravenous injection can be used, this route of administration (eg of appropriate barbiturate or other suitable agents) is recommended, since intraperitoneal injection is slower to act and might lead to irritation of the peritoneum. Other application routes for injectable anaesthetics should not be chosen except if the animals is fully anaesthetised, ie, no intracardiac injection of T61 (forbidden by law in Switzerland, for example, the EU working party also strongly discourages this application route). Gerbils can be killed by an overdose of sodium pentobarbital, for example by intraperitoneal injection (>270 mg/kg, maximum 200 mg/ml injectable solution) (Field & Sibold, 1999). Three times the anaesthetic dose is recommended. T61 must be injected intravenously very slowly, and prior sedation might be required (for exact composition of T61 see Close *et al.* 1996).

Chemical methods, inhalational agents

If inhalation anaesthesia agents such as isoflurane, halothane or enflurane are used, the animals must be left in the chamber long enough for death to be ensured, and this must be confirmed, or the animals must subsequently be killed by another method that ensures their death, for example by decapitation or exsanguination. Methoxyflurane should not be used in gerbils. Animal welfare aspects of using carbon dioxide for euthanasia have widely been discussed; see Conlee *et al.* (2005) for a review, but also Leach *et al.* (2005). Carbon dioxide is aversive, and burrow-living rodents are reported to have a high tolerance for carbon dioxide. Both the prefilled-chamber and the gradual-influx methods have their disadvantages. If the gradual-influx method is used, the home cage of the animals should be covered with a tight-fitting lid. Carbon dioxide should be introduced from the top of the cage. Structures in the cage beneath the inlet (for example a nest box) help to distribute the gas equally through turbulence. Optimal flow rate is about 13 l/min for cages type III, 6 l/min for cages type II. Solid carbon dioxide (dry ice) should not be used, since carbon dioxide concentrations cannot be controlled and the animals must be prevented from touching the dry ice (Corbach 2006).

Euthanasia of neonates

Neonates cannot be killed by carbon dioxide, since they have a high tolerance for hypoxia. Neonates can be killed by decapitation (Close *et al.* 1997).

Common welfare problems

Disease

Prophylaxis

In general, gerbils are remarkably healthy in captivity. The animals should be checked daily for their health status, and weighed at least once a week. Stressed animals are more susceptible to disease than unstressed ones. Positive reinforcement (training with treats) can be used to habituate gerbils to common handling and application procedures and reduce the impact of handling-induced stress (see Chapter 16).

Signs of disease

Diseased gerbils tend to show a reduction of activity, ruffled fur, hunched posture, diarrhoea and loss of body weight. Elderly animals tend to become emaciated (>3 years old) and to sink in at their flanks. Increased drinking might be indicative of either diabetes or renal failure.

Common diseases

Gerbils can contract Tyzzer's disease (*Bacillus piliformis*). Affected animals become apathetic and huddle in a hunched position in the corner of the cage with ruffled fur (Field & Sibold 1999). Sometimes diarrhoea can be seen. Since these animals do not feed, weight loss is quite severe, and the animals die within 1–3 days. Tyzzer's disease can be spread among animals by soiled bedding. If an outbreak occurs, affected animals, cages and rooms should be quarantined immediately. Tetracycline has been used to treat mice and might also be effective in gerbils. Oxytetracycline added to drinking water can be used, and dehydrated animals should be given rehydration therapy if they are not euthanased. Since *B. piliformis* is spore-forming, bodies, bedding, food and nesting material must be incinerated and cages, equipment and rooms thoroughly sterilised. Dihydrostreptomycin is toxic for gerbils and should therefore not be used (Field & Sibold 1999).

A much less severe condition is the red or sore nose disease sometimes observed in laboratory gerbils. The animals develop reddish sores (erythema) around the nose. Unpublished data of the author show that these sores were not caused by the animals digging in the substrate or by gnawing on the bars, since the occurrence and severity of the sore nose disease did not correlate with digging or bar-gnawing frequency. Often, red nose disease is caused by a staphylococcal infection of the nose (*Staphylococcus aureus*) (Peckham *et al.* 1974). The author used odourless topical antiseptics creams or a systemic antiobiotic treatment with good results in a non-SPF-colony (chloramphenicol 0.083 g/1100 ml water, or tetracycline 0.3 g/100 ml water for 14 days, as suggested by Field and Sibold (1999)). However, good hygiene should prevent the outbreak of this disease. As a rule, most gerbils recover from red nose disease, and only if the sores spread to larger areas of frontpaws and face, should animals be killed.

In aged animals, sebaceous gland carcinomas can occasionally be observed (Raflo & Diamond 1980; Matsuoka & Suzuki 1995; da Costa *et al.* 2007). Chronic interstitial nephritis is sometimes diagnosed in aged gerbils. Affected gerbils lose weight and exhibit polyuria and polydipsia (Johnson-Delaney 1998). Histopathological lesions of the ventral prostate have also been observed in aged gerbils (Campos *et al.* 2008).

Gerbils are prone to epileptic seizures and are used as a model to screen for antiepileptic drugs. Juveniles develop seizures at 2 months of age, by 10 months up to 80% of the animals can exhibit seizures of various degrees (Kaplan & Miezejes 1972; Loskota *et al.* 1974a; Kaplan 1975; Frey 1987; Cutler & Mackintosh 1989; Kupferberg 2001). For research not concerned with epilepsy, known seizure-eliciting stimuli such as handling stress, dangling by the tail, novelty, blasts of air or sudden noise should be avoided, as well as the use of seizure-prone strains of gerbils (Fujisawa *et al.* 2003). In the experience of the author, habituation to handling procedures reduces the incidence of epileptic seizures in gerbils, but this has not been analysed systematically so far. However, Jaworska *et al.* (2008, p. 539) mentioned having habituated gerbil pups to handling in order to reduce the frequency of seizures.

Abnormal behaviour

Laboratory gerbils commonly develop two distinct, well recognised, abnormal behaviours: stereotypic digging and bar-gnawing (Figure 23.7). These behaviours are environmentally induced. Stereotypic digging is caused by the lack of an appropriate burrow structure, either self-dug or artificial. Provision with a dark nest box and access tube can significantly reduce the incidence of this behaviour (Wiedenmayer 1996, 1997a, 1997b, 1997c). Bar-gnawing possibly has social causes. Its development can be prevented if juvenile gerbils are not separated from their parents before the next litter is born, ie, if the juveniles are left with the parents for at least 5 weeks (Wiedenmayer 1997c; Waiblinger & König 2001, 2004; Waiblinger 2002, 2003). This might present some problems with standard laboratory routine.

Most animal welfare laws state that abnormal behaviour and stereotypies are a sign of suboptimal housing or husbandry, even a welfare problem, and should therefore be prevented. The method of choice is not the physical prevention of the performance of these behaviours, in gerbils for example by denying them access to bars that might be chewed on, but the prevention of the ontogenetic development of stereotypies by removing the underlying causes of suboptimal housing or husbandry. Stereotypic behaviours in rodents originate from continuously thwarted motivations to escape or to search shelter (Würbel 2006), and therefore represent some sort of frustration and lack of control. There are strong indications that stereotypies result in CNS dysfunction (ie, recurrent perseveration and decreased dorsal striatal inhibitory behavioural control) (Garner 2006), thus making stereotypic behaviours fundamentally analogous to the repetitive behaviours associated with human pathologies such as schizophrenia and autism. Garner cautions against using such stereotyping rodents in behavioural tests in the laboratory since the underlying CNS dysfunctions might thwart their validity as animal models, at least if they are used in behavioural paradigms.

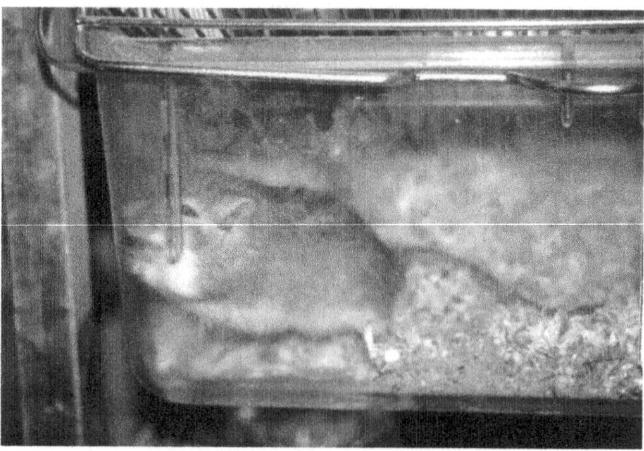

(a)

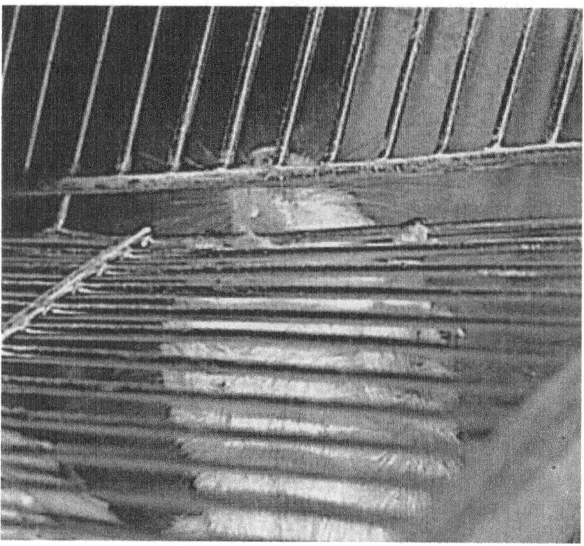

(b)

Figure 23.7 Stereotypic digging in the corner of the cage (a) and bar-gnawing (b) in laboratory gerbils.

Dedication

This chapter is dedicated to Rolf Gattermann whose premature death left a deep gap in the gerbil research community.

References

Agren, G. (1984a) Incest avoidance and bonding between siblings in gerbils. *Behavioural Ecology and Sociobiology*, **14**, 161–169

Agren, G. (1984b) Pair formation in the Mongolian gerbil. *Animal Behaviour*, **32**, 528–535

Agren, G., Zhou, Q. and Zhong, W. (1989a) Ecology and social behaviour of Mongolian gerbils, *Meriones unguiculatus*, at Xilinhot, Inner Mongolia, China. *Animal Behaviour*, **37**, 11–27

Agren, G., Zhou, Q. and Zhong, W. (1989b) Territoriality, cooperation and resource priority: hoarding in the Mongolian gerbil, *Meriones unguiculatus*. *Animal Behaviour*, **37**, 28–32

Bagorda, F., Teuchert-Noodt, G. and Lehmann, K. (2006) Isolation rearing or metamphetamine traumatisation induce a 'dysconnection' of prefrontal efferents in gerbils: implications for schizophrenia. *Journal of Neural Transmission*, **113**, 365–379

Baker, A. and Emerson, V.F. (1983) Grating acuity of the Mongolian gerbil (*Meriones unguiculatus*). *Behavioural Brain Research*, **8**, 195–209

Bannikov, A.G. (1954) The places inhabited and natural history of *Meriones unguiculatus*. Mammals of the Mongolian Peoples Republic, USSR Academy of Sciences – Committee of the Mongolian Peoples Republic. *Trudy Mongol'skoi Komissii*, **53**, 410–415

Besselmann, D. and Hatt, J.M. (2004) Diabetes mellitus in rabbits and rodents. *Tierärztliche Praxis Ausgabe Kleintiere/Heimtiere*, **32**, 370–376

Birch, D.G. and Jacobs, G.H. (1980) Light-induced damage to photopic and scotopic mechanisms in the rat depends on rearing conditions. *Experimental Neurology*, **68**, 269–283

Blottner, S., Franz, C., Rohleder, M. *et al.* (2000) Higher testicular activity in laboratory gerbils compared to wild Mongolian gerbils (*Meriones unguiculatus*). *Journal of the Zoological Society of London*, **250**, 462–466

Blottner, S. and Stuermer, I.W. (2006) Reproduction of wild gerbils bred in the laboratory in dependence on generation and season: II. Spermatogenic activity and testicular testosterone concentration. *Animal Science*, **82**, 388–395

Broom, D., Elwood, R.W., Lakin, J. *et al.* (1977) Developmental changes in several parameters of ultrasonic calling by young Mongolian gerbils (*Meriones unguiculatus*). *Journal of Zoology*, **183**, 281–290

Brummelte, S., Neddens, J. and Teuchert-Noodt, G. (2007) Alteration in the GABAergic network of the prefrontal cortex in a potential animal model of psychosis. *Journal of Neural Transmission*, **114**, 539–547

Brunner, C. (1993) The digging behaviour of the Mongolian gerbil (*Meriones unguiculatus*) in a semi-natural enclosure. Unpublished Master Thesis. Ethology and Wildlife Research, Zoologisches Institut, Universität Zürich

Buckmaster, P.S. and Wong, E.H. (2002) Evoked responses of the dentate gyrus during seizures in developing gerbils with inherited epilepsy. *Journal of Neurophysiology*, **88**, 783–793

Burley, R.A. (1979) Pre-copulatory and copulatory behaviour in relation to stages of the oestrus cycle in the female Mongolian gerbil. *Behaviour*, **72**, 211–241

Bytyqi, A. and Layer, P.G. (2005) Lamina formation in the Mongolian gerbil retina (*Meriones unguiculatus*). *Anatomy and Embryology*, **209**, 217–225

Campos, S.G.P., Zanetoni, C., Scarano, W.R. *et al.* (2008) Age-related histopathological lesions in the Mongolian gerbil ventral prostate as a good model for studies of spontaneous hormone-related disorders. *International Journal of Experimental Pathology*, **89**, 13–24

Cheal, M.L. and Foley, K. (1985) Developmental and experiential influences on ontogeny: The gerbil (*Meriones unguiculatus*) as a model. *Journal of Comparative Psychology*, **99**, 289–305

Cheal, M.L., Foley, K. and Kastenbaum, R. (1986) Brief periods of environmental enrichment facilitate adolescent development of gerbils. *Physiology & Behavior*, **36**, 1047–1051

Chevret, P. and Dobigny, G. (2005) Systematics and evolution of the subfamily *Gerbillinae* (Mammalia, Rodentia, Muridae). *Molecular Phylogenetics and Evolution*, **35**, 674–688

Clark, M.M. and Galef, B.G. (1977) The role of the physical rearing environment in the domestication of the Mongolian gerbil (*Meriones unguiculatus*). *Animal Behaviour*, **25**, 298–316

Clark, M.M. and Galef, B.G. (1979) A sensitive period for the maintenance of emotionality in Mongolian gerbils. *Journal of Comparative and Physiological Psychology*, **93**, 200–210

Clark, M.M. and Galef, B.G. (1994) A male gerbil's intrauterine position affects female response to his scent marks. *Physiology & Behavior*, **55**, 1137–1139

Clark, M.M. and Galef, B.G. (1999) A testosterone-mediated tradeoff between parental and sexual effort in male mongolian gerbils (*Meriones unguiculatus*). *Journal of Comparative Psychology*, **113**, 388–395

Clark, M.M. and Galef, B.G. (2000) Why some male Mongolian gerbils may help at the nest: testosterone, asexuality and alloparenting. *Animal Behaviour*, **59**, 801–806

Clark, M.M. and Galef, B.G. (2001a) Socially-induced infertility: Familial effects on reproductive development of female Mongolian gerbils. *Animal Behaviour*, **62**, 897–903

Clark, M.M. and Galef, B.G. (2001b) Age-related changes in paternal responses of gerbils parallel changes in their testosterone concentrations. *Developmental Psychobiology*, **39**, 179–187

Clark, M.M. and Galef, B.G. (2002) Socially induced delayed reproduction in female Mongolian gerbils (*Meriones unguiculatus*): Is there anything special about dominant females? *Journal of Comparative Psychology*, **116**, 363–368

Clark, M.M., Johnson, J. and Galef, B.G. (2004) Sexual motivation suppresses paternal behaviour of male gerbils during their mates' postpartum oestrus. *Animal Behaviour*, **67**, 49–57

Clark, M.M., Liu, C. and Galef, B.G. (2001) Effects of consanguinity, exposure to pregnant females, and stimulation from young on male gerbils' responses to pups. *Developmental Psychobiology*, **39**, 257–264

Clark, M.M., Moghaddas, M. and Galef, B.G. (2002) Age at first mating affects parental effort and fecundity of female Mongolian gerbils. *Animal Behaviour*, **63**, 1129–1134

Clark, M.M., Spencer, C.A. and Galef, B.G. (1986) Improving the productivity of breeding colonies of Mongolian gerbils (*Meriones unguiculatus*). *Laboratory Animals*, **20**, 313–315

Clark, M.M., Stiver, K., Teall, T. *et al.* (2006) Nursing one litter of Mongolian gerbils while pregnant with another: effects on daughters' mate attachment and fecundity. *Animal Behaviour*, **71**, 235–241

Clark, M.M., Tucker, L. and Galef, B.G. (1992) Stud males and dud males: intrauterine position effects on the success of male gerbils. *Animal Behaviour*, **43**, 215–221

Clark, M.M., Vonk, J.M. and Galef, B.G. (1998) Intrauterine position, parenting, and nest-site attachment in male Mongolian gerbils. *Developmental Psychobiology*, **32**, 177–181

Close, B., Banister, K., Baumans, V. *et al.* (1996) Recommendations for euthanasia of experimental animals: Part 1. *Laboratory Animals*, **30**, 293–316

Close, B., Banister, K., Baumans, V. *et al.* (1997) Recommendations for euthanasia of experimental animals: Part 2. *Laboratory Animals*, **31**, 1–32

Collins, A., Lindzey, G. and Thiessen, D.D. (1969) The regulation of cliff responses in the Mongolian gerbil (*Meriones unguiculatus*) by visual and tactual cues. *Psychonomic Science*, **16**, 227–229

Conlee, C.M., Stephens, M.L., Rowan, A.N. *et al.* (2005) Carbon dioxide for euthanasia: concerns regarding pain and distress, with special reference to mice and rats. *Laboratory Animals*, **39**, 137–161

Corbach, S. (2006) Untersuchung der CO2-Euthanasie bei Labormäusen auf Tierschutzgerechtigkeit. PhD Thesis (German), Institut für Tierschutz und Verhalten (Heim-, Labortiere und Pferde), Tierärztliche Hochschule Hannover. http://elib.tiho-hannover.de/dissertations/corbachs_ss06.pdf

Cornwell-Jones, C.A. and Azar, L.M. (1982) Olfactory development in gerbil pups. *Developmental Psychobiology*, **15**, 131–137

Council of Europe (2006) *European Convention for the Protection of Vertebrate Animals used for Experimental and other Scientific Purposes, Revised Appendix A, Guidelines on Accommodation and Care (ETS 123)* Strasbourg. http://conventions.coe.int/Treaty/EN/Treaties/PDF/123-Arev.pdf (accessed 26 October 2007)

Cutler, M.G. and Mackintosh, J.H. (1989) Epilepsy and behaviour of the Mongolian gerbil – an ethological study. *Physiology & Behavior*, **46**, 561–566

da Costa, R.M., Rema, A., Payo-Puente, P. *et al.* (2007) Immunohistochemical characterization of a sebaceous gland carcinoma in a gerbil (*Meriones unguiculatus*). *Journal of Comparative Pathology*, **137**, 130–132

Davis, S., Begon, M., De Bruyn, L. *et al.* (2004) Predictive thresholds for plague in Kazakhstan. *Science*, **304**, 736–738

De Ghett, V. (1974) Developmental changes in the rate of ultrasonic vocalization in the Mongolian gerbil. *Developmental Psychobiology*, **7**, 267–272

Dizinno, G. and Clancy, A.N. (1978) Ventral marking in black and agouti gerbils (*Meriones unguiculatus*). *Behavioural Biology*, **24**, 545–548

Eckrich, T., Foeller, E., Stuermer, I.W. *et al.* (2008) Strain-dependence of age-related cochlear hearing-loss in wild and domesticated Mongolian gerbils. *Hearing Research*, **235**, 72–79

Ellard, C.G. and Byers, R.D. (2005) The influence of the behaviour of conspecifics on responses to threat in the Mongolian gerbil, *Meriones unguiculatus*. *Animal Behaviour*, **70**, 49–58

Elwood, R.W. and Ostermeyer, M.C. (1984) The effects of food deprivation, aggression, and isolation on infanticide in the male Mongolian gerbil. *Aggressive Behavior*, **10**, 293–301

Feller, W.F. and Boretos, J. (1967) Semiautomatic apparatus for milking mice. *Journal of the National Cancer Institute*, **38**, 11

Fenske, M. (1990) Excretion of electrolytes, free cortisol and aldosterone-18-oxo-glucuronide in 24-hr urines of the Mongolian gerbil (*Meriones unguiculatus*): effect of lysine-vasopressin and adrenocorticotrophin administration, and of changes in sodium balance. *Comparative Biochemistry & Physiology A – Comparative Physiology*, **95**, 259–265

Fenske, M. (1996) Dissociation of plasma and urinary steroid values after application of stressors, insulin, vasopressin, ACTH, or dexamethasone in the Mongolian gerbil. *Experimental and Clinical Endocrinology and Diabetes*, **104**, 441–446

Field, K.J. and Sibold, A.L. (1999) *The Laboratory Hamster and Gerbil.* CRC Press Ltd., Washington, DC

Finck, A., Schneck, C.D. and Hartman, A.F. (1969) Development of auditory function in the Mongolian gerbil. *Journal of the Acoustical Society of America*, **64**, 107

Flecknell, P. (2007) Anaesthesia and peri-operative care. In: *Manual of Animal Technology*. Eds Barnett S.W. and Barley, J., pp. 399. Blackwell Publishing, Oxford

Flecknell, P.A. (2009) *Laboratory Animal Anaesthesia*, 3rd edn. Academic Press, London

Forkman, B.A. (1991) Some problems with current patch-choice theory – a study in the Mongolian gerbil. *Behaviour*, **117**, 243–254

Forkman, B.A. (1993a) Self-reinforced behavior does not explain contra-freeloading in the Mongolian gerbil. *Ethology*, **94**, 109–112

Forkman, B.A. (1993b) The effect of uncertainity on the food-intake of the Mongolian gerbil. *Behaviour*, **124**, 197–206

Forkman, B.A. (1995) The effect of hunger on the learning of new food preferences in the Mongolian gerbil. *Behaviour*, **132**, 627–639

French, J.A. (1994) Alloparents in the Mongolian gerbil: impact on long-term reproductive performance of breeders and opportunities for independent reproduction. *Behavioural Ecology*, **5**, 273–279

Frey, H.-H. (1987) Induction of seizures by air blast in gerbils: stimulus duration/effect relationship. *Epilepsy Research*, **1**, 262–264

Fujisawa, N., Maeda, Y., Yamamoto, Y. *et al.* (2003) Newly established seizure susceptible and seizure-prone inbred strains of Mongolian gerbil. *Experimental Animals*, **52**, 169–172

Galef, B.G., Rudolf, B., Whiskin, E.E. *et al.* (1998) Familiarity and relatedness: effects on social learning about foods by Norway rats and Mongolian gerbils. *Animal Learning and Behavior*, **26**, 448–454

Garner, J.P. (2006) Perseveration and stereotypy – system-level insights from clinical psychology. In: *Stereotypic Animal Behaviour*. Eds Mason, G. and Rushen, J., pp. 121–152. CAB International, Wallingford

Govardovskii, V., Röhlich, P., Szél, A. *et al.* (1992) Cones in the retina of the Mongolian gerbil (*Meriones unguiculatus*): an immunocytochemical and electrophysiological study. *Vision Research*, **32**, 19–27

Grant, M. and Thiessen, D. (1989) The possible interaction of Harderian material and saliva for thermoregulation in the Mongolian gerbil, *Meriones unguiculatus*. *Perceptual and Motor Skills*, **68**, 3–10

Gray-Allan, P. and Wong, R. (1990) Influence of coat color genes on seizure behavior in Mongolian gerbils. *Behavioural Genetics*, **20**, 481–485

Hauzenberger, A.R., Gebhardt-Henrich, S.G. and Steiger, A. (2006) The influence of bedding depth on behaviour in golden hamsters (*Mesocricetus auratus*). *Applied Animal Behaviour Science*, **100**, 280–294

Heffner, R. and Heffner, H. (1988) Sound localization and use of binaural cues by the gerbil (*Meriones unguiculatus*). *Behavioural Neuroscience*, **102**, 422–428

Hem, A., Smith, A.J. and Solberg, P. (1998) Saphenous vein puncture for blood sampling of the mouse, rat, hamster, gerbil, guinea pig, ferret and mink. *Laboratory Animals*, **32**, 364–368

Hendrie, C.A. and Pickles, A.R. (2000) Short-term individual housing in female gerbils as a putative model of depression. *Society for Neuroscience Abstracts*, **26**, Abstract No.103.12.

Henley, M. and Robinson, R. (1981) Non-agouti and pink-eyed dilution in the Mongolian gerbil. *The Journal of Heredity*, **72**, 60–61

Holman, S.D. (1980) Sexually dimorphic ultrasonic vocalizations of Mongolian gerbils. *Behavioural and Neural Biology*, **28**, 183–192

Holman, S.D. and Seale, W.T.C. (1991) Ontogeny of sexually dimorphic ultrasonic vocalisations in Mongolian gerbils. *Developmental Psychobiology*, **24**, 103–115

Ingle, D. (1981) New methods for analysis of vision in the gerbil. *Behavioural Brain Research*, **3**, 151–173

Jacobs, G. and Deegan II, J.F. (1994) Sensitivity to ultroviolet light in the gerbil (*Meriones unguiculatus*): characteristics and mechanisms. *Vision Research*, **34**, 1433–1441

Jacobs, G. and Nietz, J. (1989) Cone monochromacy and a reversed Purkinje shift in the gerbil. *Experientia*, **45**, 317–319

Jansa, S. and Weksler, M. (2003) Phylogeny of muroid rodents: relationships within and among major lineages as determined by IRBP gene sequences. *Molecular Phylogenetics and Evolution*, **31**, 256–276

Jaworska, N., Dwyer, S.M. and Rusak, B. (2008) repeated neonatal separation results in different neurochemical and behavioural changes in adult male and female Mongolian gerbils. *Pharmacology, Biochemistry and Behavior*, **88**, 533–541

Johnson-Delaney, C.A. (1998) Disease of the urinary system of commonly kept rodents: Diagnosis and treatment. *Seminars in Avian and Exotic Pet Medicine*, **7**, 81–88

Jun, L., Li, S.J., Amin, O.M. *et al.* (1993) Blood-feeding of the gerbil flea *Nosopsyllus laeviceps kuzenkovi* (Yagubyants), vector of plague in Inner Mongolia, China. *Medical and Veterinary Entomology*, **7**, 54–58

Joint Working Group on Refinement (1993) Removal of blood from laboratory mammals and birds. First Report of the BVA/FRAME/RSPCA/UFAW Joint Working Group on Refinement. *Laboratory Animals*, **27**, 1–22

Kakol Palm, D. and Hollaender, P. (2007) A procedure for intravenous injection using external jugular vein in Mongolian gerbil (*Meriones unguiculatus*). *Laboratory Animals*, **41**, 403–405

Kanarek, R.B., Ogilby J.D. and Mayer, J. (1977) Effects of dietary caloric density on feeding behavior in Mongolian gerbils (*Meriones unguiculatus*). *Physiology & Behavior*, **19**, 497–501

Kaplan, H. (1975) What triggers seizures in the gerbil, *Meriones unguiculatus*? *Life Sciences*, **17**, 693–698

Kaplan, H. and Miezejes, C. (1972) Development of seizures in Mongolian gerbils (*Meriones unguiculatus*). *Journal of Comparative and Physiological Psychology*, **81**, 267–269

Kelly, J. and Potash, M. (1986) Directional Responses to sounds in young gerbils (*Meriones unguiculatus*). *Journal of Comparative Psychology*, **100**, 37–45

Kort, W.J., Hekking-Weijma, J.M., TenKate, M.T. *et al.* (1998) A microchip implant system as a method to determine body temperature of terminally ill rats and mice. *Laboratory Animals*, **32**, 260–269

Kupferberg, H. (2001) Animal models used in the screening of antiepileptic drugs. *Epilepsia*, **42**, 7–12

Laboratory Animal Science Association (2005) Guidance on the transport of laboratory animals. Report of the Transport Working Group established by the LASA. *Laboratory Animals*, **39**, 1–39

Laidley, D., Colbourne, F. and Corbett, D. (2005) Increased behavioral and histological variability arising from changes in cerebrovascular anatomy of the Mongolian gerbil. *Current Neurovascular Research*, **2**, 410–407

Leach, M., Raj, M. and Morton, D. (2005) Aversiveness of carbon dioxide. *Laboratory Animals*, **39**, 452–453

Leclercq, G.C. and Rozenfeld, F.M. (2001) A permanent marking method to identify individual small rodents from birth to sexual maturity. *Journal of Zoology*, **254**, 203–206

Leiper, B.D. and Robinson, R. (1984) A case of dominance modification in the Mongolian gerbil. *The Journal of Heredity*, **75**, 323

Leiper, B.D. and Robinson, R. (1985) Gray mutant in the Mongolian gerbil. *The Journal of Heredity*, **76**, 473

Leiper, B.D. and Robinson, R. (1986) Linkage of albino and pink-eyed dilution genes in the Mongolian gerbil and other rodents. *The Journal of Heredity*, **77**, 207

Leont'ev, A. N. (1954) K. ekologii kogtistoi, peschanki v Buryat Mongol'skoi (Ecology of the clawed gerbil in Buryat Mongolia). *Izvestiya Irkutskogo osudarstvennyi nauchno-issledovatel'skogo protivochumnogo instituta Sibiri ii Dal'nogo Vostoka*, **12**, 137–149

Lerwill, C.J. (1974) Activity rhythms of Golden hamsters (*Mesocricetus auratus*) and Mongolian gerbils (*Meriones unguiculatus*) by direct observation. *Journal of Zoology*, **174**, 520–523

Lerwill, C.J. (1978) Ultrasound in the Mongolian gerbil, *Meriones unguiculatus*. *Journal of Zoology*, **185**, 263–266

Liu, W., Wan, X. and Zhong, W. (2007) Population dynamics of the Mongolian gerbils: Seasonal patterns and interactions among density, reproduction and climate. *Journal of Arid Environments*, **68**, 383–397

Loskota, W.J. and Lomax, P. (1974) Mongolian gerbil as an animal-model for study of epilepsies – anticonvulsant screening. *Proceedings of the Western Pharmacology Society*, **17**, 40–45

Loskota, W.J. and Lomax, P. (1975) Mongolian gerbil (*Meriones unguiculatus*) as a model for study of epilepsies – EEG records of seizures. *Electroencephalography and Clinical Neurophysiology*, **38**, 597–604

Loskota, W.J., Lomax, P. and Rich, T.S. (1972) Gerbil as a model for study of epilepsy – seizure habituation and seizure patterns. *Proceedings of the Western Pharmacology Society*, **15**, 189–195

Loskota, W.J., Lomax, P. and Rich, T.S. (1974a) Gerbil as a model for study of epilepsies – seizure patterns and ontogenesis. *Epilepsia*, **15**, 109–119

Loskota, W.J., Lomax, P. and Verity, M.A. (1974b) *A Stereotaxic Atlas of the Mongolian Gerbil Brain (Meriones unguiculatus)*. Ann Arbor Science, Ann Arbor, Michigan

Maier, J.K. and Klump, G.M. (2006) Resolution in azimuth sound localization in the Mongolian gerbil (*Meriones unguiculatus*). *Journal of the Acoustical Society of America*, **119**, 1029–1036

Marston, J.H. and Chang, M.C. (1965) The breeding, management and reproductive physiology of the Mongolian gerbil (*Meriones unguiculatus*). *Laboratory Animal Care*, **15**, 34–48

Matsuoka, K. and Suzuki, J. (1995) Spontaneous tumors in the Mongolian gerbil (*Meriones unguiculatus*). *Experimental Animals*, **43**, 755–760

Matsuzaki, T., Yasuda, Y. and Nonaka, S. (1989) The genetics of coat colors in the Mongolian gerbil (*Meriones unguiculatus*). *Experimental Animals*, **38**, 337–341

McManus, J.J. (1972a) Water relations and food consumption of the Mongolian gerbil, *Meriones unguiculatus*. *Comparative Biochemistry and Physiology*, **43**, 959–967

McManus, J.J. (1972b) Early postnatal growth and development of temperature regulation in Mongolian gerbils, *Meriones unguiculatus*. *Journal of Mammalogy*, **51**, 782

Michaux, J., Reyes, A. and Catzeflis, F. (2001) Evolutionary history of the most species mammals: molecular phylogeny of muroid rodents. *Molecular Biology and Evolution*, **18**, 2017–2031

Milne-Edwards, A. (1867) Sur quelques mammifières du nord de la chine: *Gerbillus unguiculatus*. *Annales des Science Naturelles (Zoologie)*, **7**, 375–377

Moons, C.P.H., Hermans, K., Remie, R. *et al.* (2007) Intraperitoneal versus subcutaneous telemetry devices in young Mongolian gerbils (*Meriones unguiculatus*). *Laboratory Animals*, **41**, 262–269

Naumov, N.P. and Lobachev, S.V. (1975) Ecology of the desert rodents of the USSR (Jerboas and Gerbils) In: *Rodents in Desert Environments*. Eds Prakash, I. and Gosh, P.K., pp. 529–536. Dr.W.Junk b.v. Publishers, The Hague

Neumann, K., Maak, S., Stuermer, I.W. *et al.* (2001) Low microsatellite variation in laboratory gerbils. *Journal of Heredity*, **92**, 71–74

Newsom, D.M., Bolgos, G.L., Colby, L. *et al.* (2004) Comparison of body surface temperature measurement and conventional methods for measuring temperature in the mouse. *Contemporary Topics in Laboratory Animal Science*, **43**, 13–18

Norris, M.L. (1981) Portable anaesthetic apparatus designed to induce and maintain surgical anaesthesia by methoxyflurane inhalation in the Mongolian gerbil (*Meriones unguiculatus*). *Laboratory Animals*, **15**, 153–155

Norris, M.L. (1985) Disruption of pair bonding induces pregnancy failure in newly mated Mongolian gerbils (*Meriones unguiculatus*). *Journal of Reproduction and Fertility*, **75**, 43–47

Norris, M.L. (1987) Gerbils. In: *The UFAW Handbook on the Care and Management of Laboratory Animals*, 6th edn. Ed. Poole, T., pp. 360–376. Longman, Scientific & Technical, Harlow

Norris, M.L. and Adams, C.E. (1972) Aggressive behaviour and reproduction in the Mongolian gerbil, *Meriones unguiculatus*, relative to age and sexual experience at pairing. *Journal of Reproduction and Fertility*, **31**, 447–450

Norris, M.L. and Adams, C.E. (1974) Sexual development in the Mongolian gerbil (*Meriones unguiculatus*), with particular reference to the ovary. *Journal of Reproduction and Fertility*, **36**, 245–248

Norris, M.L. and Adams, C.E. (1979a) Extroceptive factors and pregnancy block in the Mongolian gerbil, *Meriones unguiculatus*. *Journal of Reproduction and Fertility*, **57**, 401–404

Norris, M.L. and Adams, C.E. (1979b) Vaginal opening in the Mongolian gerbil, *Meriones unguiculatus*: normal data and the influence of social factors. *Laboratory Animals*, **13**, 159–162

Norris, M.L. and Adams, C.E. (1981a) Pregnancy concurrent with lactation in the Mongolian gerbils (*Meriones unguiculatus*). *Laboratory Animals*, **15**, 21–23

Norris, M.L. and Adams, C.E. (1981b) Mating post partem and length of gestation in the Mongolian gerbil (*Meriones unguiculatus*). *Laboratory Animals*, **15**, 189–191

Norris, M.L. and Adams, C.E. (1982) Lifetime reproductive performance of Mongolian gerbils (*Meriones unguiculatus*) with 1 or 2 ovaries. *Laboratory Animals*, **16**, 146–150

Norris, M.L. and Adams, C.E. (1986) Embryo transfer to Mongolian gerbils during post partum pregnancy and pseudopregnancy. *Animal Reproduction Science*, **11**, 63–67

Ostermeyer, M.C. and Elwood, R.W. (1984) Helpers(?) at the nest in the Mongolian gerbil, *Meriones unguiculatus*. *Behaviour*, **91**, 61–77

Palinov, I. (2001) Current concepts of Gerbillid phylogeny and classification. In: *African Small Mammals*, Proceedings of the 8th International Symposium on African Small Mammals, Paris, 1999. Eds Denys, C., Granjon, L. and Poulet, A., pp. 141–149. Institute de Recherche pour le Dévelopment, Paris

Payman, B.C. and Swanson, H.H. (1980) Social influence on sexual maturation and breeding in the female Mongolian gerbil (*Meriones unguculatus*). *Animal Behaviour*, **28**, 528–535

Peckham, J.C., Cole, J.R., Chapman, W.L. *et al.* (1974) Staphylococcal dermatitis in Mongolian gerbils (*Meriones unguiculatus*). *Laboratory Animal Science*, **24**, 43–47

Pendergrass, M. and Thiessen, D.D. (1983) Sandbathing is thermoregulatory in the Mongolian gerbil, *Meriones unguiculatus*. *Behavioural and Neural Biology*, **37**, 125–133

Pérez-García, C.C., Peña-Penabad, M., Cano-Rábano, M.J. *et al.* (2003) A simple procedure to perform intravenous injections in the Mongolian gerbil (*Meriones unguiculatus*). *Laboratory Animals*, **37**, 68–71

Piovanotti Arua, M.R. and Vieira, L.M. (2004) Presence of the father and parental experience have differentiated effects on pup development in Mongolian gerbils (*Meriones unguiculatus*). *Behavioural Processes*, **66**, 107–117

Prates, E.J. and Guerra, R.F. (2005) Parental care and sexual interactions in Mongolian gerbils (*Meriones unguiculatus*) during the postpartum estrus. *Behavioural Processes*, **70**, 104–112

Raffel, M. and König, B. (1999) Influence of body weight on reproduction in female house mice (*Mus domesticus*). *Zoology*, **102** (Supplement II), 33

Raflo, C.P. and Diamond, S.S. (1980) Metastatic squamous-cell carcinoma in a gerbil (*Meriones unguiculatus*). *Laboratory Animals*, **14**, 237–239

Randall, J.A. and Thiessen, D.D. (1980) Seasonal activity and thermoregulation in *Meriones unguiculatus* – a gerbil's choice. *Behavioural Ecology and Sociobiology*, **7**, 267–272

Rassin, D.K., Sturman, J.A. and Gaull, G.E. (1978) Taurine and other free amino acids in milk of man and other mammals. *Early Human Development*, **2**, 1–13

Refinetti, R. (2006) Variability in diurnality in laboratory rodents. *Journal of Comparative Physiology*, **192**, 701–714

Rich, S.T. (1968) The Mongolian gerbil (*Meriones unguiculatus*) in research. *Laboratory Animal Care*, **18**, 235–243

Rohrbach, C. (1982) Investigation of the Bruce Effect in the Mongolian gerbil (*Meriones unguiculatus*). *Journal of Reproduction and Fertility*, **65**, 411–417

Roper, T.J. and Polioudakis, E. (1977) The behaviour of Mongolian gerbils in a semi-natural environment, with special reference to ventral marking, dominance and sociability. *Behaviour*, **61**, 205–237

Ryan, A. (1976) Hearing sensitivity of the Mongolian gerbil, *Meriones unguiculatis*. *Journal of the Acoustical Society of America*, **59**, 1222–1226

Salo, A.A. and French, J.A. (1989) Early experience, reproductive success, and development of parental behaviour in Mongolian gerbils. *Animal Behaviour*, **38**, 693–702

Saltzman, W., Ahmeda, S. Fahimi, A. *et al.* (2006) Social suppression of female reproductive maturation and infanticidal behavior in cooperatively breeding Mongolian gerbils. *Hormones and Behavior*, **49**, 527–537

Scheibler, E., Weinandy, R. and Gattermann, R. (2004) Social categories in families of Mongolian gerbils. *Physiology & Behavior*, **81**, 455–464

Scheibler, E., Weinandy, R. and Gattermann, R. (2005a) Social factors affecting litters in families of Mongolian gerbils, *Meriones unguiculatus*. *Folia Zoologica*, **54**, 61–68

Scheibler, E., Weinandy, R. and Gattermann, R. (2005b) Intra-family aggression and offspring expulsion in Mongolian gerbils (*Meriones unguiculatus*) under restricted environments. *Mammalian Biology – Zeitschrift fur Säugetierkunde*, **70**, 137–146

Scheibler, E., Weinandy, R. and Gattermann, R. (2006a) Male expulsion in cooperative Mongolian gerbils (*Meriones unguiculatus*). *Physiology & Behavior*, **87**, 24–30

Scheibler, E., Liu, W., Weinandy, R. *et al.* (2006b) Burrow systems of the Mongolian gerbil (*Meriones unguiculatus* Milne Edwards, 1867). *Mammalian Biology – Zeitschrift fur Säugetierkunde*, **71**, 178–182

Schmook, M. (2004) Ursachen stereotypen Verhaltens der Mongolischen Wüstenrennmaus (*Meriones unguiculatus*). Unpublished PhD Thesis (German), Institut für Tierschutz und Verhalten (Heim-, Labortiere und Pferde), Tierärztliche Hochschule, Hannover. http://elib.tiho-hannover.de/dissertations/schmoockm_ws04.pdf

Sherwin, C.M. (1998) Voluntary wheel running: a review and novel interpretation. *Animal Behaviour*, **56**, 11–27

Shimozuru, M., Kikusui, T., Takeuchi, Y. *et al.* (2006a) Scent-marking and sexual activity may reflect social hierarchy among group-living male Mongolian gerbils (*Meriones unguiculatus*). *Physiology & Behavior*, **89**, 644–649

Shimozuru, M., Kikusui, T., Takeuchi, Y. *et al.* (2006b) Social-defeat stress suppresses scent-marking and social-approach behaviors in male Mongolian gerbils (*Meriones unguiculatus*). *Physiology & Behavior*, **88**, 620–627

Solomon, N.G. and Getz, L.L. (1996) Examination of alternative hypotheses for cooperative breeding in rodents. In: *Cooperative Breeding in Mammals*. Eds Solomon, N.G. and French, J.A., pp. 199–230. Cambridge University Press, Cambridge

Starkey, N.J. and Hendrie, C.A. (1997) Parallels between pairbond disruption in gerbils and human depression. *Behavioural Pharmacology*, **8**, 663–664

Starkey, N.J. and Hendrie, D.C. (1998a) Importance of gender for the display of social impairment in pairbond disrupted gerbils. *Neuroscience & Biobehavioral Reviews*, **23**, 273–277

Starkey, N.J. and Hendrie, C.A. (1998b) Disruption of pairs produces pair-bond disruption in male but not female Mongolian gerbils. *Physiology & Behavior*, **65**, 497–503

Starkey, N.J., Normington, G. and Bridges, N.J. (2007) The effects of individual housing on 'anxious' behaviour in male and female gerbils. *Physiology & Behavior*, **90**, 545–552

Steppan, S., Adkins, R.M. and Anderson, J. (2004) Phylogeny and divergence-date estimates of rapid radiations in muroid rodents based on multiple nuclear genes. *Systematic Biology*, **53**, 533–553

Stuermer, I.W. (1998) Reproduction and developmental differences in offspring of domesticated and wild Mongolian gerbils (*Meriones unguiculatus*). *Mammalian Biology – Zeitschrift für Säugetierkunde*, **63**, 57–58

Stuermer, I.W., Kluge, R., Nebendahl, K. *et al.* (1998) Genetic base and successful breeding of wild gerbils (*Meriones unguiculatus*) captured during an expedition to Outer Mongolia in 1995. *Mammalian Biology – Zeitschrift für Säugetierkunde*, **63**, 58–59

Stuermer, W.I., Plotz, K., Leybold, A. *et al.* (2003) Intraspecific allometric comparison of laboratory gerbils with Mongolian gerbils trapped in the wild Indicates domestication in *Meriones unguiculatus* (Milne-Edwards, 1867) (Rodentia: Gerbillinae). *Zoologischer Anzeiger – A Journal of Comparative Zoology*, **242**, 249–266

Stuermer, I.W., Tittmann, C., Schilling, C. *et al.* (2006) Reproduction of wild gerbils bred in the laboratory in dependence on generation and season: I. Morphological changes and fertility. *Animal Science*, **82**, 377–387

Stuermer, I.W. and Wetzel, W. (2006) Early experience and domestication affect auditory discrimination learning, open field behaviour and brain size in wild Mongolian gerbils and domesticated Laboratory gerbils (*Meriones unguiculatus forma domestica*). *Behavioural Brain Research*, **173**, 11–21

Susic, V. and Masirevic, G. (1986) Sleep patterns in the Mongolian gerbil, *Meriones unguiculatus*. *Physiology & Behavior*, **37**, 257–261

Swanson, H.H. & Lockley, R.M. (1977) Population growth and social structure of confined colonies of Mongolian gerbils: scent gland size and marking behaviour as indices of social status. *Aggressive Behaviour*, **4**, 57–89

Swanson, H.H. (1980) The 'hairless' gerbil: a new mutant. *Laboratory Animals*, **14**, 143–147

Tang Halpin, Z. (1975) The role of individual recognition by odours in the social interactions of the Mongolian gerbil (*Meriones unguiculatus*). *Behaviour*, **58**, 117–129

Thiessen, D., Graham, M. and Davenport, R. (1978) Ultrasonic signaling in the gerbil (*Meriones unguicululatus*): social interaction and olfactation. *Journal of Comparative Physiology and Psychology*, **92**, 1041–1049

Thiessen, D.D. and Maxwell, K.O. (1979) Glass rodent enclosure – gerbil city. *Behavior Research Methods and Instrumentation*, **11**, 535–537

Thiessen, D.D. and Yahr, P. (1977) *The Gerbil in Behavioural Investigations*. University of Texas Press, Austin, Texas

Toth, L.A. (1997) The moribund state as an experimental endpoint. *Contemporary Topics in Laboratory Animal Science*, **36**, 44–48

Toth, L.A. (2000) Defining the moribund condition as an experimental endpoint for animal research. *ILAR Journal*, **41** http://dels.nas.edu/ilar_n/ilarjournal/41_2/

Tsurim, I. and Abramsky, Z. (2004) The effect of travel costs on food hoarding in gerbils. *Journal of Mammology*, **85**, 67–71

Tumblebrook Farm Inc (1979) Physiological parameters and selected general data. *The Gerbil Digest*, **6**(2)

Tumblebrook Farm Inc (1980) The gerbil as a stroke model. *The Gerbil Digest*, **7**(2)

Tumblebrook Farm Inc (1985) The gerbil stroke model: an update. *The Gerbil Digest*, **11**(1)

Valsecchi, P., Choleris, E., Moles, A. *et al.* (1996) Kinship and familiarity as factors affecting social transfer of food preferences in adult mongolian gerbils (*Meriones unguiculatus*). *Journal of Comparative Psychology*, **110**, 243–251

Valsecchi, P., Razzoli, M. and Choleris E. (2002) Influence of kinship and familiarity on the social and reproductive behaviour of female Mongolian gerbils. *Ethology, Ecology and Evolution*, **14**, 239–253

Vandenberg, J. (1993) And brother begat nephew. *Nature*, **364**, 671–672

Waiblinger, E. and König, B. (2001) Housing and husbandry affect stereotypic behaviour in laboratory gerbils. *3R-Info-Bulletin 16 and Alternatives to Animal Experiments*, Special Issue 07, 67–69. http://www.forschung3r.ch/de/publications/bu16.html or http://www.altex.ch/resources/AltexSupl067069.pdf

Waiblinger, E. (2002) Comfortable quarters for gerbils in research institutions. In: *Comfortable Quarters for Laboratory Animals*. Eds Reinhardt, V. and Reinhardt, A. Animal Welfare Institute, Washington D.C. http://www.awionline.org/pubs/cq02/Cq-gerb.html

Waiblinger, E. (2003) *Stereotypic behaviours in laboratory gerbils: Causes and solutions*. PhD Thesis, Department of Animal Behaviour, Zoology Institute, University of Zurich.

Waiblinger, E. and König, B. (2004) Refinement of gerbil housing and husbandry in the laboratory. *Animal Welfare*, **13**, S229–235

Wallace, P., Owen, K. and Thiessen, D.D. (1973) The control and function of maternal scent marking in the Mongolian gerbil. *Physiology & Behavior*, **10**, 463–466

Wang, G. and Zhong, W. (2006) Mongolian gerbils and Daurian pikas responded differently to changes in precipitation in the Inner Mongolian grasslands. *Journal of Arid Environments*, **66**, 648–656

Wang, D.H., Pei, Y.X., Yang, J.C. *et al.* (2003) Digestive tract morphology and food habits in six species of rodents. *Folia Zoologica*, **52**, 51–55

Waring, A.D. and Perper, T. (1980) Parental behaviour in Mongolian gerbils (*Meriones unguiculatus*) II. Parental interactions. *Animal Behaviour*, **28**, 331–340

Waring, A.D. & Poole, T.W. (1980) Genetic analysis of the black pigment mutation in the Mongolian gerbil. *The Journal of Heredity*, **71**, 428–429

Waring, A.D., Poole, T.W. and Perper, T. (1978) White spotting in the Mongolian gerbil. *The Journal of Heredity*, **69**, 347–349

Weinandy, R. (1995) *Untersuchungen zur Chronobiologie, Ethologie und zu Stressreaktionen der Mongolischen Wüstenrennmaus, Meriones unguiculatus*. PhD-Thesis (German), Zoologisches Institut, Martin Luther-Universität Halle-Wittenberg

Weinandy, R., Hofmann, S. and Gattermann, R. (2001) Mating behaviour during the estrous cycle in Mongolian gerbils (*Meriones unguiculatus*). *Mammalian Biology*, **66**, 116–120

Weinandy, R., Hofmann, S. and Gattermann, R. (2002) The oestrus of female gerbils, *Meriones unguiculatus*, is indicated by locomotor activity and influenced by male presence. *Folia Zoologica*, **51**, 145–155

Weinandy, R. and Gattermann, R. (1997) Time of day and stress response to different stressors in experimental animals. 2. Mongolian gerbil (*Meriones unguiculatus* Milne Edwards, 1867). *Journal of Experimental Animal Science*, **38**, 109–122

Weinert, D., Weinandy, R. and Gattermann, R. (2007) Photic and non-photic effects on the daily activity pattern of Mongolian gerbils. *Physiology & Behavior*, **90**, 325–333

Wiedenmayer, C. (1995) *The ontogeny of stereotypies in gerbils. PhD-Thesis (partly in German)*, Zoologisches Institut, Universität Zürich

Wiedenmayer, C. (1996) Effects of cage size on the ontogeny of stereotyped behaviour in gerbils. *Applied Animal Behaviour Science*, **47**, 225–233

Wiedenmayer, C. (1997a) Causation of the ontogenetic development of stereotypic digging in gerbils. *Animal Behaviour*, **53**, 461–470

Wiedenmayer, C. (1997b) Stereotypies resulting from a deviation in the ontogenetic development of gerbils. *Behavioural Processes*, **39**, 215–221

Wiedenmayer, C. (1997c) The early ontogeny of bar-gnawing in laboratory gerbils. *Animal Welfare*, **6**, 273–277

Wilkinson, F. (1983) The development of visual acuity in the Mongolian gerbil (*Meriones unguiculatus*). *Behavioural Brain Research*, **13**, 83–94

Winterfeld, K.T., Teucert-Noodt, G. and Dawirs, R.R. (1998) Social environment alters both ontogeny of dopamine innervation of the medial prefrontal cortex and maturation of working memory in gerbils (*Meriones unguiculatus*). *Journal of Neuroscience Research*, **52**, 201–209

Wong, R., Gray-Allan, P., Chiba, C. *et al.* (1990) Social preference of female gerbils (*Meriones unguiculatus*) as influenced by coat color of males. *Behavioural and Neural Biology*, **54**, 184–190

Woolf, N.K. and Ryan, A.F. (1984) The development of auditory function in the cochlea of the Mongolian gerbil. *Hearing Research*, **13**, 277–283

Würbel, H. (2006) The motivational basis of caged rodents' stereotypies. In: *Stereotypic Animal Behaviour*. Eds Mason, G. and Rushen, J., pp. 86–120. CAB International, Wallingford

Yahr, P. (1977) Social subordination and scent-marking in male Mongolian gerbils (*Meriones unguiculatus*). *Animal Behaviour*, **25**, 292–297

Yahr, P. and Anderson-Mitchell, K. (1983) Attraction of gerbil pups to maternal nest odours: duration, soecificity and ovarian control. *Physiology & Behavior*, **31**, 241–247

Yamaguchi, H., Kikusui, T., Takeuchi, Y. *et al.* (2005) Social stress decreases marking behavior independently of testosterone in Mongolian gerbils. *Hormones & Behavior*, **47**, 549–555

Zeller, W., Weber, H., Panoussis, B. *et al.* (1998) Refinement of blood sampling from the sublingual vein of rats. *Laboratory Animals*, **32**, 369–376

Zhang, Z. and Wang, D. (2007) Seasonal changes in thermogenesis and body mass in wild Mongolian gerbils (*Meriones unguiculatus*). *Comparative Biochemistry and Physiology – Part A. Molecular & Integrative Physiology*, **148**, 346–353

van Zutphen, L.F.M., Baumans, V. and Beynen, A.C. (2001) *Principles of Laboratory Animal Science, Revised Edition: A Contribution to the Humane Use and Care of Animals and to the Quality of Experimental Results*, 2nd edn. Elsevier Health Sciences, Amsterdam

24 The Syrian hamster

David Whittaker

Biological overview

Taxonomy

Hamsters as a group can be described as stout-bodied, stubby-tailed, broad-headed, cheek-pouched, burrowing and nest building rodents. Some taxonomists (Nowak & Paradiso 1983) place hamsters in the family Muridae, whilst others (Corbet & Hill 1980; Honachi *et al.* 1982) retain them in the family of Cricetidae to which they were assigned in 1946 (Van Hoosier & McPherson 1987).

The most commonly used species in the laboratory is the Syrian hamster (*Mesocricetus auratus*), known also as the Golden Hamster. The Chinese (*Cricetus griseus*), Djungarian, or Russian (*Phodopus sungorus sungorus*), or Russian Dwarf and European hamsters (*Cricetus cricetus*) are less often used in research. For this reason, the remainder of the chapter relates to the Syrian hamster, unless otherwise indicated. A fuller account of the taxonomy of Cricetidae can be found in Van Hoosier and McPherson (1987) along with a tabulated classification scheme for 24 species in the family. Those using hamsters in research should be aware that accurate identification of the species used is essential for correct reproducibility of work and interpretation of results.

Comparative anatomy and physiology

Species within the various hamster genera vary in body size. Hamsters in the genus *Cricetus* are the largest, *Mesocricetus* are medium sized whilst *Phodopus* are dwarf, mouse-like animals. Typically, adult Syrian hamsters reach weights of 150–180 g, Chinese hamsters 120–150 g and Djungarian 100–130 g. Larger European hamsters may reach 400–500 g.

Hamsters generally have shorter lifespans than rats and mice routinely used for long-term studies; Bernfeld *et al.* (1986) provide data from over 600 control F1 hybrid Syrian hamsters. There are also marked sex and strain differences, with males tending to live longer than females. Most reports of longevity record deaths from 1 year onwards with only 50% or less survival at 2 years. Hamsters rarely survive beyond 3 years, this age being more typically reached by Chinese rather than Syrian hamsters.

Adult females (Syrian) are larger than males, and Syrian hamsters have abundant, loose skin. Both sexes possess paired, bilateral scent or flank glands, consisting of sebaceous glands, pigment cells and terminal hair. These glands are most prominent in the male, but are poorly developed in females.

The hamster's dental formula is: $I^1_1C^0_0Pm^0_0M^3_3$. They have only one set of teeth (monophyodont) and the cheek teeth are roughly quadrate and low crowned and (bunodont and brachyodont). Such teeth are characteristic of animals that have a diverse diet. The incisors are open-rooted while the molars are rooted. Primary eruption is regular. Some but not all genera possess buccal pouches extending dorso-laterally from the oral cavity on either side of the shoulder region. These structures are used experimentally as immunologically privileged sites. Hamster stomachs are divided into non-glandular and glandular segments separated by a muscular sphincter.

A detailed account of anatomy, physiology, haematology and clinical chemistry is available in Van Hoosier and McPherson (1987).

Behaviour

Syrian hamsters are terrestrial, burrow-digging rodents. Their natural habitat is dry, rocky plains or lightly vegetated slopes. They build nests within their burrows. Although primarily grain eaters, they will also eat green plant shoots and roots, insects and fruit. In the wild, adults generally inhabit lone burrows (Van Hoosier & McPherson 1987).

Some species of hamsters hibernate under certain environmental conditions. Although this is of research interest it is not an important feature with respect to their husbandry in most laboratory situations. Hibernation can be induced in hamsters by a number of environmental stimuli including low temperature, short days, solitude, nesting material and adequate food stores. Aspects of behaviour which are of importance for their husbandry include their solitary nature, propensity to burrow and nest build and their nocturnal lifestyle. These are important factors in considering their housing and husbandry.

Uses in the laboratory

Syrian hamsters have a number of unusual and unique features which make them particularly useful for certain experimental studies. The Syrian hamster has immuno-genetic characteristics that underlie marked tolerance to homologous, heterologous and human tumours, parasites, viruses and bacteria. Moreover, the presence of reversible cheek pouches, which in the Syrian hamster appear to be immunologically privileged, allow tumour grafts from other species, including man, to grow freely and symmetrically without the need to induce immunosuppression.

The Syrian hamster has also been used for dental research as the form and occlusion of their molar teeth closely resemble those of humans and the induction of lesions is possible without fracturing of the teeth, as in rats. Other areas of use include teratology and the short gestation period is advantageous for inhalation studies. The Syrian hamster has been used in thermophysiology and circadian rhythm studies. Chijioke *et al.* (1990) described the use of the Syrian hamster oocyte in assessing human spermatozoal fertilising potential. They concluded it was a relatively precise method of quantifying the effects of various factors affecting human sperm function *in vivo*. Further detailed consideration of experimental biology in all hamster species can be found in Van Hoosier and McPherson (1987).

Laboratory management and breeding

General husbandry

Housing and caging

For routine purposes, cages and equipment designed for rats can be used for housing Syrian, Chinese and Djungarian hamsters. European hamsters require more space and stronger cages due to their size and aggressiveness towards each other. Table 24.1 sets out the space requirements for Syrian hamsters according to the revised Appendix A (adopted June 2007) of the Council of Europe Convention, ETS/123 (Council of Europe 2006) and the European Directive 86/609 (European Commission 2007). Table 24.2 sets out the space requirements for Syrian hamsters according to the US Guide for the Care and Use of Laboratory Animals published by the National Research Council (1996).

The differences between these guidelines illustrate the more general point that it is difficult to specify scientifically the minimal sizes of cages for maintenance. However the European guidelines took note of research indicating that hamsters were chronically stressed when housed in small enclosures, a condition likely to affect their welfare and the quality of science obtained from these animals (Kuhnen 1999a, 1999b).

While sufficient space is needed to allow appropriate enrichment and to give the animals some control over social interactions, other aspects of housing such as material of construction, floor type, provision of furniture and bedding, as well as appropriate social enrichment are equally important. Arnold and Estep (1994) explored the caging preferences of Syrian hamsters. Whilst their research showed that most Syrian hamsters preferred solid floors with bedding, they also demonstrated that previous housing conditions can affect cage preference and behaviour. Further information on environmental enrichment for Syrian hamsters can be found *Comfortable Quarters for Laboratory Animals* (Reinhardt & Reinhardt 2002) and see Chapter 10.

The Syrian hamster does not conform to the generalisation concerning other hamsters that males are more aggressive than females. Both sexes are highly aggressive, making group housing for welfare or experimental purposes problematic. Grelk *et al.* (1974) investigated the influence of caging conditions and hormone treatments on fighting in male and female Syrian hamsters. They found that sex, hormonal state and caging condition interact in a complex manner. Arnold and Estep (1994) explored the effects of housing on social preference and behaviour in male Syrian hamsters. Their results showed that they spent more time in social proximity than out of proximity, especially if they had prior group-housing experience. In addition, singly housed animals showed more aggressive behaviour with conspecifics and lower weight gains than group-housed animals, which showed more evidence of wounding. They concluded that early housing experience can profoundly affect later social preference and behaviour.

In summary, solid-bottomed cages with bedding material are preferable and in general group housing may be preferable to individual caging so long as the groups are formed early in life and are stable and harmonious. Where this is not possible it is better to single house animals, either from the start of the study or, immediately upon arrival, if purchased from a commercial breeder. When group housing, there should be room for hiding or escaping from cage-mates.

Environmental conditions

Conditions suitable for maintaining rats and mice are also suitable for Syrian hamsters. Generally, seasonal variability in the Syrian hamster can be reduced by the provision of a constant temperature of 21–22 °C and a minimum of 14 h light. Such conditions will eliminate hibernation. Extraneous

Table 24.1 Minimum enclosure dimensions and space allowances for Syrian Hamsters according to Appendix A of the Council of Europe Convention, ETS/123 (Council of Europe 2006) and the European Directive 86/609 (European Commission 2007). Reproduced with permission of FELASA.

	Body weight (g)	*Minimum enclosure size (cm²)*	*Floor area/ animal (cm²)*	*Minimum enclosure height (cm)*
In stock and during procedures	Up to 60	800	150	14
	Over 60–100	800	200	14
	Over 100	800	250	14
Breeding		800 monogamous pair with litter		14
Stock at breeders	Less than 60	1500	100	14

Table 24.2 Minimum enclosure dimensions and space allowances for Syrian Hamsters according to the US Guide for the Care and Use of Laboratory Animals (National Research Council 1996)*.

Weight (g)	*Floor area/animal (cm²)*	*Cage height (cm)*
Less than 60	65	15
Up to 80	84	15
Up to 100	103	15
Over 100	123	15

*Dimensions in Table 24.2 are to the nearest whole number as US measurements are in inches.

noise should be kept to a minimum, consideration being given to sources of ultrasound. Excessive deviance from the normal environmental parameters should always be avoided if at all possible, especially in breeding colonies when it may contribute to lowered breeding efficiency and maternal cannibalism.

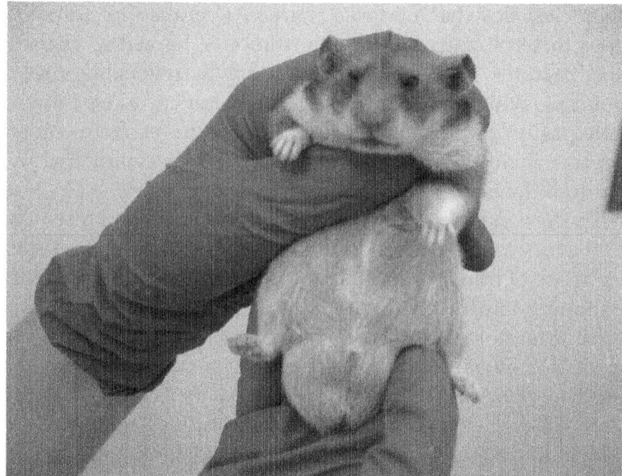

Figure 24.1 Male Syrian hamster.

Identification and sexing

The marking of individual animals (other than by using microchips) should be avoided wherever possible as no completely satisfactory method has been developed. Ear punching can be performed as in other rodents and the ears of animals without dark pigmentation can be tattooed using a fine electric vibrating tattooing machine. Microchip implants have now become the preferred method for identifying many species of animals, including Syrian hamsters. Whilst they have the distinct advantage of being a reasonably permanent means of identification, microchip implants do have some disadvantages including cost, subcutaneous migration, chip failure etc. Although the author can find no specific reference to the use of microchips in hamsters, Ball *et al.* (1991) evaluated their use in rats over a 1 year implantation period and Mrozek *et al.* (1995) evaluated the method in rabbits, guinea pigs, woodchucks and amphibians. The author also has personal experience of successfully microchipping hamsters for long-term (2 year) studies.

The gender of mature Syrian, Chinese and Djungarian hamsters can be easily distinguished by the prominent testes of the male, even in pubescent animals, and the greater anogenital distance in the male (Figures 24.1 and 24.2). Sexing the European hamster however, presents some problems during the season when sexual activity ceases – usually October to February. It is difficult to tell the sexes apart at this time as the vulva of the female is closed and the testes of the male are drawn up into the abdominal cavity. At other times the criteria used for sexing other hamster species can be used.

Transport

Transporting hamsters presents no special difficulties as long as plastic materials are used and no leading exposed edges are offered to the animals to chew. As an extra precaution when transporting European hamsters, a lining of fine wire mesh should be incorporated into the manufacture of the box. Boxes used for transporting other rodent species, made of plastic corrugated or sandwich construction with plastic formed lids and incorporating filters over wire mesh panels of an adequate size, provide good insulation whilst being adequately ventilated.

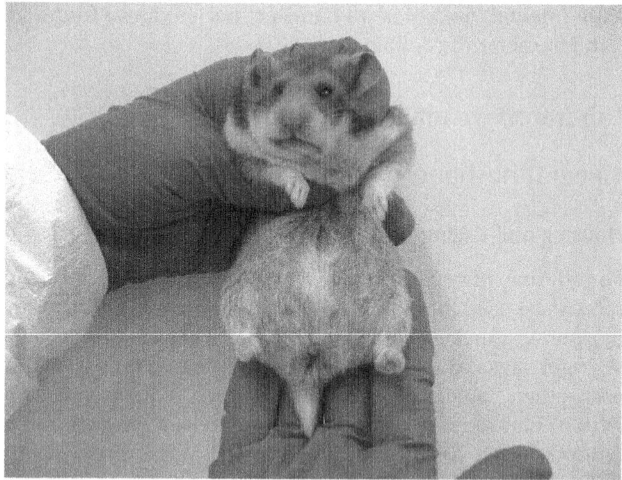

Figure 24.2 Female Syrian hamster.

Table 24.3 gives recommended stocking densities for Syrian hamsters in transit (Laboratory Animal Science Association (LASA) 2005). Optimum stocking densities are provided for non-filtered crates used during winter and for filtered crates travelling during the summer, representing the least and most demanding challenges to adequate ventilation respectively.

Breeding

The influence of parity and litter size on weaning success and offspring sex ratio in Djungarian hamsters has been reported by Lerchl (1995). Table 24.4 presents breeding data for Syrian, Chinese and Djungarian hamsters. This section will concentrate on practical aspects of hamster breeding.

Sexual maturity of the Syrian hamster is reached by 42 days of age or earlier (see later in this section) and can be confirmed using the penile smear technique to look for the presence of sperm on the glans penis. Reproductive ability at a very young age is marked in Syrian hamsters and it is not uncommon to find animals mating by 4 weeks of age. This can lead to husbandry problems with unplanned pregnancies occurring when litters are kept together post-weaning. Maximum reproductive capability is reached in Syrian hamsters by around 8–10 weeks of age for females and 10–12 weeks for males.

The oestrous cycle is regular, lasting 4 days. Two lateral pouches lined with cornified epithelial cells in the vagina of hamsters can make the vaginal cytology method of evaluating the phase of the cycle difficult. External indications of the cycle include the presence of a white, stringy, opaque discharge on the second day of the cycle followed by a waxy secretion on the third day. It is, therefore, possible to determine the day for mating by screening females for the stringy, opaque discharge. This indicates that the female reached peak oestrus the day before and therefore she can be reliably mated on the third day after disappearance of the discharge. Large groups can be selected in this way with up to 90% conception rates.

Female hamsters are relatively aggressive in the presence of unfamiliar males and generally, unless sexually receptive, will not tolerate their presence. However, at peak oestrus the female Syrian hamster tolerates the male's presence and shows lordosis. Shortly afterwards copulation will take place, lasting around 30 minutes.

Using a breeding system in which females are selected in this way, one male can serve a harem of 12 females. This is a common method of breeding Syrian hamsters but is very labour intensive. The hamsters are mated soon after dark, when they are naturally most active. The female is placed in the same cage as the male and the pair observed to ensure mating occurs. Should fighting start, the pair must be immediately separated.

Monogamous pairing of hamsters at weaning is now considered the most satisfactory and labour-efficient method of breeding Syrian hamsters. Provided they are paired at this time they are normally compatible and produce very good results with weaning rates of around 1.4 young/female/week depending upon strain, with litter intervals of around 37 days. Djungarian and Chinese hamsters can also be bred successfully using the monogamous pairing system. In addition to being more efficient, monogamous pairing allows accurate record keeping and allows post-partum mating which can occur in Djungarian, Chinese and golden hamsters. It is however, unusual for conception to take place whilst the female is lactating.

Harem mating has been used for breeding Syrian hamsters but again is labour intensive and can be stressful for

Table 24.3 Minimum floor area/animal (cm^2) for Syrian hamsters during transport. Reproduced from LASA (2005) Guidance on the Transport of Laboratory Animals. Report of the Transport Working Group established by the Laboratory Animal Science Association (LASA) *Lab Animals*, **39**, 1–39, copyright 2005 by permission of The Royal Society of Medicine Press, London.

Weight (g)	**Min. height 15 cm*	***Min. height 15 cm*
30–60	120	96
61–90	160	128
91–120	200	160
>121	240	192

*Floor area/animal in cm^2 when no active temperature control is provided throughout the journey.
**Floor area/animal in cm^2 when active temperature control is provided throughout the journey.

Table 24.4 Reproductive data for Syrian, Chinese and Djungarian hamsters. Reproduced with permission from the National Academies Press, Copyright (1996), National Academy of Sciences.

Character	*Syrian*	*Chinese*	*Djungarian*
Age at puberty	45–60 days	48–100 days	45–60 days
Min. breeding age	50 days	70–84 days	50 days
Breeding season	All year, may be a decrease in winter	All year in laboratory conditions	All year in laboratory conditions
Oestrous cycle	Polyoestrus: all year	Polyoestrus: all year	Polyoestrus: all year
Duration of oestrous cycle	4 days	4 days	4 days
Duration of oestrus	4–23 h	6–8 h	Unknown
Gestation	16 days	21 days	18 days
Average litter size	6	5	3.2
Ovulation time	Early oestrus	Shortly before oestrus	Unknown
Copulation	About 1 h after nightfall	About 1 h after nightfall	Unknown
Implantation	5 or more days	5–6 days	Unknown
Birth weight	2 g	1.5–2.5 g	1.5–2.0g
Weaned	21 days	21 days	18 days
Chromosome no.	44	22	28
Return to oestrus post partum	5–10 mins	Post-partum mating does occur	Post-partum mating does occur
No. of mammae	14–22	8	8

the animals. The usual procedure is to group one to four males with a large number of females and to separate out pregnant animals prior to parturition. Fighting will occur when the female is re-introduced into the harem.

Implantation of the fertilised ovum takes place 6 days post-coitus. It is important that at this time the animal is handled as little as possible. The Syrian hamster has a short gestation period (15.5 days) and the period is generally very regular, varying by only 2 or 3h. Pregnant females should be placed in clean cages with some form of nesting material and bedding approximately 2 days prior to parturition. Enough food should be made available in the cage to last the female 7–10 days so that there is minimal disturbance of the newborn litter. Any interference frequently results in cannibalism. Litter size normally increases with parity.

Newborn hamsters have closed eyes and ears, and are hairless but have teeth. Ears begin to open at 4 days, solids begin to be taken at 7–10 days and eyes open at 14–16 days of age. Water must be available to animals from 10 days of age. Hamsters are normally weaned around 21 days and the female re-mated. Figure 24.3 shows typical growth curves for the Syrian hamster.

The optimal reproductive life of a Syrian hamster is considered to be around 10 months and a significant reduction in reproductive capacity occurs from 1 year of age onwards. During her reproductive lifetime a female hamster will produce four to six litters.

It is commonly thought that cross-fostering is not possible, however Grainger and Plotkin (1987) investigated cross-fostering and maternal care in Syrian hamsters and concluded that it can be successfully undertaken at three different ages – soon after birth, at about 1 week of age and around 2 weeks of age. They found nest quality, survival and pup weights to correlate well. Cross-fostering could prove useful in disease control or eradication. However, the establishment of caesarean-derived, hand-reared hamster colonies has not yet been reported.

Feeding

Natural and laboratory diets

Hamsters are omnivorous and coprophagous and hoard food as a survival strategy in the wild. In the laboratory and intensive breeding situations complete diets of known formulation and quality are advised on both scientific and welfare grounds. Diets specifically formulated for rats and mice are adequate for the maintenance and breeding of hamsters (National Research Council 1978). Providing a good-quality, complete rodent diet is available, nutritional deficiencies are unlikely to occur. Vitamin E deficiency has been described by West and Mason (1958) and Keeler and Young (1979), but in both papers the deficiency was experimentally induced. More recently Mooij *et al.* (1992) described experimentally induced disturbed reproductive performance in extreme folic acid-deficient Syrian hamsters. Further information on hamster nutrition is available from Medical Research Council (1977) and National Research Council (1995).

Water

A fresh, clean, *ad libitum* supply of water must be provided to hamsters either by means of water bottles or through automatic watering devices. The average daily consumption of water by an adult Syrian hamster is 10–20ml depending upon the housing conditions, the type of feed and the hamster's physiological condition (eg, pregnancy, suckling).

Laboratory procedures

Handling

The Syrian hamster can have an unjustified reputation for being difficult to handle but this is usually due to poor or

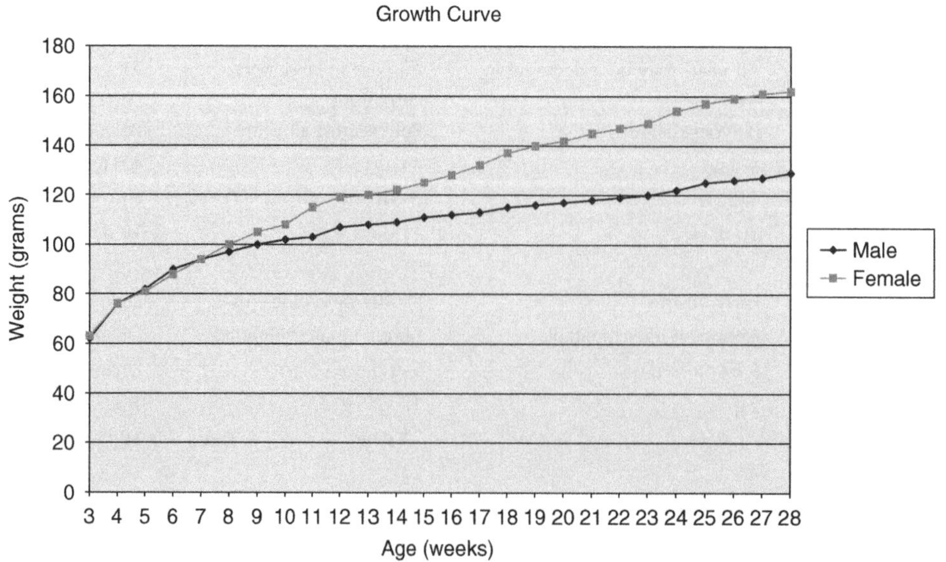

Figure 24.3 Typical growth curves for Syrian hamsters.

intensive husbandry and breeding regimes. For routine handling the Syrian hamster can be picked up by a firm but gentle grasp across the back of the animal. Picking up by placing the thumb across the abdomen enables sexing to be carried out. Turning the animal over so that it lies in the palm of the hand, ventral side up, tends to inactivate most animals and has a quietening effect. This handling technique is illustrated in Figures 24.1 and 24.2. All species of hamsters can be picked up in a similar way but the use of cupped hands is preferred when minimal restraint is required.

For oral dosing, intraperitoneal injections and other manipulations most hamsters can be held by the dorsal skin ensuring that a firm grip is made at the scruff of the neck.

Hamsters can inflict serious bites, especially during the breeding season, so it is recommended that stout protective gloves are worn to handle the European hamster. However, animals may become tamer with frequent handling. When handling hamsters, it should be remembered that, under normal conditions, they spend long periods sleeping during the day when little activity will be seen. After diurnal handling they often appear aggressive towards their cage-mates and emit loud screeching noises and aggressive movements, disproportionate to the degree of interference. Information on the recognition and assessment of the signs of pain and distress in hamsters can be found in Wallace *et al.* (1990).

Physiological monitoring

With care, a standard thermometer may be used to determine rectal temperature (37–38 °C) but it is far more convenient to use an electronic, semi-rigid probe thermometer. In addition body temperature, motor activity and heart rate can all be monitored via telemetric devices.

Blood sampling

There are no easily accessible, superficial veins in the hamster and therefore special care should be paid to the animal's welfare when collecting blood, which should be performed under general anaesthesia. Orbital venous sinus puncture, jugular access and cardiac puncture are recognised routes for blood sampling in the hamster. The circulating blood volume of the Syrian hamster is around 78 ml/kg body weight. Generally removal of no more than 10% of the circulating blood volume is advised at any one time. Further advice on the removal of blood from hamsters and other laboratory species can be found in a report by the Joint Working Group on Refinement (JWGR, 1993).

Urine, faeces and expired gases

Standard glass, metal, or plastic metabolism cages can be used to separate urine from faeces, whereas only glass is recommended for the trapping of expired respiratory gases. The nesting of hamsters in feeders or other areas of metabolism cages should be avoided when possible. Cages that provide either access for liquid diets or closure of the access to the feeder may be used.

Milk

A technique for collecting milk from mice has also been used for the collection of hamster milk, with only a minor modification to accommodate the longer nipple of the hamster. A plastic biopipette tip is placed over the nipple. Stimulants are not usually necessary to initiate milk flow. Experience shows that 0.1–0.2 ml total can be collected from two or three nipples on collections spaced a few hours apart. The use of approximately 1 USP unit of oxytocin, subcutaneously, will, however, increase milk flow if desired. No attempt has been made to collect milk more than 3 days after birth.

Various methods have been described for collecting saliva, bronchopulmonary lavage, ejaculate, vaginal mucous, urine, faeces, expired gases, milk and bile. More information on these techniques can be found in Van Hoosier and McPherson (1987).

Administration of substances

Anaesthesia

Sources of information on anaesthesia in the Syrian hamster include Ferguson (1979), Green (1979), Flecknell and Mitchell (1984), Gaertner *et al.* (1987) and most recently Flecknell (2009). It must always be remembered that whichever anaesthetic regime is chosen, the dose required to achieve the appropriate depth of anaesthesia and the subsequent sleep time will vary between strains and species of hamsters and may also be affected by other environmental factors.

Table 24.5 Provides the recommended sedatives, tranquillisers and other pre-anaesthetic medication for use in the Syrian hamster. Table 24.6 gives the anaesthetic dose

Table 24.5 Sedatives, tranquillisers and other pre-anaesthetic medication for use in the Syrian hamster. This article was published in Flecknell, P.A. (1996) *Laboratory Animal Anaesthesia*, 2nd edn, pp. 172–174, copyright Elsevier (1996). Reproduced with permission. Considerable variation in practice occurs between different strains.

Drug	*Dose rate*	*Comments*
Acepromazine	5 mg/kg ip	Light sedation
Atropine	0.04 mg/kg sc	Anticholinergic
Diazepam	5 mg/kg im, ip	Light sedation
Fentanyl/ fluanisone	0.5 ml/kg ip	Light–moderate sedation, moderate analgesia
Fentanyl/ droperidol	0.9 ml/kg im	Analgesia, unpredictable degree of sedation
Ketamine	100–200 mg/kg im	Deep sedation, mild analgesia
Medetomidine	0.1 mg/kg im, ip	Light–deep sedation, some analgesia
Midazolam	5 mg/kg im, ip	Mild–moderate sedation
Xylazine	5 mg/kg im	Light sedation, some analgesia

Table 24.6 Anaesthetic dose rates in the Syrian hamster. This article was published in Flecknell, P.A. (1996) *Laboratory Animal Anaesthesia*, 2nd edn, pp.172–174, copyright Elsevier (1996). Reproduced with permission.

Drug	*Dose rate (mg/kg)*	*Effect*	*Duration of anaesthesia (min)*	*Sleep-time (min)*
Alphachloralose	80–100 mg/kg ip	Immobilisation	–	180–240
Alphaxalone/alphadolone	150 mg/kg ip	Immobilisation/anaesthesia	20–60	120–150
Fentanyl/fluanisone + diazepam	1 ml/kg im or ip + 5 mg kg ip	Surgical anaesthesia	30–40	60–90
Fentanyl/fluanisone/midazolam	4.0 mg/kg ip*	Surgical anaesthesia	30–40	60–90
Ketamine/acepromazine	150 ml/kg + 5 mg/kg ip	Immobilisation/anaesthesia	45–120	75–180
Ketamine/diazepam	70 mg/kg + 2 mg/kg ip	Immobilisation/anaesthesia	30–45	90–120
Ketamine/medetomidine	100 mg/kg + 250 µg/kg ip	Surgical anaesthesia	30–60	60–120
Ketamine/xylazine	200 mg/kg +10 mg/kg ip	Immobilisation/anaesthesia	30–60	90–150
Pentobarbital	50–90 mg/kg ip	Immobilisation/anaesthesia	30–60	120–180
Tiletamine/zolezepam	50–80 mg/kg ip	Immobilisation/anaesthesia	20–30	30–60
Tiletamine/zolezepam/xylazine	30 mg/kg + 10 mg/kg ip		30	40–60
Urethane	1000–2000 mg/kg	Surgical anaesthesia	360–480	non-recovery only

*Dose in ml/kg of a mixture of 1 part fentanyl/fluanisone plus 2 parts water for injection, and 1 part midazolam (5 mg/ml initial concentration).
Duration of anaesthesia and sleep time (loss of righting reflex) are provided only as a general guide, since considerable between animal variation occurs. For recommended techniques see text.

rates in the Syrian hamster. Both tables are from Flecknell (1996).

Other procedures and techniques

Haisley (1980) describes the following technique for cheek pouch examination in conscious golden hamsters and which does not require forceps. The hamster is held around the body with a thumb across its chest. The fifth finger of the opposite hand is placed near the caudal end of the cheek pouch. By pushing cranially, while pulling gently at the corner of the hamster's mouth with the thumb of the free hand, the cheek pouch can be completely everted. The tissue can be manipulated gently with either index finger, and the entire surface can be examined. If the tissue is too moist to be manipulated easily, the pouch can be dried with a swab. This technique has several advantages: the hamster need not be anaesthetised; they seldom bite, since in doing so, they bite their own cheek; forceps are not needed to evert the pouch thus minimising tissue damage. Additionally, animals can be examined rapidly and frequently since no restraining devices are needed.

Ransom (1984) describes the following method for intravenous injection of unanaesthetised Syrian hamsters. A 1 ml Monoject plastic syringe with a 25.4 mm 25 G needle is filled with an appropriate solution for injection. Unanaesthetised animals are restrained by holding them by the skin of the neck and hindleg. A rubber band is then wrapped around either foreleg above the proximal joint. A small amount of 70% ethanol is applied to the lower foreleg where the cephalic vein on the ventral side is engorged by the rubber band tourniquet. The needle can be inserted easily into the vein at an approximately 10° angle to the vein, keeping the needle close to the surface of the skin after insertion through the epidermis and subcutaneous layers into the vein. If a swelling occurs at the injection site during injection, then the injection is subcutaneous. After removal of the needle, pressure is applied to the injection site to minimise haematoma formation.

With practice, it should be possible to use this procedure to perform intravenous injections in hamsters with consistent success. Care should be exercised by the person restraining the hamster to ensure that injury does not occur. Ransom (1984) reports that two injections could be made in each animal using both forelegs, but once a vein was punctured a second injection was not attempted for 24 h. Volumes of 0.1–0.3 ml were readily tolerated by both male and female hamsters.

A method for measuring cardiovascular and renal function in unrestrained hamsters is detailed by Fox *et al.* (1993), while Ohwada (1993) describes a method for calculating the body surface area of Syrian hamsters.

Euthanasia

Methods of euthanasia suitable for other small rodents can also be used for hamsters (specific methods can be found in Home Office (1997) and more extensive consideration of the various methods is given Close *et al.* (1996; 1997). See also Chapter 17. It is important to ensure that staff are competent to perform the procedure, especially when using physical methods. When using carbon dioxide, it is essential the animals are placed in a rising concentration of carbon dioxide and not a saturated atmosphere. Finally, whatever method is chosen, death must be confirmed via either severance of a major blood vessel, dislocation of the neck, or by observing rigor mortis before disposing of the carcase.

Common welfare problems

Diseases

Despite the fact that to date there has been no true caesarean derivation and hand-rearing of hamsters in order to establish true gnotobiotic or axenic stock, commercially sourced animals are typically is of a high microbiological status. Antibiotic chemotherapy, prophylaxis and improved husbandry conditions have contributed significantly to this state of affairs. There are now several established health (microbiological) monitoring schemes published for hamsters and other laboratory species. One example of such scheme is provided by Federation of European Laboratory Animal Science Associations (FELASA, 1994).

Non-infectious diseases and welfare problems

Cannibalism is common especially when hamsters are stressed. Primiparous females are renowned for their tendency to eat their young. Injuries can vary from limb amputation to death (Griffin *et al.* 1989).

Nutritional and metabolic disorders include spontaneous haemorrhagic necrosis (SHN) of the central nervous system of foetal and newborn hamsters (Keeler & Young 1979). There is a strain-related variation in susceptibility to the disease which can be induced by feeding pregnant dams a diet deficient in vitamin E. The condition can be alleviated by supplementation of the diet with vitamin E.

Environmental, genetic and other disorders include bedding-associated dermatitis (Meshorer 1976), malocclusion and periodontal disease. Diabetes mellitus is a genetically recessive disorder of Chinese hamsters. Affected individuals display classic signs of the disease (Diani & Gerritsen 1987).

Non-neoplastic age-related diseases are primarily degerative in nature and include arteriolar nephrosclerosis (hamster nephrosis), described by Slausen *et al.* (1978). Amyloidosis frequently occurs in older hamsters (Coe & Ross 1990). Atrial thrombosis is common in older hamsters in some colonies. Females are usually affected earlier than males. The syndrome is often associated with amyloidosis (McMartin & Dodds 1982) and changes also occur in coagulation and fibrinolytic parameters consistent with consumptive coagulopathy (Wechsler & Jones 1984).

Polycystic disease is characterised by multiple hepatic cysts and is occasionally seen in older hamsters at necropsy (Somvanshi *et al.* 1987). Hepatic cirrhosis is a spontaneous disorder occurring sporadically among hamsters, reaching an incidence of up to 20% in some colonies (Chesterman & Pomerance 1965). Brunnert and Altman (1991) describe the laboratory assessment of chronic hepatitis.

The incidence of neoplasms in hamsters is relatively rare but varies markedly between strains. The majority of tumours are benign and frequently arise from the endocrine system or alimentary tract. However, Brown *et al.* (1993) describe a chondroma of the foreleg in a Syrian hamster and Adaska and Carbone (1994) describe a spontaneous mesothelioma in a Syrian hamster. For extensive information on neoplasms in hamsters see Pour *et al.* (1976a, 1976b, 1976c, 1976d, 1979), Van Hoosier and Trentin (1979), Turusov and Mohr (1982), Bernfeld *et al.* (1986) and Barthold (1992).

Viral infections

Whilst hamsters are susceptible to a number of viral infections, few are of practical importance. Lymphocytic choriomeningitis virus (LCMV), whilst an important zoonosis, should now be eradicated from most, if not all, commercially sourced animals. Hotchin *et al.* (1974) describe an outbreak in hospital personnel attributable to a research colony of Syrian hamsters and Skinner and Knight (1979) review the potential role of Syrian hamsters and other small mammals as a reservoir of LCM.

Sendai virus causes clinical respiratory disease in hamsters and may reduce productivity in a breeding colony.

Coggin *et al.* (1978) reported natural horizontal transmission of lymphomas in Syrian hamsters but could find no evidence of hamster leukaemia virus. Barthold *et al.* (1987) provided evidence that a papovavirus is the probable aetiological agent of these lymphomas. However, they concluded that further study of the aetiology would be complicated due to the high degree of contagiousness, prolonged incubation period and complex epizootiology of the disease. Barthold (1992) presents a thorough review of hamster papovavirus biology.

Bacterial infections

A wide variety of pathogenic or opportunistic bacterial infections may cause disease in hamsters if predisposing factors such as concurrent viral infection, stress, immunosuppression etc are present. Case reports are too numerous to mention but Amao *et al.* (1991) reports the isolation of *Corynebacterium kutscheri* from aging Syrian hamsters and Shoji-Darkye *et al.* (1991) describe the pathogenesis of cilia-associated respiratory (CAR) bacillus in Syrian hamsters.

The most common, complex and perplexing bacterial infection in hamsters is perhaps proliferative ileitis (transmissible ileal hyperplasia). This is the most commonly recognised disease in Syrian hamsters and usually results in high morbidity and high mortality. The term 'wet-tail' should not be used because this descriptive term includes virtually all the conditions that may cause diarrhoea. *Escherichia coli, Campylobacter* spp., *Cryptosporidium* and a new species of *Chlamydia* have all been implicated in the aetiology.

Other bacteria which may give rise to enteritis include *Salmonella* spp, *Clostridia piliformis* (Tyzzer's Disease) *and Clostridium difficile* (non-antibiotic – associated). Percy and Barthold (1993) provide an excellent overview of bacterial disease in hamsters together with further references.

Parasitic infestations

Commercially sourced hamsters should for the most part be free of pathogenic parasites. Discovery of ectoparasites, nematodes and cestodes in purchased animals should trigger an investigation for alternative sources whilst intestinal protozoa are usually non-pathogenic.

Of the parasites capable of infesting hamsters those which have been reported most recently include: *Speleorodens clethrionomys* (nasal mite) (Bornstein & Iwarsson 1980), *Demodex aurati* (Skavlen & Peterson 1989), *Giardia* and *Trichomonas* (Moore 1990), *Syphacia obvelata* (Taylor 1992), *Giardia* and *Tritrichomonas* (Taylor *et al.* 1993) and *Spironucleus* sp. (Kunstyr *et al.* 1993).

Control and treatment of infections

Virus control is limited when caesarean re-derivation is not an option, however vaccination has been used against Sendai virus (Lindsey *et al.* 1991) and for some labile viruses, such as Sendai, strict quarantine and 'fire-break' techniques may be successful (Lindsey *et al.* 1991).

For a general review on the use of antibiotics to treat bacterial disease the reader is referred to Morris (1995).

La Regina *et al.* (1980) compared three antibiotics (tetracycline hydrochloride, dimetridazole and neomycin) in the treatment of proliferative ileitus. They found tetracycline hydrochloride to be the most effective whilst dimetridazole was less effective and neomycin had no effect. McNeil *et al.* (1986) reported similar success when treating wet-tail in a closed hamster colony. Isolates from affected animals included *E. coli*, *Clostridium perfringens* and *Bacteroides*. They found all three isolates were sensitive to oxytetracycline which was subsequently successfully used to treat and control the outbreak. Boss *et al.* (1994) report the successful use of oral vancomycin for the treatment of *Clostridium difficile* enteritis in Syrian hamsters while Srivastava (1988) demonstrated it was possible to eliminate the endogenous microbial flora from conventionally raised hamsters using a two-step administration of antibiotics.

Taylor (1992) describes the elimination of pinworms (*Syphacia obvelata*) using a combination of piperizine hydrate and thiabendazole.

References

Adaska, J.M. and Carbone, L.G. (1994) Spontaneous mesothelioma in a Syrian Hamster. *Laboratory Animal Science*, **44**, 383–385

Amao, H., Akimoto, T., Takahashi, W. *et al.* (1991) Isolation of *Corynebacterium kutscheri* from aged Syrian Hamsters (*Mesocricetus auratus*). *Laboratory Animal Science*, **41**, 265–268

Arnold, E.C. and Estep, Q.D. (1994) Laboratory caging preference in golden hamsters. *Laboratory Animals*, **28**, 232–238

Ball, D.J., Argentieri, G., Krause, R. *et al* (1991) Evaluation of a microchip implant system used for animal identification in rats. *Laboratory Animal Science*, **41**, 185–186

Barthold, S.W., Bhatt, P.N. and Johnson, E.A. (1987) Further evidence for papovavirus as the probable etiology of transmissible lymphoma of Syrian hamsters. *Laboratory Animal Science*, **37**, 283–288

Barthold, S.W. (1992) Haemolymphatic tumours. In: *The Pathology of Tumours of Laboratory Animals. III. Tumours of the Hamster*. Ed. Mohr, U. and Turnsov, V., pp. 318–344. IARC Scientific Publication, Lyon, France

Bernfeld, P., Homburger, F., Adams, R.A. *et al.* (1986) Base-line data in a carcinogen-susceptible first generation hybrid strain of golden hamsters: F1D Alexander. *Journal of the National Cancer Institute*, **77**, 165–171

Bornstein, S. and Iwarsson, K. (1980) Nasal mites in a colony of Syrian hamsters (*Mesocricetus auratus*). *Laboratory Animals*, **14**, 31–33

Boss, S.M., Gries, C.L., Kirchner, B.K. *et al.* (1994) Use of vancomycin hydrochloride for treatment of *Clostridium difficile* enteritis in Syrian hamsters. *Laboratory Animal Science*, **44**, 31–37

Brown, P., Henderson, J., Hilton, T. *et al.* (1993) Chondroma of the foreleg in a Syrian Hamster. *Laboratory Animals*, **27**, 391–392

Brunnert, S.R. and Altman, N. (1991) Laboratory assessment of chronic hepatitis in Syrian hamsters. *Laboratory Animal Science*, **41**, 559–562

Chesterman, F.C. and Pomerance, A. (1965) Cirrhosis and liver tumours in a closed colony of golden hamsters. *British Journal of Cancer*, **1980**, 802–811

Chijioke, C.P., Mansfield K.J. and Pearson, R.M. (1990) The reproducibility of the hamster egg penetration test for the assessment of human spermatozoal fertilising potential. *Animal Technology*, **41**, 49–58.

Close, B., Banister, K., Baumans, V. *et al.* (1996) Recommendations for euthanasia of experimental animals Part 1 Report of a Working Party. *Laboratory Animals*, **30**, 293–316

Close, B., Banister, K., Baumans, V. *et al.* (1997) Recommendations for euthanasia of experimental animals Part 2 Report of a Working Party. *Laboratory Animals*, **31**, 1–32

Coe, J.E. and Ross, J.J. (1990) Amyloidosis and female protein in the Syrian Hamster. Concurrent regulation by sex hormones. *Journal of Experimental Medicine*, **171**, 1257–1266

Coggin, J.H. Jr., Thomas, K.V. and Huebner, R. (1978) Horizontally transmitted lymphomas of Syrian hamsters. *Federation Proceedings*, **37**, 2086–2088

Corbett, G. and Hill, J. (1980) *A World List of Mammalian Species*. Comstock Publication Association, London

Council of Europe (2006) Multilateral Consultation of Parties to the European Convention for the Protection of Vertebrate Animals used for Experimental and other Scientific Purposes (ETS 123) Appendix A. *Cons 123 (2006) 3*. http://www.coe.int/t/e/legal_affairs/legal_co-operation/biological_safety,_use_of_animals/laboratory_animals/2006/Cons123(2006)3AppendixA_en.pdf (accessed 31 July 2008)

Diani, A. and Gerritsen, G. (1987) Use in research. In: *Laboratory Hamsters*. Eds Van Hoosier, G.L. Jr. and McPherson, C.W., pp 329–347. Academic Press, New York

European Commission (2007) Commission recommendations of 18 June 2007 on guidelines for the accommodation and care of animals used for experimental and other scientific purposes. Annex II to European Council Directive 86/609. See 2007/526/EC. http://eurlex.europa.eu/LexUriServ/site/en/oj/2007/l_197/l_19720070730en00010089.pdf (accessed 13 May 2008)

Ferguson, J.W. (1979) Anaesthesia in the hamster using a combination of methohexitone and diazepam. *Laboratory Animals*, **13**, 305–308

Federation of European Laboratory Animal Science Associations (1994) Report of the FELASA Working Group on Animal Health: Recommendations of the health monitoring of mouse, rat, hamster, guinea pig and rabbit breeding colonies. *Laboratory Animals*, **28**, 1–12

Flecknell, P.A. and Mitchell, M. (1984) Midazolam and fentanyl-fluanisone. Assessment of anaesthetic effects in laboratory rodents and rabbits. *Laboratory Animals*, **18**, 143–146

Flecknell, P.A. (1996) *Laboratory Animal Anaesthesia*, 2nd edn. Academic Press, London

Flecknell, P.A. (2009) *Laboratory Animal Anaesthesia*, 3rd edn. Academic Press, London

Fox, M., Vasumathi, N. and Trippodo, N.C. (1993) Measurement of cardiovascular and renal function in unrestrained hamsters. *Laboratory Animal Science*, **43**, 94–98

Gaertner, D.J., Boschert, K.R. and Schoeb, T.R. (1987) Muscle necrosis in Syrian Hamsters resulting from intramuscular injections of ketamine and xylazine. *Laboratory Animal Science*, **37**, 80–83

Grainger, L.J. and Plotkin, H.C. (1987) Cross-fostering and maternal care in Syrian Hamsters. *Animal Technology*, **38**, 25–30

Green, C.J. (1979) Animal anaesthesia. Laboratory animal handbooks no. 8. *Laboratory Animals Ltd*, London

Grelk, D.F., Papson, B.A., Cole, J.E. *et al.* (1974) The influence of caging conditions and hormone treatments on fighting in male and female hamsters. *Hormones and Behaviour*, **5**, 355–366

Griffin, H.E., Gbadamosi, S.G., Perry, R.L. *et al.* (1989) Hamster limb loss. *Laboratory Animal*, **18**, 19–20

Haisley, A.D. (1980) A technique for cheek pouch examination of Syrian Hamsters. *Laboratory Animal Science*, **30**, 107–109

Home Office (1997) *Code of Practice: The humane killing of animals under Schedule 1 to the Animals (Scientific Procedures) Act 1986.* HMSO ISBN 0102653976

Honachi, J., Kinman, K. and Koeppl, J. (1982) *Mammal Species of the World.* Allen Press Inc. and The Association of systematic Collections, Lawrence, Kansas

Hotchin, J., Sikora, E. and Kinch, W. (1974) Lymphocytic choriomeningitis in a hamster colony causes infection of hospital personnel. *Science*, **185**, 1173–1174

Joint Working Group on Refinement (1993) Removal of blood from laboratory mammals and birds. First Report of the BVA/FRAME/RSPCA/UFAW Joint Working Group on Refinement. *Laboratory Animals*, **27**, 1–22

Keeler, R.F. and Young, S. (1979) Role of vitamin E in the aetiology of spontaeous haemorrhagic necrossi of the central nervous system of foetal hamsters. *Teratology*, **20**, 127–132

Kuhnen, G. (1999a) The effect of cage size and enrichment on core temperature and febrile response of the golden hamster. *Laboratory Animals*, **33**, 221–227

Kuhnen, G. (1999b) Housing-induced changes in the febrile response of juvenile and adult golden hamsters. *Journal of Experimental Animal Science*, **39**, 151–155

Kunstyr, I., Poppinga, G. and Friedhoff, K.T. (1993) Host specificity of cloned *Spironucleus* sp originating from the European hamster. *Laboratory Animals*, **27**, 77–80

La Regina, M., Forbes, W.H. and Wagner, J.E. (1980) Effects of antibiotic treatment on the occurrence of experimentally induced proliferative ileitis of hamsters. *Laboratory Animal Science*, **30**, 38–41

Laboratory Animal Science Association (2005) Guidance on the transport of laboratory animals. Report of the Transport Working Group established by LASA. *Laboratory Animals*, **39**, 1–39

Lerchl, A. (1995) Breeding of Djungarian hamsters *(Phodopus sungorus)*: influence of parity and litter size on weaning success and offspring ratio. *Laboratory Animals*, **29**, 172–176

Lindsey, J.R., Boorman, G.A., Collins, M.J. *et al.* (1991) *Infectious Diseases of Mice and Rats.* Committee on Infectious Diseases of Mice and Rats, National Research Council, National Academic Press, Washington, DC

McMartin, D.N. and Dodds, W.J. (1982) Animal model of human disease: atrial thrombosis in ageing Syrian hamsters. *American Journal of Pathology*, **107**, 277–279

McNeil, P.E., Al-Mashat, R.R., Bradley, R.A. *et al.* (1986) Control of an outbreak of wet-tail in a closed colony of hamsters *(Mesocricetus auratus). The Veterinary Record*, **119**, 272–273

Medical Research Council (1977) *Dietary Standards for Laboratory Animals.* Report of the Laboratory Animals Centre: Diets Advisory Committee. Medical Research Council, Carshalton, Surrey

Meshorer, A. (1976) Leg lesions in hamsters caused by wood shavings. *Laboratory Animal Science*, **26**, 827–829

Mooij, P.N.M., Wouters, M.G.A.J., Thomas, C.M.G. *et al.* (1992) Disturbed reproductive performance in extreme folic acid deficient golden hamsters. *European Journal of Obstetrics, Gynaecological Reproductive Biology*, **43**, 71–75

Moore, G.J. (1990) *Giardia* and *Trichomonas* infections in Syrian hamsters. Efficacy of dimetridazole therapy and containment of infection. *Animal Technology*, **41**, 133–136

Morris, T.H. (1995) Antibiotic therapeutics in laboratory animals. *Laboratory Animals*, **29**, 16–36

Mrozek, M., Fischer, R., Trendelenburg, M. *et al.* (1995) Microchip implant system used for animal identification in laboratory rabbits, guinea pigs, woodchucks and in amphibians. *Laboratory Animals*, **29**, 339–344

National Research Council (1978) *Nutrient Requirements of Laboratory Animals.* National Research Council National Academy of Sciences, Washington, DC

National Research Council (1996) *Guide for the Care and Use of Laboratory Animals.* National Academies Press, Washington, DC. Available from URL: http://www.nap.edu/readingroom/books/labrats/

Nowak, R.M. and Paradiso, J.L. (1983) *Walker's Mammals of the World*, 4th edn. Johns Hopkins University Press, Baltimore, Maryland

National Research Council (1995) *Nutrient Requirements of Laboratory Animals*, 4th revised edn. National Academy Press, Washington, DC

Ohwada, K. (1993) A new equation for the calculation of body surface area (BSAs) in golden Syrian hamsters. *Animal Technology*, **44**, 227–232

Percy, D.H. and Barthold, S.W. (1993). Hamsters. In: *The Pathology of Laboratory Rodents and Rabbits.* pp. 115–136. Iowa State University Press, Iowa

Pour, P., Mohr, U., Cardesa, A. *et al.* (1976a) Spontaneous tumours and common diseases in two colonies of Syrian hamsters. II. Respiratory tract and digestive system. *Journal of the National Cancer Institute*, **56**, 937–948

Pour, P., Mohr, U., Althoff, J. *et al.* (1976b) Spontaneous tumours and common diseases in two colonies of Syrian hamsters. III. Urogenital system and encrodrine glands. *Journal of the National Cancer Institute*, **56**, 949–960

Pour, P., Mohr, U., Althoff, J. *et al.* (1976c) Spontaneous tumours and common diseases in two colonies of Syrian hamsters. IV. Vascular and lymphatic systems and lesions of other sites. *Journal of the National Cancer Institute*, **56**, 963–974

Pour, P., Kmoch, N., Greiser, E. *et al.* (1976d) Spontaneous tumours and common diseases in two colonies of Syrian hamsters. I. Incidence and sites. *Journal of the National Cancer Institute*, **56**, 931–935

Pour P., Mohr U., Althoff, J. *et al.* (1979) Spontaneous tumours and common diseases in three types of hamsters. *Journal of the National Cancer Institute*, **63**, 797–881

Ransom, J.H. (1984) Intravenous injection of unanesthetised hamsters *(Mesocricetus auratus). Laboratory Animal Science*, **34**, 200–201

Reinhardt, V. and Reinhardt, A. (eds) (2002) *Comfortable Quarters for Laboratory Animals.* Animal Welfare Institute, Washington, DC

Shoji-Darkye, Y., Itoh, T. and Kagiyama, N. (1991) Pathogenesis of CAR bacillus in rabbits, guinea pigs, Syrian hamsters and mice. *Laboratory Animal Science*, **41**, 567–571

Skavlen, P.A. and Peterson, M.E. (1989) Skin lesions in hamsters. *Laboratory Animal (USA)*, **16**, 17–18

Skinner, H.H. and Knight, E.H. (1979) The potential role of Syrian hamsters and other small animals as reservoire of lymphocytic choriomeningitis virus. *Journal of Small Animal Practice*, **20**, 145–161

Slausen, D.O., Hobbs, C.H. and Crain, C. (1978) Arteriolar nephrosclerosis in the Syrian Hamster. *Veterinary Pathology*, **15**, 1–11

Somvanshi, R., Iyer, P.K.R., Biswas, J.C. *et al.* (1987) Polycystic liver disease in golden hamsters. *Journal of Comparative Pathology*, **97**, 615–618

Srivastava, K.K. (1988) Elimination of microbial flora from conventionally raised Syrian hamsters by antimicrobial agents. *Laboratory Animal Science*, **38**, 169–172

Taylor, D.M. (1992) Eradication of pinworms (*Syphacia obvelata*) from Syrian Hamsters in quarantine. *Laboratory Animal Science*, **42**, 413–414

Taylor, D.M., Farquhar, C.F. and Neal, D.L. (1993) Studies on the eradication of intestinal protozoa of Syrian Hamsters in quarantine and their transfaunation to mice. *Laboratory Animal Science*, **43**, 359–360

Turusov, V.S. and Mohr, U. (1982) *Pathology of Tumours in Laboratory Animals III. Tumours of the Hamster*. IARC Scientific Publications, Lyon, France

Van Hoosier, G.L., Jr. and Trentin, J.T. (1979) Naturally occurring tumours of the Syrian Hamster. *Progress in Experimental Tumour Research*, **23**, 1–12

Van Hoosier, G.L., Jr. and McPherson, C.W. (1987) *Laboratory Hamsters*. Academic Press Inc, Orlando, Florida

Wallace, J., Sanford, J., Smith, M.W. *et al.* (1990) The assessment and control of the severity of scientific procedures on laboratory animals. Report of the LASA Working Party. *Laboratory Animals*, **24**, 97–130

Wechsler, S.J. and Jones, J. (1984) Diagnostic exercise. *Laboratory Animal Science*, **34**, 137–138

West, W.T. and Mason, K.E. (1958) Histopathology of muscular dystrophy in the vitamin E deficient hamster. *American Journal of Anatomy*, **102**, 323–363

25 The husbandry and welfare of non-traditional laboratory rodents

Chris Sherwin

Introduction

In this chapter, the physiology, behaviour, lifestyles and senses and communication of some rodent species not traditionally used in the laboratory are discussed and at the end of each section suggestions derived from these considerations are given to promote best welfare practice for these animals.

The order Rodentia is probably the most diverse taxonomic group among mammals, containing the largest number of species. Worldwide, there are approximately 2277 species of rodents, representing 42% of all mammal species (Wilson & Reeder 2005). New species continue to be discovered (eg, Werner *et al.* 2006) including, during the writing of this chapter, a giant rat from Papua New Guinea which is five times the size of a typical laboratory rat. Rodents are found around the world except in Antarctica, and in a very wide range of habitats except for the oceans and some oceanic islands. Table 25.1 presents a classification of the Rodentia adapted from Wilson and Reeder (2005), and which is regularly updated[1].

Non-traditional laboratory rodent species

The range of rodent species used in laboratories is steadily increasing as our understanding of their diversity increases and our quest for knowledge continues. Examples of these include: the Arctic porcupine (*Erethizon dorsatum*) (Folk *et al.* 2006), beaver (*Castor* spp.) (McKean 1982), capybara (*Hydrochoerus hydrochaeris*) (Labruna *et al.* 2004), chinchilla (*Chinchilla laniger*) (Burgstahler *et al.* 2008; Hamernik *et al.* 2008; Shera *et al.* 2008), collard lemming (*Dicrostonyx torquatus*) (Weil *et al.* 2006), coypu or nutria (*Myocaster coypus*) (McKean 1982; Marounek *et al.* 2005), grey squirrel (*Sciurus carolinensis*) (Van Hooser *et al.* 2005), ground squirrel (*Spermophilus* spp.) (Zhao *et al.* 2004; Mateo 2008), naked mole-rat (*Heterocephalus glaber*) (Towett *et al.* 2006; Park *et al.* 2003, 2008), southern flying squirrel (*Glaucomys volans*) (Gibbs *et al.* 2007) and zockor (*Myospalax* spp.) (Wei *et al.* 2006).

Non-traditional rodent species are increasingly being used in the following fields of research: models for human or other animal disease and other applied studies; fundamental studies; conservation research; and pest control. However, the use of less frequently used species in research requires specialist knowledge to ensure high standards of welfare.

It might be thought, due to the similar appearance of many rodents, that they have similar requirements in terms of housing and husbandry. Although some of their requirements may be similar, all species have species-specific physiology, behaviour, lifestyles and senses, which must be understood if we are to provide adequate welfare in the laboratory. It is clearly impossible to give a comprehensive review of the welfare considerations of the entire Rodentia in this single chapter, but this chapter provides a 'flavour' of the great diversity of the non-traditional laboratory rodents, and serves to highlight the need for specialist knowledge in their care. The consideration of rodent requirements taking into account their ecology, behaviour, anatomy and physiology should also help to shed light on the welfare considerations of both non-traditional and more commonly used laboratory rodents.

Physiology

Anatomy

Despite their ecological diversity, all rodents share the characteristic that their dentition is highly specialised for gnawing. It is this specialisation which gives rodents their name (from the Latin, *rodere*, to gnaw and *dens*, *dentis*, tooth). All rodents have a single pair of upper and a single pair of lower incisors, followed by a gap (diastema), and then one or more molars or premolars. Rodent incisors grow continuously and must be kept worn down by gnawing. Their anterior and lateral surfaces are covered with enamel, but the posterior surface is exposed dentine. During gnawing, the incisors grind against each other, wearing away the softer dentine leaving the enamel edge as the blade of a chisel (Hurst 1999). This 'self-sharpening' system is very effective and is one of the keys to the enormous success of rodents (Myers 2000). The diastema of the upper jaw is longer than that of the lower jaw, which allows rodents to engage their gnawing incisors while their chewing teeth (molars and premolars) are not being used. The reverse is also true;

[1] http://museum.utep.edu/mammalogy/

Table 25.1 Classification of the order Rodentia (after Wilson & Reeder 2005).

Suborder	*Superfamily*	*Family*	*Species*	*Common name*
Sciuromorpha				
		Aplodontiidae	1	Mountain beaver, boomer or sewellel
		Sciuridae	278	Tree squirrels, flying squirrels, ground squirrels, sousliks, chipmunks, marmots, prairie dogs, woodchuck
		Gliridae	28	Dormice
		Geomyidae	40	Pocket gophers
Castorimorpha				
		Castoridae	2	Beavers
		Heteromyidae	60	Pocket mice, kangaroo rats, kangaroo mice
Myomorpha				
	Dipodoidea	Dipodoidea	6	Jumping mice and jerboas
	Muroidea	Nesomyidae	61	Malagasy rats and mice, climbing mice, African rock mice, swamp mice, pouched rats, white-tailed rat
		Cricetidae	681	Hamsters, voles, lemmings, New World rats and mice
		Muridae	730	Mice, rats, gerbils
		Platacanthomyidae	2	Spiny dormice, Chinese pygmy dormice
		Spalacidae	36	Blind mole-rats, bamboo rats, root rats, zokors
		Calomyscidae	8	Mouse-like hamsters
Anomaluromorpha				
		Anomaluridae	7	Scaly-tailed squirrels
		Pedetidae	2	Springhare
Hystricomorpha				
		Ctenodactylidae	5	Gundis
		Bathyergidae	16	African mole-rats, blesmols
		Hystricidae	11	Old World porcupines
		Petromuridae	1	Dassie rat
		Ctenomyidae	60	Tuco-tucos
		Echimyidae	90	Spiny rats
		Thryonomyidae	2	Cane rats
		Erethizontidae	16	New World porcupines
		Chinchillidae	7	Chinchillas, viscachas
		Dinomyidae	1	Pacarana
		Caviidae	18	Cavies, guinea pig, mara or Patagonian hare, capybara
		Dasyproctidae	13	Agoutis, acouchis
		Cuniculidae	2	Paca
		Octodontidae	13	Degus or octodonts
		Abrocomidae	10	Chinchilla rats
		Myocastoridae	1	Coypu, nutria
		Capromyidae	20	Hutias
		Heptaxodontidae	4	Giant hutia

rodents can use their chewing teeth (also called cheek teeth) while their incisors are disengaged. No rodent has more than one incisor in each quadrant, and no rodent has canines. The entire skull structure of rodents is designed to accommodate the separate use of the different types of teeth. Rodent skulls have long snouts; the articulation of the lower jaw with the skull is orientated front-to-back rather than sideways as in other mammals; the jaw muscles (masseter complex) are extended well forward into the snout; and the number of cheek teeth is less than in most other mammals – all features unique to rodents. They have well developed muscles that move the lower jaw (pterygoid), and a long glenoid fossa which gives them the ability to move the lower jaw forward and backward. Gnawing is an essential behaviour for rodents and they should be provided with opportunities to gnaw when housed in the laboratory. Malocclusion can occur if suitable hard food and/or non-toxic chewing materials such as cardboard, hay, branches or other wood materials are not provided. Overgrowth of teeth can be a particular problem for long-lived species (Hurst 1999).

Morphology

The overall morphology of most rodents is relatively similar. Rodents tend to be small; very few weigh more than 1 kg and most weigh less than 100 g. The tiny African pygmy mouse *Mus minutoides* is only 6 cm in length and 7 g in weight. At the other extreme, the capybara can be 130 cm in length and weigh up to 66 kg (Macdonald 1984), and the extinct *Phoberomys pattersoni* is believed to have weighed 700 kg. Most rodents have short compact bodies with short legs. Some groups (jerboas Dipodidae, gerbils Gerbillinae, springhare *Pedetes capensis*) have long rear legs and feet that allow them to hop over large distances of the deserts they inhabit (the springhare can bound over 2 m). Other grassland rodents have no need for jumping and subsequently have evolved similarly sized, short front and rear limbs. The beaver, capybara, coypu and earless water rat (*Crossomys moncktoni*) have webbed, or partly webbed, feet for their aquatic lifestyle. Some rodents, particularly nocturnal species, have large eyes (dormice, hamsters) while others which have adopted a subterranean lifestyle have very small eyes, which are sometimes covered with a layer of skin making them functionally blind (blind mole-rats). Similarly, ear morphology varies amongst the rodents from being relatively large (mice, rats, springhare) to absent or invisible (blind mole-rats, earless water rat) and may have specialist structures such as a well developed cartilaginous flap (tragus) that prevents sand or soil from entering the ear during digging.

Rodents, being mammals, all possess hair, however, even this characteristic shows some remarkable adaptations. Most wild rodents are covered over their entire body with brown or grey agouti-type coloration, in which the coat might show light and dark bands for camouflage, whilst desert rodents have a more sandy appearance. The albino appearance of laboratory rodents is an artificially selected character as these mutations would be heavily selected against in the wild. Research with degus (*Octodon degus*) indicates that ultraviolet visible patterns on their coat might have a role in communication (Chavez *et al.* 2003). Some rodents are nearly completely naked (naked mole-rat), whereas others (chinchillas, beavers) have thick luxuriant coats making thermoregulation an important welfare consideration for these species when used in the laboratory – cooling may be necessary at higher ambient temperatures than for many other rodent species. Conversely, nude or less hirsute species may need to be housed in warmer than usual ambient temperatures, or at least provided with nesting materials for those species that build nests to create a suitable microclimate.

Perhaps the most varied characteristic of the rodents is their tail. Some rodents have long, nude or sparsely haired tails (mice, rats) or long, hairy tails (gerbils) which they use for balancing whilst standing running or climbing. Some species have a long prehensile tail (European harvest mouse (*Micromys minutus*)), which they use during climbing. The tail of arboreal squirrels is also used as a counterbalance and for signalling, perhaps being enhanced by its bushiness. It has been suggested that Californian ground squirrels add an infrared component from their tails when tail-flagging at infrared sensitive predatory snakes (Rundus *et al.* 2007). Some groups such as cavies (Caviidae) and hamsters (Cricetinae) have vestigial tails or no visible tail at all, whereas others, such as the beavers, have highly developed, flat muscular tails used for propulsion during swimming. Knowledge of the tail can be important for appropriate handling in the laboratory. Mice and some other small rodents are routinely picked up by the tail, however, this should not be done with gerbils and degus as the skin may tear off.

Diet

Nearly all rodents feed on plants, seeds in particular. Some species are omnivorous whereas others are exclusively herbivorous, eg, beavers, voles (Microtinae) and lemmings (Hurst 1999). Other species are highly specialised, eating, for example, only a few species of invertebrates or fungi. Some species eat fish (beavers) and some squirrels are known to eat passerine birds such as cardinals and blue jays. It has been reported that the diet of the grasshopper mouse (*Onychomys leucogaster*) is 89% animal matter (insects, scorpions, small mice) and only 11% plant matter – captive individuals are apparently especially fond of raw liver and newborn mice (Davis & Schmidley 1997). In the laboratory a suitable diet in terms of both quantity and quality must be provided. Care should be taken to avoid generalist assumptions – apparently similar species may have very different requirements for specialist diets, which must be considered before introducing the species into the laboratory.

Habitat

As might be expected from the numerous Rodentia species, they inhabit highly diverse habitats. Some are terrestrial (cotton rats (*Sigmodon* spp.), jerboas, kangaroo rats (*Dipodomys* spp.)) while others are fossorial and dig out extensive underground burrow systems (ground squirrels, mole-rats, marmots (*Marmota* spp.)). Others are largely arboreal (tree squirrels, New World porcupines (*Sphiggurus* spp.) or have become volant, (ie, they have a loose fold of furred skin (patagium) which connects the front and hindlimbs from the wrists to the ankle that allows them to glide between trees (flying squirrels)). A few have even adopted an aquatic lifestyle (beavers, capybara, coypu, water rats (*Hydromys* spp.)). Rodents are often opportunistic in their choice of habitat, but others can be highly specialist. One of the most remarkable artificially created habitats in the animal kingdom is constructed by a rodent; beavers construct their homes, or lodges, out of sticks, twigs and mud in artificial ponds they create by building dams which can be substantial structures. Clearly it would be impossible to provide or simulate many of these habitats in the laboratory, but the basic behaviours of the animals in these environments, such as burrowing, gliding, swimming, etc must be considered when designing enclosures for them. In some instances it might be possible to provide surrogate habitats, eg, pre-fabricated tunnel systems for burrowing species, small ponds or water baths for aquatic species, or construct enclosures to suit the animal's behaviour, eg, long narrow enclosures for gliding species.

Social organisation

Some rodents are highly social animals living in families (African brush-tailed porcupine *Atherurus africanus*, beavers), large groups (mice, rats), or in highly complex social systems in extensive colonies (marmots, prairie dogs (*Cynomys ludovicianus*)). The naked mole-rat and the Damaraland mole-rat (*Cryptomys damarensis*) are the only mammals currently known to be eusocial (living somewhat like termites and ants in a colony with castes) (Scantlebury *et al.* 2006). The naked mole-rat lives in subterranean colonies that commonly contain around 80 but sometimes up to 300 individuals. Reproduction is monopolised by a single dominant 'queen' and one or two males, whereas the remainder of the colony act as 'workers', maintaining the burrow system, or 'soldiers' defending the colony against foreign mole-rats or predators (Holmes *et al.* 2007). The females of the subterranean rodents, the tuco-tucos (Ctenomyidae) and degus, frequently share one burrow and nurse one another's young. Solitary ways of life are associated with species living in arid grasslands and desert areas (jerboas, marmots, Plains pocket gopher (*Geomys bursarius*), Syrian hamster *Mesocricetus auratus*, crested porcupines (*Hystrix* spp.)). Clearly, the social organisation of any species used in the laboratory needs to be considered to maintain good welfare. Unless there is evidence to the contrary, the animals should be housed as near as possible to their natural groupings, eg, individual or group housing, large or small groups, single- or mixed-sex groups.

Chronobiology

Most rodents are nocturnal or crepuscular, although some are strictly diurnal (eg, ground squirrels, tree squirrels). Some species are flexible in this regard and regulate their 24h activity around human activity (guinea pigs, coypu (Meyer *et al.* 2005)). Most rodent species are active throughout the year, but others, notably ground squirrels, may hibernate for several months (Zhao *et al.* 2004). There is a growing acceptance that gathering data from animals in the laboratory during times when they would normally be asleep is often not best practice for scientific validity or animal welfare. For example, in behavioural studies of nocturnal mice or rats, red lights are often used to allow data collection from the animals during the dark phase (their active period) without disturbing the animals. Such considerations should be extended to the choronobiology of other species brought into the laboratory.

Senses and communication

The senses of the typical laboratory rodents have been studied widely and there have been several reviews of how the laboratory environment can (adversely) affect animal welfare in this regard (eg, Olsson *et al.* 2003; Sherwin 2002, 2004). There have also been studies on the senses of non-traditional laboratory rodent species. These are discussed here, along with the welfare implications.

Pain

Rodent species are widely represented in studies of pain. All the typical laboratory species have been used: rats (eg, Dobner 2006; Vissers *et al.* 2006), mice (eg, Dobner 2006; Delporte *et al.* 2007; Marabese *et al.* 2007), gerbils (Vissers *et al.* 2006) and guinea pigs (Fox *et al.* 2003). Less well studied species used in this field include degus (Pelissier *et al.* 1989) and naked mole-rats. Rather bizarrely, the skin of African naked mole-rats lacks a key neurotransmitter called substance P that is responsible in mammals for sending burning pain signals to the central nervous system. When these animals are exposed to acid or capsaicin, it has been reported that they behave is if they feel little or no pain to these substances (Park *et al.* 2003, 2008).

Olfaction

Humans are unusual compared to other mammals because a much smaller proportion of our genome is devoted to olfaction and our vomeronasal organ is vestigial or non-existent (Burn 2008). It is therefore easy for us to under-appreciate the role that olfaction has in other species. Rodents use a variety of specialised scent glands, together with urine, faeces and vaginal secretions for olfactory communication. There is considerable diversity between the species, and between the sexes, in the location of scent glands and in their secretions, but urine is a particularly rich source of odour used by many species (Hurst 1999).

A considerable amount has been written about olfaction in the typical laboratory rodents (eg, Lonstein & Gammie 2002; Novotny 2003; Brennan & Keverne 2004; Lai *et al.* 2005; Bargmann 2006; Maras & Petrulis 2008) and some of the behavioural functions of olfaction are now understood in great detail (Humphries *et al.* 1999; Beynon & Hurst 2003; Hurst & Beynon 2004). From such studies, several welfare issues relating to olfaction in typical laboratory rodents are now recognised, eg, cleaning cages to minimise social disruption and reducing the potential for exposure to the odour of predators (please see species chapters for further information). Considerably less research has been published on the atyptical laboratory rodent species, but there are reports on olfaction in beavers (Rosell 2002; Rosell & Sanda 2006; Rosell & Thomsen 2006), chinchillas (Oikawa *et al.* 1994), flying squirrels (Pyare & Longland 2001; Borgo *et al.* 2006), lemmings (Huck & Banks 1984), mole-rats (Menzies *et al.* 1992; Zuri *et al.* 1998; Smith *et al.* 2007), tuco-tucos (Fanjul *et al.* 2003; Zenuto *et al.* 2004) and voles (Marchlewska-Koj *et al.* 2003; Wolff 2004). The blind mole-rat (*Spalax ehrenbergi*), uses its latrines in territory marking (Zuri *et al.* 1997). As with laboratory mice, removal of these markings during cleaning might have welfare implications by reducing the familiarity of the environment, and causing social disruption if dominance status is conveyed by these markings. Further research should reveal the role of olfaction in these animals, and help determine the optimum balance between cleaning whilst allowing the marks to achieve their effect.

Hearing (mechanoreception)

Many desert rodents communicate by drumming their feet on the ground to create mechanical vibrations. This is an important means of communication and occurs in a wide variety of contexts including individual-spacing, resource competition and predator defence. Foot-drumming is widespread and includes kangaroo rats from North America, and gerbils from Africa and Asia (Randall 2001; Shier & Randall 2007). All these rodents have specially adapted ears for reception of the low-frequency vibrations transmitted via both the air and seismically through the ground. A similar behaviour using head-drumming is performed by blind mole-rats (Rado *et al.* 1987). These animals possess poor auditory sensitivity, which is limited to low-frequency sounds. They detect low-frequency seismic waves using their paws, and can accurately determine the direction of the vibratory source (Kimchi *et al.* 2005). Some burrowing mole-rat species, eg, *Cryptomys hottentotus* (Muller *et al.* 1992), *Spalax ehrenbergi* and *Fukomys anselli* (Burda 2006) have ears adapted to the lower range frequencies transmitted through the ground, and have much reduced sensitivity to the higher frequencies that surface-dwelling species can hear. The welfare implications of low-frequency mechanoreceptivity have yet to be researched, but it seems likely that sources of low frequency air or seismic waves in the laboratory (eg, construction work, lifts, cages or racks being moved or knocked, items being dropped) might interfere with this sensory modality or could possibly lead to sensory overload, indicating that they should be avoided. In addition, if the animals are to be permitted to perform natural behaviours, it might be necessary to provide them with the opportunity to build tunnel systems for them to communicate effectively.

Ultrasound

Typical laboratory rodents can hear over a broad spectrum of frequencies and can hear well above the frequency of human hearing sensitivity (ultrasound). Both audible and ultrasonic calls are used by rodents in a variety of situations. Ultrasound is used in sexual communication and by pups when they have fallen out of the nest (eg, Clough 1982; Ehret 2005; Wohr & Schwarting 2008). It has even been reported that rats and shrews use ultrasound for echolocation (Kaltwasser & Schnitzler 1981; Forsman & Malmquist 1988). Some non-traditional laboratory rodents are also sensitive to ultrasound or emit these frequencies (voles, Rabon *et al.* 2001; ground squirrels, Wilson & Hare 2004; mice, Kalcounis-Rueppell *et al.* 2006; bank voles, Szentgyorgyi *et al.* 2008), although this has been considerably less well researched. Several items of common laboratory equipment such as pressure hoses, running taps, computer monitors or oscilloscopes emit ultrasound, some at very high sound pressures (Sales *et al.* 1999). These are silent to humans, but could have considerable effects on rodents and on experimental data obtained from them. Laboratory-generated ultrasound could conceivably interfere with communication between animals, cause distress or perhaps even sensory damage if severe enough. The use of bat detectors, which register ultrasonic frequencies, to detect this problem could help to improve the rodents' welfare.

Magnetoreception

It has been claimed that mole-rats (Marhold *et al.* 1997; Kimchi *et al.* 2004), Siberian hamsters (Deutschlander *et al.* 2003) and laboratory mice (Muheim *et al.* 2006) have the capacity to detect magnetic fields. Deutschlander *et al.* (2003) suggest that studies on other rodents might have incorrectly indicated that they do not possess this capability, raising the possibility that magnetoreception might be more widespread than is generally thought. Our understanding of this capability in rodents is currently limited, but sources of magnetism in the laboratory (eg, computer monitors, many items of electrical equipment) could conceivably interfere with magnetoreception.

Vision

Many rodents are nocturnal and therefore have a retina dominated by rods and which contains only a small proportion of cones. Even in these species, the cones comprise two spectral types and thus, contrary to popular belief, provide dichromatic colour vision, the most common form of mammalian colour vision (Jacobs 1993). There have been many studies on the vision of non-traditional laboratory rodents and there is considerable diversity in its physiology and function (eg, Cooper *et al.* 1993; Cernuda-Cernuda *et al.* 2002; Peichl 2005; Bobu *et al.* 2008; Lluch *et al.* 2008; Ortiz *et al.* 2008), presumably due to the diversity in lifestyles and habitats. For example, flying squirrels from both Siberia and North America no longer have colour vision, most probably as a result of switching from diurnality to a nocturnal lifestyle (Carvalho *et al.* 2006). However, the subterranean cururo (*Spalocopus cyanus*), is reported to have dichromatic colour vision with an unusually high proportion of cones in the retina, indicating adaptation to sporadic phases of diurnal surface activity, rather than to the lightless subterranean environment (Peichl *et al.* 2005). Most squirrel species are diurnal with cone-dominated retinas, similar to the primate fovea, and have excellent dichromatic colour vision that is mediated by green and blue cones (Heimel *et al.* 2005; Van Hooser & Nelson 2006). In traditional laboratory rodents, retinal functional development and visual acuity can be improved by environmental enrichment (Prusky *et al.* 2000; Landi *et al.* 2007); presumably, the same could be true of non-traditional laboratory species, indicating that enrichment should be provided to ensure appropriate development of their visual systems.

Perhaps unexpectedly, some subterranean rodents usually considered as 'blind' do respond to light (Wegner *et al.* 2006) and possess different visual capabilities and adaptations (Nemec *et al.* 2007), even if they live in apparently similar optic environments (Burda 2006). African mole-rats possess relatively well developed functional visual subsystems involved in photoperiodicity and used for form and brightness discrimination, but severely reduced subsystems involved in coordination of visuomotor reflexes, indicating the retention of only basic visual capabilities. This residual vision may enable subterranean mole-rats to find breaches in the burrows that let in light, enabling them to reseal such entry points and prevent entry of predators (Nemec *et al.* 2008). Naked mole-rats' eyes are markedly reduced in size, and generally these rodents move about with their eyes closed, suggesting they do not rely on vision. Nevertheless, they have retained most of the well characterised mammalian cell types found in the eye, although their eye's structural organisation is considerably less regular than that in more sighted mammals. The naked mole-rat reportedly cannot perceive images but can detect amorphous light (Hetling *et al.* 2005). Similarly, although the blind mole-rat has subcutaneous eyes and atrophied structures involved with image formation, the non-image-forming visual pathways involved in photoperiod perception are well developed (Xiao *et al.* 2006). The visual capabilities of non-traditional laboratory rodents should be considered by, for example, providing dim shelters or refuges for those species, which might be particularly sensitive to (strong) light. In addition, it should be remembered that even in species shown to be functionally blind, light and dark phases might be required for the animal to express behavioural and physiological periodicity.

There is growing acceptance that to gain valid data and to improve animal welfare, many studies on animals should be conducted during the animal's active phase rather than when the animal is inactive. This can pose a visibility problem for those working with nocturnal species. Dim red light is sometimes used to observe nocturnal behaviour in typical laboratory rodents because it is on the upper limit of the frequencies visible as colour to them (Jacobs *et al.* 2001) and they are thought to be insensitive to this light. However, rats' rod cells are stimulated by similar wavelengths to human rod cells, including red light (Akula *et al.* 2003). As an alternative to red light, sodium lamps, which emit very narrow peaks of yellow–orange (589 and 589.6nm) light, can be used (McLennan & Taylor-Jeffs 2004). Not only is it more visible to humans than red light, but also there were no significant long-term differences between the activity levels of mice when illuminated by this lamp or in darkness. However, if studies unequivocally require rodents to behave as if in total darkness, infrared light should be used. The lighting considerations, given above, also apply for studies using nocturnal non-traditional laboratory rodents.

Ultraviolet vision

Ultraviolet (UV) vision seems to be absent in most mammalian species (Honkavaara *et al.* 2002) although several typical and non-traditional laboratory rodent species are capable of UV vision. These include rats (Akula *et al.* 2003; Jacobs *et al.* 1991, 2001), mice (Jacobs *et al.* 1991, 2004; Szel *et al.* 1992), gerbils (Jacobs *et al.* 1991; Jacobs & Deegan 1994), hamsters (Calderone & Jacobs 1999), gophers (Jacobs *et al.* 1991) and degus (Chavez *et al.* 2003). Within the Sciurognathi (squirrels, chipmunks, beavers and many types of mice), the shortwave-sensitive visual pigments are ultraviolet-sensitive amongst the largely nocturnal murine species, whereas violet-sensitive pigments are thought to be present in diurnal ground and tree squirrels (Carvalho *et al.* 2006). The distribution of the UV-sensitive cones on the retina differs between rodent species. In rats, the cones are scattered over the entire retina, whereas in mice, the middle-wave sensitive cones occur exclusively in the dorsal half of the retina and most of the shortwave UV-sensitive cones occur in the ventral half (Szel *et al.* 1992). The function of this difference is not yet known. The functions of UV vision in rodents are not yet well understood, but include urine-mark visibility (eg, degus, Chavez *et al.* 2003; voles, Koivula *et al.* 1999; mice, Desjardins *et al.* 1973), social communication (degus, Chavez *et al.* 2003) and improved twilight ultraviolet vision (rats, Robitaille & Bovet 1976).

The human-visible spectrum is 400–700nm; the human cornea strongly absorbs in the far UV, below 310nm, and the lens has major absorption (high density) in the near UV and to a lesser extent in the visible (van de Kraats & van Norren 2007; Barber *et al.* 2006). This implies normal adult humans are visually insensitive to UV. As a consequence, artificial lights, including those used widely in laboratories, emit little or no UV. Our lack of knowledge about how rodents use UV sensitivity makes it difficult to say precisely how this lack of UV wavelengths is likely to affect the welfare of UV sensitive rodents, but potentially, it could impair communication and/or distort vision.

Acuity and depth perception

Compared to humans, laboratory rodents, especially albinos, generally have much poorer visual acuity (Creel *et al.* 1970; Prusky *et al.* 2002) and depth perception (O'Sullivan & Spear 1964; Routtenberg & Glickman 1964). It has been estimated that the visual acuity of laboratory rats[2] and gerbils is approximately twice that of mice, but 10 times less than that of humans (Artal *et al.* 1998; Prusky *et al.* 2002). Rats have an enormous depth of focus. Depth of focus is the range of distances at which an object is in equivalent focus for an unacommodated eye. In humans, the depth of focus is from 2.3m to infinity. In rats, the depth of focus is from 7cm to infinity (Powers & Green 1978; Green *et al.* 1980). A gerbil's pupil is positioned vertically in the eye. This is consistent for animals that live in desert or open steppe environments. Having vertical pupils gives the gerbil greater depth perception in the horizontal plain. This enables them to see predators both on the ground and in the air. Visual acuity in African mole-rats is thought to be low (ranging between 0.3 and 0.5 cycles/degree) (Nemec *et al.* 2008). Visual acuity should be considered during handling where a person or hand approaching the animal might very suddenly come into focus, thereby evoking a flight reaction or perhaps aggression.

Summary information for some non-traditional laboratory rodents

Tables 25.2–25.4 provide summary information for seven rodent species that have been used in the laboratory and are likely to be used in the future. The information in these tables is derived from various sources, some of which are websites that have not been peer-reviewed and independent verification has been impossible. These are not necessarily scientific reports but might include information from zoos, breeding societies, or even pet owners. These tables are meant only as an introductory guide for those considering research on the species, and researchers are strongly encouraged to seek the most recent and reliable sources of information available to them (eg, Alderton & Tanner 1999; Nowak 1999; Richardson 2003; Macdonald 2006; Begall *et al.* 2007).

---

[2]Simulated at http://www.ratbehavior.org/RatCam.htm

Table 25.2 Basic biology of some non-traditional laboratory rodents.

Common and scientific name	*Adult weight/size*	*Lifespan*	*Sociality*	*Mating*
Beaver Genus: *Castor*	15–35 kg Beavers continue to grow throughout life	Usually 6–7 years One female lived 21 years	Lives as families Three generations may occupy a single lodge	Monogamous
Naked mole-rat *Heterocephalus glaber*	30–35 g Queen is larger – up to 80 g	28 years Queen 13–18 years	Eusocial Groups of 75–80, but up to 300	Polyandry and male monogamy Single queen mates with harem of 1–3 males
Capybara 'water pig' *Hydrochaeris hydrochaeris*	Average of 40 kg but up to 66 kg. Largest living rodent	10 years in captivity	Mainly herds of 10–40. Single dominant male High incidence of infanticide in captivity	
Coypu (Nutria) 'mouse-beaver' *Myocastor coypus*	Up to 16 kg	12 years in captivity	Single dominant male Groups of approx. 11	Polygymous Induced ovulation
Degu *Octodon degu* Bite leaves an eight-sided mark	200–300 g	4–6 years in captivity	Highly social Groups of 2–5 females and 1–2 males	Harems, but also reported that degus pair for life Induced ovulation
Fat sand rat *Psammomys obesus*	14–19 cm Tail up to 15 cm		Solitary Communal nest	
Chinchilla *Chinchillidae*	600–800 g 35 cm long	15–20 years	Colony Can be kept as same-sex groups but might fight	Breed any time of the year

Table 25.3 Lifestyles of some non-traditional laboratory rodents.

Common and scientific name	*Activity*	*Habitat*	*Diet*	*Home range or territory*
Beaver Genus: *Castor*	Mainly nocturnal	Semi-aquatic Builds lodges in ponds or burrows in banks	Herbivorous (one report of opportunistically eating salmon)	Approx. 1 km of waterway
Naked mole-rat *Heterocephalus glaber*	Nocturnal	Solely subterranean Digs burrows with teeth 25% of an individual's muscle mass is involved in jaw closure	Radicivores May eat dead pups	Tunnel system can be 4 km in length, 20 football fields in area
Capybara 'water pig' *Hydrochaeris hydrochaeris*	Naturally diurnal, but nocturnal in disturbed areas	Semi-aquatic Builds burrows in banks May cover itself in mud to protect from sunburn	Herbivorous/ graminivorous Copraphagous	10–200 ha
Coypu (Nutria) 'mouse-beaver' *Myocastor coypus*	Nocturnal or crepuscular	Semi-aquatic Digs short burrows May also build floating nests of reeds and other aquatic plants	Herbivorous Reports of eating fish, earthworms, and bivalve molluscs	
Degu *Octodon degu* Bite leaves an eight-sided mark	Crepuscular in summer, diurnal in winter Diurnal in captivity	Semi-fossorial Digs burrows with teeth and front feet	Herbivorous	0.04–0.71 ha
Fat sand rat *Psammomys obesus*	Mainly diurnal	Semi-fossorial Complex burrow system	Largely herbivorous, occasional insects	75–190 m tunnel system
Chinchilla *Chinchillidae*	Crepuscular Nocturnal	Burrows or crevices in rocks Dustbathes regularly	Largely herbivorous, occasional insects	

Table 25.4 Scientific uses of some non-traditional laboratory rodents.

Common and scientific name	*Uses in science*
Beaver Genus: *Castor*	Diving physiology
Naked mole-rat *Heterocephalus glaber*	Unique metabolism Magnetoreception Nociception Only known mammals to be poikilothermic No sweat glands Does not produce the neurotransmitter substance P
Capybara 'water pig' *Hydrochaeris hydrochaeris*	Diving physiology
Coypu (Nutria) 'mouse-beaver' *Myocastor coypus*	Diving physiology
Degu *Octodon degu* Bite leaves an eight-sided mark	Prone to diabetes Cannot produce vitamin C Chronobiology
Fat sand rat *Psammomys obesus*	Prone to obesity and diabetes Highly efficient kidneys
Chinchilla *Chinchillidae*	Hearing Digestion

References

Akula, J.D., Lyubarsky, A.L. and Naarendorp, F. (2003) The sensitivity and spectral identity of the cones driving the b-wave of the rat electroretinogram. *Visual Neuroscience*, **20**, 109–117

Alderton, D. and Tanner, B. (1999) *Rodents of the World*. Cassell Illustrated, London

Artal, P, de Tejada, P.H., Tedo, C.M. *et al.* (1998) Retinal image quality in the rodent eye. *Visual Neuroscience*, **15**, 597–605

Barber, C.L., Prescott, N.B., Jarvis, J.R. *et al.* (2006) Comparative study of the photopic spectral sensitivity of domestic ducks (*Anas platyrhynchos domesticus*), turkeys (*Meleagris gallopavo gallopavo*) and humans. *British Poultry Science*, **47**, 365–374

Bargmann, C.I. (2006) Comparative chemosensation from receptors to ecology. *Nature*, **444**, 295–301

Begall, S., Burda, H. and Schleich, C.E. (2007) *Subterranean Rodents: News from Underground*. Springer, New York

Beynon, R.J. and Hurst, J.L. (2003) Multiple roles of major urinary proteins in the house mouse, *Mus domesticus*. *Biochemical Society Transactions*, **31**, 142–146

Bobu, C., Lahmam, M., Vuillez, P. *et al.* (2008) Photoreceptor organisation and phenotypic characterization in retinas of two diurnal rodent species: potential use as experimental animal models for human vision research. *Vision Research*, **48**, 424–432

Borgo, J.S., Conner, L.M. and Conover, M.R. (2006) Role of predator odor in roost site selection of southern flying squirrels. *Wildlife Society Bulletin*, **34**, 144–149

Brennan, P.A. and Keverne, E.B. (2004) Something in the air? New insights into mammalian pheromones. *Current Biology*, **14**, R81–R89

Burda, H. (2006) Ear and eye in subterranean mole-rats, *Fukomys anselli* (Bathyergidae) and *Spalax ehrenbergi* (Spalacidae): progressive specialisation or regressive degeneration? *Animal Biology*, **56**, 475–486

Burgstahler, A.W., Freeman, R.F. and Jacobs, P.N. (2008) Toxic effects of silicofluoridated water in chinchillas, caimans, alligators, and rats held in captivity. *Fluoride*, **41**, 83–88

Burn, C.C. (2008) What is it like to be a rat? Rat sensory perception and its implications for experimental design and rat welfare. *Applied Animal Behaviour Science*, **112**, 1–32

Calderone, J.B. and Jacobs, G.H. (1999) Cone receptor variations and their functional consequences in two species of hamster. *Visual Neuroscience*, **16**, 53–63

Carvalho, L.D., Cowing, J.A., Wilkie, S.E. *et al.* (2006) Shortwave visual sensitivity in tree and flying squirrels reflects changes in lifestyle *Current Biology*, **16**, R81–R83

Cernuda-Cernuda, R., DeGrip, W.J., Cooper, H.M. *et al.* (2002) The retina of Spalax ehrenbergi: novel histologic features supportive of a modified photosensory role. *Investigative Ophthalmology and Visual Science*, **43**, 2374–2383

Chavez, A.E., Bozinovic, F., Peichl, L. *et al.* (2003) Retinal spectral sensitivity, fur coloration, and urine reflectance in the genus *Octodon* (Rodentia): Implications for visual ecology. *Investigative Ophthalmology and Visual Science*, **44**, 2290–2296

Clough, G. (1982) Environmental effects on animals used in biomedical research. *Biological Reviews*, **57**, 487–523

Cooper, H.M., Herbin, M. and Nevo, E. (1993) Visual system of a naturally microphthalmic mammal: the blind mole rat, *Spalax ehrenbergi*. *Journal of Comparative Neurology*, **328**, 313–350

Creel, D.J., Dustman, R.E. and Beck, E.C. (1970) Differences in visually evoked responses in albino *versus* hooded rats. *Experimental Neurology*, **29**, 246–260

Davis, W.B. and Schmidley, D.J. (1997) Northern Grasshopper Mouse. In: *The Mammals of Texas – Online Version*. Texas Tech University, Texas http://www.nsrl.ttu.edu/tmot1/onycleuc.htm (accessed 6 August 2008)

Delporte, C., Backhouse, N., Inostroza, V. *et al.* (2007) Analgesic activity of Ugni molinae (murtilla) in mice models of acute pain. *Journal of Ethnopharmacology*, **112**, 162–165

Desjardins, C., Maruniak, J.A. and Bronson, F.H. (1973) Social rank in house mice – differentiation revealed by ultraviolet visualisation of urinary marking patterns. *Science*, **182**, 939–941

Deutschlander, M.E., Freake, M.J., Borland, S.C. *et al.* (2003) Learned magnetic compass orientation by the Siberian hamster, *Phodopus sungorus*. *Animal Behaviour*, **65**, 779–786

Dobner, P.R. (2006) Neurotensin and pain modulation. *Peptides*, **27**, 2405–2414

Ehret, G. (2005) Infant rodent ultrasounds – a gate to the understanding of sound communication. *Behavioral Genetics*, **35**, 19–29

Fanjul, M.S., Zenuto, R.R. and Busch, C. (2003) Use of olfaction for sexual recognition in the subterranean rodent *Ctenomys talarum*. *Acta Theriologica*, **48**, 35–46

Folk, G.E., Thrift, D.L., Zimmerman, M.B. *et al.* (2006) Mammalian activity–rest rhythms in Arctic continuous daylight. *Biological Rhythm Research*, **37**, 455–469

Forsman, K.A. and Malmquist, M.G. (1988) Evidence for echolocation in the common shrew. *Journal of Zoology*, **216**, 655–662

Fox, A., Gentry, C., Patel, S. *et al.* (2003) Comparative activity of the anti-convulsants oxcarbazepine, carbamazepine, lamotrigine and gabapentin in a model of neuropathic pain in the rat and guinea-pig. *Pain*, **105**, 355–362

Gibbs, S.E.B., Lea, S.E.G. and Jacobs, L.F. (2007) Flexible use of spatial cues in the southern flying squirrel (*Glaucomys volans*). *Animal Cognition*, **10**, 203–209

Green, D.G., Powers, M.K. and Banks, M.S. (1980) Depth of focus, eye size and visual acuity. *Vision Research*, **20**, 827–835

Hamernik, R.P., Qiu, W. and Davis, B. (2008) The effectiveness of N-acetyl-L-CySteine (L-NAC) in the prevention of severe noise-induced hearing loss. *Hearing Research*, **239**, 99–106

Heimel, J.A., Van Hooser, S.D. and Nelson, S.B. (2005) Laminar organization of response properties in primary visual cortex of the gray squirrel (*Sciurus carolinensis*). *Journal of Neurophysiology*, **94**, 3538–3554

Hetling, J.R., Baig-Silva, M.S., Comer, C.M. *et al.* (2005) Features of visual function in the naked mole-rat Heterocephalus glaber. *Journal of Comparative Physiology A – Sensory Neural and Behavioral Physiology*, **191**, 317–730

Holmes, M.M., Rosen, G.J., Jordan, C.L. *et al.* (2007) Social control of brain morphology in a eusocial mammal. *Proceedings of the National Academy of Sciences of the United States of America*, **104**, 10548–10552

Honkavaara, J., Koivula, M., Korpimaki, E. *et al.* (2002) Ultraviolet vision and foraging in terrestrial vertebrates. *Oikos*, **98**, 504–510

Huck, U.W. and Banks, E.M. (1984) Social olfaction in male brown lemmings (*Lemmus sibiricus*) and collared lemmings (*Dicrostonyx groenlandicus*). 1. discrimination of species, sex, and estrous condition. *Journal of Comparative Psychology*, **98**, 54–59

Humphries, R.E., Robertson, D.H.L., Beynon, R.J. *et al.* (1999) Unravelling the chemical basis of competitive scent marking in house mice. *Animal Behaviour*, **58**, 1177–1190

Hurst, J.L. (1999) Introduction to rodents. In: *The UFAW Handbook on the Care and Management of Laboratory Animals, Vol. 1, Terrestrial Vertebrates*, 7th edn. Ed. Poole, T., pp. 262–273. Blackwell Publishing, Oxford

Hurst, J.L. and Beynon, R.J. (2004) Scent wars: the chemobiology of competitive signalling in mice. *Bioessays*, **26**, 1288–1298

Jacobs, G.H. (1993) The distribution and nature of colour vision among the mammals. *Biological Reviews*, **68**, 413–471

Jacobs, G.H. and Deegan, J. (1994) Sensitivity to ultraviolet light in the gerbil (*Meriones unguiculatus*): characteristics and mechanisms. *Vision Research*, **34**, 1433–1441

Jacobs, G.H., Fenwick, J.A. and Williams, G.A. (2001) Cone-based vision of rats for ultraviolet and visible lights. *Journal of Experimental Biology*, **204**, 2439–2446

Jacobs, G.H., Neitz, J. and Deegan, J.F. (1991) Retinal receptors in rodents maximally sensitive to ultraviolet light. *Nature*, **353**, 655–656

Jacobs, G.H., Williams, G.A. and Fenwick, J.A. (2004) Influence of cone pigment coexpression on spectral sensitivity and color vision in the mouse. *Vision Research*, **44**, 1615–1622

Kalcounis-Rueppell, M.C., Metheny, J.D. and Vonhof, M.J. (2006) Production of ultrasonic vocalizations by Peromyscus mice in the wild. *Frontiers in Zoology*, **3**, 3

Kaltwasser, M.T. and Schnitzler, H.U. (1981) Echolocation signals confirmed in rats: zeitschrift für saugetierkunde. *International Journal of Mammalian Biology*, **46**, 394–395

Kimchi, T., Etienne, A.S. and Terkel, J. (2004) A subterranean mammal uses the magnetic compass for path integration. *Proceedings of the National Academy of Sciences of the United States of America*, **101**, 1105–1109

Kimchi, T., Reshef, M. and Terkel, J. (2005) Evidence for the use of reflected self-generated seismic waves for spatial orientation in a blind subterranean mammal. *Journal of Experimental Biology*, **208**, 647–659

Koivula, M., Koskela, E. and Viitala, J. (1999) Sex and age-specific differences in ultraviolet reflectance of scent marks of bank voles (*Clethrionomys glareolus*). *Journal of Comparative Physiology A – Sensory Neural and Behavioral Physiology*, **185**, 561–564

Labruna, M.B., Pinter, A. and Teixeira, R.H.F. (2004) *Life cycle of Amblyomma cooperi (Acari Ixodidae)* using capybaras (*Hydrochaeris hydrochaeris*) as hosts. *Experimental and Applied Acarology*, **32**, 79–88

Lai, W.S., Ramiro, L.L.R., Yu, H.A. *et al.* (2005) Recognition of familiar individuals in golden hamsters: A new method and functional neuroanatomy. *Journal of Neuroscience*, **25**, 11239–11247

Landi, S., Sale, A., Berardi, N. *et al.* (2007) Retinal functional development is sensitive to environmental enrichment: a role for BDNF. *The Federation of American Societies for Experimental Biology Journal*, **21**, 130–139

Lluch, S., Ventura, J. and Lopez-Fuster, M.J. (2008) Eye morphology in some wild rodents. *Anatomia Histologia Embryologia*, **37**, 41–51

Lonstein, J.S. and Gammie, S.C. (2002) Sensory, hormonal, and neural control of maternal aggression in laboratory rodents. *Neuroscience and Biobehavioral Reviews*, **26**, 869–888

Macdonald, D.W. (2006) *The Encyclopedia of Mammals*, 2nd revised edn. Oxford University Press, Oxford

Macdonald, D.W. (1984) *The Encyclopedia of Animals*, Vol **2**. George Allen and Unwin, London

Marabese, I., de Novellis, V., Palazzo, E. *et al.* (2007) Effects of (S)-3, 4-DCPG, an mGlu8 receptor agonist, on inflammatory and neuropathic pain in mice. *Neuropharmacology*, **52**, 253–262

Maras, P.M. and Petrulis, A. (2008) Olfactory experience and the development of odor preference and vaginal marking in female Syrian hamsters. *Physiology and Behavior*, **94**, 545–551

Marchlewska-Koj, A., Kruczek, M. and Olejniczak, P. (2003) Mating behaviour of bank voles (*Clethrionomys glareolus*) modified by hormonal and social factors. *Mammalian Biology*, **68**, 144–152

Marhold, S., Wiltschko, W. and Burda, H. (1997) A magnetic polarity compass for direction finding in a subterranean mammal. *Naturwissenschaften*, **84**, 421–423

Marounek, M., Skrivan, M., Brezina, P. *et al.* (2005) Digestive organs, caecal metabolites and fermentation pattern in coypus (*Myocastor coypus*) and rabbits (*Oryctolagus cuniculus*). *Acta Veterinaria Brno*, **74**, 3–7

Mateo, J.M. (2008) Inverted-U shape relationship between cortisol and learning in ground squirrels. *Neurobiology of Learning and Memory*, **8**, 582–590

McKean, T. (1982) Cardiovascular adjustments to laboratory diving in beavers and nutria. *American Journal of Physiology*, **242**, R434–R440

McLennan, I.S. and Taylor-Jeffs, J. (2004) The use of sodium lamps to brightly illuminate mouse houses during their dark phases. *Laboratory Animals*, **38**, 384–392

Menzies, R.A., Heth, G., Ikan, R. *et al.* (1992) Sexual pheromones in lipids and other fractions from urine of the male mole rat, *Spalax-ehrenbergi*. *Physiology and Behavior*, **52**, 741–747

Meyer, J., Klemann, N. and Halle, S. (2005) Diurnal activity patterns of coypu in an urban habitat. *Acta Theriologica*, **50**, 207–211

Muheim, R., Edgar, N.M., Sloan, K.A. *et al.* (2006) Magnetic compass orientation in C57BL/6J mice. *Learning and Behaviour*, **34**, 366–373

Muller, M., Laube, B., Burda, H. *et al.* (1992) Structure and function of the cochlea in the African mole rat (*Cryptomys-hottentotus*) – evidence for a low-frequency acoustic fovea. *Journal of Comparative Physiology A – Sensory and Neural Behavioural Physiology*, **171**, 469–476

Myers, P. (2000) *Rodentia* (On-line), Animal Diversity Web. http://animaldiversity.ummz.umich.edu/site/accounts/information/Rodentia.html

Nemec, P., Cvekova, P., Burda, H. *et al.* (2007) Visual Systems and the role of vision in subterranean rodents: diversity of retinal properties and visual system designs. In: *Subterranean Rodents – News from Underground*. Eds Begall, S., Burda, H. and Schleich, C.E., pp. 129–160. Springer, Heidelberg

Nemec, P., Cvekova, P., Benada, O. *et al.* (2008) The visual system in subterranean African mole-rats (Rodentia, Bathyergidae): retina, subcortical visual nuclei and primary visual cortex. *Brain Research Bulletin*, **75**, 356–364

Novotny, M.V. (2003) Pheromones, binding proteins and receptor responses in rodents. *Biochemical Society Transactions*, **31**, 117–122

Nowak, R.M. (1999) *Walker's Mammals of the World*, 6th edn. Baltimore, Johns Hopkins University Press

Oikawa, T., Shimammura, K. and Saito, T.R. (1994) Fine-structure of the vomeronasal organ in the chinchilla (*Chinchilla laniger*). *Experimental Animals*, **43**, 487–497

Olsson, I.A.S., Nevison, C.M., Patterson-Kane, E. *et al.* (2003) Understanding behaviour: the relevance of ethological approaches in laboratory animal science. *Applied Animal Behaviour Science*, **81**, 245–264

Ortiz, J.O., Rodriguez-Lanetty, M. and Bubis, J. (2008) Purification and characterization of transducin from capybara Hydrochoerus hydrochaeris. *Comparative Biochemistry and Physiology B – Biochemistry and Molecular Biology*, **149**, 22–28

O'Sullivan, D.J. and Spear, N.E. (1964) Comparison of hooded and albino rats on the visual cliff. *Psychonomic Science*, **1**, 87–88

Park, T.J., Comer, C., Carol, A. *et al.* (2003) Somatosensory organization and behavior in naked mole-rats: II. Peripheral structures, innervation, and selective lack of neuropeptides associated with thermoregulation and pain. *Journal of Comparative Neurology*, **465**, 104–120

Park, T.J., Lu, Y., Juttner, R. *et al.* (2008) Selective inflammatory pain insensitivity in the African naked mole-rat (*Heterocephalus glaber*). *Public Library of Science; Biology*, **6**, 156–170

Peichl, L. (2005) Diversity of mammalian photoreceptor properties: adaptations to habitat and lifestyle? *Anatomical Record Part A – Discoveries In Molecular Cellular And Evolutionary Biology*, **287A**, 1001–1012

Peichl, L., Chavez, A.E., Ocampo, A. *et al.* (2005) Eye and vision in the subterranean rodent cururo (*Spalacopus cyanus, Octodontidae*). *Journal of Comparative Neurology*, **486**, 197–208

Pelissier, T., Saavedra, H., Bustamante, D. *et al.* (1989) Further studies on the understanding of Octodon degus natural resistance to morphine: A comparative study with the Wistar rat. *Comparative Biochemistry and Physiology*, **92**, 319–322

Powers, M.K. and Green, D.G. (1978) Single retinal ganglion cell responses in the dark-reared rat: grating acuity, contrast sensitivity, and defocusing. *Vision Research*, **18**, 1533–1539

Prusky, G.T., Harker, K.T., Douglas, R.M. *et al.* (2002) Variation in visual acuity within pigmented, and between pigmented and albino rat strains. *Behavioural Brain Research*, **136**, 339–348

Prusky, G.T., Reidel, C. and Douglas, R.M. (2000) Environmental enrichment from birth enhances visual acuity but not place learning in mice. *Behavioural Brain Research*, **114**, 11–15

Pyare, S. and Longland, W.S. (2001) Mechanisms of truffle detection by northern flying squirrels. *Canadian Journal of Zoology – Revue Canadienne De Zoologie*, **79**, 1007–1015

Rabon, D.R., Sawrey, D.K. and Webster, W.D. (2001) Infant ultrasonic vocalizations and parental responses in two species of voles (*Microtus*). *Canadian Journal of Zoology – Revue Canadienne De Zoologie*, **79**, 830–837

Rado, R., Levi, N., Hauser, H. *et al.* (1987) Seismic signalling as a means of communication in a subterranean mammal. *Animal Behaviour*, **35**, 1249–1251

Randall, J.A. (2001) Evolution and function of drumming as communication in mammals. *American Zoologist*, **41**, 1143–1156

Richardson, V. (2003) *Diseases of Small Domestic Rodents (Library of Veterinary Practice)*. Blackwell Publishing, Oxford

Robitaille, J.A. and Bovet, J. (1976) Field observations on social behavior of Norway rat, *Rattus norvegicus* (Berkenhout). *Biology of Behaviour*, **1**, 289–308

Rosell, F. (2002) Do Eurasian beavers smear their pelage with castoreum and anal gland secretion? *Journal of Chemical Ecology*, **28**, 1697–1701

Rosell, F. and Sanda, J. (2006) Potential risks of olfactory signaling: the effect of predators on scent marking by beavers. *Behavioral Ecology*, **17**, 897–904

Rosell, F. and Thomsen, L.R. (2006) Sexual dimorphism in territorial scent marking by adult Eurasian beavers (*Castor fiber*). *Journal of Chemical Ecology*, **32**, 1301–1315

Routtenberg, A. and Glickman, S.E. (1964) Visual cliff behavior in albino and hooded rats. *Journal of Comparative Physiology and Psychology*, **58**, 140–142

Rundus, A.S., Owings, D.H., Joshi, S.S. *et al.* (2007) Ground squirrels use an infrared signal to deter rattlesnake predation. *Proceedings of the National Academy of Science of the United States of America*, **104**, 14372–14376

Sales, G.D., Milligan, S.R. and Khirnykh, K. (1999) Sources of sound in the laboratory animal environment: a survey of the sounds produced by procedures and equipment. *Animal Welfare*, **8**, 97–115

Scantlebury, M., Speakman, J.R., Oosthuizen, M.K. *et al.* (2006) Energetics reveals physiologically distinct castes in a eusocial mammal. *Nature*, **440**, 795–797

Shera, C.A., Tubis, A. and Talmadge, C.L. (2008) Testing coherent reflection in chinchilla: Auditory-nerve responses predict stimulus-frequency emissions. *Journal of the Acoustic Society of America*, **124**, 381–395

Sherwin, C.M. (2002) Comfortable quarters for mice. In: *Comfortable Quarters for Animals*. Eds Reinhardt V. and Reinhardt K., pp. 6–17. Animal Welfare Institute, Washington. http://www.awionline.org/pubs/cq02/cqindex.html (accessed 6 August 2008)

Sherwin, C.M. (2004) The influences of standard laboratory cages on rodents and the validity of research data. *Animal Welfare*, **13**, S9–15

Shier, D.M. and Randall, J.A. (2007) Use of different signaling modalities to communicate status by dominant and subordinate Heermann's kangaroo rats (*Dipodomys heermanni*). *Behavioral Ecology and Sociobiology*, **61**, 1023–1032

Smith, T.D., Bhatnagar, K.P., Dennis, J.C. *et al.* (2007) Growth-deficient vomeronasal organs in the naked mole-rat (*Heterocephalus glaber*). *Brain Research*, **1132**, 78–83

Szel, A., Rohlich, P., Caffe, A.R. *et al.* (1992) Unique topographic separation of two spectral classes of cones in the mouse retina. *Journal of Comparative Neurology*, **325**, 327–342

Szentgyorgyi, H., Kapusta, J. and Marchlewska-Koj, A. (2008) Ultrasonic calls of bank vole pups isolated and exposed to cold or to nest odor. *Physiology and Behavior*, **93**, 296–303

Towett, P.K., Kanui, T.I. and Juma, F.D. (2006) Stimulation of mu and delta opioid receptors induces hyperalgesia while stimulation of kappa receptors induces antinociception in the hot plate test in the naked mole-rat (*Heterocephalus glaber*). *Brain Research Bulletin*, **71**, 60–68

van de Kraats, J. and van Norren, D. (2007) Optical density of the aging human ocular media in the visible and the UV. *Journal of the Ophthalmology Society of America*, **24**, 1842–1857

Van Hooser, S.D., Heimel, J.A. and Nelson, S.B. (2005) Functional cell classes and functional architecture in the early visual system of a highly visual rodent. *Progress in Brain Research*, **149**, 127–145

Van Hooser, S.D. and Nelson, S.B. (2006) The squirrel as a rodent model of the human visual system. *Vision Neurobiology*, **23**, 765–778

Vissers, K.C.P., Geenen, F., Biermans, R. *et al.* (2006) Pharmacological correlation between the formalin test and the neuropathic pain behavior in different species with chronic constriction injury. *Pharmacology, Biochemistry and Behavior*, **84**, 479–486

Wegner, R.E., Begall S. and Burda, H. (2006) Light perception in 'blind' subterranean Zambian mole-rats. *Animal Behaviour*, **72**, 1021–1024

Wei, D.B., Wei, L., Zhang, J.M. *et al.* (2006) Blood-gas properties of plateau zokor (*Myospalax baileyi*). *Comparative Biochemistry and Physiology A – Molecular and Integrative Physiology*, **145**, 372–375

Weil, Z.M., Martin, L.B. and Nelson, R.J. (2006) Photoperiod differentially affects immune function and reproduction in collared lemmings (*Dicrostonyx groenlandicus*). *Journal of Biological Rhythms*, **21**, 384–393

Werner, F.A., Ledesma, K.J. and Hidalgo, R.B. (2006) Mountain vizcacha (*Lagidium* cf. *peruanum*) in Ecuador – first record of Chinchillidae from the Northern Andes. *Mastozoología Neotropical*, **13**, 271–274

Wilson, D.R. and Hare, J.F. (2004) Ground squirrel uses ultrasonic alarms. *Nature*, **430**, 523

Wilson, D.E. and Reeder, D.M. (eds) (2005) *Mammal Species of the World: A Taxonomic and Geographic Reference*, 3rd edn. Johns Hopkins University Press, Baltimore

Wohr, M. and Schwarting, R.K.W. (2008) Maternal care, isolation-induced infant ultrasonic calling, and their relations to adult anxiety-related behavior in the rat. *Behavioral Neuroscience*, **122**, 310–330

Wolff, J.O. (2004) Scent marking by voles in response to predation risk: a field-laboratory validation. *Behavioral Ecology*, **15**, 286–289

Xiao, J., Levitt, J.B. and Buffenstein, R. (2006) The use of a novel and simple method of revealing neural fibers to show the regression of the lateral geniculate nucleus in the naked mole-rat (*Heterocephalus glaber*). *Brain Research*, **1077**, 81–89

Zenuto, R.R., Fanjul, M.S. and Busch, C. (2004) Use of chemical communication by the subterranean rodent *Ctenomys talarum* (tuco-tuco) during the breeding season. *Journal of Chemical Ecology*, **30**, 2111–2126

Zhao, H., Bucci, D.J., Weltzin, M. *et al.* (2004) Effects of aversive stimuli on learning and memory in Arctic ground squirrels. *Behavioural Brain Research*, **151**, 219–224

Zuri, I., Fishelson, L. and Terkel, J. (1998) Morphology and cytology of the nasal cavity and vomeronasal organ in juvenile and adult blind mole rats (*Spalax ehrenbergi*). *Anatomical Record*, **251**, 460–471

Zuri, I., Gazit, I. and Terkel, J. (1997) Effect of scent-marking in delaying territorial invasion in the blind mole-rat, *Spalax ehrenbergi*. *Behaviour*, **134**, 867–880

26 Voles

Jonathan J. Cooper

Origins

Voles belong to the sub-family Arvicolinae (comprising voles, lemmings and muskrats) within the family Cricetedae of the Rodentia. It is thought that the Cricetids originated in the Eurasia during the mid-Miocene epoch, from ancestors that resemble modern squirrels. The voles themselves arose during the Pliocene epoch, and rapidly diversified during the Pleistocene. There are now about 70 species to be found in grassland, open forest and tundra. Voles are Paleartic and Neartic in distribution being found in Europe, Asia, Northern Africa and North America. The most numerous genus in terms of species is the Microtidae, which includes the field vole (*Microtus agrestis*), one of the most common mammals of north-west Europe and the prairie vole (*Microtus ochrogaster)* of North America (Musser & Carleton 2005). Other genera include *Avicola*, the water voles, and *Myodes* (formally *Clethrionomys*) including the red-backed voles, such as the bank vole (*Myodes glareolus*).

Biological overview

General biology

Voles are often confused with mice. Voles have been classified as Muridae (rats, mice and their relatives) (MacDonald 2001) and some species are locally described as mice. For example, the meadow vole (*Microtus pensylvanicus*) of North America is often called the field or meadow mouse. Compared with mice, voles tend to have a stouter body, a shorter hairy tail, a rounder head with a blunt snout, and smaller ears and eyes. They tend to be grey–brown to reddish brown in colour often with paler grey or silvery fur on the underside. Whilst some species such as water voles can be considerably larger, most vole species maintained under laboratory conditions are about the size of mice. For example, adult field or short-tailed voles have a body approximately 90–110 mm long and weigh between 20 and 40 g, whilst bank voles are between 80 and 120 mm long, weighing between 15 g and 40 g.

A distinguishing feature of voles is their molars which, unlike those of many rodents, are rootless and continue to grow during their entire life. Superficially many vole species appear similar, but their teeth can be used both to identify modern and ancestral species. For this reason, they can be useful to archaeologists for dating strata, in a method referred to as the 'vole clock'. The technique is based on extraction of vole teeth from substrates. Most vole species can be identified by the structure and patterns of wear on their cheek or molar teeth, and distribution of ancestral species can be used to date sediments (Jernvall *et al.* 2000). Voles are largely herbivorous and their teeth structure allows them to chew large quantities of abrasive grasses. The diet of the field vole, a largely grassland species, consists for the most part of green leaves and stems of grass, herbs, sedges and bark, whilst the bank vole, which is associated with woodland habitats, has a more varied diet of grass, flowers, fruits, seeds, leaves, roots, fungi, moss, insects and worms (Flowerdew *et al.* 1985; Harris & Yalden 2008).

Reproduction

In the wild, many vole species have a high population turnover, with few individuals surviving from one year to the next (Chitty 1952, 1996). They have a large number of natural enemies, including most carnivores, such as foxes, cats, weasels and stoats, birds of prey and owls. Average lifespan is in the order of 3–6 months and it is rare for wild voles to live for longer than 12 months, though laboratory colonies can include individuals over 18 months of age (Cooper *et al.* 1996). Voles are more active at night than during the daytime, though daytime activity can still be noticeable in the wild and the laboratory setting. Voles do not hibernate, and will continue to be active beneath lying snow. They are capable of rapid population growth in favourable conditions, and exhibit large cyclic fluctuations in population density similar to those of the closely related lemmings (Chitty 1996). Voles breed from early spring until early autumn, and their gonads are generally in a much less active state in the late autumn and winter, when they are not usually fertile. In the wild, voles do not normally have an oestrous cycle, though this can be induced under laboratory conditions by housing females in close visual contact with adult males. Ovulation in voles is normally caused by stimuli provided by mating and occurs 6–12 h later. There are normally two components of the mating process, one causing ovulation and another causing corpora lutea to become functional (Clarke 1985). Gestation lasts 16–28 days depending on species.

Vole infants or pups are altritial being born blind, hairless and heavily dependent on maternal care. Nestling voles use ultrasonic vocalisations to communicate with their mother. These signals include distress calls, which change with the developmental stage, and with ambient and body temperature (Blake 1992). Maturation is rapid with many species weaning pups within 3 weeks of age. Voles reach sexual maturity soon afterwards. For example, male field voles are sexually mature by the age of 6–7 weeks, whilst females are sexually mature by 4 weeks of age (Spears & Clarke 1987). Female field voles have, however, been known to have perforate vaginas, and to be capable of conceiving at the age of 18 days (Chitty 1952). On weaning, most vole species are solitary and do not form stable reproductive pairs. Males are promiscuous or polygamous and court females for as long as is necessary to successfully mate. There is no paternal care of the young, whereas females are highly protective of their pups.

The prairie vole is a notable exception with regard to reproduction. These voles naturally live in multigenerational family groups with a single breeding pair. The offspring remain sexually suppressed so long as they remain within their natal group, and sexual maturity in the females (rather than developing with age as with other voles) depends on exposure to chemical cues in the urine of an unrelated male. Within 24 h of this cue, repeated mating can occur and following this they form a long-lasting relationship in which they tend to be monogamous, and the males share in the raising of pups (Insel 1997; Roberts *et al.* 1998).

Sources of supply

If it is not possible to obtain breeding stock from an established laboratory colony, a new colony can be started with voles caught from the wild, though it may take about 3 months for the wild-caught animals to begin producing litters. Voles can be easily caught in their natural habitats, using 'Longworth' traps (Gurnell & Flowerdew 1982). Traps should be baited with cereals such as rolled oats or whole wheat grain, and fresh, succulent, vegetable matter such as discs of carrot. A bedding material such as hay should be provided in the trap's nest box. It is advisable to cover the traps with foliage, or if that is sparse, with a small amount of hay, to give insulation against extremes of climate. Such traps will also catch shrews which soon die unless reasonable precautions are taken. Blowfly (*Calliphora*) puparia are adequate for overnight survival of shrews, or a small hole can be made in the trap which allows escape of shrews but not the larger rodents. Such precautions are not only in the interest of animal welfare but are a legal requirement in many countries (Little & Gurnell 1989). As with any other forms of live trapping, permission should be sought from landowners, and it is advisable to liaise with local ecology or naturalist groups.

Uses in the laboratory

Whilst not as common a laboratory animal as mice and rats, voles have been housed under laboratory conditions for a number of purposes, including studies of reproductive biology, disease and behavioural biology. Voles have been used in the laboratory to investigate problems bearing on their population ecology, for example their bioenergetics as well as various aspects of their reproductive biology (Leslie & Ranson 1940; Clarke 1985). There is also considerable interest in the ecto- and endoparasites of voles (eg, Kaplan *et al.* 1980; Randolph 1995). Voles have been intensively studied since they appear to be the reservoir hosts of cowpox virus (Crouch *et al.* 1995; Burthe *et al.* 2008). The occurrence in *M. agrestis* of very large sex chromosomes has encouraged their use in studies upon heterochromatin (Kalscheuer *et al.* 1996). Voles have also been employed in the hope that they would prove useful for detecting the accumulation in herbivores of toxic minerals in herbage (Beardsley *et al.* 1978). Voles have been used to investigate rodent communication and have been used as a model to investigate the control of behaviour (Fentress 1968). Bank voles have been used in the investigation of the causes and effects of stereotypic behaviour in captive animals (Ödberg 1987).

Prairie voles and meadow voles have been used to investigate genetic and hormonal factors involved in sexual fidelity. Male prairie voles show some variation in tendency to monogamy. Extra-pair copulations can occur and the likelihood of engaging in such behaviour has been related to genetic and physiological factors (Ophir *et al.* 2008). Those males most likely to be monogamous and engage in paternal care have longer strings of repetitions of microsatellite DNA (Hammock & Young 2005). Microsatellite DNA from prairie voles has been inserted into the genome of meadow voles and found to reduce promiscuity and increase pair-bonding behaviour in males (Lim *et al.* 2004). Similarly the hormonal control of sexual fidelity involving vasopressin, oxytocin and dopamine has been investigated by manipulating their levels in male prairie voles (Cushing *et al.* 2001; Young *et al.* 2005). Finally, prairie voles have been promoted as a model for anxiety and depression (Kim & Kirkpatrick 1996; Grippo 2009) as socially isolating adult females leads to elevated corticosteroid concentrations, prolonged sensitivity to stress-inducing challenges, and affects their performance in tests of negative affective state.

Laboratory management and breeding

The bulk of this section will concentrate on laboratory management of the short-tailed field vole (*Microtus agrestis*) and the bank vole (*Myodes glareolus*). The chapter will cover their basic biology, care and management in laboratory conditions, as well as application of laboratory procedures to these species. The chapter will illustrate issues that arise from the captive rearing of rodent species which have not been intentionally selected for laboratory conditions.

Housing, environmental provisions, hygiene

Physical environment

As with other laboratory rodents it is important that voles be housed in controlled, secure, protected environments, with reliable access to food, water, shelter and/or nesting materials, where risks of infection are minimised and avoiding extremes of climatic variation. Vole rooms should be designed to provide suitable enclosures for the animals, ease of management and safety for the researchers. A well designed room should minimise disturbing noises, and be able to maintain constant temperature and humidity. A temperature of 20 °C and relative humidity of about 60%, with 15–20 changes of warm air per hour is an adequate atmosphere for a vole colony. A photoperiod of 16 h light per day is appropriate for a breeding colony. Providing access to natural daylight is appropriate so long as room temperature can be controlled to avoid hot spots within the room. To reduce noise, bins for food, sawdust and rubbish should be made of heavy-duty plastic.

The colony room should be large enough to allow cages to be placed along one wall and sufficient space for basic husbandry procedures such as washing cages or sexing pups. A room of about 4.5 m length, 3.0 m width and 2.5 m height should be adequate for colonies of 100 cages. This would provide sufficient space for a bench along one wall with sinks and the cages on shelving along the opposite wall, or fitted into racks mounted on castors. If the vole colony is housed in windowless rooms, then artificial lighting can be provided. For example, in a room laid out as above, a central 180 cm long 75 W fluorescent tube connected to a time switch, gives a light intensity of 105–735 lux at the front of cages in the absence of natural daylight. This light level seems adequate for basic husbandry procedures without flooding the cages with light, though it would be advisable to cover the top cages on a rack from direct lighting.

Housing

Voles can be housed in plastic, opaque polypropylene, or transparent polycarbonate cages designed for mice or rats. Litter can be coarse sawdust prepared commercially for use in rodent laboratory colonies or similar absorbent material. Nesting material should be provided to allow nesting behaviour. This is particularly important for pregnant or lactating females which construct spherical nests 5–10 cm in diameter in which litters are born and reared. However, all voles will build nests and provision of nesting material or other opportunities for sheltering considerably reduces the incidence of stereotypic behaviour in bank voles (Ödberg 1987; Cooper *et al.* 1996). Meadow hay makes a good nesting material, but is not suitable for systems requiring high hygiene and can evoke allergic responses in some people. In these situations, shredded paper or commercially produced rodent nesting material (eg, nestlets) may be an adequate substitute. A nest can last for a number of weeks, particularly if it is kept at the end of a cage away from the water bottle spout and can be transferred with the voles during cage cleaning.

Social grouping

It is possible to group house voles in single-sex groups following weaning, though groups should be monitored for signs of aggression (Clarke 1956; Sorensen & Randrup 1986). This is most prevalent in groups of unfamiliar males, though can arise in males housed together from weaning. Singly housed animals can be kept in standard cages such as those measuring 33 cm × 15 cm × 13 cm (l × w × h). Unless there has been significant spoilage of bedding (eg, from flooding) these can be cleaned once per week. Cages run the risk of flooding as voles are prone to rapidly emptying water bottles (possibly in association with stereotypic licking and/or locomotion) and for this reason cages should be inspected at least once every 24 h. Lactating females or breeding pairs benefit from housing in larger cages (eg, 48 cm × 15 cm × 13 cm), which again only need to be cleaned once per week unless significant spoilage has occurred. For bank voles, more frequent cleaning appears to be disturbing and may contribute to poor reproduction and infanticide. Wild-caught voles should be handled and their cages cleaned less frequently at least in the first months of introduction to the colony.

Food and water

Where problems of bulk and supply make the precise replication of wild diet impracticable for a laboratory colony, standard laboratory rodent diets can be used to meet the voles' nutritional requirements. Field voles should be given 8% or more protein in their diet, as a reduction to 4% has been shown to retard growth and sexual development (Spears & Clarke 1987). This can be provided by feeding whole oats, meadow hay, carrots and a few pellets of a rat and mouse laboratory diet. These supplies should be replenished every week or when cages are cleaned out. Field voles can be fed primarily a commercial pelleted standard rat and mouse breeding and grower diet *ad libitum*, though once per week a handful of commercial hamster food or toasted wheatgerm, should be added to each cage. Although bank voles naturally eat a more varied diet than field voles, they can also be maintained on simple diets such as whole oats augmented by pellets of rat and mouse breeding diet. Bank voles will sample from a wide range of food items and this basic diet should be supplemented by hamster mix including nuts and seeds such as rolled corn, barley, peanuts and sunflower seeds. Fresh forage can be also given to voles including chopped apples, pears and carrots, as well as meadow hay.

Water can be supplied in standard laboratory drinking bottles and should be checked daily. In addition to regular replacement with fresh tap water, water bottles and spouts should be cleaned regularly to avoid growth of algae. Voles are particularly susceptible to water shortage and total deprivation of water for 48 h will cause death. Daily water consumption is about 10 ml/24 h in both bank and field voles, so conventional water bottles should be adequate for many days. However, field vole colonies commonly water bottle siphon (Sorensen & Randrup 1986) and this behaviour is also known in other vole species (Kruckenburg *et al.* 1973). This involves the rapid emptying of water bottles, and repeated emptying of water can flood the cage and spoil litter. Voles showing this behaviour often develop the hunched posture associated with illness. This behaviour has also been termed polydipsia though evidence of over-consumption of water is sparse. Changing the drinker spout to a design less likely to allow siphoning may solve this problem, though animals that engage in this behaviour are often culled once they show overt signs of illness.

Identification and sexing

Toe clipping as a method of identification of animals is no longer either acceptable or necessary in voles as microchips can be used where individual identification is desirable. However, unless individuals need to be identified from groups then a cage card system, supported by a computer database, would be adequate for keeping records for breeding colonies and for identifying individually caged animals. Each cage should carry, in a metal holder, a card bearing the cage number and giving details of animals' identification, birth date and parents of the animals. Breeding records should be monitored to ensure that breeding stock comprise females and males descended from mothers of high fertility. Care should be taken to ensure paper cards are kept out of reach of the cage's inmates as voles have a tendency to chew these records.

The sexes can be distinguished by the greater ano-genital distance of males (about 10 mm) compared to that of females (about 5 mm). Sexually mature males have testes bulging in the perineal region to form the typical rodent scrotum. The penis is immediately anterior to the scrotum. The vaginal opening of sexually mature females has the clitoris at its anterior border. The ano-genital distance is very much smaller in newborn and sucking young of either sex, but with practice can be used to distinguish males from females. Newborn and sucking females can also be recognised by rudimentary nipples which are slightly better developed than in males. In prepubertal animals or those whose sexual development has been retarded by exposure to natural or artificial winter photoperiods, overlap in the frequency distribution of the ano-genital distance of the two sexes can cause difficulties in sexing. However, slight pressure on the lower abdomen may cause testes to descend more fully into the perineal region: they can be seen through the skin or will cause slight bulging. Females that are not yet perforate often have a small scale of skin marking the future vaginal opening.

Reproduction and breeding

If wild-caught voles are to be used to found a colony (and any local or national legal and ethical permits required for this have been obtained) they should be caught during the breeding season, though even in these situations females may take several months to produce their first laboratory conceived litter. Animals brought from the wild to create a colony should be disturbed as little as possible and, provided cages are not damp through leakage of a water bottle or are otherwise unsavoury, the cage should be cleaned infrequently. Quiet conditions in the animal room probably shorten the acclimatisision time.

Voles do not have long life expectancies, and long-term studies of their biology can be more efficiently conducted by establishing a breeding colony, than through recruitment from wild populations. A common breeding system is to house pairs permanently together until there is evidence that a pairing is not regularly producing litters or reliably rearing young: in these circumstances partners of different pairs can be swapped around. At the first and any subsequent pairing, the male can be introduced to the cage already occupied by the female. Recruitment for breeding should be reviewed once a month and animals should be removed from the breeding colony once they reach 12 months old, since by about that age fertility of females has declined. Colony records, which provide some idea of the likely fertility of stock animals, are a good guide for the recruitment of new females and males for the breeding colony.

The male and female of a pair should not be closely related and, in the field vole, it is advisable to select females and males with short upper (as well as lower) incisors. From time to time, animals of either sex may develop overgrown upper incisors. This causes difficulties in feeding, and these animals can become trapped when gnawing the wire mesh of cages. If animals with overgrown incisors are inadvertently recruited to the breeding colony or a long-term experiment, the upper incisors can be quickly clipped to a proper length with sharp fine scissors, without anaesthesia. The absence of any reflex response by voles has been taken to indicate this treatment does not cause distress, although independent measures of discomfort or pain have not been taken.

A long photoperiod consistent with natural breeding season (eg, 16L:8D for field voles) is necessary for rapid sexual development and maximum efficiency of breeding colonies of voles (Clarke 1985; Spears & Clarke 1987). Under these conditions, male field voles have spermatozoa in the testes, epididymides and vasa deferentia by the age of 42–49 days. Sexually mature males have well developed patches of sebaceous tissue on their hindquarters. These are secondary sexual characters which in laboratory stock frequently became bare, pink areas 20 × 15 mm, with folding of the skin, producing abundant sebaceous secretion giving off a musty odour and making the adjacent fur greasy. Females will develop perforate vaginas and be fertile by 28 days of age under a 16L:8D light regime, though some can be fertile by as little as 18 days of age. In an established colony, females should be recruited to breeding stock from 2 months of age, and males from about 2.5 months of age (see also Chapter 13).

Voles from laboratory colonies are generally heavier than animals from natural populations. For example by the age of 24 weeks both male and female field voles are considerably heavier than comparable wild animals, where mean maximum body weight during the breeding season has been recorded as 30 g for males and 26 g for females (Chitty 1952). The males most suitable for recruitment for breeding weigh 30–40 g and have somewhat spare bodies without much subcutaneous fat. In sexually mature males the penis is well developed, about 3 mm long within its prepuce, and the testes produce paired bulges in the perineal region, so forming a typical rodent scrotum. The scrotum may develop dark pigmentation in animals which have been sexually mature for several months, but this is not a prerequisite condition for the fertile state. Suitable sexually mature females have a perforate vagina which in the oestrous state is pink, gaping and slightly rugose. A vaginal smear made up of cornified epithelial cells is a good indication that the animal is fertile. Amongst virgin female field voles with these vaginal characteristics, those weighing from 25–35 g are usually more fertile than lighter or heavier animals. Females with abundant subcutaneous and abdominal fat (apparent from their 'feel' and conformation) tend to be less fertile than those with a more spare body.

When a sexually mature female, even one with an oestrous vaginal smear, is paired with a sexually mature male, the interaction of the animals may at first resemble that between a dominant and a subordinate male. The male may pursue the female, attempting to mount her and, at the outset, the female will often turn on the male, squeaking vigorously and lunging defensively at him. This seeming antagonism may be part of courtship behaviour. After a period ranging from a minute or two to half an hour, the squabbling interactions usually end, and copulations commence. The male usually mounts the female a number of times within a minute or two. After each mounting the female often runs ahead of the male and stops: the male follows and mounts again. Bouts of repeated leading by the female and mounting by the male are usually separated from each other by an interval of 5–15 minutes, during which the animals appear not to respond to each other (Clarke, unpublished observations).

Following copulation, a white or cream-coloured vaginal plug, formed from the male's ejaculate, can be found in the vagina, though not invariably: whether this is because it has fallen out before the female is examined, or because it has not formed, is not known. Sperm are detectable in vaginal smears for a few hours after copulation. The likelihood that a female has become pregnant or pseudopregnant can be fairly reliably gauged from the vaginal smear: the oestrous smear made up of cornified epithelial cells changes 24–48 h after mating to one consisting almost exclusively of many leucocytes, and by day 5 or day 6 after copulation there are very few cells of any sort. Pregnancy can also be reliably gauged by a gain in body weight of 2–4 g in pregnant females which occurs at about the 10th day of pregnancy, so weighing breeding females once per week (for example during cage cleaning) can avoid the need to conduct vaginal smears. Blastocysts implant 90–96 h post-coitus and pregnancy lasts 20–21 days. Pregnancy will be blocked if a female is exposed to an unfamiliar male 48–72 h after mating with a stud male. Females have a post-partum oestrus, and implantation of the resulting blastocysts is only slightly delayed by the concurrent sucking by the young.

Females in the later stages of pregnancy should be checked daily for young. By full term, pregnant female field voles may weigh between 35 and 50 g. As females are fertile post-partum and throughout lactation, and since males are normally permanently present in breeding cages, many females produce litters at 20–23-day intervals for much of their breeding lives. Disturbance during cage cleaning, or handling of litters on the day of birth and twice a week thereafter has not been found to have an adverse effect on the survival of young. However, should researchers wish to minimise disturbance then nests can be visually inspected for young with minimal disturbance using soft plastic tweezers.

Bank voles also have a breeding season lasting generally from early spring (March) until early autumn (September) so a photoperiod of 16L:8D is suitable to maintain a breeding colony. Spermatogenesis takes 31 days in males which are sexually mature. The reproductive physiology of females is, in its essentials, like that of the field vole. The general pattern of sexual behaviour in bank voles is similar to that of field voles and has been described by Christiansen and Døving (1976) and Milligan (1979). Ovulation is induced by mating and occurs 6–14 h thereafter. There is no oestrous cycle of the sort occurring in the laboratory mouse but, as in the field vole, cycles of change in the vaginal smear lasting 4–10 days, accompanied by ovulations, can occur through the remote influence of males. Compared with field voles, a smaller proportion of bank voles are likely to be in oestrus at any one time, though oestrus can be rapidly induced by nearby males. Multiple sets of corpora lutea occur in females from the wild, in young laboratory bred animals kept permanently with one male, in females mated with a succession of males at 2-day intervals, as well as through the remote influence of males. Young perforate, virgin females are less fertile than older perforate virgin animals, and bank voles take longer, generally, than field voles to become pregnant for the first time. This has been attributed to the need to have the reproductive tract primed by ovarian hormones, or the failure of corpora lutea at first mating to become functional. Implantation of blastocysts in non-lactating females occurs 105–107 h after coitus (Clarke 1985).

Pregnancy lasts 18–19 days in primigravida bank voles and a high proportion of females will be in oestrus and fertile immediately post partum, the proportion declining a day or two later and rising after the young are weaned. Permanently paired voles produce a steady stream of litters, but because implantation of blastocysts arising from post-partum mating of lactating females is delayed, their pregnancies last from 19–22 days. Although voles can deliver litters of five to six pups, smaller litter sizes (mean of 3.5 pups) are more commonly reported (Clarke 1985).

Parturition, rearing and weaning

Young are born in the nest during the day or night. Occasionally litters of permanently mated pairs are found dead and damaged. When pups are found dead or damaged it is often not clear if the pups have been attacked whilst alive, or if they have died from neglect or poor cage conditions and subsequently been eaten by the adults. Changing the pairing or removing the male before parturition can reduce this problem, but can also cause some loss of breeding efficiency since re-introduction or introduction of another male to the lactating female's cage can in itself cause the death of her young. An unpaired lactating female vole usually vigorously attacks any male added to her cage, and, in the following mayhem, young are often neglected, damaged or killed by the adults. Increasing the cage size, providing a more natural diet and nest materials (use of meadow hay) and reducing the frequency of cage cleaning may also be effective in reducing pup mortality. Randrup *et al.* (1988) reported that in bank vole colonies with little cover or nesting material, high pup mortality was associated with mothers repeatedly moving pups around the cage. Again, providing ample, suitable nesting material may reduce this problem.

Newborn vole pups are bright pink in colour, have sealed eyelids and limited capacity for movement, though development is rapid in the subsequent days and weeks (Spears &

Clarke 1987). At 2 days of age the head and back change from bright pink to grey. By about 4 days the young are able to crawl, and at 7 or 8 days they show uncoordinated walking. At this stage the coat is made up of smooth, very fine hair, brown above, light cream beneath, and the eyes have opened. When the young are 12–13 days old walking becomes coordinated as in an adult. It is possible to foster sucking young by choosing a female with a small litter of about the same age as the young to be fostered. Sucking young are quite hardy and if they are found in a cold, wet, moribund state, may revive if placed with their mother, or a suitable foster mother, in a clean, dry cage with adequate nesting material. Field voles are weaned by about 14 days, although they can be kept in the parental cage until 16 days, after which there is a small risk of juvenile females becoming fertile. At this age they have fine grey juvenile fur. From about 21 days the coarser adult coat develops on the head and then spreads down the body. It is grey with yellow–brown or reddish brown tips and black guard hairs on the upper side, and on the underside cream to pale grey.

Bank voles are born in essentially the same state as the young of field voles, and the pelage goes through the same stages as in field voles, though the hair colour is a richer brown. Because sucking bank voles develop a little more slowly than field voles, they are removed them from the parental cage at the age of 18 rather than 16 days.

Following weaning, males and females should be housed separately to avoid unwanted pregnancies. Adult females, which have been living separately, can be put together in a cage without the risk of stressful interactions, but if sexually mature males from different cages are put together they will fight vigorously, with consequent severe wounding. Even those which have been living together since weaning can start fighting when they become sexually mature.

Laboratory procedures

Transport and handling

Clear national guidelines covering transport of laboratory and other animals can be found elsewhere (eg, for UK see Laboratory Animal Science Association (LASA) 2005). This section will provide some practical advice to support these guidelines. As with other species, voles should be transported in escape-proof containers that protect the animals from unfavourable environmental conditions, ensuring they arrive alive and well at their destination. In general, voles can be transported in a similar fashion to laboratory mice. Containers should be made of rigid plastic, or similar escape-proof materials such as metal. Adequate bedding (for warmth and the absorption or containment of urine and faeces), food and a source of water must be provided, and for long journeys the container should have an inspection flap. Voles from the wild can be transported for short periods (say up to 3h) in the 'Longworth' traps in which they had been caught. Traps should always be well stocked with oats, fresh carrot and meadow hay.

For transport over long distances and lasting some hours, by road in a supervised vehicle, or by air freight, a purpose-built carrier can be used. A good practical example could consist of 12 metal boxes, each 15cm × 9cm × 8cm lightly welded together to give container of overall dimensions of about 45cm × 36cm, with a wire mesh lid (4mm square mesh). A more convenient, though less portable solution would be to use conventional cages for short distances only. In all cases, each compartment should be provided with a little sawdust and some non-absorbent cotton wool, oats and fresh carrot. In order to eliminate aggressive encounters, only one animal should be housed in each compartment, except if the animals were intended for a breeding colony, where one female and one male can travel together satisfactorily. It is said that voles are less stressed if the familiar bedding from their cage in the animal room is transferred to transport boxes, rather than if they are furnished with fresh material. If animals are to be sent abroad, a health certificate (from the relevant government department) for the animals will be needed, and the rules regulating importation into the destination country will need to be observed.

Voles are easily picked up by the loose skin of the neck. They should be quite decisively and firmly grasped, and, retaining the grip, can be cradled upside down in the palm of the hand for examination (Figure 26.1). A struggling animal, in these circumstances, can often be calmed momentarily by blowing on its nose. Under laboratory housing, bank voles are more 'lively' than field voles, even after many generations of laboratory breeding. This can make bank voles more challenging to handle. For experienced personnel, bites are very rare. Rodents can carry serious infectious diseases and careful precautions should be taken to avoid bites. As a variety of infectious and parasitic diseases can be

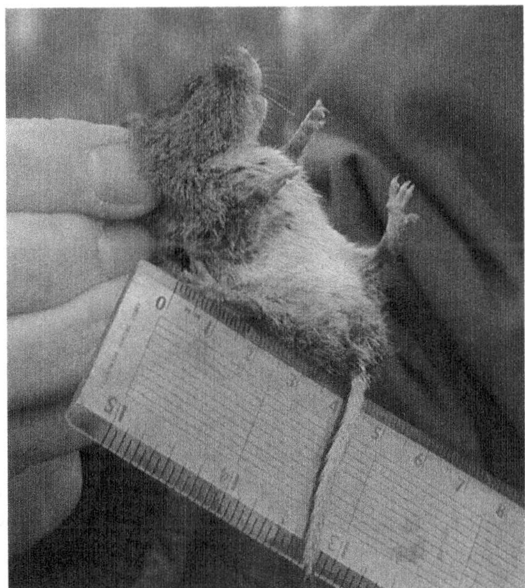

Figure 26.1 Adult female bank vole following capture in Longworth trap. Note small ano-genital distance, and restraint by firm grasp of fur at back of next, whilst supporting weight of body. (Photo: Charles Deeming.)

carried by field and bank voles, careful hygiene procedures should be followed.

Physiological monitoring

Blood samples

Some people report that (in a warm room and with practice) up to 200 µl of blood can be obtained by snipping no more than 1 mm from the tip of the tail. An analgesic or anaesthetic should be given when this method is used. Blood samples can be taken easily from the external jugular vein under alphaxalone/alphadolone anaesthesia using a 0.5 mm × 16 mm needle attached to a 1 ml plastic syringe. Clotting of blood in the syringe can be prevented by wetting the inside of the syringe with a solution of heparin (1000 U/ml, made up in 0.9% saline), shaking out fluid remaining in the nozzle. To facilitate blood collection, an incision should first be made in the neck, then fat overlying the external jugular parted, and the hypodermic needle inserted into the vein by passing it under the delicate pectoral muscle. This muscle, by its tension, serves to reduce bleeding which, with practice in delicate manipulations, becomes virtually non-existent. Nevertheless, the neck incision should be sutured, following sampling.

Terminal samples can be obtained from the heart under isoflurane anaesthesia, using an 0.8 mm × 16 mm needle, and a 1 or 2 ml syringe. It is much easier to take such samples if the manipulations are carried out while observing the site with an operating or a dissecting microscope. The needle is inserted in the midline, directly behind the sternum, at an angle of about 30° to the horizontal. It is possible routinely to get 0.75–1.25 ml of blood from field voles in this way. Taking terminal blood samples requires that an overdose of anaesthetic is given at the end of the procedure.

Valuable general information and principles about collection of blood samples is provided by Joint Working Group on Refinement (JWGR) (1993) and by the NC3Rs at their blood sampling microsite[1].

Vaginal smears

These can be easily taken using a small platinum wire loop (c.1.0 mm diameter) fixed into a glass or metal rod. After flaming the loop to remove debris, it can be used to transfer a drop of physiological saline onto a clean microscope slide, again dipped in saline and then carefully inserted into the vagina. The loop is then dabbed in the drop of saline on the slide. Cells from the vagina are thus transferred to the slide which can be immediately examined as a wet, unstained preparation with the simplest of monocular microscopes (total magnification ×60). Smears comprise: nucleated epithelial cells; or cornified epithelial cells; or leucocytes; or a mixture of two or all three cell types. Air-dried smears can be stained, for example, with 0.04% aqueous toluidine blue, and made into permanent preparations.

[1] http://www.nc3rs.org.uk/bloodsamplingmicrosite/page.asp?id=313

Administration of medicines

Anaesthesia

Alphaxalone mixed with alphadolone acetate (such as Saffan: Glaxovet Ltd, Uxbridge) is a good anaesthetic for simple surgery of field voles and bank voles (gonadectomy, vasectomy, manipulating the uterus, intravenous administration of drugs). A dose of 0.1 ml Saffan per 10 g body weight is appropriate, administered intraperitoneally. This dosage seems quite reliable with voles weighing between 20 and 30 g, though the relationship between body weight and anaesthetic dose seems more variable with larger animals. Isoflurane, administered through a mask as a vapour from a small anaesthetic machine, has been found to be a very safe anaesthetic for voles. Sodium pentobarbital, at a concentration of 72 mg/kg, has also been used (the dose for a 25 g field vole is about 0.03 ml). However this is a less safe method and success depends on the state of the animal: stressed animals can die quickly, and very active or excited animals may need a slightly higher dose (a further 0.01 ml). In simple surgical procedures, field and bank voles need be anaesthetised and immobile for no more than about half an hour. It is important to keep animals warm as they recover from anaesthesia, for example by nestling them within a cage in clean, non-absorbent cotton wool and beneath a warming light bulb. Flecknell (2009) provides general information and principles relevant to rodent anaesthesia.

Dosing and injecting

Subcutaneous injections are easily given under the skin of the neck or back. It is helpful to shave the site, or part the fur by blowing, in order more easily to guide the needle subcutaneously, to see the bleb at the injection site or to detect any leakage. Light anaesthesia makes the procedure less stressful for lively voles and the experimenter. The skin of the back or neck is held between index finger and thumb, the needle of the syringe inserted low down between finger and thumb through the fold of skin, and checked by touch and visually for correct positioning. Volumes of up to 0.2 ml can be injected in this fashion.

Intraperitoneal injections can be given by first grasping the vole by the loose skin of the back with the index finger and thumb which can then rotated so that the animal, with its belly uppermost, is supported by the palm. The needle should be inserted a couple of millimetres at an angle of about 45°, then the angle changed so that the needle is nearly parallel to the surface of the belly, and finally the needle should be pushed a little forward before discharging the fluid. Intravenous injections can be made into the external jugular vein, accessed as described above for taking a blood sample. The neck incision should be sutured following surgery. See JWGR (2001) for detailed information about administration of substances.

Euthanasia

It is possible for trained personnel to cull sick individuals in emergencies using dislocation of the neck by instantaneous sharp pressure using the index finger and thumb, though researchers and technicians may prefer euthanasia by injection or inhalation for aesthetic reasons. If inhalation is to be used the same guidelines and advice apply to voles as to similar sized mice. High concentration of carbon dioxide within a chamber connected to a carbon dioxide cylinder causes rapid loss of consciousness followed by death in voles, though it is not known how aversive they find the short exposures to this potentially noxious gas. In other rodents, euthanasia using a rising concentration of warmed hydrated carbon dioxide has been recommended as this appears to render animals unconscious before they experience highly noxious concentrations of carbon dioxide. More recent work, however has suggested that some rodents can detect carbon dioxide and find it aversive even at these low concentrations. As voles are an uncommon laboratory species no systematic research has been conducted into their perception of euthanasing agents and if small numbers of animals are to be killed, then an overdose of an injectable anaesthetic agent as a humane means of killing should be considered. Finally, if surplus stock need to be disposed of, and if local regulations permit, then it may be worthwhile considering releasing them back into the wild. However, this introduces a number of welfare and ethical issues, in particular whether captive-reared voles will be equipped with the skills required to forage and avoid predation, and also the potential disturbance to resident voles. For these reasons the matter would need to be carefully researched and it is likely also that there would be a need for careful screening for infectious diseases which might affect released animals or those with which they may come in contact. To date, no studies have tracked survival of laboratory-reared voles, following release into the wild, or their impact on resident populations.

Common welfare problems

Health, disease and zoonosis

Voles in a healthy state have a shiny coat and are vigorous. Ill animals are often hunched with fluffed-up, dull fur. It is essential that any animals showing signs of illness be examined and either treated or euthanased promptly. The abdomen of adult voles may occasionally become greatly enlarged without any matching increase in body weight, so that the females in such cases are clearly not pregnant. Such animals should be culled. *Post-mortem* examination will reveal that the small intestine is grossly distended with gas, or that the caecum is greatly engorged with digesta.

Wild voles can carry a number of ectoparasites, including fleas, ticks and mites, the human ringworm fungus, endoparasitic protozoa (including *Toxoplasma*), trematodes, cestodes and nematodes, as well as *Mycobacterium tuberculosis* and the spirochaete *Leptospira*. Tuberculosis can be endemic in wild populations of voles, and infected animals may have extensive caseous areas in subcutaneous tissue, lungs and elsewhere in the body. Antibody reacting with orthopoxvirus (cowpox virus) has been detected in both field and bank voles from the wild and both species are susceptible to a number of other viruses, including spontaneous mouse encephalomyelitis and encephalomyocarditis and various hantaviruses (Kaplan *et al.* 1980; Flowerdew *et al.* 1985; Bennett *et al.* 1997; Barnard *et al.* 2002; Harris & Yalden 2008). The latter group is responsible for important rural and sometimes urban public health problems throughout some parts of Europe and Asia (for example, Korean haemorrhagic fever, nephropathia epidemica). The infective agent(s) can occur in urban and laboratory rodents from which people have apparently become infected. The mite *Laelaps hilaris* Koch is often found in small numbers in the perineal region of field voles, feeding on host body secretion, and apparently causing little harm. Bank voles are hosts for the sheep tick (*Ixodes ricinus*) which transmits the spirochaete *Borrelia burgdorferi* responsible for Lyme disease (Randolph & Craine 1995). Infection can have arthritic, cardiac and neurological consequences for people. Bank voles are also competent hosts for the protozoan *Babesia microti* which can cause illness in people. This protozoan is transmitted by the ectoparasitic tick *Ixodes trianguliceps* (Randolph 1995).

When wild voles are brought into the laboratory for outcrossing of the breeding stock or for experimental purposes, a protocol for quarantine, screening and, where appropriate, treatment, for any parasitic or other infectious agents should be carefully devised and implemented. In order to guard against infection of laboratory workers, colonies of wild voles should be kept well separated from breeding colonies of the same or other laboratory rodent species.

Behaviour and welfare

Aggressive Interactions

Sexually mature male voles from laboratory stock are often very aggressive towards each other. This has been seen in groups of male voles housed in laboratory cages (Sorensen & Randrup 1986) as well as larger more naturalistic enclosures with high stocking densities (Clarke 1955, 1956). Sexually mature males may fight viciously if they are put together and fighting can also occur amongst sexually mature males which have cohabited since weaning (whether from the same or different litters). In cages with high levels of aggressive encounters the problem can be moderated by identifying and removing the principle aggressor(s). It may be possible to identify such individuals from size and muscle tone and also from bite marks. They will tend to be larger animals with a muscular feel when handled due to little subcutaneous or abdominal fat. They may have small wounds on the nose inflicted by the defensive actions of subordinate voles. The latter, in contrast tend to have wounds anywhere on the body but especially on the hindquarters, incurred as they flee from the aggressor. Alternatively, given the risk of aggressive encounters in group-housed males and the potential for harm, avoid group housing males in stock cages. Females do not tend to have serious aggressive interactions, except perhaps when they are pregnant or lactating, so group housing is less problematic with female voles.

Social isolation and distress

The prairie vole has been used to investigate the effects of social isolation on stress physiology (Kim & Kirkpatrick

1996). Under laboratory conditions, pairs of prairie voles develop close relationships, spending much of their time sitting side by side (Insel & Shapiro 1992; Insel 1997). This contrasts markedly with the closely related, but polygamous, montane vole (*Microtus montanus*), as well as the meadow, field and bank voles described earlier, which generally avoid contact with conspecifics in both laboratory and natural conditions except when mating. Housing adult female prairie voles in isolation causes chronic distress and has been described as leading to anxiety and depression, and consequently has been used as a model for these responses in man. Isolation leads to elevated serum corticosteroid and reduced body weight, whilst behavioural consequences of isolation include anhedonia as measured by decreased sucrose intake, a decline in swimming in a forced swimming task, which are used as measures of depression, and also reduced time in open arms of raised plus maze (Grippo 2009) which has been developed as a measure of anxiety. This extreme response to social isolation indicates the importance of maintaining prairie voles in stable pairs in breeding colonies both in terms of their welfare and in terms of successful breeding programmes.

Stereotypic behaviour

Stereotypic behaviour can be reliably induced in voles and consequently they have been used as a model species to investigate the causes and effects of repetitive, invariant apparently functionless activities. These behaviours, especially the sustained gnawing of the wire mesh of cages, as well as some weaving, jumping and somersaulting (Sorensen & Randrup 1986), have been found in field voles, but are more commonly observed in bank voles (Ödberg 1987), where they can lead to injuries such as broken tails and facial lesions due to repeated collision with cage features.

Voles readily develop stereotypies in standard laboratory conditions without the use of drug treatments. In addition, vole stereotypy can be varied by manipulation of dopamine activity, in a similar way to rat and mouse stereotypy, with dopamine antagonists blocking the performance of stereotypies, and agonists increasing their occurrence (Randrup *et al.* 1988). Stereotypic behaviour can be manipulated in bank voles by simple changes to cage conditions, for example by increasing cage size or more effectively by providing cover in the form of hay or straw (Ödberg 1987; Cooper *et al.* 1996). For example, rearing voles in 33 cm × 15 cm × 13 cm cages with sawdust litter and no bedding leads to an incidence of locomotor stereotypic behaviour approaching 100%; whereas providing a handful of bedding (eg, hay) results in only 50% of the population exhibiting the behaviour. The use of larger cages (eg, 45 cm × 28 cm × 13 cm) with ample bedding, nesting and/or sheltering substrates results in a very low incidence of stereotypic behaviour (Cooper *et al.* 1996).

The motivation underlying the performance of stereotypies in voles appears to be persistence of locomotor behaviour, possibly related to motivation to escape from the cage. Stereotypies can be initiated by an alarming stimulus (for example running a pen along the cage bars), and providing extensive shelter appears to be the most effective means of reducing the behaviour. Fine detailed observation of responses and the development of the behaviour, suggests those voles which show the highest amount of locomotor behaviour following disturbance in the absence of cover are most likely to develop stereotypies, suggesting a development from this active response. Finally, whilst environmental enrichment such as housing voles in larger cages with more shelter can prevent the performance of stereotypies, this is less effective for older voles (Cooper *et al.* 1996). It is therefore recommended that to minimise stereotypic activities, voles should be housed from weaning in large cages provided with both shelter and nesting material.

References

Barnard, C.J., Behnke, J.M., Bajer, A. *et al.* (2002) Local variation in endoparasite intensities of bank voles (*Clethrionomys glareolus*) from ecologically similar sites: morphometric and endocrine correlates. *Journal of Helminthology*, **76**, 103–112

Beardsley, A., Vagg, M.J., Beckett, P.H.T. *et al.* (1978) Use of the field vole (*M. agrestis*) for monitoring potentially harmful elements in the environment. *Environmental Pollution*, **16**, 65–71

Bennett, M., Crouch, A.J., Begon, M. *et al.* (1997) Cowpox in British voles and mice. *Journal of Comparative Pathology*, **116**, 35–44

Blake, B.H. (1992) Ultrasonic vocalization and body temperature maintenance in infant voles of three species (Rodentia: Arvicolidae). *Developmental Psychobiology*, **25**, 581–596

Burthe, S., Telfer, S., Begon, M. *et al.* (2008) Cowpox virus in natural field vole *Microtus agrestis* populations: significant negative impacts on survival. *Journal of Animal Ecology*, **77**, 110–119

Chitty, D.H. (1952) Mortality among voles (*Microtus agrestis*) at Lake Vyrnwy, Montgomeryshire in 1936–39. *Philosophical Transactions of the Royal Society B*, **236**, 505–520

Chitty, D.H. (1996) *Do Lemmings Commit Suicide? Beautiful Hypotheses and Ugly Facts*. Oxford University Press, New York

Christiansen, E. and Døving, K.B. (1976) Observations of the mating behaviour of the bank vole, *Clethrionomys glareolus*. *Behavioural Biology*, **17**, 263–266

Clarke, J.R. (1955) The influence of numbers on reproduction and survival in two experimental vole populations. *Proceedings of the Royal Society of London*, **144**, 68–85

Clarke, J.R. (1956) The aggressive behaviour of the vole. *Behaviour*, **9**, 1–23

Clarke, J.R. (1985) The reproductive biology of the bank vole (*Clethrionomys glareolus*) and the wood mouse (*Apodemus sylvaticus*). In: *The Ecology of Woodland Rodents Bank Voles and Wood Mice*. Eds Flowerdew, J.R., Gurnell, J. and Gipps, J.H.W., pp. 33–59. Symposia of the Zoological Society of London Number 55. Clarendon Press, Oxford

Cooper, J.J., Ödberg, F.O. and Nicol, C.J. (1996) Limitations on the effectiveness of environmental improvement in reducing stereotypic behaviour in bank voles (*Clethrionomys glareolus*). *Applied Animal Behaviour Science*, **48**, 237–248

Crouch, A.C., Baxby, D., McCracken, C.M. *et al.* (1995) Serological evidence for the reservoir hosts of cowpox virus in British wildlife. *Epidemiology of Infection*, **115**, 185–191

Cushing, B.S., Martin, J.O., Young, L.J. *et al.* (2001) The effects of peptides on partner preference formation are predicted by habitat in prairie voles. *Hormones and Behavior*, **39**, 48–58

Fentress, J.C. (1968) Interrupted ongoing behaviour in two species of vole (*Microtus agrestis* and *Clethrionomys brittanicus*). I. Response as a function of preceding activity and the context of an apparently 'irrelevant' motor pattern. *Animal Behaviour*, **16**, 135–153

Flecknell P.A. (2009) *Laboratory Animal Anaesthesia*, 3rd edn. Academic Press, London

Flowerdew, J.R., Gurnell, J. and Gipps, J.H.W. (Eds) (1985) *The Ecology of Woodland Rodents: Bank Voles and Wood Mice. Symposia of the Zoological Society of London* Number 55. Clarendon Press, Oxford

Grippo, A.J. (2009) Mechanisms underlying altered mood and cardiovascular dysfunction: the value of neurobiological and behavioral research with animal models. *Neuroscience and Biobehavioral Reviews*, **33**, 171–180

Gurnell, J. and Flowerdew, J.R. (1982) *Live Trapping Small Mammals: A Practical Guide*. Occasional Publications of the Mammal Society, Harvest House, Reading

Hammock, E.A.D. and Young, L.J. (2005) Microsatellite instability generates diversity in brain and sociobehavioral traits. *Science*, **308**, 1630–1634

Harris, S. and Yalden, D.W. (Eds) (2008) *Mammals of the British Isles*, 4th edn. The Mammal Society, Southampton

Insel, T.R. (1997) A neurological basis of social attachment. *American Journal of Psychiatry*, **154**, 726–735

Insel, T.R. and Shapiro, L.E. (1992) Oxytocin receptor distribution reflects social organisation in monogamous and polygamous voles. *Proceedings of the National Academy of Sciences of the United States of America*, **89**, 5981–5985

Jernvall, J., Keranen, S.V.E. and Thesleff, I. (2000) Evolutionary modification of development in mammalian teeth: quantifying gene expression patterns and topography. *Proceedings of the National Academy of Sciences of the United States of America*, **97**, 14444–14448

Joint Working Group on Refinement (1993) Removal of blood from laboratory mammals and birds. First Report of the BVA/FRAME/RSPCA/UFAW Joint Working Group on Refinement. *Laboratory Animals*, **27**, 1–22

Joint Working Group on Refinement (2001) Refining procedures for the administration of substances. Report of the BVAAWF/FRAME/RSPCA/UFAW Joint Working Group on Refinement. *Laboratory Animals*, **35**, 1–41

Kalscheuer, V., Singh, A.P., Nanda, I. *et al.* (1996) Evolution of the gonosomal heterochromatin of *Microtus agrestis*: rapid amplification of a large, multimeric, repeat unit containing a 3.0-kb $(GATA)_{11}$ – positive, middle repetitive element. *Cytogenetics and Cell Genetics*, **73**, 171–178

Kaplan, C., Healing, T.D., Evans, N. *et al.* (1980) Evidence of infection by viruses in small British field rodents. *Journal of Hygiene*, **84**, 285–294

Kim, J. and Kirkpatrick, B. (1996) Social isolation in animal models of relevance to neuropsychiatric disorders. *Biological Psychiatry*, **40**, 918–922

Kruckenburg, S.M., Gier, H.T. and Dennis, S.M. (1973) Post-natal development of the prairie vole. *Microtus ochrogaster. Laboratory Animal Science*, **23**, 53–55

Laboratory Animal Science Association (2005) Guidance on the transport of laboratory animals. Report of the Transport Working Group established by LASA. *Laboratory Animals*, **39**, 1–39

Leslie, P.H. and Ranson, R.M. (1940) The mortality, fertility and rate of natural increase of the vole (*Microtus agrestis*) as observed in the laboratory. *Journal of Animal Ecology*, **9**, 27–52

Little, J.L. and Gurnell, J. (1989) Shrew captures and rodent field studies. *Journal of Zoology*, **218**, 329–331

Lim, M.M., Wang, Z., Olazabel, D.E. *et al.* (2004) Enhaned partner preference in a promiscuous species by manipulating the expression of a single gene. *Nature*, **429**, 754–757

Macdonald, D.W. (Ed.) (2001) *The New Encyclopaedia of Mammals*: Oxford University Press, Oxford

Milligan, S.R. (1979) The copulatory pattern of the bank vole (*Clethrionomys glareolus*) and speculation on the role of penile spines. *Journal of Zoology*, **188**, 279–300

Musser, G.G. and Carleton, M.D. (2005) Superfamily muroidea. In: *Mammal Species of the World a Taxonomic and Geographic Reference*. Eds Wilson D.E. and Reeder D.M., pp. 894–1531. Johns Hopkins University Press, Baltimore

Ödberg. F.O. (1987) The influence of cage size and environmental enrichment on the development of stereotypies in bank voles (*Clethrionomys glareolus*). *Behavioural Processes*, **14**, 155–173

Ophir, A.G., Wolff, J.O. and Phelps, S.M. (2008) Variation in neural V1aR predicts sexual fidelity and space use among male prairie voles in semi-natural settings. *Proceedings of the National Academy of Sciences of the United States of America*, **105**, 1249–1254

Randolph, S.E. (1995) Quantifying parameters in the transmission of *Babesia microti* by the tick *Ixodes trianguliceps* amongst voles (*Clethrionomys glareolus*). *Parasitology*, **110**, 287–295

Randolph, S.E. and Craine, N.G. (1995) General framework for comparative quantitative studies on transmission of tick-borne diseases using Lyme borreliosis in Europe as an example. *Journal of Medical Entomology*, **32**, 765–777

Randrup, A., Sorensen, G. and Kobayashi, M. (1988) Stereotyped behaviour in animals induced by stimulant drugs or by a restricted cage environment: relation to disintegrated behaviour, brain dopamine and psychiatric disease. *Japanese Journal of Psychopharmacology*, **8**, 313–327

Roberts, R.L., Williams, J.R., Wang, A.K. *et al.* (1998) Cooperative breeding and monogamy in prairie voles; influence of the sire and geographical variation. *Animal Behaviour*, **55**, 1131–1140

Spears, N. and Clarke, J.R. (1987) Effect of nutrition, temperature and photoperiod on the rate of sexual maturation of the field vole (*Microtus agrestis*). *Journal of Reproduction and Fertility*, **80**, 175–181

Sorensen, G. and Randrup, A. (1986) Possible protective value of severe psychopathology against lethal effects of an unfavourable milieu. *Stress Medecine*, **2**, 103–105

Young, L.J., Young, A.Z.M. and Hammock, E.A.D. (2005) Anatomy and neurochemistry of the pair bond. *The Journal of Comparative Neurology*, **493**, 51–57

27 The guinea pig

Sylvia Kaiser, Christine Krüger and Norbert Sachser

Biological overview

The guinea pig (*Cavia aperea* f. *porcellus*) was domesticated about 3000–6000 years ago in the highlands of South America (Hückinghaus 1961; Gade 1967; Hyams 1972; Wing 1977; Herre & Röhrs 1990; Benecke 1994). The main aim of domestication was to provide the Indians with meat (Herre & Röhrs 1990) and guinea pigs are still one of the main sources of meat in some rural populations of South America. They have also, occasionally, been used for ritual healing (Gade 1967; Hyams 1972; Weir 1974; Wing 1977; Clutton-Brock 1989; Herre & Röhrs 1990; Benecke 1994). Guinea pigs in South America today are left to scavenge in and around the huts of the Indians, and it may be assumed that a similar husbandry has always existed (Weir 1974; Stahnke & Hendrichs 1988). In the middle of the 16th century the Spaniards discovered guinea pigs and introduced them into Europe. Within the European population, the animals rapidly became a popular pet (Gade 1967; Hyams 1972; Clutton-Brock 1989; Benecke 1994). Nowadays, guinea pigs are one of the most popular pets throughout the world, raised for fancy and companion uses.

The wild ancestor *Cavia aperea*

According to anatomical and morphological studies the domestic guinea pig derives from the subspecies *tschudii* of the wild cavy (*Cavia aperea*), which is among the most common and widespread rodents of South America (Nehring 1889; Hückinghaus 1961; Gade 1967; Rood 1972; Weir 1972; Nachtsheim & Stengel 1977; Herre & Röhrs 1990; Benecke 1994; Künzl & Sachser 1999). The wild cavy and the domestic guinea pig belong to the order Rodentia and to the family Caviidae (Figure 27.1). All cavy-like members of this family (about 14 species; Wilson & Reeder 2005) are medium-sized, tailless rodents that have four digits on the front feet and three digits on the hindfeet. All digits have claws. All forms – except the domestic guinea pig – have agouti dorsal pelage and a lighter underside (Rood 1972; Wagner 1976). The cavy-like members of the Caviidae are divided into four genera (*Cavia, Galea, Kerodon* and *Microcavia*), which are widely distributed throughout South America and inhabit a wide range of ecological niches (Mares & Ojeda 1982; Redford & Eisenberg 1992; Eisenberg & Redford 1999).

The wild cavy is a herbivorous, neotropical rodent that occurs in humid grassland habitats from Colombia through Brazil into Argentina (Mares & Ojeda 1982; Stahnke & Hendrichs 1988; Redford & Eisenberg 1992).

They live in small harem groups consisting of one adult male and one or a few females and their unweaned offspring (Rood 1972; Sachser *et al.* 1999; Asher *et al.* 2004, 2008). *C. aperea* is a crepuscular, non-climbing species, which does not dig burrows, but hides and moves through tunnels made in dense vegetation (Rood 1972; Stahnke & Hendrichs 1988; Guichón & Cassini 1998). The typical habitat of *C. aperea* contains a cover zone with high and dense vegetation, which the animals use as protection from predator attacks (Rood 1972), and an adjacent, more open zone of short vegetation where cavies forage (Cassini 1991; Cassini & Galante 1992; Guichón & Cassini 1998; Asher *et al.* 2008). *C. aperea* is a species difficult to study in the field as most social activities occur in tall vegetation (Rood 1972; Asher *et al.* 2004, 2008).

Under semi-natural and laboratory conditions adult male *C. aperea* are highly incompatible in the presence of females, whereas female *C. aperea* organise themselves into linear dominance hierarchies. The males' body mass is 11% higher than the body mass of non-pregnant females. The male–male competition brings about a polygynous mating system (Sachser *et al.* 1999). Whenever a female comes into oestrus, only one male is present. This male thus mates with several females, whereas every female mates with a single male (Sachser 1998). Females play an active role in bringing about this species' social and mating system by displaying clear preferences for single males (Adrian *et al.* 2008). Moreover, the low relative testis weights and the small epididymis size of *Cavia apera* are within the typical range of species with a single-male mating system (Kenagy & Trombulak 1986; Sachser 1998; Sachser *et al.* 1999; Cooper *et al.* 2000).

Behavioural and physiological consequences of domestication

As described above, the domestic guinea pigs derived from the wild cavy at least 3000 years ago. The process of domestication is always accompanied by distinct changes in morphology, physiology and behaviour (Darwin 1859, 1868; Hale 1969; Fox 1978; Haase & Donham 1980; Price 1984; Clutton-Brock 1989; Herre & Röhrs 1990; Künzl & Sachser 1999). As a consequence, wild and domestic animals require

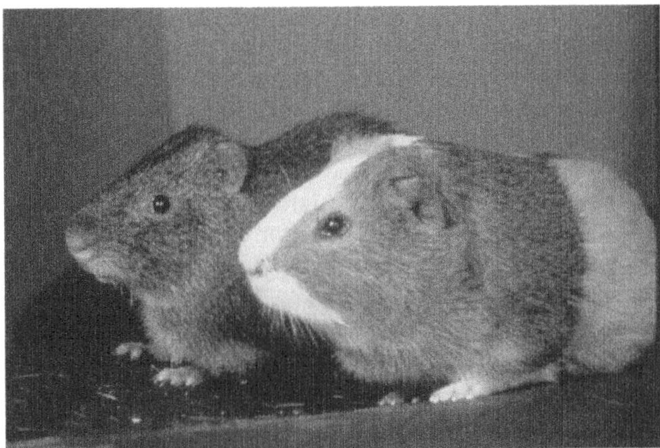

Figure 27.1 The wild cavy (*Cavia aperea*; left) and the domestic guinea pig (*Cavia aperea* f. *porcellus*, right). (Photo: M. Aulbur.)

somewhat different conditions and resources to achieve good welfare although, in a biological sense, they still belong to the same species (Sachser 2001).

Behavioural studies indicate that the repertoire of behavioural patterns is similar in domesticated and wild guinea pigs. Thus, domestication has not resulted in the loss or addition of behavioural elements (Rood 1972; Stahnke 1987; Künzl & Sachser 1999). Distinct differences have, however, developed in behavioural frequencies and thresholds (Künzl & Sachser 1999) (Table 27.1). Domestic guinea pigs display lower levels of intraspecific aggressive behaviour and higher levels of sociopositive behaviour (eg, social grooming) than the wild ancestors. They also show more frequent overt courtship behaviour and have a lower threshold for vocalisation. Finally, guinea pigs are less attentive to their physical environment and show much less exploration behaviour than their ancestors (Künzl & Sachser 1999; Künzl *et al.* 2003).

These behavioural differences are associated with marked changes in social structure compared with the wild form. When domestic guinea pigs are kept in breeding groups of one adult male and several adult females, the mature sons and daughters will integrate rather peacefully into the social system of the groups and all animals will cohabitate in a non-aggressive and non-stressful way (Sachser 1998). When adult wild cavies are kept in breeding groups of one male and several females, a completely different picture emerges: the daughters integrate into the linear dominance hierarchy of the females. In contrast, the father and his sons often become incompatible when the sons attain sexual maturity. In most cases, the sons must then be taken out of the groups, otherwise the father will injure or kill them (Sachser 1998).

Artificial selection and breeding in guinea pigs has not, however, led to degenerated animals with impaired cognitive abilities. Male and female domestic guinea pigs perform better in the Morris Water Maze (a frequently used test for the assessment of spatial learning in rodents) than their wild relatives (unpublished data of SK).

A series of experiments has been conducted to compare endocrine stress responses between wild and domestic guinea pigs (Table 27.1). Wild cavies respond with a significantly stronger increase of their serum cortisol concentrations to environmental challenge than domestic guinea pigs. Furthermore, immediately after removing animals from their home cages catecholamine concentrations are distinctly higher in the wild than in the domesticated form. In addition, significantly lower cortisol levels in response to an adrenocorticotropic hormone (ACTH) challenge indicate that there is a generalised reduction in the stress response of the domestic guinea pig (Künzl & Sachser 1999; Künzl *et al.* 2003), and this is the physiological correlate of the reduced alertness, nervousness and sensitivity of the domesticated animals. While the reduced stress response obviously helps domestic animals to live in artificial housing conditions, it would be counter-selected for by natural selection in wild animals in their natural habitats (Künzl & Sachser 1999).

Table 27.1 Physiological and behavioural consequences of domestication: comparison between domestic (*Cavia aperea* f. *porcellus*) and wild guinea pigs (*Cavia aperea*) (– rare/low; + frequent/high). For references and original data see Künzl and Sachser (1999), Künzl *et al.* (2003) and Sachser (2001).

		Domestic	*Wild*
Endocrine stress response	Adrenocortical system	–	+
	Adrenomedullary system	–	+
Behaviour	Attentive	–	+
	Vocal	+	–
	Courtship	+	–
	Sociopositive	+	–
	Aggressive	–	+

General biology

Newborn guinea pigs (body mass of about 60–100 g) are precocial, looking like small-sized adults (Table 27.2). They are fully furred, their eyes are open and the secondary teeth have already replaced the primary teeth during foetal development. On the day of birth young guinea pigs start to eat solid food and drink water, although lactation lasts for 2-3 weeks. Young males reach their sexual maturity within 2–3 months of age (body mass about 500 g), while young females may reach sexual maturity at less than 1 month of age (with a body mass of around 300 g) (Table 27.3).

Guinea pigs are fully grown at the age of 8–12 months. They live up to an age of 8 years and reach a body mass of about 800 to more than 1000 g, which is distinctly higher than in the wild form. Adult guinea pigs measure up to 30 cm in length (Sutherland & Festing 1987).

All teeth are open rooted and grow continuously throughout life. The dental formula of the guinea pig is as follows: $I^1_1C^0_0Pm^1_1M^3_3$.

Wild cavies have an agouti dorsal pelage and a lighter underside (see above), but in the domestic guinea pig there is a wide variety of colours. The coat can be unicoloured or multicoloured. The most popular breed of guinea pigs in scientific research is the short-haired English, and the most common strain is the Dunkin–Hartley (albino outbred guinea pig of the English breed). Several inbred guinea pig strains have been produced, of which strains 2 and 13 are

Table 27.2 Biological data for the guinea pig. Reprinted from North, D. (1999) with permission of Blackwell Publishing.

Parameter	*Normal value*
Lifespan (years)	2–8
Birth weight (g)	60–100
Adult weight (g)	700–1300
Food consumption (g/100g body weight per day)	6
Water consumption (ml/100g body weight per day)	10–14.5
Rectal temperature (°C)	37.2–39.8
Heart rate (beats/minute)	150–400
Blood pressure (mmHg)	
Systolic	77–94
Diastolic	47–58
Respiratory rate (breaths/minute)	42–150
Tidal volume (ml)	1.0–5.3
Total blood volume (ml/kg)	69–75
Dental formula	$I^1{}_1C^0{}_0Pm^1{}_1M^3{}_3$

Table 27.3 Reproductive data for the guinea pig.

Reproductive parameter	*Normal value*
Sexual maturity	
Female	~1 month of age
Male	2–3 months of age
Oestrous cycle	Polyoestrus, ~16 days
Gestation period	63–72 days
Lactation	~21 days
Litter size	1–7

the most widely used (North 1999). If not bred on-site in the facility, animals are obtained from commercial breeders.

Female guinea pigs exhibit a post-partum oestrus which means they become receptive immediately after giving birth. If they do not become pregnant at this time, females show periodic oestrous cycles of about 16 days (Shi *et al.* 1999). It is well known that female guinea pigs have some behavioural changes during their oestrous cycle (Birke 1981). The young are born after a gestation period of around 67 days. Usually one to four (up to a maximum of seven) young are born in one litter (Table 27.3) (Sutherland & Festing 1987; Sachser 1994a).

Guinea pigs do not show a day–night cycle of activity. Rather, they are characterised by an ultradian rhythm, that is, alternating phases of activity and rest last for about 2–3h. Thus, the activity is not dependent on the light–dark regime (Sachser *et al.* 1992).

Guinea pigs have dichromatic colour vision with a spectral neutral point centred at about 480nm (Jacobs & Deegan 1994). However, guinea pigs may have poor depth perception. Guinea pigs possess two different classes of retinal cones with peak sensitivities of about 429nm and 529nm.

The maximum auditory sensitivity is around 500 and 8000Hz. However, guinea pigs are responsive to frequencies of 125–32000 Hertz (Harper 1976). The upper limit of their hearing is probably 40000–50000Hz.

The olfactory sense is most important in social behaviour (Beauchamp *et al.* 1979, 1980, 1982; Martin & Beauchamp 1982). Male guinea pigs mark individual females with their anal glands. Guinea pigs also mark the environment with their anal glands. Urine has a high communicative value for this species. Young guinea pigs, for example, discriminate between maternal urine and urine of an unknown lactating female (Jäckel & Trillmich 2003).

Uses in the laboratory

The guinea pig is commonly used in scientific research, in areas such as toxicology, product development and medical quality control.

Laboratory management and breeding

Social life and welfare: basic research

There is a long tradition of basic research concerning the social structure and sociophysiology of guinea pigs (Kunkel & Kunkel 1964; Rood 1972; Beauchamp 1973; Berryman & Fullerton 1976; Jacobs 1976; Sachser 1986; Sachser 1994a, 1994b; Kaiser *et al.* 2003a; Hennessy & Morris 2005; Hennessy *et al.* 2006; Wallner *et al.* 2006; Bauer *et al.* 2008; Fey & Trillmich 2008). From this research, conclusions can be drawn regarding which social housing conditions can be recommended and which conditions should be avoided.

Social organisation

As for other species, the social interactions of guinea pigs are composed of agonistic behaviours and the development of dominance hierarchies, together with positive or sexual interactions, which may result in the establishment of social bonds. The overall structure of dominance relationships and social bonds constitute the animals' social organisation.

Low and high population density

The effects of increasing population density on the patterns of social interactions and reproductive success have been studied by Sachser (1986; 1994b). Four males and two females were placed in a 16m^2 enclosure and allowed to reproduce freely, so that after 20 months there were about 50 individuals in the colony. Even at this high population density the reproductive success of females (that is, the number of surviving offspring/time) did not decline, and the number of fights between individuals did not increase distinctly. So what mechanisms allow guinea pigs to cope so effectively with high population numbers? The answer is shown in Figure 27.2. As population density increases, guinea pigs change their patterns of social interactions and their social relationships, that is, their social organisation (Sachser 1986).

At low population densities (for example, three males and three females) the social organisation is characterised mainly by a linear dominance hierarchy among the adult males.

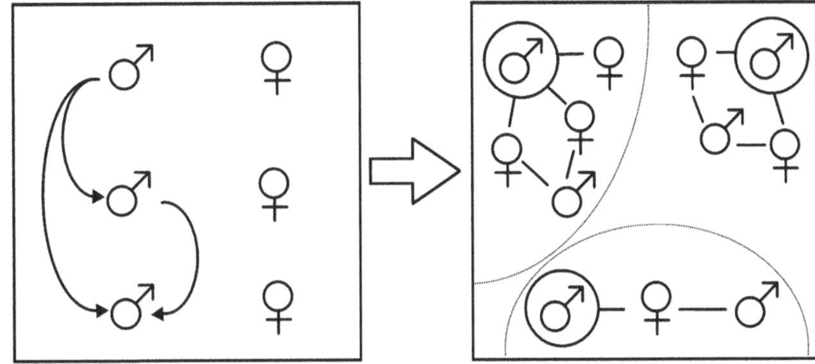

Figure 27.2 Social organisation in guinea pigs at high and low densities. Low density at the left side: arrows among males indicate direction of aggressive behaviours. High density at the right side: lines between males and females indicate individual social bonds. Alpha-males (circled males) dominate non-alpha males (non-circled males). Dotted lines represent the borders of 'territories' (Sachser 1986). Reproduced from Sachser N (1998): Of domestic and wild guinea pigs: studies in sociophysiology, domestication and social evolution, Naturwissenschaft, copyright 1998 with kind permission of Springer Science and Business Media.

Subordinate males retreat whenever a higher-ranking conspecific approaches; this largely precludes threat displays and fights. Individuals of identical rank are never found. The highest-ranking male shows much more courtship behaviour towards each of the females than any other male, and he is probably the father of the offspring. Social bonds do not exist between males and females. Among the females there is also a linear rank order (Thyen & Hendrichs 1990). However, their agonistic interactions are less pronounced than those among males. Between the sexes fighting and threat displays do not occur.

When individual numbers increase, guinea pigs change their social organisation. Groups of 10–15 or more split into subunits, each consisting of one to four males and one to seven females. The highest-ranking male of each subunit, the alpha-male, establishes long-lasting social bonds toward all females of his subunit. The alphas guard and defend their females around oestrus, and they sire more than 85% of offspring, as shown by DNA fingerprinting (Sachser 1998). The lower-ranking males also have bonds with the females of their subunits, ie, they interact predominantly with these animals. Alphas of different subunits respect each other's bonds, that is, they do not court other alphas' females even if these are receptive. In general, individuals belonging to a given subunit live in an area that does not overlap with the area of other subunits. It is in these areas that most of the social interactions are displayed, and where the individuals have their resting and sleeping places. The alphas defend the borders of these areas around the time of their females' oestrus (Sachser 1986, 1994b).

Social organisation at high population densities is therefore characterised by the following: (1) the splitting of the whole group into subunits provides all individuals with social and spatial orientation; (2) escalated fighting is rare because alphas respect the male–female bonds of other alphas; (3) the individuals' different social positions are stable over months, and the basic patterns of social organisation are independent of individual animals. Thus the change in social organisation from a strictly dominance-structured system to a system in which long-lasting bonds are predominant seems to be a mechanism for adjusting to increasing population density.

Physiological consequences of social stratification

When male guinea pigs living at different population densities are compared, those at high densities show increased activity of the sympathetic–adrenomedullary system at high densities. In contrast, the activity of the pituitary–adrenocortical system is not affected by population density. That is, a male living in a large colony does not have higher cortisol concentrations than a male living in a small group or with only one female. These endocrinological data support the behavioural findings that a change in density does not necessarily result in increased social stress for the individuals as long as a stable social environment is maintained by social mechanisms (Sachser 1990, 1994a).

At high and low population densities, males take different social positions, which are stable over months. Alphas, for example, always clearly dominate non-alphas of the same subunit. These dominance relationships are independent of place and time. Alphas bite more often and are bitten less often than non-alphas, and display far more courtship and sexual behaviour than the lower-ranking males (Sachser 1990). Surprisingly, despite these clear differences in behaviour and status, alphas and non-alphas do not differ significantly in their activity of their pituitary–adrenocortical and sympathetic–adrenomedullary systems (Sachser 1987, 1994b; Sachser *et al.* 1998); that is, having low social status does not necessarily entail a higher degree of social stress than having high social status. This is probably because of the stable social relationships which result in predictable behaviour.

Social support

In a variety of animals, the presence of specific social partners can often inhibit or ameliorate the individual's neuroendocrine responses in stressful situations; ie, the increase of the pituitary–adrenocortical and the sympathetic–adrenomedullary activities is reduced (Sachser *et al.* 1998; Kawachi & Berkman 2001). This class of effects, often referred to as social buffering of the stress response, is clearly seen in the context of the mother–infant relationship. The domestic guinea pig is one of the few animals in which social buffering effects on HPA activity have been found in both infants and adults.

Prior to weaning, guinea pig pups show evidence of a specific attachment to their mother, and the presence of the mother reduces or eliminates HPA responses in a novel environment (Hennessy & Ritchey 1987; Hennessy 1997, 1999; Hennessy *et al.* 2006). During the pre-weaning period the presence of other animals, particularly adult females, has also been found to reduce HPA activity in pups, but not as consistently as the presence of the mother (Hennessy & Ritchey 1987; Ritchey & Hennessy 1987; Sachser *et al.* 1998; Graves & Hennessy 2000; Hennessy *et al.* 2002a, 2002b). The spatial environment also seems to influence the neuroendocrine and behavioural responses of guinea pig pups to a threatening situation. For example, the pups express more distress calls in an unfamiliar than in a familiar environment irrespective of whether their mothers are present or absent (Pettijohn 1979). Furthermore, cortisol concentrations in infant guinea pigs do not increase after separation from their mother when they stay in their familiar enclosure together with familiar group members (Wewers *et al.* 2003).

Among adults, males and females form attachment-like bonds with opposite-sex partners (see earlier in this chapter) (Jacobs 1976; Sachser 1986). As regards interactions with an individual colony-living male, females can be placed in three categories: (1) his bonded females with whom most amicable interactions take place; (2) females which live in the same colony, and with whom he is familiar but has no social ties; and (3) unfamiliar females which live in a different colony, and which he has never encountered before. Interestingly, the male's endocrine stress response – ie, increase in activity of his pituitary–adrenocortical system – when placed in an unfamiliar cage is sharply reduced when a female with which he is bonded is present. In contrast, the presence of an unfamiliar female or of one with whom he is merely acquainted has little effect. Thus, the effect of various types of relationships differs remarkably, and substantial social support is given only by the bonded partner (Sachser *et al.* 1998; Hennessy *et al.* 2006).

The presence of the bonded partner also leads to a sharp reduction in the acute stress response in female guinea pigs living in large mixed-sex colonies. Thus, in guinea pigs, there is a two-way provision of social support between male and female bonded pairs. However, female guinea pigs show a different reaction to males in the presence of a familiar conspecific, who is not the bonded partner. In this case their stress response is lower than in the absence of a familiar conspecific. Thus, a familiar social partner can provide social support for females but not for males (Kaiser *et al.* 2003a).

Effects of social experiences on physiology and behaviour

Guinea pigs can co-exist in a non-stressful and non-aggressive way even at high densities. This can be attributed to three factors: (1) a greater tolerance toward conspecifics, which has been acquired during the process of domestication (see earlier in this chapter); (2) the ability to establish and to respect dominance relationships; (3) the ability to establish and to respect social bonds. However, whether these features are expressed depends on the social conditions under which the individuals were reared.

When two adult males reared in different large colonies are placed into an unfamiliar enclosure in the presence of an unfamiliar female they quickly establish stable dominance relationships without displaying overt aggression. No significant changes in pituitary–adrenocortical system or sympathetic–adrenomedullary system activities are found, either in the dominant or in the subdominant male (Sachser & Lick 1991). However, this 'peaceful' stratification into different social positions requires that the opponents, around puberty, have previously had agonistic interactions with older dominant males, which is the case in individuals reared in colonies. In these encounters as a subdominant individual, they acquire the social skills needed to adapt to conspecifics in a non-aggressive and non-stressful way (Sachser & Lick 1991; Sachser 1993; Sachser *et al.* 1994).

In contrast, a male that has grown up singly or with a female does not experience agonistic interactions around puberty (since in this species no fighting and threat displays are found between the sexes) and thus does not learn these social skills. If two of these males confront one another in the presence of an unfamiliar female in an unfamiliar enclosure, high levels of aggressive behaviour occur, and escalated fighting is frequent which, if not stopped, may lead to severe injuries or deaths. During the first days of the confrontation no stable dominance relationships are established but once this has occurred marked and persistent increases in pituitary–adrenocortical system activities occur in the subdominant males (Sachser & Lick 1991; Sachser *et al.* 1994). The evidence is that it is not fighting ability that determines the outcome of such contests, but that the winners are the males that succeed in establishing a bond toward the female.

The crucial role of social experiences has also been shown in a study taking a different approach (Sachser & Renninger 1993). Colony-reared males introduced singly into unfamiliar colonies of conspecifics easily adjust to this new social situation. They explore the new environment, but do not court any female, thereby avoiding attacks from the male residents, which have established bonds with the females. The colony-reared males gradually integrate into the social network of the established colonies and may even gain a higher social rank than they had in their native colonies. In contrast, individually reared males placed into a colony of conspecifics are frequently involved in threat displays and fights (Sachser & Lick 1991; Sachser & Renninger 1993) and may lose body weight and die, even when not injured or attacked by the residents.

In contrast, female guinea pigs reared in colonies or in pairs can adapt to introduction into a group of unfamiliar conspecifics without the occurrence of overt aggression and high degrees of social stress. Thus female guinea pigs are able to adapt to unfamiliar conspecifics independent of their social rearing conditions (Kaiser *et al.* 2003c).

Effects of the prenatal social environment on physiology and behaviour

Instability of the social environment during pregnancy and lactation (through exchange of females between groups) alters the development of guinea pig offspring. Behaviour, endocrine systems and brain development of daughters and sons, whose mothers have lived in a stable social environment during pregnancy and lactation, differ in a sex-specific fashion from those whose mothers lived in an unstable social environment during this period of life (Sachser & Kaiser 1996; Kaiser & Sachser 1998, 2005; Kaiser *et al.* 2003b, 2003d). Daughters whose mothers have lived in an unstable social environment show conspicuous behavioural masculinisation (Sachser & Kaiser 1996) displaying significantly more behaviours which are essential parts of the male courtship behaviour, such as intensive nasoanal sniffing and rumba (a swinging movement of the posterior part of the body), than daughters whose mothers have lived in a stable social environment. The behavioural masculinisation is accompanied by increased testosterone concentrations and an elevated activity of the sympathetic–adrenomedullary system as indicated by greater adrenal tyrosine hydroxylase activity (Kaiser & Sachser 1998). Daughters whose mothers have lived in an unstable social environment show an up-regulation of androgen receptors and oestrogen receptor-α in specific areas in the limbic system of the brain compared to daughters whose mothers have lived in a stable social environment (Kaiser *et al.* 2003b).

Sons of mothers from unstable social environments show a behavioural infantilisation that is accompanied by significantly decreased adrenal tyrosine hydroxylase activities and a delayed development of the adrenocortical system (Kaiser & Sachser 2001). Furthermore, these males show a down-regulation of androgen receptors and oestrogen receptor-α in specific parts of the limbic system such as the medial preoptic area of the hypothalamus and the hippocampus compared to males whose mothers have lived in a stable social environment (Kaiser *et al.* 2003d). Thus, early social stress induces changes in endocrine, autonomic and limbic brain function, which are mirrored by changes in male and female adult social behaviour.

Social housing of guinea pigs

This section provides recommendations on the social housing of guinea pigs that are based on findings from basic research into their social life and welfare. Table 27.4 summarises the housing conditions which can be recommended and those which should be avoided (see Sachser *et al.* 2004).

Table 27.4 Beneficial and detrimental housing conditions for guinea pigs. Reproduced from Sachser *et al.* (2004) The welfare of laboratory guinea pigs, In: The welfare of laboratory animals, E. Kaliste (ed.), copyright with kind permission of Springer.

Housing condition	*Recommended*	*To be avoided*
Solitary		X
Pair: 1 male, 1 female	X	
Harems (1 male, several females)	X	
Female groups: 2 females	X	
>2 females	X	
Male groups: 2 males	X	
>2 males		X
Small mixed-sex groups	X	
Large mixed-sex groups	X	

Single housing

Domestic guinea pigs still bear the heritage of their wild ancestors the cavy (*Cavia aperea*). Thus, we should not expect that they are able to adjust to any artificial housing but instead require at least some essential features of the environment in which their wild ancestors evolved (Sachser 2001). Since the ancestor of the guinea pig is a socially living wild species, it seems likely that single housing is not appropriate for its domesticated counterpart. Single-housed male guinea pigs cope with stress situations in a less effective way than guinea pigs living in social groups (Sachser 1994a).

Housing in pairs (one male, one female)

This housing condition is appropriate for guinea pigs. In this species, no fighting or threat displays are found between the sexes. Moreover, pair-reared males can cope with adversity in a much more effective way than solitary housed conspecifics.

Housing in harems

This housing system is also appropriate for guinea pigs. Agonistic interactions do occur between females, but such aggression is rare and of low intensity: escalated fights and bites almost never occur.

Female groups

Guinea pigs can be satisfactorily housed in all-female groups. The number is limited only by the enclosure size (with a maximum of about $0.25\,m^2$/animal), since females can be housed without problems in large groups. It is true that in all-female groups levels of aggression are slightly higher than in groups with one male and several females (Thyen & Hendrichs 1990) but aggression is rare and of low intensity. As in groups of one male and several females, escalated fights and bites almost never occur. Females living in large all-female groups do not experience high levels of stress.

Male groups

In groups consisting of two males, agonistic behaviour is rarely or never found. In contrast, in groups of more than two males, escalated agonistic interactions frequently occur beginning when the animals reach about 3–4 months. Additionally, animals that live in groups of two or four individuals show lower concentrations of the stress hormone cortisol than animals living in groups of six or twelve (Beer & Sachser 1992). Thus there seems to be good welfare when guinea pigs are housed in groups of two males, while indicators of social stress regularly occur in larger groups. So where mixed-sex housing is not possible we recommend keeping male guinea pigs in groups of two.

Males show courtship and sexual behaviour towards each other in the same way as males usually court females: pseudo-copulations occur including mounts and ejaculations. Specific males also display female-typical behaviour. These individuals, termed 'pseudofemales', not only tolerate the courtship and mounting by others, but also actively display defence urine-spraying, a behavioural pattern which is typical for females and usually serves to keep off courting males. The other males of the group behave towards these pseudofemales as towards real females and compete with each other for them. The pseudofemales do not take part in the aggressive conflicts. They rarely receive aggressive behaviour. Physiological stress indicators show that pseudofemales are subjected to lowest stress in the group (Beer & Sachser 1992).

Mixed-sex groups of a few males and females

Housing guinea pigs in small mixed-sex groups can also be acceptable. However, the formation of such a group with animals of unknown social rearing experience should be avoided since it frequently leads to intensive threat and fighting behaviour, extreme stress responses and injuries (see paragraph on effects of social experiences on physiology and behaviour).

Mixed-sex groups of many males and females

The housing condition, which we most favour for guinea pigs, is the large mixed-sex colony. In this, dominant as well as subordinate animals live a good life and are not subjected to high degrees of stress. All animals are able to learn the social skills which are necessary for interactions with conspecifics (see earlier). However, such a large mixed-sex group should have a varied age structure. The best system is to allow a small mixed-sex group to increase to the desired size. The assembly of a large group, using animals coming from pairs or solitary housing as well as with animals of unknown origin, should be avoided since it frequently leads to intensive threat and fighting behaviour, extreme stress responses and health problems.

Physical housing and care of guinea pigs

Housing

Guinea pigs from commercial breeders are frequently used as specific pathogen free (SPF) animals. Such guinea pigs have to be housed under barrier conditions (eg, separated positive-pressure rooms) to prevent introduction of pathogens. It is also possible to house guinea pigs in individually ventilated cages (IVCs) such as 1500 cm^2 or 2000 cm^2 cages for rats, but the space of the smaller ones does not comply with the revised Council of Europe recommendations (Appendix A, ETS 123) or the revised Annex II to the European Directive. Moreover, the 2000 cm^2 cages are very difficult to handle, and are therefore not in common use.

Guinea pigs can be kept in pens or cages (Figure 27.3). The authors also have experience with keeping guinea pigs in pens on the floor, and recommend this type of housing. In this case bedding (eg, wood shavings) is necessary. However, certain floor covering materials such as flagstones can become contaminated with uroliths because adequate cleaning at regular intervals is difficult. For this reason, rooms should be emptied periodically for cleaning, descaling and disinfection.

It is important to provide enough space. High stocking densities can lead to endocrine stress reactions and high frequencies of aggression. The recently revised Council of Europe Appendix A and the European Directive Annex II give guidelines for the accommodation and care of guinea pigs (Council of Europe 2006; European Commission 2007). These recommend a minimum enclosure size of 2500 cm^2 and a floor area per adult animal (>700 g body weight) of 900 cm^2. Sachser *et al.* (2004), however, suggest providing a floor area of about 2500 cm^2 per adult animal if possible. According to the European documents a minimum enclosure size of 1800 cm^2 for smaller animals (≤450 g body weight) is possible. However, the usual height of 20 cm in Makrolon cages type III is not sufficient, since this impairs playing behaviour ('frisky hops') of juveniles and prevents adult individuals from fully standing on their hindlegs. A minimum height of 23 cm is recommended by Appendix A, whereas Sachser *et al.* (2004) recommend 30 cm.

Specific forms of grid floors (eg, in metabolic cages) can cause problems and therefore should be used only for short periods during experiments. Grid floors are often the cause of diseases (eg, pododermatitis). Young animals' extremities are especially vulnerable if the mesh is too wide. On the other hand, openings have to be big enough to ensure the passage of faeces. If solid floors are not possible for experimental reasons, so that grids or wire mesh have to be used, then at least a solid or bedded area should be provided on which the animals can rest. Furthermore, it is important to check the grid floors closely to ensure that there is no risk of injury from loose or sharp projections. Pregnant and lactating females should always be kept on solid floors with bedding.

The most important environmental enrichment for the guinea pig is the social group. However, some physical enrichment should also be provided, eg, structural division of the environment by, for example, refuges or plastic piping into which all animals can retreat. It is important, however, to provide sufficient ventilation holes. Piping should be short enough to prevent more than two animals using it simultaneously. If more animals can enter it, a number of animals may press into the piping and there is a risk that animals in the middle will be asphyxiated. Branches for gnawing are a very easy kind of enrichment but should be autoclaved before use. Hay provides a substrate and is a useful enrichment (see section on feeding). Where hay is not used reproductive performance may be reduced.

Environmental provisions

Accommodation must provide draught-free ventilation. Relative humidity should be around 50–60%. The optimal temperature is around 18–22 °C (according to the European convention, Appendix A, 20–24 °C (Council of Europe 2006)). Guinea pigs are better able to withstand cold than heat. There are some indications that reproduction will decrease if temperature exceeds 30 °C.

Guinea pigs should be kept neither in constant light nor in constant darkness. A light–dark rhythm of about 12 h light and 12 h dark and also the natural light–dark rhythm are suitable (eg, if the animals are living in outdoor pens).

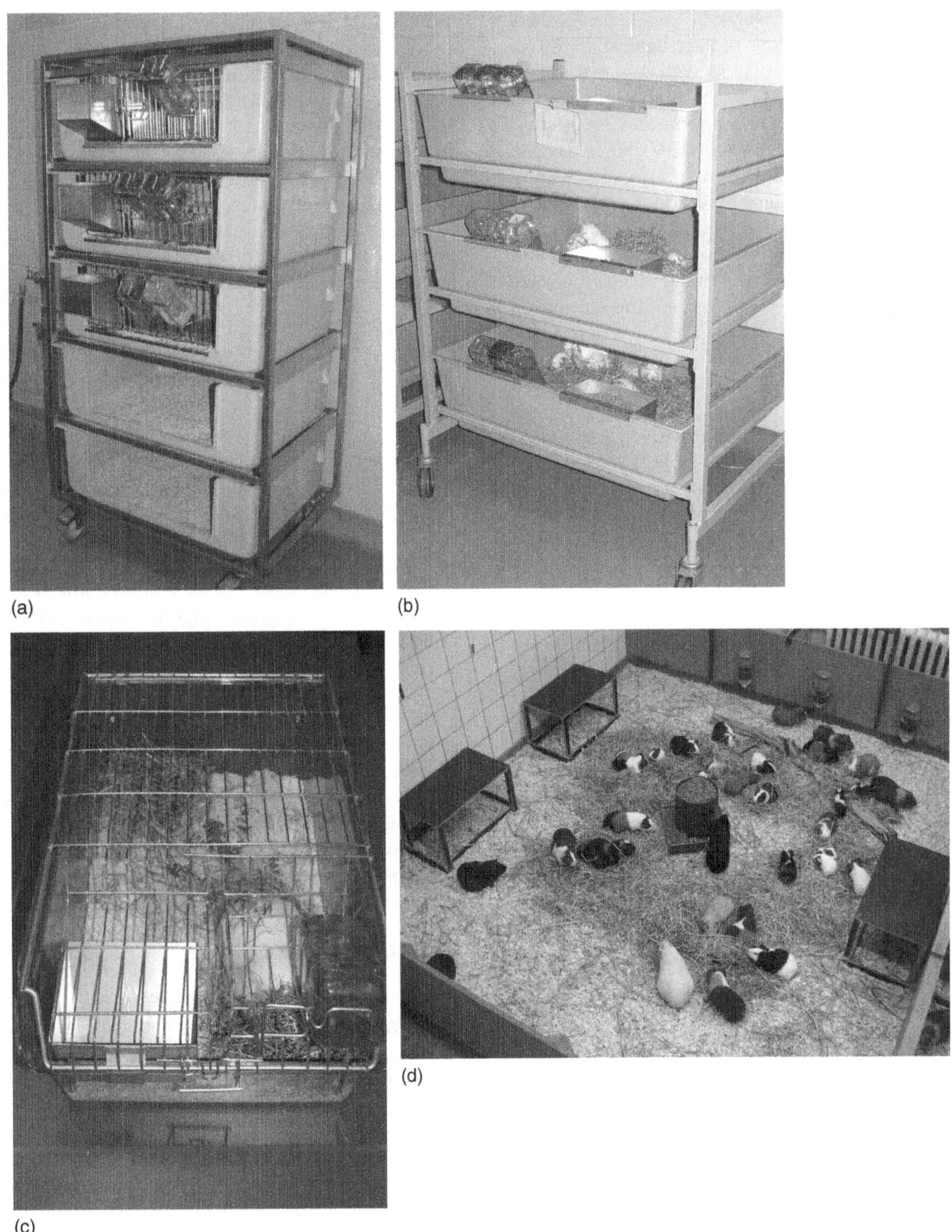

(a) (b) (c) (d)

Figure 27.3 Different types of cages suitable for housing of guinea pigs as well as floor housing.

Guinea pigs should be protected against loud noise, which can cause panic reactions, leading to injuries.

Feeding

Guinea pigs are herbivores. Their wild ancestors live on grass, roots and seeds. In the laboratory, guinea pigs are usually fed with commercial plant-based pellets. The food has to be stored in cool, dry conditions and be protected against contamination. It should be available *ad libitum*. It is essential that food is provided in such a way to ensure access by all animals. Pellets have to be small (with a diameter of about 3 mm), enabling the guinea pigs to take them directly by mouth. It is important to ensure the availability of vitamins, especially of vitamin C, since guinea pigs are susceptible to vitamin C deficiency. Signs of deficiency include: poor skin, poor haircoat, weight loss, stiffness, difficulties in walking, and even paralysis and poor bone and tooth development. If the vitamin C content in the food is insufficient (it remains active in pellets for only 90 days), ascorbic acid can be added to the drinking water (0.5 g/l). This should be freshly made as dissolved vitamin C decomposes within 24 h.

Good-quality hay should always be available. Besides diet-related benefits (eg, it may protect against digestive disturbances), hay is used for play as well as a material in which to burrow and hide. Due to the high proportion of fibre, hay also seems to prevent alopecia and teeth overgrowth (Wolf & Kamphues 2004; Wasel 2007). Since hay can represent an infection risk, heat treatment at 70 °C is recommended (autoclaving at higher temperatures may lead to injury due to hardening of the halms).

Feeding dishes or food hoppers should be designed and positioned so as to prevent animals being able to defecate or urinate into them. Guinea pigs often spill food, and on grid floors (which should be avoided, see Housing section), the food will be wasted. There are available some suitable hoppers that reduce wastage. The water supply should be spatially separated from the feeding dish because guinea pigs tend to dribble water into the feeding dish, resulting in agglutinated pellets. Guinea pigs will rapidly learn to use drinking nipples attached to bottles or automatic systems. Stainless steel sipper tubes and nipples should be used because the animals like to gnaw at them.

Bedding

The bedding material, eg wood fibres or granulate, has to be dry and absorbent. It should be free of toxic residue (eg, timber preservative), parasites and infectious agents. Dust should be kept to a minimum. The interval between cleaning depends on the kind of cage or pen used. Normally, once a week is reasonable.

Housing and change

Guinea pigs react highly sensitively to changes of environment. Thus it is important to habituate them slowly to new conditions. The combination of several factors – each of which individually would have no negative effects – may result in strong stress responses and severe health problems. For example, the simultaneous provision of a new cage and a new drinking bottle should be avoided. New drinking bottles should be offered together with the old one until the animals begin to drink from the new one. Also unfamiliar food should be mixed with the familiar food, and the portion of the old food should be reduced step-by-step. When transferring animals to a new cage, no other modifications, such as providing new food or removing a social partner, should be made simultaneously. Whether or not an animal can adjust to a new situation can be assessed reliably from its drinking and feeding behaviour. If the animals are feeding and, particularly, drinking, then they can adapt to the new situation. In contrast, refusing water and food, scrubby fur and apathy point to extremely poor welfare.

Identification and sexing

Coloured animals can be identified individually by natural markings without problems. Albino animals can be coloured, eg with food colouring on the fur. The dyes have to be renewed at regular intervals (3–4 weeks).

A frequently used method for permanent marking is ear tattooing. Another method is to implant microchips. Radio frequency identification (RFID) is a rapidly evolving technique and it is becoming an increasingly important tool in animal sciences. Even very small animals can be individually marked using small encapsulated RFID transponders. The animals can be identified with suitable readers, but only at short distances.

Guinea pigs are very easy to sex (Figure 27.4). Male and female guinea pigs can be differentiated by gentle pressing around the genital area. The penis is easily extruded. In older animals, the testes are also apparent, but can be lifted through the open inguinal ring into the abdominal cavity. In females, this technique will expose the vaginal membrane which closes the vagina (except during oestrus and parturition).

Health monitoring

Guinea pigs should undergo regular health checks: appearance should be assessed (skin state, teeth, claws, eyes, nose, anal region) and the body weight should be measured regularly. Furthermore, behavioural abnormalities should be recorded and investigated. Incoming animals should be quarantined and screened for potential infections.

When laboratory guinea pigs are kept as SPF animals, care must be taken to maintain this status for microbiological standardisation. Therefore, besides well organised housing, the colony should be involved in health-monitoring programmes. On the one hand, such programmes serve to prevent the facility from introducing pathogens by newly arrived animals; on the other hand, long-term colony health status will be monitored for accidental infections. Monitoring protocols, including the number of animals tested, can vary based upon the number of animals in the colony and the duration of their husbandry. Recommendations for reasonable monitoring design are provided by the Federation of European Laboratory Animal Science Associations (FELASA 2002) (Table 27.5).

Laboratory procedures

Handling

Guinea pigs are normally relatively docile and they bite very rarely. They should be picked up gently with both hands: one hand should hold firmly the shoulder or chest, the other hand has to support the hindquarters. In the case of pregnant guinea pigs, this is particularly important because they can become very heavy. After picking them up, guinea pigs should be held against the handler's body (Figure 27.5).

Sampling techniques

Blood collection

Choosing the right site for blood sampling depends on the size of the guinea pig and the amount of blood needed. For single blood collection no more than 10% of the total blood volume (approximately 75 ml/kg of the body mass) should be taken. Weekly collected blood volumes should not exceed 7.5% and daily collected volumes should not exceed 1% of the total blood volume (Joint Working Group on Refinement

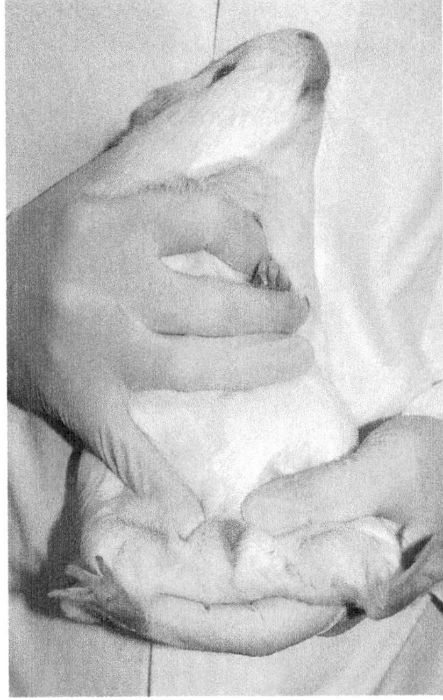

(a)

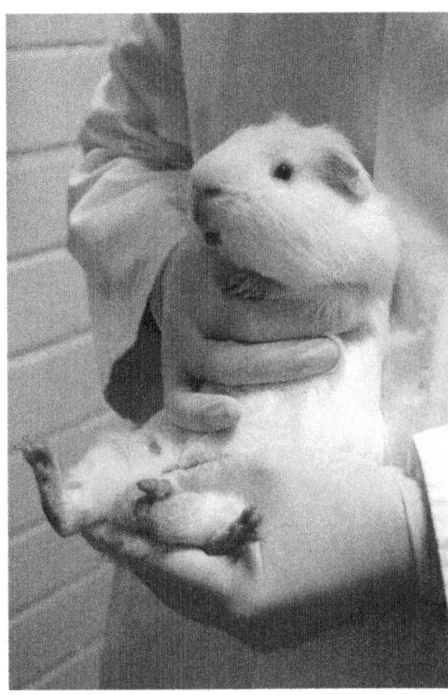

(b)

Figure 27.4 Sexing a guinea pig. (a) In the female the vaginal membrane will be exposed. (b) In the male the penis is easily extruded from the genital opening using gentle pressure.

Table 27.5 FELASA recommendations for the health monitoring of guinea pig colonies.

Disease	*Test frequency*
Viruses	
Guinea pig adenovirus	3 months
Sendai virus	3 months
Guinea pig cytomegalovirus	Annually
Bacteria, mycoplasma and fungi	
Bordetella bronchiseptica	3 months
Chlamydia psittaci	3 months
Corynebacterium kutscheri	3 months
Dermatophytes	3 months
Pasteurellaceae	3 months
Salmonella spp.	3 months
Streptobacillus moniliformis	3 months
Streptococci β-haemolytic (not group D)	3 months
Streptococcus pneumoniae	3 months
Yersinia pseudotuberculosis	3 months
Clostridium piliforme (Tyzzer's disease)	Annually
Parasites	
Ectoparasites	3 months
Endoparasites:	3 months
Encephalitozoon cuniculi	3 months
Pathological lesions observed	3 months

(JWGR) 1993). Since rodent blood often coagulates within the needle, short needles are recommended and sometimes it may be useful to remove the cone of the needle from the syringe before puncturing a vessel.

For collecting small amounts of blood, the ear vessels may be punctured (Figure 27.6). In coloured animals a cold point lamp behind the ear increases the visibility of the blood vessels. In albinos this is not necessary. To increase blood flow, the veins can be compressed manually. After disinfecting the skin the ear vessels are punctured with a sterile disposable needle (0.6 × 25 mm (23 G)) and the blood is collected, for example, in heparinised capillaries.

The lateral saphenous vein is another site for blood collection (Figure 27.6). After shaving the fur from the back of the hindlimb and disinfecting the skin, one person restrains the guinea pig with one hindlimb extended backwards. The vein runs laterally to the Achilles tendon, and the insertion site is close to the tendon in the middle third of the lower leg. Even if the vein is not visible, the needle (0.7 × 30 mm or 0.6 × 25 mm) can be inserted at a 30–45° angle from disto-caudal direction and blood can be collected in a vial.

To collect larger volumes, the jugular vein or the cranial vena cava can be used as a survival method, although there is a risk of haemorrhage or cardiac tamponade. Usually the procedure is done under anaesthesia in dorsal recumbancy. The puncture site is the thoracic inlet left or right of the sternum. A needle with a 2 ml syringe is inserted at a 45° angle while pulling back the plunger until blood appears in the syringe. After removal of the needle, pressure should be applied to the site of puncture. Hillyer *et al.* (1997) described a method to collect blood from the jugular vein without anaesthesia by restraining the animal with the forelegs extended down over a table edge and head and neck extended up. This procedure appears to be very stressful and should be done by trained personnel only, since location of the vein is often difficult.

Cardiac puncture is only recommended as terminal procedure under anaesthetic because of the comparatively high risk of cardiac tamponade. The heart can be punctured laterally in the area where the strongest heartbeat can be felt, or from a caudal direction with the insertion site behind the xiphoid.

The retro-orbital sinus may be used for blood sampling under anaesthesia, but access to the sinus is more difficult than in rats and mice and may result in severe complications (eg, exophthalmus). JWGR (1993) consider that this

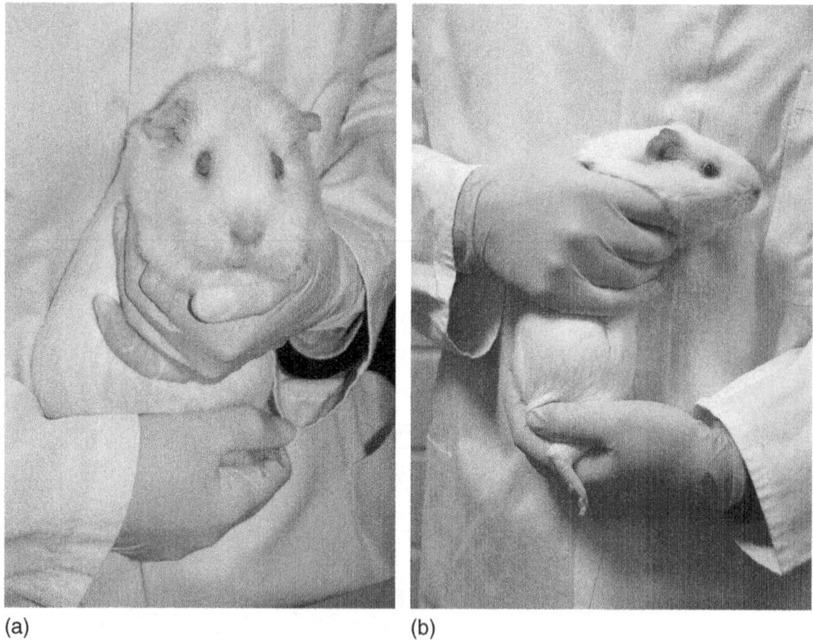

(a) (b)

Figure 27.5 Methods of handling a guinea pig.

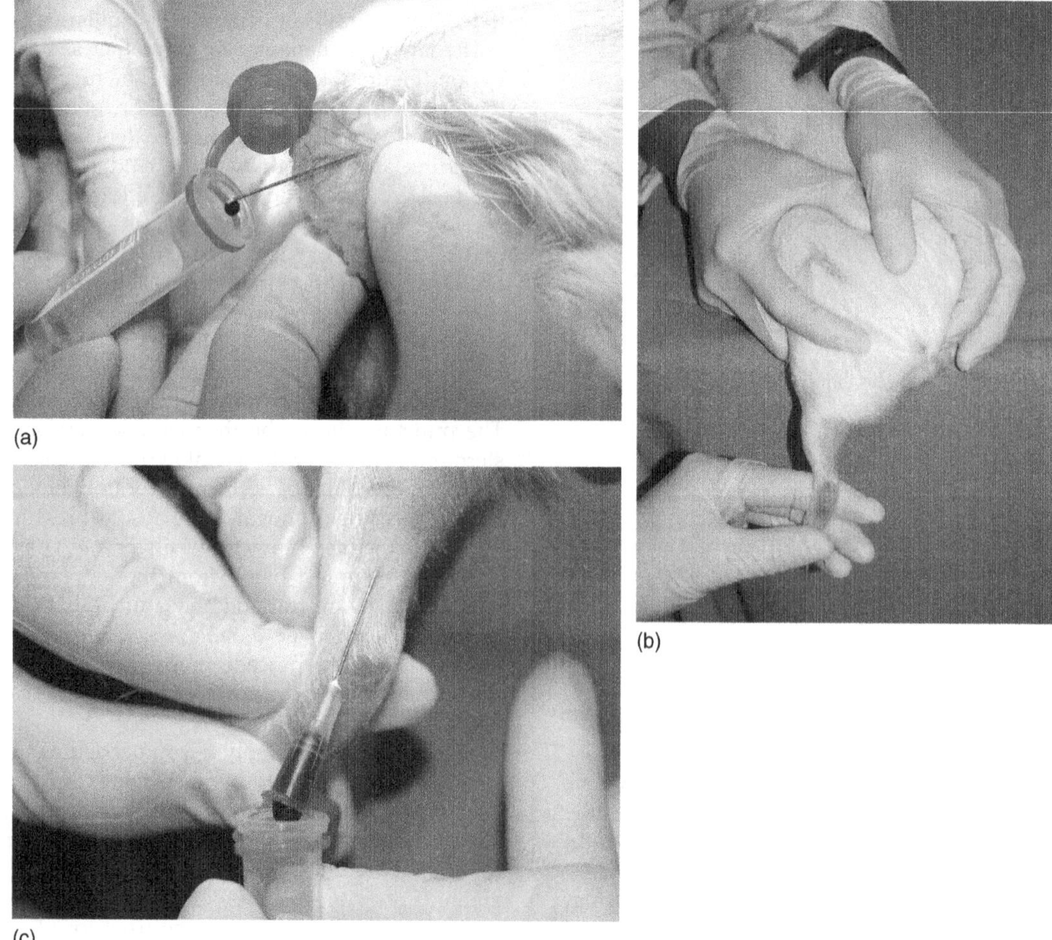

(a) (b) (c)

Figure 27.6 Blood sampling procedures. (a) Ear vessels. (b, c) Saphenous vein.

technique, which samples a mixture of blood and tissue fluid, is only appropriate under terminal anaesthesia.

Urine collection

Urine may be collected manually by applying gentle pressure over the caudal abdominal area. This method will provide a cleaner sample than collecting urine in a metabolic cage, where faeces may contaminate the urine sample. Uncontaminated urine samples can be collected via cystocentesis. For this, the guinea pig should be prepared as for surgery. Anaesthesia may be necessary for safe restraint and the bladder should be fixed manually while it is punctured with a fine needle through the abdominal wall.

A method to introduce a fine, flexible catheter into the urethra of male and female guinea pigs has been described, but there are risks of pathogen introduction into the bladder and mucosa injury, particularly in males (Ewringmann & Gloeckner 2005; Wasel 2007).

Administration of medicines

For general principles of administering substances see JWGR (2001). Oral medications can be administered by adding small quantities of liquids or solids to the feed or drinking water. However, using this method it is not possible to determine or ensure the dose consumed. Furthermore, the intake may be influenced by drug-related changes of appearance or taste of feed or water. Another method is to take a syringe or dosing needle with a rounded end to drop the liquid onto the back of the tongue. A rat dosing needle or a polyethylene catheter with outside diameter 1.0–1.3 mm can also be used. The catheter should be introduced via the interdental space. Care has to be taken that the animals have enough time to swallow during these procedures. For application of exact or larger doses of compounds, oral gavage via a gastric tube can be performed (Figure 27.7). For this, another person has to restrain the animal and a mouth gag with a hole in its middle should be placed behind the incisors to prevent the animals from biting into the tube. Subsequently, the moistened tube can be inserted carefully into the oesophagus. If coughing or dyspnoea occurs during administration of the compound, the procedure must be stopped immediately and the tube has to be reinserted.

Parenteral administration may be done in several ways. Subcutaneous or intramuscular injections (Figure 27.7) are both suitable methods, even though, depending on the agent to be administered, the subcutaneous method may be generally preferred. For administration of small volumes intramuscular injections into the thigh muscles of the hindlimbs can be performed. The needle should not be introduced too far, to avoid damage of the femur or nervus ischiadicus with associated bruising, periostitis or nerve irritation. No more than 0.3 ml should be injected into one site (Terril & Clemons 1998; North 1999) to minimise risks of muscle necrosis. Subcutaneous injections can be used for application of larger volumes (up to 3 ml per site) under the skin of the neck, back, or flanks of the animal. For intradermal injections (maximum 0.1 ml) the usual sites are the flank or the dorsum. Larger volumes of up to 10 ml can be given by intraperitoneal injection, but care has to be taken to avoid injuries to the internal organs or injecting the substance into the caecum, where it may not be absorbed. If the substance is irritant, peritonitis or adhesions of the caecum can result. Although access to superficial veins is sometimes difficult in guinea pigs, intravascular administration is also possible. The auricular veins are the most suitable. Fine needles are recommended; veins may be dilated by warming before injection; and injection must be performed very slowly by a trained person.

Injection sites should be clipped, shaved and then swabbed with a suitable antiseptic. Depending on the kind and the amount of the substance which is administered, it may be necessary to use multiple injection sites.

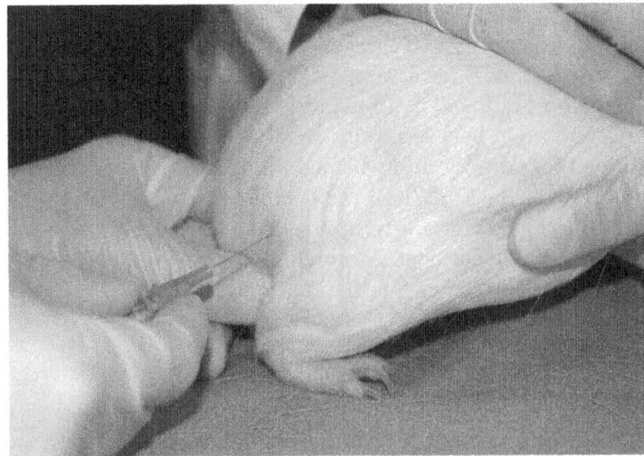

(a)

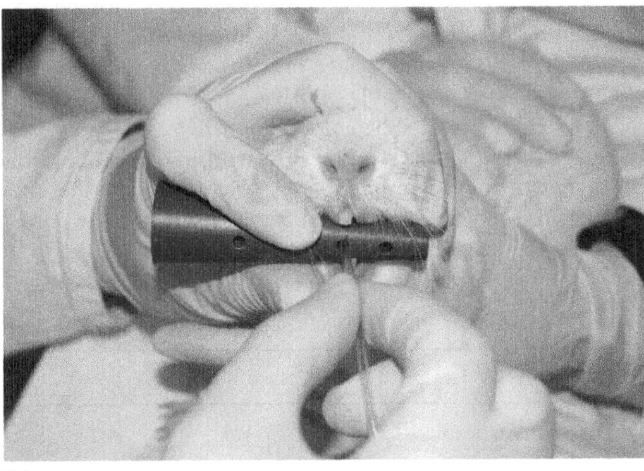

(b)

Figure 27.7 Administration techniques. (a) Intramuscular injection into the hindlimb of a guinea pig. (b) Oral gavage via gastric tube. A mouth gag prevents the guinea pig from biting into the tube.

Anaesthesia and analgesia

Anaesthesia should be used for all procedures causing more pain or stress than the anaesthesia itself. Guinea pigs, like other small rodents, have a high metabolic rate and oxygen consumption, so hypoglycaemia, dehydration, hypothermia and hypoxaemia can develop rapidly. For this reason, animals should not be fasted except for intubation or experimental reasons and oxygen should be administered if possible. If fasting is necessary, fasting time should not exceed 4 h (Abou-Madi 2006). To avoid hypothermia heating pads or lamps may be used, only small areas of fur should be clipped for surgery, and warmed fluids can be given subcutaneously (10–20 ml/kg). Anticholinergics like atropine (0.05 mg/kg sc) and glycopyrrolate (0.01–0.02 mg/kg sc) (Mason 1997) can be recommended to avoid excessive salivation, bronchial secretion and vagally induced bradycardia.

Inhalation anaesthesia

Because of its potential to induce respiratory depression as well as excessive salivation and secretion, inhalation anaesthesia alone is possible but is not the best method for general anaesthesia of guinea pigs. It is better to use a balanced technique that takes advantage of both sedative and analgesic effects of the injectable compounds. The main advantages of inhalants are their good controllability and rapid recovery of the animals. Currently, isoflurane seems to be the agent of choice for inhalants, because halothane and methoxyflurane may represent a health risk to exposed people while sevoflurane may lead to asphyxia in guinea pigs (Henke & Erhardt 2004). An anticholinergic medication should be administered before inhalation anaesthesia to decrease secretion. Some authors practise endotracheal intubation of guinea pigs with a tube size of 1.5–3.5 mm (Blouin & Cormier 1987), but long and narrow approaches to the trachea can make this difficult. In addition, food remnants stored in the cheeks may lead to obstruction or aspiration pneumonia. Therefore, intubating guinea pigs is an uncommon method and face masks are used instead. For induction 4–5% isoflurane is adequate and anaesthesia can be maintained with 2–4%.

Injectable anaesthesia

Various combinations of anaesthetics are widely used for injectable anaesthesia. Compared to inhalation anaesthesia the precise control of depth of anaesthesia and attainment of a surgical stage is more difficult when using injectable agents. Exact dosing may be difficult due to variable gastrointestinal content and its effect on body weight. Sedative and analgesic agents may be used for premedication or in combinations to induce general anaesthesia. Various anaesthetics and their dosages are summarised in Table 27.6.

Table 27.6 Sedative and anaesthetic agents for guinea pigs.

Anaesthetics	*Dosage*	*Route*	*Comments*	*Reference*
Diazepam/midazolam	2.5–5 mg/kg	im	Only sedation	Henke & Erhardt 2004, Terril & Clemons 1998
Xylazine	3–5 mg/kg	im/ip	Pre-anaesthetic, sedation	Terril & Clemons 1998
Medetomidine	0.15–0.5 mg/kg	im	Pre-anaesthetic, sedation	Henke & Erhardt 2004, North 1999
Ketamine + Xylazine	25–80 mg/kg 0.15–13 mg/kg	im/ip	Variable effect and duration, surgical anaesthesia possible	North 1999, Radde *et al.* 1996, Terril & Clemons 1998
Ketamine + Medetomidine	40–60 mg/kg 0.25–0.5 mg/kg	im/ip	Surgical anaesthesia	North 1999, Pfizer product information
Ketamine + Diazepam	44–125 mg/kg 0.1–5 mg/kg	im/ip		North 1999, Radde *et al.* 1996
Pentobarbital	15–35 mg/kg	ip	Lasts 2 h, no analgesia	Radde *et al.* 1996, Terril & Clemons 1998
Fentanyl + Midazolam + Medetomine	0.025 mg/kg 1 mg/kg 0.2 mg/kg	im	Surgical anaesthesia	Henke & Erhardt 2004
Fentanyl + Midazolam + Xylazine	0.05 mg/kg 2 mg/kg 2 mg/kg	im	Surgical anaesthesia	Henke & Erhardt 2004
Reversal agents:				
Naloxone + Flumazenile + Atipamezole	0.03 mg/kg 0.1 mg/kg 1 mg/kg	sc		Henke & Erhardt 2004
Tiletamine + Zolazepam (Zoletil®)	10–80 mg/kg	im	Minor procedures, more effective when combined with xylazine	Jacobson 2001, Terril & Clemons 1998

Increased dosages often lead to a longer anaesthetic time. In general, anaesthetics should be administered intramuscularly because subcutaneous applications often prove insufficient. Where appropriate, depending on the anaesthetic agents used, antidotes like naloxone and atipamezole should be given to promote rapid recovery.

Local anaesthetics can be used to reduce dose of general anaesthetics or for minor procedures in combination with some premedication. Usually, they are injected subcutaneously. Lidocaine 0.5–2% may be used in small volumes of 0.5–2 ml (5 mg/kg), diluted if necessary. For further advice see Flecknell (2009).

Analgesia

To control pain during and after surgery, analgesics should be administered pre-emptively, intra- and/or post-operatively, depending on the type of anaesthesia and the severity of the intervention. Different types of analgesics like NSAIDs or opiods may be used as a single treatment or combined as multimodal pain therapy. A list of analgesics and suggested dosages is provided in Table 27.7.

Euthanasia

Several methods for euthanasia are described in the literature. Currently, the American Veterinary Medical Association (AVMA) *Guidelines on Euthanasia* (2007) are considered the main reference for humane methods to euthanase animals. Furthermore, recommendations for euthanasia of laboratory animals have been published by the European Commission (Close *et al.* 1996, 1997). See also Chapter 17.

For guinea pigs, an overdose of injectable anaesthetic is preferred; the most suitable agent is sodium pentobarbital (200–400 mg/kg ip); this can be given by the intracardiac route only under anaesthesia. T-61® (a mixture of three drugs especially produced for euthanasia) should never be used without anaesthesia, due to induction of respiratory paralysis. It can be dosed intracardially or intrapulmonally. Inhalant agents like carbon dioxide or volatile anaesthetics are also commonly used, but these can be irritant to the animals. However, carbon dioxide is still widely used because it is a practical method for larger numbers of animals (and it can be an advantage in some studies that no chemical residues remain in tissues). Decapitation by guillotine and exsanguination subsequent to stunning are possible methods, but require well trained personnel. Cervical dislocation is not recommended for this species due to its short and strong neck.

Common welfare problems

Assessing welfare in guinea pigs

As for other mammals, the welfare of guinea pigs can be assessed from: (1) the guinea pig's general appearance; (2) body weight; (3) behaviour; and (4) physiological parameters (eg, Broom & Johnson 1993). See Chapter 6 for general aspects of welfare assessment.

1. General appearance of the animals: Experienced animal technicians, who know the normal appearance and behaviour of the animals, are well suited to monitor their health. The fur should be sleek and not scrubby, the claws should be short, the eyes clear and lucent, not clotted and dull, and the nose and anal region should be clean. Abnormal respiratory rate and pattern can point to disease and/or pain.
2. Body weight records: This parameter is a non-specific, but extremely reliable, indicator of welfare. Body weights of infant guinea pigs should increase regularly. In contrast, the body weights of adult animals should remain relatively constant. If there are modifications to their environment, guinea pigs can lose body weight. If an adult guinea pig loses more than 10% of its body

Table 27.7 Analgesic drug dosages for guinea pigs (NSAIDs: non-steroidal anti-inflammatory drugs).

Analgesic	*Dosage*	*Route*	*Reference*
Opioids			
Buprenorphine	0.05–0.5 mg/kg q8–12 h	sc/im	Dobromylskyj *et al.* 2000, Terril & Clemons 1998, Wasel 2007
Butorphanol	0.025–0.4 mg/kg q4 h	sc/im	Terril & Clemons 1998
Morphine	2–10 mg/kg q2–4 h	sc/im	Terril & Clemons 1998
Pethidine (meperidine)	10–20 mg/kg q2–4 h	im	Dobromylskyj *et al.* 2000, Terril & Clemons 1998
NSAIDs/mild analgesics			
Carprofen	4 mg/kg q24 h	sc/im	Henke *et al.* 2003
Flunixin	2.5 mg/kg q12–24 h	sc/im	Mason *et al.* 1997
Meloxicam	0.2 mg/kg q24 h	po/sc	Henke *et al.* 2003
Metamizol (dipyrone)	80 mg/kg q24 h	po	GV-SOLAS 2002

weight within 3 days, the former housing conditions should be restored immediately (Beer *et al.* 1994; Sachser *et al.* 2004). Weight increase in adults should be investigated as tumour growth may lead to unexpected increase in weight.

3. Behaviour: In general, normal frequencies of courtship, comfort, feeding, drinking and locomotor activity point to good welfare of the individuals. In juveniles, play behaviour ('frisky hops') should be displayed regularly. In contrast, high frequencies of aggression, apathy and absence or reduced frequencies of feeding, drinking and comfort behaviour indicate high degrees of stress. Such behavioural patterns are often paralleled by extreme neuroendocrine stress responses. Moreover, in guinea pigs there are specific vocalisations which signal stress: In juveniles the so-called 'distress call' occurs. It is a high-pitched whistle, which indicates excitement or anxiety. The distress call can be repeated several times in a bout of calls. Distress calls are most frequently encountered upon separation of the juveniles from their mothers. Frequent occurrence of the vocalisation 'chirp' is also a stress indicator. This call is emitted in situations of discomfort (Rood 1972). Chirps are a rapidly repeated series of high-pitched birdlike notes. The animal is in an alert posture and the body twitches at each note. Chirps may be given in a continuous series lasting for 10 or 15 minutes. Vocalisation in response to handling can indicate pain or stress.
4. Physiological parameters: Stress levels can be diagnosed reliably from endocrine parameters. In mammals, two stress axes exist: the pituitary–adrenocortical and the sympathetic–adrenomedullary systems (Henry & Stephens 1977; Sachser 1994a; von Holst 1998). These systems play a major role in adjusting an individual to its physical and social environment. The activation of each of these systems provides the organism with energy and shifts it into a state of heightened reactivity that is a prerequisite for responding to environmental changes in an appropriate way. Although the short-term or moderate activation of both systems represents an adaptive mechanism to cope with conflict situations, the long-term hyperactivation of both the pituitary–adrenocortical and the sympathetic–adrenomedullary systems is related to the aetiology of irreversible injury and even death (Henry & Stephens 1977; von Holst 1998). Serum glucocorticoid concentrations represent a good indication of the activity of the pituitary–adrenocortical system. Good indicators for the activity of the sympathetic–adrenomedullary system are: the serum concentrations of catecholamines (epinephrine, norepinephrine); the heart rate; and the adrenal tyrosine hydroxylase activity (Sachser 1994a; von Holst 1998). However, it should be mentioned that to determine adrenal tyrosine hydroxylase activity the animals have to be killed first. The most common method to assess stress in guinea pigs is to determine concentrations of serum cortisol (in guinea pigs cortisol is the main glucocorticoid (Jones 1974; Fujieda *et al.* 1982). Blood samples for this (about 200 µl blood) can be taken from the ear vessels (Sachser & Pröve 1984). Guinea pigs rarely struggle or vocalise during sampling with this procedure, and, since it is not necessary to anaesthetise the animals, later samples are not influenced by previous exposure to anaesthesia (Sachser 1994a). This sampling procedure is described in detail earlier in this chapter. Blood samples should to be taken within a time span of 5 minutes as glucocorticoid concentrations do not increase until 5 minutes after exposure to a stressor. Recently non-invasive techniques to assess degrees of stress have been developed. For example, glucococorticoids can be determined from saliva. In guinea pigs, saliva can be sampled very easily by putting a piece of cotton wool (eg, cotton bud) into the mouth of the animal for several minutes. Aside from endocrinological stress parameters, other indicators such as immune parameters can contribute to the diagnosis of stress and welfare in guinea pigs. Furthermore, measurements of haematological parameters as well as of blood biochemistry are helpful to indicate abnormal physiological states.

For haematological and biochemical data see Tables 27.8 and 27.9.

Disease

Details of diseases of guinea pigs are given among others in Seamer and Chesterman (1967), Wagner and Manning (1976), Harkness and Wagner (1989), Owen (1992), Huerkamp *et al.* (1996), North (1999) and Harkness *et al.* (2002). Signs of diseases may be non-specific, including symptoms like weight loss, lethargy or a rough coat. First indications of diseases are described in the section on welfare assessment. Routine checks should include observation of the behaviour, gait, urine and faeces. Animals should be regularly examined with special attention paid to their coat, eyes, nose, ears, mouth and teeth, as well as feet and nails.

Bacterial diseases, like salmonellosis, pneumonia and *Staphylococcus aureus* infections, viral diseases, like adenovirus, parainfluenza virus and herpesvirus infections, as well as parasitic diseases like mite and lice infestations can cause problems in guinea pigs. Non-infectious diseases include behavioural problems, nutritional imbalances and deficiencies (eg, hypovitaminosis C) and reproductive problems. In

Table 27.8 Guinea pig haematological data. Reprinted from North, D. (1999) with permission of Blackwell Publishing.

Haematological parameter	*Normal value*
Erythrocytes (10^6/mm^3)	4.4–8.2
Packed cell volume (haematocrit) (%)	37–48
Haemoglobin (g/dl)	11–15
Total leucocytes (10^6/mm^3)	4–18
Neutrophils (%)	17–44
Lymphocytes (%)	32–72
Eosinophils (%)	1–16
Monocytes (%)	1–12
Basophils (%)	0–3
Platelets (10^3/mm^3)	250–850
Total blood volume (ml/kg)	69–75

Table 27.9 Guinea pig biochemical data. Reprinted from North, D. (1999) with permission of Blackwell Publishing.

Blood biochemistry parameter	Normal value
Serum blood glucose (mg/dl)	60–125
Blood urea nitrogen (mg/dl)	9–31.5
Total plasma protein (g/dl)	4.2–6.5
Albumin (g/dl)	1.8–3.9
Globulin (g/dl)	0.8–2.6
Creatinine (mg/dl)	0.6–2.2
Total bilirubin (mg/dl)	0.3–0.9
Cholesterol (mg/dl)	20–43
Serum calcium (mg/dl)	4.5–12
Serum phosphate (mg/dl)	3.0–7.6

pregnant guinea pigs, especially in obese or anorexic females, toxaemia can occur during the last 2 weeks of gestation or 7–10 days after parturition. Dystocia often occurs in guinea pigs due to the large foetuses, particularly if females are bred either too young or too old for the first time. If they are older than 6–8 months, the pubic symphysis may not separate sufficiently, and obesity may furthermore obstruct the birth canal.

Tumours do not develop frequently and occur mainly in older animals. Lymphosarcoma and mammary gland tumours are the most common tumour diseases in guinea pigs and can occur both in females and males.

Table 27.10 summarises common diseases of guinea pigs. More detailed information can be taken from the cited authors as well as from North (1999).

Treatment of diseases is often difficult. First of all, sick animals have to be separated from the others. Housing conditions should be checked and optimised if necessary. The same papers cited above as well as Smith and Burgmann (1997), Ewringmann and Gloeckner (2005) and Wasel (2007) give information on treatment and drug dosages. Some bacterial diseases may be treated with antibiotics, however, antibiotic sensitivity should be tested first. Unlike most other species, the gastrointestinal flora of guinea pigs is predominated by Gram-positive bacteria. Therefore, certain antibiotics, including penicillin, ampicillin, or lincomycin cause an alteration to Gram-negative bacteria like *Escherichia coli* or *Clostridium difficile*, often resulting in severe enterotoxaemia. Broad-spectrum antibiotics such as enrofloxacin should be used for therapy, but only if really necessary.

It is often more humane and reasonable to sacrifice sick animals and above all pay attention to preventive measures.

Acknowledgements

Thanks go to Dr. Andreas Haemisch and Dr. Gero Hilken for substantial comments on aspects of care and use of guinea pigs in experimental animal sciences as well as Dr. Oliver Adrian, Dr. Philip Dammann and Dr. Ralph Waldschuetz for critical comments on the manuscript.

Table 27.10 Common diseases of guinea pigs (Noonan 1994; Schaeffer & Donnelly 1997; Wasel 2007).

Organ system	*Diseases*
Skin	Dermatophytosis (mainly *Trichophyton mentagrophytes*) Ectoparasites (mites like *Trixacarus caviae, Chirodiscoides caviae*, lice like *Gliricola porcelli, Gyropus ovalis*) Pododermatitis Endocrine alopecia (gestational, ovarian cysts) Bite wounds Barbering
Gastrointestinal tract	Malocclusion (incisors as well as back teeth) Antibiotic-associated enterotoxaemia Bacterial enteritis (*Salmonella* sp., *Clostridium* sp., *Escherichia coli, Yersinia pseudotuberculosis, Clostridium piliforme* etc) Parasitic diarrhoea (*Eimeria caviae, Paraspidodera uncinata*)
Respiratory tract	Bacterial pneumonia (*Bordetella bronchiseptica, Streptococcus pneumonia, Streptococcus zooepidemicus, Pasteurella multocida, Klebsiella pneumoniae*) Viral pneumonia (adenovirus)
Urogenital tract	Cystitis Urolithiasis Chronic interstitial nephritis (found in older animals) Ovarian cysts Endometritis Dystocia Pregnancy toxaemia Mastitis
Nervous system	Lymphocytic choriomeningitis (LCM virus), zoonotic disease! Torticollis (caused by progressive otitis media/interna, *Streptococcus pneumonia, Streptococcus zooepidemicus, Bordetella bronchiseptica*, etc)

References

Abou-Madi, N. (2006) Anesthesia and analgesia of small mammals. In: *Recent Advances in Veterinary Anesthesia and Analgesia: Companion Animals*. Eds. Gleed, R.D. and Ludders, J.W. http://www.ivis.org/advances/Anesthesia_Gleed/toc.asp. International Veterinary Information Service, Ithaca NY

Adrian, O., Dekomien, G., Epplen, J.T. *et al.* (2008) Body weight and rearing conditions of males, female choice and paternities in a small mammal, *Cavia aperea*. *Ethology*, **114**, 897–906

American Veterinary Medical Association Panel on Euthanasia (2007) AVMA Guidelines on Euthanasia. http://www.avma.org/issues/animal_welfare/euthanasia.pdf

Asher, M., Lippmann, T., Epplen, J.T. *et al.* (2008) Large males dominate: ecology, social organization, and mating system of wild cavies, the ancestors of the guinea pig. *Behavioral Ecology and Sociobiology*, **62**, 1509–1521

Asher, M., Oliveira, E.S. and Sachser, N. (2004) Social system and spatial organization of wild guinea pigs (*Cavia aperea*) in a natural population. *Journal of Mammalogy*, **85**, 788–796

Bauer, B., Womastek, I., Dittami, J. *et al.* (2008) The effects of early environmental conditions on the reproductive and somatic development of juvenile guinea pigs (*Cavia aperea* f. *porcellus*). *General and Comparative Endocrinology*, **155**, 680–685

Beauchamp, G.K. (1973) Attraction of male guinea pigs to conspecific urine. *Physiology and Behavior*, **10**, 589–594

Beauchamp, G.K., Criss, B.R. and Wellington, J.L. (1979) Chemical communication in *Cavia*: responses of wild (*C. aperea*), domestic (*C. porcellus*) and F1 males to urine. *Animal Behaviour*, **27**, 1066–1072

Beauchamp, G.K., Martin, I.G., Wysocki, C.J. *et al.* (1982) Chemoinvestigatory and sexual behaviour of male guinea pigs following vomeronasal organ removal. *Physiology and Behavior*, **29**, 329–336

Beauchamp, G.K., Wellington, J.L., Wysocki, C.J. *et al.* (1980) Chemical communication in the guinea pig: urinary components of low volatility and their access to the vomeronasal organ. In: *Chemical Signals: Vertebrates and Aquatic Invertebrates*. Eds Müller-Schwarze D. and Silverstein R., pp. 327–339. Plenum Press, New York

Beer, R., Kaiser, S., Sachser, N. *et al.* (1994) *Merkblatt zur tierschutzgerechten Haltung von Versuchstieren: Meerschweinchen*. Tierärztliche Vereinigung für Tierschutz e.V., Bramsche

Beer, R. and Sachser, N. (1992) Sozialstruktur und Wohlergehen in Männchengruppen des Hausmeerschweinchens. In: *Aktuelle Arbeiten zur artgemäßen Tierhaltung* 1991, KTBL-Schrift 351 (eds Kuratorium für Technik und Bauwesen in der Landwirtschaft e.V. & Deutsche Veterinärmedizinische Gesellschaft e.V.) pp. 158–167. KTBL-Schriften-Vertrieb im Landwirtschaftsverlag GmbH, Darmstadt

Benecke, N. (1994) *Der Mensch und seine Haustiere*. Konrad Theiss Verlag GmbH & Co, Stuttgart

Berryman, J.C. and Fullerton, C. (1976) A developmental study of interactions between young and adult guinea pigs. *Behaviour*, **59**, 22–39

Birke, L.I.A. (1981) Some behavioural changes associated with the guinea-pig oestrus cycle. *Zeitschrift für Tierpsychologie*, **55**, 79–89

Blouin, A. and Cormier, Y. (1987) Endotracheal intubation in guinea pigs by direct laryngoscopy. *Laboratory Animal Science*, **37**, 244–245

Broom, D.M. and Johnson, K.G. (1993) *Stress and Animal Welfare*. Chapman & Hall, London

Cassini, M.H. (1991) Foraging under predation risk in the wild guinea pig *Cavia aperea*. *Oikos*, **62**, 20–24

Cassini, M.H. and Galante, M.L. (1992) Foraging under predation risk in the wild guinea pig: the effect of vegetation height on habitat utilization. *Annales Zoologici Fennici*, **29**, 285–290

Close, B., Banister, K., Baumans, V. *et al.* (1996) Recommendations for euthanasia of experimental animals: Part 1. DGXI of the European Commission. *Laboratory Animals*, **30**, 293–316

Close, B., Banister, K., Baumans, V. *et al.* (1997) Recommendations for euthanasia of experimental animals: Part 2. DGXI of the European Commission. *Laboratory Animals*, **31**, 1–32

Clutton-Brock, J. (1989) *A Natural History of Domesticated Mammals*. Cambridge University Press, Cambridge

Cooper, T.G., Weydert, S., Yeung, C.H. *et al.* (2000) Maturation of epididymal spermatozoa in the non-domesticated guinea pigs *Cavia aperea* and *Galea musteloides*. *Journal of Andrology*, **21**, 154–163

Council of Europe (2006) Multilateral Consultation of Parties to the European Convention for the Protection of Vertebrate Animals used for Experimental and other Scientific Purposes (ETS 123) Appendix A. *Cons 123 (2006) 3*. Available from URL: http://www.coe.int/t/e/legal_affairs/legal_co-operation/biological_safety,_use_of_animals/laboratory_animals/2006/Cons123(2006)3AppendixA_en.pdf (accessed 31 July 2008)

Darwin, C. (1859) *On the Origin of Species by Means of Natural Selection*. John Murray, London

Darwin, C. (1868) *The Variation of Animals and Plants under Domestication*. John Murray, London

Dobromylskyj, P., Flecknell, P.A., Lascelles, B.D. *et al.* (2000) Management of postoperative and other acute pain. In: *Pain Management in Animals*. Eds Flecknell, P.A. and Waterman-Pearson, A., pp. 81–145. W.B. Saunders, London

Eisenberg, J.F. and Redford, K.H. (1999) *Mammals of the Neotropices*, Vol. **3**, The Central Neotropics. University of Chicago Press, Chicago

European Commission (2007) *Commission recommendations of 18 June 2007 on guidelines for the accommodation and care of animals used for experimental and other scientific purposes*. Annex II to European Council Directive 86/609. See 2007/526/EC. http://eurlex.europa.eu/LexUriServ/site/en/oj/2007/l_197/l_19720070730en00010089.pdf (accessed 13 May 2008)

Ewringmann, A. and Gloeckner, B. (2005) *Leitsymptome bei Meerschweinchen, Chinchilla und Degu*. Enke Verlag, Stuttgart

Federation of European Laboratory Animal Science Associations (2002) FELASA recommendations for the health monitoring of rodent and rabbit colonies in breeding and experimental units. *Laboratory Animals*, **36**, 20–42

Fey, K. and Trillmich, F. (2008) Sibling competition in guinea pigs (*Cavia aperea* f. *porcellus*): scrambling for mother's teats is stressful. *Behavioral Ecology and Sociobiology*, **62**, 321–329

Flecknell, P.A. (2009) *Laboratory Animal Anaesthesia*, 3rd edn. Academic Press, London

Fox, M.W. (1978) Effects of domestication in animals: A review. In: *The Dog: Its Domestication and Behaviour*. Ed. Fox, M.W., pp. 3–19. Garland STPM Press, New York

Fujieda, K., Goff, A.K., Pugeat, M. et al. (1982) Regulation of the pituitary-adrenal axis and corticosteroid-binding globulin-cortisol interaction in the guinea pig. *Endocrinology*, **111**, 1944–1949

Gade, D.W. (1967) The guinea pig in Andean folk culture. *Geographical Review*, **57**, 213–224

Gesellschaft für Versuchstierkunde (GV-SOLAS) Ausschuss für Anaesthesiologie (2002) Schmerztherapie bei Versuchstieren. http://www.gv-solas.de/auss/ana/schmerzen.pdf

Graves, F.C. and Hennessy, M.B. (2000) Comparison of the effects of the mother and an unfamiliar adult female on cortisol and behavioral responses of preweaning and postweaning guinea pigs. *Developmental Psychobiology*, **36**, 91–100

Guichón, M.L. and Cassini, M.H. (1998) Role of diet selection in the use of habitat by pampas cavies *Cavia aperea pamparum* (Mammalia, Rodentia). *Mammalia*, **62**, 23–35

Haase, E. and Donham, R.S. (1980) Hormones and domestication. In: *Avian Endocrinology*. Eds Epple, A. and Stetson, M.H., pp. 549–565. Academic Press, New York

Hale, E.B. (1969) Domestication and the evolution of behaviour. In: *Behaviour of Domestic Animals*, 2nd edn. Ed. Hafez, E.S.E., pp. 22–42. Williams and Wilkings, Baltimore

Harkness, J.E., Murray, K.A. and Wagner, J.E. (2002) Biology and diseases of guinea pigs. In: *Laboratory Animal Medicine*, 2nd edn. Eds Fox, J.G., Anderson, L., Loew, F. *et al.*, pp. 203–246. Academic Press, New York

Harkness, J.E. and Wagner, J.E. (1989) *The Biology and Medicine of Rabbits and Rodents*. Lea and Febiger, Philadelphia

Harper, L.V. (1976) Behavior. In: *The Biology of the Guinea Pig*. Eds Wagner, I.E. and Manning, P.J., pp. 31–52. Academic Press, New York

Henke, J. and Erhardt, W. (2004) Speziesspezifische Anaesthesie, Nager. In: *Anästhesie & Analgesie beim Klein- und Heimtier*. Eds

Erhardt, W., Henke, J. and Haberstroh, J., pp. 642–663. Schattauer GmbH, Stuttgart

Henke, J., Faltermeier, C. and Erhardt, W. (2003) Anaesthesie, Analgesie und Euthanasie bei kleinen heimtieren. *Tierärztliche Praxis (K)*, **31**, 394–397

Hennessy, M.B. (1997) Hypothalamic-pituitary-adrenal responses to brief social separation. *Neuroscience and Biobehavioral Reviews*, **21**, 11–29

Hennessy, M.B. (1999) Social influences on endocrine activity in guinea pigs, with comparisons to findings in nonhuman primates. *Neuroscience and Biobehavioral Reviews*, **23**, 687–698

Hennessy, M.B., Hornschuh, G., Kaiser, S. *et al.* (2006) Cortisol responses and social buffering: a study throughout the life span. *Hormones and Behavior*, **49**, 383–390

Hennessy, M.B., Maken, D.S. and Graves, F.C. (2002a) Presence of mother and unfamiliar female alters levels of testosterone, progesterone, cortisol, adrenocorticotropin, and behavior in maturing guinea pigs. *Hormones and Behavior*, **42**, 42–52

Hennessy, M.B. and Morris, A. (2005) Passive response of young guinea pigs during exposure to a novel environment: influences of social partners and age. *Developmental Psychobiology*, **46**, 86–96

Hennessy, M.B., O'Leary, S.K., Hawke, J.L. *et al.* (2002b) Social influences on cortisol and behavioral responses of preweaning, periadolescent, and adult guinea pigs. *Physiology and Behavior*, **76**, 305–314

Hennessy, M.B. and Ritchey, R.L. (1987) Hormonal and behavioral attachment responses in infant guinea pigs. *Developmental Psychobiology*, **20**, 613–625

Henry, J.P. and Stephens, P.M. (1977) *Stress, Health and the Social Environment. A Sociobiological Approach to Medicine.* Springer, New York

Herre, W. and Röhrs, M. (1990) *Haustiere – zoologisch gesehen.* Gustav Fischer Verlag, Stuttgart

Hillyer, E.V., Quesenberry, K.E. and Donnelly, T.M. (1997) Biology, husbandry, and clinical techniques. In: *Ferrets, Rabbits, and Rodents.* Eds Hillyer, E.V. and Quesenberry, K.E., pp. 243–259. W.B. Saunders Company, Philadelphia

Huerkamp, M.J., Murray, S.E. and Orosz, S.E. (1996) Guinea pigs. In: *Handbook of Rodent and Rabbit Medicine.* Eds Laber-Laird, K.E., Swindle M.M. and Flecknell, P.A., pp. 91–149. Pergammon Press, Oxford

Hückinghaus, F. (1961) Zur Nomenklatur und Abstammung des Hausmeerschweinchens. *Zeitschrift für Säugetierkunde*, **26**, 108–111

Hyams, E. (1972) *Animals in the Service of Man: 10 000 Years of Domestication.* J.M. Dent and Sons Ltd., London

Jacobs, G.H. and Deegan, J.F. (1994) Spectral sensitivity, photopigments, and color vision in the guinea pig (*Cavia porcellus*). *Behavioral Neuroscience*, **108**, 993–1004

Jacobs, W.W. (1976) Male-female associations in the domestic guinea pig. *Animal Learning Behavior*, **4**, 77–83

Jacobson, C. (2001) A novel anaesthetic regimen for surgical procedures in guineapigs. *Laboratory Animals*, **35**, 271–276

Jäckel, M. and Trillmich, F. (2003) Olfactory individual recognition of mothers by young guinea-pigs (*Cavia porcellus*). *Ethology*, **109**, 197–208

Joint Working Group on Refinement (1993) Removal of blood from laboratory mammals and birds. First Report of the BVA/FRAME/RSPCA/UFAW Joint Working Group on Refinement. *Laboratory Animals*, **27**, 1–22

Joint Working Group on Refinement (2001) Refining procedures for the administration of substances. Report of the BVAAWF/FRAME/RSPCA/UFAW Joint Working Group on Refinement. *Laboratory Animals*, **35**, 1–41

Jones, C.T. (1974) Corticosteroid concentrations in the plasma of fetal and maternal guinea pigs during gestation. *Endocrinology*, **95**, 1129–1133

Kaiser, S., Kirtzeck, M., Hornschuh, G. *et al.* (2003a) Sex specific difference in social support – a study in female guinea pigs. *Physiology and Behavior*, **79**, 297–303.

Kaiser, S., Kruijver, F.P.M., Straub, R.H. *et al.* (2003d) Early social stress in male guinea pigs changes social behaviour, and autonomic and neuroendocrine functions. *The Journal of Neuroendocrinology*, **15**, 761–769

Kaiser, S., Kruijver, F.P.M., Swaab, D.F. *et al.* (2003b) Early social stress in female guinea pigs induces a masculinization of adult behavior and corresponding changes in brain and neuroendocrine function. *Behavioural Brain Research*, **144**, 199–210

Kaiser, S., Nübold, T., Rohlmann, I. *et al.* (2003c) Pregnant female guinea pigs adapt easily to a new social environment irrespective of their rearing conditions. *Physiology and Behavior*, **80**, 147–153

Kaiser, S. and Sachser, N. (1998) The social environment during pregnancy and lactation affects the female offsprings' endocrine status and behaviour in guinea pigs. *Physiology and Behavior*, **63**, 361–366

Kaiser, S. and Sachser, N. (2001) Social stress during pregnancy and lactation affects in guinea pigs the male offsprings' endocrine status and infantilizes their behaviour. *Psychoneuroendocrinology*, **26**, 503–519

Kaiser, S. and Sachser, N. (2005) The effects of prenatal social stress on behaviour: mechanisms and function. *Neuroscience and Biobehavioral Reviews*, **29**, 283–294

Kawachi, I. and Berkman, L.F. (2001) Social ties and mental health. *Journal of Urban Health*, **78**, 458–467

Kenagy, G.J. and Trombulak, S.C. (1986) Size and function of mammalian testes in relation to body size. *Journal of Mammalogy*, **67**, 1–22

Kunkel, P. and Kunkel, I. (1964) Beiträge zur Ethologie des Hausmeerschweinchens. *Zeitschrift für Tierpsychologie*, **21**, 602–641

Künzl, C., Kaiser, S., Meier, E. *et al.* (2003) Is a wild mammal kept and reared in captivity still a wild animal? *Hormones and Behavior*, **43**, 187–196

Künzl, C. and Sachser, N. (1999) The behavioural endocrinology of domestication: a comparison between the domestic guinea pig (*Cavia aperea* f. *porcellus*) and its wild ancestor the wild cavy (*Cavia aperea*). *Hormones and Behavior*, **35**, 28–37

Mares, M.A. and Ojeda, R.A. (1982) Patterns of diversity and adaptation in South American hystricognath rodents. In: *Mammalian Biology in South America.* Eds Mares, M.A. and Genoways, H.H., pp. 393–432. Pymatuning Laboratory of Ecology, Special Publications No. 6., Pittsburgh, Pennsylvania

Martin, I.G. and Beauchamp, G.K. (1982) Olfactory recognition of individuals by male cavies (*Cavia aperea*). *Journal of Chemical Ecology*, **8**, 1241–1249

Mason, D.E. (1997) Anesthesia, analgesia, and sedation for small mammals. In: *Ferrets, Rabbits, and Rodents.* Eds Hillyer, E.V. and Quesenberry, K.E., pp. 378–391. W.B. Saunders Company, Philadelphia

Nachtsheim, H. and Stengel, H. (1977) *Vom Wildtier zum Haustier.* Verlag Paul Parey, Berlin

Nehring, A. (1889) Über die Herkunft des Hausmeerschweinchens. *Sitzungsberichte der Gesellschaft naturforschender Freunde zu Berlin*, **1**, 1–4

North, D. (1999) The guinea-pig. In: *The UFAW Handbook on the Care and Management of Laboratory Animals, Vol 1, Terrestrial Vertebrates*, 7th edn. Ed. Poole, T., pp. 367–388. Blackwell Publishing, Oxford

Noonan, D. (1994) The guinea pig (*Cavia porcellus*). *ANZCCART News*, **7**, 1–8

Owen, D.G. (1992) *Parasites of Laboratory Animals.* Laboratory Animals Handbooks. Royal Society of Medicine Services, London

Pettijohn, T.F. (1979) Attachment and separation distress in the infant guinea pig. *Developmental Psychobiology*, **12**, 73–81

Price, E.O. (1984) Behavioral aspects of animal domestication. *The Quarterly Review of Biology*, **59**, 1–32

Radde, G.R., Hinson, A., Crenshaw, D. *et al.* (1996) Evaluation of anaesthetic regimes in guinea pigs. *Laboratory Animals*, **30**, 220–227

Redford, K.H. and Eisenberg, J.F. (1992) *Mammals of the Neotropics, Vol. 2, the Southern Cone.* University of Chicago Press, Chicago

Ritchey, R.L. and Hennessy, M.B. (1987) Cortisol and behavioral responses to separation in mother and infant guinea pigs. *Behavioral and Neural Biology*, **48**, 1–12

Rood, J.P. (1972) Ecological and behavioural comparisons of three genera of Argentine cavies. *Animal Behaviour Monographs*, **5**, 1–83

Sachser, N. (1986) Different forms of social organization at high and low population densities in guinea pigs. *Behaviour*, **97**, 253–272

Sachser, N. (1987) Short-term responses of plasma-norepinephrine, epinephrine, glucocorticoid and testosterone titers to social and non-social stressors in male guinea pigs of different social status. *Physiology and Behavior*, **39**, 11–20

Sachser, N. (1990) Social organization, social status, behavioural strategies and endocrine responses in male guinea pigs. In: *Hormones, Brain and Behavior in Vertebrates. Comparative Physiology*, Vol. 9. Ed. Balthazart, J., pp. 176–187. Karger, Basel

Sachser, N. (1993) The ability to arrange with conspecifics depends on social experiences around puberty. *Physiology and Behavior*, **53**, 539–544

Sachser, N. (1994a) *Sozialphysiologische Untersuchungen an Hausmeerschweinchen. Gruppenstrukturen, soziale Situation und Endokrinium, Wohlergehen.* Parey, Berlin

Sachser, N. (1994b) Social stratification and health in non-human mammals – a case study in guinea pigs. In: *Social Stratification and Socioeconomic Inequality*, Vol. 2. Ed. Ellis, L., pp. 113–121. Praeger, Westport

Sachser, N. (1998) Of domestic and wild guinea pigs: studies in sociophysiology, domestication, and social evolution. *Naturwissenschaften*, **85**, 307–317

Sachser, N. (2001) What is important to achieve good welfare in animals? In: *Coping with Challenge: Welfare in Animals Including Humans*, Dahlem Workshop Report 87. Ed. Broom, D.M., pp. 31–48. Dahlem University Press, Berlin

Sachser, N., Dürschlag, M. and Hirzel, D. (1998) Social relationships and the management of stress. *Psychoneuroendocrinology*, **23**, 891–904

Sachser, N. and Kaiser, S. (1996) Prenatal social stress masculinizes the females' behaviour in guinea pigs. *Physiology and Behavior*, **60**, 589–594

Sachser, N., Künzl, C. and Kaiser, S. (2004) The welfare of laboratory guinea pigs. In: *The Welfare of Laboratory Animals*. Ed. Kalista, E., pp. 181–209. Kluwer Academic Publishers, Dordrecht

Sachser, N. and Lick, C. (1991) Social experience, behavior, and stress in guinea pigs. *Physiology and Behavior*, **50**, 83–90

Sachser, N., Lick, C., Beer, R. *et al.* (1992) Tagesgang von Serum-Hormonkonzentrationen und ethologischen Parametern bei Hausmeerschweinchen. *Verhandlungen der Deutschen Zoologischen Gesellschaft*, **85**, 120

Sachser, N., Lick, C. and Stanzel, K. (1994) The environment, hormones, and aggressive behaviour: a 5-year-study in guinea pigs. *Psychoneuroendocrinology*, **19**, 697–707

Sachser, N. and Pröve, E. (1984) Short-term effects of residence on the testosterone responses to fighting in alpha male guinea pigs. *Aggressive Behaviour*, **10**, 285–292

Sachser, N. and Renninger, S.-V. (1993) Coping with new social situations: the role of social rearing in guinea pigs. *Ethology Ecology Evolution*, **5**, 65–74

Sachser, N., Schwarz-Weig, E., Keil, A. *et al.* (1999) Behavioural strategies, testis size, and reproductive success in two caviomorph rodents with different mating systems. *Behaviour*, **136**, 1203–1217

Schaeffer, D.O. and Donnelly, T.M. (1997) Disease problems of guinea pigs and chinchillas. In: *Ferrets, Rabbits, and Rodents*. Eds Hillyer, E.V. and Quesenberry, K.E., pp. 260–282. W.B. Saunders Company, Philadelphia

Seamer, J. and Chesterman, F.C. (1967) A survey of disease in laboratory animals. *Laboratory Animals*, **1**, 117–139

Shi, F.X., Ozawa, M., Komura, H. *et al.* (1999) Secretion of ovarian inhibin and its physiologic roles in the regulation of follicle-stimulating hormone secretion during the estrous cycle of the female guinea pig. *Biology of Reproduction*, **60**, 78–84

Smith, D.A., Burgmann, P.M. (1997) Formulary. In: *Ferrets, Rabbits, and Rodents*. Eds Hillyer, E.V. and Quesenberry, K.E., pp. 392–403. W.B. Saunders Company, Philadelphia

Stahnke, A. (1987) Verhaltensunterschiede zwischen Wild- und Hausmeerschweinchen. *Zeitschrift für Säugetierkunde*, **52**, 294–307

Stahnke, A. and Hendrichs, H. (1988) Meerschweinchenverwandte Nagetiere. In: *Grzimeks Enzyklopädie Säugetiere*. Ed. Grzimek, B., pp. 314–357. Kindler Verlag, München

Sutherland, S.D. and Festing, M.F.W. (1987) The guinea-pig. In: *The UFAW Handbook on the Care and Management of Laboratory Animals*, 6th edn. Ed. Poole, T.B., pp. 393–410. Churchill Livingstone, New York

Terril, L.A. and Clemons, D.J. (1998) *The Laboratory Guinea Pig*. CRC Press, Boca Raton

Thyen, Y. and Hendrichs, H. (1990) Differences in behaviour and social organization of female guinea pigs as a function of the presence of a male. *Ethology*, **85**, 25–34

von Holst, D. (1998) The concept of stress and its relevance for animal behavior. In: *Advances in the Study of Behavior*. Eds Lehman, D.S., Hinde, R. and Shaw, E., pp. 1–131. Academic Press, New York

Wagner, J.E. (1976) Introduction and taxonomy. In: *The Biology of the Guinea Pig*. Eds Wagner, J.E. and Manning, P.J., pp. 1–4. Academic Press, New York

Wagner, J.E. and Manning, P.J. (1976) *The Biology of the Guinea Pig*. Academic Press, New York

Wallner, B., Dittami, J. and Machatschke, I. (2006) Social stimuli cause changes of plasma oxytocin and behavior in guinea pigs. *Biological Research*, **39**, 251–258

Wasel, E. (2007) Meerschweinchen. In: *Krankheiten der Heimtiere*. Eds Fehr, M., Sassenburg, L. and Zwart, P., pp. 49–86. Schlütersche Verlagsgesellschaft, Hannover

Weir, B.J. (1972) Some notes on the history of the domestic guinea pig. *Guinea Pig News Letter*, **5**, 2–5

Weir, B.J. (1974) Notes on the origin of the domestic guinea-pig. *Symposium of the Zoological Society of London*, **34**, 437–446

Wewers, D., Kaiser, S. and Sachser, N. (2003) Maternal separation in guinea pigs: a study in behavioural endocrinology. *Ethology*, **109**, 443–453

Wilson, D.E. and Reeder, D.M. (2005) *Mammal Species of the World*. Vol **1**, 3rd edn. The John Hopkins University Press, Baltimore

Wing, E.S. (1977) Animal domestication in the Andes. In: *Origins of Agriculture*. Ed. Reed, C.A., pp. 837–859. Mouton Publishers, The Hague

Wolf, P. and Kamphues, J. (2004) Ernaehrung der Heimtiere – Einfluss der Fuetterung auf das Zahnwachstum. *Kleintier konkret*, 21–24

28 The laboratory rabbit

Lena Lidfors and Therese Edström

Biological overview

General biology

The laboratory rabbit is descended from the European wild rabbit (*Oryctolagus cuniculus*) (Harcourt-Brown 2002), which appears to have had a widespread distribution across Europe before the last Pleistocene glaciations 1.8 million to 10000 years ago (Flux 1994). After the last Ice Age (20000 years ago), it was confined to the Iberian Peninsula and small areas of France and northwest Africa (Parker 1990; Wilson & Reeder 1993). However, the spread of the rabbit over the world has mainly been the result of man's activities (Flux 1994). Due to the adaptability of the species the European rabbit exists in the wild on every continent except Asia and Antarctica (Parker 1990; Wilson & Reeder 1993). In many places where rabbits have been introduced, the lack of predators has lead to an explosion in the number of animals, leading them to become pests. In order to find ways to diminish the high population of wild rabbits their behaviour and reproduction have been investigated in a large number of ecological studies.

There are different views on exactly when rabbits were domesticated; from the first century BC (Nachtsheim 1949) to the sixth to the tenth century AD (Zeuner 1963). It has also been reported that rabbits were kept in fenced hunting areas by the Romans as long ago as 2000 years ago (Meredith 2000). Domestication probably occurred in the French monasteries, where several different breeds were developed (Zeuner 1963). These were further developed to create a large number of breeds for different purposes during the past century. In 2001 the British Rabbit Council[1] recognised 57 breeds of fancy fur and Rex rabbits, whereas the American Rabbit Breeders' Association in 2006 recognised 47 rabbit breeds[2].

When the behaviour of European wild rabbits has been compared with domestic strains of rabbits kept in semi-natural enclosures their behaviour has been found to be very similar in most aspects (reviewed by Bell 1984); however, there are some differences. Domestic rabbits spend more time resting above ground during the day (Stodart & Myers 1964). Bucks chin-mark more often (Kraft 1979) and will do so in unfamiliar territory (Mykytowycz 1968). Stodart and Myers (1964) found that domestic does had fewer days out of reproduction than wild does, and therefore produced more litters with a larger mean size. When European wild rabbits were brought into the laboratory they failed to breed, and females born into the laboratory as a result of egg transfer from wild to domestic mothers retained their nervous disposition and failed to mature sexually (Adams 1982). European wild rabbits may be used for experimental research, but there are several problems in keeping and breeding them (Bell 1999), and they also may bring in several infectious agents that are normally excluded in barrier housing.

Of the 12.1 million animals used for experimental and other scientific purposes in the member states of the European Union in 2005, 2.6% (314600) were rabbits (Commission of the European Communities 2003). In general, the number of rabbits used in research has declined. As an example, in Sweden the number of rabbits used has decreased from 7141 in 1993 to 1808 in 2006 (Swedish Board of Agriculture 2007).

The most common breed used for laboratory research is the New Zealand White (NZW), which was originally bred for meat production (Bennett 2001). Other breeds used include the Dutch and the Half Lop (Batchelor 1999). A major breeder in Europe is currently breeding NZW, Chinchilla Bastard and Himalyan rabbits. The Watanabe heritable hyperlipidaemic (WHHL) rabbits have been developed as a model to study hypercholesterolaemia and atherosclerosis *in vivo* (Wetterholm *et al.* 2007), and the myocardial infarction-prone Watanabe heritable hyperlipidaemic (WHHLMI) rabbits have been developed as a model to study human acute coronary syndromes (Shiomi & Jianglin 2008).

Size range and lifespan

The European wild rabbit has been reported to vary widely in both adult weight range and lifespan both within and between populations. From northern to southern Europe the body weight (Rogers *et al.* 1994) and skull size (Sharples *et al.* 1996) are reduced. It has been suggested that this is due to phenotypic rather than genetic variation (Sharples *et al.* 1996). In a long-term study the body weight of European wild rabbits in East Anglia, UK, was found to be 1.3–2.1 kg in males and 1.3–2.3 kg in females (Bell 1999). In the

[1] http://www.thebrc.org/

[2] http://www.arba.net

domesticated rabbit, differences in weight between breeds are large: from around 1 kg (Netherland Dwarfs) to 5 kg (New Zealand White) and up to 10 kg (German Grey Rabbits) (Sawin 1950; Bennett 2001). There is large variation in the size and position of ears, body conformation, fur quality and coat colour between breeds of rabbits (Sawin 1950; Bennett 2001).

The European wild rabbit has no dimorphism in adult body size (Webb 1993). The only difference in appearance between males and females is that bucks have a more rounded, broader appearance to the front of the head, whereas does have a more pointed head (Bell 1999). Domesticated rabbit breeds do not seem to have developed dimorphism in size either. The NZW rabbit should have an ideal weight of 4.5 kg in adult bucks (8 months of age and over) and 5.0 kg in adult does (Sawin 1950). When kept as laboratory rabbits NZWs tend to lay down excessive amounts of body fat in the abdominal cavity and around the chin when they grow older. This occurs irrespective of whether they are kept single housed in a cage or group housed in a pen (Batchelor 1999).

In the European wild rabbit, mortality in the wild is very high during the first year of life and can reach up to 90% (Macdonald 1984; Nowak 1999), mainly due to myxomatosis and predation (Bell & Webb 1991; Rogers *et al.* 1994). In a long-term English study maximum age of bucks was 8 years and of does 9 years (Bell 1999), whereas Gibb (1993) had rabbits living over 10 years in a study in New Zealand. Domestic rabbits have been reported to have an average lifespan of 9 years[3], and Comfort (1956) stated that lifespan can exceed 15 years and gave examples of bucks reaching 10–14 years old.

Social organisation

European wild rabbits live in small, stable, territorial breeding groups (Parer 1977; Gibb *et al.* 1978; Cowan 1987; Bell & Webb 1991). This is the social unit and consists of one to four males and one to nine females, but different breeding groups may comprise colonies of up to 70 rabbits (Meredith 2000). The breeding group defends its territory, a core area with a warren within a larger home range, by patrolling the borders and scent-marking (Bell 1999). A warren is an area of soil or sand containing underground tunnels and nests made by the rabbits. Breeding groups can either occupy single warrens (Myers & Schneider 1964; Bell 1977) or multiple warrens (Dunsmore 1974; Parer 1977; Wood 1980; Daly 1981; Cowan 1987). Each warren has several entrances which allow quick escape from predators (Cowan 1987). Neighbouring breeding groups can move out from their territories to forage in communal grazing areas at dawn and dusk (Bell 1980).

Dominance hierarchies are formed within each sex for each breeding group, and they are stable over time (Bell 1983). The hierarchy is maintained by rabbits keeping a fixed distance from one another and exhibiting submissive behaviour. The rabbit spends a rather large portion of its daily activity in either direct or indirect aggression (Mykytowycz & Rowley 1958; Mykytowycz & Fullager 1973), and this may underlie the social and territorial organisation that influence the numbers of free-living populations (Mykytowycz 1960). It is a general perception that bucks are involved in more fighting, but does have been found to be more aggressive than bucks (Southern 1948; Myers & Poole 1961), or to fight as strongly as bucks (Lockley 1961). The does mainly fight over breeding nests (Cowan & Garson 1985), and are more aggressive towards juvenile does than towards juvenile bucks (Cowan 1987). When the number of rabbits living together increases, fighting increases dramatically (Myers 1966; Myers *et al.* 1971). Young bucks normally move to a new social group before starting their first breeding season, while young does stay on to breed in their natal group (Parer 1982; Webb *et al.* 1995).

In a study of NZW rabbits kept in a semi-natural enclosure, a total of 20 different social behaviours and their changes with age were described (Lehmann 1991). Lehmann grouped the behaviours into indifferent contacts, amicable behaviour, subdominant behaviour, aggressive behaviour and actual fights. When male and female European wild rabbits and NZW rabbits were tested with paired encounters in a home pen it was found that NZW rabbits showed as much agonistic behaviour as the wild rabbits, aggression was equally prevalent in both sexes and inter-sexual fighting occurred just as frequently as fighting between members of the same sex (Mykytowycz & Hesterman 1975).

The rabbit has three specialised scent glands. These are located in the anal region, the groin and under the chin (Mykytowycz 1968). Rabbit territory is scent-marked by placing faeces in dunghills, and by pressing the under-chin against structures in the environment so that droplets from the rabbit's submandibular glands are excreted through pores of the skin (Mykytowycz 1968). Male rabbits scent-mark more intensively than females and dominant individuals more than subdominant animals; this is correlated with larger anal and submandibular glands in dominant males (Mykytowycz 1968) with the heaviest anal glands being found in the most dominant animals. Bucks also scent mark does and young rabbits of their breeding group by spraying urine on them (Mykytowycz 1968). Does scent mark their young, attack other young within the same breeding group, and may chase and even kill young from other breeding groups (Mykytowycz 1968). Does may attack even their own young if they have been smeared with foreign urine (Mykytowycz 1968).

Biological data

Basic biological data are presented in the different sections of this chapter where they are of specific interest. The data presented here may be of interest for research purposes as well as for checking animal health. Cardiovascular and respiratory functions are of great importance for anaesthesia and normal values are presented in Table 28.1. Haematology and blood chemistry parameters can be used to assess the homeostasis of the animals prior to surgery or dosing as well

[3]http://animaldiversity.umm.umich.edu/site/accounts/information/Oryctolagus_cuniculus.html

Table 28.1 Normal values of cardiovascular and respiratory functions in rabbits (Gillett 1994; Flecknell 1996).

Parameter	*Values*
Respiratory rate (breaths/min)	40–60
Heart rate (beats/min)	200–300
Tidal volume (ml/kg)	4–6
Arterial systolic pressure (mmHg)	90–130
Arterial diastolic pressure (mmHg)	80–90
Arterial blood pO_2 (kPa)	11–12.5
Arterial blood pCO_2 (kPa)	5–6.5
Arterial blood pH	7.35–7.45

Table 28.2 Normal values of haematology in rabbits (Jenkins 2008).

Parameter	*Values*
Erythrocytes (count) ($\times 10^6/mm^3$)	5.4–7.6
Haematocrit/packed cell volume (%)	33–50
Haemoglobin (g/dl)	10.0–17.4
Mean corpuscular volume (μm^3)	60–69
Mean corpuscular haemoglobin (pg)	19–22
Mean corpuscular haemoglobin concentration (%)	30–35
Leucocytes ($\times 10^3/mm^3$)	5.2–12.5
Lymphocytes (%)	30–85
Neutrophils (%)	20–75
Eosinophils (%)	1–4
Basophils (%)	1–7
Monocytes (%)	1–4
Platelets ($\times 10^3/mm^3$)	250–650

Table 28.3 Normal values of blood clinical chemistry in rabbits (Jenkins 2008).

Parameter	*Values*
Alanine aminotransferase (IU/l)	27.4–72.2
Aspartate aminotransferase (IU/l)	10.0–78.0
Creatine kinase (IU/l)	58.6–175.0
Bilirubin (mmol/l)	2.6–17.1
Blood urea nitrogen (mmol/l)	4.6–10.7
Creatinine (µmol/l)	74–171
Glucose (mmol/l)	5.5–8.2
Calcium (mmol/l)	2.2–3.9
Phosphorus (mmol/l)	1.0–2.2

as after any experimental procedure. Normal haematology values are shown in Table 28.2 and normal values of clinical blood chemistry are shown in Table 28.3.

The body temperature of rabbits varies from 38.5–39.5°C (Ruckebusch *et al.* 1991). A calm and resting rabbit has a lower body temperature than the agitated animal. Rabbits' ears are richly vascularised and are used in regulating body temperature (Kawoto *et al.* 1989).

It is normal for the urine of rabbits to vary widely in colour, from different shades of yellow, light brown and even reddish; various degrees of turbidity are also normal because of the high concentration of calcium and mucus, among other reasons (Jenkins 2008). Red coloration of urine may result from porphyrins excreted by the kidneys depending on the diet, and this may be mistaken for blood (Jenkins 2008). The urine volume produced daily is 50–75 ml/kg and the urinary pH is 8–9 (Jenkins 2008). Rabbit urine is alkaline due to the herbivorous diet although lower urinary pH can result from high protein intake and catabolic states such as starvation and severe disease (Jenkins 2008).

Reproduction

The European wild rabbit is a seasonal breeder, with seasonality determined by the interaction of day length, climate, nutrition, population density, social status and other factors (Bell & Webb 1991; Bell 1999). In Australian wild rabbits sexual maturity occurs at the age of 5–7 months in bucks and 9–12 months in does depending on climate (Myers *et al.* 1994). Domestic rabbits of medium size should be at least 5 months of age at the first mating, but they are sexually mature earlier (Bennett 2001). The smaller breeds are sexually mature earlier than the medium and larger breeds (Bennett 2001).

Before mating an elaborate courtship takes place – the rabbits circle around each other, parade side by side, jump over each other and sniff the genital region (Lehmann 1991). Hafez (1960) described seven degrees of sex drive, which ranged from aggressive with immediate mounting and ejaculation to offensive reaction with general smelling of the skin, biting and no ejaculation. When the doe allows mating she raises the hindquarters (Bennett 2001). Mating takes only a few seconds, after which the buck falls to one side or backwards (Bennett 2001). Ovulation is induced by the act of coitus and conception occurs 8–10 h after mating (Bennett 2001). The doe can mate immediately following parturition, and if the young are removed after delivery the doe will be sexually receptive for at least 36 days (Hagen 1974).

Gestation in European wild rabbits lasts 28–30 days (Bell 1999) and in domesticated rabbits 28–34 days, with most litters being born on day 31 (Bennett 2001). In nature, some days before the birth, the doe digs a short underground tunnel or stop either within the main warren or separately from it and within this constructs a nest (Bell 1999). High-ranking does often give birth in a special breeding chamber dug as an extension to the warren, whereas some of the subordinate females are chased away from the warren and forced to give birth in isolated breeding 'stops' (Mykytowycz 1968). The survival rate of the young is much higher for high-ranking than the low-ranking females (Mykytowycz 1968). Does of both European wild rabbits and NZW rabbits collect and carry grass to their burrows and shortly before giving birth pluck their own fur from the belly, sides and dewlap, which is placed on top of the grass (González-Mariscal *et al.* 1994; Bell 1999). When domestic rabbits are kept in cages, the does also construct nests as in the wild, and often, the better the construction of the nest, the higher the survival rate of the young (Canali *et al.* 1991).

Rabbits are born with no, or only little, hair cover, and are deaf and blind (Batchelor 1999). They weigh around 50 g at birth and gain about 30 g per day (Falkmer & Waller 1984). The size of the litter is five to six young for European wild rabbits (Vaughan *et al.* 2000), and four to twelve young for domesticated rabbits (Batchelor 1999). At birth, the young rabbits are very sensitive to cold but, as their fur starts to grows some days after birth, they become less sensitive (Bennett 2001). The eyes open at 10–11 days (Kersten *et al.* 1989; Batchelor 1999), and hearing develops at the same time. Once the young are born, the doe leaves the burrow and covers the entrance with soil, urine marks it, and then leaves (Mykytowycz 1968). She returns to the burrow once daily, and then digs herself into the burrow and nurses her young for just a few minutes (Bell 1999). In a study of Dutch Belted rabbits the nursing took place in the early morning and lasted for 2.7–4.5 minutes (Zarrow *et al.* 1965). The composition of the milk is very nutritious with 10% protein, 12% fat and 2% lactose (Harkness & Wagner 1995). Does do not retrieve their young if they are placed outside the nest (Ross *et al.* 1959). After 21 days, the doe ceases closing the burrow or breeding stop and the young come up to the surface (Bell 1999). In NZW does, the young are about 18 days old when she stops closing the entrance to the breeding stop and the young are nursed outside (Lehmann 1989).

At 4 weeks of age the young are very mobile, and soon after emergence they leave their breeding stop and do not return to it again (Lloyd & McCowan 1968). They start seeking forage, but continue to suckle for several more weeks. A study on NZW rabbits indicated that the mothers were not preferred social partners for the young except during suckling attempts (Lehmann 1989). Milk production reaches a maximum about 2 weeks after giving birth, then declines during the fourth week, although lactation may continue for an additional 2–4 weeks (Hagen 1974). Lehmann (1989) also found that, in NZW rabbits, nursing was uncommon after 4 weeks and the doe littered again within a few days, although suckling attempts occurred up to 60 days. At 8 weeks of age, the young consume approximately 90% of their intake in the form of plant proteins (Hagen 1974).

Normal behaviour (wild and captive)

The rabbit is a nocturnal animal, which rests in the burrows of the warren during the day, and emerges in late afternoon (Fraser 1992). The old bucks emerge first, about 4 h before sunset (Mykytowycz & Rowley 1958), and at sunset 90% of the rabbits have emerged from the burrows up to the ground (Fraser 1992). The rabbits are above ground for 11–14 h of the diurnal cycle (Mykytowycz & Rowley 1958). When they are above ground they spend about 44% of their time eating, 33% inactive, 13% moving and 10% on other activities (Gibb 1993). Young NZW rabbits were active for an average of 30% of the daytime, during which, feeding on pellets occupied one third of this time, grazing took one third of this time, and the remaining one third was spent in exploring, gnawing, intensive locomotion and, for the older rabbits, sexual behaviour (Lehmann 1989). The rabbit's choice of habitat depends on the opportunities to find shelter and protection; where the soil is loose it digs burrows, and where the soil is more compact it often seeks protection in dense vegetation (Kolb 1994).

Foraging is performed over an area known as the home-range; this is much larger than the 'territory' that breeding groups defend. The size of the home-range varies depending on food availability, number of rabbits in the group and other factors (Donnelly 1997). Wild rabbits have been found to gather in large colonies of up to hundreds of animals under good feeding conditions or at high population densities (Myers & Poole 1963). The home-range of European wild rabbits has been found to vary between studies from 5 ha (Myers *et al.* 1994), 0.4–2.0 ha (Cowan & Bell 1986) and 0.8 ha (Vastrade 1987). In nature, rabbits mainly eat grass and herbs, but also fruit, roots, leaves and bark (Cheeke 1987). Rabbits need coarse fibre for their digestion, not just lush grass (Brooks 1997; Meredith 2000). The colon of the rabbit separates faecal waste from the B vitamin-rich faecal pellets, made up of microbes that the rabbit will ingest (Björnhag 1972). These smaller, soft and green coated faecal pellets produced by the caecum 4–8 h after feed intake (Carpenter *et al.* 1995; Brooks 1997) are picked up directly from the anus, whereas the fibrous pellets are placed on specific latrines close to the territory borders (Donnelly 1997).

The rabbit is a prey animal with many enemies. When threatened, rabbits stamp with their hindfeet and show their scut, as warning signals to other rabbits. If it is too late to flee, the rabbit may freeze. Normally, rabbits do not often vocalise within the auditory spectrum of man, but if caught by a predator they may emit a high-pitched distress scream (Cowan & Bell 1986), which may cause the predator to release it. Apart from this and some low sounds during mating and mother–young care, rabbits are silent animals.

Rabbit movement consists of hopping, crawling and intensive locomotion (ie, running, start-and-stop, jumping, double and capriole) (Kraft 1979; Lehmann 1989). Hopping is used to travel longer distances; whereas crawling is performed when feeding on grass or exploring on the spot and during social encounters (Lehmann 1989). Rabbits rear when they are looking at their surroundings (Lockley 1961) The rabbit has a light and fragile skeleton that only makes up 7–8 % of the body weight (Donnelly 1997).

Rabbits have good eyesight with a maximum field of vision of almost 360° (Peiffer *et al.* 1994). They use their whiskers, the sensitive lips, scent and taste during foraging (Meredith 2000). The whiskers are also used during orientation in the burrows and dens (Meredith 2000). Scent and taste are more important than vision in identifying members of their own breeding group (Meredith 2000). Rabbits have good hearing, and the big ears make up about 12% of the total body surface area (Meredith 2000). Rabbits regularly perform comfort behaviours such as licking and scratching themselves, shaking the body, rubbing against objects and stretching their body.

Sources/supply/transport conservation status

Laboratories usually buy rabbits of defined health status from accredited breeders (Townsend 1969; Eveleigh & Pease

1976; Eveleigh *et al.* 1984). During the last 10–15 years there has been a decline in the total number of breeding units in Europe. The reason is mainly the declining use of rabbits in laboratory animal experimentation. Another reason is the higher demands on animal health and health monitoring documentation. Health screening and documentation are expensive and higher hygienic standards are required within the breeding unit. Costs and higher quality requirements have reduced the number of suppliers. The major laboratory animal breeders are somewhat reluctant to breed rabbits because they require careful management, which affects profitability. Several of these breeders have found it difficult to relocate a colony of breeding rabbits because these animals are sensitive to disturbances of their environment, and changes are immediately reflected in their breeding performance.

Most rabbits have to be transported from the breeder to the laboratory, and this may be done by car, truck, railway or plane. The rabbits should be in good condition before transport. Rabbits are most often transported in containers made of sheet metal, fibreglass, fibreboard, rigid plastic, strong welded wire mesh or wood lined with wire mesh (Swallow *et al.* 2005). The minimum stocking density in transport containers can be found in Swallow *et al.* (2005). The height of the container should be restricted to prevent back injury caused by the rabbit kicking out (Swallow *et al.* 2005). If the containers are constructed without a wire mesh liner it must have wire screening cover on all air vents (Swallow *et al.* 2005). A grid floor or area for rabbits to separate excreta from the lying area may be necessary for long journeys (Swallow *et al.* 2005). If journeys are longer than 24 h provisions for feeding and watering are needed, even though rabbits rarely eat or drink during a journey (Swallow *et al.* 2005). See also Chapter 13 for a general discussion of transport.

Transportation vehicles should be equipped with devices for monitoring temperature, and provided with ventilation that can cool the air during warm weather and provide heating during cold weather. A source of water, for example a gel, and feed, has to be provided (Batchelor 1999; Olfert *et al.* 1993). After arrival at the new animal housing the rabbits should be checked for any health problems and injuries, which could either be caused by the transport or have been acquired before the transport. Rabbits should be given time for acclimatisation after the transport before they are used for research. The time period needed for acclimatisation depends on the stress that the animals have experienced during transport, which in turn depends on many factors such as the duration of the transport, the age of the animals and the change of the social environment (European Commission 2007). It is also important to match care routines with those of the supplier.

Very little research has been done into the effect of transport on rabbits. Batchelor (1999) found considerable differences in body weight in rabbits that were housed in group pens compared to solitary in cages after transportation. The loss of weight in rabbits after transport is mostly due to a loss of gastrointestinal contents, which account for about 10% of the total body weight (Swallow 1999). These losses are probably maximal after about 15 h of transport and similar to depriving animals of food and water for the same time (Swallow 1999). It can take up to 7 days to recover the loss in live weight (Swallow 1999). Research on the effect of providing male rabbits with or without hay and with change or no change in the feed after a 10 h transport by truck, plane and truck showed that the provision of hay significantly reduced the occurrence of diarrhoea (L. Lidfors unpublished observation).

Uses in the laboratory

The use of laboratory rabbits has declined over the last decade (Swedish Board of Agriculture 2007). A database search shows a gradual and slight decline of the use of polyclonal antibodies produced in rabbits but there is still a need for these antibodies since they are quicker and easier to produce than the monoclonal antibodies (Cooper & Paterson 2008). Rabbits are still being used in pyrogen testing of intravenous fluids and other technical products intended for patients even though other test methods without live animals are being evaluated (Hoffman *et al.* 2005). Rabbits remain popular models for *in vivo* experimentation, for example in the development of bio implant products such as dental implants and devices for orthopaedic surgery (Batchelor 1999).

Rabbits are used in the study of atherosclerosis after being given high-fat and high-cholesterol diets, which lead to the development of atherosclerotic lesions in the major arteries after approximately 2 months. Rabbits of a spontaneously mutated strain called the WHHL (Watanabe heritable hyperlipidaemic) develop atherosclerotic lesions in their blood vessels even without the high-fat diet (Clarkson *et al.* 1974) and a total of 594 scientific papers on this strain of rabbit were produced during the years 2001–2008[4].

In toxicology, rabbits are used to detect teratogenic effects of candidate drugs because the embryological development of the rabbit foetus is well known, the gestation period is short and rabbits produce a fairly large number of offspring (Wooding & Burton 2008). For the same reasons, rabbits are used in experimental teratology (Hartman 1974). Rabbits have also been used for cardiac surgery and disease, joint surgery, ophthalmology and studies of hypertension.

Laboratory management and breeding

Housing

Laboratory rabbits have traditionally been housed individually in cages for up to several years, depending on the research purpose. One reason for individual housing has been the problems with aggression that may arise in group housing, especially between males. Three main types of cages have been used: (1) wire; (2) sheet metal with wire front; and (3) plastic with wire front (Stauffacher *et al.* 1994; Morton *et al.* 1993). In the past, often no enrichments were provided and the cage sizes were such that rabbits were unable to hop around or sit upright with erect ears. Cages with solid sides, back and top tend to isolate the animals,

[4]http://www.med.kobe-u.ac.jp/iea/whhl-1.html

Table 28.4 Recommendations for minimum enclosure dimensions and space allowance for one or two socially harmonious rabbits over 10 weeks of age or a doe plus litter with additional area for nest boxes, and optimum shelf size and height from the enclosure floor (Council of Europe 2006; European Commission 2007).

Final body weight (kg)	*Minimum floor area (cm²)*	*Minimum height (cm)*	*Addition for nest boxes (cm²)*	*Optimum shelf size (cm)*	*Optimum height of shelf (cm)*
<3	3500	45	1000	55 × 25	25
3–5	4200	45	1200	55 × 30	25
>5	5400	60	1400	60 × 35	30

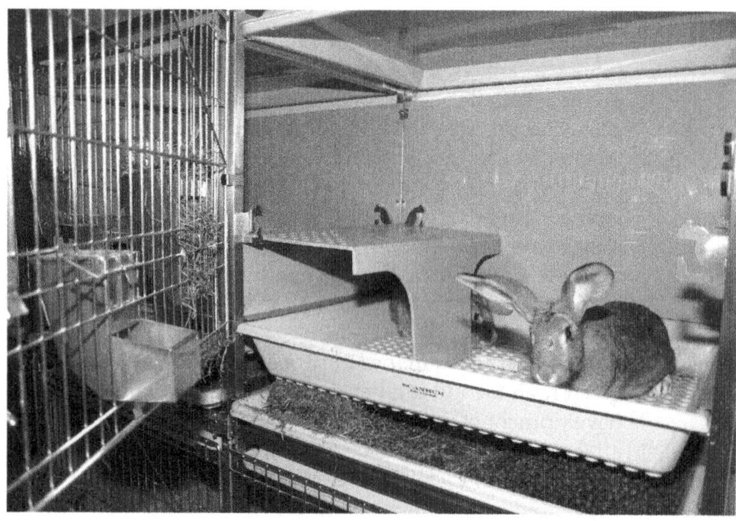

Figure 28.1 A new type of flexible rabbit cage with a pair of rabbits (Photo: Ann-Christine Nordström.)

and prevent them from seeing the source of disturbance, which may cause them to be startled, and in breeding units, lead to losses due to cannibalism (Stauffacher *et al.* 1994). It is therefore recommended that barred 'windows' occupy 30–50 % of the total wall area (Stauffacher *et al.* 1994).

In order to allow rabbits to perform normal hopping movements and to sit upright the regulations in several countries have required larger cages for over 15 years. Appendix A of the European Convention for the protection of vertebrate animals used for experimental and other scientific purposes (Council of Europe (2006) recommends larger areas and heights than in the preceding Convention from 1986, and these have been adopted by the Commission (European Commission 2007). The minimum floor area and minimum height for rabbits over 10 weeks of age and for does with a litter is presented in Table 28.4. These recommendations are for both cages and pens. The weights are for the final body weight that any rabbit will reach in the housing. The minimum floor area is for one or two socially harmonious animals. In cages, a raised area should be provided. If there are scientific or veterinary justifications for not providing a raised area then the floor area should be 33% larger for a single rabbit and 60% larger for two rabbits. Some European countries have previous stronger national regulations for housing laboratory rabbits, whereas others are currently incorporating the new minimum recommendations into their national regulations.

Improved cages have been developed and tested in parallel with the development of new regulations for housing rabbits. These cages generally have a larger floor area and greater height to enable more upright sitting, a shelf for rabbits to hop up onto or hide under, racks to make hay feeding easier and flexible cage racks so that several cages can be built together (Figure 28.1). A recent resource produced by the RSPCA and UFAW[5] provides practical suggestions on how to house and manage laboratory rabbits based on their needs. Caged rabbits use boxes and shelves as sources of enrichment and lookout posts (Hansen & Berthelsen 2000), and the presence of the shelf reduces restlessness, grooming, bar-gnawing and nervous responses when being captured (Berthelsen & Hansen 1999).

During the last 10–20 years the approach to housing rabbits has changed considerably, and group housing in floor pens has been introduced in many laboratories and countries (Figure 28.2). In the 2003 Guidelines for the Housing of Rabbits in Scientific Institutions in Australia (Animal Research Review Panel 2003)[6] two key recommendations are that *'Rabbits should be housed in groups in pens'* and *'Rabbits should not be housed singly in conventional (unenriched) cages except in exceptional circumstances …'*. European guidelines (Council of Europe 2006; European Commission 2007) also recommend that wherever it is possible, rabbits should be kept in pens. Housing in pens enables rabbits to

[5]http://www.rspca.org.uk/researchrabbits

[6]http://www.animalethics.org.au/__data/assets/pdf_file/0013/222511/housing-rabbits-scientific-institutions.pdf

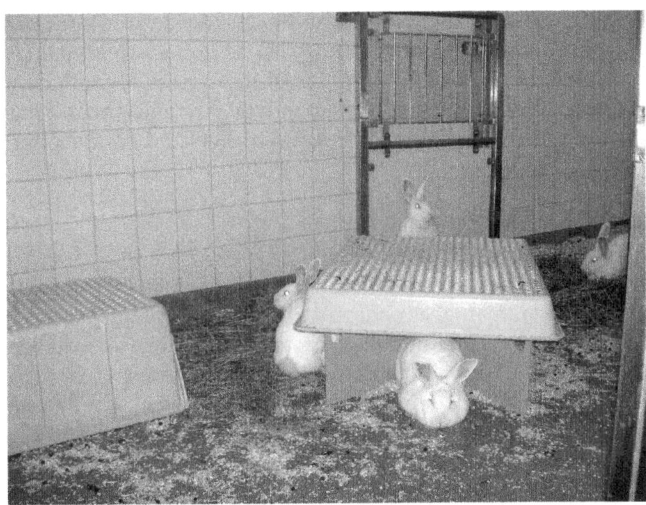

(a)

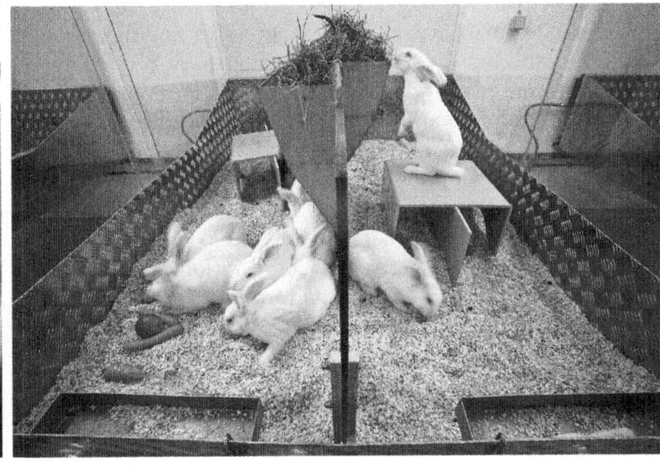

(b)

Figure 28.2 Group housing of does in a research laboratory in Sweden (a) and in a pharmaceutical company in Denmark (b) (Photos: a) Lena Lidfors, b) with kind permission of Novo Nordisk A/S.)

express social behaviours and to exercise (Heath & Stott 1990; Batchelor 1991). The RSPCA/UFAW resource recommends that young rabbits and older females should be housed in harmonious pairs or social groups unless veterinary advice or study design recommends differently. Adult entire males should, on the other hand, be singly housed due to their territorial behaviour and the consequent risks of serious injury.

Floor pens should be large enough for the rabbits to be able to carry out basic behaviours such as locomotion, rearing, grooming and avoiding cage mates, etc. European Commission (2007, Table B.1) recommends that rabbits should be provided with the same pen floor area as in cages, and an extra floor area of 3000 cm^2 per rabbit should be added for three to six rabbits and thereafter 2500 cm^2 for every additional rabbit over six. This is much less than recommended by Morton *et al.* (1993), who suggested that group houses should have a clear area of 20 000 cm^2 with an overall minimum floor area of 6000–8000 cm^2 per rabbit for groups up to six rabbits. One problem with using weight as a criterion for determining floor area is that young animals are more active and might need more space to carry out play behaviours (Stauffacher *et al.* 1994). Swiss legislation from 1991 requires that each rabbit must be able to hop for several steps or to jump up and down onto a shelf. This may help to maintain a level of fitness and reduce the occurrence of disuse osteoporosis (Morton *et al.* 1993). European Commission (2007) recommends that rabbits younger than 10 weeks should be provided with a minimum enclosure size of 4000 cm^2 and a minimum floor area per animal of 800 cm^2 from weaning to 7 weeks and 1200 cm^2 from 7–10 weeks.

The height of floor pens should be 1.25 m, and enrichment objects should be placed so that they cannot be used for jumping over walls (Morton *et al.* 1993). Table B.1 in European Commission (2007) recommends the same minimum height for pens as for cages, but this is too low to stop rabbits from jumping out of the pen. The pen should contain structures that subdivide the space so that the animals are able to initiate or avoid social contact. Examples of group housing of NZW does in a research laboratory are shown in Figure 28.2.

The floor should be solid and provided with bedding or perforated, rather than grid or wire mesh (European Commission 2007). Wire floors should not be used unless a resting area is provided which is large enough to hold all rabbits at any one time (European Commission 2007). Dimple floors were regarded as the best type of floors in metal cages by Morton *et al.* (1993).

Social housing

The major factors that need to be considered when group-housing rabbits are: compatibility of individual animals; size of pens; stocking density; husbandry practices; and environmental enrichment (Morton *et al.* 1993). Rabbits can either be group-housed in floor pens or in cages. In the latter case, weight and size limitations usually restrict this to pair-housing (Bigler & Oester 1994; Huls *et al.* 1991; Stauffacher 1993). This combines the benefits of cage-housing (eg, hygiene and experimental purposes, with animal welfare interests) and has been established in several countries (Stauffacher *et al.* 1994). While Stauffacher *et al.* (1994) report that groups of up to 20 laboratory rabbits have been successfully managed as stock and for the production of polyclonal antibodies, for monitoring and observation reasons the number of rabbits kept in group pens should not exceed six to eight mature animals (Morton *et al.* 1993; Stauffacher *et al.* 1994).

Incompatible rabbits fight when placed together in a group, and the greatest problems occur when placing adult males together (Morton *et al.* 1993). There are strain differences in aggressiveness: Dutch rabbits are more aggressive than NZW, whereas Lops are more docile (Morton *et al.*

1993). Some of the small strains of rabbits may show more aggression than the larger strains (Stauffacher *et al.* 1994). Individual animals may be highly aggressive, and fights can occur unexpectedly, even in groups that have been stable for a long time and in which an apparently stable dominance hierarchy has formed (Morton *et al.* 1993). Therefore, groups of rabbits need to be carefully selected and regularly monitored. The best option is to form female groups from litter mates which have been kept together from weaning (Zain 1988). Groups of intact, mature females not intended for breeding can be kept together (Morton *et al.* 1993). During resting, does, bucks and older young kept in mixed groups congregate and snuggle against each other or engage in mutual grooming (Stauffacher 1992). Does have demonstrated a weak preference for a large, enriched, solitary pen over a group pen, but a strong preference for a group pen over a smaller, barren, solitary pen (Held *et al.* 1995). Fighting can occur in groups of does, and a dominant female in oestrus can mount and damage the skin on the backs of other females and harass the group (Morton *et al.* 1993). The degree of compatibility of grouped rabbits depends on factors such as strain, individual characteristics, sex, age and weight, size and structuring of pens, methods of husbandry and the interest and ability of the animal care staff (Bell & Bray 1984; Zain 1988; Morton *et al.* 1993; Stauffacher 1993).

From around 10 weeks of age it may be necessary to house males individually to avoid fighting (Morton *et al.* 1993). Groups of males kept in proximity to females tend to fight and urinate more frequently (Portsmouth 1987). Castration of males kept for longer periods in the laboratory may be one solution to keeping them in groups, although this raises ethical issues, as discussed in the RSPCA/UFAW booklet[7]. The practical experience from castration of males is that aggression is reduced and stable for a long time afterwards (L. Lindberg, personal communication). Castration should be carried out only by qualified persons when the males reach sexual maturity and before they start to show aggressive behaviour, about 3–4 weeks after weaning (Morton *et al.* 1993; Stauffacher *et al.* 1994). The testicles move down during sexual maturation, but can be withdrawn again via the cremaster muscle. Another consideration is the type of research the animals will be used for, as castration has an effect on the animal's physiology and behaviour.

When establishing new groups of rabbits in floor pens, the best option is to wean and mix at the same time around 6 weeks of age and to place 6–10 rabbits preferably of the same sex in one group (Morton *et al.* 1993). The easiest approach is to group-house animals which have been kept in groups since birth (Zain 1988; Stauffacher 1993). Smaller groups may be more stable (Love & Hammond 1991). Some animals do not appear to settle well in groups, either because they are too dominant and bully the others or are too timid and prone to be bullied (Morton *et al.* 1993). When grouping rabbits that have been caged for 6 months or more it may be difficult to avoid fighting or self-inflicted injuries (Morton *et al.* 1993). However, individually caged adult female rabbits of strains that are known to be docile can be paired successfully, preferably in structured cages (Stauffacher 1993). It is very important to provide refuge and hiding places for subordinate animals (Morton *et al.* 1993).

Environmental enrichment

Abnormal behaviours in rabbits can be reduced by providing environmental enrichment in their cage or floor pen (See also Chapter 10). Roughage, hay blocks and chew sticks are recommended as suitable enrichment (Council of Europe 2006; European Commission 2007). Morton *et al.* (1993) suggested the following enrichment for caged rabbits: straw, hay, hay blocks, hydroponic grass, pieces of wood or chew sticks, hay rack, small cardboard boxes, taking them out of the cage for handling/petting or for exercise and relief of boredom, provision of bedding, vet beds for pregnant and nesting does and background noise. Gunn (1994) found that stereotypic behaviour in caged rabbits was reduced by the provision of hay, wooden sticks and wire balls. Singly housed male rabbits interacted most often with hay, less with hay blocks, even less with a plastic box and least with chewing sticks (Lidfors 1997), and showed the highest preference for hay, then hay blocks, chewing sticks and lastly a plastic box (Lidfors 1996).

The enrichment items used most often are those that the rabbits can chew on (Huls *et al.* 1991; Lidfors 1997; Berthelsen & Hansen 1999) and high-fibre objects are preferred, with hay or straw remaining effective enrichments for long periods (Brummer 1975; Lidfors 1997). If the supplementary hay is ground, it is ineffective at reducing problem behaviours, demonstrating a need for long fibre (Mulder *et al.* 1992). Hay and straw also cause less weight gain than proprietary fibre sticks or compressed grass cubes (Lidfors 1997). Studies on dietary enrichments, including the supply of fibrous food to reduce boredom, are: hay (Berthelsen & Hansen 1999); grass cubes or hay in a bottle (Lidfors 1997); and fresh grass (Leslie *et al.* 2004). Abnormal maternal behaviours and trichophagia or fur-chewing (Brummer 1975; Mulder *et al.* 1992) are eliminated in caged rabbits when hay or straw is given (Beynen *et al.* 1992).

Mirrors placed in the living area of caged rabbits increase the time they spend there, and especially the time that they spend investigating their environment and feeding (Jones & Phillips 2005). The mirrors probably stimulate activity by increasing the amount of movement perceived by the rabbit (Jones & Phillips 2005). If the racks are placed opposite to each other so that the rabbits can see other rabbits that may also be a form of enrichment (Morton *et al.* 1993).

A technique that has been used in certain Swedish animal laboratories for individually caged male rabbits that cannot be castrated, is to place them individually in an exercise arena at regular intervals. This allows them to move around on a larger floor surface, to investigate enrichment objects and to be exposed to odours from other males that have been exercised before them. To the authors' knowledge this has not been scientifically validated, and the procedure could be stimulating or stressful.

[7] http://www.rspca.org.uk/researchrabbits

Environmental provisions

Temperature and humidity

European guidelines recommend a mean room temperature for rabbits of 18°C with a range of 15–21°C (Council of Europe 2006; European Commission 2007). In rabbits the low critical temperature is –7°C and the high critical temperature is 28°C (Spector 1956). Rabbits only have sweat glands on their lips, and are less able to ventilate through their mouth than dogs (Donnelly 1997). Wild rabbits avoid high temperatures and stay away from sunshine, and during the day they stay in the cooler burrows (Gibb *et al.* 1978). The ears of the rabbit are highly vascular and can function as radiators (Harkness & Wagner 1995).

The relative humidity in rabbit facilities should not be less than 45% (European Commission 2007).

Light and noise

Batchelor (1999) recommends that the rabbit room has a regular light–dark cycle and that it is isolated from external lighting fluctuations. The lights in many laboratories are usually put on a 12h:12h light–dark cycle. Some laboratory facilities have introduced artificial dawn and dusk periods, which usually last 30 minutes. Sudden illumination of active rabbits may cause them to leap and possibly fracture the spine (Adams 1982). If there is a need to observe rabbits during the period of activity a partially reversed lighting schedule can be used, because rabbits are more nocturnal than diurnal in their activity pattern (Batchelor 1999). The normal diurnal cycle can be disrupted by noise or scheduled feeding in the laboratory (Jilge 1991).

According to Iwarsson *et al.* (1994) the optimal light intensity in rabbit rooms should be 200 lux at 1 m above the floor. However, if the illumination level is too high it can lead to retinal degeneration in some albino mammals, which may also apply to NZW rabbits (Batchelor 1999). Cages with solid sides reduce the amount of light, and cages higher up in the rack have a higher light intensity (Batchelor 1999). In floor pens, shelves and boxes may provide hiding places from high light intensity.

The rabbit's hearing threshhold has been reported to be 75–50 000 Hz with the most sensitive hearing between 2000 to about 9000 Hz (Iwarsson *et al.* 1994). The rabbit is therefore sensitive to high-pitched sounds (Milligan *et al.* 1993), but sudden noise may scare rabbits and lead to injures. A common practice is to use background music to attempt to mask sudden sounds, and this is claimed by some to result in lower excitability (Batchelor 1999).

Ventilation

European guidelines recommend 15–20 air changes per hour (Council of Europe 2006; European Commission 2007). However, it is possible to have 8–10 air changes per hour if cleaning routines are of high standard and stocking density is low (Adams 1982). There should be no draughts or turbulence in the rabbit room. If the ventilation is not working properly, high levels of ammonia and carbon dioxide may become a problem for the rabbits.

Ammonia level should never exceed 10 ppm. High ammonium levels can inactivate the cilia in the airways of rabbits.

The rabbit moults two to three times per year. Rabbit hair may also be released during handling.

Food and water

Rabbits are nocturnal and in the wild they usually graze during their active periods at dawn and dusk (Lockley 1961), or during early morning and at night (Cheeke 1987). However, laboratory rabbits in cages are almost invariably not fed the diet of grass for which they are adapted. There is little evidence that they prefer a grass diet to one based on compound feed (Leslie *et al.* 2004). Despite this, it is often beneficial to supplement their ration of proprietary compound pellets with dietary enrichment, which as well as providing adequate nutrients (National Research Council (NRC) 1966), in particular fibre (Lehmann 1990), will increase the time spent procuring food and reduce abnormal behaviours such as chewing their cage (Leslie *et al.* 2004). The visual stimulus of a varied diet is particularly important (Ruckebusch *et al.* 1971). A mixed diet is also a feature of natural herbivore feeding behaviour; due to their need to sample regularly in case of the disappearance of one feed (Parsons *et al.* 1994). Hay can make up a larger part of the feed intake of adult rabbits, and at the same time be an important enrichment (see section on Environmental enrichment).

Water should always be available *ad libitum* (Mader 1997). Rabbits fed on dry diets require approximately 120 ml water/kg body weight (Cheeke 1987), or 10% of the body weight per 24 h (Meredith 2000). More water should be provided for growing animals, pregnant and lactating females and for rabbits fed high-fibre diets (Cizek 1961).

Hygiene

Since rabbits have a sensitive digestive system with intensive interaction between the intestine and its microbiological flora, the hygiene of the cage or pen where the rabbit is held is important. Rabbits are coprophagic, but they ingest only one type of faecal pellet. The remaining faeces may contain coccidia spores and pinworm eggs that can re-infect the animal and the heavy breeds may develop cutaneous infections on their hindlegs from soiled bedding or wire floors (Bergdall & Dysko 1994).

The frequency of cleaning out and disinfection of pen floors, cage waste pans or other areas where the faeces and urine of the animals may accumulate depends on the number of animals in each cage or pen, the sizes of the animals, their diet and on other physical and practical arrangements in the animal rooms such as the efficiency of the ventilation equipment, etc. It is not possible to give specific recommendations because circumstances vary between laboratories. The room air should be perceived as fresh and clean without any smell. If there is any doubt, ammonia levels in the air can be measured. The animals should have clean fur coats and be clinically healthy. Over-zealous cleaning of any animal environment could be stressful to the animals because of changes to the olfactory environment (Batchelor 1999).

Health monitoring, barrier systems and quarantine

High health standards result in good welfare and good science. Today most breeders use barrier breeding systems with regular health monitoring. The biosafety strategy of breeders includes: control of entry of staff and goods into the breeding rooms; procedures for sterilisation of goods such as bedding, diets and other materials; and regular education and awareness training for staff. Strict barrier regimes avoid introduction of animals from elsewhere, but rely on re-deriving rabbit pups from pregnant does by caesarean section, after which the young are hand-reared. Some breeders even have regularly scheduled refurbishments of their breeding units as a part of their biohazard management.

Animal health records should show the frequency and interval of different samples taken, the result of analysis and the methods used as well as which laboratory was used. In Europe FELASA, the Federation of European Laboratory Animal Science Associations, has issued recommendations for health monitoring laboratory animals in different situations, at the breeding site and in the research laboratory (FELASA 2002).

When rabbits are introduced to a colony, quarantine can be used as a precaution if there is any doubt about their health status, but most health problems of laboratory animals nowadays are subclinical. Thus, it is unlikely that there will be clinical signs of disease during the period of quarantine. The establishment's quarantine procedures in combination with serological sampling for the more commonly occurring infectious agents could be used, but this can be time consuming and result in extra costs.

Breeding

Females can be mated for the first time at 4–5 months if they are of a small breed, 4.5–5 months if they are of a medium breed (for example NZW) and 6–9 months if they are of a large breed (Harkness & Wagner 1995). Bucks are usually used for breeding for the first time at about 6 months of age (Harkness & Wagner 1995). The decision to use a female for breeding is based on her age (4–6 months), clinical condition, weight (3–4 kg for NZW) and observation of periodic congestion of the vulva (Harkness & Wagner 1995).

Follicle-stimulating hormone (FSH) induces growth of ovarian follicles with development of ova, and the follicles produce oestrogens, which cause the female to be receptive to the male (Patton 1994). Follicular development occurs in waves, and follicles at several stages of development are always present (Patton 1994). When follicles reach mature size they produce oestrogens for 12–14 days, but if ovulation does not occur they degenerate with a corresponding reduction in blood concentration of oestrogens and sexual receptivity (Patton 1994). After about 4 days, new follicles start producing oestrogens and the doe becomes receptive again (Patton 1994). This leads to the doe having a cycle of 16–18 days during which she is receptive for 12–14 days followed by 2–4 days when she refuses to mate (Patton 1994). However, there have been several cases where does have been receptive for 14–16 days followed by a period of non-receptivity for 1–2 days (Patton 1994).

Does may vary in receptivity due to individual differences, sexual stimulation and environmental factors, such as nutrition, light and temperature (Cheeke *et al.* 1987). Sometimes does refuse to mate with a certain buck, possibly because the buck adopts a poor mounting position or because of his aggressiveness (Patton 1994). When the doe is receptive the vulva changes colour (Cheeke *et al.* 1987) and it changes to a darker pink or red and becomes swollen and moist (Patton 1994).

In captivity, the male's courtship behaviour is often restricted to tail flagging, urination and licking the genitalia (Patton 1994). A jet of urine (enurination) may also be directed at a doe (Patton 1994).

For mating, the doe should be taken to the buck's cage to avoid territorial behaviour, ie, either the doe attacking the buck or the buck showing more interest in exploring and marking the new territory (Patton 1994; Bennett 2001). If the doe is not receptive she becomes aggressive and produces a special vocalisation (B.-Å. Sandeberg, personal communication). When a receptive doe has been placed in the buck's cage she raises her hindquarters to allow copulation (see Reproduction section for more details). If copulation does not occur within 2 minutes after the doe has been placed in the buck's cage she should be removed as injuries and stress to both doe and buck may occur if they are left together too long and bucks may become poor breeders if they are repeatedly rejected by does (Patton 1994). Bucks are very fertile, even if they are used daily or several times per day (Patton 1994). If bucks are used several times in a 24 h period they are often rested on the next day, but they can also be used for multiple breeding several days in a row and then be rested for several days (Patton 1994). A common practice is to keep one buck for every 10 does, but many breeding facilities use one buck per 25 does (Patton 1994).

Ovulation is induced by mating, and occurs 10–13 h after coitus (Patton 1994); it may also be induced artificially by injecting luteinising hormone or human chorionic gonadotropin, electrical or mechanical stimulation or after contact with other does (Patton 1994). Some does may fail to ovulate after coitus, possibly as a result of a deficiency of luteinising hormone (Fox & Krinsky 1968). The number of ova released has been found to be correlated with body weight (Staples & Holtkamp 1966), so that heavier does tend to get larger litters compared to does with lighter weights. High ambient temperature has been found to depress the conception rate, especially when the temperature is high for longer periods (Sittman *et al.* 1964).

Pregnancy can be determined by palpating the developing foetuses at 12–14 days of pregnancy (Cheeke *et al.* 1987), looking at swelling of the mammary glands in late gestation (Patton 1994) or by radiographic confirmation after 11 days (Hafez 1970).

The gestation length is 31–32 days (Cheeke *et al.* 1987), and a large-scale study found that 85.5% of NZW litters were born on days 31 and 32 (Templeton 1939). Larger litters were carried for shorter times than smaller litters (Templeton

1939). Parturition usually occurs during the morning (Sawin 1950). The birth of each young takes less than 30 minutes, but young may be born several hours or days apart (3 days for live young (Patton 1994)). Foetuses older than 35 days die, and if they are not expelled can prevent future pregnancy (Adams *et al.* 1967).

Rollins *et al.* (1963) found that the most important influence on litter size was the parity of the doe, with second and third litters having the highest number of young, fewer young in fourth and fifth litters and least young in first litters. Sittman *et al.* (1964) demonstrated seasonal variation in litter size, with the highest born in February and the lowest in September.

Post-partum mating usually occurs 4–8 weeks after birth of a litter, when the young have been weaned (Patton 1994). Does will mate immediately following parturition, and if the young are removed sexual receptivity continues for at least 36 days (Patton 1994). Post-partum receptivity declines during lactation and increases again once the young are feeding themselves (Patton 1994). Females are most difficult to breed at the peak of lactation – approximately the third week (Cheeke *et al.* 1987), which may be a result of loss of body weight (Patton 1994).

Pseudo-pregnancy may be caused by an infertile mating, sexual excitement being caused by one doe mounting or being mounted by another or by injecting luteinising hormone (Patton 1994). It lasts for 16–17 days and ends when the doe attempts to make a nest at 18–22 days (Patton 1994). During pseudo-pregnancy the corpora lutea secret progesterone, which causes the uterus and mammary glands to grow (Asdell & Salisbury 1933). For more information about maternal behaviour and nursing see the section on Reproduction.

In commercial rabbit breeding, both for laboratory and food production purposes, the young are weaned and separated from the doe at 6–7 weeks of age (Hagen 1974; Bennett 2001), but some commercial breeders of laboratory NZW rabbits wean the young at 5 weeks (B.-Å. Sandeberg, personal communication).

When breeding rabbits are kept in groups, the groups should be composed of four to six females, one male and their offspring until they are weaned at 30 days of age (Stauffacher *et al.* 1994). A group breeding housing and management system has been developed in Switzerland (Stauffacher 1989) and used in agricultural rabbit farming, but not, to the authors' knowledge, for breeding laboratory rabbits.

Identification and sexing

Young rabbits are weaned at 5–7 weeks. At this time the young are also sexed and males and females placed in separate cages. This procedure requires some training. The male rabbit's penis can be extruded from the age of 2 months which is considerably later than weaning age (Harkness & Wagner 1995).

Many breeders also perform identity marking at weaning using ear tattoos, tags, etc, or subcutaneously implanted microchips. As a general principle the least invasive method, compatible with the end use, should be chosen.

Laboratory procedures

Handling

Handlers should keep in mind that rabbits, as prey animals, naturally try to flee if they perceive a threat. Rabbits are able to recognise individual humans which they can recognise by voice. Rabbits are rarely aggressive if handled in a calm and steady manner without intimidating the rabbit by unfamiliar sounds or odours.

To pick up an animal, the scruff of the neck is grasped firmly with one hand; the animal is lifted up, using the other hand to support the body, and placed on the other arm with its head in the opening between the elbow and the body of the handler (Figure 28.3). For transport over a short distance, this lets the animal rest in a normal posture on the forearm of the handler with its head hidden whilst the hand of the handler holds the scruff (Stein & Walshaw 1996). It is also possible to transport the rabbit a very short distance by holding the scruff of the neck with one hand and supporting the rabbit under the hindlegs with the other hand. While handling rabbits, it is advisable to wear long-sleeved garments because the claws of rabbits may scratch the skin of the handler's arms if they are unprotected by clothing (Suckow & Douglas 1997). Because rabbits have a fragile skeleton and strong hindleg muscles, struggling may cause fracture of the spinal vertebrae (Marston *et al.* 1965).

Training/habituation for procedures

Rabbits can be accustomed to laboratory procedures just as any other animals. It has been shown that early handling of rabbits results in more active, alert and exploratory animals, which approach novel stimuli more often (Harkness & Wagner 1995). Animals which are well acquainted with their handlers and environment are less stressed in experimental situations and this improves the outcome of the scientific work (Toth & January 1990). See also Chapter 16.

Physiological monitoring

Rabbits are often used in immunisation studies involving blood sampling. General advice on blood sampling techniques can be found in Joint Working Group on Refinement (JWGR) (1993). Blood can be taken from the marginal ear vein (Figure 28.4), from the central artery of the ear or by cardiac puncture. Cardiac puncture is carried out with the animal in dorsal recumbency and only under anaesthesia (Batchelor 1999). After cardiac puncture the animal should be immediately killed because of the risk of damage to the pericardium and subsequent heart tamponade. When using the marginal ear vein, application of a local anaesthetic ointment 15 minutes earlier facilitates the removal of blood from those animals which are distressed by the insertion of the needle into the ear vein (Batchelor 1999).

For collecting larger volumes of blood, the central ear artery is a better choice since the blood flow is stronger here but care must be taken to ensure that the puncture site is compressed afterwards in order to stop the vessel from

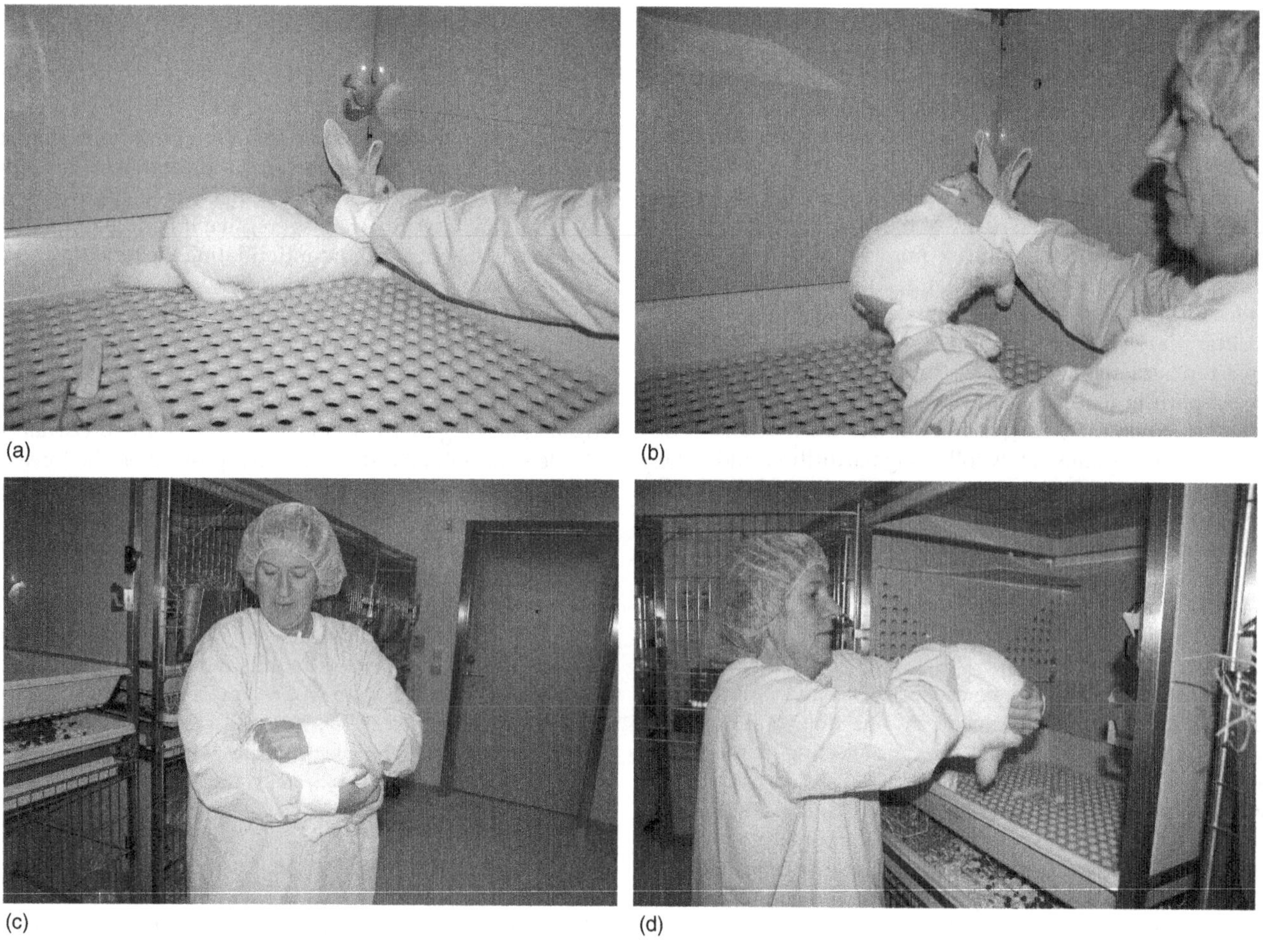

(a) (b) (c) (d)

Figure 28.3 A rabbit, its movement restrained (a), taken by the scruff with one hand and carefully moved through the air (b), and held towards the body resting on the other arm with the face tucked under the arm (c). When the rabbit is lifted back to the cage again the other hand supports the body of the rabbit (d). (Photos: Ann-Christine Nordström.)

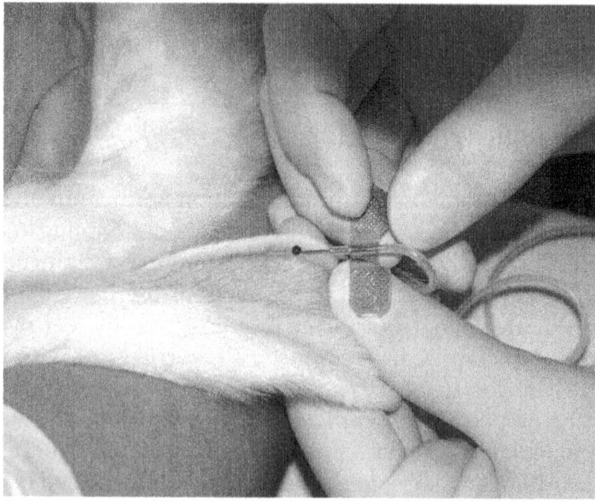

Figure 28.4 Collection of blood from the ear vein of a rabbit. (Photo: Ann-Christine Nordström.)

bleeding after sampling. This can be achieved using manual compression or a temporary compression bandage. Up to 10% of the total blood volume of the rabbit can be removed. If multiple samples are taken, the rabbit should have a recovery period of 2–3 weeks after the maximal amount of 10% of the blood volume has been sampled. Rabbits have 60–70 ml blood per kg body weight.

The body temperature of rabbits should be taken by a suitable thermometer that has been lubricated for ease of introduction into the anus (Batchelor 1999). The rabbit should be gently restrained, the tail lifted and the thermometer inserted without any force. The thermometer should be left *in situ* for 1–2 minutes. In rabbits the normal rectal temperature is 38.5–39.5°C (Ruckebusch *et al.* 1991).

Administration of medical treatment or compounds

General advice on the administration of substances can be found in JWGR (2001). Rabbits are easily dosed subcutaneously under the skin of the neck and the upper back area. The drugs or compounds given should be pH neutral because rabbits tend to develop subcutaneous abscesses after injections of irritant substances. Intramuscular injections can be given in the hindleg, in the quadriceps muscle; they can also be given into the dorsal lumbar muscles but there is a risk of damage to the ischiatic nerve running down the back and lateral part of the hindleg. In general, intramuscular injections should be avoided because they are often painful for the animal and the rate of absorption is not much quicker than from subcutaneous sites.

It is relatively easy to perform intravenous injections with a needle or infusions using an indwelling catheter placed in the marginal ear vein, and this route has many advantages such as quick onset of action of the injected compound.

Intraperitoneal (ip) injections can also be used but there is a great variability in the rate of uptake after injecting ip since there is a likelihood that at least some of the material injected will enter the gut (caecum), fatty tissue or the urinary bladder rather than the serosal cavity. Rabbits which are not trained usually struggle when restrained with their belly upwards for receiving the ip injection and this increases the risk of a less than perfect injection.

For enteral administration, gavage can be performed with a soft tube passed into the rabbit's stomach. This technique must be learnt under supervision of a person skilled in the procedure. Rabbits can be trained to ingest sweetened fluids from a syringe and it is possible to dose rabbits orally by this route, for example to provide post-surgical pain relief.

Anaesthesia/analgesia

Suitable anaesthetic and analgesic regimes should be chosen in co-operation with the laboratory animal veterinary surgeon. Depending on the equipment available, a regime based on injectables alone or a combination of injectable agents and gaseous anaesthesia may be used. Rabbits are sensitive to smells of anaesthetic gas, which renders induction of the anaesthesia difficult using gaseous agents (Svendsen 1994). Induction by injectable agents is preferable, followed by gaseous anaesthesia, which allows easy control of the depth and length of the anaesthesia (Svendsen 1994). When using only injectable agents, the use of a continuous infusion can be considered because it is easier to adjust the duration of anaesthesia to suit the length of the surgical procedure than with bolus administration (Svendsen 1994). Further advice can be found in Flecknell 2009.

Post-surgical care of rabbits includes placing them in a recovery cage, the box they were placed in before surgery or the home cage which has been lined with a tray liner (Batchelor 1999). The liner may be folded over the animal to minimise hypothermia. Commercially available veterinary bedding may also be used. The liner or bedding should be removed about 30 minutes after the animal has regained consciousness and is sitting up (Batchelor 1999).

If several group-housed animals have undergone surgery, the last animal must be completely conscious before all the animals are returned to the pen simultaneously (Batchelor 1999). If animals are returned to a group pen whilst still recovering consciousness they may be subjected to aggression (Batchelor 1999). Incision sites should be covered with a clear plastic dressing spray. Rabbits may occasionally interfere with their stitches (Batchelor 1999), and if this happens a plastic collar can be used to restrict the animal's access to the surgical wound (Batchelor 1999).

Euthanasia

Euthanasia of rabbits is most commonly performed by intravenous injection of an overdose of anaesthetic agent, such as sodium pentobarbital or anaesthetic mixtures. Captive bolt followed by exsanguination is another method for euthanasia that can be used by experienced personnel if the use of chemical euthanasia is for some reason unsuitable or contraindicated. Physical dislocation of the neck followed by exsanguination is an option for rabbits up to 1 kg body weight. Concussion and exsanguination can be done on unconscious animals. Decapitation should only be carried out on animals weighing less than 1 kg, which are already unconscious.

Common welfare problems

Health

The clinical health of modern laboratory animals is rarely a major issue; more important are subclinical infections and the ways they may affect and alter research results. For example, it is quite possible for rabbits not to show clinically obvious signs or symptoms of disease unless they are negatively influenced by multiple agents or other stressors simultaneously (Nerem 1980). However, there are some differences between rabbits and more commonly used species – mice and rats. Health management of mice and rats is an issue mainly of maintaining freedom from pathogens of viral, bacterial and more rarely parasitic origin; rabbit health management is mainly concerned with maintaining freedom from parasites and to some degree from bacteria. All major breeders of laboratory rabbits use a health-monitoring programme and these programmes comprise microbiological testing and some pathology surveillance. In Europe the Federation of European Laboratory Animal Associations (FELASA 2002) recommendations are widely accepted

A healthy rabbit has alert and clear eyes and well groomed fur. Even if the animal is well accustomed to being handled by humans, it will jump in an effort to escape if startled by a handler. A daily health check should include observation of the animal's posture, its eyes and nose to look for discharge and the state of the fur. When rabbits are group-housed, a check for wounds inflicted by other animals should also be made at least once daily. The faeces and urine should also be checked for abnormalities. Normal faeces should consist of dry pellets of a uniform size and normal urine can vary in colour from yellow to dark red and is often cloudy due to the excretion of calcium[8].

The FELASA recommendations are based on the incidence of different infections and vary depending on the size and purpose of each colony. When the FELASA guidelines for health monitoring of laboratory rabbits are followed, the animal can be called a 'health defined rabbit'. There are similar terms of earlier origin that are sometimes used for the same purpose, (SPF, specific pathogen free or VAF, virus antibody free animal). These different terms aim to provide information about the microbiological health status of the

[8] http://www.aquavet.i12.com/Rabbit.htm

rabbits in a colony. Health monitoring results are always historical and documentation should be read carefully with attention to how often the samples are taken, which method of evaluation has been used and the rationale for why certain agents are or are not evaluated in the specific colony.

Infectious diseases

Bacterial agents

The main infective causes of respiratory inflammations are *Pasteurella multocida* and *Bordetella bronchiseptica*, which cause symptoms such as sneezing, coughing, nasal discharge and lethargy. Abscesses in subcutaneous tissues, behind the eye bulb or in internal organs, as well as inflammation of the mucous membranes of the eyes and middle ear are often caused by *Pasteurella multocida* and *Staphylococcus aureus*. Bacterial eye infections by *Moraxella catarrhalis* can also occur in laboratory rabbits.

Young rabbits are particularly susceptible to bacterial imbalances within the intestine leading to conditions such as mucoid enteritis. Depression, anorexia, diarrhoea and mucus in the stool are the main symptoms; the cause is multifactorial with the bacterium *Clostridium spiroforme* being one of the major factors (Peeters 1986). Bacterial enteritis associated with diarrhoea as main symptom may also be caused by *Escherichia coli* and other strains of clostridia. Nutritional imbalance and lack of dietary fibre can predispose rabbits to enteritis.

Viral infections

Even though viral infections are not a major problem in barrier-bred laboratory rabbits, it is important to be aware of the potential of viral causes of disease. Mild diarrhoea may be caused by rotavirus and rabbit enteric coronavirus. Breeders and owners of pet rabbits fear rabbit viral hemorrhagic disease (RVHD). The symptoms of RVHD include lethargy, anorexia, diarrhoea and haemorrhage from body openings such as the nose and urogenital openings. This disease is unlikely to occur within a modern laboratory rabbit colony. Myxoma virus can be transferred to laboratory rabbits by vectors such as fleas and other insects. Because myxomatosis is common in wild rabbits it is possible for laboratory rabbit colonies located in areas with large populations of wild rabbits to be infected.

Parasites

Endoparasites (parasites inside the body) are more common than ectoparasites in laboratory rabbits; among endoparasites, coccidiosis is the greatest problem. This disease is caused by different strains of *Eimeria*. For example, *E. stiedae* is a strain infecting the liver and causes a wide range of symptoms from slight growth retardation to death. Several *Eimeria* strains such as *E. perforans* and *E. magna* affect the intestine of rabbits. The symptoms of coccidiosis depend on the location and number of coccidia in the gut and on the susceptibility of the animal. Younger animals more often show symptoms such as weight loss and mild to severe intermittent diarrhoea, whereas older animals rarely show any signs at all (Peeters 1986).

Passalurus ambiguus, the rabbit's pinworm, can colonise the caecum and colon and its eggs are passed in the faeces but these infections seldom affect the animals to such a degree that signs can be seen.

Encephalitozoon cuniculi, an intracellular protozoan, gives rise to a disease called encephalitozoonosis or nosematosis. This disease is common in pet and wild rabbits and regularly occurs in laboratory rabbits. The parasite is transmitted by the urine of infected animals via the oral route to the intestine and tissues of susceptible rabbits. Clinical signs are not always apparent, but heavy infections damage the kidneys and the brain of infected animals.

The two most common ectoparasites of pet rabbits are ear mites and fur mites, although these are rare in laboratory rabbit colonies. *Psoroptes cuniculi*, the ear mite, causes wounds on and around the ears. The fur mite, *Cheyletiella parasitivorax*, along with other mites, fleas and lice of rabbits, can cause considerable suffering and may induce self-inflicted wounds. Itching and anaemia caused by these blood-sucking insects result in poor general condition in the rabbit.

Traumatic injuries

Among animals that are housed in pairs or groups, the most common cause of traumatic injury is fighting. Both sexually mature males and females that are not acquainted with each other can fight aggressively. The likelihood of fighting increases when groups of animals are housed in overcrowded pens with too few water bottles or food hoppers. The wounds inflicted by fighting males can be severe and need suturing but may often be concealed by the fur of the animal if they are small.

The skeleton of rabbits is fragile in comparison to its muscular hindleg strength (Rothfritz *et al.* 1992), and rabbits which are not accustomed to handling by humans may struggle forcefully when picked up in the cage, resulting in vertebral fracture.

Diseases associated with housing, feeding and breeding regimes

The standards of housing, maintenance routines, hygiene measures and feeding and watering regimes all affect the health and well-being of rabbits. Animals held in pens on floor or in solid-bottom cages need management and thorough cleaning and disinfection of the pen or cage in order to minimise the spread of intestinal parasites and bacteria. Keeping the litter dry prevents coccidia from multiplying and minimises the need for frequent changes, which may then be as low as once monthly. Perforated cage floors that allow droppings to fall down onto a tray underneath help reduce the number of coccidian spores and bacteria in the immediate environment of the animal.

If larger rabbit breeds are kept in poorly designed perforated or wire mesh floors 'sore hocks' or pododermatitis can occur. Some individuals seem to be sensitive to wood shavings and other materials commonly used as bedding material in pens or solid-bottom cages. Inadequate hygiene is a predisposing factor. Symptoms include bleeding and chronic wounds on the hindfeet of affected animals. Softer bedding material and improved hygiene will be beneficial to these animals.

Dietary fibre concentration is critical for the intestinal flora and the intestinal morphology of rabbits (Tawfik *et al.* 1997). Young animals are most sensitive to imbalances caused by lack of fibre. Sufficient dietary fibre is essential to keep the animals from developing soft stools or diarrhoea.

Health problems may also arise from the feeding of modified laboratory diets during investigations, where the aim may be to produce metabolic changes in the rabbit. For example, diets containing high concentrations of fatty acids and cholesterol intended to produce atherosclerosis during long-term studies, may cause the deposition of fat in the liver and cholesterol in different parts of the body.

Behavioural abnormalities

Laboratory rabbits kept in small or barren cages may develop stereotyped behaviour, for example, wire-gnawing and excessive wall-pawing (Lehmann & Wieser 1985; Wieser 1986; Bigler & Lehmann 1991; Loeffler *et al.* 1991; Stauffacher 1992). Wall-pawing, which is derived from digging, may be constrained by the solid floor of the cage (Podberscek *et al.* 1991). Individually caged rabbits can show changes in their behaviours such as somersaulting, no full hops, less activity than group-penned rabbits, and less marking and investigatory behaviour than in group pens (Podberscek *et al.* 1991). Social isolation can induce physiological symptoms of stress, which may be relieved by the presence of conspecifics (Held *et al.* 1995). Stereotypic behaviour may indicate frustration, anxiety or boredom, and develop through a number of stages involving a progressive narrowing of the behavioural repertoire (Gunn 1994).

Singly housed laboratory rabbits in barren environments often show signs interpreted as boredom, such as hunched posture (Gunn & Morton 1995a, 1995b), inertia (Metz 1984), and a staring coat and dull eyes (Wallace *et al.* 1990). Chu *et al.* (2003) found that singly housed rabbits showed more abnormal behaviour and less movement than pair-housed rabbits. Prolonged inactivity associated with unresponsiveness may occur as well as, or in place of stereotypic behaviour, and is thought to be associated with changes in brain chemistry intended to help alleviate boredom (Broom 1988). Under-grooming may lead to development of a staring coat (Gunn & Morton 1995a), whereas over-grooming may result in development of hair-balls in the stomach (gastric trichobezoars) which in turn may cause intestinal stasis (Jackson 1991) and, if uncorrected, lead to death (Wagner *et al.* 1974). Other behavioural problems include under-eating and over-eating, associated with weight loss and obesity, respectively (Gunn & Morton 1995a).

The freedom of movement of rabbits housed in cages is very limited; for example normal hopping is impossible. This causes changes in the muscles, joints and bones (Lehmann 1989; Stauffacher 1992); and changes in the bone structure particularly evident in the femur proximalis (thinner and less strong bone) and the vertebral column (Lehmann 1989; Drescher & Loeffler 1991a, 1991b). Growing rabbits kept in cages perform almost no hopping or intensive locomotion, for example associated with play, when compared to those reared in outdoor enclosures (Lehmann 1989). The most common movement pattern, crawling, occurs at a slightly lower frequency in the cages (Lehmann 1989). In cages, rabbits often perform interrupted jumps, where the hindlegs are only lifted slightly and then put down again, so that the musculoskeletal system is not used as in normal hopping (Lehmann 1989). Rabbits may also show abnormal postures because of spatial constraints, for example when lying stretched out during resting or when performing stretching behaviour (Gunn 1994).

Rabbits may also show restlessness, such as non-functional bouts of activity with disconnected elements of feeding, comfort, resting, alertness and withdrawal behaviour alternating with locomotion with social and temporal disorder in behaviour, and panic (Lehmann & Wieser 1985; Bigler & Lehmann 1991; Stauffacher 1992).

A variety of disturbances to sexual behaviour have been described, some of which may lead to low conception rates (30–70 %) (Stauffacher 1992). For example, abnormal mating behaviour following placement of the doe into the buck's cage has been described as rape (Stauffacher 1992). The doe may show disturbed nesting behaviour and nesting stereotypies which may lead to rearing losses (Wieser 1986; Wullschleger 1987; Loeffler *et al.* 1991). In addition, the doe may show disturbed nursing and cannibalism associated with restlessness which may also increase rearing losses (Bigler 1986; Brummer 1986; Stauffacher 1992).

Acknowledgements

The authors want to thank AstraZeneca R&D Mölndal for letting Lena Lidfors carry out research on improving the housing of laboratory rabbits and for financing the time for Therese Edström to write this chapter. They also want to thank the Department of Animal Environment and Health for financing the time Lena Lidfors has used to write this chapter. They send a special thanks to Bengt-Åke Sandeberg at KB Lidköpings Rabbit Farm for sharing his knowledge on breeding laboratory rabbits with them. Special thanks are also sent to Ann-Christine Nordström at Astra Zeneca for taking some of the photos for this chapter.

References

Adams, C.E. (1982) Artificial insemination in the rabbit: the technique and application to practice. *Journal of Applied Rabbit Research*, **4**, 10–13

Adams, C.E., Atkins, F.C. and Worden, A.N. (1967) The rabbit. In: *The UFAW Handbook on the Care and Management of Laboratory Animals*, 3rd edn. Eds UFAW staff, pp. 396–448. E & S Livingstone Ltd, Edinburgh

Animal Research Review Panel (2003) *Guidelines for the Housing of Rabbits in Scientific Institutions*. ARRP Guideline 18. Animal Welfare Unit, New South Wales Agriculture, Sydney, Australia

Asdell, A.S. and Salisbury, G.W. (1933) The cause of mammary development during pseudopregnancy in the rabbits. *American Journal of Physiology*, **103**, 595–599

Batchelor, G.R. (1991) Group housing on floor pens and environmental enrichment in sandy lop rabbits (I). *Animal Technology*, **42**, 109–120

Batchelor, G.R. (1999) The laboratory rabbit. In: *The UFAW Handbook on the Care and Management of Laboratory Animals*, 7th edn. Ed. Poole, T., pp. 395–408. Blackwell Publishing, Oxford

Bell, D.J. (1977) *Aspects of the Social Behaviour of Wild and Domesticated Rabbits Oryctolagus cuniculus L.* Unpublished PhD thesis, University of Wales

Bell, D.J. (1980) Social olfaction in lagomorphs. In: *Symposia of the Zoological Society of London*, **45**, 141–164

Bell, D.J. (1983) Mate choice in the European rabbit. In: *Mate Choice.* Ed. Bateson, P.P.G., pp. 211–223. Cambridge University Press, Cambridge

Bell, D.J. (1984) The behaviour of rabbits: implications for their laboratory management. In: *Proceedings of UFAW/LASA Joint Symposium. Standards in Laboratory Animal Management, Part II.* pp. 151–162. Universities Federation for Animal Welfare, Potters Bar

Bell, D.J. (1999) The European wild rabbit. In: *The UFAW Handbook on the Care and Management of Laboratory Animals*, 7th edn. Ed. Poole, T., pp. 389–394. Blackwell Publishing, Oxford

Bell, D.J. and Bray, G.C. (1984) Effects of single- and mixed-sex caging on post-weaning development in the rabbit. *Laboratory Animals*, **18**, 267–270

Bell, D.J. and Webb, N.J. (1991) Effects of climate on reproduction in the European wild rabbit *Oryctolagus cuniculus*. *Journal of Zoology*, **224**, 639–648

Bennett, B. (2001) *Storey's Guide to Raising Rabbits*. Eds Burns D. and Salter M. Storey Communications Inc, USA

Berthelsen, H. and Hansen, L.T. (1999) The effect of hay on the behaviour of caged rabbits (*Oryctolagus cuniculus*). *Animal Welfare*, **8**, 149–157

Bergdall, V.K. and Dysko, R.C. (1994) Metabolic, traumatic and miscellaneous diseases in rabbits. In: *The Biology of the Laboratory Rabbit*, 2nd edn. Eds Manning, P.J., Ringler, D.H. and Newcomer, C.E., pp. 335–353. Academic Press, San Diego

Beynen, A.C., Mulder, A., Nieuwenkamp, A.E. *et al.* (1992) Loose grass hay as a supplement to a pelleted diet reduces fur chewing in rabbits. *Journal of Animal Physiology and Animal Nutrition*, **68**, 226–234

Bigler, L. (1986) *Mutter-Kind-Beziehung beim Hauskaninchen.* Lizentiatsarbeit, Universität Berne

Bigler, L. and Lehmann, M. (1991) *Schlussbericht ueber die Pruefung der Tiergerechtheit eines Festwandkaefigs fuer Hauskaninchen-Zibben.* Report Swiss Federal Veterinary Office, Berne

Bigler, L. and Oester, H. (1994) Paarhaltung nicht reproduzierender Zibben im Käfig. *Berliner und Münchener tierärztliche Wochenschrift*, **107**, 202–205

Björnhag, G. (1972) Separation and delay of contents in the rabbit colon. *Swedish Journal of Agriculture Research*, **11**, 25–136

Brooks, D.L. (1997) Nutrition and gastrointestinal physiology. In: *Ferrets, Rabbits and Rodents – Clinical Medicine and Surgery*. Eds Hillyer, E.W. and Quesenberry, K.E., pp. 169–175. WB Saunders, London

Broom, D.M. (1988) The scientific assessment of animal welfare. *Applied Animal Behaviour Sciences*, **20**, 5–19

Brummer, H. (1975) Trichophagia: a behavioural disorder in the domestic rabbit. *Deutsche Tierarztliche Wochenschrift*, **82**, 350–351

Brummer, H. (1986) Symptome des Wohlbefindens und des Unwohlseins beim Kaninchen unter besonderer Beruecksichtigung der Ethopathien. In: *Wege zur Beurteilung tiergerechter Haltung bei Labor-, Zoo- und Haustieren*. Ed. Militzer, K., pp. 44–53. Parey Schriften Versuchstierkunde

Canali, E., Ferrante, V., Todeschini, R. *et al.* (1991) Rabbit nest construction and its relationship with litter development. *Applied Animal Behaviour Sciences*, **31**, 259–266

Carpenter, J.W., Mashima, T.Y., Gentz, E.J. *et al.* (1995) Caring for rabbits: An overview and formulary. *Veterinary Medicine*, **90**, 340–364

Cheeke, P.R. (1987) *Rabbit Feeding and Nutrition*. Academic Press, New York

Cheeke, P.R., Patton, N.M., Lukefahr, S.D. *et al.* (1987) *Rabbit Production*, 6th edn. Interstate Printers and Publishers, Danville, Illinois

Chu, L., Garner, J.P. and Mench, J.A. (2003) A behavioural comparison of New Zealand White rabbits (*Oryctolagus cuniculus*) housed individually or in pairs in conventional laboratory cages. *Applied Animal Behaviour Science*, **85**, 121–139

Cizek, L.J. (1961) Relationship between food and water ingestion in the rabbit. *American Journal of Physiology*, **201**, 557–566

Clarkson, T.B., Lehner, N.D.M. and Bullock, B.C. (1974) Arteriosclerosis research. In: *The Biology of the Laboratory Rabbit.* Eds Weisbroth, S.H., Flatt, R.E. and Kraus, A.L., pp. 155. Academic Press, New York

Comfort, A. (1956) *The Biology of Senescence*. Routledge and Kegan Paul, London

Commission of the European Communities (2003) Third report from the Commission to the Council and the European Parliament on the statistics on the number of animals used for experimental and other scientific purposes in the member states of the European Union, Brussels 22.01.2003, COM (2003) 19 final

Cooper, H.M. and Paterson, Y. (2008) Production of polyclonal antisera. In: *Current Protocols in Molecular Biology*. Ed. Ausubel, F.M., pp. 11.12.1–11.12.10. John Wiley & Sons, New York

Council of Europe (2006) Multilateral Consultation of Parties to the European Convention for the Protection of Vertebrate Animals used for Experimental and other Scientific Purposes (ETS 123) Appendix A. *Cons 123 (2006) 3.* Available from URL: http://www.coe.int/t/e/legal_affairs/legal_co-operation/biological_safety,_use_of_animals/laboratory_animals/2006/Cons123(2006)3AppendixA_en.pdf (accessed 31 July 2008)

Cowan, D.P. (1987) Aspects of the social organisation of the European wild rabbit (*Oryctolagus cuniculus*). *Ethology*, **75**, 197–210

Cowan, D.P. and Bell, D.J. (1986) Leporid social behaviour and social organization. *Mammal Review*, **16**, 169–179

Cowan, D.P. and Garson, P.J. (1985) Variations in the social structure of rabbit populations: causes and demographic consequences. In: *Behavioural Ecology: the Ecological Consequences of Adaptive Behaviour*. Eds Sibly R.M. and Smith R.H., pp. 537–555. Blackwell Publishing, Oxford

Daly, J.C. (1981) Effects of social organisation and environmental diversity on determining the genetic structure of a population of the wild rabbit (*Oryctolagus cuniculus*). *Evolution*, **35**, 689–706

Donnelly, T.M. (1997) Basic anatomy, physiology and husbandry. In: *Ferrets, Rabbits and Rodents – Clinical Medicine and Surgery*. Eds Hillyer, E.W. and Quesenberry, K.E., pp. 147–159. WB Saunders, London

Drescher, B. and Loeffler, K. (1991a) Einfluss unterschiedlicher Haltungsverfahren und Bewegungsmöglichkeiten auf die Kompakta der Röhrenknochen von Versuchs – und Fleischkaninchen. *Tierärztliche Umschau*, **46**, 736–741

Drescher, B. and Loeffler, K. (1991b) Einfluss unterschiedlicher Haltungsverfahren und Bewegungsmöglichkeiten auf die Kompakta der Röhrenknochen von Mastkaninschen. *Tierärztliche Umschau*, **47**, 175–179

Dunsmore, J.D. (1974) The rabbit in subalpine south-eastern Australia, 1. Population structure and productivity. *Australian Wildlife Research*, **1**, 1–16

European Commission (2007) Commission recommendations of 18 June 2007 on guidelines for the accommodation and care of animals used for experimental and other scientific purposes. Annex II to European Council Directive 86/609. See 2007/526/EC. http://eurlex.europa.eu/LexUriServ/site/en/oj/2007/l_197/l_19720070730en00010089.pdf (accessed 13 May 2008)

Eveleigh, J.R. and Pease, S.S. (1976) The establishment of a breeding nucleus of category 4. *Dutch Rabbits*, **10**, 297–303

Eveleigh, J.R., Taylor, W.T.C. and Cheeseman, R.F. (1984) The production of specific pathogen free rabbits. *Animal Technology*, **35**, 1–12

Flecknell, P.A. (2009) *Laboratory Animal Anaesthesia*, 3rd edn. Academic Press, London

Fraser, K.W. (1992) Emergence behaviour of rabbits, *Oryctolagus cuniculus*, in Central Otago, New Zealand. *Journal of Zoology*, **228**, 615–623

Falkmer, S. and Waller, T. (1984) *Försöksdjursteknik- en praktisk handledning*, 2nd edn. pp. 87–106. Liber utbildning AB, Falköping

Federation of European Laboratory Animal Science Associations (2002) FELASA recommendations for the health monitoring of rodent and rabbit colonies in breeding and experimental units. *Laboratory Animals*, **36**(1), 20–42

Flux, J.E.C. (1994) World distribution. In: *The European Rabbit – The History and Biology of a Successful Colonizer*. Eds Thompson H.V. and King C.M., pp. 8–21. Oxford University Press, Oxford

Fox, P.R. and Krinsky, W.L. (1968) Ovulation in the rabbit related to dosage of human chorionic gonadotrophin and pregnant mare's serum. *Proceedings of the Social Experimental Biological Medicine*, **127**, 1222–1227

Gibb, J.A. (1993) Sociality, time and space in a sparse population of rabbits (*Oryctolagus cuniculus*). *Journal of Zoology*, **229**, 581–607

Gibb, J.A., Ward, C.P. and Ward, G.D. (1978) Natural control of a population of rabbit, *Oryctolagus cuniculus* L. for 10 years in the Kourarau enclosure North Island New Zealand. *New Zealand Department of Scientific and Industrial Research Bulletin*, **223**, 6–89

Gillett, C.S. (1994) Selected drug dosages and clinical reference data. In: *The Biology of the Laboratory Rabbit*, 2nd edn. Eds Manning, P.J., Ringler, D.H. and Newcomer, C.E., pp. 496–492. Academic Press, San Diego

González-Mariscal, G., Díaz-Sánchez, V., Melo, A.I. *et al*. (1994) Maternal behaviour in New Zealand White rabbits: quantification of somatic events, motor pattern, and steroid plasma levels. *Physiology and Behaviour*, **55**, 1081–1089

Gunn, D. (1994) *Evaluation on Welfare in the Husbandry of Laboratory Rabbits*. PhD Thesis University of Birmingham

Gunn, D. and Morton, D.B. (1995a) Rabbits. In: *Environmental Enrichment Information Resources for Laboratory Animals*. Eds Smith C.P. and Taylor V., pp. 127–143. Virginia-Maryland Regional College of Veterinary Medicine, Place of publication?

Gunn, D. and Morton, D.B. (1995b) Inventory of the behaviour of New Zealand White rabbits in laboratory cages. *Applied Animal Behaviour Sciences*, **45**, 277–292

Hafez, E.S.E. (1960) Sex drive in rabbits. *Southwestern Veterinarian*, **14**, 46–49

Hafez, E.S.E. (1970) Rabbits. In: *Reproduction and Breeding Techniques for Laboratory Animals*. Ed. Hafez, E.S.E., pp. 273–298. Lea and Febiger, Philadelphia

Hagen, K.W. (1974) Colony husbandry. In: *The Biology of the Laboratory Rabbit*. Eds Weisbroth, S.H., Flatt, R.E. and Kraus, A.L., pp. 23–47. Academic Press Inc, New York

Hansen, L.T. and Berthelsen, H. (2000) The effect of environmental enrichment on the behaviour of caged rabbits (*Oryctolagus cuniculus*). *Applied Animal Behaviour Sciences*, **68**, 163–178

Harcourt-Brown, F. (2002) *Textbook of Rabbit Medicine*. Butterworth-Heineman, Oxford

Harkness, J.E. and Wagner, J.E. (1995) *The Biology and Medicine of Rabbits and Rodents*, 4th edn. Williams and Wilkins, Baltimore

Hartman, H.A. (1974) The foetus in experimental teratology. In: *The Biology of the Laboratory Rabbit*. Eds Weisbroth, S.H., Flatt, R.E. and Kraus, A.L., pp. 92–134. Academic Press, New York

Heath, M. and Stott, E. (1990) Housing rabbits the unconventional way. *Animal Technology*, **41**, 13–25

Held, S.D.E., Turner, R.J. and Wootton, R.J. (1995) Choices of laboratory rabbits for individual or group-housing. *Applied Animal Behaviour Sciences*, **46**, 81–91

Hoffman, S., Peterbauer, A., Schindler, S. *et al*. (2005) International validation of novel pyrogen tests based on human monocytoid cells. *Journal of Immunological Methods*, **298**, 161–173

Huls, W.L., Brooks, D.L. and Bean-Knudsen, D. (1991) Responses of adult New Zealand White rabbits to enrichment objects and paired housing. *Laboratory Animal Science*, **41**, 609–612

Iwarsson, K., Lindberg, L. and Waller, T. (1994) Common nonsurgical techniques and procedures. In: *Handbook of Laboratory Animal Science*. Eds Svendsen, P. and Hau, J., pp. 229–272. CRC Press, Boca Raton

Jackson, G. (1991) Intestinal stasis and rupture in rabbits. *Veterinary Record*, **129**, 287–289

Jenkins, J.R. (2008) Rabbit diagnostic testing. *Journal of Exotic Pet Medicine*, **17**, 4–15

Jilge, B. (1991) The rabbit: a diurnal or nocturnal animal? *Journal of Experimental Animal Science*, **34**, 170–183

Jones, S.E. and Phillips, C.J.C. (2005) The effects of mirrors on the welfare of caged rabbits. *Animal Welfare*, **14**, 195–202

Joint Working Group on Refinement (1993) Removal of blood from laboratory mammals and birds. First Report of the BVA/FRAME/RSPCA/UFAW Joint Working Group on Refinement. *Laboratory Animals*, **27**, 1–22

Joint Working Group on Refinement (2001) Refining procedures for the administration of substances. Report of the BVAAWF/FRAME/RSPCA/UFAW Joint Working Group on Refinement. *Laboratory Animals*, **35**, 1–41

Kawoto, F., Kouno, T. and Harada, Y. (1989) A scanning electron microscopic study of the arteriovenous anastomoses of rabbit ear using corrosive rein casts. *Kaibogaku Zasshi*, **64**, 185–195 (in Japanese with English abstract)

Kraft, R. (1979) Vergleichende Verhaltensstudien an Wild- und Hauskaninchen. *Zeitschrift für Tierzuechtungsbiologie*, **95**, 165–179

Kersten, A.M., Meijsser, F.M. and Metz, J.H. (1989) Effects of early handling on later open-field behaviour in rabbits. *Applied Animal Behaviour Sciences*, **24**, 157–167

Kolb, H.H. (1994) The use of cover and burrows by a population of rabbits (Mammalia: *Oryctolagus cuniculus*) in eastern Scotland. *Journal of Zoology*, **233**, 9–17

Lehmann, M. (1989) *Das verhalten junger hauskaninchen unter verschieden umgebungsbedingungen*. PhD Thesis, Universität Berne

Lehmann, M. (1990) Activity requirement for young domestic rabbits: raw fibre consumption and animal welfare. *Schweiz Archiv Tierheilkeld*, **132**, 375–381

Lehmann, M. (1991) Social behaviour in young domestic rabbits under semi-natural conditions. *Applied Animal Behaviour Science*, **32**, 269–292

Lehmann, M. and Wieser, R.V. (1985) Indikatoren für mangeinde Tiergerechtheit sonie Verhaltensstorugen bei Hauskaninchen. *KTBL – Schrift*, **307**, 96–107

Leslie, T.K., Dalton, L. and Phillips, C.J.C. (2004) Preference of domestic rabbits for grass or coarse mix feeds. *Animal Welfare*, **13**, 57–62

Lidfors, L. (1996) Behaviour of male laboratory rabbits given environmental enrichment in a preference test and in an individual cage. In: *Proceedings of the 30th International Congress of the International Society for Applied Ethology*. Eds Duncan, I.J.H., Widowski, T.M. and Haley, D.B., p. 67. Guelph, Canada

Lidfors, L. (1997) Behavioural effects of environmental enrichment for individually caged rabbits. *Applied Animal Behaviour Sciences*, **52**, 157–169

Lloyd, H.G. and McCowan, D. (1968) Some observations on the breeding burrows of the wild rabbit on the island of Skokholm. *Journal of Zoology*, **156**, 540–549

Lockley, R.M. (1961) Social structure and stress in the rabbit warren. *Journal of Animal Ecology*, **30**, 385–423

Loeffler, K., Drescher, B. and Schulze, G. (1991) Einfluss unterschiedlicher Haltungsverfahren auf das Verhalten von Versuchs- und Fleischkaninchen. *Tieraerztliche Umschau*, **46**, 471–478

Love, J.A. and Hammond, K. (1991) Group-housing rabbits. *Laboratory Animals*, **20**, 37–43

Macdonald, D.W. (1984) *The Encyclopedia of Mammals*, Vol. 2. George Allen and Unwin, London

Mader, D.R. (1997) Basic approach to veterinary care. In: *Ferrets, Rabbits and Rodents – Clinical Medicine and Surgery*. Eds Hillyer, E.W. and Quesenberry, K.E., pp. 160–168. WB Saunders, London

Marston, H.H., Rand, G. and Chang, M.C. (1965) The care, handling and anaesthesia of the snowshoe hare (*Lepus americanus*). *Laboratory Animal Care*, **15**, 325–327

Meredith, A. (2000) General biology and husbandry. In: *Manual of Rabbit Medicine and Surgery*. Ed. Flecknell, P., pp. 13–23. British Small Animal Veterinary Association, Goucester

Metz, J.H.M. (1984) Effects of early handling in the domestic rabbit. *Applied Animal Ethology*, **11**, 71–87

Milligan, S.R., Sales, G.D. and Khirnykh, K. (1993) Sound levels in rooms housing laboratory animals: an uncontrolled daily variable. *Physiology and Behavior*, **53**, 1067–1076

Morton, D.B., Jennings, M., Batchelor, G.R. *et al.* (1993) Refinement in rabbit husbandry. *Laboratory Animals*, **27**, 301–329

Mulder, A., Nieuwenkamp, A.E., van der Palen, J.G. *et al.* (1992) Supplementary hay reduces fur-chewing in rabbits. *Tijdschrift fur Diergeneeskunde*, **117**, 655–658

Myers, K. (1966) The effects of density on sociality and health in mammals. Proceedings of the Ecological Society of Australia, 40–64

Myers, K., Hale, C.S., Mykytowycz, R. *et al.* (1971) The effects of varying density and space on sociality and health in animals. In: *Behaviour and Environment*. Ed. Esser, A.H., 148–187. Plenum Press, New York

Myers, K., Parer, I., Wood, D. *et al.* (1994) The rabbit in Australia. In: *The European Rabbit: The History and Biology of a Successful Coloniser*. Eds Thompson, H.V. and King, C.M., pp. 108–157. Oxford University Press, Oxford

Myers, K. and Poole, W.E. (1961) A study of the biology of the wild rabbit, *Oryctolagus cuniculus* (L.), in confined populations II. The effects of season and population increase on behaviour. *CSIRO Wildlife Research*, **6**, 1–41

Myers, K. and Poole, W.E. (1963) A study of the biology of the wild rabbit, *Oryctolagus cuniculus* (L.), in confined populations. V. Population dynamics. *CSIRO Wildlife Research*, **8**, 166–203

Myers, K. and Schneider, E.C. (1964) Observations on reproduction, mortality and behaviour in a small, free-living population of wild rabbits. *CSIRO Wildlife Research*, **9**, 138–143

Mykytowycz, R. (1960) Social behaviour of an experimental colony of wild rabbits, *Oryctolagus cuniculus* (L.), III second breeding season. *CSIRO Wildlife Research*, **5**, 1–20

Mykytowycz, R. (1968) Territorial marking by rabbits. *Scientific American*, **218**, 116–126

Mykytowycz, R. and Fullager, P.J. (1973) Effect of social environment on reproduction in the rabbit, *Oryctolagus cuniculus* (L.). *Journal of Reproduction and Fertility*, **19** (Suppl.), 503–522

Mykytowycz, R. and Hesterman, E.R. (1975) An experimental study of aggression in captive European rabbits, *Oryctolagus cuniculus* (L.). *Behaviour*, LII **1–2**, 104–123

Mykytowycz, R. and Rowley, I. (1958) Continuous observations of the activity of the wild rabbit, *Oryctolagus cuniculus* (L.) during 24-hour periods. *CSIRO Wildlife Research*, **3**, 26–31

Nachtsheim, H. (1949) *Vom Wildtier zum Haustier*, 2nd edn. Parey, Berlin

National Research Council (NRC) (1966) *Nutrient Requirements of Rabbits*. National Academy of Sciences, Washington, DC

Nerem, R.M. (1980) Social environment as a factor in diet-induced atherosclerosis. *Science*, **208**, 1475–1476

Nowak, R. (1999) *Walker's Mammals of the World*, 6th edn. The John's Hopkins University Press, Baltimore

Olfert, E.D., Cross, B.M. and McWilliam, A.A. (1993) *Guide to the Care and Use of Experimental Animals*, Vol. 2, 2nd edn. Canadian Council on Animal Care, Ottawa, Ontario

Parer, I. (1977) The population ecology of the wild rabbit, *Oryctolagus cuniculus* L., in a Mediterranean-type climate in New South Wales. *Australian Wildlife Research*, **4**, 171–205

Parer, I. (1982) Dispersal of the wild rabbit, *Oryctolagus cuniculus*, at Urana in New South Wales. *Australian Wildlife Research*, **9**, 427–441

Parker, S. (1990) *Grzimek's Encyclopedia of Mammals*. McGraw-Hill Inc, New York

Parsons, A.J., Newman, J.A., Penning, P.D. *et al.* (1994) Diet preference of sheep – effects of recent diet, physiological state and species abundance. *Journal of Animal Ecology*, **63**, 465–478

Patton, N.M. (1994) Colony husbandry. In: *The Biology of the Laboratory Rabbit*, 2nd edn. Eds Manning, P.J., Ringler, D.H. and Newcomer, C.E., pp. 27–45. Academic Press, New York

Peeters, J.E. (1986) Etiology and pathology of diarrhea in weanling rabbits. Agriculturae, In: *Rabbit Production Systems including Welfare*, A seminar in the community program for the coordination of agricultural research, 6–7 November 1986, pp. 128–131

Peiffer Jr, R.L., Pohm-Thorsen, L. and Corcoran, K. (1994) Models in ophthalmology and vision research. In: *The Biology of the Laboratory Rabbit*, 2nd edn. Eds Manning, P.J., Ringler, D.H. and Newcomer, C.E., pp. 409–433. Academic Press, New York

Podberscek, A.L., Blackshaw, J.K. and Beattie, A.W. (1991) The behaviour of group penned and individually caged laboratory rabbits. *Applied Animal Behaviour Science*, **28**, 353–363

Portsmouth, J. (1987) *Commercial Rabbit Keeping*, 3rd edn. Nimrod Press Ltd, Alton

Rogers, P.M., Arthur, C.P. and Soriguer, R.C. (1994) The rabbit in continental Europe. In: *The European Rabbit: The History and Biology of a Successful Coloniser*. Eds Thompson, H.V. and King, C.M., pp. 22–63. Oxford University Press, Oxford

Rollins, W.D., Casady, R.B., Sittman, K. *et al.* (1963) Genetic variance components analysis of litter size and weaning weight of New Zealand White rabbits. *Journal of Animal Science*, **22**, 654–654

Ross, S., Denenberg, V.H., Frommer, G.P. *et al.* (1959) Genetic, physiological and behavioural background of reproduction in the rabbit. V. Nonretrieving of neonates. *Journal of Mammals*, **40**, 91–96

Rothfritz, P., Loeffler, K. and Drescher, B. (1992) Einfluss unterschiedlicher Haltungsverfaren und Bewegungsmöglichkeiten auf die Spongiosastruktur der Rippen sowie Brust- und Lendenwirbel von Versuchs- und Fleischkaninchen. *Tierärztliche Umschau*, **47**, 758–768

Ruckebusch, Y., Grivel, M.L. and Fargeas, M.J. (1971) Electrical activity of the intestine and feeding associated with a visual conditioning in the rabbit. *Physiology and Behaviour*, **6**, 359–365

Ruckebusch, Y., Phaneuf, L.P. and Dunlop, R. (1991) *Physiology of Small and Large Animals*. Dekker, Philadelphia

Sawin, P.B. (1950) The rabbit. In: *The Care and Breeding of Laboratory Animals*. Ed. Farris, E.J., pp. 153–181. John Wiley & Sons, New York

Sharples, C.M., Fa, J.E. and Bell, D.J. (1996) Geographical variation in size in the European rabbit Oryctolagus cuniculus (*Lagomorpha: Leporidae*) in Western Europe and North Africa. *Zoological Journal of the Linnean Society*, **117**, 141–158

Shiomi, M. and Jianglin, F. (2008) Unstable coronary plaques and cardiac events in myocardial infarction-prone Watanabe heritable hyperlipidemic rabbits: questions and quandaries. *Current Opinion in Lipidology*, **19**, 631–636

Sittman, D.B., Rollins, W.C., Sittman, K. *et al.* (1964) Seasonal variation in reproductive traits of New Zealand White rabbits. *Journal of Reproductive Fertility*, **8**, 29–37

Staples, R.E. and Holtkamp, D.E. (1966) Influence of body weight upon corpus luteum formation and maintenance of pregnancy in the rabbit. *Journal of Reproductive Fertility*, **12**, 221–224

Southern, H.N. (1948) Sexual and aggressive behaviour in the wild rabbit. *Behaviour*, **1**, 173–194

Spector, W. (1956) *Handbook of Biological Data*. WB Saunders, Philadelphia

Stauffacher, M. (1989) Kaninchenhaltung in Zucht und Mastgruppen – ein neues tiergerechtes haltungskonzept fuer Hauskaninchen. *Schweizer Tierschutz*, **116**, 20–35

Stauffacher, M. (1992) Group housing and enrichment cages for breeding, fattening and laboratory rabbits. *Animal Welfare*, **1**, 105–125

Stauffacher, M. (1993) Tierschutzorientierte Labortierethologie in der Tiermedizin und in der Versuchtstierkunde – ein Beitrag zum Refinement bei der haltung und im Umgang mit Versuchstieren. In: *Ersatz- und Ergänzungsmethoden zu Tierversuchen*, Vol. 2. Eds Schöffl, H., Spielmann, H., Gruber, F. *et al.*, pp. 6–21. Springer, Wien

Stauffacher, M., Bell, D.J. and Schulz, K.-D. (1994) Rabbits. In: *The Accommodation of Laboratory Animals in Accordance with Animal Welfare Requirements*. Ed. O'Donoghue P.N., pp. 15–30. Proceedings the International Workshop Bundesgesundheitsamt, Berlin 17–19 May 1993

Stein, S. and Walshaw, S. (1996) Rabbits. In: *Rodent and Rabbit Medicine*. Eds Laber-Laird, K., Swindle, M.M. and Flecknell, P., pp. 183–211. Elsevier, Oxford

Stodart, E. and Myers, K. (1964) A comparison of behaviour, reproduction and mortality of wild and domestic rabbits in confined populations. *C.S.I.R.O. Wildlife Research*, **9**, 144–159

Suckow, M.A. and Douglas, F.A. (1997) The laboratory rabbit. In: *The Laboratory Animal Pocket Reference Series*. Ed. Suckow, M., pp. 71–74. CRC Press LLC, Boca Raton

Svendsen, P. (1994) Laboratory animal anesthesia. In: *Handbook of Laboratory Animal Science*. Eds Svendsen, P. and Hau, J., pp. 311–337. CRC Press, Boca Raton

Swallow, J.J. (1999) Transporting animals. In: *The UFAW Handbook on the Care and Management of Laboratory Animals*, 7th edn. Ed. Poole, T., pp. 171–187. Blackwell Publishing, Oxford

Swallow, J., Anderson, D., Buckwell, A.C. *et al.* (2005) Guidance on the transport of laboratory animals. *Laboratory Animals*, **39**, 1–39

Swedish Board of Agriculture (2007) Statistics. http://www.sjv.se (accessed 23 January 2009)

Tawfik, E.S., Sherif, S.Y., El-Hindawy, M. *et al.* (1997) The role of fibre in rabbit nutrition. *Der Tropenlan, Beitrage zur Tropischen Landwirtschaft und Veternarmedizin*, **98**, 73–81

Templeton, B.S. (1939) Length of gestation period in domestic rabbits. *Small Stock Magazine*, **23**, 3

Toth, L.A. and January, B. (1990) Physiological stabilisation of rabbits after shipping. *Laboratory Animal Science*, **40**, 384–387

Townsend, G.M. (1969) The grading of commercially bred laboratory animals. *Veterinary Record*, **85**, 225–226

Vastrade, M. (1987) Spacing behaviour of free-ranging domestic rabbits, *Oryctolagus cuniculus* L. *Applied Animal Behaviour Sciences*, **18**, 185–195

Vaughan, T., Ryan, J. and Czaplewski, N. (2000) *Mammalogy*. Harcourt Inc, New York

Wagner, J.L., Hackel, D.B. and Samsell, A.G. (1974) Spontaneous deaths in rabbits resulting from trichobezoars. *Laboratory Animal Science*, **24**, 826–830

Wallace, J., Sanford, J., Smith, M.W. *et al.* (1990) The assessment and control of the severity of scientific procedures on laboratory animals. Report of the Laboratory Animal Science Association Working Party. *Laboratory Animals*, **24**, 97–130

Webb, N.J. (1993) Growth and mortality in juvenile European wild rabbits *Oryctolagus cuniculus*. *Journal of Zoology*, **230**, 665–677

Webb, N.J., Ibrahim, K.M., Bell, D.J. *et al.* (1995) Natal dispersal and genetic structure in a population of the European wild rabbit (*Oryctolagus cuniculus*). *Molecular Ecology*, **4**, 239–247

Wetterholm, R., Caidahl, K., Volkmann, R. *et al.* (2007) Imaging of atherosclerosis in WHHL rabbits using high-resolution ultrasound. *Ultrasound Medical Biology*, **33**, 720–726

Wieser, R.V. (1986) *Funktionale analyse des verhalten als grundlage zur beurteilung der tiergerechtheit. Eine untersuchung zu normalverhalten und verhaltensstoerungen bei hauskaninchen-zibben*. PhD Thesis, University of Berne

Wilson, D. and Reeder, D. (1993) *Mammal Species of the World: A Taxonomic and Geographic Reference*. The Smithsonian Institution, Washington, DC

Wood, D.H. (1980) The demography of a rabbit population in an arid region of New South Wales, Australia. *Journal of Animal Ecology*, **49**, 55–80

Wooding, P. and Burton, G. (2008) *Comparative Placentation: Structures, Functions and Evolution*. SpringerLink. Heidelberg

Wullschleger, M. (1987) Nestbeschaeftigung bei saeugenden Hauskaninchenzibben. *Revue Suisse de Zoologie*, **94**, 553–562

Zain, K. (1988) *Effects of early social environment on physical and behavioural development in the rabbit*. PhD Thesis, University of East Anglia

Zarrow, M.X., Denenberg, V.H. and Anderson, C.O. (1965) Rabbit: frequency of suckling in the pup. *Science*, **150**, 1835–1836

Zeuner, F.E. (1963) *A History of Domestic Animals*. Hutchinson, London

29 The ferret

Michael Plant and Maggie Lloyd

Biological overview

General biology

The domestic ferret belongs to the family Mustelidae which includes stoats, weasels, badgers and mink. All mustelids secrete a strong-smelling musk from their anal glands, and ferrets are no exception. They have the Latin name *Mustela putorius furo*, which translates as 'stinky raging thief'.

Ferrets are thought to be a domesticated form of the European polecat (*Mustela putorius putorius*), with which they can interbreed, although their masks are different and polecats have darker fur (Ryland & Gorham 1978). Ferrets are more docile than polecats, but have retained many of their natural behaviour patterns. Different varieties of domestic ferret can be distinguished based on fur coloration. The most common or wild type variety is known as 'fitch' or 'polecat' (black guard hair, cream undercoat, black points, lighter facial fur with dark mask, dark brown or black eyes). This fur pattern is very similar to that of the wild European polecat, and has led to confusion between feral pigmented ferrets and wild polecats. Other colours include cinnamon (beige guard hair, cream undercoat, no mask) and the albino, or English ferret. Albinos have yellow or white fur and pink eyes. The albino variety is genetically recessive to the pigmented wild type.

Both male and female ferrets show marked seasonal variations in coat and body weight (Lloyd 1999). The overall coat colour and pigment distribution are similar throughout the year, although under natural lighting conditions they moult in the autumn. The coat in males is usually not fully replaced until the end of the breeding season. In females, a moult follows the first ovulation of the season and usually subsequent ones, but may be delayed during lactation. Moulting can sometimes result in marked alopecia.

The natural history of the domestic ferret is uncertain due to the lack of written records, but it is likely that ferrets have been domesticated for at least 2500 years (Lloyd 1999; Porter & Brown 1997). Early Greek and Roman records describe an animal that was almost certainly the ferret, and pictures have been found in Egyptian tombs of ferret-like animals on leads. It is not certain for what purpose the ferret was originally domesticated, but they have been used for hunting small game such as rabbits, and for the control of rodents and snakes. The general external morphology of the ferret resembles that of other members of the family Mustelidae, having the typical characteristics of a sleek, flexible, elongated tubular body, relatively short legs and small rounded ears. These characteristics allow the animal to work in confined spaces, as they can move freely and turn round in narrow tunnels. Ferrets can be trained to work on leads or lines and to come to call and have been used to lay cables. They have also been bred for their fur, known as fitch. Ferrets are still used for hunting today but increasingly are kept simply as pets.

Ferrets are highly intelligent, agile, lively, playful and curious. Their natural instinct is to explore and, if kept and handled appropriately, they do not develop a fear of humans or human environments (Porter & Brown 1997). Their motivation to explore needs to be taken into consideration when designing cages and pens, as the curious nature of these animals leads them to test all avenues of escape and adventure. Any hole large enough to get a head through will allow the animal to escape, with potentially tragic consequences for the ferret itself or neighbouring rodent or bird populations (Lewington 2000). Cage furniture should also take this inquisitiveness into account. Tubes, tunnels, boxes and paper bags can all help to provide a more interesting and stimulating environment, which is essential for the well-being of ferrets, but must be designed such that the animals cannot chew and swallow them, leading to gastrointestinal foreign bodies.

Ferrets have an undeserved reputation for being aggressive. Ferrets certainly play roughly with each other, dragging other ferrets by the neck and ears with lots of squealing, and may mistake a tentatively approaching hand for food, but they respond well to frequent handling and rapidly become friendly. Properly handled and well kept ferrets are neither smelly nor aggressive.

Size range and lifespan

Ferrets vary considerably in size according to season, sex and reproductive status. Both sexes show seasonal fluctuations in body weight of up to 30–40%, as subcutaneous fat is laid down in the autumn and shed in the spring (Burke 1988; Lloyd 1999). They range from 0.5 kg (females) to 2.5 kg (males) (see Table 29.1). They measure between 44 cm and 60 cm in length, including their tails. Their normal lifespan is 5–10 years but under favourable conditions some may live considerably longer.

Table 29.1 Standard biological data for the ferret (Fox 1998; Lloyd 1999).

Parameter	*Value*
Adult weight[a]	
Male (kg)	1–2
Female (g)	600–900
Life-span (average) (years)	5–11
Body temperature (°C)	38.8 (37.8–40)
Chromosome number (diploid)	40
Blood pressure systole (mmHg)	140 +/– 35
Blood pressure diastole (mmHg)	110 +/– 31 Mean diastolic
Heart rate (beats/min)	110–125 (anaesthetised)
Cardiac output (ml/mm)	200–400
Circulation time (s)	139
Blood volume (ml/kg)	45–70
Male	60
Female	40
Respiratory frequency (breaths/ min)	33–36
Dental formula	
Permanent	$I^3{}_3C^1{}_1Pm^3{}_3M^1{}_2$
Deciduous	$I^4{}_3C^1{}_1Pm^3{}_3$
Vertebral formula	C7, T15, L5(6), S3, Cy18
Puberty (months)	8–12
Length of breeding life (years)	2–5
Gestation (days)	42 ± 2
Litter size	
Average	8
Range	1–14
Birth weight (g)	6–12
Eyes open (days)	34
Onset of hearing (days)	32
Weaning (weeks)	6–8
Food consumption (g/24 h)[b]	50–75
Water intake (ml/24 h)	75–100
Urine volume (ml/24 h)	26–28
Urine pH	6.5–7.5

[a] Both sexes show seasonal weight fluctuation of 30–40%. Fat is laid down in autumn and lost in winter.
[b] Dry carnivore pelleted diet. Soak in hot water to form a paste, give 140–190 g daily.

Social organisation

Ferrets are domesticated animals, and are not generally found in the wild. Being closely related to polecats, ferrets can interbreed with them, and this has occasionally resulted in feral colonies of ferret–polecat hybrids. What is known of the natural social organisation of ferrets comes from studies of these feral ferrets and of the European polecat. These studies lead to the conclusion that wild ferrets are largely solitary (Clapperton 2001). The males, or hobs, occupy large territories, which usually include those of several females, or jills with whom he mates. Young ferrets are born in the spring or summer, and initially accompany their mother on hunting expeditions. They may remain together as a group after weaning until they finally disperse in the spring following their birth and establish their own territories. However, domestic ferrets are sociable and gregarious, and seem to benefit from being kept in compatible groups in captivity, where interaction with other animals provides environmental enrichment. Groups of jills without litters, young animals and castrated males (hobbles) can be kept together, although group housing is not advisable for adult hobs, jills with litters and females that are in oestrus or have been mated, which should be kept separately.

Standard biological data

Standard biological data for ferrets is shown in Table 29.1.

Reproduction

Ferrets, like wild polecats, are seasonal breeders. They become sexually mature in the spring following birth, at between 8 and 12 months of age (Burke 1988). The breeding season is determined by photoperiod, responses being mediated via the pineal body. Males are light-negative: they begin coming into season as the day shortens, whereas females are light-positive, responding to increasing day length. In the northern hemisphere, males are in breeding condition between December and July, and females between March and September. The seasonal nature of breeding means that ferrets generally have one litter per year, in the late spring or early summer, and may sometimes have a second litter at the end of the summer, although first litters are generally superior in vigour to subsequent ones.

Females in oestrus develop vulval swelling which peaks 1 month after the onset of oestrus and is easily identified. Ferrets are induced ovulators, and remain in oestrus until mated, or until the end of the breeding season when the days begin to shorten, causing them to enter a period of anoestrus. Oestrous females are exposed to prolonged high oestrogen levels, which lead to weight loss, alopecia and even bone marrow depression. All bone marrow blood cell series may be affected, causing leucopenia, thrombocytopenia, or anaemia. It is recommended that females which are not to be used for breeding are spayed at 6–8 months of age (Burke 1988; Lloyd 1999).

During the non-breeding season, the testes of the male recede into his body, becoming almost invisible under the heavy winter coat. About the time of the shortest day, they begin to move back into the scrotum. The males need to come into season about 4 weeks prior to the females to allow for sperm maturation. The male reaches his sexual peak in March or April as the females begin to come into season, remaining in breeding condition until the end of the summer, when the testes begin to withdraw back into the body cavity.

The female is responsive to the male when there are about 14–15 h of daylight. Conception can occur soon after the onset of vulval swelling, but the optimum time is 14 days after vulval swelling appears. Mating is vigorous, prolonged and noisy. The male will grasp the jill by the scruff of the neck and drag her around for up to 1 hour before coitus, which can then take up to a further 3h. Ovulation occurs 30–35h after mating. The vulval swelling recedes within a few days of mating.

Gestation lasts for 40–44 days and, assuming an early mating, litters are born in early summer when the days are at their longest and warmest. Up to 14 young can be produced, the average litter being seven, each kit weighing around 6–12g. All kits have white hair regardless of their eventual coat colour. Jills have eight nipples but can feed more kits if the milk supply is good. Ferret milk contains 23.5% solids, composed of 34% fat, 25.5% protein and 16.2% carbohydrate (Lloyd 1999). Kits have voracious appetites, and they develop rapidly, doubling their birth weight in 5 days. Although their eyes are closed until around 34 days, they are active from about 14–21 days. At this point they start to eat solids, and the jill can be seen taking food to the kits. Growth is gradual up to weaning at about 6–8 weeks of age, when body weight reaches at least 200–250g. At this point kits fed *ad libitum* eat approximately 30g of solid food and drink about 125ml daily. The kits are weaned at the end of the summer and can build up their supply of body fat during the autumn for the coming winter. Adult weight is reached at approximately 16 weeks.

Breeding performance declines after approximately 3 years of age in males, or after three or four litters in females.

Normal behaviour

Ferrets spend up to 75% of the day asleep, and typically are very active for short periods then sleep soundly for several hours. They are more active at night (Hillyer & Quesenberry, 1997).They like to sleep in dark, enclosed areas such as wooden or cardboard boxes, and will even sleep in paper bags. The remainder of their time is spent actively exploring the environment and playing and interacting with other ferrets. They spend much time burrowing through their bedding, which often leads to bouts of sneezing, which is normal unless persistent. Exercise periods often coincide with feeding time.

Young ferrets play constantly. Mock aggression, play chasing, wrestling and pouncing may be commonly observed. They will nip at anything and often bite when first handled, but become more friendly if handled frequently.

Ferrets are able to vocalise and produce a number of different sounds. When playing, they may hiss and chuckle, and when frightened or threatened they may scream. When foraging, they may produce a low-pitched grumble.

Sources of supply

The best sources of ferrets are specialist laboratory animal breeders or other laboratories. Although they are also available through the pet trade, from specialist breeders of working ferrets and private owners, such sources are not recommended for laboratories as there may be little quality control with regard to pedigree and disease status (see section on common diseases). In the UK it is a requirement that ferrets are obtained only from breeders or suppliers designated under the Animals (Scientific Procedures) Act 1986.

Uses in the laboratory

The ferret is not commonly used in the laboratory. Uses of the ferret include research into viral diseases such as influenza, gastrointestinal disorders, neuroscience and auditory physiology, and pharmacological studies for which rodents are not suitable, such as emesis. The ferret has also been used in toxicology and teratology.

Laboratory management and breeding

General husbandry

Housing

When designing housing for ferrets, as natural an environment as possible should be provided, with sufficient room for all their different needs. Given the choice, a ferret will build a burrow incorporating a sleeping area, a larder for food storage, several escape holes and a latrine area, usually a vertical surface against which defecation takes place.

Ferrets are inquisitive animals with an amazing ability to escape, and will readily destroy a cage which has any holes or edges unprotected (Moody *et al.* 1985). Cages can be made from various materials, for example wood, plastic, metal (sheet or wire) or fibreglass, with solid floors. Ferrets adapt very well to floor pens, which allow for a far more varied environment. Enclosures should have a minimum height of 50cm and a floor area of 4500cm^2, depending on the number and type of animals held (see Table 29.2). Solid floors should be provided wherever possible, to allow for the provision of bedding material. In cages with wire fronts, a strip of solid edging around the cage may help to retain the bedding, which is otherwise likely to be thrown out of the cage during normal burrowing behaviour.

Ferrets are intelligent and inquisitive and their housing needs a sufficient degree of complexity to cater for their needs. Failure to provide for these needs results in poor psychological well-being and ferrets may develop stereotypic behaviour. The inclusion of cardboard or rigid plastic tubes, containers of various materials and paper bags provides interest and stimulates both investigation and play.

Table 29.2 Minimum space recommendations for ferrets (European Commission 2007).

Animals	*Minimum enclosure size (cm^2)*	*Minimum floor area per animal (cm^2)*
Animals up to 600g	4500	1500
Animals over 600g	4500	3000
Adult male*	6000	6000
Jill and litter*	5400	5400

*Single housing recommended

Deep littering of group animals can also provide a stimulating and hygienic environment. Although ferrets spend a large proportion of the day sleeping, the active periods can be frantic times, even in adult animals, and an imaginative approach on the part of the carers can improve the welfare of the animals.

Taking into account that hobs can be twice the size of jills, the housing must provide adequate space for movement and ample height to allow the animal to stand on its back legs. The minimum height recommended in the revised European Directive Annex II is 50 cm (European Commission 2007).

Environmental provisions

The ferret is a resilient animal that can tolerate a wide range of temperatures, although because ferrets have poorly developed sweat glands they tolerate extreme heat poorly and they are susceptible to heat exhaustion when exposed to very high temperatures. Experience suggests that a temperature range of 15–24 °C with approximately 10–15 air changes per hour and a relative humidity range of 40–60% are satisfactory. Unweaned young should be kept above 15 °C.

Identification

Ferrets can be identified using a number of different methods. Collars can be used for short-term identification, but the narrow head of the ferret makes it difficult to keep collars in place. Tattooing provides a permanent method if identification, and the best site is on the inside of the thigh. Young animals (6–8 weeks) can be tattooed when conscious. Electronic microchips are probably the most effective method for identification, and these can be inserted at any age without sedation or anaesthesia. There are numerous systems available.

The ears of ferrets are small and so do not lend themselves to tattooing and ear tags are liable to tear out. Albino ferrets may be identified using dyes, but dyes have to be renewed on a regular basis, and care must be taken when animals are in moult.

Sexing

Males are usually called hobs, and females jills. Sexing mature ferrets is relatively easy. In mature male animals the tip of the penis opens onto the abdominal surface at a point about 5 cm from the base of the tail. This opening is usually obvious, but in animals with particularly long fur it may be partially obscured. As with other mustelidae, the male ferret has a penile bone (baculum) which is about 3–4 cm long in the adult animal. The testes become enlarged during the mating season and are visible for 5–6 months starting in late winter. In anoestrous females the anogenital distance is about 1–2 cm. Females in oestrus exhibit a significantly enlarged vulva.

Transport

A major consideration when transporting ferrets is their susceptibility to heat exhaustion. Their bodies can only be cooled by heat loss from respiration, therefore air-conditioned vehicles may be required in hot weather to prevent heat stroke.

Travel boxes with adequate ventilation must be provided, and care should be taken when stacking boxes to allow air circulation. Commercial plastic boxes with mesh liners provide adequate transport accommodation for one adult ferret, and single housed animals will invariably travel without problems, whereas multiple housed animals may fight or be unlikely to settle on a journey. It is important that a mesh liner is used to cover all vents, because ferrets will chew any material to assist escape.

Current International Air Transport Association Live Animal Regulations suggest the density guidelines given in Table 29.3. See also Chapter 13.

Table 29.3 Transport containers for ferrets.

Weight of animals (g)	*<2000*	*2001–5000*
Maximum number per compartment	4	2
Space per animal (cm^2)	770	970–1160
Height of box (cm)	20	25

Breeding

Ferrets reach sexual maturity at 8–12 months and are then seasonal breeders, however this can be altered by manipulating the light cycle. Care must be taken to provide an appropriate light cycle however, or problems may ensue. Rearing females from birth in short day conditions until 90 days then exposing them to long days can induce them to reach sexual maturity by as early as 4–5 months of age. If reared on long days, the onset of oestrus can be delayed until the animal is around 1 year old, although some females may remain anoestrous thereafter. Adult females kept continually in stimulatory photoperiods (14 h light) will have three or four litters in succession, then reproductive performance declines and eventually they fail to conceive. A period of 5–6 weeks in a winter photoperiod (6–8 h light) is then required. Mated and lactating females need to be maintained on long day cycles, otherwise the animals will fail to reproduce or maintain lactation. Males kept on short days of around 8 h light may remain in breeding condition for more than a year, but they then need a rest period of 5–6 weeks in a long photoperiod to maintain breeding efficiency.

Ferret breeding can be maintained throughout the year by careful manipulation of the lighting. Maintaining males in short photoperiods (8 h) ensures they are available for breeding throughout the year. Each male should have an annual period of rest for 5–6 weeks in a long photoperiod (14 h). Females can also be kept in short photoperiod, and moved into long photoperiod to bring them into season as required. Females begin their season after 6–8 weeks on long days. Having two ferret breeding rooms, one on northern hemisphere light cycles and one on southern hemisphere light cycles or one winter and one summer, allows for year-round breeding.

The condition of the jill should always be checked prior to mating, and only animals in good condition should be mated. The birth process is particularly demanding on jills, and an unfit female is more likely to have problems during pregnancy and birth, and as a result produce small, weak young.

The female should be taken to the male and left for 2 days. Mating is a very noisy and prolonged affair, with the male biting the female's neck and dragging her around. This is entirely natural and the skin on the back of the jill's neck is sufficiently thick to withstand this behaviour, but injuries may be inflicted on occasion.

After mating, jills should be housed away from stud males, to reduce the risk of disturbance to the jill leading to cannibalism of the young, and they should not return to the same enclosure as unmated cage mates, as this can cause pseudopregnancy in the unmated females. Pregnant females should be moved into their littering cages about 2–3 weeks prior to parturition. They should be provided with a nest box and suitable nesting material such as shredded paper, wood shavings or soft straw. Jills lose their winter coat and may look rather scruffy during gestation, and it is important that they get adequate nutrition. She should be fed *ad libitum* a diet of 35–40% protein and 18–20% fat during pregnancy, increasing the fat content to 30% during lactation. Nutritional supplementation may be required (Besch-Williford 1987).

Technicians should be wary when handling pregnant females, as they become more aggressive as gestation progresses. Jills are very protective of their young.

Dystocia is common, and neonatal mortality can reach 8–10%, due to stillbirths, congenital defects and cannibalism (Besch-Williford 1987; Lewington 2000). Cannibalism is common with larger litters, but can also be an inherited trait. Hypothermia or bloat caused by poor hygiene or overeating may also lead to neonatal death. Mortality declines after 5 days, and deaths after this time may be due to maternal neglect or agalactia, often caused by a return to oestrus. With litters larger than five, oestrus is usually suppressed, but with small litters the jill may return to oestrus before weaning. In this case she should be mated again, as high oestrogen levels suppress the milk supply. The jill may also kill a small litter, allowing her to return into season.

Good management can reduce problems encountered in the periparturient period. The jill should be left undisturbed for several days post-partum, and given adequate nutrition, with increasing quantities of food offered from 2–3 days after birth. Calcium supplementation may be needed to prevent hypocalcaemia, which can occur at peak lactation 3–4 weeks after birth.

Nutrition

The ferret is an obligate carnivore, their natural diet consisting mainly of small mammals, with some fish, birds, amphibia and even invertebrates. Under natural conditions they may eat up to nine or ten small meals a day, although twice daily feeding is adequate. Little research has been done on their exact nutritional needs, but important considerations seem to be the energy concentration of the diet, the amino acid composition and the digestibility of dietary protein (Porter & Brown 1997). Ferrets need a diet high in protein and fat but low in fibre, and have little absolute requirement for carbohydrate provided there is sufficient protein and fat to provide substrates for gluconeogenesis. They have little capacity to digest complex carbohydrates. They eat to calorie requirements, and their short gut transit time means they need highly digestible diets with high energy density and protein levels (Porter & Brown 1997; Lloyd 1999; Lewington 2000). Requirements for a typical ferret diet are shown in Table 29.4.

Commercial ferret diets are available. Ferrets need 840–1260 kJ/kg body weight (200–300 kcal/kg) daily, and diets with up to 21 000 kJ/kg diet (500 kcal/kg) may be needed for growth and reproduction. The diet should contain 30–40% protein, with a minimum level of 35% protein for breeding and young animals. The primary protein should be of animal origin, as the ferret digestive system is relatively inefficient at absorbing vegetable protein, and plant-derived proteins are associated with the formation of uroliths in mustelids. Breeding animals may fail to conceive or may suffer from lactation failure following parturition if fed insufficient animal protein (Burke 1988; Lloyd 1999).

A fat content of 18–20% is sufficient, and linoleic acid should account for 7–15% of total fat (Fox 1998). Unsaturated fats have a tendency to become rancid, which reduces palatability and leads to destruction of vitamin E, so ferret diets should contain adequate levels of vitamin E and be stored correctly to prevent this. A ratio of tocopherol (vitamin E): polyunsaturates (mg:g) of at least 0.5 is recommended to prevent vitamin E deficiency. Vitamin E deficiency leads to steatitis (yellow fat disease).

Table 29.4 Requirements for a typical ferret diet (Lloyd 1999; Fox 1998).

Diet component	*Quantity*
Energy (kJ/kg diet)	21 000
Protein (%)	30–40 (min 35% for production)
Fibre (%)	2 (low level required)
Carbohydrate (%)	22–44 (no absolute requirement)
Fat (%)	18–20
Vitamin A (IU/kg)	33 600
Vitamin D3 (IU/kg)	3667 (depends on Ca and P levels and exposure to UV light)
Vitamin E (IU/kg)	125 (need at least 0.5 mg vitamin E per g unsaturated fat in diet)
Thiamine (B1) (mg/kg)	8.4–97.8
Riboflavin (B2) (mg/kg)	1.5–3
Niacin (B3) (mg/kg)	80
Calcium (%)	1.1–2.2
Phosphorus (%)	0.9–1.2 (need Ca:P of at least 1:2 and adequate vitamin D)
Sodium chloride (%)	≤1
Zinc (mg/kg)	105–215 (deficiency can lead to skin lesions in kits, excess causes toxicity)
Copper (mg/kg)	15

Ferrets can do well on pelleted cat or kitten food with an appropriate protein level, which can be soaked and fed as a stiff paste. Tinned diets may also be used, provided that the protein content is derived from animal protein and the total protein level is in excess of 30%. Raw fish and eggs should be avoided, because they contain an excess of thiaminase and may predispose the ferret to thiamine deficiency. Raw fish may also contain high levels of nitrates. Feeding utensils should be in good condition, and the use of galvanised bowls should be avoided, as ferrets are susceptible to zinc toxicity.

For pregnant and lactating females, commercial pelleted diets may be supplemented with tinned food to give a higher level of nutrition and allow for weanling animals to feed at 3–4 weeks of age. Females take meat to the litter to encourage feeding, and weanling animals may not easily consume pelleted diet. Soaking pelleted diets in clean water and presenting it as a mash may enable weanlings to increase their food intake. Dead mice, pinkies or day-old chicks may also be offered in addition to commercial diet, but care must be taken to ensure that any uneaten carcases are removed, as ferrets are notorious hoarders of food and will bury them in the bedding.

Laboratory procedures

Handling and training

Ferrets are considered to be fairly placid and friendly animals that respond well to frequent handling. It is important that ferrets are handled sensitively and frequently from an early age. Ferrets are hunters with relatively poor eyesight, and their reactions are reflex and instant. They may mistake a hesitantly approaching finger for prey, and are likely to bite it, but a well handled ferret approached correctly will not bite. The important rules when handling ferrets are:

1. Be positive, calm and confident.
2. Know what you are doing.
3. Keep movements smooth and decisive.
4. Use your voice as well as your hands (Lloyd 2002a).

This way, the ferret will not be startled. All movements should be confident, steady and deliberate.

Two main methods are used for picking the animals up. Ferrets that have often been handled may be restrained by simply slipping a hand under the animal just behind the forelegs, supporting the rump with the other hand once the animal is away from the surface. Alternatively, distract the ferret with one hand and then quickly place the other hand over its shoulders and place a finger under the jaw to provide additional control. Again, support the animal's weight by placing a hand under the rump.

When dealing with unknown or frightened animals it may be advisable to wear protective gloves. Females with young and sick animals are more likely to bite and should always be treated with care. From the handler's point of view practice makes perfect, and from the animal's point of view frequent handling decreases the likelihood of an aggressive response. A ferret's bite can easily penetrate down to the bone. Ferrets have a tenacious grip and do not let go easily, especially if their feet are not touching the ground. If this occurs, place the animal's feet onto a solid surface and try to prise the jaws apart. If this fails, apply gentle pressure on the bridge of the nose, place some isopropyl alcohol on the gum, pinch the foot pad, or in extreme cases place the animal's head under cold running water to encourage them to let go.

Ferrets handled regularly can become really affectionate and amply repay the time and effort spent on them. Ferrets also respond well to positive reinforcement: food, treats or interaction with the handler can be used as rewards when training ferrets to co-operate with the handler.

Physiological monitoring

Temperature

Core temperature can be monitored by the insertion of a thermometer into the rectum, but the probe should be less than 3 mm in diameter and penetration should be no more than 1–2 cm. Larger probes can cause discomfort and may elicit retching and defecation. Ferrets generally struggle when having their temperature taken and readings may be artificially elevated.

Collection of samples

Blood

Small volumes can be collected by clipping a toenail or pricking a footpad (local anaesthetic cream or spray may be applied first) and collecting the blood in a capillary tube. When clipping the toenail, ensure that only the very end of the quick is cut. The use of local anaesthetic is advised for this. Alternatively, the cephalic or saphenous veins can be used (Lloyd 1999; Lloyd 2002a; Hillyer & Quesenberry 1997; Joint Working Group on Refinement (JWGR) 1993).

The cephalic vein is located on the upper surface of the forelimb and is one of the most accessible veins in the conscious ferret. The procedure is best performed by three people, one to hold the ferret by the neck and abdomen, one to hold one forelimb and the third to hold the other forelimb and take the sample. The limb should be shaved and swabbed. Small scissors are more suitable than clippers, which are noisy and tend to agitate the animal. Raise the vein by applying gentle pressure on the proximal part of the dorsal surface of the limb. This can be difficult because of the short legs of the ferret, and it may be most effectively achieved by using a quick-release tourniquet. The vein should then be palpable and a 25G or 27G needle or 24G over-the-needle cannula can be inserted.

The saphenous vein is found on the lateral surface of the distal hindleg. The overlying fur should be shaved, then the vessel can be raised by applying a quick-release tourniquet above the stifle. A 23G or 25G needle can then be inserted into the vein. Alternatively the vein can be cannulated with a 24G over-the-needle cannula. This is made easier if the skin over the vein is nicked with a needle or scalpel blade before trying to insert the cannula.

Larger samples can be taken from the jugular or tail veins. Jugular venepuncture is usually best achieved by having the person performing the technique standing with the animal's head facing towards them, and an assistant restraining the animal in dorsal recumbency. The animal is firmly grasped around the anterior thorax and the forelegs extended down along its body, then a towel is tightly wound around the body, leaving the head and neck uncovered so the head can be extended backwards. Alternatively, the animal can be held prone with neck extended upwards to access the vein. The vein is raised by supporting the animal's neck and applying pressure at the thoracic inlet. The vessels run craniolaterally from the midline at the thoracic inlet to a point just below the base of the ears. A 21 G or 23 G needle can then be inserted into the vein facing towards the heart. The skin is very thick and venepuncture may be facilitated by bending the needle upwards by approximately 30°, and by putting the needle through the skin lateral to the vein first and then into the vein itself.

The ventral tail vein and artery can be accessed by restraining the ferret in dorsal recumbency (this can be facilitated using a restraining tube). The ventral aspect of the proximal tail is shaved. The tail has a flattened area on the ventral side for the first 4–5 cm, representing the ventral concavity of the caudal vertebrae. The artery lies 2–3 mm beneath the surface, flanked by two smaller veins. The skin is swabbed, then the tail is held in one hand and a 23 or 21 G needle inserted at a shallow angle towards the body in the midline, 3–4 cm from the base of the tail. As the needle enters the vessel, blood appears in the hub of the needle.

Ferrets have a high packed cell volume (PCV) and a slow erythrocyte sedimentation rate. When collecting serum or plasma or measuring the PCV, the blood must be centrifuged for 20% longer than for other species, and three times the required plasma volume must be collected. Normal values for haematology and biochemistry and sample volumes may be found in Table 29.5.

Table 29.5 Haematological and biochemical parameters (Fox *et al.* 1984; Fox 1998; Lloyd 1999).

Parameter	Value
PCV (%)	42–61 (varies with sex and strain of animal)
Haemoglobin (g/dl)	12.0–18.2
RBC (10^6/mm^3)	6.77–13.2
Platelets (10^3/mm^3)	297–910
WBC (10^3/mm^3)	4.4–19.1
Reticulocytes (%)	1–14
Neutrophils (%)	11–84
Lymphocytes (%)	12–69
Monocytes (%)	0–8
Eosinophils (%)	0–7
Basophils (%)	0–2
Blood volume (ml/kg)	70
Safe volume of single bleed (ml/kg)	7
Sodium (mmol/l)	137–162
Potassium (mmol/l)	4.5–7.7
Chloride (mmol/l)	102–125
Calcium (mg/dl)	8–11.8
Phosphorous (mg/dl)	4–9.5
Glucose (mg/dl)	62–207
Urea nitrogen (mg/dl)	10–45
Creatinine (mg/dl)	0.2–0.6
Total protein (g/dl)	3.5–7.4
Albumin (g/dl)	2.6–4.1
Globulin (g/dl)	2.5–4.8
Total bilirubin (mg/dl)	0–0.4
Cholesterol (mg/dl)	34–296
ALP (iu/l)	9–120
ALT (iu/l)	82–289
AST (iu/l)	28–248

Faeces and urine

The ferret normally defecates in one particular corner of its cage, and this facilitates collection of faecal samples. If fresh specimens are required, defecation can be readily stimulated by the insertion of a small blunt probe into the rectum. Ferrets can be induced to urinate in the same manner as the rat (ie, by gentle pressure on the abdomen overlying the bladder). Faeces-free urine samples may also be obtained by placing the animal in a metabolism cage. Sterile urine samples can be obtained by cystocentesis in the sedated or anaesthetised animal.

Administration of substances

This section draws on Hillyer and Quesenberry (1997); Fox (1998); and Lloyd (1999). See also JWGR (2001).

Intravenous administration

Intravenous injections can be made into the cephalic, saphenous, jugular or tail veins, as described for blood sample collection above.

Intramuscular and subcutaneous injection

Small volumes can be given into the quadriceps muscle on the anterior aspect of the hindleg, or into the muscles each side of the lumbar spine using a 25 G needle. Subcutaneous injections can be given under the skin of the scruff of the neck. The skin of the ferret is particularly thick in this area and a 23 G or even 21 G needle may be required.

Intraperitoneal

This route of administration is particularly useful when it is necessary to administer the drug in a large volume. With the animal held firmly, a 23 G 2.5 cm needle is inserted at a shallow angle into the caudal abdomen, 6–8 cm below the xiphisternum, slightly to one side of the midline. The needle should penetrate no more than 2 cm.

Oral

Ferrets will readily accept palatable medicines in feed or dissolved in milk. Liquids or suspensions can be administered by holding the animal vertically or in dorsal recumbency, and inserting a suitable strong pipette into the angle of the mouth between the upper teeth and the dorsal surface of the tongue. Fluids may be given directly orally into the stomach by inserting a gastric tube through a hole in a spatula inserted between the jaws. The diameter of the gastric tube used should not exceed 5 mm. Ferrets retch readily and occasionally vomit on insertion of a tube into the oesophagus, and it may be necessary to sedate the animal to minimise trauma and facilitate administration. A maximum volume of 100 ml can be administered by this method.

Intranasal

The animal is held in a vertical position using the usual grip around the neck, and the substance is placed drop by drop in the nose. Administration must be slow and in small drops, or the animal will sneeze. This method can be used on conscious animals if they are accustomed to handling, but anaesthetic can be given in case of difficulty. Aerosols can be administered either directly via a face mask, or indirectly by placing the animal in a closed environment to which the aerosol has been added. With the latter method it is difficult to administer a standard dose.

Anaesthesia

Pre-anaesthetic considerations

In healthy ferrets, anaesthesia should not be difficult or risky. First the cardiovascular and respiratory systems should be checked, and an accurate weight obtained, since a thick coat may lead to over-estimation of body weight and overdose of anaesthetic. Ferrets vomit readily, and should be fasted for up to 4 h prior to anaesthesia. Due to the short gut transit time, longer periods of fasting may lead to hypoglycaemia. Free access to water should be given until immediately prior to induction.

The animal should be calm before anaesthesia; premedicants can be used if required, as stress increases the risk of problems. For short, non-painful procedures, diazepam may be sufficient. For major surgical procedures, combinations including an analgesic are recommended. Since the airways are small and easily blocked, drying agents should be given before general anaesthesia. Table 29.6 gives suggested doses of sedatives and premedicants.

Table 29.6 Sedatives and premedicants. Note that these doses are only intended as a guideline and there may be considerable variation between animals depending on their body weight, sex and general health (Lloyd 1999; Marini & Fox 1998; Hillyer & Quesenberry 1997). These products may not have licences for use in ferrets. Rules regarding their use should be checked with the relevant competent authority.

Drug	*Dose*	*Comments*
Midazolam with ketamine	0.2 mg/kg with 10 mg/kg im	Mix in same syringe. Short-term sedation with relaxation
Medetomidine	0.1 mg/kg iv, im or sc	Reverse with atipamezole. Useful for minor procedures or premedication
Diazepam or midazolam	2 mg/kg im	Reduces anxiety and produces relaxation. Can be hypotensive
Xylazine	1 mg/kg iv, im or sc	Hypotensive. Not recommended for use alone
Ketamine	20–30 mg/kg im	Poor muscle relaxation if used alone
Fentanyl/ fluanisone	0.5 ml/kg im	Neuroleptanalgesia with poor muscle relaxation. Can reverse with opioid antagonists/ partial agonists
Acepromazine	0.05–0.5 mg/kg sc or im	Hypotensive
Atropine	0.05 mg/kg sc	Dries airway secretions
Glycopyrolate	0.01 mg/kg sc	As above

General anaesthesia

General anaesthesia may be induced by intravenous or intramuscular injection. Administration by intravenous injection can be difficult in the conscious animal, and therefore preference is usually given to agents that can be administered by a different route. Injectable agents should be dosed by weight, but account should be taken of the time of year, since in the winter ferrets accumulate fat and may require relatively more anaesthetic. Always administer oxygen, since many anaesthetics cause respiratory depression. Respiratory failure is a common cause of anaesthetic emergencies in ferrets. Suitable drug combinations for anaesthesia are given in Table 29.7. See also Flecknell (2009).

Anaesthesia can be induced in friendly or sedated ferrets by intravenous injection of alphaxolone or propofol. Alternatively, intramuscular injection of ketamine in combination with xylazine, medetomidine, diazepam or acepromazine can produce 20–30 minutes of surgical anaesthesia.

Volatile anaesthetics can be used for both induction (after sedation if required) and maintenance. Isoflurane is recommended, with nitrous oxide for additional analgesia. If using an induction chamber, the same chamber that is used for rodents should not be used, since the smell of the ferret will cause distress to any rodents placed in the chamber subsequently. Induction takes 1–2 minutes. Anaesthesia is maintained using a low-resistance circuit, such as a T-piece. For short procedures a face mask can be used for maintenance of anaesthesia, but for longer procedures, endotracheal intubation is recommended using a 2.5–4 mm tube or a modified urinary catheter. The animal is placed in sternal recumbency and an assistant bends the head upwards as far as possible by placing thumb and forefinger in the corners of the mouth. The tongue is pulled forwards and over the lower incisors to depress the mandible. The lubricated tube

Table 29.7 Drug combinations suitable for anaesthesia in ferrets (Lloyd 2002b). The doses may have to be modified if given after premedication. All the times are approximate. These products may not have licences for use in ferrets. Rules regarding their use should be checked with the relevant competent authority.

Drug	*Dose*	*Comments*
Isoflurane	3–4% induction, 1.5–3% for maintenance	
Halothane	2–4% induction, 0.8–2% for maintenance	
Medetomidine with ketamine	50–100 μg/kg with 4–8 mg/kg	Mix in same syringe, administer im for 30–60 minutes surgical anaesthesia. Can reverse with atipamezole, 0.25–0.5 mg/kg im
Xylazine with ketamine	1–4 mg/kg with 25 mg/kg im	As above but with more respiratory depression
Alphaxalone	8.2–11 mg/kg im or iv	Premedicate with diazepam. Short anaesthesia with good relaxation. Incremental doses 6–8 mg/kg iv for prolonged anaesthesia
Ketamine with diazepam	25 mg/kg with 2 mg/kg im	Surgical anaesthesia for approx. 30 minutes. Less respiratory depression than with α_2 agonists
Ketamine with acepromazine	25 mg/kg with 0.25 mg/kg im	As above
Propofol	10 mg/kg iv	Can be used for total intravenous anaesthesia

is advanced into the mouth (a laryngoscope may help to visualise the larynx) and the tube is gently slid through the glottis.

At the conclusion of the procedure, the animal should be allowed to breathe oxygen only for a few minutes to flush out the nitrous oxide. Animals usually recover consciousness in about 5 minutes.

Surgery

Ferrets have thick skin and thin abdominal musculature. They are keen suture chewers and are unforgiving if sutures are uncomfortable so care must be taken to ensure that the sutures are secure. Wounds in the neck appear to irritate more than abdominal ones, although ferrets are prone to the development of a serosanguinous discharge from the wound following abdominal surgery, which is normally self-limiting (Hillyer & Quesenberry 1997; Lloyd 1999). It is recommended that subcuticular sutures using fine synthetic absorbable suture materials are placed in the skin to reduce the likelihood of wound breakdown.

Antibiotic therapy should not normally be required after surgery provided aseptic techniques are employed. If required, treatment with clavulanate/amoxicillin (12.5/50 mg/ml) (0.2 ml/kg oral suspension twice daily), amoxicillin (10–25 mg/kg orally or by subcutaneous injection once daily), or enrofloxacin (3–5 mg/kg orally twice daily) can be given.

Table 29.8 Analgesics (Lloyd 1999; Lloyd 2002a). These products may not have licences for use in ferrets. Rules regarding their use should be checked with the relevant competent authority.

Drug	*Dose*	*Comments*
Buprenorphine	0.05 mg/kg sc or im	Lasts up to 12 h
Butorphanol	0.25 mg/kg sc or im	Lasts 2–4 h
Morphine	0.5–2 mg/kg sc or im, 1 mg/kg iv	Lasts 3–4 h
Carprofen	1 mg/kg po or sc	Repeat after 12–24 h
Meloxicam	0.2 mg/kg sc or im, 0.3 mg/kg po	Lasts 24 h
Ketoprofen	2 mg/kg sc	Administer once daily
Flunixin	0.5–2 mg/kg sc	Do not administer under anaesthesia
Aspirin	200 mg/kg po	

Post-operative care and analgesia

Hypothermia under anaesthesia is common. The animal should be kept warm throughout the procedure by wrapping it up and providing supplementary heating if necessary. Following surgery, the body temperature should be kept up until the animal has fully regained consciousness. It is also important to maintain fluid balance to prevent dehydration. The daily fluid requirement is approximately 75–100 ml/kg and, in addition, any blood or fluid losses during surgery should be replaced. Warmed fluids can be given by slow intravenous injection into the cephalic or saphenous veins.

Ferrets are stoic animals and will mask signs of pain, so they should be given the benefit of the doubt and analgesics should be administered routinely after surgery to avoid unnecessary pain. Doses of suitable analgesics are given in Table 29.8.

Post-operatively the appetite may be decreased, and solid food may be refused. Small amounts of liquid diet, soaked maintenance diet or convalescent diet for dogs and cats should be offered. Anorexic animals may need to be force-fed meat-based baby food or convalescent diet or given nutritional supplements until the appetite has returned to normal. After abdominal surgery, food should be given in small amounts until digestive functions have returned to normal.

Common disease problems

Disease control, vaccinations and routine health checks

A programme of routine preventive care should be implemented, to allow for prevention and early detection of diseases. Young ferrets should be given a health check and first vaccination at 6–8 weeks of age, and then an annual check until 4–5 years old. Older animals are more prone to diseases, and benefit from twice-yearly health checks. Table 29.9 gives an example of a health monitoring protocol for ferrets.

It is recommended that ferrets acquired from dealers or other laboratories should be quarantined for 40 days before introduction to a colony, to minimise the risk of introducing infections.

Ferrets should be vaccinated against canine distemper (Burke 1988; Oxenham 1990; Lloyd 1999). No vaccines are currently licensed for use in ferrets in the UK. Vaccine production changes continually and it is wise to check with the manufacturer, since insufficiently attenuated vaccines may cause disease. Ferrets are not susceptible to feline panleucopenia, canine parvovirus, leptospirosis or mink enteritis.

Ferrets of unknown health status should be tested on acquisition for Aleutian disease. Positive animals should not enter a colony since they present a health risk for the other animals, even if overtly well.

Signs of disease

Ferrets are stoic animals and often do not show clinical signs until a disease has reached an advanced stage. It is important that handlers can recognise the slightest changes. Diseased animals become lethargic, uninterested in their surroundings and have a reduced food intake. Grooming behaviour may decrease and as a result the animal may appear dishevelled. The animal will offer little resistance to being handled, unless there is a tumour or abscess, which is sensitive to touch. Weight loss is also a sign of disease and can be confirmed by weighing the animal over several days. It is possible for the animal to lose weight if it is diseased (for example with a tumour) even with a normal food intake. Vomiting does not appear to be a commonly observed symptom of disease, however a sudden change in the bulk, colour or consistency of the faeces not associated with a change in diet may indicate illness.

Table 29.9 Routine health monitoring schedule. Routine health checks are recommended annually until 4–5 years of age, then every 6 months. Animals of unknown origin should be tested for Aleutian disease virus (Lloyd 2002a).

Age (weeks)	*Procedure*
6 or 8*	First distemper vaccine if needed (endemic areas), faecal screen
10–12*	Second distemper vaccine if needed
12–14	First (or third) distemper vaccine, rabies vaccine if required, faecal screen
26–32	Spay or castrate, faecal screen
1 year	Rabies booster if required (annual)
3 years	Distemper booster (every 1–3 years)

*Earlier vaccination for kits of non-vaccinated dams and in endemic areas.

Animals should first be inspected in their home cages for observation of natural behaviour and signs of illness, before being removed from the cage to make an assessment of provoked behaviour. Normal ferrets exhibit exploratory behaviour: if this is absent it may be a sign of illness. The gait of the animal can also be observed for hindlimb paresis and other musculoskeletal or neurological disturbances such as generalised tremor.

Viral diseases

Ferrets are prone to several viral diseases, the most significant of which are Aleutian disease, canine distemper and influenza.

Aleutian disease

Aleutian disease is caused by a parvovirus, and although originally a disease of mink it is increasingly diagnosed in ferrets (Welchman *et al.* 1993). Following infection there is persistent viraemia and hypergammaglobulinaemia, leading to immune complex deposition in many organs including liver, kidneys, spleen and thyroid. Clinical signs depend on the organs most affected. Frequently, there is central nervous involvement, with a non-suppurative encephalomyelitis. The virus can spread both vertically and horizontally, although the transmission rate appears to be low.

There may be no clinical signs, or variable signs including anorexia, posterior paralysis and ataxia, quadriplegia, chronic wasting, cachexia, melaena, ill-thrift, poor reproductive performance, collapse and sudden death. Animals may have repeated episodes of posterior paresis but remain bright and alert and otherwise unaffected. Clinical disease can be precipitated by stress. Infection may also increase the animal's susceptibility to other diseases. Animals of any age may be affected, and the signs may develop over 24h or progress over several months.

Diagnosis can be made by counter-immunoelectrophoresis (CIEP) on a sample of plasma, raised plasma globulin, or by histopathology of affected tissues. However, there may be no histopathological changes, and there are no consistent haematological changes.

There is no treatment. Animals may respond to supportive therapy, corticosteroids and antibiotics although they will remain infected and present a risk to other animals. Culling of infected animals is recommended. Since the transmission rate is low, it is possible to test individual animals, and cull those testing positive. Two tests 3 weeks apart should allow the virus to be eradicated from a colony.

Canine distemper virus

Canine distemper virus (CDV) produces an acute disease with nearly 100% mortality (Burke 1988; Lloyd 1999). Transmission is by contact or droplet infection, with an incubation period of 10–12 days. There is fever, loss of appetite, and an initially serous then mucopurulent ocular and nasal discharge, which can stick the eyelids together. There may be photophobia and blepharospasm. A rash develops under the chin and in the inguinal area on day 10–12, and there may be keratitis of the footpads producing classical hardpad. The disease progresses to tracheitis, bronchitis and severe bronchopneumonia. Death usually follows on day 12–25 depending on the strain. If animals survive this phase, they develop a central nervous system (CNS) phase within a few weeks, characterised by hyperexciteability, excess salivation, muscle tremor, convulsion, coma and death. Vomiting and diarrhoea are uncommon. CDV causes suppression of cell-mediated immunity, predisposing to secondary bacterial infection.

CDV should be suspected in unvaccinated ferrets showing the typical signs. This can be confirmed by virus isolation, immunofluorescence on smears of conjunctival epithelium, blood, lymph node, bladder epithelium or cerebellum or examination of conjunctival, bladder or tracheal epithelium for typical distemper inclusion bodies.

There is no treatment, and affected animals should be euthanased. In the face of an outbreak, affected animals should be separated and healthy animals vaccinated immediately. The virus is labile and easily destroyed by disinfecting the environment. Cages, equipment and rooms should be disinfected and sterilised, and the source of infection identified and eliminated.

Influenza

Ferrets can catch influenza from people, and it can then be spread by droplets from ferret to ferret, or back to people. The disease in adult ferrets is usually mild, but it can cause mortality in kits. The virus causes catarrhal inflammation in the upper respiratory tract leading to congestion, oedema and some necrosis in the nasal mucosa.

Clinical signs may develop within 48h. Affected animals develop a biphasic fever (40–41°C), they become anorexic and listless, then begin sneezing and coughing, with a nasal discharge. There may be sensitivity to light. The disease rarely progresses further, and recovery usually begins after the second pyrexic episode. Supportive therapy and occasionally antibiotics may be needed to control secondary infection. Recovery is followed by a short-lived period of immunity to reinfection by the same strain of virus. Occasionally, the disease may progress to pneumonia.

Diagnosis can be confirmed by virus isolation or rising antibody titres. Vaccination is not indicated, since protection is short lived and there are many antigenically distinct strains of the virus.

Bacterial diseases

Helicobacter mustelae and gastroduodenal ulcers

H. mustelae is increasingly implicated in gastroduodenal ulceration in ferrets (Lloyd 1999). It is found in the pyloric area in up to 100% of animals, and although clinical disease is rare it can produce ulceration and death, particularly at times of stress. Large ulcers can erode into submucosal blood vessels causing rapid death. Ulcers cause anorexia and stress, leading to further development of the disease and a progressive deterioration in the animal's condition.

Clinical signs include lethargy, anorexia and weight loss, vomiting, ptyalism and tooth grinding. Chronic cases may be dehydrated. There may also be melaena, peripheral lymphocytosis and regenerative anaemia. The presence of black tarry stools with tooth grinding are highly suggestive of gastroduodenal ulceration.

If the animal is not vomiting, frequent, small meals of a bland, highly digestible diet can encourage the animal to eat and break the cycle that allows ulcers to form. If the animal is vomiting, food should first be withheld for 6–12h until vomiting ceases. Parenteral fluids and electrolytes may be needed. *Helicobacter mustelae* can be treated using a combination of antimicrobials and bismuth subsalicylate for at least 14 days. It may take 4 weeks or more for ulcers to heal completely and recurrence is common.

Botulism

Ferrets are susceptible to botulism, and care must be taken in feeding raw meat (Ryland & Bernard 1983). The disease is usually fatal. The symptoms of muscular stiffness and coordination appear 12–96h after eating contaminated food. The animal eventually dies of anoxia due to paralysis of the respiratory muscles.

Abscesses

Subcutaneous abscesses in group-housed ferrets are common and are often associated with staphylococcal or streptococcal infections in skin wounds resulting from neck biting during the early breeding season (Burke 1988). Abscesses seen in this region are manifested by large swellings that may involve the salivary glands and even erosion of bone at the base of the skull.

Vaginitis and pyometra

Vaginitis and pyometra may be seen in oestrous females, secondary to immune suppression (Burke 1988; Lloyd 1999). Jills produce a mucoserous discharge during oestrus which causes the perineal area to become wet, predisposing to infection. Vaginitis may also be caused by irritation from bedding adhering to the vulva. Pyometra leads to lethargy, and there may be a purulent discharge from the vagina and enlarged uterine horns. Treatment consists of removal of the source of irritation, and the use of broad-spectrum antibiotics.

Mastitis

Mastitis is quite common in ferrets, occurring immediately after parturition or at peak lactation. It can manifest as cellulitis, mammary abscesses, necrotic mastitis or chronic mastitis. Necrotic mastitis presents rapidly with large areas of liquefactive necrosis extending into surrounding tissues. Affected areas can become gangrenous within hours of infection and the jill can become very ill. Immediate surgical treatment may be required to remove the affected areas. In chronic mastitis, mammary tissue is gradually replaced by fibrous tissue and milk production falls, resulting in the loss of the litter and possibly the jill herself. Antibiotic therapy and possibly surgical removal of the affected glands may be necessary. Mastitis is usually very infectious, and sucking kits can transfer infection from one gland to another. Affected jills should be isolated from the remainder of the colony to avoid spreading infection, and should not be used for breeding again. Kits should be left with their mother while she is undergoing treatment: fostering them may spread the infection to other jills, and removing the milk from affected glands aids recovery.

Parasitic diseases

Ear mites

Otodectes cynotis is common in ferrets, particularly young kits and old animals. The adult mite spreads by direct contact. Often, there are no signs, or there may be pruritus, rubbing the ears or head shaking, leading to reddening and ulceration of the pinna. Secondary bacterial infection can lead to otitis media and a head tilt. There is inflammation of the ear canal with a thick, brown or black waxy exudate. Adult mites, larvae and eggs are visible in the exudate under a microscope.

All susceptible animals should be treated concurrently. The ears of affected animals should be cleaned using a proprietary cleaner (usually under general anaesthesia) before using an insecticide such as ivermectin, topically or by parenteral administration. Eradication of *Otodectes cynotis* from a ferret colony can be achieved by treatment of all individuals in the colony with ivermectin every 3 weeks for three or four treatments (authors).

Endoparasites

In general endoparasitic infestation is comparatively rare in the ferret under hygienic conditions. Ferrets may be experimentally infected with *Dirofilaria immitis* (dog heart worm) (Burke 1988), and coccidiosis, *Toxoplasma gondii* and various gastrointestinal helminths have been reported in ferrets (Thornton & Cook 1986; Rehg *et al.* 1988; Lewington 2000).

Non-infectious diseases

Hyperoestrogenism

Jills are induced ovulators, and if not bred may remain in oestrus for the duration of the breeding season. The high levels of oestrogens produced may cause bone marrow depression, with leucopenia, thrombocytopenia and aplastic anaemia. All jills develop a mild anaemia during oestrus at some point, and up to 50% of jills with prolonged oestrus will develop aplastic anaemia. If animals remain in oestrus for more than 2 months, the reduction in platelet count may lead to haemorrhage and death (Lloyd 1999; Hillyer & Quesenberry 1997; Lewington 2000).

The signs include a bilaterally symmetrical alopecia on the ventral abdomen and tail, weight loss, enlarged vulva and a serous or mucopurulent vaginal discharge. This may progress to anorexia, depression and lethargy, and generalised weakness. There may be pale mucous membranes, haemorrhages, a systolic murmur and secondary bacterial infections. Subdural haematomas may lead to posterior paralysis.

The diagnosis can be made on history and clinical signs, and confirmed by haematology. A PCV of less than 20% with depression of all blood cell series is highly indicative.

Ovariohysterectomy is the fastest way to remove the source of oestrogens, although initial treatment must be dictated by the PCV. In severe cases, a blood transfusion may be required first. Ferrets have no detectable blood groups, and there is little risk of a transfusion reaction. In milder cases, hormone treatments (such as proligestone (Delvosteron, Intervet) 0.5 ml sc) can be used to induce ovulation before ovariohysterectomy. The vulva will soften within 3–4 days and all signs of oestrus will then abate usually within 10–11 days, sometimes up to 3–4 weeks. Supportive treatments may be necessary, and it may take up to 4 months for the anaemia to resolve.

The prognosis depends on the length of time the animal has been in oestrus, and on the PCV on presentation. If the PCV is 25% or above, the prognosis is good. If it is below 15%, the outlook is poor and very intensive therapy including multiple blood transfusions will be required for several months.

To prevent a recurrence, females should not remain in heat for longer than 1 month. Ovariohysterectomy at 6–8 months of age is recommended for jills that are not to be bred. Ovulation can be induced by mating jills in oestrus with a vasectomised male. Hormone treatments can also be used to postpone oestrus until the following breeding season.

Dilated/congestive cardiomyopathy

This is increasingly recognised in middle-aged to older animals (Lloyd 2002b). Affected animals develop lethargy, weight loss, anorexia, depression, exercise intolerance and respiratory distress over a period of several months. The condition can be diagnosed by radiography, ultrasound or on electrocardiogram (ECG).

Treatment is aimed at maintaining cardiac output. Oxygen, vasodilators, positive inotropes and diuretics may be beneficial, and thoracocentesis may be required to remove pleural fluid. A low salt diet and exercise restriction can be of benefit. Treatment failure is not uncommon.

Foreign bodies

Intestinal foreign bodies are common in ferrets, because they are inquisitive and playful. Gastric foreign bodies may cause lethargy, inappetence, diarrhoea with or without tarry stools, weakness and dehydration. Vomiting is uncommon, although nausea can lead to ptyalism and face rubbing. Foreign bodies lodged at the pylorus can ulcerate through the stomach wall. Intestinal foreign bodies may cause sudden collapse with a painful abdomen.

The diagnosis may be made on the history, clinical signs and a careful clinical examination. Radiography is essential.

Foreign bodies rarely pass unaided and removal under general anaesthesia is usually required after the animal has been stabilised. Prevention of a recurrence may be achieved by 'ferret-proofing' the environment carefully, and by the regular use of a palatable cat laxative if necessary to reduce the formation of hairballs.

Posterior paresis and ataxia

Posterior paresis and ataxia are common in ferrets. The animal presents with abducted, uncoordinated hindlimbs, or a frog-legged appearance. The body may lose its curved appearance as the animal is unable to flex the spine as much as usual. The withdrawal and placing reflexes may be absent, and the animal may be incontinent. Often, the animal remains bright and alert and otherwise normal. There are many possible causes, including neurological conditions (eg, intervertebral disc disease or Aleutian disease), diseases causing generalised weakness, cardiac disease, abdominal pain, and metabolic diseases (eg, hypocalcaemia, thiamine deficiency and hypoglycaemia).

Specific treatment depends on the diagnosis. Non-specific supportive therapy, cage rest and prednisolone may be effective in cases of disc disease, or viral myelitis. However, recurrence is common and the prognosis is guarded.

Milk fever

Milk fever may occur at peak lactation, 3–4 weeks postpartum. It can lead to posterior paralysis and convulsions. Treatment with calcium borogluconate is usually successful.

Neoplasia

Reports of neoplasia in ferrets are increasing (Beach & Greenwood 1993; Lloyd 1999). Primary neoplasms have been reported in all organ systems except the cardiovascular system, although tumours of the respiratory tract and CNS are extremely rare. Tumours of the reproductive tract and lymphoid system occur most commonly in the UK. It is quite common for two or more different neoplasms to be found in the same animal. Nearly half of all tumours reported have been malignant.

Most cases occur in ferrets between 4 and 7 years of age, but some have occurred in younger animals. Any neoplasm may metastasise, although it is rare for abdominal tumours to spread into the chest cavity, and vice versa. Resection of the tumour is usually the best treatment, however recurrences at the site or in local lymph nodes may occur. Neoplasms in the distal forelimb may best be treated by amputation, and ferrets can do well with only three legs.

Lymphosarcoma

Lymphosarcoma is relatively common in ferrets, and there may be solid tumours in parenchymal organs, disseminated lesions throughout the body, or leukaemic spread (Fox 1998). Animals less than 1 year old tend to develop an acute lymphoblastic form with thymic involvement, and animals over 2 years old tend to develop a more chronic lymphocytic disease with lymphadenopathy. Males and females are equally affected, as are neutered and entire animals. The leukaemic form is relatively rare, but may be seen in the later stages of both juvenile and adult forms of the disease.

The clinical signs depend upon the site of the lesion and are often non-specific. In the acute lymphoblastic form, animals exhibit a rapidly progressive loss of condition, with anorexia, weakness and lethargy. Dyspnoea is common, but lymphadenopathy is rare. Young animals are more likely to die from the disease than adults are.

In adults, there is usually peripheral and visceral lymphadenopathy, with some organ involvement later in the course of disease. Animals may have cycles of non-specific signs such as recurrent infections, anorexia, weight loss and lethargy over months or years. Splenomegaly is common.

Diagnosis can be difficult. Lymphosarcoma may be diagnosed provisionally on the history and clinical signs, and confirmed by cytology or histology on blood, tissue aspirates or biopsies.

The choices for treatment are surgery, chemotherapy, radiotherapy or combinations of these. However, the prognosis is guarded since, even if there appears to be only one organ affected, the disease is likely to be systemic.

Insulinoma

Tumours of the β-cells of the islets of Langerhans are reportedly common in the USA. They produce excess insulin, leading to hypoglycaemia. It is commonly seen in animals of 4–5 years. Animals present with variable neurological signs caused by hypoglycaemia, such as weakness, apparent blindness, muscle twitches, or seizures. Signs are intermittent initially and may become more prolonged as the disease progresses. Diagnosis is made on clinical signs and on measurement of blood sugar. Medical treatments can be used in older animals or those with intercurrent disease, although surgical removal is indicated in young animals (Lewington 2000).

Adrenal-related endocrinopathy

Adrenal tumours are again reportedly common in the USA but are rare in Europe. This may be due to differences in husbandry: early neutering and housing in artificial light cycles appear to predispose to the condition. Animals over 2 years of age are typically affected. One or both adrenals may be affected, and tumours typically secrete androgens, oestrogens or progestagens, rather than glucocorticoids, so the signs are similar to those of hyperoestrogenism rather than typical Cushing's syndrome (Hillyer & Quesenberry 1997). Increased aggression, bilaterally symmetrical alopecia and pruritus are common. Females may develop vulval swelling, and males stranguria due to prostatic cysts. Vulval swelling that does not respond to hormone treatment may be due to an adrenal tumour rather than hyperoestrogenism.

Diagnosis can be made on clinical signs and analysis of hormone levels. Surgery to remove the affected glands is recommended in young animals, older animals may be treated medically.

References

Beach, J.E. and Greenwood, B. (1993) Spontaneous neoplasia in the ferret (*Mustela putorius furo*). *Journal of Comparative Pathology*, **108**, 133–147

Besch-Williford, C.L. (1987) Biology and medicine of the ferret. *Veterinary Clinics of North America: Small Animal Practice*, **17**, 1155–1183

Burke, T.J. (1988) Common diseases and medical management of ferrets. In: *Exotic Animals*. Eds Jacobson, E.R. and Kollias, G.V., pp. 247–260. Churchill Livingstone, New York

Clapperton, B.K. (2001) Advances in New Zealand mammalogy 1990-2000: feral ferret. *Journal of the Royal Society of New Zealand*, **31**, 185–203

European Commission (2007) *Commission recommendations of 18 June 2007 on guidelines for the accommodation and care of animals used for experimental and other scientific purposes*. Annex II to European Council Directive 86/609. See 2007/526/EC. http://eurlex.europa.eu/LexUriServ/site/en/oj/2007/l_197/l_19720070730en00010089.pdf (accessed 13 May 2008)

Flecknell, P.A. (2009) *Laboratory Animal Anaesthesia*, 3rd edn. Academic Press, London

Fox, J.G. (1998) *Biology and Diseases of the Ferret*, 2nd edn. Williams and Wilkins, Baltimore

Fox, J.G., Cohen, B.J. and Loew, F.M. (1984) *Laboratory Animal Medicine*. Academic Press, Orlando

Hillyer, E.V. and Quesenberry, K.E. (1997) *Ferrets, Rabbits and Rodents: Clinical Medicine and Surgery*. W.B. Saunders Company, Philadelphia

Joint Working Group on Refinement (1993) Removal of blood from laboratory mammals and birds. First Report of the BVA/FRAME/RSPCA/UFAW Joint Working Group on Refinement. *Laboratory Animals*, **27**, 1–22

Joint Working Group on Refinement (2001) Refining procedures for the administration of substances. Report of the BVAAWF/FRAME/RSPCA/UFAW Joint Working Group on Refinement. *Laboratory Animals*, **35**, 1–41

Lewington, J.H. (2000) *Ferret Husbandry, Medicine and Surgery*. Butterworth Heinemann, Oxford

Lloyd, M. (1999) *Ferrets: Health Husbandry and Diseases*. Blackwell Publishing, Oxford

Lloyd, M. (2002a) Veterinary care of ferrets 1. Clinical examination and routine procedures. *In Practice*, **24**, 90–95

Lloyd, M. (2002b) Veterinary care of ferrets 2. Common clinical conditions. *In Practice*, **24**, 136–145

Marini, R.P. and Fox, J.G. (1998) Anaesthesia, surgery and biomethodology. In: *Biology and Diseases of the Ferret*, 2nd edn. Ed. Fox, J.G., pp. 449–484. Williams and Wilkins, Baltimore

Moody, K.D., Bowman, T.A. and Lang, C.M. (1985) Laboratory management of the ferret for biomedical research. *Laboratory Animal Science*, **35**, 272–279

Oxenham, M. (1990) Distemper vaccination in ferrets. *(Letter) Veterinary Record*, **126**, 67

Porter, V. and Brown, N. (1997) *The Complete Book of Ferrets*. DandM Publications, Bedford

Rehg, J.E., Gigliotti, F. and Stokes, D.C. (1988) Cryptosporidiosis in ferrets. *Laboratory Animal Science*, **38**, 155–158

Ryland, L.M. and Bernard, S.L. (1983) A clinical guide to the pet ferret. *Compendium on Continuing Education for the Practising Veterinarian*, **5**, 25–32

Ryland, L.M. and Gorham, J.R. (1978) The ferret and its diseases. *Journal of the American Veterinary Medical Association*, **173**, 1154–1158

Thornton, R.N, and Cook, T.G. (1986) A congenital Toxoplasma-like disease in ferrets (*Mustela putorius furo*). *New Zealand Veterinary Journal*, **34**, 31–33

Welchman, D. de B., Oxenham, M. and Done, S.H. (1993) Aleutian disease in domestic ferrets: diagnostic findings and survey results. *Veterinary Record*, **132**, 479–484

30 The laboratory dog

Judy MacArthur Clark and C. Jane Pomeroy

Biological overview

General biology

The dog (*Canis familiaris*), which has been domesticated for at least 14 000 years (Clutton-Brock 1995), is a monogastric carnivore, capable of exploiting a wide range of food types. As a result of selection by man, the species has diversified immensely from its assumed ancestor, the Asiatic wolf (*Canis lupus pallipes*).

The anatomy of the dog is comprehensively described by Evans (1993). The purebred dog population consists of over 300 partially inbred genetic isolates known as breeds. A comprehensive review of the genetics of different breeds and strains is provided by Willis (1989). The canine karyotype consists of 78 chromosomes.

Size range and lifespan

The life expectancy of a dog is around 12–16 years with larger breeds tending to have a shorter lifespan. The purpose-bred beagle is most commonly used in research owing to its compact shape and size (adult weight is generally between 7 and 17 kg), short coat, co-operative and docile nature, proclivity for large kennel environments, regulatory requirements regarding its use for toxicology studies and because of the wealth of background data on this breed.

Social organisation

Dogs are highly gregarious mammals with complex social behaviour (Serpell 1995). Most breeds of domesticated dog have a looser pack structure than their wild predecessors (Boitani *et al.* 1995; MacDonald & Carr 1995) and are able to readily form social relationships with human beings as well as with conspecifics (Fox 1975).

Communication is important in developing social relationships in a kennel environment and consideration should be given to allowing this through appropriate housing design Joint Working Group on Refinement (JWGR 2004). Auditory signals are important and a dog's hearing may be particularly sensitive to the frequency range of maximum energy in the bark (Sales *et al.* 1996). It also appears that visual signals are important in canine communication, and ensuring that dogs in a kennel environment have clear lines of sight to each other may reduce barking. In addition to being a nuisance and a health hazard for people, barking can be an indication that a dog is anxious about a potential threat.

The significance of olfactory signals, including urination, which dogs use to communicate sexual and social status and to mark territory, is often underestimated (Sommerville & Broom 1998).

Standard biological data

A wealth of biological data can be found in Altman and Dittmer (1972, 1973, 1974). Some of the more commonly needed values are shown in Table 30.1. Values for haematology can be found in Spurling (1977), while Kaneko *et al.* (2008) and Loeb and Quimby (1989) have provided comprehensive reference values for the clinical chemistry of canine body fluids. An analysis of cerebrospinal fluid can be found in Rushton (1981). Wherever possible, reference values derived from the source colony and analysing laboratory should be used for comparison.

Reproduction

Some reproduction data for the laboratory beagle are summarised in Table 30.2. Allen (1992) provides a detailed review of fertility and obstetrics in the dog. Pre-weaning losses in beagles (including stillbirths and neonatal losses) should be less than 12% of all births.

Normal behaviour

Dogs have a rich repertoire of visual and vocal displays. These are illustrated in Shepherd (2002) and handlers should become familiar with the patterns of behaviour associated with greeting, sexual behaviour, nervousness, submission and aggression. Similar signals are used towards both humans and conspecifics and the displays are good predictors of future behaviour. For example, a young dog that comes forward confidently to greet human visitors to its kennel is likely to adapt well to a laboratory environment.

It is now well accepted that there is a critical period between 3 and 13 weeks of age during which puppies should

Table 30.1 Some typical physiological values for the laboratory beagle.

Parameter	*Normal value*
Adult weight (kg)	7–17
Life span (years)	10–15
Rectal temperature	37.5–39.2 °C (99.5–102.5 °F)
Mean heart rate (beats per minute)	60–120
Mean arterial blood pressure (mmHg)	90–120
Arterial blood pH	7.36–7.46
PaO_2 (mmHg)	85–105
$PaCO_2$ (mmHg)	30–44
Respiratory rate (breaths per minute)	10–30
Tidal volume (ml/kg)	10–15

Table 30.2 Breeding data for the laboratory beagle.

Parameter	*Normal value*
Age at puberty (months):	
Male	7–8
Female	8–14
Gestation period (days)	63 ± 4
Oestrus interval (months)	7–8
Average litters born per bitch per year	1.3
Average litter size (puppies):	
Born	6.6
Weaned	6.2

be familiarised with humans. Handling and socialisation should start from birth and training for experimental procedures from about 3 weeks of age (Boxall *et al.* 2004) including exposure to novel toys, brushes, bins, coverall suits, clippers and handlers with glasses. By 14 weeks, a dog deprived of such socialisation may show fear-motivated aggression, timidity or hyperactivity and may become stressed and experience poor welfare when subjected to even simple, non-invasive procedures (reviewed in Hubrecht 1995). Physiological values in such dogs may fall outside normal limits (Vanderlip *et al.* 1985a, 1985b).

Sources of supply

Dogs are, by nature, pack animals and usually live well in a kennel environment with a defined social order. Purpose-bred animals develop within this background and are likely to be, temperamentally, more suited to the laboratory environment than those with either a free-ranging or domestic history such as stray animals or pets. For the most part, purpose-bred animals are used, particularly for pharmacological and toxicological experiments. For example, a total of 4271 dogs were used in the UK in 2008 of which 4240 were purpose-bred beagles, and only 31 were other breeds which may not have been purpose-bred (Home Office 2009).

The number of dogs used in research has been on a downward trend over the last 20 years. Figures for the UK show some 20 500 procedures performed on carnivores (the majority being dogs) in 1988 compared with 9000 in 2007 and a similar decline in numbers is also seen in the USA. An estimated 140 000 dogs are used worldwide in research and testing every year (JWGR 2004). Nevertheless, the species represents a very small proportion of overall animals used – less than 0.25% in the UK (Home Office 2009). This probably reflects the widespread view, also embodied in many regulatory systems, that alternative species should be used wherever possible.

In Europe, there is a legal requirement that prevents the use of non-purpose bred animals unless the proposed use is carefully justified on scientific and welfare grounds (European Community 1986, 2008). In the USA, a committee of the Institute for Laboratory Animal Research (ILAR) concluded that, under some circumstances, dogs with qualities of random source animals may be desirable and necessary. However, it was not necessary to obtain such dogs from dealers since direct acquisition from breeders, individual owners, or from shelters was both preferable and feasible as an option (National Research Council 2009). JWGR (2004) provide a helpful comparison of the benefits of purpose-bred dogs over dogs from random sources.

If it is proposed to use non-purpose-bred animals, there should be strong justification for this use, such as in the study of a genetic defect only seen in a breed not available from a purpose-bred colony. Economic reasons alone are not sufficient. It is advisable to obtain written confirmation from the supplier that the animal has been obtained legally. Even so, it is important to appreciate the reasons for widespread public concern surrounding such acquisitions.

The option of homing dogs at the end of their experimental use is being increasingly considered, although experience has shown that this is not always an easy task. It is important to consider the temperament of each individual in deciding whether this is feasible. A veterinary certificate of health and suitability is desirable and, in some countries, may be a legal requirement. After selection, a socialisation programme should be used to prepare the animal psychologically for its new environment (Laboratory Animal Science Association (LASA) 2004).

Transport

General advice on transport is provided in LASA (2005), and see also Chapter 13. Transport of animals causes stress and ideally only healthy subjects should be moved, even for short distances. Prior to their journey, dogs should be habituated to their crate to minimise fear and apprehension. This can be done by placing the crate in the dog's pen. Social groupings can be conserved by selecting dogs to travel in compatible pairs or small groups, although it may be safer to transport each dog in its own crate.

Acceptable designs and dimensions for crates for transport by air are detailed in International Air Transport Association (IATA) Live Animals Regulations (2009), which take the size of dog into account in their recommendations. These standards may also be suitable for dogs travelling by sea, road or rail. It is generally recommended that any crate used for transport, no matter how brief the journey, should be large enough to allow the dog to stand in a natural position, turn around and lie down (Animal Transportation Association 2000).

Glass fibre and rigid plastic are the best materials for transport crates. Commercially manufactured models are available that come in a range of sizes, are designed for the purpose and can be readily sanitised. Particular care should be taken to ensure adequate ventilation, usually by making the whole of one end of the crate open with a mesh door that is nose and paw proof. The crate should be designed to prevent adjacent crates being stacked too close together and there should be side ventilation.

Road vehicles, trains and boats should be ventilated with air of adequate quality. Airlines should always place dogs in pressurised compartments. Prolonged exposure to temperatures below 7°C or above 29°C should be avoided during transport, ideally by using temperature-controlled vehicles.

In many countries, it is illegal to transport puppies under 8 weeks of age without their mother. With this exception, puppies under 4 months old should not be transported in the same primary container as adult dogs. Pregnant bitches should not normally be more than two thirds of the way through pregnancy and should be accompanied by a veterinary certificate stating that there is no expectation of birth occurring during transit. It is advisable that all transported dogs should undergo a veterinary examination within a few days beforehand to ensure they are fit for the proposed journey. For international transportation, this examination is often specified by the importing country's regulations. A journey plan should be prepared, and it is advisable, and in some countries mandatory, to use an authorised animal transporter.

Adult dogs should be fed about 2h before despatch and gently exercised to encourage defecation before being placed in the crate. An interval of up to 24h can elapse between feeds for adult dogs but puppies require feeding at shorter intervals (up to 12h depending on age) and this should be taken into account when planning journeys of more than 8h duration.

For long journeys, water should be offered at intervals or provided in a spill-proof container. Written instructions for feeding and watering in transit, together with any instructions for special care, should be attached to the primary container in such a way that they can be easily seen and read. Food and water deprivation are major contributors to the accumulated stress of transport.

Uses in the laboratory

The Committee on Dogs of the US National Research Council has reviewed a range of research areas in which the dog is commonly used (National Research Council 1994). The review not only expands on the uses, but also on the special considerations for husbandry and veterinary care of dogs during such studies.

The dog has many physiological functions similar to those of humans and so can be used as a model for many conditions including those associated with complex genetic traits. Mapping techniques, such as linkage disequilibrium and whole-genome radiation hybrids, have identified some 724 markers (235 genes and 489 microsatellites) (Ostrander & Wayne 2005). Over 360 genetic disorders in dogs have been described, at least half of which resemble specific human disorders (Patterson 2000).

Among those disorders for which the mode of inheritance is known, over 70% are inherited as autosomal recessive, X-linked, or genetically complex traits and 46% are believed to occur predominantly or exclusively in one or a few breeds. This is the largest set of genetic disorders in any non-human species and, together with the mapping information, presents opportunities for research relevant to human disease (Switonski 2004).

The range of research areas in which the dog has played a role is very extensive, including studies of:

- degenerative problems and carcinogenesis;
- aging and its associated disorders;
- cardiovascular diseases, both congenital and induced, including hypertension and heart failure;
- haematological disorders and immunodeficiencies, including autoimmune diseases;
- organ transplantation and open-heart surgery;
- neurological, ophthalmological and orthopaedic disorders;
- radiation-induced injuries;
- early studies of gene transfer and genetic modification which have paved the way for human clinical gene therapy.

Laboratory dogs are also used to develop and test veterinary products for companion dogs such as vaccines, worming and flea treatments, antibiotics, non-steroidal anti-inflammatory drugs (NSAIDs), cardiac drugs and prescription diets.

Increasing pressure to justify the selection of the dog in all research means that other species such as the minipig are being selected where appropriate. In the UK, over 80% of procedures using dogs are for toxicology tests, most of which are performed to satisfy legislative requirements. In a recent study (Olson *et al.* 2000), it was found that non-rodents (primarily dogs) predicted 63% of human toxicities observed in clinical studies for pharmaceuticals compared with only 43% in rodents.

Laboratory management and breeding

General husbandry

Enclosures

Housing systems in Europe have undergone significant change over the last two decades based upon greater understanding of the natural behaviour of the laboratory dog. These changes have been reflected in new guidelines and regulations (Council of Europe 2006; European Community 2008). Hubrecht and Buckwell (2004) provide extensive information about appropriate housing and care systems for laboratory dogs, largely based upon behavioural considerations. In addition, JWGR (2004) describe a range of refinements to dog husbandry and care and provide a number of recommendations that are now becoming widely accepted.

In general, dogs should be housed in indoor pens, preferably with adjacent outdoor runs for exercise. Where the exercise run is outdoors and in a populated area, consideration should be given to the noise nuisance in the neighbourhood. Such a problem is not sufficient grounds for 'debarking' dogs. Some recent facility designs based upon indoor housing also offer secure outdoor exercise areas by locating them within the perimeter of the building (Figure 30.1).

Outdoor access helps to provide a stimulating environment for dogs so it is unfortunate that the actions of extremists in some countries (or the fears of such action) have led to the common practice of housing dogs entirely indoors. In such situations, some access to daylight is desirable, either through windows or skylights, and access to an indoor run, in which individuals or small groups of dogs can regularly exercise, is essential.

Exercise runs, whether indoors or outdoors, should be designed to provide a stimulating environment (Figure 30.2), and human contact during exercise periods should be encouraged. In some countries, climates are sufficiently mild that dogs can be housed almost entirely outdoors, nonetheless, they should still be given access to protective shelter at all times.

Floor materials for dog facilities are often a problem. These should be smooth and resistant to corrosion, denting, cracking or chipping. Sealed junctions between floor and walls are important with coving to ensure dirt traps are avoided. Modern epoxy finishes can be ideal but, if inadequately installed, may cause costly long-term problems.

Bare solid floors, particularly with under-floor heating, may present a cleaning problem since faeces and urine will accumulate. Experience has shown that even a small amount of substrate, such as sawdust or woodchips scattered on a solid floor, will help with cleaning and assist the animal in maintaining a healthy coat and paws.

Open flooring (perforated, grids or mesh) has been subject to criticism since the animal's weight is borne on a relatively small area of the foot pad. Such flooring should not be used without strong justification and never for pre-weaning pups, lactating or periparturient bitches. If its use can be justified, it is generally accepted that it should be covered with smooth, soft plastic for tactile warmth as well as improved cleanliness and dogs should also have access to a solid floor over part of the available living area.

Environmental provisions and enrichment

Modern dog pens are designed to allow flexibility with respect to pen size and interconnections between pens. Thus pens designed to separate single animals for short periods (eg, for feeding) can be readily reconnected to maintain social groups. Stainless steel is generally used for structural frames in preference to galvanised metal which may have toxic effects due to the surface zinc.

Materials used in panels between pens may consist of stainless steel rods, strengthened glass, or plastics (which must be of Food Grade Approved standard), which are warmer to touch and absorb some of the noise generated by barking. Horizontal bars are preferred in panels over mesh (which creates a visual barrier) or vertical bars (which provide no support for the dogs' paws, and which reduce lateral visibility through the bars).

It is important to ensure that each pen has sufficient space and resources to provide for all the functional requirements of the occupants. This should include separate areas for urination and defecation, for resting or sleeping, for breeding where appropriate, and for social interaction such as play. Good modern dog enclosures are sub-divided and furniture is provided. These allow for normal behaviour patterns (see Figures 30.2 and 30.3) including avoidance of aggressive encounters and play behaviour.

Hubrecht and Buckwell (2004) have suggested that practical experience indicates that a dog pen of 4.5 m^2 (as used in the UK at the time of writing) provides sufficient space for

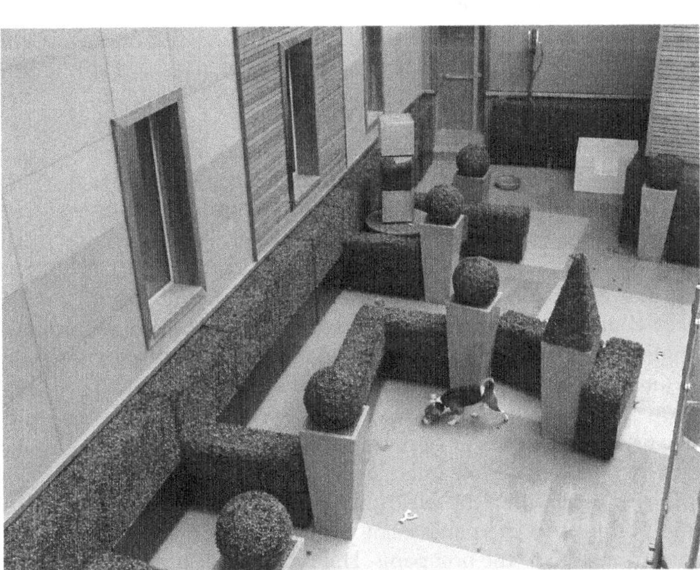

Figure 30.1 A secure outdoor run provided within the perimeter of the surrounding building. (Reproduced with permission of Astra Zeneca.)

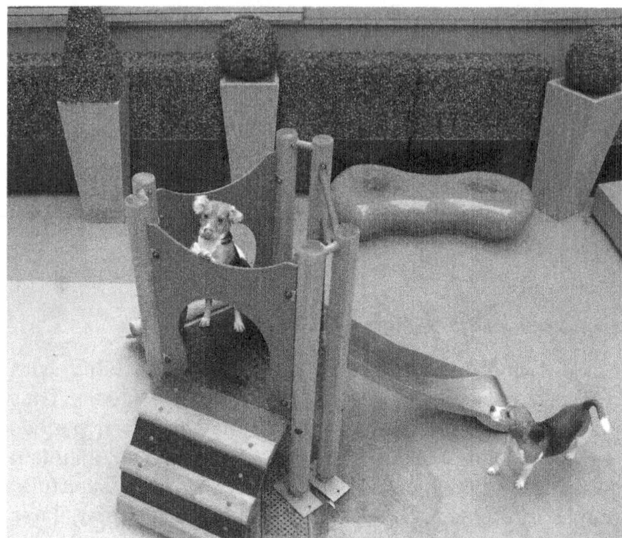

Figure 30.2 Suitable equipment in an exercise area will stimulate play behaviour. Active human contact is also important. (Reproduced with permission of Astra Zeneca.)

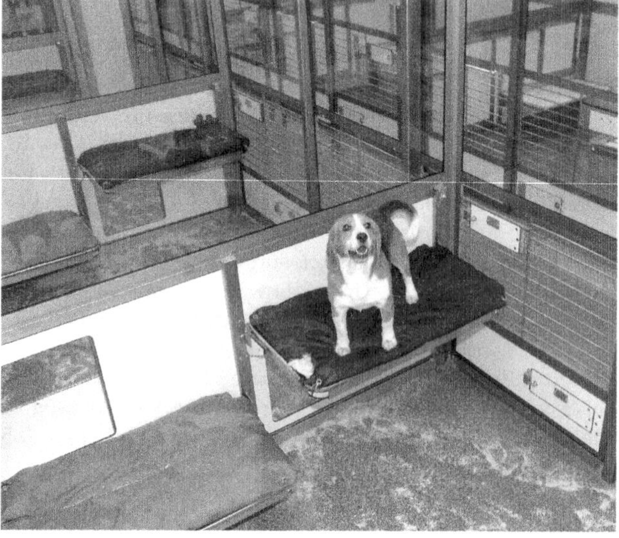

Figure 30.3 Glass panels between pens can improve overall visibility and reduce levels of barking. (Reproduced with permission of Astra Zeneca.)

sub-division and enrichment to allow functional use of space for two adult beagle dogs. Within Europe somewhat smaller minimum dimensions of 4 m^2 (representing a doubling of the existing single housing) have been recommended for one or two dogs in order to encourage social housing without requiring an increase in existing building sizes (European Commission 2007). If an animal must be single-housed, it should be provided with the same space (Council of Europe 2006). It should also be remembered that these are minimum dimensions and it is possible that dogs benefit from the greater opportunities for enrichment and activity that are possible in larger enclosures.

Enrichment within the enclosure is critically important. It is important that the pen design incorporates features that are stimulating to the occupants. Hubrecht (1993) has demonstrated the clear benefits of enriched environments for dogs, including the desirability of providing raised platforms in pens and areas of restricted visibility into which dogs can withdraw or hide. These allow the occupants to make choices in relation to the complexity of their environment, permit use of the third dimension of height, and can be designed to not disrupt routine husbandry practices and animal observation.

Dogs are naturally inquisitive and actively seek information about their environment. The use of a raised platform and ramp is especially beneficial allowing some privacy from neighbouring dogs but also allowing good vision of the surroundings (Figure 30.3). Since dogs naturally chew, objects which are safe and possibly flavoured, such as rawhide or other commercially produced chews, may be suspended within the pen enclosure (Hubrecht 1993, 1995) avoiding monopolisation, soiling or the blocking of drains.

Dogs need a warm dry area for sleeping. In pens with under-floor heating this may be an intrinsic part of the design. In other housing systems a raised bed should be provided, preferably made of a plastic material such as polyethylene or polypropylene, or a high-quality compacted building panel which is resistant to chemicals. Wood can be difficult to sanitise but, in some situations, it may be acceptable to provide wooden beds that are routinely replaced. If wood is used, the life may be extended by framing the edges of the beds in stainless steel to reduce damage from chewing. The size of the bed will vary with the size of the dog but it is not normally necessary to allow for the dog to fully stretch out. Thus a bed area of 0.5 m^2 is adequate for an adult beagle. Soft veterinary bedding material may be appropriate but it will be damaged by chewing and need to be regularly cleaned. An alternative is commercially available shredded paper bedding.

Although dogs may have been kept in cages in the past, such conditions are not able to meet their essential needs in relation to space for locomotion, social contact with conspecifics and environmental enrichment. Dogs are members of a family of active, cursorial mammals so should preferably be housed in floor pens with environmental choice incorporated into their design. Bebak and Beck (1993) have looked at the effect of cage size on play and aggression and shown the benefits of spacious environments for beagles. If dogs must be caged for anything more than the briefest of periods, there should be an opportunity for vigorous activity at least once a day for not less than 30 minutes (O'Donoghue 1993).

Visual contact with other dogs and humans is very important and singly housed or caged dogs should be visited and handled regularly throughout the day to reduce the development of stereotypical behaviour which may persist even after the animal is returned to its pen. Strict limits should always apply to the maximum acceptable periods in single housing or cages and this should be considered as part of the 'cost' to the animals in a cost–benefit analysis.

Metabolism cages for dogs allow separate collection of faeces and urine but inevitably restrict the animal's movement and use of space. Recent moves toward larger cage areas have lead to designs for folding metabolism cages which provide more generous space for the dog (up to 2 m^2) yet can be moved through doorways and packed away when not in use. These larger folding cages can often be located in the animal's home pen so that visual contact with familiar animals is maintained. Alternatively it may be possible to locate metabolism cages within a laboratory area so dogs have human company for large parts of the day or are within sight of other dogs in similar cages.

Facilities must also be available for the isolation of sick animals or those needing special attention. These are normally cages made of fibreglass or similar warm material with a mesh front to permit easy observation. Cages designed for clinical veterinary practice are suitable.

Feeding and watering

Dogs vary enormously in both adult size and in absolute growth rate but most will grow to at least 40 times their birth weight during their first year. Beagles, and dogs of similar size, reach their mature weight at about 18 months of age, so experimental animals below this age will require a diet capable of supporting growth during the experiment. Pregnant and lactating bitches have special nutritional requirements but a carefully balanced diet is also needed during the non-productive periods if the bitch is to achieve her full breeding potential.

Natural and laboratory diets

Most laboratory dogs have all their dietary needs provided in the form of a commercially prepared dried diet. The dried diets are generally produced in an expanded form and should be fed with free access to drinking water since they themselves contribute negligible water. Ideally, dried diets should be available *ad libitum* enabling the animal to develop a nibbling pattern of feeding. In many dogs, this leads to obesity so that restricted meals offered once or twice daily become preferable (Markwell & Butterwick 1994). Dried diet has the advantage that it can be fed from a hopper where it will remain fresh for several days.

Alternatively, a satisfactory diet can be provided in canned or semi-moist form. Some canned diets contain added cereals so that they constitute a complete diet, whilst others with a higher protein content are intended to be fed together with a cereal biscuit. The semi-moist diets usually constitute a complete diet and should be fed with an ample supply of drinking water. Both canned and semi-moist diets have the disadvantage of being perishable so that they must be provided fresh each day. Diets should be fed according to the manufacturers' recommendations with regular body condition scoring to ensure optimal weight.

The nature of the diet may influence the incidence of dental disease with the accumulation of tartar. This can be a significant problem in dogs in colonies from as early as 1 year of age with a reported 84% incidence in beagles aged more than 3 years (Kortegaard *et al.* 2008). Problems occur both directly through dental disease and indirectly through possible systemic effects leading to histopathological changes in kidney, myocardium and liver (DeBowes *et al.* 1996). Regular dental checks should be performed.

Dietary requirements

The dietary requirements of dogs are detailed by the US National Research Council (1985) together with specific procedures to be followed to ensure that foods do not become nutritionally deficient during storage. Essentially, a maintenance diet should provide 22% digestible protein and 5% fat, when calculated on a dry matter basis.

Because the dog is an extremely adaptable animal, deficiencies of nutrients are unusual except in highly productive or rapidly growing animals. For example, the dog can use over 96% of its dietary fat and the essential fatty acids are all interconvertible in the tissues. Therapeutic diets are available for dogs with special nutrient requirements caused by disease but these should only be used under veterinary direction. For example, low-salt diets are useful in the management of experimentally hypertensive dogs. Simpson and Anderson (1993) describe clinical aspects of nutrition in the dog.

Water

The water content of the diet will vary between about 80% in canned diets and less than 10% in dried diets. Thus the need for drinking water will vary not only with the size of the dog and its water loss through urine, faeces and expired air, but also with its type of food. The total daily water requirement in a temperate environment is 70–80 ml/kg body weight. It is essential to provide unrestricted drinking water.

Presentation of food and water

Feeding bowls should have broad flat bases for stability and be made of a material that will resist chewing. Stainless steel is the most satisfactory. A metal retaining device can be used to prevent movement of the bowl during eating. Alternatively, a stainless steel food hopper can be incorporated into the design of the pen. Food dispensers should be positioned so as to prevent soiling. Hoppers should be inspected at least daily to ensure they do not contain caked or unfit food. This creates a useful opportunity to socialise with the dogs associated with feeding. Hoppers should also be emptied and thoroughly cleaned at least twice weekly.

Dried diet can be fed *ad libitum* from a food hopper but this may promote obesity and increased oral bacterial growth and tartar production. In the wild or feral state, a significant proportion of a dog's day might be spent acquiring food by hunting and scavenging. It may be beneficial in the captive environment to simulate this, for example with pet toys made of natural rubber into which food can be inserted, since it may reduce boredom. However these products may be rapidly destroyed by chewing. It is also important to avoid competitive aggression over restricted food supplies and careful supervision during feeding times is important. Pen mates may need to be separated during feeding. Diet aversion can occur if a diet becomes associated with negative physiological effects, such as with a drug dose with unpleasant consequences (JWGR 2004).

Water should be constantly available either from a fixed water bowl, or preferably from an automatic drinking system. Dogs will rapidly learn to drink from such a system, which has the advantage of avoiding static water in bowls which may become soiled. Pipework used for drinking water systems should be of high-quality stainless steel to prevent corrosion and contamination of the water. Drinking valves are generally reliable and rarely block or leak but it is essential to check the operation of each valve at least twice daily, and always when dogs are placed in a previously vacant pen to ensure that an intact water supply exists.

Social housing

Social housing is always preferable to single housing. Hetts *et al.* (1992) examined the influence of single housing conditions on beagle behaviour and found that solitary dogs have a reduced behavioural repertoire, sleep less and tend to vocalise more than dogs with social contact.

Puppies should be reared in groups which provide both the opportunity to interact with peers and a situation in which they can indulge in complex social play. Being naturally gregarious animals, older dogs should be kept in pairs or small groups though separation may be necessary during feeding unless the diet is supplied *ad libitum*. Male dogs are generally more aggressive than bitches and as they pass through puberty they may become more hostile to other males. Different breeds of dog vary in their reactions to other dogs and in some cases unfamiliar adults are hostile and cannot easily be introduced into a group without fighting. When dogs are kept socially, care should be taken to ensure that low-ranking individuals are not deprived of resources such as food or access to a resting area.

In some experimental situations it may be useful to be aware of the individual's social status as this can affect physiological measures such as corticosteroid levels and resting heart rate. Klumpp *et al.* (2006) showed that housing with a familiar conspecific resulted in lower haemodynamic parameters and fewer vocalisations.

Dogs should not be housed singly unless there is strong scientific justification or in the interests of animal welfare (eg, following anaesthesia and surgery). Where it is necessary to singly house a dog, the housing should be designed so that the isolated animal is always able to choose visual contact with other dogs and receives regular contact with humans. A good relationship with humans will be invaluable during experimental procedures.

Surgically prepared dogs with exteriorised implanted devices may need to be isolated although totally implantable devices are now available and should be used wherever possible. If this is not possible, other means of protecting the protruding devices, such as tethers or jackets, should be used if necessary.

In toxicity trials, dogs are usually housed in pairs or small groups though separation for short periods (4 h or less is common practice) should be feasible for feeding and dosing and for individual observation. However, it is preferable not to separate dogs for individual food and water consumption unless absolutely necessary. In many cases, comparative consumption data across entire dose groups can be used.

Identification

In the past, puppies have been permanently marked at 4–6 weeks of age using tattooing forceps on the ear flap. This causes significant discomfort and the technique has been superseded by microchipping.

Electronic microchips have been shown to provide reliable identification over prolonged periods. Microchips can be obtained pre-programmed with identification codes, or can be programmed at the time of insertion. Special chips are also available which indicate the dog's body temperature in addition to its unique identifier. These may be useful during clinical examinations and during surgery. Microchips are inserted subcutaneously, usually in the scruff of the neck between the shoulder blades, without the need for anaesthesia. A reader is used to scan the microchip. There are occasional problems of migration or chip failure that make scanning difficult or impossible. However, the incidence of total loss of microchips is very low making this the method of choice for identification.

Physical environment

Temperature

Dogs are extremely adaptable with regard to their temperature requirements and thrive in climatic conditions ranging from the arctic to the tropics. Dramatic changes in the ambient temperature should be avoided. At lower temperatures it is important that dogs should have access to a shelter, preferably with a source of heat. In hot environments, access to a shaded shelter is essential.

The temperature of indoor dog pens is usually kept between 18 °C and 21 °C. It is important to avoid extreme fluctuations in the temperature though grouped animals in pens will usually be better able to cope with lower temperatures than animals housed singly.

Ventilation and relative humidity

A ventilation rate of 10–12 air changes per hour should be provided in all indoor accommodation. Provided the air is evenly distributed, this will prevent unacceptable build-up of foul odours at recommended stocking densities. Air-handling devices should be designed to avoid draughts and to distribute the air evenly to all of the animal area. It is best to provide 100% fresh air to the ventilation system. If recirculation units are used, effective air cleaning and filtration should take place to remove smell, moisture and chemicals such as ammonia, as well as potential pathogens.

Extremes of humidity should be avoided but this may be difficult during cold weather where cleaning is performed by hosing down. Not only will high levels of humidity predispose dogs to respiratory infections, but the effects of condensation on the building structure can also be very damaging.

Lighting

Lighting systems should provide sufficient illumination for easy observation of animals and a safe working environment for personnel performing husbandry and hygiene tasks (National Research Council 1996). Natural lighting, with its seasonal variation, is normally acceptable though this may affect breeding patterns. In artificial lighting, the daylight period should be at least 10 h and normally 12 h in duration. Simulating dawn and dusk by slowly increasing or decreasing light intensity can avoid startling dogs with sudden changes.

A thoughtful approach to the use of lighting, which is functional yet attractive, can provide a congenial environment both for staff and animals. This can be important to create good staff morale which may reflect a more caring approach to husbandry. Attractive features such as bright wall colours, decorative tiles, glass and colourful plastic panels, skylights, murals and appropriately placed vegetation can all be used to good effect without major additional cost. Such an approach has been exemplified very well by Loveridge (1994).

Noise

There is currently a lack of adequate guidelines for noise in dog kennels in spite of the recognition that noise levels regularly reach values between 85 and 122 decibels throughout a working day. These levels will cause annoyance, stress and damage to human hearing and personal protective equipment should be provided for personnel. There is increasing evidence that excessive noise in the kennel environment may be a welfare issue (Sales *et al.* 1997). Hubrecht *et al.* (1997) measured noise levels and made some useful recommendations to reduce levels in kennels using sound-absorbent materials and small group sizes.

Barking is often triggered by human activity and changes to husbandry practices may reduce noise levels. Recent experience using glass partitions that allow dogs to have clear vision of the activity of humans and of other dogs across an entire kennel area suggest that barking is reduced in such environments (Figure 30.3). Herringbone patterns allow dogs to see activity in the room from within the pen and may reduce barking. Further studies need to be done to confirm these approaches, which may result from animals not being surprised by events in their surroundings.

Hygiene

Faecal material should be regularly removed throughout the day from indoor pens. Dogs tend to defecate shortly after feeding and so removal is especially required during this period. Thorough washing of the pen should also be carried out daily. Where possible, pen washing, particularly where pressure hoses are used, should be performed when dogs are outside the pen, either socialising or undergoing procedures. If sawdust is used on the floor, this should be swept up prior to washing and replaced after the pen is dry.

Disinfectants should be chosen and used carefully to avoid skin irritation. Ideally, complete rooms of dog pens should be emptied periodically, deep cleaned and disinfected thoroughly. This may be feasible between studies especially in toxicology facilities.

If access to the outside is constantly available, an adult dog will usually not soil its indoor pen. Faecal material should be removed from the outside run regularly throughout the day and the floor and walls should be washed daily. Puppies are less fastidious in their habits and a pen containing a group of weanling animals may need to be thoroughly cleaned many times during the day.

Health monitoring, quarantine and barrier systems

Laboratory dog colonies can be divided into two main categories with regard to health monitoring and disease control. The first, and most common, is the closed or semi-closed colony (eg, a breeding colony or a long-term experimental colony) where few introductions of new animals occur and always from reliable sources. In such a colony, the major threat is from new dogs, which should always have been effectively immunised against the common canine infectious diseases in compliance with the vaccine manufacturers' data sheets or according to the WSAVA Guidelines for the Vaccination of Dogs and Cats (Day *et al.* 2007). A well managed personnel barrier, involving at least a change of outer clothing and hand-washing, is also important to avoid humans acting as vectors of disease.

Some infectious pathogens are of particular concern to breeding colonies such as canine herpesvirus (CHV) which can cause abortions and neonatal deaths and *Brucella canis* which is also a zoonosis. Since no vaccine is available against the latter, a serological sample collected on arrival may be checked for antibodies.

The second type of colony receives frequent introductions of new dogs, some of which may be from sources where the health status is unreliable. Effective quarantine may be very difficult but should always be the aim. Newly arrived dogs should be housed in groups according to their source and receive a veterinary examination soon after arrival. Unvaccinated dogs should not normally be accepted and must be kept in strict isolation and immunised as soon as possible.

Health monitoring of established colonies should follow a defined programme of sample collection including faecal and blood samples (Federation of European Laboratory Animal Science Associations (FELASA) 1998). In a breeding colony, careful examination of breeding and puppy growth data is also important.

A health programme should also be implemented to protect personnel based upon medical advice. As a minimum, this should include tetanus vaccination for all personnel. In countries where rabies occurs, vaccination against rabies should also be considered, and special attention should be paid to any scratch or bite injuries to ensure personnel receive prompt medical attention.

A quarantine facility should be designed to provide physical barriers to disease spread, including the possibility of air-borne spread, and should preferably have its own animal care staff. Dogs should be checked at regular intervals throughout the day (*Department for Environment, Food and Rural Affairs* (DEFRA) 2007).

Breeding

Identifying the fertile state

Dogs become sexually mature at 6–12 months of age; small breeds normally reach puberty earlier than large breeds. Following puberty in the bitch, oestrous cycles continue throughout life, each cycle being divided into four stages: pro-oestrus, the beginning of the sexual season; oestrus, the period of receptivity; metoestrus, the period of subsiding activity; and anoestrus, the period of quiescence.

The bitch is monoestrous since several months of sexual inactivity elapse between breeding periods regardless of pregnancy. The concept of two oestrous cycles a year is erroneous since most reports give an average oestrous interval of 7–8 months, but with a variation ranging from 4–14 months reported.

Colony breeding data tend to show some seasonal influence, with increased incidence of oestrus in late winter and spring. This implies that either light intensity or duration affects the breeding cycle of the bitch.

Pro-oestrus is flagged by enlargement of the external genitalia. Within 2–4 days a sanguinous discharge appears from the vulva, usually regarded as the first day of pro-oestrus. Discharge continues for 6–10 days during which the female is attractive to, but will not accept, the male. When oestrus commences, the female will accept the male showing a characteristic stance of arched back and elevated tail. At the same time, the sanguinous discharge begins to subside. Following acceptance of the male with intromission, the two usually remain 'tied' in the coital lock for 10–40 minutes.

Oestrus lasts from 6–12 days during which time the female may continue to allow coitus. Ovulation normally occurs within 1–2 days after first acceptance of the male and is spontaneous. The female refusing coitus marks the start of metoestrus and is characterised by a gradual decrease in size and turgidity of the vulva. A portion of the metoestrus may be associated with pregnancy or pseudopregnancy and anoestrus commences when the desquamated endometrial lining has been regenerated.

The female, when approaching puberty, may occasionally show an episode of false pro-oestrus with an increase in turgidity of the vestibular wall sometimes accompanied by a slight sanguinous discharge. Acceptance of the male does not occur and it is usually several weeks before true pro-oestrus begins. The condition does not recur at later oestruses and fertility is not affected (Harvey 1998).

Vaginal cytology can be used to estimate the best time for breeding. The technique has been described by Concannon and DiGregorio (1986) and the following microscopical features may be seen:

- pro-oestrus – abundant erythrocytes and 'cornified' cells with pyknotic nuclei, leucocytes sparse;
- oestrus – abundant 'cornified' cells, many without nuclei, and a moderate number of erythrocytes, few leucocytes;
- metoestrus – epithelial cells of varying size and shape, variable number of leucocytes and debris;
- anoestrus – epithelial cells with cytoplasmic granules or vacuoles, variable number of leucocytes.

Additionally, plasma progesterone concentrations can be used to augment the assessment of vaginal cytology; concentration is low during anoestrus and pro-oestrus, increasing when pre-ovulatory follicular luteinisation occurs, followed by a rapid rise after ovulation (England 1998a).

Breeding systems

Dogs will breed in groups of one stud male with up to 12 bitches. If several bitches are in oestrus simultaneously, the male may be unable to impregnate all of them. Once each bitch is obviously pregnant she should be removed to separate accommodation for whelping. This system has the advantage that oestrus detection by animal care staff is unnecessary.

An alternative system involves examining each bitch daily for signs of pro-oestrus. A bitch is then put with a male on about the 10th day following pro-oestrus detection and remains for about 5 days. Bitches normally ovulate about 2 days after a surge of luteinising hormone which may occur as early as 5 days after the onset of pro-oestrus or as late as 21 days (Wright & Watts 1998). To address this variation, introductions can be made daily over this period, lasting for about 1 hour each day, until a successful mating has been observed on at least two occasions.

A variation of this system would involve housing the bitch with the male from the onset of pro-oestrus until several matings have been observed. Some bitches have a short interval from onset of observable pro-oestrus to their fertile period so that waiting until 10 days after the start of pro-oestrus may result in no pregnancy. However this system has the disadvantage that a stud male can cover only one bitch at a time.

Conception and pregnancy

Canine spermatozoa can survive for many days in the uterus and are only able to fertilise the ovum some 2–3 days following ovulation.

The preferred imaging technique for pregnancy detection is ultrasonography, which allows foetuses to be seen from 15 days after ovulation (England 1998a). It is difficult to count foetuses precisely ultrasonographically but this can best be done about 1 month after conception with significantly lower accuracy in late pregnancy. The gestation period in the bitch, if measured from mating to parturition, is variable due to the delay which occurs between insemination and fertilisation. Yeager and Concannon (1990) demonstrated ultrasonographic detection of pregnancy from day 16 and noted that gestational age was best estimated based upon the day of the preovulatory surge of luteinising hormone. Embryonic mass and heart beat were first detected at 23–25 days after the LH surge. Kutzler *et al.* (2003) were able to predict parturition date very accurately (85% accuracy within ±2 days) using foetal measurements obtained by ultrasonography.

Manual palpation of the standing bitch can be used at 28–32 days after ovulation when foetuses may be felt as a chain of discrete firm swellings, each about 2 cm in diameter. After 32 days, palpation becomes increasingly difficult until very late in pregnancy when the foetal heads may be felt. By this time, mammary development is also obvious.

There is little difference in progesterone concentration between pregnant and non-pregnant bitches (England 1998a).

Parturition

Signs of impending parturition (whelping) in the bitch have been described by Johnson (1986). A fall in body temperature to less than 37.2 °C normally occurs within 24 h before parturition accompanied by palpable relaxation of pelvic and abdominal musculature. Increased friendliness, restlessness and loss of appetite may also occur. For several days prior to expected parturition, a bed should be provided using a bedding material that is designed to drain fluid to the base of the bed leaving the bitch and puppies relatively dry.

Jones and Joshua (1988) have described the pattern of normal whelping together with excellent advice on coping with problems which may arise. The first stage of parturition begins with the onset of uterine contractions. This may last for 6–12 h during which time the bitch may appear agitated.

Stage two commences when the cervix is fully dilated. The allantochorion or 'water bag' of the first foetus appears at the vulva and is often ruptured by the bitch. By now, the bitch is exerting obvious abdominal contractions. Shortly after, the first foetus is presented in the cervix and expulsion may take from only a few minutes to a couple of hours. It is natural for the bitch to chew the umbilical cord and eat the placenta. Her continual licking of the puppy stimulates respiration during the first few minutes of independent life. Further puppies will follow at intervals of 20–60 minutes (maybe as long as 2 h). A non-purulent greenish discharge may precede the first and subsequent foetuses.

Stage three begins after delivery of the puppies and ends with the passage of all placentae. A bitch with multiple puppies may alternate between stages two and three.

Commonly the foetal head will present towards the maternal pelvis, although many foetuses in other presentations are delivered unassisted and should not be considered abnormal. Difficulties may be encountered if the first foetus is in posterior presentation since the dilating affect of the head on the cervix and vagina will be absent. The following are indications of a difficult birth (dystocia) that may require intervention (Tilley & Smith 2004b):

- 30 minutes of strong persistent abdominal contractions or straining without delivering a puppy;
- more than 4 h from the onset of stage two to the delivery of the first puppy;
- more than 2 h between the birth of each puppy;
- failure to deliver more than 24 h after the rectal temperature falls to less than 37.2 °C or within 36 h of serum progesterone being less than 2 ng/ml;
- the bitch shows visible signs of pain or is constantly licking the vulva while attempting to deliver;
- prolonged gestation – greater than 70 days from first mating, or 59 days from first day of cytological dioestrus, or 66+ days from the luteinising hormone peak.

Nutrition during pregnancy and lactation

During the first 5–6 weeks of pregnancy, a bitch can be fed the same amount as before mating. During the last 3–4 weeks, the foetal puppies are growing very rapidly and the diet must be increased according to the manufacturers' recommendations. The gravid uterus often limits intake so this should be provided in small frequent meals.

Lactation is nutritionally very demanding and the bitch will require 3–4 times her maintenance level of food when milk production reaches its peak 3–4 weeks post-partum. This should be fed as frequent small meals.

Reproductive problems

Pseudopregnancy is a common reproductive problem, occurring in about 16% of bitches during metoestrus, the incidence increasing with age. It is characterised by a varying degree of abdominal distension and mammary development, some bitches actually lactating about 60 days after ovulation. It is thought that falling progesterone precipitates a rise in prolactin in affected animals. The condition is self-limiting and does not usually require intervention (Feldman & Nelson 1987). Cabergoline can be used to selectively inhibit prolactin in bitches distressed by false pregnancy.

False oestrus has been reported (Shille *et al.* 1984) in which the bitch will mate but fail to conceive since no ovulation occurs. This may be followed a few weeks later by true oestrus. Bitches which repeatedly show this pattern can have a very disruptive effect on a breeding colony and should normally be culled, unless of special value. Culling based on small litter size, problems with whelping or maternal behaviour, chronic infertility, age or persistent anoestrus is also appropriate.

Methods for the assessment and treatment of infertility in both the male and female dog have been reviewed by Johnston and Romagnoli (1991).

Rearing the young

Early development

Cannibalism of puppies is unusual though a bitch will often reject a weak or 'runted' offspring, thus allowing it to die. Primigravid bitches are sometimes apprehensive of their litter initially, but usually settle down once the puppies start sucking. Sedation (eg, acepromazine) may be useful for these first hours, once parturition has been completed.

Newborn puppies do not have fully developed temperature control and require a higher ambient temperature than adults to avoid hypothermia. Some of this warmth can be provided by the bitch and littermates but an ambient temperature of 26–28 °C will be needed for at least the first 5–10 days. Local heat, using an infra-red lamp, is suitable but the lamp and flex should be hung out of reach of the bitch and at least 1 m above the litter.

Newborn puppies commence sucking immediately after they have been licked clean by the bitch. During the first week, sucking occurs about every 2h after which the frequency reduces to every 4h. It is very important that puppies feed adequately during the first 24h of life as it is during this time that they receive high levels of colostrum which provides important passive immunity. Puppies are born with their eyes and ears closed. The eyelids gradually separate until the eyes are fully open by day 10–14. By this time the ears are also patent. Puppies are usually able to stand by day 10 and walk steadily by day 21. Voluntary control of micturition and defecation begins between days 16 and 21.

Hand rearing

By far the best method of hand rearing puppies is by fostering onto a lactating female. Docile bitches with a litter of similar age and size, or a pseudopregnant bitch, will often accept one or more foster puppies. Puppies can be successfully hand reared using a commercial milk substitute formulated for dogs.

It is vital to provide an environmental temperature of 30–32°C for newborn orphan puppies. After 7 days this can gradually be lowered to about 24°C by 4 weeks of age. At these temperatures, the puppy should be fed at 3-hourly intervals between 08.00 and midnight for the first 3 weeks. At lower temperatures, an overnight feed will be necessary. Thereafter feeds should be reduced in frequency to four times daily by 6 weeks of age. Solid food should be offered from 4 weeks of age. A detailed review of rearing orphaned puppies is given by Edney (1982).

Weaning and rearing

Puppies will start eating solid food at about 3 weeks of age and can be separated from the bitch at 7–8 weeks. The nutrient requirements of the weaned puppy are about double those of an adult dog of the same weight. This food should be given in several small meals as shown in Table 30.3. Commercial puppy foods should be fed according to the manufacturer's recommendations. Acceptability and palatability of the food is most important during this period of rapid growth and, if biscuit or a dried diet is used it may be moistened to soften it prior to feeding.

Selection of breeding stock

Future breeders should be selected on the basis of parental performance, temperament and conformation. Litters from primiparous females should be avoided since parental performance will not yet have been adequately assessed. Detailed records must be maintained for each breeding animal showing date and size of litters born, stillbirths, neonatal deaths, size of litters weaned, sex of offspring and identity of the sire. If oestrus detection is being practised, the frequency of oestrus must be recorded together with dates of mating. All these records must be considered in assessing parental performance when selecting bitches.

Table 30.3 Frequency of meals for puppies after weaning.

Age (months)	*Meals per day*
1½–3	4
3–4	3
4–6	2
Over 6	1 or 2

Standard growth curves[1] of a colony can be maintained to ensure selection from healthy stock of near average weight. Individual examination is of paramount importance to assess the temperament of the animal and to ensure good health and avoid detectable inherited defects.

Selection of good-quality stud males is of even greater importance due to the wider impact on the colony compared with bitch selection. In addition to many of the selection criteria mentioned above, potential studs can have semen samples collected by manual ejaculation and testicular ultrasound can also be performed to evaluate fertility. Once selected, the libido of a stud male should be assessed at regular intervals.

Care must be taken to avoid unintentional inbreeding, particularly in a small breeding colony where random mating would lead to a significant increase in inbreeding coefficient. It has been estimated that a ratio greater than two males for each 10 females is needed to prevent an increase in the coefficient of inbreeding (Shultz 1970). Unrelated stud dogs should also be selected to mitigate against this effect.

The ability of female beagles to breed reaches a peak at 3 years of age and then wanes from 4–8 years of age (Andersen & Simpson 1973). During this latter period there is an increase in the number of mated females who fail to whelp, a decrease in the number of pups born per litter and an increase in the pre-weaning losses. Extended oestrous cycles, 1 year or more in length, are common in beagles over 8 years of age.

Production of gnotobiotic and specific pathogen free (SPF) stock

Griesemar and Gibson (1963) have described techniques for obtaining gnotobiotic puppies. It would appear that the last few days *in utero* are important for the production of vigorous puppies. Therefore the accurate detection of imminent parturition is essential to ensure correct timing of the hysterectomy. Gnotobiotic puppies are commonly infected with the roundworm *Toxocara canis* and, in countries where it is endemic, the hookworm *Ancylostoma caninum* but this should be a limited contamination if appropriate sterile hysterectomy techniques are used. Dosing with an appropriate anthelmintic (eg, fenbendazole 50 mg/kg/day) during pregnancy will significantly reduce this parasite burden in the puppies after the hysterectomy (Burke & Roberson 1983; Fisher 2001).

Since they have never been exposed, either naturally or through vaccination, to the relevant infectious agents, SPF dogs can be used for research into canine infectious diseases and for vaccine development and testing. It may also be preferable to use SPF dogs in transplantation studies since

[1] http://www.marshallbio.com/docs/pub/Refdata/Reference_b_growth.pdf

latent viruses in non-SPF dogs may be activated during profound immunosuppression and cause disease.

Artificial insemination

Methods of collection, storage and insemination of canine semen have been described by Farstad (1998). Semen samples can be evaluated for a variety of characteristics including motility, sperm count, pH and live to dead ratio. Canine semen is ejaculated in three fractions: the second, the sperm-rich fraction, is used for insemination. Fresh semen can be stored at 4 °C. If appropriately diluted, sperm motility remains almost normal for 3–4 days and for 1 day if stored undiluted (Morton & Bruce 1989). Alternatively, semen can be stored frozen. Freezing techniques have stringent requirements for rate of thawing, dilution and site of deposition which must be followed (England 1993). Sperm normally die within a few hours of thawing so precise timing of insemination is critical to success.

In nature, the semen is deposited into the anterior vagina, but reaches the uterus and oviducts within 1–2 minutes post-coitus. Concannon and Battista (1989) have described a technique of intrauterine artificial insemination with a 50–90% conception rate. Kim *et al.* (2007) compared intrauterine and intratubal insemination and showed low conception rates (20%) with the latter technique. The best time for insemination is usually shortly after oocyte maturation which occurs 5–6 days after the initial rise in progesterone and around the time of the surge in luteinising hormone. Most successful inseminations take place 2–4 days before the decrease in vaginal cornification.

Oestrus control and impact on research

England (1998b) has comprehensively reviewed the pharmacological control of oestrus in the bitch. Oestrus can be postponed or prevented in the bitch. Progesterone or progestagens are most commonly used and are available in a variety of formulations, including depot preparations and tablets, to be given orally. Androgens may also be given in anoestrus to prevent the return to cyclical activity, either as a prolonged release implant or as a depot injection of mixed testosterone esters. The mechanism of action of androgens is not clear.

Kutzler (2005) reviewed methods of oestrus induction and synchronisation of ovulation for embryo transfer programmes. He concluded that methods vary widely in efficacy of inducing oestrus as well as fertility. Chandra and Adler (2008) reviewed the frequency of different oestrus stages to permit interpretation of morphological changes in toxicity studies. They found that more than 80% of the animals studied were in the anoestrus–dioestrus stage at the time of autopsy.

Laboratory procedures

Handling and training

Puppies should be handled frequently to accustom them to human company. Purchased animals should be given similar attention in their breeding facility and during quarantine when they are adapting to their new environment. Dogs are generally amenable creatures and any tendency to aggression is usually due to nervousness. A quiet, gentle approach will frequently overcome any problems. Rarely, nervous dogs may snap at their handlers and need to be muzzled for minor procedures. Use of such dogs should be avoided, especially for long-term procedures. If a dog develops nervousness over time, sensitive remedial training may be able to resolve the problem.

Dogs can easily be trained to walk on a lead and this experience is beneficial in bonding the dog with its handlers. This may be facilitated by use of head collars designed to prevent pulling. Dogs not so trained, and weighing up to about 15 kg, may be carried (Figure 30.4). Larger animals should be moved in a wheeled box or crate to which they should be habituated.

In addition to lead training, dogs can readily be trained to relax in a body sling or small study cubicle for periods of 8 h or more. This is important where animals have been surgically instrumented to permit monitoring of physiological parameters whilst fully conscious. These and other forms of training, including habituation to electric clippers, and sitting still for blood sampling, provide environmental enrichment for these intelligent animals and give opportunities for close human contact. JWGR (2004) provide useful advice on socialisation, habituation and training of laboratory dogs and the benefits which accrue.

Physiological monitoring

Recording body temperatures

Rectal temperature can be measured with a digital or mercury thermometer. The normal range is 38–39 °C. The

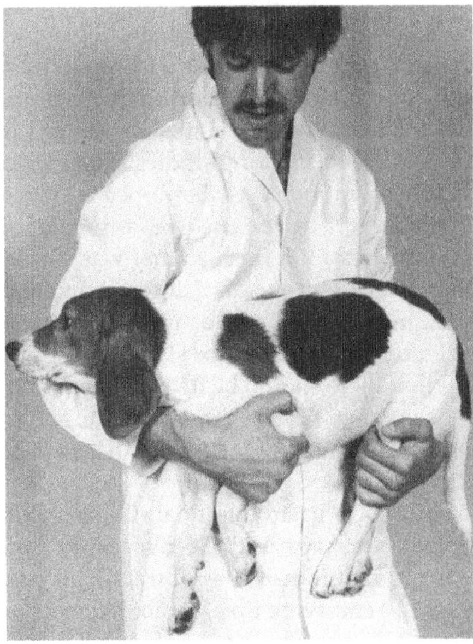

Figure 30.4 The correct way of carrying a medium-sized dog. (Crown copyright.)

technique is slow since the thermometer should be placed in the rectum for at least 2 minutes before being read. Continuous or remote recordings are not possible by this method. Microchips which include a temperature sensor are available for subdermal implantation but may be less reliable than rectal probes due to their peripheral position.

In anaesthetised animals, temperature probes may be sited in the rectum or lower oesophagus for core temperature measurements. A nasopharyngeal reading can be taken as an estimate of brain temperature. Inspired and expired air temperature can be measured by a probe placed in the trachea.

Telemetry

Telemetric devices can be surgically implanted for recording physiological values such as body temperature, electrocardiogram (ECG), blood pressure (arterial, venous and left ventricular), intraocular pressure, kidney pressure, electromyogram, electroencephalogram (EEG), electro-oculogram, respiratory rate and motor activity in the conscious dog. Texts are available to assist the interpretation of these recordings including for ECGs (Tilley 1992) and EEGs (Redding & Knecht 1983).

Telemetric methods are used widely to monitor cardiovascular and neurobehavioural effects of potential pharmaceuticals (Tontodonati *et al.* 2007). By mounting the receiver above the pen, recovered animals can move freely whilst continuous remote recordings are taken. A significant advantage is that results are not masked by the effects of handling stress. Recording can also be conducted for prolonged periods without human presence.

Careful consideration should be given to housing a companion animal with the telemetered animal for social enrichment and to inhibit development of stereotypic behaviour. Many modern telemetry devices have batteries which can be switched on and off giving 3–5 years' service before the implant fails. Repeat surgery for battery replacement may become necessary but strict limits should be applied to the number of times this may be done with up to two replacement surgeries normally considered to be maximum.

In many countries it is permitted to re-use animals in telemetry and other monitoring studies under strict regulatory controls. The rationale is that, once a dog has been surgically prepared, it can be used for a number of studies with minimal distress. If a fresh animal was surgically prepared for each use, the overall distress would be greater. Furthermore, an animal can act as its own control, thereby reducing the number required for statistical significance. It is important that there should be frequent veterinary checks to ensure dogs remain fit for subsequent use, and only dogs selected for a temperament which suits them for laboratory life should be used.

A new approach to gastrointestinal (GI) monitoring uses an ingestible wireless capsule that can measure pressure, pH and temperature as it transits the GI tract. This can be used to provide gastric emptying time, combined small and large intestine transit time, pressure contraction patterns and motility indices. The data receiver can be fitted into a jacket for protection.

Collection of specimens

Blood

General advice on blood sampling is available in JWGR (1993). Blood samples may be conveniently and safely taken from three veins in the dog, namely, the cephalic, external jugular and lateral saphenous veins.

The cephalic vein runs along the dorsal surface of the forelimb from the medial to the lateral side. It can be dilated by compressing the upper surface of the limb at the elbow as shown in Figure 30.5. Blood can be collected by syringe and needle (0.6 mm outside diameter (od) × 16 mm or 0.8 mm × 16 mm) using a steady gentle pull on the plunger. Compression of the vessel should be maintained during collection of the sample, but relaxed before the needle is withdrawn. Compression should then be applied over the puncture site for about a minute to prevent haemorrhage and haematoma formation. When repeated samples are required it is better to place a flexible cannula in the vein. This can be fixed in place with adhesive tape and, provided it is flushed with heparinised saline (5 IU/ml) about every 4 h, it will remain patent for 24 h or more. Bandaging may prevent some dogs removing the cannula but must not tightly encircle the limb as venous drainage will be occluded. Alternatively, a dog can be fitted with a protective plastic collar and singly housed to prevent itself or other dogs chewing the cannula.

The external jugular vein is a larger vessel and is appropriate for routine blood sampling as well as catheterisation of the right heart and pulmonary artery. The dog is held either sitting or standing as in Figure 30.6 and the vessel is dilated by applying pressure in the jugular furrow at the base of the neck. Venepuncture is made from the lateral side directed cranially for a venous sample or caudally for catheterisation.

The lateral saphenous vein is less easily stabilised for puncture but is a useful alternative for single samples. The animal is held as in Figure 30.7. It is also useful for catheterisation, especially for dogs supported in slings.

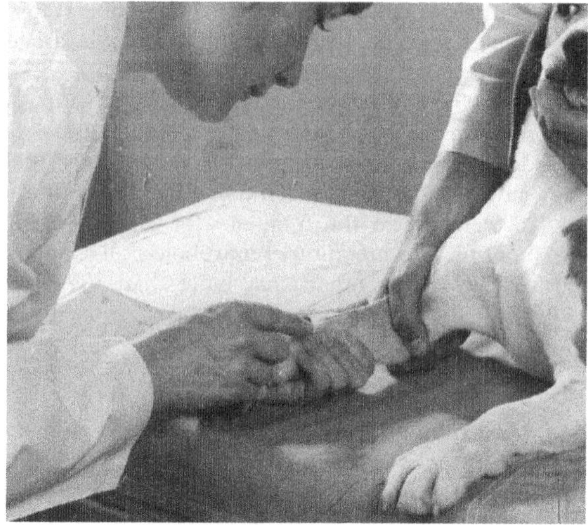

Figure 30.5 Collection of blood from the cephalic vein. (Crown copyright.)

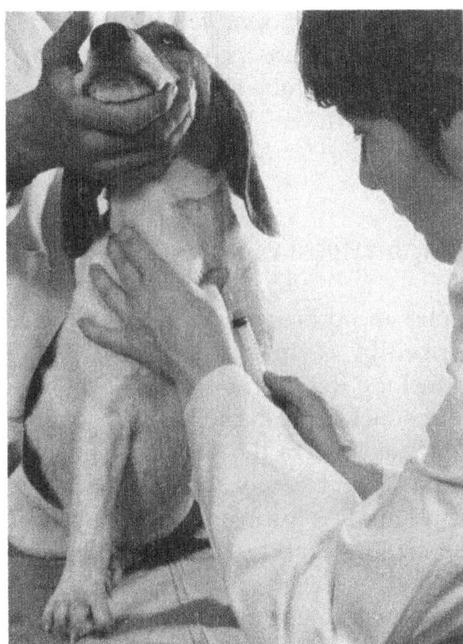

Figure 30.6 Collection of blood from the external jugular vein. (Crown copyright.)

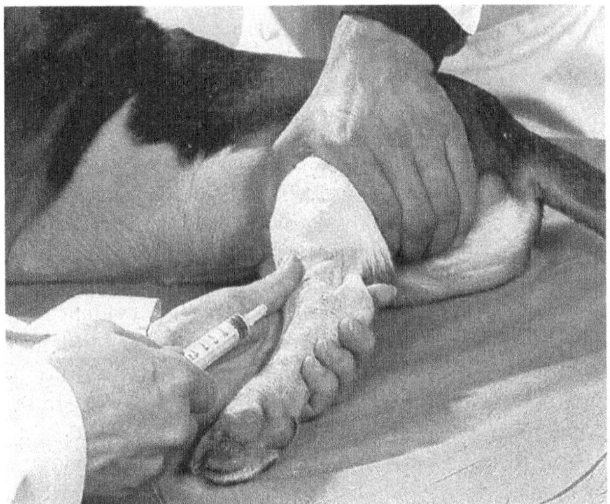

Figure 30.7 Collection of blood from the lateral saphenous vein. (Crown copyright.)

Venepuncture should normally be performed under aseptic conditions. This would usually involve careful clipping and antiseptic swabbing of the puncture area and the use of sterile syringes, needles and catheters. If repeated samples are required, it is preferable to insert a catheter to avoid repeated application of antiseptic and venepuncture, both of which may cause irritation.

Bone marrow

Bone marrow can be removed under general anaesthesia or sedation with local anaesthesia, normally from the dorsal iliac crest. Full surgical asepsis is essential which includes clipping the site, scrubbing and draping. A bone marrow biopsy needle 25–45 mm long and about 2.5 mm internal diameter is used. The technique is described in detail by Raskin (1993).

Urine

A metabolism cage which incorporates adequate separation of faeces and urine should be used for the collection of a 24 h urine sample. However, it will not be suitable for bacteriological examination, this requiring a sample obtained by cystocentesis to ensure no contamination. Sterile plastic catheters are available for both the dog and the bitch and should be used with full aseptic technique to prevent infection of the urinary tract. Repeated catheterisation is unwise as the abrasive effect on the urethra may predispose to pain and infection.

Faeces

Faeces can be collected in a metabolism cage, or from the floor of an ordinary cage or pen soon after defecation. Alternatively, a spatula or gloved finger can be used to gently ease faeces out of the rectum.

Abdominal organ biopsy

A percutaneous method of sampling one or more abdominal organs under ultrasound guidance is described by Barr (1995). Tissue core samples of good quality can be obtained from both liver and kidney. Endoscopic biopsy of the small intestine is described by Hall (1994) but is prone to artefacts due to the small sample size which may include only mucosa and submucosa. Biopsy of the intestine by laparotomy allows full-thickness samples to be obtained (Tobias 2007) and visual inspection of the alimentary tract and other organs.

Administration of substances

See JWGR (2001) for general advice on the administration of substances.

Intravenous route

The techniques for intravenous injections are similar to those described for blood sampling. Compression of the vessel should be relaxed prior to injecting the material.

Intramuscular route

Intramuscular injection can be made into the quadriceps muscle of the hindleg or the lumbar musculature, pushing the needle (0.8 mm od × 16 mm or 25 mm) into the body of the muscle before injecting the material. Kruesi (2004) describes the lumbar technique with helpful photographs.

Subcutaneous route

Subcutaneous injection is made under the loose skin above the shoulder blades. A three-cornered fold of skin is raised with the thumb and two fingers. The needle (0.8 mm od × 16 mm) penetrates the dog's skin under the thumb, pointing towards the two fingers and slightly downwards (Figure 30.8). This technique avoids the possibility of double penetration of a simple skin fold which would result in loss of injected material.

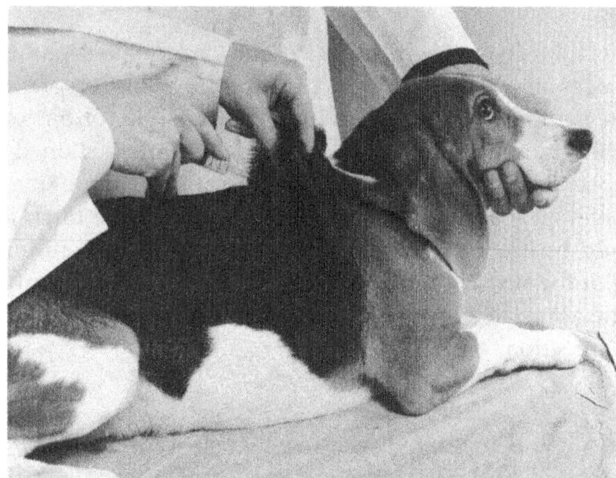

Figure 30.8 Raising a three-cornered fold of skin for a subcutaneous injection. (Crown copyright.)

Intraperitoneal route

The intraperitoneal route is not commonly used and is not normally recommended in the dog. The site for injection is 2–3 cm lateral to the umbilicus with the animal standing or in dorsal recumbency. The needle should be introduced at least 2 cm and the syringe plunger pulled back to ensure no blood, urine or other fluid enters the barrel. If this occurs, reposition the needle before injecting. It is unwise to attempt intraperitoneal injections in bitches during the last 2 weeks of pregnancy.

Oral route

If the pharmacokinetics of the product allow, oral doses can often be administered by mixing the dose with the normal diet without altering acceptability, or by concealing it within a treat. The giving of treats may, of course, be impractical if it is in conflict with an experimental protocol. If this is not possible, tablets or capsules can be placed on the back of the dog's tongue and will be swallowed if the jaw is held closed. Swallowing can be induced by massaging the dog's throat. This procedure is more stressful to both animal and handler particularly in nervous animals.

Fluids can be poured into the labial pouch at the angle of the jaw with the muzzle held upwards. The fluid should be given in small aliquots to permit swallowing and avoid choking.

Alternatively, fluids can be orally administered by stomach tube which may be passed easily in trained dogs. A flexible rubber or plastic tube (9 mm od) should be used in animals weighing over 6 kg. The length is marked in advance by measuring the distance from the nose, via the acromion of the shoulder, to the tenth costochondral junction. The first few centimetres of the tube should be lubricated with an appropriate water-soluble jelly.

The muzzle of the dog is lifted to point upwards and the jaws opened. The tube will then pass easily over the back of the tongue and into the oesophagus until the mark is level with the incisors. If there is any resistance, the tube should be withdrawn and the procedure repeated. When the tube is correctly placed, the odour of gastric contents will be easily smelt. A small amount of fluid should initially be administered and, in the absence of any choking, the remainder given steadily. The tube should then be flushed before being gently withdrawn to avoid reflex vomiting or regurgitation.

Anaesthesia, analgesia and post-operative care

Basic principles and procedures for anaesthesia and analgesia are described by Seymour and Gleed (1999) while Hall *et al.* (2001) include descriptions of anaesthesia for specialised techniques such as obstetrics and intrathoracic surgery. Flecknell (2009) considers the particular anaesthetic needs of the laboratory dog. Healthy dogs can readily be anaesthetised and present few problems. Anaesthetic techniques require considerable expertise and should not be contemplated by an inexperienced anaesthetist.

Prior to administering a general anaesthetic, a thorough pre-operative assessment should be carried out to ensure the dog is fit for anaesthesia. Food should be withheld for at least 6 h beforehand to reduce the risk of regurgitation.

Pre-anaesthetic medication is advisable, even in quiet animals, for the following reasons:

- to alleviate anxiety;
- to provide muscle relaxation and analgesia;
- to suppress vomiting and regurgitation;
- to provide smoother induction and recovery;
- to reduce the dose of anaesthetic required.

A premedicant combination of an opioid analgesic and a sedative may also produce moderate to deep sedation enabling minor procedures such as radiography to be undertaken. Opioid analgesics are best administered pre-operatively prior to more major surgery since evidence suggests that pain, once experienced, becomes more difficult to control. The analgesic effect may also continue into the immediate post-surgery period thus aiding a smooth recovery.

General anaesthesia can be maintained by intravenous and inhaled agents either separately or in combination. The former are usually administered via an in-dwelling cannula placed in the cephalic, external jugular or lateral saphenous vein (Figures 30.5, 30.6 and 30.7). Table 30.4 lists anaesthetic agents and adjuncts suitable for the dog with their doses, routes of administration and special considerations.

The anaesthetist should also be responsible for monitoring and maintaining body temperature during the procedure. Heat loss is especially significant in small breeds, immature subjects or during prolonged anaesthesia and recovery. Maintenance fluids appropriate to the procedure should be given and fluid loss by bleeding should be monitored and appropriately replaced. Tear formation may be reduced so it is beneficial to protect the animal's eyes with sterile lubricant.

Post-operative analgesia must be provided for as long as is needed. The opioid analgesics, for example buprenorphine, are suitable with the first dose being given as part of the pre-medicant. Individual responses to all opioids are variable, making ongoing assessment of pain imperative to inform subsequent requirements. Opioid analgesics can also

Table 30.4 Some anaesthetic agents and adjuncts suitable for the laboratory dog.

Agent	*Dose*	*Route*	*Effect*	*Comment*
Acepromazine	0.01–0.1 mg/kg	im, sc or slow iv	Sedative	Dose dependent on route. Onset 20–30 mins after im administration
Morphine	0.5 mg/kg	im, iv	Opioid analgesic	Continuous rate infusion 0.15–0.2 mg/kg/hr iv
Methadone	0.1–0.5 mg/kg	im	Opioid analgesic	Duration of action 3–4 h
Buprenorphine	5–20 µg/kg	im, iv or sc	Opioid analgesic	Duration ~6 h but individual variation
Medetomidine	10–30 µg/kg	iv, im or sc	Premedicant, sedative	Used alone or in combination with an opioid analgesic
Propofol	1–4 mg/kg in premedicated animal	iv	Induction agent	Can be used to maintain anaesthesia by continuous infusion or intermittent boluses. Smooth, rapid recovery
Alfaxolone	2 mg/kg in premedicated animal	Slow iv	Induction agent	Can be used to maintain anaesthesia by continuous infusion or intermittent boluses
Sevoflurane	7–8% for induction; 2–3% for maintenance	Inhaled	Fully potent anaesthetic	Good analgesia and muscle relaxation. Use dedicated calibrated vaporisers
Isoflurane	4–5% for induction; 2–3% for maintenance	Inhaled	Fully potent anaesthetic	Good analgesia and muscle relaxation. Use dedicated calibrated vaporisers
Pancuronium	0.06 mg/kg	iv	Non-depolarising muscle relaxant	May require specific licence authority; demands skilled assessment of anaesthesia and analgesia
Alphachloralose	80 mg/kg	Slow iv	Long-lasting anaesthetic	Duration 6–10 h. **Non-recovery only**
Urethane	1000 mg/kg	Slow iv	Long-lasting anaesthetic	Duration 6–10 h. **Non-recovery only**

be injected epidurally (Campoy 2004) to control post-surgical pain for extended periods, for example, after thoracotomy, with minimal systemic effects (Popilskis *et al.* 1991). Modern NSAIDs such as meloxicam, ketoprofen and carprofen can provide excellent relief of post-operative pain (Lascelles *et al.* 1994) and can be used either alone or in combination with opioids. Tramadol is an opioid agonist that inhibits the reuptake of noradrenaline and 5-HT, and stimulates pre-synaptic 5-HT release. It provides an alternative pathway for analgesia involving the descending inhibitory pathways within the spinal cord. It is available in a variety of formulations for human use but not yet widely used in dogs. However, it may be useful for the control of post-operative and chronic pain and avoid some of the side effects of NSAIDs.

An animal that has undergone surgery is vulnerable during the immediate post-operative period and it is essential that adequate facilities and care are available at this time. Even in the absence of emergencies, each animal should receive individual attention to ensure its safe recovery. Of paramount importance is the provision of warmth in the pen or cage. Adult dogs require an ambient temperature of 25 °C and puppies 32 °C and a heated mat may be used to provide local warmth. Food and water bowls should not be placed in the pen until the dog is aware of its surroundings, and no other animal should be present to interfere with the patient during the recovery period.

If an endotracheal tube has been used, this should be left in place until the swallowing reflex has returned, when it can be gently withdrawn. If recovery is prolonged, the animal should be turned from side to side every 30 minutes to prevent postural hypostatic lung congestion.

Regional nerve blocks can be used both during and after surgery to decrease the amount of other anaesthetic drugs needed and to lower the post-operative requirement for analgesics. Many minor surgical procedures can be performed under local or regional analgesia although it is usually necessary to provide sedation as an adjunct. Specific techniques for regional anaesthesia are described by Hall *et al.* (2001).

In the days following surgery, the dog should be observed to ensure that it is eating, drinking, defecating and urinating normally. Pain control should be carefully assessed. The surgical wound should be inspected daily and any sutures or staples removed 10 days post-operatively. Exercise should be restricted until this time.

Euthanasia

Euthanasia should be performed in the most humane manner possible to minimise both mental and physical suffering and should be carried out by trained and experienced personnel, preferably familiar with the animal to minimise the distress of being handled by a stranger. The bereavement distress to handlers can be considerable and should not be ignored (Arluke 1988). The World Society for the Protection of Animals (WSPA) provides excellent guidance on methods of euthanasia suitable for dogs (WSPA 2005) indicating those which are recommended, acceptable, conditionally acceptable and not acceptable. Any method used should produce rapid unconsciousness and subsequent death without evidence of pain or distress. It should be safe for the handlers, easy to perform and cause death without producing changes in tissues that might interfere with experimental results.

Intravenous injection of a lethal dose of barbiturate is the most common method of euthanasia of conscious dogs, normally by using a 20% pentobarbital solution rapidly injected at 150 mg/kg. The animal becomes anaesthetised within seconds and undergoes no pain or distress. Venepuncture is easily performed on most reasonably docile dogs by trained and experienced personnel. In anaesthetised animals, euthanasia can be carried out by overdose of barbiturates as above or by increasing the anaesthetic dose to a lethal level.

Physical methods of euthanasia such as shooting and electrocution are distasteful and dangerous to the operator and are no longer considered acceptable. Decapitation and drowning are not acceptable, even for very young puppies, and both are illegal in many countries.

Following euthanasia, death should always be verified (if necessary by waiting for rigor mortis to set in) before disposing of the carcase.

Common welfare problems

Health and disease

Prophylaxis

Dogs that are not in good health are always unsuitable for experimental work except in the investigation of naturally acquired or induced disease.

Dogs should be visually assessed daily to look for signs of health or disease (Table 30.5). It is important that carers are aware of differences in temperament and behaviour between individual dogs so that deviations from the norm are promptly recognised.

Regular, more detailed, health checks may be performed by trained technical staff and might include body weight, body condition, nail clipping, dental checks and ear cleaning. Blood samples might be taken for biochemical and haematological examination to assess health status. Routine prophylactic treatments might accompany such examinations and any necessary vaccinations administered and recorded.

In the event of concern, a veterinary surgeon should be consulted. This is important not only for the welfare of the animals involved, but also to prevent the spread of disease to other animals. In addition, the veterinary surgeon should regularly visit all areas to assure the quality of health and welfare of the dogs. The veterinary surgeon should also be responsible for the maintenance of comprehensive and accurate clinical records.

In addition, the environment should also be checked daily and recorded eg, temperature, humidity and effectiveness of ventilation.

Common diseases

Table 30.6 summarises significant infectious diseases in the dog. Clinical texts (Chandler 1994; Ettinger & Feldman 1994; Gaskell & Bennett 1996; Ramsey & Tennant 2001) should be consulted for a more comprehensive description including methods of diagnosis, prevention and treatment whilst Tilley and Smith (2004a) provide a simple reference handbook. Many diseases can vary in the severity of their clinical signs and thus in the presenting picture. Hence, an early diagnosis may be difficult but is essential if spread of disease to neighbouring animals is to be avoided. The diagnosis must normally be confirmed by laboratory tests and treatment and a strategy for control implemented immediately. For these reasons, laboratory dogs, whether in a breeding colony or involved in an experiment, should always be under the care of a veterinary surgeon with direct responsibility for their health and welfare.

These infectious diseases are generally of low incidence in well managed laboratory dog colonies. More common clinical problems may include fight wounds, lameness, dental disease, ear inflammation, hernias, histiocytomas and cryptorchidism as well as complications from experimental procedures. It is important that all such conditions are promptly identified as part of routine health checks and appropriately treated. Diarrhoea is a common clinical sign with a multitude of possible causes including a wide range of infectious agents as well as stressors, such as change of diet or accommodation, and experimental procedures –

Table 30.5 Signs of health in the dog.

Sign	*Description*
General appearance	Active, alert, responds to presence of humans and conspecifics. Stands on all four limbs evenly and is neither lame nor stiff, especially after rest. Responds normally to being handled. No uncharacteristic vocalisations
Appetite and weight	Good appetite. Some dogs are slow eaters whilst others consume their ration immediately. Not obese or thin. Normal water requirement varies (eg, with diet). Beware of sudden changes in weight, drinking or eating behaviour
Mouth	Teeth firm and clean. Gums pink, smooth and moist. Inflammation absent especially at gum margins. Absence of offensive smell
Eyes	Bright, clear; symmetrical appearance; absence of inflammation, discharge, irritation or opacities of the cornea or lens
Ears	Clean, non-irritant; absence of inflammation and offensive smell or discharge
Skin	Freely moveable, ribs and spine easily felt. No scratching; inflammation and lesions absent. Coat clean, unmatted and free from parasites and excessive scurf. No swellings or masses. No areas of hair loss
Respiration	Regular, effortless even after moderate exercise. Absence of cough. No nasal discharge
Urine	Clean, straw coloured. Pus and blood absent. No pain or straining or altered frequency of urination. Normal urine marking behaviour
Faeces	Firm, dark brown (colour and consistency varies with diet but should not be pale and bulky). Free from blood or mucus. No pain or straining on defecation

Table 30.6 Infectious diseases of the laboratory dog.

Name	*Causal agent*	*Clinical picture*	*Prevention*	*Comment*
Infectious canine hepatitis (ICH)	Adenovirus	Pyrexia, anorexia, vomiting and diarrhoea, general malaise. Congested mucosae, leucopenia; raised liver enzymes. Late stage 'blue-eye'	Vaccination	Following recovery, virus is eliminated in urine for several months
Canine distemper	Morbillivirus (paramyxovirus)	Pyrexia, oculonasal discharge, anorexia and diarrhoea. May be secondary pneumonia. Enamel hypoplasia; hardening of footpads and nose	Vaccination	Neurological signs may appear in adults following an earlier episode of the generalised disease
Canine parvovirus	Parvovirus	Vomiting, diarrhoea and dysentery with rapid dehydration	Vaccination	Disease not seen prior to 1978. Susceptible very young puppies may develop myocarditis with acute heart failure
Infectious canine tracheobronchitis (kennel cough)	*Bordetella bronchiseptica*, several viruses, ?*Mycoplasma* spp.	Sporadic outbreaks of mild respiratory disease with coughing	Vaccination available for *B. bronchiseptica* and parainfluenza virus	Occurs in kennels when dogs from different sources are mixed
Canine herpes virus (CHV)	Herpesvirus	Infertility, abortions, stillbirths. Neonatal neurological signs and death	Vaccination of bitch to protect puppies	Clinical disease rare in dogs older than 3–4 weeks
Rabies	Rhabdovirus	Usual route of infection via bite; neurological signs; fits or moroseness	Vaccination	Fatal zoonosis; invariably fatal in dogs
Leptospirosis	*Leptospira* serovars inc. *L. canicola* & *L. icterohaemorrhagiae*	Acute or chronic renal failure. Jaundice, severe depression and death	Vaccination together with rodent control	Chronic disease may occur following an earlier acute episode. Organism may be carried by rats
Brucellosis	*Brucella canis*	Abortion in female; orchitis in male	Screen new breeders	Zoonosis reported. Uncommon but problematical in a breeding colony
Ascariasis	Helminths, mainly *Toxacara canis*	Unthriftiness and diarrhoea in puppies. Abdominal distension	Regular anthelmintic treatment	Zoonotic. Treat pregnant and lactating bitch. Other helminths such as hookworm and lungworm as well as tapeworm also occur
Mange	Various mites inc. *Sarcoptes scabiei, Cheyletiella* spp. *Otodectes cynotis* and *Demodex canis*	Pruritis, alopecia and skin thickening. May become pustular. Infestation of ear causes severe irritation	Strict hygiene together with rodent and fox control. Topically applied acaricides	May be zoonotic. Examine incoming dogs very carefully to avoid introduction of mites
Ringworm	*Microsporum canis* & *Trichophyton* spp.	Discrete areas of alopecia and broken hairs	Isolation and disinfection	May be zoonotic. Treat systemically or topically

notably toxicology studies. Faecal examination may be revealing but the problem will often resolve spontaneously or with removal of the stressor.

Several spontaneously occurring disorders occur among laboratory dogs and are considered to have a genetic basis, including hypothyroidism due to lymphocytic thyroiditis, beagle neck pain syndrome (also known as neck pain syndrome, steroid responsive meningitis and necrotising vasculitis), distichiasis, cryptorchidism, prolapse of the gland of the third eyelid, idiopathic epilepsy and factor VII deficiency (Mustard *et al.* 2008).

Behavioural problems

It has been recognised for many years that dogs housed in restricted environments tend to develop behavioural abnormalities (stereotypies) generally considered indicative of poor welfare (Luescher *et al.* 1991). Such environments may be restricted either in the overall space available, or equally in the lack of stimulating features.

Hubrecht *et al.* (1992) studied various different types of housing in which dogs were spending substantial proportions of their time in stereotypic behaviour including repetitive jumping so the hindlegs leave the ground, circling around the pen, pacing usually along a fence, and social pacing in parallel with another dog on the other side of the fence. Whilst barking may be normal for the dog, in a colony situation some dogs develop a repetitive staccato barking which appears to have no communicative purpose and is often linked with other stereotypic behaviours.

Single housing of dogs is associated with passive and non-social repetitive behaviour probably due to the dog's efforts to offset boredom. Housing dogs in groups tends to be associated with non-repetitive social behaviour, high activity and investigation, together with low levels of aberrant repetitive behaviour. This is considered to be due to 'social buffering' associated with factors such as the complexity of the environment (Kikusui *et al.* 2006).

Provision of human contact may be of even greater social value than canine contact (Wolfle 1990) although it may only require a relatively small amount of time. Hubrecht (1995) tested the effect on young puppies of human socialisation and environmental enrichment with toys on ultimate adult behaviour. He found that human socialisation and even simple toys were enjoyed by puppies with benefits in adulthood. Means of managing behavioural problems in dogs are described by Horwitz *et al.* (2002).

Further reading

The range of manuals published by the British Small Animal Veterinary Association (BSAVA) provides excellent background information and clinical details for the dog including haematology (Day *et al.* 2000), urology (Elliott & Graver 2007), endocrinology (Mooney & Peterson 2004) and neurology (Platt & Olby 2004).

References

Animal Transportation Association (2000) *AATA Manual for the Transport of Live Animals*, 2nd edn. Animal Transportation Association, Redhill

Altman, P.L. and Dittmer, D.S. (1972, 1973 and 1974) *Biology Data Book*. 2nd edn. Vols. I–III. Federation of American Societies for Experimental Biology, Bethesda

Allen, W.E. (1992) *Fertility and Obstetrics in the Dog*. Blackwell Publishing, Oxford

Andersen, A.C. and Simpson, M.E. (1973) *The Ovary and Reproductive Cycle of the Dog (Beagle)*. Geron-x Inc, Los Altos, California

Arluke, A.B. (1988) Sacrificial symbolism in animal experimentation. Object or pet? *Anthrozoos*, **2**, 98–117

Barr, F. (1995) Percutaneous biopsy of abdominal organs under ultrasound guidance. *Journal of Small Animal Practice*, **36**, 105–113

Bebak, J. and Beck, A.M. (1993) The effect of cage size on play and aggression in purpose-bred beagles. *Laboratory Animal Science*, **43**, 457–459

Boitani, L., Francisci, F., Ciucci, P. *et al.* (1995) Population biology and ecology of feral dogs in central Italy. In: *The Domestic Dog: Evolution, Behaviour, and Interactions with People*. Ed. Serpell, J., pp. 217–244. Cambridge University Press, Cambridge

Boxall, J., Heath, S. and Brautigam, J. (2004) Modern concepts of socialisation for dogs: implications for their behaviour and use in procedures. *Alternatives to Laboratory Animals*, **32** (Suppl. 2), 81–93

Burke, T.M. and Roberson, E.L. (1983) Fenbendazole treatment of pregnant bitches to reduce prenatal and lactogenic infections of Toxacara canis and Ancylostoma caninum in pups. *Journal of the American Veterinary Medical Association*, **183**, 987–990

Campoy, L. (2004) Epidural and spinal anaesthesia in the dog. *In Practice*, **26**, 262–269

Chandler, E.A. (ed.) (1994) *Canine Medicine and Therapeutics*. Blackwell Publishing, Oxford

Chandra, S.A. and Adler, R.R. (2008) Frequency of different estrous stages in purpose-bred beagles: a retrospective study. *Journal of Toxiocological Pathology*, **36**, 944–949

Clutton-Brock, J. (1995) Origins of the dog: domestication and early history. In: *The Domestic Dog: Evolution, Behaviour and Interactions with People*. Ed. Serpell, J., pp. 7–20. Cambridge University Press, Cambridge

Concannon, P.W. and Battista, M. (1989) Canine semen freezing and artificial insemination. In: *Current Veterinary Therapy: Small Animal Practice, Vol. X*. Ed. Kirk, R.W., pp. 1247–1259. WB Saunders, Philadelphia

Concannon, P.W. and DiGregorio, G.B. (1986) Canine vaginal cytology. In: *Small Animal Reproduction and Infertility*. Ed. Burke, T., pp. 96–111. Lea and Febiger, Philadelphia

Council of Europe (2006) Multilateral Consultation of Parties to the European Convention for the Protection of Vertebrate Animals used for Experimental and other Scientific Purposes (ETS 123) Appendix A. *Cons 123 (2006) 3*. Available from URL: http://www.coe.int/t/e/legal_affairs/legal_co-operation/biological_safety,_use_of_animals/laboratory_animals/2006/Cons123(2006)3AppendixA_en.pdf (accessed 31 July 2008)

Day, M., Mackin, A. and Littlewood, J. (2000) *BSAVA Manual of Canine and Feline Haematology and Transfusion*. BSAVA, Cheltenham

Day, M.J., Horzinek, M.C. and Schultz, R.D. (2007) World Small Animal Veterinary Association Guidelines for the vaccination of dogs and cats. *Journal of Small Animal Practice*. http://www.wsava.org/PDF/Misc/VGG_09_2007.pdf (accessed 25 May 2009)

DeBowes, L.J., Mosier, D., Logan, E. *et al.* (1996) Association of periodontal disease and histologic lesions in multiple organs from 45 dogs. *Journal of Veterinary Dentistry*, **13**, 57–60

Department for Environment, Food and Rural Affairs (2007) Code of Practice for Quarantine Kennels and Catteries. http://www.defra.gov.uk/animalh/quarantine/quarantine/welfare/code-practice.htm (accessed 31 January 2009)

Edney, A.T.B. (1982) *Dog and Cat Nutrition*. Pergamon Press, Oxford

Elliott, J. and Graver, G.F. (2007) *BSAVA Manual of Canine and Feline Nephrology and Urology*, 2nd edn. BSAVA, Gloucester

England, G. (1993) Cryopreservation of dog semen: a review. *Journal of Reproduction and Fertility*, **47**, 243–255

England, G.C.W. (1998a) Pregnancy diagnosis, abnormalities of pregnancy and pregnancy termination. In: *BSAVA Manual of Small Animal Reproduction and Neonatology*. Eds Simpson, G., England, G. and Harvey, M., pp. 113–125. BSAVA, Gloucester

England, G.C.W. (1998b) Pharmacological control of reproduction in the dog and bitch. In: *BSAVA Manual of Small Animal Reproduction and Neonatology*. Eds Simpson, G., England, G. and Harvey, M., pp. 197–218. BSAVA, Gloucester

Ettinger, S.J. and Feldman, E.C. (eds) (1994) *Textbook of Veterinary Internal Medicine: Diseases of the Dog and Cat*. W.B. Saunders, London

European Commission (2007) Commission recommendations of 18 June 2007 on guidelines for the accommodation and care of animals used for experimental and other scientific purposes. Annex II to European Council Directive 86/609. See 2007/526/EC. http://eurlex.europa.eu/LexUriServ/site/en/oj/2007/l_197/l_19720070730en00010089.pdf (accessed 13 May 2008)

European Community (1986) Council Directive 86/609/EEC on the Approximation of Laws, Regulations and Administrative

Provisions of the Member States regarding the Protection of Animals used for Experimental and other Scientific Purposes. *Official Journal L358*. Official Journal of the European Communities, Luxembourg

European Community (2008) Proposal to revise Directive 86/609/EEC. http://eur-lex.europa.eu/LexUriServ/LexUriServ.do?uri=CELEX:52008PC0543:EN:NOT (accessed 15 February 2009)

Evans, H.E. (1993) *Miller's Anatomy of the Dog*, 3rd edn. WB Saunders, London

Farstad, W. (1998) Mating and artificial insemination in the dog. In: *BSAVA Manual of Small Animal Reproduction and Neonatology*. Eds Simpson, G., England, G. and Harvey, M., pp. 95–103. BSAVA, Gloucester

Federation of European Laboratory Animal Science Associations (1998) FELASA recommendations for the health monitoring of breeding colonies and experimental units of cats, dogs and pigs. *Laboratory Animals*, **32**, 1–17

Feldman, E.C. and Nelson, R.W. (1987) *Canine and Feline Endocrinology and Reproduction*. W.B. Saunders, Philadelphia

Fisher, M. (2001) Endoparasites in the dog and cat: 1. Helminths. *In Practice*, **23**, 462–471

Flecknell, P.A. (2009) *Laboratory Animal Anaesthesia*, 3rd edn. Academic Press, London

Fox, M.W. (1975) Evolution of social behaviour in canids. In: *The Wild Canids*. Ed. Fox M.W., pp. 429–460. Van Nostrand Reinhold, New York

Gaskell, R.M. and Bennett, M. (1996) *Feline and Canine Infectious Diseases*. Blackwell Publishing, Oxford

Griesemar, R.A. and Gibson, J.P. (1963) The gnotobiotic dog. *Laboratory Animal Science*, **13**, 643–649

Hall, E.J. (1994) Small intestinal disease – is endoscopic biopsy the answer? *Journal of Small Animal Practice*, **35**, 408–414

Hall, L.W., Clarke, K.W. and Trim, C.M. (2001) *Veterinary Anaesthesia*, 10th edn. Elsevier Science B.V., The Netherlands

Harvey, M. (1998) Conditions of the non-pregnant female. In: *BSAVA Manual of Small Animal Reproduction and Neonatology*. Eds Simpson, G., England, G. and Harvey, M., pp. 35–51. BSAVA, Gloucester

Hetts, S., Clark, J.D., Calpin, J.P. *et al.* (1992) Influence of housing conditions on beagle behaviour. *Applied Animal Behaviour Science*, **34**, 137–155

Home Office (2009) *Statistics of Scientific Procedures on Living Animals in Great Britain 2008*. http://rds.homeoffice.gov.uk/rds/scientific1.html (accessed 17 November 2009)

Horwitz, D., Mills, D. and Heath, S. (2002) *BSAVA Manual of Canine and Feline Behavioural Medicine*. BSAVA, Gloucester

Hubrecht, R.C. (1993) A comparison of social and environmental enrichment methods for laboratory housed dogs. *Applied Animal Behavioural Science*, **37**, 345–361

Hubrecht, R.C. (1995) Enrichment in puppyhood and its effects on later behavior of dogs *Laboratory Animal Science*, **45**, 70–75

Hubrecht, R.C. and Buckwell, A.C. (2004) The welfare of laboratory dogs. In: *The Welfare of Laboratory Animals*. Ed. Kaliste, E., pp. 245–273. Kluwer Academic Publishers, The Netherlands

Hubrecht, R.C., Sales, G., Peyvandi, A. *et al.* (1997) Noise in dog kennels; effects of design and husbandry. In: *Animal Alternatives, Welfare and Ethics*. Eds. van Zutphen, L.F.M and Balls, M., pp. 215–220. Elsevier Science B.V., The Netherlands

Hubrecht, R.C., Serpell, J.A. and Poole, T.B. (1992) Correlates of pen size and housing conditions on the behaviour of kennelled dogs. *Applied Animal Behavioural Science*, **34**, 365–383

International Air Transport Association (2009) *Live Animals Regulations*, 36th edn. IATA, Montreal, Quebec

Johnson, C.A. (1986) Reproduction and periparturient care. *Veterinary Clinics of North America*, **16**, 1–605

Johnston, S.D. and Romagnoli, S.E. (1991) Canine reproduction. *Veterinary Clinics of North America*, **21**, 421–640

Joint Working Group on Refinement (1993) Removal of blood from laboratory mammals and birds. First Report of the BVA/FRAME/RSPCA/UFAW Joint Working Group on Refinement. *Laboratory Animals*, **27**, 1–22

Joint Working Group on Refinement (2001) Refining procedures for the administration of substances. Report of the BVAAWF/FRAME/RSPCA/UFAW Joint Working Group on Refinement. *Laboratory Animals*, **35**, 1–41

Joint Working Group on Refinement (2004) Refining dog husbandry and care: Eighth report of the BVAAWF/FRAME/RSPCA/UFAW Joint Working Group on Refinement. *Laboratory Animals*, **38** (Suppl. 1), 1–94

Jones, D.E. and Joshua, J.O. (1988) *Reproductive Clinical Problems in the Dog*, 2nd edn. Wright, London, UK

Kaneko, J.J., Harvey, J.W. and Bruss, M.L. (2008) *Clinical Biochemistry of Domestic Animals*, 6th edn. Academic Press, San Diego

Kikusui, T., Winslow, J.T. and Mori, Y. (2006) Social buffering: relief from stress and anxiety. *Philosophical Transactions of the Royal Society*, **361**, 2215–2228

Kim, H.J., Oh, H.J., Jang, G. *et al.* (2007) Birth of puppies after intrauterine and intratubal insemination with frozen-thawed canine semen. *Journal of Veterinary Science*, **8**, 75–80

Klumpp, A., Trautmann, T., Markert, M. *et al.* (2006) Optimizing the experimental environment for dog telemetry studies. *Journal of Pharmacological and Toxicological Methods*, **54**, 141–149

Kortegaard, H.E., Eriksen, T. and Baelum, V. (2008) Periodontal disease in research beagle dogs – an epidemiological study. *Journal of Small Animal Practice*, **49**, 610–616

Kruesi, W.K. (2004) How to administer an intramuscular injection. http://www.crvetcenter.com/injection.htm (accessed 15 February 2009)

Kutzler, M. (2005) Induction and synchronisation of estrus in dogs. *Theriogenology*, **64**, 766–775

Kutzler, M.A., Yeager, A.E., Mohammed, H.O. *et al.* (2003) Accuracy of canine parturition date prediction using fetal measurements obtained by ultrasonography. *Theriogenology*, **60**, 1309–1317

Laboratory Animal Science Association (2004) *LASA Guidance on the Rehoming of Laboratory Dogs*. Eds. Jennings, M. and Howard, B. http://www.lasa.co.uk/synopsis_%20LASA_guidance_on_rehoming_dogs.html (accessed 25 May 2009)

Laboratory Animal Science Association (2005) Guidance on the transport of laboratory animals. Report of the Transport Working Group established by the Laboratory Animal Science Association (LASA). *Laboratory Animals*, **39**, 1–39

Lascelles, B.D.X., Butterworth, S.J. and Waterman, A.E. (1994) Postoperative analgesic and sedative effects of carprofen and pethidine in dogs. *Veterinary Record*, **134**, 187–191

Loeb, W.F. and Quimby, F.W. (1989) *The Clinical Chemistry of Laboratory Animals*. Pergamon Press, New York

Loveridge, G. (1994) Provision of environmentally enriched housing for dogs. *Animal Technology*, **45**, 1–19

Luescher, U.A., McKeown, D.B. and Halip, J. (1991) Stereotypic or obsessive-compulsive disorders in dogs and cats. Advances in companion animal behaviour. *Veterinary Clinics of North America Small Animal Practice*, **21**, 401–413

Macdonald, D.W. and Carr, G.M. (1995) Variation in dog society: between resource dispersion and social flux. In: *The Domestic Dog: Evolution, Behaviour, and Interactions with People*. Ed. Serpell, J., pp. 199–216. Cambridge University Press, Cambridge

Markwell, P.J. and Butterwick, R.F. (1994) Obesity. In: *The Waltham Book of Clinical Nutrition of the Dog and Cat*. Eds Wills, J.M. and Simpson, K.W., pp. 131–148. Pergamon Press, Oxford

Mooney, C. and Peterson, M. (2004) *BSAVA Manual of Canine and Feline Endocrinology*. BSAVA, Gloucester

Morton, D.B. and Bruce, S.G. (1989) Semen evaluation, cryopreservation and factors relevant to the use of frozen semen in dogs. *Journal of Reproduction and Fertility*, **39** (Suppl.), 311–316

Mustard, J.F., Secord, D., Hoeksma, T.D. *et al.* (2008) Canine factor-VII deficiency. *British Journal of Haematology*, **8**, 43–47
National Research Council, Board on Agriculture, Subcommittee on Dog Nutrition, Committee on Animal Nutrition (1985) *Nutrient Requirements of Dogs*. National Academy Press, Washington, DC
National Research Council, Institute of Laboratory Animal Resources, Committee on Dogs (1994) *Laboratory Animal Management; Dogs*. National Academy Press, Washington, DC
National Research Council, Institute of Laboratory Animal Resources, Commission on Life Sciences (1996) *Guide for the Care and Use of Laboratory Animals*. National Academy Press, Washington, DC
National Research Council, Institute of Laboratory Animal Resources, Committee on Scientific and Humane Issues in the Use of Random Source Dogs and Cats in Research (2009) *Scientific and Humane Issues in the Use of Random Source Dogs and Cats in Research*. National Academy Press, Washington, DC
O'Donoghue, P.N. (1993) *The Accommodation of Laboratory Animals in Accordance with Animal Welfare Requirements*. Proceedings of an international workshop held at the Bundesgesundheitsamt, Berlin 17–19 May 1993
Olson, H., Betton, G., Robinson, D. *et al.* (2000) Concordance of the toxicity of pharmaceuticals in humans and in animals. *Regulatory Toxicology and Pharmacology*, **32**, 56–67
Ostrander, E.A. and Wayne, R.K. (2005) The canine genome. *Genome Research*, **15**, 1706–1716
Patterson, D.F. (2000) *Canine Genetic Disease Information System: A Computerized Knowledge Base of Genetic Diseases in the Dog*. Mosby-Harcourt, St Louis
Platt, S. and Olby N. (2004) *BSAVA Manual of Canine and Feline Neurology*, 3rd edn. BSAVA, Gloucester
Popilskis, S., Kohn, D., Sanchez, J.A. *et al.* (1991) Epidural versus intramuscular oxymorphone analgesia after thoracotomy in dogs. *Veterinary Surgery*, **20**, 462–467
Ramsey, I. and Tennant, B. (2001) *BSAVA Manual of Canine and Feline Infectious Diseases*. BSAVA, Gloucester
Raskin, R.E. (1993) Bone marrow. In: *Textbook of Small Animal Surgery*, 2nd edn. Ed. Slatter, D., pp. 942–948. W.B. Saunders Company, Philadelphia
Redding, R.W. and Knecht, C.E. (1983) *An Atlas of Electroencephalography in the Dog and Cat*. Praeger Scientific, New York
Rushton, B. (1981) *Veterinary Laboratory Data*. British Veterinary Association, London
Sales, G., Hubrecht, R.C. and Peyvandi, A. (1996) Noise in dog kennelling: a survey of noise levels and the causes of noise in animal shelters, training establishments and research institutions. *Animal Welfare Research Report No. 9*. Universities Federation for Animal Welfare, Potters Bar
Sales, G., Hubrecht, R.C., Peyvandi, A. *et al.* (1997) Noise in dog kennelling: Is barking a welfare problem for dogs? *Applied Animal Behaviour Science*, **52**, 321–329
Serpell, J. (1995) *The Domestic Dog: Evolution, Behaviour, and Interactions with People*. Cambridge University Press, Cambridge
Seymour, C. and Gleed, R. (Eds) (1999) *BSAVA Manual of Small Animal Anaesthesia and Analgesia*. pp. 312. BSAVA, Cheltenham
Shepherd, K (2002) Development of behaviour, social behaviour and communication in dogs. In: *BSAVA Manual of Canine and Feline Behavioural Medicine*. Eds. Horwitz, D.F., Mills, D.S. and Heath, S., pp. 8–20. BSAVA, Gloucester
Shille, V.M., Calderwood-Mays, M.B. and Thatcher, M.J. (1984) Infertility in a bitch associated with short interestrous intervals and cystic follicles: a case report. *Journal of the American Animal Hospitals Association*, **20**, 171–176
Shultz, F.T. (1970) Genetics. In: *The Beagle as an Experimental Dog*. Ed. Andersen, A.C., pp. 489–509. Iowa State University Press, Ames, Iowa
Simpson, J.W. and Anderson, R.S. (1993) *Clinical Nutrition of the Dog and Cat*. Blackwell Publishing, Oxford
Sommerville, B.A. and Broom, D.M. (1998) Olfactory awareness. *Applied Animal Behavioural Science*, **57**, 269–286
Spurling, N.W. (1977) Haematology of the dog. In: *Comparative Clinical Haematology*. Eds. Archer, R.K. and Jeffcott, L.B., pp. 365–440. Blackwell Publishing, Oxford
Switonski, M. (2004) Gene mutations causing hereditary diseases in dogs. *Animal Science Papers and Reports*, **22**, 131–134
Tilley, L.P. (ed) (1992) *Essentials of Canine and Feline Electrocardiography*. Lea and Febiger, Philadelphia
Tilley, L.P. and Smith, F.W.K. (2004a) *The 5-Minute Veterinary Consult: Canine and Feline*, 3rd edn. Lippincott Williams and Wilkins, Philadelphia
Tilley, L.P. and Smith, F.W.K. (2004b) Dystocia. In: *The 5-Minute Veterinary Consult: Canine and Feline*, 3rd edn. pp. 382–383. Lippincott Williams and Wilkins, Philadelphia
Tobias, K. (2007) How I obtain surgical gastrointestinal biopsy specimens. In: *Scientific Proceedings of BSAVA Congress, April 2007*. BSAVA, Gloucester
Tontodonati, M., Fasdelli, N., Moscardo, E. *et al.* (2007) A canine model used to simultaneously assess potential neurobehavioural and cardiovascular effects of candidate drugs. *Journal of Pharmacological and Toxicological Methods*, **56**, 265–275
Vanderlip, S.L., Vanderlip, J.E. and Myles, S. (1985a) A socializing program for laboratory raised canines. *Lab Animal*, **14**, 33–36
Vanderlip, S.L., Vanderlip, J.E. and Myles, S. (1985b) A socializing program for laboratory raised canines. Part 2: The puppy socialization schedule. *Lab Animal*, **14**, 27–36
Willis, M.B. (1989) *Genetics of the Dog*. H. F. and G. Witherby, London
Wolfle, T.L. (1990) Policy, program and people; the three P's to well-being. In: *Canine Research Environment*. Eds Mench, J.A. and Krulisch, L., pp. 41–47. Scientists Center for Animal Welfare, Bethesda
World Society for the Protection of Animals (2005) Methods for the euthanasia of dogs and cats: comparison and recommendations. http://www.icam-coalition.org/downloads/Methods%20for%20the%20euthanasia%20of%20dogs%20and%20cats-%20English.pdf (accessed 15 February 2009)
Wright, P. and Watts, J.R. (1998) The infertile female. In: *BSAVA Manual of Small Animal Reproduction and Neonatology*. Eds Simpson, G., England, G. and Harvey, M., pp. 17–33. BSAVA, Gloucester
Yeager, A.E. and Concannon, P.W. (1990) Association between the preovulatory luteinizing hormone surge and the early ultrasonographic detection of pregnancy and fetal heartbeats in beagle dogs. *Theriogenology*, **34**, 655–665

31 The domestic cat

Sandra McCune

Biological overview

General biology

The domestic cat *Felis silvestris catus* used in laboratories is the same species that is commonly kept as a companion animal and which exists in substantial numbers in a feral state. Cats are intelligent, highly specialised mammals that have evolved a range of morphological adaptations and sensory abilities to suit their exclusively carnivorous lifestyle (reviewed by Bradshaw 1992). A cat's perception of the world is therefore different from ours. Hunting by sight at night means they see in lower light intensities than we can and are particularly sensitive to rapid movement. They are not, however, able to see in fine detail or to discriminate clearly between shades of colour (Bradshaw 1992). They also hunt by sound and are very sensitive to the ultrasonic frequencies that rodents use to communicate. Their sensitive sense of smell helps them to locate prey although, in the final stages of a kill, touch is the dominant sense. Smell is also used to select food while a second olfactory system (the vomeronasal organ) is used in social communication. Sebaceous glands are located throughout the body, especially on the head and the peri-anal area, and between the digits. Scratching, which deposits scent from the interdigital glands, is a marking behaviour which leaves visual and olfactory signals, and helps to maintain the claws in good shape (Rochlitz 2005). The deposition of urine and faeces, and rubbing of the body against objects, may also be used in olfactory signalling. Allo-rubbing, where cats rub their face and body against each other and intertwine their tails, serves to exchange scent profiles between cats.

Standard biological data are listed in Table 31.1.

Size range and lifespan

Average domestic cats weigh between 2 and 5 kg. Males are significantly heavier than females. There are breed differences; American Ragdolls or Maine Coons can be three times heavier than the average, whilst the small Singapura weighs a mere 2–3 kg. Well cared for domestic cats can, on average, expect to live for about 12 years and many cats live into their twenties.

Social organisation of free-ranging cats

Cats can adapt to a wide range of population densities. Feral cat populations range from densities of 1–2000/km^2 (Izawa *et al.* 1982; Izawa 1984; Kerby & Macdonald 1988). The social system feral cats adopt depends upon the distribution and availability of resources. The home ranges of breeding males are usually much larger than those of females. The sizes of their home ranges are determined by both food supply and social considerations (including availability of breeding females, whether females are solitary or social and the degree of competition for females). Male home ranges encompass the territories of several breeding females. The home ranges of females are determined by the needs for shelter and food both for themselves and for any dependent young. Where cats have to support themselves solely by hunting, they are often solitary as their prey is unlikely to be sufficiently abundant to sustain a social group. If food is more common but patchily distributed, then the home ranges of cats may overlap though they would rarely hunt in the same area at the same time.

Social groups exist where food is locally concentrated; usually as a result of human activities (Kerby & Macdonald 1988). These groups are basically matrilineal, consisting of females, usually related, and their offspring (including immature males). The size of the groups is very variable and seems to be determined largely by food availability, mortality amongst kittens from a range of infectious diseases and extermination by humans. Females are tolerant of other members in the group but defend their communal core area (containing their den and major source of food) aggressively against intruders. Their aggression intensifies if there are young kittens in the group. This exclusion of outsiders makes it difficult for females to move between groups. Males tend to disperse away from their mother's home range when they are 2 or 3 years old. Initially they avoid contact with all other cats but as they mature and get stronger they will challenge other males for access to females. Mature males are only loosely associated with any group but in areas where most females are group-living, a particular male may concentrate his mating efforts within a single group. Further information on cat behaviour can be found in Thorne (1992); Beaver (2003) and in the American

Table 31.1 Standard biological data for the cat (after Hurni & Rossbach 1987).

Parameter	Value
Age of replacement of deciduous dentition (months)	3.5–6
Life expectancy (years)	9–14 (over 20 has been recorded)
Body weight:	
Female (non-breeding) (kg)	3–4
Male (kg)	3–7
Birth (g)	110 ± 20
Respiration rate (/min)	16–40
Volume (ml)	12–15 (0.3–0.4l/min)
Arterial blood pressure (mmHg)	120/75
pH	7.35
Blood volume:	
Total (ml/kg body weight)	75
Maximum single sample (ml/kg body weight)	7
Pulse rate (/min)	150–200 (range 120–220)
Body temperature (°C)	38–39.5
Dental formulae:	
Deciduous	$2\ (I^3{}_3C^1{}_1Pm^3{}_2) = 26$
Permanent	$2\ (I^3{}_3C^1{}_1Pm^3{}_2M^1{}_1) = 30$
Oestrous cycle (days)	14 (anovular)
Gestation (days)	65.5 ± 1.7
Litter size	3–6 (range 1–10)
Lactation (weeks)	7
Weaning (weeks)	4–7

Association of Feline Practitioners Feline Behaviour Guidelines[1].

Reproduction

Under optimum conditions, females become sexually mature at around 9 months (range 4–18 months). Males (toms) are sexually mature by 8 months though some may be fertile earlier. Cats are normally seasonal breeders in temperate climates. Toms are most sexually active in spring though they can sire kittens at any time of the year. Females will breed all year round if they are kept indoors with no exposure to sunlight and with a 12:12 hour light–dark regime. Most oestrous cycles last between 18 and 24 days. Oestrus lasts about 4 days if mating occurs but otherwise between 5 and 10 days. Cats are induced ovulators (although see Lawler *et al.* 1991), with foreplay and coitus stimulating ovulation. Sterile copulation may result in pseudopregnancy which lasts about 36 days. Successful pregnancies last about 63 days (range 58–72 days). Females are capable of coming into oestrus 3–4 weeks after a litter is weaned.

The average litter size is 4 (typical range 3–10), with 104 males born to every 100 females. Maximum litter size is usually reached by the third litter. Females are optimally fertile between the ages of 1 and 8; subsequently their oestrous cycles may become irregular and litters are fewer and smaller. Although sperm quality declines with age, males can remain fertile into their twenties.

[1]http://www.aafponline.org/resources/guidelines/Feline_Behavior_Guidelines.pdf

Breeds, strains and genetics

A recent genetic assessment of 979 domestic cats and their wild progenitors – *Felis silvestris silvestris* (European wildcat), *F. s. lybica* (Near Eastern/north African wildcat), *F. s. ornata* (central Asian wildcat), *F. s. cafra* (southern African wildcat) and *F. s. bieti* (Chinese desert cat) – indicates that each wild group represents a distinctive subspecies of *Felis silvestris* (Driscoll *et al.* 2007). As *F. s. lybica* and domestic cats fall into the same genetic clade (a group of species with the same ancestor), it is likely that the *lybica* subspecies gave rise to the genetic lineage that eventually produced all domesticated cats. Cats were domesticated in the Fertile Crescent of the Near East and north Africa, probably coincident with the development of agricultural villages where cats fed on the rodents that infested the grain stores of the first farmers. The first evidence of cat remains buried together with human remains was found in Cyprus, and determined to be 9500 years old (Vigne *et al.* 2004). The earliest evidence for domestication comes from Egypt in the third millennium BC (Linseele *et al.* 2007)

Cats have not been subject to intensive selective breeding programmes with most breeds originating in single gene mutations or a few combinations. The concept of cat breeds dates from the nineteenth century. Breeds are classified into British (European or American) and Foreign on the basis of head shape, body conformation and coat quality. British types are stocky with a heavier coat. Foreign types are slender and smooth coated. Breeds are also classified by hair length; Short-hairs and Long-hairs. The difference is due to a single gene, the allele for long coat being recessive. A more recent hair mutation has resulted in three new breeds; the Cornish Rex, the Devon Rex and the American Wire-hair. Colour varieties are caused by less than a dozen mutations. Most seem to affect only pigmentation but that producing blue-eyed white cats is linked with timidity, deafness, elevated mortality and poor mothering ability. Breeders are now producing breeds in several colours; blurring the distinction between breeds and varieties (a full account of breeds and varieties is provided by Vella *et al.* 1999).

Sources of supply

It is good practice, and a legal requirement in some countries (eg, in the European Union), for cats to be bred and obtained from approved establishments. Many laboratories use specific pathogen free (SPF) cats which will need to come from recognised SPF sources. These cats should be free from viral and chlamydial upper respiratory disease, FeLV (feline leukaemia virus), FIV (feline immunodeficiency virus), coronavirus and both ectoparasites and endoparasites. Cats should be quarantined for at least 3 weeks before joining the colony. Cats from random sources would need a 6 week quarantine as their disease status would be unknown. They might also have behavioural and handling problems.

Management and breeding

General husbandry

Husbandry systems should use best health care practices, which emphasise good welfare and meet the animals' behavioural needs. Systems should provide safe, comfortable, animal-friendly conditions, environmental choice for the animal, sensory stimulation, physical and mental exercise and should minimise disease. Detailed recommendations for cat housing exist (eg, Home Office 1989; European Commission 2007) and provide guidelines on the design, construction and security of animal facilities; and on the environmental conditions within the facility, encompassing guidelines for temperature, relative humidity, ventilation and lighting). There are examples of innovative design incorporating elements intended to meet cats' behavioural needs (Loveridge 1994; Loveridge *et al.* 1995).

Housing

Cats can be kept outdoors or indoors. Considerations of environmental control, costs and disease transmission mean most colonies are kept in closed indoor accommodation. Housing needs to be easy to clean and maintain, and compatible with the requirements of laboratory studies. Using several individual buildings reduces the potential for disease to spread throughout a colony (Hawthorne *et al.* 1995).

Group housing

Groupings should take account of density recommendations. In the UK for group-housed cats, recommended minimum floor area per cat is 3300 cm^2 for cats weighing up to 3 kg and 5000 cm^2 for cats weighing over 3 kg (Home Office 1989). This rises to 5000 cm^2 and 7500 cm^2 respectively when cats are housed singly. The revised guidelines of the European Convention for the Protection of Vertebrate Animals used for Experimental and Other Scientific Purposes (ETS 123), Appendix A (Council of Europe 2006), and the revised Annex II to the European Directive 86/609 (European Commission 2007) require a minimum floor area of 1.5 m^2 and shelving of 0.5 m^2, with another 0.75 m^2 of floor space and 0.25 m^2 of shelf space for every additional cat; and that the cage should be 2 m high.

A critical minimum cage size has not been established for cats. Some cats will show behaviour problems when confined in cages with the dimensions given above. Indeed, some free-ranging cats will show behaviour problems. However, cats with restricted access to outdoors are more commonly presented with behaviour problems than free-ranging cats so it appears that space is limiting to some individuals even in relatively enriched home settings. The response of the individual to confinement varies widely and is based on many factors. The most important of these is likely to be quality of the confined space and the cat's previous experience. Investing in the quality of the space rather than the quantity may often result in a better outcome for the cat.

The cat, having originated from a largely solitary-living species, has not developed the complex visual signalling that is typical of species that have had a long evolutionary history of social living, such as the domestic dog. As a result, lacking or having limited signals for avoiding conflict such as appeasement (Casey 2007b), and post-conflict mechanisms such as reconciliation (van den Bos 1998), they do not form distinct dominance hierarchies. Usually, cats will avoid physical confrontation by using behaviours to maintain distance, such as olfactory marking, posturing and vocalisation. Alternatively, they may try to evade threats from other cats by hiding or fleeing to elevated locations. If housing conditions in the laboratory do not provide for these responses, cats may end up in aggressive encounters with each other.

The maintenance of groups is influenced by factors that include familiarity, stability, socialisation to other cats and availability of resources. Sibling pairs of cats have more amicable relationships than unrelated cats living together (Bradshaw & Hall 1999), and close social bonds may also develop between unrelated kittens that are raised together. Attention to the socialisation of cats with other cats at a young age will make them more tolerant of others in adulthood. Optimal socialisation to humans occurs if kittens are handled between the second and seventh week of life (Karsh & Turner 1988), and it is generally accepted that the period of socialisation of kittens to other cats also occurs during this time (Rochlitz 2005).

Housing cats at high densities increases the likelihood of their being stressed. While housing in groups provides opportunities for complex social interactions and so increases mental and physical stimulation (Figure 31.1), group composition should be kept fairly constant to avoid disrupting established group dynamics. Social cohesion is maintained through behaviours such as allo-rubbing, which involves tactile communication and the mixing and exchange of scent, such that all individuals in the group have a shared scent profile. The frequent addition of new cats into a group disrupts relationships and introduces new olfactory profiles that interfere with social cohesion.

When cats are housed in groups, attention should be paid to the availability of resources (food, toileting sites, resting and hiding areas). Resources should be distributed in a number of places to prevent certain animals from monopolising one area, and to enable them to avoid conflict with others when accessing these resources. Cats which fail to adapt to a particular social group, for example those which avoid contact with all other group members, should be rehoused, either with a smaller group or singly.

Individual housing

Sometimes cats need to be housed individually. For instance; post-/pre-parturition females; mature males; sick, injured or quarantined individuals; or as a necessary part of a specific research programme. The most specialised or extreme form of single housing is probably the metabolism cage which is used, for example, to facilitate the reliable collection and assessment of faeces. These cages are usually made of metal

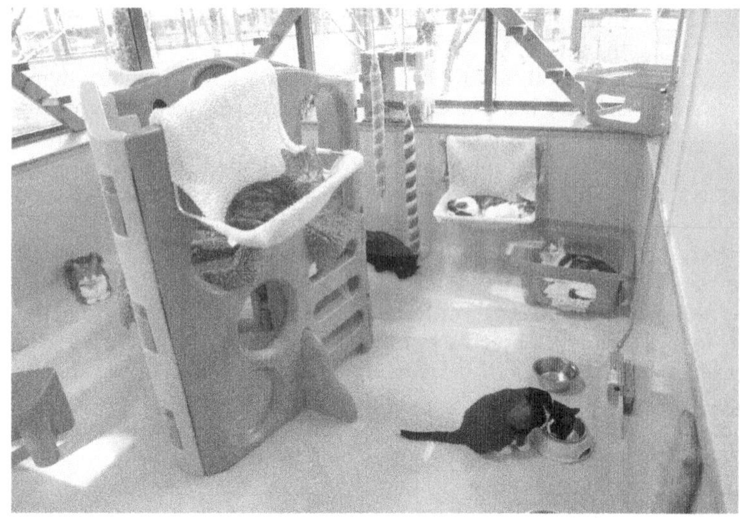

Figure 31.1 Enriched housing provides opportunities for play, social contact and privacy.

(often stainless steel) with mesh floors. They can be stressful to the cats confined in them in many ways. The accommodation may be unfamiliar to the animal if it is normally group-housed. The cages are usually small and so lack space for normal movement. They provide only a barren environment; devoid of comfort and facilities providing physical and mental stimulation. The enforced social isolation may also cause stress to cats that are used to social contact with others. These cages should be made as appealing as possible with the addition of resting boards with covers, toys and visual observation of other cats and should be used for as short a time as possible.

In response to the need to improve upon such cages, Loveridge and co-workers (1995) developed a system of two-roomed lodges which provide individually housed cats with an enriched environment, freedom of choice, mental and physical stimulation and conditions as similar as possible to those in the main colony (Figure 31.2). Extensive use of glass throughout the building allows the individually housed animals to be visually stimulated by those on either side, by human and cat activity within the colony, and by activity in the grounds outside the colony building. Individually housed cats should have access to a larger exercise area space and be given some personal attention every day (Figure 31.3). Even more recently, an organisation has developed a mechanical litter tray system that allows urine and faeces to be collected from specific cats housed in their normal group housing. Users should explore the possibilities of these techniques before resorting to metabolism cages.

Environmental provisions

An important objective of good housing is to improve welfare by giving the animal a degree of control over its environment and the opportunity to make choices (Broom & Johnson 1993). Good laboratory housing for cats should include a range of shelving at different heights, and a choice of resting and hiding places. Timid cats and those less well integrated into the social group will occupy the higher shelves (Rochlitz *et al.* 1995), particularly those in corners as

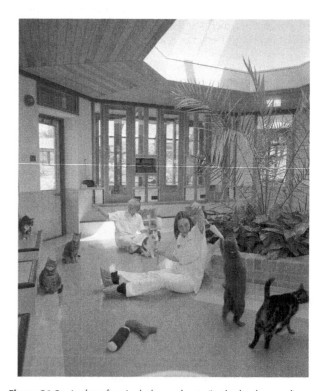

Figure 31.2 Lodges for singly housed cats (in the background) can be built around central areas of activity to provide visual stimulation.

they provide the best vantage points and protect the cat from being approached from behind. Cats spend a large portion of their day either resting or sleeping, so it is important that there are plenty of rest areas with comfortable surfaces.

Hiding is a coping behaviour that cats often show in response to stimuli or changes in their environment (Rochlitz 2005). It is commonly seen when cats want to avoid interactions with other cats or people, and in response to other potentially stressful situations. A recent study investigated the effect of hiding enrichment on stress and behaviour of kennelled cats (Kry & Casey 2007). The hiding enrichment

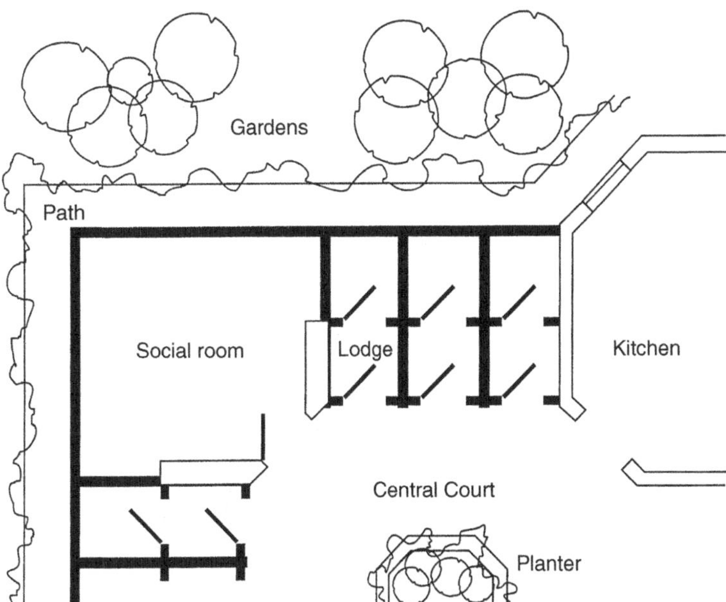

Figure 31.3 Section through a facility providing single and group housing for cats (from Loveridge *et al.* 1995). Reproduced with kind permission of Waltham Centre for Pet Nutrition.

consisted of a cardboard box (Hide, Perch and Go® box, British Columbia SPCA), whilst control animals were provided with an open bed. A significant reduction in stress was noted in the enriched group: these cats were more likely to approach humans and displayed relaxed behaviours much more frequently.

Visual barriers can be useful, to enable cats to get out of sight of others and also to break up the three-dimensional space into sections or compartments, making it more complex and giving the cat more choice about where it wants to be (Rochlitz 2005). Housing should incorporate features to provide opportunities for stimulation, and for environmental and social choice. For example: provision of internal windows to enable cats to watch other cats and human activity; internal arrangement of pens incorporating different levels to increase usable space and give opportunities for climbing, for example by imaginative use of shelving, climbing poles and ropes; semi-hidden spaces to explore or to withdraw from the group, for example, plastic hollow cubes, large children's toys etc which can be moved from group to group; experience of the natural environment either by direct access (which may not be possible in a minimal disease system) or through glass.

Olfactory enrichment is relatively underused in animal housing, perhaps because of the relatively poor sense of smell of humans compared with many other species. Surfaces for the deposition of olfactory and visual signals and for claw abrasion, such as scratch posts, rush matting, pieces of carpet and wood, should be provided.

Presentation of food and water

Fresh water should always be available and, ideally, replenished constantly from a chlorinated mains supply. Some cats prefer to drink from a water fountain. Food should be kept fresh. Removing food for a period each day seems to renew the cats' interest.

Identification and sexing

In small colonies cats can be identified by their markings and other characteristics. Microchip implants provide a secure, safe and permanent method of identifying individuals. Insertion of the microchips is less painful than tattooing. Collars can be used but their fit needs to be checked regularly and they are unsuitable for very young kittens. Cats can be sexed at birth from the ano-genital distance (about 6 mm in females and 13 mm in males).

Physical environment and hygiene

The physical environment should be monitored, and ambient temperature and humidity adjusted for comfort (15–24 °C and 55% ± 10% relative humidity are recommended by the UK Home Office (1989)). Rather than having a homogeneous environment, creating a range of micro-environments is preferable as this provides a cat with some choice, for example: heated beds; sun-warmed ledges; and shaded lying areas. Even in single metabolism cages, a single shelf at least provides some choice of location for the individual. Good ventilation is important to dilute and remove air-borne pathogens and to disperse heat produced by animals and equipment. Cats need protection from extremes of heat and housing will need extractor fans, blinds or solar-absorbing glass and reflective film.

The combination of good design and an effective cleaning regimen will minimise disease transmission. All rooms and litter trays, 'furniture' and other surfaces within, need daily cleaning with detergent and disinfectant. Cleaning materials need to be chosen carefully as cats are particularly sensitive to phenolic compounds. Aerosolisation of phenolics can result in corneal lesions if the cats remain in the room during cleaning. Chlorhexidine appears to be a safe and effective disinfectant for cat rooms (suggestions in Hawthorne *et al.* 1995). Bedding should be disposable or washable. Only small quantities of food should be stored within the buildings to avoid attracting vermin and this should be kept in vermin-proof containers. Every care should be taken to avoid any wild, stray or pet animals entering the animal facility. Particular care needs to be taken with drains and other services that penetrate the fabric of the building and so allow a potential route into the animal rooms.

Health monitoring, quarantine and barrier systems

Cats should be handled frequently and checked daily; handling and restraint techniques were reviewed by Wills, J. (1993). Every week they should have a specific health check (ears, eyes, nose, genitalia and general body condition), be groomed and weighed (Figure 31.4). Twice a year they should have a dental examination and a haematology and biochemistry screen. Colonies should be screened for viruses, bacteria and parasites. Viral screening should occur on an epidemiological basis. Assuming a low incidence of disease a large number of cats may need to be screened to find a problem. Any unexpected death should be thoroughly investigated.

The probability of cats contracting an infectious disease depends on a number of factors, including: age; genetic predisposition; nutritional status; levels of stress; concurrent illness; level of infectious disease challenge and virulence of the infectious organism.

Separate facilities should be provided for the isolation of suspected infected cats and for those in quarantine. Isolation facilities should be completely self-contained and, ideally, in a separate building from the main colony. Disease transmission can be limited further by housing all cats according to their susceptibility. Preferably each susceptibility group should be handled by different personnel, otherwise the sequence in which they are handled should be on a susceptibility basis from most to least susceptible, eg: early-weaned kittens; queens with kittens; older cats; quarantine cats; and finally sick cats. Further details are given by Hawthorne *et al.* (1995).

Transport

Cats are not good travellers. Travel causes stress in many individuals and therefore should be kept to a minimum (McCune 1994). Journeys of over 10h duration appear to be especially stressful (Bradshaw & Holloran 2005). Preferably cats should be accompanied to ensure their safety and welfare. If cats are to travel unaccompanied, across borders, or by air, sea or rail then special regulations will probably apply. Each country and carrier will have its own regulations regarding animal transport. Cats appreciate being able to look out of their carrier. SPF cats will need to be protected from infection during transit. Cats travelling by air will require containers approved by the *International Air Transport Association* (*IATA*) who revise their regulations annually (see also Chapter 13 and Laboratory Animal Science Association (LASA) 2005).

Breeding

For general advice see Wills, M.B. (1993).

Condition of adults

Cats are sexually mature at 8–9 months of age. Cats that begin to cycle and are not bred are likely to develop uterine pathology that decreases reproductive performance. Therefore, if the colony has reproduction as a goal, queens should be placed into a harem in their first year. At the Waltham Centre for Pet Nutrition queens are retired at 8 years and toms are retired at 10 years, but other breeders may continue to use their breeding animals for longer than this if they remain in good health.

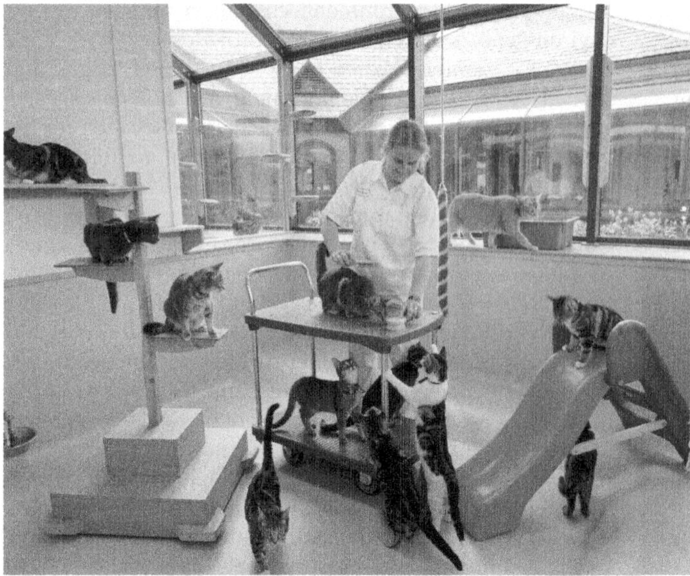

Figure 31.4 Regular health checks and grooming are essential to ensure the well-being of individuals.

Identifying the fertile state

Anoestrous females will respond aggressively to any sexual approach by a male. Females in pro-oestrus show subtle changes in their behaviour; they tend to be rather restless and rub up against objects. They allow males to approach but prolonged contact is not tolerated. Over the next 24 h the females rub their head and flank against objects with increasing intensity, they roll on the floor, stretch, purr and rhythmically open and close their paws, flexing their claws. At this stage they will tolerate grooming by the male but not mounting. Full sexual receptivity is indicated by females adopting the lordosis position; the female crouches with her head close to the ground, her hindlegs treading and partly extended, and her tail laterally displaced to expose the perineum (UK Cat Behaviour Working Group 1995).

Mating systems

In the harem or group mating system, ideally one male cat is kept in a group of females. The dominant male will usually mate with more than 80% of the females. A potential difficulty with this system is that the exact date of mating is not known and pregnancy is determined by the female gaining weight (Figure 31.5). The female should be moved to kittening accommodation 10–14 days before birth is due to allow her to habituate to the new surroundings.

A second, but perhaps less welfare friendly, system is to house females together in groups and to accommodate the males in individual housing. When signs of oestrus are observed, the female is taken to the chosen male and mated a number of times. Males need to be replaced regularly to avoid inbreeding. The advantage of this system is that parentage and date of mating are known. The disadvantage for the singly housed males is they have relatively little social contact with other cats.

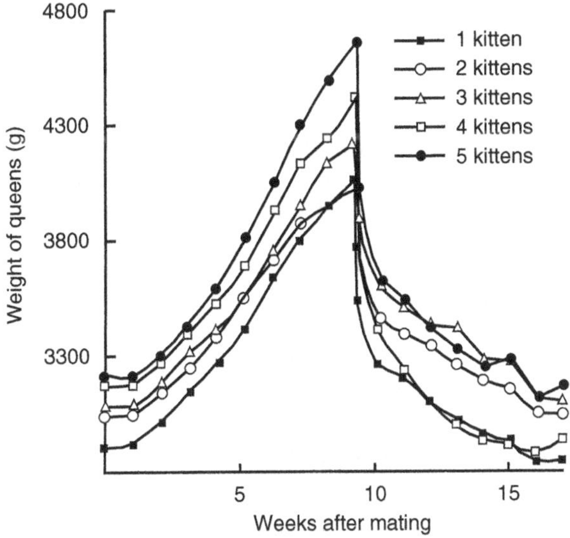

Figure 31.5 Weight changes during gestation and lactation in queens with different litter sizes (group size = 15) (from Loveridge & Rivers 1989). Reproduced with kind permission of Waltham Centre for Pet Nutrition.

Conception and pregnancy

Ovulation is triggered by mating, possibly from the stimulation of the tom withdrawing his barbed penis. After copulation both cats wash their urinogenital area, the female continues to roll for about 30 minutes before they mate again. Multiple copulations are normally required to trigger ovulation. Females may mate many times and with different males. Pregnancy can be reliably diagnosed by palpation at 21–28 days, by ultrasound after 21 days and by radiography after 40–45 days. Pregnancy can be assessed by monitoring weight gain, and weight gain also gives some indication of the size of the litter (Loveridge 1986).

Nesting

Cats do not usually build nests but make use of whatever protective shelter is available; they will usually make use of boxes, newspaper, cardboard or other forms of bedding if provided. They like to choose where to give birth, and may visit suitable sites several times before coming to a decision. Some cats prefer dark, quiet places; a box provided in the breeding area will generally be used. Occasionally cats will transfer their kittens to a new nest site.

Parturition

Group-housed pregnant cats are moved to separate accommodation about 10 days before parturition to protect the newborn kittens from attack. Feral queens living in social groups do use communal dens and collaborate to nurse each other's offspring; in large groups it tends to be mothers and daughters co-operating but in small groups all adult females may nurse each other's offspring, (Bradshaw 1992). Confined females have been known to kill newborn kittens. Infanticide by tomcats has also been recorded.

Before giving birth the queen cleans herself thoroughly, particularly her ventrum around the nipples, and her anogenital area. Parturition is usually uneventful. The kittens are born at 2–30-minute intervals. After the birth the queen removes the amniotic sac from around the kitten, severs the umbilical cord, eats the placenta and licks the kitten clean which stimulates its breathing. After delivery of the last kitten, the queen then encircles her litter and encourages them to suckle by nuzzling and licking them. Kittens find the nipple and suckle spontaneously using innate reflexes. Suckling must be established promptly as neonatal kittens cannot withstand even short periods without food and need to acquire maternal antibodies from the milk. The mother will remain in contact with the kittens for at least the first 24 h. For the first month the queen spends about 70% of her time in the nest caring for her kittens; initiating feeding bouts, grooming, and stimulating their perineal area to encourage urination and defecation (this must be done until they are about 7 weeks old).

Development of the young

Sensory development

Sensory systems are not fully operational in the newborn kitten. They are born blind, virtually deaf and completely dependent. They have a fully developed sense of touch, and can detect and respond to temperature gradients. Olfaction is fully developed by 3 weeks and hearing by 4 weeks. Kittens' eyes open at about 6 days. They can follow visual cues by 3–4 weeks. Thereafter their visual acuity improves and is fully developed by about 16 weeks. Internal control of body temperature is not fully developed until 7 weeks.

Physical development

Motor skills develop in parallel with sensory abilities. Newborn kittens can only move by wriggling against a substrate but by the third week they can stand, though their balance is poor, and by 5 weeks they are attempting complex movements. Motor control is fully developed by 11 weeks. Predatory behaviour is observed in cats with no experience of prey but they require experience to become efficient hunters. Feral kittens learn by interacting with prey brought to the nest by their mothers. Pet kittens learn by interacting with toys, litter mates and their mothers.

Kittens' milk teeth begin to appear about 14 days after birth. Initially they are not very interested in solid food but by week 5 are consuming substantial quantities. Kittens can be weaned at 8 weeks. Sensory and physical development are reviewed in Robinson (1992a).

Behavioural development

In the first 2 weeks, kittens mainly sleep and eat. The sensitive period for socialisation to people lies between the end of the second and seventh weeks. This is the period when contact with people has the greatest influence on a kitten's development of friendliness to people. Kittens should be given plenty of opportunity to socialise with other cats and humans, to play and experience colony routines. Older kittens should continue to be given a wide range of experiences as this will help them to accept novel events as adults. Cats that are handled from birth show more rapid physical development and, as adults, are more responsive to humans and to novel events (McCune 1992). Their friendliness to people is affected by the quality and quantity of handling they receive (reviewed in McCune *et al.* 1995) but is also dependent on their parent's temperament (McCune 1995a). Kittens from confident fathers are more confident themselves and cope better when faced with unfamiliar situations such as being handled by strangers or being caged (McCune 1992). Consequently, it is important to consider temperament when selecting individuals for a breeding programme.

Weaning and rearing

The queen begins weaning by spending more time away from her kittens and by adopting postures which make her nipples inaccessible. Weaning can be encouraged by providing shelving to which queens can retreat and by removing queens for increasingly longer periods. The kittens are encouraged to eat solid food from approximately 3 weeks of age, which helps to reduce their dependence on mothers' milk. Weaning is usually complete at 8 weeks of age.

In breeding colonies, weaned kittens are usually housed separately from their mothers. Housing kittens aged 8–18 weeks together widens their social experience and increases their sociability to other cats. Young toms can be allowed supervised socialisation with groups of kittens. This provides stimulation and activity for the tom and teaches kittens how to interact with adults. Older kittens are usually grouped with others of a similar age.

Selection of breeding stock

Cats used for breeding should be free from detectable abnormalities, have a good temperament, and be fastidiously clean. Breeding females should be good mothers and have produced good-sized litters with an even sex ratio and good-sized offspring. Immunodeficiencies may occur in inbred lines.

Special systems – barrier colonies

A successful barrier colony can be established using simple and straightforward procedures (Loveridge 1984). The colony is set up using SPF cats and accommodated away from existing non-SPF catteries. Access is limited, and personnel shower and dress in a separate set of clean clothing before entering and only handle the barrier colony cats. Goods and equipment are disinfected by immersion in a tank containing aldehyde-based disinfectant, delicate items are wiped with disinfectant.

Feeding

Cats are solitary hunters and tend to take prey that is considerably smaller than themselves. Although their natural feeding behaviour is to eat small meals through the 24 h day, cats are opportunistic feeders and will adjust their patterns of activity to suit the frequency with which food becomes available. Adult cats at maintenance can adapt to being fed once or twice a day but growing kittens and lactating queens require more frequent feeds. Confined cats are generally given food *ad libitum* and eat small quantities at frequent intervals. Cats are highly selective feeders and require their food to be highly palatable and fresh. Odour and texture play an important part in diet selection by cats. Careful observation is required to establish individual preferences and the correct level of feeding. Most cats seem to be able to monitor, and therefore adjust, their own calorie intake to match their energy requirements quite accurately. Good nutrition during pregnancy and lactation will give kittens the best start in life.

Natural and prepared diets

Cats are obligate carnivores: they must eat meat products. Free-living cats eat most parts of their prey (small vertebrates and insects) including skin, bones and viscera. Most confined cats are fed solely on commercially prepared canned or complete dry cat foods. These diets have been designed to supply all the key nutrients and energy needed and have been tested for digestibility and palatability. Many come in a range of types and flavours since cats are known to appreciate variety in their diet (Bradshaw 1992). Canned food is a heat-sterilised moist food and, as such, is a safe product with a very long storage life and so requires no special storage conditions. Good-quality complete dry food made specifically for cats can also be used as the sole source of nutrition. Dry food can be kept for many months providing it is stored in dry cool conditions. Offering some dry food maintains oral hygiene in cats. Its natural abrasive action helps to prevent build-up of plaque and reduces gum disease. Another advantage is that it can be left out longer than canned food, which allows the cats to adopt a more natural feeding pattern of many small meals throughout both the day and night. However, in general, most cats find dry foods less palatable than moist foods like meat or canned foods.

Diets can be made directly from raw ingredients. The National Research Council (NRC) (2006) gives dietary guidelines for cats, both minimum requirements and maximum tolerable levels, and lists the composition of a wide range of ingredients from which diets can be formulated to meet the cat's nutritional requirements. Further information can be found in Burger (1993) and Markwell (1994).

Water

The requirement for fresh clean water is at least as important as that for other nutrients. The water content of the diet affects the amount of water cats drink.

Dietary requirements

Dietary requirements are listed in Tables 31.2 and 31.3. These will change with life stage as does the way in which the food should be presented.

The NRC (2006) estimate energy requirements in normal adult cats using an exponential equation of $100\,BW^{0.67}$ kcal per day (BW = bodyweight in kg), which is based on data from lean cats using indirect calorimetry (Nguyen *et al.* 2001). For overweight cats the suggested equation is $130\,BW^{0.4}$ kcal per day (Table 31.2).

Pregnant and lactating queens

Pregnant and lactating queens should be fed *ad libitum* on a balanced diet (Figure 31.6). Specially formulated diets are available and supplements should be avoided as they can result in nutritional imbalances (reviewed by Legrand-Defretin & Munday 1993). The NRC (2006) recommends the equation for energy requirements for gestation to be $ME = 140\,BW^{0.67}$ kcal/day (Table 31.2).

Cats increase their food intake from the first day of pregnancy and, on average, gain about 39% of their pre-mating weight during pregnancy (reviewed in Loveridge & Rivers 1989). Weight gain varies with the size of the litter (according to the equation: weight gain (g) = 888.9 + 106.5 N, where N is the number of kittens in the litter) (Loveridge & Rivers 1989). Some of the weight queens accumulate is lost at parturition, the rest acts as an energy reserve for lactation (Loveridge 1986). In the first 4 weeks of lactation queens expend more energy than they can take in. They continue to

Table 31.2 Energy requirements of growing cats (from the NRC Guidelines 2006).

Lifestage	*Energy measurement*	*Notes*
Adult maintenance		
Normal	100 kcal/kg $BW^{0.67}$/day	
Overweight/low activity	130 kcal/kg $BW^{0.4}$/day	
Pregnancy	ME 140 $BW^{0.67}$ kcal/day	
Lactation		
<3 kittens	ME kcal = maintenance + 18 × BW × L	L = stage of lactation from week 1 to week 7 where *Week 1* = 0.9 *Week 2* = 0.9 *Week 3* = 1.2 *Week 4* = 1.2 *Week 5* = 1.1 *Week 6* = 1.0 *Week 7* = 0.8
3–4 kittens	ME kcal = maintenance + 60 × BW × L	As above
>4 kittens	MEkcal = maintenance + 70 × BW × L	As above
Growth[+]	$100 \times BW_a^{0.67} \times 6.7 \times (e^{(-0.189p)} - 0.66)$	where *p* = BWa/BWm *BWa* = actual body weight (kg) *BWm* = expected mature bodyweight *E* = base of natural log ~2.718

[+] The age at which a cat's energy requirement settles to the adult level is around 40 weeks, although actual bodily development may continue to 12 months – especially for a large male cat.

Table 31.3 Nutrient requirements of cats (From the NRC Guidelines 2006). Nutrient requirements/1000 kcal.

Nutrient	*Units*	*Cat requirement*
Protein	g	50.00
Arginine	g	1.93
Histidine	g	0.65
Isoleucine	g	1.08
Leucine	g	2.55
Lysine	g	0.85
Methionine and cystine	g	0.85
Phenylaline and tyrosine	g	3.83
Threonine	g	1.30
Tryptophan	g	0.33
Valine	g	1.28
Taurine	g	0.10
Fat	g	22.50
Linoleic acid		1.40
Arachidonic acid		0.015
Minerals		
Calcium	g	0.72
Phosphorus	g	0.64
Potassium	g	1.30
Sodium	mg	170.00
Chloride	mg	240.00
Magnesium	mg	100.00
Iron	mg	20.00
Zinc	mg	18.50
Copper	mg	1.20
Manganese	mg	1.20
Iodine	μg	350.00
Selenium	μg	75.00
Vitamins		
Vitamin A (retinol)	μg	250.00
Vitamin D (cholecalciferol)	μg	1.75
Vitamin E (α-tocopherol)	mg	10.00
Vitamin K (phylloquinone)	mg	0.25
Thiamin	mg	1.40
Riboflavin	mg	1.00
Pantothenic acid	mg	1.44
Niacin	mg	10.00
Pyridoxine	mg	0.625
Folic acid	μg	188.00
Vitamin B_{12}	μg	5.60
Choline	mg	637.00
Biotin	μg	18.75

need extra energy whilst they suckle and rebuild body reserves. The amount of energy required depends on the number and age of the kittens. The NRC (2006) recommendation for ME in lactating cats is based on the maintenance requirement increased by a factor determined by the number of kittens in the litter and the stage of lactation (Table 31.2).

Growing kittens

Nutrition is one of the major determinants of kittens' growth rate, along with freedom from disease, good husbandry, maternal weight and the kitten's sex (Loveridge 1987). During a kitten's first few weeks it is entirely dependent on its mother's milk to achieve the desired growth rate of nearly 100 g a week. If the queen's milk is insufficient, or kittens are being hand reared, specially manufactured milk replacers should be given at frequent intervals. Milk replacers mimic the composition of queen's milk, are highly digestible and may include a probiotic to help establish a healthy gut flora. NRC (2006) recommends a factorial equation to estimate the energy requirements for kittens (Table 31.2).

Although deciduous teeth appear about 14 days after birth, very young kittens are not very interested in solid food. From about 3–4 weeks, they become increasingly interested in the solid food that their mother is eating. By week 6, kittens are eating for 50 minutes a day (Robinson 1992a) and should be given finely chopped or moistened food. Commercial food specifically formulated for kittens is available; it has a higher concentration of energy and some nutrients than food formulated for adult cats. The amount of food kittens can ingest at one meal is limited and, ideally, they should be fed *ad libitum*. Weaned kittens do not need milk and become less able to digest lactose as their gut matures. At 6 months of age most kittens have gained 75% of their final adult weight and can be given food formulated for adult cats.

Older cats

Most colony cats are retired when they are around 8 years old. If studies require geriatric cats some changes in feeding regimens may be required. Geriatric cats require small but regular feeds of a high-energy, highly palatable and digestible diet (feeding frequently rather than *ad libitum* allows food intake to be monitored). Recent research has shown that their ability to digest fat, protein and energy declines with

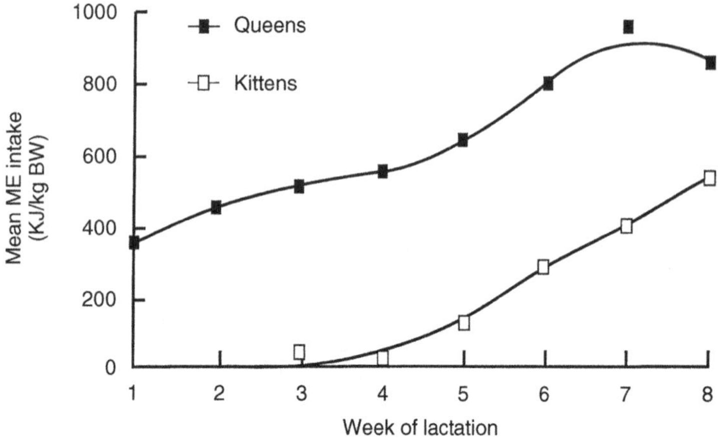

Figure 31.6 Energy intakes of queens and kittens during lactation (mean of three kittens/litter).

age (Taylor *et al.* 1995), whilst energy requirements remain constant. It may be necessary to offer finely chopped or moistened food if they have poor dentition. It is particularly important that elderly cats have easy access to a supply of fresh clean drinking water. They are inclined to become dehydrated because they are less sensitive to thirst and are less efficient thermoregulators (Markham & Hodgkins 1989).

Laboratory procedures

Handling and training

Cats that have been handled and well socialised as kittens are much easier to handle and train as adults. Good handling techniques help cats feel comfortable and secure. Grown cats can be picked up with one hand under the chest, just behind the front paws, and the other under the hindquarters (Wills, J. 1993). Once picked up, the cat will probably be most comfortable sitting in the crook of the handler's arm, with its forepaws either leaning against the handler's shoulder or held in the handler's other hand. Most of the cat's weight should be taken on the handler's arms. Young kittens should be picked up with one hand under the chest and the other under the hindlegs. A young kitten will be small enough to sit on a palm as long as the handler supports its head with the other hand.

Manual restraint

The usual method of restraining a calm cat is to sit the cat on a surface and hold its front legs. The jaw can be gently but firmly held in the other hand to control its head. Alternatively, it can be wrapped securely in a blanket (reviewed by Wills, J. 1993). Further restraint may be necessary for agitated or nervous cats, for example the use of an extending collar on a rod or crush cages. Sedation is the preferred method of restraint for any cat with a history of being fractious. In the case of blood parameters, it greatly diminishes the effect of stimulating the fight or flight response on blood values.

A handling technique called 'clipnosis' or 'clipthesia' has been described (Pozza *et al.* 2008), which is used to immobilise cats for nail clipping, blood sampling and other minor procedures. The application of spring paper clips or clothes pegs that gently grasp the skin along the dorsal midline of the neck and cranial thorax renders the cat immobile. Although the technique's effectiveness varies between individuals, it appears to be useful for providing gentle restraint in most cats (Pozza *et al.* 2008). Based on their behavioural responses, the application of the clips does not appear to be aversive to most cats.

Training

Kittens will learn from their mother to use a litter tray. Hand-reared kittens need to be trained to use one by putting them on the tray frequently, particularly when they look ready to urinate or defecate. Consideration should be given to exposing kittens to minor procedures that will be part of the routine in the future (eg, use of clippers and being gently restrained on an examination table).

Physiological monitoring

To maximise welfare and data reliability, monitoring methods should be as non-invasive as possible. Procedures are easier with two experienced handlers; one restrains the cat while the other performs the procedure. The more relaxed the handlers and the cat are, the easier and less distressing the procedure.

Recording body temperatures

Most cats can simply be held while their rectal temperature is taken. Cats that do object will need to be restrained.

Collection of specimens

Blood

Samples of 1–2 ml are most easily obtained from the front leg: from the antebrachial cephalic vein. For smaller samples, blood can be collected directly by letting it drop out through the needle into the collection vessel rather than being drawn out by syringe. Larger samples are easier to obtain from the jugular veins. See Joint Working Group on Refinement (JWGR) (1993) for general guidance, and limits to blood volume that can be acceptably withdrawn.

Urine

Many of the methods used to collect urine (cystocentesis, catherisation, manual transabdominal expression) are invasive and may be traumatic, particularly when testing is repeated or long-term. They also interfere with the cat's normal urination pattern (as can keeping cats on mesh floors through which urine drains). Most cats can be trained to urinate in a clean tray: cats accustomed to urinating and defecating in a litter tray can be trained to use decreasing amounts of litter until the tray is empty. The outlet of the tray can be connected to a collection vessel outside the pen, enabling urine to be collected separately from faeces. Markwell and Smith (1993) describe a non-invasive collection system whereby urine can be continuously monitored (Figure 31.7).

Milk

Milk can be manually expressed with some difficulty from lactating queens by gentle massaging of the teats after the administration of 5 IU of oxytocin (im) to stimulate milk flow (Keen *et al.* 1982).

Administration of medicines

General advice on the administration of substances can be found in JWGR (2001). Most cats will detect drugs mixed in their food and will refuse to eat.

Dosing and injection procedures

Oral dosing is best carried out with two handlers, one restrains the cat while the other gives the medicine. To give

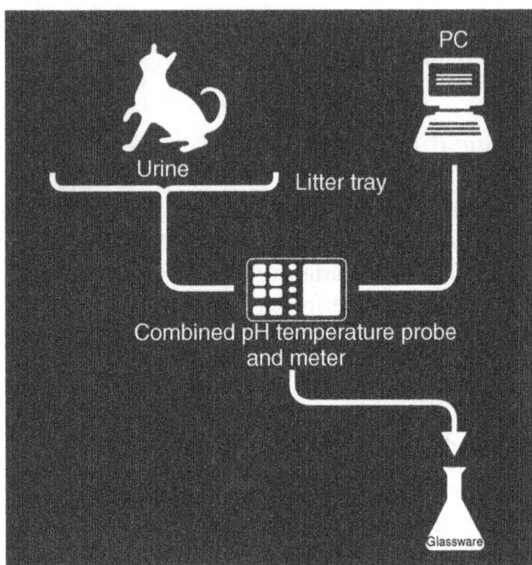

Figure 31.7 Non-invasive collection system for urine (after Markwell & Smith 1993). Reproduced with kind permission of Waltham Centre for Pet Nutrition.

a tablet grasp the cat's head from above, at the points where the jaws meet, with forefinger and thumb, tip the head back and press in with thumb and finger. Push on the lower jaw with the index finger of the other hand to open the animal's mouth and drop the tablet far back on the middle of the tongue. Push it quickly and gently so it moves over the back of the tongue. Close the mouth and gently stroke the throat to encourage swallowing. Large tablets have to be broken into smaller pieces. When giving liquid medicines let the liquid run down the tongue drop by drop, allowing the cat to swallow after every two to three drops or it may choke.

Cats need to be restrained for the application of eye and ear drops. To give ear drops hold the cat's head to one side and put the drops in, externally massaging the ear canal helps the drops to penetrate. Apply eye drops to the inner corner of the eye and keep the head back for a while to allow the drops to cover the eye's surface.

Injections are given when the cat is restrained. Subcutaneous injections are usually given into the scruff of the neck, intramuscular injections into the muscle (quadriceps) overlying the femur of the hindleg or, for small volumes, into the paralumbar (epaxial) muscles. Absorption can be accelerated by gentle massage. Cats which require routine subcutaneous injections (eg, diabetics) can be trained to accept injection without restraint by associating the procedure with a highly palatable food treat.

Anaesthesia and analgesia

General advice can be found in Hall and Taylor (1994) and Flecknell (2009).

Pre-anaesthesia

Preparation

Prior to administering an anaesthetic, food should be withheld for 12h (there is no need to withhold water). This will reduce the risk of vomiting during induction or during the recovery period.

Cats object to aggressive restraint, particularly if they are not sedated. It is always better to give them the benefit of the doubt by first handling them with the minimum restraint. If stronger restraint is required, then premedication and anaesthesia may be used.

Premedication

Agents and dosages are given in Table 31.4. Premedication with a sedative is advisable, even in placid cats, as it reduces struggling during induction. A less stressful induction has several advantages: a reduced dose of induction agent and maintenance agent is required; recovery is smoother; and analgesia is more effective.

Pain

Pain can be difficult to recognise in cats, as their behavioural responses may not be as overt as in other species such as the dog. Behaviours indicating pain can be subtle and easily overlooked, and there may be individual variation. Several studies have examined the behavioural indicators of post-operative pain; these indicators include the inhibition or loss of normal behaviour (such as decreased grooming or failure to eat), the expression of abnormal behaviours (such as altered posture or aggression) (Waran *et al.* 2007) and increased reaction or sensitivity to touch (Taylor & Robertson 2004). Chronic long-term pain, such as that caused by degenerative joint disease, is likely to have a more significant impact on the welfare of cats than is currently recognised. Typical signs of chronic pain include reduced activity, hiding, decreased interest and decreased response to surroundings; there may be inappetance leading to weight loss. Proper assessment of pain in cats will require the development and validation of behaviour-based, multidimensional pain measurement tools. These are available for dogs (Holton *et al.* 2001) but are in their infancy for cats. Guidelines on pain management in cats have recently been published (Hellyer *et al.* 2007).

Analgesia

Safe and effective methods of analgesia are now available. Pain should be prevented whenever possible. Pain can be managed more effectively if analgesia is given before the pain occurs. It is particularly important to consider any requirements for analgesia in sedated cats as they may be unable to demonstrate in any observable way the true level of pain they are experiencing. If a procedure or a disease is known to cause pain in other species, or it seems probable that it might be painful, then analgesia should be given. Analgesics should not be given 'as needed', rather they should be administered on a fixed schedule which can be re-evaluated and changed as necessary. There should be a scale of assessment that all workers can use.

There are two approaches to analgesia:

1. Non-pharmaceutical (see Post anaesthesia section);
2. Pharmaceutical:
    - Opioids – morphine, oxymorphone, buprenorphine, fentanyl;

Table 31.4 Sedatives, tranquillisers, analgesics, pre-anaesthetic and anaesthetic medication for use in cats (derived from BSAVA Small Animal Formulary 2005, National Office of Animal Health 2006, Flecknell 1996). See also Flecknell (2009). Data sheets should be consulted for the various drugs, combinations with other drugs and their dosages and route of administration.

Drug	*Dosage*	*Route*	*Comments*
Atropine sulphate	0.03–0.05 mg/kg	sc	
Acepromazine	0.03–0.125 mg/kg	sc, im	
Diazepam	0.1–0.3 mg/kg	iv	
	0.2–0.4 mg/kg	im	
Opioids			
Buprenorphine	0.01–0.02 mg/kg	sc, im. or sublingually	Lasts 6–8 h
Morphine	0.1–0.2 mg/kg	sc, im	Lasts 6–8 h
Oxymorphone	0.02–0.1 mg/kg	im, sc	Lasts 2–6 h
Fentanyl: skin patch	0.025 mg/h patch for cats weighing 3–5 kg; in smaller cats only half the protective liner should be removed	Applied to clipped and shaved chest wall, and covered with a light dressing	Replace every 2–3 days
Non-steroidal anti-inflammatory drugs (NSAIDs)			
Carprofen	4 mg/kg	sc or iv	Lasts 24 h, given as a single dose; one single further dose at 2 mg/kg may be given
Meloxicam	0.3 mg/kg	sc	Lasts 24 h, given as a single dose
	0.05 mg/kg	Orally	Once daily, following initial 0.1 mg/kg loading dose orally
Ketoprofen	2 mg/kg	iv, im, sc	Every 24 h for up to 3 days
	2 mg/kg	iv, im, sc	Given once, followed by 1 mg/kg orally every 24 h for 4 further days
	1 mg/kg	orally	Every 24 h for up to 5 days
Local anaesthetics			
Bupivacaine 0.5%	Up to 1 mg/kg	Perineural	Duration 2–6 h
Lidocaine 2%	Up to 4 mg/kg	Perineural	Duration 1–2 h
Sedatives and anaesthetics			
Ketamine	1–2 mg/kg	im	Analgesia
	11 mg/kg	im	Minor restraint (in lower doses and with fewer side effects if combined with other drugs)
	22–33 mg/kg	im	Minor surgery (in lower doses and with fewer side effects if combined with other drugs)
	2.2–4.4 mg/kg	iv	
Ketamine	5–10 mg/kg	im	Sedation
Midazolam	0.2 mg/kg		
Ketamine	100 mg/kg	im	Anaesthesia; xylazine and atropine are administered first, followed by ketamine 20 minutes later
Xylazine	1.1 mg/kg		
Atropine	0.03 mg/kg		
Ketamine	5–20 mg/kg	im	Sedation or anaesthesia depending on dose
Medetomidine	40–100 µg/kg		
Ketamine	5 mg/kg	im	Anaesthesia
Medetomidine	80 µg/kg		
Butorphanol	0.4 mg/kg		

- Local anaesthesia – lidocaine, bupivacaine;
- NSAIDs (non-steroidal anti-inflammatory drugs) – carprofen; meloxicam, ketoprofen.

Prolonged, effective analgesia is best achieved by using a combination of these drugs with non-pharmaceutical techniques. The effect of opioid analgesia can be optimised by sedatives.

Anaesthesia

For procedures lasting 20 minutes or less, or for minor surgery (eg, suturing small skin wounds), cats are often given intravenous general anaesthetics or heavy sedation with analgesia (xylazine, medetomidine or ketamine). For longer procedures or major surgery, general anaesthesia is usually induced with intravenous agents and then maintained with a gaseous anaesthetic. The preferred route for intravenous administration is into the cephalic vein in the foreleg (using a 0.6 mm or 0.5 mm (24–25 G), 16 mm needle). If this is not possible, the injection can be made into the medial vein of the hindleg or jugular veins.

For intubation, a selection of endotracheal tubes, from 3.0–5.5 mm, should be available. Cats have a very sensitive laryngeal reflex. To prevent laryngeal spasm, the larynx is sprayed with 2% lidocaine and the endotracheal tube is lubricated with lidocaine gel. The formulation of some local anaesthetic sprays can cause laryngeal oedema in cats, and the spray should be checked before use to ensure it is safe for use in cats. A semi-rigid wire in the lumen of the endotracheal tube can facilitate tracheal intubation. The end of the tube should not pass further than the point of the shoulder.

Intravenous agents and dosages

Agents used routinely for intravenous induction of anaesthesia are: 2.5% thiopental (10 mg/kg iv) or propofol, 10 mg/ml emulsion (6 mg/kg iv for a premedicated cat).

Gaseous agents

Gaseous agents include isoflurane, sevoflurane and halothane. Isoflurane is considered to have several benefits over halothane. Sevoflurane is relatively new to the veterinary market, but appears to have benefits over halothane and to be similar to isoflurane (Hammond 2007).

Muscle relaxants

With modern anaesthetics, muscle relaxants are not usually necessary. Their use is not recommended unless the anaesthetist is very experienced with feline anaesthetics.

Anaesthetic protocol – best practice

A best practice protocol for routine surgery would be: acepromazine; buprenorphine; carprofen or meloxicam; intravenous propofol; isoflurane; and with application of local anaesthetic into the wound.

Post anaesthesia

A variety of non-pharmaceutical techniques can be used to create the optimum conditions in the cat's external and internal environments. Cats should be allowed to recover from anaesthesia in a quiet warm room. They should be nursed on soft bedding and kept clean and comfortable. A semi-enclosed box or high-sided soft bed where the cat can feel secure and still be monitored can be useful. Cats that are used to contact with humans can be given plenty of reassuring verbal and physical contact. Frightening noise and smells should be excluded from the recovery area. Any painful tissues should be immobilised using splints or bandages. The cat should be carefully monitored throughout the post-anaesthesia recovery period, as it is during this time that complications are most likely to occur.

Euthanasia

Euthanasia should be performed in a dignified manner, minimising any mental or physical suffering to the cat, (see also Chapter 17). The method of choice is injection of an anaesthetic agent sufficient to cause rapid unconsciousness and a certain death. A common method is to give a high overdose (about 200 mg/kg) of pentobarbital by intravenous injection. This results in an immediate loss of consciousness, rapidly followed by deep narcosis and respiratory and cardiac arrest. The cat dies within a few seconds apparently without pain or distress. If a cat is difficult to handle, it may need to be sedated before being euthanased.

Common welfare problems

Disease

This section summarises the diseases that most commonly threaten laboratory cats. More detailed reviews are provided by Chandler *et al.* (2007) and Sherding (2008). See also King and Boag (2007).

Prophylaxis

Cats are susceptible to a number of viral, bacterial and parasitic diseases. Colony cats should be vaccinated from the age of 9–12 weeks against feline viral rhinotracheitis, feline calicivirus and feline infectious enteritis. It is important to use a killed vaccine in an SPF-derived cat to minimise the risk of experiencing full-blown disease. Closed colonies are unlikely to be exposed to the feline leukaemia virus. Cats entering the colony should be treated to eliminate all parasites; in a closed colony reinfestation is unlikely.

Signs of diseases

A cat's behaviour and appearance reflect its state of health. A healthy cat will have an alert bearing and move easily and confidently about its accommodation. It will be interested in its surroundings and its food, and groom frequently. It will have clean ears, eyes, mouth and skin. Animals that show any deviations from these signs should be observed and examined carefully to investigate the cause. Any cat exhibiting watery lacrimation, purulent discharges from eyes, nose, or ears, excessive salivation, vomiting or diarrhoea should be isolated immediately.

Viral diseases

Feline immunodeficiency virus (FIV)

FIV is a lentivirus that shares many characteristics of other lentiviruses, such as human immunodeficiency virus. FIV is transmitted primarily by parenteral inoculation of virus present in saliva or blood, via bite and fight wounds. This accounts for the higher prevalence of the virus in adult male cats. Occasional transmission of virus *in utero* and post parturition via the milk may occur.

FIV infection progresses through several stages: an acute phase; a clinically asymptomatic phase of variable duration; and a terminal phase of infection often referred to as feline acquired immunodeficiency syndrome (Sellon & Hartmann 2006). The hallmark of FIV pathogenesis is progressive disruption of normal immune function. During the last stages of infection, clinical signs are often a reflection of opportunistic infections, neoplasia, myelosuppression and neurological disease. However, with proper care some FIV-infected cats can live for many years with a good quality of life, and may die in old age from causes unrelated to FIV infection.

Diagnosis of FIV infection is made most commonly by detection of FIV-specific antibodies in blood by either enzyme-linked immunosorbent assay (ELISA) or rapid immunomigration-type assays (Sellon & Hartmann 2006). An FIV vaccine is available commercially (Fel-O-Vax®, Fort Dodge); because the vaccine contains whole virus, cats respond to vaccination by producing antibodies that are indistinguishable from those produced during natural infection.

Feline leukaemia virus (FeLV)

The prevalence and importance of FeLV as a pathogen in cats are decreasing, primarily because of testing and eradication programmes and the routine use of FeLV vaccines. FeLV, a retrovirus and member of the Oncornavirus subfamily, causes clinical illness related to the haemopoeitic and immune systems and neoplasia. The three most important FeLV subgroups are FeLV-A, FeLV-B and FeLV-C; only FeLV-A is contagious and passed horizontally from cat to cat in nature. Subgroups FeLV-B and FeLV-C evolve *de novo* in an FeLV-A-infected cat by mutation and recombination between FeLV-A and cellular or endogenous retroviral sequences contained in normal feline DNA (Hartmann 2006).

FeLV spreads between susceptible cats primarily via saliva, where virus concentration is higher than in plasma. Vertical transmission can also occur: kittens can be infected transplacentally or when the queen licks and nurses them. Susceptibility to infection is highest in young kittens. The outcome of FeLV infection mainly depends on immune status and age of the cat, but is also affected by virus pathogenicity, infection pressure and virus concentration. Guidelines for testing cats for FeLV have been published (American Association of Feline Practitioners and Academy of Feline Medicine (AAFP/AFM) 2001). While persistently viraemic cats have a decreased life expectancy, treatments for the many clinical syndromes that accompany infection are available. A discussion of FeLV infection and outcome, testing and treatment can be found in Hartmann (2006).

FeLV vaccines are available but the relative efficacy of the vaccines is controversial. Vaccine efficacy testing protocols vary widely between studies and are complicated by the natural resistance of cats (especially older cats) to FeLV infection; none of the licensed vaccines are 100% effective.

An epidemiological association exists between FeLV (and rabies) vaccination and the later development of soft tissue sarcomas at the injection site, referred to as injection site sarcomas, vaccine-associated sarcomas and vaccine site-associated sarcomas (Hartmann 2006).

Feline infectious peritonitis (FIP)

FIP is an infrequent virus infection, which is almost invariably fatal. It is caused by feline infectious peritonitis virus (FIPV), which is generally accepted to be a mutation of feline enteric coronavirus (FECV) (Addie & Jarrett 2006). The latter is common in the domestic cat population, particularly in multicat households or where cats are kept in crowded conditions. Transmission is primarily indirect through contact with virus-containing faeces or fomites, for example contaminated litter trays.

The mutation enables FIPV to infect macrophages and monocytes, and spread throughout the body. The damage caused by the virus is due to the intense immune reaction, localised inflammatory response and vasculitis at the site of virus colonisation.

Two basic forms of FIP, effusive (wet) and non-effusive (dry) are recognised. Approximately half the cats with FIP are less than 2 years of age, although all age groups can be affected (Addie & Jarrett 2006). The risk factors for FIP development are age and crowding, with young cats in crowded catteries being most at risk. Good husbandry is particularly important in controlling FIP. When establishing a colony a decision must be made on whether to focus on FIP or the coronavirus family. If it is the broader family, then the goal should be to maintain the cats free of antibodies to coronaviruses. This would require a different level of surveillance and then the use of vaccines.

An intranasal vaccine, given to cats over 16 weeks of age, has been developed but it is not effective if the cat has already been exposed to the virus. Definitive diagnosis of FIP is by *post-mortem* examination or by using DNA sequencing to detect FIP virus genes in blood, peritoneal fluid or tissue biopsy.

Feline infectious enteritis or panleucopenia (FIE)

Feline panleucopenia is a parvovirus; it is shed in all body secretions during acute stages of disease, but mainly in the vomitus and faeces. It has a short shedding period but long survival in the environment (Greene & Addie 2006), where it is resistant to heat and to many disinfectants. FIE is a highly infectious disease with a high mortality rate. The virus is usually transmitted by indirect contact of susceptible animals with contaminated premises; *in utero* transmission does occur, and may cause early foetal death and resorption or result in the birth of live kittens with varying degrees of neurological damage.

Subclinical cases of infection, more common in older cats, may go unrecognised, while severe clinical illness is the rule in young kittens; sudden death may occur. A presumptive diagnosis is usually made based on clinical signs and the presence of leucopenia. With appropriate symptomatic therapy and nursing care, cats may recover from infection. Immunisation has been very effective at reducing the incidence of this disease.

Feline viral upper respiratory infection (cat 'flu)

Between 85% and 90% of cases are caused by either feline herpesvirus (which causes feline viral rhinotracheitis) or feline calicivirus. Feline herpesvirus (FHV) generally causes more severe disease than feline calicivirus (FCV), but FCV appears to be relatively more common. The viruses are shed mainly in ocular, nasal and oral secretions, and transmission is largely by direct contact from infected to susceptible cat.

After FHV infection virtually all recovered cats become latently infected carriers, with intermittent episodes of virus shedding, particularly after periods of stress. FCV carriers shed virus more or less continuously; in some cats the carrier state appears to be lifelong, but most cats at some point spontaneously recover and appear to eliminate the virus.

Bordetella bronchiseptica is also recognised as a primary pathogen to the feline respiratory tract, although its precise contribution to disease in the field is not yet fully established (Gaskell *et al.* 2006).

Although immunisation cannot guarantee complete protection from upper respiratory infection nor from the development of latent infection, routine vaccination of kittens using a modified live or killed bivalent vaccine, and regular booster vaccination, is recommended.

Cats can carry zoonotic diseases that may be a risk to people (reviewed by Greene & Levy 2006).

Reproductive problems

Major causes of infertility in both toms and queens include inbreeding, poor husbandry, disease, anatomical or reproductive defects and social stress. Investigation should first eliminate any non-reproductive disorders by a thorough physical, haematological and biochemical examination, followed by a thorough evaluation of the reproductive system and semen.

Prolonged anoestrus is usually a management problem. The cats' general health and nutrition should be optimised, and they should be exposed to 14–16h of light per day and to reproductively active cats. Some queens cycle but do not show any oestrous behaviour (silent heat). They may breed if housed with a male.

Failure to mate may be caused by inexperience. Virgins should be partnered with an amenable, experienced mate. Immature toms can lack libido, some may respond after visual exposure to breeding males, others may need more time to mature. Toms should mate in familiar surroundings otherwise they may concentrate on territory marking instead of mating. Mating may fail because the cats are incompatible; the cats may have definite mating preferences, or some physical incompatibility may prevent intromission.

Queens may not conceive after mating. Failure to conceive following breeding is occasionally caused by vaginal or, more commonly, by uterine disease. Ovulation may fail because of inadequate vaginal stimulation or hormonal insufficiencies. Toms may fail to inseminate; their fertility declines if they are mated too frequently. Failure to carry a pregnancy to term has been associated with environmental stress, dietary insufficiencies, or failure of extraovarian progesterone.

Effects of neutering

Neutering eliminates sexual behaviour in males and females, and maternal behaviour in females. It reduces the incidence of behaviours such as urine marking in both sexes, and increases tolerance towards cats from outside the social group (Bradshaw 1992). However, neutering predisposes to obesity by causing a reduction in energy expenditure. While a cat may adapt its food intake in accordance with this, the adaptation may take 9–10 weeks, by which time its body weight would have increased. The risk of obesity is greatly increased if the cat is confined in a small enclosure and is inactive.

Abnormal behaviour

Specific problems associated with confinement include boredom, aggression to people and cats, fearfulness, behavioural inhibition, withdrawal, escape behaviour, hiding, poor reproductive success, anorexia, weight loss, tail chasing, stereotypies, fabric eating and self-mutilation (reviewed in McCune 1995b). Introducing a new cat into a stable colony produces conflict in the group until both newcomer and residents habituate to the new social hierarchy. Studies of stray cats housed communally at a shelter have shown that most overt aggression occurs within the first 4 days and that mutual toleration is established after 2 weeks (Bradshaw 1992). However, although many of these cats will appear to have behaviourally habituated to confinement at this stage, a recent study has shown that cats were still showing abnormally high urinary cortisol levels (indicative of increased stress) up to 5 weeks after entry to a quarantine cattery (Rochlitz *et al.* 1995). Behavioural inhibition is commonly the response of cats to confinement. Unlike the more overt forms of distress like vocalising, spitting, hissing and growling, behavioural inhibition is easy to miss unless detailed observation is made of the cat (McCune 1992).

Preventing problems

Research animals without behavioural problems are likely to have better welfare and be better for research purposes. Many problems associated with confinement can be prevented by adequate early socialisation and careful selection of cats for suitable temperament (Robinson 1992b; McCune *et al.* 1995). Siegford *et al.* (2003) developed and validated a test to evaluate temperament in cats. These authors found that cats could be ranked, using an easily scored feline temperament profile (FTP), as being more or less sociable toward people, and that FTP scores were fairly consistent over time and circumstance and correlated positively with responses of cats to animal care staff and unfamiliar humans. Cats with timid temperament, extremes of age and restricted experience are more likely to have problems adjusting to confinement and responding to novelty.

There are three approaches to preventing stress in confined cats: (1) selective breeding of the most suitable individuals; (2) an investment of time and effort in the early development phase of kittens; and (3) maintaining a varied and stimulating environment which offers cats choices about what they do and where they do it.

All these approaches have been touched on earlier in this chapter. The benefits of breeding from healthy, confident, well socialised, unrelated parents will help preserve the quality of a cat colony. Early socialisation is a critical time in the development of kittens and, if handled sensitively, will produce cats that are more tractable and pleasant to work with. The quality of the environment is also critical to a cat's well-being. With a little imagination, there can be many opportunities for providing variety and reducing stress (reviewed in McCune 1997). Enriching the environment through the provision of social contact, toys and food presented in novel ways will help to ensure good welfare.

Keeping groups stable reduces conflict. Where cats cannot be group-housed they can be given visual, olfactory and auditory contact by using glass partitions with nose-height holes drilled between adjacent pens. They can be given access to a communal room on a rota basis, each cat leaving olfactory and sometimes visible messages for the next occupant. Likewise, scratch posts can be moved from one pen to another (these posts carry interesting olfactory information).

Although cats normally spend a large part of their day asleep or resting, they can become bored. They should be given opportunities for play, exercise and predatory behaviour. Food is often used as an enrichment device. Dry food is particularly suitable for hiding in pens or for placing inside containers which the cat has to work at to extract individual pieces. Puzzle boxes are now commercially available and can extend the handling time of the food. Small pieces of dry food (or toys) can be pawed through irregular openings in the lid of the box (Figure 31.8).

Cats socialised to humans find human company stimulating and have been found to show signs of stress when the caretaking style becomes less interactive (Carlstead *et al.* 1993). A range of activities can be engaged in, from talking quietly to interactive play with a range of toys. Activities can be selected to suit the personality and response of the individual cat. Cats will play with toys. They show most interest in toys that mimic prey but toys need to be changed frequently and offered in randomised rotation to sustain long-term interest. Rods attached to toy fish that can be jiggled to stimulate play seem particularly popular with younger cats.

In addition to providing an enriched environment, fearfulness can be significantly reduced by consistent, positive handling (Gourkow & Fraser 2006). Animal care staff should handle the cats under their care daily, at times that are not part of routine caretaking procedures such as feeding or cleaning (Rochlitz 2000). Hoskins (1995) examined the effect of human contact on the reactions of cats in a rescue shelter: cats that received additional handling sessions, where they interacted closely with a familiar person, could subsequently be held for longer by an unfamiliar person than cats that did not receive additional handling sessions.

Older cats

A range of medical and behavioural conditions is recognised in older cats. Common medical conditions associated with aging include renal disease, dental disease, hyperthyroidism, diabetes mellitus and osteoarthritis. Sensory loss, such as deafness, and signs of cognitive impairment may become evident (Bowen & Heath 2005). Signs of cognitive impairment may include disorientation, altered interaction with others, sleep problems (usually associated with vocalisation), house soiling and failure of appetite. A number of treatment approaches may be used. Environmental modification, by making the environment more accessible to the cat (for example, providing additional, lower resting and hiding places), exposure to play and increased social contact, will stimulate and maintain mental processes. Dietary supplementation with a range of antioxidants, essential fatty acids and other additives has been shown to improve neuronal metabolic function and boost central nervous system antioxidant reserve. While environmental enrichment and dietary modification should be the mainstay therapies to delay progression of cognitive decline, and where euthanasia is not indicated because of the nature of the research, some psychoactive drugs may also be useful (Bowen & Heath 2005).

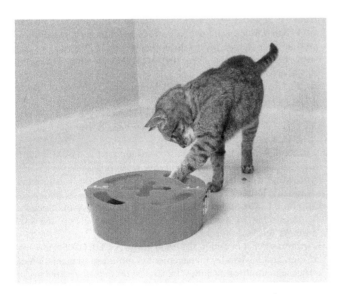

Figure 31.8 Presenting part of the food ration in a puzzle can provide a rewarding challenge.

Feline facial pheromones

A range of pheromones has been isolated from feline facial secretions (Mills 2005), and two fractions are available commercially: F3 and F4. The F3 fraction can be used to have a calming effect on cats and facilitate their adaptation to new environments, such as new housing or hospitalisation for veterinary treatment (Griffith *et al.* 2000), or during transport. It is also used in the treatment of behavioural problems such as urine marking and spraying, and scratching of objects. It is available as a spray for application onto cages, tables and blankets and as a plug-in diffuser for rooms or treatment areas. The F4 fraction reduces the cat's wariness of unfamiliar people, and is used to reduce the risk of aggression due to handling in the veterinary hospital. It is available as a spray that is applied to the environment or to the person's hands prior to handling the cat.

Monitoring welfare

The effect of changes made to relieve stress and enrich the captive environment can be assessed by looking for a decrease in abnormal behaviours associated with long-term stress (Bradshaw 1992) and for a behavioural repertoire which more closely resembles that of free-ranging cats (UK Cat Behaviour Working Group 1995; see also Chapter 6). Changes over time can be assessed quickly by using a scoring system. A composite behavioural scale for quantifying stress in confined cats was devised by McCune (1992) and had 10 levels, which were later reduced to seven (McCune 1994). This scale was refined by Kessler and Turner (1997) by adding more postural elements to form the cat stress score (CSS), still with seven levels. This behavioural score correlates well with many indicators of stress (McCune 1992), although there is not always agreement between it and some physiological measures of stress (McCobb *et al.* 2005). Casey (2007a) found a negative correlation between the rate of decline of the CSS and the rate of decline of urinary cortisol to creatinine ratios for cats newly admitted to an animal shelter. This implies the presence of different 'coping styles' in cats, where some actively respond to stress and adapt to the unfamiliar surrounding physiologically, while others appear to be more passive but change little physiologically.

All workers in an establishment should ensure they are using the score in the same way and are being consistent over time in their scoring. Although such a score does require training, once learnt it is a powerful means of assessment as it summarises so much fine detail and can be quickly applied.

A combination of good innovative design and thoughtful husbandry enables confined cats to be kept in conditions where the demands on their welfare and the laboratory's work schedule can be harmoniously balanced.

Quality of life

Quality of life is an abstract construct that has been formally recognised and widely used in human medicine. In recent years there has been much discussion about the concept of quality of life and its application to companion animals. While it is generally accepted that quality of life has to do with the animal's feelings, how it can be defined, measured and reported in animals is currently being explored (McMillan 2005; Scott *et al.* 2007). Approaches include the observation and interpretation of the animal's behaviour, and the use of questionnaires directed at the person most closely involved with the animal's care (see also Chapter 6).

References

Addie, D. and Jarrett, O. (2006) Feline coronavirus infections. In: *Infectious Diseases of the Dog and Cat*, 3rd edn. Ed. Greene, C.E., pp. 88–102. Elsevier Inc, St. Louis, Missouri

American Association of Feline Practitioners and Academy of Feline Medicine (AAFP/AFM): Advisory Panel Report on Feline Retrovirus Testing and Management (2001) Feline retrovirus testing and management. *Compendium on Continuing Education for the Practising Veterinarian*, **23**, 652–692

Beaver B.V. (2003) *Feline Behaviour: A Guide for Veterinarians*, 2nd edn. Saunders, St. Louis, Missouri

Bowen, J. and Heath, S. (2005) Geriatric behavioural issues. In: *Behaviour Problems in Small Animals: Practical Advice for the Veterinary Team*. pp. 59–69. Elsevier Limited, London

Bradshaw, J.W.S. (1992) *The Behaviour of the Domestic Cat*. CAB International, Wallingford

Bradshaw, J.W.S. and Hall, S.L. (1999) Affiliative behaviour of related and unrelated pairs of cats in catteries: a preliminary report. *Applied Animal Behaviour Science*, **63**, 251–255

Bradshaw, J.W.S. and Holloran, D. (2005) Effects of air transportation on behavioural signs of stress in cats. Scientific Proceedings of the BSAVA Congress 2005, p. 537

Broom, D.M. and Johnson, K.G. (1993) *Stress and Animal Welfare*. Chapman and Hall Limited, London

British Small Animal Veterinary Association (2005) *Small Animal Formulary*, 5th edn. Ed. Tennant, B. BSAVA, Gloucester

Burger I. (1993) *The Waltham Book of Companion Animal Nutrition*. Pergamon Press, Oxford

Carlstead, K., Brown, J.L. and Strawn, W. (1993) Behavioural and physiological correlates of stress in laboratory cats. *Applied Animal Behaviour Science*, **38**, 143–158

Casey, R. (2007a) Do I look like I'm bothered – recognition of stress in cats. *Scientific Proceedings of the European Society of Feline Medicine Congress 2007*, Prague, pp. 95–97

Casey, R. (2007b) From the cat's perspective – how to readjust your thinking. *Scientific Proceedings of the European Society of Feline Medicine Congress 2007*, Prague, pp. 9–14

Chandler, E.A., Gaskell, C.J. and Gaskell, R.M. (2007) *Feline medicine and therapeutics*, 3rd edn. Blackwell Publising, Oxford

Council of Europe. (2006) Multilateral Consultation of Parties to the European Convention for the Protection of Vertebrate Animals used for Experimental and other Scientific Purposes (ETS 123) Appendix A. *Cons 123 (2006) 3*. Available from URL: http://www.coe.int/t/e/legal_affairs/legal_co-operation/biological_safety,_use_of_animals/laboratory_animals/2006/Cons123(2006)3AppendixA_en.pdf (accessed 31 July 2008)

Driscoll, C.A., Menotti-Raymond, M., Roca, A.L. *et al.* (2007) The near eastern origin of cat domestication. *Science*, **317**, 519–523

European Commission (2007) Commission recommendations of 18 June 2007 on guidelines for the accommodation and care of animals used for experimental and other scientific purposes. Annex II to European Council Directive 86/609. See 2007/526/EC. http://eurlex.europa.eu/LexUriServ/site/en/oj/2007/l_197/l_19720070730en00010089.pdf (accessed 13 May 2008)

Flecknell, P.A. (1996) *Laboratory Animal Anaesthesia: A Practical Introduction for Research Workers and Technicians*, 2nd edn. Academic Press, London

Flecknell, P.A. (2009) *Laboratory Animal Anaesthesia*, 3rd edn. Academic Press, London

Gaskell, R.M., Dawson, S. and Radford, A. (2006) Feline respiratory disease. In: *Infectious Diseases of the Dog and Cat*, 3rd edn. Ed. Greene C.E., pp. 145–153. Elsevier Inc, St. Louis, Missouri

Gourkow, N. and Fraser, D. (2006) The effect of housing and handling practices on the welfare, behaviour and selection of domestic cats (*Felis sylvestris catus*) by adopters in an animal shelter. *Animal Welfare*, **15**, 371–377

Greene, C.E. and Addie, D. (2006) Feline parvovirus infection. In: *Infectious Diseases of the Dog and Cat*, 3rd edn. Ed. Greene C.E., pp. 78–87. Elsevier Inc, St. Louis, Missouri

Greene, C.E. and Levy, J.K. (2006) Immunocompromised people and shared human and animal infections: zoonosees, sapronoses, and anthroponoses. In: *Infectious Diseases of the Dog and Cat*, 3rd edn. Ed. Greene C.E., pp. 1051–1068. Elsevier Inc, St. Louis, Missouri

Griffith, C.A., Steigerwald, E.S. and Buffington, C.A.T. (2000) Effects of a synthetic facial pheromone on behavior of cats. *Journal of the American Veterinary Medical Association*, **217**, 1154–1156

Hall L.W. and Taylor P.M. (1994) *Anaesthesia of the Cat*. Balliére Tindall, London

Hammond, R. (2007) Anaesthesia and sedation in the critical patient. In: *BSAVA Manual of Canine and Feline Emergency and Critical Care*, 2nd edn. Eds King L.G. and Boag A., pp. 309–319. British Small Animal Veterinary Association, Gloucester

Hartmann, K. (2006) Feline leukaemia virus infection. In: *Infectious Diseases of the Dog and Cat*, 3rd edn. Ed. Greene C.E., pp. 105–131. Elsevier Inc, St. Louis, Missouri

Hawthorne, A.J., Loveridge, G.G. and Horrocks, L.J. (1995) Housing design and husbandry management to minimise transmission of disease in multi-cat facilities. In: *Cats on the Capital. Proceedings of 1995 Symposium on Feline Infectious Disease*. pp. 97–107 American Association of Feline Practitioners Academy of Feline Medicine, Washington, DC

Home Office (1989) *Code of Practice for the Housing and Care of Animals Used in Scientific Procedures*. Her Majesty's Stationery Office, London

Hellyer, P., Rodan, I., Brunt, J. *et al.* (2007) AAHA/AAFP pain management guidelines for dogs and cats. *Journal of the American Animal Hospital Association*, **43**, 235–248

Holton, L., Reid, J., Scott, E.M. *et al.* (2001) Development of a behaviour-based scale to measure acute pain in dogs. *Veterinary Record*, **148**, 525–531

Hoskins, C.M. (1995) *The effects of positive handling on the behaviour of domestic cats in rescue centres*. MSc thesis, University of Edinburgh

Hurni, H. and Rossbach, W. (1987) The laboratory cat. In: *The UFAW Handbook on the Care and Management of Laboratory Animals*, 6th edn. Ed. Poole, T.B., pp. 476–492. Longman Scientific & Technical, Harlow

Izawa, M. (1984) *Ecology and social systems of the feral cat (Felis catus Linn.)*. PhD thesis, Kuyshu University

Izawa, M., Doi, T. and Ono, Y. (1982) Grouping patterns of feral cats (*Felis catus*) living on a small island in Japan. *Japanese Journal of Ecology*, **32**, 373–382

Joint Working Group on Refinement (2001) Refining procedures for the administration of substances. Report of the BVAAWF/FRAME/RSPCA/UFAW Joint Working Group on Refinement. *Laboratory Animals*, **35**, 1–41

Karsh, E.B. and Turner, D.C. (1988) The human-cat relationship. In: *The Domestic Cat: the Biology of its Behaviour*. Ed. Turner, D.C. and Bateson, P.P.G., pp. 159–177. Cambridge University Press, Cambridge

Keen, C.L., Lonnerdal, B., Clegg, M.S. *et al.* (1982) Developmental changes in composition of cats' milk: trace elements, minerals, protein, carbohydrate and fat. *Journal of Nutrition*, **112**, 1763–1769

Kerby, G. and Macdonald, D.W. (1988) Cat society and the consequences of colony size. In: *The Domestic Cat: the Biology of its Behaviour*. Ed. Turner, D.C. and Bateson, P.P.G., pp. 67–81. Cambridge University Press, Cambridge

Kessler, M.R. and Turner, D.C. (1997) Stress and adaptation of cats (*Felis silvestris catus*) housed singly, in pairs and in groups in boarding catteries. *Animal Welfare*, **6**, 243–254

King, L.G. and Boag, A. (2007) *Manual of Canine and Feline Emergency and Critical Care*, 2nd edition. British Small Animal Veterinary Association, Gloucester

Kry, K. and Casey, R. (2007) The effect of hiding enrichment on stress levels and behaviour of domestic cats in a shelter setting and the implications for adoption potential. *Animal Welfare*, **16**, 375–383

Laboratory Animal Science Association (2005) Guidance on the transport of laboratory animals. Report of the Transport Working Group established by the Laboratory Animal Science Association (LASA) *Lab Animals*, **39**, 1–39

Lawler, D.F., Evans, R.H., Reimers, T.J. *et al.* (1991) Histopathologic features, environmental factors, and serum estrogen, progesterone, and prolactin values associated with ovarian phase and inflammatory uterine disease in cats. *American Journal of Veterinary Research*, **52**, 1747–1753

Legrand-Defretin, V. and Munday, H.S. (1993) Feeding dogs and cats for life. In: *The Waltham Book of Companion Animal Nutrition*. Ed. Burger, I., pp. 57–68. Pergamon Press, Oxford

Linseele, V., Van neer, W. and Hendrickx, S. (2007) Evidence for early cat taming in Egypt. *Journal of Archaeological Science*, **34**, 2081–2090

Loveridge, G.G. (1984) The establishment of a barriered respiratory disease-free cat breeding colony. *Animal Technology*, **35**, 83–92

Loveridge, G.G. (1986) Bodyweight changes and energy intakes of cats during gestation and lactation. *Animal Technology*, **37**, 7–15

Loveridge, G.G. (1987) Some factors affecting kitten growth. *Animal Technology*, **38**, 9–18

Loveridge, G.G. (1994) Provision of environmentally enriched housing for cats. *Animal Technology*, **45**, 69–87

Loveridge, G.G., Horrocks, L.J. and Hawthorne, A.J. (1995) Environmentally enriched housing for cats when housed singly. *Animal Welfare*, **4**, 135–141

Loveridge, G.G. and Rivers, J.P.W. (1989) Bodyweight changes and energy intakes of cats during pregnancy and lactation. In: *Nutrition of the Dog and Cat*. Eds Burger, I.H. and Rivers, J., pp. 113–132. Cambridge University Press, Cambridge

Markham, R.W. and Hodgkins, E.M. (1989) Geriatric nutrition. *Veterinary Clinics of North America: Small Animal Practice*, **19**, 165–185

Markwell P.J. (1994) *Applied Clinical Nutrition of the Dog and Cat*. Waltham Centre for Pet Nutrition, Waltham-on-the-Wolds

Markwell, P.J. and Smith, B.H.E. (1993) An effective urine pH monitoring system for cats. *Animal Technology*, **44**, 239–245

McCobb, E.C., Patronek, G.J., Marder, A. *et al.* (2005) Assessment of stress levels among cats in four animal shelters. *Journal of the American Veterinary Medical Association*, **226**, 548–555

McCune, S. (1992) *Temperament and the welfare of caged cats*. PhD thesis, University of Cambridge.

McCune, S. (1994) Caged cats: avoiding problems and providing solutions. *Newsletter of the Companion Animal Behaviour Study Group*, *7*

McCune, S. (1995a) The impact of paternity and early socialisation on the development of cats' behaviour to people and novel objects. *Applied Animal Behaviour Science*, **45**, 111–126

McCune, S. (1995b) Environmental enrichment for the laboratory cat. In: *Environmental Enrichment Information Resources for Laboratory Animals: Birds, Cats, Dogs, Farm Animals, Ferrets, Rabbits, and Rodents, AWIC Resources Series No. 2*. Animal Welfare Information Centre/Universities Federation for Animal Welfare, Maryland

McCune, S. (1997) Environmental enrichment for confined cats – a review. In: *Proceedings of the Second International Conference on Environmental Enrichment*. Ed. Holst, B., pp. 103–117. Copenhagen Zoo, Copenhagen

McCune, S., McPherson, J.A. and Bradshaw, J.W.S. (1995) Avoiding problems: the importance of socialization. In: *The Waltham Book of Human-Animal Interaction: Benefits and Responsibilities of Pet Ownership*. Ed. Robinson, I., pp. 71–86. Pergamon Press, Oxford

McMillan, F.D. (2005) *Mental Health and Well-being in Animals*. Blackwell Publishing, Ames, Iowa

Mills, D. (2005) Pheromonotherapy: theory and applications. *In Practice*, **27**, 368–373

National Office for Animal Health (2006) *Compendium of Data Sheets for Animal Medicines*. NOAH, Enfield

National Research Council (2006) *Nutrient Requirements of Dogs and Cats*. National Academies Press, Washington, DC

Nguyen, P., Dumon, H., Frenais, R. *et al.* (2001) Energy expenditure and requirement assessed using three different methods in adult cats. *Supplement to Compendium on Continuing Education for the Practicing Veterinarian*, **23**, 86

Pozza, M.E., Stella, J.L., Chappuis-Gagnon, A.-C. *et al.* (2008) Pinch-induced behavioral inhibition ('clipnosis') in domestic cats. *Journal of Feline Medicine and Surgery*, **10**, 82–87

Robinson, I. (1992a) Behavioural development of the cat. In: *The Waltham Book of Dog and Cat Behaviour*. Ed. Thorne, C., pp. 53–64. Pergamon Press, Oxford

Robinson, I. (1992b) Social behaviour of the cat. In: *The Waltham Book of Dog and Cat Behaviour*. Ed. Thorne, C., pp. 79–95. Pergamon Press, Oxford

Rochlitz, I. (2000) Recommendations for the housing and care of domestic cats in laboratories. *Laboratory Animals*, **34**, 1–9

Rochlitz, I. (2005) Housing and welfare. In: *The Welfare of Cats*. Ed. Rochlitz, I., pp. 177–203. Springer, Dordrecht

Rochlitz, I., Podberscek, A.L. and Broom, D.M. (1995) The behaviour and welfare of cats in a quarantine cattery. In: *Proceedings of the 29th International Congress of the International Society for Applied Ethology*. Eds Rutter, S.M., Rushen, H.D., Randle, H.D. *et al.*, pp. 125–126. UFAW, Potters Bar

Sherding, R.G. (2008) *The Cat: Diseases and Clinical Management*, 3rd edn. Saunders, Philadelphia

Scott, E.M., Nolan, A.M., Reid, J. *et al.* (2007) Can we really measure quality of life? Methodologies for measuring quality of life in people and other animals. *Animal Welfare*, **16**, 17–24

Sellon, R.K. and Hartmann, K. (2006) Feline immunodeficiency virus infection. In: *Infectious Diseases of the Dog and Cat*, 3rd edn. Ed. Greene C.E., pp. 131–143. Elsevier Inc, St. Louis, Missouri

Siegford, J.M., Walshaw, S.O., Brunner, P. *et al.* (2003) Validation of a temperament test for domestic cats. *Anthrozoös*, **16**, 332–351

Taylor, E.J., Adams, C. and Neville, R. (1995) Some nutritional aspects of ageing in dogs and cats. *Proceedings of the Nutrition Society*, **54**, 645–656

Taylor, P.A. and Robertson, S.A. (2004) Pain management in cats-past, present and future. Part 1. The cat is unique. *Journal of Feline Medicine and Surgery*, **6**, 313–320

Thorne C.J. (1992) *The Waltham Book of Dog and Cat Behaviour*. Pergamon Press, Oxford

UK Cat Behaviour Working Group (1995) *An Ethogram for Behavioural Studies of the Domestic Cat (Felis silvestris catus L.)*. Universities Federation for Animal Welfare, Potters Bar

van den Bos, R. (1998) Post-conflict stress-response in confined group-living cats (*Felis silvestris catus*). *Applied Animal Behaviour Science*, **59**, 323–330

Vella, C.M., Shelton, L.M., McGonagle, J.J. *et al.* (1999) *Robinson's Genetics for Cat Breeders and Veterinarians*, 4th edn. Butterworth-Heinemann, Oxford

Vigne, J.D., Guilane, J., Debue, K. *et al.* (2004) Early taming of the cat in Cyprus. *Science*, **304**, 259

Waran, N., Best, L., Williams, V. *et al.* (2007) A preliminary study of behaviour-based indicators of pain in cats. *Animal Welfare*, **16**, 105–108

Wills, J. (1993) Handling. In: *Handbook of Feline Medicine*. Eds Wills, J. and Wolf, A., pp. 1–11. Pergamon Press, Oxford

Wills, M.B. (1993) *Dalton's Introduction to Animal Breeding*, 3rd edn. Blackwell Publishing, Oxford

32 Pigs and minipigs

Wolfgang Holtz

Biological overview

General biology

Pigs are found in almost every part of the world. Within the order Artiodactyla (even-toed ungulates) the Suiformes, encompassing pigs, peccaries and hippopotamuses, form a suborder of animals with a single stomach. There are two families: Tayassuidae (Central and South American pigs) and Suidae (true pigs). Within the the Suidae are the genera: *Potamochoerus* (bush pigs), *Phacochoerus* (wart hogs), *Hylochoerus* (forest hogs), *Babirussa* (Celebes hogs) and *Sus* (European pigs).

All modern domestic pigs are varieties of the species *Sus scrofa* and have 38 (2N) chromosomes. They are omnivorous mammals with a high degree of adaptability and intelligence, a lively temperament and high fecundity. The anatomy and physiology of pigs is thoroughly covered in a range of veterinary textbooks, most comprehensively in Pond & Mersmann (2001). Most of the information is also applicable to miniature pigs (minipigs), which are often used in biomedical research as an alternative to larger breeds. Minipigs are smaller than large domestic pigs, but there is close resemblance with regard to proportions and functions. Texts covering various aspects of minipigs are Glodek & Oldigs (1981), Leucht *et al.* (1982) and Svendsen (1998).

Size range and lifespan

The typical body masses of farm and miniature pigs (Goettingen strain) at various ages is presented in Table 32.1. The growth curve of farm pigs follows the classical sigmoid pattern (Figure 32.1), whereas in minipigs it is more linear, with the point of inflection appearing at about 250–300 days of age (Brandt *et al.* 1997; Koehn *et al.* 2008). Farm pigs reach their adult body mass of 180–250 kg, or sometimes more, at an age of 3 years. According to information compiled by Swindle (2007), amongst the miniature pig breeds the Goettingen miniature pig is the lightest, approaching 35–45 kg at the age of 2 years. In order of increasing adult mass, other breeds are the Yucatan micro, Sinclair, Yucatan and Hanford. Adult pigs fed a high-energy diet while not breeding tend to grow excessively obese. The average life expectancy is 10–20 years.

Social organisation

Wild pig social groups consist of small numbers of females and their offspring. Adult males tend to be solitary except during the mating season. In groups of domestic pigs, a social dominance order is quickly established. Generally, the level of aggression, mainly expressed by butting and biting the neck and ears, soon subsides. Rarely, fighting continues to the state of total exhaustion. Sexually mature males may fight fiercely, especially in the presence of females.

Within a litter of newborn piglets a social hierarchy is established within 3–4 days after birth. From then on each piglet suckles its individual teat, with dominant piglets usually gaining the more productive anterior teats. When piglets from different litters are mixed after weaning, they establish a new dominance hierarchy. Usually, ranking is established through aggressive interaction, but may take place without overt aggression. Dominant–subordinate relationships remain unchanged as long as a group stays together. Subordinates that have been separated from a group will be attacked after reintroduction, whereas reintroduction of dominant animals rarely results in aggression.

Reproduction

Domestic pigs are prolific and reproduce at all times of the year. They are polytocous and the uterus consists of two long convoluted horns. The oestrous cycle averages 21 (17–25) days. First signs of heat (pro-oestrus) make their appearance 2–3 days before the onset of oestrus. Oestrus, which is characterised by the standing reflex, lasts for 2.5 (1–5) days, and within another 2–3 days the symptoms gradually subside (post- or metoestrus). Ovulation occurs early in the second half of standing oestrus (Figure 32.2) and extends over 1–4 h. Signs of oestrus include swelling and reddening of the vulva, restlessness, increased interest in other animals, especially males, mounting of other animals, occasionally growling sounds and, eventually, display of the standing reflex in the presence of a male or if mounted by another female.

Mating is preceded by foreplay: the male circling, sniffing and nudging the female and attempting to mount. If the sow displays the standing reflex, intromission occurs and the corkscrew-shaped tip of the penis is locked into the cervix

Table 32.1 Typical body masses (kg) of female breeding stock of farm pigs (ad libitum feeding, figures assembled from several sources) and Goettingen miniature pigs (restricted feeding, figures from the breeding herd at Dalmose/Denmark).

Age	*Farm pigs*	*Miniature pigs*
Newborn	1.3	0.45
4 weeks (weaning)	7.5	2.5
3 months	33	7
6 months	90	13
1 year	150	26
2 years	200	35
3 years	230	45

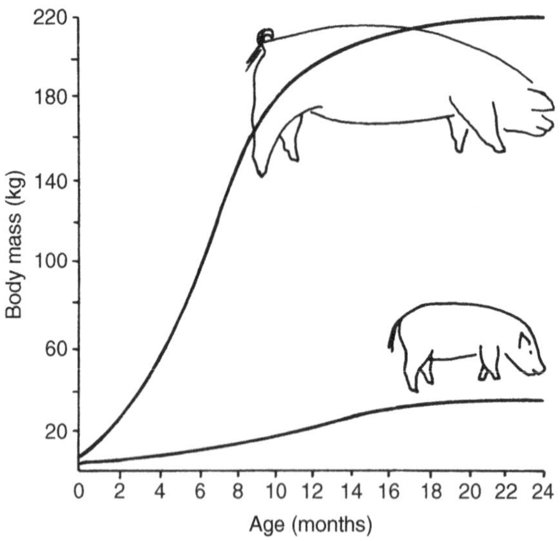

Figure 32.1 Growth curves for farm pigs and Goettingen miniature pigs. Whereas the former shows the classical sigmoid pattern, the latter is almost linear.

of the sow. Copulation lasts 3–10 minutes and the semen is deposited in the uterus. Intrauterine sperm transport is rapid and fertilisation occurs in the ampullar segment of the oviduct. Embryos enter the uterus 2–3 days after fertilisation at the four-cell stage. Six days after fertilisation the blastocysts hatch from the zona pellucida, start migrating throughout both uterine horns and are eventually evenly distributed. Attachment to the endometrium begins 2 weeks after conception. There are no specialised areas of contact (*placenta diffusa*) and, compared with primates, attachment is rather superficial (epitheliochorial). The average length of the gestation period is 115 days in farm pigs and 114 days in minipigs, plus or minus 3 days. Small litters are carried a day or two longer than larger ones. The embryology of the pig is described in great detail in Patten (1948) and Marrable (1971). Corresponding information on minipigs may be found in Glodek & Oldigs (1981).

In most domestic farm breeds 11–16 ovulations are typical for primiparous and 14–18 for pluriparous females. Typically more than 90% of the ova are fertilised, but early embryonic mortality, occurring within the first 30 days of pregnancy, generally amounts to 30–40%. In well managed herds, typical pregnancy rates are 80–90% with litter sizes of 9–12 piglets born to primiparous and 11–14 to pluriparous females. In Goettingen, our experience with miniature pigs is that litter size for both primiparous and pluriparous females is much less (five to eight and six to eight, respectively). Typical reproductive parameters are summarised in Table 32.2.

Sows produce milk rich in dry matter, containing about 9% fat, 6% protein, 5% lactose and 0.7% minerals. Colostrum contains close to 20% protein, comprising mainly gammaglobulins that act as antibodies. These need to be imbibed by the piglets within the first few hours after parturition to cross the wall of the alimentary tract and provide passive immunity. Milk production of suckling sows increases up to the third week of lactation and declines gradually thereafter. The daily milk production of a sow suckling 10 piglets is about 8 l. Data on milk production in minipigs are not avail-

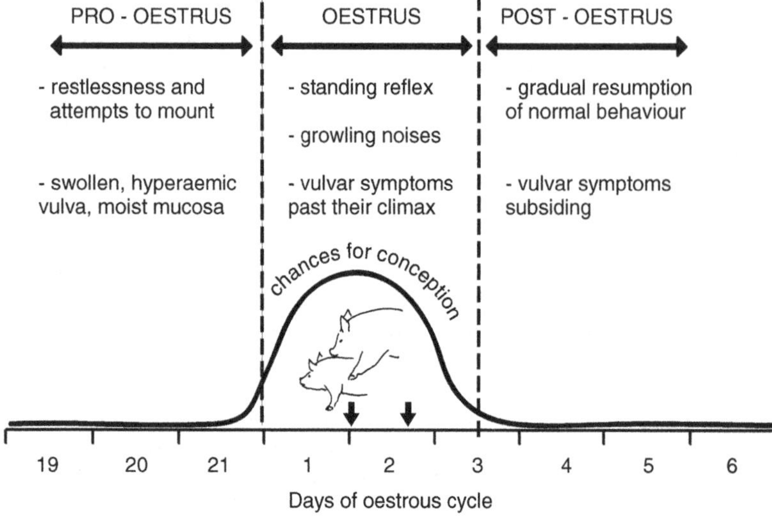

Figure 32.2 Oestrous symptoms and the best time for having sows mated or inseminated (arrows). The oestrous cycle of approximately 21 days is divided up into 2–3 days of pro-oestrus, 2–3 days of 'standing' oestrus, 2–3 days of post-oestrus and the inter-oestrous period. In the absence of a boar the standing reflex will be elicited 12 h later than indicated in the diagram.

able. The natural suckling period may extend to 10 weeks, and in extreme cases up to 17 weeks. In commercial production units piglets are usually weaned at around 4 weeks, but sometimes at 5 or 6 weeks of age. While suckling, sows usually do not come into oestrus. The first post-partum oestrus, which is accompanied by ovulation, is usually recorded 4–8 days after weaning. In primiparous sows and under unfavourable environmental conditions the return to oestrus may be delayed. Heat symptoms that are observed about 3 days after parturition in many animals are not associated with ovarian function and ovulation.

Standard biological data

Published information on biological parameters of the pig is inconsistent. Reference values for cardiovascular, respiratory, haematological and clinical chemical parameters vary within a wide range. Some variation may be explained by genetic differences; however, age, reproductive status and a variety of environmental factors such as husbandry system, microbiological status and conditions under which the information was obtained have a much greater impact. Differences between various pig breeds and among farm pigs and miniature pigs at a comparable stage of development are comparatively minor. Differences between adult miniature pigs and weight-matched farm piglets, however, may be substantial because of the difference in the physiological state of maturity. Likewise, biological parameters originating from anaesthetised animals do not necessarily agree with those of conscious animals, depending on the anaesthetic used. Factors that may be responsible for variability include: immobilisation, transportation or fasting of the animals, sampling site and method (venepuncture or permanently indwelling catheter).

Table 32.3 provides some values for vital functions and Table 32.4 provides physiological means and ranges of relevant blood parameters typical for farm and miniature pigs.

Table 32.2 Typical reproductive data for adult farm pigs (figures from various sources) and miniature pigs (Goettingen strain, figures from Goettingen, Germany and Dalmose, Denmark).

Parameter	*Farm pig*	*Minipig (Goettingen strain)*
Age at puberty (months)	7	4
Minimum breeding age (months)	8	5
Length of oestrous cycle (days)	21	19.5
Duration of oestrus (days)	2.5	2.9
Number of ovulations	20	11
Gestation period(days)	115	114
Litter size	11	6
Birth weight/piglet (g)	1300	450
Interval weaning-oestrus (days)	5	7
Ejaculate volume (ml)	250	90
Spermatozoa/ejaculate (10^9)	50	10
Spermatozoan motility (%)	75	75

Breeds, strains and genetics

There are close to 100 known breeds of pigs mostly reared for pork and bacon production. Breeding stock have been selected with an emphasis on growth rate, feed conversion and lean content, as well as fecundity and mothering ability. The most common domestic breeds are Yorkshire and Landrace (white), Pietrain and Hampshire (spotted or belted) and Duroc (red). In commercial pork production, hybrid crosses of two, three or more breeds are common.

Miniature pig breeds were established for the purpose of biomedical research. They are smaller than farm pigs, but resemble them in proportion and physiology. Many of the present breeds of miniature pigs have their origin in the Minnesota (Hormel) minipig, which was developed in 1949 at the Hormel Institute in Austin, USA. Miniature pigs derived from this population are the Goettingen minipig, developed in 1961, the NIH (Beltsville) minipig and the Sinclair minipig. Others are the Pitman-Moore and the Hanford (derived from the Pitman-Moore). A Mexican feral pig was used in research in 1960 and later referred to as Yucatan mini- and micropig. In addition, breeds such as the Minisib minipig (Siberia), Ohmini and Clawn minipigs (Japan) and several other breeds have been established.

Colonies bred for biomedical research may be randombred, outbred or (partially) inbred. In commercial pig farming, random breeding and crossing are typical. Purpose-bred pigs and minipigs for biomedical research typically originate from colonies with outbred genetics.

Pigs have 18 autosomal chromosome pairs plus the X and Y chromosomes. A map of the entire genome is close to being fully established (Swine Genome Sequencing

Table 32.3 Typical resting values for some vital functions for farm and miniature pigs (figures assembled from several sources).

Age (weeks)	*Heart rate (beats/min)*	*Mean arterial blood pressure (mmHg)*	*Respiratory rate (breaths/min)*	*Rectal. temperature (°C)*
1	220	–	50	39.5
3	150	–	40	39.5
6	120	120	30	39.5
12	100	135	25	39.0
52	70	150	15	38.9

Consortium (SGSC) 2009), which will facilitate research on locating genes associated with traits of economic or disease importance. The similarity of the human and porcine genome maps suggests that there will be further development of the pig as a model for human diseases and in xenotransplantation research.

Sources of supply

Pigs from random-bred sources are typically of farmed strains, whose breeding has been focused on production rather than family genetics. In these populations individual genetic and phenotypic variation is high, and such animals may not be suited for certain experiments. Purpose-bred pigs and minipigs for biomedical research typically originate from a closed colony with outbred genetics. These populations require genetic management to ensure continued genetic variability. Monitoring may involve biomedical, immunologic or DNA markers or quantitative genetic analysis of physiological variables. Some minipigs are partially inbred as a result of selection for a specific phenotype, such as expression for major histocompatibility complex (MHC) homozygosis (eg, the NIH minipig).

Pigs and minipigs may be sourced from breeders with different health status, such as conventional, minimal disease (MD), specific pathogen free (SPF) and microbiologically defined. Whereas MD, SPF and biologically defined pigs are produced under barrier protection with increasing security (Table 32.5), conventional pigs are kept in a less rigidly controlled environment with a regular health monitoring schedule and thus have a largely unknown microbiological status.

Table 32.4 Physiological values of some haematological and clinical chemical parameters for adult farm and miniature pigs (values assembled from various sources).

Parameter	*Mean*	*Range*
Blood volume (ml/kg)	65	55–75
Erythrocyte count (10^9/ml)	7	5–9
Haematocrit (%)	33	30–50
Haemoglobin (mg/ml)	125	90–180
Leucocyte count (10^6/ml)	13	12–17
Neutrophils (%)	48	40–55
Eosinophils (%)	1.5	0–4
Basophils (%)	0.5	0–1
Monocytes (%)	3.5	1–7
Lymphocytes (%)	50	35–60
Thrombocytes (10^6/ml)	450	200–500
Total protein (g/dl)	7	6–9
Albumin (g/dl)	4	3–5
Aspartate aminotransferase(AST) (U/l)	38	20–200
Creatine kinase (CK) (U/l)	450	100–3000
Alkaline phosphatase (AP) (U/l)	60	30–130

Uses in the laboratory

Pigs and minipigs are valuable models in various areas of biomedical research, including: physiology, pharmacology, toxicology, radiology, surgery and organ transplantation, traumatology, pathology, embryology and paediatrics. Characteristics that make them particularly suitable for research include:

1. a convenient body size for most clinical and surgical experiments or trials involving repeated collection of blood samples, biopsies, etc;
2. many similarities with the human, in particular, skin, skeleton and joints, teeth, gastointestinal tract, pancreas, liver and kidney, cardiovascular system, lung, immune system and physiological state of the newborn;
3. the ease and safety of handling and housing under confined conditions;
4. the relatively low price of acquisition and maintenance;
5. a vast literature extending from embryonic development to modern genomics as well as the expertise of highly specialised commercial farmers and veterinarians;
6. the availability of reproductive technologies, including collection, storage and manipulation of gametes, well in advance of what is available for most other laboratory species.

Table 32.5 Conditions for accommodation of various categories of pigs for experimental purposes (Hansen 1997).

Condition	*Conventional*	*SPF or MD*	*Microbiologically defined*
Caesarean originated	–	+	+
Quarantine regulation	–	+	+
Change of dress	–	+	+
Shower in	–	+	+
Decontamination of:			
Diet	–	–	+
Equipment	–	–	+
Water	–	–	+
Absolute filter ventilation	–	–	+
Health monitored	–	+	+

Laboratory management and breeding

General husbandry

Housing

Wild pigs roam in forests with no permanent retreat except when they build a nest to raise a litter. Their domesticated descendents are less hardy and, in cold climates, are kept indoors during the winter months. All year round indoor housing is also a common practice to protect the herd from parasites and epidemics. This, however, can conflict with the pig's natural qualities of alertness and curiosity and restricts activity. In regions with mild climatic conditions (eg, UK and France), the use of huts or kennels on pasture for breeding sows has gained some popularity.

Detailed information on the housing of farm pigs may be found in husbandry texts (see Further reading section). In a typical commercial piggery, separate quarters are provided for:

1. young stock from weaning to breeding age (growing quarters);
2. weaned sows and gilts that are to be mated and are, therefore, kept in close proximity to a boar (mating quarters);
3. pregnant sows (gestation quarters);
4. parturient and nursing sows (farrowing quarters).

Young gilts and pregnant sows are usually housed in groups. During the first 4 weeks and at an advanced stage of gestation sows should be able to enter a protected area, especially when feeding, otherwise fighting and crushing against rails can lead to abortion. When farrowing, sows have traditionally been caged in special farrowing crates (Figure 32.3). The crates are equipped with rails to prevent the sows from the lying on and crushing their young. They also provide hygienic conditions and protect the stock person from sow aggression while managing the litter. Farrowing crates, however, seriously compromise sow welfare by restricting nest building behaviour and other periparturient behavioural patterns and are, therefore, much disputed and banned in some countries. Loose farrowing and other pen systems under investigation have, under most practical farming conditions, failed to provide viable alternatives as far as piglet losses (Cronin & Smith 1992; Kamphues *et al.* 2003) and other economic considerations such as barn space and labour requirements are concerned. If crates are to be abandoned, pen systems must be devised that provide most of the benefits of farrowing crates. From a welfare point of view ideally the sow should have enough space to turn around and the floor should be, at least in part, solid and covered with shavings or chaff. Anti-crushing rails and a separate heated creep area for the protection of the piglets and provision for temporary fixation of the sow are necessary. Ideally, the sow should be able to leave her nest to move to a separate dunging area as was possible with early farrowing crates when the sows were group-fed twice daily outside the farrowing area. Until more suitable systems have been devised the period of confinement in a farrowing crate should be limited to the period of 3–4 days from the onset of parturition (when the urge for nest building has

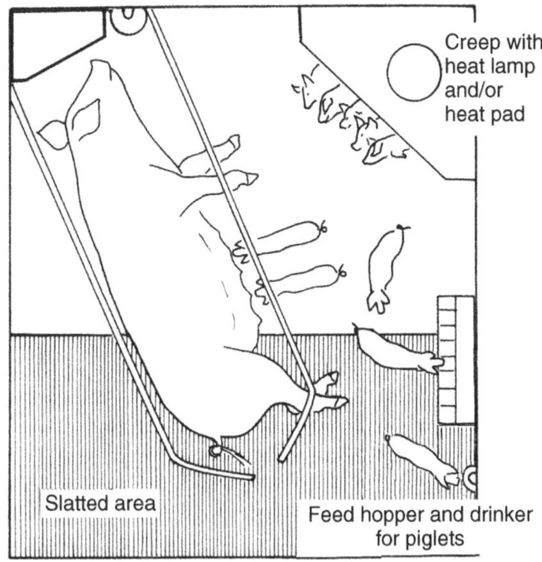

Figure 32.3 Top view of a traditional farrowing crate. Confinement of the sow should preferably be restricted to the 3–4 days following commencement of parturition. Loose housing farrowing systems favour the well-being of the sow, though usually at the price of increased piglet losses.

subsided) until the danger of crushing is over. Various farrowing and nursing pen types are dealt with in a report by European Food Safety Authority (EFSA 2007).

For experimental purposes pigs are occasionally housed in special crates or cages. Up to a body mass of 30 kg they may be kept on perforated or wire mesh floors for limited periods (at the most for a few weeks), provided the cages are located in a room with perfectly controlled climate and ventilation. However, since pigs lack an insulating coat, cage-rearing is a vulnerable system requiring constant care. Several manufacturers supply special miniature-pig cages, including metabolism cages that permit collection of urine and faeces. Dog facilities can usually be modified to house young pigs or minipigs. Partitions between cages should be 1.00–1.10 m high. Individually penned pigs must be in visual or olfactory contact with other pigs. Cages should be large enough for the confined animal to turn around and should have separate sleeping and dunging areas. Minimum floor space recommended by various sources varies considerably. The most recent proposal of the Commission of the European Community in the Directive of the European Parliament and of the Council on the Protection of Animals Used for Scientific Purposes[1], to take effect in 2017, calls for a minimum pen size of 2 m^2. Guidelines for minimum floor space per animal are provided in Table 32.6. They represent a reasonable compromise between the requirements of the animals and practical and economic considerations of space limitation. More confined enclosures may be justified for limited periods to serve special experimental conditions, for example, when monitoring individual feed consumption, or

[1]http://eur-lex.europa.eu/LexUriServ/LexUriServ.do?uri=CELEX:52008PC0543:EN:NOT

Table 32.6 Recommended minimum enclosure dimensions and space allowances for the accommodation of farm and miniature pigs. Figures were assembled from various sources, in particular the commission recommendations of the European Convention (2007) (http://eurlex.europa.eu/LexUriServ/site/en/oj/2007/l_197/l_19720070730en00010089.pdf) and the Council of Europe (2006) Multilateral Consultation of Parties to the European Convention for the Protection of Vertebrate Animals used for Experimental and other Scientific Purposes (ETS 123) Appendix A. Cons 123 (2006) 3 (http://www.coe.int/t/e/legal_affairs/legal_cooperation/biological_safety,_use_of_animals/laboratory_animals/2006/Cons123(2006)3AppendixAen.pdf).

Body mass (kg)	*Pen length (m)*	*Enclosure size (m^2)*	*Floor area (m^2/animal)*	*Lying space** (m^2/animal)*
≤10	1.0	2.0	0.25	0.11
11–20	1.4	2.0	0.35	0.18
21–30	1.6	2.0	0.50	0.24
31–50	1.8	2.0	0.70	0.33
51–70	2.0	3.0	0.80	0.41
71–100	2.1	3.0	1.00	0.53
101–150	2.5	4.0	1.35	0.70
>150	2.5	5.0	2.50	0.95
Adult boar*	2.7	7.5	7.50	1.30

*Miniature pig boars require half the space at the most
**Thermoneutral conditions

taking serial samples. As a rule of thumb, adult miniature pigs require about half the space of adult farm pigs.

Physical environment and hygiene

With their scanty hair covering and lack of sweat glands, pigs are sensitive to temperature extremes. A particularly efficient heating and ventilation system is required when they are kept on perforated floors. Optimum environmental temperatures for pigs vary with age. Newborns thrive best at temperatures of 30–32 °C. The temperature may be lowered by 1 °C for every day of the first week and by 1 °C each week for the second, third and fourth weeks of age. Adult animals housed singly and without bedding feel comfortable at 20 °C or more. With an insulated floor and abundant bedding, they will tolerate temperatures as low as 10 °C without ill effect, especially in a group-housing system where they are able to huddle. In order to satisfy the special temperature needs of the young without exposing the mother to heat stress, farrowing pens should be provided with a heated creep area (Figure 32.3). In hot climates, the lack of shade and of wallows or sprinklers may lead to sunburn or heat stroke.

The favourite relative humidity for pigs is around 60–70%. It should not range beyond extremes of 50% or 90%. Ventilation is critical to keep the concentration of potentially harmful gases low, especially in densely stocked quarters. Concentrations of 10 ppm for ammonia, 0.15 vol% for carbon dioxide and 5 ppm for hydrogen sulphide should not be exceeded. Air speed must not exceed 0.2–0.3 m/s for adult animals and 0.1 m/s for piglets.

Pens should be cleaned out frequently, and on concrete floors dry bedding is most desirable. The daily excretions of an adult farm pig amount to 0.5–3.0 kg faeces (water content 55–75%) and up to 6 l of urine. Once a month, pens should be emptied for thorough cleaning and disinfection. Floors, walls and caging utensils should be soaked and scrubbed or washed down with a high-velocity water jet and treated with a disinfectant. The animals should be returned to the pens once they are dry.

Environmental provisions

Like their wild ancestors, domestic pigs and minipigs are sociable, lively and exploratory animals. They spend 70–80% of their time lying or sleeping; during the remaining time they like to romp, wallow and root in soil or bedding. When given the opportunity, pigs are clean, choosing specific sites for defecation and urination, and keeping their sleeping area dry. In modern pig farming, however, animals are commonly kept in less welfare-friendly conditions such as single stalls or crowded pens, on slatted floors with no bedding. Moreover these environments are often deficient in external stimuli and objects to keep them occupied. Tethering of sows used to be common but is now banned. Pigs, being curious and agile animals, will suffer from boredom if not given the opportunity to perform a range of activities (Wemelsfelder 2005). Common enrichment items include the provision of hanging chains or objects in the pens. Straw provides comfortable bedding, keeps the animals occupied with rooting and chewing activities, and serves as low-calorie fodder, providing a feeling of satiation without leading to obesity. Therefore, clean, dry straw may contribute substantially to the well-being of pigs. Unless experimental conditions require otherwise, the best way of accommodating pigs or minipigs is by housing them in groups of up to 10 or 15 in spacious pens with straw-covered floors. In a number of countries, rules and regulations are laid down to improve husbandry conditions for pigs (eg, European Council 1991; European Commission 1997; New Zealand National Animal Welfare Advisory Committee 2005; EFSA 2007).

Social grouping

Socialisation within groups and the establishment of a social hierarchy are behavioural traits typical of free-ranging pigs. These behavioural patterns should be taken into account when housing pigs in pens. Isolated housing of individuals should be avoided, with the exception of adult males and farrowing sows. When animals are grouped, they should be of similar size and, if feed is restricted, trough space should be sufficient to permit all animals to feed at the same time. Ideally, partitions should be provided, enabling weaker animals to evade aggression from others. If group size exceeds 10–15, agonistic behaviour tends to be increased because no lasting hierarchy is established. This is not always the case, however, because in addition to the amount of space, the quality of space is also important (pen divisions, availability of substrates, feeding places etc). If possible, stable groups should remain together. When animals are mixed from different pens, fighting can be minimised by grouping them just before feeding or sleeping time, preferably in an unfamiliar pen. The animals' individual scent may be camouflaged by sprinkling the animals with anything from cresol to eau-de-cologne. In critical cases, the injection of a tranquillising agent may be necessary.

Adult boars tend to live a solitary life when given the opportunity. Therefore, for them, individual housing is appropriate. Nonetheless, it is possible to group-house boars, with the exception of particularly aggressive individuals, provided they have been reared together or given the opportunity to get accustomed to each other under unconfined conditions, such as on pasture or in a yard. The level of aggressiveness in males is reduced to that of females if they are castrated at an early age (barrows).

Presentation of food and water

Pigs are generally fed once or twice a day. Dry pelleted rations may be presented on the bare, clean concrete floor as long as there is a sufficient distance from the dunging area. More commonly, the feed is presented in a trough or bowl of non-corrosive material installed at or close to ground level. Trough space per animal should be 20–40 cm depending on body size. The feed may be dry or mixed with water or whey to make a gruel or soup. Self-feed hoppers for concentrates, sometimes equipped with a built-in spray nipple for moisturising the feed, are also common. When dry feed is not provided, troughs need to be cleaned daily. Stale feed may lead to digestive disorders. As adult pigs tend to put on excessive fat, transponder systems with computer-controlled feeding stations have been designed. One of these stations will serve 40–50 animals. A hayrack with freshly cut green fodder, hay or straw is valuable from a nutritional and behavioural point of view.

Clean drinking water should be available at all times, so automatic drinkers (nipple or bowl type) are recommended. Nipples should be installed at an adjustable height of 15–50 cm, depending on the size of the animals, preferably above the trough or, otherwise, in the pen area where the animals are expected to defecate and urinate. If automatic drinkers are not available, the usual practice is to mix water with the feed and refill the trough with water after the pigs have finished eating (see Feeding section). Farrowing pens should be equipped with an extra easy-to-operate automatic drinker for the piglets (Figure 32.3).

Health monitoring, quarantine and barrier systems

Existing systems for disease control in pigs are generally aimed at improving the economy of farming operations. Specific pathogen free (SPF) or minimal disease (MD) animals may be infected with pathogens which, although of little economic relevance, could interfere with experiments by changing physiological responses through: immunosuppression, contamination of biological products, anaesthetic death, etc. Therefore, pigs bred for biomedical research should ideally originate from a caesarean-derived colony, be kept in a protected environment (see Sources of supply) and have a regular health-monitoring programme; as is common practice in laboratory rodent colonies (Table 32.5). Staff should not have contact with other pigs, and all materials, including feed, bedding and equipment, needs to be sterilised (autoclaved, fumigated or otherwise). Embryo transfer is an important technique for introducing genetic material into a closed unit.

The Scandinavian Federation for Laboratory Animal Science (Scand-LAS) has published guidelines for health monitoring of pigs (Hem *et al.* 1994), and the Federation of European Laboratory Animal Science Associations (FELASA) has a working group on animal health establishing similar guidelines (Rehbinder *et al.* 1998).

Transport

Transportation is stressful for pigs. To reduce physical strain the animals should be deprived of feed for at least 12 h beforehand. Hot, humid conditions should be avoided, as should extremely low temperatures and draught.

Large pigs are generally transported by truck or trailer. A space of $0.5\,m^2/100\,kg$ body mass should be allowed. Floors must not be slippery and should be fitted with battens or covered with a deep layer of sand. Large loading surfaces should be subdivided by partitions. When driving or loading animals, it is important to understand that they are bewildered and anxious, rather than stubborn. Therefore, be patient, determined and firm, but never rough. Pigs are apprehensive of sloping surfaces, especially if these are unstable or slippery, and do not like entering dark or brightly lit areas.

Miniature pigs and young farm pigs may be transported in portable dog kennels or custom-made durable crates. The floor and bottom part of the sides must be closely boarded to avoid spillage of excreta. Ample straw or shavings must be provided to furnish soft bedding and absorb moisture. There should be openings for fresh air and sufficient space for all animals to lie down comfortably. Feed should be made available at least once, and water at least twice daily. Under certain conditions, the use of a tranquillising agent may be useful. Additional information may be obtained from the latest issue of Live Animals Regulations by the International Air Transport Association (IATA)[2].

Microbiologically defined or SPF pigs or minipigs should preferably be transported in air-conditioned vans equipped with filtered ventilation to prevent infection.

Within the laboratory, animals may either be walked from one place to another, or transported in a trolley; the sides of which should be high enough to prevent the animals from jumping out, but not too high to make it impractical to lift them in and out. When driving pigs, a group always handles better than single individuals. Training the animals by rewarding them with tasty morsels will make operations easier and faster.

[2]http://www.iata.org.

Identification and sexing

Ear tattoos are the most common method of permanently identifying pigs. With pigmented breeds or those with small, cartilaginous ears, such as certain minipig breeds, it may be necessary to resort to notching or ear tagging (Figure 32.4). However, where possible the least invasive method of marking should always be used. Nowadays, electronic identification systems are available, consisting of transponders that are attached to the ear or injected into the tissue at the base of the ear. Recently, injectable microchips have been successfully implanted into unborn piglets (Birck *et al.* 2008). Stationary or portable readers can be used to read the transponders. For temporary marking, special colour markers or sprayers with water-soluble dye are available. Pigs with a light complexion may be given lasting body tattoos applied with a slap marker or an electric tattooing device.

Sexing of pigs presents no problem as they have clearly discernible sex organs from birth.

Breeding

Condition of adults

In contrast to their feral ancestors, reproductive activity in the domestic pig is not seasonal. Normally sows ovulate every 21 days. Males are always ready to mate. Ovulation is accompanied by characteristic oestrous symptoms climaxing in the standing reflex.

Heat checks should be performed at least once daily at a time when animals are not occupied by feeding or the like. Vulvar and behavioural signs are used for testing for oestrus. When there is no teaser boar available, tactile and olfactory stimuli can be imitated by applying manual pressure to the sow's back and by spraying synthetic boar taint (Figure 32.5). Standing heat lasts longer when the boar is present.

The optimal time to have a sow mated or inseminated is about 24h after the onset of standing oestrus if oestrus is detected with the aid of a boar and about 12h after the onset of oestrus in the absence of a boar. Additional matings at about 16h intervals should be allowed as long as sexual receptivity persists.

It is possible to avoid having to detect oestrus by controlling the oestrous cycle and conducting fixed-time insemination. In prepubertal gilts and freshly weaned sows this is done by injecting equine and human chorionic gonadotropins (eCG and hCG), in cycling females, by oral administration of the progestagenic compound altrenogest, followed by withdrawal and an eCG injection (Wallenhorst *et al.* 2000).

As previously mentioned, well managed pig herds achieve farrowing rates of 80–90%. The average gestation period in pigs and Goettingen miniature pigs is 114–115 days (see Reproduction).

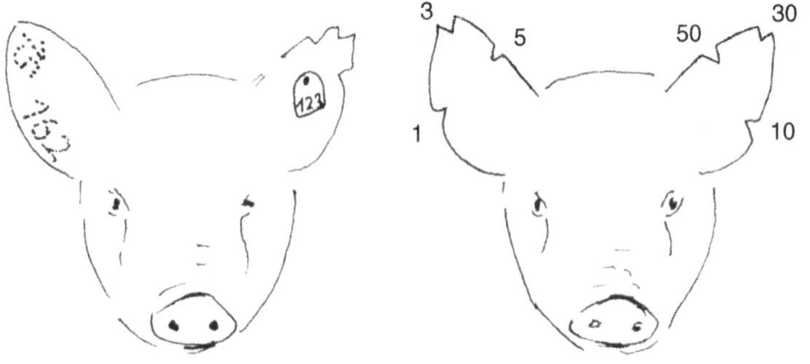

Figure 32.4 Pigs are commonly identified by ear tattoo, ear tag or notches in the ears (notching key used for Goettingen miniature pigs worldwide on the right).

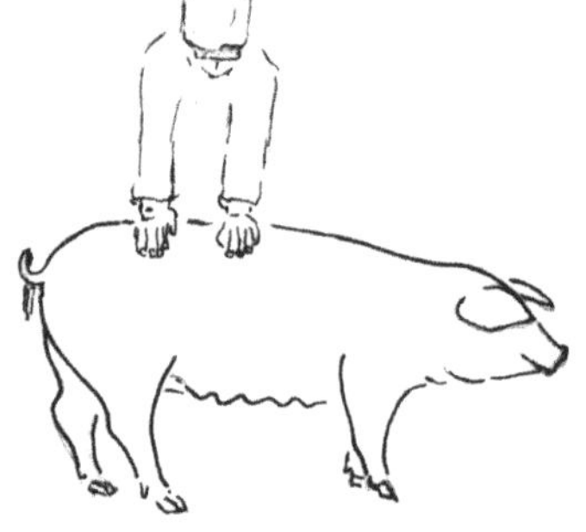

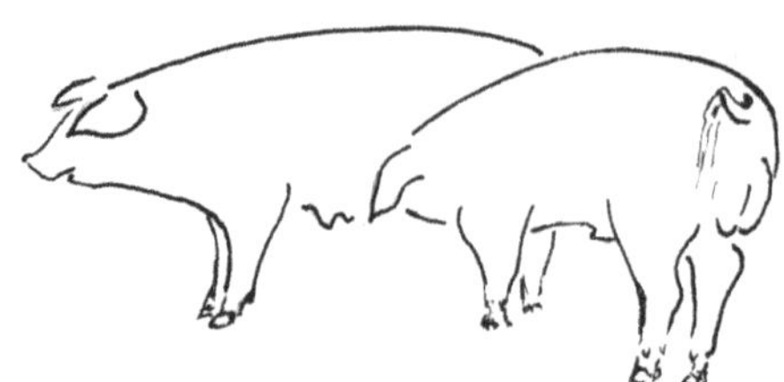

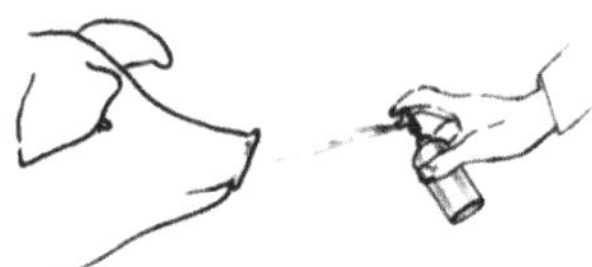

Figure 32.5 Oestrus detection in pigs with the aid of a teaser boar or by manual back pressure and commercially available boar taint.

Artificial insemination has become standard in modern pig farming, and can also be used with minipigs. Semen collection and insemination are easy to conduct, and, with experienced personnel, success rates are comparable with natural mating. Semen can be stored in a commercially available diluent at 15–18 °C for 3–4 days. Conception rate and litter size after insemination with cryopreserved semen is usually unsatisfactory.

There are reasonable success rates for transfer of pre-implantatory embryos, usually flushed from superovulated donors around day 7 after conception (Bruessow *et al.* 2000). Existing techniques for cryopreservation of embryos are unsatisfactory and, at present, embryo transfer must be looked upon as a technique for special situations and experimental purposes.

The traditional method of pregnancy detection is to carefully observe the sows for oestrous signs around the 3rd and 6th week (one and two cycles) after insemination. In modern farming operations ultrasonic equipment is available: the A-mode pulse echo system produces reliable results between 28 and 85 days of pregnancy; the more elaborate and time-consuming Doppler system can be used to detect pregnancy as early as day 16; and real-time echography enables visualisation of foetuses by day 23 of pregnancy. The latter system requires specially trained operators. Rectal palpation, serum progesterone, urinary oestrogens or histological examination of vaginal biopsies are feasible alternatives, but are rarely applied.

Approximately 1 week before they are due to farrow, sows should be moved to the farrowing quarters where they are kept in farrowing crates (Figure 32.3). Under conventional (non-barrier) housing conditions, they should be wormed, scrubbed down with soap and water and treated with a parasiticide. The crates are equipped with rails controlling the movement of the sow to protect the piglets from being crushed and with a heat pad and/or creep area with overhead heat lamp to provide them with a suitable microclimate. If no heat source is available, ample straw bedding must be provided to enable the piglets to burrow into it, huddling together for warmth.

During the 2–3 days prior to farrowing, feed supply to the sow should be reduced to half. Components rich in crude fibre, such as bran, are increased, water is supplied *ad libitum* and sometimes 1 or 2 tablespoons of Epsom or Glauber's salt are added. These measures help to reduce the incidence of constipation and parturient infection of uterus and mammary glands, commonly termed metritis–mastitis–agalactia (MMA) or post-partum dysgalactia (PPD) syndrome.

About 1 day before parturition, sows will display nest-building behaviour when given the opportunity. They will carry grass and other nesting material in their mouth to a shallow pit and with snout and forelimbs arrange it in a cup-shaped nest of more than 2 m^2. The young are born into the nest. Sows penned in a conventional farrowing crate will start getting restless, repeatedly change their posture, paw and root the floor, gnaw and tear on the confining rails or boards and defecate frequently. This behaviour may be interpreted as displacement nest-building behaviour, or as symptomatic of frustration.

Signs of approaching parturition are enlargement of the vulva and swelling of the mammary glands with the presence of colostrum, restlessness and nest-building behaviour. Eventually the sow lies down on her side and the piglets are delivered at intervals of 10–30 minutes, the fetal membrane being expelled between births or within 2–3 h after the birth of the last piglet. Although birth is usually trouble free, supervising parturition can minimise piglet losses. It may be necessary to free newborn pigs from the enveloping membranes, remove mucus from mouth and nose to help them start breathing, help weaker ones to reach the udder or the heated creep area, and rescue them from being crushed by overlying, trampling or savaging by the sow. With weak and underweight piglets, stomach tube feeding of colostrum substitute will improve survival. As a general rule, intervention should be limited to a minimum. Occasionally, savaging of piglets becomes a problem. In these cases piglets should be removed from the sow and placed back as soon as she has finished farrowing. If the sow does not quieten down, a small dose of tranquilliser will usually help.

If labour lasts for more than 45 minutes without visible progress, assistance should be given by inserting a clean, preferably gloved, and lubricated hand into the vagina, gently correcting the condition preventing delivery. In nulliparous gilts and minipigs where the vagina is too narrow, the use of gynaecological forceps is necessary. If inertia of the uterus is the problem, one or several injections of 1–2 IU oxytocin and infusion of 30–40 ml of a 50% calcium gluconate solution are indicated. Large doses of oxytocin tend to cause spasm and even rupture of the uterus. As a last resort a caesarean section should be performed without unnecessary delay, because more than 24 h after the onset of labour the piglets are usually dead.

Parturition may be induced prematurely to facilitate supervision and cross-fostering of piglets ('batch-farrowing'). Induction can be achieved by injecting prostaglandin $F_{2\alpha}$ or one of its analogues. Normally, delivery commences 24–30 h after prostaglandin injection. Parturition should never be induced before 111–112 days after the last mating, otherwise premature piglets will be born that have reduced chances of survival. Individual variation in response to the prostaglandin treatment can be further reduced by following the prostaglandin injection, about 20 h later, with a long-acting oxytocin preparation.

The young

Pigs produce precocial offspring born with all sense organs functioning. The newborn immediately start seeking the udder and generally achieve their first successful suckle within about 45 minutes. Baby pigs need antibody-containing colostrum within the first few hours. The energy reserves of newborn piglets are limited and they rely heavily on a warm, protected environment and frequent milk feeds. Young piglets suckle at less than 1 h intervals; later the frequency declines. Soon after birth, piglets fight fiercely until a teat order is established. The teat order arrived at about 4 days after parturition is adhered to until weaning.

When nursing, the sow lies down on her side calling her litter with a series of grunts. The piglets start nosing the udder vigorously until the milk let-down reflex is elicited. After 15–20 seconds, during which the sow gives a series of low grunts in quick succession, the milk flow ceases. Young piglets fall asleep at the udder; as they grow older they move back to the creep area. Neonatal mortality averages 10–15%, 80% of which occurs within the first week. Most losses occur during the first 24h after birth, especially if the birth mass is low and litter size exceeds the number of functional teats. The primary causes of death are crushing by the mother (almost half of the losses), chilling and starvation.

Fostering piglets from one sow to another (eg, in the case of extranumerary piglets, agalactia or loss of a sow) is not a major problem and works best within the first 2 days after birth among sows that have farrowed within a day or so of each other. Unsuckled mammary glands dry up after about 3 days. When adjusting unequally sized litters, a measure facilitated by batch farrowing, the most vigorous members of a litter should be fostered, especially if the offspring of the host are older and stronger. When cross-fostering older piglets, it is important to camouflage their individual scent and mix the foster piglets with the original litter for 2–3h before presenting them to the new mother. The piglets to be fostered may be rubbed, particularly in the perineal region, with dung from the sow's own litter.

During the suckling period it is important to consider the following issues relating to health and well-being of sow and litter:

1. Parturient infection of uterus and mammary glands, often accompanied by agalactia, may pose a major problem in some herds. Therefore, it is advisable to monitor body temperature of the sow for the first 3 days after parturition, to immediately take action in terms of suitable antibiotic treatment and support of the piglets.
2. Newborn piglets can injure the sow's teats with their needle-sharp canines. This is commonly an indication of a deficiency in the amount of milk produced by the sow. The piglets' teeth may be blunted with the aid of an electric tooth grinder. Care should be taken not to expose the pulp and clippers are not recommended as their use may lead to pulp infection.
3. In commercial breeding units where the intestinal threadworm *Strongyloides ransomi* may occur, piglets have to be wormed within the first 3–4 days after birth.
4. Within 1 week after birth, piglets having no access to soil or another source of iron must be given an intramuscular injection or oral medication of an iron preparation because they are born with a very limited store of iron and the iron content of the sow's milk is low. After 2–3 weeks the treatment should be repeated.
5. Where males are neutered, this has to be done in the period between birth and 8 weeks. Within the first week bleeding and pain are thought to be less than in older animals. The testes are removed via two incisions in the ventral scrotum. The incisions should remain unsutured to facilitate drainage. Strict hygiene must be observed to prevent infection, especially since at age 3–6 weeks piglets have low antibody titre. Anaesthesia, as well as administration of a long-acting analgesic, is recommended.
6. For older animals, and where tail-biting is a problem, amputation of the caudal third of the tail within 3 days after birth may be necessary. The remaining part of the tail is more sensitive to pain, so the animal will not tolerate others to gnaw on it. Once they sense blood, other piglets will mercilessly pursue the victim and may inflict potentially fatal injuries. Tail-biting commonly is a consequence of suboptimal husbandry conditions. Reducing light intensity may attenuate this behaviour. Keeping pigs in permanent darkness, however, is prohibited by law.
7. After parturition, the amount of feed provided to the sow must be gradually increased to reach *ad libitum* levels within 1 week (Table 32.7, Figure 32.6).

Table 32.7 Basic nutrient requirements of farm pigs (NRC, 1998 and other sources) and miniature pigs (GV-SOLAS, 1999b) at various ages and reproductive states.

Category	*Metabolisable energy (MJ/day)*	*Crude protein (%)*	*Maximum crude fibre (%)*
Piglet			
3–5 kg	2–5	25	2
6–10 kg	6–8	22	6
11–20 kg	10–13	20	6
21–50 kg	18–24	18	6
51–120 kg	25–40	14	7
Pregnant sow			
<12 weeks	28	12	14
>12 weeks	35	16	7
Lactating sow (10 piglets @ 5 kg)	80*	16	7
Breeding boar	33	16	7
Adult maintenance	16–28**	12	14
Minipig (20–40 kg)			
Breeding	12–19	12–15	6–8
Maintenance	4–6	12	14

*17 MJ for maintenance of sow + 5.8 MJ per piglet
**$0.44 \times BM^{0.75}$

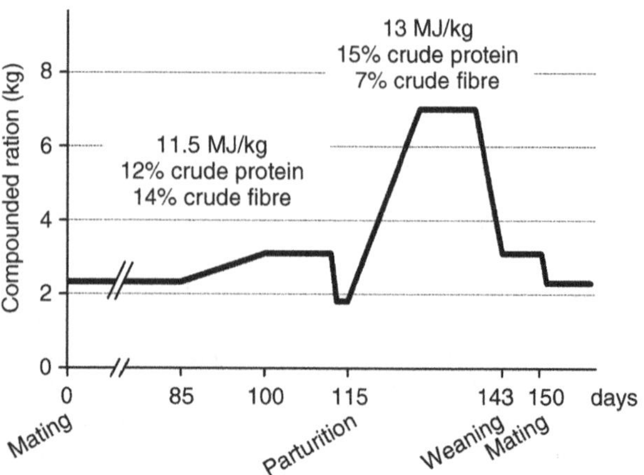

Figure 32.6 Average daily amount of a complete compounded ration fed to a sow of 200 kg at various reproductive states (litter size: 10; suckling period: 4 weeks).

In conventional production units, piglets are usually weaned at about 4 weeks of age. At that stage they weigh 7–8kg and are strong enough, and are able from an immunological point of view, to cope with the harsh environment of modern rearing units (eg, flat-deck cages). Moreover, by that time the reproductive tract of the sow has recovered to the extent that normal fertility has been regained. This system of early weaning was originally adopted to yield more piglets per sow and year. The younger the piglets are at weaning, the more vulnerable they are, consequently more attention must be given to environmental control. When post-weaning rearing conditions are suboptimal, piglets should be weaned at an age of 6–8 weeks. As long as the weaners are accustomed to creep feed, they will readily take to solid food and water. The average daily weight gain in pigs increases from 150g after weaning to 700–800g or more for body weights between 40 and 80kg.

When a mother dies or suffers from agalactia, or if more young are born than there are functional teats, piglets have to be either fostered onto another sow or reared artificially. The latter is labour-intensive and time-consuming, and the following provisions must be made.

The accommodation must supply protection from draught; temperatures should be around 30°C at the beginning and may be gradually reduced to 20–22°C at 3 weeks of age; relative humidity should not exceed 60–70%. A suitable substitute for sows' milk has to be provided. This may consist of a commercially available substitute, cow colostrum, condensed cows' milk fortified with minerals and vitamins or slurry made up of 20% starter creep in water. Each feeding must be freshly and hygienically prepared and provided in portions small enough to be consumed at once. During the first few days the feed must be warm; after this, a gradual decline to room temperature is acceptable. For hand feeding, there should be four to six feeds of about 100ml each, preferably offered in a shallow bowl. Today reliable automatic feeders are available that may be programmed or sensor-run.

If possible, piglets should obtain colostrum (sow or cow) during the first 6–12h of their life to provide them with protection from infection. In the event of scouring, feed intake should be reduced drastically for at least 24h, and fluid intake should be encouraged and a suitable therapy, if necessary, with antimicrobial agents (oral or parenteral), should be put into effect. Transfer to solid feed (initially milk-based, later cereal-based) should take place at 2–3 weeks of age (about 3kg body mass).

Breeding programmes

The selection of breeding stock has to comply with the breeding goal in question, and this may differ for farm and research pigs. Miniature pigs have been selected for low body mass (Koehn *et al.* 2008). The original breeding policy of the Goettingen miniature pig has been described in Glodek & Oldigs (1981) and Glodek *et al.* (1977). Special breeding programmes, such as selection for larger ear veins (to enable better access to the blood system) are used at Dalmose, Denmark, where Goettingen miniature pigs are being bred. Attempts to select strains for hereditary diseases, such as diabetes mellitus, arteriosclerosis, cutaneous melanoma and congenital ventricular septum defect, to generate genetic models of human disease, tend to fail because most defects have a multifactorial genetic background (Hand *et al.* 1987).

Feeding

Natural and laboratory diets

Wild and domesticated pigs are truly omnivorous, consuming and digesting anything from grass to highly concentrated food of plant or animal origin. Their ability to break down and utilise raw fibre, however, is limited. Although a large proportion of the nutrient requirements can be provided by good pasture, it is more common to keep domestic pigs indoors throughout the year and feed them on concentrates. These usually consist of ground cereals supplemented with protein (fish meal, soybean meal, milk by-products), essential amino acids (mostly L-lysine, D-methionine, L-threonine, L-tryptophan), vitamins (A, D_2, D_3, E, several B vitamins) and minerals. Standard diets may be obtained from commercial producers as meal or in pelleted form. They may be fed as complete rations, or in combination with several kinds of roughage or by-products such as brewers' grains or whey. If roughage is supplied, it may consist of grass, lucerne, clover, hay, silage or root and tuber crops.

Meal or pelleted feed may be offered dry or mixed with water or whey to make a mash. For young stock and animals kept on a maintenance diet, a single feed per day suffices; lactating animals should be fed more than once. Where computer-controlled feed dispensers are available, transponders, usually attached to the ear, make sure each individual receives the appropriate amount.

Laboratory diets for pigs and minipigs are based on natural ingredients, and are usually fixed-formula diets. They are available from specialised commercial producers as diets for growth or maintenance. Some producers offer expanded diets that have been heat-treated with steam. This process is claimed to give a better availability of nutrients, a low microbial count and good acceptability by the animals. Laboratory diets should be batch controlled for nutrient content and contaminants as variation in nutrients may produce unexpected experimental results. Contaminants such as heavy metals, fungal toxins or pesticides may also seriously impair the health status of animals and interact with drugs.

Before introduction into an SPF environment, diets may be sterilised by autoclaving or irradiation. In general, expanded diets have a low microbial count, and may be introduced into a barrier after decontamination of the feed containers.

Water

Since most diets are offered in a dry form, clean drinking water must be constantly available, even though pigs drink mainly after eating. The average daily water demand of adult pigs varies between 10l and 30l (nursing sows). The individual demand is quite variable as for lactating sows between 10 and 78l have been recorded. Under high temperature conditions the demand may be substantially increased. Therefore, functioning automatic drinkers are the best solution. Usually, but not always, water from the public supply is of good quality. If necessary, water may be decontaminated with chlorine or ultraviolet light.

Dietary requirements

Nutrient requirements for animals of different ages and reproductive status differ, especially with regard to protein, energy and crude fibre content. Under farming conditions, generally three types of rations are supplied: (1) creep feed for suckling and newly weaned piglets (at least 20% crude protein, not more than 7–8% crude fibre); (2) production rations for growing, late pregnant or nursing animals (16–18% crude protein, not more than 7–8% crude fibre); (3) maintenance rations for mature animals (12% crude protein, 14% crude fibre). The lipid content (ether extract) of most rations is in the range 3–3.5%. Changes from one type of ration to another should occur gradually. Dietary requirements for pigs are given in detail by the National Research Council (NRC 1998) and *DLG-Futterwerttabellen Schweine* (DLG 1991). Despite the fact that these are minimum requirements to prevent deficiencies, the National Research Council guidelines are based on maximum growth and, when keeping mature animals on a maintenance ration, may lead to obesity. Table 32.7 lists lower energy requirements for pigs of 21–120 kg. Since sows that are hungry tend to be restless and aggressive, it is advisable to feed rations with high crude fibre content or include good-quality hay or straw with the ration. Note that a high level of crude fibre will impair feed efficiency.

Figure 32.6 summarises a typical feeding strategy for sows fed exclusively on a commercially available complete compounded ration. As obesity predisposes to birth difficulties, postpartum metabolic disorders and low milk yield, the feed supply for dry sows has to be strictly limited. Only during the last third of pregnancy should the ration be gradually increased. By reducing the feed supply 2 or 3 days before expected parturition, commonly encountered problems with constipation and postpartum complications may be averted. After farrowing, the level of feeding is gradually stepped up at a rate of 400 g per day to the maximum amount of wholesome feed the sow will consume. As a rule of thumb, suckling sows should be provided with 1% of their body mass plus 0.5 kg per piglet of a concentrated ration each day. Three or four days before weaning, the feed supply is gradually cut back to pre-parturient level, and is further reduced as soon as the sow has been re-mated. After mating, the original system of restricted feeding is resumed.

This highly controlled feeding regimen necessitates individual feeding facilities; otherwise slow eaters and weaker animals will not get their share, while others grow fat. By monitoring the appetite and condition of the animals, individual requirements must be recognised and met by adjusting the amount of feed accordingly.

The growth rate of suckling piglets is such that, with large litters, after about 2 weeks the mother's milk will not satisfy their nutritional demand. Thus, piglets should have free access to palatable creep feed of high digestibility and protein, vitamin and mineral content from 1 week after parturition onward. After weaning, farm pigs are fed *ad libitum* until reaching a body mass of 80–90 kg. Thereafter feed intake has to be restricted; in the case of concentrates to about 80% of the unrestricted intake. More detailed information on the nutrition of domestic pigs is provided in standard texts (NRC 1998; Lewis & Southern 2000; Lindberg & Ogle 2001; Kirchgessner *et al.* 2008; Jeroch *et al.* 2008).

The nutritional requirements of miniature pigs closely resemble those of farm pigs. The daily energy requirement for maintenance is about 0.4 MJ/kg body weight$^{0.75}$; during the growth phase it approaches 1.2 MJ/ kg body weight$^{0.75}$. A major problem in feeding adult miniature pigs is the avoidance of obesity, particularly in females not producing offspring. Restricted feeding imposes a perpetual feeling of hunger, with obvious animal welfare implications. Therefore, it is better to provide a voluminous, low energy density, maintenance ration with high fibre content (14% or more) with an adequate vitamin and mineral content. The ration should contain components such as bran, sugar beet pulp, green fodder, hay or straw. At Dalmose, Denmark, Goettingen miniature pigs beyond 6 months of age receive their daily ration in just one feeding. This way they remain sedate throughout the day. The German Society for Laboratory Animal Science (GV-SOLAS 1999b) has published the dietary requirements for miniature pigs. Although the recommendations are based on empirical results, they will lead to satisfactory growth, good fertility and the avoidance of obesity.

Laboratory procedures

Handling and training

Pigs that are not used to being handled are shy and excitable. When anxious or confined they tend to panic. They scream, struggle and may even succumb to circulatory collapse. Force or subjugation will aggravate the situation, where patience, a handful of feed, a chip of apple or a lump of sugar will render a pig tame and co-operative. When handled gently and patiently, pigs become affectionate and usually relish a back scratch or stroking behind their ears or on their bellies. Vietnamese potbellied pigs are more reluctant to overcome their fear of humans. Adult boars should be approached with due respect as they can inflict serious injury with their tusks. But they, too, will grow tame and easy to handle, provided the person working with them always remains calm, though firm. To avoid injury it is advisable, under anaesthesia, to cut the tusks of adult males close to the gums with a wire saw. Sows rearing litters will sometimes be aggressive if they deem their young in danger.

Up to 5 kg, piglets can be picked up by the hindlegs, but a better method, resulting in less stress, is to lift them on the arm, as with a small dog. Heavier animals up to 20 kg can be held tucked under the arm. For certain procedures, such as taking faecal samples or blood from the jugular vein, smaller animals may be held on the lap or placed legs up in a V-trough (Figure 32.7). Another method of immobilisation is to move them into a special restraint box or place them in a hammock-like sling with holes for the legs. Animals too

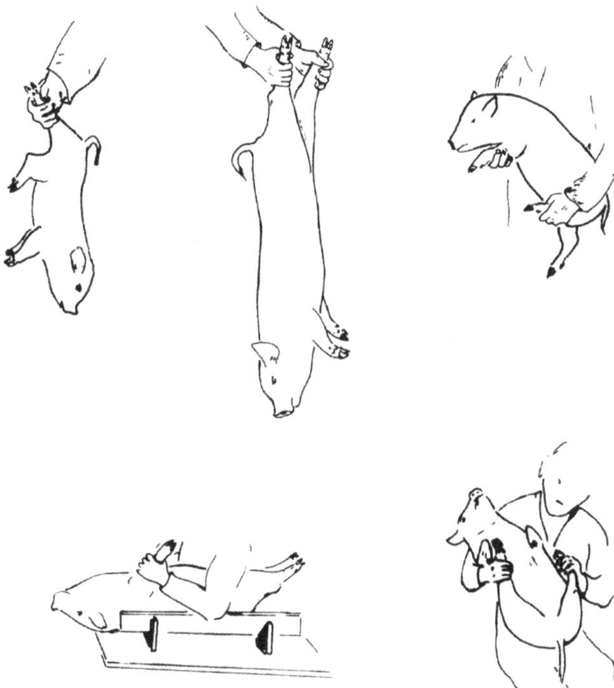

Figure 32.7 Handling and restraining of light farm pigs or miniature pigs. Piglets may be picked up by the hindlegs but should only be held like that for short periods.

heavy to be held can be restrained using the agricultural practice of slipping a wire snare over their upper jaw and positioning it behind the canines. In this situation the reaction of the pig is to pull back (Figure 32.8). If this is executed skilfully, the floor is not slippery and the animal is able to rest its rear against a wall, then not much force needs to be exerted and the animals are not overly stressed. Whereas a wire snare has to be held continuously, a rope noose may be tied to a pole or fence. This means of restraint is commonly applied for brief manipulations on conscious animals such as administration of an injection or collection of blood or a faecal sample. Miniature pigs sometimes behave differently: jumping and turning around instead of pulling back. A more gentle approach would be to train the animal to walk into a large sling with some method of elevating it. The best alternative, though time consuming, is for the handler to establish a relationship with the animal that will enable him or her to train the pig to accept regular routine procedures such as injections or blood sampling, using appropriate positive reinforcement.

When moving individual pigs or groups of pigs, light boards or hurdles are useful. Single animals may also be driven by walking behind them, directing them with a cane or paddle (Figure 32.8). Pigs are quick to learn and easy to train. They will perform routine acts such as entering a restraint box or keeping to a certain order. Tasty rewards are a sure way to success, whereas the use of force or punishment is counterproductive.

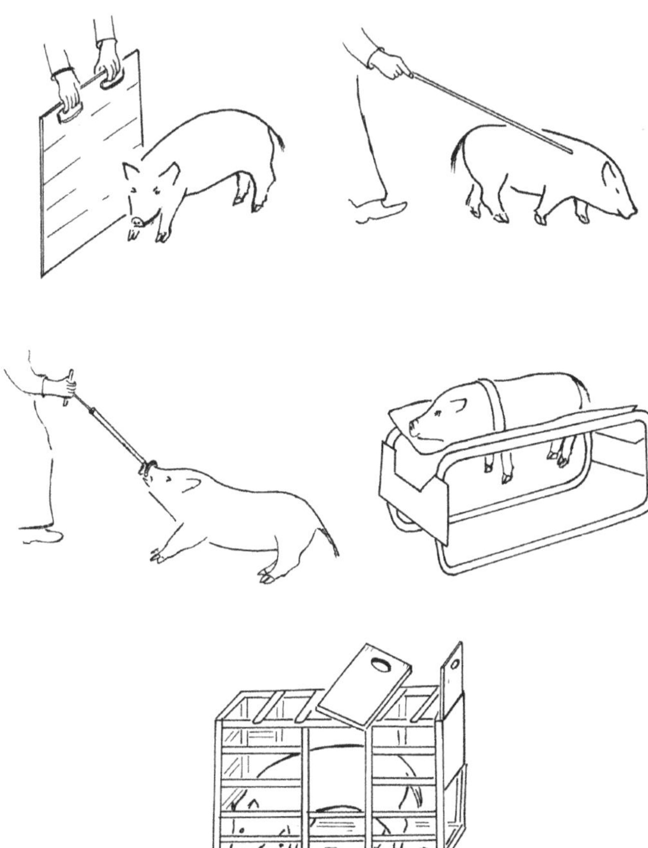

Figure 32.8 For moving pigs or miniature pigs about, light boards or a cane are useful. For immobilising them, an upper jaw snare, a sling with holes for the legs or a restraint box are expedient.

Physiological monitoring

Recording body temperature, cardiac and pulmonary functions

Body temperature in pigs is measured by inserting a thermometer 5–6 cm deep into the rectum or vagina. The pulse may be taken by placing the palm of the hand (or a stethoscope) against the thoracic wall under the left elbow or on the inside of the thigh where the femoral artery is close to the skin. Alternatively an artery on the rostral rim of the ear or the coccygeal artery on the underside of the tail may be palpated (Figure 32.9). Careful auscultation of heart and lung has to be carried out with a stethoscope as described in Straw *et al.* (2006). Percussion is described in Jaksch and Glawischnik (1990). Blood pressure may be approximated by palpation of the pulse on the underside of the tail. A more accurate estimate may be obtained by applying the inflatable cuff method after Riva-Rocci in the coccygeal artery at the base of the tail. Direct measurement of arterial and venous pressures requires introduction of catheters or probes into blood vessels (Marshall *et al.* 1972; Neundorf & Seidel 1977). To obtain an electrocardiogram, the electrodes of the recording unit may be attached to the trunk of the animal to approximate an Einthoven's triangle with the heart in its centre (Neundorf & Seidel 1977), referred to as the Nehb-Spoerri method, or to the extremities (Hoeller 1959). The latter approach provides poorer wave amplitudes. The animals must be kept off the ground and should, therefore, be placed in a sling (Figure 32.8). A long-term electrocardiogram recording system for miniature pigs has been described by Suzuki *et al.* (1998) and a range of electrophysiological and other recording procedures may be found in Swindle (2007).

Procedural information on a range of electrophysiological, haemodynamic and other procedures can be found in Heinritzi *et al.* (2006) and Swindle (2007).

Collection of specimens

Blood

General advice on blood collection can be found in Joint Working Group on Refinement (JWGR) (1993). In the pig there are not many easily accessible blood vessels. Depending on the quantity desired, several approaches may be taken. To obtain just a few drops or up to 1 ml of blood it is easiest to nick an ear vein with the tip of a scalpel blade. Up to 5 ml may be collected by puncturing the distended marginal ear vein with a hypodermic needle. The procedure resembles an intravenous injection. Larger volumes are drawn from the cranial vena cava, the brachiocephalic or the external jugular vein. The cranial vena cava extends from the heart to the cranial tip of the sternum, where it branches into the brachiocephalics, which branch again to form the external and internal jugular veins running toward the head on both sides of the trachea. To draw blood from the vena cava or the brachiocephalic veins of animals weighing up to 30 kg, the animals are held in a supine position, preferably in a V-trough, head and neck straightened out and front limbs drawn backwards (Figure 32.7). In farm and minipigs up to 25 kg, a 20 G hypodermic needle (0.9 × 40 mm), in adult miniature and farm pigs a larger cannula (1.5 × 100 and 1.5 × 150 mm, respectively) is inserted cranial to the sternum slightly lateral to the midline. While advancing the needle in a caudal-dorso-medial direction, a vacuum is maintained in the syringe so blood starts streaming in as soon as the vessel is punctured. The use of vacutainers or monovettes facilitates the operation. In minipigs the cannula should be inserted on the midline just cranial to the sternum, at an angle of 60°. To find the external jugular vein further up the neck, the jugular fossa may be used for orientation. In heavier animals, the same procedure is followed while they are standing up with the head pulled forward and slightly upward by an upper jaw snare (Figure 32.8). A way of col-

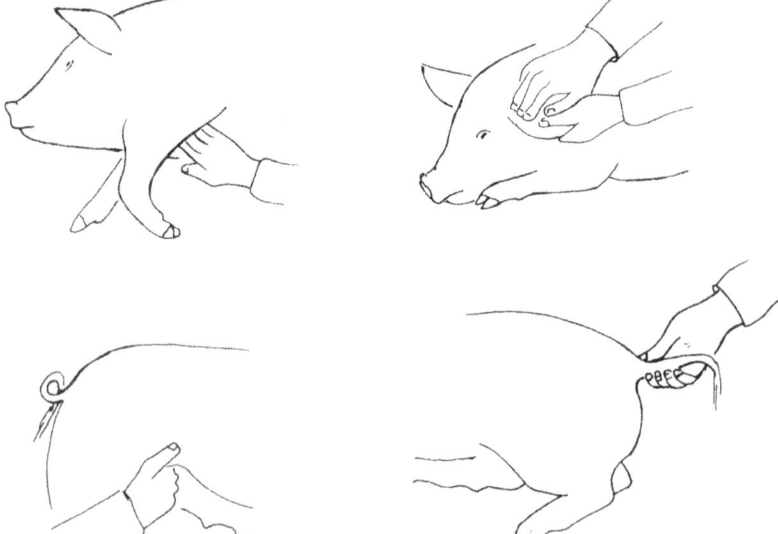

Figure 32.9 Pulse rate may be monitored by placing the palm of the hand under the left elbow or by palpitating auricular, femoral or coccygeal vessels.

lecting venous blood from the sinus ophthalmicus is described in Huhn *et al.* (1969) and Leucht *et al.* (1982) and from the tail vein by Muirhead (1981). Arterial blood may be collected from the brachiocephalic artery (Neundorf & Seidel 1977).

Excitement before or during the collection of blood can induce contraction of the spleen, resulting in an increase in packed cell volume of more than 10%. It is also likely to result in a neuro-endocrine response. Therefore, permanently indwelling catheters may be used for repeated blood collection. Adult domestic pigs, that have big enough ear veins, may be fitted with ear vein catheters. The animal is immobilised by an upper jaw snare and, after thorough cleaning of the ear, a tourniquet is placed around its base. A sharp, thin-walled 14G hypodermic needle is inserted into the marginal (*V. auricularis lateralis*) or central (*V. auricularis intermedia*) ear vein. After releasing the tourniquet, approximately 60cm of tubing (PE 100, 0.86 and 1.52mm internal and external diameters) is threaded through the needle which then is removed. Occasionally some resistance is met at the ear base. A small zippered purse, sutured to the ear with two stitches or a pocket of adhesive tape enveloping the ear, contains the curled-up free end of the stoppered catheter.

In young farm pigs and minipigs, with small ear veins, it is best to resort to jugular catheters. These may be fitted by non-surgical means as described by Carroll *et al.* (1999) for young pigs and Damm *et al.* (2000) for adult animals. For long-term catheterisation a surgical approach is preferable because the catheter may be secured by a retention cuff to prevent it from being pulled out. A thick-walled silicone catheter (1.0mm internal diameter, 2.4mm external diameter) with a retention cuff, 10–15mm in diameter consisting of 1mm thick extra firm grade silicone rubber sheeting attached with silicone adhesive 8–14cm from the tip, is fitted as follows. Under anaesthesia the external jugular is exposed caudal to the larynx via a small skin incision lateral to the *musculus sternomastoideus*, followed by blunt dissection. The vessel is liberated from surrounding tissue for a length of 3–4cm and the blood flow is blocked at both ends with the aid of suture material. A puncture hole is inflicted with a sharp lancet and spread with two loops of fine thumb forceps to permit insertion of the non-bevelled catheter which is filled with sterile physiological saline. The catheter is advanced 6–12cm (depending on the size of the animal) so the tip gets located close to the junction of cranial and caudal *vena cava*. Only on occasion a purse string suture is required to prevent haemorrhage. With the aid of a long stainless steel probe the free end of the catheter is routed to the back of the neck subcutaneously and brought out through a stab wound in the dorsal neck region. About 10cm protruding from the neck is left unrestrained and stoppered with a tight fitting plug. Before suturing the ventral incision, the wound is thoroughly rinsed with sterile saline containing a few drops of iodine, which helps to avoid local infection.

Catheterised animals have to be kept in a clean environment and the catheter exteriorisation site should be dressed with antibiotic powder or ointment on a daily basis. Between samplings, catheters must be filled with sterile saline containing an anticoagulant (100IU/ml heparin) and be tightly stoppered to prevent blood from entering and occluding it. Daily replacement of the saline is advisable. Provided strict hygienic principles are followed, both ear vein and jugular catheters may remain functional for many weeks. Bilateral jugular catheterisation, even if resulting in complete occlusion of both veins, is well tolerated by the animals. Instead of the jugular, the cephalic vein may be used by making an incision halfway between shoulder joint and *manubrium sterni*.

Arterial catheters may be inserted in the carotid artery, which is easily localised dorsal to the jugular vein by digital palpation of the pulse.

Serial blood sampling in conscious pigs may also be accomplished by implanting a vascular access port (VAP) consisting of a reservoir with self-sealing rubber septum and a silicone catheter. The catheter is introduced into a vein and its free end is attached to the VAP reservoir located in a subcutaneous pocket made, for example, in the dorsolateral neck region. The port can be accessed through the skin with a needle for withdrawal or infusion. VAPs are easy to implant (Baille *et al.* 1986; Palmisano *et al.* 1989) and allow for group housing, which is not possible with animals with a protruding catheter.

Porcine erythrocytes are fragile and excessive turbulence and agitation during blood collecting and processing will bring about haemolysis. Coagulation of porcine blood is rapid, and to avoid clotting, the collecting vials must contain an anti-coagulant (Straw *et al.* 2006).

Urine

The easiest way to obtain urine from a pig is to keep it in a metabolism cage, however this is a restricted environment for the pig. Collecting urine during spontaneous micturition is best done after making the animals get up from a resting position, as they will usually urinate soon afterwards. Collection directly from the urinary bladder may be carried out in the female by introducing a catheter of no more than 2mm external diameter into the urethral orifice with the aid of a vaginal speculum. In the male, the urethral approach is not feasible and urine specimens can only be obtained by turning the animal on its back and piercing the abdominal wall cranial to the pubic arch with a long cannula. For repeated collection a flexible catheter is introduced via an incision in the pubic area. This technique has been described by Marshall *et al.* (1972).

Faeces

Specimens may be collected by introducing one or two gloved fingers into the rectum. The faecal sample is grasped with one hand, while the other hand pulls down the plastic glove, everts it and ties the top of the glove to a knot, thus sealing the sample. The use of positive reinforcement techniques might be an option in some studies. If large amounts of faeces are to be collected, animals must be placed in a metabolism cage.

Milk

Milk may be stripped from the teat of a lactating sow. If the sows are trained they will readily present their udder for manual massage and stripping. In some cases oxytocin has to be administered intravenously. For experimental purposes special milking machines have been designed. These are operated in conjunction with oxytocin treatment.

Biopsies

Biopsies have been taken from the testes, skin and other organs, usually under full anaesthesia or after tranquillisation and local anaesthesia. Special equipment has been developed for the taking of back fat and muscle biopsies from pigs without anaesthesia causing neither distress nor pain (Lahucky *et al.* 1982).

Other specimens

To obtain information on the collection of specimens not covered in this chapter, such as lymph, bile, bone marrow, stomach or intestinal contents, skin scrapings, biopsies or entire organs, the following sources may be consulted: Mount & Ingram (1971); Marshall *et al.* (1972); Neundorf & Seidel (1977); Glodek & Oldigs (1981); Leucht *et al.* (1982); Heinritzi *et al.* (2006); Swindle (2007). A system for continual perfusion or dialysis of internal organs in freely moving miniature pigs has been described by Jarry *et al.* (1990) and van Kleef (1996).

Administration of substances

General advice on the administration of substances is provided in JWGR (2001).

Tablets, pills and capsules

Administration of drugs often involves restraint of the animals. Tablets, pills or capsules may be deposited deep in the buccal cavity with the aid of a balling gun. When offered concealed in a morsel of tasty feed, they may be taken voluntarily. In order to circumvent hepatic passage, rectal suppositories may be inserted.

Liquids

Small amounts of liquids may be squirted into the back of the mouth with the aid of a syringe. For large amounts, animals have to be restrained and a mouth gag made of wood or non-toxic hard plastic, with a hole in the centre, is wedged between the jaws. A lubricated stomach tube (0.8–1.7 cm outside diameter) with rounded tip is introduced through the hole into the oesophagus. It will meet elastic resistance, especially when passing the cardiac notch. The pig will vocalise strongly. A smell of acid is indicative of arrival in the gastric lumen. If the tube does not meet resistance, the animal does not scream and breathing is detected, it will have been inserted into the trachea.

In young piglets the tip of a syringe may be introduced into a nostril and pressed firmly against it. If fluid is gradually introduced, it will be swallowed.

Injections

The most common routes of injection (Fig. 32.10) are:

- Intradermal (id, intracutaneous). These injections usually involve very small volumes (2–4 µl) and are administered to the corium layer of the skin on the ear or the back of the animal with a fine (0.6 mm) hypodermic needle.
- Subcutaneous (sc). In animals up to 25 kg such injections are most conveniently administered by lifting them up by the hindlegs, gripping the skin fold between flank and hind leg and introducing the needle (0.9 mm) between the two layers of skin. In animals too heavy to be picked up the needle is introduced caudal to the base of the ear in a perpendicular direction. Dziuk (1991) reports that *'with a little patience and some dexterity'* it is possible, even in unrestrained pigs, to place an injection under the thin, loose and relatively insensitive skin area of the chest just behind the elbow.
- Intramuscular (im). Usually, these injections are administered by inserting the needle (0.9 mm) 1 or 2 cm caudal to the base of the ear in a ventromedial direction. Alternatively, the musculature of the dorsal neck or the thigh may be used. The volume administered should be small, though large enough that there is not a risk of depositing the drug in a fat layer where absorption is poor. Peak blood and tissue levels for most drugs will be reached within about 2 h.
- Intraperitoneal (ip). Usually intraperitoneal (abdominal) injections are applied to animals light enough to be picked up. When held head-down by the hindlegs, an injection caudal to the navel will not cause injury to inner organs. Distribution of the drug throughout the body is faster than with im injections.
- Intravenous (iv) These injections are usually given into an ear vein. For that purpose, the head of the animal has to be fixed, usually with the aid of an upper jaw snare, and the veins are raised by rubbing or slapping the ear and tying a string or rubber band around its base. After the needle (0.7–0.9 mm) has been inserted, the tourniquet is released and infusion can commence. Most minipigs have small, sometimes pigmented ears, with the consequence that the veins can only be identified with the aid of a torch. Other reasonably accessible superficial vessels are the cephalic vein near the forearm, and the femoral and caudal epigastric veins on the inside of the hindlimb. In conscious animals, however, it is very difficult to introduce a needle into these; therefore most people prefer to use the jugular or the cranial vena cava. The procedure resembles that of blood collection (Figure 32.10).

Injection volumes considered to be good practice and maximum acceptable doses are summarised in Table 32.8. The figures refer to aqueous solutions, not to solvents such as dimethyl sulfoxide (DMSO), carboxymethylcellulose (CMC) or oily suspensions. If the administration of larger volumes is unavoidable, multiple injection sites may be indicated. It should be kept in mind that injections might cause pain and tissue damage and should, where possible, be replaced by other routes of administra-

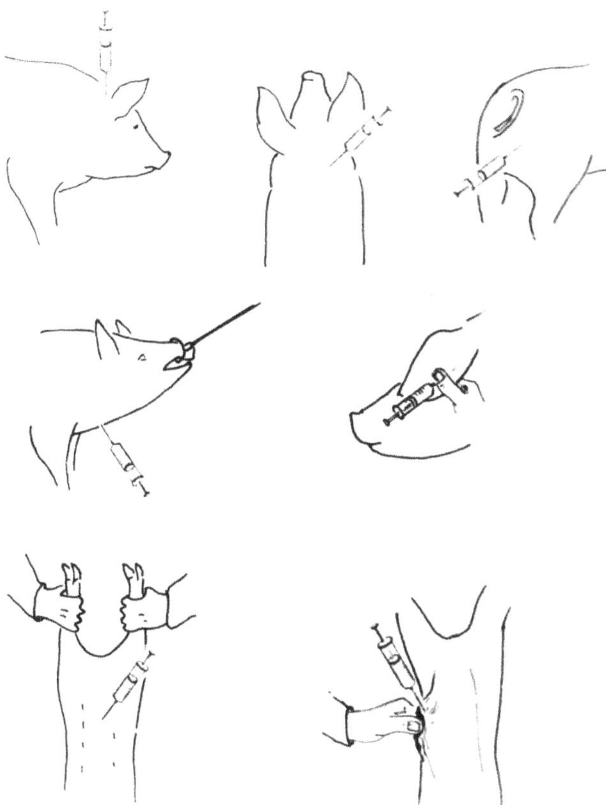

Figure 32.10 Typical injection sites: intramuscular (top), intravenous (middle), intraperitoneal (bottom left) and subcutaneous (top left and bottom right).

Table 32.8 Good practice dose volumes for injecting miniature pigs of 25–40 kg body mass (GV-SOLAS, 1999a; Dorsch, 1999). For lighter pigs smaller volumes are recommended; however, for heavier pigs approximately similar volumes are appropriate.

Dose volumes	*ml/injection site*			*ml/kg body weight*		
				ip	*iv*	
	id	*sc*	*im*		*Bolus*	*Slow injection*
Recommended	0.2	10	5	1	1	2
Maximum	0.4	20	10	20	2	5

tion. In the case of antibiotics administration *per os* is usually possible.

For continuous drug administration, permanently indwelling catheters or ambulatory infusion pumps positioned, for example, in a pocket of a specially tailored vest, might be employed. An alternative approach is to implant an osmotic pump.

Anaesthesia and analgesia

Sedation

Pigs that are to be anaesthetised should be deprived of feed, but not water, for at least 12 h. To minimise stress, it is advisable to sedate them by administering an intramuscular injection of a tranquillising agent in familiar surroundings. The needle can be prevented from being pulled out, if the animal moves, if the hypodermic needle and syringe are connected with flexible tubing. The most commonly applied tranquillising drug is azaperone (1–4 mg/kg) sometimes combined with midazolam (0.5–1 mg/kg) or ketamine (5–20 mg/kg). Azaperone has a wide tolerance range and few side effects and produces sedation, indifference and drowsiness, but not analgesia. Atropine (0.05 mg/kg im or sc, 0.02 mg/kg iv) should generally be included as it cuts down on profuse salivation and bronchial secretion and stabilises the heart action. Animals should be left alone for 5–15 minutes, preferably in dark surroundings, for the sedative to take full action. The animals will remain sensitive to acoustic stimuli and body temperature will drop.

Surgical anaesthesia

No anaesthetic satisfies all possible requirements (ie, sedation, hypnosis, analgesia and muscular relaxation). Therefore, depending on the type and duration of the surgical intervention intended, combinations of various agents may be indicated. Minor surgery may be performed by combining sedation with local anaesthesia using, for example, procaine or lidocaine. For longer interventions it is recommended to place an indwelling catheter in the lateral ear vein for intravenous injection and intubation of the animal.

Injectable anaesthesia

Ketamine is commonly used as a replacement for metomidate, which is no longer available. As ketamine tends to increase muscle tone and exerts little visceral analgesia, it is usually combined with other agents such as azaperone, droperidol, acepromazine, diazepam, midazolam, fentanyl, telazol or xylazine. According to Green and Benson (2002) the group of tranquillisers that is most effective in pigs is the butyrophenone class. Azaperone is a member of this group that is specifically approved for use in pigs by the Center for Veterinary Medicine (CVM) of the Food and Drug Administration (FDA). Phenothiazine tranquillisers are less effective but are also commonly used when butyrophenone tranquillisers are not available. Alpha-2-agonist sedatives are useful, especially in combination with other agents, but relatively high doses must be used (eg, 2.2 mg/kg xylazine). Various laboratories have established protocols of their own depending on the purpose of study. A protocol found to be effective, safe and both clinically and economically sound (Erhardt *et al.* 2004) consists of an intramuscular injection of a mixture of azaperone (2 mg/kg), ketamine (15 mg/kg) and atropine (0.02 mg/kg) followed, 10 minutes later, by an intravenous injection of either the barbiturate thiamylal (5–15 mg/kg) or propofol (4 mg/kg). Propofol is metabolised rapidly, whereas thiamylal, as it is redistributed in the body, will remain present somewhat longer. For extension of anaesthesia, additional amounts of barbiturate or propofol may be infused and an analgesic has to be administered. The amount required may vary considerably.

Inhalation anaesthesia

Anaesthesia may be accomplished with the aid of an inhalation drug, but surgical interventions should not be carried out under inhalation anaesthesia alone. An analgesic such as metamizole or fentanyl should be used in combination. For inhalation anaesthesia halothane or another flurane (sevoflurane, isoflurane) is recommended. Sedated animals rapidly pass into deep anaesthesia without excitation if they inhale 4% halothane in oxygen at a flow rate of 6–8 l/min via a face mask or via an endotracheal tube. Once surgical anaesthesia has been reached, the halothane concentration may be reduced to 1.5 or 2%. In a closed circuit, requiring a tracheal cannula or nose tubes (Bolin *et al.* 1992), surgical anaesthesia will be maintained at concentrations as low as 0.5–1.5%. A further reduction in halothane concentration to 0.4–1.0% may be accomplished by replacing pure oxygen with a mixture of one-half to two-thirds nitrous oxide (laughing gas). An asset of halothane is the quick recovery of the animals and the lack of adverse after effects, even after several hours of anaesthesia. Other fluranes are more expensive than halothane but, according to Smith *et al.* (1997), safer for the personnel. With some susceptible breeds (Pietrain, Poland China and their crossbred offspring) the use of fluranes is not advised as they can induce malignant hyperthermia syndrome; this is characterised by a rapid increase in body temperature, hyperventilation, muscle rigidity and sudden death. The heritable condition is transmitted by a single dominant gene and it is associated with general susceptibility to stress. Breeding programmes are conducted aimed at eliminating the trait from the population. In miniature pigs the condition is unknown.

Finding face masks for pigs that fit snugly and have little dead space is a problem. Shape and size of the pigs' heads varies depending on breed and age. Sometimes commercially available dog masks, consisting of a plexiglas dome fitted with a rubber diaphragm with a central opening for the snout, may be suitable. Improvised masks can also be used, for example, a deflated punch ball, with the bottom cut off, which can be drawn over the pig's snout with the gas supply provided via the blow-tube. Small-animal endotracheal tubes of 5–12 mm outer diameter may be used for nose tubes. They are lubricated and inserted about 4–5 cm into the nares. A broad rubber band tied around the upper jaw just behind the tip of the snout secures the tube in position (Bolin *et al.* 1992).

Endotracheal intubation requires experience. Pigs need to be sedated and anaesthetised (usually via a mask) and treated with atropine. They are placed in lateral or ventral recumbency, the neck is extended and the jaws are opened as wide as possible so the larynx can be seen with the aid of a laryngoscope. The tongue is pulled forward and a long spatula, the first 5–15 cm of which is slightly bent, is inserted between the vocal cords to serve as a guide for the endotracheal tube. The tube should ideally be lubricated with gel containing a local anaesthetic. It must be carefully inserted into the trachea during an inspiratory movement, and is held in position by an inflatable cuff. The tube may be fixed to the upper jaw with adhesive tape or a gauze bandage. Depending on the body weight, the outer diameter of the tube should be between 9 and 12 mm. For miniature pigs, normal oral paediatric endotracheal tubes of 6–8 mm outer diameter without a cuff proved to be suitable. According to Becker & Stauffer (1974) these can be introduced without the use of a spatula. Detailed descriptions of the procedure may be found in Svendsen & Rasmussen (1998); Erhardt *et al.* (2004) and Swindle (2007).

As an alternative to endotracheal intubation a laryngeal mask airway (LMA), designed for use in humans, may be inserted into the hypopharynx of a pig. Once inflated, it will provide an airtight seal around the laryngeal inlet and proved to be efficient in both spontaneously breathing (Wemyss-Holden *et al.* 1999) and mechanically ventilated pigs (Goldmann *et al.* 2005). The system proved to be convenient and efficient even when applied by relatively inexperienced personnel.

Epidural anaesthesia

If surgery is to be performed caudal to the umbilicus, epidural anaesthesia may be applied. Animals are tranquillised and procaine or lidocaine is infused into the spinal canal by inserting a long 20–22 G hypodermic needle through the lumbosacral aperture as described by Neundorf & Seidel (1977), Bolin *et al.* (1992), Heinritzi *et al.* (2006) and Swindle (2007).

Peri- and post-operative care

Most precautions taken to maintain anaesthetised animals in a state of near homeostasis are the same for most mammals. Pigs, lacking a dense hair coat, are particularly prone to hypothermia. To aid in body heat retention it helps to drape them and/or place them on a heating pad both during anaesthesia and the recovery phase. Recuperating pigs should at least be bedded on a thick straw mattress and covered with an armful or two of clean dry straw. During extended interventions additional care might be warranted, including administration of parenteral fluids for maintenance of water and electrolyte balance, analgesics and other drugs. Depending on the situation it may be indicated to monitor respiration, heart rate, body temperature, blood pressure, blood gases or EEC. Appropriate ways of accomplishing this are to be found in Swindle (2007).

Intra- and post-operative analgesia may be provided by using non-steroidal anti-inflammatory drugs (NSAIDs) such as carprofen or meloxicam, metamizole and/or an opiate like fentanyl, remifentanyl or buprenorphine (Preissel, personal communication). The effect of analgesics lasts between a few hours and a whole day depending on the substance used (e.g. the NSAIDs carprofen or flunixine provide analgesia for 24 h whereas the pyrazole derivative, metamizole, needs to be administered every 6 h). The combination of an anti-inflammatory NSAID and the spasmolytic agent metamizole appears suitable (Steffen *et al.* 2002). Carprofen has the advantage that it can be administered as a tasty chewable tablet instead of having to be injected. The use of opiates for bolus administration or continuous infusion during surgery requires intubation because of the opiate's respiratory depressive action. For post-operative analgesia buprenorphine is to be administered at 8–12 h intervals. The use of a fentanyl (an opiate) patch, attached to the shaven skin behind the ear, has been found to be useful (Malavasi *et al.* 2005; Stubhan *et al.* 2008).

Emergencies

The mild respiratory depression caused by barbiturates is easily controlled. If respiration fails, animals that are intubated must be connected to a respirator. It may be necessary to intubate them at this point. Usually it suffices, however, to place them in lateral recumbency, and compress the thorax rhythmically with both hands 10–20 times per minute. Oxygen may be offered, if available. As long as the heart is beating, artificial respiration should be maintained, as the animal has a good chance of recovery. Artificial respiration should be interrupted, from time to time, to reactivate the respiratory centre. In severe cases, especially when working with barbiturates, an intravenous application of a heart stabilising agent, such as lidocaine or, as a last resort, adrenalin may be indicated.

Detailed treatises covering anaesthesia in the pig are to be found in Riebold (1995); Thurmon & Benson (1996); Svendsen & Rasmussen (1998); Erhardt *et al.* (2004) and Swindle (2007). See also Flecknell (2009).

Euthanasia

Euthanasia should be accomplished by methods that induce rapid unconsciousness and death of the animal without pain or distress (see Chapter 17). Generally, inhalant or non-inhalant chemical agents (such as barbiturates, inhalant anaesthetics and carbon dioxide) are preferable to physical methods such as a penetrating captive bolt. However, there might be reasons against using chemical agents. Pigs destined for consumption and slaughter are killed by stunning them with electric current, captive bolts or carbon dioxide, and then bleeding them to death by stabbing with a long knife cranial to the sternum to sever the great blood vessels at the base of the heart. In exceptional cases a free bullet may be used instead of a captive bolt. Very young animals may be killed with a strong blow on the head, but generally an overdose of anaesthetic is preferable. Pigs that are not to be consumed may be killed by intravenous or intraperitoneal injection of a large overdose of an anaesthetic or toxic substance (eg, more than 150 mg/kg pentobarbital). In anaesthetised animals, intravenous infusion of 2 mmol/kg potassium chloride or terminal exsanguination are acceptable.

Common welfare problems

Disease

Prophylaxis

Pathogenic microbes travel with airborne particles or droplets, but more commonly they are transmitted via animal vectors. The most important of these are infected pigs. Other vectors include domestic animals such as cats and dogs, vermin, such as rats and mice, birds, insects and, most frequently, humans. Therefore, good barrier systems should ideally be employed. Principles and procedures of such systems are described in the section on health monitoring, quarantine and barrier systems. When the establishment of a barrier system is not feasible, precautions must be taken to minimise the risk of infectious disease. A few basic principles to be considered are the provision of appropriate housing, husbandry and feeding conditions, a good sanitation programme and, as far as possible, prevention of the introduction of infectious agents.

Before moving animals into quarters formerly occupied by others, the rooms must be thoroughly cleaned and scrubbed with antiseptic solution, preferably with a high pressure jet and hot water or steam. Complete units should be evacuated, cleaned and restocked (all-in, all-out). Animals should be treated for internal and external parasites before being introduced to sanitised housing especially when they had been run on pastures or dirt lots. Animal traffic and visits by people who have been in contact with other pigs within the last 48 h should not be permitted. Foot dips and changing of clothes should be mandatory. Health control specialists advocate a shower to be taken before entering a unit. The origin and quality of biological material (feed, bedding, experimental materials) and equipment should be controlled to prevent the introduction of infectious agents. A rodent and insect barrier should be part of the disease-control programme.

Depending on the source of the pigs and the diseases prevalent in the area, vaccination protocols have to be established. It should be kept in mind that vaccination will protect against disease, but will not usually prevent the transmission of pathogens. Furthermore, vaccinated pigs will be seropositive, which may interfere with health monitoring. Prophylactic antibiotic treatment may control bacterial propagation and enable the host to develop immunity, but will not eliminate the pathogen. Animals to be introduced into the herd should originate from suppliers providing a high standard of hygiene (preferably with SPF or MD status) and a defined disease-control system. It is good practice to quarantine new arrivals for at least 3, preferably 6, weeks before integrating them into the herd. The first 3 weeks are a period of isolation, the animals being monitored, wormed, vaccinated etc; during the following 3 weeks animals from the herd they are to be integrated in are introduced so they may adapt immunologically.

Signs of poor health

General symptoms indicating poor health in adult pigs are emaciation; listlessness and lack of appetite; increased body temperature; discoloration (cyanosis) of skin areas; stiffness of limbs; diarrhoea; snuffling and coughing; in certain conditions hyperactivity, excitability, frequent change of posture and convulsions. Typical symptoms of diseased young piglets are: wasting; listlessness; rough coat; abnormal posture and behaviour; diarrhoea; sneezing, coughing and laboured breathing ('pumping'); swollen joints; increased body temperature and skin conditions.

In addition, there will generally be specific symptoms indicative of the particular ailment involved.

Common diseases

In commercial pig husbandry usually large numbers of animals are kept under confined conditions, facilitating rapid spreading of infectious diseases.

The most important viral diseases affecting pigs are foot and mouth disease, hog cholera (swine fever), porcine influenza, porcine rotavirus, porcine parvovirus, porcine reproductive and respiratory syndrome (PRRS), transmissible gastroenteritis (TGE)/porcine endemic diarrhoea, pseudorabies (Aujeszky's disease) and circovirosis. As some are brought under control (eg, pseudorabies) new ones are cropping up (eg, circovirosis).

Bacterial and fungal infections may cause enteric (*Escherichia coli*, *Isospora suis*, *Clostridium perfringens*, *Brachyspina hyodesenteria*, *Salmonella* spp., *Campylobacter* spp., *Yersinia enterocolitica*), or respiratory diseases (*Mycoplasma hyopneumoniae*, *Pasteurella* spp., *Actinobacillus pleuropneumoniae*, *Streptococcus pneumoniae*, *Bordetella bronchiseptica*) or diseases affecting the skin (*Microsporum* spp., *Trichophyton* spp.), renal system (*Actinobaculum suis*) or a range of other organ systems (*Haemophilus parasuis*, *Erysipelothrix rhusiopathiae*, *Staphylococcus hyicus* and *aureus*, *Streptococcus suis*).

Endoparasites that might give reason for concern even under well managed indoor husbandry conditions are the nematodes *Ascaris suum*, *Strongyloides ransomi* and *Trichuris suis* as well as the protozoan parasites *Isospora suis*, *Eimeria* spp. and – where cats are permitted – *Toxoplasma gondii*, a zoonosis.

Useful handbooks covering diseases in pigs are Taylor (1999), Prange (2004), Waldmann & Wendt (2004), Heinritzi *et al.* (2006) and Straw *et al.* (2006).

Abnormal behaviour

Prevailing husbandry conditions for many farmed pigs are notoriously deficient in providing a complex enriched environment (see Environmental provisions) and high-quality individual attention (see Handling). Under farming conditions breeding stock is usually slightly better off than fattening animals, though, with increasing herd size and growing economic pressures, even these are increasingly reduced to anonymous production units. Unfortunately more acceptable production systems have usually turned out to be less economically viable.

These unfavourable conditions facilitate behavioural aberrations, the most commonly observed of which being:

1. Bar biting. The animals take horizontal bars in their mouth and either bite on it with a chewing motion or just hold it in their mouth for extended periods. This behaviour is commonly observed in sows kept in single crates on concrete floors without litter, and is an expression of boredom and frustration.
2. Vacuum chewing. Animals chew with an empty mouth, froth dripping from the lips and the corners of the mouth. Sometimes the chewing motion is interrupted by gaping. As in the case of bar biting, this behaviour is associated with isolation and boredom.
3. Dog-sitting (German: trauern). Animals spend extended periods in a dog-sitting posture with a sad and distracted look on their faces. This behaviour is usually associated with stimulus-poor situations under conditions of single housing and cold floors.
4. Cannibalism. This usually begins with a non-injurious sucking and nibbling of the ears, legs and, most commonly, the tail of another animal. Typically the tail is taken into the mouth crosswise and bitten playfully; first gently, then harder until blood is drawn. Now all other animals join in and the injured animal becomes the object of a hunt. Once the tail is bitten off, the ears and other parts of the body are mutilated. Eventually the victim becomes apathetic and will usually succumb to bacterial infection. Another variation on the theme is the continued forceful massage of the anal region with the snout. This, too, may lead to injury, inflammation and eventually death.
5. Piglet savaging. This abnormality is usually limited to sows giving birth for the first time. Sometimes the newborn are killed immediately after birth. This might be related to pain and anxiety associated with parturition. Occasionally a sow savages her young after initially accepting them. In some cases this occurs following severe disturbance and turmoil. The occasional consumption of dead piglets by the mother is not directly associated with killing.

With the possible exception of piglet savaging, all the abnormal behaviours mentioned are related to environmental deficiencies such as lack of space, exercise and distraction (see section on environmental provisions), unsuitable floor construction, microclimate or ventilation, insufficient access to feed and water, no means of social interaction, large group size, high stocking density and lack of ability to evade aggressive pen members.

Reproductive problems

Reproductive problems are not common in pigs and minipigs. If they occur, it is usually due to shortcomings in housing, feeding, health status or management. Pigs may produce more than two litters per year and have been selected for centuries to have a high rate of reproduction. Oestrus detection may pose a problem when applying artificial insemination, especially in the absence of a teaser boar. Newly mated sows are sensitive to environmental changes around the time of implantation. During that time shipping or changes in diet should be avoided, otherwise embryo survival is impaired and sows will return to oestrus. In some herds, puerperal infection is an issue and may assume epidemic dimensions. The so-called MMA syndrome is a combination of metritis, mastitis and, as a sequel of the latter, agalactia. Rigorous hygiene programmes and antibiotic therapy may help to alleviate the problem. Abortion and stillbirths may occur and are usually caused by infections such as parvovirus.

Further reading

Further information of relevance for pig experimenters are to be found in specialised texts covering the fields of porcine anatomy (Sack 1982), physiology (Pond & Mersmann 2001; McGlone & Pond 2002), nutrition (Kyriazakis & Whittemore

2006), husbandry and breeding (Glodek 1992; EFSA 2007), behaviour and welfare (Report of the Scientific Veterinary Committee1997; Kaliste, 2004; Broom & Fraser 2007) and experimentation (Stanton & Mersman 1986; Tumbleson 1986; Tumbleson & Schook 1996; Bollen *et al.* 2000; Swindle 2007). Texts focusing specifically on miniature pigs are Glodek and Oldigs (1981), Leucht *et al.* (1982) and Fisher (1993). In addition, attention should be given to websites such as those offered by breeders on handling of miniature pigs, anaesthesia and surgical techniques and to the RETHINK project on the use of minipigs in toxicity testing[3].

References

Baille, M., Wixson S. and Landi, M. (1986) Vascular-access-port implantation for serial blood sampling in conscious swine. *Laboratory Animal Science*, **36**, 431–433

Becker, M. and Stauffer, U.G. (1974) The role of general anaesthesia in experimental surgery on young minipigs. *Journal of Pediatric Surgery*, **9**, 515–519

Birck, M.M., Iburg, T., Schmidt, M. *et al.* (2008) A novel method for transuterine identification of piglets. *Laboratory Animals*, **42**, 331–337

Bolin, S.R., Runnels, L.J. and Bane, D.P. (1992) Chemical restraint and anesthesia. In: *Diseases of Swine*, 7th edn. Eds Leman, A.D., Straw, B.E., Mengeling, W.L. *et al.*, pp. 933–942. Iowa State University Press, Ames, Iowa

Bollen, P.J.A., Hansen, A.K. and Rasmussen, H.J. (2000) *The Laboratory Swine*. CRC Press, Boca Raton

Brandt, H., Moellers, B. and Glodek, P. (1997) Prospects for a genetically very small minipig. In: *The Minipig in Toxicology*. Ed Svendsen, O., pp. 93–96. Satellite Symposium to Eurotox, Aarhus, Denmark

Broom, D.M. and Fraser, A.F. (2007) *Domestic Animal Behaviour and Welfare*. Oxford University Press, Oxford

Bruessow, K.P., Torner, H., Kanitz, W. *et al.* (2000) In vitro technologies related to pig embryo transfer. *Reproduction, Nutrition and Development*, **40**, 469–480

Carroll, J.A., Daniel, J.A., Keisler, D.H. *et al.* (1999) Non-surgical catheterization of the jugular vein in young pigs. *Laboratory Animals*, **33**, 129–134

Cronin, G.M. and Smith, J.A. (1992) Effects of accommodation type and straw bedding around parturition and during lactation on the behaviour of primiparous sows and survival and growth of piglets to weaning. *Applied Animal Behaviour Science*, **33**, 191–208

Damm, B.I., Pedersen, J.L., Ladewig, J. *et al.* (2000) A simplified technique for non-surgical catheterization of the vena cava cranialis in pigs and an evaluation of the method. *Laboratory Animals*, **34**, 182–188

DLG (1991) *DLG-Futterwerttabellen Schweine*, 6th edn. DLG-Verlag, Frankfurt

Dorsch, M. (1999) Applikation von Substanzen. http://www.tierschutz-tvt.de/merkblatt76.pdf.f.

Dziuk, P. (1991) Subcutaneous and intramuscular injection. In: *Handbook of Methods for Study of Reproductive Physiology in Domestic Animals Section 9B, 1 Pig*. Eds Dziuk, P. and Wheeler, M. Dept. of Animal Science, Urbana

European Commission (1997) The Welfare of Intensively Kept Pigs. Report of the Scientific Veterinary Committee: Adopted 30 September 1997. http://ec.europa.eu/food/fs/sc/oldcomm4/out17_en.pdf (accessed 19 March 2009)

[3]www.rethink-eu.dk

European Council (1991) COUNCIL DIRECTIVE 19 November 1991 laying down minimum standards for the protection of pigs (91/630/EEC). http://eur-lex.europa.eu/LexUriServ/LexUriServ.do?uri=CELEX:31991L0630:EN:HTML (accessed 19 March 2009)

European Food Safety Authority (2007) Scientific report on animal health and welfare aspects of different housing and husbandry systems for adult breeding boars, pregnant, farrowing sows and unweaned piglets. *Annex to the EFSA Journal*, **572**, 1–13 http://www.efsa.europa.eu/EFSA/efsa_locale-1178620753812_1178655708740.htm

Erhardt, W., Henke, J. and Haberstroh, J. (2004) *Anaesthesie und Analgesie beim Klein- und Heimtier*. Schattauer Verlag, Stuttgart

Fisher, T.F. (1993) Miniature swine in biomedical research – applications and husbandry considerations. *Lab Animal*, **22**, 47–50

Flecknell, P.A. (2009) *Laboratory Animal Anaesthesia*, 3rd edn. Academic Press, London

Glodek, P. (1992) *Schweinezucht*. Eugen Ulmer Verlag, Stuttgart

Glodek, P., Bruns, E., Oldigs, B. *et al.* (1977) Das Goettinger Miniaturschwein – ein Laboratoriumstier mit weltweiter Bedeutung. *Zuechtungskunde*, **49**, 21–32

Glodek, P. and Oldigs, B. (1981) *Das Goettinger Miniaturschwein*. Paul Parey Verlag, Berlin

Goldmann, K., Kalinowski, M. and Kraft, S. (2005) Airway management under general anaesthesia in pigs using the LMA-ProSeal: a pilot study. *Veterinary Anaesthesia and Analgesia*, **32**, 308–313

Green, S.A. and Benson, G.J. (2002) Porcine Anaesthesia. In: *Veterinary Anaesthesia and Pain Management Secrets*, Vol. **45**. Ed. Green, S.A., pp. 273–275. Hanley and Belfus, Philadelphia

GV-SOLAS (German Society for Laboratory Animal Science) (1999a) Ausschuss fuer Tierschutzbeauftragte: Empfohlene maximale Injektionsvolumina bei Versuchstieren. http://www.tierschutz-tvt.de/merkblatt76.pdf

GV-SOLAS (German Society for Laboratory Animal Science) (1999b) Ausschuss der Ernaehrung der Versuchstiere: Fuetterungskonzepte und –methoden in der Versuchstierhaltung und im Tierversuch: MiniPig. http://www.tiho-hannover.de/einricht/itv/gvsolas/auss/ern/fuetterung_minipig.pdf (Accessed 7 July 2009)

Hand, M.S., Surwit, R.D., Rodin, J. *et al.* (1987) Failure of genetically selected miniature swine to model NIDDM. *Diabetes*, **36**, 284–287

Hansen, A.K. (1997) Health status of experimental pigs. *Pharmacology and Toxicology*, **80** (Suppl 2), 10–15

Heinritzi, K., Gindele, H.R., Reiner, G. *et al.* (2006) *Schweinekrankheiten*. Uni-Taschenbücher, Stuttgart

Hem, A., Hansen, A.K., Rehbinder, C. *et al.* (1994) Recommendations for health monitoring of pig, cat, dog and gerbil breeding colonies. Report of the Scandinavian Federation for Laboratory Animal Science (Scand-LAS) Working Group of Animal Health. *Scandinavian Journal of Laboratory Animal Science*, **21**, 97–115

Hoeller, H. (1959) Vergleichende elektrocardiographische Untersuchungen an normal gefütterten und eiweissmangelernäherten Schweinen. *Berliner und Münchener Tierärztliche Wochenschrift*, **73**, 265–269

Huhn, R.G., Osweiler, G.D. and Switzer,W.P. (1969) Application of the orbital sinus bleeding technique to swine. *Laboratory Animal Care*, **19**, 403–405

Jaksch, W. and Glawischnik, E (1990) *Klinische Propaedeutik der inneren Krankheiten und Hautkrankheiten der Haustiere*, 3rd edn. Paul Parey Verlag, Berlin

Jarry, H., Einspanier, A., Kanngiesser, L. *et al.* (1990) Release and effects of oxytocin on estradiol and progesterone secretion in porcine corpora lutea as measured by an in vivo microdialysis system. *Endocrinology*, **126**, 2352–2358

Jeroch, H., Drochner, W. and Simon, O. (2008) *Ernährung landwirtschaftlicher Nutztiere*. Uni Taschenbuecher fuer die Wissenschaft, Ulmer Verlag, Stuttgart

Joint Working Group on Refinement (1993) Removal of blood from laboratory mammals and birds. First Report of the BVA/FRAME/RSPCA/UFAW Joint Working Group on Refinement. *Laboratory Animals*, **27**, 1–22

Joint Working Group on Refinement (2001) Refining procedures for the administration of substances. Report of the BVAAWF/FRAME/RSPCA/UFAW Joint Working Group on Refinement. *Laboratory Animals*, **35**, 1–41

Kaliste, E. (2004) *The Welfare of Laboratory Animals*. Kluwer Academic Publishers, New York

Kamphues, B., Snell, H., Hessel, E. *et al.* (2003) Litterless housing systems in the farrowing area – ethological and pathological criteria as well as biological performance. *Agrartechnische Forschung*, **9**, E63–E69

Kirchgessner, A., Roth, F.X., Schwarz, F.J. *et al.* (2008) *Tierernaehrung*, 12th edn. DLG-Verlag, Frankfurt

Koehn, F., Sharifi, A.R., Taeubert, H. *et al.* (2008) Breeding for low body weight in Goettingen minipigs. *Journal of Animal Breeding and Genetics*, **125**, 20–28

Kyriazakis, I. and Whittemore, C.T. (2006) *Whittemore's Science and Practice of Pig Production*, 2nd edn. Blackwell Publishing, Oxford

Lahucky, R., Fischer, K. and Augustin, C. (1982) Zur Vorhersage der Fleischbeschaffenheit am lebenden Tier mit Hilfe der Schussbiopsie. *Fleischwirtschaft*, **62**, 1323–1326

Leucht, W., Gregor, G. and Stier, H. (1982) *Einfuehrung in die Versuchstierkunde, Band 4: Das Miniaturschwein*. VEB Gustav Fischer Verlag, Jena

Lewis, A.J. and Southern, L.E. (2000) *Swine Nutrition*. CRC Press, Cleveland

Lindberg, J.E. and Ogle, B. (2001) *Digestive Physiology of Pigs*. CABI Publishers, New York

Malavasi, L.M., Augustsson, H., Jensen-Waern, M. *et al.* (2005) The effect of transdermal delivery of fentanyl on activity in growing pigs. *Acta Veterinaria Scandinavica*, **46**, 149–157

Marrable, A.W. (1971) *The Embryonic Pig*. Pitman Medical, London

Marshall, M., Lydtin, H., Krawitz, W. *et al.* (1972) Das Miniaturschwein als Versuchstier in der experimentellen Medizin. *Research in Experimental Medicine*, **157**, 300–316

McGlone, J. and Pond, W.G. (2002) *Pig Production: Biological Principles and Applications*. Cengage Learning, Boston

Mount, L.E. and Ingram, D.L. (1971) *The Pig as Laboratory Animal*. Academic Press, London

Muirhead, M.R. (1981) Blood sampling in pigs. *In Practice*, **3**, 16–20

National Research Council (1998) *Nutrient Requirements of Swine*, 10th edn. National Academic Press, Washington, DC

Neundorf, R. and Seidel, H. (1977) *Schweinekrankheiten*. Gustav Fischer Verlag, Jena

New Zealand National Animal Welfare Advisory Committee (2005): *Animal Welfare (Pigs) Code of Welfare 2005*. www.biosecurity.govt.nz/files/regs/animal-welfare/req/codes/pigs/pigs-code-of-welfare.pdf (accessed 19 March 2009)

Palmisano, B.W., Clifford, P.S. and Coon, R.L. (1989) Chronic vascular catheters in growing piglets. *Journal of Developmental Physiology (Eynsham)*, **12**, 363–367

Patten, B.M. (1948) *Embryology of the Pig*. Blakiston, Philadelphia

Pond, W.G. and Mersmann, H.J. (2001) *Biology of the Domestic Pig*. Comstock Publishing Associates, Ithaca

Prange, H. (2004) *Gesundheitsmanagement in der Schweinehaltung*. Eugen Ulmer Verlag, Stuttgart

Preissel, A.-K., Centre of Preclinical Research, Klinikum Rechts der Isar, Munich (2009) Personal communication

Rehbinder, C., Baneux, P., Forbes, D. *et al.* (1998) FELASA recommendations for the health monitoring of breeding colonies and experimental units of cats, dogs and pigs. Report of the Federation of European Laboratory Animal Science Associations (FELASA). *Laboratory Animals*, **32**, 1–17

Report of the Scientific Veterinary Committee (1997) *The Welfare of Intensively Kept Pigs*. http://ec.europa.eu/food/fs/sc/oldcomm4/out17_en.pdf

Riebold, T.W. (1995) *Large Animal Anaesthesia: Principles and Techniques*, 2nd edn. Iowa State University Press, Ames

Sack, W.O. (1982) *Essentials of Pig Anatomy*. Veterinary Textbook, Ithaca

Smith, A.C., Ehler, W. and Swindle, M.M. (1997) Anaesthesia and Analgesia in Swine. In: *Anaesthesia and Analgesia in Laboratory Animals*. Eds Kohn, D.H., Wixson, S.K., White, W.J. *et al.*, pp. 313–336. Academic Press, New York

Stanton, H.C. and Mersmann, J.H. (1986) *Swine in Cardiovascular Research, Vol. 1 and 2*. CRC Press, Boca Raton

Steffen, P., Krinn, E., Moeller, A. *et al.* (2002) Metamizole and diclofenac profoundly reduce opioid consumption after minor trauma surgery. *Acute Pain*, **4**, 71–75

Straw, B.E., Zimmerman, J.J., D'Allaire, S. *et al.* (2006) *Diseases of Swine*, 9th edn. Blackwell Publishing, Oxford

Stubhan, M., Markert, M., Mayer, K. *et al.* (2008) Evaluation of cardiovascular and ECG parameters in the normal, freely moving Göttingen Minipig. *Journal of Pharmacological and Toxicological Methods*, **57**, 202–211

Suzuki, A., Tsutsumi, H., Kusakabe, K. *et al.* (1998) Establishment of a 24-hour electrocardiogram recording system using a Holter recorder for miniature swine. *Laboratory Animals*, **32**, 165–172

Svendsen, O. (1998) The minipig in toxicology. Proceedings of the Satellite Symposium to Eurotox, Aarhus, Denmark, 24–25 June 1997. *Scandinavian Journal of Laboratory Animal Science*, **25** (Suppl 1), 1–243

Svendsen, P. and Rasmussen, A. (1998) Anaesthesia of minipigs and basic surgical techniques. *Scandinavian Journal of Laboratory Animal Science*, **25** (Suppl 1), 31–43

Swine Genome Sequencing Consortium (SGSC) (2009) www.animalgenome.org/pigs/genomesequence/ (accessed 20 March 2009)

Swindle, M.M. (2007) *Swine in the Laboratory*, 2nd edn. CRC Press, Boca Raton

Taylor, D.J. (1999) *Pig Diseases*, 8th edn. D.J. Taylor, Glasgow

Thurmon, J.C. and Benson, G.J. (1996) *Lumb and Jones Veterinary Anaesthesia*, 3rd edn. Williams and Wilkins, Baltimore

Tumbleson, M.E. (1986) *Swine in Biomedical Research, Vol. 1–3*. Plenum Press, New York

Tumbleson, M.E. and Schook, L.B. (1996) *Advances in Swine in Biomedical Research, Vol. 1 and 2*. Plenum Press, New York

van Kleef, D.J. (1996) A new system for continuous intravenous infusion in pigs. *Laboratory Animals*, **30**, 75–78

Waldmann, K.-H. and Wendt, M. (2004) *Lehrbuch der Schweinekrankheiten*, 4th edn. Parey Verlag, Berlin

Wallenhorst, S., Wallenhorst, C.K. and Holtz, W. (2000) Steuerung des Reproduktionsgeschehens beim Schwein durch Verabreichung von Gestagenen, Gonadotropinen oder Gonadotropin-Releasing-Hormon – eine Bestandsaufnahme. *Zuechtungskunde*, **72**, 28–42

Wemelsfelder, F. (2005) Animal boredom: Understanding the tedium of confined lives. In: *Mental Health and Well-Being in Animals*. Ed. McMillan, F.D., pp. 79–84. Blackwell Publishing, Ames, Iowa

Wemyss-Holden, S.A., Porter, K.J., Baxter, P. *et al.* (1999) The laryngeal mask airway in experimental pig anaesthesia. *Laboratory Animals*, **33**, 30–34

33 Cattle

Roger Ewbank

Introduction

Although there are many papers, books and reports on the husbandry, management and agricultural use of cattle, there has been relatively little published on their care and use in biomedical research. Publications that do exist include: a series of chapters in the various editions since 1967 of this volume; Doyle *et al.* (1968) produced a review article on the use of domestic farm animals in medical research; the guidelines published by the US National Academy of Sciences (1974); the 1st edition of The Canadian Council on Animal Care *Guide to the Care and Use of Experimental Animals* contained a short section on the specific environmental needs of cattle (Canadian Council on Animal Care 1980)[1]; a chapter by Brooks *et al.* (1984) on ungulates as laboratory animals; in 1988 a USA Consortium of universities, land grant colleges and concerned professional organisations (now the Federation of Animal Science Societies) produced the first edition of their full and detailed *Guide for the Care and Use of Agricultural Animals in Agricultural Research and Teaching* (Consortium 1988); recommended pen sizes for the accommodation of cattle are provided by the Home Office (1989) and Institute of Laboratory Animal Resources (1996); Swanson (1998) discussed the place of farm animals in biomedical research and (Barnett 2007) provided a relatively short but up-to-date care and husbandry chapter.

The proceedings of two conferences on the general theme of farm animals and their use in the biomedical and agricultural sciences have been issued (Mench *et al.* 1992; Baker *et al.* 1996); and a substantial book on cattle welfare has recently been published (Rushen *et al.* 2008).

Much of the material contained in these proceedings, articles and books is relevant to the humane, efficient and wise employment of cattle as experimental animals.

Biological overview

General biology

Most breeds of cattle are large and horned, although a few small and/or naturally polled breeds do occur. Cattle are, even-toed, hoofed, ruminant mammals (ungulates) possessing a four-chambered stomach, and with upper incisor teeth replaced by a thickened layer of the hard palate, the dental pad. They belong to the genus *Bos* within the family Bovidae (suborder Ruminantia, order Artiodactyla). They were domesticated some 8000–10 000 years ago, and they are now used for the production of milk and meat and, in certain areas, for draught purposes. Their current world population is put at some 1370 million (Food and Agricultural Organization 2004).

The care and management of domesticated cattle should present few problems. Due to their extensive commercial use, farmers, agriculturalists and stockmen are well versed in the practicalities of their care. Veterinarians are familiar with their diseases and know how to treat and/or prevent them, while nutritionists understand their dietary requirements. Buildings, fittings, equipment, feed etc are commercially available and realistically priced.

Social organisation

Cattle are a group-living species. Farmers tend to limit the number of males which are allowed to grow to sexual maturity, and the traditional domesticated cattle breeding herd is (or was) a group of females with one attendant bull. Due to the ease and efficiency of artificial insemination in bovines, commercial dairy cattle groups are sometimes totally female. The behavioural organisation of cattle groups is based on a number of co-existing social hierarchies of which the dominance hierarchy (bunt order) seems the most important. Large (older) animals tend to occupy the top places in the hierarchies while smaller (younger) animals fill the lower positions. The well known entry-order of cows into the milking parlour is not strongly related to social hierarchy – high-yielding cows tend to enter first and, during grazing, it is not necessarily the most dominant animals that lead the herd (Hall 2002). For full accounts of the behaviour of cattle see Albright & Arave (1997), Hall (2002) and Phillips (2002).

Breeds and types

Cattle are classified into numerous breeds and types: some have been developed for the production of milk, some primarily as producers of meat, whilst others are essentially

[1]The CCAC 1993 Guide is available at: http://www.ccac.ca/en/CCAC_Programs/Guidelines_Policies/GUIDES/ENGLISH/V1_93/CHAP/CHIV.HTM#4B1

Table 33.1 Biological data for cattle. For further information see Allen (1991), Feldman *et al.* (2000), Kerr (2002) and Reece (2004).

Parameter	*Normal value*
Age adult weight attained (years)	3–4
Adult weights (kg) (depends on breed)	
Males	600–1000
Females	400–800
Total lifespan (years)	15–20
Body temperature (°C)	38.5 ± 1.0
Pulse rate (beats/minute)	50–70
Respiration rate (breaths/minute)	15–30
Blood volume (ml/kg body weight)	57–62

draught animals. Not all breeds are as specialised, and dual-purpose and even triple-purpose breeds and types are recognised. From the biological point of view, however, most breeds of cattle can be placed into one of two groups: those mainly derived from Asiatic stock, the humped (Zebu) (*Bos indicus)* type animals, and those developed mainly from European stock, the non-humped (*Bos taurus*) cattle (Epstein & Mason 1984). Interbreeding between the groups results in fully fertile offspring. There are some anatomical, physiological and behavioural differences between the two groups, such as the presence or absence of humps or pronounced dewlaps, the smaller digestive tract capacity in Asiatic derived cattle, differing water needs, differing behavioural reactions to environmental heat and differences in disease susceptibility. Although for most practical purposes both species can be considered as one kind of animal, there are differences. Therefore, the following account is mainly directed towards European cattle – for details of the husbandry of Asiatic group animals see Payne and Wilson (1999) and Fielding & Matthewman (2004).

Standard biological data for cattle, including size range and life-span, are shown in Table 33.1.

Sources of supply

Cattle required for experimental purposes can be obtained as follows:

(1) by purchase, at any age, from a public market;
(2) by purchase, at any age, direct from an established breeder, rearer or contract supplier who has genetically defined animals which are known to be healthy and disease free and who allows his premises to be inspected and, where appropriate, selected animals to be blood tested and/or vaccinated or treated prior to transport to the research establishment;
(3) by breeding at the research establishment.

Cattle bred at a research establishment have the advantages that they are of known health and rearing history and have usually been handled from an early age. Unfortunately, this ideal approach demands substantial resources of land, buildings and staff, and is often only practical at the larger institutes.

Most research establishments purchase their animals from an established breeder, rearer or contract supplier. Depending on the nature of the scientific investigation, the cattle may be examined/sampled on the farm of origin to assess suitability and, if necessary, vaccinated against respiratory disease (particularly if they are going to be mixed with other cattle). After transportation to the research establishment they will probably be placed in quarantine for further tests, etc, if necessary. In other cases the animals may be transported directly into quarantine and all the tests/treatments etc, carried out there.

Whatever the source, the overall strategy should be to ensure that the biosecurity of the institute is maintained, and that the condition/health status of the cattle is suitable for the management system in which they will be kept and the experiments to which they will be subjected.

Uses in the laboratory

Because of their great economic importance, cattle have been the subjects of scientific study in many agricultural and veterinary research institutes. Most investigations have been in the fields of bovine nutritional, environmental, reproductive and lactation physiology, or on cattle diseases. They are not often used as a model for human conditions although Leathers (1990) has listed some 18 human diseases for which cattle have been useful biological models. Kues & Niemann (2004) have also reviewed the contribution of farm animals to human health following recent developments in transgenic technology. There has also been research into zoonoses such as tuberculosis and brucellosis and in conditions such as bovine spongiform encephalopathy (BSE), which are of considerable interest with respect to public health.

Use of cattle twins in scientific work

It is possible, using like-sex twin cattle, to considerably reduce the numbers of animals used in studies which seem to involve a high environment/treatment/genetic interaction, without lowering the statistical significance of the results (Rowan 1989). Identical (one-egg) twins are best for this purpose, but like-sex non-identical (two-egg) twins can be of value.

The logistical problems of locating, identifying and collecting naturally occurring identical twin calves has largely resulted in the abandonment of this somewhat novel approach to reducing the size – and thus the cost – of certain kinds of cattle experiments.

Relatively recently hormonal methods have been developed to produce multiple ova and embryos, and these can result in the birth of multiple viable offspring. Live embryos can be surgically harvested and transferred to recipient cows; and harvesting micromanipulation and subsequent implantation of fertile zygotes can result in the birth of monozygotic twins. These techniques may result in a further look into the use of genetically similar cattle in experimental work. For details of these various twin producing techniques see Gordon (2003, 2004) and Ball & Peters (2004).

Laboratory management and breeding

General husbandry

Environmental conditions and housing

If healthy and well fed, cattle can cope with wide extremes of climatic conditions, and can be kept outside all the year round in most parts of the temperate and sub-tropical parts of the world. It is widely held – without much in the way of quoted scientific evidence – that there is breed and/type variation in adaptability; beef cattle seem to stand cold better than dairy cows and Asiatic (Zebu) type cattle tolerate high temperatures more readily than European type animals. Whatever the breed, all animals must be protected against extremes of weather, shade or windbreaks must be provided as appropriate, and the animals should always have access to food and water.

Cattle used for scientific purposes should be kept in comfortable quarters (Reinhardt & Reinhardt 2002). The type of housing used is dictated by the type of investigatory work to be undertaken; the need to monitor the welfare of the cattle and the disease security required. Sometimes no housing is provided and the animals are kept outside on pasture or even under extensive range conditions but it is more likely that cattle kept for experimental purposes will be accommodated in one of the following:

1. Small paddocks close to the laboratories.
2. Open-sided buildings with strawed (deep litter) or slatted-floors or containing lines of cubicles.
3. Enclosed buildings, for example, loose boxes or enclosed sheds. For study of infectious diseases these may include barriered buildings with bird proofing, and for contagious diseases sophisticated buildings with negative pressure air regimes and waste containment equipment.
4. Special facilities within a building, such as metabolism or feeding trial crates (Figure 33.1) or individual tie-up standings (Figure 33.2).

Indoor facilities and even some outdoor paddocks can be equipped with closed-circuit television to record animal behaviour.

Within open-sided buildings, loose boxes and enclosed sheds there should, as a general rule, be at least sufficient

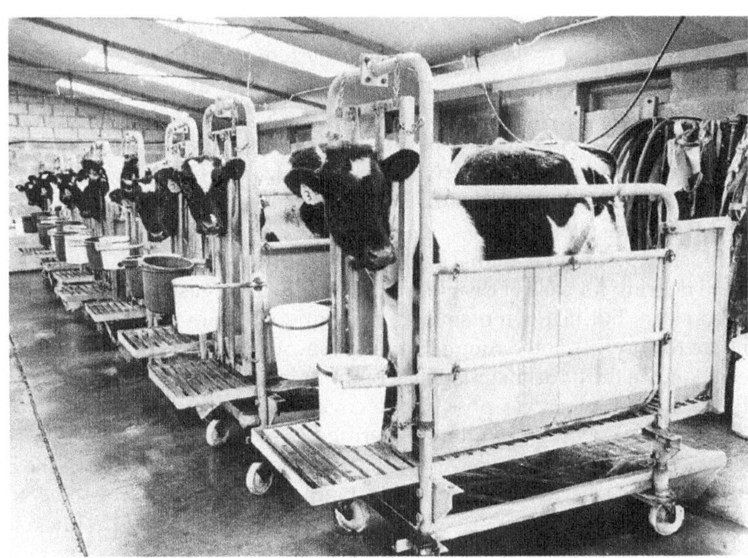

Figure 33.1 Young cattle confined in feeding trial crates.

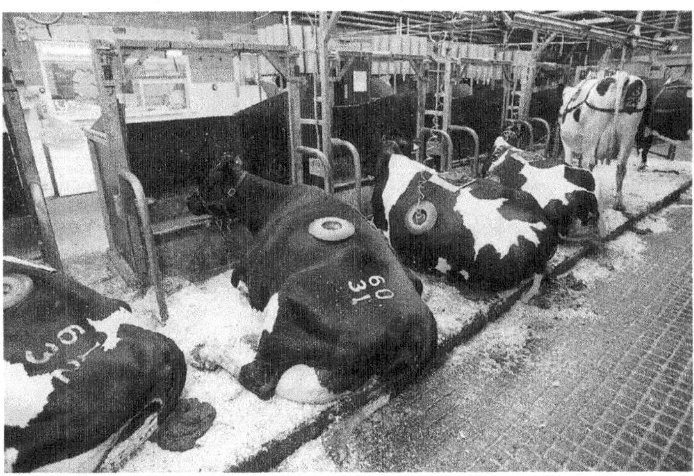

Figure 33.2 Individual tie-up standings contained within a building.

space for each animal to readily stand up, lie down, turn round, stretch its limbs and groom itself (Table 33.2). The animals should, if appropriate to the experiment, have continuous access to individual cow cubicles or to a communal dry bedded-down lying area and to a water supply (trough or water bowls). They should, wherever possible, be housed in sight of each other – as cattle are herd animals, visual contact is important and is a major component of environmental enrichment. There are tables giving the recommended minimum pen sizes for the accommodation of laboratory cattle in the UK *Code of Practice for the Housing and Care of Animals in Scientific Procedures* (Home Office 1989) and in the American *Guide for the Care and Use of Laboratory Animals* (Institute of Laboratory Animal Resources 1996) and the figures in Table 33.2 are based on them. The European Commission has recently adopted minimum enclosure dimensions (European Commission 2007).

Accommodation for dairy cattle must provide facilities where they can be milked. The development of the portable milking machine means that animals kept in isolated places can be milked mechanically, reducing the demand for time-consuming hand milking. To milk larger numbers of cattle a special milking parlour can be used but, of course, the cows have to be moved to the parlour and then returned to their living quarters. A vacuum pump system capable of maintaining a negative pressure of about half an atmosphere (approximately 35 cmHg) must be provided, as must equipment for cooling the milk for storage; for details of milking techniques etc see McNitt (1983) and Leaver (1999). For further information on cattle housing see Blowey (1994) and Lawrence (1994).

Much experimental animal accommodation has solid concrete flooring for ease of disinfection. This is usually easy to keep clean, but if it is too smooth, the cattle may slip and injure themselves; if too rough, it may be uncomfortable and can damage the udder, legs and feet of the animals. Concrete floors should, wherever possible, be covered with either a deep layer of straw over a thin scattering of sand, or ample shredded newspaper. In most bedding systems the soiled bedding must be removed and fresh bedding added each day.

One of the best types of bedding for cattle is deep litter (thick straw and /or shavings and/or sawdust). This is usually used in cattle yards or loose boxes. It must be kept dry and there must be no real contact, in the case of dairy animals, between udders and dung (faeces). If well managed, this bedding provides some warmth (from bacterial action occurring deep in the bed) and much comfort.

The choice of bedding will depend on the design of the building, the availability of suitable material and the nature of the experiment. Typical considerations affecting the choice may be experimental restrictions on cattle eating it or contamination on its disposal due to disease or toxin. Whenever possible, preference should be given to bedding that offers comfort, as indicated by maximum lying time.

Exercise helps to maintain the health and welfare of cattle. Animals accommodated outside in grassed paddocks or kept together with others in yards will usually take sufficient exercise of their own volition. The space allocated for group-housed cattle is generally sufficient for them to exercise. However cattle held singly for lengthy periods of time in loose boxes or other restrictions should, wherever possible, be exercised daily. This can be done by either releasing them for set periods into exercise yards or paddocks (small groups work best); or by walking them out individually on hand-held halters on dry, firm ground or non-stony soft-surface roadways (purpose-built cow tracks are even better); or by attaching them by halter to a mechanically operated horizontally rotating 'bull-walker'.

Presentation of food and water

Food is usually presented to cattle in raised troughs. The troughs ideally should be designed, constructed and sited so that:

- they are not readily contaminated with faeces;
- they are easily cleaned;
- they are not likely to injure the animals in any way;
- they do not allow the cattle to waste their food.

Water can be piped to bowls which are automatically kept at a constant water level or which are operated by the cow when it pushes its muzzle against a shaped flange (tongue) in the bowl. Water meters can readily be fitted to piped supplies to monitor consumption. Water can also be offered in buckets (generally within fittings to stop them being knocked over) but this is labour intensive and tends to be used for calves or loose-box housed animals but does allow water consumption to be measured. Water sources should be positioned so as to minimise contamination by faeces, food or

Table 33.2 Minimum space requirements for loose housed cattle. Adapted from Home Office (1989), Institute of Laboratory Resources (1996) and Council of Europe (2006).

Weight of animal (kg)	*Min. enclosure (ie, single housing) size (m²)*	*Min. floor area/animal (m²/animal)*	*Trough space (or feed rack length) for ad libitum feeding of polled cattle (m/animal)*	*Trough space (or feed rack length) for restricted feeding of polled cattle (m/animal)*
Up to 100	2.50	2.30	0.10	0.30
100–200	4.25	4.00	0.15	0.50
200–400	7.00	4.80	0.18	0.60
400–600	8.00	7.50	0.21	0.70
600–800	11.0	8.75	0.24	0.80
Over 800	16.0	10.0	0.30	1.00

bedding and, ideally, the water should be placed near a floor drain so that spilt water does not lie about and/or wet the bedding.

Identification

Cattle which are kept in small numbers and which are frequently handled will be individually recognised by care staff. However, many countries have statutory requirement that all cattle should be permanently, individually and uniquely marked. They can be permanently marked by having tattooed numbers or 'tamper-proof' numbered tags placed in their ears. (It should be noted that 'tamper-proof' tags, once correctly placed fully into position, cannot be removed without either mutilating the ear and/or damaging the tag.)

If it is important that animals should be identifiable from a distance, for example where groups of cattle are kept at grass or housed in yards, then they should have one of the following:

- large coloured and/or numbered plastic tags placed in their ears;
- coloured and numbered plastic collars placed round their necks;
- large numbers or letters freeze-branded on to a pigmented area of their skin (the intense cold of the freeze-branding process permanently damages the pigment-forming cells and white hairs grow in the treated areas);
- large numbers or letters marked on non-pigmented areas of their skin by application of hair dyes; these marks have to be renewed as the hairs grow and are replaced.

There is increasing use of implanted microchips and bar codes on eartags – both these methods of identification require the use of an electronic reading device. Some commercial systems have microchips placed in neck collars for ration management (they may, for example, control access to a feeding station). Microchips may also be placed in eartags or foot bands to assist with recording the production performance of dairy cows.

The marking system chosen should be the least invasive method, consistent with the husbandry system and the aims of the research. No matter what type of individual identification is used, it is good practice to have a database containing information on individual animals. The data retained should trace key life events and list any interventions that the animal has been subjected to.

Physical environment

Ideally, the environment inside buildings should be kept at about 17–18°C (range 10–24°C) and a relative humidity of about 50% (range 25–75%). Enclosed buildings should have a ventilating capacity of at least 5 air changes per hour in winter and up to 25 air changes per hour in the summer, in the hotter parts of the world. Background lighting of 200 lux or above should be provided for not less than 12 h each day. The light:dark ratio should be about 1:1 and additional artificial light of not less than 500 lux must always be available, so that animals can be closely inspected at any time of the day or night.

Health monitoring, quarantine and biosecurity

A health plan should be drawn up by the institute veterinary surgeon in consultation with the stock managers for all the cattle held and used on the experimental station. The plan will vary with the type of cattle involved, the environment and the experimental design.

As for all animals used in experiments that may impact on their health and welfare, clinical signs should be regularly monitored and clear guidelines provided regarding actions to be taken. Records should be kept of all veterinary treatments and operations. All animals that die should be examined post mortem, and the reasons for their deaths determined and recorded. There should be health and welfare meetings between all staff involved in a particular experiment prior to starting as well as review meetings at the end. There also should be regular and, if necessary, frequent meetings during the span of an experiment, to review the on-going health and well-being of the animals. This is especially important for long drawn-out investigations.

Quarantine and biosecurity

One of the major health risks is the introduction of new animals into an establishment or even, at times, between different groups within the same establishment.

Animals arriving at the experimental farm should be placed into rodent-, and wild bird-free, easily disinfected quarantine premises. The quarantine facility should be separate from the main animal buildings and should have its own food and bedding stores and its own handling facilities. It should be surrounded by its own double, stock-proof fence. The manure from the quarantined cattle should be kept adjacent to the quarantine quarters. The quarantine area should have its own separate drainage and waste product disposal system.

The whole experimental farm should be surrounded by a stock-proof and, ideally, vermin-proof ring fence to prevent contact with ground-dwelling animals living outside the unit. This is best if it is double: the two fences should be at least 1 m and preferably 3 m apart, particularly if there are cattle in adjacent properties. It is important to control visitors and deliveries to the unit. The entrance should be gated and provided with a shallow drive-through disinfection bath for vehicles – for use should the need (local disease situation) dictate.

The road to the reception area should be concreted, short in length and not in close proximity to the animal accommodation or grazing paddocks and the parking area for visitors' cars and delivery lorries should be of concrete and easily washed down. Goods should be received into a secure, clean 'bonded' store and only issued after due inspection and verification that they are indeed what was ordered and do not pose a risk of introducing disease into the unit. All visitors should report to reception and be provided with institute-owned rubber boots and protective clothing before they are allowed access to other parts of the establishment. Isolation and other 'sensitive' areas may require special visitor access procedures and facilities. All persons entering or working in quarantine or isolation areas should wear colour-coded overalls etc, unique to the particular area.

All material moved within the unit as well as waste material leaving the unit should be risk assessed regarding potential release of infectious organisms or toxins. It may be necessary to arrange sterilisation and/or safe disposal.

For further details on farm animal biosecurity etc, see Gibson and Andrews (2000); Belk *et al.* (2007).

Transport

For long-distance movements, cattle should be carried in specially designed animal transport lorries. Stock trailers towed behind a van or tractor can be used for short local journeys and within the institute. These trailers and trucks should be designed, constructed and maintained so that they are easily cleaned and disinfected, and do not injure the animals transported within them. Care must be taken in loading and unloading animals from these transport vehicles; non-slip loading and unloading ramps must be used.

For further details of cattle transportation see Grandin & Gallo (2007) and Grandin (2009).

Breeding

The adults

Cows, which are on heat (oestrus), tend to show characteristic behaviour such as head rubbing, mounting, standing to be mounted, vocalisation (bellowing) and more general activity (restlessness) than is usual. Signs that cows have been mounted include soiling of the flanks and tail/head rubbing. A clear, viscous (the latter may be more definitive) discharge may be seen issuing from the vulva. Swollen vulval lips tend not to be a feature of cattle in oestrus. Groups of cows must be observed several times a day if all the heat periods are to be detected.

Cows, under normal conditions, are capable of producing, on average, one calf per year (see Table 33.3 for reproductive data) and most management systems are based on this. The simplest way of producing a calf crop is to run a known fertile bull with a group of cows and/or heifers. A crayon marker, which can have its colour changed at 14-day intervals, can be placed on the sternal region (brisket) of the bull. Daily observation of the cows will then indicate which ones have mated and which, if any, have to be returned to service (ie, have been mated but have not conceived). From this information the approximate date of parturition of each cow can be calculated.

Alternative artificial insemination (AI) is generally used for dairy cattle. The cows should be served by AI approximately 12 h after the heat is first detected. The insemination is usually done by inserting a long sterile plastic pipette into the vagina and depositing semen either on to the cervix, or better still, into the cervical canal. This is a skilled job done by trained technicians generally using semen that has been stored in liquid nitrogen. In many countries there are licensed commercial and/or governmental agencies that undertake a travelling cattle AI service. Travelling AI services may be a significant factor in the introduction of disease (eg bovine viral diarrhoea, *Salmonella*, Johne's disease).

Table 33.3 Reproductive data for cattle.

Parameter	*Normal value*
Onset of puberty (months)	12–15
Length of reproductive life (years)	12–15
Type of oestrus cycle	Polyoestrus
Duration of oestrus (heat)(h)	12–14 (shorter duration in the winter)
Frequency	Every 20–21 days
Seasonality	Oestrus occurs all the year round but most strongly in the summer; herds running all the year with a bull tend to calve in the spring
Length of gestation (days)	c 280 (about 7 less for twins)
Number of calves born	1–2; occasionally 3 or more; twinning rate in cattle about 2–3%
Average weight of calf at birth (kg)	23–45; much breed variation; males tend to be slightly heavier than females of the same breed/type
Post-partum oestrus	30–60 days after parturition

It is possible to synchronise the heat periods in a group of reproductively active cattle by means of prostaglandins (for details see Roche 1989). It is usual in these circumstances for two inseminations to be performed on each of the animals on two successive days. The advantage of this synchronisation technique is that a number of inseminations can be carried out at one time, and it also means that the synchronised group will usually all calve down at approximately the same time.

Determination of conception ('pregnancy diagnosis') can be carried out at:

- 21–26 days after insemination, by estimating the progesterone content of the cow/s milk (a cow-side test is available);
- 6–8 weeks after insemination by palpation per rectum of the reproductive tract, by a veterinary surgeon or specially trained technician.

As the pregnancy progresses there is an increase in the size of the abdomen and after about the 6th month an increase in the size of the mammary gland. These changes are more readily detected in heifers than in cows. The signs of imminent parturition are as follows:

1. behavioural changes such as restlessness, seeking solitary areas, vocalisation;

2. increasing distension of the udder and stiffening of the teats;
3. slackening of the pelvic ligaments each side of the tail, which may appear some 3–4 days before calving;
4. the vulva may become swollen;
5. drops of honey-coloured colostrum (first milk) may appear some 6–8 h before the birth;
6. abdominal discomfort with possible straining

Most cows and heifers deliver their offspring without any real difficulty and should, wherever possible, be allowed to calve without human interference.

Parturition can be induced in cattle, in the last 2–3 weeks of their pregnancies, by the injection of short acting corticosteroids and/or prostaglandin $F_{2\alpha}$. The drug or drug combination used depends upon the nearness of the normal delivery date. If induction is required 2–3 weeks before the normal delivery date, long-acting corticosteroids can be used alone. Within a week of delivery, short-acting corticosteroids with prostaglandin $F_{2\alpha}$ will be effective and, within 1–2 days of parturition, prostaglandin $F_{2\alpha}$ alone will often be adequate.

The calves produced under these induction regimes may initially need greater care on the part of the animal attendant. The earlier the induction, the greater the need for such care. There is also a tendency for induced cows to retain their placentas (for details see Hartigan 1995).

Parturition should be allowed to take place either inside a clean draught-free loose box or, weather conditions permitting, outside in a field. The animal should not be tied by its neck and should have sufficient space to turn round easily, stand up and lie down at will. The loose box should have a well bedded non-slip floor; water should be provided and there should be a good source of artificial light. Once abdominal contractions (second-stage labour) have started the calf should be born in under 4 h. Expulsion of the placenta (afterbirth) is usually completed within 30 minutes to 12 h.

The young

In beef suckler herds, the newborn calf is left with its dam until natural weaning occurs at 6–8 months of age. In dairy herds, calves are removed at birth or some 48 h later and placed on milk replacer foods. Whichever system is adopted, it is essential that the calf takes in up to 4 l of colostrum as soon as possible. The immunity of the newborn calf towards infectious diseases is largely dependent upon its absorbing, within the first 6 h of birth, the antibodies contained in high concentrations in its dam's colostrum. The abdomen of the newborn calf can be palpated around 6 h after birth to check if it has a full stomach. If it does not, colostrum should be milked from the dam and fed (stomach tubed) to the calf. Calves weaned at birth will need to have their dam's colostrum collected (hand milked) from the udder and fed to them using a teated bottle. The level of circulating antibodies in the calf's blood can be estimated by a number of simple tests (for example the zinc sulphate turbidity test for serum globulin) carried out on the calf's serum.

Calves which have been deliberately separated from their dams, or purchased at an early age, should be accommodated in clean, dry draught-free straw-bedded pens. They should be kept in buildings with an air temperature of about 20°C and relative humidity not greater than 70%. Calves should have clean water and good quality hay available at all times. All calves should have frequent human contact during their first 6 months. This makes them easy to manage throughout their lives, reducing stress for both the animal and care staff (see section on handling and training).

Calves can be fed on liquid food (milk or milk replacers) two or three times a day or *ad libitum* for at least the first 3 weeks of life. Young calves start picking at hay in the first few days after birth; they start eating small quantities of palatable early-weaning mixtures from the first week onwards. They can show signs of rumination from 1–2 weeks of age, and can be weaned from liquid food when they are eating 1 kg/day of a suitable concentrate ration. This may be as early as 3 weeks, but it is preferable to leave them on liquids for at least 3 weeks longer as there is usually a general setback to their health on weaning. Calves normally obtain their ruminal micro-organisms from being in close contact with their dams.

For further information on feeding, housing and health of calves see Roy (1990), Thickett *et al.* (2003) and Allen (2004).

Breeding systems

Breeding stock must have the desired genetic and physical characteristics and should also, where possible, have a long history of freedom from disease and be docile in temperament.

Feeding

Diets

Cattle are essentially grazing and browsing animals, and if allowed to roam freely will consume considerable quantities (up to 90 kg in total) of forage material (grass, clover or browse) each day.

Cattle spend an average of 8 out of each 24 h grazing (range 4–14 h); usually in four to five bouts during the hours of daylight. During this time they may walk a distance of up to 2 km. In very hot conditions, cattle will graze at night and lie and ruminate during the day. It is important from the point of view of environmental enrichment that, wherever possible, the diet offered to cattle should contain sufficient forage material to allow a normal duration of rumination. Total ruminating time is usually some three quarters of normal grazing time (ie, about 6 h). If the herbage is succulent, ruminating time is reduced in relation to grazing; if it is coarse and fibrous the animals will ruminate for longer.

Because of their great economic importance, and because their growth and production are largely dependent upon how they are fed, a large body of theoretical knowledge and practical experience exists on cattle nutrition (see Agriculture and Food Research Council 1993; Owen 1995; Greenhalgh *et al.* 2002). Modern feeding systems for cattle are designed to first meet the nutritional needs of the cow's ruminal micro-organisms and then to supply the requirements of the cow with metabolisable energy and metabolisable protein from the products of ruminal and post-ruminal digestion. Agriculturalists and nutritionists can give advice on the design of cattle feeding regimes based on the body size and physiological needs of the cow (eg, growth rate, stage of pregnancy or lactation), and veterinarians are used to dealing with the diseases associated with faulty feeding. There are many commercial firms that can provide an efficient advisory service and which can contract to supply correctly balanced cattle rations.

Dietary requirements

The theoretical background to the nutrition of cattle has traditionally been approached by first finding their energy requirement, then their need for protein and finally by considering the intake of dry matter which they are capable of taking in (Table 33.4). These needs have then to be matched with the energy values and the protein and dry matter contents of the foods available (see Table 33.5 for examples). Finally, the ration has to be examined to see if it is likely to contain adequate amounts of essential vitamins and minerals.

This simple approach to calculating the dietary requirements of cattle is being replaced, in the UK, by more complex systems using concepts such as: is the diet likely to contain adequate amounts of the essential vitamins and minerals; and does it provide fermentable metabolisable energy (energy available for the ruminal micro-organisms) and effective ruminal degradable crude protein (the protein available for the ruminal micro-organisms). For details of systems that take into account these and other factors and for outline accounts of other systems used outside the UK, see Greenhalgh *et al.* (2002).

The main parts of the daily ration of a ruminant consist of:

1. bulk food – supplying energy, some protein and fibre;
2. concentrate food – supplying extra protein and/or energy, additional vitamins and minerals;
3. water.

Cattle out on good-quality grassland can sometimes take in all their daily needs by grazing up to 90 kg of grass per day.

Table 33.4 Energy and protein requirements for maintenance* and dry matter intake limits of cattle.

Body weight of animal (kg)	*Metabolic energy (ME) (MJ/day)*	*Digestible crude protein (DCP) (g/day)*	*Limit of dry matter intake (kg/day)*
200	27	150	5.0
300	36	200	7.5
400	45	250	10.0
500	54	300	12.5
600	63	350	15.0

*For production each kilogram of live weight gain requires a further 34 MJ of ME and 320 g of DCP. The additional ME required by animals in lactation can be calculated from the formula 1.694(0.0386 BF + 0.0205 SNF – 0.236), where BF is butterfat and SNF is solids not fat (both in grams per kilogram of milk).

However, most modern high-yielding dairy cows, often require far higher levels of energy, protein and fibre than can be provided by grass alone – in itself a crop varying in analysis from region to region and season to season. Many cattle in modern intensive systems are fed a total mixed ration of grass by (grazing) or as grass silage/maize silage/straw (hay) plus some sort of concentrate – the whole being designed to fulfil the specific nutritional requirement of the particular production system.

Cattle indoors may be given their bulk ration as silage (up to 70 kg a day) or hay (10–15 kg a day), and this is often supplemented with relatively small quantities of high-protein concentrate foods. Water must be supplied. Cattle need 40–50 l/day and, if they are lactating, they need additionally about five times the volume of milk produced. If they are being milked there will also be a requirement for additional water to keep clean the milking stall, to wash and sterilise the milking equipment and to cool the milk.

Whatever the system or means by which cattle are fed, the end results can be judged by the body condition, weight, health and production of the animals. These must be monitored at frequent and regular intervals and any loss of condition etc, must be assessed and, if necessary, action must be taken to overcome the cause. Sometimes all that is needed is a gradual increase in the quantity and/or quality of the food provided.

A body condition scoring scheme can be useful. In these, an assessment is made, on a scale of 1–5 (or 8), of the weight for age and the relative proportions of muscle to fat of cattle using a graded set of photographs or drawings (Figure 33.3) of scored animals; see Bazeley & Hayton (2007) for further details.

Table 33.5 Typical metabolic energy (ME), digestible crude protein (DCP) and dry matter (DM) contents of some common foods.

Food	*ME (MJ/kg DM)*	*DCP (g/kg DM)*	*DM (g/kg)*
Succulents and roughages			
Swedes/turnips	12.8	91	120
Kale	11.0	110	140
Grazing (rotational)	12.1	225	200
Grazing (extensive)	10.0	170	200
Grass silage (good)	9.3	107	200
Maize silage	11.2	70	250
Meadow hay (good)	9.0	58	850
Dried grass	10.6	120	900
Barley straw	7.3	8	860
Concentrate foods			
Barley	13.7	84	860
Maize	14.2	70	860
Oats	11.5	77	860
Soyabean cake	12.3	405	900
Decorticated cottonseed cake	12.3	365	900
Decorticated groundnut cake	11.7	427	900
Linseed cake	13.4	300	900
Sugar beet pulp, dried	12.7	59	900

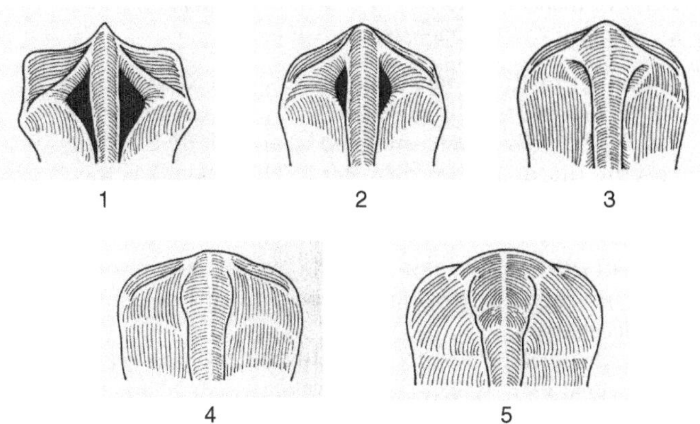

Figure 33.3 Condition score of cows assessed for fat cover over tailhead and loin area. 5, grossly fat; 4, fat; 3, good, 2, moderate; 1, very poor. Drawing: J. Webster (from Webster 1993).

Laboratory procedures

Handling and training

Cattle reared from a young age with human contact are usually quiet and easy to manage. They respond well to a calm but firm approach. There are many advantages in having experimental subjects exposed to a minimum of non-experimental (and usually non-quantifiable) stressors. See Stookey & Watts (2007) for a general account of low-stress restraint and handling of cattle.

When handling cattle all staff should be aware of the risks. Mature bulls should never be handled by one person alone; they are often large, sometimes bad tempered, quick in action, and are not to be trusted. Accommodation for this type of animal should be designed with safe refuges for staff. Cows with young calves at foot can sometimes be very protective towards their young and must also be handled with care.

Most cattle can be trained to tolerate many minor routine experimental procedures, such as blood sampling, injections etc, with the minimum of physical restraint: see Dickfos (1991).

Depending upon their size and situation the subject animals are usually tied by the neck (chain or yoke; see Figure 33.1), tied and/or held by means of a leather head-collar (head stall) or rope halter or restrained in a cattle crush (squeeze). Under the direction of the unit veterinarian, sedative type drugs can be given (such as xylazine intramuscularly at 5–30 mg/100 kg body weight, chloral hydrate by mouth at 6–12 g/100 kg body weight to nervous animals or in anticipation of a potentially stressful procedure.

Within a research establishment, cattle can be moved in small groups by being quietly driven by one or two handlers. It must be made obvious to the animals which way they are expected to go by the correct deployment of handlers and barriers and by opening and closing gates in the correct sequence. It is not usual to employ cattle dogs to move experimental stock, but it may occasionally be necessary, for example, on extensive grazing trials. Where dogs are used they must be quiet and well under control.

In an emergency it may be necessary to restrain cattle by holding them with a finger and thumb in the nostril pressing on the nasal septum or by grasping them in the same place using a metal pincer device ('bulldog'). A looped cotton rope tightened round the abdomen just in front of the udder generally prevents cattle kicking with the hindlegs, and thus can make it easier to examine and/or manipulate the hind end of the animal. It must be emphasised that it should not be necessary, except in an emergency, to use these physical means of restraint when carrying out routine procedures on trained cattle.

There are advantages to the safety of both handlers and other cattle with which naturally horned breeds may be in contact if they have had their horns removed. This can be done once they are adults, but it is better to remove the horn buds of 1–2-week-old calves by firstly anaesthetising the horn buds and then burning them out with a hot disbudding iron.

For further information on cattle handling see Holmes (1991); Fowler (1995); Albright & Fulwider (2007); Ewbank & Parker (2007); Grandin (2007a, 2007b); Humane Slaughter Association (2008).

Physiological monitoring

The body temperature of cattle is readily taken by carefully inserting a lubricated blunt-ended clinical, or digital thermometer, into the rectum and holding it there for 1 minute while, at the same time, ensuring that the thermometer is touching the rectal wall.

Depending upon the nature of the scientific investigation other measurements that can be made include: weight and condition score for general health; respiration rate; the presence or absence of nasal discharge if respiratory disease is being studied; and rumination rate if digestive function is of concern.

Collection of specimens

Blood

General advice on blood sampling techniques can be found in the report by the Joint Working Group on Refinement (JWGR, 1993). Blood can be readily obtained from the jugular or coccygeal veins of cattle. As long as the animals are used to being handled, a very sharp and appropriately sized bleeding needle is used and a precise technique employed; very little restraint is usually required. The skin over the vein site should be clipped (if necessary) and then cleaned and, if thought necessary, disinfected.

- Jugular vein: this large, external vessel is a ready source of blood. The vein is raised either by the use of a neck rope or by digital pressure and a large cattle-bleeding needle (up to 1.5 mm diameter × 20 mm long) is then inserted with, usually, the point directed towards the head. A local analgesic can be injected by means of a fine needle into the skin over the jugular vein prior to the insertion of the large needle, but this is usually unnecessary.
- Coccygeal vein: blood can readily be taken from the coccygeal vein, which lies on the underside of the tail. There are advantages in using single-use disposable needles. Coccygeal vein blood sampling is a particularly convenient technique when the animal is restrained in a cattle crush, which has easy rear access.

Milk

Mixed samples from the udder can be obtained from the milking-machine bucket. An individual sample from a teat (quarter sample) can be collected by first cleaning and disinfecting the teat end and then squeezing out, by a stripping action of the first finger and thumb, the contents of the lumen of the teat into its own small collecting vial. To reduce contamination it is usual to discard the first five squirts and then collect the sample into the vial. The end of the teat should then be disinfected and the cow allowed (or persuaded) to stand for 30 minutes in order for the teat to reseal properly.

Faeces

These can be collected from the floor behind tied-up cattle or from a special bag fitting over the hindquarters, or removed manually from the rectum.

Ruminal contents

A rounded-end 'stomach' tube is passed via the mouth and oesophagus into the rumen, and the ruminal contents are then drawn out by a hand-operated pump, or large veterinary 'syringe' attached to the stomach tube.

For details of experimental techniques used with cattle see Grassland Research Institute (1961), Chapman (1969), Wood (1975) and Leaver (1982). Guidance as to the care, management and welfare of the cattle confined in metabolic cages can be found in Olfert *et al.* (1993), and Harrison (1995) provides a detailed account of surgical techniques used on experimental farm animals, including cattle.

Administration of medicines and test substances

General advice on the administration of substances can be found in JWGR (2001).

Dosing and injection procedures

Non-bitter tasting, non-volatile medicines which are active in the alimentary tract or which are absorbed by the oral route can, if suitably formulated, be given in the food – a good, if variable way of dosing a large group of animals. If accurate dosing is required then one of the following methods may have to be used:

- making the dose up as a drench (usually with water) and giving by means of a specially designed drenching 'gun' or, where very large volumes are required, by stomach tube;
- putting the substance into gelatine capsules and placing them far back in the mouth of the animal by means of a specially designed balling gun.

Many medicines are precisely and easily given by injection via the appropriate intravenous, intramuscular, subcutaneous, or intraperitoneal routes. For more details of the various techniques see McNitt (1983), Holmes (1991), Fowler (1995) and appropriate chapters in Battaglia (1998).

Anaesthesia and analgesia

Cattle are very suitable subjects for regional analgesia, for example paravertebral blocks, caudal epidurals or perineural blocks. They can be given general anaesthetics but must first be starved of concentrate food overnight and forage should be removed a few hours prior to induction. They are then sedated with a drug such as xylazine (iv or im) and induced using a quick-acting intravenous anaesthetic agent. They should then have a cuffed tube placed in the trachea to allow the administration of gaseous anaesthetic and to stop inhalation of regurgitated rumen contents. They should also have their front end propped upright on their sternums so that dangerous levels of gas do not accumulate in the rumen interfering with venous return. Alternatively local analgesics can be injected at or close to the operation site. See Hall *et al.* (2001) for more detailed descriptions of these various techniques.

A recent and full account of the anaesthetic agents and methods which can be used on ruminants can be found in Riebold (2007).

Euthanasia

The act of euthanasia is most easily and humanely carried out on quiet co-operating animals. It may be possible and indeed desirable to sedate 'non-co-operating' cattle, when the experimental protocol allows this, by the use of an injectable sedative.

The most humane and efficient way to kill cattle is to first render them unconscious by means of a captive-bolt stunner or a specially designed free-bullet humane killer, and then to cut their throats. In the case of the captive-bolt stunner, death occurs through blood loss, resulting from the throat cut; in the case of the free-bullet humane killer, from damage to the brain.

The muzzle of the captive-bolt stunner or the specially designed free-bullet humane killer should be placed in contact with, and at approximately right angles to, the forehead of the animal at the crossing over point of two imaginary lines joining the eyes of the animal with the base of the ears on the opposite sides (Figure 33.4). The point of aim for calves should be slightly lower. In old heavy-headed animals the aiming point should be 1 cm to the right or left of the cross-over point. Once the animal has fallen to the ground it can be pithed (ie, a cane or piece of wire can be inserted into the hole in the skull and moved around to destroy the brain). Pithing is not allowed if the carcase is to enter the food chain. The animal usually kicks out when this is done. Once it is still its throat can be cut to sever the carotid arteries and jugular veins.

In an emergency, a standard shotgun, handgun or rifle may have to be used. The shotgun is the best for use under farm conditions. The muzzles of these standard weapons should not be placed in contact with the animal; they should be fired with the muzzle some 8–10 cm away from the point of aim. The animal's throat is then cut.

An overdose of an intravenous anaesthetic agent can be used to kill experimental stock. This technique preserves the brain for pathological examination, but it usually leaves drug residues in the tissues and renders the carcase unsuitable for some chemical analyses, or for human or animal consumption. For practical details of cattle slaughter see Sibley (1995) and Humane Slaughter Association (2005, 2006).

Common welfare problems

Prophylaxis and disease control

Cattle obtained from a known good source, which are in a stable social group, fed and housed correctly, and which are well looked after by their attendants, usually remain disease free. There may, however, be a need for the routine prophylactic use of vaccines, regular treatment for parasites and drying-off mastitis control. This should be part of the health plan agreed with the unit veterinarian.

In long-term cattle projects, attention should be paid to the feet and the diet. Commercial diets are usually designed to feed growing beef cattle or productive dairy cows; long-term cattle which have reached maturity need a diet which maintains their weight and provides them with suitable amounts of vitamins and minerals. It is important to prevent the development of urolithiasis in entire and castrated males.

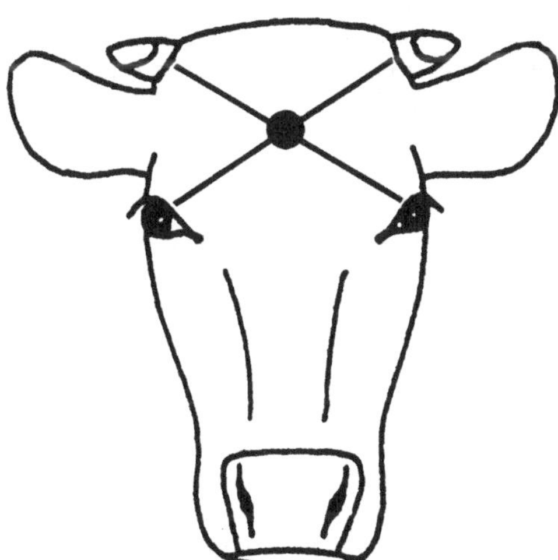

Figure 33.4 Diagram of the head showing the point of aim when using a captive-bolt stunner or free-bullet humane killer.

Signs of health and disease

Healthy cattle usually graze for about 8 h a day and ruminate for a further 6–7 h. They should chew their cud without difficulty and have a normal rumen turnover rate of about three times in 2 minutes. They should have a rumen fill (concavity of left paralumbar fossa) and a body condition score appropriate to the nature of the experiment they are on. About half of every 24 h is spent lying down. Cattle stretch themselves when they get up. They usually have a moist cool muzzle and a sweet smelling breath, and generally have a shiny coat, which they lick. They should be free from lameness, excessive salivation and from nasal eye discharges; they should only cough occasionally. Cattle should urinate and defaecate without any signs of distress, and the consistency of their faeces should be appropriate to the nature of the bulky part of their daily ration. If, for example, they are eating grass their faeces should be fairly loose, whereas when fed on hay their faeces should be firm. Their respiration and pulse rate and their body temperature should be within the normal range (see Table 33.1).

The more obvious signs of ill health in cattle are the following:

- loss of appetite;
- separation from the group or herd;
- fall in milk yield;
- loss of body condition;
- cessation of rumination;
- rise in body temperature;
- lameness, salivation, excessive coughing;
- sudden change in consistency of faeces.

Many countries have statutory schemes as listed in the Office International des Epizooties's (2009) manual for the control of the important infectious diseases of cattle, such as anthrax, brucellosis, rabies, foot and mouth disease, bluetongue, tuberculosis, rinderpest and BSE. There may be duty in law for the owners and/or keepers of cattle to know about the common symptoms of these diseases, and to report to the appropriate government authorities when they suspect that their animals may be suffering from them.

The control of infectious disease usually depends upon some or all of the following actions:

1. Early recognition of the disease.
2. Treatment (ideally to cure) or disposal of infected animals (and possibly in-contact stock).
3. Cleaning and appropriate disinfection of the premises in which they were kept.
4. Testing of the remaining animals for disease-carrier status, and the isolation and possible disposal of positive reactors.
5. Vaccination (when appropriate) of susceptible animals.

6. Taking care not to re-introduce the disease, for example by setting up barrier fences, controlling pest rodents and birds and establishing quarantine facilities.

Common diseases

Some diseases are of common occurrence and/or zoonotic. Keepers of experimental cattle should be acquainted with their characteristics.

Bovine viral diarrhoea (BVD)

A viral disease causing infertility, poor-doing calves and, in some cases, fatal diarrhoea. Carrier animals occur in some herds. Vaccines are available.

Ectoparasites

Lice can be a problem in housed cattle. They can be treated with an appropriate non-toxic injectable or pour-on insecticide. Ticks are important as transmitters of viral and rickettsial diseases. Cattle kept outside in some tick-infested areas may have to be regularly treated.

Endoparasites

Gastrointestinal parasites are a cause of diarrhoea, debility and loss in young cattle, but can be treated with anthelmintics. Many oral and pour-on preparations are available. There is an increasing problem with certain parasitic worm populations showing a resistance to many of the currently used drugs. Veterinary advice should always be sought when setting up a control and treatment programme.

Liver fluke causes a persistent wasting disease but can be treated. Control programmes are mainly based on eradicating the intermediate hosts (a snail) by draining the cattle-grazing areas and the by use of molluscicides. Lungworm causes coughing and debility in young animals. A vaccine is available and a control and treatment programme should be instigated based on regular dosing with suitable medicaments, pasture control of the parasite and, where appropriate, the use of a vaccine.

Johne's disease

This is a disease caused by *Mycoplasma avium paratuberculosis*. It commonly affects adult cattle and is characterised by chronic wasting and profuse diarrhoea. It is untreatable. Clinically affected animals should be disposed of and, under veterinary guidance, an effective preventative control scheme should be started.

Lameness

There are many causes of lameness in cattle, such as injury, overgrown feet and specific bacterial infections. Individual cases should be treated, and if the problem is common veterinary advice will be needed. Preventive measures (attention to floor surfaces, routine trimming of feet, the regular use of footbaths etc) should be undertaken.

Leptospirosis

Leptospirosis is an important and sometimes common cause of abortion. The disease is transmissible to humans. Carrier animals can be detected by blood test and should be eliminated. Vaccines are available.

Mastitis

This is caused by a variety of bacteria; but in many instances there may be predisposing building and environmental factors. Individual cases can be treated with antibiotics but preventive programmes should first be set up (attention to environments and buildings; hygiene at milking time; ensuring the milking machine is working correctly; post-milking teat dipping; the rational use of intra-mammary antibiotic treatments; the possible use of vaccines) after taking veterinary advice.

Metabolic diseases

These are caused by the breakdown of internal metabolic processes, and their development is influenced by environmental stress, the nutritional state of the animal and the production demands being made of it. A preventive programme can be set up, taking veterinary and nutritional advice.

Pneumonia

There are many causes of pneumonia in cattle, both bacterial and viral, and it is particularly prevalent and severe in young cattle when they are mixed from various sources. There can be a wide range of bacteria and viruses involved and vaccines are available, although to be effective, they need to be combined with suitable management and husbandry practices (eg vaccination prior to mixing; logical antibiotic treatment of individual clinical cases; buildings designed to allow suitable ventilation).

Ringworm

This specific fungal infection is indicated by round, raised whitish lesions on the skin of young cattle. Vaccines and treatment regimes are available, but even untreated animals usually recover. The disease is transmissible to humans.

Salmonellosis

This is a bacterial infection mainly affecting calves and young cattle, which causes diarrhoea and dysentery. A vaccine is available. The condition is usually responsive to antibiotic treatment, although multidrug resistance is an increasing problem. Some strains of *Salmonella* can be transmitted to humans.

Scours (diarrhoea)

Many diseases may produce scour in calves and adult cattle. Most of these may be related to the animals' environment. Sufficient good quality colostrum given soon after birth will often considerably reduce the problem in calves.

Common causes may include rotavirus, coliform bacteria, coccidiosis, *Cryptosporidium*, endoparasites, BVD and Johne's disease.

Tuberculosis

This is a notifiable, infectious bacterial disease and a zoonosis. Cattle should be tested for tuberculosis regularly (dependent on country disease status) and removed if they are infected. Only animals shown to be free from the disease should be kept.

Currently uncommon but still important diseases

Anthrax

This is an acute infectious bacterial disease causing sudden death in cattle; it is a zoonosis and is notifiable in many countries. All cases of sudden death should be investigated by a veterinary surgeon. Prophylactic vaccines are available for use, under licence, in anthrax areas.

Bluetongue

Bluetongue is a notifiable disease and on the increase in Europe. It is vector-borne (by a *Culicoides* midge) viral infection. Prevention may involve substantial biosecurity measures to protect cattle against midge bites as well as routine annual vaccination.

Brucellosis

Brucellosis is an infectious bacterial disease causing abortion and infertility; it is a zoonosis and is notifiable in many countries. All cases of abortion should be investigated by a veterinarian. Cattle should only be used if a blood test has shown them to be free from the disease.

Standard texts, for example Blowey (1999), Andrews *et al.* (2004) and Divers & Peek (2007) should be consulted for details of these and other cattle diseases.

Abnormal behaviour

Cattle kept outdoors on pasture or fed large quantities of silage, hay or other bulky fodders do not usually show abnormal behaviours. This is thought to be a result of them spending some 8h out of the 24 consuming grass, or somewhat less time eating hay, and a further 6–7h ruminating – so that they are 'gainfully occupied' during most of the day. As herd animals, an important component of providing an appropriately enriched environment is the presence of other cattle.

However, cattle kept tied up for long periods of time, or confined within metabolism crates, sometimes show oral stereotypies such as compulsive licking, tongue sucking, tongue rolling and horizontal bar grasping. Once established these behavioural abnormalities are very difficult to eliminate, but they largely disappear once the animal is turned out to graze.

Reproductive problems

Infertility is an important source of economic loss in cattle and has many causes. The causes of infertility can be usually identified by an experienced veterinarian and a control programme instigated.

Dystocia

If a cow's normal calving behaviour ceases and, on physical examination there is no sign that the calving is progressing normally, then it should be considered as a dystocia. There are many potential causes and veterinary advice should be taken.

Metritis

This is characterised by infection of the uterus and is usually seen in the post-parturient period. A foul-smelling discharge from the vulva is observed. It may be predisposed to when foetal membranes are retained and metritis has occurred previously in the cow. Treatment should be undertaken by a veterinary surgeon.

For details of the prevention, control and treatment of reproductive problems see the appropriate chapters of Meredith (1995), Noakes *et al.* (2001) and Ball & Peters (2004).

Cattle are delightful creatures to work with. They respond well to gentle treatment; they can be readily trained to cooperate in many scientific procedures but they are big, sometimes a little clumsy and obstinate and, of course, they are expensive to keep. The latter fact has probably been instrumental in the decline in their use as an experimental animal.

The validity and usefulness of the results obtained from animal experimentation depends upon many factors, not least of which is the quality of life being experienced by the subject animals. Animals which are healthy, thriving and contented and which are kindly handled are most likely to yield sound data. Cattle are no exception to this – they give the best experimental results when they are humanely husbanded and treated with care and consideration.

Further reading

The literature relating to the care and management of cattle is immense. One of the best general introductions is Webster (1993) *Understanding the Dairy Cow*. There is much relevant material in the husbandry section of Andrews *et al.* (2004) *Bovine Medicine: Diseases and Husbandry of Cattle*. There are useful chapters on dairy cattle (Leaver 1999) and on beef cattle and veal calves (Webster 1999) in Ewbank *et al.* (1999) *Management and Welfare of Farm Animals*. Blowey (1999) *A Veterinary Book for Dairy Farmers* provides an excellent general introduction to cattle disease, welfare and the health aspects of husbandry. A recent book (Bazeley & Hayton 2007) deals in detail with many practical aspects of cattle care and management. The UK Department for Environment, Food and Rural Affairs issues in 2003 the most recent version of its useful *Codes of Recommendations for the Welfare of*

Livestock – Cattle. Similar codes of practice have been produced by the Ministry of Agriculture and Fisheries of New Zealand (1992) and for Australia by Primary Industries Standing Committee (2004). There has recently been published a substantial and most useful book entitled *The Welfare of Cattle* (Rushen *et al.* 2008) and the US Federation of Animal Science Societies has issued the 2009 edition of its *Guide for the Care and Use of Agricultural Animals in Research and Teaching*.

References

Agriculture and Food Research Council (1993) *Energy and Protein Requirements of Ruminants.* An advisory manual prepared by the AFRC Technical Committee on Responses to Nutrients. CAB International, Wallingford

Albright, J.L. and Arave, C.W. (1997) *The Behaviour of Cattle.* CAB International, Wallingford

Albright, J.L. and Fulwider, W.K. (2007) Dairy cattle behaviour, facilities, handling, transport, automation and well-being. In: *Livestock Handling and Transport*, 3rd edn. Ed. Grandin, T., pp. 109–133. CAB International, Wallingford

Allen, D.M. (2004) Calf rearing. In: *Bovine Medicine: Diseases and Husbandry of Cattle,* 2nd edn. Eds Andrew, A.H., Blowey, R.H., Boyd, H. *et al.*, pp. 3–6. Blackwell Publishing, Oxford

Allen, W. (1991) *Veterinary Laboratory Data,* 2nd edn. British Veterinary Association, London

Andrews, A.H., Blowey, R.H., Boyd, H. *et al.* (Eds) (2004) *Bovine Medicine: Diseases and Husbandry of Cattle*, 2nd edn. Blackwell Publishing, Oxford

Baker, K.C., Einstein, R. and Mellor, D. (eds) (1996) *Farm Animals in Biomedical and Agricultural Research.* Proceedings of Conference, Wellington, NZ. 1995. Australia, Glen Osmond

Ball, P.J.H. and Peters, A.R. (2004) *Reproduction in Cattle,* 3rd edn. Blackwell Publishing, Oxford

Barnett, S.W. (2007) Cattle. In: *Manual of Animal Technology*. Ed. Barnett, S.W., pp. 118–130. Blackwell Publishing, Oxford

Battaglia, R.A. (1998) Handbook of Livestock Management Techniques, 3rd edn. Upper Saddle River, NJ

Bazeley, K. and Hayton, K. (2007) *Practical Cattle Farming.* Crowood Press, Ramsbury, Wiltshire

Belk, K.E., Scanga, J.A. and Grandin, T. (2007) Biosecurity for animal health and food safety. In: *Livestock Handling and Transport*, 3rd edn. Ed. Grandin, T., pp. 354–369. CAB International, Wallingford

Blowey, R. (1994) Dairy cattle housing. In: *Livestock Housing.* Eds Wathes, C.M. and Charles, D.R., pp. 305–337. CAB International, Wallingford

Blowey, R.W. (1999) *A Veterinary Book for Dairy Farmers*, 3rd edn. Farming Press, Ipswich

Brooks, D.L., Tillman, P.C. and Niemi, S.M. (1984) Ungulates as laboratory animals. In: *Laboratory Animal Medicine.* Eds Fox, J.G., Cohen, B.E. and Loew, F.M., pp. 273–295. Academic Press, San Diego

Canadian Council on Animal Care (1980) *Guide to the Care and Use of Experimental Animals*, Vol 1. CCAC, Ottawa

Chapman, A.B. (1969) *Techniques and Procedures in Animal Production Research.* Revised edn. American Society for Animal Science, Albany

Consortium (1988) *Guide for the Care and Use of Agricultural Animals in Agricultural Research and Teaching.* Consortium for Developing a Guide for the Care and Use of Agricultural Animals in Agricultural Research and Teaching, Champaign, Illinois. (The 1999 edition is listed under Federation of Animal Science Societies)

Council of Europe (2006) Multilateral Consultation of Parties to the European Convention for the Protection of Vertebrate Animals used for Experimental and other Scientific Purposes (ETS 123) Appendix A. *Cons 123 (2006) 3.* Available from URL: http://www.coe.int/t/e/legal_affairs/legal_co-operation/biological_safety,_use_of_animals/laboratory_animals/2006/Cons123(2006)3AppendixA_en.pdf (accessed 31 July 2008)

Department for Environment, Food and Rural Affairs (2003) *Code of Recommendations for the Welfare of Livestock: Cattle (PB 7949).* DEFRA Publications, London

Dickfos, J.A. (1991) *Training Cattle for Scientific Experiments.* Commonwealth Scientific and Industrial Research Organisation, Rockhampton, Queensland

Divers, T.J. and Peek, S.F. (Eds) (2007) *Rebhun's Diseases of Dairy Cattle*, 2nd edn. Saunders Elsevier, St.Louis

Doyle, R.E., Garb, S., Davis, S.E. *et al.* (1968) Domesticated farm animals in medical research. *Annals of the New York Academy of Sciences*, **147**, 129–204

Epstein, H. and Mason, I.L. (1984) Cattle. In: *Evolution of Domesticated Animals.* Ed Mason, I.L., pp. 6–27. Longman, London

European Commission (2007) Commission recommendations of 18 June 2007 on guidelines for the accommodation and care of animals used for experimental and other scientific purposes. Annex II to European Council Directive 86/609. See 2007/526/EC.

http://eurlex.europa.eu/LexUriServ/site/en/oj/2007/l_197/l_19720070730en00010089.pdf (accessed 13 May 2008)

Ewbank, R., Kim-Madslien, F. and Hart, C.B. (Eds) (1999) *Management and Welfare of Farm Animals, The UFAW Farm Handbook*, 4th edn. Universities Federation for Animal Welfare, Wheathampstead

Ewbank, R. and Parker, M. (2007) Handling cattle raised in close association with people. In: *Livestock Handling and Transport*, 3rd edn. Ed. Grandin, T., pp. 76–89. CAB International, Wallingford

Federation of Animal Science Societies (2009) *Guide for the Care and Use of Agricultural Animals in Research and Teaching*, 3rd edn. FASS, Champaign, Illinois

Feldman, B.F., Zinkl, J.G. and Jain, N.C. (eds) (2000) *Schalm's Veterinary Hematology*, 5th edn. Lippincott Williams and Wilkins, Savoy, Illinois

Fielding, R.D. and Matthewman, R.W. (2004) Tropical cattle management. In: *Bovine Medicine: Diseases and Husbandry of Cattle*, 2nd edn. Eds Andrew, A.H., Blowey, R.H., Boyd, H. *et al.*, pp. 68–82. Blackwell, Oxford

Food and Agriculture Organization (2004) *FAO Production Yearbook for 2003*, Vol. 50, p. 210. FAO of the United Nations, Rome

Fowler, M.E. (1995) *Restraint and Handling of Wild and Domestic Animals*, 3rd edn. Saunders, Philadelphia

Gibson, L.A.S. and Andrews, A.H. (2000) Disease security. In: *The Health of Dairy Cattle.* Ed. Andrews, A.H., pp. 328–350. Blackwell Publishing, Oxford

Gordon, I. (2003) *Laboratory Production of Cattle Embryos*, 2nd edn. CAB International, Wallingford

Gordon, I. (2004) *Reproductive Technologies in Farm Animals* CAB International, Wallingford

Grandin, T. (2007a) Behavioural principles of handling cattle and other grazing animals under extensive conditions. In: *Livestock Handling and Transport*, 3rd edn. Ed. Grandin, T., pp. 44–64. CAB International, Wallingford

Grandin, T. (2007b) Handling facilities and restraint of range cattle. In: *Livestock Handling and Transport*, 3rd edn. Ed. Grandin, T., pp. 90–108. CAB International, Wallingford

Grandin, T. (2009) Handling and transport of agricultural animals used in research and teaching. *SCAW Newsletter* **31**(2) 6–12 and (3) 14–21

Grandin, T. and Gallo, C. (2007) Cattle transport. In: *Livestock Handling and Transport*, 3rd edn. Ed. Grandin, T., pp. 134–154. CAB International, Wallingford

Grassland Research Institute (1961) *Research Techniques in Use at the Grassland Research Institute.* Bulletin No 45. Commonwealth Agricultural Bureau, Farnham Royal

Greenhalgh, J.F.D., Morgan, C.A., Edwards, R.A. *et al.* (2002) *Animal Nutrition*, 6th edn. Pearson Education Ltd, Harlow

Hall, L.W., Clarke, K.W. and Trim, C.W. (2001) *Veterinary Anaesthesia*, 10th edn. Saunders, London

Hall, S.J.G. (2002) Behaviour of cattle. In: *The Ethology of Domestic Animals. An Introductory Text.* Ed. Jensen, P., pp. 131–143. CABI Publishing, Wallingford

Harrison, F.A. (1995) *Surgical Techniques in Experimental Farm Animals.* Oxford University Press, Oxford

Hartigan, P.J. (1995) Cattle breeding and infertility. In: *Animal Breeding and Infertility.* Ed Meredith, M.J., pp. 1–75. Blackwell Publishing, Oxford

Holmes, R.J. (1991) Cattle. In: *Practical Animal Handling.* Eds Anderson, R.S. and Edney, A.T.B., pp. 15–38. Pergamon Press, Oxford

Home Office (1989) *Animals (Scientific Procedures) Act 1986: Code of Practice for the Housing and Care of Animals Used in Scientific Procedures* (HC 107). HMSO, London

Humane Slaughter Association (2005) *Humane Killing of Livestock Using Firearms*, 2nd edn. HSA, Wheathampstead

Humane Slaughter Association (2006) *Captive-Bolt Stunning of Livestock*, 4th edn. HSA, Wheathampstead

Humane Slaughter Association (2008) *Humane Handling of Livestock.* HSA, Wheathampstead

Institute of Laboratory Animal Resources (1996) *Guide for the Care and Use of Laboratory Animals.* National Academy Press, Washington, DC

Joint Working Group on Refinement (1993) Removal of blood from laboratory mammals and birds. First Report of the BVA/FRAME/RSPCA/UFAW Joint Working Group on Refinement. *Laboratory Animals*, **27**, 1–22

Joint Working Group on Refinement (2001) Refining procedures for the administration of substances. Report of the BVAAWF/FRAME/RSPCA/UFAW Joint Working Group on Refinement. *Laboratory Animals*, **35**, 1–41

Kerr, M.G. (2002) *Veterinary Laboratory Medicine*, 2nd edn. Blackwell Publishing, Oxford

Kues, W.A. and Niemann, H. (2004) The contribution of farm animals to human health. *Trends in Biotechnology*, **22**, 286–294

Lawrence, N.G. (1994) Beef cattle housing. In: *Livestock Housing.* Eds Wathes, C.M. and Charles, D.R., pp. 339–357. CAB International, Wallingford

Leathers, C.W. (1990) Choosing the animals – reasons, excuses and welfare. In: *The Experimental Animal in Biomedical Research*, Vol. 1. Eds Rollin, B.E. and Kessel, M.L., pp. 67–79. CRC Press, Boca Raton

Leaver, J.D. (1982) *Herbage Intake Handbook.* British Grassland Society, Hurley

Leaver, J.D. (1999) Dairy cattle. In: *Management and Welfare of Farm Animals*, 4th edn. Eds Ewbank R., Kim-Madslien, F. and Hart, C.B., pp. 17–47. Universities Federation for Animal Welfare, Wheathampstead

McNitt, J.I. (1983) *Livestock Husbandry Techniques.* Granada, London

Mench, J.A., Mayer, S.A. and Krulish, L. (eds) (1992) *The Well-being of Agricultural Animals in Biomedical and Agricultural Research.* Proceedings of a symposium. Scientists Center for Animal Welfare, Bethesda

Meredeth, M.J. (ed) (1995) *Animal Breeding and Infertility.* Blackwell Publishing, Oxford

Ministry of Agriculture and Fisheries (1992) *Codes of Recommendations and Minimum Standards for The Welfare of Dairy Cattle*, (Code of Welfare No.4). MAF, Wellington

National Academy of Sciences (1974) *Ruminants: Cattle, Sheep and Goats. Guidelines for Breeding, Care and Management of Laboratory Animals.* NAS, Washington, DC

Noakes, D.E., Parkinson, T.J. and England, G.C.W. (Eds) (2001) *Arthur's Veterinary Reproduction and Obstetrics*, 8th edn. Saunders, Edinburgh

Office International des Epizooties (2008) *Terrestial Animal Health Code.* 17th edn OIE, Paris

Olfert, E.D., Cross, B.M. and McWilliam, A.A. (1993) *Guide to the Care and Use of Experimental Animals* Vol. 1, 2nd edn. Canadian Council on Animal Care, Ottawa

Owen, J. (1995) *Cattle Feeding*, 2nd edn. (with revisions). Farming Press, Ipswich

Payne, W.J.A. and Wilson, R.T. (1999) *An Introduction to Animal Husbandry in the Tropics*, 5th edn. Blackwell Publishing, Oxford

Phillips, C. (2002) *Cattle Behaviour and Welfare*, 2nd edn. Blackwell Publishing, Oxford

Primary Industries Standing Committee (2004) *Model Code of Practice for the Welfare of Animals. Cattle*, 2nd edn. (PISC Report – No.85). CSIRO Publishing, Collingwood

Reece, W.O. (ed) (2004) *Duke's Physiology of Domestic Animals*, 12th edn. Cornell University Press, Ithaca

Reinhardt, V. and Reinhardt, A. (2002) Comfortable quarters for cattle in research institutions. In: *Comfortable Quarters for Laboratory Animals*, 9th edn. Eds Reinhardt V. and Reinhardt A., pp. 89–95. Animal Welfare Institute, Washington, DC

Riebold, T.W. (2007) Ruminants. In: *Lumb and Jones' Veterinary Anesthesia and Analgesia*, 4th edn. Eds Tranquilli, W.J., Thurmon, J.C. and Grim, K.A., pp. 731–736. Blackwell Publishing, Oxford

Roche, J.F. (1989) New techniques in hormonal manipulation of cattle production. In: *New Techniques in Cattle Production.* Ed. Phillips, C.J.C., pp. 48–60. Butterworths, London

Rowan, T.G. (1989) Identical twins – their value in research. *Proceedings of the British Cattle Veterinary Association for 1988–89.* pp. 49–53. BCVA, Frampton-on-Severn

Rushen, J., Passille, A.M.D., Keyserlingk, M.A.G.V. *et al.* (2008) *The Welfare of Cattle.* Springer, Amsterdam

Roy, J.H.B. (1990) *The Calf, Vol. 1. Management of Health*, 5th edn. Butterworths, London.

Sibley, R.J. (1995) *Casualty Slaughter.* British Cattle Veterinary Association, Frampton-on-Severn

Stookey, J.M. and Watts, J.M. (2007) Low-stress restraint, handling and weaning of cattle. In: *Livestock Handling and Transport*, 3rd edn. Ed. Grandin, T., pp. 65–75. CAB International, Wallingford

Swanson, J.C. (1998) Oversight of farm animals in research. *Lab Animals*, **27**, 28–31.

Thickett, B., Mitchell, D. and Hallows, B. (2003) *Calf Rearing*, 3rd edn. Crowood Press, Marlborough

Webster, J. (1993) *Understanding the Dairy Cow*, 2nd edn. Blackwell Publishing, Oxford

Webster, A.J.F. (1999) Beef cattle and veal calves. In: *Management and Welfare of Farm Animals*, 4th edn. Eds Ewbank R., Kim-Madslien, F. and Hart, C.B., pp. 49–82. Universities Federation for Animal Welfare, Wheathampstead

Wood, P.D.P. (Ed.) (1975) Considerations for the design and interpretation of cattle experiments. Proceedings of Symposium of British Society of Animal Production. *British Society of Animal Production, London*

34 Sheep and goats

Colin L. Gilbert and Keith M. Kendrick

Biological overview

Introduction

Sheep and goats have been domesticated by man and used for meat, milk and wool for several thousand years. It may therefore seem somewhat surprising that behavioural traits such as flocking for protection and running from humans remain so well defined. The likely reason for this is that these instincts have been exploited rather than repressed through the ages to facilitate animal management and handling in groups. The same instincts can and should be used in the laboratory environment when working with groups of animals, but it may also be necessary to work with separated individuals. It is always important to remember that sheep and goats are gregarious by nature, and isolation will result in stress (Parrott 1988). However, sheep and particularly goats, respond very well to gentle handling over a period of time, and in most cases will eventually lose their flight instinct even when penned singly. This accommodation to environment should be the first objective of all laboratory users of small ruminants for medium- to long-term experiments. Benefits will accrue to animal handlers, the quality of data, and most importantly to the animals themselves.

Perceptual and cognitive abilities of sheep and goats – social organisation

It is entirely wrong to equate the strong retention of flight instincts in these animals with a lack of intelligence. Indeed, behavioural and neurobiological studies of the perceptual and cognitive abilities of sheep and goats have revealed that they make sophisticated use of both visual and olfactory cues from their environment to enable them to rapidly learn to recognise individual offspring, flock members and humans as well as palatable and unpalatable foods. Their ability to do this almost rivals that seen in higher primates including man; and one obvious conclusion that must be drawn from such studies is that, if they need to be able to recognise a number of specific individuals and objects and, if their brains are specialised for carrying out this process, then their social requirements and interactions must be far more complex than a cursory view of their behaviour within a flock might suggest. Research has also shown that sheep have individual personality traits. Therefore, as an intelligent species with a degree of sentience, the use of sheep in experimental procedures should be undertaken thoughtfully and only when specific need arises.

There has been a tendency to overlook the possibility that sheep and goats, or for that matter other domestic ungulates, use vision to learn about and interact with their environment. While they lack an accommodation reflex, their visual acuity in the frontal eye field is very good and probably lies somewhere between that of a cat and a monkey (Piggins 1992). They are capable of recognising individuals from visual cues from the face region and are able to visually discriminate between different types of grass, clover and concentrates (Kendrick 1992; Kendrick *et al.* 2001; Tate *et al.* 2006). Indeed, sheep can identify and remember at least 50 different sheep and 10 different human faces and even after long periods of absence (Kendrick *et al.* 2001; Peirce *et al.* 2000). For this reason, it is important to take care that fleece or horn growth does not significantly interfere with an animal's line of sight. Both sheep and goats can be trained to perform operant tasks (eg, choices indicated by pressing panels with their nose); to discriminate between different faces or other visual stimuli (Baldwin 1979, 1981; Tate *et al.* 2006); or to choose between faces or geometrical stimuli in a Y-maze (Kendrick *et al.* 1995, 1996; Tate *et al.* 2006). Animals can be easily trained to use this apparatus either for food or social rewards.

Faces clearly have an important emotional significance for sheep. Studies have shown that when they are exposed to social isolation stress, the sight of pictures of familiar sheep can alleviate behavioural, autonomic and endocrine indices of stress and reduce activation of brain centres controlling stress and fear responses (Da Costa *et al.* 2004). Showing animals video sequences depicting other sheep can also evoke profound interest and relieve stress (Elliker 2006). Recent work has also shown that sheep can detect and respond to human face expressions (smiling and angry) and emotion cues in sheep faces (fearful vs calm) (Kendrick 2004; Elliker 2006; Tate *et al.* 2006) and that they may be able to form and use mental images of faces (Tate *et al.* 2006).

Both sheep and goats also have a remarkably acute sense of smell and can discriminate between a large number of biological and chemical odours in operant experiments (Baldwin & Meese 1977). However, in spite of possessing a highly developed sense of smell they do not appear to need it for food recognition or even individual recognition in most cases, although it is entirely possible that olfactory cues might complement visual ones to speed up recognition or improve its accuracy. The main exception to the predominance of vision over olfaction is the selective olfactory recognition of offspring which develops in both species very quickly after they have given birth and which seems to be essential since accurate visual and vocal discrimination of offspring develops much more slowly (Kendrick *et al.* 1996). Another context in which olfactory cues are important appears to be synchronisation of oestrus which occurs in response to odours from the fleece of a male – the so-called 'ram effect'.

The hearing sensitivities of sheep and goats are broadly similar to those of humans with the exception that they can hear frequencies above the human upper limit of hearing (ultrasonics). However, their ability to localise sounds is relatively poor compared to that of some other mammals (Heffner & Heffner 1992) and may reflect their greater reliance on vision. Sheep also only have a limited vocal repertoire which essentially falls into three different types. These include a high-pitched or protest bleat which can be used to signify anything from slight agitation or mild impatience to extreme fear; a low-pitched more rumbling bleat used specifically by maternal ewes to call their lambs; and a similar type of low-pitched vocalisation sometimes used by rams engaged in courtship with ewes. While there is evidence that maternal ewes can learn to recognise their lambs' voices, and vice versa (Shillito & Alexander 1975), the ability of sheep to recognise individual members of the flock from their high-pitched bleats has yet to be demonstrated convincingly (Kendrick *et al.* 1995; Elliker 2006), although sound spectrograms show clear individual differences in sheep voices. It seems fair to conclude at this stage that the main function of the high-pitched bleats is for an individual to express some degree of concern or impatience and, in certain circumstances, to warn other flock members of some impending danger.

The cognitive abilities of sheep and goats enable them to cope successfully with changing environments. Abilities to follow rules and abstract ideas are more limited although they do show some capacity to form concepts. For example, sheep are capable of discerning that there is a physical barrier between them and a human no matter what form that barrier may take (wire fence, chain fence, gate etc). Even with a single-stranded electric fence a sheep appears to know that what keeps it in will also keep humans out. Thus a sheep will often tolerate the presence of humans at much smaller distances to themselves when there is an intervening fence and will often not show an alerting response when a human approaches the fence. However, in other respects their conceptualisation does show clear limitations. For example, whereas sheep will normally run away from a human walking towards them when the human is 10 m or more away from them, they will often let a human crawl in amongst them providing that he or she keeps their eyes averted downwards. Thus their concept of a human shape appears rather limited.

Learning skills of sheep are also dependent, to some extent, on the type of objects that they are being trained to visually discriminate. Thus when they are trained to discriminate between totally unfamiliar geometrical symbols (triangles, squares, circles, lines etc) they are relatively slow at learning (Baldwin 1981; Kendrick *et al.* 1996). However, if they are required to discriminate between familiar types of real object, such as faces, they can learn very rapidly (Kendrick *et al.* 1996; Peirce *et al.* 2000), and have been shown to recognise and remember at least 50 different sheep and 10 different human faces for up to 2 years. Thus an important consideration with these species is to use familiar types of objects as discriminanda or reinforcement signals if speed of learning is an important issue. They also clearly have a long-term memory for both other sheep and humans who interact with them.

One other important aspect of behaviour in sheep and goats that should not be overlooked is developmental influences on learning and preferences. While such influences are still poorly understood, certain principles have nevertheless emerged which have direct bearing upon how experimental animals should be reared. In both sheep and goats, where a selective and initially exclusive bond exists between mother and offspring, the mother is an enormously influential role model. There is evidence, for example, that dietary preferences learned from the mother can be retained for periods in excess of 3 years. Moreover, work on the effects of cross-fostering between sheep and goats has shown that the mother rather than the genetic species dictates social and sexual preferences in adulthood and that her influence appears to be practically irreversible in this respect (Kendrick *et al.* 1998). Therefore, it is clearly preferable to rear infant kids and lambs with a mother since this close emotional mother–infant relationship is of great importance to their normal social and emotional development. In addition, it is important to recognise that trying to make an animal do something which goes against what it has learned from its mother is always going to be difficult or even impossible. This might simply involve the effects of changing diets but can also extend to attitudes towards humans. Lambs will learn to avoid humans from the actions of their mothers within a few days of birth and this attitude can be extremely difficult to overcome, even with the best possible interactions between them and humans. Conversely, adult sheep that were reared by hand as orphan lambs tend to be less fearful of humans. For experimental purposes that require close interactions between sheep and humans, it is preferable to ensure that a positive initial attitude to humans is passed on from mother to offspring by attempting to create a positive attitude in the mother first. With goats this is not so much of a problem since most breeds are tolerant of, and even interact with, humans. Nonetheless, even with this species positive human interactions with the mothers may result in easier interactions with their young.

Standard biological data

Standard biological data for sheep and goats are shown in Table 34.1 and comprehensive haematological and biochemical data for these species may be found in Wolfensohn and Lloyd (2003) and Aitken (2007).

Choice of breed

This is to some extent dictated by climatic conditions and availability. Theoretically almost any breed of sheep should

Table 34.1 Some standard biological data for sheep and goats.

Parameters	Sheep	Goats
Normal temperature (°C)	38.5–39.5	38.5–39.5
Chromosome number	54	60
Lifespan (years)	10–15	10–15
Heart rate (beats/minute)	65–110	70–120
Resting respiratory rate (breaths/minute)	15–20	15–25
Dental formula	$I^0_3\ C^0_1\ P^3_3\ M^3_3$	$I^0_3\ C^0_1\ P^3_3\ M^3_3$

readily adapt to most experimental conditions provided that they are treated correctly, although an exception to this would be feral breeds. However, a number of criteria should be assessed when deciding which breed is suitable for a particular research project. There are over 200 breeds of sheep worldwide, many of which are localised to specific countries or conditions and are rare elsewhere. The most numerous breed internationally is the Merino, which is kept for wool production and is found predominantly in Australia and South Island, New Zealand. New Zealand also has a number of meat-producing or dual-purpose breeds, such as the Romney, the Perendale and the Drysdale. In the UK, lowland sheep breeds such as Dorset, Suffolk and Friesland, together with most breeds of goat tend to settle more quickly to individual penning and handling than do upland or hill breeds, such as the Scottish Blackface, Cheviot and Welsh Mountain, although these breeds may also adapt eventually. However, lowland breeds may become very large and heavy (80 kg or more) when compared to hill breeds (35–50 kg), or indeed the Soay (15–20 kg); so whilst lowland breeds may be easier to catch they often prove to be more difficult to move or carry and may become overweight when penned indoors for extended periods. Saanen and Anglo-Nubian goats are usually considerably larger than British Alpine or Bagot. Larger animals require more floor space and food.

Reproductive characteristics such as strong seasonality driven by day length (most breeds), a longer breeding season (Dorset) or large litter sizes (Finn or Boroolla Merino) may be important. Most breeds of goat and milking breeds of sheep such as Friesland lend themselves to lactation studies. Other special considerations might include growth rate, carcase quality, wool or coat colour. Using a purebred has advantages over using a crossbred ewe since buying in breeding stock can be minimised.

Some researchers find horns useful for attaching equipment although the horns should never be used as a sole means of restraint. The presence of horns can be a potential hazard to both handlers and other animals, and this should be part of the decision-making process on whether they should be removed. Horn buds may be removed safely between 3 and 7 days of age. Adequate anaesthesia and analgesia are essential during removal and providing the right balance of drugs for different circumstances requires experience. Sensory innervation to the horns varies between species. The removal of horn buds, particularly in kid goats, requires both skill and experience. The use of a hot disbudding iron in goats can easily result in brain damage as the thin cranial vault offers little thermal protection to neural tissues. In the UK disbudding goat kids may only be performed by a veterinary surgeon. The UK goat veterinary society[1] has produced a DVD on the subject, for distribution to veterinary surgeons. The method of Boyd (1988), using general anaesthesia, is also reliable.

Source of animals

Ideally an on-site breeding flock/herd should be maintained. This allows for continuity of supply, standardisation of genetic background and maintenance of a health barrier (see below). If maintaining flocks on-site is impractical then animals may be bought in, bearing in mind that known single sources of supply are generally better and more accountable than open markets, and that availability of animals is likely to be seasonal.

Uses in the laboratory

Current areas of research that routinely use sheep and goats as experimental animals include studies into the seasonal control of reproductive activity, parturition, neonatal care and reproduction in general, lactation, growth, ruminant metabolism and physiology, and behavioural and neurobiological studies of cognitive and motivational processes. They have also been used as large-scale producers of antibodies in blood and trialled for synthesising bioactive compounds in milk through transgenic manipulation. Other studies include those related directly to disease conditions which cause harm to sheep (such as foot and mouth disease and bluetongue). A particular recent interest has been the transmissible spongiform encephalopathies (TSEs). Models of human disease include bone metabolism studies and polycystic ovarian disease.

Management and breeding

General husbandry

Housing

Generally speaking, well fleeced sheep are very tolerant of low temperatures providing that the fleece is dry. Hill breeds of sheep are more tolerant of poor weather than lowland breeds, but even the hardiest animals require some protection from wind and rain. Goats are also fairly tolerant to cold weather providing they are dry, but prefer warmer climates and should have access to shelter at all times. Shelters can take the form of small huts in pastures during the summer time (with the entrance way sheltered from prevailing winds), but these can be inadequate in the winter. Both sheep and goats benefit from access to shade during the summer to prevent heat stress. Goats have a tendency to eat their shade, which may constitute an enrichment in

[1]http://www.goatvetsoc.co.uk

the short term but can then contribute to both overheating and poisoning, so should be monitored carefully. A key enrichment is the presence of other animals with which to form stable social groups. A dry lying area should always be made available. Animals at pasture need to be protected from predators and harassment by dogs.

Group housing

Where possible, sheep and goats should be kept in groups of two or more animals (species and sexes are normally kept separate). An open-plan floor area which can be partitioned off with hurdles under a high roof provides a versatile solution to varying group sizes (Figure 34.1). The use of straw bales can complement the hurdles. In this system, a floor of rammed chalk or similar is ideal to provide natural drainage on top of which a deep-litter bed of straw can be laid. Impervious floors such as concrete are an alternative and can be more easily decontaminated between groups, but must be sloped to prevent pooling of liquids. The system depends absolutely on sufficient straw laid often enough to provide a dry layer on top in which animals can make themselves comfortable. Inadequate drainage leads to waterlogged pens, damp fleeces and skins, a humid atmosphere, condensation, chilling of animals and compromised well-being. An increase in respiratory disease may also result.

Animals may also be group-housed on wooden slats, through which urine and faeces fall to a collecting pit below. This system has the advantage that animals are always dry, and need less labour in the winter. However the slats are less comfortable than a straw bed, are expensive to maintain and, if allowed to deteriorate, can result in severe leg injuries to sheep (especially fine-boned breeds) treading on broken slats or into gaps. The belly draughts which rise through the slats make these systems unsuitable for goats and for parturient animals. Recent guidance within the Council of Europe ETS 123 revised appendix A for sheep and goats (Council of Europe 2006), and which has been adopted by the European Commission (2007) that the entire enclosure should have a '*solid floor with appropriate bedding provided*' indicates that slatted floors systems may be superseded by more modern alternatives.

Good ventilation is the key to successful housing of sheep and goats. Inadequate air movement produces similar problems to those encountered by poor drainage. In high-ceilinged barns the walls need not be solid and may consist of hit and miss boarding or heavy duty netting in temperate climates to reduce the effect of prevailing winds. Netting is very versatile if kept on a roller blind apparatus, so that it can be easily lifted clear during fine weather. In buildings with low ceilings or solid sides, adequate ventilation will require the provision of ceiling-mounted extractor fans (with a reliable power supply) and wall air inlets above animal height. High-roofed buildings should have a gap running along the roof apex to allow warm humid air to escape. This is helped by providing insulation on the underside of a sloping roof, particularly if the roof is metal, preventing the warm air from cooling and falling back, forming condensation and a stagnant atmosphere.

Group housing of laboratory sheep and goats depends absolutely on a reliable method of identification (see later in this chapter). Adequate trough space must be supplied to allow all animals to feed together when concentrates are offered (Table 34.2). Less space may be needed when food is offered *ad libitum*, but close observation is required to ensure that no bullying occurs at the food rack, especially if a fine mesh is used for the rack (see section on feeding for more details), or if some of the animals have horns.

Individual penning

Experimental demands may require sheep or goats to be housed individually. Researchers must always critically review the need for single housing before imposing it. Animals with long-term surgical preparations may need to be singly housed to prevent damage to implants from curious pen-mates. Sexually active males may require single penning to avoid fighting. Singly penned sheep and goats should always be able to see and hear companions. Prior to any experimental procedure animals require a period of acclimatisation to a new environment, routines and staff.

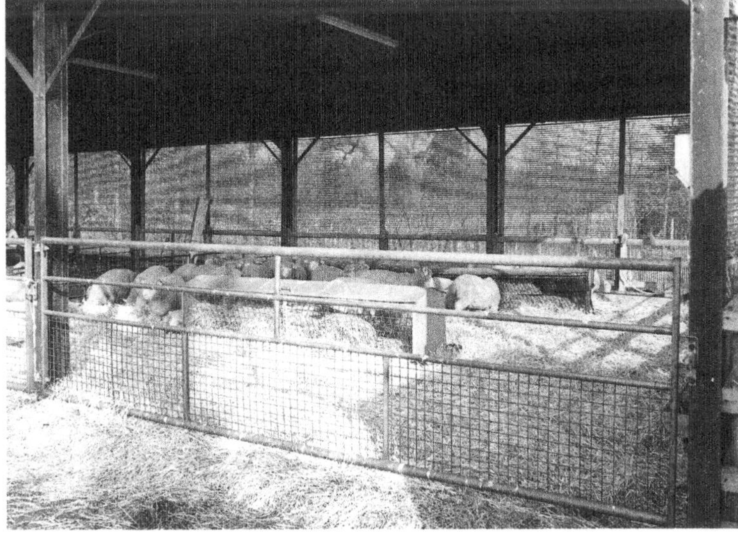

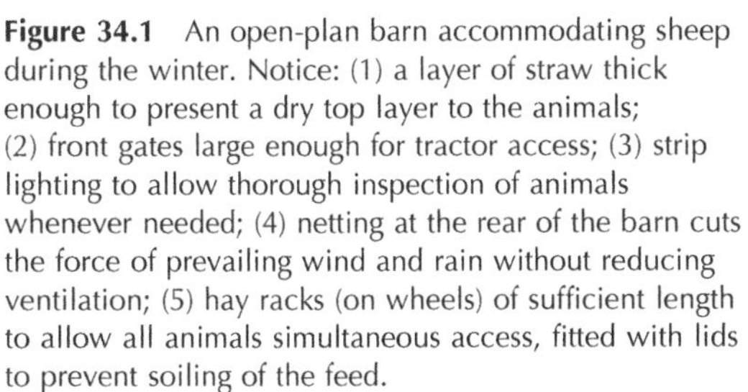

Figure 34.1 An open-plan barn accommodating sheep during the winter. Notice: (1) a layer of straw thick enough to present a dry top layer to the animals; (2) front gates large enough for tractor access; (3) strip lighting to allow thorough inspection of animals whenever needed; (4) netting at the rear of the barn cuts the force of prevailing wind and rain without reducing ventilation; (5) hay racks (on wheels) of sufficient length to allow all animals simultaneous access, fitted with lids to prevent soiling of the feed.

Table 34.2 Recommended minimum pen dimensions for sheep and goats being used for scientific procedures. From Appendix A of the European Convention for the protection of vertebrate animals used for experimental and other scientific purposes (ETS 123) (Council of Europe 2006).

Animal weight (kg)	*Minimum individual enclosure size (m^2)*	*Minimum floor area/animal (m^2)*	*Minimum partition height (m)**	*Minimum length of ad libitum feeding space (m/animal)*	*Minimum length of restricted feeding space (m/animal)*
<20	1.0	0.7	1.0	0.1	0.25
20–34	1.5	1.0	1.2	0.1	0.3
35–59	2.0	1.5	1.2	0.12	0.4
>60	3.0	1.8	1.5	0.12	0.5

*May need to be higher for goats

Goats tend to adapt more rapidly to penning than do sheep and generally show fewer escape behaviours when being caught and handled.

Table 34.2 shows minimum space allowances under European Union recommendations for laboratory sheep and goats. Floors for permanent indoor single housing of sheep and goats should normally be of an impervious material such as concrete or tiles, with at least a 1 in 15 slope to provide drainage. Floor texture needs to achieve a compromise between minimal abrasion to exposed skin and good grip to hooves. Warmth from radiant heat or underfloor heating may be of value for young, sick or infirm animals, or in a surgical recovery area especially for goats or shorn sheep. Gentle underfloor heating can also help to maintain a dry floor and reduce humidity in buildings of low volume, but is costly both to install and maintain. Straw bedding or wood shavings may be provided, although shavings achieve little more than to absorb urine and do not otherwise add to comfort. Bedding in individual pens needs to be changed very regularly, preferably daily.

Pen walls can be solid and impervious to fluids to animal head height, above which a barred arrangement may continue, or barred to floor level to keep animals in but allowing easy observation by staff and between animals. Horizontal bars near floor level are dangerous as limbs may poke underneath when animals lie down and then break when they attempt to rise. All pens must be free from projections such as bolts or sharp metal edges. Concentrate food may be provided in free-standing plastic bins or troughs. Built in metal troughs tend to be cumbersome, are difficult to clean *in situ*, hard to replace when they rust or rot and can cause pain when kicked by either sheep or handler. Removable hayracks can be hung from partitions. Water may be provided in automatic drinkers or in bowls that hang from the gate, filled by hoses. The latter are preferable in being easy to remove when necessary for cleaning, or to deprive animals of water prior to surgery; and when in use give the animal technician an immediate indication of individual water intake. Individual drinkers of whatever type should be cleaned and checked daily and under normal circumstances should never be allowed to become empty. In exposed locations, the pipes may need frost protection. A typical individual sheep or goat pen is shown in Figure 34.2.

Occasionally it is necessary to hold sheep in metabolism cages or slings. The former are used when collection of urine and faeces is required and the latter for behavioural testing, visual discrimination experiments or similar. Due to their restrictive nature both of these holding methods should only be used when a clear scientific need arises for which normal penning would be inadequate. When using metabolism crates a minimum of a week of acclimatisation is recommended prior to experimentation and in slings the same period is necessary with animals only spending 6–8h per day in slings, under constant supervision. Both systems should use animals already familiarised to human contact and a laboratory environment.

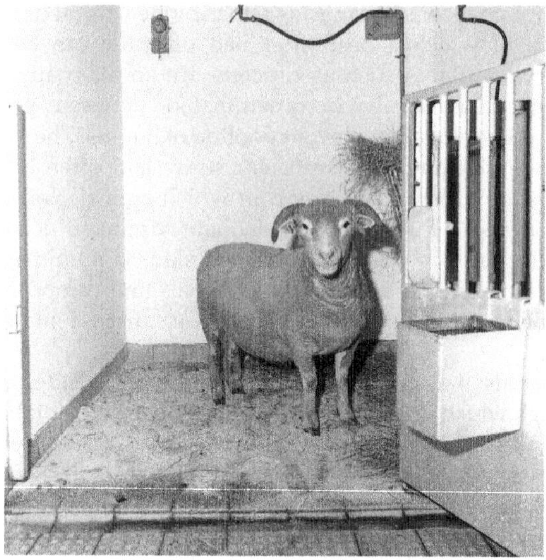

Figure 34.2 A pen suitable for individual housing of sheep or goats in a research environment. Notice: (1) a water bowl, mineral lick and hay rack are all provided but easily removable, the free-standing plastic food trough has been removed; (2) the floor consists of a textured tile which is non-abrasive but gives good grip even when wet, a covering of sawdust helps to maintain dryness; (3) the floor slopes gently to a drain in front of the gate; (4) the bars in the gate allow singly penned animals to see adjacent companions; (5) a convenient electricity supply is provided.

In order to induce out-of-season breeding or to study other light-related phenomena, controlled lighting rooms may be required, but a light-tight space must not be achieved at the expense of compromised ventilation. When lights are turned off the light level must be less than 3 lux to be considered as 'dark' by the day length detection systems used by sheep.

In a large laboratory it may be useful to set aside a separate area or building for special care and quarantine of sick, injured or convalescent animals.

Identification

A reliable and easily read method of identification is vital for animals kept in groups. Ear-tagging is popular and generally effective, but two tags should be used to mitigate against the likelihood of one being lost. Poorly designed tags with sharp edges or protruding surfaces can catch in fencing and tear out of the ear, causing pain and potential infection. A non-toxic spray applied to the flanks allows animals to be identified over a considerable distance but must be regularly renewed and is lost at shearing. Electronic identification devices (EIDs) in rumenal bullets or subcutaneous implants are becoming more popular, especially for valuable individuals. An ear tattoo can be useful for animals with white ears, although these tend to fade and become difficult to decipher with time.

Maintenance of health

Keeping stock healthy is more difficult to achieve in open flocks than closed (those with a non buying-in policy). Veterinary advice should be sought in advance of acquiring new animals. Any bought-in stock must be quarantined for at least 4 weeks on a pasture or in a building well away (more than 100 m) from other stock. Bought-in animals should come with a comprehensive clinical history of the flock from which they originate. On arrival, the animals should be carefully and individually examined for signs of ill-health (see later) by a veterinary surgeon and animals suspected of having particular problems rejected. Further investigation may include serological testing for diseases such as border disease, chlamydophilia or toxoplasmosis using blood samples taken after 2 weeks of quarantine to allow for seroconversion to diseases experienced immediately prior to purchase. During quarantine, routine measures such as vaccinations, treatment against parasitic worms and immersion dipping (or the use of suitable pour-on agents) to control ectoparasites, should be undertaken as necessary to correct for any imbalance between the health status of incoming animals and that of the parent stock. Despite these precautions it is still possible to import disease with new animals. A closed flock is therefore highly desirable.

Sheep intended for research are no less susceptible to disease than stock in commercial flocks. Maintenance of a high health status amongst research animals is an important ethical responsibility for research groups and will also improve data quality through minimising intercurrent, and possibly subclinical disease, during procedures and reducing between-animal variation. Strategies to exclude disease include: membership of national disease eradication or notification schemes; local barriers such as quarantining and well maintained fencing; and use of disease prevention measures such as vaccinations and strict worming policies. Veterinary advice should be taken on these matters, bearing in mind the geographical location and standard practice routines built into the annual cycles of flock management. It is also important to maintain disease prevention routines when an animal leaves the stock pool and enters a laboratory.

Transport

Never begin to move animals from place to place until adequately staffed and fully prepared. The vast majority of sheep will try to run from humans, and animals which are surprised and excited by an impatient handler will run sooner and more quickly. 'Stampedes' of animals may result in self-inflicted injury to animals or handlers and must be avoided. Animals move more easily from place to place in groups. All routes except the desired route should be closed, and then the animals should be allowed to go at a steady walk with gentle encouragement from behind. Single animals are very difficult to move by this method and should be loaded into some form of crate or transporter (Figure 34.3). A very confined transporter is best for this purpose as it prevents a frightened animal from accelerating into an obstruction. For moving flocks over longer distances, specialised animal wagons are required and national regulations regarding animal transport apply. Loading ramps must have barriered sides and ridged walkways. All transporters and transport procedures should comply with current animal transport legislation requirements.

Breeding

Sheep and goats are both seasonally polyoestrous, with shortening day length inducing oestrous cyclical activity in females. Ewe lambs and kids may be large enough to be mated in the autumn of their first year if born early in the season with no subsequent growth check (75% or more of final adult weight). It is preferable not to breed from the smaller ewe lambs or from goats until the following season when they will be at least 1 year old. The rearing conditions used for prospective working rams are also important since there is evidence that rearing rams together from weaning in single sex groups with no access to females can lead to a

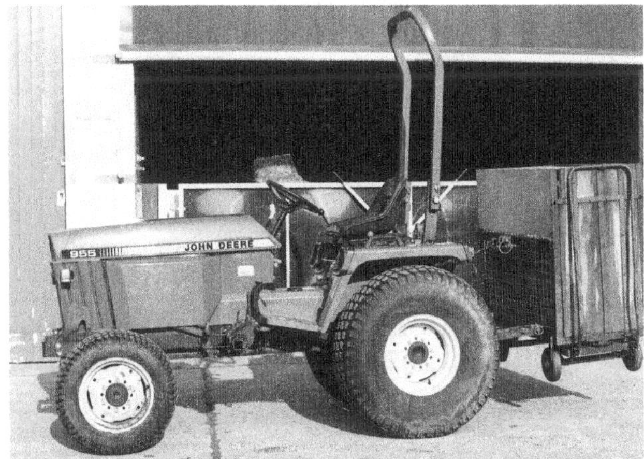

Figure 34.3 A home-made crate suitable for transporting one or two sheep or goats. Notice the couplings to allow carriage by tractor, plus the wheels and handle for manual pulling. Both ends can be lowered to form a stepped ramp, and the top can be lifted to access the animal.

high incidence of homosexual rather than heterosexual preferences. It is, therefore, better to let the ram lambs run with the ewes for as long as possible whilst the ewes and any ewe lambs remain in anoestrus. A good introduction to reproduction in the sheep and goat is provided by *Salamon's Artificial Insemination of Sheep and Goats* (Evans and Maxwell 1988).

Behavioural changes in oestrous ewes are difficult to detect under farm conditions, so rams or teasers (vasectomised males) usually wear coloured crayons on their brisket which leave a mark on a ewe's rump following service. Some goats show inappetance, a drop in milk yield, restlessness and increased vocalisation during oestrus but these signs are not reliable, and willingness to accept the billy is the only sure indicator. Under laboratory or controlled field conditions it is possible to show that female sheep and goats can display a number of proceptive (invitational) and receptive behaviours which can be quantified for experimental purposes to produce an overall receptivity index (Fabre-Nys and Venier 1987).

Although the normal reproductive pattern of sheep and goats leads to the production of one set of offspring in the spring of each year, some breeds, such as the Dorset or the Finnish Landrace, are capable of producing offspring more frequently than this. However, this requires early weaning of the lambs and places pressure on husbandry systems and maternal physiology. A realistic target for more frequent breeding is for the ewe to produce three sets of offspring over 2 years, or five over 3 years. Exceeding this rate is not recommended and such systems are rarely required in a research environment.

At different periods of the reproductive cycle, nutritional requirements are higher. Ewes from mid-pregnancy (especially late gestation) and during lactation need a higher energy intake, and diets may need to be adjusted to give more energy per unit of bulk to supply sufficient nutrition at the limit of appetite. Both rams and ewes may require supplementary feeds in the pre-mating period, to help the rams through to the end of mating and to improve ovulation rate in females (a practice known as 'flushing'). A body condition score of 3 (Figure 34.4) is ideal for a ewe at mating, on a rising plane of nutrition.

Melatonin implants may be used to advance the onset of the breeding season. Strategies for encouraging oestrus early in the breeding season include the use of teaser (vasectomised) rams, intra-vaginal progesterone sponges and

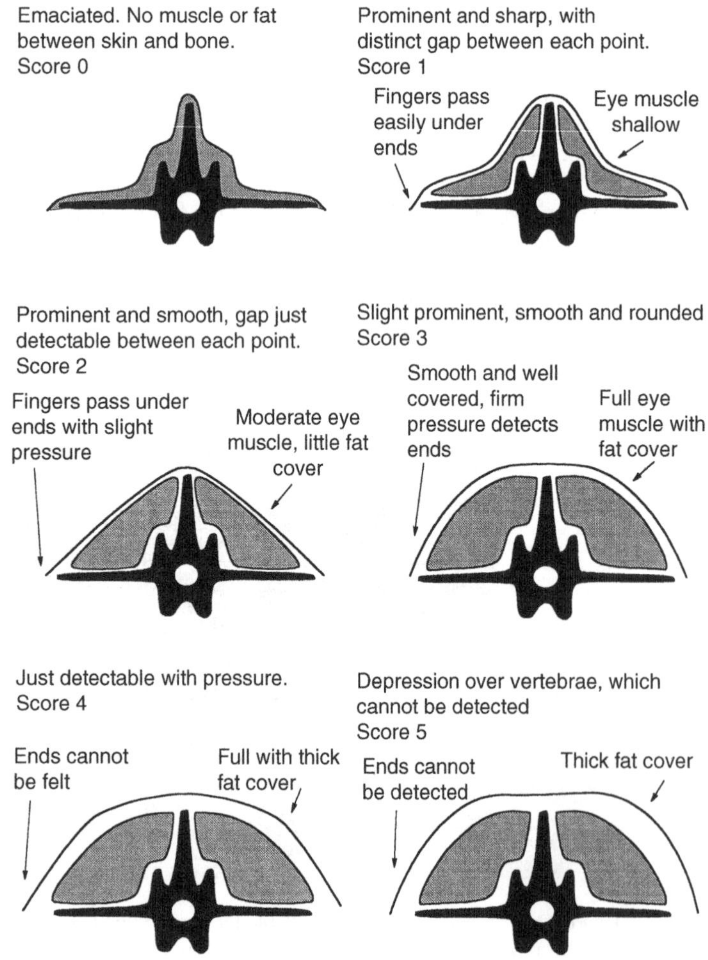

Figure 34.4 Drawings of transverse sections through the lumbar spine of sheep with different body scores. Reproduced with permission from Hindson, J. (1989) *In Practice*, **11**, 152.

injections of gonadotropin-releasing hormone (GnRH) analogues or pregnant mare serum gonadotrophin, although none of these are wholly reliable.

The inter-oestrous period is 16.5 days in the sheep and 21 days in the goat. A number of management strategies exist to synchronise oestrous activity in females in order to produce tight lambing/kidding patterns, including the use of intra-vaginal progesterone sponges or by giving intramuscular injections of prostaglandin $F_{2\alpha}$ or an analogue. A disadvantage of synchronising oestrus is that more rams are needed per ewe. A good-quality fertile ram may be able to serve up to 50 unsynchronised ewes, but only 10–12 ewes in a synchronised flock.

Pregnancy is indicated by non-return to oestrus, and may be confirmed using blood or milk progesterone assays in goats, or through the use of ultrasound scanning, which carries the additional advantage of determining the number of offspring. A skilled interpreter of ultrasound images can identify a pregnancy at 30 days but more usually ewes are scanned at 50–90 days post mating. Other methods, now mostly superseded, include vaginal biopsy, X-rays and abdominal ballottement.

The gestation period is normally 145 days in the sheep and 150 days in the goat with 5 days variation in either direction being normal. Signs of imminent parturition include: seeking isolation from the main group, restlessness including circling and pawing the ground, mammary development, the ability of handlers to express milk from the teats, lifting of the head with licking of the lips and, finally, powerful abdominal contractions. If some control over lambing is required for experimental reasons then an intravenous injection of dexamethasone (0.25 mg/kg) can be given between days 140 and 142 of gestation and ewes will give birth around 48 h later (usually between 40 and 54 h). Intramuscular administration of dexamethasone is not nearly as reliable in this respect. Earlier induction of parturition is not recommended as lambs will be progressively weaker with more respiratory problems.

Clear and simple guides to obstetrics in sheep are provided by Eales and Small (2004) and Winter and Hill (2003). Knowing when to intervene in lambing or kidding requires considerable experience, and the novice should never be put in a position of supervising lambings without skilled backup. As a general rule of thumb, ewes or nannies which do not produce young within 1 hour after the appearance of fluid-filled membranes or a rush of fluid from the vagina may need assistance. Earlier intervention may be required if the animals become weak or unwell. Ewes or nannies which show just a head or one limb protruding from the vagina need assistance immediately. A number of diseases causing abortion are zoonotic, and human contact with parturient ewes should be strictly controlled.

Normally, ewes and nannies will stand following birth, consume the foetal membranes as they are expelled, and bond with their offspring. Following birth the ewe's udder should be checked to ensure that milk is normal and abundant. The majority of lambs and kids are able to stand and feed soon after birth. Weak newborn animals need special attention, particularly warmth, dryness and food. Initial feeds must be given as colostrum (or a colostrum replacer) at 50 ml/kg within 6 h of birth, repeated at 6–8-hourly intervals for the first day if artificial rearing is needed. Colostrum from donor ewes can be frozen and stored for up to 12 months. Stomach tubing may be necessary for neonates that will not suck but should be performed only by a competent person. In severe, hypothermic cases an intraperitoneal injection of a calculated dose of warm sterile isotonic fluid containing glucose may be life saving. Dams and offspring should only be separated if this is essential for their well-being as hand rearing is time consuming and affects behaviour when lambs reach adulthood.

Maternal behaviour and selective bonding

Sheep and goats do not normally show maternal behaviour towards lambs and kids respectively until they give birth, although some stealing of young can occur in experienced mothers towards the end of their pregnancies. When they give birth, maternal behaviour and selective bonding are triggered by feedback to the brain from receptors in the vagina and cervix activated during labour contractions and the expulsion of the foetus. Thus lambs delivered from pregnant ewes by caesarean section or following an epidural anaesthetic block are often not mothered. Birth also triggers selective bonding behaviour with offspring in both sheep and goats, whereby the mother rapidly learns to recognise the odour signatures of its individual lambs or kids and will subsequently refuse suckling attempts from offspring other than its own. In sheep, this process of selective bonding generally occurs within 1 hour post-partum, although with Saanen goats as little as 15 minutes may be sufficient in some cases. Primiparous ewes and nannies take longer to bond with their offspring, often 4 h or more (Kendrick 1994), since maternal experience is required to alter the brain to respond to the feedback from the vagina and cervix during birth. This then promotes changes in olfactory processing structures that underlie the bonding process. Thus, bonding between first-time mothers and their young relies almost exclusively on physical interactions between mother and offspring and removal of the offspring for even short lengths of time or contaminating them with strange odours (including human ones) may result in the mother rejecting her own young.

While selective bonding may ensure the offspring an exclusive milk supply and, for that matter, an individual role model, this has caused farmers problems for hundreds of years when they want to foster orphan or triplet/quadruplet lambs. Where large numbers of animals are giving birth in the same period then 'wet' fostering becomes possible since both maternal ewes and nannies will accept other young prior to forming a selective bond with their own. Once the bond has formed however, the authors have found that its selectivity can be overcome by manually stimulating the vagina and cervix of a post-partum mother for 2 minutes even up to 3 days after she has given birth. To do this the ewe's or nanny's own offspring are temporarily removed from her to a warm place and out of earshot. The stock person then dons lubricated sterile elbow gloves (to prevent transmission of potential zoonotic pathogens eg, *Chlamydophila*, orf etc), and using light restraint, a gloved hand is inserted into the vagina and rhythmically pushed up to the neck of the cervix and withdrawn over a period of

2 minutes. The animal will usually push backwards onto the hand to help the procedure and will normally lie down and exhibit behavioural signs of being in labour. If a strange lamb or kid is then introduced the ewe or nanny will, in around 80% of cases, accept it and their own offspring can be re-introduced to them within 15–30 minutes. This process works since it merely mimics nature in convincing the mother that she has given birth again and has been successfully used by farmers in the UK and other European countries during the last few years. It is also possible to treat multiparous non-pregnant ewes and nannies with vaginal sponges containing oestradiol and progesterone to induce lactation (including colostrum formation) and they can be induced to mother orphan or triplet lambs or kids by the same process of stimulation of the vagina and cervix (Kendrick *et al.* 1992). It is not recommended to use this latter procedure in nulliparous ewes or nannies.

While there are other methods used to promote fostering in maternal animals after they have bonded these are either not very effective (using added artificial odours, for example) or represent poor welfare (physically restraining/yoking the mother so she cannot reject the offpring, which may be needed for up to a week or more to be successful).

Weaning and rearing

Once lambs and kids have received colostrum, it is possible to rear them artificially 'on the bottle' using milk replacer powders, introducing solids from 7 days of age. Such lambs should be abruptly weaned no later than 6 weeks old to avoid problems of abomasal bloat, from too rapid ingestion of milk substitute.

Lambs and kids reared naturally normally start the process of weaning themselves at 3 weeks of age and can be offered specialised creep feed from 2 weeks old, in addition to the milk from their mothers. This creep feed should be given in a feeder which restricts access to the lambs or kids and does not allow the mothers to eat it. While it is possible to leave offspring with their mothers indefinitely, it is usual to wean lambs and kids completely onto solid food at around 16 weeks of age. This allows the mother to recover fully prior to the next breeding season. If a schedule of enforced weaning is not used, especially with prolific breeds, the condition of the mothers can deteriorate markedly as a result of persistent suckling by the offspring. In frequent-breeding systems, where an earlier than usual return to sexual receptivity and pregnancy is required, early weaning at 6–8 weeks is necessary as lactating ewes rarely undergo oestrous cycles.

Acute weaning is best carried out by separating a group of lambs/kids from their mothers at the same time. It is best to relocate the ewes/nannies rather than take the offspring to new accommodation, because the young then remain familiar with their surroundings and can easily find water and feed hoppers. The ewes/nannies should be removed to a location out of earshot and regular checks should be made to ensure that none of them develop mastitis. The lambs/kids can be fed on creep feed and hay or grass during this time and if necessary can be re-introduced to the flock after 3–4 weeks, at which time their mothers will not accept any suckling attempts.

Feeding

The feeding of sheep and goats for maximum productivity and health is a large and complex field beyond the scope of this article. Bretzlaff *et al.* (1991) and Calhoun (1991) provide reviews on this topic for goats and sheep respectively and numerous publications are available from agricultural advisory services and colleges. Sheep and goats are ruminant animals which possess a digestive system and physiology that is highly specialised and adapted to the extraction and metabolism of usable nutrients from plants, and in particular the cellulose in plant cell walls. The rumen is little more than a fermentation vat where a delicate mix of micro-organisms is provided with the right conditions and substrates from which to produce short chain fatty acids from cellulose; the adapted biochemical systems of the adult ruminant are able to use these as an energy source or as a substrate from which to manufacture glucose. Rapid changes to diet, particularly a sudden excess of nutrient- rich food, are likely to upset the fermentation process with disastrous and potentially fatal consequences. It therefore follows that dietary stability should be a prime feature of any feeding regime, and any changes in either quality or quantity must be introduced gradually.

In the wild, the natural food of the sheep is grass, whereas goats tend to browse on the leaves of bushes and trees. The inquisitive feeding habit of goats is well known and care must be taken to keep poisonous plants, for example, yew trees, and dangerous objects, such as electric cables, out of reach of a goat even at full stretch. Presentation of strictly limited quantities of safe hedge trimmings or freshly fallen branches with leaves can be a treat for goats.

Sheep and goats kept indoors can be fed fresh cut grass (but not lawn mowings), but more usually are given hay, which is readily but slowly broken down in the rumen and helps to maintain rumenal stability. Mouldy or rotten hay will be rejected. Goats tend to be more selective than sheep with hay, and will eat the leafy parts and seed heads at the expense of the stalks. Silage is an acceptable alternative to hay for sheep and goats, but is less palatable for some animals and all stock adapt to it with some hesitation. Silage is heavy and more difficult to manhandle in a laboratory environment. Poor-quality silage will be rejected.

The design of fodder racks is an important consideration, particularly with goats. Goats are agile climbers and will readily stand on their hindlegs to pull down fodder. They will also climb onto racks if allowed to, and subsequent contamination of feed with urine and faeces will cause much wastage. Feed racks should therefore be designed with a cover.

A fine mesh (1.5 cm square) for hay racks is preferable since it increases feeding time and slows intake to more closely match time spent grazing. This increase in time spent acquiring food may also be considered as a welfare refinement, especially for singly housed animals. It also reduces waste. Sufficient rack space is essential to avoid bullying.

Other bulk foods used for sheep include good-quality barley straw, chopped maize and roots such as mangolds. These foods are only generally suitable as part of a balanced diet that also includes forage and concentrates. Bulky foods are useful to control obesity when animals have limited opportunities for exercise. Sugar beets may be used as a treat for penned animals. Roots may be inedible to animals with poor front teeth and may accelerate tooth wear if fed for long periods.

Concentrate foods are widely available as proprietary products with 'guaranteed' nutritional content shown on the food bag label. The actual constituents of these diets may vary seasonally. Vitamins may 'go off' in the bag so freshness and a dry cool food storage area are important: always observe any 'use by' dates. Animals kept indoors for prolonged periods should be supplied with mineral licks to provide supplementary metal ions and minerals. Particular attention should be paid to copper, selenium and cobalt levels, and to vitamin D in animals with no access to natural daylight. Copper and selenium, in excessive quantities, are toxic to sheep and goats. Licks and concentrate feeds should always be specific for the species concerned as some foods for eg, cattle and pigs may contain inappropriate amounts of copper.

As both pasture-grass and hay have variable nutritional values, animals should be regularly assessed for body condition score, and the quantity of supplementary feeds such as proprietary concentrates adjusted accordingly. A body condition score scale of 1–5 is universally employed in sheep, with the muscle and fat coverage of transverse processes of the cranial lumbar vertebrae used as the criteria for determining the score (see Figure 34.4). Sheep with a thick fleece are impossible to condition score properly without being caught and palpated. It is normal for healthy goats to carry relatively less external body fat than sheep.

The diets for lambs and kids need special attention, particularly when they are newly weaned. A careful balance needs to be drawn between providing sufficient nutrient-rich food for rapid growth and avoiding over-feeding which can lead to diarrhoea and acidosis.

Given the variables outlined above it will be clear that there are no universally reliable rules by which to calculate how much food to offer any one animal. A starting point might be that individually housed ewes at maintenance only will receive 1.5–2.5 kg of fresh good-quality hay and 0–150 g of 16% protein concentrate food daily, depending on condition score. All animals should have constant access to clean fresh water.

Laboratory procedures

Handling and training

The key to catching and handling sheep and goats in a confined space is to move calmly and confidently. Once acclimatised to humans, the animals should be handled with the minimum frequency that is compatible with experimental success. The increasing use of telemetry for physiological monitoring and even blood sampling which requires minimal restraint and creates animals who are their own 'mobile labs' is to be greatly encouraged, although the cost of such systems is high.

Nervous animals may need two catchers in a large pen. Guide the animal into a high-walled corner with no protrusions. Reduce freedom of movement gradually until the animal can be grasped firmly with one hand under the chin and the other used to draw the body against the handler's legs. Resist the temptation to make a wild lunge if an animal tries to escape, but rather let it go and begin again. Do not grab or hold animals by the fleece, ears or tail, as they will struggle and injure themselves. Goats are so inquisitive that they often approach handlers (especially those with a food bucket) and can be caught easily. Once the head is held, the body of a sheep or goat can be pressed gently against a wall with one knee against the lumbar vertebrae in front of the hip and the animal thus restrained by one person.

Some procedures may require an animal to be cast (tipped over onto its rump). To cast a sheep or goat first turn the head round horizontally using mild to moderate force until the neck is bent and the head faces towards the tail. Then apply moderate downward pressure on the rump, back and turn the animal away from the head around a bent knee, and the animal should fall to the ground. The head and shoulders may then be lifted and held between the handler's knees with the animal on its back (Figure 34.5).

Beware rams and billy goats! These animals are larger than ewes and nannies and may elect to charge rather than run, especially when sexually active. Horned males are potentially dangerous.

Sheep and goats which have been treated gently by diligent staff using positive reinforcement techniques respond well to regular handling and this facilitates efficient and stress-free completion of tasks. Nervous or newly acquired animals require particular patience which will eventually benefit all. Comprehensive guides to shepherding sheep and handling goats are provided by Holmes (1991) and Mews and Mowlem (1991).

Recording body temperatures

Measurement of an animal's temperature is usually done using a lubricated clinical thermometer inserted into the rectum.

Administration of medicines

Oral

Liquids can be given to sheep and goats using a strong smooth-sided bottle or dosing gun introduced gently into the diastema (the gap rostral to the premolars). A calibrated dosing gun may also be used. Plastic syringes are easily chewed and destroyed. The head should be held steadily and tilted slightly upward. Liquids should be dribbled in slowly and animals allowed to swallow. The process must be stopped at the first sign of choking. This method always results in some spillage. Stomach tubing requires a mouth gag and is a skilled procedure. Some substances may be delivered in accurate dosages using rumenal boluses.

Injections

Subcutaneous injections should be given under the loose skin above or behind the scapulae. Short needles (less than 25 mm with a diameter 0.4–1.2 mm, 23–18 G (for oily liquids)) are suitable. Intramuscular injections may be given into the

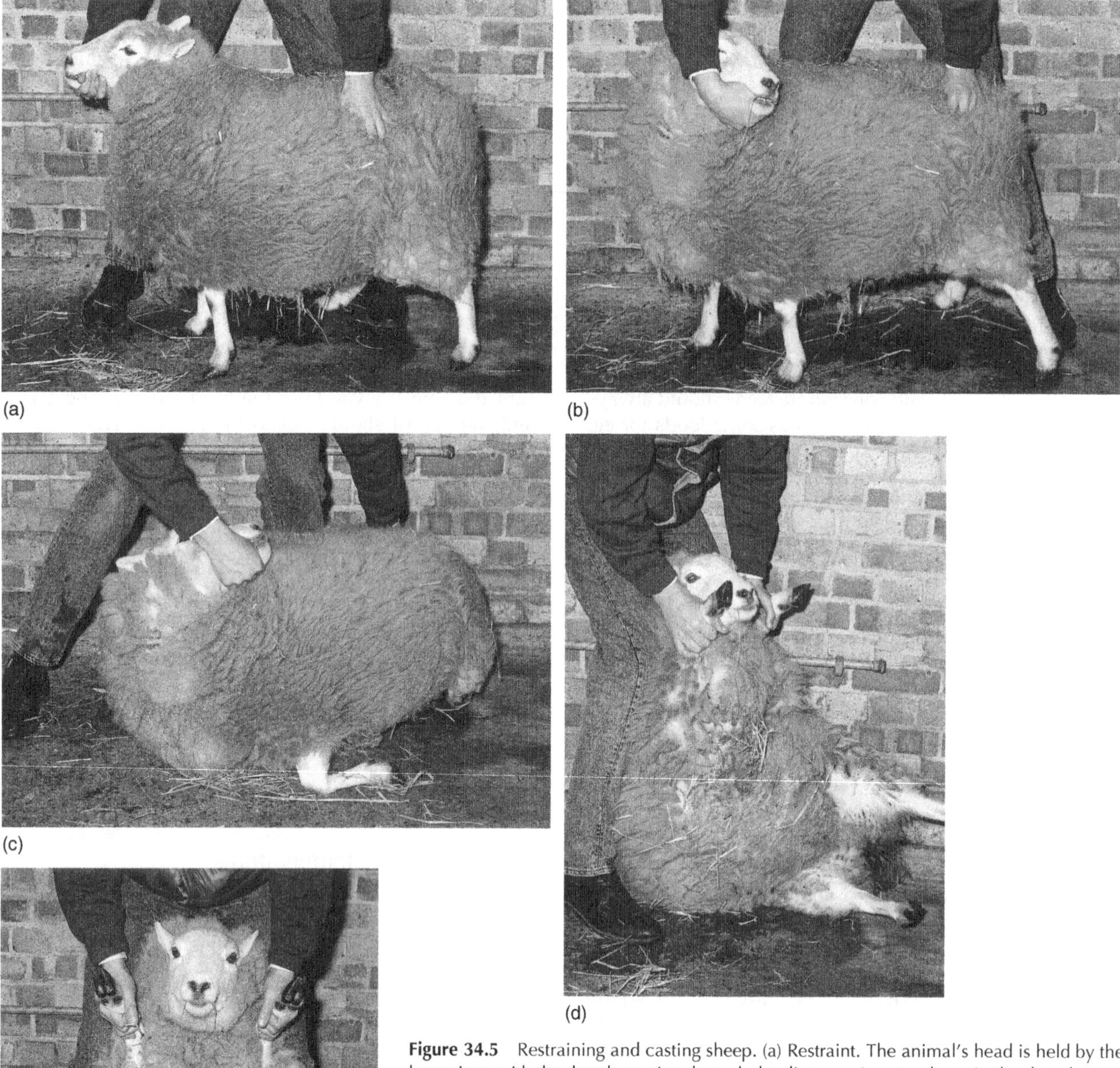

Figure 34.5 Restraining and casting sheep. (a) Restraint. The animal's head is held by the lower jaw, with the thumb passing through the diastema (a natural gap in the dental arcades behind the incisors and before the premolars). The body is restrained between the handler's knee and firm pressure from the hand in opposing sublumbar fossae (the depressions in the flanks behind the ribcage and in front of the hip bones). For additional control the animal may be backed into a corner or gently pressed against a wall with a knee in one sublumbar fossa. (b) Casting. The animal's head is turned away from the handler in a horizontal plane so that it points towards the tail, using moderate force. The hindquarters are kept under control using the knees and the spare hand without pulling on the wool. (c) The animal is pushed backwards using the hand controlling the head, and rotating the body in a horizontal plane around the knee in the sublumbar fossa, using downwards pressure with the hand placed on the animal's flanks. The sheep will collapse to the ground. It is important that this stage is performed quickly to prevent the animal from adjusting the position of its feet, which will enable it to remain standing. Practice is required. (d) The grip is transferred to the forelegs (moving the hand that was on the flanks first) and lifting the ewe's forequarters. The animal is lifted using the knees and not the back. (e) The animal is held resting on its tail with the shoulders gripped between the handler's knees. Inspections of the animal's feet and undersurface are now possible.

gluteal muscles caudal to the tuber coxae, the quadriceps muscle groups in front of the femur or the muscle bellies dorsal to the neck vertebrae in the midpoint of the neck; 25 mm needles of 0.8–1.2 mm diameter (21–18 G) are suitable. Injections into the muscle behind the femur should be avoided as there is a risk of damaging the sciatic nerve. Intravenous injections may be given and intermittent blood samples withdrawn using a 0.8 mm, 21 G (small volume) to 1.6 mm 16 G (large volume) needle inserted into the jugular vein. Vacutainer systems can be a convenient alternative for taking blood samples, and also allow immediate mixing with anti-coagulants if required.

If repeated access to the blood stream is required an indwelling catheter should be placed in the jugular vein using a sterile technique under local anaesthesia. By far the best method is that described by Seldinger (1953) and Harrison (1995), which involves passing a wire through a needle and into the vein, which, after withdrawal of the needle, acts as a guide over which a nylon, vinyl or silastic catheter may be passed and sutured in placed. See Joint Working Group on Refinement (JWGR) (1993) for guidance on limits to blood volume that can be acceptably withdrawn.

Anaesthesia and surgery

Anaesthesia of sheep and goats, including premedication and post-operative analgesia has been described by Flecknell (2009). Due to the large capacity of the gastrointestinal tract, it may be necessary to deprive animals of food for 24–48 h and water for 12–24 h prior to surgery. This reduces gas formation in the rumen and passive regurgitation of fluids when the animals are lying prone. Hungry animals may eat their straw bedding during the pre-surgical phase, so this should be removed.

A cuffed endotracheal tube must always be used when sheep or goats are kept under general anaesthesia, to prevent rumenal fluids or saliva (which is copiously secreted) from entering the trachea. A laryngoscope is necessary to visualise the larynx over the large dorsum of the tongue. After intubation a slight incline to the surgical table allows the head to be lower than the body and will help secretions to drain from the mouth.

Pressure on the diaphragm and the great veins due to the weight of the rumen contents or from the accumulation of rumenal gas (bloat) is a hazard of all ruminant anaesthesia. It may be helpful to pass a stomach tube into the rumen to reduce this risk during long operations. Surgical preparations commonly used in research are described by Harrison (1995). Techniques for placement of probes or cannulae into specific areas of the central nervous system and making electrophysiological recordings or measuring *in vivo* transmitter release have been described in detail elsewhere (Fabre-Nys *et al.* 1991; Kendrick 1991; Kendrick & Baldwin 1991).

Euthanasia

Sheep and goats may be humanely killed using an intravenous injection of pentobarbital (150 mg or more/kg body weight). If suitable equipment and expertise is available then shooting a captive bolt directly into the brain is an acceptable alternative, bearing in mind that the approach must be from directly above or behind the skull, not between the eyes (Humane Slaughter Association, 2006). Once unconscious, great vessels should be severed. The booklet *The Casualty Sheep* (Sheep Veterinary Society 1994) provides further details of all methods of euthanasia, and see also Chapter 17.

Common welfare problems

Assessing the health and welfare of any stock must be based upon a sound knowledge and experience of what is normal. Signs of ill-health might include an elevated temperature (over 40°C is a cause for concern), reduction in appetite, changes in behaviour, colour change of the mucous membranes (pale pink is normal), a cessation of rumination or abnormal discharges from mouth, nose, eyes, ears, anus or genitalia. Sheep and goats lagging behind the flock when driven should be caught and examined. Animals in pain or distress may be reluctant to rise, display an abnormal posture and often grind their teeth noisily. Although harsh and laboured breathing is an indication of respiratory disease, moderate hyperventilation can be deceiving in the sheep as healthy animals tend to breathe more rapidly than other species, especially when being handled. Likewise, the heart rate may be considerably elevated in a normal but nervous animal.

Common diseases

Sheep and goats are susceptible to a wide variety of diseases. Many of the more common diseases are preventable using vaccination (for example clostridiosis, pasteurellosis, contagious pustular dermatitis (orf), and infectious abortion caused by *Chlamydophilia* and *Toxoplasma*) or prophylaxis (for parasitic infestations including coccidiosis). Wherever a particular disease is known to occur, preventative steps should be taken in preference to treatment after the disease appears. Contagious pustular dermatitis and chlamydiophilial abortion are amongst the more worrying zoonoses transmissable to humans. Other potential zoonoses include toxoplasmosis, louping ill, listeriosis, campylobacteriosis, leptospirosis, Q fever and salmonellosis.

The following brief outline of the more common clinical signs and diseases of sheep and goats is intended only to introduce the reader to the complexity of the subject. For a general introduction to sheep management and disease, *The Veterinary Book for Sheep Farmers* (Henderson 1990) is useful, whilst *Diseases of Sheep* (Aitken 2007) is the standard reference work in the UK. Amateur diagnosis and treatments should never be attempted: a veterinary surgeon should be consulted.

Weight loss

Weight loss in a group of animals is usually due to poor diet, poor teeth or parasitism by intestinal nematodes or liver flukes. Nutritional deficiencies may occur as a result of diets with insufficient carbohydrates, proteins, minerals such as cobalt, or vitamins, or a combination of these. Weight loss may, of course, also occur if the diet has an adequate composition but is fed in inadequate amounts The dietary requirements of growth and pregnancy must be considered. Weight loss in individuals may be the result of any chronic condition; for example, lameness, abcessation, maedi-visna, Johne's disease, caseous lymphadenitis, ovine pulmonary adenomatosis or rarely a tumour.

Diarrhoea

Diarrhoea is usually a consequence of over-feeding, intestinal parasitism or coccidiosis. Diarrhoea in lambs is frequently associated with bacterial infections and can result in a rapid deterioration in condition due primarily to dehydration. Bacterial infections are less commonly a primary cause in adult sheep. It is important to encourage fluid intake whilst awaiting a diagnosis.

Nervous signs

Nervous signs and ataxia owing to disease processes are relatively common in sheep and goats of any age. A wide variety of causes exist, such as thiamine deficiency, copper deficiency, scrapie, listeriosis, plant or chemical poisoning, brain space-occupying lesions due to tapeworm cysts, abscesses or tumours, louping ill, metabolic disorders, etc. Some conditions may progress to convulsions or coma (see later). Accurate and early diagnosis is essential.

Intestinal worms and liver flukes

Most adult sheep and goats carry a limited burden of these parasites, which with proper treatment and management are not clinically significant. Clinical disease is more often seen in young stock. In all cases, to minimise the impact of worms on animal health it is necessary to pay careful attention to pasture maintenance. Significant numbers of infective nematode larvae can develop, even on fields used only for occasional grazing, if the adult stock are inadequately wormed, pasture access is not properly rotated or stocking density is too high when animals are allowed access. This can make small paddocks adjacent to research facilities which are used for animal exercise potentially dangerous locations for unprotected grazing animals. Nematode resistance to wormers (anthelmintics) is an increasing problem worldwide, and appears to be particularly prevalent in goats. A strategic control programme should be developed. Boggy areas of pasture should be drained to discourage the snails that act as intermediate hosts for liver flukes.

Foot care

Animals housed indoors for prolonged periods tend to develop overgrown hooves. Overgrown hooves lead to lameness, bad posture, cracking of the hoof wall and infection running into damaged white line areas. Animals at pasture are susceptible to damaged feet produced by poached soils, sharp stones and the like. Such damage predisposes to interdigital dermatitis (scald) and to footrot, caused by *Dichelobacter nodosus*, which is a common and debilitating problem worldwide. All sheep and goats should therefore be turned regularly (see the section on handling for techniques) the feet cleaned and hoof walls pared as necessary by a skilled person. Beware over-paring and causing damage to the sensitive structures of the hoof, as this can lead to permanent lameness. Standing sheep and goats with clean feet three to four times a year in shallow non-irritant footbaths containing 10% zinc sulphate solution (followed by a period on concrete to allow the chemicals to dry) helps to maintain strong disease-free hooves. The likelihood of wet and damaged pastures precipitating foot problems is particularly high in areas of high rainfall, and strong consideration should be given to housing animals indoors over winter in such locations.

If access to the outside is intended to be for exercise only on a daily basis, and space is limited, a concrete floored yard may be better than a pasture. These are washable, will help to stop hooves becoming overgrown and will not retain a significant worm burden. Pasture is of course preferable but needs more work and a bigger area to keep a given number of animals healthy and contented. Further information on the important topic of foot care in sheep can be found in *Lameness in Sheep* (Winter 2004).

Shearing and fleece care

Sheep are normally shorn annually in the late spring. It is advisable for animals with surgical preparations, such as rumen fistulae, cranial implants or blood vessel loops, to be shorn separately from the main flock and with great care. Policies of regular control measures should be put in place to control or prevent skin parasites, especially sheep scab (caused by a *Psoroptes* mange mite), and blowfly larvae (maggots) which are prevalent during the summer. As with worming and foot care, animals under experiment or permanently housed indoors should not be excluded from routine skincare treatments. Housed sheep and goats are particularly susceptible to infestations by lice.

Special health problems

Occasionally sheep and goats will present with veterinary problems with a rapid onset that are immediately life-threatening or very serious.

1. Rumenal bloat. A grossly dilated abdomen is seen, accompanied by rapid shallow breathing and eventual collapse.
2. Urolithiasis. This is particularly common in young male kids and rams. A rigid stance and inability to urinate freely are characteristic. Sometimes urine can escape in small quantities which stains the coat around the penile sheath. Excessive straining may cause a rectal prolapse and if this is seen in a male animal urolithiasis should always be suspected.
3. Poisoning or metabolic disorders caused by ion imbalance. These diseases may be difficult to distinguish. Signs including hyperexcitability or deep depression, tremors and convulsions may all be seen in one or more individuals.

4. Diseases caused by clostridial organisms. Very high rectal temperatures (42°C or more) and rapid deterioration in condition are seen, leading to recumbency and death.
5. Obstetrical problems.
6. Acute mastitis. Signs are a discoloured udder, thin, blood-coloured milk, high temperature and a very sick animal.
7. Acute pneumonia. Often occurs following stress, with *Mannheimia* (formerly *Pasteurella*) species predominating. Animals have a high temperature and severe respiratory distress. This can be confused with heat stress following transport in a poorly ventilated vehicle.

Extreme clinical signs of these types should be recognisable to technicians and help sought immediately.

Acknowledgement

The authors would like to thank Chris Trower, secretary of the Laboratory Animals Veterinary Association and past President of the Sheep Veterinary Society (both organisations affiliated to the British Veterinary Association) for his helpful comments and amendments to the text.

References

Aitken, I.D. (2007) *Diseases of Sheep*. Blackwell Publishing, Oxford

Baldwin, B.A. (1979) Operant studies on shape discrimination in goats. *Physiology and Behaviour*, **23**, 455-459.

Baldwin, B.A. (1981) Shape discrimination in sheep and calves. *Animal Behaviour*, **29**, 830–834

Baldwin, B.A. and Meese, G.B. (1977) The ability of sheep to distinguish between conspecifics by means of olfaction. *Physiology and Behaviour*, **18**, 803–808

Boyd J.H. (1988) Disbudding goat kids. *Veterinary Record*, **122**, 494

Bretzlaff, K., Haenlein, G. and Hutson, E. (1991) The goat industry: feeding for optimal production. In: *Large Animal Clinical Nutrition*. Eds Naylor J.M. and Ralston S.L., pp. 339–350. Mosby-Year Book Inc, St. Louis

Calhoun, M. (1991) Feeding sheep for optimal production. In: *Large Animal Clinical Nutrition*. Eds Naylor, J.M. and Ralston,S.L., pp. 367–383. Mosby-Year Book Inc, St. Louis

Council of Europe (2006) Multilateral Consultation of Parties to the European Convention for the Protection of Vertebrate Animals used for Experimental and other Scientific Purposes (ETS 123) Appendix A. *Cons 123 (2006) 3*. Available from URL: http://www.coe.int/t/e/legal_affairs/legal_co-operation/biological_safety,_use_of_animals/laboratory_animals/2006/Cons123(2006)3AppendixA_en.pdf (accessed 31 July 2008)

Da Costa, A.P., Leigh, A.E., Man, M-S. *et al.* (2004) Face pictures reduce behavioural, autonomic, endocrine and neural indices of stress and fear in sheep. *Proceedings of the Royal Society Biology B*, **271**, 2077–2084

Eales, A. and Small, J. (2004) *Practical Lambing – A Guide to Veterinary Care at Lambing*. Blackwell Publishing, Oxford

Elliker, K. (2006) *Recognition of Emotion in Sheep*. PhD Thesis, University of Cambridge

European Commission (2007) Commission recommendations of 18 June 2007 on guidelines for the accommodation and care of animals used for experimental and other scientific purposes. Annex II to European Council Directive 86/609. See 2007/526/EC. http://eurlex.europa.eu/LexUriServ/site/en/oj/2007/l_197/l_19720070730en00010089.pdf (accessed 13 May 2008)

Evans, G. and Maxwell, W.M.C. (1988) *Salamon's Artificial Insemination of Sheep and Goats*. Butterworth, Sydney

Fabre-Nys, C., Blache, D. and Lavenet, C. (1991) A method for accurate implantation in the sheep brain. In: *Neuroendocrine Research Methods: Implantation and Transfection Procedures*. Ed Greenstein, B., pp. 295–314. Harwood, Chur

Fabre-Nys, C. and Venier, G. (1987) Development and use of a method for quantifying female sexual behaviour through the breeding season in two breeds of sheep. *Animal Reproduction Science*, **21**, 37–51

Flecknell, P.A. (2009) *Laboratory Animal Anaesthesia*, 3rd edn. Academic Press, London

Harrison, F. (1995) *Surgical Techniques in Experimental Farm Animals*. Oxford University Press, Oxford

Henderson, D.C. (1990) *The Veterinary Book for Sheep Farmers*. Old Pond Publishing, Ipswich

Heffner, H.E. and Heffner, R.S. (1992) Auditory perception. In: *Farm Animals and the Environment*. Eds Phillips, C. and Piggins, D., pp. 159–184. CAB International, Wallingford

Hindson, J. (1989) Examinations of the sheep flock before tupping. *In Practice*, **11**, 149–155

Holmes, R.J. (1991) Sheep. In: *Practical Animal Handling*. Eds Anderson, R.S. and Edney, A.T.B., pp. 39–49. Pergamon Press, Oxford

Humane Slaughter Association (2006) *Captive-bolt Stunning of Livestock*, 4th edn. Humane Slaughter Association, Wheathampstead

Joint Working Group on Refinement (1993) Removal of blood from laboratory mammals and birds. First Report of the BVA/FRAME/RSPCA/UFAW Joint Working Group on Refinement. *Laboratory Animals*, **27**, 1–22

Kendrick, K.M. (1991) Microdialysis in large unrestrained animals: neuroendocrine and behavioural studies of acetylcholine, amino acid, monoamine and neuropeptide release in the sheep. In: *Microdialysis in the Neurosciences*. Eds Robinson, T.E. and Justice, J.B., Jr., pp. 327–348. Elsevier, Amsterdam

Kendrick, K.M. (1992) Cognition. In: *Farm Animals and the Environment*. Eds Phillips, C. and Piggins, D., pp. 209–234. CAB International, Wallingford

Kendrick, K.M. (1994) Neurobiological correlates of visual and olfactory recognition in sheep. *Behavioural Processes*, **33**, 89–112

Kendrick, K.M. (2004) Faces in the flock: implications for understanding animal minds. *New Scientist*, **182**, 48–49

Kendrick, K.M., Atkins, K., Hinton, M.R. *et al.* (1995) Facial and vocal discrimination in sheep. *Animal Behaviour*, **49**, 1665–1676

Kendrick, K.M., Atkins, K., Hinton, M.R. *et al.* (1996) Are faces special for sheep? Evidence from facial and object discrimination learning tests showing effects of inversion and social familiarity. *Behavioural Processes*, **38**, 19–35

Kendrick, K.M. and Baldwin, B.A. (1991) Single-unit recording in conscious sheep. In: *Methods in Neurosciences: Electrophysiology and Microinjection*, Vol 4. Ed. Conn, P.M., pp. 3–14. Academic Press, San Diego

Kendrick, K.M., Da Costa, A.P., Hinton, M.R. *et al.* (1992) A simple method for fostering anoestrus ewes with artificially induced lactation and maternal behaviour. *Applied Animal Behaviour Science*, **34**, 345–357

Kendrick, K.M., Da Costa, A.P., Hinton, M.R. *et al.* (2001) Sheep don't forget a face. *Nature*, **414**, 165–166

Kendrick, K.M., Hinton, M.R., Atkins, K. *et al.* (1998) Mothers make sexual preferences. *Nature*, **395**, 229–230

Mews, A.R. and Mowlem, A. (1991) Goats. In: *Practical Animal Handling*. Eds Anderson, R.S. and Edney, A.T.B., pp. 51–55. Pergamon Press, Oxford

Parrott, R.F. (1988) Physiological responses to isolation in sheep. In: *Social Stress in Domestic Animal*. Eds Zayan R. and Dantzer R., pp. 212–226. Kluwer Academic Publishers, Dordrecht

Peirce, J.W., Leigh, A.E. and Kendrick, K.M. (2000) Configurational coding, familiarity and the right hemisphere advantage for face recognition in sheep. *Neuropsychologia*, **38**, 475–483

Piggins, D. (1992) Visual perception. In: *Farm Animals and the Environment*. Eds Phillips, C. and Piggins, D., pp. 131–158. CAB International, Wallingford

Seldinger, S.I. (1953) Catheter replacement of the needle in percutaneous arteriography. *Acta Radiologica*, **39**, 368–376

Sheep Veterinary Society (1994) *The Casualty Sheep*. British Veterinary Association Animal Welfare Foundation, Swindon Press, Swindon

Shillito, E. and Alexander, G. (1975) Mutual recognition amongst ewes and lambs of four breeds of sheep (*Ovis aries*). *Applied Animal Ethology*, **1**, 151–165

Tate, A.J., Fischer, H., Leigh, A.E. *et al.* (2006) Behavioural and neurophysiological evidence for face identity and face emotion processing in animals. *Philosophical Transactions of the Royal Society London B-Biological Sciences*, **361**, 2155–2172

Wolfensohn, S. and Lloyd, M. (2003) *Handbook of Laboratory Animal Management and Welfare*. Blackwell Publishing, Oxford

Winter, A.C. (2004) *Lameness in Sheep*. The Crowood Press, Marlborough

Winter, A.C. and Hill, C.W. (2003) *A Manual of Lambing Techniques*. The Crowood Press, Marlborough

35 The horse

Fernando Montesso

Biological overview

Introduction

The horse was domesticated around 2500 BC. Its relatively compliant behaviour, together with its speed, agility and strength, gave it a unique role amongst domesticated animals. Because it could be trained to harness or the saddle, the horse provided humans with a means of transport and traction for work, war or recreation.

With the increasing use of the internal combustion engine in the early part of the twentieth century, the number of horses declined and, with it, equine research. However, over the past 50 years, horse numbers have steadily increased because of the renewed interest in using horses for recreational purposes. This has led to greater equine research into diverse areas such as nutrition, reproduction, sports injuries, infectious diseases and welfare. Although the ultimate beneficiary of this research is the horse, horses are also used for the production of hyperimmune antiserum for humans and animals and also for production of conjugated oestrogens for use in human medicine.

Social organisation

Horses are herd animals and, in the feral state, live in small family groups with a clearly defined hierarchy. Social facilitation (same, or similar, behaviour initiated as a response to the occurrence of a behaviour by another animal within the social group) is common both within and between groups, and the pattern of behaviour involved includes resting, grazing, walking, rolling, eliminative behaviour (defecation and urination) and sucking. Mutual grooming, although usually a response to the irritation caused by ectoparasites or coat shedding, is also an important form of social contact (Tyler 1972; Crowell-Davis 1986).

The individually stabled horse is denied these social interactions, and this may contribute to the development of abnormal behaviour such as box walking and weaving. However, the attention given to stabled horses, for example daily grooming by knowledgeable and sympathetic stable attendants, may provide some compensation to horses for the reduced social interaction with their own species, but are not complete substitutes.

When kept at pasture or housed in groups, the group size is often larger than in a typical horse herd, and is not a family group, but consists of horses introduced as adults. This results in social reorganisation, and on occasion, to fighting when the groups are first formed or when they are crowded together. Injuries are likely if there is no room to escape, and at feeding times subordinate horses may be denied access to food (Houpt 1991).

Biological data

Normal biological values are summarised in Table 35.1. The first, second and third permanent incisors erupt at 2.5 years, 3.5 years and 4.5 years, respectively. All permanent teeth (incisors, premolar and molars) are present by 4.5 years. A horse's height is traditionally measured in hands, one hand being equal to 4 inches (1 inch = 2.54 cm). The measurement is taken from the ground level to the highest point on the horse's withers. Horses range in height from about 60 cm (6 hands) to more than 173 cm (>17 hands). They frequently remain fit and active into their twenties and some will live in excess of 30 years.

Because of the stay apparatus of the hindlimbs, adult horses can rest and sleep while standing, but rapid eye movement sleep can only occur when the horse is in sternal or lateral recumbency. They enjoy rolling, especially in mud and dust, and stabled horses will frequently roll in their beds if still warm and sweaty from exercise.

They change their coat twice yearly in the spring and autumn. The winter coat usually provides sufficient protection from inclement weather for most native breed horses not in work in northern temperate areas, though field shelters or wind breaks should be available. If living out, the winter coat should not be groomed as this would remove secretions which assist in keeping the animal warm and dry. In more extreme climates, horses are usually housed during the winter months. A full winter coat would result in excessive sweating during ridden work, and so it is customary to clip the winter coat off and rug the horse. Clipped horses should also be housed, though they can be turned out, suitably rugged, into paddocks for a short period every day during the winter months.

Reproduction

Mares first show signs of oestrus at puberty (about 18–24 months of age) and continue to cycle until 20–30 years old.

Table 35.1 Normal biological values for horses.

Parameter	*Value*
Rectal temperature (°C)	38 ± 0.5
Resting pulse (beats/minute)	25–45
Respiratory rate (breaths/minute)	8–12
Permanent teeth	$I^3_3\ C^{*1}_1\ P^{3or4\dagger}_3\ M^3_3$
Deciduous teeth	$I^3_3\ C^0_0\ P^3_3\ M^0_0$

* Rare or rRudimentary in mares.
† First premolar (wolf tooth) is vestige and remnant of a tooth well developed in ancestors of the horse. Often shed, but if retained and thought to be associated with biting problems, it is usually removed by a veterinarian.

The majority (80%) of mares are seasonally polyoestrous with regular cycles during the breeding season (spring–summer) and a period of sexual quiescence in the winter months. Daylight length (photoperiod) is the most important regulating factor, increasing daylight length in the spring in temperate regions being the main stimulus for the initiation of ovarian activity. However, even at the equator, where day length is approximately 12h throughout the year, mares show a definite seasonal pattern to oestrus. Good nutrition and housing to protect mares from harsh weather conditions will increase the likelihood that they cycle and ovulate normally at the beginning of the breeding season (van Niekerk 1992). The breeding season, under natural conditions, for example in pony herds, is usually later than that artificially imposed on Thoroughbreds where the idea of producing foals as near as possible to January 1st, the official birthday of all Thoroughbred racehorses, is aimed for at stud farms.

Spermatogenesis starts during the second year of life in colts receiving adequate nutrition, and the testes are usually functional by 2 years of age. Colts of less than 2 years of age have lower sperm production rates than older stallions, and rates in the non-breeding season are about 75% of that in the breeding season (Thompson 1992).

Normal behaviour

Healthy equids are active and alert. When stabled they frequently nicker or whinny to their attendant, particularly at feeding time. They are usually keen to eat, and some will paw or kick at the stable door whilst waiting to be fed. Some horses will also weave (see Abnormal behaviour) whilst waiting for feed. Some horses, especially entire males, will lay their ears back and swish their tails as the attendant enters the box with feed. This aggression may be feigned or real: if the latter, care must be taken when feeding the horse if injury to the attendant is to be avoided, and the reasons why this behaviour is being displayed should be investigated. Horses urinate about six times daily and defecate approximately every 2h. Attendants should check faecal consistency and quantity automatically as they clean the stable, as any changes from the normal pattern could be indicative of illness. They should also note the state of the bedding: evidence of excess activity could indicate distress, for example due to colic. Alternatively, the bed may be relatively undisturbed, indicating that the horse had not lain down in sternal or lateral recumbency to rest.

When at pasture, horses usually graze as a group and an animal separated from the group may be unwell. When resting, at least one number of the group often remains standing whilst the remainder rest in sternal or, if warm and sunny, in lateral recumbency. Before getting up, horses frequently roll. Once up, they will often stretch and shake themselves before moving off to start grazing. Whilst in groups at pasture, the affiliations between pairs of horses will become obvious, as they usually graze together and mutually groom. Attendants should be aware of these relationships so that they are allowed to continue during the winter housing period: accidental splitting up of these affiliations can be stressful and so should be avoided.

Uses of horses in research

The majority of equids used in research are bought in from outside sources. However, there is occasionally a need to breed them within an institute, for example, when helminth-free foals and weanlings or horses with a specific blood type are required. Sound, ex-racehorses are a good source of animals for use in exercise physiology research, as they are adjusted to stable routines and training procedures. Having been handled frequently since the early stages of life, they are usually amenable to most minimally invasive procedures such as the collection of blood samples.

Ponies are frequently used in behavioural studies, in reproductive physiology, pharmaceutical, infectious diseases and nutritional research. The Welsh Mountain pony is a well established breed used in research. These ponies are small, hardy and overall have a very good and easy temperament, adapting quickly to new routines and procedures. As they are usually obtained directly from breeders or dealers, they may have had minimal exposure to humans and will need regular handling and training to ensure they accept being restrained during common procedures, including routine husbandry measures such as farriery.

Blood and serum production horses are usually former recreational horses, which may not be able to work at the level expected of them because of an irreversible injury such as a tendon strain or joint damage. They should, however, be healthy and capable of light exercise without discomfort.

General husbandry

Housing

Traditionally the horse has been housed individually in loose boxes or communally. A modern variation on the individual loose box is the American barn style of housing (Figure 35.1), which comprises rows of individual loose boxes under a single roof. Unlike the traditional loose box where the partitions between the boxes are usually solid from floor to ceiling, the upper half of the boxes in the

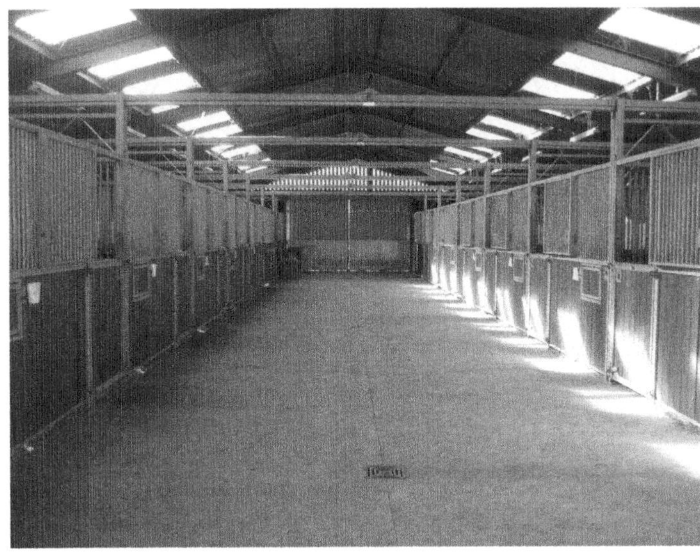

Figure 35.1 American barn.

Table 35.2 Types of housing suitable for horses and their advantages and disadvantages.

Type of housing	*Advantages*	*Disadvantages*
Loose box	Freedom of movement Individual air space Visual contact if top half door open Can provide thermal comfort and good ventilation	Solitary confinement Reduced visual contact Labour intensive Extensive use of bedding material
American style barns	Freedom of movement Easier working conditions for staff Visual and some social contact (through bars)	Shared air space Ventilation often inadequate
Loose yarding	Freedom of movement Full socialisation possible Less labour intensive	Shared air space Aggression especially at feeding may lead to injuries. Timid horses may be denied food

American barn are not usually solid and comprise vertical bars or metal mesh. Horses can also be kept loose in groups, in barns similar to those used for cattle. The advantages and disadvantages of the various types of housing are summarised in Table 35.2.

Statutory recommended minimum floor areas for individually housed horses are illustrated in Table 35.3. These are minimum permitted dimensions in the UK listed by the Home Office (1989). For the revised guidelines for accommodation and care of animals used for experimental and other scientific purposes from the European Commission (2007) please refer to Annex II of European Council Directive 86/609 (see 2007/526/EC) (European Commission 2007, also Council of Europe 2006).

Table 35.3 Dimensions recommended for housing horses in loose boxes (Home Office, 1989). Note that housing may be subject to statutory requirements in some countries.

Height of horse at withers	*Minimum floor area when housed individually*
Up to 147 cm	12 m^2
148–160 cm	17 m^2
>160 cm	20 m^2

Three-sided field shelters should be provided for horses and ponies at pasture and 1.6–2.5 m^2 of space should be allowed in these per 100 kg liveweight. The shelter should face the sun and be bedded in cold regions, and should face away from the sun in hot regions. Feeding racks should be situated outside the shelters in a protected position. Four-sided windbreaks (Figure 35.2) or natural hedging sufficient to supply shelter from driving weather and the prevailing wind can be used for native ponies kept outside.

Housing and respiratory disease

A major drawback of all housing for horses is the potential for respiratory disease. The stabled horse is exposed to a variety of airborne contaminants (viruses, bacteria, fungal and actinomycete spores, dust mites, noxious gases such as ammonia, and plant material). Infectious causes of respiratory disease can spread rapidly through a population of housed horses, particularly when they share air space, and although vaccines are available, they are limited in their spectrum and duration of effect. Lower airway inflammation can affect young and old animals. Recurrent airway obstruction (RAO) – referred in the past as chronic obstructive pulmonary disease (COPD) – usually affects middle-aged animals (7 years old or more). Inflammatory airway disease (IAD) affects horses of any age. In young horses it is usually associated with bacterial infection, however, non-infectious IAD can occur in horses of all ages and ways of life (Allen & Franklin 2007). RAO is a pulmonary hypersen-

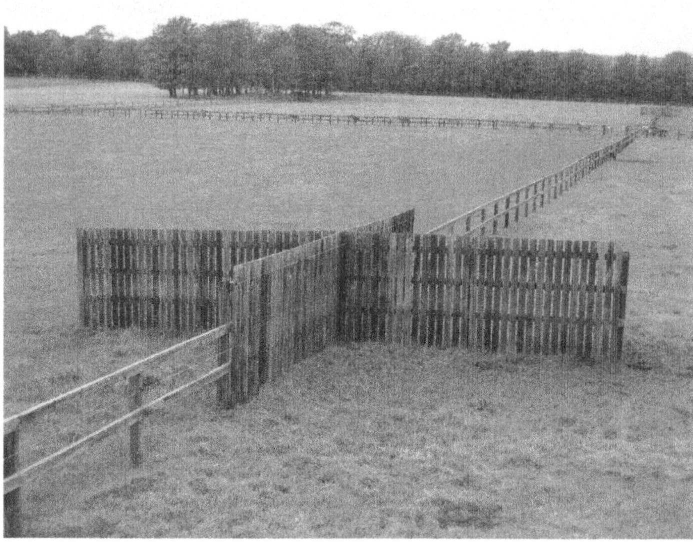

Figure 35.2 Four-sided windbreak to shelter animals kept outside.

sitivity to inhaled allergens present in hay and straw. The allergens are the spores of fungi and actinomycetes, and these are the major constituents of respirable dust in stables. They are usually less than 5 μm in diameter, and remain antigenic after death. Concentrations of airborne pollutants can be reduced by increasing clearance rates (mainly by ventilation) and by reducing release rates, by modifying the source materials, namely hay and straw. Ideally both approaches should be used. The specific cause of IAD is still unclear and it is likely that several factors are involved.

Optimising air quality in stables

When bedding management is good, a minimum of four air changes per hour, under still air conditions, is required to ensure optimal ventilation (Webster *et al.* 1987). Well designed loose boxes, with the top half of the stable door open, provide this. In very cold weather, it is better to provide the horse with extra rugs and to resist the temptation to shut the top door, as the number of air changes per hour will drop to dangerously low levels. Ventilation rates in barns are usually poorer, but can be improved by either providing draught-free inlets (at least $0.3\,m^2$) on the outside wall of each box, or by using spaced vertical boarding (Yorkshire boarding) along the walls starting 2 m above the ground.

Modifying source materials, such as hay and bedding, is the second important means of optimising air quality. Some degree of fungal contamination is present in all hays. Lucerne and clover hays, despite the high price they command, can be heavily contaminated. Totally immersing the hay, contained either in a haynet or other suitable receptacle, in water for 12 h will minimise the respirable challenge, though any spores present will still be ingested. Cleaner alternatives to hay are haylage and silage, both of which must be packed airtight at harvesting, and used within a few days of opening. These alternatives are to be recommended if hay quality is suspect, and for routine use in animals with respiratory disease. Feeding hay from floor level is the most natural way for the horse to eat, encouraging good natural posture. The other major source of fungal spores is bedding. Straw baled when damp is as dangerous as heated hay. Horses prefer straw bedding and it may act as a stimulant for investigatory behaviour. Alternatives to straw, such as wood shavings, peat moss and shredded paper, may be poorer in terms of enrichment. Whilst these are practically free of fungi when fresh, they too can become heavily contaminated in poorly ventilated stables and in deep litter systems. Commercially available non-biological bedding material such as rubber matting is clean, thermally efficient and does not provide a medium for fungi, but is even more barren behaviourally. The risk of stabled horses developing allergic respiratory disease and the recovery time from infectious causes of respiratory diseases can be reduced by ensuring ventilation is optimal, by feeding good-quality dust-free hay, silage or haylage, by managing bedding well (daily removal of dropped hay, faeces and urine-soiled straw) and by avoiding 'dust raising' procedures, for example shaking out fresh straw bedding while the horse is in the stable.

Exercise

Horses and ponies not in work, but kept at pasture or loose yarded when housed, will usually get sufficient exercise for their needs. The individually stabled horse in work will benefit from being kept loose in a paddock or arena for as much time as practicable. However, there are situations where specific provision must be made for some form of daily exercise: for example for horses used for serum and/or blood production and which are individually housed during the winter months, and horses or ponies being raised helminth-free and thus denied access to pasture. For these animals it is just as important that exercise and social interaction are part of the daily routine, and they can be turned out in small groups into winter grass paddocks, sand or peat arenas for at least 1 h daily. This will allow them to have complete freedom of movement and to interact socially with each other, although care must be taken to ensure compatible grouping if injuries are to be avoided. Other forms of non-ridden exercise are lungeing, where the horse is exercised on grass or other suitable surface on a circle at the end of a long lead, or the use of horsewalker machines. Lungeing is labour intensive, whereas horse walkers allow several horses to be exercised at once. Both, however, are poor substitutes for the freedom provided when the horse is turned out loose.

Hoof care

The growth rate of horses' hooves depends on age, season and nutritional status, and is normally faster in young horses and in the spring. The average rate of growth is about 10mm/month (Butler 1992). The feet should be inspected daily and trimming should be done as regularly and as often as is necessary. Although a 6-week interval is the average for many horses, it can vary from 2 weeks to 2 months. Horses in work require shoeing, as they invariably have to exercise on hard surfaces. However, serum-producing horses and ponies rarely require shoeing and, if being kept in groups, should never have hind shoes on because of the risk of causing serious injury from kicks. Foals should start to have their feet trimmed when about 1 month old, or earlier if they have limb deformities, many of which can be corrected by foot trimming and exercise alone. During dry weather, horses at pasture may develop vertical cracks in the feet and require regular foot rasping or even the application of a light shoe to limit damage. Stabled horses should have their feet cleaned and examined at least once daily.

Puncture wounds of the foot with the subsequent development of a subsolar abscess are a common cause of acute lameness, and require immediate treatment by a farrier or a veterinarian.

Identification

Horses usually differ sufficiently in their colour, markings and conformation for individuals to be recognised, even within a breed. Under current European Union legislation, all horses, ponies and donkeys must have a horse passport which is a permanent record of colour distribution, together with the position of whorls (areas where the hairs are radially arranged). Other permanent methods of identification, which can act as a deterrent to thieves, are freeze branding and microchips.

Management of newcomers

All newcomers should be isolated from the resident horse population for a minimum quarantine period of 3–4 weeks before they join the resident population. A full clinical examination, including a routine blood examination, should be conducted as soon as possible after arrival. The collection of nasopharyngeal swabs once a week for three consecutive weeks for *Streptococcus equi* profile is recommended as 'strangles' is common in animals being sourced from dealers. Teeth should be checked and rasped if necessary. Hooves should be checked and the hind shoes removed if the horse is to be group housed or at pasture with others. Vaccination against tetanus is essential. The administration of other vaccines will depend on the research programme the horse is entering; for example it would be contraindicated in vaccine research. Unless there is specific reason for not doing so, incoming animals should be treated for endo- and ectoparasite infections. Colts may need to be castrated if they are to be group managed.

Transportation

Horses and ponies are usually transported in purpose-built motorised horse boxes or trailers, though they may also be transported in modified cattle lorries. Broken, adult horses should be fitted with a strong, properly fitting headcollar (halter) and are usually loosely tethered. If shod, their lower limbs should be protected from tread injuries by the application of either woollen bandages (stable bandages) on top of cotton wool or a similar material or purpose-made padded leggings, from below the knee or hock to the coronet. Kneecaps will protect them from injury should they stumble and fall during loading and unloading, and poll guards, hock guards and tail guards are other protective items of clothing that may be used. When transporting mares and foals, each mare and foal usually occupy the area needed for two adult horses. The mare is usually loosely tethered, the foal not. Foals adapt remarkably well to being transported so long as they are in close proximity to their dam and they frequently suck during travel. Short rest periods (10 minutes for every hour of the journey) should be provided during longer journeys. Unbroken ponies are best transported loose in small groups.

Patience and care are needed when loading and unloading both experienced travellers and unbroken animals if injuries are to be avoided. The ramps of the vehicles should have a non-slip surface and sidewings to ensure that the horse walks down the middle of the ramp: as horses have an aversion to stepping on such surfaces, the floor of the box should be covered with straw or other suitable material. Studies have been undertaken to try to clarify the effects of forward and rear-facing travel. Works from Clark *et al.* (1993), Smith *et al.* (1994) and Waran *et al.* (1996) found that there was some benefit from rear-facing travel for some horses. Later studies by Collins *et al.* (2000) and Toscano and Friend (2001) found that neither orientation when travelling had a clear overall effect. The individual preference to which direction to face when being transported seems to play a part but the reasons for their choices are not clear.

Breeding

General reproductive features of the mare (average values) are summarised in Table 35.4.

Stallions are used to detect oestrus in mares, though some mares will indicate receptivity to geldings grazing with them. Teasing can either be done on an individual or group basis. With the former, the mare is separated from the stallion by a padded, solid barrier. The barrier should be about

Table 35.4 Reproductive features of the mare.

Parameter	*Normal value*
Onset of puberty (months)	18–24
Oestrus cycle (days)	
In spring	25 (range 9–50)
In late spring/summer	20.9
Duration of oestrus (days)	5–7
Duration of dioestrus (days)	14–16
Ovulation (days before end of oestrus)	1–2
Foal heat (first oestrus post-partum) (days)	9 (range 5–18)

the same height as the withers, so that limited physical contact is possible. With the latter, the stallion can be led past the paddocks where the mares are grazing. Alternatively the stallion can be placed in a small pen near the paddock.

The mare in oestrus adopts an urination posture where the hindlegs are extended backward and the tail is raised. Small amounts of urine are expelled and the clitoris is exposed in a rhythmic fashion ('winking'). The intensity of the signs of oestrus varies considerably between animals. They increase progressively during oestrus and are maximal as ovulation approaches; some mares are very reluctant to be separated from the stallion at this time. In contrast to this, the mare in dioestrus shows hostility to the stallion by biting, kicking and laying her ears back. Mares which are overly protective of their foals, even when in oestrus, will sometimes display hostility to the stallion, particularly if their foal is within earshot.

Mating ('covering') is usually carried out with the mare and stallion suitably restrained. Both should be bridled, and covering should be done in an enclosed area with a good surface so that neither the mare nor the stallion are likely to slip. Hind shoes should always be removed from the mare. When using valuable stallions, it is customary to fit felt boots to the hindfeet of the mare to prevent injury to the stallion. A nose twitch may be applied for additional restraint if necessary (Figure 35.3). If the mare has a foal at foot, it should be kept out of sight and earshot during mating, in a loose box with the top half of the door shut. As the results of teasing are not always conclusive, the optimum time for mating can be determined by veterinary examinations per rectum where the ovaries, uterus and cervix are palpated, and/or by scanning using ultrasonography, or by vaginal examination using a speculum where the colour and state of relaxation of the cervix are determined.

Pregnancy can be confirmed using several techniques. Ultrasound echography, using an ultrasound probe carried into the rectum and directed over the uterus, can be used to detect pregnancy as early as 14–16 days post-conception. Repeated scans are essential, as early pregnancy failures can occur. Scanning should be used in conjunction with the other methods of pregnancy diagnosis, for example manual palpation, per rectum, of the uterus. The changes experienced with manual palpation are described in a review by Sharp (1992). This examination should only be performed by trained personnel. Biochemical tests for pregnancy are available commercially if the technology and/or expertise for ultrasound and palpation techniques are not available. The most useful test is the measurement of equine chorionic gonadotrophin (eCG) in the plasma. This test can only be done after day 40 of pregnancy and is not effective after day 120. False positives can also occur. Although not as infallible as a pregnancy test, teasing of pregnant mares can be used.

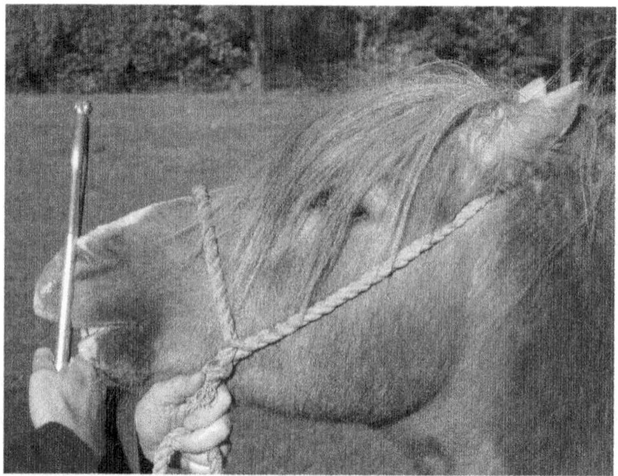

Figure 35.3 Nose twitch for restraining. Other types of twitch with rope or chain loop can also be used.

Management of the in-foal mare

In-foal mares should lead as natural a life as possible. In temperate areas, they are usually at pasture by day and housed by night. In warmer climates, they can remain at pasture 24 h per day. Shelter from sun and insects may be required. Their nutritional needs will increase as the pregnancy progresses, and increasing amounts of concentrates are usually fed to meet these, particularly in the latter third of pregnancy. However, they should not be allowed to become fat as over-fat pony mares, in particular, run the risk of developing hyperlipaemia in late pregnancy if their management is suddenly changed; for example, a sudden fall in energy intake. They should be up to date with their tetanus and influenza vaccinations. Mares should also be vaccinated against equine herpesvirus 1 and 4 according to the manufacturer's recommendation, to help reduce clinical signs of respiratory disease and abortion caused by this virus. Routine anthelmintic treatments should also be given (see later).

Preparation for foaling

In temperate climates, mares are normally foaled indoors where they can be observed frequently and easily, and given assistance if needed. Pony mares and mares in warmer climates are often left to foal outside. They should still be closely observed as parturition approaches, and lights can be used to provide some illumination of the foaling paddocks. Mares foaling inside should be provided with as large a loose box as possible (a minimum of 30 m^2): it should have a deep, clean bed, and the bedding should be extended and banked up along each wall to provide further protection. Hay should be fed off the ground and mangers and water buckets are better at chest height. Small red light bulbs (10 Watts) will provide sufficient light for observation without disturbing the mare. Closed circuit television can be used to observe when the mare or mares are due to foal at the same time. Foaling alarms are available commercially and can work as an aid to alert the staff when birth is imminent.

Parturition

Mares usually foal at night, and seem to be able to delay foaling until conditions are right for them, for example when the stable yard is quiet. They seem to prefer to foal unobserved: hence any lighting should be dim. Signs of impending parturition are not consistent and can only serve as a rough guide. Udder development starts 3–6 weeks pre-foaling, and distension of the udder with colostrum occurs in the last 2–3 days. When colostrum begins to ooze from the teats and forms honey-coloured wax-like beads at the teat orifice ('waxing'), foaling is imminent. Mares can deviate from the predicted foaling date by 1–2 weeks or more. This is quite normal and does not require veterinary intervention: each pregnancy is a unique combination of maternal and foetal traits, and will be terminated at the appropriate time (Sharp 1992). The various stages of parturition and their main presenting signs are given in Table 35.5.

Foaling is a normal physiological process, and attendants should be sufficiently acquainted with the normal pattern of foaling and resist the temptation to interfere unnecessarily. However, as parturition is very rapid in the mare compared with other domestic animals, experienced veterinary help should be readily available should it not proceed normally. Swift intervention is necessary if premature separation of the allantochorion is likely, as may occur if delivery is delayed. Any traction applied to the foal should coincide with the mare's own efforts at expulsion. The amniotic sac may be manually ruptured if it has failed to do so after the foal is delivered. The mare should be left undisturbed and allowed to rest after foaling. The umbilical cord should be left to break naturally to allow passage of placental blood to the foal; this could take several minutes. Excessive human activity will stimulate the mare to rise too soon, and in nervous primiparous mares this could interfere with the normal bonding between the mare and her foal. The establishment of the bond between the mare and her foal is triggered by hormonal changes, which may be based on olfaction, as the mare licks the newborn for a few hours after parturition.

The normal healthy foal is in sternal recumbency within 1–2 minutes of delivery and a suck reflex is present within 2–20 minutes. On average, a healthy foal will take up to 1 h to stand and up to 2 h to suck. By 12 h of age it is able to walk, trot and gallop.

Post-foaling activities

In the immediate postpartum period, the foal's navel should be dressed with 2% potassium iodide solution to reduce the chance of bacterial infection; this should continue twice daily until the navel is dry (about 48 h). It is important that the foal suckles as soon as possible (within 2 h) as absorption of protective immunoglobulins present in the colostrum is maximal at birth, marginal by 15 h and has ceased by 24 h post-partum.

Primiparous mares, in particular, may not accept their foals and may not allow them to suckle, either because of udder distension or possibly because of an association with pain at parturition. Occasionally these mares will attack their foals in addition to refusing to let them suckle. Assuming that no mastitis is present, they should he held by an attendant, with or without prior sedation, whilst another attendant helps the foal to suck.

The mare should be provided with a warm bran mash as laxative and her water buckets kept full. Tetanus antitoxin must be given to both mare and foal if the mare is unvaccinated. The mare should be checked for foaling injuries which should be stitched and repaired as necessary. The

Table 35.5 Stages of parturition in the mare and their main presenting signs.

	Stage		
	1	*2*	*3*
	Up to time of rupture of allantochorionic membranes	*Delivery of foal*	*Expulsion of placenta*
Duration	Approx. 1 h	<30 min	Approx. 1 h
Activity	Uterine contractions begin; foal rotates head and forelimbs into dorsal position; allantochorion ruptures releasing fluid; amniotic membranes and forelimbs appear in birth canal	Foal completes its rotation, assumes diving position and passes through the birth canal	Continuing uterine contractions to expel the placenta
Behavioural signs	Mare increasingly restless; box walking; rolling/gazing at flanks; patchy sweating; often runs milk	Powerful abdominal contractions, usually when in lateral recumbency; may get up and down, adjusting position before the final push to give birth; profuse sweating	Mild colic signs and some straining; may move into sternal recumbency prior to expelling the placenta

foetal membranes should be examined to ensure they are complete and intact. If the foal is straining and having difficulty in passing meconium (the first faeces), proprietary enemas should be given *per rectum*. If in doubt about colostrum intake, the foal's blood IgG levels should be tested. If the weather is suitable, the foal should be haltered and led out to pasture with the mare: if not, the mare and foal should he turned into a covered arena for exercise.

If a mare dies at foaling, the foal should be given colostrum by stomach tube as soon as possible after birth. Most breeding studs keep deep-frozen supplies of mare colostrum for such emergencies. Rearing is best done using a foster mother, though foals can be reared artificially using commercially available mare milk replacers. Foals reared artificially may not grow as well as those raised by the mare, and so every effort should he made to find a foster mother. Mare's milk is lower in both protein and fat content than cow's milk, but higher in lactose. The milk replacer should be fed at a temperature of approximately 37.5°C. All utensils must be thoroughly washed and sterilised before and after use. The teat should he introduced carefully to the side of the foal's mouth and care must be taken to ensure that milk is not inhaled. The foal must therefore be given frequent opportunities to rest during feeding.

Post-parturient behaviour

For the first few days following parturition mares are extremely protective of their offspring. Stabled mares will rapidly circle their foals and even threaten their attendants. When outside, they will drive away other mares and foals, even if they have previously had an affiliative relationship with another mare. This protectiveness may be related to the fact that the young foal takes about a week to visually recognise its mother (Houpt 1992). A human–foal bond can be usefully established during the first few days of life, and is best done by an attendant with whom the mare is familiar and trusts.

Foal behaviour: early handling and training

Foals nurse about four times per hour in the first week of life: the duration of nursing increases as the foal becomes older, but the frequency of nursing decreases. If separated from their mother, even briefly, or if frightened, they will immediately nurse. Foals spend 70–80% of their time resting when very young. When they get up to nurse they generally stretch their limbs and arch their neck and back before going to the mare to feed. Since so much time is spent resting, usually lying down, it is important that young foals are not left outside in inclement weather, as they would then only rest standing. A healthy foal is normally very active, and within a few days of birth will be confidently galloping and bucking round its mother. As they get older they soon start to play with their mother and, if allowed to do so, play with other foals in the group.

Foals less than 4 weeks of age will often nibble at their mother's freshly passed faeces: this is normal behaviour thought to be important in the establishment of bowel flora and presents no hazard to the foal. The first faeces passed by foals, the meconium, are frequently difficult to pass. However, once the foal has nursed, the laxative effect of the colostrum usually ensures no further problems. A transient diarrhoea often occurs on the foal at the time of the foal heat, the first oestrus after foaling; this usually resolves without treatment.

When first approached by humans, young foals will be nervous, try to evade being caught and may start snapping (also referred as 'champing' or mouthing). This is a submissive gesture and usually indicates fear: the foal's ears turn back slightly, the neck is stretched out, the corner of the mouth is drawn back and the jaws start to move vertically in a rhythmical fashion. This gesture is adopted by young animals when approaching older ones, including their mothers. A short time spent every day quietly talking to young foals and gently scratching their crest and along their spine will help them to relax and accept being handled. Their hooves should be picked up daily so that they habituate to the procedure. This will minimise problems with the farrier at a later stage. They should also accept being cleaned with a soft cloth all over their body in preparation for grooming when older. Handling the muzzle area and habituating the nose to a finger will help with tubing later in life. Special lightweight foal headcollars (foal slips) should be put on daily from birth onwards before the mare and foal go to pasture, and the foal taught to be led. A foal is usually led from its left side and close to its mother's left shoulder. A long piece of rope should be looped through the ring on the foal slip: if the foal should escape the handler, the rope will then pull free and not get entangled round the foal's legs.

Verbal commands should precede the physical commands so that, eventually, the voice alone is sufficient. Foals should be rewarded by scratching the withers rather than patting anywhere. If they misbehave and kick or try to kick, they should be discouraged immediately. In most cases this can be achieved by voice alone; alternatively use a slap across the pectorals accompanied by an appropriate verbal message. Other behaviour management techniques should be explored as an alternative to punishment. Colt foals, in particular, will strike out with the front feet, this should be discouraged promptly. It is better to spend time disciplining and teaching a foal 'manners' when it is small and manageable than to leave this initial training until it is 500 kg and unmanageable.

Weaning

As some mares will be in foal again within a few months of parturition, it is customary to wean the foals when they are about 4–5 months of age. By this age the foals are already physically fairly independent of their dams, will be grazing like adult horses, and have usually been introduced to concentrate feeding ahead of the anticipated weaning date. Thus, they have little, if any, setback. The time of weaning is a period of peak growth and a time when stereotypical behaviours can start. Post-weaning concentrates can be introduced 4–6 weeks prior to the foal being separated from its dam.

At weaning it is important that the mare is moved out of sight and earshot of the foal. The foal is usually kept in a loose box with the top door shut until it has settled down, which is usually within a few hours of separation. Being able to see other foals will minimise stress at this time. Weanlings are usually turned out into a securely fenced paddock with the other weanlings within 24h of being separated from their mothers. If other foals are not available, quiet mares or geldings can serve as suitable companions. Alternatively, the mares may be moved from the paddocks one by one over a period of time leaving the foals with their usual companions. Gradual weaning is also an alternative method, where the time of separation is increased gradually over a period of days, either by placing the mare and foal in adjacent boxes, or adjacent small paddocks, allowing only visual contact. It is an area where more welfare research is needed.

Mares usually settle down quickly after the foals have been weaned. Their udders are usually distended for a few days but soon start to dry off. It is customary to cut back the amount of concentrate feed and ensure the mare can take exercise until the udder has 'dried off'. The milk should not be stripped off during this phase.

Management of stallions

Stallions, like brood mares, should be allowed to lead as natural a life as possible. Pony stallions can be left to run out with their mares. However, because of the risk of injury and the greater value of the animal, non-pony stallions are individually stabled, and when turned out to graze, this is also on an individual basis. It is beneficial for them to see other horses, but they should not be able to make physical contact with them. The fencing surrounding stallion paddocks must be robust and sufficiently high to deter them from jumping out. They need to be fit for the breeding season if they have many mares to cover: regular exercise (ridden or in-hand) is required in the preceding months. They are less predictable than mares or geldings, and it is important for their optimum performance that they are not badly or roughly handled: hence the necessity for experienced handlers.

Feeding management

The individually stabled horse

It has been shown that visual contact and the smell or noise of adjacent horses encourage horses to eat (Sweeting *et al.* 1985; Houpt 1991). The provision of a small window or grille in the partition between loose boxes and the repositioning of the manger may be sufficient to encourage shy feeders to eat. As a horse becomes fitter it may not finish its early morning feed, so the size of the individual concentrate meal should be adjusted down to what the horse is willing to consume at that meal; an extra feed can be included later in the day. Turning stabled horses in work out in a paddock or sand arena for a short period daily is invariably beneficial for the overall well-being of the horse, and is to be encouraged.

Groups of horses

The main problem of group feeding is ensuring that the more timid horses in the group get sufficient feed. If at pasture, feed racks should be located in a sheltered position, not in a field shelter, on a well drained surface and in sufficient number to ensure that all horses get access without fighting. Group housing may aggravate the situation because of the greater restriction in space. Group-managed horses should be examined carefully daily, as long winter coats may mask thinness. Timid horses may need to be removed to a smaller group to ensure that they get sufficient feed.

Feeding

The horse is a non-ruminant herbivore with significant microbial fermentation occurring in the caecum and colon. The stomach is only about 8% of the capacity of the total digestive tract, and is relatively small in relation to body size. In contrast, the hindgut comprises 62% of the capacity of the total digestive tract. The sacculations of the colon are thought likely to reduce the rate of passage of digesta, leading to enhanced microbial fermentation and digestion (Hintz & Cymbaluk 1994). As a herbivore, the horse is accustomed to continuous feeding, and in the feral state ponies spend most of their time grazing or browsing, particularly in the winter months when grazing is scarce and of poor nutritive value (Tyler 1972). By individually stabling horses, their movements are restricted and socialisation is reduced. Managing these horses, when they are in work and on a diet high in concentrates but low in roughage, is challenging. There is an increased possibility of both gastrointestinal (for example, colic) and behavioural problems arising from individual housing and intermittent feeding. Because of changing patterns in agriculture, the traditional horse feeds of hay and oats are not necessarily always readily available.

Concentrates

Alternatives to oats are barley and maize, both of which have higher energy density than oats. In view of this, when they are substituted for oats, it should be on a basis of energy and not volume (see Table 35.6). Oats can be fed whole, crimped, rolled or ground. Maize can be fed whole, cracked, flaked or ground, but processing is probably only advantageous for very young animals, those with poor chewing habits or poor teeth. Barley should be processed (steam or dry rolled) in order to expose the barley kernel.

In addition to grains, there are now various proprietary horse feeds available in the form of pellets or as coarse mixtures. These are specially formulated to meet the needs of horses and ponies of different ages and at varying activity levels, and are very simple to use. It is always best to reduce

Table 35.6 Oats and substitute grains suitable for feeding to horses, based on digestible energy values (after Cuddeford, 1986).

Feed	*Replacement rate for 1 kg oats DM (kg)*
Oats	1.000
Barley	0.930
Maize	0.869

the energy from carbohydrate and increase the amount from fats and oils.

Despite vitamin supplementation being heavily promoted commercially, it remains a controversial subject to how beneficial the effects of supplementation in exercising horses are. Salt (about 50g/day) is probably the cheapest and most useful supplement for all horses and is commercially available in the form of mineralised salt blocks. These provide salt and essential trace elements and should be provided all year round.

Dried sugarbeet pulp, as pellets or shredded, can be usefully added to the concentrate ration, but must be thoroughly soaked before use or else there is the risk of oesophageal obstruction (choke). Wheat bran and dried brewers grains can also be fed, but both have high phosphorus levels and should be used with discretion.

The concentrate ration is usually fed in mangers, which can be at chest height or on the ground. However, there is greater risk of fouling if mangers are at ground level. They should be kept clean, and rejected food should be removed before fresh feed is put in.

Roughages

The hay requirements of horses range between 0.5 and 1.0 kg per 100 kg liveweight per day. Horses in intensive work that are fed large quantities of concentrate may only consume the lower amount of roughage. In this situation, the main function of the hay is mechanical to ensure normal gut function. Although it could be replaced by other sources of long fibre such as chaffed straw, hay occupies the horses' attention, which is an important consideration in avoiding behavioural problems in stabled horses. Where hay provides most of the dietary intake (for example, adult horses on maintenance rations and ponies during the winter months) any alternatives must provide both fibre and nutrients.

Silage, especially big bale silage, is now more readily available; if harvested at the correct stage of growth and stored properly, it should be superior to hay as it is not field cured for long periods. The risk of botulism can be minimised by ensuring that the bags are air-tight, that there is no smell of ammonia when they are opened, that the pH is less than 5, and there is no contamination with soil. It is also important that the dry matter content is not too low, to avoid horses in hard work having to consume inappropriately large quantities. Haylage, high dry matter silage, is another excellent (but expensive) product available for horses. Both silage and haylage are excellent alternatives to hay for horses with respiratory allergies.

In comparison with good or average hay, straws have low densities of energy, protein and minerals. Wheat and rye straw are not suitable for feeding to horses because of their high lignin content, which makes them indigestible, but spring sown oat or barley straw, which have been under sown with grass, are good feeding straws. However, they need to be supplemented with protein, energy and minerals. Treatment of the straw with ammonia improves energy values and significantly reduces fungal contamination. Ammonia-treated straw can be fed at up to 1.5 kg per 100 kg live weight, and used to replace hay on a kg/kg dry matter basis, although it will still be necessary to provide a vitamin and mineral supplement (Cuddeford 1986).

Grass cubes, manufactured from chopped and not ground grass, and lucerne cubes usually provide sufficient protein and calcium, and could be fed exclusively to horses. However, these products and other 'complete cubed' diets have a major disadvantage in that they are usually consumed quickly and thus encourage the development of behavioural problems in stabled horses. Good-quality chaffed hay or straw with added molasses and minerals can be fed in place of hay on a weight for weight basis. They are frequently mixed with the grain ration to discourage too rapid consumption of the feed. Roughages can be fed off the floor, which is more wasteful but more natural. By lowering the head the tracheal mucociliary clearance is accelerated which contributes in avoiding lower respiratory tract disease (Raidal 1996). Alternatively hay can be fed in wall-mounted racks or in hay nets. Racks and hay nets should be at an appropriate height (head height) so that there is no risk of a hoof becoming entrapped. Hay nets should not be available for foals because of the risk of injury.

Energy requirements

The energy requirements of horses vary according to size, activity level, ambient temperature and individual metabolic activity. The digestible energy (DE) requirements for the maintenance of horses weighing up to 600 kg liveweight can be calculated using the following formula (Hintz & Cymbaluk 1994):

$$\mathrm{DE\,(MJ/day)} = 5.8 + (0.03 \times \mathrm{LW})$$

where LW is the liveweight in kilograms.

DE requirements increase by 25–100% for mature horses in light to intensive work. These increases, including those required as a result of growth, pregnancy and lactation, are usually met by the introduction of concentrates (grain) into the diet. The energy requirements of the pregnant mare may increase to 110%, 113% and 120% of maintenance during the 9th, 10th and 11th months of pregnancy, respectively.

Requirements during lactation depend on milk yield, but can be double those required for maintenance. Horses in heavy training may require more energy than they can consume on a conventional diet. Increasing the energy density of the diet has been achieved by the addition of fat at levels of between 6 and 12% of the total diet. Supplementing protein as a means of increasing energy is not efficient, and there is no evidence of any benefits of vitamin supplementation above the required levels. For more detailed information on the nutritional needs of growing, breeding and exercising horses the reader is referred to an excellent review by Ott (1992).

Cold weather increases DE requirements. These requirements are best met by feeding good-quality hay (at least 50% of the ration), *ad libitum*. This encourages high voluntary intake of a feed with a good energy content and a high heat increment (HI). (HI is the heat of nutrition, metabolism, digestion and muscular activity involved during digestion.) In hot weather, the diet should not include excessive levels of feeds with a high HI such as hay, as this would aggravate heat stress. The HI of grains or fat is lower than that of fibrous feeds.

Water requirements

Whether stabled or at pasture, horses should have constant access to clean water. When housed in groups, the water supply should be sufficiently large to allow several horses to drink at one time. Cattle troughs are quite satisfactory for this purpose. Care should be taken to ensure that there are no sharp edges which could cause injury. When on a predominantly hay diet, stabled horses require 5l of water per 100kg liveweight per day; when on a hay and grain diet, 3l of water per 100kg liveweight per day should suffice (Cymbaluk & Chrislison 1990). Voluntary water intake is reduced in cold weather, so it is importan t that horses kept outside are provided with highly digestible feeds in order to minimise the risk of intestinal impaction. In cold weather water temperature should be 2–10°C in order to optimise intake (Cymhaluk & Christison 1990). Water can be supplied in plastic buckets or via automatic drinkers. The former, though more laborious, are to be preferred, as monitoring of water intake is possible. Water buckets should be scrubbed out daily.

Laboratory procedures

Restraint

Most horses and ponies will accept being restrained for various procedures if they have been well handled since birth. The voice should be used to calm them and they should be approached, in a firm and confident manner, from the shoulder area. A headcollar, with or without a bit attachment, should then be put on and a long lead, preferably with a quick release catch, attached to the centre back loop of the headcollar. Short-term, relatively painless procedures, such as the collection of venous blood samples, usually do not require additional control in a horse accustomed to the procedure. If more control is needed, then grasping a fold of skin in the neck with one or both hands and twisting it (neck twitch) is usually sufficient to keep the horse still until the sample is collected. Alternatively the lead rope can be wound round the front of the headcollar to provide more control. Grasping the ear is not to be recommended, as it could make the horse head shy. For more fractious animals, a twitch can be applied to the upper lip (Figure 35.3), although specific training should be considered as a long-term alternative. Twitches should only be applied by staff experienced in their use, and should only be used for a short period of time. Picking up and minimally supporting one front foot facilitates simple procedures at the hind end of the animal in many cases, for example, recording of rectal temperature and collection of feacal samples.

Young foals should be restrained by one arm around the front of the chest and the other around the back of the hindquarters, and held against a wall in the loose box: they should not be held round the chest/abdomen. If very unruly, they can be held round the front of the chest with one arm whilst the tail is grasped firmly at the root with the free hand.

All the physical methods of restraint are suitable for short-term procedures in relatively amenable horses and ponies. The horse or pony should always be rewarded with a rub of the withers after all procedures and, on occasions, with a small handful of its favourite feed, particularly when it is being trained.

Special frames (stocks) designed to restrain horses for veterinary examinations are particularly useful during time-consuming procedures, for example, gynaecological examinations, biopsy collection and tracheal washes (Figure 35.4). They should have no sharp projections. The horizontal bars should be well rounded and the floor surface non-slip when wet or dry. Some means of quick side release should be available should a horse slip and go down. Chemical restraint is often advisable for longer term, more invasive procedures in both co-operative and uncooperative animals, for example, standing castration under local anaesthesia and stitching of wounds.

Handling and training

The adult horse is potentially dangerous because of its size, strength and agility, together with its ability to bite and to kick with both front and hindlegs. Therefore, it is essential that it is handled and trained by experienced people. The very young foal should be introduced to normal stable procedures and trained to accept simple procedures by its handler as soon after birth as possible (see Foal behaviour). If more invasive procedures (for example, the collection of blood samples) are necessary, it is important that the foal is

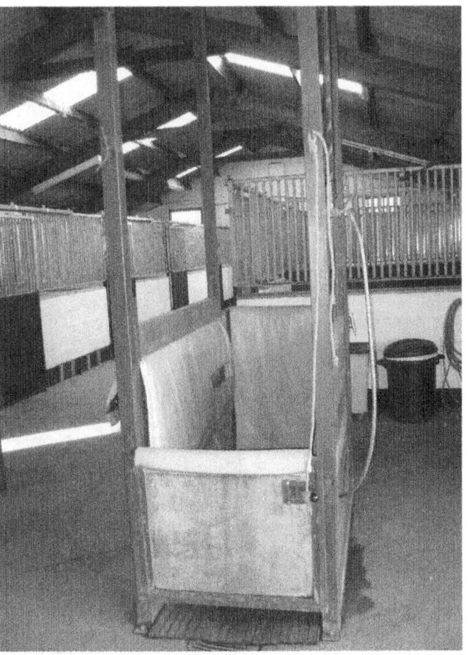

Figure 35.4 Rear view of type of stocks used for restraining horses for veterinary examinations and procedures. The boards on the sides can be removed if access is needed.

restrained by experienced, strong handlers, and that the person collecting the sample is adept at venepuncture. This will minimise stress, and with time and subsequent exposure to the procedure, the foal will usually accept it. Training a horse to be ridden does not normally begin until it is 3–4 years old, except in the case of the racing Thoroughbred. This is skilled work and should only be done by people with training and experience. If not required to be ridden, the basic training such as acceptance of normal husbandry procedures and being restrained in or out of stocks for different procedures should continue. Additionally, horses should be trained to accept the bit and should be taught to exercise on the lunge. The horse should always be rewarded when it has behaved well during procedures. Corrective action should be imposed at the time of the misdemeanour and not hours later. For safety reasons, during all the procedures described below, the horse should have an experienced handler present to restrain it if and when it is necessary. The person carrying out the procedures should have been correctly trained and be experienced in the techniques.

For large numbers of ponies a system of race and crush is advisable to use to facilitate the handling and the procedures (Figure 35.5). The ponies should be slowly introduced to this system from a young age. They are restrained in the crush and procedures like measuring body temperature, taking faeces samples and bleeding can be easily performed.

Physiological monitoring

Recording of body temperature

Temperatures are taken per rectum under suitable restraint. If necessary, the handler can hold up a front foot, thus making it difficult for the horse to use its hindfoot to kick the person recording the temperature.

Collection of blood samples

These are usually collected from the jugular vein which is readily visible when the vein is raised by manual pressure in the jugular groove. Horses accustomed to the procedure require minimal restraint. Foals are more unruly, but experienced attendants can usually restrain them sufficiently for a sample to be collected. If large volumes of blood are to be collected, large-gauge needles (minimum 2 mm) or sterile indwelling catheters are to be recommended. In this case the skin over the injection site is infiltrated with local anaesthetic first.

If frequent blood sampling is required, for example in a pharmacokinetic study, it may be better to insert an indwelling cannula under local anaesthesia, and suture it in place. The cannula is kept patent with sterile heparinised saline. With care, good technique and adequate supervision cannulae can be left *in situ* for several days. There is frequently a local reaction to their presence, but this subsides rapidly once they are removed. The decision to cannulate or not will depend on the number of samples, the temperament of the horse and how stoical it is to repeated injections (see also Joint Working Group on Refinement (JWGR) 1993).

Virus isolation from the upper respiratory tract

A nasopharyngeal swab is inserted into the pharynx via the ventral meatus of the nares and rubbed carefully against the pharyngeal mucosa. Prior sedation is not usually needed, but the horse should be restrained in stocks and a nose twitch applied if necessary. If the twitch is necessary, and the process is to be repeated, consider whether there would be a welfare benefit in habituating the horse to the technique.

Tracheal washes

This procedure may be carried out by percutaneous puncture or endoscopically. The latter is less invasive and is

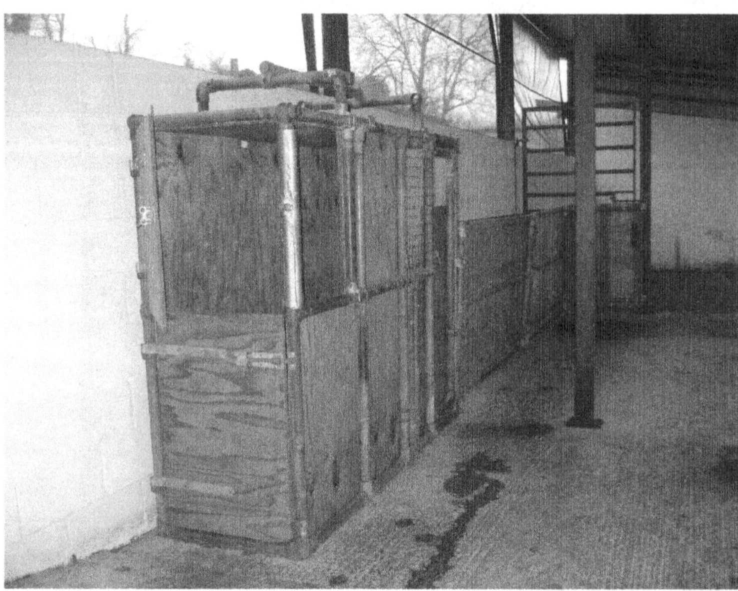

Figure 35.5 System of race and crush for handling large numbers of ponies.

preferable for multiple sampling. A catheter is directed down the biopsy channel of an endoscope which has been inserted via the external nares and pharynx. Sedation may be required. It is best if the horse is restrained in stocks.

Genital swabs/uterine biopsy

Swabs are routinely collected from breeding mares and stallions to check for the presence of infection, specifically venereal pathogens. Cervical and clitoral swabs can be taken with the aid of a speculum to dilate the vagina if necessary; the swab is passed into and through the cervix of the mare and rubbed against the mucosa of the uterus. Uterine biopsies are done to evaluate the histological structure of the uterus, particularly in relation to the mare's ability to successfully conceive and carry a foal to term. Mares should be restrained in stocks prior to carrying out these procedures. The sites for examination in the stallion are the urethral fossa, the sheath and the urethra.

Urine samples

Catheterisation of the bladder can be performed on mares: for male animals samples are collected at urination. Horse nappies may be an alternative collection technique.

Faecal samples

If collection from the floor will not suffice for the purpose required, faecal samples are best collected carefully per rectum: lubrication should be used, as horses have tight anal sphincters. Extra restraint may be necessary, such as picking up a front foot.

Administration of medicines

Oral (pastes, suspension, granules, powders)

If they are palatable, administration of medicines in the feed is easy and involves no restraint of the horse. However, if large volumes of fluid have to be administered, this should be done, using a nasogastric tube, by operators correctly trained in the procedure, in order to avoid accidental introduction of fluid into the lungs. This procedure can be carried out in most horses without prior sedation. Paste formulations are usually administered directly into the oral cavity.

Parenteral

Many drugs are designed to be administered parenterally. The muscles of the neck, pectoral or gluteal muscles can be used for intramuscular injections. The risk of the operator being kicked is greater with the use of the gluteals. When several days' treatment are necessary the injection site should be varied. Occasionally horses will develop stiffness following intramuscular injection into the neck, despite it being correctly sited: care should be taken to ensure horses can reach their water buckets and feed mangers during this time. Injection into the pectorals may lead to dependent swellings, and occasionally the horse is stiff when asked to move forward. The gluteal area is well muscled, has a good blood supply and is a good site for intramuscular injection despite the extra risk to the operator. Any complication here, such as abscess formation, would drain better than in the neck area.

Chemical restraint: sedation, analgesia and anaesthesia

General anaesthesia in the horse carries a slightly greater risk than for other domestic animals (Jones 2001), and should only be undertaken by a veterinarian assisted by trained staff. A major problem is the possibility of ischaemic muscle necrosis associated with the prolonged pressure of recumbency. However, the introduction of safer, effective and more reliable drugs allows many of the procedures which previously required general anaesthesia to be done in the standing horse using a combination of sedatives and analgesics together with local or regional anaesthesia. Before any central nervous depressant drug is administered, a full clinical examination should be carried out, in order to detect any pre-existing condition that may be exacerbated by the use of the drug or may potentiate the side effects of the drug. The patient should be kept in quiet surroundings before drug administration and while sedation is allowed to develop. Although some of the drugs may be given by the intramuscular route, the intravenous route is the most rapidly effective and reliable. The manufacturer's datasheets should always be consulted beforehand, as there are important contraindications and possible side effects to be considered. The various drugs used for chemical restraint are well reviewed by Munro and Young (1991) and are summarised in Table 35.7. Although acepromazine may be used to sedate horses, they still respond to visual and aural stimuli and so arousal during sedation is possible. Other more serious side effects are priapism and paraphimosis.

Analgesics

Analgesics commonly used in horses are summarised in Table 35.8. Several are controlled drugs.

Anaesthesia

Xylazine, detomidine and romifidine can be used in combination with ketamine or sodium thiopental for short-term anaesthesia. The use of an intravenous cannula is essential in case of emergencies during anaesthesia, and to reduce the risk of accidental perivascular administration of sodium thiopental which would cause tissue damage and sloughing. Induction of anaesthesia is normally done in a padded induction and recovery room, the anaesthetised horse is then transported to an adjacent operating theatre where there is specialist equipment for the maintenance of long-term anaesthesia. However, short-term anaesthesia using intravenously administered drugs is possible under field conditions and is acceptable for minor surgical procedures, provided supplemental oxygen can be provided. A well-bedded cattle pen with straw bales lining the walls would be a suitable place to carry out the procedure.

Table 35.7 Sedative properties.

Active ingredient	*Dose[†]/route*	*Onset of peak sedation*	*Duration of useful sedation (dose dependent)*
Xylazine*	0.6–1 mg/kg slow iv	Within 5 min	Approx. 20 min
Detomidine*	10–80 μg/kg slow iv	1–3 min	Approx. 30–60 min
Romifidine	40–120 μg/kg iv only	5 min	Approx. 30–180 min
Butorphanol in combination with detomidine or in combination with romifidine	20–25 μg/kg iv 12 μg/kg iv 40–120 μg/kg iv	5 min	Approx. 30–60 min

*Xylazine and Detomidine may also be given im.
[†]Based on manufacturer's data sheet.

Table 35.8 Analgesics suitable for use in horses.

Active ingredient	*Route of administration*	*Use*	
		Musculoskeletal pain	*Visceral pain*
Butorphanol*	iv	x	√
Flunixin	iv/oral (up to 5 days)	√	√
Detomidine	iv/im	x	√
Romifidine	iv only	x	√
Xylazine	iv/im	x	√
Phenylbutazone	iv/oral (long term)	√	√
Pethidine	im	x	√

*Can be used in combination with xylazine and detomidine

Euthanasia

A free-bullet humane killer or pistol of 0.32 calibre is the traditional way of euthanasing horses. In the hands of an experienced person it is fast and efficient, and disposal of the carcase is not complicated by the presence of chemical agents used for euthanasia. The weapon is aimed just above the point of intersection of lines joining the lateral canthus of the eye to the base of the opposite ear (the intersection is usually under the forelock at its base). There are chemical alternatives to shooting which may be more suitable under some circumstances. A new combination product containing quinalbarbitone and cinchocaine hydrochloride (Somulose, Arnolds Veterinary, UK) would appear to have considerable advantages over the use of anaesthetic overdoses. All chemical methods of euthanasia render the carcase unsuitable for pet food manufacture. For further reading on euthanasia of horses see Knottenbelt (1995).

Common welfare problems

Significant diseases

Some of the more common diseases relevant to horses entering or participating in research programmes are listed in the following paragraphs. Some, for example colic, are often a consequence of poor management; others can be controlled by vaccination, for example tetanus and equine influenza, or, in the case of endoparasitism, by the use of an effective worm control programme. Others, such as amyloidosis, are generally specific to hyperimmune serum producing horses. It is important that stable staff are aware of the main clinical signs of the more common diseases so that veterinary advice is sought promptly, thus limiting the disease. The salient features of the diseases are briefly reviewed below. More information can be found in *The Equine Manual* (Higgins & Snyder 2006).

Tetanus (lock jaw)

The causal agent is *Clostridium tetani*, a Gram-positive spore-forming bacillus present in soil and as a commensal in the gastrointestinal tract. The spores can survive for years in the environment. The disease is mainly seen following puncture wounds, as the anaerobic conditions in devitalised tissue provide the ideal environment for the spores to generate and release a neurotoxin. Treatment is often difficult and unsuccessful. It is imperative to vaccinate horses against the disease, and in countries where vaccination is common the disease is rare. It is essential that antitoxin is administered following injury if the horse's vaccination history is unknown. Mares are usually given a booster vaccination 1 month prior to the anticipated date of foaling: their foals are then passively protected from infection via antibodies in the colostrum for about 3 months, after which they can start their active immunisation programme. Foals born to unvaccinated mares should be given tetanus antitoxin at birth and 6 weeks later. The timing of the start of a foal's active immunisation programme will depend on the vaccine being used. The manufacturer's datasheet should be consulted for the optimum time to start. After the initial vaccine course, booster vaccinations are usually given every 2–3 years.

Colic

Colic is the term used to describe pain arising from the gastrointestinal tract. All cases of colic should be regarded as potentially serious and, as 6–10% will require surgical intervention, it is essential that a diagnosis is made swiftly and the appropriate treatment initiated. Most cases of colic are related to the effects of intestinal parasites, or diet and feeding practices. Signs will vary according to the type of colic, for example whether impactive or spasmodic, and will also vary in intensity. Signs include inappetence, scant faeces, restlessness, rolling, scraping the floor with a foreleg, gazing at the flanks, patchy sweating and kicking at the abdomen. Affected horses should be housed in a large loose box or cattle pen with a deep bed, the sides of which should be banked up along the walls. There should be no sharp projections. It is important to monitor frequently and record the vital signs (normal values in Table 35.1) so any deterioration can be detected in the early stages. Treatment consists of the control of pain with the use of non-steroidal anti-inflammatory drugs (NSAIDs) or using compounds such as xylazine alone or in combination with synthetic opioids such as butorphanol, together with any specific therapy indicated by the cause of the colic. Pethidine has excellent spasmolytic properties and is a cheaper alternative to synthetic opioids, but is a controlled drug in some countries. The underlying causes, for example endoparasitism or nutritional upset, should be rectified.

Respiratory infections

Bacteria and viruses may cause upper and lower respiratory tract infections, the former playing a more predominant role now than was previously thought. Infection with equine influenza and equine herpesvirus (EHV) 1 and 4 are the more common causes of acute upper respiratory tract disease. Influenza occurs in susceptible horses of all ages, whereas herpesvirus infection is more common in young horses. Treatment includes rest, good nursing and antibiotics if bacterial infection, primary or secondary, is involved. Prevention of influenza and EHV is possible by vaccination, though EHV vaccines are not universally available.

Strangles

This is a bacterial infection of the upper respiratory tract caused by *Streptococcus equi*. The infection is often introduced when young horses and ponies from varying sources are bought in. Recovered animals may remain carriers for long periods of time, and they are an important source of infection for in-contact animals. Hence the importance of isolation and a thorough clinical examination of all newcomers. The main clinical signs of infection are loss of appetite, pyrexia and depression, bilateral or serous purulent nasal discharge, and swelling and abscessation of the lymph nodes of the head and neck. Horses in contact with an affected horse and those in the very early stages of the disease (within 24 h of onset of pyrexia) can be treated with benzyl penicillin in large doses to prevent progression of the disease; otherwise it is generally better to allow the infection to run its course. Good nursing is essential, and lancing and draining lymph node abscesses should be done as necessary. Following a disease outbreak, because the organism is able to survive for weeks in pus, disinfection of stabling, feeding and watering equipment, and tack and grooming equipment is essential. Vaccines are available in some countries but they have been of poor efficacy.

Allergic respiratory disease

This is an important and frequent cause of disease, particularly in stabled horses. See Housing and respiratory disease section for details on prevention and management.

Internal parasites

All grazing horses are infected with internal parasites. These include roundworms, tapeworms and bots (larvae of the bot fly, *Gasterophilus* spp.). Some roundworms are specific to unweaned foals and yearlings, for example *Strongyloides westeri* (threadworm) and *Parascaris equorum* (the large roundworm). However, the large and small strongyles (redworm) are found in horses of all ages, and are potentially very pathogenic. Migrating larvae of the large redworm *Strongylus vulgaris* cause arteritis and thrombus formation, which can result in ischaemia and necrosis of part of the large intestine. However, with the introduction of broad-spectrum anthelmintics over the last three decades, the prevalence of *S. vulgaris* has declined dramatically, whilst that of the small strongyles (cyathostomes) has increased. Cyathostome larvae undergo a prolonged period of development in the large intestinal mucosa, and are increasingly being associated with several clinical syndromes such as diarrhoea and weight loss which have a seasonal pattern. Tapeworm infections are also common, and there is a tenuous association with infection and the incidence of ileocaecal colic.

Traditional control programmes based on treatments every 2 months are now insufficient, and an integrated approach to control is necessary. This encompasses the use of the appropriate wormer at the correct time of the year for the particular target parasite, together with good pasture management. None of the available equine anthelmintics is effective against the full spectrum of endoparasites infecting horses, but each class of anthelmintic has a specific unique indication (Table 35.9). The manufacturers' datasheets should be read carefully prior to selection of an anthelmintic.

Mares should be treated in the last month of pregnancy to limit contamination of the pastures used by them and their foals: all the modern broad spectrum wormers can be used during pregnancy. Foals should be introduced into the worm control programme when about 6 weeks of age, and both they and their dams should be treated regularly throughout the rearing period. All horses grazing the same pasture should be treated with the same anthelmintic at the same time. Specific treatments for bots, tapeworms, mucosal cyathostome larvae and migrating large redworm larvae should be given at the appropriate time of the year for the climatic region. In general terms, in northern temperate regions, treatment for mucosal cyathostome larvae, tissue stages of large strongyles and bots is given in the autumn and/or winter months. In the warmer southern regions, treatment for these parasites may extend into the late spring and may require to be done twice yearly. Tapeworm treatments should be given twice yearly, in the late summer and again 6 months later. All newcomers should be treated with a larvicidal dose of fenbendazole followed by a double dose of pyrantel and kept housed for 48 h after last treatment,

Table 35.9 Modern broad-spectrum anthelmintics commonly used in the horse and efficacy spectrum.

Chemical group	*Lumen adults/Larvae*	*Mucosal larvae*[a]	*Arterial/tissue larvae*[b]	*Tapeworms*
Benzimidazoles				
Fenbendazole	√/√	√[c] (all stages)	√[c]	X
Oxibendazole	√/√	X	X	X
Mebendazole	√/X	X	X	X
Macrocyclic lactones				
Ivermectin	√/√	X	√	X
Moxidectin	√/√	√ (late stages only)	√	X
Tetrahydropyrimidines				
Pyrantel salts	√/√	X	X	√[d]

√, Activity; X, no activity.
[a] Cyathosomes (small strongyles).
[b] Large strongyles.
[c] Larvicidal dose rate.
[d] Double routine dose rate.

before turning them out to graze with the resident population. Anthelmintics used routinely during the grazing season should be rotated on an annual basis to reduce the likelihood of the development of resistant strains of parasites.

Large paddocks should be subdivided so that they can be more easily managed: special electric fencing material is available for doing this cost effectively. Broad electric tape, easily visible, should be used when first introducing the horses to this area. Faeces should be removed twice weekly, particularly in warm moist periods when conditions are optimal for larval development on pasture. Machines are available which will both collect faeces and debris and harrow the pasture. Mixed grazing with cattle (or sheep) will reduce pasture infectivity, as the main parasites are host specific.

Pasture quality and palatability are also improved by mixed grazing, as ruminants will graze areas rejected by horses. Pasture should not be overstocked, and attempts should be made to ensure that young horses get the cleanest and best pasture. It is recommended to have 1 acre of grazing per horse and 0.5 acre per pony (1 UK acre = 4047 m^2). This can be affected by a number of factors such as: length of time spent stabled, time of year, pasture quality and number of animals on the pasture.

Laminitis ('founder')

Laminitis is a common cause of lameness and disability in horses and ponies. It can affect both forefeet, both hindfeet, all of the feet or just one foot. The disease is metabolic in origin and is associated with overfeeding of grain and concentrates to stabled horses, and with over-fat, under-exercised ponies grazing lush pasture. It can also be a consequence of corticosteroid therapy and a sequel to systemic infections such as endometritis and enteritis. The extreme pain seen in the acute stage of the disease is caused by ischaemia of digital dermal tissue (Eustace 1990). Affected animals throw their weight back on their heels and are very reluctant to move. If permanent damage is to be avoided, veterinary assistance should be sought as soon as the lameness is noticed. If a systemic illness such as endometritis is involved, then this must be treated. Additionally, drugs to reduce hypertension and anxiety, such as acepromazine, are given together with analgesics such as phenylbutazone. Good nursing and the provision of quality roughages together with supplemental methionine and biotin are essential (Eustace 1990). Affected animals must be confined in a well bedded loose box and provided with frog support. Prevention is by sensible feeding and grazing management. Further information can be found in Eustace (1992).

Hyperlipaemia

This is a disorder of lipid metabolism particularly common in pony breeds, especially Shetland ponies. It is characterised by gross lipaemia, elevated plasma triglyceride concentrations and fatty infiltration of body tissues leading to organ failure, especially of the liver and kidneys. The most common clinical signs are anorexia and lethargy, and the mortality rate is high, commonly 60–85%. Stress and obesity are important risk factors. Stressors include transportation, inclement weather and changes in management. The majority of affected ponies are in good or fat condition, and pregnant mares seem to be particularly susceptible. Diagnosis can be confirmed by measuring plasma triglyceride concentrations. Values in excess of 5 mmol/l indicate disease. Treatment involves identifying and treating any underlying disease. High-energy diets should be fed, as the animals are in negative energy balance. Intravenous fluids should be given to maintain circulatory volume and to correct electrolyte and acid–base balance. Intramuscular insulin, in conjunction with oral or intravenous glucose or galactose, may reduce mobilisation of free fatty acids from adipose tissue and intravenous heparin may increase the activity of enzymes responsible for the clearance of lipoproteins from circulation.

Skin infections

The more common skin infections are summarised in Table 35.10.

Table 35.10 Common skin infections of horses.

Common name/incidence	*Cause*	*Lesions/signs*	*Treatment and control*
Ringworm; mainly stabled horses	*Trichophyton* and *Microsporum* species of fungi	Small tufts of hair agglutinated with serum especially in harness-abraded areas	Topical or systemic treatments available. Disinfection of buildings, trailers, tack, clothing and grooming equipment used by infected horses
Rain scald (body) and mud fever (legs); pastured ponies and horses in the winter months	*Dermatophilus congolensis*	Tufts of hair over crusts of exudate; pus underneath. Usually bilateral and symmetrical on back	House affected animals or provide with waterproof rugs if to remain at pasture
Sweet itch/summer itch; mainly ponies, sporadic cases in summer	Hypersensitivity to midge bites	Lesions at base of mane and tail head. Intense rubbing of affected areas	Topical insect repellents. House at dusk when midges are out; run a fan in the stable
Pediculosis; all horses and ponies susceptible mainly in winter/late spring	Sucking and biting lice	Intense rubbing of infected areas (chest/hindlegs/neck)	Control with pour-on synthetic pyrethroid; repeat every 14 days until cured. BHC powder, if available

Amyloidosis

Although a rare clinical entity in the general horse population, amyloidosis is a frequent *post-mortem* finding in horses used for hyperimmune serum production, the liver and the spleen being the more commonly affected organs. Since liver rupture is a common cause of death in such horses, on welfare and economic grounds, regular monitoring of gamma glutamyl transferase (GGT) activity in serum would seem to be advisable. Studies in hyperimmune serum producing horses over a 5-year period have shown that GGT levels increase within 6–7 years of first starting the immunisation procedure, and that constantly high values seemed to correlate with advanced liver amyloidosis (Abdelkader *et al.* 1991).

Abnormal behaviour

Ideally, management systems for equines should accommodate their natural behaviour, in particular the need to graze, exercise and socialise. They are flight animals and hence easily startled and this should also be taken into account (European Commission 2007). One of the most effective management strategies for reducing abnormal behaviour is to increase turnout time. Equines should be kept at pasture or have access to pasture for at least 6 h a day. This encourages social contact, and also increases the amounts of time spent eating.

Weaving/box (stall) walking

Weaving, where the horse sways from side to side on its forelimbs, and box or stall walking where it endlessly walks round its box, are typical examples of behavioural stereotypies. They are usually the consequence of the stress, or thwarted motivation for locomotory behaviour, experienced by an open-country animal being kept isolated in a restricted area such as a stall or loose box (Houpt 1992). Endorphins are released from the central nervous system during stereotypic behaviour, possibly encouraging the horse to persist in the behaviour. Amelioration can be achieved by providing the horse with sufficient windows or openings to enable it to see its companions and its immediate environment at all times. Placing mirrors in the stables of weavers significantly reduces this abnormal behaviour. The mirror is believed to mimic visual contact providing environmental distraction (McAfee *et al.* 2002).

Biting and kicking

Biting and kicking, or threatening to do so, are the horse's main ways of showing aggression. Normally this is reserved for other horses, especially at feeding time or to newcomers to a group. However, horses which have been maltreated will also threaten their attendants. With time, patience, experienced handling and expert advice, most of these horses can be retrained to trust their handlers.

Wood chewing

As mentioned earlier (see Roughages), low-roughage diets in stabled horses can encourage wood chewing; this can be rectified by providing more hay in the diet but it may also be necessary to apply creosote to chewed areas to discourage further wood chewing in the short term.

Crib-biting/wind-sucking

Crib-biting and wind-sucking are common oral stereotypes and both are perceived as detrimental to the horses' health.

Crib-biting is an oral stereotype where a fixed object is grasped with the incisors, the lower neck muscles contract to retract the larynx caudally; air is drawn into the cranial oesophagus, which produces the characteristic grunt (Nicol *et al.* 2002). No air is swallowed (McGreevy *et al.* 1995) but there is a view that this type of behaviour could be harmful. In wind-sucking the same posture and grunt are adopted but without grasping a fixed object.

The exact causes behind these two stereotypes remain unclear. Heritability, management, feeding practices, social contact, crowding and many more have all been suggested as being responsible for their development or have been shown to increase the risk of them happening. A permanent cure is yet to be found and attempts to prevent it occurring have included surgery, acupuncture, environmental enrichment and others (McGreevy & Nicol 1998).

Acknowledgement

This chapter is updated, but based considerably on the chapter previously written by Elizabeth Abbott published in the 7th edition of the handbook. Her substantial contribution is gratefully acknowledged.

Further reading

Useful sources of general information on equine behaviour, care and breeding can be found in Houpt and Wolski (1982); Warren Evans (1992) Mills and Nankervis (1999) and Higgins and Snyder (2006).

References

Abdelkader, S.V., Gudding, R.J. and Nordstoga, K. (1991) Clinical chemical constituents in relation to liver amyloidosis in serum-producing horses. *Journal of Comparative Pathology*, **105**, 203–211

Allen, K. and Franklin, S. (2007) RAO and IAD: respiratory disease in horses revisited. *In Practice*, **29**, 76–82

Butler, K.D. (1992) Foot care. In: *Horse Breeding and Management*. Ed. Warren Evans, J., pp. 177–205. Elsevier, London

Collins, M.N., Friend, T.H., Jousan, F.D. *et al.* (2000) *Applied Animal Behaviour Science*, **67**, 169–179

Clark, D. K., Friend, T.H. and Dellmeier, G. (1993) The effect of orientation during trailer transport on heart rate, cortisol, and balance in horses. *Applied Animal Behaviour Science*, **38**, 179–189

Council of Europe (2006) Multilateral Consultation of Parties to the European Convention for the Protection of Vertebrate Animals used for Experimental and other Scientific Purposes (ETS 123) Appendix A. *Cons 123 (2006) 3.* Available from URL: http://www.coe.int/t/e/legal_affairs/legal_co-operation/biological_safety,_use_of_animals/laboratory_animals/2006/Cons123(2006)3AppendixA_en.pdf (accessed 31 July 2008)

Crowell-Davis, S.L. (1986) Developmental behaviour. In: *Veterinary Clinics of North America: Equine Practice*, **2**, 573–590

Cuddeford, D. (1986) Alternative feedstuffs for horses. *In Practice*, **8**, 68–70

Cymbaluk, N.F. and Christison, G.I. (1990) Environmental effects on thermoregulation and nutrition of horses. *Veterinary Clinics of North America: Equine Practice*, **6**, 355–372

European Commission (2007) Commission recommendations of 18 June 2007 on guidelines for the accommodation and care of animals used for experimental and other scientific purposes. Annex II to European Council Directive 86/609. See 2007/526/EC. http://eurlex.europa.eu/LexUriServ/site/en/oj/2007/l_197/l_19720070730en00010089.pdf (accessed 13 May 2008)

Eustace, R.A. (1990) Equine laminitis. *In Practice*, **12**, 156–161

Eustace, R. A. (1992) *Explaining Laminitis and its Prevention*. R.A. Eustace, Bristol

Higgins, A. J. and Snyder, J. R. (2006) *The Equine Manual*. Saunders Elsevier, Philadelphia

Hintz, H.F. and Cymbaluk, N.R. (1994) Nutrition of the horse. *Annual Reviews of Nutrition*, **14**, 243–267

Home Office (1989) *Home Office Code of Practice for the Housing and Care of Animals in Designated Scientific Procedure Establishments*. HMSO London. 2005 update available at http://scienceandresearch.homeoffice.gov.uk/animal-research/publications/publications/code-of-practice/ (accessed 15th October 2009)

Houpt, K.A. (1991) Animal behaviour and animal welfare. *Journal of the American Veterinary Medical Association*, **198**, 1355–1360

Houpt, K.A. (1992) Horse behaviour. In: *Horse Breeding and Management*. Ed. Warren Evans, J., pp. 63–83. Elsevier, London

Houpt, K. A. and Wolski, T. R. (1982) *Domestic Animal Behaviour for Veterinarians and Animal Scientists*. pp. 172–176. Iowa State University Press, Ames

Jones, R.S. (2001) Editorial II. *British Journal of Anaesthesia*, **87**, 813–815

Joint Working Group on Refinement (1993) First Report of the BVA/FRAME/RSPCA/UFAW Joint Working Group on Refinement. *Laboratory Animals*, **27**, 1–22

Knottenbelt, D. (1995) Euthanasia of horses – alternatives to the bullet. *In Practice*, **17**, 464–465

McAfee, L.M., Mills, D.S. and Cooper, J.J. (2002) The use of mirrors for the control of stereotypic weaving behaviour in the stabled horse. *Applied Animal Behaviour Science*, **78**, 159–173

McGreevy, P.D., Richardson, J.D., Nicol, C.J. *et al.* (1995) Radiographic and endoscopic study of horses performing and oral based stereotypy. *Equine Veterinary Journal*, **27**, 92–95

McGreevy, P.D. and Nicol, C.J. (1998) Prevention of crib-biting: a review. *Equine Veterinary Journal Supplement*, **27**, 35–38

Mills, D.S. and Nankervis, K.J. (1999) *Equine Behaviour: Principles and Practice*. Blackwell Publishing, Oxford

Munro, G. and Young, L. (1991) Standing chemical restraint in the horse. *In Practice*, **13**, 163–166

Nicol, C.J., Davidson, H.P.D., Harris, P.A. *et al.* (2002) Study of crib-biting and gastric inflammation and ulceration in young horses. *The Veterinary Record*, **151**, 658–662

Ott, E.A. (1992) Nutrition. In: *Horse Breeding and Management*. Ed. Warren Evans, J., pp. 337–368. Elsevier, London

Raidal, S.E., Love, D.N. and Bailey, G.D. (1996) Effects of posture and accumulated airway secretions on tracheal mucociliary transport in the horse. *Autralian Veterinary Journal*, **73**, 45–49

Sharp, D.C. (1992) Pregnant mare and Jenny. In: *Horse Breeding and Management*. Ed. Warren Evans, J., pp. 299–323. Elsevier, London

Smith, B.L., Jones, J.H., Carlson, G.P. *et al.* (1994) Body position and direction preferences in horses during road transport. *Equine Veterinary Journal*, **26**, 374–377

Sweeting, M.P., Houpt, C.E. and Houpt, K.A. (1985) Social facilitation of feeding and time budgets in stabled ponies. *Journal of Animal Science*, **60**, 369–374

Toscano, M.J. and Friend, T.H. (2001) A note on the effects of forward and rear-facing orientations on movement of horses during transport. *Applied Animal Behaviour Science*, **73**, 281–287

Thompson, D.L. (1992) Reproductive physiology of the stallions and jack. In: *Horse Breeding and Management*. Ed. Warren Evans, J., pp. 237–261. Elsevier, London

Tyler, S.J. (1972) The behaviour and social organization of the New Forest Ponies. *Animal Behaviour Monograph*, **5**, 5–196

van NieKerk, C.H. (1992) Non pregnant mare and jenny. In: *Horse Breeding and Management*. Ed. Warren Evans, J., pp. 263–297. Elsevier, London

Waran, N.K., Robertson, V., Cuddeford., D. *et al.* (1996) Effects of transporting horses facing either forwards or backwards on their behavior and heart rate. *The Veterinary Record*, **139**, 7–11

Warren Evans, J. (ed) (1992) *Horse Breeding and Management*. Elsevier, London

Webster, A.J.F., Clarke, A.F., Madelin, T.M. *et al.* (1987) Air hygiene in stables I: Effects of stable design, ventilation and management on the concentration of respirable dust. *Equine Veteterinary Journal*, **19**, 448–453

36 Marmosets and tamarins

Hannah M. Buchanan-Smith

Biological overview

General biology

The New World monkeys, of the family Callitrichidae, subfamily Callitrichinae, have seven distinct genera, and include the marmosets and tamarins. These species show a range of interesting pelage forms and colorations; some have ear tufts, others white crests on their heads or a large moustache, and some sport a golden fringe about the face. Why many of these small primates, which are vulnerable to predation by birds, snakes and mammals, are brightly coloured rather than cryptic, is poorly understood. Their small size, combined with their breeding success when housed in an appropriate environment, and easy handling make them a comparatively inexpensive primate to maintain in laboratories. Understanding the natural history and basic adaptations of any species is critical for providing appropriate captive environments, and Rylands (1993) provides excellent reviews of callitrichine ecology, mating systems and behaviour.

Marmoset species

There are 22 species of marmosets in four genera; six species from the Atlantic forest (*Callithrix*), 14 from the Amazonian forest (*Mico*), one species of pygmy marmoset (*Cebuella pygmaea*) and one species of dwarf marmoset (*Callibella humilis*), also from Amazonia (Rylands *et al.* 2000) (Table 36.1). The common marmoset, *Callithrix jacchus*, is the most extensively used callitrichine monkey in laboratory research (eg, Abbott *et al.* 2003; Mansfield 2003), and is therefore discussed in more detail. A full behavioural ethogram has been compiled for this species (Stevenson & Poole 1976; Stevenson & Rylands 1988) and should be consulted.

C. jacchus have large white ear tufts, a brindled black, brown and dark yellow pelage on their back and alternating wide dark and narrow pale bands on the tail. Young animals lack the adult body markings. This arboreal (tree-dwelling) species lives in north-eastern Brazil, occupying a wide variety of habitats such as the lower strata of gallery forests, secondary forests, scrubs, swamps and tree plantations (Hershkowitz 1977; Stevenson & Rylands 1988). Wild marmoset groups occupy a home range of 0.5–6.5 ha, which overlaps with neighbouring groups (Hubrecht 1985; Stevenson & Rylands 1988; Alonso & Langguth 1989; Scanlon *et al.* 1989; Ferrari & Digby 1996). They are classified as Least Concern by the International Union for the Conservation of Nature and Natural Resources (IUCN 2009). Habitat destruction has reduced their original distribution and their numbers have declined (Mittermeier *et al.* 1981, cited in Rylands 1993). However, as they are adaptable, introduced populations are establishing themselves in areas outwith their original range (Rylands 1993).

All marmosets have specialised teeth for gouging trees, by using the lower teeth as a cutting-scoop (Coimbra-Filho & Mittermeier 1976). This enables them to consume the exudates from trees. Tree exudates are a major part of their diet and they have a specialised digestive system adapted for absorbing gum (Power 1996). *C. jacchus* spend up to 15–29% of their daily activity feeding on tree exudate (Maier *et al.* 1982; Alonso & Langguth 1989). In addition, marmosets eat fruits, flowers, insects and other small animals such as spiders, lizards, frogs and snails (Stevenson 1978; Stevenson & Rylands 1988; Rylands & de Faria 1993; Ferrari & Digby 1996). When foraging for insects, marmosets use a stealthy stalk and pounce technique. This foraging style allows them to glean foliage for insects (Rylands & de Faria 1993). Although primarily arboreal, *C. jacchus* will descend to the ground to cross forest clearings and pick up fallen fruits (Stevenson & Rylands 1988).

Tamarin species

Tamarins are distributed throughout the Atlantic and Amazonian rainforest and in the forests of northern South America and southern Middle America. There are four species of lion tamarins (*Leontopithecus*) living in the Atlantic forests and 15 species of tamarins (*Saguinus*) (Rylands *et al.* 2000) (Table 36.1) of which the saddle back tamarins (*S. fuscicollis*), the red bellied tamarin (*S. labiatus*), the moustached tamarin (*S. mystax*) and the cotton top tamarin (*S. oedipus*) are the most frequently used in laboratory experimentation (Rensing & Oerke 2005). These tamarin species are therefore the focus of this chapter. *Saguinus* can be divided into the Amazonian species, and those found in Panama and Colombia. They inhabit primarily tropical lowland humid forests, although some extend into highland forests, and most species adapt well to secondary forests (Snowdon & Soini 1988).

Tamarins are insectivore–frugivores and as such their dentition is not adapted for gnawing like the marmosets, and although they may consume tree exudates they lack the

Table 36.1 Latin name, common name, and conservation status of members the Callitrichidae (from Rylands *et al.* 2000; Groves 2001).

Latin name	*Common name (English)*	*Conservation status*[1,2]
Cebuella pygmaea	Pygmy marmoset	LC
Callibella humilis[3]	Black-crowned dwarf marmoset	VU
Callithrix aurita	Buffy-tufted-ear marmoset	VU
Callithrix flaviceps	Buffy-headed marmoset	EN
Callithrix geoffroyi	Geoffroy's marmoset	LC
Callithrix jacchus	Common marmoset	LC
Callithrix kuhlii	Wied's black-tufted-ear marmoset	NT
Callithrix penicillata	Black-pencilled marmoset	LC
Mico acariensis	Rio Acarí marmoset	DD
Mico argentatus	Silvery marmoset	LC
Mico chrysoleucus	Golden-white tassel-ear marmoset	DD
Mico emiliae	Snethlage's marmoset	DD
Mico cf. *emiliae*[4]	Rondônia marmoset	VU
Mico humeralifer	Black and white tassel-ear marmoset	DD
Mico intermedius	Aripuanã marmoset	LC
Mico leucippe	Golden-white bare-ear marmoset	VU
Mico manicorensis	Manicoré marmoset	DD
Mico marcai	Marca's marmoset	DD
Mico mauesi	Maués marmoset	LC
Mico nigriceps	Black-headed marmoset	DD
Mico saterei	Sateré marmoset	DD
Saguinus bicolor	Brazilian bare-faced tamarin	EN
Saguinus fuscicollis	Saddle back tamarin	LC
Saguinus geoffroyi	Geoffroy's tamarin	LC
Saguinus imperator	Emperor tamarin	LC
Saguinus inustus	Mottle-face tamarin	LC
Saguinus labiatus	Red bellied tamarin	LC
Saguinus leucopus	Silvery-brown bare-face tamarin	EN
Saguinus martinsi	Martin's bare-face tamarin	LC
Saguinus melanoleucus	White saddle back tamarin	LC
Saguinus midas	Golden-handed tamarin	LC
Saguinus mystax	Black-chested moustached tamarin	LC
Saguinus niger	Black-handed tamarin	VU
Saguinus nigricollis	Black-mantled tamarin	LC
Saguinus oedipus	Cotton top tamarin	CR
Saguinus tripartitus	Golden-mantled saddle back tamarin	NT
Leontopithecus caissara	Black-faced lion tamarin	CR
Leontopithecus chrysomelas	Golden-headed lion tamarin	EN
Leontopithecus chrysopygus	Black lion tamarin	EN
Leontopithecus rosalia	Golden lion tamarin	EN
Callimico goeldii	Goeldi's monkey	VU

[1] CR = critically endangered; EN = endangered; VU = vulnerable; NT = near threatened; LC = least concern; DD = data deficient (See IUCN, 2009 for full definitions)

[2] Rylands (2007).

[3] First described as a member of the genus *Callithrix* by van Roosmalen *et al.* (1998) but subsequently placed in its own genus *Callibella* (van Roosmalen & van Roosmalen 2003).

[4] de Vivo (1985, 1991) considered this marmoset from the state of Rondônia to be *Callithrix emiliae* (Thomas 1904). It is in fact distinct and geographically separated (Ferrari *et al.*1999). It is being re-described with a new name (S.F. Ferrari, personal communication).

necessary digestive system adaptations to exploit its nutritional value fully. There are differences in foraging strategies amongst *Saguinus*. Three distinct insect foraging patterns have been described (Garber 1993). The first pattern is shown by *S. oedipus* and *S. geoffroyi* who hunt for insects on thin flexible branches in the low shrub layer of the forest understorey. The second is shown by *S. labiatus*, *S. mystax*, *S. imperator* and possibly *S. midas* who have a similar insect foraging style to the marmosets, exploiting insects on leaves and branches in the lower and middle levels of the forest. Visual scanning plays an important role in the detection of their prey. The third pattern is shown by *S. fuscicollis* and possibly *S. nigricollis* and *S. bicolor*. These species are predominantly manipulative, specific site foragers, concentrating their feeding efforts on relatively large cryptic prey (Garber 1993). For example, orthopteran insects, have been found to make up to 61–67% of the volume of the stomach ingesta in *S. fuscicollis* (Garber 1993). In addition, ripe fruits have been found to account for 20–65% of total feeding time in those species of tamarin studied in the wild (Garber 1993). Plant exudates and nectar are also consumed, the latter principally in the dry season (Garber 1993).

Tamarins, like marmosets, are arboreal, but they are more reluctant to go to the ground. The home ranges vary from 8–120 ha (*S. fuscicollis* – 16–120 ha, *S. mystax* – 30–40 ha, *S. labiatus* – 23–41 ha, *S. oedipus* – 8–10 ha). Their home ranges overlap with neighbouring groups from 13–83% (reviewed in Garber 1993). Classification by the IUCN is Least Concern for *S. fuscicollis*, *S. labiatus* and *S. mystax*, but *S. oedipus* is critically endangered (Table 36.1). Figure 36.1 illustrates *C. jacchus* and the *Saguinus* spp. that are most frequently held in captivity.

Goeldi's monkey

The jet black Goeldi's monkey (*Callimico goeldi*) also belongs to the Callitrichinae, but they differ from marmosets and tamarins in several ways. For example, they have 36 teeth (marmosets and tamarins have 32), and like *Callibella* (van Roosmalen & van Roosmalen 2003) they give birth to just one infant, whilst the norm of other members of the family is twins. As they are not considered to be true marmosets or tamarins they are not discussed further.

Size range and lifespan

The Amazonian pygmy marmoset (*Cebuella*) is the smallest higher primate with both males and females weighing around 128 g (Ford 1994), *Callibella* weighs 150–185 g (van Roosmalen & van Roosmalen 2003), whilst wild-caught *Mico* and *Callithrix* are heavier, weighing 182–357 g (Ford 1994). In the wild, male and female *C. jacchus* weigh approximately 317 g and 322 g respectively (Araũjo *et al.* 2000), but captive individuals have weighed as much as 600 g (Poole *et al.* 1999 and see Prescott & Buchanan-Smith 2004). *C. jacchus* reach puberty before 1 year of age and are skeletally and sexually mature by 2 years (Tardif *et al.* 2006). *Saguinus* are slightly heavier; the average adult body weight for both males and females is 387–560 g (Ford 1994) and can be up to 700 g for captive-bred *S. oedipus* (Savage *et al.* 1993). *Leontopithecus rosalia* weigh from 361–794 g (Ford & Davis 1992). It is not known how long callitrichines live in the wild, but in captivity they have lived to 18 years (Poole *et al.* 1999). However, the average lifespan of *C. jacchus* and *C. kuhli* that lived to weaning in the laboratory is only around 5.7–7.5 years (Tardif *et al.* 2003; Smucny *et al.* 2004; Ross *et al.* 2007a). The age of sexual maturity depends upon sex and species, but is usually 12–24 months (Yamamoto 1993).

Social organisation and reproduction

In the wild, groups of *C. jacchus* usually contain between 3 and 15 individuals (Hubrecht 1984; Scanlon *et al.* 1989; Digby & Barreto 1993; Pontes & Da Cruz 1995). Groups are relatively stable (Ferrari & Lopes Ferrari 1989), although there are immigrations, emigrations, births and disappearances (Arruda *et al.* 2005). Females cycle throughout the year and males copulate with females, even during pregnancy. They ovulate soon after parturition, and can conceive again shortly after birth, when they are still lactating.

In captivity, *C. jacchus* groups are most stable when they consist of a monogamously breeding pair (eg, Gerber *et al.* 2002a, 2002b), and sexual behaviour is inhibited in subordinate females by pheromones, visual stimuli and aggression from the breeding female (eg, Saltzman *et al.* 1997). Occasionally, polygynous mating has been observed in captivity but the groups are less stable than those that consist of monogamous pairs (Rothe & Koenig 1991). In wild populations, monogamous groups have been documented (Albuquerque *et al.* 2001). There have also been numerous cases of two reproductive females in one group (Digby & Ferrari 1994; Digby 1995; Ferrari & Digby 1996; Roda & Mendes Pontes 1998; Arruda *et al.* 2005; de Sousa *et al.* 2005), although breeding is often alternated or one set of offspring does not survive, sometimes due to infanticide by the other breeding female (Digby 1995; Roda & Mendes Pontes 1998). Comparative data on key reproductive parameters for *C. jacchus*, *S. fuscicollis* and *S. oedipus* are shown in Table 36.2. Although some species breed seasonally in the wild (eg, *S. oedipus*) (Neyman 1977), they breed all year round in captivity. There appears to be no menopause, and females will continue to breed throughout their lives. *C. jacchus* that first breed at a later age (>4 years) have better survivorship than those first reproducing when younger (<2.5 years) (Jaquish *et al.* 1991; Smucny *et al.* 2004).

Twin offspring are the norm in the wild, and in addition to the mother, the father and other group members help rear the young by carrying, except for *Callibella* (van Roosmalen & van Roosmalen 2003). They may also provision the young with solid food, a behaviour that may be passive (all species studied) or active as recorded in *S. oedipus*, *Cebuella pygmaea*, *C. flaviceps*, *L. rosalia* and *L. chrysomelas* (see Feistner & Price 1991).

A fascinating twist that may underpin the evolution of co-operative rearing has recently been discovered (Ross *et al.* 2007b) and awaits confirmation. Due to genetic chimerism (when an animal has genetically distinct cells that come from different zygotes and are created by fertilised eggs or embryos fusing together) the patterns of relatedness between twins, and between other family members change. This chimerism applies to marmosets and tamarins with multiple births because in the womb, placentas grow quickly and fuse, creating a network of blood vessels through which cells can travel from one twin to the other. Chimeras may exist in almost any part of the body – blood, hair, liver, and even in sperm and eggs. Therefore, one brother may contribute the genetic makeup of his twin brother's offspring, effectively fathering nephews or nieces! The full implications of this phenomenon have yet to be explored, but in addition to the scientific interest in its role in the evolution of the co-operative rearing system, it may have implications for managing studbooks for optimal outbreeding, and in the selection of individuals for experimental protocols.

Biological data

Rensing and Oerke (2005) provide a thorough overview of basic biological data (including reproductive, physiological, normative haematological and blood chemistry values) in a range of callitrichines. Table 36.3 provides a summary of key data for *C. jacchus*. Infant weights vary depending upon litter size, with mean values of 34.7 g +/− 3.81 (n = 5),

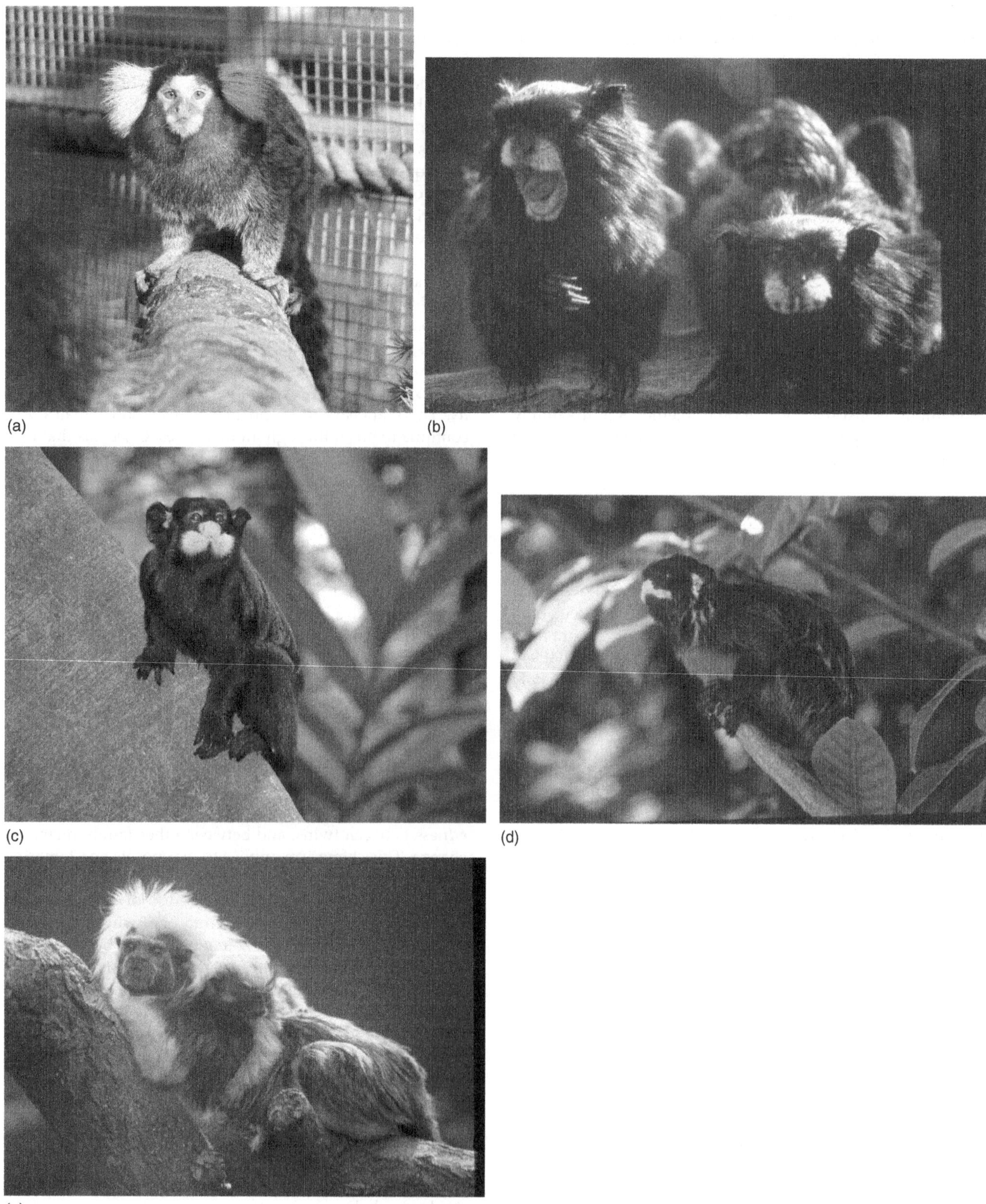

Figure 36.1 Photographs of species of callitrichines most commonly used in the laboratory. (a) *Callithrix jacchus* (common marmoset); (b) *Saguinus fuscicollis* (saddle back tamarin); (c) *Saguinus mystax* (black-chested moustached tamarin); (d) *Saguinus labiatus* (red bellied tamarin); (e) *Saguinus oedipus* (cotton top tamarin). (All photos by Hannah Buchanan-Smith, except (c), courtesy of Julia Diegmann.)

Table 36.2 Comparative reproductive data for *C. jacchus, S. fuscicollis* and *S. oedipus* (Savage 1995; Fortman *et al.* 2002; Rensing & Oerke 2005).

	C. jacchus	*S. fuscicollis*	*S. oedipus*
Sexual maturity (months)	24	26	24
Oestrous cycle length (days)	28	26	21
Gestation (days)	144	150–155	180–185
Post-partum ovulation (days)	10	17–18	17–18

Table 36.3 Summary of key biological data for *C. jacchus* (Ludlage & Mansfield 2003; Rensing & Oerke 2005; Wolfensohn & Honess 2005).

Biological data	*Normal values*
Rectal temperature (°C)	38.6 (day) 36.3 (night)
Heart rate (beats per minute)	230–312 (sedation) 348 +/– 51 (restrained) 230 +/– 26 (unrestrained)
Mean arterial pressure (mmHg) under sedation	65–100 (day) 50–95 (night)
Blood volume (ml/kg)	70
Haematological data	*Normal values*
Red blood cells (RBC) ($\times10^6$/mm^3)	5.7–6.95
Packed cell volume (PCV) (%)	45–52
Haemoglobin (Hb) (g/dl)	14.9–17
White blood cells (WBC) ($\times10^3$/mm^3)	7.3–12.8
Neutrophils (%)	26–62
Lymphocytes (%)	30–67
Eosinophils (%)	0.6–4.2
Monocytes (%)	0.4–5
Basophils (%)	0.1–1.1
Platelets ($\times10^3$/mm^3)	490
Biochemical data	*Normal values*
Serum protein (g/dl)	6.6–7.1
Albumen (g/dl)	3.8
Globulin (g/dl)	2.7–3.9
Glucose (mg/dl)	126–228
Blood urea nitrogen (mg/dl)	51.8
Creatinine (mg/dl)	0.9–1.2
Gamma glutamyl transferase (IU/l)[1]	1.7–9.1 (<2 years) 2.5–10.3 (♂ > 2 years) 0.5–13.3 (♀ > 2 years)
Total bilirubin (mg/dl)	0.4–0.6

[1] Brok, personal communication

30.24 +/– 3.33 (n = 59) and 27.73 +/– 2.03 (n = 30) for singletons, twins and triplets respectively (Tardif & Bales 2004). Growth rates of infants can be divided into an early stage of rapid growth, with a weight gain of around 1.15 g/day for all infants regardless of litter size, followed by a slower, later growth rate which is more variable but averages at 0.81 g/day (Tardif & Bales 2004). Factors affecting growth rates of infants and their adult weight are numerous and interrelated. They include maternal age and weight, and also litter size (Tardif & Bales 2004). Large litters result in high mortality; a meta-analysis of data from five colonies in the Americas (n = 625 dams) reported a mean of 50% loss between number of infants produced, and weaned at 3 months (Smucny *et al.* 2004). A very robust finding is that that triplets and quadruplets, especially if very small (<20 g) have significantly lower survival compared to twins and very large (>35 g) infants which are often singletons (Jaquish *et al.* 1991, 1997). Infant weight has also been shown to be related to abuse (defined as physical injury by other members of the group); abused infants have lower birth weights than non-abused infants (Tardif *et al.* 1998).

Normal behaviour (wild and captive)

All animals should be allowed to express their natural patterns of behaviour in the captive environment. For callitrichines, this includes a range of locomotor and positional behaviours in relation to foraging strategies (eg, gnawing for tree exudate, food capture and processing), social activities (eg, resting, grooming, playing), the opportunity to explore novelty (either new environments, or objects) and having safe and comfortable places to sleep. The type of cage (construction materials and dimensions) and furnishings (substrate types, orientation and its placement) should be designed to allow and encourage specific-specific postures, behaviours and space-use preferences (Buchanan-Smith 2001).

Detailed descriptions of the development of young callitrichines have been described for *C. jacchus* (Stevenson 1976) and *S. oedipus* (Cleveland & Snowdon 1984). Yamamoto (1993) compares behavioural ontogeny across genera. Until infants are 3 weeks old, they are carried all of the time, usually by all group members, but often exclusively by the mother in *Leontopithecus*. By week 4 the infants are showing interest in their environments and beginning to explore, to touch, lick and smell objects, and they leave the carriers' backs for increasing periods of time. If startled, young will try to climb back onto carriers for protection. The first social interactions occur whilst the infants are still on their carrier's backs but after week 8 (week 12 in *Leontopithecus*) they are only carried occasionally. Weaning from lactation occurs from weeks 8–15, although infants taste solid food earlier. Infant development is affected by enrichment (an artificial gum tree, additional shelves, a hanging cloth and a variety of manipulable objects on rotation), with the appearance of certain behaviours (chewing wood, begging towards animal care staff, solitary play, exploration and scent marking) occurring earlier in enriched environments (Ventura & Buchanan-Smith 2003; see also Chapter 10).

Senses and communication

Like other simians, vision is the dominant sensory modality of callitrichines. As both predators and prey, they use sight to detect prey items and potential threats. Their vigilance in captivity likely reflects that care staff may be seen as threats, and alertness has been found to increase after stressful events (Bassett *et al.* 2003). Callitrichines have binocular vision, with overlapping visual fields, and good visual acuity allowing them to manoeuvre themselves safely through complex three-dimensional worlds, judging depth and distance, and to respond to visual stimuli, be they potential threats, conspecifics, or prey items, such as insects. Marmosets perform headcocking where they move their heads in the lateral direction. Young *C. jacchus* headcock more than older marmosets, and often this is in the context of novelty (Stevenson & Rylands 1988). *Saguinus* perform a behaviour termed head flicking by Snowdon and Soini (1988) but it should not be confused with headcocking – head flicking is directed towards conspecifics as a hostile display. *Leontopithecus* will sometimes bob and up and down when staring threateningly (Kleiman *et al.* 1988).

Whilst the Old World monkeys and apes have colour vision that is similar to our own (trichromacy, based on three classes of cone receptors) (Jacobs 1996), callitrichines are polymorphic and show a wide variety of colour vision phenotypes. Females have either trichromatic or dichromatic vision (based on two classes of cone receptors, like humans with red–green 'colour blindness') (Jacobs *et al.* 1993). However, all males are dichromatic. Trichromatic colour vision has been shown to be useful for selecting ripe fruits from unripe and semi-ripe ones, and may also be advantageous for the detection of insect prey and predators (Regan *et al.* 2001; Smith *et al.* 2003; Buchanan-Smith 2005; Jacobs 2007). Individuals with dichromatic vision may not be able to differentiate well between yellows, greens, browns and reds. This has implications for choice of colour stimuli in experiments (Waitt & Buchanan-Smith 2006) and for choosing target colours for positive reinforcement training (Buchanan-Smith 2005).

All callitrichines have a well developed sense of smell, possess specialised scent organs, and have a rich repertoire of chemosignalling behaviours (eg, Epple *et al.* 1993). The most conspicuous of these are scent marking patterns involving the circumgenital and subrapubic glands. Scent marking itself and the chemical signals deposited are important in many areas of their behavioural biology. They contain information on individual identity, rank and reproductive status, and play a role in reproductive suppression of subordinate females. It may also aid territorial defence, intergroup spacing and provide cues as to mate quality (Epple *et al.* 1993). The rate of scent marking in wild *C. jacchus* ranges from 0.19–0.45 scent marks/hour (Lazaro-Perea *et al.* 1999), much lower than is seen in captive conditions, where it exceeds 40 scent marks/hour post-stressor (Bassett *et al.* 2003). Adults scent mark more frequently than young in captivity (de Sousa *et al.* 2006).

Their acute sense of smell, together with taste, assists in food identification and selection. Callitrichines have a very varied diet (eg, Smith *et al.* 2003 found that two mixed-species groups of *Saguinus* consumed fruits from 833 plants from 167 species in 87 genera and 50 families during 164 days of observation!). Providing a variety of nutritional and appetising food is likely to be beneficial for their psychological well-being and is often used as enrichment, but may lead to nutrition-related illnesses in the long term (Plesker & Schuhmacher 2006) (see Feeding/watering).

Callitrichines have a range of high-pitched vocalisations. Several vocal ethograms have been published including that of *C. jacchus* (Stevenson & Rylands 1988); *S. oedipus* (Cleveland & Snowdon 1982); *Leontopithecus* (Kleiman *et al.* 1988); and *Cebuella* (Soini 1988). The long calls, which serve many possible functions, including group defence against intruders, maintenance of group cohesion (eg, reuniting separated group members), and mate attraction, have been studied extensively (Pook 1977; Cleveland & Snowdon 1982; Snowdon 1993). Vocalisations are also important indicators in welfare assessment (Jones 1997). Callitrichines can hear higher frequencies than humans (see Heffner 2004 for a review). Ultrasonic frequencies present in the captive environment, such as a dripping tap, trolley wheels or computer monitors may adversely affect welfare (Clough 1982).

The sensory receptors in the epithelial and connective tissues of callitrichines respond to changes in temperature, touch, pressure and pain. These sensations then guide them in their behaviour. For example, Rumble and colleagues (2005) found that *C. jacchus* choose warmer, 'softer' wooden and plastic nest boxes over metal next boxes. Providing different textures appears to be very rewarding for them (eg, when given a fleece-like hammock, or a technician's lap (Figure 36.2), they will often roll around in it. Tactile contact, through huddling and grooming, develops and maintains affiliative bonds, and may help individuals to cope with stressors (Schaffner & Smith 2005). Grooming plays a role in keeping a healthy skin and coat. Tactile contact when young may be particularly critical and it is known that repeated early parental deprivation of infant *C. jacchus* can have long-term effects on their behaviour and physiology (Dettling *et al.* 2002a, 2002b).

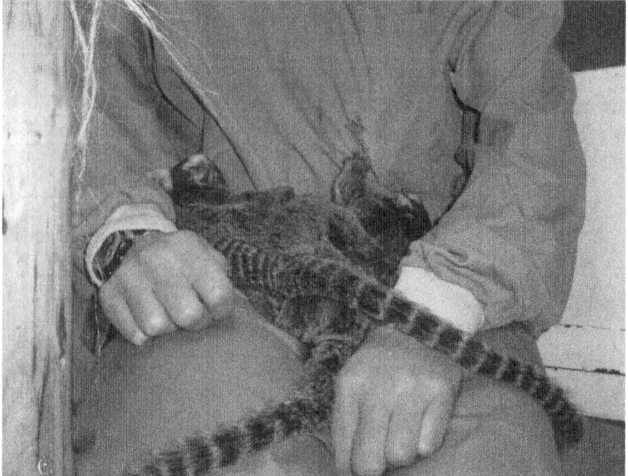

Figure 36.2 Encouraging positive interactions between the monkeys and technicians can be rewarding for both parties. Hands would normally be latex-gloved. (Photo: Hannah Buchanan-Smith.)

Behavioural welfare indicators

Behaviour, postures and vocalisations are the most immediate way to determine good and poor welfare, and it is critical that staff are trained to accurately recognise and assess key indicators, not only to recognise pain and distress, but also to recognise happy healthy animals. It is important that staff are familiar with natural behaviour as a reference point. Significant increases or decreases in natural behaviour should be noted (ie, abnormally high or low) as should the performance of unnatural behaviours. Although there has been a focus on poor welfare indicators in the literature, a callitrichine monkey could be assessed as having good welfare if it appears relaxed (in his/her social group and in the presence of humans) and engages in calm allogrooming, play and exploration. He or she should interact with other group members affiliatively and in social support. A few non-injurious aggressive threats and physical contact may be expected from time to time.

In *C. jacchus*, increases in calm locomotion (relaxed gait) and exploration, and decreased scent marking, scratching, agitated locomotion (but not in play context – may be fast like Stevenson and Rylands' (1988) gallop, or slow, but with piloerection) and inactive inalert behaviour are seen when conditions are improved (eg, access from laboratory cages to outdoor runs) (Badihi 2006). Furthermore, scent marking, scratching, inactive alert (vigilance) and locomotion are known to increase following stressful events (Cilia & Piper 1997; Bassett *et al.* 2003) and these increases are key indicators of reduced welfare. Inappropriate social behaviour, such as excessive grooming, or infanticide, are causes for concern. Abnormal unnatural behaviours exhibited by callitrichines include locomotor stereotypies such as circling and weaving (Hubrecht 1995), head bobbing and self-injurious behaviour (Box & Rohrhuber 1993).

Tail raised-present is displayed in marmosets when threatened (Figure 36.3), and other postures and facial expressions (eg, movements of the ear-tufts and baring of the teeth in open-mouth displays) serve as communication and can be used to monitor welfare (Stevenson & Poole 1976; Stevenson & Rylands 1988). If these behaviours and vocalisations are directed towards care staff on a regular basis, the staff are probably being viewed as predators and efforts should be made to improve the human–monkey relationship as this is arguably one of the most critical factors influencing welfare (Rennie & Buchanan-Smith 2006a).

Sources, supply and transport

There are breeding programmes set up for all callitrichines used commonly in biological and biomedical research. These breeding programmes are often in-house, obviating the need for potentially stressful transport, quarantine and adaptation to a new colony. Breeding in-house also allows socialisation and training specific to their intended future use to begin early. However, some facilities may be too small, or lack expertise required for breeding, and therefore the primates must be transported to them. In these cases, legislation following the international trade in and transport of primates should be followed. A number of publications provide useful information on transport and should be consulted (Wolfensohn & Honess 2005; Joint Working Group on Refinement (JWGR) 2009).

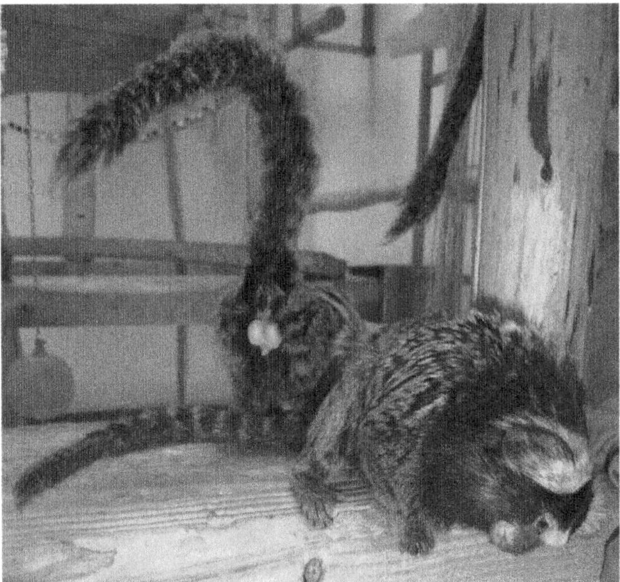

Figure 36.3 A male common marmoset performing a tail-raised present as a threat. (Photo: Hannah Buchanan-Smith.)

If transport between facilities is required, callitrichines should be placed in a ventilated wooden box (a softer quieter environment than metal) with some soft substrate (Poole *et al.* 1999). There should be moist food available (eg, fruit and vegetables) and a window to allow monitoring and to supplement food and water on longer journeys. Familiar conspecifics should be transported together. It poses a serious welfare risk to transport females in late pregnancy. Moreover, females with young infants may attack them, so transportation is not advised. In addition, the separation of offspring under 5 months from their parents is not acceptable during transport (Poole *et al.* 1999). For further information see Chapter 13.

Use in research

Callitrichines are used in a wide range of studies, including: behavioural, reproductive physiology, neuroscience, obesity, ageing, infectious disease, drug development and safety assessment (Abbott *et al.* 2003; Mansfield 2003). *C. jacchus* are frequently used for research on Parkinson's disease (Eslamboli 2005), and *S. oedipus* is used to study colon adenocarcinoma as these animals spontaneously develop colitis and/or colon cancer (Saunders *et al.* 1999).

Laboratory husbandry, management and breeding

Enclosures

Callitrichines need sufficient space to exhibit species-typical locomotor patterns, and to use the vertical dimension, as in the wild they are arboreal and rarely come to the ground. In two-tier cages, monkeys in lower tiers are, by design, denied the use of the vertical dimension. Although few differences have been found in the behaviour of *C. jacchus* housed in upper and lower tier cages measuring 55 cm wide × 95 cm high × 110 cm deep (Buchanan-Smith *et al.* 2002; Badihi 2006), others have reported some differences. Activity is higher in upper-tier *C. jacchus* (Scott 1991) and *S. oedipus* (Box & Rohrhuber 1993) than lower-tier, with the tamarins also exhibiting more close physical contact. Furthermore, the behaviour of *C. jacchus* pairs improves (increases in calm locomotion and inactive rest behaviours and lower levels of agitated locomotion, inactive alert behaviours and watch observer) when they have access to a double enclosure incorporating both upper and lower tiers (Badihi 2006). Numerous other researchers have found behaviour indicative of improved welfare (such as increased play and exploration, and decreased stress-related behaviours) to be present in larger cages (eg, *S. oedipus*, Box & Rohrhuber 1993; *C. jacchus*, Schoenfeld 1989; Kitchen & Martin 1996; Gaspari *et al.* 2000; Pines *et al.* 2002). Given these findings, callitrichines should not be housed in two-tier cages.

Furthermore, light intensity in the lower tiers is reduced in comparison to the upper tiers (Scott 1991; Schapiro *et al.* 2000). Light intensity is known to impact behaviour and to improve reproduction. For example, Hampton and colleagues (1966) found that *S. oedipus* had markedly reduced activity when the light was dimmed, and Badihi (2006) found improvements in the behaviour of *C. jacchus* (eg, increased levels of calm locomotion and social play in youngsters) at higher light intensities. There has also been one report that reproduction in *C. jacchus* decreases at the very low light intensity of 20 lux (Heger *et al.* 1986).

Cages in laboratories generally consist of mobile enclosures (cages mounted on wheels), that can be autoclaved (Figure 36.4). The cages are often made of stainless steel, yet wooden cages provide a quieter environment, and although the wood can be protected from gnawing by wire mesh, they will require more frequent replacement. Ensuring the space is fully utilisable is of critical importance, and thus providing mesh or some climbing structures on solid walls is important. This also applies to the ceiling material, so that the monkeys can hang down and play. A mesh ceiling also allows a greater variety of enrichment to be attached, for example using cable ties or karabiner-type clips. Enclosures that have slide dividers can be very useful as they allow animals to be temporarily separated (for example for veterinary treatment or experiments) whilst maintaining the familiarity within the cage and close contact with the group.

Solid cage floors with sawdust/wood shavings/wood chips are often recommended, as callitrichines will often drop food, but later forage through the substrate for it. Care must be taken to ensure these do not harbour pathogens that might be transmitted between cages. A biofloor, which consists of a 25 cm covering of woodchips over a filterpad, with a concrete floor and drain, functions as a biological system to prevent build-up of pathogens or parasite infestation (Carroll 2002). Faeces may need to be spot cleaned, but urine drains away. The biofloor requires total replacement every 3–4 years and provides excellent continuity of familiar scents for the monkeys and minimises the disruption of regular cleaning.

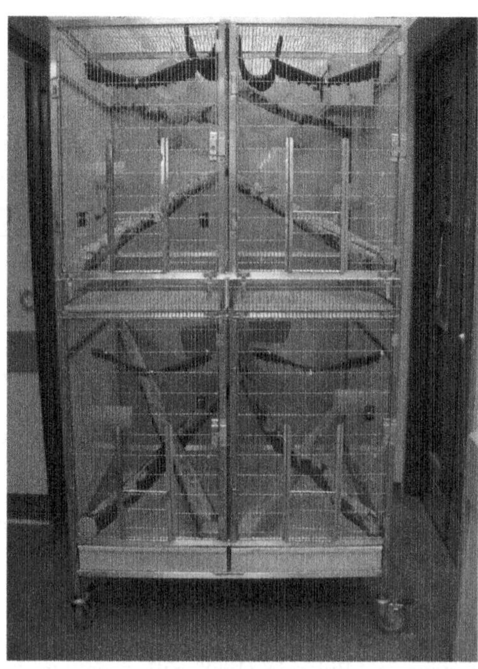

Figure 36.4 Cages on wheels that can be autoclaved easily. Note the rubber matting shelves at the front of the cage, which provide marmosets with good grip and a comfortable place to sit. The nest box is mounted on runners and slides into the cage in the corner. Food dishes are placed on the shelf at the front. (Photo: Keith Morris.)

Specifying cage sizes is highly controversial, given the financial implications. Marmosets and tamarins are generally treated the same, as cage size is usually based upon their body weight (<1 kg; Buchanan-Smith *et al.* 2004; Prescott & Buchanan-Smith 2004). Poole and co-authors (1994) specified a minimum of 1 m^2 floor area for two animals and 0.25 m^2 for each additional animal, excluding carried infants (ie, a floor area of 2 m^2 for a group of eight). The minimum cage height they specified was 1.5 m. However, marmosets and tamarins differ in some critical ways that impact on their welfare and captive conditions (Prescott & Buchanan-Smith 2004). Tamarins are slightly heavier, have larger home ranges (up to 50–100 ha), and longer daily path lengths related to a more frugivorous diet and less dependence on gum-feeding. *Saguinus* have an even greater tendency than marmosets to avoid the ground where they behave nervously. Furthermore, *Saguinus* seem to be more susceptible to developing locomotor stereotypies and to self-injure than marmosets (reviewed in Prescott & Buchanan-Smith 2004). Prescott and Buchanan-Smith (2004) have argued that based on this suite of characteristics, *Saguinus* species should have larger minimum cages sizes in the laboratory than *C. jacchus*. Council of Europe Convention ETS 123 (Appendix A 2006) and the European Commission (2007) have taken this into account specifying a floor area of 0.5 m^2 for *Callithrix* and 1.5 m^2 for *Saguinus* (for one to two animals over 5 months), with a minimum height of 1.5 m, and the top of the enclosure should be at least 1.8 m from the floor. Each additional monkey over 5 months requires an extra 0.2 m^3.

Although prescribed minimum cage sizes are increasing, as noted above, those exceeding current minimum size have been found to improve welfare (eg, *S. oedipus*, Box & Rohrhuber 1993; *C. jacchus*, Schoenfeld 1989; Kitchen & Martin 1996; Gaspari *et al.* 2000; Pines *et al.* 2002). An example of a larger walk in cage is shown in Figure 36.5. The opportunities to engage in locomotion are far greater and the monkeys are known to engage in more solitary play and exploration (Badihi *et al.* 2007). However, care should be taken to ensure continuity for animals who are given larger enclosures, as if animals have to be moved to smaller enclosures there are severe welfare consequences (Schoenfeld 1989; Badihi *et al.* 2007).

Callitrichines scent mark territories and are aggressive to neighbouring groups, so physical or close (<1 m) visual contact between captive groups should be avoided. At the very least, the monkeys should be given choice to avoid visual contact with group mates and neighbouring groups should they wish to, and stability within a colony room should be maintained, so individuals may become familiar with each other. This can be done by providing visual barriers, such as hanging screens within the cage (McKenzie *et al.* 1986). An alternative is to allow monkeys an opportunity to peep through a small hole at a neighbouring group (Moore *et al.* 1991). As the neighbours do not know they are being watched it is unlikely to have any detrimental effects on them.

Turrets or verandas have been used in several colonies, with mixed success. These are mesh additions to the enclosures that permit the monkeys to extend their visual field. Initial use may cause disturbances as animals unfamiliar with each other are able to directly threaten each other visually and vocally. They should not be placed too close so monkeys can physically touch each other. They may have some benefits in increasing predictability of negative events (see Bassett & Buchanan-Smith 2007), as the marmosets will have a better view of what care staff are doing (in relation to cleaning, capture for procedures etc).

Empirical studies have shown that access to outdoor environments has a positive effect the welfare of primates in captivity (eg, Novak & Suomi 1988) and the International Primatological Society (IPS) guidelines (2007) recommend a combination of indoor and outdoor housing, including exercise areas, where possible. Seasonal fluctuations in light and climate may contribute positively to the animals' welfare and allow animals a choice to experience a wider range of sensory stimulation such as sunshine and greater opportunities for exploration and manipulation (eg, Novak & Suomi 1988; Pereira *et al.* 1989; Buchanan-Smith 1998; Pines *et al.* 2007). Free access to warm indoor or sheltered facilities is critical whenever outdoor enclosures are used. *C. jacchus* prefer to spend time outside than in a large indoor enriched enclosure when given access from their home cage (Pines *et al.* 2007) and they engage in more positive welfare behaviours outdoors (including increased play, allogrooming, exploration, rest relaxed and calm locomotion and decreased stress-related scratching and scent-marking) than when housed indoors (Badihi 2006). Care must be taken to minimise the risk of disease transmission from outside vectors.

Environmental provisions

A number of key aspects of the environment promote good welfare. These include the ability to express natural behaviour, and unpredictable positive environmental changes which can elicit an adaptive response from the animal, the opportunities for animals to choose and to facilitate change in the environment, and the perception of control (Sambrook & Buchanan-Smith 1997; IPS 2007; JWGR 2009; and reviewed in Rennie & Buchanan-Smith 2006b).

All callitrichines have claw-like nails to facilitate grip and all cage furnishings should take grip into account (eg, rough surfaces). Locomotion is primarily quadrupedal, but vertical clinging and leaping is seen in several species. Positioning of vertical supports is particularly important for *S. fuscicollis*

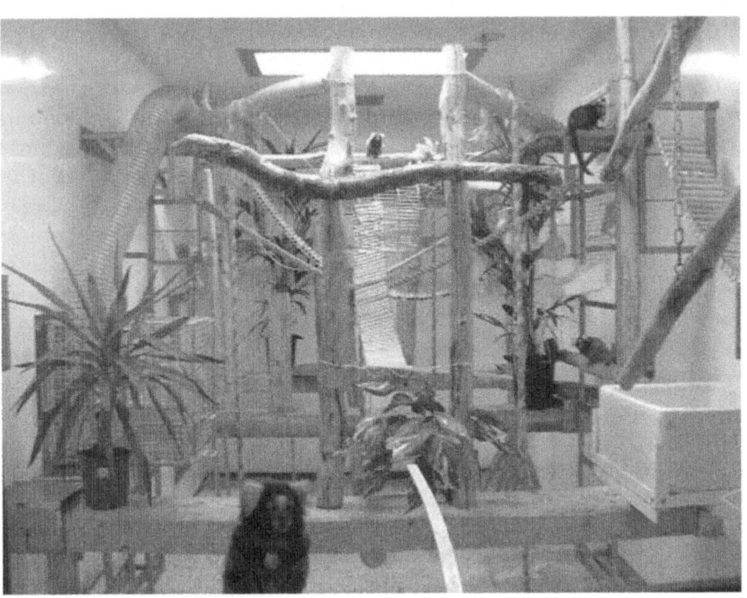

Figure 36.5 An example of a large walk-in enclosure for marmosets. (Photo: Keith Morris)

which locomote extensively by vertical clinging and leaping. To allow full resting, huddling and grooming postures, flat surfaces which several individuals may occupy simultaneously should be provided. These may contain holes, to provide extra grip, and to prevent any puddles of urine from forming.

In the wild, most callitrichines sleep huddled together in tree forks or in dense tangles of vines and leaves and a secure place for sleeping is important in captivity. *Leontopithecus* are unusual in that they primarily use holes in tree trunks and branches as sleeping sites; therefore providing nesting 'holes' in captivity is appropriate. Nest boxes should be provided as they provide comfort and security, as evidenced by reduced vigilance (*S. labiatus*) (Caine *et al.* 1992). Rumble and colleagues (2005) showed that *C. jacchus* prefer wooden and plastic nest boxes over metal ones which may be related to comfort and temperature. They should be placed high in the enclosure. Nest boxes should be well ventilated so that moisture from breathing does not condense and so there is no risk of suffocation.

Feeding/watering

Nutritional status influences growth, reproduction and longevity, as well as resistance to disease and environmental stressors (Knapka *et al.* 1995). Callitrichines have a very varied natural diet, that they have to work hard to get; getting access to food (eg, gnawing at trees to get exudates in marmosets, or removing inedible outer skin of fruits) and using memory (spatial, temporal and seasonal) for returning to fruiting trees. In the wild, they rarely encounter food in great abundance, and often they must search for it, with foraging occupying up to 50–60% of waking time, throughout the day (Garber 1984; Yoneda 1984). Providing a varied, appetitive and nutritionally balanced diet, and ensuring that foraging takes up a significant proportion of the day as it does in the wild, is critical. Food should therefore be made more difficult to find and process, and be provided at several times over the course of the day, taking their natural activity patterns into account. It is especially important to feed in the early morning, and early afternoon as they would in the wild.

Cafeteria-style diets in which commercially available pellets containing the required nutritional constituents are augmented with a range of additional food items, such as fresh or dried fruit, vegetables, seeds, nuts and animal protein (eg, insects, mealworms, hard-boiled eggs and boiled chicken) are often considered to cater well for psychological well-being, being varied and palatable. However, such a diet may lead to nutritional imbalance as pellets are generally not appetitive and callitrichids often avoid them in preference to the other food being offered. One solution to maintain the variability, but reduce nutritional imbalance is to soak the pellets in milk or flavoured juice to soften them and make them more palatable. Another solution is to use agar-based purified diets which are more appetising to marmosets, and have been used successfully (Layne & Power 2003). The National Research Council (NRC) (2003) provides a thorough review of nutrient requirements for primates, and Rensing and Oerke (2005) summarise the key points for callitrichine nutrition. Vitamin D3 is a critical supplement for callitrichines who cannot synthesise it without access to ultraviolet light. Feed supplements, such as yoghurt, are often provided to females in late pregnancy and who are lactating, but there is no evidence that this benefits their offspring. Infants from mothers fed a higher protein diet did not have higher survival, nor growth. Indeed, at 42 days the mean infant body weight of supplemented mothers was less than that of infants of non-supplemented mothers (Layne & Power 2003).

Care should be taken on placement of food dishes. In *S. oedipus*, group members carrying infants were reluctant to approach food dishes placed near floor level. This was remedied by placing food dishes at least 1 m from floor level, whereupon group members carrying infants readily approached food dishes and fed (Snowdon & Savage 1989). Furthermore, by providing a meal in two or more sets of dishes in larger groups, competition between group members may be reduced, and each individual is more likely to get a more varied diet and an equal share of the preferred food items (Price & McGrew 1990).

Food choice and presentation should take their natural feeding adaptations into account. For example *Leontopithecus* and some *Saguinus* species are described as being extractive foragers, and feeding devices fashioned to stimulate these particular foraging skills can be used (eg, hiding food in bromeliads such as pineapple tops). Insects should be included as part of the diet if possible. Given the dental and intestinal adaptation to gum feeding, it is recommended that marmosets are given gum in such a way to encourage gnawing. It is easy to buy commercial gum Arabic that can be syringed onto branches in the enclosure and requires little time to prepare or administer (Kelly 1993).

Fruit is often chopped to ensure an even distribution amongst group members, but leaving skin on bananas, oranges and other fruits increases animal processing time (although fruit should be washed prior to presentation to remove pesticides). Spearing whole fruits on bamboo encourages callitrichines to hang upside down and spend time picking off bits of apple or orange (personal observation) in a similar fashion to how they would forage naturally. A similar technique is to suspend plastic film cases filled with small food pieces on string from the top of the cage.

These foraging techniques are preferable to scattering food items in the wood shavings or other floor coverings, as callitrichines do not go to the ground regularly in the wild, or if they do they are especially cautious as they may be more vulnerable to predation. However, foraging boxes containing a mixture of sawdust with dried fruits, such as raisins, bananas, or mealworms, attached higher in the enclosure work well. Fresh water should be available *ad libitum*, preferably from an automated watering system, as normal laboratory water bottles are potentially a source of infections such as *Pseudomonas* spp. (Brok, personal communication).

Social housing

Housing callitrichines in harmonious social groups is fundamental to their welfare as it allows them to carry out species-specific behaviours and buffers the effects of stressful situations (Schaffner & Smith 2005). Callitrichines (with the exception of *Callibella*) have a co-operative rearing system where the mother generally gives birth to usually twin offspring, and the father and other group members care for the young by carrying, food sharing and perhaps by looking out for predators (Buchanan-Smith 1984; Cleveland & Snowdon 1984; Price 1992). There are many published reports that if offspring are removed from their group before they have had experience with rearing infants, they have a much lower likelihood of raising offspring themselves (*S. fuscicollis*, Epple 1978; *L. rosalia*, Hoage 1977; *S. oedipus*, Cleveland & Snowdon 1984; Snowdon *et al.* 1985; Tardif *et al.* 1984a; *C. jacchus* Tardif *et al.* 1984a). It is recommended that callitrichines should have experience with at least two sets of rearing episodes; otherwise they will not make good parents themselves (Snowdon & Savage 1989). This applies to sons as well as daughters, because fathers as well as mothers care for the young and may be even more important for tamarins than for marmosets (Tardif *et al.* 1984a).

Optimal housing in captivity is in large family groups (up to 8–10 individuals if space allows), giving the offspring the opportunity for good social development. Offspring should not be removed until they are sexually mature. Pairing unfamiliar male and female callitrichines is usually a smooth process, but certain guidelines should be followed carefully (see JWGR 2009). With particular reference to callitrichines, the newly formed pair should be some distance away from the family as reproductive suppression through olfactory cues may still occur. If individuals have to be housed in pairs for experimental reasons, housing familiar siblings or vasectomised male or contracepted female pairs increases the likelihood of compatibility. Unrelated same-sex pairs of *C. jacchus* are often difficult to pair, unless one individual is younger (Majolo *et al.* 2003), or if in same-sexed rooms (Brok personal communication). However, as often they do not affiliate, unrelated same-sex pairs are not recommended (Majolo *et al.* 2003). Disturbance within a colony room should be kept to a very minimum, as the presence of unfamiliar individuals may cause anxiety and even redirected aggression towards group mates. If a parent dies, it is possible to introduce a step-parent, but care should be taken, and the step-parent should be allowed to interact with his/her intended pair mate in the absence of other family members, who may mob the unfamiliar group member (Tardif *et al.* 2003).

Single housing of callitrichines is never recommended unless it is unavoidable for justifiable veterinary or human health reasons. It should be kept to a minimum time and the monkey should be able to see, hear and smell familiar group mates. Although weaning to large same-sex 'gang groups' is relatively common, primarily for ease of management (Buchanan-Smith 2006), this practice is not recommended as it is an unnatural social grouping, and can lead to serious fighting.

Identification and sexing

International guidelines (IPS 2007) recommend that all primates have permanent identification to ensure accuracy as staff change and to permit matching with medical and research records. The best method to permanently identify a primate is using a microchip (Rennie & Buchanan-Smith 2006c; JWGR 2009). The microchip is implanted subcutaneously and holds a unique code which must be read using a scanner. Monkeys previously required sedation before the microchip was inserted under the skin using a specially designed hypodermic needle, usually supplied ready loaded with a microchip. However, the chips are now so small that sedation is not required (Morris, personal communication). For callitrichines, the chip is placed under the interscapular skin. The scanner wand needs to be 5–10 cm away from the chip (Poole *et al.* 1999) for reading. Callitrichids can easily be trained to stay still whilst the microchip is scanned (Savastano *et al.* 2003). Microchips have been known to migrate under the skin leading to a potential reduction in efficiency of identification.

Although marmosets and tamarins may all look pretty identical to the untrained observer, careful observation soon allows individuals to be identified by facial characteristics, size differences and markings. However, in large groups, or in facilities where a large number of callitrichines are kept, and there are regular staff changes, an easy method of accurately identifying individuals is strongly recommended (Fortman *et al.* 2002; Rennie & Buchanan-Smith 2006c). In addition to the benefits of immediate identification to assist with behavioural welfare assessment, it encourages naming individuals which facilitates positive staff–animal relationships to develop (Rennie & Buchanan-Smith 2006a). There are many different methods of temporary identification, including hair dyes, fur clipping (often done on the tail), and high-quality stainless steel ball chain collars with identity tags (Rennie & Buchanan-Smith 2006c). Tags/discs can be coloured and numbered. Dyes must be chosen so as not to cause irritation, especially to youngsters, and care taken to avoid injury with clipping. These methods may last less than a month, but dye can be re-applied without the need for capture and handling (Halloren *et al.* 1989). Collars and tags cannot be used until the animal has stopped growing. Collars and tags must be kept clean, and callitrichines may be trained to accept collar and tag cleaning without restraint.

Sexing of adult callitrichines is easy as males have prominent scrotal sacks, although females also have a pale glandular area around the genitalia and this should not be confused. Sexing young infants is more difficult, but the key differences are illustrated in Figure 36.6.

Record keeping

In order to provide the best care, each monkey should have an individual file or 'passport'. This should include details of their biography (date of birth, sire, dam etc) and their prior experiences (eg, transport history, social groups, training, husbandry system, type of environmental enrichment, research project history and medical history) (see JWGR 2009). This information will assist with analyses of primate care, use and breeding, and to review the adequacy of systems in order to develop good practice (JWGR 2009).

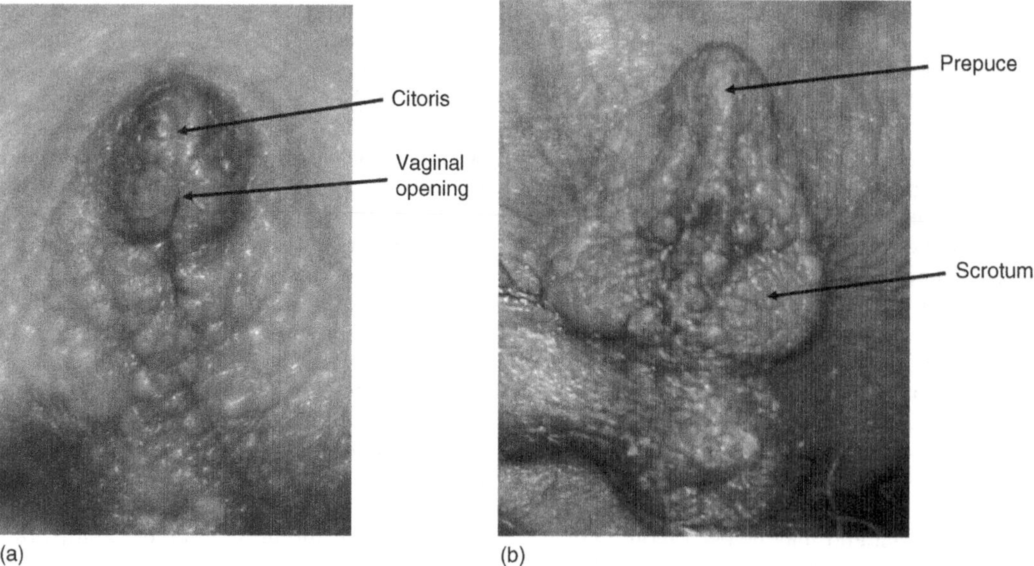

Figure 36.6 The external genitalia of (a) female and (b) male infant common marmosets. (Photos: Hannah Buchanan-Smith.)

Physical environment and hygiene

As callitrichines are tropical primates, they require an ambient temperature of around 23°C (range of 23–28°C) and humidity of 40–70% (Council of Europe 2006). However, they will choose to go outside, often in much cooler temperatures, especially if the sun is shining and they have shelter from the wind. Fluctuations in humidity are not well tolerated by marmosets and tamarins and humidity should be kept higher than 40% as respiratory disorders may result. Callitrichines respond adversely to noise (eg, construction noise). The level of background noise should be kept low and if it is absolutely necessary to exceed 65dBA, it should only be for short periods.

Callitrichines should be kept in hygienic conditions, with regular cleaning to remove stale food, and excreta. Scent marking leads to sticky substrates that can lead to oily coats. A complete cage clean, by autoclave, or by scrubbing using a hot water, domestic detergent and bleach, together with thorough rinsing, should only occur at 1–2-month intervals. Because of the role of scent marking in territorial behaviour, in modulating reproductive physiology and their importance in social interactions, familiar scents should not be totally removed from the captive environments during cleaning. Alternating cleaning and sanitation of enclosures and substrates and enrichment devices will have beneficial effects by maintaining familiarity and reducing over-stimulated scent marking (Prescott 2006).

Health monitoring and quarantine and barrier systems

It is important that callitrichines are checked at least twice daily for changes in behaviour, inactivity, nasal discharge and signs of diarrhoea. Deviations from normality should be marked on a standardised scale to ensure records are accurately kept; Wolfensohn and Honess (2005) provide scales that may be modified to suit callitrichines. Veterinary advice should be sought if non-normal patterns persist, or if the monkeys are listless, remain in their nest boxes, or do not eat. Infants who have fallen to the floor, and have not been picked up by group members, should be examined carefully for injury and disease, but the decision to hand rear should not be made lightly as there are potential problems associated with this (Kirkwood & Stathatos 1992), and hand-reared individuals are unlikely to be suitable breeders or good models for scientific research.

Although callitrichines are commonly bred in-house (Rennie & Buchanan-Smith 2005), occasionally relocation is required. The animal passport should be available to the new facility before the monkeys arrive and every effort should be made to achieve continuity (or in some cases improvement) of care and also help to ensure rapid acclimatisation to the new facility (JWGR 2009). Food should initially be identical or similar to that of the source colony, and changes introduced slowly (Tardif *et al.* 2003). Individuals newly acquired from elsewhere must be quarantined for at least 30 days. The transport to the facility will have caused stress, and extra care must be taken upon arrival to ensure the monkeys are not dehydrated. It also important to ensure continuity of water supply as some animals may not learn a new method of acquiring water (Tardif *et al.* 2003). During quarantine they should receive a thorough health check, including haematology and radiography to check for skeletal problems and tuberculosis (TB) (Poole *et al.* 1999).

There are no national or international standards of personal protective equipment (PPE) for humans interacting with callitrichines, although facilities usually develop their own. The health status/infectious state of the callitrichine dictates the level of PPE, but there are also a number of other considerations, including level of physical contact, staff experience, etc. Staff should wear protective clothing, including face masks if they display any sign of a cough or cold. Particular care should be made to prevent contact with any human with cold sores, due to the herpes virus that can prove fatal.

Breeding

The method of pregnancy testing is generally by abdominal palpation, and pregnancy can be detected from 5 weeks post conception (Kirkwood & Stathatos 1992), although as this can be disruptive and is not recommended on a regular basis. Weight gain and abdominal distension are clear signs of pregnancy in later stages. Ultrasound and urinary hormone measurement may also be used; callitrichines can be trained to accept ultrasound (Savastano *et al.* 2003). Marmosets and tamarins usually give birth at night (between 20.00 h and 07.00 h); if the female shows signs of labour during the day, veterinary intervention may required. During birth the group members gather around the mother and may share in eating the placenta (Stevenson 1976; Price 1990). Although twins are the norm, *C. jacchus* are increasingly producing triplets (or even quadruplets) in captivity, due to their rich diet. This creates some problems for rearing them (see Reproductive problems).

Reproductive success and infant mortality vary quite substantially between facilities, suggesting there are numerous factors associated with successful breeding, including genetic factors, early rearing history, temperament, housing, husbandry and diet. *C. jacchus* are now successfully bred in many facilities, with mortality rates of less than 20% (Prescott & Buchanan-Smith 2004) although a meta-analysis of data from five colonies in the Americas (n = 625 dams) reported a mean of 50% loss between number of infants produced, and weaned at 3 months (Smucny *et al.* 2004). *Saguinus* are more difficult to breed (Tardif *et al.* 1984b), but there is a strong link between quality of captive conditions and breeding success; when they are housed in large complex enclosures and with a group composition resembling those in the wild, they have greater success (reviewed in Prescott & Buchanan-Smith 2004).

Laboratory procedures

Handling

Marmosets and tamarins generally do not like being handled, although with extensive gentle handling and desensitising (with small pieces of treat foods such as gum arabic, grape, raisin or marshmallow) some will tolerate it and a latex-gloved hand can be used. However, to avoid handling they can be trained using positive reinforcement techniques (see Chapter 16) to co-operate with routine husbandry procedures such as capture, weighing, veterinary procedures, oral administration or palpation, or to provide samples for analysis (such as saliva or urine). If there is good reason why they need to be handled, a firm but gentle approach is critical. When possible, callitrichines should be trained, using positive reinforcement techniques, to enter a transport box or Perspex cylinder, and capture by gloved hand from the box will be substantially easier than capture from within the home cage. A detailed illustrated account of how to train marmosets to enter a transport box is provided by Prescott *et al.* (2005). Chasing individuals into nest boxes for capture is not recommended as the nest box should be seen as a safe place to rest, and not associated with any potential stressor (Rennie & Buchanan-Smith 2006c). Removal of a callitrichine from the transport box is best done by opening the door slowly and grasping the monkey around the shoulders as he/she exits. If heavy, the weight of the body should be supported with the other hand and the monkey should remain in an upright position so it can look around, as he/she will likely feel less vulnerable than in a supine position. Movements should be slow, and voices muted. When catching by hand the weight of the glove used must be carefully gauged to ensure that excessive pressure is not applied to the animal and that the handler is sufficiently well protected (Sainsbury *et al.* 1989). Callitrichines may bite the glove, and this has been known to cause dental problems (eg, broken teeth). They should not be left in a transport box for any longer than is absolutely necessary. The monkeys should be returned to their home cage as soon as possible following handling.

If monkeys are being caught within the home cage, the handler should approach calmly and wait until they are stationary, and then grip the part of the tail nearest the body whilst the other hand is placed around the shoulders. This approach is not recommended unless monkeys have been very well habituated to it. If they are being removed from wire mesh great care must be taken to remove their tight grip from the mesh as injuries can occur to their claws. Capture by net is not recommended as it causes fear and distress, can result in injury when the animals are chased around and entanglement during removal from the net. Great care should be taken not to allow individuals to escape as this creates disruption as individuals in other cages in the colony room may attempt to bite them (and have been known to bite off digits). Swift return to the cage should be a priority; if animals are trained they can be enticed back into their home cages with food rewards. However, if they are not, a net may be required as a last resort.

Training/habituation for procedures

Although all methods of restraint can be highly stressful, much of this stress can be eliminated if the method is used sensitively (Fortman *et al.* 2002), and if the callitrichines are desensitised to the procedure, by pairing it with food rewards, and by making the procedure predictable, so they are familiar with what is going to happen.

There is now very good evidence that callitrichines can be trained for a variety of tasks related to husbandry, veterinary treatment, scientific studies and tests of cognitive ability with no need for food or water management (eg, McKinley *et al.* 2003; Savastano *et al.* 2003; Scott *et al.* 2003; Smith *et al.* 2004 and see Prescott *et al.* 2005). Cognitive testing within the home cage is preferred, for welfare and scientific reasons (Scott *et al.* 2003). Temperature is an important indicator of health, and callitrichines can be trained to accept a tympanic thermometer without restraint (Savastano *et al.* 2003). Temperature can also be read remotely in telemetric microchips (reviewed in Rennie & Buchanan-Smith 2006c).

C. jacchus have been trained to stand on a balance for weighing in the home cage (McKinley *et al.* 2003). The initial time investment is not high for this training (between two and twelve, 10-minute training sessions per pair, with a mean of six sessions, see Figure 36.7). If the marmosets were already taking food from the trainer's hand, it took a mean of just two, 10-minute sessions per pair. A comparison with the standard weighing procedure showed that this initial time investment can be quickly recouped. One of the many advantages of training for in-home cage weighing is that it avoids the need for capture and restraint. Poole and colleagues (1999) have suggested that even the weights of carried young can be measured in this way, by weighing the carrier with and without a single youngster on his/her back. Schultz-Darken and co-workers (2004) have described habituation of *C. jacchus* to sling harness restraint for neuroendocrine experiments, and Ferris and colleagues (2001) described habituation for functional magnetic imaging experiments. Restraint devices for sample collection are described later in this chapter.

Monitoring methods

Surgically implanted telemetric devices have been used successfully in non-human primates to collect cardiovascular, blood pressure, temperature, motor, vocalisation, locomotion and pH data, and to record electrocardiograms (ECG), electromyograms (EMG), electroencephalograms (EEG) and electrocorticograms (ECoG) (Kinter & Johnson 1999). There are advantages and disadvantages to the non-invasive externally worn telemetry devices, and partially and fully surgically implanted devices (reviewed in Rennie & Buchanan-Smith 2006c). Fully implanted devices allow multiple subjects to be housed in pairs or groups; working instrumentation has been successfully maintained in *C. jacchus* for up to 2 years (Crofts *et al.* 2001), and used to monitor responses to a range of environments and events (eg, Gerber *et al.* 2002a).

Urine samples allow analyses of accumulation of metabolites, are easy to collect and provide sufficient volume. Marmosets can be trained, in a short period of time, to urinate into a collection vial on request (McKinley *et al.* 2003), or using a similar technique to provide a sample scent mark for analysis (Schultz-Darken 2003). Other methods of urine collection that do not necessitate social isolation have also been documented (Anzenberger & Gossweiler 1993; Smith *et al.* 2004). Steroid and protein metabolites can also be measured in faeces, but lag times must be well understood. Saliva has also been validated for cortisol in *C. jacchus* (Cross *et al.* 2004). The ease with which it is collected from known individuals, and the fact that it allows measurement of currently circulating cortisol, and may be collected at very regular intervals may make it the preferred method of cortisol analysis.

Training callitrichines to accept venepuncture has not been achieved, partially because their small size makes it difficult to access blood vessels, and because of the precision required. However, with training and desensitisation, the stress of capture and restraint can be minimised and thus the overall stress of routine procedures can also be reduced (Greig *et al.* 2006). Restraint devices offer some benefits over conventional handling techniques. First, they allow the procedure to be carried out by just a single person whereas sometimes two or three technicians are involved in manual restraint, one to restrain and the other(s) to carry out the procedure (eg, Hearn 1977; Buchanan-Smith, personal observation). Second, with the restraint device, the animal's movement is quite restricted, for a short period, and the chance of a haematoma and bruising is decreased. There is good back support, and the marmoset is held in an upright position allowing him/her to look around. Third, most marmosets habituate to the device; they appear comfortable and without obvious signs of stress. They accept a food reward following the procedure (Greig *et al.* 2006), and indeed food rewards should be offered following all procedures to desensitise them. Figure 36.8 shows *C. jacchus* in a restraint device.

Blood sampling requires a short, 0.4–0.5 mm diameter (25–27 g) needle, with a small 1–2.5 ml syringe (Poole *et al.* 1999). Single blood samples of up to 0.5 ml/100 g body

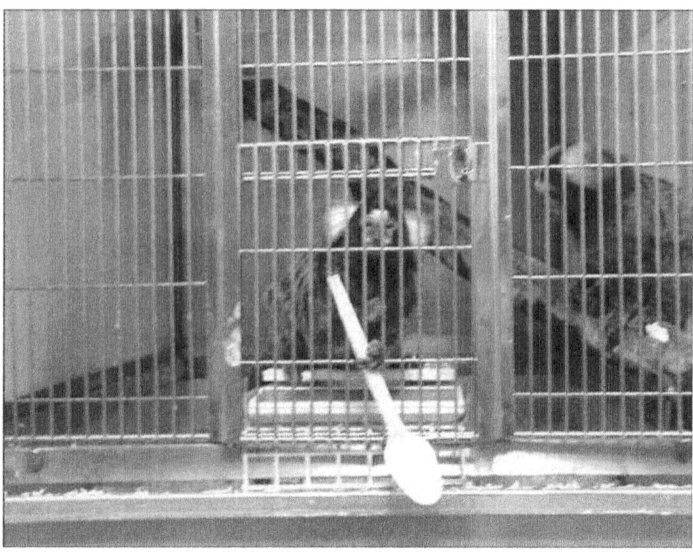

Figure 36.7 A marmoset holding a target (plastic spoon), whilst sitting on scales for in-home cage weighing. (Photo: Jean McKinley.)

weight can be taken safely (Poole *et al.* 1999). If repeated sampling is required, no more than 15% of total blood volume should be taken per month (Diehl *et al.* 2001), approximating to 3.7ml per month for a 350g marmoset (Poole *et al.* 1999). However, this must be monitored closely to check for normal cell composition and haemoglobin concentration, and iron supplements should be given (Poole *et al.* 1999).

Greig and co-workers (2006) describe the procedure for blood collection from the femoral vein. The leg should be held straight by curling fingers around the length of the leg to ensure that the animal cannot bend at the knee or kick. The thumb provides extra restraint and support to the syringe. The syringe needle should be inserted at an angle of approximately 15° into the groove midway down the leg, the thumb can be used as a guide. The vein or the groove is not always visible in heavier animals so the midpoint should be used. The syringe plunger should be slowly pulled back just after insertion of the needle point, to ensure that it has entered the vein. If correctly inserted blood should flow back into the syringe, if not then the needle should be inserted further until blood is seen entering the needle hub. There should be no further insertion of the needle at this point. The plunger should be pulled slowly until the appropriate volume is acquired. Schultz-Darken (2003) also provides details of blood sampling from a restraint device, and advice on an intravenous femoral catheter for repeated blood sampling and a jugular vein catheter for longer-term sampling over several hours.

A restraint device can also be used for collection of semen from mated females (details in Greig *et al.* 2006), and is seen as a refinement over other methods of sperm collection such as electro-ejaculation. Schultz-Darken (2003) describes a procedure for collecting semen using vibratory stimulation whilst the male marmoset is restrained.

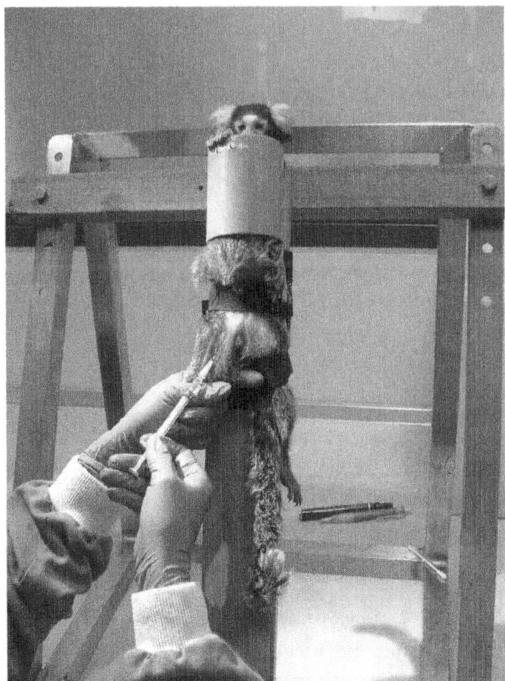

Figure 36.8 A marmoset in a restraint device, showing the plastic tube and Velcro straps, having a blood sample taken from the femoral vein. (Photo: by Keith Morris, from Greig *et al.* 2006.)

Administration of substances

The substance to be administered and the route of its administration are determined to a great extent by the objectives of the experimental procedure concerned. A thorough review of refinement techniques for administration of substances has been provided by the BVAAWF/FRAME/RSPCA/UFAW working party (JWGR 2001). Oral administration by gavage requires careful restraint because poor placement of the tube (into the trachea rather than the oesophagus or the top of the stomach) has the potential to harm or kill the subject animal, and marmoset teeth are delicate and easily damaged. A small soft plastic tube can be used to keep the mouth open. It is preferable to incorporate substances into treat feeds (such as marshmallows) or favoured fluids, a method considered to have minimal impact on the animal (JWGR 2001). If the callitrichine will not eat, the solution can be fed into the mouth with syringe. Subcutaneous injections are best administered into the loose skin above the shoulders, and the upper thigh is suitable for intramuscular injection (Poole *et al.* 1999). Intravenous injections should be performed into the saphenous vein (or caudal vein) which are preferred over the femoral vein as the neighbouring femoral artery can be injected accidentally; Bakker, personal communication).

Anaesthesia/analgesia

Ketamine (a dissociative anaesthetic) is the most commonly used anaesthetic agent for marmosets and tamarins. Dosage depends upon depth of anaesthesia required. Poole and colleagues (1999) recommend 5–15mg/kg by intramuscular injection for mild restraint such as fitting identity collars, although muscle relaxation is often poor. Rensing and Oerke (2005 and Rensing, personal communication), recommend up to 50mg/kg for surgical procedures (combined with a potent analgesic) with a maximum of 25mg/animal due to myotoxicity. To improve muscle relaxation, Poole and colleagues (1999) recommend a combination of ketamine and xylazine at a dose rate of 10–15mg/kg ketamine and 1.5mg/kg xylazine. Further they and Rensing (personal communication) recommend a ketamine/medetomidine mixture (3mg/kg ketamine with 0.05mg/kg medetomidine given intramuscularly) as this has the advantage of being reversed by administration of atipamezole intravenously or intramuscularly. In order to maintain general anesthesia, inhalation of the narcotic gaseous anaesthetic isofluorane can be used, delivered via a modified endotracheal tube (2.0mm) or with a face mask (Rensing & Oerke 2005). Recovery time is fast (Morris, personal communication).

Rensing and Oerke (2005) recommend Saffan® (new trade name is Alfaxan-CD RTU), of which the active constituents are alphaxalone and alphadolone, as a safer alternative to ketamine (dose rate: 18mg/kg) to induce anaesthesia. Poole and co-authors (1999) note this has to be incremented at 30–60-minute intervals to maintain effect. For longer surgery

Rensing and Oerke (2005) note that a combination of Saffan® (8mg/kg) and diazepam (0.25mg/animal) is reliable in *C. jacchus*; and ketamine (25mg/kg) and midazolam (25mg/kg) can be used for *S. oedipus*. Morris (personal communication) recommends buprenorphine (10–20μg/kg or 0.03–0.06ml/kg) for longer analgesia and post-operative pain relief and carpofen (4mg/kg administered subcutaneously) for short-term analgesia before surgery. It is important to keep the monkey warm during anaesthesia and surgery. This can be achieved using heat lamps or heat pads, or using an operating table with a built-in thermoregulator in the table surface. It is critical to monitor anaesthesia carefully to prevent deaths and ensure safe recovery. For further advice see Flecknell (2009).

Euthanasia

Euthanasia is required if animals are found to experience an unacceptable level of pain or suffering (specified humane endpoints), when the project requires pathology or histology examination of organs or tissues, or at the end of an experiment if they cannot be re-used (as outlined in the project licence). An overdose of an anaesthetic agent, pentobarbital (also known as sodium pentobarbital, a barbiturate formulated for euthanasia) by intraveneous injection is the only acceptable method for the euthanasia of marmosets and tamarins (Poole *et al.* 1999; Rennie & Buchanan-Smith 2006c; IPS 2007). It is recommended that animals lose consciousness rapidly following injection, prior to the loss of motor function, and that no signs of pain, distress or panic should be observed (JWGR 2009). This is the case when using intraveneously injected pentobarbital. Poole and coworkers (1999) and Morris (personal communication) recommend that ketamine is injected intramuscularly, to induce anaesthesia, and to mitigate the stress of handling for intravenous injection of pentobarbital. Suitable prior anaesthesia will facilitate accurate administration of pentobarbital, as extravascular injection causes irritation and may be painful. Under certain circumstances such as severe cardiac or circulatory deficiencies (eg, shock, intensive blood sampling prior to euthanasia), intracardiac injection on a deeply sedated animal may be preferred to intravenous injection (Bakker, personal communication).

Common welfare problems

Health

If kept permanently indoors, immunoprophylaxis is generally not required for animals if housing and husbandry are appropriate and they are provided with nutritionally balanced diets. If callitrichines have access to outside runs, they will require protection against *Yersinia* and *Salmonella* bacteria and other infections which can be carried in bird droppings (Poole *et al.* 1999).

Signs of illness include changes in activity, often listlessness including lack of alertness, a reduction in body weight, poor coat condition, diarrhoea and withdrawal from group mates. In relation to body weight, in a study of the effects of chronic psychosocial stress in *C. jacchus*, Johnson and colleagues (1996) observed a 10% drop in body weight in individuals taken from stable pairings and placed in isolation and considered this to be indicative of considerable social stress. This was accompanied by an increase in locomotion and cringing behaviours and in crying vocalisations. Acceptable boundaries of weight loss or gain, within which the welfare of the individual is protected have not been deduced specifically for marmosets. However, persistent anorexia resulting in a loss of 10% or more of the animal's original weight is considered to signify unacceptable suffering and has been used as a humane endpoint in parasitological studies in baboons (Farah *et al.* 2001). Fluctuating body weight (in contrast to a stable body weight) in adults is also a useful indicator of poor welfare.

Callitrichines can be infected with a range of parasites, gut bacterial and viral infections and well as non-infections diseases. A very brief summary of the main diseases is provided here; further details can be found in Bennett *et al.* (1998) and Potkay (1992). Rensing and Oerke (2005) provide a summary of symptoms and details of treatment.

In the wild, callitrichines may have several parasitic infections, but these are rarely seen in captivity. Acanthocephala (*Prosthenorchis* spp.) is an exception, in colonies where cockroaches are present. It can be fatal. Other parasites reported include *Rictulria nycticebus*, *Giardia lamblia*, *Balantidium* and *Entamoeba* spp., and *Toxoplasma gondii*. Of the bacterial diseases, *Shigella*, *Yersina pseudotuberculosis* and *Y. enterocolitica*, *Klebsiella* spp. and *Bordetella bronchiseptica* are those that cause the greatest concern. *Campylobacter* spp., *Salmonella* spp. and *Escherichia coli* can also have severe consequences. As mentioned above, the viral infection of the human herpes simpex or hominis virus can be fatal. Herpes saimiri and tamarinus have squirrel monkeys (*Saimiri*) as reservoir hosts and great care should be taken to avoid exposure (eg, though saliva, bite wounds, and on capture nets and gloves).

Wasting marmoset syndrome (WMS) used to be a common killer of captive marmosets, but is no longer frequently observed. Its aetiology is still poorly understood but it may be associated with stress, malnutrition (too much fruit, protein deficiency), parasitic, bacterial, viral infections or colitis (Sainsbury *et al.* 1987; Rensing & Oerke 2005). Haemosiderosis (a deposit of iron pigment haemosiderin in the liver) has been found in marmosets with WMS (Miller *at al.* 1997).

Behavioural

If physical and social housing conditions are good, callitrichines rarely behave abnormally. However, hand-rearing may lead to a variety of behavioural abnormalities (Kirkwood & Stathatos 1992), and single housing may lead to locomotor stereotypies such as circling or weaving in *C. jacchus* (Hubrecht 1995). Prescott and Buchanan-Smith (2004) argue that *Saguinus* may be more predisposed to develop such abnormal behaviour than marmosets; head bobbing and self-inflicted trauma has been reported in *S. oedipus* (Box & Rohrhuber 1993; Savage 1995) and *S. labiatus* (Buchanan-Smith, personal observation).

Reproductive problems

The increase in triplet and quadruplet births in captivity is potentially problematic. The increase in multiple births is related to weight gain in *C. jacchus* although the mechanism is not understood (Tardif & Jaquish 1997). Multiple births can lead to problems during pregnancy and birth complications (such as transverse presentation of the foetus, lameness in the pregnant female, hydrocephalus or a dead embryo blocking the cervix) (Poole *et al.* 1999). Infanticide rarely occurs in captivity, although occasionally part of an infant's tail will be bitten off. Breeding should cease from tail-biters as this behaviour appears to be passed from generation to generation.

Although, occasionally, the family will rear triplets without human intervention, often this is not the case and the weakest may fall to the floor. Hand rearing of infants is possible but the infants must be reintroduced into a conspecific group as soon as possible to minimise the serious adverse effects of separation from their natal groups. The practice of rotational hand rearing, when two infants are reared by the family group and one is human reared, has been used to reduce mortality. However it requires the animal care staff to disturb the group on a regular basis, to replace and remove an infant, and each offspring will be subjected to period of separation, which is known to influence behaviour and physiology (Dettling *et al.* 2002a, 2002b). The impact of this practice on future reproductive success, and on the suitability as models for scientific research has not been determined but it is likely to have an adverse effect (Buchanan-Smith 2006). A better practice for successfully rearing triplets may be to provide supplementary feeding to the infants whilst they remain in the family group, or to cross-foster the infants to surrogate *C. jacchus* parents, who are well experienced and on contraception. This latter practice has proved highly successful in one laboratory, reducing mortality (Morris, personal communication).

Acknowledgments

The author would like to thank the many people who have discussed issues concerning keeping marmosets and tamarins in captivity, but in particular Hilary Box, Robert Hubrecht, Mark Prescott, Rob Rumble, Herbert Brok, Jaco Bakker, Susanne Rensing, Jean McKinley, Lois Bassett and Keith Morris and his staff at the MRC Human Reproductive Sciences Unit, Edinburgh, where several of the photos were taken. The author is most grateful to Anthony Rylands who provided to most up-to-date advice on taxonomy and to the anonymous reviewers whose constructive comments improved the chapter. Thanks also go to Lou Tasker and Inbal Badihi for their excellent editorial help.

References

Abbott, D.H., Barnett, D.K., Colman, R.J. *et al.* (2003) Aspects of common marmoset basic biology and life history important for biomedical research. *Comparative Medicine*, **53**, 339–350

Albuquerque, A.C.S.R., Sousa, M.B.C., Santos, H.M. *et al.* (2001) Behavioral and hormonal analysis of social relationships between oldest females in a wild monogamous group of common marmosets (*Callithrix jacchus*). *International Journal of Primatology*, **22**, 631–645

Alonso, C. and Langguth, A. (1989) Ecology and behavior of *Callithrix jacchus* (Primates: Callitrichidae) living on an Atlantic forest island. *Revista Nordestina de Biologia*, **6**, 105–137

Anzenberger, G. and Gossweiler, H. (1993) How to obtain individual urine samples from undisturbed marmoset families. *American Journal of Primatology*, **31**, 223–230

Ara jo, A., Arruda, M.F., Alencar, A.I. *et al.* (2000) Body weight of wild and captive common marmosets (*Callithrix jacchus*). *International Journal of Primatology*, **21**, 317–324

Arruda, M.F., Araujo, A., Sousa, M.B.C. *et al.* (2005) Two breeding females within free-living groups may not always indicate polygyny: alternative subordinate female strategies in common marmosets (*Callithrix jacchus*). *Folia Primatologica*, **76**, 10–20

Badihi, I. (2006) The effect of complexity, choice and control on the behaviour and the welfare of captive common marmosets (*Callithrix jacchus*). PhD thesis, University of Stirling, Scotland, https://dspace.stir.ac.uk/dspace/bitstream/1893/120/1/Badihi%20PhD.pdf (accessed 30 April 2008)

Badihi, I., Morris, K. and Buchanan-Smith, H.M. (2007) The effects of increased space, complexity, and choice, together with their loss, on the behavior of a family group of *Callithrix jacchus*: a case study. *Laboratory Primate Newsletter*, **46**, 1–5

Bassett, L. and Buchanan-Smith, H.M. (2007) Effects of predictability on the welfare of captive primates. In: *Animal Behaviour, Conservation and Enrichment*. Ed. Swaisgood, R.R. *Applied Animal Behaviour Science*, **102**, 223–245

Bassett, L., Buchanan-Smith, H.M., McKinley, J. *et al.* (2003) Effects of training on stress-related behavior of the common marmoset (*Callithrix jacchus*) in relation to coping with routine husbandry procedures. *Journal of Applied Animal Welfare Science*, **6**, 221–233

Bennett, B.T., Abee, C.R, and Henrickson, R. (eds) (1998) *Non-Human Primates in Biomedical Research*, Vol. II (Diseases). Academic Press, San Diego

Box, H.O. and Rohrhuber, B. (1993) Differences in behaviour among adult male, female pairs of cotton-top tamarins (*Saguinus oedipus*) in different conditions of housing. *Animal Technology*, **44**, 19–30

Buchanan-Smith, H.M. (1984) Preliminary report on infant development of the black-tailed marmoset *Callithrix argentata melanura* at the Jersey Wildlife Preservation Trust. *Dodo: Journal of the Jersey Wildlife Preservation Trust*, **21**, 57–67

Buchanan-Smith, H. M. (1998) Enrichment of marmosets and tamarins – considerations for the care of captive callitrichids. In: *Guidelines for Environmental Enrichment*. Ed. Field, D.A., pp. 183–201. Top Copy, Bristol

Buchanan-Smith, H.M. (2001) Species-specific housing and husbandry for marmosets and tamarins (Callitrichinae). *Proceedings of the 4th International Conference on Environmental Enrichment*, pp. 95–105. The Shape of Enrichment Inc., San Diego

Buchanan-Smith, H.M. (2005) Recent advances in color vision research. *American Journal of Primatology*, **67**, 393–398

Buchanan-Smith, H.M. (2006) Primates in laboratories: standardisation, harmonisation, variation and Science. *ALTEX – Alternatives to Animal Experimentation*, **23**, 115–119

Buchanan-Smith, H.M., Prescott, M.J. and Cross, N.J. (2004) What factors should determine cage sizes for primates in the laboratory? *Animal Welfare*, **13**, S197–S201

Buchanan-Smith, H.M., Shand, C. and Morris, K. (2002) Cage use and feeding height preferences of captive common marmosets (*Callithrix jacchus*) in two-tier cages. *Journal of Applied Animal Welfare Science*, **5**, 139–149

Caine, N.G., Potter, M.P. and Mayer, K.E. (1992) Sleeping site selection by captive tamarins (*Saguinus labiatus*). *Ethology*, **90**, 63–71

Carroll, B. (Ed.) (2002) *EAZA Husbandry Guidelines for the Callitrichidae.* Bristol Zoo Gardens, Bristol

Cilia, J. and Piper, D.C. (1997) Marmoset conspecific confrontation: an ethologically-based model of anxiety. *Pharmacology Biochemistry and Behavior*, **58**, 85–91

Cleveland, J. and Snowdon, C.T. (1982) The complex vocal repertoire of the adult cotton-top tamarin (*Saguinus oedipus oedipus*). *Zeitschrift Fuer Tierpsychologie*, **58**, 231–270

Cleveland, J. and Snowdon, C.T. (1984) Social development during the first twenty weeks in the cotton-top tamarin (*Saguinus o. oedipus*). *Animal Behaviour*, **32**, 432–444

Clough, G. (1982) Environmental effects on animals used in biomedical research. *Biological Reviews of the Cambridge Philosophical Society*, **57**, 487–523

Coimbra-Filho, A.F. and Mittermeier, R.A. (1976) Exudate-eating and tree-gouging in marmosets. *Nature*, **262**, 630

Council of Europe (2006) *Multilateral Consultation of Parties to the European Convention for the Protection of Vertebrate Animals used for Experimental and other Scientific Purposes (ETS 123) Appendix A. Cons 123 (2006) 3.* Available from URL: http://www.coe.int/t/e/legal_affairs/legal_co-operation/biological_safety,_use_of_animals/laboratory_animals/2006/Cons123(2006)3AppendixA_en.pdf (accessed 30 April 2008)

Crofts, H.S., Wilson, S., Muggleton, N.G. *et al.*. (2001) Investigation of the sleep electrocorticogram of the common marmoset (*Callithrix jacchus*) using radiotelemetry. *Clinical Neurophysiology*, **112**, 2265–2273

Cross, N., Pines, M.K. and Rogers, L.J. (2004) Saliva sampling to assess cortisol levels in unrestrained common marmosets and the effect of behavioral stress. *American Journal of Primatology*, **62**, 107–114

Dettling, A.C., Feldon, J. and Pryce, C.R. (2002a) Repeated parental deprivation in the infant common marmoset (*Callithrix jacchus*, Primates) and analysis of its effects on early development. *Biological Psychiatry*, **52**, 1037–1046

Dettling, A.C., Feldon, J. and Pryce, C.R. (2002b) Early deprivation and behavioral and physiological responses to social separation/novelty in the marmoset. *Pharmacology, Biochemistry and Behavior*, **73**, 259–269

de Vivo, M. (1985) On some monkeys from Rondônia, Brasil (Primates: Callitrichidae, Cebidae). *Papéis Avulsos de Zoologia (São Paulo)*, **4**, 1–31

de Vivo, M. (1991) *Taxonomia de Callithrix Erxleben, 1777 (Callitrichidae, Primates).* Fundação Biodiversitas, Belo Horizonte

Diehl, K.H., Hull , R., Morton, D. *et al.* (2001) A good practice guide to the administration of substances and removal of blood, including routes and volumes. *Journal of Applied Toxicology*, **21**, 15–23

Digby, L. (1995) Infant care, infanticide, and female reproductive strategies in polygynous groups of common marmosets (*Callithrix jacchus*). *Behavioral Ecology and Sociobiology*, **37**, 51–61

Digby, L.J. and Barreto, C.E. (1993) Social organization in a wild population of *Callithrix jacchus*. I. Group composition and dynamics. *Folia Primatologica*, **61**, 123–134

Digby, L.J. and Ferrari, S.F. (1994) Multiple breeding females in free-ranging groups of *Callithrix jacchus*. *International Journal of Primatology*, **15**, 389–397

Epple, G. (1978) Reproductive and social behavior of marmosets with special reference to captive breeding. *Primates in Medicine*, **10**, 50–62

Epple, G., Belcher, A.M., Kuederling, I. *et al.* (1993) Making sense out of scents: species differences in scent glands, scent-marking behaviour, and scent-mark composition in the Callitrichidae. In: *Marmosets and Tamarins: Systematics, Behaviour, and Ecology*. Ed. Rylands A.B., pp. 123–151. Oxford University Press, Oxford

Eslamboli, A. (2005) Marmoset monkey models of Parkinson's disease: which model, when and why? *Brain Research Bulletin*, **68**, 140–149

European Commission (2007) Commission recommendations of 18 June 2007 on guidelines for the accommodation and care of animals used for experimental and other scientific purposes. Annex II to European Council Directive 86/609 See 2007/526/EC. http://eurlex.europa.eu/LexUriServ/site/en/oj/2007/l_197/l_19720070730en00010089.pdf (accessed 13 May 2008)

Farah, I.O., Kariuki, T.M., King, C.L. *et al.* (2001) An overview of animal models in experimental schistosomiasis and refinements in the use of non-human primates. *Laboratory Animals*, **35**, 205–212

Feistner, A.T.C. and Price, E.C. (1991) *Food offering in New World primates: two species added. Folia Primatologica*, **57**, 165–168

Ferrari, S.F. and Digby, L.J. (1996) Wild *Callithrix* groups: stable extended families? *American Journal of Primatology*, **38**, 19–27

Ferrari, S.F. and Lopes Ferrari, M.A. (1989) A re-evaluation of the social organization of the Callitrichidae, with reference to the ecological differences between genera. *Folia Primatologica*, **52**, 132–147.

Ferrari, S. F., Sena, L. and Schneider, M.P.C. (1999). Definition of a new species of marmoset (Primates: Callithrichinae) from southwestern Amazonia based on molecular, ecological, and zoogeographic evidence. In: *Livro de Resumos, IX Congresso Brasileiro de Primatologia*, pp. 80–81. Santa Teresa, Espírito Santo, Brazil, 25–30 July 1999

Ferris, C.F., Snowdon, C.T., King, J.A., *et al.* (2001) Functional imaging of brain activity in conscious monkeys responding to sexually arousing cues. *Neuroreport*, **12**, 2231–2236

Flecknell, P.A. (2009) *Laboratory Animal Anaesthesia*, 3rd edn. Academic Press, London

Ford, S.M. (1994) Evolution of sexual dimorphism in body weight in platyrrhines. *American Journal of Primatology*, **34**, 221–244

Ford, S.M. and Davis, L.C. (1992) Systematics and body size: implications for feeding adaptations in New World monkeys. *American Journal of Physical Anthropology*, **88**, 415–468

Fortman, J.D., Hewett, T.A. and Taylor-Bennet, B. (2002) *The Laboratory Non-human Primate*. CRC Press Ltd, Florida

Garber, P.A. (1984). Use of habitat and positional behavior in a neotropical primate, *Saguinus oedipus*. In: *Adaptations for Foraging in Nonhuman Primates*. Eds Rodman P.S. and Cant J.G.H., pp. 112–133. Columbia University Press, New York

Garber, P.A. (1993) Feeding ecology and behaviour of the genus *Saguinus*. In: *Marmosets and Tamarins: Systematics, Behaviour, and Ecology*. Ed. Rylands A.B., pp. 273–295. Oxford University Press, Oxford

Gaspari, F., Perretta, G. and Schino, G. (2000) Effects of different housing systems on the behaviour of the common marmoset (*Callithrix jacchus*). *Folia Primatologica*, **71**, 291 (abstract)

Gerber, P., Schnell, C.R. and Anzenberger, G. (2002a) Behavioral and cardiophysiological responses of common marmosets (*Callithrix jacchus*) to social and environmental changes. *Primates*, **43**, 201–216

Gerber, P., Schnell, C.R. and Anzenberger, G. (2002b) Comparison of a beholder's response to confrontations involving its pairmate or two unfamiliar conspecifics in common marmosets (*Callithrix jacchus*). *Evolutionary Anthropology*, **11** (Suppl. 1), 117–121

Greig, I., Morris, K.D., Mathiesen, E. *et al.* (2006) An improved restraint device for infections and collection of samples from marmosets. *Laboratory Primate Newsletter*, **45**, 1–5

Groves, C.P. (2001) *Primate Taxonomy*. Smithsonian Institution Press, Washington, DC

Halloren, E., Price, E.C. and McGrew, W.C. (1989) Technique for non-invasive marking of infant primates. *Laboratory Primate Newsletter*, **28**, 13–15

Hampton, J.K., Hampton, S.H. and Landwehr, B.T. (1966) Observations on a successful breeding colony of the marmoset, *Oedipomidas oedipus*. *Folia Primatologica*, **4**, 265–287

Hearn, J.P. (1977) Restraining device for small monkeys. *Laboratory Animals*, **11**, 261–262

Heffner, R.S. (2004) Primate hearing from a mammalian perspective. *Anatomical Record*, **281A**, 1111–1122

Heger, W., Merker, H.J. and Neubert, D. (1986) Low light intensity decreases the fertility of *Callithrix jacchus*. *Primate Report*, **14**, 260 (abstract)

Hershkowitz, P. (1977) *Living New World Monkeys (Platyrrhini) with an Introduction to Primates*, Vol. 1. The University of Chicago Press, Chicago

Hoage, R.J. (1977) Parental care in *Leontopithecus rosalia rosalia*: Sex and age differences in carrying behavior and the role of prior experience. In: *The Biology and Conservation of the Callitrichidae*. Ed. Kleiman, D.G., pp. 293–305. Smithsonian Institution Press, Washington, DC

Hubrecht, R.C. (1984) Field observations on group size and composition of the common marmoset (*Callithrix jacchus jacchus*), at Tapacura, Brazil. *Primates*, **25**, 13–21

Hubrecht, R.C. (1985) Home-range size and use and territorial behavior in the common marmoset, *Callithrix jacchus jacchus*, at the Tapacura Field Station, Recife, Brazil. *International Journal of Primatology*, **6**, 533–550

Hubrecht, R. (1995) *Report on a UK survey of Housing Husbandry and Welfare provision for Animals used in Toxicology studies by the Toxicology and Welfare Working Group (abstract)* The Implications of Non-Invasive and Remote Monitoring Techniques for Non-Human Primate Research and Husbandry: EUPREN/EMRG Meeting, Goettingen, http://www.emrg.org/Activities/emrgwws1.htm (accessed 30 April 2008)

International Primatological Society (2007) International Primatological Society Captive Care Committee. *International Guidelines for the Acquisition, Care and Breeding of Nonhuman Primates*, http://www.internationalprimatologicalsociety.org/docs/IPS_International_Guidelines_for_the_Acquisition_Care_and_Breeding_of_Nonhuman_Primates_Second_Edition_2007.pdf (accessed 30 April 2008)

International Union for the Conservation of Nature and Natural Resources (2009) *IUCN Red List of Threatened Species. Version 2009.1.* www.iucnredlist.org (accessed 30 September 2009)

Jacobs, G.H. (1996) Primate photopigments and primate color vision. *Proceedings of the National Academy of Sciences of the USA*, **93**, 577–581

Jacobs, G.H. (2007) New World Monkeys and Color. *International Journal of Primatology*, **28**, 729–759.

Jacobs, G.H., Neitz, J. and Neitz, M. (1993) Genetic basis of polymorphism in the color vision of platyrrhine monkeys. *Vision Research*, **33**, 269–274

Jaquish, C., Gage, T. B. and Tardif, S.D. (1991) Reproductive factors affecting survivorship in captive Callitrichidae. *American Journal of Physical Anthropology*, **84**, 291–305

Jaquish, C., Tardif, S. D. and Cheverud, J. M. (1997) Interactions between infant growth and survival: Evidence for selection on age-specific body weight in captive common marmosets (*Callithrix jacchus*). *American Journal of Primatology*, **42**, 269–280

Johnson, E.O., Kamilaris, T.C., Carter, A.E. *et al.* (1996). The biobehavioral consequences of psychogenic stress in a small, social primate (*Callithrix jacchus jacchus*). *Biological Psychiatry*, **40**, 317–337

Jones, B.S. (1997) Quantitative analysis of marmoset vocal communication. In: *Handbook: Marmosets and Tamarins in Biological and Biomedical Research*. Eds Pryce, C., Scott, L. and C. Schnell, C., pp. 145–151. DSSD Imagery, Salisbury

Joint Working Group on Refinement (2001) Refining procedures for the administration of substances. Report of the BVAAWF/FRAME/RSPCA/UFAW Joint Working Group on Refinement. *Laboratory Animals*, **35**, 1–41

Joint Working Group on Refinement (2009) Refinements in husbandry, care and common procedures for non-human primates. Ninth report of the BVAAWF/FRAME/RSPCA/UFAW Joint Working Group on Refinement. *Laboratory Animals*, **43**, S1:1–S1:47

Kelly K. (1993) Environmental enrichment for captive wildlife through the simulation of gum feeding. *Animal Welfare Information Center Newsletter*, **4**, 5–10

Kinter, L.B. and Johnson, D.K. (1999) Remote monitoring of experimental endpoints in animals using radiotelemetry and bioimpedance technologies. In: *Humane Endpoints in Animal Experiments for Biomedical Research*. Eds Hendriksen, C.F.M. and Morton, D.B., pp. 58–65. Proceedings of the International Conference. Royal Society of Medicine Press, London

Kirkwood, J.K. and Stathatos, K. (1992) *Biology, Rearing, and Care of Young Primates*. Oxford University Press, Oxford

Kitchen, A.M. and Martin, A.A. (1996) The effects of cage size and complexity on the behaviour of captive common marmosets, *Callithrix jacchus jacchus*. *Laboratory Animals*, **30**, 317–326

Kleiman, D.G., Hoage, R.J. and Green, K.M. (1988) The lion tamarins, genus *Leontopithecus*. In: *Ecology and Behavior of Neotropical Primates*, Vol. 2. Eds Mittermeier, R.A., Rylands, A.B., Coimbra-Filho, A.F. *et al.*, pp. 299–347. World Wildlife Fund, Washington, DC

Knapka, J.J., Barnard, D.E., Bayne, K.A.L. *et al.* (1995) Nutrition. In: *Nonhuman Primates in Biomedical Research*. Eds Bennett, B.T., Abee, C.R. and Henrickson, R., pp. 211–248. Academic Press, San Diego

Layne, D.G. and Power, R.A. (2003) Husbandry, handling, and nutrition for marmosets. *Comparative Medicine*, **53**, 351–359

Lazaro-Perea, C., Snowdon, C.T. and Arruda, M.F. (1999) Scent-marking behavior in wild groups of common marmosets *(Callithrix jacchus)*. *Behavioral Ecology and Sociobiology*, **46**, 313–324

Ludlage, E. and Mansfield, K. (2003) Clinical care and diseases of the common marmoset (*Callithrix jacchus*). *Comparative Medicine*, **53**, 369–382

McKenzie, S.M., Chamove, A.S. and Feistner, A.T.C. (1986) Floor-coverings and hanging screens alter arboreal monkey behavior. *Zoo Biology*, **5**, 339–348

Maier, W., Alonso, C. and Langguth, A. (1982) Field observations on *Callithrix jacchus jacchus*. *L. Zeitschrift Fuer Saeugetierkunde*, **47**, 334–346

Majolo, B., Buchanan-Smith, H.M. and Morris, K. (2003) Factors affecting the successful pairing of unfamiliar common marmoset (*Callithrix jacchus*) females: preliminary results. *Animal Welfare*, **12**, 327–337

Mansfield, K. (2003) Marmoset models commonly used in biomedical research. *Comparative Medicine*, **53**, 383–392

McKinley, J., Buchanan-Smith, H.M., Bassett, L. *et al.* (2003) Training common marmosets (*Callithrix jacchus*) to co-operate during routine laboratory procedures: ease of training and time investment. *Journal of Applied Animal Welfare Science*, **6**, 209–220

Miller, G.F., Barnard, D.E., Woodward, R.A. *et al.* (1997) Hepatic hemosiderosis in common marmosets, *Callithrix jacchus*: effect of diet on incidence and severity. *Laboratory Animal Science*, **47**, 138–142

Mittermeier, R.A., Coimbra-Filho, A.F. and Constable, I. (1981) Conservation of eastern Brazilian primates. Unpublished report for the period 1979/1980, Project No. 1614, World Wildlife Fund, Washington D.C. 39 pp.

Moore, K., Cleland, J. and McGrew, W.C. (1991) Visual encounters between families of cotton-top tamarins, *Saguinus oedipus*. *Primates*, **32**, 23–33

National Research Council, Committee on Animal Nutrition (2003) *Nutrient Requirements of Non-human Primates*. National Academy of Science, Washington, DC

Neyman, P.F. (1977) Aspects of the ecology and social organization of free-ranging cotton-top tamarins (*Saguinus oedipus*) and the conservation status of the species. In: *The Biology and Conservation of the Callitrichidae*. Ed. Kleiman, D.G., pp. 39–71. Smithsonian Institution Press, Washington, DC

Novak, M.A. and Suomi, S.J. (1988) Psychological well-being of primates in captivity. *American Psychologist*, **43**, 765–773

Pereira, M.E., Macedonia, J.M., Haring, D.M. *et al.* (1989) Maintenance of primates in captivity for research: The need for naturalistic environments. In: *Housing, Care and Psychological Wellbeing of Captive and Laboratory Primates*. Ed. Segal, E.F., pp. 40–60. Noyes Publications, New Jersey

Pines, M.K., Kaplan, G. and Rogers, L.J. (2002) Comparison of behaviour changes and cortisol levels of common marmosets (*Callithrix jacchus jacchus*) to indoor and outdoor cages. The XIXth Congress of the International Primatological Society, Beijing, China (abstract)

Pines, M. K., Kaplan, G. and Rogers, L. J. (2007) A note on indoor and outdoor housing preferences of common marmosets (*Callithrix jacchus*). *Applied Animal Behaviour Science*, **108**, 348–353

Plesker, R. and Schuhmacher, A. (2006) Feeding fruits and vegetables to nonhuman primates can lead to nutritional deficiencies. *Laboratory Primate Newsletter*, **45**, 1–5

Pontes, M.A.R. and da Cruz, M.M.A.O. (1995) Home range intergroup transfers, and reproductive status of common marmosets *Callithrix jacchus* in a forest fragment in north-eastern Brazil. *Primates*, **36**, 335–347

Pook, A.G. (1977) A comparative study of the use of contact calls in *Saguinus fuscicollis* and *Callithrix jacchus*. In: *The Biology and Conservation of the Callitrichidae*. Ed. Kleiman, D.G., pp. 271–280. Smithsonian Institution Press, Washington, DC

Poole, T.B., Costa, P., Netto, W.J. *et al.* (1994) Non-human primates. In: *The Accommodation of Laboratory Animals in Accordance With Animal Welfare Requirements*. Ed. O'Donoghue, P.N., pp. 81–86. Proceedings of an International Workshop Held at the Bundesgesundheitsamt, Berlin (The Berlin Workshop). Bundesministerium für Ernährung, Landwirtschaft und Forsten, Bonn, Germany

Poole, T., Hubrecht, R. and Kirkwood, J.K. (1999) Marmosets and tamarins. In: *The UFAW Handbook on the Care and Management of Laboratory Animals*, 7th edn. Ed Poole, T., pp. 559–573. Blackwell Publishing, Oxford

Potkay, S. (1992) Diseases of the Callitrichidae: a review. *Journal of Medical Primatology*, **21**, 189–236

Power, M.L. (1996) The other side of Callitrichine gummivory: digestibility and nutritional value. In: *Adaptive Radiations of Neotropical Primates*. Eds Norconk, M.A., Rosenberger, A.L. and Garber, P.A.), pp. 97–110 and 535–536. Plenum Press, New York

Prescott, M. (2006) Primate sensory capabilities and communication signals: implications for care and use in the laboratory. *NC3Rs*, London, http://www.nc3rs.org.uk/primatesenses (accessed 30 April 2008)

Prescott, M.J., Bowell, V.A. and Buchanan-Smith, H.M. (2005) Training of laboratory-housed non-human primates, part 2: Resources for developing and implementing training programmes. *Animal Technology and Welfare*, **4**, 133–148

Prescott, M.J. and Buchanan-Smith, H.M. (2004) Cage sizes for tamarins in the laboratory. *Animal Welfare*, **13**, 151–158

Price, E.C. (1990) Parturition and perinatal behaviour in captive cotton-top tamarins (*Saguinus oedipus*). *Primates*, **31**, 523–535

Price, E.C. (1992) The benefits of helpers: Effects of group and litter size on infant care in tamarins (*Saguinus oedipus*). *American Journal of Primatology*, **26**, 179–190

Price, E.C. and McGrew, W.C. (1990). Cotton-top tamarins (*Saguinus o. oedipus*) in a semi-naturalistic captive colony. *American Journal of Primatology*, **20**, 1–12

Regan, B.C., Julliot, C., Simmen, B. *et al.* (2001) Fruits, foliage and the evolution of primate colour vision. *Philosophical Transactions of the Royal Society of London*, **B356**, 229–283

Rennie, A. and Buchanan-Smith, H.M. (2005) Report on the extent and character of primate use in scientific procedures across Europe in 2001. *Laboratory Primate Newsletter*, **44**, 6–12

Rennie, A.E. and Buchanan-Smith, H.M. (2006a) Refinement of the use of non-human primates in scientific research. Part I: The influence of humans. *Animal Welfare*, **15**, 203–213

Rennie A.E. and Buchanan-Smith, H.M. (2006b) Refinement of the use of non-human primates in scientific research. Part II: Housing, husbandry and acquisition. *Animal Welfare*, **15**, 215–238

Rennie A.E. and Buchanan-Smith, H.M. (2006c) Refinement of the use of non-human primates in scientific research. Part III: Refinement of procedures. *Animal Welfare*, **15**, 239–261

Rensing, S. and Oerke, A.K. (2005) Husbandry and management of New World species: marmosets and tamarins. In: The Laboratory Primate. Ed. Wolfe-Coote, S., pp. 145–162. Elsevier Academic Press, San Diego

Roda, S.A. and Mendes Pontes, A.R. (1998) Polygyny and infanticide in common marmosets in a fragment of the Atlantic forest of Brazil. *Folia Primatologica*, **69**, 372–376

Ross, C.N., Fite, J.E., Jensen, H. *et al.* (2007a) Demographic review of a captive colony of callitrichids (*Callithrix kuhlii*). *American Journal of Primatology*, **69**, 234–240

Ross, C.N., French, J.A. and Ortí G. (2007b) Germ-line chimerism and paternal care in marmosets (*Callithrix kuhlii*). *Proceedings of the National Academy of Sciences*, **104**, 6278–6282

Rothe, H. and Koenig, A. (1991) Variability of social organization in captive common marmosets (*Callithrix jacchus*). *Folia Primatologica*, **57**, 28–33

Rumble, R., Saville, M., Simmons, L. *et al.* (2005) The preference of the common marmoset for nest boxes made from three different materials: wood, plastic, metal. *Animal Technology and Welfare*, **4**, 185–187

Rylands, A.B. (1993) *Marmosets and Tamarins: Systematics, Behaviour, and Ecology*. Oxford University Press, Oxford

Rylands, A.B. (2007) Provisional results of the IUCN/SSC Red List Assessment Workshop for the Neotropical Primates, Disney Institute, Orlando, Florida, 27 November–2 December 2007. Personal communication. Final assessments will be available in October 2008, http://www.iucnredlist.org/

Rylands, A.B. and de Faria, D.S. (1993) Habitats, feeding ecology, and home range size in the genus Callithrix. In: *Marmosets and Tamarins: Systematics, Behaviour, and Ecology*. Ed. Rylands A.B., pp. 262–272. Oxford University Press, Oxford

Rylands, A.B., Schneider, H., Langguth, A. *et al.* (2000) An assessment of the diversity of New World primates. *Neotropical Primates*, **8**, 61–93

Sainsbury, A.W., Eaton, B.D. and Cooper, J.E. (1989) Restraint and anaesthesia of primates. *Veterinary Record*, **125**, 640–644

Sainsbury, A.W., Kirkwood, J.K. and Appleby, E.C. (1987) Chronic colitis in common marmosets (*Callithrix jacchus*) and cotton-top tamarins (*Saguinus oedipus*). *Veterinary Record*, **121**, 329–330

Saltzman, W., Schultz-Darken, N.J. and Abbott, D.H. (1997) Familial influences on ovulatory function in common marmosets (*Callithrix jacchus*). *American Journal of Primatology*, **41**, 159–177

Sambrook, T.D. and Buchanan-Smith, H.M. (1997) Control and complexity in novel object enrichment. *Animal Welfare*, **6**, 207–216

Saunders, K.E., Shen, Z., Dewhirst, F.E. *et al.* (1999) Novel intestinal *Helicobacter* species isolated from cotton-top tamarins (*Saguinus oedipus*) with chronic colitis. *Journal of Clinical Microbiology*, **37**, 146–151

Savage, A. (1995) The cotton-top tamarin SSP husbandry manual. Available at: http://www.csew.com/cottontop/ (accessed 30 April 2008)

Savage, A., Giraldo, L.H., Blumer, E.S. *et al.* (1993) Field techniques for monitoring cotton-top tamarins (*Saguinus oedipus oedipus*) in Colombia. *American Journal of Primatology*, **31**, 189–196

Savastano, G., Hanson, A. and McCann, C. (2003) The development of an operant conditioning training program for New World primates at the Bronx Zoo. *Journal of Applied Animal Welfare Science*, **6**, 247–261

Scanlon, C.E., Chalmers, N.R. and Monteiro da Cruz, M.A.O. (1989) Home range use and the exploitation of gum in the marmoset *Callithrix jacchus jacchus*. *International Journal of Primatology*, **10**, 123–136

Schaffner, C.M. and Smith, T.E. (2005) Familiarity may buffer the adverse effects of relocation on marmosets (*Callithrix kuhlii*): preliminary evidence. *Zoo Biology*, **24**, 93–100

Schapiro, S.J., Stavisky, R. and Hook, M. (2000) The lower-row cage may be dark, but behavior does not appear to be affected. *Laboratory Primate Newsletter*, **39**, 4–6

Schoenfeld, D. (1989) Effects of environmental impoverishment on the social behavior of marmosets (*Callithrix jacchus*). *American Journal of Primatology*, Suppl. **1**, 45–51

Scott, L. (1991) Environmental enrichment for single housed common marmosets. In: *Primate Responses to Environmental Change*. Ed. Box, H.O., pp. 265–274. Chapman and Hall, London

Scott, L., Pearce, P., Fairhall, S. *et al.* (2003) Training nonhuman primates to cooperate with scientific procedures in applied biomedical research. *Journal of Applied Animal Welfare Science*, **6**, 199–207

Schultz-Darken, N.J. (2003) Sample collection and restraint techniques used for common marmosets (*Callithrix jacchus*). *Comparative Medicine*, **53**, 360–363

Schultz-Darken, N.J., Pape, R.M., Tannenbaum, P.L. *et al.* (2004) Novel restraint system for neuroendocrine studies of socially living common marmoset monkeys. *Laboratory Animals*, **38**, 393–405

Smith, A.C., Buchanan-Smith, H.M., Surridge, A.K. *et al.* (2003) The effect of colour vision status on the detection and selection of fruits by tamarins (*Saguinus* spp.). *Journal of Experimental Biology*, **206**, 3159–3165

Smith, T.E., McCallister, J.M., Gordon, S.J. *et al.* (2004) Quantitative data on training New World primates to urinate. *American Journal of Primatology*, **64**, 83–93

Smucny, D.A., Abbott, D.H., Mansfield, K.G. *et al.* (2004) Reproductive output, maternal age, and survivorship in captive common marmoset females (*Callithrix jacchus*). *American Journal of Primatology*, **64**, 107–121

Snowdon, C.T. (1993) A vocal taxonomy of the callitrichids. In: *Marmosets and Tamarins: Systematics, Behaviour, and Ecology*. Ed. Rylands A.B., pp. 78–94. Oxford University Press, Oxford

Snowdon, C.T. and Savage, A. (1989) Psychological well-being of captive primates: General considerations and examples from callitrichids. In: *Housing, Care and Psychological Wellbeing of Captive and Laboratory Primates*. Ed Segal, E.F., pp. 75–88. Noyes Publications, New Jersey

Snowdon, C.T., Savage, A. and McConnell, P.B. (1985) A breeding colony of cotton-top tamarins (*Saguinus oedipus*). *Laboratory Animal Science*, **35**, 477–480

Snowdon, C.T. and Soini, P. (1988) The tamarins, genus *Saguinus*. In: *Ecology and Behavior of Neotropical Primates*, Vol. 2. Eds Mittermeier, R.A., Rylands, A.B., Coimbra-Filho, A.F. *et al.*, pp. 223–298. World Wildlife Fund, Washington, DC

Soini, P. (1988) The pygmy marmoset, genus *Cebuella*. In: *Ecology and Behavior of Neotropical Primates*, Vol. 2. Eds Mittermeier, R.A., Rylands, A.B., Coimbra-Filho, A.F. *et al.*, pp. 79–129. World Wildlife Fund, Washington, DC

de Sousa, M.B.C., Albuquerque, A.C.S.R., Albuquerque, F.S. *et al.* (2005) Behavioral strategies and hormonal profiles of dominant and subordinate common marmoset (*Callithrix jacchus*) females in wild monogamous groups. *American Journal of Primatology*, **67**, 37–50

de Sousa, M.B.C., Nogueira Moura, S.L. and Menezes, A.A.L. (2006) Circadian variation with a diurnal bimodal profile on scent-marking behavior in captive common marmosets (*Callithrix jacchus*). *International Journal of Primatology*, **27**, 263–272

Stevenson, M.F. (1976) Birth and perinatal behaviour in family groups of the common marmoset (*Callithrix jacchus jacchus*), compared to other primates. *Journal of Human Evolution*, **5**, 365–381

Stevenson, M.F. (1978) The ontogeny of playful behaviour in family groups of the common marmoset. In: *Recent Advances in Primatology*, Vol. 1. (Behaviour). Eds Chivers, D.J. and Herbert, J., pp. 139–143. Academic Press, New York

Stevenson, M. F. and Poole, T. B. (1976) An ethogram of the common marmoset (*Callithrix jacchus jacchus*): General behavioural repertoire. *Animal Behaviour*, **24**, 428–451

Stevenson, M.F. and Rylands, A.B. (1988) The marmosets, genus *Callithrix*. In: *Ecology and Behavior of Neotropical Primates*, Vol. 2. Eds Mittermeier, R.A., Rylands, A.B., Coimbra-Filho, A.F. *et al.*, pp. 131–222. World Wildlife Fund, Washington, DC

Tardif, S.D. and Bales, K.L. (2004) Relations among birth condition, maternal condition, and postnatal growth in captive common marmoset monkeys (*Callithrix jacchus*). *American Journal of Primatology*, **62**, 83–94

Tardif, S., Bales, K., Williams, L. *et al.* (2006) Preparing New World monkeys for laboratory research. *ILAR Journal*, **47**, 307–315

Tardif, S.D. and Jaquish, C.E. (1997) Number of ovulations in the marmoset monkey (*Callithrix jacchus*): Relation to body weight, age and repeatability. *American Journal of Primatology*, **42**, 323–329

Tardif, S.D., Jaquish, C., Layne, D. *et al.* (1998) Growth variation in common marmoset monkeys (*Callithrix jacchus*) fed a purified diet: relation to care-giving and weaning behaviors. *Laboratory Animal Science*, **48**, 264–269

Tardif, S.D., Richter, C.B. and Carson, R.L. (1984a) Effects of sibling-rearing experience on future reproductive success in two species of Callitrichidae. *American Journal of Primatology*, **6**, 377–380

Tardif, S.D., Richter, C.B. and Carson, R.L. (1984b) Reproductive performance of three species of Callitrichidae. *Laboratory Animal Science*, **34**, 272–275

Tardif, S.D., Smucny, D.A., Abbott, D.H. *et al.* (2003) Reproduction in captive common marmosets (*Callithrix jacchus*). *Comparative Medicine*, **53**, 364–368

Thomas, O. (1904) New *Callithrix*, *Midas*, *Felis*, *Rhipidomys*, and *Proechimys* from Brazil and Ecuador. *Annals and Magazine of Natural History*, **14**, 188–196

van Roosmalen, M.G.M. and van Roosmalen, T. (2003). The description of a new marmoset genus, *Callibella* (Callitrichinae, Primates), including its molecular phylogenetic status. *Neotropical Primates*, **11**, 1–10

van Roosmalen, M.G.M., van Roosmalen, T., Mittermeier, R.A. *et al.* (1998). A new and distinctive species of marmoset (Callitrichidae, Primates) from the lower Rio Aripuanã, state of Amazonas, central Brazilian Amazonia. *Goeldiana Zoologia*, **22**, 1–27

Ventura, R. and Buchanan-Smith, H.M. (2003) Physical environment effects on infant care and infant development in captive common marmosets *Callithrix jacchus*. *International Journal of Primatology*, **24**, 399–413

Waitt, C. and Buchanan-Smith, H.M. (2006) Perceptual considerations in the use of colored artificial visual stimuli to study nonhuman primate behavior. *American Journal of Primatology*, **68**, 1054–1067

Wolfensohn, S. and Honess, P. (2005) *Handbook of Primate Husbandry and Welfare*. Blackwell Publishing, Oxford

Yamamoto, M.E. (1993) From dependence to sexual maturity: The behavioural ontogeny of Callitrichidae. In: *Marmosets and Tamarins: Systematics, Behaviour, and Ecology*. Ed. Rylands A.B., pp. 235–254. Oxford University Press, Oxford

Yoneda, M. (1984) Ecological study of the saddle backed tamarin (*Saguinus fuscicollis*) in northern Bolivia. *Primates*, **25**, 1–12

37 Squirrel monkeys

Lawrence E. Williams, Alan G. Brady and Christian R. Abee

Biological overview

Taxonomy

All squirrel monkeys were once considered to be a single species *(Saimiri sciureus)* with several geographically separated subspecies. However, karyotypic and phenotypic information gathered in the early 1980s led Hershkovitz (1984) to the conclusion that squirrel monkeys should be classified as a single genus with four species (*Saimiri boliviensis, S. oerstedii, S. sciureus and S. ustus*) and nine subspecies. Studies conducted by Assis and Barros (1987), da Silva *et al.* (1987), VandeBerg *et al.* (1990) and Cropp and Boinski (2000) support the taxonomic classification of Hershkovitz. Ayres (1985) has described a fifth species, *Saimiri vanzolinii* that is found in central Brazil along the south bank of the Amazon River. Cropp and Boinski (2000) present evidence that *Saimiri oerstedii,* indigenous to parts of Central America (primarily Costa Rica), is a genetically distinct population and not the result of human introduction.

Squirrel monkeys are divided into two groups based on the shape of the patch of nonpigmented hair above the eyes (Figure 37.1). The use of this phenotypic characteristic for identifying species and subspecies of squirrel monkeys was first described by MacLean (1964) and later by Cooper (1968), and its usefulness confirmed by Hershkovitz (1984). Monkeys belonging to the *S. sciureus* and *vanzolinii* groups are classified as 'gothic arch' squirrel monkeys and possess a pointed arch of whitish hair above each eye. Those belonging to the *S. boliviensis* group are referred to as 'roman arch' squirrel monkeys and are characterised by more shallow semicircular patterns above the eyes. Additional phenotypic characteristics include differences in coloration of the hair on the head and body, which can range from subtle to obvious. Squirrel monkeys of the roman arch variety usually have black hair crowning their heads, although exceptions exist (Hershkovitz 1984); and gothic arch squirrel monkeys usually have a grey–green agouti coloration. *S. sciureus sciureus,* the Guyanese squirrel monkey, also possesses a pattern of pigmented hairs within the patch of whitish hair above each eye, resembling an eyebrow (Ariga *et al.* 1978).

Precise identification of squirrel monkeys often requires both phenotypic and karyotypic examination. All squirrel monkey species and subspecies that have been examined, thus far, have 44 (diploid) chromosomes; however, they vary in their number of acrocentric autosomes from five to seven. More certain identification can be made by counting the number of acrocentric autosomes and observing the periocular patches (Ariga *et al.* 1978). Squirrel monkeys are sexually dimorphic, although sex differences are less distinct than in many Old World primates. Male squirrel monkeys weigh 25–30% more than females, and canine teeth are larger and longer in males. In Table 37.1, the species and subspecies of squirrel monkeys are listed using the nomenclature suggested by Hershkovitz (1984).

Taxonomy is an important issue for those using squirrel monkeys in research, as a substantial body of information has accumulated over the past 30 years, providing convincing evidence that species and subspecies of squirrel monkeys vary in their susceptibility to both naturally occurring and experimentally induced diseases (Portman *et al.* 1980; Martin & McNease, 1982; Ausman *et al.* 1985; Coe *et al.* 1985).

The karyotypic variations observed in squirrel monkeys are thought to be due to pericentric inversions in the ancestral karyotype (Jones *et al.* 1973). Failure to identify and separate Peruvian, Bolivian and Guyanese squirrel monkeys in breeding colonies may result in interbreeding. Progeny of squirrel monkeys that interbreed will be heterozygous for the inversion, which may lead to the production of non-viable gametes due to crossovers at the inversion loop during meiosis. Theoretically, 50% of conceptions in hybrid squirrel monkeys may be non-viable, reducing reproductive efficiency in breeding colonies that mix species and subspecies. Furthermore, mixing species and subspecies within experimental groups may create confounding variables. There are, therefore good reasons to carefully identify and separate species and subspecies of squirrel monkeys in both breeding and experimental colonies.

Ecology

In the wild, squirrel monkeys inhabit most types of tropical forest including both wet and dry forest, continuous and secondary forest, mangrove swamps, riparian habitat and forest fragments (Hernandez-Camacho & Cooper 1976; Terborgh 1983; Baldwin 1985; Boinski 1987b). They appear highly flexible in their ability to adapt to different environments, and in some geographic areas appear to prefer disturbed habitats (Konstant & Mittermeier 1982; Boinski 1987b). They are omnivores, eating insects when they are available but also include fruit, flowers, bird eggs, and

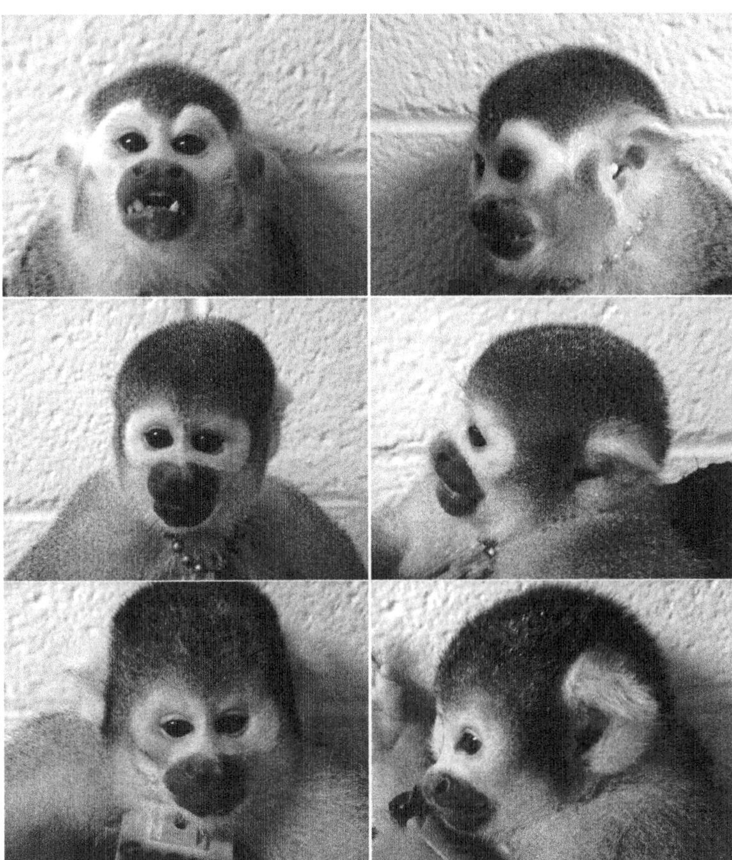

Figure 37.1 Photograph of the faces of three types of squirrel monkeys; *Saimiri sciureus sciureus* (Guyanese) top, *Saimiri boliviensis peruviensis* (Peruvian) middle and *Saimiri boliviensis boliviensis* (Bolivian) bottom. The Peruvian and Bolivian squirrel monkeys have 'Roman' or rounded periorbital arches, while the Guyanese has the 'gothic' or peaked arches.

Table 37.1 Selected taxonomic characteristics of the squirrel monkey. Adapted from Hershkovitz (1984) and Costello *et al.* (1993).

Scientific name	*Chromosome no. (diploid)*	*Variety*	*Acrocentric autosomes*
Saimiri sciureus sciureus	44	Gothic	7
S. sciureus macrodon	44	Gothic	6
S. sciureus cassiquiarensis	44	Gothic	?
S. sciureus abigena	44	Gothic	?
Saimiri oerstedii oerstedii	44	Gothic	5
S. oerstedii citrineflis	44	Gothic	5
Saimiri ustus	44	Gothic	5
Saimiri boliviensis boliviensis	44	Roman	6
S. boliviensis peruviensis	44	Roman	5
Saimiri vanzolinii	44	Roman	?

occasionally vertebrates in their diet when necessary or readily available (Thorington 1967; Baldwin & Baldwin 1972; Jones *et al.* 1973; Izawa 1975; Mittermeier & van Roosmalen 1981; Scollay & Judge 1981; Mitchell *et al.* 1991). Lima & Ferrari (2003) reported that the diet of *Saimiri sciureus* in eastern Brazil shifted from 80% animal to 80% plant depending on the availability of insects.

Social structure

In the wild, squirrel monkeys are found in large multi-male/multi-female social groups of between 20 and 50 animals, with unconfirmed reports of up to 300 monkeys in a group (Thorington 1967; Baldwin & Baldwin 1971a; Baldwin 1985; Boinski 1987b). Group size may vary somewhat depending on habitat type (Baldwin & Baldwin 1971b; Scollay & Judge 1981). In the 1960s it was thought that groups tended to break into smaller groups for foraging, rejoined for a time during the day for a rest period, and then continued foraging separately until coming back together for the night (Thorington 1967). More recent studies have found that members of social groups tend to forage as a unit, and the earlier reports are explained as observations of one troop using several large fruiting trees (Mitchell 1990). Boinski (1987b) found that Costa Rican squirrel monkeys tend to forage more widely and rest less when food is scarce during the peak wet season and travel least during the birth season.

In captivity, age/sex ratio differs depending on the type of social grouping that can be maintained in the available housing. Generally, social groups are maintained in captivity with only one or two males per group; as male–male aggression has occurred when more than two males are maintained within a social group. Groups which have access to a more semi-natural living situation within a larger living space are able to accommodate more males within the same groupings due to the increased complexity of the environment and the possibility of escape from social conflicts. In captivity, social group size can range from a single pair up to 35–50 animals per group depending on available housing. For smaller populations, one male for every three to four females is recommended. Squirrel monkeys are very social animals and should be maintained in species-typical social groupings as much as possible.

Female squirrel monkeys reach maturity and begin breeding at around 2.5–3 years of age. In the wild, the frequency of female inter-troop transfer differs among groups from differing geographical regions. A high rate of female transfer occurs in *Saimiri oerstedii* with males remaining in their natal groups, compared to a low rate of female transfer in *Saimiri sciureus* and *boliviensis* spp., which have relatively high rates of male transfer (Boinski 1987c). Males reach sub-adult age by the time they are 2.5–3 years old and generally transfer from the natal group at that time. They may then join an all male group of juveniles and sub-adults until they become fully adult at about the age of 5 years and are able to work their way into the male dominance hierarchy of an established group (Roder & Timmermans 2002). Both social patterns provide a mechanism for maintaining genetic variability in wild populations.

Social organisation

Squirrel monkey societies are generally kept stable by the adult females. All age–sex classes except fully adult males have been shown to be more attracted to adult females than to any other age–sex class (Baldwin 1969, 1985; Strayer & Harris 1979; Scollay & Judge 1981). Sexual segregation occurs on a seasonal basis as a unique feature of social organisation in this species. Males remain near the periphery of the group in the non-breeding season, and the majority of social interactions between the sexes take place during the breeding season (Du Mond 1967; Baldwin 1968; Mason & Epple 1969; Baldwin & Baldwin 1972; Candland *et al.* 1973; Coe & Rosenblum 1974, 1978; Strayer *et al.* 1975; Kaplan 1977; Vaitl 1977b; Vaitl *et al.* 1978; Hopf 1978; Mendoza *et al.* 1978b; Leger *et al.* 1981; Lyons *et al.* 1992; Boinski & Mitchell 1994).

The behaviour of populations from different geographical regions appears to differ (Mendoza *et al.* 1978a; Gonzalez *et al.* 1981; Mitchell *et al.* 1991). There is strong sexual segregation in *Saimiri boliviensis*, whereas *Saimiri sciureus* spp. and *Saimiri oerstedii* spp. societies are more sexually integrated (Mendoza *et al.* 1978a; Boinski 1987c). Some studies have found evidence that this sexual segregation may be female initiated through active exclusion of the males (Du Mond 1968; Baldwin & Baldwin 1972; Fairbanks 1974; Vaitl 1977a; Mendoza *et al.* 1978a). Other studies have found that the segregation may be due to inter-male social dynamics instead of female agonism (Strayer and Harris 1979; Lyons *et al.* 1992). Boinski *et al.* (2002) suggests that the amount of female–female bonding within *Saimiri* species is related to their ecology. *Saimiri sciureus* in Suriname exhibited weaker social bonds and rarely formed coalitions with other females, when compared to *Saimiri boliviensis boliviensis*. They relate this difference to the fact that in Suriname the food patches are small and dense unlike the western South American forest. Hence, one female can dominate the food patch making any coalition unstable.

Dominance hierarchies within squirrel monkey groups differ between species. *Saimiri boliviensis boliviensis* have a high degree of sexual segregation, and also possess linear male dominance hierarchies, in which dominance is associated with higher testosterone levels and copulatory frequency. A less distinct dominance hierarchy is seen among females of this species (Mendoza *et al.* 1978a). The linear dominance hierarchies of *Saimiri sciureus* spp., which are more sexually integrated within social groups, include both sexes, with all males being dominant over all females (Mendoza *et al.* 1978a; Mitchell *et al.* 1991). *Saimiri oerstedii* spp. in the wild do not have dominance hierarchies amongst either sex; and males may co-operatively mob females to establish their state of oestrus from olfactory cues during the breeding season (Boinski 1987c; Mitchell *et al.* 1991).

Allomaternal care, or infant care by social group members other than the birth mother, has been documented in field studies (Ploog 1967; Du Mond 1968; Baldwin 1969; Hunt *et al.* 1978; Morton 2000) and in the laboratory (Williams *et al.* 1988, 1994; Soltis *et al.* 2005). Infant squirrel monkeys may spend as much as 30% of their time on allomothers during the first 6 months of their lives (Baldwin 1969; Williams *et al.* 1994). Allomothering usually begins during the first 2 weeks of life (Williams *et al.* 1994). In the wild, allomothers are usually juvenile females (Du Mond 1968). In captivity, reports have shown that one half (53%) of the allomothering is performed by young adult females, aged 4–6 years, whereas adult females, age 7–9 years, provided about 20% of the allomaternal care (Williams *et al.* 1994). Females which have experienced a reproductive failure during the year (Williams *et al.* 1988) performed almost all of the allonursing. This proclivity can be used to foster orphan infants in captivity.

Breeding and reproduction

Squirrel monkeys have an annual reproductive cycle, with a distinct 3-month breeding season followed about 5 months later by a birth season (Du Mond 1967, 1968; Goss *et al.* 1968; Rosenblum & Cooper 1968; Baldwin 1969; Michael & Zumpe 1971; Coe & Rosenblum 1978; Boinski 1987c; Trevino 2007). A feature of this yearly cycle is reproductive seasonality in breeding males as well as the females (Du Mond 1967; Du Mond & Hutchinson 1967; Baldwin 1969; Kaplan 1977; Coe & Rosenblum 1978; Mendoza 1987; Williams *et al.* 1986b; Boinski 1987c). The 'fatted male' condition is a component of this reproductive cycle. Both sexes gain weight throughout the pre-breeding season, attaining peak weights prior to breeding. Weight gain in males is associated with increased spermatogenesis in preparation for breeding (Du Mond &

Hutchinson 1967; Coe & Rosenblum 1978; Williams *et al.* 1986b). Nadler and Rosenblum (1972) and Chen *et al.* (1981) demonstrated that male fattening is closely related to circulating levels of testosterone.

The yearly cycle has been shown, in some field studies, to be related to seasonal food availability (Du Mond & Hutchinson 1967; Baldwin 1968; Du Mond 1968; Thorington 1968; Baldwin & Baldwin 1981; Boinski 1987a). Changes in light cycles have also been shown to be associated with the timing of the reproductive cycle (Rosenblum & Cooper 1968) as has humidity level (Du Mond 1968). Boinski (1987a), in her field studies in Costa Rica, found a strong tendency towards birth synchrony in *Saimiri oerstedii* which she suggested might be an anti-predator adaptation.

Oestrous cycle lengths have been estimated to be around 8–12 days (Rosenblum & Cooper 1968; Wolf *et al.* 1975; Kaplan 1977; Diamond *et al.* 1984; Yeoman *et al.* 2000). Cycle length can be affected by social conditions (Hutchinson 1970; Wolf *et al.* 1975) and light cycles (Rosenblum & Cooper 1968).

The breeding season in squirrel monkeys shows a shift when animals are moved into the northern hemisphere (Lehner *et al.* 1967; Du Mond 1968; Rosenblum & Cooper 1968; Kaplan 1977). Several studies have linked this breeding season shift to humidity factors (Du Mond 1968; Baldwin & Baldwin 1971a; Harrison & Dukelow 1973). It has also been linked to the photoperiod by other authors (Coe & Levine 1981; Trevino 2007). The breeding season in captive squirrel monkeys is probably controlled by a combination of environmental factors, including photoperiod and humidity, that correspond with environmental changes experienced by the monkeys in their natural habitat (Dukelow 1985; Trevino 2007).

Sources and conservation

Once plentiful and available at modest cost, squirrel monkeys were imported to the United States and Europe in large numbers in the 1960s (Cooper 1968). However, the governments of South America began banning export of primates indigenous to their countries in the 1970s. The exportation of the Bolivian squirrel monkey (*S. boliviensis boliviensis*), a species considered especially suitable for malaria vaccine studies, was banned by the Bolivian government in 1983. Thus, by the late 1980s, only Peruvian squirrel monkeys (*S. boliviensis peruviensis*) were available from the wild.

Saimiri oerstedii citrinellus is an endangered subspecies of which fewer than 1000 are believed to exist in the wild (Boinski 1985). These animals are not available for export; however, non-invasive field research and research aimed at improving their chances for survival are possible (Rodriguez-Vargas 2003; Sierra *et al.* 2003). Wild-caught Guyanese squirrel monkeys (*S. sciureus*) are available from Guyana and Suriname through commercial exporters. Also, Peruvian squirrel monkeys (*S. boliviensis peruviensis*) continue to be available through the Peruvian Primatology Project (PPP) in Iquitos, Peru.

There are major disadvantages to using feral-origin squirrel monkeys in research: they are of unknown age, medical history, genetic background and reproductive history. Wild-caught animals are likely to be stressed by the process of capture and captive housing (Joint Working Group on Refinement (JWGR) 2009). Furthermore, feral animals frequently have parasitic infections, which reduce their desirability for some types of research (Abee 1985). For example, squirrel monkeys naturally infected with malaria, are not suitable for malaria vaccine development studies.

Uses in the laboratory

The squirrel monkey as a research subject

Squirrel monkeys (*Saimiri* spp.) are the most commonly used neotropical primates in biomedical research in the United States, whereas in Europe the predominant New World monkey used in research is the marmoset. Squirrel monkeys and marmosets share many physical characteristics, including small size and ease of handling that contribute to their desirability as research subjects. The mean body weight of adult squirrel monkeys is less than 1 kg compared with female rhesus monkeys, which usually weigh 4–5 kg. As a result, much smaller doses of synthesised compounds are necessary when using squirrel monkeys to test new drugs. This can be an important advantage when studies require administration of expensive compounds. Squirrel monkeys easily adapt to laboratory housing and can be maintained in smaller spaces and less expensive cages than larger primates, such as macaques and baboons. This characteristic is especially important in facilities with space limitations.

Interest in using squirrel monkeys instead of macaques has increased following the tragic deaths of laboratory workers after exposure to macaques shedding Cercopithecine herpesvirus 1 (B virus) in Florida (Centers for Disease Control and Prevention (CDC) 1987), Michigan (CDC 1989) Texas and Georgia (CDC 1998). There is less risk of serious zoonotic disease transmission with squirrel monkeys and other neotropical primates than with macaques and other Old World primates. Additionally, accidental exposures from bites and scratches can be managed in a manner similar to those from dogs and cats, and personal protective equipment required for handling squirrel monkeys is less extensive. The reduced risk to laboratory workers combined with ease of handling, allow more procedures to be carried out without chemical restraint or expensive handling equipment. In addition, squirrel monkeys are easily habituated to handling, which further reduces stress from manipulation. For these reasons, experimental procedures that must be performed without sedation can be carried out relatively easily in squirrel monkeys.

Research models

The squirrel monkey has proven to be valuable in a number of areas of biomedical research as demonstrated by the publication of two textbooks devoted entirely to the squirrel monkey (Rosenblum & Cooper 1968; Rosenblum & Coe 1985). See also reviews by Brady (2000); Galland (2000);

Scammell (2000); Williams and Glasgow (2000) on further important uses of the squirrel monkey.

Although the virtues of the squirrel monkey as a research subject were described as early as the 1930s (Kluver 1933), it was not until the late 1950s that interest in its use in biomedical science really started to develop. Their small size, ease of handling and ability to tolerate high gravitational forces resulted in their use for physiological studies of the effects of space flight (Beischer 1968). The findings that squirrel monkeys maintained under laboratory conditions had fatty streaks and plaques in their aortas resembling human atherosclerosis (Middleton, *et al.* 1964), and that wild squirrel monkeys also have naturally occurring atherosclerotic lesions (Middleton *et al.* 1967), has led to their use in atherosclerosis research (reviewed by Strickland & Clarkson 1985).

Squirrel monkeys have been the subject of research involving the experimental induction of cholelithiasis (Lofland 1975; Osuga and Portman 1971) and into reproductive biology (Bennett 1967a, 1967b). The squirrel monkey is an important animal model for malaria vaccine development studies. *Plasmodium* spp. are host specific; therefore the animals used for studies of human malaria must be susceptible to the same strains of *Plasmodium* that cause disease in humans. The Bolivian squirrel monkey has been shown to be a superior model than the Guyanese squirrel monkeys *(S. sciureus sciureus)* for studies of the pathogenesis of *Plasmodium falciparum* Indochina I (Whiteley *et al.* 1987). Differences in susceptibility to experimental malaria infections emphasise the importance of species identification when using squirrel monkeys.

The squirrel monkey is one of the most susceptible non-human primate species to experimental infection with Creutzfeldt-Jakob disease (CJD) and other transmissible spongiform encephalopathies (Zlotnik *et al.* 1974; Brown *et al.* 1994; Schätzl *et al.* 1995; Marsh *et al.* 2005). Williams *et al.* (2007) reported on behavioural changes seen in squirrel monkeys that were associated with experimental transmission of both variant CJD and sporadic CJD.

Foetal rotation resembling that seen during labour and delivery in women has been observed in the squirrel monkey. The implications of this for obstetric evaluation of fossil hominid pelves may prompt re-evaluation of currently accepted views of labour and delivery in these species (Stoller 1995). A report of lesions consistent with pelvic organ prolapse (POP) in a small group of aged squirrel monkeys from the Scott & White Clinic and Hospital in Temple, Texas (Coates *et al.* 1995), suggested that the squirrel monkey might be a model for the disease. (Shull *et al.* 1992). It was subsequently confirmed that multiparous squirrel monkeys develop lesions resembling POP in women.

Laboratory management

General husbandry

Housing, food and water

General advice on husbandry, care and common procedures for non-human primates can be found in JWGR (2009). Squirrel monkeys are social animals and all efforts should be made to house them in social groups or, at least, in pairs. Figures 37.2 and 37.3 illustrate a large social group pen and smaller cages that can be used for single- or pair-housed animals. The European standard for squirrel monkey caging calls for a minimum floor space of $2\,m^2$ for up to two animals, with an additional $0.5\,m^2$ for each additional animal (European Commission 2007). The US standards classify squirrel monkeys as type 2 primates, requiring $3\,ft^2$ ($0.28\,m^2$) for each animal (National Research Council 1996). All squirrel monkeys should be housed with a temperature range of around 24–27 °C (75–82 °F) and with a relative humidity of 40–60%. Lower temperatures or humidity levels can lead to upper respiratory problems (Abee 1985).

Squirrel monkeys do well when exposed to natural lighting (Srivastava *et al.* 1970; Williams *et al.* 1986a) with the breeding season shifted toward the period of short days. A 12 h light–dark cycle is appropriate for indoor-housed animals, although light cycles can vary somewhat. There is anecdotal evidence that when housed indoors for extended periods, time-limited exposure to UV lamps may be helpful for vitamin D3 synthesis.

Squirrel monkeys should be fed a nutritionally balanced diet such as commercially available monkey chows, specifically formulated for New World primates. *Ad libitum* feeding should be supplemented with fresh vegetables, fruit slices and mealworms periodically. Non-carbonated sports drinks and yogurt should be considered for animals that are ill or debilitated. Feeding each morning following completion of the cage sanitation procedures and again in the afternoon will ensure food is continuously available.

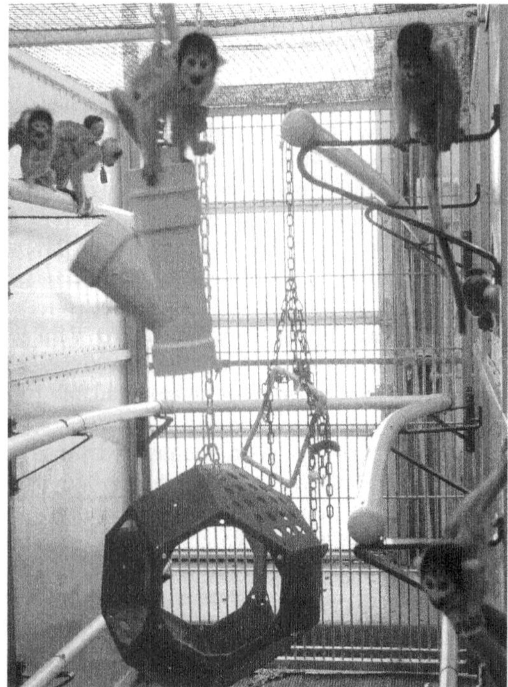

Figure 37.2 Socially housed squirrel monkeys in an indoor facility. Note the use of vertical space and multiple travel paths throughout the cage. The animal on the middle-right is coming through a doorway from a second cage.

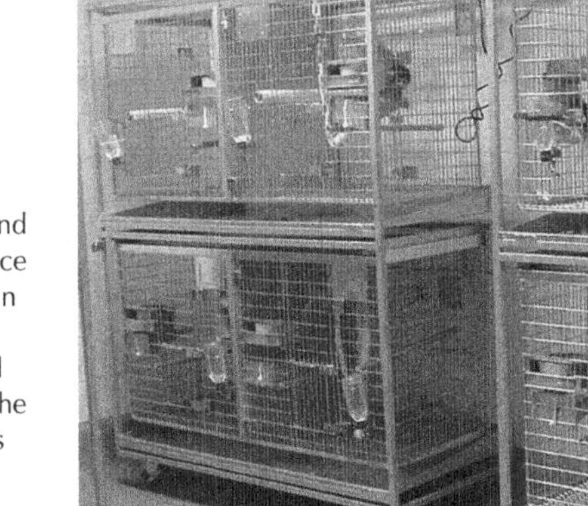

Figure 37.3 Individually housed squirrel monkeys in enriched cages. There are multiple levels of perching and plastic chain used to increase access to the vertical space in the cage. Small enrichment devices are hung either in the cage or on the outside wire mesh. These cages conform to the US standard of 3 ft^2 (0.28 m^2) per animal floor space with 30 inches (0.76 m) minimum height. The European standard is 2 m^2 for either one or two animals (an additional 0.5 m^2 for each animal over two) with 1.8 m^2 minimum height.

Animal feeds should be stored on pallets in a clean, dry, vermin-free environment. Milling dates should be monitored as a standard procedure to make certain that fresh feed is used. Those commercial diets made in the US with milling dates of more than 90 days (180 days for feeds certified to maintain vitamin C levels for that period of time) should be discarded. Since group-housed animals may fight over feed, sufficient food should be provided at multiple sites in the cage to allow *ad libitum* feeding throughout the daylight hours. Broadcasting diet pellets within group pens will encourage foraging behaviour and discourage food guarding by dominant animals (see general recommendations for feeding primates in European Commission 2007). This method should be considered for larger pens with solid floors.

Water may be provided from bottles with sipper tubes or by automatic watering devices, which consist of low-pressure water pipes equipped with watering valves. Monkeys unaccustomed to these devices may need to be shown how they operate to avoid dehydration. Animals housed in pens or cage/rack units should be provided with water continuously. Watering bottles should be changed no less than three times per week and should always contain water.

Environmental provisions

In nature, squirrel monkeys live in large social groups containing 20–200 animals (Baldwin & Baldwin 1971a) with multiple males and females of different ages. Efforts should be made to house them in social groups where possible. Animals born into a social group should be maintained within their social group as long as possible. In the South American species of squirrel monkeys, females typically stay within the social group and males emigrate after age 1.5–2 years. Squirrel monkeys will fight with unfamiliar conspecifics (Williams & Abee 1988) so frequent movement of animals between social groups should be avoided. Squirrel monkeys that must be held separate from their social group for experimental or clinical purposes should be pair-housed. If that is not possible they should be given visual or auditory access to other animals (Schuler & Abee 2005).

Since squirrel monkeys are arboreal, perch arrangements can be used to vary the cage environments and increase the activity of the animals. Figures 37.2 and 37.3 illustrate caging and enrichment. Rearranging the perches and providing new materials is an easy way to provide novelty. Notice the extensive use of three-dimensional spaces. Squirrel monkeys are arboreal and will use vertical space if it is available.

Squirrel monkeys are naturally curious and will manually probe objects hung in their cages. Hanging objects such as practice golf balls, infant toys, and polyvinyl chloride (PVC) plumbing joints can be used with or without food enrichment to increase activity rates. However, using foraging (Fekete *et. al.* 2000) and other devices (Spring *et al.* 1997) to ameliorate stereotypical behaviour has not been successful. See also Chapter 10.

Cleaning, sanitation and personnel hygiene

The maintenance of monkeys in cages limits their living space to a relatively small area. This results in concentration of faeces and urine within the animals' immediate living area. Many pathogens in otherwise healthy animals are shed in large numbers in faeces. Therefore, daily cleaning of cages and contact surfaces is an essential part of the preventive medicine programme. Animal husbandry and cage sanitation schedules should include routine sanitising of contact surface areas consistent with guidelines, such as those provided in National Research Council (1996). For squirrel monkeys maintained in Europe, the Commission Recommendations (European Commission 2007) serve as guidelines for the accommodation and care of animals for experimental and other scientific purposes, and may shortly become mandatory.

Group pens should be cleaned daily. Pens should be scrubbed every 2 weeks with a detergent–disinfectant. Cages and racks should be changed and sanitised every 2 weeks. Excreta pans should be flushed daily. Accessory items, such as catch gloves, should be dedicated to specific areas to prevent fomite transmission of pathogens and should be cleaned or replaced regularly. Bedding materials, when used, should be emptied into plastic bin liners.

Technicians and other personnel working with monkeys should be provided with clean protective clothing daily.

Personnel should be required to wear a surgical mask or respirator and gloves when handling primates. Persons developing positive tuberculin reactions should not be permitted to work with monkeys until a sufficient period of treatment has elapsed or medical evaluation has been carried out. Examination gloves, leather catch gloves, face masks, dedicated uniforms and head covers should be worn whenever animals or their wastes are handled. Staff showers and locker rooms should be provided for bathing and staff should change into street clothes before leaving the facility.

Identification of animals

Several methods are available for identification of squirrel monkeys. When properly applied, tattoos provide a durable method of identification. Recommended tattoo sites are on the chest, abdomen, or the medial thigh. Neck tags that can be read from a distance are advantageous when animals are group-housed. Modified livestock tags, cut down in size or coloured beads (Soltis *et al.* 2005) can be used to identify individuals. Neck chains for identification tags must be carefully fitted. A chain that is too loose may slip over the animal's mandible or catch on parts of the cage. If it fits too tightly, it may cause skin lesions or, in extreme cases, impede respiration. Neck chains should be rechecked for proper fit whenever animals are handled because weight loss or gain may mean that they need resizing.

Implantable microchip transponders that broadcast a unique identifying number to an external receiver provide a reliable means of identification. When choosing a method of identification consideration should be given to using the least invasive technique.

Age determination

One major advantage of using purpose-bred squirrel monkeys for research is that the age of an animal will be known. If animals with unknown birthdates are used, an estimate of the animal's age may be made by examining dentition and general physical appearance (Galliari & Colillas 1985; Long and Cooper 1968; Smith *et al.* 1994; Tappen & Severson 1971). Williams and Gibson (2004) provide a useful chart for aging female Guyanese squirrel monkeys (*Saimiri sciureus*) using the length of the black 'sideburns' seen only on the females. There is a high correlation (r = 0.97) between the length of the sideburn and the age of the female.

Health monitoring

Daily observation of all squirrel monkeys is an important husbandry and veterinary support procedure. Serious health problems can progress rapidly in squirrel monkeys so that an animal overlooked during the morning observations could die before being discovered later in the day. Observations of all animals should be carried out at least twice daily. The first observation should be made before cages are cleaned in the morning. The floor of the cage should be observed for signs of blood, aborted or stillborn foetuses (during the birth season), and for animals sitting or lying on the floor of the cage. An estimation of the feed consumed should also be made at this time. If water bottles are being used, the water consumed should be also estimated. A second observation is made late in the day. Animals that do not appear interested in eating should be observed for signs of injury or disease. During the birth season, observations are often useful in determining which females are nearing parturition and whether labour is beginning or whether there is an abnormal foetal presentation. The veterinary staff should be consulted immediately if unproductive labour is observed. Unproductive labour exceeding 1 h requires immediate veterinary attention.

Biosafety considerations

Squirrel monkeys are carriers of herpesvirus saimiri 2, which is known to be oncogenic in other primates and can infect and transform human T-lymphocytes *in vitro* (Mansfield & King 1998). Although there are no data which would indicate that Herpesvirus saimiri 2 can cause disease in humans, its ability to cause disease in other animals and to replicate in human issues is sufficient reason to counsel persons who work with squirrel monkeys to use appropriate procedures to minimise potential risk of transmission of the virus from the animals to themselves.

They are also carriers for herpesvirus saimiri 1, which is known to cause fatal disease in *Aotus* and some other species of New World primates (Mansfield & King 1998). Biosafety precautions should always be followed with squirrel monkeys. A sensible approach is to follow the *Update: Universal Precautions for Workers Handling Human Blood, Body Fluids and Tissue in the Workplace* (CDC 1988) when working with squirrel monkeys, their tissues and their body fluids.

Squirrel monkeys are not considered to be carriers of Cercopithecine herpesvirus 1, CHV-1 (also known as B virus), which can cause deadly central nervous system disease in humans. Therefore, the stringent testing and treatment techniques required for bites, scratches and splashes on humans when inflicted by macaques from B-virus positive colonies are not required for cases involving squirrel monkeys (Holmes *et al.* 1995). Squirrel monkeys are also thought to be less likely to contract tuberculosis than macaques (Osborn & Lowenstine 1998).

Laboratory procedures

Restraint techniques

Manual and chair restraint methods may be used for squirrel monkeys. Techniques of restraint may have important effects on certain types of studies. Both capture and chair restraint can cause adrenal cortical activation and growth hormone release (Brown *et al.* 1971b, 1971a). Manual restraint can cause elevation in glucagon (Myers *et al.* 1988). Ketamine anaesthesia has been postulated to cause changes in glucose tolerance test results in other non-human primates (Streett & Jonas 1982); however, this belief has been disputed by others (Brady & Koritnik 1985; Castro *et al.* 1981); Kemnitz & Kraemer 1982). The ultrashort-acting barbiturate anaesthetic sodium thiopental can cause premature ventricular contractions in squirrel monkeys (Wolf *et al.* 1969) and should be used with caution.

Gastric intubation and vascular access

Gastric intubation and vascular access techniques are useful for a variety of studies. Gastric intubation may be performed by the orogastric or nasogastric route. Both may be performed using a number 5 French infant feeding tube (Abee 1985). Orogastric intubation requires the use of a speculum in awake animals to prevent the animal from chewing the tube. Nasogastric intubation requires some practice to be performed properly in the squirrel monkey. After marking the distance to the stomach on the tube, a small amount of sterile lubricant jelly is applied to the tip, and the tube is gently inserted into the nares. The tube must be directed medially to avoid the blind pouch in the nasal cavity (Abee 1985). When the tube has been inserted to the previously made mark, it should be dipped in water to form a meniscus on the luer adapter. This meniscus should then be observed for respiratory movement because such movement suggests that the tube may have been inserted into the trachea and it should be repositioned before use to prevent accidental aspiration. Epistaxis may occasionally occur as a result of nasogastric intubation, but it is usually mild and self-limiting when the technique is performed properly.

Blood sampling and parenteral injections

General advice on blood sampling techniques can be obtained from JWGR (1993). Venous sampling and intravenous injection are best performed with 23–27G needles. Large samples (>0.25ml) may be taken from the femoral vein at the femoral triangle or the lateral tail vein. These sites are also suitable for injection. The saphenous veins located on the dorsal surface of the leg below the knee may be used for intravenous injections and small blood volume collections. These sites are generally suitable only for smaller samples because veins at these sites collapse easily. Blood sample volumes are limited by the size of squirrel monkeys. As a general rule, no more than 3–4ml of blood per kilogram of body weight should be obtained at one time. Animals from which samples are taken repeatedly should have periodic haematocrits to monitor for anaemia. The following protocol can be used to treat adult squirrel monkeys that have anaemia associated with blood loss or that are included on experimental protocols requiring frequent blood sampling: (1) iron as iron dextran: 50mg intramuscularly, once; (2) folic acid: 2.5mg subcutaneously, twice weekly; and (3) vitamin B complex includes cyanocobalamin, riboflavin (B2), and pyridoxine (B6): dose depends on formulation, subcutaneously, twice weekly. Once the hematocrit reaches 40%, treatment should stop.

General advice on the administration of substances can be found in JWGR (2001). Subcutaneous injections in squirrel monkeys may be performed dorsally between the scapulae. Caution should be used when intramuscular injections into the thigh are performed because the ischiatic nerve is easily damaged by needle penetration of the leg (Abee 1985).

Anaesthesia and analgesia

Anaesthesia may be performed in squirrel monkeys with many of the same agents used in other primate species (Brady 2000; Horne 2001). The discussions later in the chapter, regarding hypothermia and hypoglycaemia in squirrel monkeys, are directly applicable to animals that are anaesthetised, and especially those animals anaesthetised for prolonged periods. Appropriate precautions should be taken to prevent hypothermia and hypoglycaemia.

The use of a long-acting barbiturate such as sodium pentobarbital is recommended in squirrel monkeys only for terminal procedures because long-acting barbiturates cause respiratory depression (Flecknell 2009) and prolonged recovery in squirrel monkeys. If sodium pentobarbital is used at the standard 50mg/ml concentration, it should be diluted 1:1 with saline before use.

Isoflurane is an excellent agent for inhalation anaesthesia of squirrel monkeys. Mask induction may be rapidly performed in animals that are manually restrained, or animals may be induced with an injectable agent, intubated, and maintained under anaesthesia with isoflurane. Morris *et al.* (1997) have described a technique for intubation of squirrel monkeys. Dead space, resistance to flow, and heat and humidity loss in anaesthesia circuits are important considerations due to the small size of the squirrel monkey (Hartsfield 1996). A non-rebreathing anaesthesia circuit is recommended for inhalation anaesthesia.

Experimental work with pregnant squirrel monkeys anaesthetised for extended periods has shown the value of careful anaesthesia monitoring, and 'balanced anaesthesia' technique, where multiple drugs are used with each agent directed at a different component of the anaesthetic state (consciousness, analgesia, autonomic reflexes, muscle relaxation) (Thurmon *et al.* 1996). End-tidal carbon dioxide and blood pressure/heart rate are especially useful parameters for managing squirrel monkeys during anaesthesia. Drugs to consider for this balanced approach may include isoflurane, nitrous oxide and thiopental (Avidan, personal communication).

Mechanical ventilation can be performed in squirrel monkeys under anaesthesia. A neurophysiology study of five adult squirrel monkeys used an estimated tidal volume of 6–8ml/kg with a respiratory rate of 70/minute as initial settings. These volumes were then adjusted to give an end-tidal carbon dioxide (collected through a catheter inserted through the endotracheal tube to midtrachea) of 3.5–3.8% (Maier *et al.* 1997; Morris, personal communication).

Analgesics should be used in squirrel monkeys during and after recovery from surgical procedures unless specifically contraindicated by experimental protocol or the medical condition of the animal. Buprenorphine at a dose of 0.01mg/kg intramuscularly or intravenously causes little sedation in squirrel monkeys and is an effective analgesic that may be given every 12h (Jenkins, 1987).

Euthanasia

Euthanasia should be performed in accordance with established humane procedures (American Veterinary Medical

Association (AVMA) 2007) in the US. European laboratories with squirrel monkeys should comply with the principles set by the European Commission Recommendations for euthanasia of experimental animals (Part 1 and Part 2) (European Commission 2007) or local national regulations.

Common welfare problems

Hypothermia and hypoglycaemia

Investigators accustomed to using rodents and larger primates in their research should be aware of squirrel monkey characteristics that may require alteration of experimental procedures. Their small size, low body fat reserve and long extremities all contribute to rapid heat loss when they are anaesthetised or debilitated. At-risk animals should be monitored for body temperature on a regular basis. Awake, restrained squirrel monkeys normally have a temperature of 38–39.5 °C. Healthy, active, struggling animals may rapidly increase their body temperatures as high as 41 °C. Temperatures of less than 37.7 °C are seen with seriously ill animals and should be investigated immediately. In general, electronic thermometers designed for use on humans and animals may be used with squirrel monkeys. Tympanic membrane thermometers register temperatures much faster than most rectal thermometers, and can be used with adult squirrel monkeys. These thermometers are especially useful for rapidly estimating temperatures on multiple animals. Williams (unpublished data) has found an 85% correlation between the two methods, with the tympanic membrane thermometer registering 0.2–0.6 °C lower than the mercury rectal thermometer. Careful positioning of these thermometers over the tympanic membrane is important. These thermometers may not work well for infant or smaller juvenile squirrel monkeys.

For hypothermic animals, supplemental heat may be provided in a variety of ways. Awake animals may be housed in incubator-type enclosures or on warm water recirculating pads. Recirculating pads may also be used for anaesthetised animals. Heat packs that use a controlled exothermic chemical reaction can provide a convenient, portable, temporary source of warmth for anaesthetised and recovering animals. Electrical heating pads should not be used with squirrel monkeys due to the danger of burns and electrical shock. Convection warmers are effective for maintaining body temperature in anaesthetised squirrel monkeys.

Squirrel monkeys are predisposed to hypoglycaemia (Abee 1985; Brady *et al.* 1990, 1991). The normal blood glucose concentration for adult squirrel monkeys is 80 ± 28 mg/dL (Loeb & Quimby 1989). Prolonged research procedures, fasting, or debilitating conditions that result in anorexia may place animals at risk for a hypoglycaemic crisis. Dry reagent strips for determining blood glucose concentration and meters that accurately read these strips are available from most pharmacies. These strips are inexpensive and useful tools for monitoring squirrel monkeys. Hypoglycaemic animals that are still conscious should be given glucose or sucrose solution orally. Unconscious animals should be given sterile 20% dextrose solution by nasogastric tube (discussed earlier in this chapter). Infants should be given 1 ml, juveniles 3–5 ml, and adults 10 ml. Use of concentrated intravenous glucose solutions to treat hypoglycaemia is not recommended.

Selected diseases and injuries

Infection of squirrel monkeys with herpesvirus saimiri 1 and 2 (HS-1 and –2) is widespread, with most infected animals having no clinical signs. Squirrel monkeys infected with HS-1 that are stressed or immunosuppressed may have oral–pharyngeal lesions that resemble human cold sores. The lesions usually resolve within a few days without treatment, but animals may require hand-feeding during this period due to difficulty eating. (Gibson, personal communication).

Yersinia enterocolitica and *Yersinia pseudotuberculosis* are aetiological agents for the disease known as pseudotuberculosis in squirrel monkeys and other non-human primates. Infection can result in septicaemia. Animals are often not diagnosed until the disease is severe, or animals are simply found dead with no prior clinical signs. This makes treatment of pseudotuberculosis difficult. Visceral abscesses are commonly seen at necropsy. Feral rodents and birds are reservoirs for the causative agents. Squirrel monkeys can also be silent carriers. Cultures of rectal swabs under the required conditions may identify monkeys that carry these agents (Brady & Morton 1998). *Pasteurella*, *Bordetella*, *Staphylococcus* and *Klebsiella* have caused bacterial disease in squirrel monkeys.

Heart disease is frequent in older squirrel monkeys (Brady *et al.* 2003). In one study, 23 of 88 adult squirrel monkeys necropsied over a 4-year period had a diagnosis of heart failure or had lesions consistent with heart disease. Heart disease is most often seen in multiparous older females, but may also be seen in peripartum females of any age and in older males (Gibson, personal communication). Most heart disease in squirrel monkeys is cardiomyopathic. Clinical signs may include laboured respiration, ascites, hepatomegaly and cyanosis. Diagnosis is best accomplished by echocardiography. Although successful protocols have been developed for treatment of other New World primates (Brady *et al.* 2005), squirrel monkeys with cardiomyopathy have been relatively refractory to treatment.

Renal disease

Renal disease has long been recognised as a major cause of morbidity and mortality in older squirrel monkeys, especially those of feral origin. Glomerulonephritis, pyelonephritis and renal lithiasis have been reported (Stills & Bullock 1981). Affected animals may have weight loss, lethargy, a characteristic foul odour and, in advanced cases, subcutaneous oedema (Abee 1985). Serum chemistry generally demonstrates elevated blood urea nitrogen (BUN) and creatinine with low serum albumen. Haematology test results may reveal anaemia (see Tables 37.2 and 37.3). Animals with acute renal disease may respond to supportive care and fluid therapy. However, chronic renal disease with clinical signs noted above is often refractory to treat-

Table 37.2 Reference haematology values taken at the Center for Neotropical Primate Research and Resources. Assays were performed on blood collected in EDTA. Blood samples were collected from juvenile and adult Bolivian squirrel monkeys, most of which were colony born. Values from pregnant monkeys were included. CBCs were performed using an Abaxis VetScan® Hematology System. (WBC: white blood cell count; RBC: red blood cell count; MCV: mean corpuscular volume; HCT: haematocrit; MCH: mean corpuscular haemoglobin; MCHC: mean corpuscular haemoglobin concentration; RDW: red blood cell distribution width; HB (HGB): haemoglobin; MPV: mean platelet volume).

	Units	*N*	*Mean*	*SD*	*Minimum*	*Maximum*	*25th percentile*	*50th percentile*	*75th percentile*
WBC	$10^3/mm^3$	267	8.3	2.5	2.6	17.6	6.7	7.9	9.8
RBC	$10^6/mm^3$	267	6.4	0.8	2.9	7.96	6.2	6.7	6.9
MCV	fl	267	60.0	3.2	50.3	70.8	58.0	60.0	62.2
HCT	%	267	38.5	5.5	15.4	49.8	36.2	39.7	42
MCH	pg	267	19.8	2.4	13.7	49.1	18.7	19.6	20.7
MCHC	g/dl	267	33.1	4.7	21.7	92.8	30.9	33.1	34.4
RDW	%	267	10.6	2.3	7.1	18.4	8.8	10.2	11.3
HB	gm/dl	267	12.6	1.6	6.1	15.7	12.0	13.0	13.7
MPV	fl	267	9.0	1.7	6.3	16.1	8.1	8.5	8.9

Table 37.3 Reference serum chemistry values collected at the Center for Neotropical Primate Research and Resources. Assays were performed on serum samples from juvenile and adult Bolivian squirrel monkeys, the majority of which were colony born. Values from pregnant monkeys were included. All assays were performed using an Abaxis VetScan® Chemistry System Analyzer using the Comprehensive Diagnostic rotor for small animals.

Parameter	*Units*	*N*	*Mean*	*SD*	*Minimum*	*Maximum*	*25th percentile*	*50th percentile*	*75th percentile*
Albumin*	g/dl	256	2.4	0.2	1.8	3.0	2.3	2.4	2.6
Alanine aminotransferase ALT (SGOT)	u/l	52	181	78	82	502	128	171	211
Alkaline phosphatase Adult, (4 yrs of age	u/l	153	389	159	98	1103	288	357	466
Alkaline phosphatase Juvenile, <4 yrs of age	u/l	90	919	441	228	2400	616	843	1101
Amylase	u/l	203	54	96	10	943	31	37	46
Total bilirubin	mg/dl	243	0.4	0.2	0.1	1.3	0.3	0.4	0.5
Urea nitrogen (BUN)	mg/dl	256	34	10	18	147	30	34	38
Calcium	mg/dl	243	10.0	0.8	8.1	12.7	9.5	10.0	10.7
Phosphorus (adult)	mg/dl	128	4.6	1.5	1.6	9.0	3.3	4.3	5.5
Phosphorus (juvenile)	mg/dl	64	6.8	1.7	3.7	12.0	5.7	6.7	7.8
Creatinine	mg/dl	256	0.6	0.2	0.2	1.5	0.4	0.6	0.7
Glucose	mg/dl	256	109	28	51	201	89	104	129
Potassium	mmol/l	252	5.3	1.0	3.0	9.8	4.7	5.4	6.0
Sodium	mmol/l	256	149	6	130	170	145	149	153
Total protein	g/dl	255	6.7	0.5	5.2	8.3	6.3	6.7	7.1
Globulin	g/dl	202	4.2	0.4	3.2	5.3	4.0	4.3	4.6

*Albumin levels are low due to test methodology (dry substrate bromidene green) and under-represent actual values.

ment. Ensuring adequate hydration at all times is the best method for preventing and managing renal disease.

Periodontal disease

Dental disease, especially periodontal disease, has been reported in captive colonies of squirrel monkeys (Clark *et al.* 1988; Brady *et al.* 2000). Periodontal disease can lead to dental abscesses and reduced food intake due to painful eating, especially in older animals. It can also cause systemic bacteraemia, with associated health problems. Increased diet supplementation with vegetables as opposed to fruits may be of some benefit in preventing periodontal disease (Williams *et al.* 1992). Sodium hexametaphosphate as a feed additive has been proposed as a means to prevent dental calculus formation that is thought to predispose squirrel monkeys to periodontal disease. Unfortunately, the diet with this additive does not appear to be effective in reducing existing calculus (Brady *et al.* 2000). All squirrel monkey colonies should have programmes for routine dental examination and cleaning and be equipped to treat dental problems such as dental abscesses.

Fight-related injuries

Although social housing of squirrel monkeys is desirable, fight-related injuries are common in such housing, especially when social groups are first established. Close attention to group compatibility, careful supervision of newly established groups and provision of hiding places in animal enclosures can help reduce such injuries or prevent them altogether (Williams & Abee 1988). When wounds do occur, they can usually be divided into crushing-type injuries (more commonly inflicted by female squirrel monkeys) or lacerations (commonly inflicted by males) (Ruiz *et al.* 2005). To treat wounds, surrounding hair should be clipped, the wound cleaned and debrided as needed and the wound dressed and/or sutured at the discretion of the attending veterinarian. Care should be used when deciding to suture fight wounds, especially the crushing-type of injuries. Many of these wounds will heal better by second intention rather than suturing. Absorbent dressings may be useful with suppurative wounds as these dressings will serve as a wick to draw the infection out of the wound.

Failure-to-thrive syndrome

A syndrome resembling human failure-to-thrive syndrome (FTT) has been described in squirrel monkey infants. In one colony, 3% of live-born infants showed signs of FTT. It was characterised by premature thymic involution, poor weight gain and increased number of opportunist infections. Most of the infants died before they reached 6 months of age (Gibson *et al.* 1998). No effective treatment has been developed for FTT in squirrel monkeys.

References

Abee, C.R. (1985) Medical care and management of the squirrel monkey. *Handbook of Squirrel Monkey Research.* Plenum Press, New York

Ariga, S., Dukelow, W.R., Emley, G.S. *et al.* (1978) Possible errors in identification of squirrel monkeys (*Saimiri sciureus*) from different South American points of export. *Journal of Medical Primatology*, **7**, 129–135

Assis, M.F.L. and Barros, R. (1987) Karyotype pattern of *Saimiri ustus. International Journal of Primatology*, **8**, 552

Ausman, L.M., Gallina, D.L. and Nicolosi, R.J. (1985) Nutrition and metabolism of the squirrel monkey. In: *Handbook of Squirrel Monkey Research.* Eds Rosenblum, L. and Coe, C., pp. 349–378. Plenum Press, New York

American Veterinary Medical Association (2007) AVMA Guidelines on Euthanasia American June 2007 (formerly Report of the AMVA Panel on Euthanasia). http://www.avma.org/issues/animal_welfare/euthanasia.pdf (accessed 16 April 2009)

Ayres, J. (1985) On a new species of squirrel monkey, genus Samiri, from Brazilian Amazonia (Primates, Cebidae). *Papéis Avulsos Zool. São Paulo*, **36**, 147–164.

Baldwin, J.D. (1968) The social behavior of adult male squirrel monkeys (*Saimiri sciureus*) in a seminatural environment. *Folia Primatologica*, **9**, 281–314

Baldwin, J.D. (1969) The ontogeny of social behavior of squirrel monkeys (*Saimiri sciureus*) in a seminatural environment. *Folia Primatologica*, **11**, 35–79

Baldwin, J.D. (1985) The behavior of squirrel monkeys (*Saimiri*) in natural environments. In: *Handbook of Squirrel Monkey Research.* Eds Rosenblum, L. and Coe, C., pp. 35–54. Plenum Press, New York

Baldwin, J.D. and Baldwin, J.I. (1971a) Squirrel monkeys (*Saimiri*) in natural habitats in Panama, Colombia, Brazil, and Peru. *Primates*, **12**, 45–61

Baldwin, J.D. and Baldwin, J.I. (1971b) The ecology and behavior of squirrel monkeys (*Saimiri oerstedii*) in a natural forest in western Panama. *Folia Primatologica*, **18**, 161–184

Baldwin, J.D. and Baldwin, J. (1972) The ecology and behavior of squirrel monkeys (*Saimiri oerstedi*) in a natural forest in western Panama. *Folia Primatologica*, **18**, 161–184

Baldwin, J.D. and Baldwin, J.I. (1981) The squirrel monkeys, genus *Saimiri*. In: *Ecology and Behavior of Neotropical Primates*, Vol. 1. Eds Coimbra-Filho, A. and Mittermeier, R., pp. 227–330. Academia Brasileira de Ciencias, Rio de Janeiro

Beischer, D.E. (1968) *Vectorcardiogram and Aortic Blood Flow of Squirrel Monkeys (Saimiri sciureus) in a Strong Superconductive Electromagnet.* Pensacola, Florida

Bennett, J.P. (1967a) Artificial insemination of the squirrel monkey. *Journal of Endocrinology*, **37**, 473–474

Bennett, J.P. (1967b) The induction of ovulation in the squirrel monkey (*Saimiri sciureus*) with pregnant mares serum (PMS) and human chorionic gonadotrophin (HCG). *Journal of Reproduction and Fertility*, **13**, 357–359

Boinski, S. (1985) Status of the squirrel monkey *Saimiri oerstedi* in Costa Rica. *Primate Conservation*, **6**, 15–16

Boinski, S. (1987a) Birth synchrony in squirrel monkeys (*Saimiri oerstedi*): a strategy to reduce neonatal predation. *Behavioural Ecology and Sociobiology*, **21**, 393–400

Boinski, S. (1987b) Habitat use by squirrel monkeys (*Saimiri oerstedi*) in Costa Rica. *Folia Primatologica*, **49**, 151–167.

Boinski, S. (1987c) Mating patterns in squirrel monkeys (*Saimiri oerstedi*): implications for seasonal sexual dimorphism. *Behavioural Ecology and Sociobiology*, **21**, 13–21

Boinski, S. and Mitchell, C.L. (1994) Male residence and association patterns in Costa Rican squirrel monkeys (*Saimiri oerstedi*). *American Journal of Primatology*, **34**, 157–169

Boinski, S., Sughrue, K., Selvaggi, L. *et al.* (2002) An expanded test of the ecological model of primate social evolution: competitive regimes and female bonding in three species of squirrel monkeys (*Saimiri oerstedii, S. boliviensis, and S. sciureus*). *Behaviour*, **139**, 227–261

Brady, A.G. (2000) Research techniques for the squirrel monkey (*Saimiri* sp.). *ILAR Journal*, **41**, 10–18

Brady, A.G., Hutto, G.E., Williams, L.E. *et al.* (1991) Comparison of two tests for identifying squirrel monkey infants at risk for hypoglycemia. *AALAS Bulletin*, **30**, 28–29

Brady, A.G. and Koritnik, D. (1985) The effects of ketamine anesthesia on glucose clearance in African green monkeys. *Journal of Medical Primatology*, **14**, 99–107

Brady, A. and Morton, D.G. (1998) Digestive system. In: *Nonhuman Primates in Biomedical Research, Diseases.* Eds Bennett, B., Abee, C. and Hendrickson, R., pp. 377–414. Academic Press, San Diego

Brady, A.G., Parks, V.L., Gibson, S.V. *et al.* (2005) Cardiomyopathy of owl monkeys: a study of seven cases. *Contemporary Topics in Laboratory Animal Science*, **44**, 57

Brady, A.G., Watford, J.W., Massey, C.V. *et al.* (2003) Studies of heart disease and failure in aged female squirrel monkeys (*Saimiri* sp.). *Comparative Medicine*, **53**, 657–662

Brady, A.G., Williams, L.E. and Abee, C.R. (1990) Hypoglycemia of squirrel monkey neonates: implications for infant survival. *Laboratory Animal Science*, **40**, 262–265

Brady, A.G., Williams, L.E., Haught, D. *et al.* (2000) Use of the feed additive sodium hexametaphosphate to prevent dental calculus in squirrel monkeys (*Saimiri* spp.). *Contemporary Topics in Laboratory Animal Science*, **39**, 27–29

Brown, G.M., Schalch, D.S. and Reichlin, S. (1971a) Hypothalamic mediation of growth hormone and adrenal stress response in the squirrel monkey. *Endocrinology*, **89**, 694–703

Brown, G.M., Schalch, D.S. and Reichlin, S. (1971b) Patterns of growth hormone and cortisol responses to psychological stress in the squirrel monkey. *Endocrinology*, **88**, 956–963

Brown, P., Gibbs, C.J., Rodgers-Johnson, P. *et al.* (1994) Human spongiform encephalopathy: The National Institutes of Health series of 300 cases of experimentally transmitted disease. *Annals of Neurology*, **35**, 513–529

Candland, D.K., Dresdale, L., Leiphart, J. *et al.* (1973) Social structure of the squirrel monkey (*Saimiri sciureus*, Iquitos): relationship among behavior, heart rate and physical distance. *Folia Primatologica*, **20**, 211–240

Castro, M.I., Rose, J., Green, W. *et al.* (1981) Ketamine-HCl as a suitable anesthetic for endocrine, metabolic, and cardiovascular studies in Macaca fascicularis monkeys. *Proceedings of the Society for Experimental Biology and Medicine*, **168**, 389–394

Centers for Disease Control and Prevention (1987) B-virus infection in humans – Pensacola, Florida. *Morbidity And Mortality Weekly Report*, **36**, 289–290, 295–296

Centers for Disease Control and Prevention (1988) Update: universal precautions for prevention of transmission of human immunodeficiency virus, hepatitis B virus, and other bloodborne pathogens in health-care settings. *Morbidity Mortality Weekly Report*, **37**, 377–382, 387–388

Centers for Disease Control and Prevention (1989) B-virus infections in humans – Michigan. *Morbidity And Mortality Weekly Report*, **38**, 453–454

Centers for Disease Control and Prevention (1998) Fatal Cercopithecine herpesvirus 1 (B Virus) infection following a mucocutaneous exposure and interim recommendations for worker protection. *Morbidity And Mortality Weekly Report*, **47**,1073–1076, 1083

Chen, J., Smith, E., Gray, G. *et al.* (1981) Seasonal changes in plasma testosterone and ejaculatory capacity in squirrel monkeys (*Saimiri sciureus*). *Primates*, **22**, 253–260

Clark, W.B., Magnusson, I., Abee, C. *et al.* (1988) Natural occurrence of black-pigmented *Bacteroides* species in the gingival crevice of the squirrel monkey. *Infection and Immunity*, **56**, 2392–2399

Coates, K.W., Galan, H.L., Shull, B.L. *et al.* (1995) The squirrel monkey: an animal model of pelvic relaxation. *American Journal of Obstetrics and Gynecology*, **172**, 588–593

Coe, C.L. and Levine, S. (1981) Psychoendocrine relationships underlying reproductive behavior in the squirrel monkey. *International Journal of Mental Health*, **10**, 22–42

Coe, C.L. and Rosenblum, L.A. (1974) Sexual segregation and its ontogeny in squirrel monkey social structure. *Journal of Human Evolution*, **3**, 551–561

Coe, C.L. and Rosenblum, L.A. (1978) Annual reproductive strategy of the squirrel monkey (*Saimiri sciureus*). *Folia Primatologica*, **29**, 19–42

Coe, C.L., Wiener, S.G., Rosenberg, L.T. *et al.* (1985) Endocrine and immune responses to separation and maternal loss in nonhuman primates. In: *The Psychobiology of Attachment and Separation*. Eds. Reite, M. and Field, T., pp. 163–199. Academic Press, Orlando

Cooper, R.W. (1968) Squirrel monkey taxonomy and supply. In: *The Squirrel Monkey*. Eds. Rosenblum, L. and Cooper, R., pp. 1–29. Academic Press, New York

Costello, R.K., Dickinson, C., Rosenberger, A.L. *et al.* (1993) Squirrel monkey (genus *Saimiri*) taxonomy: a multidisciplinary study of the biology of species. In: *Species, Species Concepts and Primate Evolution*. Eds. Kibel, W. and Martin, L., pp. 177–210. Plenum Press, New York

Cropp, S. and Boinski, S. (2000) The central American squirrel monkey (*Saimiri oerstedii*): introduced hybrid or endemic species? *Molecular Phylogenetics and Evolution*, **16**, 350–365

da Silva, B., Sampico, M.I.C., Scheider, M.P.C. *et al.* (1987) Preliminary analysis of genetic distance between squirrel monkeys. *International Journal of Primatology*, **8**, 828

Diamond, E.J., Aksel, S., Hazelton, J.M. *et al.* (1984) Seasonal changes of serum concentrations of estradiol and progesterone in Bolivian squirrel monkeys (*Saimiri sciureus*). *American Journal of Primatology*, **6**, 103–113

Dukelow, R. (1985) Reproductive cyclicity and breeding in the squirrel monkey. In: *Handbook of Squirrel Monkey Research*. Eds Rosenblum, L. and Coe, C., pp. 169–190. Plenum Press, New York

Du Mond, F.V. (1967) Semi-free-ranging colonies of monkeys at Goulds Monkey Jungle. *International Zoo Yearbook*, **7**, 202–207

Du Mond, F.V. (1968) The squirrel monkey in a semi-natural environment. In: *The Squirrel Monkey*. Eds. Rosenblum, L. and Cooper, R., pp. 87–145. Academic Press, New York

Du Mond, F.V. and Hutchinson, T.C. (1967) Squirrel monkey reproduction: the 'fatted' male phenomenon and seasonal spermatogenesis. *Science*, **158**, 1067–1070

European Commission (2007) Commission recommendations of 18 June 2007 on guidelines for the accommodation and care of animals used for experimental and other scientific purposes. Annex II to European Council Directive 86/609. See 2007/526/EC. http://eurlex.europa.eu/LexUriServ/site/en/oj/2007/l_197/l_19720070730en00010089.pdf (accessed 13 May 2008)

Fairbanks, L. (1974) An analysis of subgroup structure and process in a captive squirrel monkey (*Saimiri sciureus*) colony. *Folia Primatologica*, **21**, 209–224

Fekete, J., Norcross, J.L. and Newman, J.D. (2000) Artificial turf foraging boards as environmental enrichment for pair-housed female squirrel monkeys. *Contemporary Topics in Laboratory Animal Science*, **39**, 22–26

Flecknell, P.A. (2009) *Laboratory Animal Anaesthesia*, 3rd edn. Academic Press, London

Galland, G.G. (2000) Role of the squirrel monkey in parasitic disease research. *ILAR Journal*, **41**, 37–43

Galliari, C.A. and Colillas, O.J. (1985) Sequences and timing of dental eruption in Bolivian captive-born squirrel monkeys. *American Journal of Primatology*, **8**, 195–204

Gibson, S., Williams, L., Brady, A. *et al.* (1998) Failure to thrive syndrome in squirrel monkey infants (*Saimiri* spp.). *American Journal of Primatology*, **45**, 181–182

Gonzalez, C.A., Hennessy, M.B. and Levine, S. (1981) Subspecies differences in hormonal and behavioral responses after group formation in squirrel monkeys. *American Journal of Primatology*, **1**, 439–452

Goss, C.M., Popejoy, L.T., II, Fusiler, J.L. *et al.* (1968) Observations on the relationship between embryological development, time of conception, and gestation. In: *The Squirrel Monkey*. Eds. Rosenblum, L. and Cooper, R., pp. 171–191. Academic Press, New York

Harrison, R.M. and Dukelow, W.R. (1973) Seasonal adaption of laboratory-maintained squirrel monkeys (*Saimiri sciureus*). *Journal of Medical Primatology*, **2**, 277–283

Hartsfield, S. (1996) Anesthetic machines and breathing systems. In: *Lumb & Jones' Veterinary Anesthesia*. Eds Thurmon, J., Tranquilli, T.W. and Benson, G., pp. 336–408. Williams & Wilkins, Baltimore

Hernandez-Camacho, J. and Cooper, R.W. (1976) The nonhuman primates of Colombia. In: *Neotropical Primates: Field Studies and*

Conservation. Eds. Thorington, R. and Heltne, P., pp. 35–60. National Academy of Sciences, Washington, DC

Hershkovitz, P. (1984) Taxonomy of squirrel monkeys genus *Saimiri* (Cebidae, platyrrhini): a preliminary report with description of a hitherto unnamed form. *American Journal of Primatology*, **7**, 155–210

Holmes, G.P., Chapman, L.E., Stewart, J.A. *et al.* (1995) Guidelines for the prevention and treatment of B-virus infections in exposed persons. *Clinical Infectious Diseases*, **20**, 421–439

Hopf, S. (1978) Huddling subgroups in captive squirrel monkeys and their changes in relation to ontogeney. *Biology of Behaviour*, **3**, 147–162

Horne, W. A. (2001). Primate anesthesia. *Veterinary Clinics of North America: Exotic Animal Practice*, **4**, 239–266, viii–ix

Hunt, S.M., Gamache, K.M. and Lockard, J.S. (1978) Babysitting behavior by age/sex classification in squirrel monkeys (*Saimiri sciureus*). *Primates*, **19**, 179–186

Hutchinson, T.C. (1970) Vaginal cytology and reproduction in the squirrel monkey (*Saimiri sciureus*). *Folia Primatologica*, **12**, 212–223

Izawa, K. (1975) Foods and feeding behavior of monkeys in the upper Amazon basin. *Primates*, **16**, 295–316

Jenkins, W.L. (1987) Pharmacologic aspects of analgesic drugs in animals: An overview. *Journal of the American Veterinary Medical Association*, **191**, 1231–1240

Joint Working Group on Refinement (1993) Removal of blood from laboratory mammals and birds. First Report of the BVA/FRAME/RSPCA/UFAW Joint Working Group on Refinement. *Laboratory Animals*, **27**, 1–22

Joint Working Group on Refinement (2001) Refining procedures for the administration of substances. Report of the BVAAWF/FRAME/RSPCA/UFAW Joint Working Group on Refinement. *Laboratory Animals*, **35**, 1–41

Joint Working Group on Refinement (2009) Refinements in husbandry, care and common procedures for non-human primates. Ninth report of the BVAAWF/FRAME/RSPCA/UFAW Joint Working Group on Refinement. *Laboratory Animals*, **43**, S1:1–S1:47

Jones, T.C., Thorington, R.W., Hu, M.M. *et al.* (1973) Karyotypes of squirrel monkeys (*Saimiri sciureus*) from different geographic regions. *American Journal of Physical Anthropology*, **38**, 269–277

Kaplan, J.N. (1977) Breeding and rearing squirrel monkeys (*Saimiri sciureus*) in captivity. *Laboratory Animal Science*, **27**, 557–567

Kemnitz, J.W. and Kraemer, G.W. (1982) Assessment of glucoregulation in rhesus monkeys sedated with ketamine. *American Journal of Primatology*, **3**, 201–210

Kluver, H. (1933) *Behavior Mechanisms in Monkeys*. University of Chicago Press, Chicago

Konstant, W.R. and Mittermeier, R.A. (1982) Introduction, reintroduction and translocation of neotropical primates: past experiences and future possibilities. *International Zoo Yearbook*, **22**, 69–77

Leger, D.W., Mason, W.A. and Fragaszy, D.M. (1981) Sexual segregation, cliques, and social power in squirrel monkey (*Saimiri*) groups. *Behaviour*, **76**, 163–181

Lehner, N.D.M., Bullock, B.C., Clarkson, T.B. *et al.* (1967) Biological activities of vitamins D-2 and D-3 for growing squirrel monkeys. *Laboratory Animal Care*, **17**, 483–493

Lima, E.M. and Ferrari, S.F. (2003) Diet of a free-ranging group of squirrel monkeys (*Saimiri sciureus*) in Eastern Brazilian Amazonia. *Folia Primatologica*, **74**, 150–158

Loeb, W.F. and Quimby, F.W.E. (1989) *The Clinical Chemistry of Laboratory Animals*. Pergamon Press, New York

Lofland, H. (1975) Animal model of human disease. *American Journal of Pathology*, **79**, 619–622

Long, J.O. and Cooper, R.W. (1968) Physical growth and dental eruption in captive-bred squirrel monkeys, *Saimiri sciureus* (Letica, Colombia). In: *The Squirrel Monkey*. Eds. Rosenblum, L. and Cooper, R., pp. 193–205. Academic Press, New York

Lyons, D.M., Mendoza, S.P. and Mason, W.A. (1992) Sexual segregation in squirrel monkeys (*Saimiri sciureus*): A transactional analysis of adult social dynamics. *Journal of Comparative Psychology*, **106**, 323–330

MacLean, P.D. (1964) Mirror display in the squirrel monkey, *Saimiri sciureus*. *Science*, **146**, 950–952

Maier, M.A., Olivier, E., Baker, S.N. *et al.* (1997) Direct and indirect corticospinal control of arm and hand motoneurons in the squirrel monkey (*Saimiri sciureus*). *Journal of Neurophysiology*, **78**, 721–733

Mansfield, K. and King, N. (1998) Viral diseases. In: *Nonhuman Primates in Biomedical Research, Diseases*. Eds Bennett, B., Abee, C. and Hendrickson, R., pp. 1–48. Academic Press, San Diego

Marsh, R.F., Kincaid, A.E., Bessen, R.A. *et al.* (2005) Interspecies transmission of chronic wasting disease prions to squirrel monkeys. *Journal of Virology*, **79**, 13497–13796

Martin, L.N. and McNease, P.E. (1982) Genetically determined antigens of squirrel monkey (*Saimiri sciureus*) IgG. *Journal of Medical Primatology*, **11**, 272–290

Mason, W.A. & Epple, G. (1969) Social organization in experimental groups of *Saimiri* and *Callicebus*. Proceedings of the Second International Congress of Primatology, Vol. 1: Behavior. Karger, Basel

Mendoza, S.P. (1987) Breeding in groups: the influence of social context on the reproductive potential of squirrel monkeys. *International Journal of Primatology*, **8**, 459

Mendoza, S.P., Lowe, E.L. and Levine, S. (1978a) Social organization and social behavior in two subspecies of squirrel monkeys (*Saimiri sciureus*). *Folia Primatologica*, **30**, 126–144

Mendoza, S.P., Lowe, E.L., Resko, J.A. *et al.* (1978b) Seasonal variations in gonadal hormones and social behavior in squirrel monkeys. *Physiology and Behavior*, **20**, 515–522

Michael, R.P. and Zumpe, D. (1971) Patterns of reproductive behavior. In: *Comparative Reproduction of Nonhuman Primates*. Ed. Hafez, E.S.E., pp. 205–242. Charles C Thomas, Springfield

Middleton, C.C., Clarkson, T.B., Lofland, H.B. *et al.* (1964) Atherosclerosis in the squirrel monkey. Naturally occurring lesions of the aorta and coronary arteries. *Archives of Pathology*, **78**, 16–23

Middleton, C.C., Clarkson, T.B., Lofland, H.B. *et al.* (1967) Diet and atherosclerosis of squirrel monkeys. *Archives of Pathology*, **83**, 145–153

Mitchell, C.L. (1990) The ecological basis for female social dominance: a behavioral study of the squirrel monkey (*Saimiri sciureus*) in the wild. *Dissertation Abstracts International*, **B51**, 1614

Mitchell, C.L., Boinski, S. and Van Schaik, C.P. (1991) Competitive regimes and female bonding in two species of squirrel monkeys (*Saimiri oerstedi* and *S. sciureus*). *Behavioral Ecology and Sociobiology*, **28**, 55–60

Mittermeier, R.A. and van Roosmalen, M.G. (1981) Preliminary observations on habitat utilization and diet in eight Surinam monkeys. *Folia Primatologica*, **36**, 1–39

Morris, T.H., Jackson, R.K., Acker, W.R. *et al.* (1997) An illustrated guide to endotracheal intubation in small non-human primates. *Laboratory Animals*, **31**, 157–162

Morton, L.S. (2000) Maternal and non-maternal contributions to infant caregiving in wild and captive Peruvian squirrel monkeys (*Saimiri* spp.). *Dissertation Abstracts International*, **B61**, 1819

Myers, B.A., Mendoza, S.P. and Cornelius, C.E. (1988) Elevation in plasma glucagon levels in response to stress in squirrel monkeys: Comparisons of two subspecies (*Saimiri sciureus boliviensis* and *Saimiri sciureus sciureus*). *Journal of Medical Primatology*, **17**, 205–214

Nadler, R.D. and Rosenblum, L.A. (1972) Hormonal regulation of the 'fatted' phenomenon in squirrel monkeys. *Anatomical Record*, **173**, 181–187

National Research Council (1996) *Guide for the Care and Use of Laboratory Animals*. National Academy Press, Washington, DC

Osborn, K.G. and Lowenstine, L.J. (1998) Respiratory system. In: *Nonhuman Primates in Biomedical Research, Diseases*. Eds Bennett, B., Abee, C. and Hendrickson, R., pp. 245–262. Academic Press, San Diego

Osuga, T. and Portman, O.W. (1971) Experimental formation of gallstones in the squirrel monkey. *Proceedings of the Society for Experimental Biology and Medicine*, **136**, 722–726

Ploog, D.W. (1967) The behavior of squirrel monkeys (*Saimiri sciureus*) as revealed by sociometry, bioacoustics, and brain stimulation. In: *Social Communication Among Primates*. Ed. Altman, S.A., pp. 149–184. University of Chicago Press, Chicago

Portman, O.W., Alexander, M., Tanaka, N. *et al.* (1980) Relationships between cholesterol gallstones, biliary function, and plasma lipoproteins in squirrel monkeys. *Journal of Laboratory and Clinical Medicine*, **96**, 90–101

Roder, E.L. and Timmermans, P.J.A. (2002) Housing and care of monkeys and apes in laboratories: Adaptations allowing essential species-specific behaviour. *Lab Animal*, **36**, 221–242

Rodriguez-Vargas, A.R. (2003) Analysis of the hypothetical population structure of the squirrel monkey *(Saimiri oerstedii)* in Panama. In: *Primates in Fragments: Ecology and Conservation*. Ed. Marsh, L.K., pp. 53–62. Kluwer Academic/Plenum Publishers, New York

Rosenblum, L.A. and Coe, C.L.E. (1985) *Handbook of Squirrel Monkey Research*. Plenum Press, New York

Rosenblum, L.A. and Cooper, R.W.E. (1968) *The Squirrel Monkey*. Academic Press, New York

Ruiz, J.C., Brady, A.G., Gibson, S.L. *et al.* (2005) Morbidity and mortality of adult female Bolivian squirrel monkeys in a 10-year-period. *Contemporary Topics in Laboratory Animal Science*, **44**, 74

Scammell, J.G. (2000) Steroid resistance in the squirrel monkey: an old subject revisited. *ILAR Journal*, **41**, 19–25

Schätzl, H.M., Da Costa, M., Taylor, L. *et al.* (1995) Prion protein gene variation among primates. *Journal of Molecular Biology*, **245**, 362–374

Schuler, A.M. and Abee, C.R. (2005) *Squirrel monkeys (Saimiri), Enrichment for Non-human Primates*, NIH Pub No. 05-5749. NIH Office of Laboratory Animal Welfare, Bethesda. pp. 20

Scollay, P.A. and Judge, P. (1981) The dynamics of social organization in a population of squirrel monkeys (*Saimiri sciureus*) in a seminatural environment. *Primates*, **22**, 60–69

Shull, B.L., Capen, C.V., Riggs, M.W. *et al.* (1992) Preoperative and postoperative analysis of site-specific pelvic support defects in 81 women treated with sacrospinous ligament suspension and pelvic reconstruction. *American Journal of Obstetrics and Gynecology*, **166**, 1764–1771

Sierra, C., Jimenez, I., Altrichter, M. *et al.* (2003) New data on the distribution and abundance of *Saimiri oerstedii citrinellus*. *Primate Conservation*, **19**, 5–9

Smith, B.H., Crummett, T.L. and Brandt, K.L. (1994) Ages of eruption of primate teeth: a compendium for aging individuals and comparing life histories. *Yearbook of Physical Anthropology*, **37**, 177–231

Soltis, J., Wegner, F.H. and Newman, J.D. (2005) Urinary prolactin is correlated with mothering and allo-mothering in squirrel monkeys. *Physiology & Behavior*, **84**, 295–301

Spring, S.E., Clifford, J.O. and Tomiko, D.L. (1997) Effect of environmental enrichment devices on behaviors of single- and group-housed squirrel monkeys (*Saimiri sciureus*). *Contemporary Topics in Laboratory Animal Science*, **36**, 72–75

Srivastava, P.K., Cavazos, F. and Lucas, F.V. (1970) Biology of reproduction in the squirrel monkey (Saimiri sciureus): I. The estrus cycle. *Primates*, **11**, 125–134

Stills, H.F. Jr &and Bullock, B.C. (1981) Congenital defects of squirrel monkeys (*Saimiri sciureus*). *Veterinary Pathology*, **18**, 29–36

Stoller, M.K. (1995) The obstetric pelvis and mechanism of labor in nonhuman primates. *American Journal of Physical Anthropology*, **20**, 204

Strayer, F.F. and Harris, P.J. (1979) Social cohesion among captive squirrel monkeys (*Saimiri Sciureus*). *Behavioral Ecology and Sociobiology*, **5**, 93–110

Strayer, F.F., Taylor, M. and Yanciw, P. (1975) Group composition effects on social behavior of captive squirrel monkeys (*Saimiri sciureus*). *Primates*, **16**, 253–260

Streett, J.W. and Jonas, A.M. (1982) Differential effects of chemical and physical restraint on carbohydrate tolerance testing in nonhuman primates. *Laboratory Animal Science*, **32**, 263–266

Strickland, H.L. and Clarkson, T.B. (1985) Use of squirrel monkeys in cardiovascular research. In: *Handbook of Squirrel Monkey Research*. Eds Rosenblum, L. and Coe, C., pp. 295–314. Plenum Press, New York

Tappen, N.C. and Severson, A. (1971) Sequence of eruption of permanent teeth and epiphyseal union in New World monkeys. *Folia Primatologica*, **15**, 293–310

Terborgh, J. (1983) *Five New World Primates: A Study in Comparative Ecology*. Princeton University Press, Princeton, New Jersey

Thorington, R.W. Jr. (1967) Feeding and activity of *Cebus* and *Saimiri* in a Columbian forest. In: *Neue Ergenbisse der Primatologie*. Eds. Starck, D., Schneider, R. and Kuhn, H.J., pp. 180–184. Gustav Fischer Verlag, Stuttgart

Thorington, R.W. Jr. (1968) Observations of squirrel monkeys in a Columbian forest. In: *The Squirrel Monkey*. Eds. Rosenblum, L. and Cooper, R., pp. 69–85. Academic Press, New York

Thurmon, J.C.T., W.J. Tranquilli and Benson, G.J. (1996) *Lumb and Jones' Veterinary Anesthesia*. Williams & Wilkins, Baltimore

Trevino, H.S. (2007) Seasonality of reproduction in captive squirrel monkeys (*Saimiri Sciureus*). *American Journal of Primatology*, **69**, 1001–1012

Vaitl, E.A. (1977a) Experimental analysis of the nature of social context in captive groups of squirrel monkeys (*Saimiri sciureus*). *Primates*, **18**, 849–859

Vaitl, E.A. (1977b) Social context as a structuring mechanism in captive groups of squirrel monkeys (*Saimiri sciureus*). *Primates*, **18**, 861–874

Vaitl, E.A., Mason, W.A., Taub, D.M. *et al.* (1978) Contrasting effects of living in heterosexual pairs and mixed groups on the structure of social attraction in squirrel monkeys (*Saimiri*). *Animal Behaviour*, **26**, 358–367

VandeBerg, J.L., Williams-Blangero, S., Moore, C.M. *et al.* (1990) Genetic relationships among three squirrel monkey types: implications for taxonomy, biomedical research, and captive breeding. *American Journal of Primatology*, **22**, 101–111

Whiteley, H.E., Everitt, J.I., Kakoma, I. *et al.* (1987) Pathologic changes associated with fatal *Plasmodium falciparum* infection in the Bolivian squirrel monkey (*Saimiri sciureus boliviensis*). *American Journal of Tropical Medicine and Hygiene*, **37**, 1–8

Williams, L.E. and Abee, C.R. (1988) Aggression with mixed age-sex groups of Bolivian squirrel monkeys following single animal introductions and new group formations. *Zoo Biology*, **7**, 139–145

Williams, L.E., Abee, C.R. and Barnes, S. (1988) Allo-maternal behavior in *Saimiri boliviensis*. *American Journal of Primatology*, **14**, 452

Williams, L., Brown, P., Ironside, J. *et al.* (2007) Clinical, neuropathological and immunohistochemical features of sporadic and variant forms of Creutzfeldt-Jakob disease in the squirrel monkey (*Saimiri sciureus*). *Journal of General Virology*, **88**, 688–695

Williams, L. and Gibson, S. (2004) Sideburn size as a measurement of sex and age in *Saimiri sciureus sciureus*. *Laboratory Primate Newsletter*, **43**, 10–11

Williams, L., Gibson, S., McDaniel, M. *et al.* (1994) Allomaternal interactions in the Bolivian squirrel monkey (*Saimiri boliviensis boliviensis*). *American Journal of Primatology*, **34**, 145–156

Williams, L. and Glasgow, M. (2000) Squirrel monkey behavior in research. *ILAR Journal*, **41**, 26–36

Williams, L.E., Palughi, P.J., Cushman, A. *et al.* (1992) Vegetables as dietary enrichment for *Saimiri*. *American Journal of Primatology*, **27**, 63–64

Williams, L., Vitulli, W., Mcelhinney, T. *et al.* (1986a) Male behavior through the breeding season in *Saimiri boliviensis boliviensis*. *American Journal of Primatology*, **11**, 27–35

Williams, L.E., Yeoman, R.R. and Abee, C.R. (1986b) Estrus cycle influences on mating behavior in *Saimiri boliviensis*. *Primate Report*, **14**, 112–113

Wolf, R.H., Harrison, R.M. and Martin, T.W. (1975) A review of reproductive patterns in New World monkeys. *Laboratory Animal Science*, **25**, 814–821

Wolf, R.H., Lehner, N.D.M., Miller, E.C. *et al.* (1969) Electrocardiogram of the squirrel monkey, *Saimiri sciureus*. *Journal of Applied Physiology*, **26**, 346–351

Yeoman, R.R., Wegner, F.H., Gibson, S.V. *et al.* (2000) Midcycle and luteal elevations of follicle stimulating hormone in squirrel monkeys (*Saimiri boliviensis*) during the estrous cycle. *American Journal of Primatology*, **52**, 207–211

Zlotnik, I., Grant, D.P., Dayan, A.D. *et al.* (1974) Transmission of Creutzfeldt-Jakob disease from man to squirrel monkey. *Lancet*, **2**, 435–438

38 Capuchin monkeys

James R. Anderson and Elisabetta Visalberghi

Biological overview

Recent revisions of the taxonomy of the genus *Cebus* have identified between 7 and 11 species (see overview in Fragaszy *et al.* 2004b). In addition to the long-recognised four species (white-fronted capuchin, *C. albifrons*; black-capped, brown or tufted capuchin, *C. apella*; white-faced or white-throated capuchin, *C. capucinus*; and weeper or wedge-capped capuchin, *C. olivaceus*), the following are now increasingly accorded full species status: the yellow-breasted capuchin (*C. xanthosternos*), the Ka'apor capuchin (*Cebus kaapori*), the black-striped or bearded capuchin (*C. libidinosus*), and the black or black horned capuchin (*C. nigritus*). However, more systematic and comprehensive studies of morphology, anatomy and molecular biology are needed in order to base taxonomic revisions on solid evidence.

Notwithstanding the new revisions, almost all the literature concerning capuchin monkeys follows the 'traditional' taxonomic four-species split. This is especially true for studies carried out in captivity on the tufted species, the former *C. apella*; most researchers have not known the geographical origin of the founders of the colony and it is likely that interbreeding of *C. apella*, *C. libidinosus* and *C. nigritus* has occurred. In this chapter we refer to the four traditional species except in cases where one of the recently designated species (such as *C. xanthosternos*) has been explicitly identified.

It is clear that the genus *Cebus* is a successful and adaptable one, with representatives widely distributed throughout Central and South America. Capuchin monkeys are not particularly rare; in fact *C. xanthosternos* is the only species listed as 'critically endangered' in the 2007 International Union for the Conservation of Nature and Natural Resources (IUCN) Red list, but this probably reflects a lack of adequate information on some of the other species; see Rylands *et al.* (1995, 2005) for discussions of taxonomy and distribution of capuchin monkeys). Most information about behavioural biology, and how best to keep capuchins in captivity, comes from studies of *C. albifrons*, *C. capucinus* and *C. olivaceus*, and especially *C. apella*, but taxonomic misidentifications seem likely throughout much of the earlier literature.

Social organisation

Capuchins live in groups, typically ranging in size from around 12–35 individuals (Fragaszy *et al.* 2004b). Although group size is variable across populations and species, groups typically contain at least one adult male and several adult females, juveniles and infants. Males, but not females, typically emigrate from their natal group, and they may emigrate more than once in their lifetime. Some aspects of social organisation may vary across species, but there is usually a clearly dominant male (often larger and stronger than the other males, but in captivity at least it is not always so) and a dominant female.

Although group members can be categorised into different dominance classes, this can be difficult below alpha status, as social relations are characterised by a high degree of inter-individual tolerance and low rates of aggression. In captive groups of *C. apella*, sometimes one individual can become the target of harassment or aggression by many of the other group members, thus becoming a scapegoat. In the wild, such a subordinate would be better able to avoid others by staying on the periphery of the group, possibly even leaving the group altogether. Agonistic interactions do not usually escalate to involve two competing factions, but instead consist of one or more individuals pitted against another individual. Agonistic coalitions may occur, reflecting kinship or rank relations (Ferreira *et al.* 2006). The extent of post-conflict reconciliation in the different species remains an open question, but the behaviour may be more common in captivity (*C. capucinus*, Leca *et al.* 2002), and influenced by early experience (*C. apella*, Weaver & de Waal 2003).

Feeding habits

Capuchins live in a wide variety of habitats from sea level to above 2500 m altitude, mostly but not exclusively in forests (Fragaszy *et al.* 2004b). Some groups inhabit forest patches surrounded by large open areas and secondary vegetation, and some may be commensal with humans, living close to urban areas and coming into daily contact with people (Sabbatini *et al.* 2006). They spend most of their time in trees, especially in middle layers of the canopy, but depending on local habitat conditions they also exploit resources on the ground, for feeding (including crop raiding), drinking, playing, or crossing gaps between patches of forest.

Capuchins are omnivores. They eat mostly fruits, but include varying proportions of other vegetable items (shoots, flowers, buds, leaves etc), invertebrates (molluscs, insects, worms, etc) and vertebrates (for example, birds and their eggs, snakes, lizards, small mammals including bats) in their diet. Some groups also exploit human garbage. Many other South American monkeys eat the same items as capuchins, but the latter are distinguished by their 'destructive' manner of foraging. They are 'extractive' foragers, meaning that they exploit hidden and encased foods. Fragaszy and Boinski (1995) describe the wide diversity of capuchins' foraging styles, including the following 'strenuous' foraging actions, which may be combined: dig, rip, bite, bang, grab, break, carry, tap, roll, scrape, chase. 'Quiet' foraging actions, which may also be combined, include pick, visually examine, lick, mouth, sniff, manually examine, sift, take, feel, scoop, turn over, masticate, open by peeling.

One particular combination of strenuous foraging activities typifies wild capuchins: breaking open hard-shelled fruits or nuts. For example, *C. apella* pluck hard-shelled cumare fruits by biting through the stem, then repeatedly bang the fruit against the tree trunk or a branch until cracks appear on the fruit. They then peel the cracked rind with their teeth and then bang the nut again until the husk breaks and the kernels can be extracted. Combined foraging actions are also evident in searching for edible items among the debris to be found in palm fronds, and in breaking off palm leaves and peeling off the stems. Another foraging category, long known in captive groups but recently confirmed in the wild, is tool-assisted extractive foraging, notably using sticks to dig, and nut cracking using natural hammers and anvils (*C. libidinosus*, Fragaszy *et al.* 2004a; Moura & Lee 2004).

Standard biological data

Table 38.1 presents information on a number of important aspects of growth and development of *C. apella*. Data are provided on this species because it is by far the most commonly studied species in captivity. Blood biochemistry, haematological and serum protein parameters for adult males and females, and juveniles, are reported in Appendix III of Fragaszy *et al.* (2004b). Recent information on reproductive biology (including hormonal profiles) can be found in Carosi *et al.* (2005) and Carnegie *et al.* (2005a). Ankel-Simons (2007) presents anatomical data.

In addition to some distinctive physical biological traits (see later), a number of behavioural features combine to make capuchins unique among New World monkeys. They have the same variety of facial displays as Old World monkeys, with displays emerging at different points in development (Visalberghi *et al.* 2006; De Marco & Visalberghi 2007) (Figure 38.1). Lip-smacking (an affiliative display) appears near the end of the first month; the open-mouth threat face is the last to emerge, between 4.5 and 10 months of age. Capuchins also possess a rich vocal repertoire – still to be thoroughly studied – and great manual dexterity that includes precision grips and diverse tool-using behaviours (Fragaszy *et al.* 2004a, 2004b; Spinozzi & Truppa 1999; Visalberghi 1990).

C. apella show highly elaborate sexual behaviour. Females in oestrus actively solicit males, who may be at least initially reluctant (Phillips *et al.* 1994; Carosi & Visalberghi 2002; Carosi *et al.* 2005). Females' soliciting behaviour includes facial expressions such as eyebrow raise, vocalisations, gestures, such as head tilting and chest rubbing, and active following. This female 'proceptivity' is pronounced, and though the component behaviours may be used in other social contexts, when the female persistently shows them in

Table 38.1 Reproduction, growth and development of Cebus apella.

Parameter	*Normal value*	*Source*
Gestation	Captive capuchins, 160 days	Fragaszy & Adams-Curtis, 1998
Birth seasonality	Not marked. Peak birth period may coincide with increased availability of food	Di Bitetti & Janson, 2000
Interbirth interval	Captive capuchins, 20.6 months	Fragaszy & Adams-Curtis, 1998
	Wild capuchins, 19.4 months;	Di Bitetti & Janson, 2001
	Wild capuchins, 22 months	Robinson & Janson, 1987
Birth weight	170–260 g 220–270 g [1]	Fragaszy & Adams-Curtis, 1998
Ovarian cycle	20.8 ± 1.2 days[2]	
External signs of oestrus	Female proceptive behaviour	
Age at sexual maturity	Males are fertile: 4–5 years	
	Females give birth: 3 yr 10 mth (earliest)	Zunino, 1990
	Females give birth: 5 yr 7 mth (average)	Fragaszy & Adams-Curtis, 1998
Age at weaning	416 days	Fragaszy & Bard, 1997
Adult weight	Males: 3.3 ± 0.5 kg; (max >6 kg) Females: 2.4 ± 0.4 kg; (max 4 kg)	Growth curves for males and females from birth to over 20 years are available in Carosi *et al.* (2005)
Dental formula	$I^2{}_2C^1{}_1P^3{}_3M^3{}_3 = 36$	Napier & Napier, 1967
Age at gingival eruption	1st molar 1.2 years; 2nd molar 2.2 years	Galliari, 1985
Longevity	Max 53 years[3]	

[1] Data from the Primate Center of the Istituto di Scienze e Tecnologie della Cognizione in Rome concerning living newborns.
[2] Data based on measurements of hormonal levels (Linn *et al.* 1995; Nagle & Denari, 1983; Carosi *et al.* 1999).
[3] Bartus (personal communication).

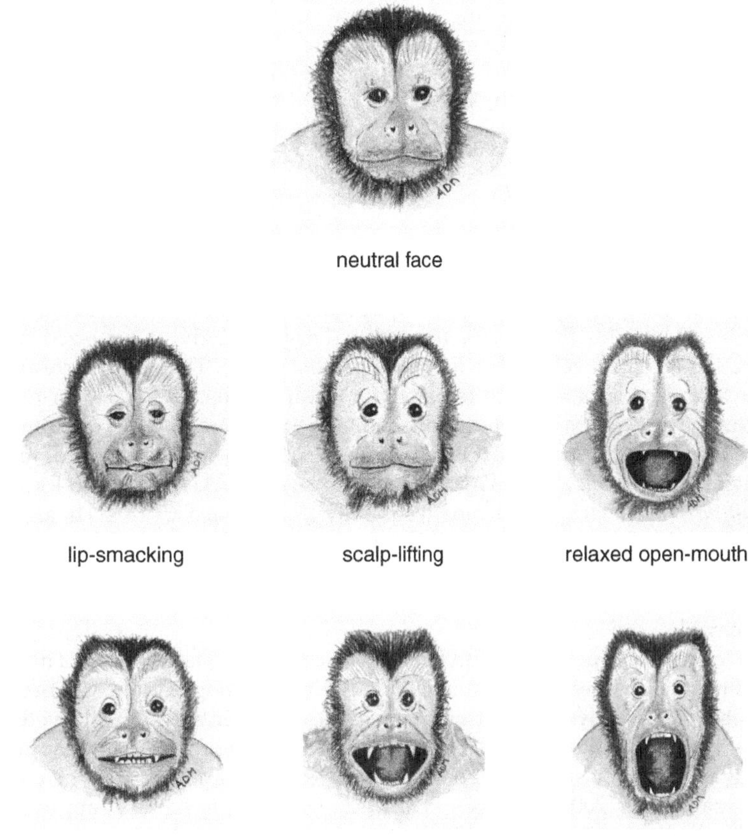

Figure 38.1 Example of facial displays in young *Cebus apella*. Top: neutral face. Middle: lip-smacking (left), scalp lifting (middle), relaxed open-mouth (right). Bottom: silent bared-teeth (left), open-mouth silent bared-teeth (middle), open-mouth threat-face (right). (Drawings: Arianna De Marco)

combination it signals that she is in the periovulatory phase. Although copulation is mostly dorso-ventral, ventro-ventral posturing with mutual gaze is common. The sexual behaviour of the other *Cebus* species has not been so closely investigated, but good field data exist for *C. capucinus* (Manson *et al.* 1997; Carnegie *et al.* 2005b). In this species chemical communication has a greater role, as indicated by male interest in females' urine.

It is easy to mistake male and female newborns and infants because the external sex organ of the female resembles that of the male in size, general shape and mobility (Figure 38.2); only close examination allows detection in females of a fissure instead of a hole at the tip of the genitalia and sex differences in shape. For good illustrations of the genitalia of both sexes, see Fragaszy *et al.* (2004b).

Like other New World primates, capuchins show sex-linked colour vision polymorphism. Some females have trichromatic vision, whereas all other individuals have dichromatic vision. Several studies have attempted to link this polymorphism to differences in wild monkeys' foraging strategies or efficiency, with little overall success. However, a recent study on wild *C. capucinus* reported differential success in preying upon camouflaged insects (Melin *et al.* 2007). A study on captive *C. apella* also reported an advantage of dichromacy compared to trichromacy for detecting camouflaged stimuli (Saito *et al.* 2005). The fact that there will probably be different colour vision abilities within a given captive group should always be borne in mind, as this may influence choice of enrichment devices and feeding techniques.

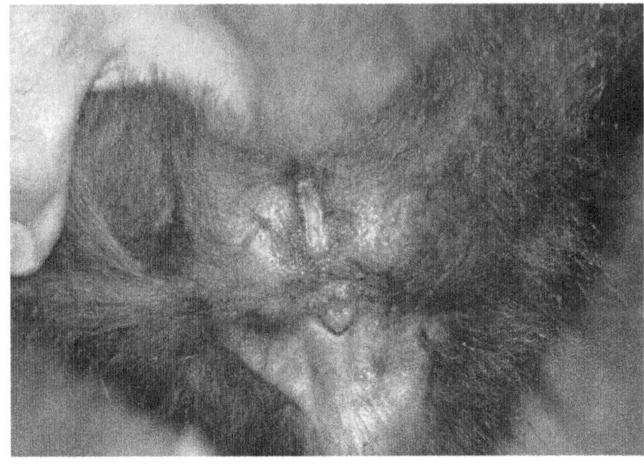

Figure 38.2 Clitoris of 1-day-old female *Cebus apella*. In females the tip of the genitalia has a fissure, whereas in males there is a hole. (Photo: E. Visalberghi)

Sources of supply

Capuchins are widely distributed in the wild and breed very well in captive conditions. They are quite hardy and resistant to disease (see later), although intestinal parasites (worms) may be present. Laboratories and zoos have often a surplus of animals, leading to the use of birth control methods. Captive-bred specimens can be found through the Primate Resource Referral Service (Washington National Primate Research Center, USA).

Uses in the laboratory

Due to their fascinating biological and behavioural features, capuchins have become very popular in behavioural studies both in the wild and captivity. This popularity seems likely to increase, with the first *in vivo* brain imaging study a notable recent development (eg, Phillips *et al.* 2007). They are also used in biomedical research; for example, pharmacology, *Trypanosoma cruzi* infection, genital herpes II, reproductive biology and neuroscience, but to a much lesser extent than other New World monkeys such as *Aotus, Callithrix or Saimiri.* Capuchins (especially *C. apella and C. albifrons*) have been used to provide 'simian helpers' to paraplegics in North America, Israel and France, but the cost effectiveness and welfare implications of these projects are debatable.

However, capuchins are probably considered especially interesting for their cognitive abilities. Their psychological traits are currently studied from many perspectives including tool use (Anderson 2002; Fujita *et al.* 2003; Visalberghi & Fragaszy 2006); visual perception and visuo-spatial learning (Fragaszy *et al.* 2003; Anderson *et al.* 2005; Fujita & Giersch 2005; Rosengart & Fragaszy 2005), visual search, memory, and metacognition, (Tavares & Tomaz 2002; Spinozzi *et al.* 2003; Paukner *et al.* 2006; De Lillo *et al.* 2007), co-operation, exchange, and symbolic representation (Brosnan & de Waal 2004; Addessi *et al.* 2007a, 2007b), judgements of quantity (Addessi *et al.* 2007b; Beran *et al.* 2007), use of social and non-social cues for finding food (Vick & Anderson 2000; Visalberghi & Neel 2003; Hattori *et al.* 2007; Sabbatini & Visalberghi 2008), face processing (Dufour *et al.* 2006) and self-recognition (Paukner *et al.* 2004; de Waal *et al.* 2005; Roma *et al.* 2007). Despite the fact that fieldwork has been done on all four traditionally recognised *Cebus* species and is now extending to other species, the laboratory population consists almost entirely of tufted capuchins (*C. apella*), while zoos host also *C. capucinus, C. albifrons, C. olivaceus* and *C. xanthosternos.* It should be noted that captive capuchins may live for well over 40 years, and one specimen reportedly lived up to 53 years (Bartus, personal communication). Any planning of research should take this extended longevity into consideration.

Laboratory management and breeding

General husbandry

General advice on husbandry, care, and common procedures for non-human primates can be found in a report by the Joint Working Group on Refinement (JWGR) (2009). Many of the safety- and hygiene-related requirements for the transportation, housing and handling of capuchins are identical to those that apply when dealing with other non-human primate species (see the Primate Info Net website[1]). In this chapter we focus particularly on aspects of welfare that might concern capuchins more specifically, given their somewhat unique biological and behavioural profiles.

Although they may spend much time on the ground, capuchins are primarily arboreal, and they employ their semi-prehensile tail during above ground locomotion and posturing. The height of cages or enclosures should reflect these adaptations and, for example, allow the monkeys to perch above human eye level. Prior to its revision in June 2007, Annex II to the European Directive 86/609 EEC specified a minimum floor area of 0.5 m^2 for individual capuchin-sized monkeys and a cage height of 0.8 m. This and the corresponding US stipulations are, in the authors' views, over-restrictive (Reinhardt *et al.* 1996a). The revised Annex II (European Commission 2007) does not provide specific recommendations for capuchins but does provide general performance standards that can be applied for this species. There are not yet any published guidelines regarding increasing space requirements as a function of group size. For example, the ISTC-CNR, Rome, keeps groups of five to ten capuchins in indoor/outdoor enclosures of 374 m^3 (outdoors) and 25.3 m^3 (indoors), and 106.5 m^3 (outdoors) and 24.4 m^3 (indoors), respectively. In the Strasbourg Primate Centre, different groups of 14+ *C. apella* and *C. capucinus* thrived in a complex three-structure indoor/outdoor facility of approximately 180 m^2 (height 3 m). In a recent study, when capuchins' normal indoor area was reduced by approximately half, the monkeys coped by avoiding social encounters and by increasing self-grooming, which may reduce arousal (van Wolkenten *et al.* 2006). In laboratories, where space is more restricted, the following minimum cage dimensions are suitable for capuchins: each monkey should have at least 1 m^2 floor area, and the cage should be at least 2 m high. If a capuchin needs to be housed singly, the minimum available floor area should be 2 m^2, and the height, 2 m. For a typical captive group of 10 individuals, the recommended minimum space allowances (floor area 10 m^2, height 2 m) will allow expression of the full locomotor repertoire (including leaping, running and climbing) and sitting or hanging by the tail above human eye level.

Environmental provisions

Promoting the psychological well-being of captive primates is important for ethical and scientific as well as legal reasons. Of course, it is not feasible, nor indeed desirable for a laboratory or zoo to attempt to meticulously reproduce all aspects of natural settings. However, appropriate compromises are feasible. This involves focusing on features of the environment that can be either recreated or simulated in order to elicit a similar range of social and non-social activities as seen in the wild. For example, it would be hopeless to try to provide exactly the same foods as capuchins eat in the wild, but it is important to give adequate proportions of proteins, carbohydrates, vitamins, minerals, etc, as well as variety, and to do so through situations that encourage the kinds of

[1]http://pin.primate.wisc.edu/research/vet/

manipulatory, locomotor and temporal patterns of feeding-related activities seen in wild capuchins (see later in this chapter).

In view of their highly developed manipulatory propensities, broad repertoire of object-orientated actions and their curiosity and sustained interest in objects, providing capuchins with a stimulating environment is not only a requisite of good husbandry, but also relatively easy and gratifying to do. Many potential enrichment techniques exist, ranging from increasing the diversity and processing requirements of food (to simulate aspects of foraging), improving furnishing of the cage or enclosure (to improve locomotor possibilities and provide cover) and providing stimulating sensory events including objects to explore, play with or destroy. Recommendations given here are based upon species-typical behaviour in the wild or, in a few cases, outcomes of enrichment studies in captivity.

One important goal of the care and management of captive primates is the reduction of excessive inactivity in the animals, that is, to reduce boredom and its negative consequences, such as lethargy and abnormal behaviours. The following aspects are addressed from this perspective in the rest of this chapter: the social and physical environment, and routine capture and handling techniques.

Capuchins are arboreal quadrupedalists that locomote on surfaces which are vertical and horizontal, but mostly oblique. Therefore, capuchins should be provided with oblique structures in addition to the more obvious vertical and horizontal ones. Panels, hanging screens, branches, slides, swings, ropes, crates, frames, poles and PVC pipes and plastic mats are all potentially suitable structures. Some such structures should be selected to allow monkeys to avoid others if they so choose, as well as to provide shade and shelter (if outdoors) and appropriate substrates for resting and sleeping. See Anderson (2000), for environmental factors influencing sleep. Visalberghi, (personal observation) has seen wild capuchins use caves to shelter from inclement weather. Such structures can also be excellent stimuli for promoting physical exercise and play and for better exploiting available cage space.

Another effective way of increasing use of available cage space is to make the floor more attractive. Plants may be a feasible addition to some enclosures (Figure 38.3), although in relatively small spaces capuchins are likely to eventually destroy all or most of them, except for stinging nettles or toxic varieties (eg, Solanaceae). (Note: the authors do not advocate giving captive animals access to toxic plants.) More plants are likely to survive in very large enclosures, especially if they are already well established before the capuchins arrive. Many laboratories and zoos use deep litter such as woodchips, woodwool, straw, or bark chips (eg, Ludes & Anderson 1996); there is adequate scope for trying other potentially suitable materials. The best litters encourage locomotion and foraging activities and sometimes play; they also afford some protection if an animal falls from an elevated position. Furthermore, concerns regarding possible hygienic disadvantages of using deep litter have so far proved to be unfounded; litter may be safely left for several weeks without hosing or disinfecting. However, the removal of heavily soiled parts of the litter or rotten food is advisable, especially if there is the chance that rodents might be attracted.

Capuchins will readily manipulate and do their best to break open almost any object given. (They can learn to open cage doors or partitions that are secured only by simple latches or dog clips, so padlocks are advised.) Discarded children's toys, tennis balls, plastic and cardboard boxes, wooden blocks, rubber tubing, plastic mirrors are all examples of good, readily available and affordable enrichment objects. They must be checked carefully and all potentially dangerous parts (protruding wires, nails, sharp edges etc) removed. The most effective strategy for maintaining the monkeys' interest is to replace objects every few days. Certain types of objects (eg, a puppet) may initially elicit alarm and mobbing by the capuchins, especially upon first introduction. It has been suggested that occasional brief challenging events of this type may be beneficial to the animals, allowing them to express natural behavioural and physiological responses without undue risk. Capuchins do not readily enter deep

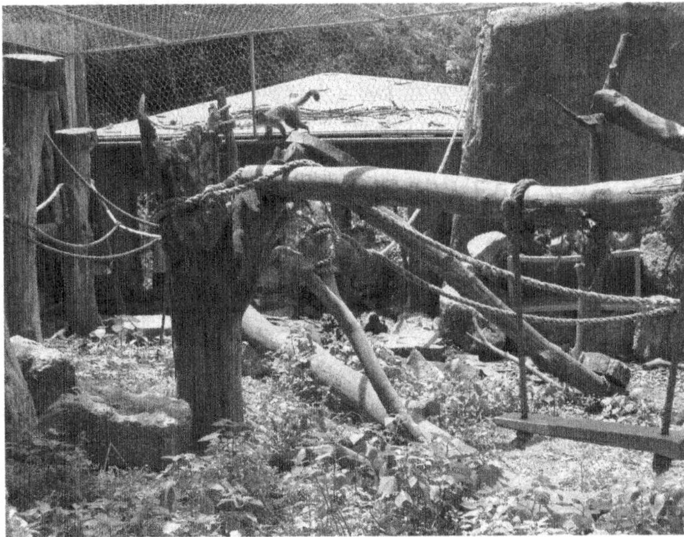

Figure 38.3 Outdoor enclosure in the Primate Center of the Istituto di Scienze e Tecnologie della Cognizione hosted by the Bioparco of Rome (Italy). Members of the public (in the background) can observe the capuchin monkeys; the latter are also used for research. (Photo: Valentina Truppa)

water, but a plastic container filled with shallow water undoubtedly stimulates exploratory and playful activities, especially in hot weather.

In summary, there are many different ways in which the physical environment can be enriched. The choices need not be mutually exclusive. For example, simple objects can be baited with food treats to elicit specific feeding techniques. When deep litters contain buried food, animals devote much time to sifting and searching through the litter (Westergaard & Fragaszy 1985). Finally, furnishings may well include structures with holes or openings containing treats (syrup, honey, raisins, etc) to encourage extractive techniques, including tool use.

In the wild, capuchin monkeys have been observed rubbing leaves, fruits and even ants and millipedes into their fur (sometimes referred to as 'anointing') (see Baker 1996). The monkeys sometimes appear highly motivated to do this and the significance of the behaviour may be related to skin/pelage maintenance, and to repel insects. Captive capuchins also readily engage in this behaviour. There may be species and individual preferences for which substances may be rubbed into the fur, but the authors have seen onions, citrus fruits, garlic, peat, tobacco, and even tobacco smoke used for this purpose (the authors do not advocate the use of tobacco products). At least two independent observations have suggested that such fur-rubbing activities may reduce the incidence of skin sores (Ludes and Anderson 1995a). Given the high motivation of capuchins for this activity, the authors recommend that trial and error be used to identify appropriate fur-rubbing-eliciting objects or substances, and that the capuchins are allowed to perform this behaviour periodically. It should be noted that both wild and captive capuchin monkeys also frequently rub their bodies with urine, which they collect on the hands and feet and tip of the tail. The functions of 'urine washing' are not fully understood, but it is a normal behaviour, possibly with a thermoregulatory function (Roeder & Anderson 1991).

Social grouping

Capuchin monkeys demonstrably prefer to be in contact with at least one familiar social partner (Dettmer & Fragaszy 2000). The optimal social grouping for captive capuchins is undoubtedly one that would contain proportions of age- and sex-classes as seen in natural conditions. However, capuchins' social structure is quite variable, so this principle can be implemented with some flexibility, depending on space limitations and on the purpose for which the monkeys are maintained. In any case, except under truly exceptional circumstances, capuchin monkeys should be kept socially, as social companions are excellent sources of interactive and ever-changing stimulation (Visalberghi & Anderson 1993).

As already mentioned, in some groups the lowest-ranking individual can become the target of repeated aggression. This is obviously a stressful situation for the victim, and in extreme cases removal of the unfortunate individual may be the best solution. However, unless serious injury or depression results from such bullying, removal can have some considerable drawbacks: it results in isolation and possible problematic (re-)integration for a socially rejected individual. Furthermore, there is no guarantee that the remaining group members will not start to redirect their aggression upon another individual. The physical and psychological health of the victimised individual should be carefully monitored, and temporary relief and food supplements provided during temporary separations, if necessary. The authors are not aware of any cases in which a subordinate individual has been harassed to the point of death; indeed, they have noticed that not only physical but also social wounds usually heal with time. For example, in the Rome colony a female who was a scapegoat at 3 years of age rose to become the dominant female of her group a few years later. It should be ensured that subordinates have adequate access to resources, including shelter. Facilities should be designed such that subordinates cannot easily be trapped or cornered during aggression. It should also be noted that haematological, physiological and immunological parameters of severely bullied or otherwise stressed animals might be outside the normal range of values.

If two or more groups are housed in the same facility, care should be taken to prevent direct physical contact between them. A single wire mesh partition is not sufficient for separating neighbouring groups; fingers, toes, and tips of tails can easily be bitten off. Groups in visual or auditory contact may react to each other, but if managed properly this should give rise to no negative consequences. Several zoos have successfully kept capuchins in mixed-species exhibits; compatible mixed-species groups can be enriching not only for the species involved but also for visitors.

It is advisable to allow animals some choice regarding whom to be with in the group, and whether to be in visual contact with a neighbouring group (International Primatological Society 2007). This can be achieved by providing 'privacy' panels or other structures inside the cage(s) or, even better, housing groups in interconnecting rooms or cages, preferably with more than one connecting door or hatch between them.

Experimental testing sometimes requires working with a single subject at a time, leading to the question of how to separate the subject from the group while minimising stress. A tried and tested solution is to have the test apparatus in or alongside a cage or room connected to the colony quarters by sliding doors. The authors strongly recommend the use of horizontally or upward sliding doors instead of the traditional guillotine door, to reduce the risk of injury to monkeys. For most individuals, gradual habituation to increasingly long periods of separation associated with positive reinforcement, inherent interest of the tasks (using only positive reinforcement, never punishment) and subsequent reunion, are sufficient to overcome the initial reluctance to be separated.

As a general rule, a well established stable group will pose fewer problems than the process of forming a new group or of introducing unfamiliar individuals into an established group. The latter two scenarios are focused upon in the next section, drawing upon the authors' personal experiences and those of colleagues to suggest some procedures, as well as some pitfalls to avoid. It should be noted that most of the authors' knowledge on how to form or modify capuchin groups comes not from systematic experimental manipulations but from experience gained through husbandry challenges faced occasionally by laboratories and zoos. Overall, group formation is a stressful procedure both for the animals and the care staff, and although cumulative experience may help to reduce the risks of failure, the outcome can never be predicted with absolute certainty (Visalberghi & Anderson 1993).

Introduction and re-introduction

Since an individually housed monkey is *de facto* living in impoverished conditions and therefore psychologically deprived, all efforts should be made towards compatible social housing. Sometimes, this may be feasible even shortly after major veterinary treatment; for an example with a newborn infant see Anderson *et al.* (1995). Hand-reared (ages ranging from 5–9 months) and mother-reared (8–12 months) infants were successfully introduced to a group when full integration was preceded by a period of visual contact, allowing mutual familiarisation at a safe distance (Visalberghi & Riviello 1987; Riviello 1992). In order to integrate single adult females, initial visual contact was followed by periods in which the female was together with the dominant male and then together with him and each of the other group members, before being housed permanently with the entire group (Anderson *et al.* 1991; Ludes & Anderson 1995b). In the most extensive report on introduction and integration of strangers into captive groups of tufted capuchins, Fragaszy *et al.* (1994) describe the successful introduction of two to four individuals (adult males, females and juveniles) into three established groups of six to nine capuchins. This report is useful as it provides several behavioural categories that can be employed in both monitoring and predicting the success of introductions. First, the newcomers were familiarised with the resident group's living quarters, and only then were residents and newcomers mixed. No serious aggression-related injuries occurred at the time of introductions or during the following months. When one or more individuals persistently chased a new female, partial separations were used to form mixed subgroups of newcomers and residents for overnight housing.

Concerning the introduction of adult males, one adult male (more than 10 years old), previously kept in a zoo, was successfully introduced to a group in which the dominant male was only 4 years old. The procedure included a quicker progression through stages similar to those just described for adult females, and with contact between the newcomer and the dominant resident male left until last. Strikingly, these two males immediately came into contact and performed joint threats, towards no particular target. They quickly developed a positive relationship, the newcomer being alpha male. Although all introductions are likely to involve some degree of stress, in none of the above cases did the introduced monkey need to be removed from the group due to aggression or stress-related ill-health. Two introduction scenarios did result in severe aggression: unfamiliar adult males going into a group with no resident adult male, and males familiar with each other going into a group containing an elderly resident male (Cooper *et al.* 2001). In contrast, moving two males familiar with each other into a group with no resident male was peaceful.

Overall, the risks associated with introductions appear greatly outweighed by the disadvantages of solitary housing. No foolproof recipe is yet available for group formation or introduction procedures, but the chances of success can be increased by having a good knowledge of the animals involved, careful monitoring before and after the introduction, and by taking into account factors such as sex, age and experience of the newcomers (Visalberghi & Anderson 1993). Given a few recent reports of male-perpetrated infanticide in the wild (Fragaszy *et al.* 2004b), introduction of a fully adult male into a group containing neonates should be considered risky. Also, the introduction of an adult female in a group containing more than one adult male may lead to a violent attempt by a subordinate to overthrow the dominant male, especially if the latter is old.

Identification

Tattooing with an electric pen and ink is still the most commonly used method, and the authors are aware of no ill effects. Identification collars are not advised, as capuchins will try their best to destroy them. Implanted microchips are becoming increasingly popular for individual identification of captive New World primates (Savastano *et al.* 2003), including some pet capuchins. However, the use of microchips is not problem-free; cost, equipment incompatibility and possible migration of the microchip are all potential compromising factors (Rennie & Buchanan-Smith 2006). The authors know of no published reports on their use in capuchins kept in laboratories or zoos.

The physical environment

Capuchins are quite hardy animals provided that they have constant access to heated indoor quarters. They may occasionally venture outdoors in temperatures close to freezing; however, they do not appear to enjoy walking on frozen surfaces. In enclosed environments, a temperature of around 23 °C, humidity of 50–60% and a ventilation rate of 4–5 air changes per hour are recommended. Rooms without natural light are typically kept on a 12h–12h artificial light cycle. Although no scientific data are available, gradual light changes to simulate natural changes at dawn and dusk may be beneficial. Natural light from windows or skylights will provide low levels of light at night, similar to the situation in the wild. There is little systematic work on the influence of auditory environments on captive primates, but excessive noise should be avoided.

Quarantine

Quarantine procedures are broadly similar to those for other primates. Duration ranges from 40–90 days, during which time repeated tuberculin skin tests, serology and stool analyses are performed. Prophylactic treatment varies across institutions; for groups with access to outdoor areas vaccination against tetanus is recommended. A zoo-housed colony was successfully protected against rabies using a human non-vaccinated exposure protocol consisting of periodic intramuscular doses of killed rabies (between possible post-exposure days 2–33) and a single dose of human rabies immune globulin (at possible post-exposure day 5) (Kenny *et al.* 2001).

Breeding

Pregnancy and newborns

The authors do not recommend separating pregnant females from their group, even though dead neonates are occasionally recovered. Greater importance is attached to maintaining the complex network of intra-group social relations than to episodic breeding success if the latter implies stress due to lengthy separation and later reintegration of the mother–infant pair into the group. As in other primates, most births occur at night. Also as in other primates, maternal performance may differ between primiparous and multiparous mothers, and the former may abandon their infants. Conceivably, delivery for primiparous females is particularly long and/or tiring, and the infant may be compromised after a lengthy delivery. Some females with inadequate early social experience might kill their newborn. If an abandoned or abused neonate is recovered in time, hand rearing is a viable possibility (see below). However, after initial incompetence, capuchin females may become competent mothers with subsequent offspring. While it is not clear why this improvement occurs, age, previous experience of hormonal changes, higher social status of the female and the presence of other mothers with infants may be contributing factors.

In a recent analysis of breeding records of four American and European colonies of tufted capuchins, 2.4% of pregnancies gave rise to twins, a higher incidence than previously estimated, and not dissimilar to human twinning rates (Leighty *et al.* 2004). If twins survived the first day of postnatal life (45% did not, compared to 16% of singletons), then subsequent survival was similar to that of singletons. Three complete sets of twins out of 10 sets recorded survived beyond 30 days, while another three individuals whose twin died survived beyond the first month.

Infant transfer is common in capuchins. Young infants, even newborns, may be held or transported (and, rarely, nursed) by individuals other than their mother. Infant white-faced and tufted capuchins may be carried by adult males for long periods. This is usually safe, but it may carry risks if the infant is very young and/or when the mother does not retrieve it. The infant may take the initiative in transferring from the mother onto a nearby individual, or the other individual may solicit the transfer by adopting an inviting posture. The non-maternal carrier is rarely aggressive, but infants up to about 8 weeks run the risk of dehydration/starvation if they are unable to transfer back to the mother, so surveillance is recommended. Some mothers do not attempt to get their infant back; sometimes, but not always, this is due to the mother's subordinate status. In such cases intervention may become necessary. This can involve either bringing the mother and the carrier into close proximity, for example by offering a non-transportable treat such as juice, or by restraining them in a restricted space. If these procedures fail, the carrier may need to be captured and the infant returned to its mother, with follow-up monitoring for adequacy of maternal care. Sometimes during this process the carrier (even the mother) will forcefully dislodge the infant by rough pulling or even biting. Care should be taken to keep the capture process calm so as not to endanger the infant.

Hand rearing

Viable infants abandoned at birth can be successfully hand reared. Commercially available human infant milk formulas generally work well for common laboratory primate species. Following an initial few feeds consisting of warmed rehydration fluid or 5% glucose, the authors recommend bottle-feeding newborns every 3h with artificial milk, for example, Similac (Ross Laboratories, Columbus, OH), SMA (Wyeth Laboratories), or S-26 powdered baby milk. The interval between feedings can be gradually increased, especially during the night. The concentration of the milk substitute can also be progressively increased, until full strength is reached by 24–36h. Usually the infant vocalises when hungry. The hole in the nipple should be small enough to prevent excessively fast ingestion. The monkey stops drinking when satiated and it is advisable to keep it upright for a few minutes to facilitate burping and avoid regurgitation. Based on what happens in the wild, the authors recommend giving small pieces of solid foods (eg, cookies, banana or apple) to infant capuchins as early as 3–4 weeks. Not much is consumed at this age, but the animals lick or mouth it.

According to Lehner (1984) nursery-reared infants ingest about 175kcal/kg per day during the first week. The amount peaks at around 400kcal/kg per day at 2 months, then declines to a stable level of around 300kcal/kg for rest of the first year. They grow rapidly, gaining about 100g per month for the first 10 months. By 1 year of age, the infant will have reached more than 50% of the mother's non-pregnant body weight (Fragaszy & Adams-Curtis 1998). Like other New World monkeys, capuchins require vitamin D3 for adequate skeletal growth, especially if the monkeys have no access to unfiltered sunlight. Vitamin D3 is available in pelleted diets and vitamin/mineral supplements. Sainsbury (1991) gives 100IU/kg body weight as sufficient for young animals.

Feeding

Mann (1970) traces the development of diets for captive *Cebus*, and describes some common nutritional deficiency states including rickets. For a recent detailed overview of primate nutrition see National Research Council of the National Academies (2003). Commercially available New World monkey food supplemented with fresh vegetables and fruits satisfies the general requirements of captive capuchins. However, pellets are not among capuchins' preferred foods (Addessi *et al.* 2005), despite containing all the requirements for physical health. Furthermore, given wild capuchins' wide variety of foods and feeding techniques (see overview earlier in this chapter), it is highly recommended to attempt to simulate some aspects of this diversity. For example, capuchins like to break open and peel fruits, so it is rarely necessary to peel and chop such items into fine pieces. Whole fruits allow them to spend more time in species-typical feeding behaviour. Food can be placed in locations to encourage arboreality and increase search time; for example if the top of the cage or enclosure is of wire mesh, foods big enough not to drop directly through the holes can be spread there to encourage a variety of food-gathering techniques. Food can also be hidden in a variety of ways and locations so as to stimulate searching. For example, when capuchins were presented with food treats dispersed in bins full of sawdust or water (the food could be reached only by inserting an arm through holes in the bins), they spent considerable time engaged in tactile search. Specially constructed containers containing straw or wood-chips and food treats can used to elicit a range of species-typical foraging activities. Extensive picking activities including fine precision grips are easily elicited by synthetic 'grass' secured to a board outside the cage and filled with grains or other small edible items. Variability can also be made a feature of the timing of feeding, although whether this has observable beneficial effects for capuchins requires confirmation.

Raw and unprocessed foods are an obvious way of challenging capuchins' natural extractive propensities. Unshelled nuts can be made even more of a challenge to manual or tool-assisted cracking techniques by increasing the resistance of their shells (Visalberghi & Vitale 1990). Every region has products suitable for capuchin 'treatment': corn on the cob, unshelled beans and nuts, coconuts and unhusked cereals are good examples, and all are excellent supplements to the staple balanced diet. Raw eggs are a preferred treat, although there may be an associated risk of salmonellosis, and of restricted biotin uptake due to the uncooked avidin. Commercial pellets for South American monkeys appear nutritionally ideal, although as mentioned above, they are not particularly appreciated (Addessi *et al.* 2005). Such diets are prepared to include requisite proportions of proteins, amino acids and minerals, etc. Especially when commercial food is not given, mealworms, cheese, yoghurt etc, should be added to the regime to provide animal proteins. Obese capuchins are rare, even among those known to eat rich, processed human foods, therefore some food can be given almost *ad libitum*. It is advisable to provide a highly preferred mixture (cottage cheese, eggs, cereals, etc) a few times a week and to use this occasion to administer medicines by mixing them with the food.

Laboratory procedures

Handling and training

The traditional way of capturing group-living capuchins is with a net and/or protective gloves. The chasing involved in this method is extremely stressful, and the method is not without risk of injury to the animal(s). Some of the stress and most of the risk of injury can be eliminated by shepherding the animal through a system of tunnels that lead the animal into a squeeze cage where it can be restrained for examination or treatment. In either case, the expertise of the person doing the capture is paramount. Since stress increases over time if its source persists, rapid, efficient netting may be preferable to a prolonged wait for a frightened animal to enter the tunnel (Linn *et al.* 1995). Nets should have padded rims to prevent injury to the animal (especially to its teeth) during capture. Capture-related stress can be reduced by giving piece of banana or grape containing a few drops of diazepam (2 mg/kg, C. Tomaz, personal communication).

Capture may be made less stressful by habituating the monkeys to sights and sounds associated with capture from an early age. Even so, capture typically results in the colony being highly aroused for some time afterward, although this may be alleviated by providing distracting foraging opportunities immediately after the event (Landau & Fragaszy, unpublished, cited in Fragaszy *et al.* 2004b). The authors have noticed that events typically occurring on capture days often become associated with the stressful experience. For example the arrival of the veterinarian, or the sight or noise of capture equipment (gloves, tunnel-cages, etc), give rise to tension and/or fear. Therefore, it may be advisable for those whose research activity involves direct observation of spontaneous behaviour not to be involved in capturing the animals. Capuchins have extremely powerful jaws and can inflict serious bite wounds, so personnel should guard against being bitten (or scratched), for example by wearing protective gloves.

Transport boxes are commonly used to take individual monkeys from their home cage to an experimental room, for example to administer Wisconsin General Test Apparatus- or video-based tasks. Initial coaxing of the animal to enter the box may require any of a number of strategems of varying forcefulness, ranging from attracting it into the box using treats to chasing it in by blocking all escape routes except the entrance to the box. Capuchins can distinguish between different tones of voice and possibly words; this can be used in training. However, positive reinforcement is essential. Once the transport procedure becomes routine, the monkeys often start to enter the transport cage spontaneously, sometimes even in absence of food reward. Indeed it is common for a reliable order to emerge, often dominance-related, in which group members vie to be given access to the test apparatus.

Physiological monitoring

For general advice see JWGR (1993, 2009). In zoos and laboratories, positive reinforcement training is becoming popular as an alternative to capturing monkeys for collecting vaginal swabs or blood (Prescott *et al.* 2005). However, there are still very few examples with capuchins; it is possible that capuchins are harder to train than macaques for such procedures (see Fragaszy *et al.* 2004b). Drug treatments can also be administered to co-operative animals in this way, thus circumventing the problem of rejection of food or liquid laced with the substance to be administered. Females can be trained to sit on a plastic bin for increasingly long periods and to urinate while seated. It took less than 1 month to fully train a female to urinate on the bin within a few minutes of taking up position. However, such training does not succeed with all animals.

It is increasingly common for physiological data to be collected by implantation of telemetry devices that weigh only a few grams or by equipping the subject with a jacket containing a measuring device. Jackets have been also used with *Cebus apella* (Vitale *et al.* 1994). However, those that fitted well were bitten and torn apart by the animals, and tighter jackets appeared to restrict the animal's locomotor behaviour; currently available jackets are not well suited to the body shape or the behavioural tendencies of this species.

Administration of medicines

For general advice see JWGR (2001, 2009). Oral doses can readily be given either in fruit juice or concealed in a preferred small fruit, such as a grape. Intravenous injections should be given in either the femoral or saphenous veins, although the latter may be more difficult.

Diseases and treatments

As in other primates, behavioural changes may be the last signs of underlying illness to appear, so regular careful monitoring (including weighing) is advised. Lehner (1984) and Sainsbury (1991) give summaries of diseases to which capuchins and other members of the Cebidae are susceptible. These include the common human cold and other viral diseases (eg, measles, chicken pox). Tuberculosis appears to be the most important of the bacterial diseases, although capuchins are quite resistant and diagnosis may be difficult. Among parasitic diseases, malarial infection (*Plasmodium brazilianum*) and haemo-flagellate infection (*Trypanosoma cruzi*) have sometimes been fatal. Lehner (1984) describes the various signs of these diseases and others, such as rickettsial and viral, along with treatments and prognoses.

Three cases of tetanus have occurred in Italian colonies and two of them were successfully treated. The animals (all adults) were found rigid and presented marked locomotor impairment and 'lockjaw'. One died after several hours; the others were treated as humans with the same disease. Medical care consisted of immunoglobulin, diazepam, antibiotics and rehydration therapy with physiological solution, and vitamins were administered in doses appropriate for the monkeys' body weights. They were kept in a warm, dimly lit environment and fed by hand four times a day. Treatment lasted between 20 and 30 days, after which the animal slowly recovered and was able to return to its group (Lorenzo De Marco, Massimilaino Bianchi and Fabio Faiola, personal communication). A 32-year-old *C. capucinus* was successfully treated for *Toxoplasma* meningitis using clindamycin and trimethaprim-sulfamethoxazole (Fiorello *et al.* 2006).

Diarrhoea may occur in response to stress, incorrect diet, or infection. Sainsbury (1991) indicates fenbendazole, mebendazole and ivermectin for the treatment of nematode parasites, and dichlorophen and niclosamide for the treatment of cestodes. Nagle and Denari (1983) describe the treatment of respiratory tract infections and diarrhoea in recently captured capuchins using penicillin, chloramphenicol and electrolytes with 5% dextrose solution. They state that thiabendazole is effective against nematodes. Wolff (1990) provides an extensive table of internal and external parasites of cebid monkeys, along with host location, disease signs and diagnostic and treatment procedures. Information on miscellaneous health problems including fractures, dental disease and soft tissue injuries can be found in Sainsbury (1991).

Anaesthesia

Short-term sedation can be induced with ketamine (10 mg/kg). In order to treat a sick infant every 2–3 days, the authors first lightly anaesthetised the mother with intramuscular ketamine 10 mg/kg. Inhalation anaesthetics and endotracheal techniques are indicated for surgical procedures. Specialised information on anaesthesia and analgesia can be found in Sedgwick (1986), Sainsbury (1991), Flecknell (2009) and Popilskis and Kohn (1997); the last authors also address intra-operative monitoring and support, and special anaesthetic considerations, although no specific recommendations are made for capuchin monkeys.

Care must be taken to ensure that a captured animal is unable to reach the needle of the syringe. Capuchins are extremely swift and capable of exploiting any possibility to prevent capture, injections and so on, unless specifically trained. Training, however, may require patience. Dettmer *et al.* (1996) reported that repeated capture and venepuncture procedures in *C. apella* resulted in raised cortisol levels, before a reduction in week 7 brought them back down to week 1 levels. After this phase, however, behaviourally habituated animals no longer showed this physiological stress response to venepuncture, whereas non-habituated animals did.

The post-anaesthesia recovery period should follow standard monitoring and hygiene-related protocols, ensuring adequate warmth, freedom from potential injury, and rapid return to the social group as soon as possible.

Euthanasia

If euthanasia is necessary, the animal should be anaesthetised and then injected intravenously with an overdose of pentobarbital. See also Chapter 17.

References

Addessi, E., Stammati, M., Sabbatini, G. *et al.* (2005) How tufted capuchin monkeys (*Cebus apella*) rank monkey chow in relation to other foods. *Animal Welfare*, **14**, 215–222

Addessi, E., Crescimene, L. and Visalberghi, E. (2007a) Do capuchin monkeys (*Cebus apella*) use tokens as symbols? *Proceedings of the Royal Society of London, B*, **274**, 2579–2585

Addessi, E., Crescimene, L. and Visalberghi, E. (2007b) Food and token quantity discrimination in capuchin monkeys (*Cebus apella*). *Animal Cognition*, **11**, 275–282

Anderson, J.R. (2000) Sleep-related behavioural adaptations in free-ranging anthropoid primates. *Sleep Medicine Reviews*, **4**, 355–373

Anderson, J.R. (2002) Tool-use, manipulation and cognition in capuchin monkeys (*Cebus*). In: *New Perspectives in Primate Evolution and Behaviour*. Eds Harcourt C.S. and Sherwood B.R., pp. 127–146. Westbury, Otley

Anderson J.R., Andre A. and Wolf P. (1995) Successful mother- and group rearing of a newborn capuchin monkey (*Cebus apella*) following emergency major surgery. *Animal Welfare*, **4**, 171–182

Anderson J.R., Combette C. and Roeder J.-J. (1991) Integration of a tame adult female capuchin monkey (*Cebus apella*) into a captive group. *Primate Report*, **31**, 87–94

Anderson, J.R., Kuwahata, H., Kuroshima, K. *et al.* (2005) Are monkeys aesthetists? Rensch (1957) revisited. *Journal of Experimental Psychology: Animal Behavior Processes*, **31**, 71–78

Ankel-Simons, F. (2007) *Primate Anatomy: An Introduction*. Academic Press, New York

Baker, M. (1996) Fur rubbing: use of medicinal plants by capuchin monkeys (*Cebus capucinus*). *American Journal of Primatology*, **38**, 263–270

Beran, M.J., Evans, T.A., Leighty, K.A. *et al.* (2007) Summation and quantity judgments of sequentially presented sets by capuchin monkeys (*Cebus apella*). *American Journal of Primatology*, **70**, 191–194.

Brosnan, S.F. and de Waal, F.B.M. (2004) A concept of value during experimental exchange in brown capuchin monkeys. *Folia Primatologica*, **75**, 317–330

Carnegie, S.D., Fedigan, L.M. and Ziegler, T.E. (2005a) Behavioral indicators of ovarian phase in white-faced capuchins (*Cebus capucinus*). *American Journal of Primatology*, **67**, 51–68

Carnegie, S.D., Fedigan, L.M. and Ziegler, T.E. (2005b) Post-conceptive mating in white-faced capuchins, *Cebus capucinus*: Hormonal and sociosexual patterns of cycling, noncycling and pregnant females. In: *New Perspectives in the Study of Mesoamerican Primates: Distribution, Ecology, Behavior, and Evolution*. Eds Estrada, A., Garber, P., Pavelka, M. *et al.*, pp. 387–409. Springer, New York

Carosi, M., Heistermann, M. and Visalberghi, E. (1999) Display of proceptive behaviors in relation to urinary and fecal progestin levels over the ovarian cycle in female tufted capuchin monkeys. *Hormones and Behavior*, **36**, 252–265

Carosi, M. and Visalberghi, E. (2002). Analysis of tufted capuchin (*Cebus apella*) courtship and sexual behavior repertoire: changes throughout the female cycle and female interindividual differences. *American Journal of Physical Anthropology*, **118**, 11–24

Carosi, M., Linn, G.R. and Visalberghi, E. (2005) The sexual behavior and breeding system of tufted capuchin monkeys (*Cebus apella*). *Advances in the Study of Behavior*, **35**, 105–149

Cooper, M.A., Bernstein, I.S., Fragaszy, D.M. *et al.* (2001) Integration of new males into four social groups of tufted capuchins (*Cebus apella*). *International Journal of Primatology*, **22**, 663–683

De Lillo, C., Spinozzi, G. and Truppa, V. (2007) Pattern recognition in tufted capuchin monkeys (*Cebus apella*): the role of spatial organisation of stimulus parts. *Behavioural Brain Research*, **181**, 96–109

De Marco, A. and Visalberghi, E. (2007) Facial displays in young tufted capuchin monkeys (*Cebus apella*): appearance, meaning, context and target. *Folia Primatologica*, **78**, 118–137

Dettmer, E. and Fragaszy, D. (2000) Determining the value of social companionship to captive capuchin monkeys (*Cebus apella*). *Journal of Applied Animal Welfare Science*, **3**, 293–304

Dettmer, E.R., Phillips, K.A., Rager, D.R. *et al.* (1996) Behavioral and cortisol responses to repeated capture and venipuncture in *Cebus apella*. *American Journal of Primatology*, **38**, 357–362

de Waal, F.B.M., Dindo, M., Freeman, C.A. *et al.* (2005) The monkey in the mirror: Hardly a stranger. *Proceedings of the National Academy of Sciences USA*, **102**, 11140–11147

Di Bitetti, M.S. and Janson C.H. (2000) When will the stork arrive? Patterns of birth seasonality in neotropical primates. *American Journal of Primatology*, **50**, 109–130

Di Bitetti, M.S. and Janson, C.H. (2001) Reproductive socioecology of tufted capuchins (*Cebus apella nigritus*) in northeastern Argentina. *International Journal of Primatology*, **22**, 127–142

Dufour, V., Pascalis, O. and Petit, O. (2006) Face processing limitation to own species in primates: a comparative study in brown capuchins, Tonkean macaques and humans. *Behavioural Processes*, **73**, 107–113

European Commission (2007) Commission recommendations of 18 June 2007 on guidelines for the accommodation and care of animals used for experimental and other scientific purposes. Annex II to European Council Directive 86/609 See 2007/526/EC. http://eurlex.europa.eu/LexUriServ/site/en/oj/2007/l_197/l_19720070730en00010089.pdf (accessed 13 May 2008)

Ferreira, R.G., Izar, P. and Lee, P.C. (2006) Exchange, affiliation, and protective interventions in semifree-ranging brown capuchin monkeys (*Cebus apella*). *American Journal of Primatology*, **68**, 765–766

Fiorello, C.V., Heard, D.J., Barnes Heller, H.L. *et al.* (2006) Medical management of *Toxoplasma* meningitis in a white-throated capuchin (*Cebus capucinus*). *Journal of Zoo and Wildlife Medicine*, **37**, 409–412

Flecknell, P.A. (2009) *Laboratory Animal Anaesthesia*, 3rd edn. Academic Press, London

Fragaszy, D.M. and Adams-Curtis, L.E. (1998) Growth and reproduction in captive capuchins (*Cebus apella*). *American Journal of Primatology*, **44**, 197–213

Fragaszy, D.M., Baer J. and Adams-Curtis L. (1994) Introduction and integration of strangers into captive groups of tufted capuchin monkeys (*Cebus apella*). *International Journal of Primatology*, **15**, 399–420

Fragaszy D. and Bard, K. (1997) Comparison of development and life history in *Pan* and *Cebus*. *International Journal of Primatology*, **18**, 683–701

Fragaszy, D.M. and Boinski, S. (1995) Patterns of individual diet choice and efficiency of foraging in wedge-capped capuchin monkeys (*Cebus olivaceus*). *Journal of Comparative Psychology*, **109**, 339–348

Fragaszy, D., Izar, P., Visalberghi, E. *et al.* (2004a) Wild capuchin monkeys (*Cebus libidinosus*) use anvils and stone pounding tools. *American Journal of Primatology*, **64**, 359–366

Fragaszy, D., Johnson-Pynn, J., Hirsh, E. *et al.* (2003) Strategic navigation of two-dimensional alley mazes: comparing capuchin monkeys and chimpanzees. *Animal Cognition*, **6**, 137–139

Fragaszy, D.M., Visalberghi, E. and Fedigan, L.M. (2004b) *The Complete Capuchin*. Cambridge University Press, Cambridge

Fujita, K. and Giersch, A. (2005) What perceptual rules do capuchin monkeys (*Cebus apella*) follow in completing partly occluded figures? *Journal of Experimental Psychology: Animal Behavior Processes*, **31**, 387–398

Fujita, K., Kuroshima, H. and Asai, S. (2003) How do tufted capuchin monkeys (*Cebus apella*) understand causality involved in tool use? *Journal of Experimental Psychology: Animal Behavior Processes*, **29**, 233–242

Galliari, C.A. (1985) Dental eruption in captive born *Cebus apella*: from birth to 30 months old. *Primates*, **26**, 506–510

Hattori, Y., Kuroshima, H. and Fujita, K. (2007) I know you are not looking at me: capuchin monkeys' (*Cebus apella*) sensitivity to human attentional states. *Animal Cognition*, **10**, 141–148

International Primatological Society (2007) *IPS International Guidelines for the Acquisition, Care and Breeding of Nonhuman Primates*, 2nd edn. www.internationalprimatologicalsociety.org (accessed 16 July 2009)

Joint Working Group on Refinement (1993) Removal of blood from laboratory mammals and birds. First Report of the BVA/FRAME/RSPCA/UFAW Joint Working Group on Refinement. *Laboratory Animals*, **27**, 1–22

Joint Working Group on Refinement (2001) Refining procedures for the administration of substances. Report of the BVAAWF/FRAME/RSPCA/UFAW Joint Working Group on Refinement. *Laboratory Animals*, **35**, 1–41

Joint Working Group on Refinement (2009) Refinements in husbandry, care and common procedures for non-human primates. Ninth report of the BVAAWF/FRAME/RSPCA/UFAW Joint Working Group on Refinement. *Laboratory Animals*, **43**, S1:1–S1:47

Kenny, D.E., Knightly, F., Baier, J. *et al.* (2001) Exposure of hooded capuchin monkeys (*Cebus apella cay*) to a rabid bat at a zoological park. *Journal of Zoo and Wildlife Medicine*, **32**, 123–126

Leca, J.-B., Fornasieri, I. and Petit, O. (2002) Aggression and reconciliation in *Cebus capucinus*. *International Journal of Primatology*, **23**, 979–998

Lehner, N.D.M. (1984) Biology and diseases of Cebidae. In: *Laboratory Animal Medicine*. Eds Fox J.F., Cohen, B.J. and Loew, F., pp. 321–353. Academic Press, Orlando

Leighty, K.A., Byrne, G., Fragaszy, D.M. *et al.* (2004) Twinning in tufted capuchins (*Cebus apella*): rate, survivorship, and weight gain. *Folia Primatologica*, **75**, 14–18

Linn, G.S., Mase, D., Lafrancois, D. *et al.* (1995) Social and mentrual cycle phase influences on the behavior of group housed *Cebus apella*. *American Journal of Primatology*, **35**, 41–57

Ludes, E. and Anderson, J. R. (1995a) 'Peat bathing' by captive white-faced capuchin monkeys (*Cebus capucinus*). *Folia Primatologica*, **65**, 38–42

Ludes E. and Anderson J.R. (1995b) Introduction d'une nouvelle femelle singe capucin (*Cebus apella*) dans un groupe en captivité. *Mammalia*, **59**, 303–313

Ludes E. and Anderson J.R. (1996) Comparison of the behaviour of captive white-faced capuchin monkeys (*Cebus capucinus*) in the presence of four kinds of deep litter. *Applied Animal Behaviour Science*, **49**, 293–303

Mann, G.V. (1970) Nutritional requirements of Cebus monkeys. In: *Feeding and Nutrition of Nonhuman Primates*. Ed, Harris, R.S., pp. 143–157. Academic Press, New York

Manson, J.H., Perry, S. and Parish, A.R. (1997) Nonconceptive sexual behavior in bonobos and capuchins. *International Journal of Primatology*, **18**, 767–786

Melin, A., Fedigan, L.M., Hiramatsu, C. *et al.* (2007) Effects of colour vision phenotype on insect capture by a free-ranging population of white-faced capuchins, *Cebus capucinus*. *Animal Behaviour*, **73**, 205–214

Moura, A.C.A. and Lee, P.C. (2004) Capuchin stone tool use in Caatinga dry forest. *Science*, **306**, 1909

Nagle, C.A. and Denari, J.H. (1983) The Cebus monkey (*Cebus apella*). In: *Reproduction in New World Primates*. Ed. Hearn, J., pp. 41–67. MTP Press, Hingham

Napier, J.R. and Napier, P. (1967) *A Handbook of Living Primates*. Academic Press, London

National Research Council of the National Academies (2003) *Nutrient Requirements of Nonhuman Primates, Second Revised Edition*. National Academies Press, Washington, DC

Paukner, A., Anderson, J.R. and Fujita, K. (2004) Reactions of capuchin monkeys (*Cebus apella*) to multiple mirrors. *Behavioural Processes*, **66**, 1–6

Paukner, A., Anderson, J.R. and Fujita, K. (2006) Redundant food searches by capuchin monkeys (*Cebus apella*): a failure of metacognition? *Animal Cognition*, **9**,110–117

Phillips K.A., Bernstein I.S., Dettmer, E.L. *et al.* (1994) Sexual behavior in brown capuchins (*Cebus apella*). *International Journal of Primatology*, **15**, 907–917

Phillips, K.A., Sherwood, C.C. and Lilak, A.L. (2007) Corpus callosum morphology in capuchin monkeys is influenced by sex and handedness. *PLoS ONE*, **8**, e792

Popilskis, S.J. and Kohn, D.F. (1997) Anesthesia and analgesia in nonhuman primates. In: *Anesthesia and Analgesia in Laboratory Animals*. Eds Kohn, D.F., Wixson, S.K., White, W.J. *et al.*, pp. 233–255. Academic Press, New York

Prescott, M.J., Bowell, V.A. and Buchanan-Smith, H.M. (2005) Training laboratory-housed non-human primates, part 2: Resources for developing and implementing training programmes. *Animal Technology and Welfare*, **4**, 133–148

Reinhardt, V., Liss, C. and Stevens, C. (1996a) Comparing cage size requirements for nonhuman primates in the United States and Europe. *Animal Welfare Information Center Newsletter*, **7**, 12–13

Rennie, A.E. and Buchanan-Smith, H.M. (2006) Refinement of the use of non-human primates in scientific research. Part III: refinement of procedures. *Animal Welfare*, **15**, 239–261

Riviello, M.C. (1992) Introduction of two infant capuchin monkeys (*Cebus apella*) in a captive group: analysis of their behavior. *Laboratory Primate Newsletter*, **31**, 17–18

Roeder, J.-J. and Anderson, J.R. (1991) Urine washing in brown capuchin monkeys (*Cebus apella*): testing social and non-social hypotheses. *American Journal of Primatology*, **24**, 55–60

Robinson J.G. and Janson C.H. (1987) Capuchins, squirrel monkeys, and atelines: socioecological convergence with Old World primates. In: *Primate Societies*. Eds Smuts, B.B., Cheney, D.L., Seyfarth, R.M. *et al.*, pp. 69–82. University of Chicago Press, Chicago

Roma, A., Silberberg, A., Huntsberry, M.E. *et al.* (2007) Mark tests for self-recognition in capuchin monkeys (*Cebus apella*) trained to touch marks. *American Journal of Primatology*, **69**, 989–1000

Rosengart, C.R. and Fragaszy, D.M. (2005) Experience and materials affect combinatorial construction in tufted capuchin monkeys (*Cebus apella*). *Journal of Comparative Psychology*, **119**, 166–178

Rylands, A.B., Kierulff, M.C.M. and Mittermeier, R.A. (2005) Notes on the taxonomy and distributions of the tufted capuchin monkeys (*Cebus*, Cebidae) of South America. *Lundiana*, **6** (suppl.), 97–110

Rylands, A.B. Mittermeier, R.A. and Luna E.R. (1995) A species list for the New World Primates (Platyrrhini): Distribution by country, endemism, and conservation status according to the Mace-Land System. *Neotropical Primates*, **3** (suppl.), 113–160

Sabbatini, G., Stammati, M., Tavares, M.C.H. *et al.* (2006) Interactions between humans and capuchin monkeys (*Cebus libidinosus*) in the Parque Nacional de Brasilia, Brazil. *Applied Animal Behaviour Science*, **97**, 272–283

Sabbatini, G. and Visalberghi, E. (2008) Inferences about the location of food in capuchin monkeys (*Cebus apella*) in two sensory modalities. *Journal of Comparative Psychology*, **122**, 156–166

Sainsbury, A.W. (1991) Primates. In: *Manual of Exotic Pets*, 3rd edn. Eds Benyon, P.H. and Cooper, J.E., pp. 111–121. British Small Animal Veterinary Association, Cheltenham

Saito, A., Mikami, A., Kawamura, S. *et al.* (2005) Advantage of dichromats over trichromats in discrimination of color-camouflaged stimuli in non-human primates. *American Journal of Primatology*, **67**, 425–436

Savastano, G., Hanson, A. and McCann, C. (2003) The development of an operant conditioning training program for New World primates at the Bronx Zoo. *Journal of Applied Animal Welfare Science*, **6**, 247–261

Sedgwick, C.J. (1986) Scaling and anesthesia for primates. In: *Primates: The Road to Self-Sustaining Populations*. Ed. Benirschke, K., pp. 815–822. Springer-Verlag, New York

Spinozzi, G., De Lillo, C. and Truppa, V. (2003). Global and local processing of hierarchical visual stimuli in tufted capuchin monkeys (*Cebus apella*). *Journal of Comparative Psychology*, **117**, 15–23

Spinozzi, G. and Truppa, V. (1999) Hand preference in different tasks by tufted capuchin monkeys, *Cebus apella*. *International Journal of Primatology*, **20**, 827–849

Tavares, M.C.H. and Tomaz, C. (2002) Working memory in capuchin monkeys (*Cebus apella*). *Behavioural Brain Research*, **131**, 131–137

van Wolkenten, M.L., Davis, J.M., Gong, M.L. *et al.* (2006) Coping with acute crowding by *Cebus apella*. *International Journal of Primatology*, **27**, 1241–1256

Vick, S.-J. and Anderson, J.R. (2000) Learning and limits of use of eye gaze by capuchin monkeys (*Cebus apella*) in an object-choice task. *Journal of Comparative Psychology*, **114**, 200–207

Visalberghi, E. (1990) Tool use in *Cebus*. *Folia Primatologica*, **54**, 146–154

Visalberghi, E. and Anderson, J.R. (1993) Reasons and risks associated with manipulating captive primates' social environments. *Animal Welfare*, **2**, 3–15

Visalberghi, E. and Fragaszy, D. (2006) What is challenging about tool use? The capuchin's perspective. In: *Comparative Cognition: Experimental Explorations of Animal Intelligence*. Eds Wasserman, E.A. and Zentall, T.R., pp. 529–552. Oxford University Press, New York

Visalberghi, E. and Neel, C. (2003) Tufted capuchins (*Cebus apella*) use weight and sound to choose between full and empty nuts. *Ecological Psychology*, **15**, 215–228

Visalberghi, E. and Riviello M.C. (1987) The integration into a social group of a hand-reared brown capuchin, *Cebus apella*. *International Zoo Yearbook*, **26**, 232–236

Visalberghi, E., Valenzano, D.R. and Preuschoft, S (2006) Facial displays in *Cebus apella*. *International Journal of Primatology*, **27**, 1689–1707

Visalberghi, E. and Vitale, A. (1990) Coated nuts as an enrichment device to elicit tool use in *Cebus*. *Zoo Biology*, **9**, 65–71

Vitale A., Barbaro V., Bartolini P. *et al.* (1994) Effects of wearing a jacket on the behavior of socially housed tufted capuchins (*Cebus apella*). In: *Current Primatology, Vol. 3: Behavioural Neuroscience, Physiology and Reproduction*. Eds Anderson, J.R., Roeder, J.-J., Thierry, B. *et al.*, pp. 279–284. Université Louis Pasteur, Strasbourg

Weaver, A. and de Waal, F.B.M. (2003) The mother–offspring relationship as a template in social development: reconciliation in captive brown capuchins (*Cebus apella*). *Journal of Comparative Psychology*, **117**, 101–110

Westergaard G.C. and Fragaszy D.M. (1985) Effects of manipulatable objects on the activity of captive capuchin monkeys (*Cebus apella*). *Zoo Biology*, **4**, 317–327

Wolff, P.L. (1990) The parasites of New World monkeys: a review. *Proceedings, American Association of Zoo Veterinarians*, 87–94

Zunino, G.E. (1990) Reproduction and mortality of *Saimiri boliviensis* and *Cebus apella* in captivity. *Boletin Primatologico Latinamericano*, **2**, 23–28

39 Old World monkeys

Sarah Wolfensohn

General biology

Natural history

St. George Mivart (1873) defined the order Primates as

> *Unguiculate claviculate placental mammals, with orbits encircled by bone; three kinds of teeth, at least at one time of life; brain always with a posterior lobe and calcarine fissure; the innermost digits of at least one pair of extremities opposable; hallux with a flat nail or none; a well-developed caecum; penis pendulous, testes scrotal; always two pectoral mammae.*

Primate taxonomy and definitions of particular species now go beyond simple anatomical parameters and includes considerations such as: genetics, population biology, ecology and biodiversity. There is disagreement over precisely what constitutes a particular species and definitions shift slightly over time. A more modern, lengthy definition of primate may be found in Martin (1990). However, a simplified classification of living primates is shown in Figure 39.1 (adapted from Wolfensohn & Honess 2005). The term 'Old World monkeys', indicates a geographical origin from Asia and Africa, as opposed to the Americas. They are generally accepted to be monkeys from the superfamily Cercopithecoidea; all lack prehensile tails and have some degree of callus over the ischial tuberosities. Many have cheek pouches, all have a narrow nasal septum and opposable thumbs. They may be divided into two subfamilies – the *Cercopithecine* and the *Colobinae*. The genera in the *Cercopithecine* subfamily fall more or less into two groups – the African long-tailed monkeys (such as vervets, guenons, talapoins and patas monkeys), and the macaques, baboons and mangabeys. The genera of the *Colobine* subfamily are the colobine monkeys, langurs and other leaf eaters.

This chapter will only deal with selected species from the *Cercopithecine* subfamily which are commonly used in research programmes, that is *Macaca mulatta* (rhesus macaque), *Macaca fascicularis* (long-tailed, crab-eating or cynomolgus macaque), *Chlorocebus* sp. (formerly *Cercopithecus* sp. (Groves 2001)) (sometimes called the African green monkey or the vervet monkey) and *Papio* species (baboons). Old World primates includes many species that vary widely in social structure, ecology, reproduction, etc. It would be cumbersome in this chapter to continually refer to the rhesus, cynomolgus, vervet and baboon either as a list or as 'Old World primates commonly used in research'. Therefore, in this chapter the term Old World primates is used to refer only to these species, except where otherwise stated. Moreover, the emphasis of this chapter is on the rhesus and cynomolgus macaque as these are, by far, the most commonly used Old World primates.

Biological data

See Table 39.1 (reproduced from Wolfensohn and Lloyd 1998 and 2003).

Social organisation and normal behaviour

The literature on primate biology, ecology and behaviour is extensive from both field and laboratory studies, eg, Smuts *et al.* (1987); Mittermeier *et al.* (1988); Lindburg (1991); Bennett *et al.* (1995); Fa and Lindburg (1996); Fleagle (1999); Cowlishaw and Dunbar (2000); Strier (2000); Röder and Timmermans (2002).

The primate species commonly used in research are highly social animals. There are both costs and benefits from living in a group (Lee 1994; Strier 2000). The potential negative consequences of group living such as competition for food or mates, or increased likelihood of parasitism or predation, are offset by co-operation resulting in the improved survival of individuals with shared genes (Krebs & Davies 1993). This is achieved by living with close relatives, described as kin-bonded groups, which in Old World primates are typically female kin-bonded groups with the distribution of males superimposed on to that of the females. Group structure varies according to differences in the quality and density of resources and incidence of disease and level of predation. An excellent treatment of the variation in primate societies and the different strategies adopted by different species in balancing the costs and benefits of group living with attempts to maximise individual reproductive success and inclusive fitness is presented by the authors in Smuts *et al.* (1987).

The macaque genus has a wide range, extending from Morocco and Gibraltar through the Indian subcontinent up through China and Japan and down through the Philippines, Java and Sumatra. This range includes a wide variation in environmental temperatures and diets, and the macaques have adapted to a variety of ecological niches. This is

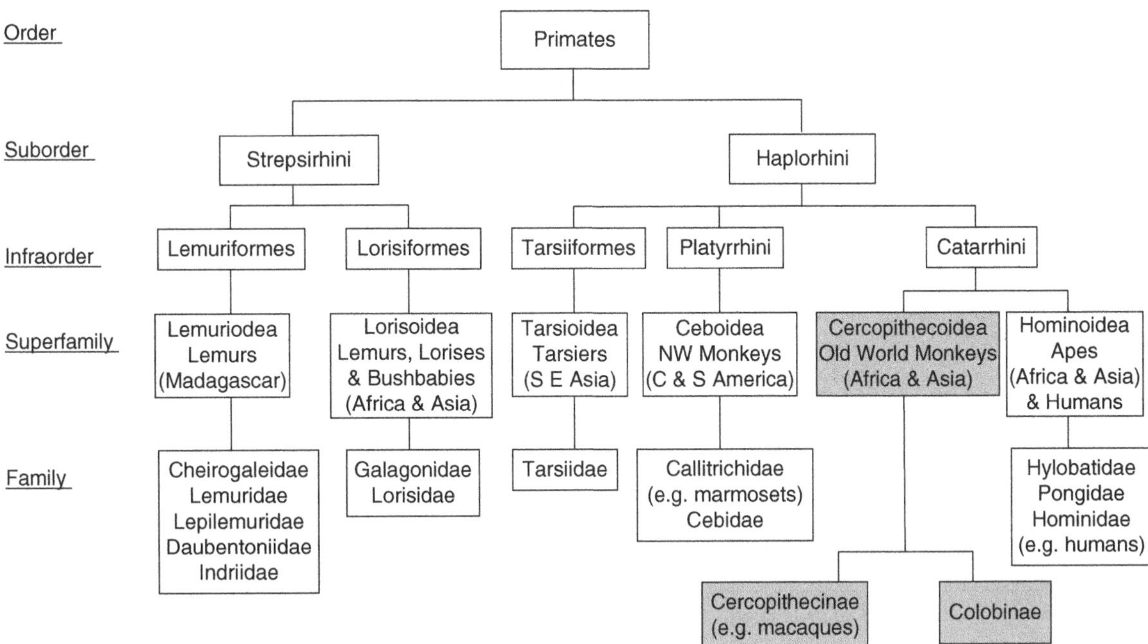

Figure 39.1 A simplified classification of primates.

reflected in normal variations in patterns of behaviour and interactions with humans, for example foraging around urban environments (Honess *et al.* 2006) to foraging in remote areas. The components of a wild macaque's diet typically come in small aliquots (eg, seeds, buds and flowers), dispersed over a wide area, so the process of gathering them is very time consuming and demands much energy. The daily activity cycle reflects this as a macaque troop typically spends the morning foraging, followed by a rest period, then another bout of food gathering through the afternoon, finally moving to a sleeping site for grooming and sleep. Of the two macaque species commonly used in research, the cynomolgus monkey spends more of its time in the trees whereas the rhesus is a ground-dwelling monkey that forages on the floor and takes to the trees for safety and to sleep. Macaques also appear to enjoy playing in water and, although they do not actively swim, they will forage for food in shallow water and use water for thermoregulation.

Reproduction and rearing

There are a several types of captive breeding systems for primates including free-ranging island colonies, semi-free-ranging corral colonies and enclosure or pen pairs or harems. A description of each is provided in a report by the Scientific Committee on Animal Health and Welfare (SCAHAW) (2002). Kirkwood and Stathatos (1992) provide a list of primate reproduction parameters such as the duration of events, adult and neonate weights, growth curves, infant feeding, weaning and physical and behavioural development.

Reproductive success depends on four key elements. Firstly, the individual must be able to survive to breeding age, which depends on the health and condition of the mother, the growth rate of the infant and the incidence of predation, disease and accidental death. Second, is the duration of the reproductive lifespan. Thirdly, productivity depends on fertility which can be affected by environmental, social, lactational and genetic factors. Finally, to ensure their genetic contribution to succeeding generations any offspring produced must, themselves, be able to survive to reproductive age.

Assuming that resources are sufficient, the major recurring influence on female fertility is lactation through the inhibition of ovulation and the negative effect on maternal condition (Lee 1987). There are also social influences on the fertility of primate species that live in groups, since Old World primates moderate the potentially negative process of competing for resources, such as food, nest sites or mates, through the development of dominance hierarchies. Dominance rank is maintained through displays of strength, or in some macaque species through the inheritance of maternal rank thus reducing the incidence of aggressive competition for limited resources. A number of primate species use social dominance and status to improve their reproductive success and females with higher dominance rank breed earlier and produce more offspring per year (Harcourt 1987).

The period of oestrus is indicated by changes in the female's behaviour; olfactory cues and swelling and reddening of the perineal skin may occur to a varying degree. Sexual activity peaks around the time of ovulation and the frequency of aggressive episodes also increases during mating periods. Fraser and Lunn (1999) present a detailed

Table 39.1 Biological data.

	Rhesus macaque (Macaca mulatta)	*Cynomolgus macaque* (Macaca fascicularis)	*Baboon* (Papio *sp.)*
Biological data			
Adult weight (kg)	Male 6–11 Female 4–9	Male 4–8 Female 2–6	Male 22–30 Female 11–15
Diploid number	42	42	42
Food intake	420 J/kg for maintenance, 525–630 J/kg for production, 840 J/kg for neonates		
Water intake	*Ad libitum*, 40–80 ml/kg daily		
Natural lifespan (years)	20–30	15–25	Up to 28
Temperature (°C)	36–40	37–40	36–39
Heart rate/min	120–180*	240	75–200
Blood pressure systole (mmHg)	125	As rhesus	135
Blood pressure diastole (mmHg)	75	As rhesus	80
Blood volume (ml/kg)	55–80	50–96	62–65
Respiratory rate/min	32–50*		29
Breeding data			
Age at puberty	Male 3–4 years Female 2–3 years	3–4 years	2.5–3 years
Age to breed	Male 4–5 years Female 3–5 years	4–5 years	Male 4.5–5 years Female 3.5–4 years
Gestation (days)	146–180, average 164	153–179, average 167	164–186, average 170
Litter size	1	1	1
Birth weight (kg)	0.4–0.55	0.33–0.35	0.87–0.94
Weaning age	12 months	12 months	12 months
Breeding cycle	Menstrual cycle 28 days	Menstrual cycle 31 days	Menstrual cycle 36 days
Comments	Seasonal breeding September to January	Non-seasonal breeding	Non-seasonal breeding
Haematological data			
RBC (× 10^6/mm^3)	3.56–6.95	4.8	
PCV (%)	26–48	35–40	
Hb (g/dl)	8.8–16.5	11.9–12.7	
WBC (× 10^3/mm^3)	2.5–26.7	7.5–9.6	
Neutrophils (%)	5–88	51	
Lymphocytes (%)	8–92	43	
Eosinophils (%)	0–14	3	
Monocytes (%)	0–11	2–8	
Basophils (%)	0–6	0.2	
Platelets (× 10^3/mm^3)	109–597		
Biochemical data			
Serum protein (g/dl)	4.9–9.3	6.6	
Albumin (g/dl)	2.8–5.2	3.8	
Globulin (g/dl)	1.2–5.8	2.8	
Glucose (mg/dl)	46–178	95.9	
Blood urea nitrogen (mg/dl)	8–40	12	
Creatinine (mg/dl)	0.1–2.8	1.28	
Total bilirubin (mg/dl)	0.1–2	0.33	
Cholesterol (mg/dl)	108–263		

*values determined under sedation

description of the physiological features of reproduction in female primates. Data on primate ovarian cycle length are given in Hendrickx and Dukelow (1995a). Dixson (1998) describes in detail the differences between primate taxa in reproductive anatomy, both internal and external, and also provides detail on the menstrual cycle of the rhesus macaque. The size and colour of the sexual skin in Old World primates may not only indicate the occurrence of ovulation but may also be associated with attractiveness in the context of mate choice, both of females to males and *vice versa*, eg, in rhesus macaques (Waitt *et al.* 2003). In females the anogenital region is frequently the primary site of sexual skin, but it may occur in other areas, such as the side of the thigh in rhesus macaques. The presence of sexual skin in male primates may also be dramatic and brightly coloured, eg, the blue of the scrotum of the vervet monkey (*Chlorocebus aethiops*). In addition to visual signals of reproductive state, communication via auditory and olfactory routes is extremely important in many primate species.

Primate groups are not simply convenient aggregations of individuals for breeding purposes (Dixson 1998); even seasonal breeders will form groups all year-round, so it is necessary to distinguish between grouping or social systems, and breeding or mating systems. The reproductive behaviour of male and female primates may vary considerably with the stage of the ovarian cycle, for example in the frequency of ejaculatory mounts in males and the proceptiveness and receptiveness of females. Evidence suggests that changes in the proceptivity behaviour of females, in initiating copulations, may serve as a useful predictor of the day of conception in some species (eg, rhesus macaque, *Macaca mulatta* (Zehr *et al.* 2000)), and this may be very valuable for studies where accurate aging of embryos is required. The rhesus macaque is a seasonal breeder in which reproduction appears to be triggered by changes in day length. The importance of day length in this context is supported by observations of a captive rhesus population in Brazil, in the southern hemisphere, outside the natural range of this species which is totally in the northern hemisphere. In this colony there is an inversion of the breeding season, with births occurring between October and April compared to March to September in the northern hemisphere (Gomes & Bicca-Marques 2003).

In some cases contraceptive strategies may be required. Permanent sterility can be ensured by surgical means, but a reversible solution may be preferred. Useful information on contraception can be found in the 2003 AZA Contraception Advisory Group Recommendations[1]. There can be complications associated with the use of contraceptives. Implants may be lost, or new ones may not be administered soon enough, resulting in pregnancies. In some cases there can be permanent sterility; and a predisposition to simian immunodeficiency virus (SIV) infection by sexual transmission, possibly due to a thinning of the vaginal epithelium, has been associated with the use of progesterone implants in macaques (Marx *et al.* 1996). Contraceptive strategies for some primates are aimed at prevention of implantation (Sengupta *et al.* 2003).

[1]http://www.stlzoo.org/animals/scienceresearch/contraceptioncenter/

Artificial insemination is generally unnecessary as part of a breeding management strategy in the normal captive breeding of primates. It has been undertaken successfully in various Old World primate species (Gould & Martin 1986), including the rhesus macaque (Dede & Plentl 1966). The diagnosis of pregnancy in primates can be made by manual palpation, detection of hormonal changes in the urine and serum (Kirkwood & Stathatos 1992; Hendrickx & Dukelow 1995b) and the use of ultrasound imaging. Data on embryonic and foetal development of commonly used Old World species are given by Fortman *et al.* (2002). Morphological and endocrine diagnosis can be used to determine the early loss of pregnancy (Hendrickx *et al.* 1999). See Table 39.1 for data on duration of gestation.

Hendrickx & Dukelow (1995a) detail many of the hormonal changes that occur during pregnancy and parturition. In most primates, parturition takes place at night or in the early morning. If delivery takes in excess of three hours it will require careful monitoring and may need veterinary intervention (Kirkwood & Stathatos 1992). Multiple births are rare in Old World Monkeys (0.06% to 0.5% of births in macaques (Canfield *et al.* 2000)), though twins are known to occur (eg, in the stump-tailed macaque, *Macaca arctoides;* (Schrier & Povar 1984)). Complications such as the production of conjoined twins are even rarer, but reports do exist (eg, in the rhesus macaque (Canfield *et al.* 2000)).

The production of milk and suckling behaviour is a vital part of the reproductive cycle of primates. It performs several important functions, providing nourishment and early immune protection of the infant; establishing and maintaining the maternal–infant bond; and causing lactational amenorrhoea – a period after the birth which impedes the ovarian cycle and prevents the mother becoming pregnant again for a period after the birth. Data on the length of the lactation period, as well as information on milk composition for many species are presented in Hendrickx and Dukelow (1995a).

Sometimes it is necessary to consider hand rearing of infants, due to human interference by taking neonatal primates for scientific procedures, or due to maternal neglect or death or because the mother has an inadequate supply of milk. In the latter case it may be possible to leave the infant with the mother for nurturing and care, and simply provide supplementary feeding until the infant is able to take food for itself. This is the preferred option since it will develop within its natal and peer group and the risk of any consequential behavioural abnormalities will be reduced. However, if it is established that an infant should be removed from its mother for hand rearing, it should be placed in a cage with some type of surrogate mother. This should be soft to touch, warm and, if possible, should move gently. Each day the infant's body weight is recorded and its physical state monitored. Other parameters to be monitored include level of activity and general alertness, body tone, quality and quantity of faecal output, peripheral perfusion and weight gain. Hand feeding is not a precise activity and the timing of feeds and quantity of feed given may be varied according to the viability of the infant, but all information on the infant's food intake should be recorded. It may sometimes be necessary to foster or hand rear young primates but they should not be maintained in isolation. For a protocol for hand rearing see Wolfensohn and Honess (2005).

Lactation in the macaque has all but finished by 10–11 months so that the infants would be fully weaned before the birth of the next, and at this stage they do not depend on their mother for nutrition. Confusion arises over the use of the term 'weaning' to describe both the cessation of suckling by the mother, in unmanaged populations, as well as the removal of offspring in captive populations as part of a breeding management or supply strategy. The conflicting interests of the mother (to accelerate weaning) and offspring (to prolong suckling) result in the mother terminating suckling at a point determined by the metabolic independence of the offspring, this being a factor of the offspring's body weight at birth and at weaning – the 'metabolic weaning weight'. In rhesus macaques the threshold weaning weight is 1.34 kg (with a range of 1.0–1.6 kg), which reflects a constant multiple 3.4 times the neonate's birth weight (Lee 1999).

Natural weaning is not an abrupt event but a process lasting several months. Most infants can feed themselves at 6 months but remain socially dependent on their mothers and return to them when disturbed and to sleep. This period of suckling and gradual increasing independence is an important time in the development of the infants. It is during this time, and shortly after, that they begin to learn from their mother and to refine food selection, acquisition and processing skills (Altmann 1980; Janson & van Schaik 2002). After the first year, juvenile animals, especially males, become more and more involved in peer group activities. Stimulus deprivation in infancy has a dramatic impact on the development of young macaques, making them less active, more withdrawn, with more stereotypic behaviour (Harlow *et al.* 1965), higher basal cortisol levels and showing more fear–disturbance–emotional behaviour than non-deprived control animals (Sacket *et al.* 1973). The importance of social stimulation during infancy is well established, but considerably less is known about the influence of social contact during juvenile and adolescent stages of development (National Research Council (NRC) 1998). It is therefore important to monitor each animal and if the assessments indicate an incidence of behavioural problems, then management regimes, such as age of separation from the natal group, should be reviewed. Continual assessment of behaviour and welfare is more important than sticking to rigid temporal criteria, and each animal should be considered individually.

Since many managers have tried to use temporal criteria for separating infants from mothers in captive breeding colonies, opinions differ on the ideal time (Goo & Fugate 1984; Home Office 1995; Wallis & Valentine 2001; Reinhardt 2002; International Primatological Society (IPS) 2007). However, forced weaning appears to have no appreciable benefit in terms of increased production, and account must be taken of the welfare aspects on the psychological well-being of the mother and the infant. If young monkeys are reared with an inappropriate social background they will show indicators of poor welfare such as a restricted repertoire of behaviours, an abnormal activity pattern, inadequate social behaviour and/or abnormal behaviours such as self-injury. Monkeys raised without appropriate social stimulation tend to be dysfunctional in their reproductive behaviour (Goldfoot 1977). Socially deprived male rhesus do not develop the full double foot-clasp mating stance adopted by undeprived animals (Goy *et al.* 1974) and there is a higher rate of rejection of infants in primiparous socially deprived females (Suomi 1986).

Sufficient outbreeding helps to avoid some hereditary conditions or familial predispositions to diseases such as metabolic bone disease (Wolfensohn 2003). Researchers working in immunology may prefer animals of a specific type of major histocompatability complex (MHC) but those individuals with a greater variety of MHC alleles will have more protection from a corresponding diversity of possible diseases (Strier 2000). Knapp *et al.* (1996) demonstrated, in pig-tailed macaques (*Macaca nemestrina*), that mates sharing the same MHC type suffered significantly more spontaneous abortions than those with different MHC types, and the olfactory recognition of MHC type among animals (Brown & Eklund 1994) avoids this kind of reproductive wastage, while at the same time maximising MHC allele diversity. In addition to considering genetic profile, breeding facilities that supply animals for research may wish to select animals based on aspects of their behaviour, such as temperament or learning ability. Tracking the performance of animals during training within both the breeding facility and the experimental facility will help to identify individuals that produce offspring that are more likely to be easily trainable and to co-operate with research protocols. This will contribute, when coupled with the highest welfare standards in housing and husbandry, to a reduction in the stress of primates maintained for research.

Sources, supply, conservation status, transportation

In the USA and Europe, although there are some facilities for breeding macaques for research use, these do not yet supply adequate numbers to match the demand in these countries. Most jurisdictions either do not permit, or discourage the use of wild-caught primates in research and some are encouraging moves to the use of F2 animals (ie, ones that are second-generation captive bred). The current text of article 7(3) of EU Directive 86/609/EEC states, '*experiments on animals taken from the wild may not be carried out unless experiments on other animals would not suffice for the aims of the experiment*' (European Council 1986).

A substantial number of macaques are, therefore, imported into the USA and Europe from countries of origin where they are purpose-bred. Cynomolgus macaques may be sourced from China, the Philippines, Mauritius, Indonesia and Israel; and rhesus macaques may be sourced from China, Vietnam and Cambodia. The majority of primates used in scientific procedures are purpose bred, but at present a number of the breeding animals from which they are derived are still sourced from the wild in some facilities. Some breeding establishments are now introducing programmes to move to use of F1 or subsequent generation animals for breeding, with the aim of avoiding the need over the next decade or so to take animals from the wild and enabling them to supply F2 or subsequent generation animals for use in research from self-sustaining captive colonies. However, ongoing pilot projects evaluating the impact of self-sustaining breeding and inbreeding show there may be a significant impact on fertility rates and other physiological parameters. At this time, it is not yet possible to assess the impact of these changes on availability of animals for research. The feasibility and impact of these moves towards self-sustaining breeding is being monitored to inform future decisions about moving exclusively to use of self-sustaining breeding colonies.

When breeding stock is sourced from the wild conservation status has to be carefully taken into account. However, there is no evidence that the trapping of the cynomolgus macaque in controlled conditions for breeding purposes, is necessarily a conservation issue and in Mauritius the cynomolgus macaque has been implicated as a predator of other species that are endangered (Carter & Bright 2002). Indeed, in some areas the cynomolgus monkey is considered a pest, causing significant damage to agricultural crop production. Sourcing from the wild is also associated with potential health risks and these must be controlled by appropriate quarantine procedures.

There is debate about the merits of obtaining primates from overseas breeding centres rather than from national breeding centres. This has been prompted partly by findings about the stress that primates respond to during international air transport (Wolfensohn 1997; Prescott 2001; SCAHAW 2002; Honess *et al.* 2004).

Macaques come from a wide range of natural habitats, and it seems likely that the genetic backgrounds and responses to experimental procedures may also be variable for macaques from different populations. For example, rhesus macaques from India and China can show very different responses to experimental infections (Smith 2005). However, without better knowledge of this variation it is possible that crucial characteristics for future experimental models may be lost if they are not present in the limited number of parents from which self-sustaining colonies are derived. Therefore, wild animals are an important reservoir of genetic characteristics that may be of prime importance for the study of diseases in the future. For other species, recent legislation against the exportation of wildlife in a number of source countries has affected supply. Even where the export of captive-bred representatives of indigenous species is permitted, this is often under a quota system. Wild-caught olive baboons (*Papio hamadryas anubis*) have been exported from African countries (eg, Kenya) for research use, but the trade in this species from Tanzania and Ethiopia is now subject to CITES export quotas (Prescott 2001).

The Convention on International Trade in Endangered Species of Wild Fauna and Flora (CITES) regulates international trade in endangered species, live or dead, or any parts or products of them. Species listed in Appendix I are considered the most endangered. Currently, all primates are listed as being in either Appendix I (threatened with extinction) or Appendix II (could become endangered without control of trade). CITES permits must be obtained for all movements (import and export) of CITES listed species between countries that have signed the Convention. These CITES management authorities are listed in the International Air Transport Association (IATA) Live Animal Regulations which are published annually in several languages (English, Spanish and French). The IATA regulations set out minimum conditions for the air transport of live animals and provide essential information for all those seeking to transport live primates. Further information relating to transport has been provided by the Laboratory Animal Science Association (LASA) (2005), IPS (2007) and see also Chapter 13.

When primates are transported to research facilities, they are usually shipped while still juvenile, so that the total weight and cost of the consignment is reduced. Juvenile animals may be shipped in pairs within the transport container, and pairing animals allows for mutual support during stressful events. Evidence suggests that when primates are subjected to a stressful event, such as transportation, signs of physiological stress are markedly reduced when in the presence of other individuals (Honess & Marin 2006a). The compatibility of paired animals can be ensured by studying the interactions of the animals in their social groups prior to being transported; animals which show affiliation can be assigned to travel together. This approach should extend beyond the transport phase and efforts should be made to ensure that groups which will be housed together at their destination are socially stable and, where possible, from the same breeding group. In this way, relationships and social status will have already been established in natal groups, reducing the likelihood and intensity of conflict. This makes future veterinary and behavioural management of the animals easier.

A change in diet can affect the gut flora and, with all the other changes involved in transportation, will add to the animals' stress. A gradual change to a new diet over 4–5 days will reduce the incidence of diarrhoea. Communication between shipper and recipient, prior to shipping, should ensure that a list of the animals' favoured and acceptable foods is passed on so that these can be available on arrival.

There may also be disease risks associated with the transportation of primates, both between the animals and handling staff and between consignments of animals, particularly if the health status of the animals is unknown. They may be carrying zoonotic diseases, and disease could also pass from the shipment handlers to the primates. Rhesus, long-tailed, bonnet and pig-tailed macaques show distinct and consistent differences in behavioural and adrenocortical responses to stress induced by confinement in a transport cage, and by a cage and room change (Clarke *et al.* 1988; Crockett *et al.* 1995, 2000). It is frequently difficult, if not impossible, to separate the effect of the transport element of their journey from the effect on the animals of other changes that may accompany this: changes in accommodation, animal care staff, diet, climatic conditions etc. (Honess *et al.* 2004).

General husbandry

Enclosures

The physical environment in which captive primates are housed is an essential element of the conditions that contribute to the physical and psychological health of the animals. When designing accommodation in which to keep primates, the starting point is to examine the ecological requirements of the species, consider its habitat in the wild and what features of that environment can be replicated in the captive setting. Not all features of the wild environment are in the animal's welfare interest; for example, food resources may be scarce, competition from conspecifics and prevalence of predation and disease may be high in the wild. In captivity, on the other hand, there may be plentiful provision of food and effective disease control; but there may be a reduction in activity leading to boredom and obesity with resultant poor health, both physical and psychological. Replication of the natural environment in the captive situation must be balanced to ensure that the animals' health is maximised.

While there may be similar trends in many species, the details may differ for some with variation in social relationships, anatomical and ecological adaptations, use of space, level of activity and time and energy budgets, and in aspects of infant rearing, feeding and foraging (Honess & Marin 2006b). Thus, some practices suitable for one species may have unforeseen and potentially disastrous consequences when applied to another. Recommendations for captive maintenance, therefore, need to take into account knowledge of species-specific behavioural responses, life history patterns and clinical tendencies.

There are many imperfections in current guidelines on the housing of primates kept for research, and there are inconsistencies between countries in regulations (Poole 1995). Sometimes, specific space guidelines (eg, NRC 1996) may be incompatible with the recommendation that behavioural needs should be met (NRC 1998) and the wide discrepancies in the recommended space allowances (Terao 2005) can throw doubt on their credibility. It is, therefore, important that these guidelines should be scrutinised and revised regularly, using a harmonised approach that will best serve the interests of the animals. The most recent recommendations are those published by the European Commission (2007).

Existing recommendations for primate housing, particularly in research facilities, are generally inadequate from the animal welfare perspective. Most are based solely on the weight of an animal without reference to linear dimensions. This can result in recommended cage sizes which are actually smaller in the vertical dimension than the head to tail length of the monkey so that the animals cannot perch in the cage with the tail freely suspended, as they do in nature. The sizes of cages are sometimes too small to meet the behavioural needs of the animals; providing neither adequate space for exercise nor room for environmental enrichment (Crockett *et al.* 1995). The assumption is made that heavier individuals require more space than lighter ones, although in practice light, young animals are usually more active than the heavier adults (Wolfensohn & Honess 2005). Rather than basing cage size on parameters such as body weight or crown to rump length, it is better to use performance standards which assess the ability of the animal to express its species-typical behaviours and which will vary depending on species, age, sex, individual temperament, group composition and dynamics (Honess & Marin 2006b). It is important to appreciate that most recommendations for cage sizes represent *minimum* dimensions for animals of all ages. The duration of stay of the animal is also relevant. Where primates are to be kept for a period of years, the necessity for housing them in an environment that better satisfies their needs is even more important than for those animals which will only stay for a short while.

Cages are frequently constructed of metal with wire mesh walls, or parallel metal bars. Such cages are not only expensive but cold to touch, noisy and not very animal friendly. Metal is easy to clean but materials that are warmer to the touch, chewable, and which provide a quieter environment than the clanking of metal cages are preferable. The structural division of space in primate enclosures is of paramount importance. It is essential that the animals should be able to utilise as much of the volume as possible because, being arboreal, they occupy a three-dimensional space. To make this possible, perches, swings and climbing structures should be provided. Visual barriers, which allow the animals to be out of sight of one another, are important in group housing and multiple escape routes provide opportunities to avoid attacks and also prevent dominant individuals from restricting access of subordinates to other parts of the cage (National Centre for the Replacement, Refinement and Reduction of Animals used in Research (NC3Rs) 2007). Where individuals may need to be treated individually, as in some toxicology experiments, areas with a partition to allow separation or varying degrees of social contact is required. Flexibility of use should be incorporated into the design of the housing.

In a research setting, a design that combines cages with a larger enclosed area is a flexible and useful solution to the conflict between wishing to give the animal free access to space and wishing to keep it in a cage to make it more accessible. This permits the retention of a number of standard cages allowing the animals to be removed into transport chairs for testing, dosing or sampling; but at the same time allowing them access to a much larger and more complex space when not in use. In this setting, the animals will show an extensive range of natural behaviours, little aggression and will move readily into chairs or boxes. There is an ethical obligation to house and maintain animals used in research in the best conditions that can be provided. So, as 'best practice' evolves it is necessary to continually re-evaluate whether the facilities and their operation and management can be improved.

Foraging is a natural and desirable behaviour which can occupy a significant period of time, reducing boredom and the incidence of stereotypic behaviours. Therefore, a substrate such as woodchips, hemp or shavings should be provided in which forage can be scattered. Hay, straw or other material such as shredded paper may be provided for environmental enrichment. Careful design and positioning of drains and air vents are required to ensure they do not become blocked, or can be readily cleared.

In addition to animal holding areas, a primate facility should be equipped with many functional support areas (see Chapter 9). The kinds of support areas needed will depend on the purpose of the facility and the use to which the primates are put, but all should receive due consideration in the planning stages.

Social housing

All species of primates used in the laboratory are social animals that live in family groups or large troops and it is widely accepted that housing individuals on their own is a major stressor (Joint Working Group on Refinement (JWGR) 2009). Knowledge of the normal social structure (including how groups are constituted and dominance hierarchies established) should be used to inform how they should be group-housed in captivity. This is important in determining group size and structure, defining socialisation programmes, managing aggression, promoting natural behaviour, optimising reproductive success, where appropriate, and of course initially in the design of housing and husbandry systems (Wolfensohn 2004).

The Old World primates described in this chapter live in social hierarchies in which there are inevitable conflicts and fights which may result in some animals being injured or even killed. A singly housed animal may be in excellent physical health because it is not exposed to the risk of infections from other animals, there is no competition for food and no chance of wounding by companions. Furthermore, although it will suffer the stress of social deprivation, it will not have to try to maintain its position in a social hierarchy. However, such animals frequently show a poor behavioural repertoire with abnormal and even self-harming behaviours and do not have well developed coping skills. The benefit of social housing is that the environment is dynamic, variable and unpredictable so there is little habituation, but on the other hand, there may be increased risks of infection, wounding and competition for food. With good management strategies these risks can be minimised but not altogether removed. Because of the overall welfare benefits, it is widely accepted that monkeys should be kept in groups. There will, however, be the occasional social misfit who will have to be removed either for their own safety or for the benefit of the remainder of that group. It is important to maintain a flexible approach to the management and use of monkey colonies to ensure that such individuals are used to maximum benefit, and are neither wasted nor left to suffer social deprivation simply because they do not fit in. The size of the group is important, and arguably more important than the amount of space per animal. In nature, many primates live in fairly large groups (for macaques around 50 in a troop) and while putting a small group of animals or a pair together will give them company, there appears to be a higher incidence of fights and unsettled behaviour in these than in larger groups, even if floor space per monkey is lower in the latter case.

Provision of foraging opportunities in an adequate amount of space is a way of offering a socially sanctioned method of establishing the hierarchy that does not result in significant wounding and injury. The damage caused to an animal by individual housing may not be immediately apparent as the changes in behaviour may at first be very subtle, but in the long term there may be self-mutilation and more obvious damage. The animal's individual experiences will modify its development since there is a dynamic process that determines its later behaviour. For example, sucking and clinging, which should be directed toward the mother, may become directed toward other available objects or even the individual's own body. Although this does not provide the nutrition and contact that should come from the natural mother-directed behaviour, it continues to provide a state of a psycho-physiological arousal. Thus digit sucking or self-hugging will occur when an individual is anxious or distressed; the same circumstances in which an animal will return to its mother. Stimulation-seeking behaviours manifest themselves in a variety of ways depending on the available options afforded by the environment.

Evaluation of the psychological condition of the animal should take into account its physical health, its behavioural repertoire and an assessment of its coping skills when presented with novelty. The latter will evaluate normal inquisitive and explorative behaviour or any abnormal response and how long the animal takes to return to baseline level of behavioural repertoire.

Environmental enrichment

Establishments wishing to demonstrate best practice should endeavour to produce conditions for their animals which provide key safe features of a naturalistic environment that will contribute to encouraging as natural a range and rate of behaviours as possible. Environmental enrichment is essential for captive non-human primates to meet their ethological and psychological needs (Young 2003). It should provide the animals with the opportunity to carry out a sufficiently varied daily programme of activity (see Chapter 10). The actual enrichment provided will vary, but there is now a large literature offering a wide variety of options. The effectiveness of many is reviewed in Honess and Marin (2006b).

Opportunities for the animals to exercise a full locomotory repertoire should be provided in the living area. To allow this, the cage must be sufficiently large and contain adequate furnishings. Cage furniture itself can provide opportunities for a wide repertoire of behaviour. Perches, ladders, swings, plastic chains, car tyres etc. are all of value, and allow the animals plenty of places to sit without having to squabble. This allows a social hierarchy to develop with less aggressive encounters. Devices to encourage foraging (ranging from food scattered in the substrate to puzzle feeders) have also proved effective. Some practical methods include the use of wire grids over food hoppers rather than expensive manufactured food puzzles, ice cubes of frozen juice, frozen grapes or melon cubes, food on top of the enclosure to encourage animals to forage upwards through the mesh, wrapping or boxing of treats, empty diet bags or cardboard boxes, and foraging boxes full of hay or sawdust (Dean 1999). Novelty is important so the items should be changed frequently to avoid habituation and a programme of rotation of items of environmental enrichment should be recorded.

Reducing the incidence of aggressive encounters by resorting to long-term single housing of animals is not acceptable; the environment and the group composition need to be actively managed to ensure maintenance of social stability. A key component in a successful strategy is to start with the right compatible grouping, which may require coordination and effective communication with the source breeding colony which establishes the groups at weaning. Training animals to co-operate with carers and experimenters also helps to enrich the animals' lives and reduces handling stress (Reinhardt & Reinhardt 2000). It is vital to remember that the animal's principal purpose is for a scientific procedure and the animal model must be valid in terms of normality and reproducibility. The environmental enrichment programme should be reviewed to consider of any effect (positive or negative) on the quality of the scientific data generated.

Physical environment

The environmental sensitivity of primates varies considerably between species, some being more tolerant of environmental change than others. In the wild, rhesus macaques (*M. mulatta*) occur across a wide range of altitudes from sea level to 3000 metres (Rowe 1996) indicating a tolerance of a substantial temperature range. Long-tailed macaques (*M. fascicularis*), on the other hand, may be less tolerant, being found in habitats from sea level to 2000 metres.

Temperature

The recommended temperature regimes for Old World primates relate to differences in the natural habitats to which they have adapted. In the UK codes of practice for users and breeders, 15–24°C is required for Old World monkeys reflecting their tropical to subtropical natural habitat (Home Office 1989, 1995). In the USA the recommended temperature range is 18–24°C for all primates (NRC 1996). Depending on the location and ambient temperature of the facility housing primates these recommended temperatures will be achieved and maintained either through a system of heating or cooling. Stocking density will affect the temperature in each room, so leading to significant temperature variation between rooms with the same heating/cooling system where stocking density varies significantly. Rapid fluctuations in housing temperature are undesirable, but appropriate dampened temperature fluctuation on a 24h cycle that mimics natural temperature may help encourage natural behaviour, such as taking a siesta during the hot part of the day and huddling at nights when it is cooler (Honess *et al.* 2004).

Where no indoor housing is provided, it is vital that sufficient shelter is available to protect animals from climatic extremes. If an outside run is provided, the interior accommodation should be sufficiently attractive that animals do not seek all their stimulation outside, particularly during periods of inclement weather. Outside caging can be protected with natural vegetation or roofing; during seasonally bad weather, sides and a ceiling can be attached to the caging for extra shelter and to allow heating of the interior. Where excessive heat may be a problem, this can be alleviated by providing a pool for recreational use and behavioural thermoregulation or by thermostatically controlled spraying of a fine mist of water droplets that can reduce the ambient temperature by about 5°C (Honess *et al.* 2004). Under certain experimental regimes and containment levels it may be important to ensure negative air pressure in the animal rooms. In the UK 10–12 air changes per hour are required (Home Office 1989, 1995) while 10–15 air changes per hour are recommended in the USA and recycled air should contain at least 50% fresh air (NRC 1996). It is important, however, to prevent draughts.

Relative humidity

In the UK relative humidity levels are required to be 45–65% in areas where primates are used in scientific procedures (Home Office 1989); or 40–70% where they are kept for breeding (Home Office 1995). In the USA the recommended range is 30–70% for all primates (NRC 1996). Efforts should be made to reduce the impact of husbandry practices, such as extensive cage/housing washing, on conditions such as humidity levels. Extensive daily washing, such as pressure-hosing, may result in surfaces which remain permanently wet, resulting in elevated humidity levels and also presenting a potential health risk to the animals as many pathogens remain viable in a warm, wet environment.

Lighting

Where animals have access to daylight and are not maintained in a region where day lengths are the same as, or very similar to, those in the natural geographical range of the species it will be necessary to regulate lighting regimes. Where access to daylight is not available a lighting regime of 12h light, 12h dark is typically provided, in which case efforts should be made to replicate dawn and dusk gradations in light intensity. In the wild, primates rely on the ultra violet (UV) in daylight to produce vitamin D_3. Care should be taken to ensure that, particularly in the absence of natural light, artificial light is provided using daylight spectrum tubes or bulbs, rather than standard fluorescent lighting. This is of particular importance where there may be a familial predisposition to metabolic bone disease or an even minor deficit in dietary vitamin D_3 (Wolfensohn 2003). Artificial lighting typically lacks a UV component; where this is the case and access to daylight is limited, specific provision of UV light is recommended, and vitamin D_3 should be supplied as a supplement in the animals' diet.

Care should be taken in the positioning and intensity of artificial lighting in interior accommodation. Highly engineered caging, such as that found in experimental facilities, is frequently made of galvanised steel. Poorly positioned and overly intense lighting can intensify the glare from highly polished metal surfaces. This can be reduced by using more sympathetic, better placed lighting and the use of more natural caging materials such as wood and wire. The lighting system is also important in preventing the creation of dark areas of the caging, such as the lower levels or corners of shelved caging, in which animals may hide from view. A facility can be designed to maximise daylight by the incorporation of windows; and if the configuration of the building offers a choice between a place in a sunny/cool window region and a more controlled environment within the inner confines of the building this will allow the animals to select their own thermal environment.

Noise

There are four primary sources of noise: the primates themselves (eg, vocalisations); the physical environment (eg, caging, extractors, pumps, doors); the staff (overshoes, shouting, husbandry procedures); alarms, public address and entertainment systems (for staff and animals). High noise levels may intimidate many animals and have a negative effect on their psychological well-being. Primates are highly social animals and one of their primary modes of communication is vocal. Dominance can be asserted through vocalisations and therefore care needs to be taken in placement of overly assertive animals in proximity to those that may be negatively affected by vocal bullying.

The design of the physical environment and materials used in its construction can be responsible for substantial noise pollution. If cages are constructed using metal sheeting and heavy meshing with metal furniture, such as swings, noise production can be substantial particularly when larger primates display. The use of more natural caging construction and furnishing materials such as wood will help reduce noise, as will the provision of a solid, rather than grid, floor covered with sound dampening forage substrate such as wood chips. Other sources such as air extractors and pumps also need to be considered when trying to minimise noise.

The people working around the primates, as well as those who visit the facility, can generate considerable noise. It may be reassuring for the animals to hear the voices of familiar care staff but not all staff are viewed as friendly by the animals and their voices may, particularly when loud, produce a response suggesting stress or anxiety. Staff should be encouraged to keep voices down and to work around the animals in a way that reduces unnecessary loud noises. Heavy metal modular caging is noisy to manipulate during cleaning or when catching animals for treatment, research procedures or husbandry changes. Trolleys that are used to move animals, food and bedding can be noisy especially if they collide with walls and doors. Other noise-generating factors such as slamming doors and clothing, including plastic overshoes, should be included in reviews of noise production and its prevention around captive primates.

Accommodation design

Laboratory primates are often kept in cages or rooms, but some larger species may be kept in outside pens or corrals, with free access to a heated indoor area. There is a perception that there is a welfare advantage to all primates associated with the provision of external accommodation. However, it is the quality of the accommodation and the handling of the animals which matters most in terms of animal welfare and outdoor accommodation is not necessarily in itself a benefit. External accommodation carries with it risks from exposure to wildlife (small birds, rodents, insects), disease transmission from outside vectors (eg, *Mycobacterium*, *Salmonella*, *Yersinia*), and damage due to adverse climate conditions (eg, frost injuries). In the laboratory setting where disease-free animals are required, these factors may reduce the supposed welfare gain of external accommodation over a good quality internal exercise area.

The choice of internal accommodation will also facilitate animal handling and may influence the extent to which the primates become accustomed to human contact and socialisation. Achieving this with a potentially aggressive species depends not only on staff education and training, but also on the configuration of the facilities, including plentiful enrichment, and accommodation which allows the animal refuge points from where it can interact with humans without feeling threatened. In the development of non-stressful and safe means of capture, and in the training of animals, there should be dual emphasis on animal welfare and staff health and safety. These developments are only practicable in a building which allows for the seclusion of the occasional aggressive animal (sub-division of areas) for the protection of staff and other animals, and within which it is possible to train animals to come forward for capture and for simple interventions. Capture by means of netting (as is often used in large outside runs) is both stressful for the animals and may be source of minor injuries. The stress of handling for minor procedures can be greatly reduced by training, and monkeys are capable of learning to volunteer for these interventions (see Chapter 16). The extent of the human–monkey interaction bears directly on intended end-use; familiarity with human handling is valuable in preparing animals for work in some studies. Initial profiling and training has potential benefits in selecting animals for different end-uses. This is more difficult to deliver without the kind of close contact which is possible in an internal facility. However, for other types of study (such as studies of natural behaviour) it is necessary to have large naturalistic social groups (depending on the species) with diversity of demography and social and genetic relationships which are more achievable in a parkland type setting. The final decision on whether to choose an internal, external or mixed facility will depend on factors including the use of the animals (laboratory, zoo, sanctuary, conservation study prior to returning to the wild), the species, the local climate and cost. The facility must be 'fit for purpose' but there should be no underlying assumption that outside living areas are somehow automatically better. A well designed facility is critical to be able to deliver a successful animal care programme and behavioural management.

Building a new facility takes a long time from conception to completion and there will be many factors and details to consider (see Chapter 9). Cost, design, materials and utilities will be high on the list of priorities for the build management team, however the species-specific behaviours of the animals to be housed in it should take an equally high priority in the design criteria. Finally, managers will often require husbandry duties to be carried out in a way that optimises the efficient use of staff time and as a result it is easy to overlook the effect their methods of working have on the animals. Wherever possible, husbandry duties should be carried out to minimise the impact on the animals being cared for, even if this may be at the cost of working efficiency. Husbandry regimes that may be more labour-intensive but have a reduced impact on the animals should be used. It may well be that there will be cost savings elsewhere; for example, through less aggression leading to less traumatic injuries, easier training producing a more valid research model and ultimately a more effective use of research funds.

Feeding/watering

Food

Analysis of wild primate activity budgets has shown that more time is given to foraging than to any other activity

(Lindburg 1991), and arguably food gathering is the most profoundly affected activity of a captive existence. Since many primates choose to spend a substantial amount of their time foraging, anything that may restrict this should be regarded as potentially detrimental to their welfare. In captivity, providing food removes the need to forage and food tends to be presented to a predictable schedule. It is better to provide small portions and with an unpredictable schedule to satisfy the animal's behavioural needs than to provide the quantity required to satisfy the daily nutritional requirements in just one feed.

Nutrient intake cannot be assessed adequately just in terms of grams of food taken. It is necessary to consider the metabolisable energy (ME) value and the nutrient content of the food so as to take into account variations in water content and digestibility. Macaques require approximately 420 kJ ME/kg daily for maintenance, 525–630 kJ/kg if pregnant or lactating, and 840 kJ/kg for neonatal growth. Commercial Old World monkey diets that have a protein density of 15–25% are used, with supplements of fruit and nuts. Foraging mix can be scattered through the substrate of the enclosure adding interest to the diet as well as providing environmental enrichment. Very useful tables of the nutrient contents of foods commonly used to feed primates are published by the NRC (2003).

Dietary intake is affected by the colour, smell and taste of the food. Most species prefer sweet foods, but its hardness and density will also affect intake. The food pieces need to be of a size such as to be held easily so the primate can manipulate its food, but it is not necessary to chop foods into very small pieces. Food may be offered *ad libitum* or given in a fixed amount. If fed *ad libitum*, primates eat to their energy requirements but can become obese if fed on palatable foods, this applies especially to dominant animals who may monopolise favoured foods.

An overview of energy requirements and how these are calculated is given in Chapter 4 of Wolfensohn and Honess (2005). This energy requirement is met by a combination of commercial primate diet, a selection of fruit and vegetables and forage mix, but variety is essential and, when adding any supplements such as fruit, care must be taken not to upset the nutrient balance. Amounts fed will also need to be adjusted according to levels of activity and weight gain/loss must be evaluated regularly. Recommended dietary levels of minerals and vitamins are given in Table 39.2.

Supplements are generally given for environmental enrichment or as part of positive reinforcement training, rather then primarily for nutrition, but they may have the undesired effect of distorting the balance of the nutrition provided. It is therefore important to use items that are nutritionally complete or which are high in moisture and low in calories – such as fresh fruit and vegetables – rather than offering energy-dense but nutritionally incomplete foods such as nuts and raisins. Since fresh fruit and vegetables are 80–90% moisture, if these make up less than 40% of the wet weight of the diet, they will be providing less than 10% of the total dietary dry matter and therefore will minimally distort the nutrient balance.

Data on composition of foods and feed ingredients, including details of dry matter, energy, protein and other nutrient densities are essential for formulating feeds and diets that meet requirements (see NRC 2003). The exact analysis of fruits will vary depending on the condition of the particular batch, the season and the source. Animals should be fed according to their individual needs, and these will depend on species, age, sex, physiological and reproductive status, health and environmental conditions. Estimates of energy requirements are usually related to the stage of life cycle – maintenance, growth, pregnancy or lactation – and are often expressed as multiples of the maintenance requirement. Over-consumption of calories by immature animals will lead to excess weight gain, affect age of sexual maturity and adult weight, and predispose to obesity. Energy requirements during pregnancy and lactation are substantially increased, with lactation being the most energetically demanding phase of reproduction (NRC 2003).

Growth can be measured in various ways such as body weight, crown–rump length, limb length, or head circumference. The linear measurements are not distorted by accumulations of body fat in the way that body weight may be. Growth rate will vary depending on genetic background, maternal nutrition in pregnancy and lactation, availability of supplementary weaning foods and rearing practices.

Table 39.2 Recommended dietary concentration and levels of minerals and vitamins.

Mineral	*Concentration*
Calcium	0.8%
Phosphorus	0.6%
Magnesium	0.08%
Potassium	0.4%
Sodium	0.2%
Chloride	0.2%
Iron	100 mg/kg
Copper	20 mg/kg
Manganese	20 mg/kg
Zinc	100 mg/kg
Iodine	0.35 mg/kg
Selenium	0.3 mg/kg
Vitamin	*Level*
Vitamin A	12 000 IU/kg DM
Vitamin D	1000–3000 IU/kg DM
Vitamin E: (α-tocopherol)	50 mg/kg DM
Vitamin K	2 μg/kg body weight/day
Thiamine	1.1 mg/kg DM
Riboflavin	1.7 mg/kg DM
Niacin	16–56 mg/kg DM
Vitamin B6	4.4 mg/kg DM
Biotin	110 μg/kg DM
Folic acid	2.55–5.61 mg/kg DM
Vitamin B12	11 μg/kg DM
Vitamin C	55–110 mg/kg DM

Water

The amount of water drunk to satisfy physiological needs will depend on many factors such as the water and electrolyte content of the food eaten, the ambient temperature and humidity and activity level of the animal. The mean total water intake in cynomolgus monkeys has been found to be 76 ± 35 ml/kg/day for males and 100 ± 51 ml/kg/day for females, of which drinking water comprised 50 ± 33 ml/kg /day for males and 49 ± 48 ml/kg/day for females – other water being derived from food (Suzuki *et al.* 1989). Even moderate restriction of water will reduce food consumption.

Identification

All primates should be uniquely identifiable, and this is a legal requirement in some countries (eg, European Commission 2007). In some establishments this is done by a tattoo, and some animals may receive two or more of these if they are marked at both the breeding and the using establishment. A number of other methods can be used (Honess & Macdonald 2003). Animals that are individually recognisable can be given names since this helps to increase recognition of their individuality, facilitate recall of the animal's history, and encourage appropriate attitudes to the animal (Segal 1989; Reinhardt 2003a). Names can be a useful aid in training, particularly when animals are in groups. Variations in fur colour or pattern, ridges, wrinkles, pigmentation, flaps of skin or other physical traits can be permanently recorded by photographs, drawings or written descriptions. The disadvantage of this method is that it can be difficult to identify individuals in large groups and may not comply with regulation of some studies. Coloured collars may be used, but should be monitored regularly to ensure that they do not abrade the skin or become too tight. Non-toxic dyes such as 'permanent' hair dye for human use are a useful minimally invasive method to mark animals for short-term needs but most dyes last less than 1 month and animals will have to be captured for re-application for longer-term marking. Temporary marking can be achieved by clipping patches of fur and this can last up to 4 months before re-clipping is necessary.

Microchips are electronic implants that provide unique permanent identification. However, they give no external indication of the animal's identity and so may be unsuitable for some applications. In the UK and Europe, most microchips and readers comply with ISO (International Standards Organisation) Standards (ie, ISO 11784 and 11785). The USA and Canada have different microchips that necessitate use of different readers. If animals are to be supplied microchipped to a different world region, the appropriate reader should be supplied with the animals and the location of the microchip specified. Tattoos are also permanent, though ink may diffuse over time and become unreadable. Invasive methods of identification (microchipping and tattooing) should always be carried out by competent, trained staff. Ideally, the method used should: not be painful, not cause an adverse reaction, not be uncomfortable and not be likely to cause injury, and must also be appropriate to the study.

Health monitoring and quarantine

When new monkeys are brought into a facility, basic information about them is necessary in order to be able to design the quarantine programme and establish the health-screening programme. The first consideration is the source of the animals. The choice of where they are bought from may be imposed simply by availability, but this will have profound effects on the design of the quarantine and health-screening programmes. It is necessary to establish how the animals were kept at the source establishment, or if they were of wild origin. Details should be obtained of the groups in which they were kept (eg, peer groups or family groups) and how long they had been established. If they were weaned at an early age (less than 12 months) they will be more likely to be stressed and more likely to be carrying subclinical infections, such as shigellosis, which may then become a clinical problem when they arrive. Previous exposure to some infections, such as *Yersinia* from birds or avian mycobacteria, will depend on whether they have been housed with access to the outside, and may interfere with the interpretation of the tuberculin test. Information should be obtained on the standards of care in the source establishment and the background health status of the source colony, taking note of the time period over which this been established.

Lists of pathogens for which the animals have been tested should be examined closely, an unlisted pathogen may mean it is not tested for, rather than that the colony has a negative status. Samples from individual animals may be unhelpful without details of the full colony history. If screening results are available, it is important to determine which tests were carried out, where the laboratory processing was done, the method of quality control and whether or not any independent checks were made.

Once the source of the monkeys has been decided, they then have to be transported. If they are only coming a short distance, the impact of transportation will be much less than if they are coming half way round the world and stopping at airports in various countries where they may potentially encounter pathogens from other animals in airport holding areas. It is important to determine how they are to be transported, what will be the prevailing environmental conditions and how this may result in pathological changes in the animal affecting its health and welfare. Additional factors such as whether the monkeys travel alone, or in pairs or with another from its peer group, or with a stranger, will influence the degree of stress and the likelihood of fight wounds and of transmitting infections. All these parameters will influence the interpretation of signs that may seen in the quarantine period.

During the quarantine period incoming monkeys need to be isolated from existing stock. This could be in a different building or in a separate area within the same building. Staff working practices must be such that they do not risk spreading infection to existing stock (or vice versa). There should be adequate provision of protective clothing and changing areas, and methods to prevent spread of disease by rodents or insects. Access to monkeys in quarantine should be limited. In research establishments, scientists may want to start work on the animal from the moment it arrives. However, it is vital to set aside enough time to allow for observation of these new animals, building up a picture of each one's normal behavioural repertoire, so that changes due to illness or experimental stress may be spotted rapidly. The key here is good-quality staff and good technician training. It has been demonstrated that the behaviour of juvenile long-tailed macaques does not settle to pre-transport levels even 1 month after international transport and relocation to a new unit (Honess *et al.* 2004).

Quarantine can have a considerable impact on animal welfare through the way that animals are housed and handled, particularly if there is separation by single housing and a poor physical environment due to small cage sizes, lack of enrichment, isolation from former social companions, and fear of unfamiliar animals and humans in close proximity. Since some forms of quarantine or conditioning can have serious consequences for animal welfare, it is important for everyone to be clear about what is required and why, in order to avoid unnecessary constraints on the animals' husbandry and care.

The length of the quarantine period also depends on the source. In the UK, under the Rabies (Importation of dogs, cats and other mammals) Order 1974, if the animal comes from overseas it will have to be held under rabies quarantine for 6 months. If there is any risk of filovirus, then an absolute minimum of 31 days quarantine should be applied. If there are doubts about simian herpesvirus (herpesvirus simiae, B virus) and tuberculosis (TB) status then it will take 3 months to establish these. If the source is one for which there is 100% certainty of the health status of the animals then they can be moved sooner, depending on the use to which they will be put. 'Conditioning' is a particular form of quarantine which covers the processes often used in source countries. This may be used to ensure that animals are in good condition and physical health before transport and relocation, or may be to 'prepackage' and stress habituate the animals.

Health-screening programme

It is preferable to prevent diseases than to have to deal with them when they arise. Several infectious diseases of primates are potentially zoonotic so health-screening programmes can not only improve animal health and welfare but will also contribute to the occupational health programme of the institute in which they are kept. The health programme should also take into account any necessity to screen staff to prevent spread of infections from humans to monkeys.

Monkeys can carry a number of potentially serious infectious diseases: some bacterial, ranging from salmonellosis to tuberculosis, and some viral. The UK Advisory Committee on Dangerous Pathogens has made particular recommendations with respect to simian herpesvirus (herpesvirus simiae, B virus) and simian retroviruses (Advisory Committee on Dangerous Pathogens 1998). Cohen *et al.* (2002) give recommendations for prevention of and therapy for exposure to B virus. A health-screening programme should be drawn up for every facility holding primates which should take account of the source of the animals, the use to which they are put (eg, breeding/experimental, long term/short term, immunology/neuroscience), and the resources available for testing.

A health-monitoring programme must define what samples to take (how many and how much) and how the samples will be stored and then processed. All animals that die unexpectedly for whatever reason should be subjected to full *post-mortem* examination including routine monitoring of enteric organisms, even if the cause of unexpected death is obvious, such as traumatic wounding. The cause of death should be established on the basis of facts, not based on circumstantial and anecdotal evidence from care staff. In a research environment there may be plenty of available data from animals at the end of experiments. The opportunity should be taken to use this and carry out a complete routine *post-mortem* examination on as many subjects as possible. Given the problems of false positives (and negatives) with tuberculin testing this may be an additional method for screening for tuberculosis. This opportunity can be taken to check for changing antibiotic resistance of normal gut bacterial flora, particularly if there are antibiotics used routinely post-operatively following experimental surgery.

Random sampling for haematology, clinical biochemistry and faecal bacteriology and parasitology will all yield useful background information about a colony. Ensuring full investigation of any clinical disease may reveal background health problems that might be affecting the health of the colony, such as marginal nutritional deficiencies. There should also be in place an annual screening programme for selected diseases. As an absolute minimum, the screening history for B virus should be available for Old World monkeys and faecal bacteriology/parasitology should be carried out annually. Every such primate over 12 months of age should have the following checked annually:

- clinical assessment (weight, review growth, condition score, alopecia);
- dentistry/oral examination;
- fingers/toes/tail examination;
- thoracic auscultation;
- abdominal palpation;
- assessment of psychological health;
- serum sample to check B virus serology;
- other tests as necessary.

A regular health-screening programme of a colony of animals should be maintained to cover some or all of the following:

- B virus;
- simian immunodeficiency virus (SIV);
- simian T-lymphotrophic virus (STLV-1);
- simian retroviruses;
- foamy virus;
- SV 40;
- hepatitis A;
- filoviruses;
- tuberculosis;
- faecal pathogens:
    - *Campylobacter* spp.;
    - *Salmonella* spp.;
    - *Shigella* spp.;
    - *Yersinia pseudotuberculosis*;
    - *Entamoeba histolytica*;
    - *Trichuris*.

The number of animals to be sampled (the sample size) should be as appropriate for the pathogens under investigation, taking into account that the probability of detecting infection will depend on the infection rate and other factors (ILAR 1976; Weber *et al.* 1999).

The health monitoring report should contain information on:

- species, breed and unit to which the report applies;
- date the colony was established;
- list of organisms monitored;
- date of latest investigation, diagnostic test used and identification of the testing laboratory;
- results of latest investigation, number of positive/negative animals and number tested;
- dates, test method, testing laboratory and results of the two preceding investigations;
- any additional information of other investigations not included in the standard report such as investigations of sick animals.

All animals should undergo a full *post-mortem* examination as soon as possible after death. If they are found out of normal working hours the carcase should be kept in a refrigerator at 4°C, not frozen, so as not to damage tissues that may be required for histological examination, and examined as soon as possible (within a day).

Animals used in experiments should, wherever possible, be from herpes B virus (BV)-free colonies, particularly where animals are handled under conditions of close contact, in long term studies or for neurological surgery, or for work where a latent infection may be reactivated. Examples of such procedures are those involving psychological stress or immunosuppression, the establishment of tissue culture or cell lines, surgery of the brain or oropharyngeal region, the genital region or the neural ganglia related to these areas. A comprehensive programme of testing in the source colony over many years will enable interpretation of the results in individual animals from that source colony with more confidence. Unless full background information is provided, testing of single specimens may not be diagnostic and interpretation of the result is not possible (Kalter *et al.* 1997). The animals should come from regularly monitored BV-negative stocks, from breeding colonies free of BV or by serologically testing each animal. All animals used to start a breeding colony should be screened and all Old World monkeys should be tested annually. All incidents should be taken seriously and guidelines should be in place to deal with potential transmissions of infection.

Use in research

Primates should only be used in research programmes where there is particular need in justified research programmes and where it can be demonstrated that the benefits to society outweigh the harms inflicted on the animals that are used (Wetherall 2006). While this principle applies to the use of all animals used in research, there is a particular societal concern and uncertainty over the acceptability of using primates in research, principally because of their evolutionary proximity to human beings. It is also considered by some that they may have a greater capacity for suffering than other animals because of their more developed cognitive abilities (Summerhoff 1990). It is therefore particularly necessary when considering the use of primates in research to consider the ethical issues as well as the merely practical ones.

The total number of primates used in research worldwide is estimated at between 100 000 and 200 000, with 64.7% involving Old World monkeys (Carlsson *et al.* 2004). Most (up to 70%) are used in regulatory toxicology.

The most common research areas for which primates are used are: infectious diseases (including HIV/AIDS) 26%, neuroscience 19%, biochemistry 12% and pharmacology/physiology 11%, in addition to their use in regulatory toxicology. The use of non-human primates in research in the UK has recently been comprehensively reviewed by Wetherall (2006).

The responses of different species of macaques to environmental stressors varies and this is reflected in their response to minor procedures such as routine capture, when compared with rhesus. Cynomolgus macaques tend to be more stressed (Clarke *et al.* 1988), and the animals' responses to stress can have implications for research (Boccia *et al.* 1995).

Laboratory procedures

Handling, restraint and training

Particular care must be taken when handling primates because of the danger of transmitting potentially zoonotic diseases. Appropriate protective clothing must be worn. For quarantine animals, this should include cap, gown, mask, boots and gloves. For other animals, gloves and protective gowns may be sufficient but there will be local safety rules for each institution which must be followed. These rules will take into account the origin of the animal and the results of health screening.

Many experimental procedures require gaining access to the individual animal but since primates are intelligent they can readily be trained to co-operate, even when they are living in social groups. Training is encouraged by the use of positive reinforcement, which may be in the form of a favourite food or drink which does not form part of their normal diet, so they are not habituated to it. Rhesus monkeys respond very well to being trained to co-operate using voice commands, which will not distort their nutrition.

In order to carry out a full examination of a primate it may be necessary to sedate it in order to reduce the risk of injury to the handler (eg, in experiments involving the use of infectious agents), to reduce the stress to the animal and also to enable the examination to be carried out thoroughly to yield the maximum possible information. A 'restraint' cage may be used for this in which the back is pulled gently forward or the front pushed gently backwards. Most animals find this procedure very stressful and there are better ways to handle most monkeys. The animal may also be netted but this is a significant stress factor and most animals will not respond well to this method of capture. It is much better to spend time training the monkey to present its hindquarters for injection of sedative, which can then be carried out without stress to animal or handler (Wolfensohn & Finnemore 2006). Even if a macaque is sedated it should be held by the upper arms, to keep its face away from the handler. Even better is to train the animal for manual capture and restraint since sedatives themselves are stressors (Honess & Marin 2006a). The most humane method of capture for macaques is to train animals to enter a transport container. Other methods used to catch laboratory primates include net-catching (see Luttrell *et al.* 1994), catching animals in a nest box or transport container, and, for macaques, use of a pole and collar. These methods all have advantages and disadvantages and a useful discussion of the welfare implications of the various techniques is contained in Rennie and Buchanan-Smith (2006). Whatever the method of capture, macaques should be safely restrained and their body weight supported when they are carried.

It is important to recognise that restraint for any purpose and whether for short duration or longer may induce fear and stress responses, such as physical resistance to handling, alarm vocalisations, defensive threatening and aggression, urination and defecation, and that there are also likely to be physiological responses that will increase unwanted data variability (Reinhardt *et al.* 1995; Honess & Marin 2006b). These fear and stress responses should be recognised as indicative of a serious welfare problem that must be properly addressed. It may be that restraint itself can be avoided. Habituation and socialisation, together with training animals to co-operate with procedures using positive reinforcement techniques, can obviate the need for physical or chemical restraint. For example, macaques can quite quickly and easily be trained to present their hindquarters for injection or present a limb for blood sampling, and this avoids the need to catch them or to use a squeeze-back mechanism (Reinhardt *et al.* 1995; Reinhardt 2003b; Sauceda & Schmidt 2000; Wolfensohn and Finnemore 2006).

If restraint is required to control a primate during a scientific procedure, then the method used should provide the least level of restraint for the minimum frequency and duration necessary consistent with achieving the experimental aims. It should protect both primate and personnel from harm and should avoid causing unnecessary distress or discomfort.

Restraint chairs are used to support primates in a sitting position when it is deemed necessary to restrain them for prolonged periods, such as for single cell recording within the CNS or chronic infusion when they may be required to remain in one position for several hours. Chair restraint can affect the animal's physiology (Norman & Smith 1992; Norman *et al.* 1994) and can severely compromise their welfare (Klein & Murray 1995; Morton *et al.* 1987).

All primates can and will, on occasion, bite. They are very quick, surprisingly strong and will snatch and grab at such things as jewellery and loose clothing. Injuries can be prevented by knowledge of the particular species and the individual, including knowledge and interpretation of the posture and expression of the animal. Primates communicate in a variety of ways using sounds, facial expressions and postural changes. Many signals can be easily interpreted. For example, shaking a tree is a sign of aggression which, in a captive environment, translates to rattling the cage. A low-grade threat can be communicated in some primates with a brief 'eyebrow flash' which in humans is an indication of recognition and may form part of ritualised flirting behaviour. Raised eyebrows combined with lip-smacking are used as a social appeasement signal in macaques. Other facial expressions may communicate quite different meaning to non-human primates than to humans. For example, the grimace, or silent bared-teeth face, indicates uncertainty or submission in many primates but, as a smile in humans, can be seen as an expression of friendliness. Another common source of confusion is the human 'stare'. A person may stare at an animal out of interest, but most primates will interpret this as an aggressive threat and respond accordingly. This 'miscommunication' is a common problem when people who have no experience of interacting with primates visit animal units.

One of the most effective ways to minimise stress for primates in the laboratory is to ensure that they are handled in a competent and empathetic way, and that they react well to this, without trying to assert dominance over staff members. The aim should be for the animals to feel unafraid, at ease and comfortable when they are approached, handled, carried and restrained. Major improvements in this respect have been achieved in many laboratories in recent years (JWGR 2009).

All staff–animal interactions should be based on an understanding of species-typical behaviour patterns and communication systems, such that these are interpreted correctly and responded to appropriately. Direct eye contact and potentially threatening body postures should be avoided. Animals should be adequately habituated and socialised to humans early in life, so breeders and users of primates should liaise closely to ensure that good practice in handling and restraint procedures is harmonised between facilities. Good training can enable less invasive restraint procedures to be used. All methods of capture, handling and restraint require experience and skill and should therefore be included as an integral part of staff training programmes. Methods used should safeguard the health and welfare of both animals and staff.

Training animals to co-operate with scientific, veterinary and husbandry procedures helps to reduce the stress that may be caused to both the animal and the laboratory staff (see Chapter 16). However, in order to start a programme of training with laboratory primates it is first necessary to train the people to communicate and interact positively with primates through recognition and interpretation of primate signals, and to help the primates to respond positively to humans through habituation and socialisation. Primates are not domesticated animals and contact with humans can be extremely stressful, especially where the primates are not in control of the level and intensity of that contact, which is a particular problem in the laboratory (SCAHAW 2002). Habituating and socialising captive primates to the presence (sight, sound, smell) and behaviour of humans as early as possible in their lives is essential. If the need to do this is not taken seriously, both animal welfare and the science can be seriously affected.

Early habituation reduces any fear or distress the animals may experience when confronted with new situations as adults. It can also facilitate handling and restraint and training of animals, and may reduce the need for sedation and personal protective equipment when carrying out procedures (Reinhardt *et al.* 1995). It also allows staff to observe behaviour patterns which are relatively unaffected by their own presence, and this helps them to assess the welfare of the animals more effectively.

There should be a formal habituation and socialisation programme, based on the principles of positive reinforcement (Prescott & Buchanan-Smith 2007). In addition, all staff that come into contact with the animals should understand the need to ensure that their own actions make a positive and consistent contribution to the habituation and socialisation programme, and everyone should be trained accordingly.

Training primates has significant benefits for animal welfare, science and staff, especially when combined with appropriate socialisation, habituation and desensitisation. This is additional to the training required for primates to carry out specific tasks in some areas of research. Accordingly, training is recommended as good practice by many legislative and professional guidelines (Home Office 1989; NRC 1998; IPS 2007). Training methods should be based on positive reinforcement techniques, which reward desired behaviour, since this method of training is considered to be the most humane (see Chapter 16; Laule *et al.* 2003; Pryor 2002). Negative reinforcement should only be used when positive alternatives have been exhausted (eg, training for aversive procedures), and it should only be used in combination with positive reinforcement.

Positive reinforcement training is the preferred method of training animals. It refers to any form of training that is based on rewards rather than punishment. The animal is rewarded with some treat, such as a morsel of food, for a job well done. Negative reinforcement is the opposite of positive reinforcement and involves a punishment for less than favourable performances and usually implies some kind of fear, pain or discomfort for the animal being trained. Another way to get an animal to perform a task is to motivate it by withholding food or water and it has to perform the task in order to obtain food or water. As the intake of water is essential for survival, water deprivation is a stronger motivator than food deprivation and will achieve faster results since an animal will become physiologically compromised quicker with water deprivation than with food deprivation. Access to fluid in these conditions cannot be described as 'positive reward'.

Some research protocols require the regulation of the food or fluid intake. This regulation may simply involve strict scheduling of the access to water, or may involve restriction in which the total amount of water is strictly controlled, so that thirst becomes the motivator for performance of certain tasks. With limited access to water, food consumption also decreases and these protocols are often associated with weight loss and associated stress. Pre-screening should be conducted to determine whether the particular animal's temperament is conducive to training and to performing the tasks required. On such protocols the amount of fluid consumed and a hydration assessment should be recorded daily for each animal. Variables that can be used to assess hydration status include the body weight, food intake, skin turgor, urine output, moistness of faeces, general appearance and demeanour. It is important to evaluate the health and welfare of each animal individually (Smith *et al.* 2006). Animals should generally be given free access to water for some period of time on days when there are no experimental sessions (NRC 2003). There is currently much debate over the use of water restriction paradigms and guidelines have been issued by the UK Home Office (2003) and Prescott *et al.* (in prep).

Administration of substances, blood sampling

Some recent reviews have been published which provide detailed advice on refinements for the administration of substances and of sampling (JWGR 1993, 2001, 2009; Diehl *et al.* 2001).

Factors to consider include whether the particular individual or species is the most appropriate for the study or whether it is too easily stressed by handling and requires further time to acclimatise to the procedures. The use of sedatives may or may not reduce stress (Honess & Marin 2006a), but may confound the experiment and not be feasible. If possible, animals should be trained to co-operate with the procedures to avoid the need for physical restraint. Staff should be competent to carry out the procedure and post-administration monitoring.

Telemetry

Telemetry is frequently used in studies involving primates, including those carried out to fulfil the requirements of regulatory bodies. Telemetry is widely viewed as benefiting science and animal welfare because it can reduce stress caused to animals (eg, by restraint), enable reductions in animal numbers and provide indicators of animal well-being to help implement humane endpoints. However, telemetry can require invasive procedures such as implantation surgery, single housing and use of jackets, which can cause pain and distress. Although telemetry is often described as a refinement, this will not be the case unless the technique itself has been fully refined.

Detailed advice on refinements in telemetry can be found in JWGR (2003 and 2004), including maintaining stable group housing, and behavioural pre-screening to ensure that individuals are suitable for projects and are not implanted unnecessarily. In particular, the reports explain how to pair- or group-house animals implanted with devices that transmit at the same frequency, eg, by housing an implanted animal with a naïve 'buddy' or using devices that can be turned on and off one at a time or by using developing devices which transmit at different frequencies.

Anaesthesia, analgesia and post-operative care

A selection of drugs that may be used to sedate primates to facilitate handling are listed here. Veterinary advice should be sought on the use of these but some further information is provided by Foster *et al.* (1996); Sun *et al.* (2003) and Flecknell (2009). In the UK, all these drugs are prescription-only medicines and therefore must only be used under veterinary direction.

- Ketamine (5–25 mg/kg im) is the drug of choice to produce tranquillisation to facilitate handling. Peak effect is reached in 5–10 minutes and lasts 30–60 minutes.
- Medetomidine can be used to produce moderate sedation which can be reversed with atipamezole. Use medetomidine at 50–100 µg/kg im; reverse with atipamezole at 250–500 µg/kg im.
- Ketamine can be used in combination with medetomidine to produce anaesthesia.
- Acepromazine (0.2 mg/kg im) produces sedation but this is insufficient for safe handling.
- Diazepam (1 mg/kg im) also produces insufficient sedation for handling of larger primates, but may be used in combination with ketamine.

Once the animal can be handled, anaesthesia for surgical interventions should be of the highest standard. Induction (and maintenance) of anaesthesia can be by intravenous infusion of propofol. Barbiturates are associated with respiratory depression and resultant hypercapnia. Initial trials with Alfaxan indicate that it may be suitable for use in primates, but further work is necessary to substantiate this. Primates should be intubated, having first sprayed the larynx with local anaesthetic to prevent the occurrence of larygospasm. Prior to intubation, administration of oxygen by face mask is advisable. Maintenance of anaesthesia using isoflurane or sevoflurane is most satisfactory and gives a good quality of recovery.

During anaesthesia, it is vital to monitor the vital signs including, temperature, blood pressure, oxygen and carbon dioxide levels and to maintain physiological stability with administration of fluids. This will assist the quality of the animal's recovery. Post-operatively, analgesia can be provided with opioids or non-steroidal anti inflammatory drugs. Post-operative gastritis and vomiting can be controlled using metoclopramide. Selection of the appropriate regime will also depend on the area of scientific investigation as some anaesthetics may affect the area under study (Culley *et al.* 2007).

Husbandry following surgery

Primates have traditionally been housed singly after surgery because it has been thought that otherwise animals will interfere with the other's sutures or equipment, such as cranial implants, or that animals which are slower to recover than others could be at risk of bullying or aggression. Clearly, animals need to be allowed to recover separately in the immediate post-operative period. However, it has been successfully demonstrated that surgically treated animals can be pair- or group-housed soon after recovery (Wolfensohn & Peters 2005).

Interrupted subcuticular sutures, with the possible additional use of tissue adhesives, should be sufficient to maintain the integrity of a surgical wound such that removal of sutures by the individual or cage mates is not a problem. Adequate perioperative analgesia will prevent animals from paying untoward attention to their own wound sites and attracting the attention of others. It has also been shown that primates with surgical implants, for example cranial implants, can successfully be kept in social groups (Wolfensohn & Peters 2005). For work on extremities and limbs primates will tolerate bandaging to provide protection and support of the affected area provided the dressing is carefully applied.

When planning housing for the recovery period, it should be remembered that primates may climb before they are fully recovered from anaesthesia, and may fall and injure themselves. A purpose-built recovery enclosure may be used, or a temporary reduction in the height of the home area may be implemented. If a recovery enclosure is used, it should be constructed so that the primate does not have to be physically caught in order to be returned to the home cage, or animals should be trained to enter and leave a transport cage. Animals should be allowed to recover in proximity to others from their social group, not in social isolation. If surgery involves producing neurological lesions, the home area may need to be adapted to take account of any possible long-term side effects. If single housing following surgery can be justified, individual animals should have visual, auditory and, if possible, tactile contact with other primates.

Welfare

Assessment of welfare

Primates are highly intelligent, sentient and social animals with a complex range of physical as well as psychological needs. There is no doubt that they experience pain and that they experience a range of negative psychological states, such as anxiety, apprehension, fear, frustration and boredom, as well as a range of positive states (JWGR 2009). It should be assumed that procedures that cause pain and distress in humans will probably cause pain or distress in other primates (Organisation for Economic Co-operation and Development (OECD) 2001; Soulsby & Morton 2001). A monkey in pain may show a generally miserable appearance, and may adopt a huddled position or crouch with head forwards and arms across the body. It will tend to refuse food and drink and to avoid companions, although monkeys that are unwell may attract extra attention from cage mates, varying from social grooming to attack. Vocalisation is more likely to indicate anger than pain.

Good animal welfare may be defined according to the five freedoms:

1. Freedom from hunger and thirst.
2. Freedom from discomfort.
3. Freedom from pain, injury and disease.
4. Freedom to express normal behaviours.
5. Freedom from fear and distress.

Research using primates has the ability to impact on these five freedoms in some of the following ways, depending on the types of procedure being used:

- Freedom 1: use of food/fluid regulation paradigms.
- Freedom 2: keeping animals in metal cages on grid floors.

- Freedom 3: carrying out surgery, placement of implants with subsequent chronic infections.
- Freedom 4: use of single housing and restricted availability of space.
- Freedom 5: use of handling methods and procedural techniques which do not use reinforcement training but use aversive methods such as squeeze cages.

The welfare of primates will be maximised by keeping the animals in good health. This applies not just to their physical health but also to their psychological health. It has been demonstrated that cynomolgus macaques have the capacity for depression and that there is a relationship between social status and mood-related behaviours in this species (Shively 2006). The health should be evaluated regularly and records kept and a programme to review and improve physical and mental health applied where necessary. Quantitative assessment of the animal's well-being can be usefully recorded with a clinical score sheet. The animal should be reassessed at appropriate intervals in order to monitor its progress and check on the responses to any treatment given or changes in management. Good clinical score sheets remove the variation in interpretation of clinical signs which is frequently found between animal care staff and research staff; and the criteria for intervention are clearly defined before the animal's condition deteriorates (Wolfensohn & Lloyd 2003). The recognition of animals suffering pain or psychological distress is important, as it is the first step to avoiding or alleviating such conditions.

There are several parameters that can be used to assess welfare, which may be behavioural, physiological or biochemical (Table 39.3). The most readily accessible and commonly used index for assessing well-being in primates is behaviour.

Table 39.3 Parameters used to assess welfare.

Behavioural parameters	*Physiological parameters*	*Biochemical parameters*
Time budgets	Body weight	Corticosteroids
Play	Condition scoring*	Reproductive hormones
Allogrooming	Alopecia scoring***	Leucocyte activity**
Locomotion	Heart rate	
Posture	Blood pressure	
Social interactions	Body temperature	
Sleep		
Self-scratching		
Stereotypical behaviours		

*Wolfensohn & Honess (2005);
**Honess *et al.* (2005a);
***Honess *et al.* (2005b).
For general information see Novak and Suomi 1988, Boccia *et al.* (1995), Mendoza *et al.* (2000), Honess and Marin (2006a).

Clinical scoring systems are usually used for monitoring of single incidents but there should also be some assessment of the cumulative suffering and the lifetime experience of the animal. This will include direct suffering from the procedure as well as contingent suffering (Russell & Burch 1959) as a result of transport, housing, the environment and injuries from caging or conspecifics, to name just a few examples. The lifespan of primates, compared with other laboratory animal species, is relatively long. They are valuable animals, have long breeding lives and are likely to be used in long-term experiments. Some primates may therefore be housed in the laboratory for many years. In such circumstances, there are particular welfare issues that must be addressed (JWGR 2003, 2004). A welfare assessment matrix can be used to give a pictorial view of welfare and is based on Wolfensohn and Honess (2007). The matrix consist of axes relating to the following basic parameters:

- clinical condition (physical well-being);
- behavioural deviations (psychological well-being);
- the time frame of incident (duration);
- harm: benefit (justification).

This produces a basic four-axes matrix to which additional axes may be added (Wolfensohn & Honess submitted). The use of this type of matrix allows comparison of one animal at different time points or allows comparison between groups of animals. It also allows estimation of cumulative suffering and, by giving a pictorial representation, may be very useful for ethical review committees, particularly where there is lay representation.

Behavioural monitoring

When assessing welfare using behavioural parameters it is important to assess the animals at various times. The animal's behaviour should be noted on the approach of the observer. Observations should then be repeated after the animal has had time to habituate to the presence of the observer. The use of space and structures, any self-maintenance behaviour, social behaviour, as well as the animal's disposition and interaction with observers are all recorded. An example of a behavioural assessment table is shown in Table 39.4, which demonstrates a difference in the behavioural repertoire between the two groups, the cause of which can then be investigated.

An awareness of the normal behavioural repertoire for the species is important to enable provision of appropriate care and management and for assessing their physical and psychological well-being. Knowledge of the behaviour of individual animals is also essential since primates show a high degree of individuality. Any deviations from normal must also be recognised to enable evaluation of refinements such as changes in cage design or environmental enrichment.

The advice of a primate behaviour specialist is invaluable in training both care staff and research staff to recognise and interpret deviations from normal behaviour and to assist in developing programmes to ensure good psychological health.

Table 39.4 Example of behavioural assessment table.

Parameter	Group A	Group B
Confidence in approaching observer	Confident	Huddled at back of cage
Use of all levels of enclosure	Used all	Remained at highest level
Use of foraging	Used	Did not use
Use of environmental enrichment	Used them	Occasionally biting at objects
Manipulation of objects	Yes	No manipulation
Social interaction	Normal auto- and allogrooming	Hugging, no grooming
Dominance behaviour	No aggression	Aggression and chasing
Alopecia score	9 animals, total score 11	13 animals, total score 35

Physical health

The first step in assessment of the monkey's physical health is to observe the animal in its home cage and evaluate its appearance, behaviour and general demeanour. In order to do this it is vital that the observer has some experience of the animal (both the species and the individual) in order to be able to judge whether the animal is exhibiting a normal behavioural repertoire. Just like humans some individual non-human primates exhibit behavioural patterns that are specific for that individual, but do not necessarily reflect poor well-being. Only after completing the examination from a distance and noting the behavioural responses, should the animal be caught in order to look at it more closely. Catching it will markedly affect its behaviour, whether or not sedatives are used, which it why it is important to make a full evaluation, before disturbing it other than by one's presence. For a full description of clinical assessment of a monkey see Wolfensohn and Honess (2005) and Smith *et al.* (2006).

The animal's weight should be recorded and its body condition noted as in Figures 39.2 and 39.3. This may be scored in a similar way to condition scoring of sheep (Ministry of Agriculture, Fisheries & Food 1994). It is assessed by palpating the monkey over its thoracic and lumbar vertebrae (at the level of the last rib) and making a judgment as to the amount of fat and muscle covering the bony prominences of the vertebrae and giving a quantitative score. Condition scoring at weaning and during the post-weaning period, combined with regular weight measurements, is important to ensure that the animal is receiving adequate nutrition and growing properly.

Diseases

The potential of primates to carry serious zoonotic diseases should not be underestimated (Advisory Committee on Dangerous Pathogens 1998). Captive-bred animals of known health status are less of a risk, and these should now comprise the majority of animals used. Monkeys are susceptible to many diseases carried by humans, such as colds and flu, tuberculosis, measles and many others. Therefore it is important to exclude casual visitors or at least wear a suitable face mask to reduce the risk of spreading such infections to the monkeys if appropriate occupational health surveillance has not been established. It is important to wear appropriate protective clothing and use good hygiene, to protect us from them, and them from us. Power hoses promote the formation of aerosols, which may allow transmission of zoonotic diseases, so suitable protective clothing must be worn when operating these.

There are many diseases which should be included in a regular screening programme as discussed above. Full details on the diseases of primates and their management can be found in Bennett *et al.* (1998) and Wolfe-Coote (2005); only a brief resumé is presented here.

Tuberculosis causes a chronic fatal disease in monkeys, and can pass from monkey to man and vice versa. It can be screened for using an intradermal skin test, commonly in the skin of the eyelid. Alternatively there are enzyme-linked immunosorbent assay (ELISA) tests available to detect antibody (Brusasca *et al.* 2003; Kanaujia *et al.* 2003). The disease in monkeys can remain subclinical for 6 months or more, and indeed may be latent until the animal is terminally ill. To prevent the disease from entering the colony, all new animals should come with a health profile which indicates they have been screened prior to arrival. Personnel intending to work with monkeys should be vaccinated or screened regularly for the disease. Any animal which has contacted a known human case should be effectively quarantined for at least 6 months until it is proved not to have contracted the disease. The important points about tuberculosis in primates are:

- skin tests are not 100% reliable;
- infectivity precedes radiographic or clinical signs or positive tuberculin test;
- radiographic signs precede clinical signs;
- coughing is the most common clinical sign;
- no single test is reliable – use combinations;
- take sequential chest X-rays of coughing monkeys;
- routine *post-mortem* examinations will add to the available screening data.

Enteric disease may be caused by a number of factors including pathogenic organisms. Monkeys will pass loose stools if they are frightened, or if there are changes in their environment or diet. Stress, such after weaning, transportation, surgery or due to changes in social hierarchy, can also cause sub-clinical infections to become clinical, so any case of diarrhoea should be investigated to eliminate infectious causes. Zoonoses such as *Shigella*, *Salmonella*, *Campylobacter* and *Yersinia* are common bacterial pathogens, and protozoa such as *Entamoeba* or helminth parasites may also pose a risk. Some of these organisms can cause explosive outbreaks of disease and death if not controlled immediately. Regular screening and treatment will reduce the level of infection, and must be combined with strict hygiene and good husbandry to prevent transmission between animals and to personnel. Husbandry and environmental factors may also

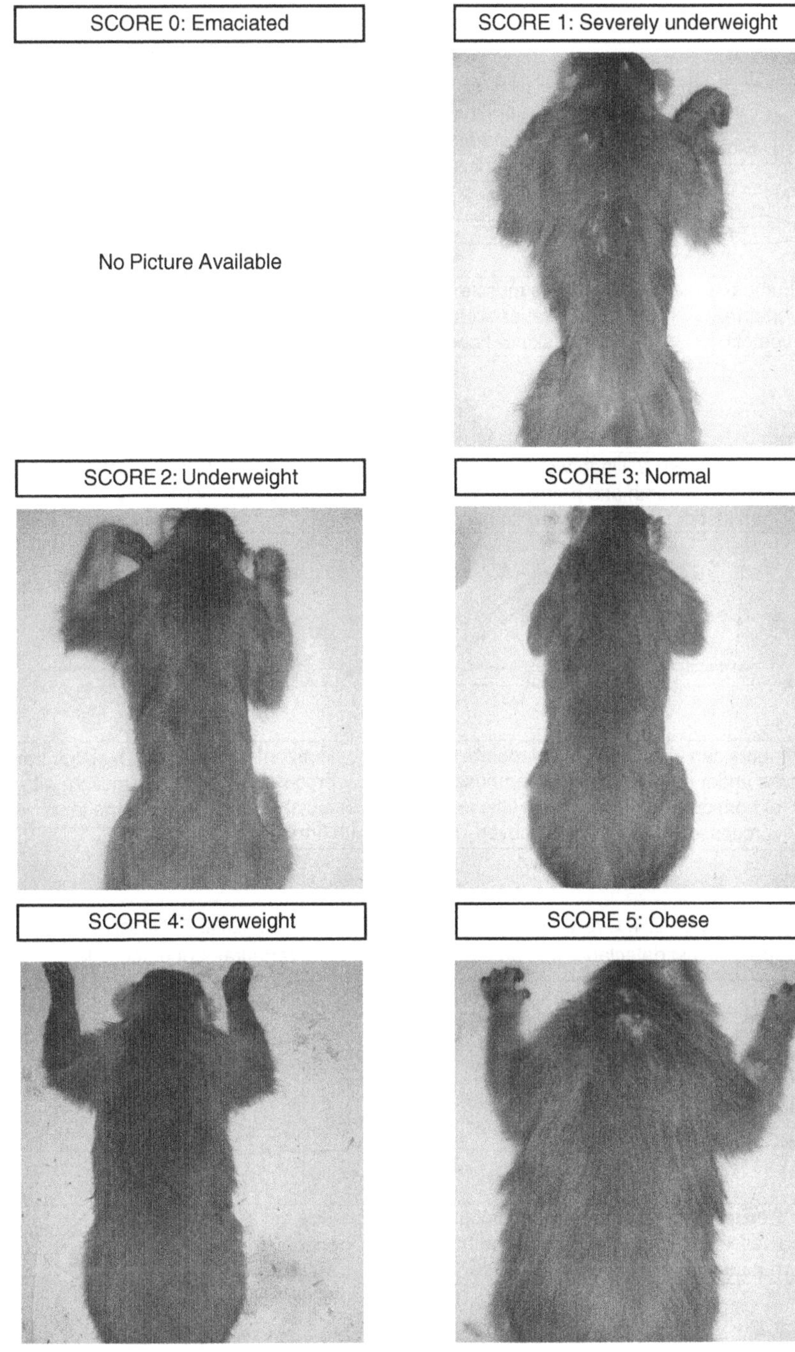

Figure 39.2 Condition scoring: whole primates.

contribute to the development of enteric disease, as will the presence of parasites or viruses such as rotavirus, retroviruses and haemorrhagic viruses. Therefore, prompt and accurate diagnosis of the aetiology of the enteritis is important so that a specific therapy can be instituted.

Eradication will depend on a prolonged programme to break the cycles of infection and transmission by improving hygiene and detecting and treating carriers (Wolfensohn 1998). In some units, the presence of *Shigella* is accepted, since with good husbandry, control is possible even with healthy carriers in the colony, provided the animals are not subjected to undue levels of stress, which may precipitate clinical disease. However, given the zoonotic potential, consideration must be given to the assessment of risk to staff and, since the secondary complications possible from the type of pathology induced by shigellosis could be numerous and serious, it is important to keep animals free from disease wherever possible.

Post-weaning chronic diarrhoea is significantly associated with body weight at weaning rather than age (Munoz-Zanzi *et al.* 1999). An episode of pre-weaning diarrhoea is a good predictor for the occurrence of post-weaning diarrhoea, possibly since this may alter the function of intestinal mucosa and thus reduce the absorption of nutrients. This leads to reduced growth, smaller weight, impaired immune function and consequently post-weaning diarrhoea.

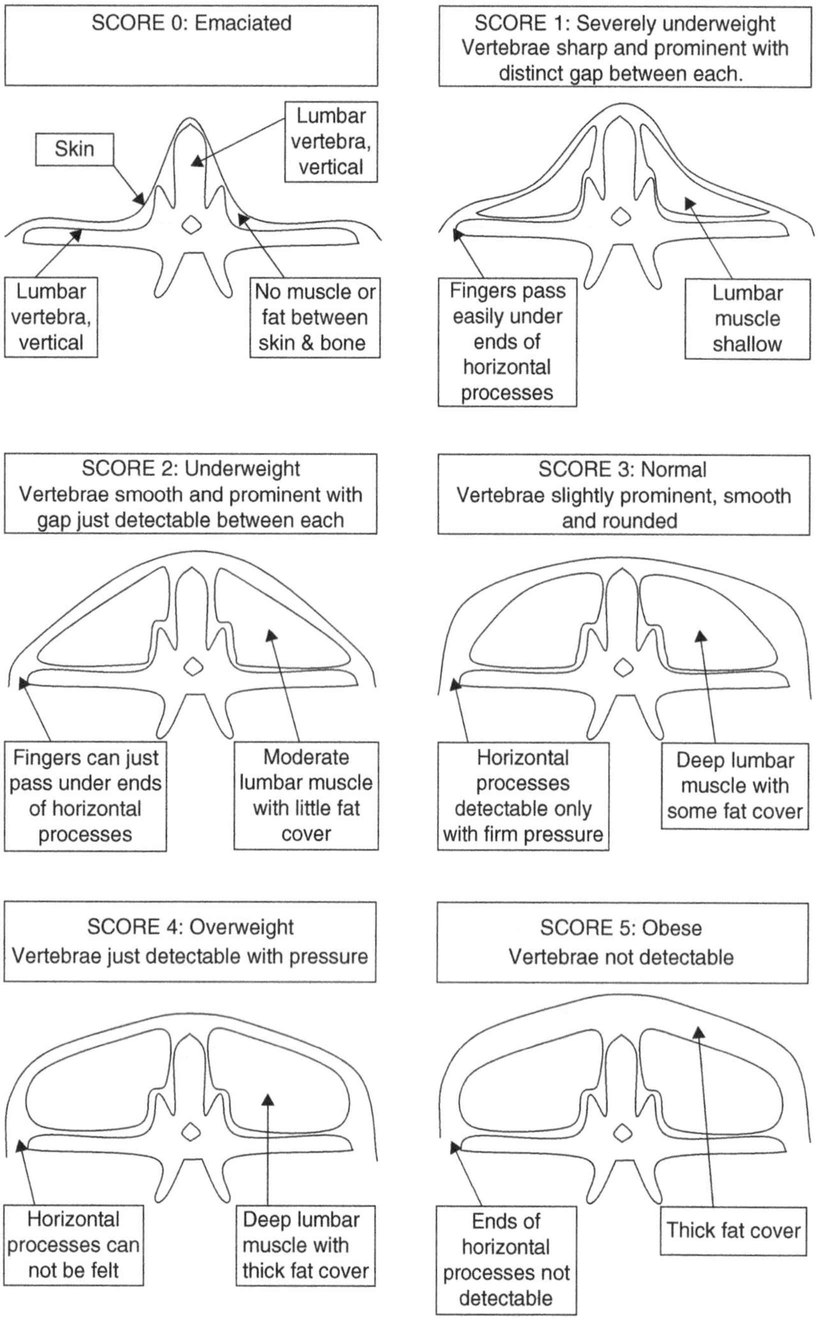

SCORE 0: Emaciated

Skin

Lumbar vertebra, vertical

Lumbar vertebra, vertical

No muscle or fat between skin & bone

SCORE 1: Severely underweight
Vertebrae sharp and prominent with distinct gap between each.

Fingers pass easily under ends of horizontal processes

Lumbar muscle shallow

SCORE 2: Underweight
Vertebrae smooth and prominent with gap just detectable between each

Fingers can just pass under ends of horizontal processes

Moderate lumbar muscle with little fat cover

SCORE 3: Normal
Vertebrae slightly prominent, smooth and rounded

Horizontal processes detectable only with firm pressure

Deep lumbar muscle with some fat cover

SCORE 4: Overweight
Vertebrae just detectable with pressure

Horizontal processes can not be felt

Deep lumbar muscle with thick fat cover

SCORE 5: Obese
Vertebrae not detectable

Ends of horizontal processes not detectable

Thick fat cover

Figure 39.3 Condition scoring: vertebrae.

There are many enteric parasitic infections of primates, many are non-pathogenic, some are zoonotic, a few require diagnosis and treatment. Full details may be found in Owen (1992). The important ones to consider are the protozoans, *Giardia* spp., *Trichomonas* spp., *Entamoeba histolytica*, *Cryptosporidium* spp., *Balantidium* spp., and the metazoans, *Strongyloides* spp. and *Trichuris* spp. The protozoa may be treated with agents such as metronidazole and the metazoans with ivermectin.

For further information on screening of primate colonies see Weber *et al.* (1999).

Husbandry-related diseases

A management strategy for dealing with such problems as fight injuries or nutritional imbalances which may be encountered with increasing use of foraging and group housing should be developed and built into any primate health-management programme. The benefit of social housing is that the environment is dynamic, unpredictable and variable so there is little habituation, but there are increased risks of infection, wounding and competition for food. With good management strategies, such as appropriate housing, these risks can be minimised but not altogether removed.

Clinical problems may be brought about by the increasing provision of forage mix in addition to normal pelleted diet. Although the forage mixes are all well balanced nutritionally, this assumes that the monkey will not pick out its favourite bits and leave the rest. By introducing an element of choice the diet may become unbalanced and problems, such as rickets in juvenile animals, may arise from this.

Age-related disorders

These are frequently linked to nutrition; dietary restriction (but without essential nutrient deficiencies) will increase survival and delay the onset of degenerative aging conditions. A persistently positive energy balance will lead to accumulations of adipose tissue with increasing body weight and obesity.

$$\text{Obesity index for rhesus} = \frac{\text{Weight (kg)}}{(\text{Crown–rump length (cm)})^2}$$

(Jen *et al.* 1985)

Social rank may be associated with obesity (Kemnitz 1984) since the dominant animal determines feeding time and the subordinates eat afterwards, depending on spatial distribution of food and the mix of food types. Chronic dietary restriction also protects against the development of diabetes in aging rhesus monkeys since, although it is not the sole causal agent, obesity is necessary for diabetes to develop.

Euthanasia

The principles of euthanasia are set out in Chapter 17 and in Close *et al.* (1996, 1997) and American Veterinary Medical Association (AVMA) (2001); all of which refer to the animal welfare concerns with respect to carrying out of euthanasia. Having to kill a primate may be a more emotionally challenging experience for staff than having to kill some other species. Staff who carry out this procedure must not only competent in the appropriate methods, but it is essential that they receive good training, adequate supervision and any necessary empathetic support.

Appropriate methods of euthanasia should be selected after discussion with veterinary staff and with due regard for the collection of scientific data. The most common methods for killing primates is an overdose of an anaesthetic, such as sodium pentobarbital (at 100 mg/kg) administered intravenously. For larger primates it will be necessary to sedate the individual before attempting an intravenous injection.

When primates are euthanased, every effort should be made to make full use of their tissues and blood, particularly if this will minimise the number of animals having to be used. This requires good mechanisms for communication to match supply and demand both within and between establishments. Establishing tissue banks and data exchange networks is one means of coordinating, optimising, reducing and refining primate use. In the USA Primate Info Net[2] achieves this objective and in Europe, EUPRIM-NET offers a tissue/gene bank[3].

Record keeping

A file or 'passport' giving full details on each individual primate should be maintained (JWGR 2009). It should keep the details of their biography, enabling a full picture of previous experiences to be established. For example, it should include details of transport history, social grouping from birth through weaning to set up of experimental or breeding group, training records, husbandry system and type of environmental enrichment. This is in addition to reproductive history and full details of medical conditions (physical health and psychological health assessment details and screening records) and, of course, full details of any use in a research project.

The file should be sent with the animal if it is moved between institutions, together with general information on the establishment of origin, such as details of animal care and routine procedures, in order to assist in continuity of care and to ensure successful acclimatisation to the new facility.

Future developments

It is very important to maintain current knowledge of technical developments that could benefit animal welfare. While a good deal is known about the needs of non-human primates in captivity, there are several aspects where more scientifically validated information would be welcome to supplement the experience on which the present recommendations are largely based.

Little is known of the effects of transportation on primates (Wolfensohn 1997). While it may seem ideal for primates to be bred in Europe, breeding in source countries may have some advantages for the animals in terms of climate. These advantages, however, need to be balanced against any stress the animals may be subjected to as a result of the additional transportation. The increases in cage sizes and use of enclosures and social housing that are now recommended produce more efficient use of space and cost savings over single housing of individuals, thus promoting the keeping of animals in groups. However, this leads to a necessity for more research to develop improved techniques for handling and training primates to facilitate their research use in this type of housing. This will encourage the development of humane techniques to facilitate the movement of primates from one cage to another or to a particular area of the home cage.

The use of sound through music or television as environmental enrichment is anecdotally reported to be beneficial, but this may be of more direct benefit to staff. While good well-being of staff may improve the well-being of the animals under their care, the provision of such aural enrichment requires evaluation, as does the use of water as enrichment in water features and provision of bathing. The provision of drinking water from bottles or automatic drinkers or from the water enrichment is another variable that requires assessment.

The validation of different methods of monitoring and quantifying stress and development of new parameters that are simple to measure would greatly benefit the debate on primate welfare and the impact of housing, husbandry and use in scientific procedures. Further work of this nature needs to be conducted on a routine basis as part of the continuing assessment of the welfare of primates held in captivity. It could also enable the identification of specific

[2]http://pin.primate.wisc.edu/

[3]http://www.euprim-net.eu/

behaviours, in which changes might provide an early indication of compromised animal welfare. Such tools would allow planning for the alleviation of any stress caused to the animal. For efficient, rigorous and objective studies of this nature it is important that a professional primatologist is involved in the planning. Perhaps with the increasing requirement that primate facilities include a primatologist on their staff, the objective study of the welfare of captive primates will become more commonplace and incorporated into research funding.

References

Advisory Committee on Dangerous Pathogens (1998) *Working Safely with Simians: Management of Infection Risks*. Specialist supplement to Health and Safety Commission's Advisory Committee on Dangerous Pathogens *Working safely with research animals: management of infection risks*. HSE Books, London

Altmann, J. (1980) *Baboon Mothers and Infants*. University of Chicago Press, Chicago

American Veterinary Medical Association (2001) AVMA 2000 Report of the AMVA panel on euthanasia. *Journal of the American Veterinary Medical Association*, **218**, 669–696

Bennett, B.T., Abee, C.R. and Hendrickson, R. (1995) *Nonhuman Primates in Biomedical Research: Biology and Management*. American College of Laboratory Animal Medicine Series. Academic Press, San Diego

Bennett, B.T., Abee, C.R. and Hendrickson, R. (1998) *Nonhuman Primates in Biomedical Research: Diseases*. Academic Press, San Diego

Boccia, M.L., Laudenslager, M.L. and Reite, M.L. (1995) Individual differences in macaques' responses to stressor levels based on social and physiological factors: Implications for primate welfare research outcomes. *Laboratory Animals*, **29**, 250–257

Brown, J.L. and Eklund, A. (1994) Kin recognition and the major histocompatability complex: an integrative review. *American Naturalist*, **143**, 435–461

Brusasca, P.N., Peters, R.L., Motzel, S.L. *et al.* (2003) Antigen recognition by serum antibodies in non human primates experimentally infected with Mycobacterium tuberculosis. *Comparative Medicine*, **53**, 165–172

Canfield, D., Brignolo, L., Peterson, P.E. *et al.* (2000) Conjoined twins in a rhesus monkey (*Macaca mulatta*). *Journal of Medical Primatology*, **29**, 427–430

Carlsson, H.E., Schapiro, S.J., Farah, I. *et al.* (2004) Use of primates in research: a global overview. *American Journal of Primatology*, **63**, 225–237

Carter, S.P. and Bright, P.W. (2002) Habitat refuges as alternatives to predator control for conservation of endangered Mauritian birds. In: *Turning the Tide: The Eradication of Invasive Species*. Eds Veitch, C.R. and Clout, M.N., pp. 71–78. IUCN SSC Invasive Species Specialist Group. IUCN, Gland, Switzerland and Cambridge, UK

Clarke, A.S., Mason, W.A. and Moberg, G.P. (1988) Differential behavioural and adrenocortical responses to stress among three macaque species. *American Journal of Primatology*, **14**, 37–52

Close, B., Banister, K., Baumans, V. *et al.* (1996) Recommendations for euthanasia of experimental animals Part 1 Report of a Working Party. *Laboratory Animals*, **30**, 293–316

Close, B., Banister, K., Baumans, V. *et al.* (1997) Recommendations for euthanasia of experimental animals Part 2 Report of a Working Party. *Laboratory Animals*, **31**, 1–32

Cohen, J.I., Davenport, D.S., Stewart, J.A. *et al.* (2002) Recommendations for prevention of and therapy for exposure to B virus *(Cercopethicine Herpesvirus 1). Clinical Infectious Disease*, **35**, 1191–1203

Cowlishaw, G. and Dunbar, R.I.M. (2000) *Primate Conservation Biology*. Chicago University Press, Chicago

Crockett, C.M., Bowers, C.L., Shimoji, M. *et al.* (1995) Behavioural responses of long tailed macaques to different cage size and common laboratory experiences. *Journal of Comparative Psychology*, **109**, 368–383

Crockett, C.M., Shimoji, M. and Bowden, D.M. (2000) Behaviour, appetite and urinary cortisol responses by adult pigtailed macaques to cage size, cage level, room change and ketamine sedation. *American Journal of Primatology*, **52**, 63–80

Culley, D.J., Raghavan, S.V., Waly, M. *et al.* (2007) Nitrous oxide decreases cortical methionine synthase transiently but produces lasting memory impairment in aged rats. *Anesthesia and Analgesia*, **105**, 83–88

Dean, S.W. (1999) Environmental enrichment of laboratory animals used in regulatory toxicology studies. *Laboratory Animals*, **33**, 309–327

Dede, J.A. and Plentl, A.A. (1966) Induced ovulation and artificial insemination in a rhesus colony. *Fertility and Sterility*, **17**, 757–764

Diehl, K-H., Hull, R., Morton, D.B. *et al.* (2001) A good practice guide to the administration of substances and removal of blood, including routes and volumes. *Journal of Applied Toxicology*, **21**, 15–23

Dixson, A.F. (1998) *Primate Sexuality: Comparative Studies of the Prosimians, Monkeys, Apes and Human Beings*. Oxford University Press, Oxford

European Commission (2007) Commission recommendations of 18 June 2007 on guidelines for the accommodation and care of animals used for experimental and other scientific purposes. Annex II to European Council Directive 86/609 See 2007/526/EC. http://eurlex.europa.eu/LexUriServ/site/en/oj/2007/l_197/l_19720070730en00010089.pdf (accessed 13 May 2008)

European Council (1986) COUNCIL DIRECTIVE of 24 November 1986 on the approximation of laws, regulations and administrative provisions of the Member States regarding the protection of animals used for experimental and other scientific purposes (86/609/EEC). http://ec.europa.eu/food/fs/aw/aw_legislation/scientific/86-609-eec_en.pdf (accessed 16 May 2008)

Fa, J.E. and Lindburg, D.G. (1996) *Evolution and Ecology of Macaque Societies*. Cambridge University Press, Cambridge

Fleagle, J.G. (1999) *Primate Adaptation and Evolution*, 2nd edn. Academic Press, San Diego

Flecknell, P.A. (2009) *Laboratory Animal Anaesthesia*, 3rd edn. Academic Press, London

Fortman J.D., Hewett, T.A. and Bennett B.T. (2002) *The Laboratory Non-Human Primate*. CRC Press, Boca Raton

Foster, A., Zeller, W. and Pfannkuche, H-J. (1996) Effect of thiopental, saffan and propofol anaesthesia on cardiovascular parameters and bronchial smooth muscle in the rhesus monkey. *Laboratory Animal Science*, **46**, 327–334

Fraser, H.M. and Lunn, S.F. (1999) Nonhuman primates and female reproductive medicine. In: *Reproduction in Nonhuman Primates: A Model System for Human Reproductive Physiology and Toxicology*. Eds Weinbauer, G.F. and Korte, R., pp. 27–59. Waxmann Münster, New York

Goldfoot, D.A. (1977) Rearing conditions which support or inhibit later sexual potential of laboratory-born rhesus monkeys: hypotheses and diagnostic behaviours. *Laboratory Animal Science*, **27**, 548–556

Gomes, D.F. and Bicca-Marques, J.C. (2003) An inversion in the timing of reproduction of captive *Macaca mulatta* in the southern hemisphere. *Laboratory Primate Newsletter*, **42**, 6

Goo, G.P. and Fugate, J.K. (1984) Effects of weaning age on maternal reproduction and offspring health in rhesus monkeys (*Macaca mulatta*). *Laboratory Animal Science*, **34**, 66–69

Gould, K.G. and Martin, D.E. (1986) Artificial insemination in nonhuman primates. In: *Primates: The Road to Self-sustaining Populations*. Ed. Benirschke, K., pp. 425–443. Springer-Verlag, New York

Goy, R.W., Wallen, K. and Goldfoot, D.A. (1974) Social factors affecting the development of mounting behaviour in male rhesus monkeys. In: *Reproductive Behaviour*. Eds Montagna, W. and Sadler, W.A., pp. 223–247. Plenum Publishing, New York

Groves, C. (2001) *Primate Taxonomy*. Smithsonian Series in Comparative Evolutionary Biology, Smithsonian Books. Smithsonian Institution Press, Washington

Harcourt, A.H. (1987) Dominance and fertility among female primates. *Journal of Zoology, London*, **213**, 471–487

Harlow, H.F., Dodsworth, R.O. and Harlow, M.K. (1965) Total social isolation in monkeys. *Proceedings of the National Academy of Sciences*, **54**, 90–97

Hendrickx, A.G. and Dukelow, W.R. (1995a) Reproductive biology. In: *Nonhuman Primates in Biomedical Research: Biology and Management*. Eds Bennett, T.B., Abee, C.R. and Hendrickson, R., pp. 365–374. American College of Laboratory Animal Medicine Series. Academic Press, San Diego

Hendrickx, A.G. and Dukelow, W.R. (1995b) Breeding. In: *Nonhuman Primates in Biomedical Research: Biology and Management*. Eds Bennett, T.B., Abee, C.R. and Hendrickson, R., pp. 147–191. American College of Laboratory Animal Medicine Series. Academic Press, San Diego

Hendrickx, A.G., Peterson, P.E., Otianga-Owiti, G.E. *et al.* (1999) Endocrine and morphological biomarkers of early pregnancy loss in macaques. In: *Reproduction in Nonhuman Primates: A Model System for Human Reproductive Physiology and Toxicology*. Eds Weinbauer, G.F. and Korte, R., pp. 111–135. Waxmann Münster, New York

Home Office (1989) *Code of Practice for the Housing and Care of Animals in Designated Scientific Procedure Establishments*. HMSO, London

Home Office (1995) *Code of Practice for the Housing and Care of Animals in Designated Breeding and Supplying Establishments*. HMSO, London

Home Office (2003) *Guidance Note. Water and food restriction for scientific purposes*. http://scienceandresearch.homeoffice.gov.uk/animal-research/publications-and-reference/publications/code-of-practice/housing-of-animals-breeding/waterfoodguidance.pdf?view=Binary (accessed 10 November 2009)

Honess, P.E., Gimpel, J.L., Wolfensohn, S.E. *et al.* (2005b) Alopecia scoring: the quantitative assessment of hair loss in captive macaques. *Alternatives to Laboratory Animals*, **33**, 193–206

Honess P., Johnson P. and Wolfensohn S. (2004) A study of behavioural responses of non-human primates to air transport and re-housing. *Laboratory Animals*, **38**, 119–132

Honess P.E. and Macdonald, D.W. (2003) Marking and radio tracking primates. In: *Field and Laboratory Methods in Primatology: a Practical Guide*. Eds Curtis, D. and Setchell, J., pp. 158–173. Cambridge University Press, Cambridge

Honess, P.E. and Marin, C. (2006a) Behavioural and physiological aspects of stress and aggression in nonhuman primates. *Neuroscience and Biobehavioural Reviews*, **30**, 390–412

Honess, P.E. and Marin, C. (2006b) Enrichment and aggression in primates: a review. *Neuroscience and Biobehavioural Reviews*, **30**, 413–436

Honess, P.E., Marin, C., Brown, A.P. *et al.* (2005a) Assessment of stress in non-human primates: application of the neutrophil activation test. *Animal Welfare*, **14**, 291–295

Honess, P.E., Pizarro, M., Sene, N.N. *et al.* (2006) Disease transmission in Barbary and other macaques: risks and implications for management and conservation. In: *The Barbary Macaque: Biology and Conservation*. Eds Hodges, J.K. and Cortes, J., pp. 149–168. Nottingham University Press, Nottingham

Institute of Laboratory Animal Resources (1976) Long term holding of laboratory rodents. *ILAR News*, **19**, L1–L25

International Primatological Society (2007) International Primatological Society. *International Guidelines for the Acquisition, Care and Breeding of Non-human Primates*. http://www.internationalprimatologicalsociety.org/publications.cfm (accessed 10th November 2009)

Janson, C.H. and van Schaik, C.P. (2002) Ecological risk aversion in juvenile primates: slow and steady wins the race. In: *Juvenile Primates: Life History, Development, and Behavior*. Eds Pereira, M.E. and Fairbanks, L.A., pp. 57–74. University of Chicago Press, Chicago

Jen, K.L.C., Hansen, B.C. and Metzger, B.L. (1985) Adiposity, anthropometric measures and plasma insulin levels of rhesus monkeys. *International Journal of Obesity*, **17**, 597–604

Joint Working Group on Refinement (1993) Removal of blood from laboratory mammals and birds. First Report of the BVA/FRAME/RSPCA/UFAW Joint Working Group on Refinement. *Laboratory Animals*, **27**, 1–22

Joint Working Group on Refinement (2001) Refining procedures for the administration of substances. Report of the BVAAWF/FRAME/RSPCA/UFAW Joint Working Group on Refinement. *Laboratory Animals*, **35**, 1–41

Joint Working Group on Refinement (2003) Refinements in telemetry procedures. Seventh report of the BVAAWF/FRAME/RSPCA/UFAW Joint Working Group on Refinement. Part A. *Laboratory Animals*, **37**, 261–299

Joint Working Group on Refinement (2004) Husbandry refinements for rats, mice, dogs and non-human primates used in telemetry procedures. Seventh report of the BVAAWF/FRAME/RSPCA/UFAW Joint Working Group on Refinement. Part B. *Laboratory Animals*, **38**, 1–10

Joint Working Group on Refinement (2009) Refinements in husbandry, care and common procedures for non-human primates. Ninth report of the BVAAWF/FRAME/RSPCA/UFAW Joint Working Group on Refinement. *Laboratory Animals*, **43**, S1:1–S1:47

Kalter, S.S., Heberling, R.L., Cooke, A.W. *et al.* (1997) Viral infections of nonhuman primates: overview of data from Viral Reference Laboratory San Antonio on results from 53,000 tests. *Laboratory Animal Science*, **47**, 461–467

Kanaujia, G.V., Garcia, M.A., Bouley, D.M. *et al.* (2003) Detection of early secretory antigenic target-6 antibody for diagnosis of tuberculosis in non human primates. *Comparative Medicine*, **53**, 602–606

Kemnitz, J.W. (1984) Obesity in macaques: spontaneous and induced. *Advances in Veterinary Science and Comparative Medicine*, **28**, 81–114

Kirkwood, J.K. and Stathatos, K. (1992) *Biology, Rearing and Care of Young Primates*. Blackwell Publishing, Oxford

Klein, H.J. and Murray, K.A. (1995) Restraint. In: *Nonhuman Primates in Biomedical Research: Biology and Management*. Eds Bennett, T.B., Abee, C.R. and Hendrickson, R., pp. 286–297. Academic Press, San Diego

Knapp, L.A., Ha, J.C. and Sackett, G.P. (1996) Parental MHC antigen sharing and pregnancy wastage in captive pig-tailed macaques. *Journal of Reproductive Immunology*, **32**, 73–88

Krebs, J.R. and Davies, N.B. (1993) *An Introduction to Behavioural Ecology*, 3rd edn. Blackwell Publishing, Oxford

Laboratory Animal Science Association (2005) Guidance on the transport of laboratory animals. *Laboratory Animals*, **39**, 1–39

Laule, G.E., Bloomsmith, M.A. and Schapiro, S.J. (2003) The use of positive reinforcement training techniques to enhance the care, management, and welfare of laboratory primates. *Journal of Applied Animal Welfare Science*, **6**, 163–174

Lee, P.C. (1987) Nutrition, fertility and maternal investment in primates. *Journal of Zoology, London*, **213**, 409–422

Lee, P.C. (1994) Social structure and evolution. In: *Behaviour and Evolution*. Eds Slater, P.J.B. and Halliday, T.R., pp. 266–303. Cambridge University Press, Cambridge

Lee, P.C. (1999) Comparative ecology of postnatal growth and weaning among haplorhine primates. In: *Comparative Primate Socioecology*. Ed. Lee, P.C., pp. 111–136. Cambridge University Press, Cambridge

Lindburg, D.G. (1991) Ecological requirements of macaques. *Laboratory Animal Science*, **41**, 315–322

Luttrell, L., Acker, L., Urben, M. *et al.* (1994) Training a large troop of rhesus macaques to cooperate during catching: analysis of time investment. *Animal Welfare*, **3**, 135–140

Ministry of Agriculture, Fisheries & Food (1994) *Condition Scoring of Sheep: Action on Animal Welfare*. MAFF Publications, London

Martin, R.D. (1990) *Primate Origins and Evolution, a Phylogenetic Reconstruction*. Chapman and Hall, London

Marx, P.A., Spira, A.I., Gettie, A. *et al.* (1996) Progesterone implants enhances SIV vaginal transmission and early virus load. *Nature Medicine*, **2**, 1084–1089

Mendoza, S., Capitanio, J. and Mason, W. (2000) Chronic social stress: studies in non-human primates. In: *The Biology of Animal Stress: Basic Principles and Implications for Animal Welfare*. Eds Moberg, G. and Mench, J., pp. 227–248. CAB International, Wallingford

Mittermeier, R.A., Rylands, A.B., Coimbra-Filho, A.F. *et al.* (1988) *Ecology and Behaviour of Neotropical Primates*, Vol. 2. World Wildlife Fund, Washington, DC

Mivart, St G. (1873) On *Lepilemur* and *Cheirogaleus*, and on the zoological rank of the *Lemuroidea*. *Proceedings of Scientific Meeting, Zoological Society, London*, 484–510

Morton, W.R., Knitter, G.H., Smith, P.M. *et al.* (1987) Alternatives to chronic restraint of nonhuman-primates. *Journal of the American Veterinary Medical Association*, **191**, 1282–1286

Munoz-Zanzi, C.A., Thurmond, M.C., Hird, D.W. *et al.* (1999) Effect of weaning time and associated management practices on postweaning chronic diarrhoea in captive rhesus monkeys (*Macaca mulatta*). *Laboratory Animal Science*, **49**, 617–621

National Centre for the Replacement, Refinement and Reduction of Animals used in Research (NC3Rs) (2007) National Centre for the 3 Rs. *Guidelines on Primate Accommodation, Care and Use*. Available from http://www.nc3rs.org.uk/page.asp?id=277 (accessed 10th November 2009)

National Research Council (NRC) (1996) National Research Council. *Guide for the Care and Use of Laboratory Animals*. National Academy Press, Washington, DC

National Research Council (NRC) (1998) National Research Council. *The Psychological Well-Being of Non-Human Primates*. National Academy Press, Washington, DC

National Research Council (NRC) (2003) National Research Council. *Nutrient Requirements of Nonhuman Primates*. The National Academies Press, Washington, DC

Norman, R.L., McGlone, J. and Smith, C.J. (1994) Restraint inhibits lutenizing hormone secretion in the follicular phase of the menstrual cycle in rhesus macaques. *Biology of Reproduction*, **50**, 16–26

Norman, R.L. and Smith, C.J. (1992) Restraint inhibits lutenizing hormone and testosterone secretion in intact male rhesus macaques: effects of concurrent naloxone administration. *Neuroendocrinology*, **55**, 405–415

Novak, M.A. and Suomi, S.J. (1988) Psychological well-being of primates in captivity. *The American Psychologist*, **40**, 765–773

Organisation for Economic Co-operation and Development (2001) *Guidance Document on the Recognition, Assessment, and Use of Clinical Signs as Humane Endpoints for Experimental Animals used in Safety Evaluation*. Environment Directorate, OECD, Paris

Owen, D.G. (1992) *Parasites of Laboratory Animals*. Laboratory Animal Handbooks No. 12. Royal Society of Medicine Press, London

Poole, T. (1995) Guidelines and legal codes for the welfare of non-human primates in biomedical research. *Laboratory Animals*, **29**, 244–249

Prescott, M.J. (2001) *Counting the Cost: Welfare Implications of the Supply and Transport of Non-Human Primates for Use in Research and Testing*. Royal Society for the Prevention of Cruelty to Animals, Horsham, West Sussex

Prescott, M.J. and Buchanan-Smith, H.M. (2007) Training laboratory-housed non-human primates, Part 1: A survey of current practice in the UK. *Animal Welfare*, **16**, 21–36

Prescott, M., Brown, V., Flecknell, P. *et al.* (in prep) Refinement of food and fluid control as motivational tools for macaques used in behavioural neuroscience research: Report of a Working Group of the NC3Rs.

Pryor, K. (2002) *Don't Shoot the Dog!: The New Art of Teaching and Training*. Revised edn. Ringpress Books, Gloucestershire

Reinhardt, V. and Reinhardt, A. (2000) Social enhancement for adult non human primates in research laboratories. *Lab Animal*, **29**, 34–41

Reinhardt, V. (2002) Artificial weaning of Old World monkeys: benefits and costs. *Journal of Applied Animal Welfare Science*, **5**, 149–154

Reinhardt, V. (2003a) Compassion for animals in the laboratory: Impairment or refinement of research methodology? *Journal of Applied Animal Welfare Science*, **6**, 123–130

Reinhardt, V. (2003b) Working with rather than against macaques during blood collection. *Journal of Applied Animal Welfare Science*, **6**, 189–197

Reinhardt, V., Liss, C. and Stevens, C. (1995) Restraint methods of laboratory nonhuman primates: a critical review. *Animal Welfare*, **4**, 221–238

Rennie, A.E. and Buchanan-Smith, H.M. (2006) Refinement of the use of non-human primates in scientific research. Part III: refinement of procedures. *Animal Welfare*, **15**, 239–261

Röder, E.L. and Timmermans, P.J.A. (2002) Housing and care of monkeys and apes in laboratories: adaptations allowing essential species-specific behaviour. *Laboratory Animals*, **36**, 221–242

Rowe, N. (1996) *A Pictorial Guide to the Living Primates*. Pogonias Press, East Hampton, New York

Russell, W.M.S. and Burch, R.L. (1959) *The Principles of Humane Experimental Technique*. 1992 Special Edition, UFAW, Potters Bar

Sacket, G.P., Bowman, R.E., Meyer, J.S. *et al.* (1973) Adrenocortical and behavioural reactions by differentially raised rhesus monkeys. *Physiological Psychology*, **1**, 209–212

Sauceda, R. and Schmidt, M.G. (2000) Refining macaque handling and restraint techniques. *Lab Animal*, **29**, 47–49

Scientific Committee on Animal Health and Welfare (2002) *The Welfare of Non-Human Primates Used in Research*. Scientific Committee on Animal Health and Welfare, Health and Consumer Protection Directorate-General, European Commission. http://europa.eu.int/comm/food/fs/sc/scah/out83_en.pdf

Schrier, A.M. and Povar, M.L. (1984) Twin stumptailed monkeys born in laboratory. *Laboratory Primate Newsletter*, **23**, 18

Segal, E.F. (1989) *Housing, Care and Psychological Well-being of Captive and Laboratory Primates*. Noyes Publications, New York

Sengupta, J., Dhawan, L., Lalitkumar, P.G.L. *et al.* (2003) A multiparametric study of the action of mifepristone used in emergency contraception using the rhesus monkey as a primate model. *Contraception*, **68**, 453–469

Shively, C.A., Friedman, D.P., Gage, H.D. *et al.* (2006) Behavioural depression and positron emission tomography-determined serotonin 1A receptor binding potential in cynomolgus monkeys. *Archives of General Psychiatry*, **63**, 396–403

Smith, D.G. (2005) Genetic Characterization of Indian-origin and Chinese-origin rhesus macaques (*Macaca mulatta*). *Comparative Medicine*, **55**, 227–230

Smith, J.J., Hadzic, V., Li, X. *et al.* (2006) Objective measures of health and well-being in laboratory rhesus monkeys (*Macaca mulatta*). *Journal of Medical Primatology*, **35**, 388–396

Smuts, B.B., Cheney, D.L., Seyfarth, R.M. *et al.* (1987) *Primate Societies*. University of Chicago Press, Chicago

Soulsby, L. and Morton, D.B. (2001) *Pain: Its Nature and Management in Man and Animals*. Royal Society of Medicine, London

Strier, K.B. (2000) *Primate Behavioural Ecology*. Allyn and Bacon, Boston

Summerhoff, G. (1990) *Life, Brain and Consciousness*. North Holland, Amsterdam

Sun, F.J., Wright, D.E. and Pinson, D.M. (2003) Comparison of ketamine versus combination of ketamine and medetomidine in injectable anaesthetic protocols: chemical immobilization in macaques and tissue reaction in rats. *Contemporary Topics*, **42**, 32–37

Suomi, S.J. (1986) Behavioural aspects of successful reproduction in primates. In: *Primates: The Road to Self-sustaining Populations*. Ed Benirschke, K., pp. 331–340. Springer-Verlag, New York

Suzuki, M.T., Hamano, M., Cho, F. *et al.* (1989) Food and water intake, urinary and faecal output, and urinalysis in the wild originated cynomolgus monkey (*Macaca fascicularis*) under individually caged conditions. *Experimental Animal*, **38**, 71–74

Terao, K. (2005) Management of Old World Primates (Table 11.1). In: *The Laboratory Primate*. Ed, Wolfe-Coote S., pp. 163–173. Elsevier Academic Press, London

Waitt, C., Little, A., Wolfensohn, S. *et al.* (2003) Evidence from rhesus macaques suggests that male colouration plays a role in female mate choice. *Proceedings of the Royal Society of London B*, **270**, 144–146

Wallis, J. and Valentine, B. (2001) Early vs. natural weaning in captive baboons: The effect on timing of postpartum estrus and next conception. *Laboratory Primate Newsletter*, **40**, 10–13

Weber, H., Berge, E., Finch, J. *et al.* (1999) FELASA (Federation of Laboratory Animal Science Associations) Working Group on Non-Human Primate Health. Health monitoring of non-human primate colonies. *Laboratory Animals*, **33** (Suppl 1), S1:3–S1:18

Wetherall, D. (2006) *The Use of Non-human Primates in Research*. A report sponsored by the Academy of Medical Sciences, the Medical Research Council, The Royal Society and The Wellcome Trust. Available from http://www.acmedsci.ac.uk/images/project/nhpdownl.pdf (accessed 10 November 2009)

Wolfe-Coote, S. (2005) *The Laboratory Primate*. Elsevier Academic Press, London

Wolfensohn, S.E. (1997) Brief review of scientific studies of the welfare implications of transporting primates. *Laboratory Animals*, **31**, 303–305

Wolfensohn, S.E. (1998) *Shigella* infection in macaque colonies: case report of an eradication and control program. *Laboratory Animal Science*, **48**, 330–333

Wolfensohn, S.E. (2003) Case report of a possible familial predisposition to metabolic bone disease in juvenile rhesus macaques. *Laboratory Animals*, **37**, 139–144

Wolfensohn, S. (2004) Social housing of large primates: Methodology for refinement of husbandry and management. *Alternatives to Laboratory Animals*, **32** (suppl 1), 149–151

Wolfensohn, S. and Finnemore, P.F. (2006) *Refinements in Primate Husbandry*: a DVD training resource. Available from http://www.oxforduniversityshops.co.uk/store/shop/products.asp?func=prodvar&compid=14&deptid=33&prodtypeid=16&prodID=63

Wolfensohn, S. and Honess, P. (2005) *Handbook of Primate Husbandry and Welfare*. Blackwell Publishing, Oxford

Wolfensohn, S. and Honess, P. (2007) Laboratory animal, pet animal, farm animal, wild animal: Who gets the best deal? UFAW Symposium: Quality of Life: The Heart of the Matter. *Animal Welfare*, **16** (suppl 1), 17–123

Wolfensohn, S. and Honess, P. (submitted) The extended welfare assessment grid: A matrix for the assessment of welfare and cumulative suffering in experimental animals. *Alternatives to Laboratory Animals*

Wolfensohn, S.E. and Lloyd, M.H. (1998) *Handbook of Laboratory Animal Management and Welfare*, 2nd edn. Blackwell Publishing, Oxford

Wolfensohn, S.E. and Lloyd, M.H. (2003) *Handbook of Laboratory Animal Management and Welfare*, 3rd edn. Blackwell Publishing, Oxford

Wolfensohn, S. and Peters, A. (2005) Refinement of neuroscience procedures using non human primates. *Animal Technology and Welfare*, **4**, 49–50

Young, R.J. (2003) *Environmental Enrichment for Captive Animals*. Blackwell Publishing, Oxford

Zehr, J.L., Tannenbaum, P.L., Jones, B. *et al.* (2000) Peak occurrence of female sexual initiation predicts day of conception in rhesus monkeys (*Macaca mulatta*). *Reproduction, Fertility and Development*, **12**, 397–404

40 Chimpanzees

Steven J. Schapiro and Susan P. Lambeth

Introduction

Entire volumes have been devoted to the care and management of captive chimpanzees (eg, Brent 2001a), so this chapter will not attempt to provide all the information necessary for the those involved in the care of chimpanzees. Instead, the aim of this chapter is to draw attention to those aspects of chimpanzee biology, care and management that have significantly changed since the last edition of the UFAW Handbook (Poole 1999).

Biological overview

The previous edition of this Handbook contained an excellent treatment of chimpanzee biology (Fritz *et al.* 1999) as does the book by Brent (2001a) on management of captive chimpanzees. There has not been much change in knowledge of the basic biology of chimpanzees since the last edition of the UFAW Handbook. They are Great Apes and are among the most intelligent primates. Their similarities to humans make them, both an extremely attractive model for biomedical research (VandeBerg *et al.* 2005; Varki 2007) and, an extremely problematic model for many types of investigations (Knight 2007; Rowan 2007). Many readers will neither be able to fathom the need for using chimpanzees in research nor, the moral justification for doing so. On the other hand, many readers will understand that the value of the research can be more than adequate justification for the use of a species so similar to our own.

Taxonomy

The taxonomy of the common chimpanzee (*Pan troglodytes*) is still being debated. Three subspecies are normally proposed (*P. t. troglodytes*, *P. t. verus* and *P. t. schweinfurthii*), and considerable academic discussion is currently devoted to the clarification of this issue (Gonder *et al.* 2006; Becquet *et al.* 2007). There does not appear to be much drive for maintaining distinct subspecies in the captive chimpanzee population in contrast to the situation for orangutans and certain other primate species (Groves 2005).

Genetics

Chimpanzee genetics is an area in which substantial and important progress has been made since the last edition of this handbook. Specifically, both the human genome (Venter *et al.* 2001) and the chimpanzee genome (The Chimpanzee Sequencing and Analysis Consortium 2005) have been sequenced since 2001. As should be obvious, substantial similarities exist between the two genomes, providing opportunities to further exploit the genetic, physiological, behavioural and social similarities as well as the differences between the two species to learn more about both species (Varki & Nelson 2007). The high degree of genetic similarity between chimpanzees and humans highlights both the importance of chimpanzees as animal models in human-focused research as well as the problems associated with conducting research with such close relatives (VandeBerg *et al.* 2005; Rowan 2007; Varki 2007).

Social organisation

Chimpanzees are usually described as living in fission–fusion societies consisting of up to 100 members per community (Wrangham *et al.* 1994). Fission–fusion societies are frequently characterized by fairly fluid social relationships within the community; with subgroup composition varying considerably on a day-to-day basis. Unlike many other species of non-human primates that live in multimale–multifemale groups, male–male bonds (rather than female–female bonds) are the most important social factor in chimpanzee groups (Goodall 1986). Although chimpanzee social relationships are fluid within the group, relationships between communities of chimpanzees can be extremely aggressive (Mitani & Watts 2005). Multiple reports have described fatal encounters between individuals of different chimpanzee communities (Watts *et al.* 2006; Boesch *et al.* 2007, 2008). Females exhibiting maximal oestrous swellings appear to be the age–sex class of individuals that is least likely to receive high levels of aggression in intergroup encounters (Deschner & Boesch 2007).

The fission–fusion societies of wild chimpanzees include regular and frequent social separations and re-introductions. It is therefore somewhat surprising that it is so difficult to re-introduce captive chimpanzees back into their social groups, even after only a short absence, such as for an annual physical examination. Development and use of appropriate standard operating procedures (SOP) for group formations and re-introductions are critical for the successful management of captive chimpanzees (Bloomsmith & Baker 2001; Fritz & Howell 2001; Lambeth personal observation). Since natural chimpanzee sociality in the wild includes repeated separations and re-introductions that are under the animals' control, it has been suggested that re-introduction difficulties may arise from the fact that separations and re-introductions in captivity are under the control of human care staff, rather than the chimpanzees themselves. Certainly, gradual, systematic and sometimes individualised re-introductions are necessary to minimise damaging aggression (Fritz & Howell 2001).

Reproduction

Chimpanzees are a slow-producing, slow-maturing species (traits characteristic of a K-selected species). Under natural conditions, the average length of gestation is difficult to accurately determine, but the mean is estimated at 228 days (Tutin 1994) and females do not give birth to their first infant until around 11 years of age (Fritz *et al.* 1999). Females nurse their offspring for several years, with interbirth intervals ranging from 36–84 months (Fritz *et al.* 1999). Infants and juveniles remain in the company of their mothers and maternal kin for years, often forming reasonably stable subgroups within the fission–fusion community. In addition, young chimpanzees typically learn many foraging skills from their mothers, especially those that involve the use of tools, such as termite fishing and nut cracking (Biro *et al.* 2006). Captivity can influence virtually all aspects of this pattern of reproduction and development, with captive females giving birth for the first time earlier and having shorter interbirth intervals on average (Roof *et al.* 2005).

The female reproductive cycle lasts approximately 34 days and is characterised by conspicuous swelling of the perineal area leading up to a maximum on the day of ovulation (Wrangham 1994). The patterns of social interactions of an adult female with other females and with adult males differ according to the state of her oestrous swelling (Wallis 1992). Males will attempt to mate with females throughout their oestrous cycles, but male interest increases as swelling size increases. Maximally swollen females are able to move between social groups in the wild, whereas most other age–sex classes are not (Deschner & Boesch 2007). This fact can be used to advantage in captivity when attempting to introduce a new animal (swollen female) to other animals.

Physiological parameters

Since the publication of the 7th edition of the UFAW Handbook (Poole 1999), several papers have been published that contain normal values for a variety of physiological parameters for captive chimpanzees. Many of these primary publications present normal ranges differentiated by the age and sex of the chimpanzee. The reader can find the original sources for complete sets of normal ranges in Herndon and Tigges (2001); Ihrig *et al.* (2001); Lee and Guhad (2001); Howell *et al.* (2003); Lamperez and Rowell (2005); Videan *et al.* (2008). Representative values for adult males, adult females, aged males and aged females, the most common age–sex classes of animals currently in research colonies, are included in Table 40.1 (adapted from Herndon and Tigges 2001; Ihrig *et al.* 2001; Lee and Guhad 2001; Howell *et al.* 2003; Lamperez and Rowell 2005; Videan *et al.* 2008). It is important to note that the values in the table represent normal ranges; it is not necessarily correct to assume that animals displaying values outside of the normal range are clinically ill and/or in need of treatment.

Most physiological data obtained from adult chimpanzee blood samples come from anaesthetised animals. It is well known that ketamine and telazol, two of the most frequently used anaesthetics for captive chimpanzees, influence many of these physiological parameters in non-human primates (Woodward & Weld 1997). Efforts are currently underway to establish unanaesthetised normal ranges from samples obtained from adult chimpanzees that will voluntarily present their arms for conscious venepuncture (Schapiro *et al.* 2006b). Whether these unanaesthetised normal ranges will differ significantly from anaesthetised normal ranges has yet to be determined. Additionally, data are accumulating to establish normal ranges for several immunological parameters (eg, lymphocyte subsets, cytokine production, natural killer cell activity) for both anaesthetised and unanaesthetised chimpanzees (Schapiro *et al.* 2006a).

Conservation and ecology

Threats

Clearly, there are many factors that are threatening the survival of chimpanzees in their natural settings. Destruction of habitat, logging, disease and hunting for bushmeat are probably the biggest threats (Kormos *et al.* 2003; Fa *et al.* 2005; Arnhem *et al.* 2008; Hanamura *et al.* 2008; Kondgen *et al.* 2008). These factors are all interrelated and can in general be attributed to increased human encroachment into chimpanzee habitat. It is extremely unlikely that any of these threats will diminish in the near (or distant) future, leaving the chimpanzee at considerable risk of extinction in the not-so-distant future. It is unlikely that the captive population of laboratory chimpanzees, for whom a breeding moratorium is in effect, will play any role (positive or negative) in the conservation of the species. Zoo chimpanzees may play a small positive role, given the limited amount of breeding (zero population growth) that is permitted in the zoo population.

Recent findings

Despite fairly gloomy news concerning the ultimate survival of chimpanzees in the wild, recent field studies of populations of chimpanzees (Pruetz 2007; Boesch *et al.* 2008; Stanford 2008) have yielded some extremely interesting findings. While most findings from field studies have implications for the captive management of chimpanzees, the

Table 40.1 Physiological parameters for adult chimpanzees (values taken from Herndon & Tigges 2001; Ihrig *et al.* 2001; Lee & Guhad 2001; Howell *et al.* 2003; Lamperez & Rowell 2005; Videan *et al.* 2008).

Analyte	*Units*	*Adult males*	*Adult females*	*Aged males*	*Aged females*
Haematocrit	%	44.09–46.50	41.27–42.05	45.00–52.80	37.00–43.40
Haemoglobin	g/dl	14.39–15.51	13.40–13.86	15.00–16.50	11.78–14.00
RBC count	$\times 10^6/mm^3$	5.31–5.65	5.03–5.14	5.00–6.14	4.38–5.50
WBC	$\times 10^3/mm^3$	11.17–11.37	10.62–12.88	10.07–10.30	10.83–14.42
Neutrophils segmented	$\times 10^3/mm^3$	6.15–6.70	5.42–7.49	3.61–5.69	5.19–9.51
Lymphocytes	$\times 10^3/mm^3$	3.88–4.58	4.61–4.72	3.90–6.39	4.23–6.32
Monocytes	$\times 10^3/mm^3$	0.31–0.33	0.25–0.32	0.26–0.31	0.15–0.33
Platelets	$\times 10^3/mm^3$	231.93–258.94	242.64–255.13	226.90–270.00	240.84–299.28
Total bilirubin	mg/dl	0.36–0.37	0.28–0.33	0.20–0.27	0.22–0.27
AST	U/l	25.99–35.79	18.33–25.01	27.50–33.36	26.13–31.44
ALT	U/l	37.13–42.28	26.49–32.57	41.50–43.85	29.92–47.49
Alkaline phosphatase	U/l	85.22–93.02	95.67–100.70	91.00–111.00	98.00–107.79
Glucose	mg/dl	85.14–100.33	83.6–92.11	98.50–101.98	104.24–121.72
BUN	mg/dl	13.14–13.59	11.15–12.15		
Creatinine	mg/dl	1.09–1.12	0.86–1.00	1.00–1.20	0.99–1.15
Total protein	g/dl	7.33–7.80	7.33–7.59	7.20–7.39	7.28–7.40
Albumin	g/dl	3.36–4.10	3.34–3.70	3.45–3.69	3.26–3.52
Globulin	g/dl	3.40–4.06	3.70–3.95	3.75–4.00	3.48–4.02
Cholesterol	mg/dl	179.50–222.58	212.20–228.52	211.23–235.50	225.75–263.39
HDL	mg/dl	49.81 ± 11.74	55.68 ± 14.34		
LDL	mg/dl	143.61 ± 26.63	154.88 ± 34.84		
Triglycerides	mg/dl	82.62–93.67	84.00–109.74	69.84–119.50	75.2–109.12
Creatine kinase	U/l	270.67–379.63	213.54–335.42	351.88–361.50	242.75–452.18
C-reactive protein	mg/dl	0.86 ± 0.74	1.08 ± 0.99		

findings from savannah chimpanzees in Senegal are among the most interesting and the most relevant. Pruetz and her colleagues (Pruetz 2007; Pruetz & Bertolani 2007; Stewart *et al.* 2007; Roach 2008) have demonstrated that wild chimpanzees will play in water, live in caves, make comfortable nests and hunt for bushbabies in holes in trees using tools (modified and sharpened sticks). The implications for the management of captive chimpanzees should be clear; small pools, nesting material, and food stuffed into holes in structures that can be speared with sticks should be useful, naturalistic forms of environmental enrichment.

Uses in the laboratory

Biomedical research

When chimpanzees are used in infectious disease research, they are usually involved in studies of hepatitis viruses. In the past, chimpanzees had been infected with human immunodeficiency virus (HIV), but only a single chimpanzee may have developed AIDS, making them a less than ideal model for this type of research (Stump & VandeWoude 2007). They are a far superior model for hepatitis research; in fact vaccines for hepatitis B were successfully developed in chimpanzees and potential vaccines for hepatitis C are currently being tested and evaluated using chimpanzees (Elmowalid *et al.* 2007). An analysis of primate use in biomedical research (Carlsson *et al.* 2004) revealed that members of the genus *Pan* were used in 4.9% of studies involving primates published in 2001, and infectious disease was among the most common topics of investigation involving chimpanzees.

Chimpanzees are also used in assessments of the efficacy of a variety of novel therapeutic approaches, including analyses of monoclonal antibodies as treatments for cancer (VandeBerg *et al.* 2005). Although mice are useful models for many aspects of biomedical research, they are not valid models for all aspects. For some investigations, it may be that chimpanzees are the most valid model. Use of words like test article suggests that a regulatory process is involved, and in fact, the United States Food and Drug Administration (FDA) often requires that compounds be tested in appropriate non-human primate models, using good laboratory practices (GLP), prior to approving the compound for the next stages of evaluation and/or use in humans. However decisions to use chimpanzees should always include a full consideration of ethical and welfare issues. Performing GLP studies with chimpanzees presents a series of significant management challenges for those responsible for the care and well-being of the animals. While it is difficult to bring a non-GLP-compliant chimpanzee programme up to GLP standards, once GLP-compliant protocols and record keeping practices become part of normal operating procedures, multiple benefits accrue for the research and care staff and for the chimpanzees used in research. Most of these benefits are related to: (1) the establishment of SOPs which promote consistent care and treatment of the animals and (2) enhanced record keeping systems that promote the systematic collection of health, behavioural and research data.

Behavioural research

Applied research

The primary goal of most applied laboratory chimpanzee behavioural research projects is to improve the welfare, while simultaneously enhancing the definition of chimpanzees as animal models for biomedical research (Bloomsmith & Else 2005; Videan & Fritz 2007; Coleman *et al.* 2008). Such efforts should result in improvements in the quality and utility of the chimpanzee as a research model. A typical focus in applied research programmes is to 'refine' (one of the Three Rs as discussed by Russell and Burch (1959), see also Chapter 2) management and handling techniques so as to minimise psychological/behavioural confounds that might adversely affect subjects, research protocols and/or results. More specifically, attempts are being made to minimise the stress experienced by chimpanzees in an effort to limit interindividual variation in the measures typically assessed by investigators working with chimpanzees as subjects (Lambeth *et al.* 2006; Bloomsmith *et al.* 2006b; Schapiro *et al.* 2007). Reducing inter-animal variability should make it possible to reduce the number of subjects required for experimental comparisons without diminishing the power of experimental designs. This addresses 'reduction', another of Russell's and Burch's Three Rs (Russell & Burch 1959); one that is of great relevance when dealing with an animal model as complex as the chimpanzee.

There are considerably fewer applied research projects focusing on factors that influence the quality and utility of chimpanzees as models in the zoo setting. However, findings from applied investigations that delineate beneficial management strategies for chimpanzees used in research can, should be and, in most cases, are, adapted to zoo settings. Similarly, findings from investigations conducted on chimpanzees in zoos that identify beneficial management strategies are adapted to laboratory settings whenever possible.

Various welfare-enhancing techniques have been developed, and are in use, to manage the behaviour and the psychological environments of captive chimpanzees (Bloomsmith & Else 2005; Videan & Fritz, 2007; Coleman *et al.* 2008). These techniques are designed to functionally simulate important components of the animals' natural environment/habitat, thereby providing them with opportunities to express species-typical behaviours and some degree of choice and control over what they experience. Conventional wisdom suggests that 'normally' behaving laboratory animals are likely to make better models than animals that behave abnormally. Since wild chimpanzees are able to control many aspects of their existence in their natural environments, providing laboratory chimpanzees with opportunities to choose should promote normal behaviour in the non-natural laboratory setting. Studies of behavioural management strategies are designed to empirically address the question of whether such procedures influence behavioural and physiological variables of interest to those working with and studying captive chimpanzees.

Basic research

Captive chimpanzees are ideal subjects for both simple and complex investigations of learning, hemispheric specialisation, cultural transmission, behavioural economics, language development, cognition, facial expressions and prosociality (Silk *et al.* 2005; Hopkins *et al.* 2005, 2007; Brosnan *et al.* 2007; Hopper *et al.* 2007; Parr *et al.* 2007; Whiten *et al.* 2007), just to name a few. Many of these investigations can be combined with non-invasive imaging techniques to gather even more data to test critical hypotheses (Cohen 2007a). In addition, many of the procedures used to generate the data are quite stimulating, challenging and enriching for the participating chimpanzees.

Laboratory management and breeding (or non-breeding)

Intelligent, powerful animals like chimpanzees present a number of management challenges for those charged with providing them with optimal care in captivity. Nothing is simple when managing chimpanzees and the volume edited by Brent (2001a) addresses many aspects of their management. Techniques for managing the successful breeding of captive chimpanzees are not of great concern at the time of writing, as the National Institutes of Health of the United States is maintaining the moratorium on the breeding of research chimpanzees (Cohen 2007b). This moratorium has been in effect for over a decade and was recommended by the advisory committee of the National Research Council (National Research Council 1997). Obviously, the indefinite continuation of this breeding moratorium will result in the eventual extinction of the population of captive research chimpanzees. This strategy is in harmony with legislation designed to outlaw invasive research on Great Apes that is currently under consideration in the United States (the only country that still allows and conducts 'invasive' research with Great Apes). As mentioned several times previously, some readers will find this an appropriate and commendable outcome, while others will find it extremely short-sighted and objectionable.

The main thrust of the rest of this section will be the breeding moratorium that is in effect for captive research chimpanzees in the US (National Research Council 1997; Cohen 2007b). Most female chimpanzees of breeding age in both the zoo and laboratory populations in the US are given some form of contraception to prevent the unplanned birth of additional chimpanzees (Bettinger & DeMatteo 2001). Different facilities are using oral birth control pills, intrauterine devices (IUD), hormonal implants, sexual segregation and/or surgical interventions to prevent additional chimpanzee births. Regardless of the technique, the overall goal is to prevent the addition of any new chimpanzees to the population of research chimpanzees (Cohen 2007b) and to maintain zero population growth among the zoo chimpanzees (Ross, personal communication). Given the slow reproductive rate, long interbirth intervals and the long lifespan of chimpanzees, it would be extremely difficult to rapidly produce a new set of subjects for an emerging health-related crisis that required the use of chimpanzees (VandeBerg *et al.* 2005).

For a number of reasons, reversible contraceptive techniques that allow reasonably normal oestrous cycles are preferred for chimpanzees. First, the possibility exists (VandeBerg *et al.* 2005) that the breeding moratorium will be at least partially lifted at some point in the near future. Reversible forms of contraception, such as sexual segregation, oral contraceptives, intrauterine devices and hormonal implants, are thus favoured. While there are few empirical data that guarantee that IUD and hormonal implants are completely reversible forms of contraception, the occasional failures of these contraceptives (in chimpanzees and humans) and the reversibility in humans suggest that reproduction could be effectively re-started in chimpanzees, even after a fairly long period of contraception.

Secondly, IUD and certain hormonal implants in particular, seem to minimally disrupt the oestrous cycling of mature female chimpanzees; many animals appear to swell and detumesce in patterns that are similar to female chimpanzees that are not on contraceptives (Bettinger *et al.* 1997). Given the importance that reproductive cycles play in the social dynamics of chimpanzee groups, where females are treated differently by other members of the group depending on the stage of their cycles (Wallis 1992; Wrangham *et al.* 1994; Deschner & Boesch 2007), it is important to maintain reproductive swelling cycles in order to maintain cyclical patterns of social activity as well. This aspect of the interplay between contraception, reproductive cycles and social behaviour is important in both the zoo and the laboratory, regardless of whether births are allowed to take place and animals are replaced or not.

Preliminary observations of animals with some of the newer hormonal implant contraceptives suggest that these contraceptives do disrupt normal oestrous cycles (Lambeth, personal observation). While this is clearly undesirable in terms of maintaining normal patterns of social interaction, there may be at least one circumstance in which the smaller and shorter swellings observed in females on the implantable contraceptive is an advantage. Aggression and wounding among males in social groups that are housed in proximity to, but not in contact with, adult females, increases when female(s) are maximally swollen. Aggression among males in groups housed in proximity to females with the new implants has decreased, as has the amount of time that the females are swollen (Lambeth, personal observation). Currently, this relationship is only correlational and needs further investigation.

Finally, evidence is accumulating that males that have been vasectomised are still occasionally impregnating females (Noon, personal communication). Preliminary investigations suggest that the vasectomies are being performed properly, but for reasons yet to be determined, the long-term effectiveness of the procedures has been less than desired.

Husbandry

Cleaning and hygiene

As with any species of laboratory animal, it is imperative that chimpanzees are maintained in sanitary conditions that enhance their welfare and do not compromise their health and safety. Aside from the chapters contained in the Brent (2001a) book on captive care, little new chimpanzee husbandry information has been published since the last edition of the UFAW Handbook (Poole 1999). The book by Brent (2001a), the chapter by Fritz and colleagues (1999) in the seventh edition of the UFAW Handbook (1999), and the husbandry manual edited by Fulk and Garland (1992) are likely to remain the most useful guides to chimpanzee husbandry until the imminent publication of the new AZA (Association of Zoos and Aquariums) chimpanzee care manual (Ross, in press). The second edition of the International Primatological Society captive care guidelines are also available (International Primatological Society Captive Care Committee 2007), but they primarily provide general guidance for caring for non-human primates, rather than information specific to the care of chimpanzees. A much abbreviated discussion of selected aspects of chimpanzee husbandry follows.

A variety of different husbandry schemes are used with chimpanzees, including both 'wet' and 'dry' systems. In a dry system, some type of bedding (ie, shredded paper, hay, straw, wood chips) is typically used, and cleaning involves the removal of soiled bedding on a regular basis without using water (bedding would be shovelled, scooped, or vacuumed out). As the name implies, cages/enclosures maintained by a wet system are cleaned on a regular basis using water hoses (often high-pressure) and chemicals (ie, bleach, disinfectants, degreasers). In wet systems, drains are critical factors in the 'performance' of the facility and are often a limiting factor in determining what types of enrichment are regularly used. Drain placement, drain function and drain covers are critical variables in the effective management of captive chimpanzees using wet systems.

In both wet and dry systems, maintenance of the animals in multiroom 'suites' significantly enhances the ability to clean and sanitise cages/enclosures properly. When chimpanzees have access to more than one room, the animals can be securely excluded from Room 1 when it is being cleaned and then moved back into Room 1 so that Rooms 2, 3, etc can be cleaned. This removes the need to 'clean around' animals or 'jump' animals into transport boxes as may occur for other non-human primate species. However, this process works best when some effort is devoted to training the animals to shift on command, preferably using positive reinforcement training techniques (Laule & Whittaker 2001), see also Chapter 16. Since chimpanzees are so strong and are potentially dangerous, appropriate shifting and cleaning SOPs must be in place and rigorously adhered to, to minimise the risk of accidents in both zoo and laboratory settings.

Environmental enrichment devices often complicate the cleaning and sanitation processes of both types of husbandry schemes (including clogging drains in wet systems). The ideal environmental enrichment device from a husbandry perspective, is one that does not have to be put up and taken down frequently, does not clog drains, and can be easily sanitised while in place.

Veterinary management and geriatric care

Veterinary management (Lee & Guhad 2001) has always been a critical component of the proper maintenance of chimpanzees in captivity, but as the captive population ages, it will take on even greater significance. Middle-aged and older chimpanzees require considerably more care than do young to prime-aged chimpanzees, especially in the area of preventive medicine (Lammey *et al.* 2008). As animals age, biannual physical examinations are likely to replace the current practice of annual examinations. Echocardiograms should be added to health maintenance SOPs for older or 'at-risk' animals (Doane *et al.* 2006), although there may be some diagnostic limitations of echocardiograms conducted on anaesthetised chimpanzees (Bernacky personal communication).

Assessments of physiological parameters, usually through bodily fluid samples (blood, urine, saliva, semen) are routinely made to not only aid in the diagnosis of acute conditions, but also to provide a comparative database for assessments of chronic health conditions (Videan *et al.* 2008). Normal ranges (differentiated by age class and sex) for a variety of physiological parameters in captive chimpanzees have been published (Ihrig *et al.* 2001; Lamperez & Rowell 2005) (Table 40.1). Occasionally, clinical pathologists, veterinarians and behavioural scientists encounter animals whose physiological measures are outside the published normal ranges. This can lead to lively discussions concerning the health and/or welfare of the animals (young or old) when the numbers on paper do not agree with the clinical signs and behavioural observations. Frequently, chimpanzees with 'poor' readouts on paper appear to be in much better overall health than the readouts would suggest.

In addition to enhancements to monitoring and other types of preventive medicine procedures as the population of captive chimpanzees ages, other modifications to their veterinary care and management may become necessary. If advancing age is accompanied by non-lethal sensory, motor, cognitive, or health-related impairments, then animals may have to be removed from their 'normal' groups or enclosures and placed in other groups or enclosures that minimise the potential for injury and other negative consequences due to their impairment(s). Even though an older female may be an important participant in the social interactions of her group, if a bad hip or impaired vision limits her ability to escape from an aggressive member of her group, then she may need to be removed and placed in a safer situation. The question then arises as to when an animal is too impaired to safely or usefully remain within the colony. The next obvious question is what is to become of an animal that is to be removed. Retirement is one obvious option and a number of sanctuaries do exist to house chimpanzees no longer 'useful' for research or exhibition (Brent 2007). Euthanasia of chimpanzees to solve management problems is not permitted (National Research Council 1997), although euthanasia of an animal that is suffering is clearly acceptable. There is still an ongoing debate over the definition of the terms that are critical to this discussion, including impairment thresholds, usefulness and suffering.

Housing

Chimpanzees should be housed in physical and social conditions that: (1) functionally simulate natural conditions; (2) stimulate naturalistic behaviour patterns; (3) are safe; (4) can be sanitised; and (5) are functional for humans (Brent 2001b). Housing conditions for captive chimpanzees range from small cages (3.25 m^2, 35 ft^2) for a single animal up to 5-acre (20 324 m^2) corrals (Brent 2007) for groups of as many as 34 animals, and can include almost anything in between (Figure 40.1). Given the social tendencies of chimpanzees in their natural environment and the behavioural data demonstrating the value of social partners to captive chimpanzees (Bloomsmith & Baker 2001), social housing must be the default option in captivity. Single housing should be an infrequent and short-term condition in all but the most well justified situations (ie, recovery from injury or experimental manipulation; some infectious disease research; social incompatibility). As mentioned above, older and/or mildly impaired animals may need to be transferred from their normal groups to modified groups or enclosures for safety reasons.

While captive housing regulations typically focus on delineating minimum floor areas (National Research Council

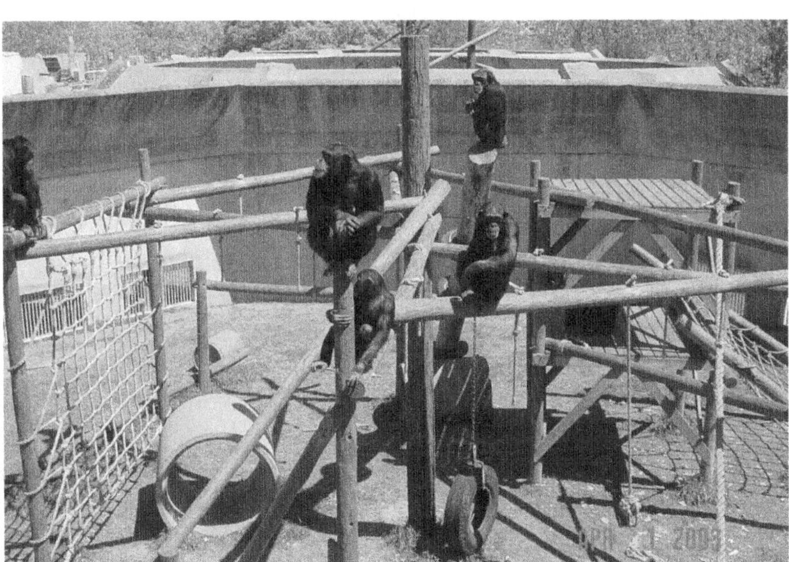

Figure 40.1 Chimpanzee enclosure (corral) at The University of Texas M. D. Anderson Cancer Center, Bastrop, TX USA.

1996), three-dimensional volume is probably a more useful 'engineering' measure for the chimpanzee, a species that spends a considerable portion of its day (and all of its night) above the ground. Single cages may be 1.8 m (6 ft) tall, while outdoor enclosures may include towers that are as high as 15.2 m (50 ft) (Figure 40.2). As with most non-human primates maintained in captivity, performance standards are usually more useful than engineering standards.

No chimpanzee enclosure is escape-proof and escapes do occur (no fewer than six escapes from all types of facilities across the globe have been reported in the popular media in 2006, 2007, and the first half of 2008 according to a Google search of the term 'chimpanzee escape'), so SOPs that minimise the risk of escapes must be developed and stringently followed. In addition, safe capture SOPs in the event of an escape must be developed and practised, for the safety of both the animals and the people involved in the capture process. Although chimpanzees have occasionally escaped from their enclosures through unanticipated feats of athleticism, the majority of escapes occur through human error – the failure of care staff to properly lock or secure doors, gates or chutes (Schapiro & Lambeth personal observation).

Behavioural management

Behavioural management is a critical component of the captive care of all laboratory animals, and is especially important for the care of non-human primates (National Research Council 1998), and even more so for the care of chimpanzees (Bloomsmith & Else 2005). Behavioural management is typically described as an approach that integrates behavioural strategies (environmental enrichment, socialisation and training) designed to functionally simulate natural conditions with more traditional husbandry and veterinary management programmes. The general goal of most chimpanzee behavioural management programmes is to maintain and enhance the welfare/psychological well-being of captive chimpanzees by providing them with opportunities to express species-typical activity patterns (Bloomsmith & Else 2005; Schapiro *et al.* 2007). This is usually discussed in terms of providing the chimpanzees with opportunities to control or to choose what happens to them (Schapiro & Lambeth 2007) and may be formalised in a facility's 'environmental enhancement plan' (see Table 40.2 for a sample environmental enhancement plan). The provision of bedding material (hay, blankets, excelsior, shredded paper, etc) each evening to stimulate nest-building behaviour is a clear example of providing the animals with opportunities to choose to perform naturalistic behaviours (Stewart *et al.* 2007) in the captive setting.

Behavioural management programmes are in operation at most primate facilities (Baker *et al.* 2007), although the maturity of the programmes differs considerably across facilities. The ultimate goal of most behavioural management programmes is to include all animal care staff as participants in the specialised functions of the behavioural-management team. However, during the early stages of the development of a behavioural-management programme, it is often more effective to identify a specific subgroup of people that is responsible for the training, enrichment and handling procedures that comprise the specialised behavioural-management duties. As the programme matures, these duties and responsibilities can then be distributed among all animal care staff.

A considerable amount of empirical data has been published that addresses how enrichment, socialisation and training can influence the welfare of captive animals (see Chapters 10 and 16), with a reasonable number of these publications focusing on chimpanzees (eg, Bloomsmith & Baker 2001; Baker 2005; Bloomsmith & Else 2005; Schapiro & Lambeth 2007; Schapiro *et al.* 2007). Many of these reports focus on the behavioural effects of these types of manipulations, but assessments of physiological effects are available as well (Lambeth *et al.* 2006).

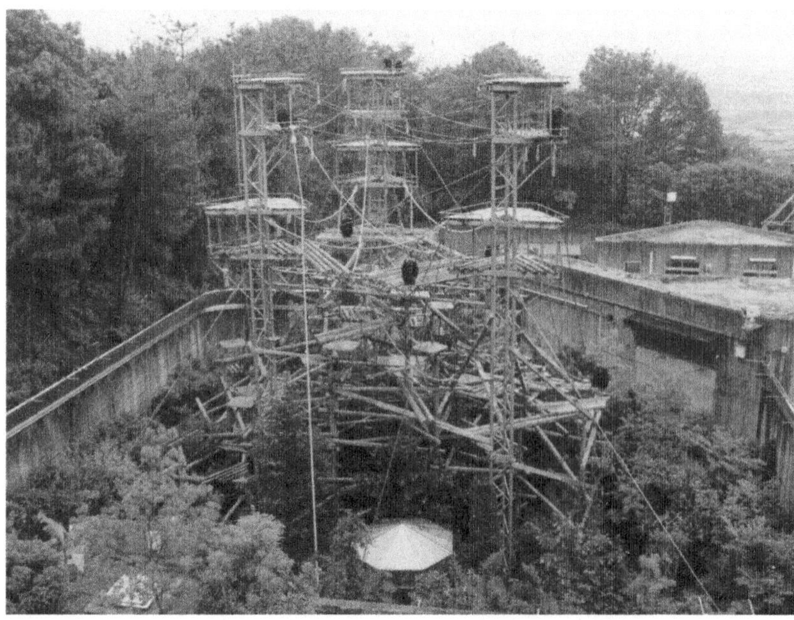

Figure 40.2 Chimpanzee housing (Triple Tower) at the Primate Research Institute, Kyoto, Japan. Reproduced with permission of Tetsuro Matsuzawa.

Table 40.2 A sample environmental enrichment plan for research chimpanzees. The last four columns refer to the description of the chimpanzees depending on their housing situation. This table presents the temporal frequency of enrichment, which may be available on a 'continuous' or 'occasional' basis, or at a specific daily frequency.

Enrichment type	*Corral-housed*	*Indoor/outdoor run*	*Biomedical study groups*	*Biomedical study singles*	
				Outside	*Inside*
SOCIAL					
Conspecific contact	Continuous	Continuous	Continuous		
Human contact[8]	Daily	Daily	Daily	Daily	Daily
Conspecific non-contact	Continuous	Continuous	Continuous	Continuous	Continuous
PHYSICAL					
Ropes	Continuous		Continuous	Continuous	
Fire hose[1]		Continuous			
Swings	Continuous		Continuous		
Climbing structure	Continuous	Continuous[3]	Continuous[3]	Continuous[3]	
Overhead brachiation bars	Continuous	Continuous	Continuous	Continuous	Continuous
Grass (ground cover)	Continuous	Continuous[3]	Continuous[3]	Continuous[3]	
Cargo nets	Continuous	Continuous[3]	Continuous[3]		
Culverts	Continuous	Continuous[3]	Continuous[3]	Continuous[3]	
Tires	Continuous	Continuous[3]	Continuous[3]	Continuous[3]	
Plastic milk crates	Continuous	Continuous	Continuous	Continuous	
Sturdy latex tubing	Continuous	Continuous	Continuous	Continuous	Continuous
55-gallon barrels	Continuous	Continuous	Continuous[3]	Continuous	
FEEDING	*3/week*	*3/week*	*7/week*	*7/week*	*7/week*
Forage mix[4]	Occasional	Occasional	Occasional	Occasional	Occasional
Novel food items	Occasional	Occasional	Occasional	Occasional	Occasional
Frozen produce[2]	Occasional	Occasional	Occasional	Occasional	Occasional
Stuffed chow bags	Occasional	Occasional	Occasional	Occasional	Occasional
Frozen milk cartons[2]			Occasional	Occasional	Occasional
Frozen soda bottles[2]			Occasional	Occasional	Occasional
Brent puzzle			Occasional	Occasional	Occasional
Forage trough	Occasional	Occasional	Occasional	Occasional	Occasional
Stuffed paper bags	Occasional	Occasional	Occasional	Occasional	Occasional
Crate puzzle/double crate	Occasional	Occasional	Occasional	Occasional	
Browse (leaves, bamboo, vine, etc.)[7]	Occasional	Occasional	Occasional	Occasional	Occasional
Frozen juice cups	Occasional[2]	Occasional[2]	Occasional[2]	Occasional[2]	Occasional
Food PVC tubes	Occasional	Occasional	Occasional	Occasional	Occasional
Smeared forage lids/boards		Occasional[2]	Occasional[2]	Occasional[2]	Occasional[2]
Toilet paper rolls			Occasional	Occasional	Occasional
Reel in feed		Occasional	Occasional	Occasional	Occasional
Goodie box			Occasional	Occasional	
OCCUPATIONAL	*3/week*	*3/week*	*4/week*	*5/week*	*5/week*
Pipefeeder (termite) puzzle[6]	Occasional	Occasional	Occasional	Occasional	Occasional
Raisin board puzzle		Occasional	Occasional	Occasional	Occasional
PVC puzzle	Occasional	Occasional	Occasional	Occasional	Occasional
Banana puzzle	Occasional	Occasional	Occasional	Occasional	Occasional
Ball puzzle		Occasional	Occasional	Occasional	Occasional
Peanut puzzle	Occasional	Occasional			
Three-level puzzle	Occasional	Occasional	Occasional	Occasional	Occasional
Astroturf forage board (hanging)	Occasional	Occasional	Occasional	Occasional	Occasional
Astroturf hanging tubes	Occasional	Occasional	Occasional	Occasional	Occasional
Cap puzzle	Occasional	Occasional	Occasional	Occasional	Occasional

Table 40.2 *Continued*

Enrichment type	*Corral-housed*	*Indoor/outdoor run*	*Biomedical study groups*	*Biomedical study singles*	
				Outside	*Inside*
Forage bleach bottle	Occasional	Occasional	Occasional	Occasional	Occasional
Frozen fruit buckets/tubs[2]	Occasional	Occasional	Occasional	Occasional	
Food-stuffed Kong Toys™		Occasional	Occasional	Occasional	Occasional
Wadger (trough on the outside of the cage mesh containing diluted fruit juice, in which the animals dip sponges of paper)	Occasional	Occasional	Occasional	Occasional	Occasional
Frozen vertical PVC puzzle			Occasional	Occasional	Occasional
Chalk/drawing/paint	Occasional	Occasional	Occasional	Occasional	Occasional
Boomer Ball™	Continuous	Continuous	Continuous	Continuous	Occasional
Other toys[9]	Occasional	Occasional	Occasional	Occasional	Occasional
NESTING MATERIALS	*5/week*	*5/week*	*5/week*	*5/week*	*5/week*
Excelsior	Regular	Regular	Occasional	Occasional	Occasional
Fleece/blankets/clothes	Occasional	Occasional	Occasional	Occasional	Occasional
Butcher paper	Occasional	Occasional	Occasional	Occasional	Occasional
Cardboard boxes	Occasional[2]	Occasional[2]	Occasional[2]	Occasional[2]	Occasional
Shredded paper	Occasional	Occasional	Occasional	Occasional	Occasional
SENSORY	*5/week*	*5/week*	*5/week*	*7/week*	*7/week*
Television/videotapes	Occasional	Occasional	Occasional	Occasional	Occasional
Radio/music	Occasional	Occasional	Occasional	Occasional	Occasional
Visual items[5]	Continuous	Continuous	Occasional	Occasional	Occasional
Nature sounds	Occasional	Occasional	Occasional	Occasional	Occasional
Olfactory	Occasional	Occasional	Occasional	Occasional	Occasional
Rattle ball			Occasional	Occasional	Occasional
Water in barrels[2]		Occasional	Occasional	Occasional	
Transport cage 'ride'	Occasional	Occasional	Occasional	Occasional	Occasional
Tug-of-war	Continuous		Continuous	Occasional	Occasional
Water sprinkler/misters[2]	Daily	Daily	Daily	Daily	
Bubbles	Occasional	Occasional	Occasional	Occasional	Occasional
Destructible items[10]	Occasional	Occasional	Occasional	Occasional	Occasional
Mirror	Continuous	Continuous	Continuous	Continuous	Continuous
Triangle noisemakers	Continuous	Continuous	Continuous	Continuous	Continuous

1. Young animals and some adult groups in the indoor/outdoor runs.
2. During warm weather only.
3. Animals with access to Primadomes®.
4. Forage mix can consist of popcorn, raisins, dry cereals, nuts and graham crackers.
5. Visual items include windmills, birdfeeders, balloons, painted murals, decorative shower curtain, etc.
6. Pipe feeders are filled with liquid and semi-liquid foods (apple sauce, syrup, jelly, or tomato sauce, etc)
7. All browse (leaves, stick, roots, vines, plants) must be approved by the veterinarian.
8. Human interactions or training with the chimps is conducted regularly through the wire mesh. All precautions are taken to ensure human safety.
9. Other toys include, but not limited to Kongs, Dental Devices, Havaballs, Gumabones, Dumbbells, etc.
10. Destructible items include magazines, boxes, etc.

Environmental enrichment

Captive chimpanzees respond well to a variety of environmental enrichment strategies and procedures (Brent 2001b; Baker 2005). Social enrichment opportunities typically work the best; these options will be discussed in more detail in the Socialisation section. This section will focus on inanimate enrichment strategies, including brief treatments of physical, sensory, foraging and occupational enhancement approaches (Figure 40.3).

Enclosures for captive chimpanzees should be physically complex enough to stimulate species-typical levels and

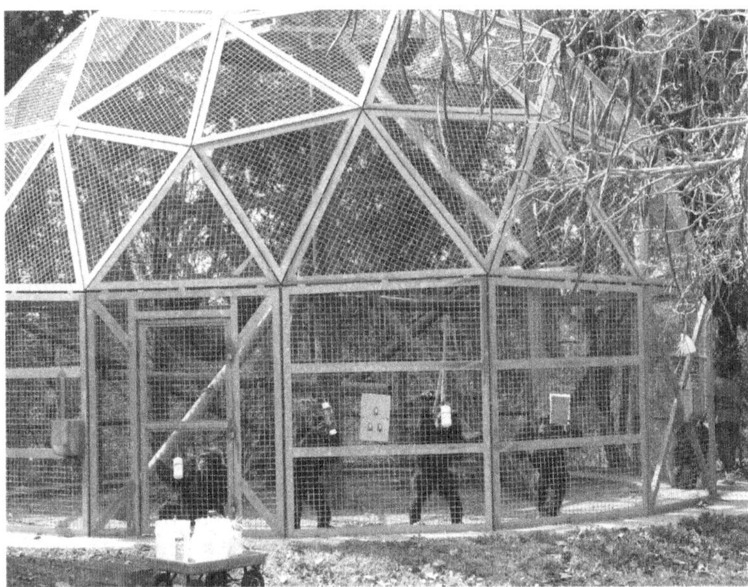

Figure 40.3 Foraging enrichment for chimpanzees in a Primadome at The University of Texas M. D. Anderson Cancer Center, Bastrop, TX, USA.

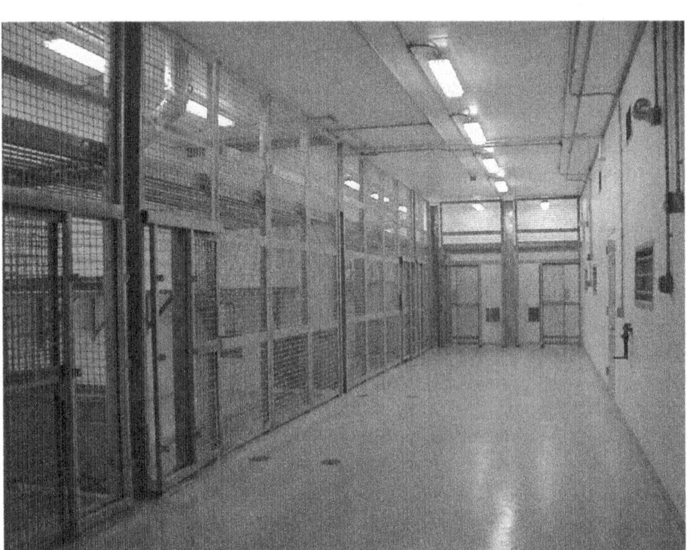

Figure 40.4 Indoor portion of enclosure with barred ceilings for brachiation at The University of Texas M. D. Anderson Cancer Center, Bastrop, TX, USA.

types of locomotor activity. While this can usually be achieved in situations where the enclosures include an outdoor component, it is somewhat more difficult when access to the outside is not possible. For animals maintained only indoors, it is especially important to provide opportunities for brachiation (typically using barred ceilings see Figure 40.4). Since young chimpanzees are considerably more physically active than older chimpanzees, physical enhancements that promote running, jumping, swinging etc may be more important for younger animals. However, since older captive chimpanzees may develop and exhibit health problems related to weight gain and a lack of physical activity, it may be important to provide an environment that also stimulates physical exercise in this age group (it would not be appropriate however, to house geriatric, mobility-impaired animals in environments that require high levels of exercise). As the number of young chimpanzees in research settings continues to decrease, enhancements that promote physical activity in older, mobile chimpanzees may be the most practical and valuable to implement.

While open-topped enclosures may provide especially naturalistic and functional environments for larger groups of chimpanzees, they also provide an additional opportunity for chimpanzees to escape. Complex climbing structures are typically provided in all outdoor chimpanzee enclosures – it is especially important when designing the structures to make sure that it is 'impossible' for the chimpanzees to jump out. Factors that require significant scrutiny include the distance (horizontal and vertical) between the structure and the top of the external wall and the availability of smaller items that could be stacked and used as ladders, or as poles for vaulting. Additionally, sufficient space must be provided between the walls and any overhanging objects outside the enclosure.

Sensory enrichment is most important for captive chimpanzees maintained in settings where there are limited opportunities for species-typical sensory stimulation. This would apply primarily to chimpanzees housed by themselves or in small groups in potentially static or sterile indoor environments. For animals living under these conditions, auditory (CDs), visual (videos or TV), olfactory and tactile (contact comfort items such as blankets) stimuli can serve as options for sensory enrichment (Bloomsmith & Lambeth 2000; Sak *et al.* 2005; Videan *et al.* 2007). The empirical data are not particularly convincing concerning the value of these types of enrichment for socially housed chimpanzees, and many of the studies on the topic have used sensory stimuli that are probably not 'species-typical' (music, cartoons, bubbles, etc). Overall though, sensory enrichment is reasonably inexpensive and easy to provide in many captive circumstances, so the inclusion of such stimuli, especially species-typical stimuli (sounds, videos or odours of conspecifics), in a comprehensive enrichment programme should be worthwhile. The value of sensory enrichment can be significantly enhanced by providing chimpanzees with the opportunity to control the sensory stimuli; to turn lights, TVs, radios, fans, etc on and off or to change the type of stimulus (eg, classical vs rock music; cartoons vs live action video) that they are experiencing (Bloomsmith *et al.* 2001; Schapiro & Lambeth 2007).

Since wild chimpanzees spend up to 60% of their waking day searching for, finding, processing and eating food items (Goodall 1986), it is imperative that the captive environment includes opportunities for the animals to work (forage) for their food. In the past, in many captive situations, highly nutritious, though frequently heavily processed food (chow, pellets or biscuits) was simply presented to the chimpanzees on a scheduled basis, at times that were convenient for those providing the food. Current feeding practices for captive chimpanzees are much better simulations (although still far from perfect) of natural chimpanzee feeding and foraging behaviour: (1) various types of food are distributed so that they must be searched for and located by the animals; (2) food items are presented in forms in which the animals have to work to get to the edible portions (whole fruits, food puzzles, foraging devices); and (3) multiple small meals are fed, rather than one or two large meals (Bloomsmith & Else 2005; Bloomsmith 2007). These types of foraging enrichment strategies can be implemented with both unprocessed foods (fruits, vegetables, seeds, etc) and processed foods (biscuits, chow or pellets) and can involve the construction and use of tools, an important component of natural chimpanzee foraging behaviour.

Chimpanzees have considerable cognitive abilities and occupational enrichment is typically designed and implemented to provide the animals with opportunities to use their cognitive skills (Bloomsmith & Else 2005). Computers with levers, joysticks or touch screens can be used for occupational enrichment, although any piece of apparatus (enrichment-related or research-related) used, must be made as 'chimp-proof' as possible (no device or apparatus is completely chimp-proof). Occupational enrichment will occasionally include the provision of food rewards, however occupational enrichment differs from foraging enrichment in that the occupational enrichment task is more important than the reward. It is not unreasonable to consider the tasks performed by chimpanzees maintained for cognitive experiments, primarily apparatus-based operant conditioning procedures, as occupational enrichment. Additionally, many of the tasks that comprise studies of cultural transmission, social learning, problem solving, laterality and behavioural economics (Silk *et al.* 2005; Hopkins *et al.* 2005, 2007; Brosnan *et al.* 2007; Hopper *et al.* 2007; Whiten *et al.* 2007) are also likely to function as occupational enrichment. Many of these techniques could serve as ideal behavioural assays of the effects of aging on cognitive function in the captive chimpanzee population.

Socialisation

Captive chimpanzees should be maintained in social groupings that promote naturalistic social behaviours, are stimulating, are safe and can be managed. The typical fission–fusion community of chimpanzees in the wild (Goodall 1986; Wrangham *et al.* 1994) is an extremely difficult type of social organisation to simulate in captivity. This is partially due to space limitations, but is also due, in part, to the potential for damaging aggressive episodes when chimpanzees are improperly introduced or re-introduced to one another (Fritz & Howell 2001). In the wild, the space available to animals and their 'flight' options are significantly greater than they are in the laboratory or zoo. Although in captivity (and on many research protocols) it is not possible to maintain chimpanzees in a fission–fusion community of 100 animals, it is possible functionally to simulate other aspects of their natural social organisation (Bloomsmith & Baker 2001). Specifically, captive managers of chimpanzees have had good success maintaining chimpanzees in multimale–multifemale groups of between eight and 20 animals, where male–male social behaviour can be expressed in a manner similar to that seen in the wild. One specific example of such interactions would be the post-aggression reconciliation, which is observed in both wild and captive groups of chimpanzees (Koski *et al.* 2007). Although multimale groups may result in infrequent outbreaks of aggression (as may unimale groups; Alford *et al.* 1995), the daily positive consequences of male–male affiliative and agonistic interactions are typically thought to outweigh the rare negative consequences of aggressive interactions.

The social development of juvenile and adolescent female chimpanzees is another potentially critical aspect of captive chimpanzee socialisation that merits discussion. The moratorium on breeding of research chimpanzees is likely to have long-term social consequences, beyond the reduction in size of the chimpanzee population. Currently, young female chimpanzees have few opportunities to allomother younger chimpanzees and these opportunities are progressively declining over time. While many of these females will have been raised by their own mothers, data from Bloomsmith and colleagues (2006) suggest that opportunities to 'aunt' infants should increase the probability that young females will be competent mothers when (and if) they give birth and a lack of such opportunities should decrease the probability. However, their data also suggest that about one third of females that are not raised by their mothers should still become competent mothers themselves (Bloomsmith *et al.* 2006). These findings could be important for understanding and assessing maternal competence, if the breeding moratorium is eventually lifted.

Positive reinforcement training

Positive reinforcement training (PRT) can be profitably employed in a number of ways in the management of captive chimpanzees. Animals can be trained to voluntarily participate in husbandry, veterinary and research procedures (Laule & Whittaker 2001; Lambeth *et al.* 2006; Schapiro & Lambeth 2007; Coleman *et al.* 2008), dramatically increasing the amount of control and choice available to them. This volume contains an entire chapter on PRT (Chapter 16), so only a few chimpanzee-specific highlights will be addressed here.

Chimpanzees have been trained to voluntarily present for injections (Lambeth *et al.* 2006). There are many benefits to having this behaviour under stimulus control, not the least of which is being able to administer a dose of anaesthetic (or antibiotic) in a manner that is as minimally stressful as possible. Recent studies have shown that numerous haematological and chemistry parameters obtained when chimpanzees voluntarily presented for an anaesthetic injection prior to a blood sample differed significantly from parameters obtained from samples in which subjects were non-voluntarily anaesthetised (Lambeth *et al.* 2006). This was true for comparisons across different subjects, but more importantly, was also true for within-subjects comparisons, in which the same subjects were non-voluntarily anaesthetised on one occasion and voluntarily presented for an anaesthetic injection on another occasion.

Chimpanzees have also been trained to voluntarily present for an unanaesthetised venepuncture and blood sample (Coleman *et al.* 2008). Among the small number of chimpanzees that have been trained to reliably perform this complex and difficult behaviour, the pattern of physiological results obtained is similar to that reported for present for injection above; haematology and chemistry parameters differed significantly between blood samples obtained voluntarily without anaesthesia and blood samples obtained from the same animals 2–3 days later when anaesthetised (Schapiro *et al.* 2006b).

PRT has been used to decrease food stealing and animal chasing during feeding times in relatively large (n = 8–16) social groups of chimpanzees (Bloomsmith *et al.* 1994). Briefly, chimpanzees that usually chased other animals and stole their food were trained using PRT techniques to perform a behaviour that was incompatible with chasing and stealing; namely, sitting in one place. Many management benefits were gained once the animals had been trained to feed in this 'co-operative' fashion, including a more equal distribution of food items (especially highly desirable food items) across all members of the group and the necessity of using fewer food items in order to make certain that each animal received the minimum portion.

Feeding

Wild chimpanzees spend much of their time searching for, working for, processing and eating food items, including constructing tools to obtain food. Captive chimpanzees should be fed in a manner that promotes foraging and tool use. Since wild chimpanzees tend to eat a wide variety of food items during foraging bouts throughout the day rather than large, human-like 'meals' of only one or two food items, captive chimpanzees should be encouraged to forage/feed on many foods in a number of bouts across the day to achieve a balanced diet (the National Research Council (2003) has published nutrient requirements for captive non-human primates, however this volume contains surprisingly little information of direct value to managers of captive chimpanzees). This is obviously a more work-intensive and potentially more costly approach for animal care staff than is feeding a few large, discrete meals of a limited number of foods. But the benefits to the animals of a more naturalistic feeding regimen are quantifiable (Bloomsmith 2007) and address the achievement of the general goal of functionally simulating natural conditions. Many of the strategies used to feed captive chimpanzees are predicated on issues of convenience, cost effectiveness and manageability for the care staff. Clearly, certain accommodations for such issues have to be made, but integrative strategies that take into account both human-related and chimpanzee-related factors are in use and are constantly being updated. As one example, by using small meals as positive reinforcement for the performance of timely shifting behaviour, the initial commitment of additional effort to the feeding of a larger number of smaller meals can ultimately reduce the amount of time required to get animals to voluntarily move from place to place.

Safety

The importance of maintaining a safe environment for chimpanzees and those working with them in captivity cannot be overemphasised. Chimpanzees can be dangerous to those who work with them (care staff, researchers, veterinarians) and to one another. Housing, handling and research protocols must take into account the animals' strength, health, social relationships and cognitive capabilities. Additionally, the potential for humans to make mistakes must be factored into all aspects of chimpanzee care and management. Effective and efficient SOPs must be developed and implemented to promote a safe environment for the animals and those responsible for them. While it is essential to have SOPs for working with chimpanzees, it is also critical that SOPs are followed with little or no deviation. If aspects of SOPs are unmanageable or inappropriate, then the SOPs need to be modified. Even seemingly harmless enrichment tools and devices need to be 'safety-assessed' as chimpanzees will often use them for unintended (but no doubt enriching) purposes, such as using foraging tubes as projectiles and foraging sticks as weapons.

Retirement and sanctuaries

As the population of laboratory (and zoo) chimpanzees continues to age, it will be necessary to retire some of the animals (Figure 40.5). Primary candidates for retirement include those animals that are deemed no longer 'useful' for research (or exhibition in the zoo). 'Useful' can be defined in a number of different ways, some of which are quite contentious, especially if animals have to be removed from social groups at their research facility and placed in one of

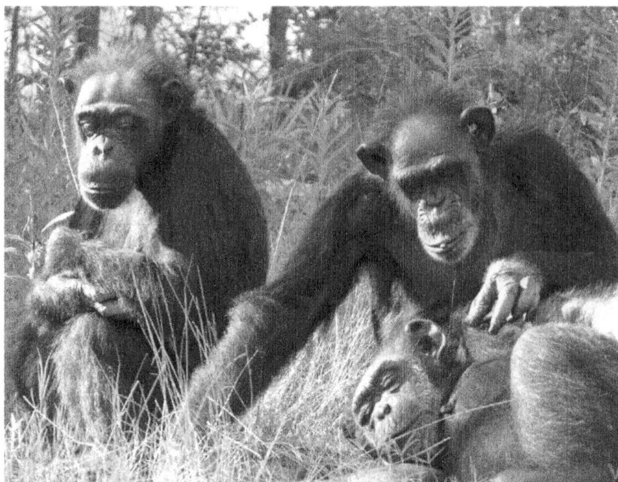

Figure 40.5 Former laboratory chimpanzees in the 5-acre natural enclosure at Chimp Haven, Keithsville, LA, USA. Reproduced with permission of Chimp Haven.

the small number of credible chimpanzee sanctuaries. Many of these sanctuaries do not permit even non-invasive manipulations of their retired residents, a reasonable policy in certain circumstances, but one that may also prevent the non-invasive collection of extremely valuable research data, especially data related to the aging process.

Common welfare problems

Most of the chapters in this Handbook include a section on common welfare problems, including disease issues and behavioural factors, and how to deal with them. Virtually everything contained in the present chapter has been written to address common welfare issues that must be considered and managed when housing chimpanzees in captivity; essentially all aspects of the management of captive chimpanzees have been designed and are updated to provide continual enhancements to the welfare of the animals.

Priorities and future directions

While captive chimpanzees have been reasonably well studied in the past and new publications are accruing at a steady rate, there are still areas of investigation where additional important data should be collected. Management-orientated research questions that should receive considerable attention in the near future include: long-term consequences of developmental, management and reproductive schemes; captive techniques that optimally simulate natural conditions; and physiological consequences of providing control and choice, just to name a few. Additionally, a number of non-invasive imaging techniques should be more widely adapted and routinely used to collect dependent measures in investigations focusing on chimpanzee behaviour, cognition and physiology. Where possible, animals should be trained to participate voluntarily in these procedures without anaesthesia.

The amount of space 'required' by captive chimpanzees is another question that needs to be empirically investigated. Space per animal is one variable that is regularly 'addressed' by rules, regulations and/or regulatory bodies (International Primatological Society Captive Care Committee 2007), and may turn out to be a critical aspect in the performance of GLP studies with chimpanzees. GLP studies have additional experimental and documentation requirements compared to non-GLP studies, and often result in subjects living in more restricted housing conditions. It would be quite useful to have some objective criteria by which to determine how much space a chimpanzee (or other non-human primate) 'needs' as a study subject or simply as a member of a resource colony. While it is quite clear that the quality of the space and who else is occupying it are more important than the quantity of space for most captive non-human primates (in laboratories or zoos), empirically determined space guidelines would benefit both animals and humans. These are difficult and expensive investigations to perform however, requiring evaluation of a wide array of housing options, not just cages/enclosures that are slightly smaller or slightly larger than those recommended in the current and relevant guidelines (Crockett *et al.* 2000).

Concluding remarks

Chimpanzees are extremely valuable animals that present a number of very significant moral, ethical and practical challenges for those involved with their management and use in captivity. Their many similarities to humans make them of great interest to all people and important models for a variety of investigations. However, these similarities also create dilemmas related to their appropriate care and use. Those responsible for the welfare of captive chimpanzees must continuously strive to provide them with safe environments that stimulate the performance of a wide range of species-typical behaviours. Those responsible for studying captive chimpanzees must continuously strive to develop innovative research procedures that refine the ways that these animals are handled in captivity.

Acknowledgements

The time to prepare this chapter was supported in part by NIH/NCRR U42-RR15090.

References

Alford, P.L., Bloomsmith, M.A., Keeling, M.E. *et al.* (1995) Wounding aggression during the formation and maintenance of captive multimale chimpanzee groups. *Zoo Biology*, **14**, 347–359

Arnhem, E., Dupain, J., Vercauteren Drubbel, R. *et al.* (2008) Selective logging, habitat quality and home range use by sympatric gorillas and chimpanzees: a case study from an active logging concession in Southeast Cameroon. *Folia Primatologica*, **79**, 1–14

Baker, K. (2005) Chimpanzees. In: *Enrichment for Nonhuman Primates*. pp. 28–42. NIH Office of Laboratory Animal Welfare, Bethesda

Baker, K.C., Weed, J.L., Crockett, C.M. *et al.* (2007) Survey of environmental enhancement programs for laboratory primates. *American Journal of Primatology*, **69**, 377–394

Becquet, C., Patterson, N., Stone, A.C. *et al.* (2007) Genetic structure of chimpanzee populations. *PLoS Genetics*, **3**, e66. doi:10.1371/journal.pgen.0030066

Bettinger, T.L. and DeMatteo, K.E. (2001) Reproductive management of captive chimpanzees: Contraceptive decisions. In: *The Care and Management of Captive Chimpanzees, Special Topics in Primatology*, Vol. 2. Ed Brent, L., pp. 119–145. American Society of Primatologists, San Antonio

Bettinger, T., Cougar, D., Lee, D.R. *et al.* (1997) Ovarian hormone concentrations and genital swelling patterns in female chimpanzees with Norplant implants. *Zoo Biology*, **16**, 209–223

Biro, D., Sousa, C. and Matsuzawa, T. (2006) Ontogeny and cultural propagation of tool use by wild chimpanzees at Bossou, Guinea: Case studies in nut cracking and leaf folding. In: *Cognitive Development in Chimpanzees*. Eds Matsuzawa, T., Tomonaga, M. and Tanaka, M., pp. 476–508. Springer, New York

Bloomsmith, M. (2007) Feeding enrichment for chimpanzees (*Pan troglodytes*): twenty years later. *American Journal of Primatology*, **69** (Suppl 1), 124

Bloomsmith, M.A. and Baker, K.C. (2001) Social management of captive chimpanzees. In: *The Care and Management of Captive Chimpanzees, Special Topics in Primatology*, Vol. 2. Ed Brent, L., pp. 205–241. American Society of Primatologists, San Antonio

Bloomsmith, M.A., Baker, K.C., Lambeth, S.P. *et al.* (2001) Is giving chimpanzees control over environmental enrichment a good idea? In: *The Apes: Challenges for the 21st Century. Conference Proceedings*. pp. 88–89. Brookfield Zoo, Brookfield

Bloomsmith, M.A., Baker, K.C., Ross, S.R. *et al.* (2006a) Early rearing conditions and captive chimpanzee behavior: some surprising findings. In: *Nursery Rearing of Nonhuman Primates in the 21st Century*. Eds Sackett, G.P., Ruppenthal, G.C. and Elias, D., pp. 289–312. Springer, New York

Bloomsmith, M.A. and Else, J.G. (2005) Behavioral management of chimpanzees in biomedical research facilities: The state of the science. *ILAR Journal*, **46**, 192–201

Bloomsmith, M.A. and Lambeth, S.P. (2000) Videotapes as enrichment for captive chimpanzees (*Pan troglodytes*). *Zoo Biology*, **19**, 541–551

Bloomsmith, M.A., Laule, G.E., Alford, P.L. *et al.* (1994) Using training to moderate chimpanzee aggression during feeding. *Zoo Biology*, **13**, 557–566

Bloomsmith, M.A., Schapiro, S.J. and Strobert, E.A. (2006b) Preparing chimpanzees for laboratory research. *ILAR Journal*, **47**, 316–325

Boesch, C., Crockford, C., Herbinger, I. *et al.* (2008) Intergroup conflicts among chimpanzees in Taï National Park: lethal violence and the female perspective. *American Journal of Primatology*, **70**, 519–532

Boesch, C., Head, J., Tagg, N. *et al.* (2007) Fatal chimpanzee attack in Loango National Park, Gabon. *International Journal of Primatology*, **28**, 1025–1034

Brent, L. (2001a) *The Care and Management of Captive Chimpanzees: Special Topics in Primatology*, Vol. 2. Ed. Brent, L. American Society of Primatologists, San Antonio

Brent, L. (2001b) Behavior and environmental enrichment of individually housed chimpanzees. In: *The Care and Management of Captive Chimpanzees, Special Topics in Primatology*, Vol. 2. Ed Brent, L., pp. 147–171. American Society of Primatologists, San Antonio

Brent, L. (2007) Life-long well being: Applying animal welfare science to nonhuman primates in sanctuaries. *Journal of Applied Animal Welfare Science*, **10**, 55–61

Brosnan, S.F., Jones, O.D., Lambeth, S.P. *et al.* (2007) Endowment effects in chimpanzees. *Current Biology*, **17**, 1704–1707

Carlsson, H-E., Schapiro, S.J., Farah, I. *et al.* (2004) Use of primates in research: A global overview. *American Journal of Primatology*, **63**, 225–237

Cohen, J. (2007a) The endangered lab chimp. *Science*, **315**, 450–452

Cohen, J. (2007b) NIH to end chimp breeding for research. *Science*, **316**, 1265

Coleman, K., Pranger, L., Maier, A. *et al.* (2008) Training rhesus macaques for venipuncture using positive reinforcement techniques: a comparison with chimpanzees. *Journal of the American Association for Laboratory Animal Science*, **47**, 37–41

Crockett, C.M., Shimoji, M. and Bowden, D.M. (2000) Behavior, appetite, and urinary cortisol responses by adult female pigtailed macaques to cage size, cage level, room change, and ketamine sedation. *American Journal of Primatology*, **52**, 63–80

Deschner, T. and Boesch, C. (2007) Can the patterns of sexual swelling cycles in female Tai chimpanzees be explained by the cost-of-sexual-attraction hypothesis? *International Journal of Primatology*, **28**, 389–406

Doane, C.J., Lee, D.R. and Sleeper, M.M. (2006) Electrocardiogram abnormalities in captive chimpanzees (*Pan troglodytes*). *Comparative Medicine*, **56**, 512–518.

Elmowalid, G.A., Qiao, M., Jeong, S.H., *et al.* (2007) Immunization with hepatitis C virus-like particles results in control of hepatitis C virus infection in chimpanzees. *Proceedings of the National Academy of Sciences of the USA*, **104**, 8427–8432

Fa, J.D., Ryan, S.F. and Bell, D.J. (2005) Hunting vulnerability, ecological characteristics and harvest rates of bushmeat species in afrotropical forests. *Biological Conservation*, **121**, 167–176

Fritz, J. and Howell, S. (2001) Captive chimpanzee social group formation. In: *The Care and Management of Captive Chimpanzees, Special Topics in Primatology*, Vol. 2. Ed Brent, L., pp. 173–203. American Society of Primatologists, San Antonio

Fritz, J., Wolfle, T.L. and Howell, S. (1999) Chimpanzees. In: *The UFAW Handbook on the Care and Management of Laboratory Animals*, Vol. 1 *Terrestrial Vertebrates*, 7th edn. Ed. Poole, T., pp. 643–658. UFAW, Potters Bar

Fulk, R. and Garland, C. (1992) *The Care and Management of Chimpanzees (Pan troglodytes) in Captive Environments: A Husbandry Manual Developed for the Chimpanzee Species Survival Plan.* North Carolina Zoological Park, Asheboro

Gonder, M.K., Disotell, T.R. and Oates, J.F. (2006) New genetic evidence on the evolution of chimpanzee populations and implications for taxonomy. *International Journal of Primatology*, **27**, 1103–1127

Goodall, J. (1986) *The Chimpanzees of Gombe, Patterns of Behaviour*. The Belknap Press of Harvard University, Cambridge

Groves, C. (2005) The taxonomy of primates in the laboratory context. In: *The Laboratory Primate*. Ed. Wolfe-Coote, S., pp. 3–15, Elsevier, San Diego

Hanamura, S., Kiyono, M., Lukasik-Braum, M., *et al.* (2008) Chimpanzee deaths at Mahale caused by a flu-like disease. *Primates*, **49**, 77–80

Herndon, J.G. and Tigges, J. (2001) Hematologic and blood biochemical variables of captive chimpanzees: cross-sectional and longitudinal analyses. *Comparative Medicine*, **51**, 60–69

Hopkins, W.D., Russell, J., Freeman, H. *et al.* (2005) The distribution and development of handedness for manual gestures in captive chimpanzees (*Pan troglodytes*). *Psychological Science*, **16**, 487–493

Hopkins, W.D., Russell, J.L., Remkus, M. *et al.* (2007) Handedness and grooming in *Pan troglodytes*: comparative analysis between findings in captive and wild individuals. *International Journal of Primatology*, **28**, 1315–1326

Hopper, L.M., Spiteri, A., Lambeth, S.P. *et al.* (2007) Experimental studies of traditions and underlying transmission processes in chimpanzees. *Animal Behaviour*, **73**, 1021–1032

Howell, S., Hoffman, K., Bartel, L. *et al.* (2003) Normal hematological and serum clinical chemistry values for captive chimpanzees (*Pan troglodytes*). *Comparative Medicine*, **53**, 413–423

Ihrig, M., Tassinary, L.G., Bernacky, B. *et al.* (2001) Hematologic and serum biochemistry reference intervals for the chimpanzee (*Pan troglodytes*) categorized by age and sex. *Comparative Medicine*, **51**, 30–37

International Primatological Society Captive Care Committee (2007) *IPS International Guidelines for the Acquisition, Care and Breeding of Nonhuman Primates*. IPS, Orlando

Knight, A. (2007) The poor contribution of chimpanzee experiments to biomedical progress. *Journal of Applied Animal Welfare Science*, **10**, 281–308

Kondgen, S., Kuhl, H., N'Goran, P.K. *et al.* (2008) Pandemic human viruses cause decline of endangered great apes. *Current Biology*, **18**, 260–264

Kormos, R., Bakarr, M.I., Bonnehin, L. *et al.* (2003) Bushmeat hunting as a threat to chimpanzees in West Africa. In: *West African Chimpanzees: Status Survey and Conservation Action Plan*. Eds Kormos, R., Boesch, C., Bakarr, M.I. *et al.*, pp. 151-155. IUCN – World Conservation Union, Gland, Switzerland

Koski, S.E., Koops, K. and Sterck, E.H.M. (2007) Reconciliation, relationship quality, and postconflict anxiety: testing the integrated hypothesis in captive chimpanzees. *American Journal of Primatology*, **69**, 158–172

Lambeth, S.P., Hau, J., Perlman, J.E. *et al.* (2006) Positive reinforcement training affects hematologic and serum chemistry values in captive chimpanzees (*Pan troglodytes*). *American Journal of Primatology*, **68**, 245–256

Lammey, M.L., Lee, D.R., Ely, J.J. *et al.* (2008) Sudden cardiac death in 13 captive chimpanzees (*Pan troglodytes*). *Journal of Medical Primatology*, **37** (Suppl 1), 39–43

Lamperez, A.J. and Rowell, T.J. (2005) Normal C-reactive protein values for captive chimpanzees (*Pan troglodytes*). *Contemporary Topics in Laboratory Animal Science*, **44**, 25–26

Laule, G. and Whittaker, M. (2001) Training for cooperative behaviors and enrichment. In: *The Care and Management of Captive Chimpanzees, Special Topics in Primatology*, Vol. 2. Ed Brent, L., pp. 243–265. American Society of Primatologists, San Antonio

Lee, D.R. and Guhad, F.A. (2001) Chimpanzee health care and medicine program. In: *The Care and Management of Captive Chimpanzees, Special Topics in Primatology*, Vol. 2. Ed Brent, L., pp. 83–117. American Society of Primatologists, San Antonio

Mitani, J.C. and Watts, D.P. (2005) Correlates of territorial boundary patrol behaviour in wild chimpanzees. *Animal Behaviour*, **70**, 1079–1086

National Research Council (1996) *Guide for the Care and Use of Laboratory Animals*, 7th edn. National Academy Press, Washington, DC

National Research Council (1997) *Chimpanzees in Research. Strategies for Their Ethical Care, Management, and Use*. National Academy Press, Washington, DC

National Research Council (1998) *Psychological Well-being of Nonhuman Primates*. National Academy Press, Washington, DC

National Research Council (2003) *Nutrient Requirements of Nonhuman Primates*, 2nd edn. National Academy Press, Washington, DC

Parr, L.A., Waller, B.M., Vick, S.J. *et al.* (2007) Classifying chimpanzee facial expressions using muscle action. *Emotion*, **7**, 172–181

Poole, T. (1999) *The UFAW Handbook on the Care and Management of Laboratory Animals, Vol. 1 Terrestrial Vertebrates*, 7th edn. UFAW, Potters Bar

Pruetz, J.D. (2007) Evidence of cave use by savanna chimpanzees (*Pan troglodytes verus*) at Fongoli, Senegal: implications for thermoregulatory behavior. *Primates*, **48**, 316–319

Pruetz, J.D. and Bertolani, P. (2007) Savannah chimpanzees, *Pan troglodytes verus*, hunt with tools. *Current Biology*, **17**, 412–417

Roach, M. (2008) Almost human. *National Geographic*, **213**, 124–145

Roof, K.A., Hopkins, W.D., Izard, M.K *et al.* (2005) Maternal age, parity, and reproductive outcome in captive chimpanzees (*Pan troglodytes*). *American Journal of Primatology*, **67**, 199–207

Ross, S.R. (in press) *Chimpanzee Animal Care Manual*. Association of Zoos and Aquariums, Silver Spring

Rowan, A. (2007) Letter to the editor. *Science*, **315**, 1493

Russell, W.M.S. and Burch, R.L. (1959) *The Principles of Humane Experimental Technique*. Methuen and Co Ltd, London

Sak, A., Videan, E. and Fritz, J. (2005) The effects of aromatherapy on the behavior and psychological well-being of captive chimpanzees (*Pan troglodytes*). *American Journal of Primatology*, **66** (Suppl 1), 146

Schapiro, S.J. and Lambeth, S.P. (2007) Control, choice, and assessments of the value of behavioral management to nonhuman primates in captivity. *Journal of Applied Animal Welfare Science*, **10**, 39–47

Schapiro, S.J., Lambeth, S.P., Perlman, J.E. *et al.* (2006a) Immunological responses and captive procedures in rhesus monkeys and chimpanzees. *International Journal of Primatology*, **27** (Suppl 1), 25

Schapiro, S.J., Lambeth, S.P., Perlman, J.E. *et al.* (2006b) Positive reinforcement training may diminish interindividual variation in physiological parameters among captive chimpanzees (*Pan troglodytes*). *International Journal of Primatology*, **27** (Suppl 1), 72

Schapiro, S.J., Lambeth, S.P., Thiele, E. *et al.* (2007) The effects of behavioral management programs on dependent measures in biomedical research. *American Journal of Primatology*, **69** (Suppl 1), 115

Silk, J.B., Brosnan, S.F., Vonk, J. *et al.* (2005) Chimpanzees are indifferent to the welfare of unrelated group members. *Nature*, **437**, 1357–1359

Stanford, C. (2008) *Apes of the Impenetrable Forest: The Behavioral Ecology of Sympatric Chimpanzees and Gorillas*. Pearson/Prentice Hall, Upper Saddle River

Stewart, F.A., Pruetz, J.D. and Hansell, H.M. (2007) Do chimpanzees build comfortable nests? *American Journal of Primatology*, **69**, 930–939

Stump, D.S. and VandeWoude, S. (2007) Animal models for HIV AIDS: a comparative review. *Comparative Medicine*, **57**, 33–43

The Chimpanzee Sequencing and Analysis Consortium (2005) Initial sequence of the chimpanzee genome and comparison with the human genome. *Nature*, **437**, 69–87

Tutin, C.E.G. (1994) Reproductive success story: variability among chimpanzees and comparisons with gorillas. In: *Chimpanzee Cultures*. Eds Wrangham, R.W., McGrew, W.C., deWaal, F.B.M. *et al.*, pp. 181–194. Harvard University Press, Cambridge

VandeBerg, J.L., Zola, S.M., Fritz, J. *et al.* (2005) A unique biomedical resource at risk. *Nature*, **437**, 30–32

Varki, A. (2007) Letter to the Editor. *Science*, **315**, 1493

Varki, A. and Nelson, D.L. (2007) Genomic comparisons of humans and chimpanzees. *Annual Review of Anthropology*, **36**, 191–209

Venter, J.C., Adams, M.D., Myers, E.W. *et al.* (2001) The sequence of the human genome. *Science*, **291**, 1304–1351

Videan, E.N. and Fritz, J. (2007) Effects of short- and long-term changes in spatial density on the social behavior of captive chimpanzees (*Pan troglodytes*). *Applied Animal Behaviour Science*, **102**, 95–105

Videan, E.N., Fritz, J., Howell, S. *et al.* (2007) Effects of two types and two genre of music on social behavior in captive chimpanzees (*Pan troglodytes*). *Journal of the American Association for Laboratory Animal Science*, **46**, 66–70

Videan, E.N., Fritz, J. and Murphy, J. (2008) Effects of aging on hematology and serum clinical chemistry in chimpanzees (*Pan troglodytes*). *American Journal of Primatology*, **70**, 327–338

Wallis, J. (1992) Chimpanzee genital swelling and its role in the pattern of sociosexual behavior. *American Journal of Primatology*, **28**, 101–113

Watts, D.P., Muller, M., Amsler, S.J. *et al.* (2006) Lethal intergroup aggression by chimpanzees in Kibale National Park, Uganda. *American Journal of Primatology*, **68**, 161–180

Whiten, A., Spiteri, A., Horner, V. *et al.* (2007) Transmission of multiple traditions with and between chimpanzee groups. *Current Biology*, **17**, 1038–1043

Woodward, R.A. and Weld, K.P. (1997) A comparison of ketamine, ketamine-acepromazine, and tiletamine-zolazepam on various hematologic parameters in rhesus monkeys (*Macaca mulatta*). *Contemporary Topics in Laboratory Animal Science*, **36**, 55–57

Wrangham, R.W. (1994) The evolution of sexuality in chimpanzees and bonobos. *Human Nature*, **4**, 47–79

Wrangham, R.W., McGrew, W.C., de Waal, F.B.M. *et al.* (1994) *Chimpanzee Cultures*. Harvard University Press, Cambridge

Birds

41 The domestic fowl

Ian J.H. Duncan

Biological overview

Origins

The domestic fowl is derived from the junglefowl, probably mainly from the Burmese red junglefowl (*Gallus gallus spadiceous*, Bonnaterre), but possibly with contributions from the other three junglefowl species (Siegel *et al.* 1992). The junglefowl is a ground-dwelling, gallinaceous bird with territorial males looking after small harems of two to ten females with their offspring. Junglefowl are considered graminivorous, feeding on leafy material, seeds and grains, but, as with many gallinaceous species, the young chicks require a higher-quality diet than this and feed on insects and other invertebrates for the first few weeks of life. Junglefowl are extremely timid and secretive and therefore difficult to study in the wild. They can fly reasonably and roost in trees at night and occasionally through the day. Otherwise they spend most of their time on the ground and tend to run from frightening stimuli.

Domestic fowl have probably been domesticated for about 5000 years but early archaeological records are scant. Two features of their early history are of note. The first is that it seems likely the original relationship between human beings and the progenitors of chickens was a predator–prey one. The usual reaction of prey species to predators is a fearful one and the evidence suggests that domestication has not removed this completely (Duncan 1990). The second is that during much of their domestication, chickens were selected for fighting ability, not for their egg- or meat-producing capabilities (Wood-Gush 1959), and this probably accounts for the aggressiveness of some modern strains.

Lifespan

Domestic fowl have a life span of 5–8 years. Commercially, egg-laying hens are kept for only 1 or 2 laying years, because egg production declines rather rapidly after this. Breeding birds of egg-laying strains are also kept for 1 or 2 years. Breeding stock for broilers are kept for less than a full laying year because fertility declines so quickly that it is not worthwhile keeping them longer. Broilers themselves, of course, are killed at ages ranging from 32–70 days depending on what final product is required.

The unnaturally short lives of commercial chickens should not necessarily set the pattern for laboratories. Chickens can live healthy lives for at least 4–6 years, and this should be made use of if possible.

Social organisation

The basic social unit of jungle fowl consists of about 4–12 females accompanied by a dominant male and their subadult offspring. Dominant males establish and defend territories (Collias *et al.* 1966). From the scant information that is available, it appears that domestic fowl that have gone feral, have a very similar organisation (McBride *et al.* 1969). When in a group, domestic fowl form a social hierarchy. Males and females do not generally interact agonistically, although males tend to dominate females passively. Male and female hierarchies are separate. Once formed, the social hierarchy is fairly stable with little social friction. On the other hand, mixing strangers together leads to a lot of fighting.

Under commercial or laboratory conditions, domestic fowl are fairly adaptable. In order to control disease transmission, they are normally kept in single-age groups and this is not a problem for them. Newly hatched chicks are precocial and develop normally without contact with their dam. They are also able to adapt easily to being kept in single- or mixed-sex groups. As males approach sexual maturity, they may become very aggressive to each other. This is generally not a problem if they are in mixed-sex groups and the sex ratio is kept at 10 or more females per male. However, in all-male groups, the aggression may lead to injury, and it may be necessary to house males individually. In general, domestic fowl will adapt to the range of group sizes normally found in a laboratory, (ie, from three to four to several hundred).

Breeds, strains and genetics

Chickens kept for commercial purposes can generally be divided into three main types, two of which are kept for eggs and one for meat production. In Europe and North America, white-egg-laying strains are derived from the White Leghorn breed, whereas brown-egg-laying strains are derived from a variety of breeds but usually include some Light Sussex and Rhode Island Red or Rhode Island White blood. Elsewhere in the world, there may be incorporation of local genetic material such as the Australorp breed in Australia. Meat-producing strains (usually referred to as 'broilers') are derived from many different breeds including Cornish and White Rock. Primary breeding companies keep selected inbred lines which produce grandparent, parent, and eventually three- or four-way cross hybrid chicks which are sold on the commercial market. This method exploits hybrid vigour and gives an extremely productive and uniform final product, the hybrid chicken. This structure in the poultry industry also separates breeding from commercial production which provides good biological security. It also, of course, provides great genetic security to the primary breeding companies, since the result of breeding commercial stock would be genetic segregation and recombination and a whole mixture of genotypes of little value.

Reproduction

Reproductive function in domestic fowl is at least partly controlled by day length. Commercially, egg-laying strains and breeders are kept under short day conditions (often 8 h light and 16 h dark or 10 h light and 14 h dark) until they are about 16 weeks of age in the case of laying strains and 20–22 weeks of age in the case of broiler breeders. They are then photo-stimulated by increasing day length by about 1 h per week to 20–22 weeks (in the case of laying strains) to 14 L : 10 D or 15 L : 9 D. Thereafter, day length usually remains constant. There are various modifications that can be made (see, for example, Lewis & Morris 2006), but this basic lighting programme works well. For ease of management, males and females of the same age are usually used, although it would be possible to successfully photo-stimulate males earlier.

When hens of laying strains are photo-stimulated in week 16, the first egg is usually laid in week 18, the birds reach 5% production in week 20 and peak production, which should be well over 90% (90 eggs per 100 birds per day), is reached in weeks 26–28. There is then a gradual decline in egg production until at week 72 or 74 the birds should be laying at about 70%. Commercially, day length is often gradually increased through the laying year but there is no good evidence that this actually stimulates more production. A long day of only 14 or 15 h (in contrast to a very long day of 16 or 18 h) may have more welfare advantages for the hens, in that it provides them with plenty of rest and they do not have an exceptionally long day to fill with activities. With broiler breeders, egg production is delayed by 2–3 weeks and is lower.

It should be remembered that birds differ from mammals in that the male is the homogametic sex carrying two similar sex chromosomes designated ZZ, with females being heterogametic and designated ZW. The fowl has some useful sex-linked traits such as silver (S) and gold (s) down colour, and slow (K) and fast (k) feathering. These traits enable chicks to be sexed easily at hatching.

Behaviour

The behaviour of the domestic fowl has been well studied and reported (eg, Wood-Gush 1971; Duncan 1980; Appleby *et al.* 2004). Chickens spend a considerable part of the day foraging for food. This is true even if food is provided in a very concentrated and highly nutritious form so that they can consume their requirements in a short time; they still spend many hours pecking, probing and flicking with their beaks and scratching with their feet. A good husbandry system should allow this foraging behaviour to occur unimpeded. Chickens can adapt their drinking behaviour to different sources of water such as troughs, cups or nipples. However, if they have learned to obtain water from one source, they may not recognise it if it is offered from another source.

Other maintenance behaviour includes preening and other activities associated with feather care. Domestic fowl do not bathe in water, but show dust-bathing behaviour which functions to rid the feathers of excess lipids. Sleeping and resting are normally done in a perching position but domestic fowl seem able to adapt to flat-footed resting and sleeping.

As mentioned previously, chickens are highly social animals. They also tend to synchronise their activities and do things together as a flock. It is therefore important that the facilities provided allow them to do this. The only activity in which chickens will take turns, is drinking at a limited water source. All these social activities, both agonistic and associative, are organised by a rich repertoire of visual and vocal signals.

Domestic chicks are precocial when they hatch. Although the mother hen would normally be responsible for showing chicks sources of food and water, they are quite able to learn to feed and drink on their own when food and water are obvious. The one function they cannot manage well is thermoregulation; young chicks, therefore, have to be kept in a warm environment for the first few weeks of life.

Mating behaviour is preceded by elaborate courtship with the male being the initiator and main actor. Once inseminated, the hen remains fertile for about 14 days although fertility drops quickly after 7 days. Nesting behaviour is complex and involves both nest site selection and nest building and may occupy 60–90 minutes every time an egg is laid. The evidence suggests that the performance of this behaviour is very important to the hen (Follensbee *et al.* 1992).

One other behaviour pattern requires special mention, and that is feather pecking and cannibalism which can be a problem in some strains of laying fowl. Outbreaks of feather pecking and cannibalism can occur at any time in a chicken's life but the common times are from 6–12 weeks and at point-of-lay. This behaviour has nothing to do with aggression and is probably some form of foraging behaviour directed at other birds' feathers rather than a potential food source (Blokhuis & Arkes 1984; Blokhuis 1986). It is likely that many factors contribute to an outbreak of feather pecking, including large group size, wire floor housing and bright lighting (Kjaer & Vestergaard 1999). Feather pecking behaviour varies substantially between strains of domestic fowl and it has been shown to be a heritable trait (Kjaer & Sørensen 1997) which can be selected against (Muir & Craig 1998).

The most effective way to reduce the effects of feather pecking is to debeak (beak trim) the birds. However, there is strong evidence that this causes both acute and chronic pain and therefore reduces the welfare of the birds (Duncan *et al.* 1989; Gentle *et al.* 1990). Therefore, where possible, strains with low tendencies to feather peck should be chosen; if the chosen strain has a bad reputation for feather pecking, then the chicks should be precision debeaked at the hatchery – a procedure which is less traumatic than later debeaking (Gentle *et al.* 1997).

Standard biological data

Body weights for various strains of domestic fowl are shown in Table 41.1. Growth rate depends on the strain of chicken being used. The primary breeding companies produce 'Management Guides' with growth curves for each of their hybrids. As an example, females of a light hybrid strain should weigh around 450, 900 and 1350 g at 6, 12 and 18 weeks of age. If reproductive fitness is important for the research being undertaken, then it is essential that chickens reach the correct weight for age as they are growing. There is usually no problem with light hybrids which can be fed *ad libitum*. Medium hybrids have a slight tendency to gain weight too rapidly, so growth rate must be checked regularly during the rearing period. Moderate food rationing can easily correct any tendency for the birds to gain too much weight. Broiler breeders, on the other hand, have enormous appetites and have to be very severely food restricted in order to be reproductively fit later in life. This is a big animal welfare problem in the poultry industry. There is no easy solution; the short-term welfare of broiler breeding fowl must be reduced by keeping them on severe food restriction so that they suffer from extreme hunger every day, or they suffer later in life from diseases of excessive weigh gain, including abnormalities of limb bone development (leg weakness) and obesity. For this reason, laboratories should avoid using broiler breeding fowl if at all possible. Of course this may not be possible if the birds are being used as a model in obesity or pathological bone growth studies.

Chickens have a core temperature of about 41.5 °C (Whittow 1986). Like many avian species, they have good control over blood flow to the lower, unfeathered part of the leg and the feet and can use this to conserve or dissipate heat. The resting heart rate of adult fowl is about 230 beats/min and this increases to about 280–320 beats/min in active but undisturbed birds. When frightened, the heart rate can rise to 460 beats/min (range 380–460) (Duncan 1981).

Table 41.1 Average body weights of various types of domestic fowl.

Type of bird	*Average weight (kg)*
Light[a] hybrid adult females	1.3–1.8
Light[a] hybrid adult males	2.0–2.6
Medium[a] hybrid adult females	1.5–2.2
Medium[a] hybrid adult males	3.0–3.6
Female broilers at 42 days	1.9
Male broilers at 42 days	2.2
Broiler breeder adult females[b]	3.0
Broiler breeder adult males[b]	4.0

[a] 'Light' and 'medium' refer to light and medium body weight birds, the two common types of fowl kept for table egg production.
[b] These weights refer to birds which are food-restricted according to the management guidelines.

Uses in the Laboratory

The domestic fowl (*Gallus gallus domesticus*) continues to be a popular laboratory animal. It is small and comparatively cheap and easy to maintain. It also has several biological features that make it the species of choice for several avenues of research. For example, there is still great interest in immune function in chickens. B lymphocytes were first described in chickens, the 'B' referring to the bursa of Fabricius. The chicken is also often preferred for classical studies in developmental biology. It lost ground to the mouse some years ago when mouse genetics surged ahead, but the convenience of having the embryo on hand outside the mother has meant that many laboratories have continued to work with chick embryos. The chicken is also favoured for certain oncological studies probably because the avian leucosis viruses are amongst the better characterised tumour-forming viruses. The chick embryo is also used fairly widely in general virus research and toxicology studies. Of course, in addition to being used as models for other species and for some general biological principles, chickens are also used in agricultural laboratories specialising in chickens.

Sources of supply

Laboratories using domestic fowl can buy day-old chicks from commercial hatcheries each time more birds are required. A commercial type can be selected to suit the requirements of the particular lines of research. Moreover, the sex of bird required can be specified. This strategy will result in a dependable source of uniform birds. Over the short term, it will also result in birds with a very similar genetic make-up. However, the primary breeding companies are constantly striving for improvement, and, every few years, introduce new hybrids and discontinue old ones. If genetic similarity is important for the research over an extended period, then a different strategy should be adopted. Many countries have specialised non-commercial lines of poultry available. These may be research lines maintained by other laboratories, or pure breeds maintained by local fanciers. Information on these sources can usually be obtained from government agricultural departments/ministries, university animal science departments, or poultry research institutes/centres. Pure breeds may be of interest because they carry particular genes such as the gene for polydactyly carried by the Silkie breed. Another solution is to maintain breeding stock, but this tends to be expensive. The minimum number of breeding birds required to avoid inbreeding problems is about 20 males and 20 females in each generation. This assumes that all 40 birds will contribute to the next generation, which implies the use of artificial insemination. It should be remembered that if the research to be carried out involves chick embryos, then the source of the eggs is very important. For example, certain research projects might require background information on the disease status and vaccination programme of the parent flock; such information may or may not be available for fertile eggs purchased from a commercial hatchery.

Laboratory management and breeding

Housing

Any well designed laboratory animal house can be used for chickens. There is advantage in having rooms of sufficient size such that commercial poultry equipment can be used. This would include a ceiling height of 2.5 m. Large rooms also allow for flexibility in the configuration of penning or caging. The surfaces of rooms should be of some impervious material that can be thoroughly cleaned and disinfected. There are various plastic laminates available which, although expensive, serve this purpose extremely well and these should cover the walls and ceiling. The floors of rooms should slope to drains and be of sealed concrete. If possible, all electrical fittings should be sealed so that each room can be pressure-washed. The lights in each room should be fitted with a timer and dimmer so that the length and level of illumination can be controlled automatically. Incandescent or fluorescent lights can be used but fluorescent lights, although more efficient, are difficult to dim at the present time (although this is likely to change in the near future).

A system for the removal of manure should be incorporated. As a rough guide, 100 light hybrid laying hens produce about 12 kg manure per day. Also, local authority rules and regulations governing the disposal of waste water should be carefully observed. It may be necessary to provide a large settling tank within the building to remove the bulk of the solids. Ideally, advice from an architect and sewage engineer, who are familiar with local by-laws, should be sought during the design phase of the building. These people should also be consulted if an existing building is being converted to hold chickens.

Environmental provisions

General advice on environmental requirements can be found in the report on birds by the Joint Working Group on Refinement (JWGR 2001). The ventilation system should have sufficient capacity to cope with the local climatic conditions and the maximum numbers of birds held in each room. The main purpose of a ventilating system is to remove excess heat and water vapour from the building. It is unlikely that bird density in a laboratory setting will ever be so high as to constitute an over-heating problem, but it should be noted that a light hybrid, medium hybrid and broiler breeding hen produce about 42, 48 and 59 kJ of heat per hour. With regard to water production, 100 light hybrid laying hens at normal room temperature produce 11.4 kg respiratory water per day and 8.8 kg faecal water per day, giving a total of 20.2 kg water per day. The ventilation system has to remove much of this water and the efficiency of the system will depend on the relative humidity of the air at the time. The usual formula for calculating fan capacity is to allow 0.17 m^3 air per bird per minute. If the laboratory is located in an area where summer temperatures of over 30 °C are common, then an air-conditioning system should be installed.

It is essential that the whole building is fitted with an alarm system which will give warning if there is a power failure to any room. The building should have an emergency generator which switches in automatically in the event of a power failure and, in addition, an alarm system which will notify a responsible person that there is an emergency. Systems are available whereby the alarm will ring a series of telephone numbers until one is answered.

Pens or cages?

Probably the first important decision to be made is whether birds can be kept on the floor or if they must be housed in some form of cage. The nature of the research will probably determine which route must be followed. In general, it is possible to provide the birds with a better, more appropriate environment if they are kept on the floor. However, the fact that a cage environment separates the bird from its faeces, means that cages are more hygienic although more restrictive. There may also be many good scientific reasons for deciding on cages, such as projects requiring faecal collection or if the nature of the research precludes medication with a coccidiostat. It should also be remembered that conventional battery cages will be banned for commercial use in the European Union (EU) from January 2012. Moreover, the EU has recently adopted recommendations for animals used in research that provide advice on housing and husbandry, including enrichment (European Commission 2007). These recommendations (portions of which may become compulsory within the EU) also provide minimum enclosure dimensions and space allowances that are substantially greater than previous recommendations (eg, a minimum enclosure size of 2 m^2 for birds above 600 g). It may also be possible to brood the chicks and rear the young stock on the floor, while keeping the adult stock in cages. It may even be possible to keep all stock on the floor and move birds into cages for the duration of an experiment. Of course, there are not the same financial constraints on the keeping of birds in a laboratory. So, for example, it may be perfectly feasible to keep laboratory hens in a small floor pen on litter and maintain hygiene by cleaning the pen out each week which would be totally unacceptable financially in commercial practice.

Equipment

The equipment selected will depend very much on the nature of the research being carried out. For many research projects, commercial equipment may be used. In other cases, for example in nutritional studies into trace elements, specialised equipment made of stainless steel or special plastics, may be needed.

Brooding phase

Chicks may be brooded on the floor or in tier brooders. They are not able to regulate their body temperature very well for the first few weeks of life and require warmth. It is usually best to raise the temperature of the room in which chicks are being brooded to say, 24–26 °C, and to provide some supplemental heat.

If chicks are brooded on the floor, the extra heat is most easily provided by a suspended electrical heater. More powerful commercial brooders operated by natural gas and other fuels are available if large numbers of chicks are being brooded. For a laboratory, electrical brooders are probably more convenient. It is recommended that dull emitter heaters are used rather than heating lamps since this means that the lighting and heating programmes can be controlled independently. The heater should be suspended above the floor of the pen with some means of adjusting the height, since this is how temperature is controlled. The heater should be switched on 24 h before the chicks are due. A thermometer can be used to check the temperature before the chicks arrive. It should be about 32 °C 15 cm outside the brooder canopy or reflector and 5 cm above the floor. However, the main guide to brooder temperature should be the chicks themselves. When they are placed, they should arrange themselves in a ring below where the brooder is radiating heat. If they huddle directly below the brooder, then they are cold and the brooder should be lowered. If they are spread out as far from the brooder as possible, then they are hot and the brooder should be raised. Dull emitter heaters are capable of brooding a few hundred chicks. Supplemental heat is gradually reduced through the brooding period by raising the height of the brooder.

For the first few days, chicks are usually not allowed access to the whole pen, but are confined to a smaller area, about 1.5 m in diameter, under the brooder using a brooder guard. This is simply a temporary construction made out of a roll of corrugated cardboard, perhaps 30–40 cm high with the ends clipped together to make a circle. It is scrapped after a few days.

Some form of litter with good insulating and absorbing properties should be placed on the floor to a depth of about 3–5 cm. Wood shavings are common but many other materials can be used. If wood shavings are used, they should be from untreated wood.

Water can be provided in various ways. Chick founts, with a large glass or plastic jar inverted in a plastic or metal dish, are common (Figure 41.1). Automatic drinking nipples, cups and bells also work well. A bell drinker is a plastic bell-shaped container suspended from the ceiling and supplied with water via a flexible water line from above. Water flows over the outside of the bell and is held in an upturned rim. When a set amount of water is in the rim, the weight of the water operates a stop valve in the supply line. As the birds drink the water, the weight decreases and the valve opens allowing water to flow again (Figure 41.2). There is some advantage to using nipples since they often have a drop of water hanging from the nipple and this attracts chicks which have a natural tendency to peck at bright shiny objects. Allow 1.5 cm/chick of water trough access, 1.3 cm/chick if pans or bells are used, four automatic cups/100 chicks, or eight automatic nipples/100 chicks. There should be a daily inspection of all drinkers to ensure there is an unimpeded supply of water.

There is also a variety of feeders available in metal and plastic. Allow 5 cm/chick of trough access or 4 cm/chick if round pans are used. In addition, some extra food should be provided on 'scratch trays' for the first few days. Cardboard trays used for egg storage are ideal for this purpose.

Tier brooders are cages for groups of chicks. Each cage is commonly divided into an enclosed section which is heated electrically with the heat being controlled by a thermostat, and a more open section which allows for inspection. Food and water are supplied from troughs running round the outside of the cage (Figure 41.3). Tier brooders save space and are often on wheels so they can easily be moved between rooms. The thermostat should be adjusted to provide a temperature of about 32 °C in the enclosed section of the brooder.

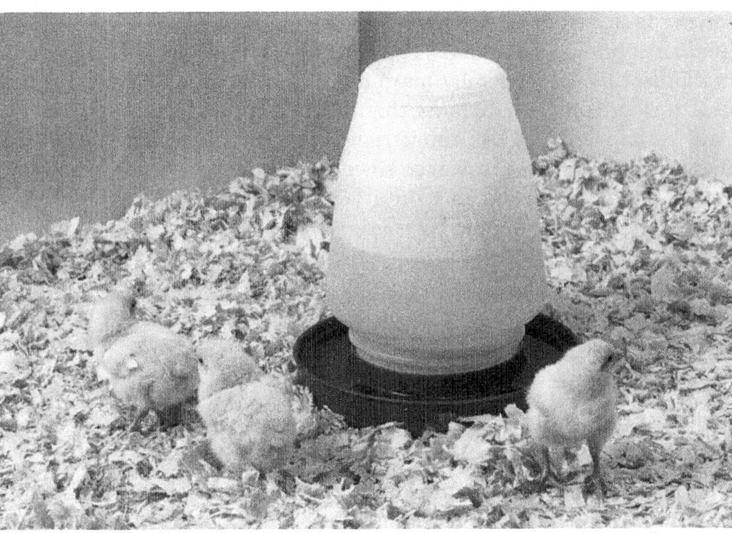

Figure 41.1 A chick fount suitable for supplying chicks with water for the first few weeks of life.

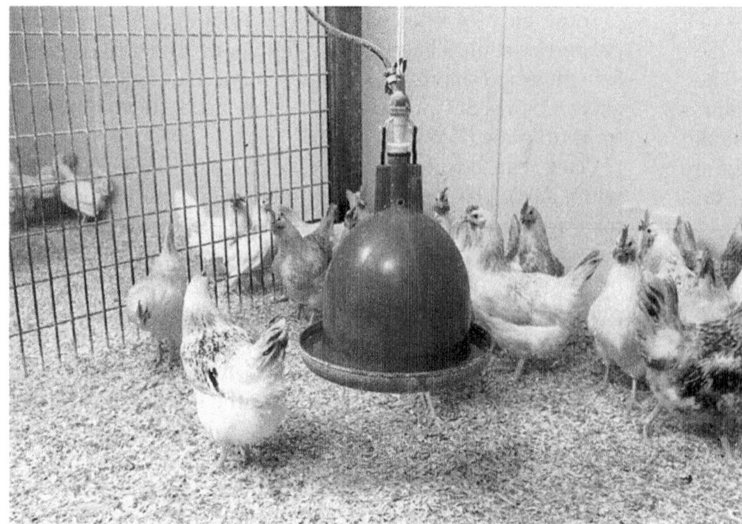

Figure 41.2 A drinking bell suitable for supplying water to all growing and adult birds on the floor.

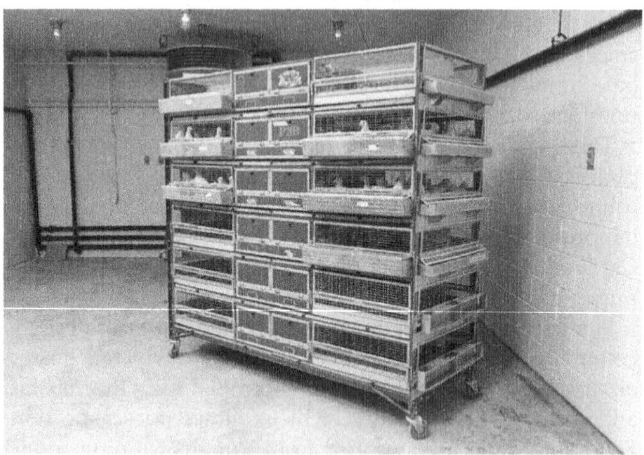

Figure 41.3 A tier brooder.

As with all neonates, rest and sleep are extremely important for chicks (Malleau *et al.* 2007). Therefore, chicks should be given at least 8h of darkness every 24h. When the lights are on, the level of illumination should be fairly high (40 lux) for the first 3–5 days. After this, birds should go on to a lifetime lighting programme. For laying hens and all breeding birds, this will generally mean that, from about 5 days until they are photo-stimulated, they will be kept on a short day, perhaps 8L:16D. Commercially, chickens are kept under very dim light. However, since they are very visual animals, it is suggested that, in a laboratory setting, the level of illumination should be as bright as possible, at least 20 lux.

Rearing phase

After about 4 weeks, young birds generally do not require supplemental heat. The phase that follows brooding until they reach sexual maturity at 19–24 weeks is considered the rearing phase. The optimum room temperature is about 20 °C, but growing birds can easily cope with a range of 18–26°C. Birds can be reared on the floor or in cages. Once again, the nature of the research will determine which husbandry method is selected. If they are destined to become breeding stock, breeding naturally, then they should be reared on the floor.

Birds should be given plenty of space. If they are being reared in cages, each bird will require a minimum of about 600 cm^2 as they approach sexual maturity, so this capacity should be available. They can be kept at a higher density when they are young, and then be split into smaller groups at a lower density as they grow. If they are reared on the floor on litter, the space required as they approach maturity is about 5 birds/m^2. Once again they can be kept more densely than this when young and the groups sub-divided as they grow.

There are many different kinds of commercial feeders available for floor rearing. Allow 9 cm/bird of trough access or 4 cm/bird if large-diameter (120 cm) tube feeders are used. Of course, if any type of food restriction is going to be practised, then these allowances must be greatly increased to 15 cm/bird for troughs and 8 cm/bird for tube feeders, to ensure that all the birds can very easily feed at once. For cage-reared birds, towards the end of the rearing period, allow 9–10 cm/bird of trough space.

Water can be provided by means of troughs, bells, automatic cups or nipples, with cups and nipples being more hygienic. Allow 2.5 cm/bird of water trough access, 2.0 cm/bird of bell access, nine automatic cups/100 birds, or 12 automatic nipples/100 birds. Birds should be monitored closely if the type of drinker is changed between phases. For example, chicks that have been brooded with nipple drinkers may not recognise water when it is presented in a trough or bell drinker. There should be a daily inspection of all drinkers to ensure there is an unimpeded supply of water. Drinking troughs require frequent cleaning. Bells and cups also require cleaning but less frequently than troughs.

Since domestic fowl learn to perch at an early age, and since, if given the opportunity, they rest in a perching posture and are strongly motivated to do so (Olsson & Keeling 2002), it is recommended that perches be provided. These should be round, or round with a flattened top, of about 25 mm in diameter for younger birds, and made of reasonably hard wood. As the birds approach adulthood, the perches should be exchanged for ones with a diameter of about 36 mm (Tauson & Abrahamsson 1994). It is recommended that perches be provided at different heights, one at 5–10 cm above the floor, and at least one other at about 30 cm above the floor. Allow about 30 cm perch length per bird at each level so that the birds can perch communally.

Adult phase

Birds should be moved to their adult quarters at about 16 weeks of age so that they can settle down before the first egg is produced. The optimum temperature for adult chickens is 20–21 °C but the range 16–26 °C is satisfactory. Below 16 °C birds will eat considerably more food to keep warm, and above 27 °C hens may not eat enough to maintain a high level of egg production. At 28–29 °C they begin to encounter heat stress problems.

It is the housing of adult chickens that raises the most animal welfare concerns. The traditional battery cage, although being a hygienic and profitable husbandry system commercially, is much less than ideal from a welfare point of view. It should also be remembered that conventional cages will be banned in the EU from January 2012. Standards of care in a laboratory should be higher than those in commercial conditions. Laboratories should, therefore, make every attempt to find an alternative, more welfare-friendly husbandry system for keeping adult chickens.

If some type of conventional cage is essential for the research, then it must be of the best possible design. Tauson (1980, 1985) describes how design features of conventional cages may be modified to improve welfare. For some years Sweden has insisted on this improved cage design, therefore a cage manufacturer supplying the Swedish commercial market should be sought. If some form of conventional cage in a special material such as stainless steel or plastic is necessary, then the cages may have to be built to order. Once again, the modifications suggested by Tauson (1980, 1985) should be incorporated into the design, including an absence of V-shaped spaces where birds can be trapped, a floor slope of no more than 8°, and an appropriate distance that the bird has to stretch to the bottom of the food trough. Cage height should be at least 40 cm throughout the cage. If possible, birds should be kept in small groups of three or four with 800 cm^2 floor space per bird or at least 600 cm^2 if the birds are small. If birds must be kept in single-bird cages these should allow about 1200 cm^2 floor space per bird. If birds are kept in pairs, each cage should have at least 1800 cm^2 floor space. The minimum feeding space should be 12 cm per bird. In multi-bird cages, birds retain better plumage condition if there are solid rather than wire mesh divisions between cages.

Conventional cages, even those with all the improvements described above, are not suitable for males. It will not generally be possible to keep more than one male to a cage because of the risk of fighting and injury. Cages for males should be 60 cm in height and a space allowance of about 2500 cm^2 is recommended. Since there are no eggs to roll away, the floor should be level.

The simplest and most hygienic method of supplying water to cages is by means of nipples or cups. One nipple or cup per cage of three to four birds is sufficient. However, since chickens do not compete over water, a better configuration is to locate nipples or cups at cage junctions so that two or four cages can share the facility. This means that birds in each cage will have access to more than one water outlet. There should be a daily inspection of all drinkers to ensure there is an unimpeded supply of water. Drinking cups also require periodic cleaning.

If the type of research being conducted by the laboratory allows alternatives to cages, then there are many systems to choose from. The past 20 years has seen a burgeoning of alternative commercial systems (eg, Appleby *et al.* 2004) and a laboratory could easily adopt one of these, either in its commercial form or as a modified scaled-down version. There are two main types of system, one based on floor-housing and the other on modified cages. A good housing system should include the following essential features:

1. The birds should be in reasonably small groups. There is no hard evidence on what the upper threshold might be, above which welfare is reduced, but it is likely that a group size of 15–20 is ideal and that problems may arise with groups over 40. Maintaining birds in appropriately sized groups should not be a problem for most laboratories. Within the group, each bird should have 800 cm^2 of space. Since, in many of these systems, more use is made of vertical space, and birds may 'share' floor space by being at different levels, it is sometimes difficult to make this calculation. As a general rule, laboratories should be generous with space allowances.
2. The birds should be able to feed at the same time; this means that at least 10 cm feed trough space per bird is required, slightly less than this if food is provided from a round pan.
3. Birds should have access to water at all times. Any of the previously described drinkers is suitable. Allow about one cup for 12 hens or one nipple for eight hens.
4. Hens should have access to a suitable nesting place. Single- or pair-housed birds should each have access to a nest box, with a ratio of at least one nest box per two birds provided in larger groups (European Commission 2007). The nest should be secluded but not necessarily dark. It should allow the hen to express the various nest-building motor patterns. Loose nesting material is not essential but a round cup-shaped nest is preferred (Duncan & Kite 1989). It is possible to collect eggs automatically from a nest of this type. If individual nest boxes are used, then allow one nest box for five hens.
5. Perches should be available for roosting at night and for resting through the day. The best perch designed so far (a perfect perch has not yet been designed) is of reasonably hard wood, circular in profile, 36 mm in diameter and flattened on the top and bottom giving a vertical cross-section of 31 mm (Tauson & Abrahamsson 1994). If perches are provided at different levels, there should be sufficient length of perch to allow all the birds in a group to perch at the same level. This will require about 15 cm of perch per bird. It should be pointed out that,

although on balance, the provision of perches increases welfare, they do have some costs. Perches increase the incidence of bumble foot (an inflammatory infection of the foot pad) and keel bone deformations, compared with birds kept without perches. On the other hand, perches decrease the incidence of toe pad hyperkeratosis when they are added to conventional battery cages (Tauson & Abrahamsson 1994).

The best alternative systems, whether based on floor-housing or cage-housing, incorporate all these features. The following features are not equally available in the two types of system:

1. It is much easier to provide opportunities for foraging in floor-based housing systems. Since foraging normally occupies a great deal of time, it is probably very important to the chicken. It is not impossible to allow hens in cage-based environments to forage, but it takes some ingenuity and stamina on the part of the animal care staff. For example, some type of fresh green material, such as a cabbage or piece of cabbage or net filled with clover could be hung in the cage. The hygiene associated with a mesh floor would thus be maintained. However, the labour involved in such a scheme would be considerable and if fresh greens are not provided after the chickens have become used the routine, there would then be a grave risk of the chickens starting to featherpeck. Therefore, if foraging behaviour is considered essential, a floor-based system should be selected.
2. Dustbathing behaviour can be encouraged in cage-based systems by the provision of sand boxes. However, there have been problems associated with these, notably hens laying in the sand boxes, probably because the design was not ideal. On the other hand, dusty locations quickly develop in the litter of floor-based systems and these are used for dustbathing.

Fowl are highly motivated to perform 'comfort behaviour' such as wing flapping, feather ruffling and leg stretching, which help to maintain strong leg bones. Birds should therefore be housed in enclosures large enough to permit all of these behaviours whenever possible (European Commission 2007). There are so many housing systems available that it is impossible to describe each. One that is showing considerable promise is a type of modified cage called the 'Edinburgh modified cage' (Appleby & Hughes 1995) or the 'modified and enriched cage' (Abrahamsson *et al.* 1996). This is essentially a cage for four to six hens with a perch, nest box and sand box for dustbathing. These cages can be tiered to save space, and feeding, drinking and egg collection can be automated. They also provide a fairly high standard of hygiene.

Hygiene

It is essential that newly hatched chicks go into a clean environment. In a laboratory the best way to achieve this is to copy commercial husbandry and operate an 'all-in, all-out' system. Of course, in a laboratory, all-in, all-out will apply to individual rooms and not to the whole establishment. When each room becomes empty of birds, the room and all the equipment in it, should be thoroughly cleaned and disinfected. If individual rooms can be hermetically sealed, then they should also be fumigated at this time. There may be some advantage in rotating disinfectants and in allowing rooms to stand empty for some days after disinfection. All the equipment in the room should be cleaned and disinfected at the same time as the room is being treated.

It is also good practice to have disinfectant foot baths outside each room so that diseases are not spread inadvertently by the animal care staff. Of course, if the laboratory is dealing with diseases, then much more stringent precautions will have to be taken such as specialist protective clothing and apparatus, and showering in to and out of each room or unit.

Identification and sexing

Small, numbered, metal or plastic wing-tags can be used to give day-old chicks a unique, lifetime identification. A special tool is used to clip the tags through the wing-web on the front edge of the wing taking care not to pierce any muscle tissue. These wing-tags seem to have minimal adverse effects.

Commercial breeding companies often arrange their day-old chicks to be auto-sexed. Use is made of certain genes carried on the sex chromosomes, such as silver down colour, barring, or fast feathering. In the case of silver down colour for example, cocks (the homogametic sex) which are homozygous recessive for the trait (and gold) are mated with females which are hemizygous dominant (and silver). This results in male progeny in which the males are all heterozygous (and silver) and the females are all hemizygous (and gold). If breeding companies cannot arrange for auto-sexing then they use vent-sexing in which highly trained personnel are able to sex the chicks using differences in genital papillae.

It is thus simple for a laboratory to buy day-old chicks of the required sex but not so easy to arrange auto-sexing or vent-sexing within the laboratory. If birds of a certain sex are required, the solution may be to rear all the chicks until feather differences become obvious. These differences can usually be identified at a few weeks of age.

Natural breeding

Domestic fowl will breed easily if kept in floor pens. If the experimental procedures dictate that the breeding birds should be kept in cages, then it is advisable to use artificial insemination, since cage breeding is never very successful. Birds are usually photo-stimulated to bring them into breeding condition at around 17–21 weeks of age (a few weeks later for meat-type birds). Rapid growth and reddening of the comb is characteristic of birds coming into breeding condition. In hens, the vent becomes moist and red a few days before the first egg is due and the pubic bones separate from about 1 finger-width to about three finger-widths.

A sex ratio of about one male to ten females usually works well. Eggs laid 2 days after the sexes are mixed should be fertile. If the laboratory is practising some form of pedigreed mating system, then it should be remembered that hens remain fertile for 7–10 days after one successful copulation. Fertility then drops quite quickly and few fertile eggs should be produced 15 days after the sexes are separated.

Fertile eggs should be collected often in order to get them into ideal storage conditions as quickly as possible. They should be stored, blunt end up, in egg trays, in an egg storage room designed for the purpose, with a temperature of about 16–18 °C and a relative humidity of 75%. Fertile eggs may be stored for 1 week but hatchability will decrease after longer storage times.

It is best to warm hatching eggs at room temperature (20–22 °C) for 4–6 h before setting them in the incubator. The incubation period for domestic fowl is 21 days. Optimal incubation conditions are a temperature of 37.5–37.7 °C and a relative humidity of 60% for the first 19 days and a temperature 36.1–37.2 °C and a relative humidity of 75% for the final 2 days. This is normally achieved by moving the trays from the setter to the hatcher on day 19 of incubation; if the chicks are to be pedigreed, the hatcher must have individual boxes for each egg/chick. The eggs must be turned regularly (commercially they are turned every hour) during the first 19 days. If incubation is going to be carried out regularly in a laboratory, then papers which cover the topic such as Hulet (2007), Fasenko (2007) and Decuypere and Bruggeman (2007) should be consulted.

Artificial insemination

Artificial insemination may be necessary because, for example, of a scientific requirement for individually housed hens, or when natural mating results in low fertility, or if specific pedigreed matings are required. The technique is straightforward. For best results, males should be housed individually, otherwise homosexual mating may deplete semen yields. Males can be photo-stimulated to produce semen at a fairly young age but it is normal to do this at about 18 weeks for laying-type males and 20 weeks for meat-type males. They will then start to produce semen at about 20 weeks and 22 weeks respectively, and collection of semen should start at that time. The procedure for semen collection is well described by Etches (1996) but requires a highly skilled technician for best results. The male is held with his feet at right angles to his body, and his belly and back stroked towards the tail with quick firm strokes. This stimulates erection of the phallic folds. When stimulated, the hand massaging the back is then transferred to the cloacal area with the thumb and index finger located on the lateral aspects of the cloaca and slightly anterior to the vent. Gentle pressure can then be used to expel semen from the ductus deferens. The flow of semen can then be collected by aspiration into a collecting ampoule. Care should be taken to collect semen only and avoid urates and faeces. Males should be handled gently and consistently. They become accustomed to being milked by the same operator and changes of personnel should be avoided if possible. A collecting schedule of three times per week (Mondays, Wednesdays and Fridays) will yield good volumes (0.15–0.35 ml) of semen. Etches (1996) recommends collecting the semen into semen diluent at 15°C, evaluating the semen for sperm density and quality, then arranging the rate of dilution such that each hen gets a standard insemination volume of 0.05 ml containing 100 million sperm cells.

Females can be inseminated as soon as they are in lay and it is better to inseminate later in the day when there is not a hard-shelled egg in the shell gland. The hen is held in the palm of the left hand facing left with the thighs held by the thumb and index finger. Gentle pressure is then exerted in a posterior direction with the left hand as the tail is pressed in an anterior direction with the right hand. This everts the hen's cloaca. A second person then inserts the inseminating pipette into the oviduct to a depth of about 3 cm. The first person releases the pressure on the body cavity allowing the cloaca to return to its natural position and the second person inseminates and withdraws the pipette. Inseminating hens every 5 days will usually maintain a high fertility rate.

Inspection of birds

All birds in a laboratory should be inspected at least twice a day, first thing in the morning and again later in the day. The inspection should be carried out by personnel who are familiar with the healthy appearance and normal behaviour of various classes of domestic fowl. It is good laboratory practice to have check sheets in every bird room on which any departure from normal appearance or behaviour can be recorded. Of course, if birds are subjected to any experimental treatment that might jeopardise their welfare, then inspections should be more frequent than this. During routine inspections of the birds, equipment such as feeders and drinkers should be checked. This is also a good opportunity to monitor and record environmental variables such as temperature and ventilation.

Feeding

Commercial poultry rations are formulated to very high standards and laboratories can have confidence in buying these. Complete balanced rations are usually fed, either as a dry mash, pellets or crumbles, which are partially ground-up pellets. The steam and pressure used in pelleting increase the digestibility of a ration so that weight-for-weight, pellets and crumbles are slightly more nutritious than the same ration in mash form. It is advantageous to feed chicks crumbles; the particle size of crumbles is very attractive to chicks and ensures that they ingest plenty of food in the first few days. In the rearing and adult stages, it is usual to choose a mash ration if over-consumption is a problem or if it is necessary to occupy the birds with feeding through a large part of the day and essential if feather pecking is likely to be a problem. (Birds take longer to eat the same quantity of mash compared with pellets or crumbles.) If high consumption and quick growth are necessary, or if under-consumption is a problem, then pellets or crumbles should be fed.

The energy in poultry diets normally comes from a cereal, often maize, wheat or barley or a mixture of these, sometimes boosted with tallow. The protein comes from a source of vegetable protein such as soybean meal supplemented with animal protein or individual synthetic amino acids. To this is added a pre-mix containing minerals, vitamins and possibly some additives such as an anti-oxidant, a coccidiostat, xanthophylls to give yolk colour, etc.

Different ages and types of bird have different nutritional requirements which means that, in a laboratory housing chickens with a range of ages and types, several rations have to be fed. The specifications for the most commonly fed chicken rations are shown in Tables 41.2–41.8.

It should be noted that if hens are producing fertile eggs for hatching, then it is usual to increase the nutrient density of the diet slightly. In addition, special attention is paid to minerals, vitamins and essential amino acids in breeder diets. It is normal for the males in a breeder flock to receive the same ration as the hens. However they should receive less calcium (<1.0%). If artificial insemination is being practised and the males are separate from the females, this can be arranged. It can also occur in broiler breeder flocks in which the sexes are fed separately.

It is usual to include a coccidiostat in the rations of young birds being kept on the floor. Rations containing tallow should also have an anti-oxidant, such as ethoxyquin, to prevent the fat going rancid.

More information on poultry nutrition can be obtained from Leeson & Summers (1997).

If commercial poultry rations are not available, then there are other possibilities which, although not ideal, will provide the essential nutrients. However if standardised commercial

Table 41.2 Chick starter diet specifications for egg-type strains (from day-old to week 5). The quality of the protein must be high and this can be verified by checking the levels of certain amino acids which should be present at least at the level shown.

Diet specification	*Value*
Metabolisable energy (ME) (MJ/kg)	12.13
Protein (%)	18–20
Arginine (%)	1.0
Lysine (%)	0.9
Methionine (%)	0.4
Tryptophan (%)	0.18
Fibre (%) (upper limit)	3–4
Calcium (%)	1.0
Phosphorus (%)	0.45
Plus a good vitamin and mineral supplement at the recommended level	

Table 41.3 Grower diet specifications for egg-type strains (from week 5 to week 16/17).

Diet specification	*Value*
ME (MJ/kg)	11.71
Protein (%)	14
Calcium (%)	0.8
Phosphorus (%)	0.4
Plus a good vitamin and mineral supplement at the recommended level	

Table 41.4 Two-phase grower diet specifications for egg-type strains.

Diet specification	*Week 5–11*	*Week 12–16/17*
ME (MJ/kg)	11.92	11.50
Protein (%)	15	13
Calcium (%)	0.8	0.8
Phosphorus (%)	0.4	0.4
Plus a good vitamin and mineral supplement at the recommended level		

Table 41.5 Layer diet specifications for egg-type strains.

Diet specification	*Value*
ME (MJ/kg)	11.50
Protein (%)	16
Calcium (%)	3.5
Phosphorus (%)	0.4
Plus a good vitamin and mineral supplement at the recommended level	

Table 41.6 Breeder diet specifications for egg-type strains.

Diet specification	*Value*
ME (MJ/kg)	11.71
Protein (%)	17
Calcium (%)	3.7
Phosphorus (%)	0.44
Plus a good vitamin and mineral supplement at the recommended level	

Table 41.7 Three-phase broiler diet specifications.

Diet specification	*Starter (days 1–24)*	*Grower (days 25–35)*	*Finisher (days 36–42)*
ME (MJ/kg)	12.75	13.18	13.38
Protein (%)	22	20	18
Calcium (%)	1.0	0.95	0.95
Phosphorus (%)	0.42	0.4	0.4
Plus a good vitamin and mineral supplement at the recommended level			

Table 41.8 Broiler breeder diet specifications.

Diet specification	*Value*
ME (MJ/kg)	12.13
Protein (%)	16.5
Calcium (%)	3.7
Phosphorus (%)	0.45
Plus a good vitamin and mineral supplement at the recommended level	

rations are not available, then consider whether it is worthwhile performing research that may not be replicable.

1. Any other commercial laboratory animal ration may be fed (eg, rat chow or dog chow). If the birds are hens in laying condition, this type of diet should be supplemented with a source of calcium such as oyster shell or ground limestone sprinkled over the food.
2. Birds are very good at balancing their own diet if provided with a variety of ingredients (Dove 1935). Therefore, they could be given a selection of locally available seeds and grains. The local ingredients should be checked against tables of nutrient composition (in any good nutrition textbook) to ensure that they are likely to provide sufficient energy and protein. Leeson and Summers (1997, pp. 61–62) provide tables of ingredient constraints showing the maximum amount of various ingredients that should be included in diets for different classes of domestic fowl. If soluble vitamins and minerals are available, they could be supplied in the water to supplement local rations. Again, if the birds are laying hens, then some form of supplemental calcium will be required. Also, if whole grains are being fed, then the birds should have access to some form of insoluble grit which is needed to grind the grains in the gizzard.

Laboratory procedures

Handling

As pointed out previously, many strains of domestic fowl have retained their ancestral fear of human beings. They should therefore be handled gently but firmly in order that fear responses are not exacerbated. There is little problem with very young chicks, since fear responses to human beings only develop over the first few days after hatching. There may be some advantage for laboratory managers to habituate birds to human beings and to handling early in life. There is evidence that early handling reduces fearful responses to human beings later (Hughes & Black 1976; Jones & Faure 1981) although some particularly flighty strains may not show much improvement (Murphy & Duncan 1978). Birds should be caught using both hands to pin the bird's wings against its sides. When held firmly like this, birds usually settle down very quickly, and they can be transported over short distances, say between a pen and an examination table within a room. For transporting between rooms, a carrying crate is recommended. Disposable cardboard carrying crates are ideal for this purpose. If birds are difficult to catch because they show excessive avoidance behaviour, dimming the lights usually helps.

Restraint and blood sampling

Birds may be restrained on their backs, say for examination, with one hand gripping both legs firmly, leaving the other hand free for manipulation. Blood samples are usually drawn from the brachial vein close to where it passes over the ulna and radius just distal to the joint with the humerus. The easiest method is for one person to restrain the bird on its side using one hand to hold both legs with the other hand over the breast pinning the lower wing to the bird's side. The person taking the sample can then use one hand to extend the other wing. The axillary feathers should be removed from the site and the skin swabbed with spirit. Whether the needle is inserted into the vein towards or away from the heart is a matter of personal preference. The following sizes of needles are recommended for blood sampling; 0.7 mm × 15 mm long needle (22 G) for 0–2-week-old chicks, 0.7 mm × 19 mm (21 G) for 2–6-week-old chicks, 0.8 mm × 38 mm (20 G) for 6–18-week-old birds, and 0.9 mm × 38 mm for adults.

Monitoring physiological variables

The fact that restraint is an extremely stressful procedure for domestic fowl means that obtaining undisturbed physiological data can be a challenge. Birds are also very intolerant of leads or catheters running from the skin surface. With a great deal of patience birds can sometimes be habituated to the presence of leads or catheters, but one would then need to question how normal their behaviour was. Birds have extremely flexible necks and can reach almost every part of their bodies with their beaks, which are usually very efficient at removing attachments. The upper neck and head, which cannot be reached by the beak, can be very effectively scratched by the bird's feet. A solution to this problem could be bio-telemetry, by which physiological variables are sent from a radio transmitter on (Duncan *et al.* 1975) or in the bird (Filshie *et al.* 1980; Duncan and Filshie 1980) to a receiver some distance away. A bird will habituate to a small device strapped to its back whereas it is very intolerant of attached leads. Once a bird with an implanted device has recovered from anaesthesia, it is free to move about unencumbered. Biotelemetry techniques have improved in the past 30 years and now multichannel devices are available which can transmit up to nine variables simultaneously and even have a two-way capability by which the implanted device can accept commands to perform various tasks within the animal (Axelsson *et al.* 2007).

Injections and dosing

Intravenous injections are usually given in the brachial vein (see Restraint and blood sampling). Intramuscular injections are usually given in the muscles of the upper leg. Subcutaneous injections can be given in the web of the wing or, with the bird restrained on its back, into a patch of loose bare skin at the junction of the breast and leg which makes a very convenient site.

Birds can be dosed orally very easily. With the bird restrained in an upright position and the beak held open, pills can be gently pushed to the back of the mouth with a finger. When the head is released the pill will be swallowed. Liquids can be injected into the crop by way of the oesophagus (taking care to avoid the trachea) by means of a syringe and a flexible plastic tube and with the bird restrained as described above. For best practice, after insertion the correct position of the tube should be confirmed by ensuring it can be felt within the oesophagus.

Anaesthesia and analgesia

Birds are not the easiest class of animals to anaesthetise and those administering anaesthetics to chickens should be properly trained. Specialist texts that should be consulted include Sinn (1994), Schaeffer (1994) and Lawton (2008).

Chickens should be fasted sufficiently to empty the crop before proceeding with anaesthesia. This will vary from an hour or two with young chicks to overnight for adult birds. It should also be remembered that birds can quickly become hypothermic. Therefore, a warming pad should be used during anaesthesia and some provision should be made to provide heat during recovery, such as a heating lamp over the recovery cage.

With regard to pre-anaesthetics, atropine is generally not used in birds; diazepam (0.5–1.5 mg/kg im or iv) is the pre-anaesthetic of choice.

Isoflurane is the best anaesthetic agent for chickens. They can be induced in a chamber or by means of a mask with 3–5% isoflurane. They may then be intubated with a non-cuffed endotracheal tube and maintained on 1.0–1.5% isoflurane. Halothane and methoxyflurane may also be used as anaesthetics but are more likely to produce undesirable side effects.

For short-term procedures, an injectable mixture of ketamine and xylazine may be used to anaesthetise chickens. The required dosage is about 20 mg/kg ketamine and 2 mg/kg xylazine both given im. This anaesthesia may be partially reversed by yohimbine injected iv at a rate of 0.1 mg/kg.

There is very little information available on analgesics for chickens (see Howlett (2008) for brief review of local anaesthesia and analgesia in birds). It is thought that butorphanol at a dosage rate of 0.2–2.0 mg/kg im and buprenorphine at a rate of 0.01–0.05 mg/kg im have good analgesic effects. Lame broilers will self-medicate with the anti-inflammatory drug carprofen sufficiently to reduce their lameness, which suggests that this drug is an effective analgesic for joint pain (Danbury *et al.* 2000).

Euthanasia

When chickens are to be killed, the method must be humane; that is, it must be painless and must minimise fear and anxiety (see Chapter 17). It must also be reliable, reproducible, irreversible, simple, safe and rapid (Canadian Council on Animal Care 1993; Close *et al.* 1996; 1997; Humane Slaughter Association, 2001). The recommended method for humanely killing chickens is by overdose of an injectable anaesthetic, such as a barbiturate, given intravenously. Laboratory managers should ensure that a suitably qualified person is readily available to carry out this procedure in emergencies as well as in planned procedures. In an emergency, if barbiturates are available but the carer is inexperienced in intravenous injection, then it can be administered by intraperitoneal injection at about 1.0–1.5 ml/kg of 20% pentobarbital sodium solution. This causes very little distress, and death occurs quietly after a slightly longer period. In every case after euthanasia by injection, the body should be kept until *rigor mortis* has occurred before disposal of the body.

In cases of emergency when someone with authority to use barbiturates is not available, it is preferable to kill a chicken by cervical dislocation rather than let it suffer for long, even though this may not be an approved method of killing in some countries. Cervical dislocation can be carried out manually, but requires a little training on cadavers. In young chicks, the neck may be dislocated by using the thumb to press the neck against the sharp edge of a table or bench. An older bird is held by the legs with the head downwards. The other hand is then placed with the head between the index and second fingers so that the other fingers are under the jaw. By applying pressure downwards with the knuckle of the index finger while simultaneously pulling the jaw upwards, the neck can be dislocated. In the case of large birds, the neck can be dislocated using mechanical dislocators or Burdizzo forceps. If cervical dislocation is used, the dislocation should be at as high a level as possible, preferably at the atlas (C1) and axis (C2) joint.

Common welfare problems

Disease

Chickens suffer from a variety of infectious diseases caused by viruses, bacteria, mycoplasma and larger parasitic organisms as well as several metabolic diseases. Birds in a laboratory should be monitored regularly for signs of sickness. Symptoms are usually fairly obvious and would include lethargy, poor appetite, loss of condition, hens going out of lay, production of malformed eggs, coughing, wheezing, blood in faeces, etc.

It is beyond the scope of this chapter to describe each disease in detail and for more information a standard text should be consulted such as Saif *et al.* (2003), Jordan (1990) or Sainsbury (1992). Neither is this text meant as a diagnostic tool; birds which die or are sick should always be sent to a pathology laboratory for proper diagnosis. What follows is simply a rough guide to the more important diseases. The mode of transmission is given; 'vertical transmission' means that the organism is passed from generation to generation via the egg; 'horizontal transmission' means that the organism is passed from bird to bird by a variety of routes.

Bacterial diseases

There are several *Salmonella* diseases of poultry.

Pullorum disease (Salmonella pullorum)

Symptoms This is a disease of all poultry and some wild birds with acute white diarrhoea and deaths (up to 50%) in young chicks. If chicks have become infected through the hatching egg, then symptoms, including huddling, can start very early (2nd day). Survivors can be chronically infected with few symptoms. In older birds, there are few symptoms except green–brown diarrhoea.

Transmission Vertical through the hatching egg (this is the most important).

Horizontal:

- in the hatcher, debris and dust from infected eggs;
- through the droppings (into feed and water);
- cannibalism, birds eating infected blood and tissues;
- birds eating infected eggs;
- from infected equipment eg, debeakers;

Diagnosis Bacteria are isolated and can be cultured in the laboratory.

Treatment None is practised. The idea is to eradicate the disease and this is done by blood-testing breeders for antibodies.

Prevention Breeders should be blood-tested for the presence of pullorum antibodies and reactors eliminated.

Fowl typhoid (S. gallinarum)

Symptoms This is a slow-spreading disease of all poultry of all ages. Birds show loss of appetite, green diarrhoea, with pale combs and wattles in adults. Mortality can eventually reach 50%.

Diagnosis Bacteria are isolated and can be cultured in the laboratory.

Transmission Exactly the same as for pullorum disease.

Treatment None is practised and, as for pullorum, eradication is the answer.

Prevention Breeders should be blood-tested using an agglutination test.

Paratyphoid (*eg,* S. typhimurium, S. montevideo, S. derby)

These are important infections because of the risk of food poisoning to humans.

Symptoms There are often no symptoms in the birds, sometimes diarrhoea.

Diagnosis Bacteria are isolated and cultured in laboratory.

Transmission Spread is mainly horizontal through droppings, equipment and people.

Treatment This is not a major disease of poultry and treatment is not usually required. However, sulfadimethoxine, furazolidone and tetracycline are all quite effective.

Prevention Cleaning and disinfection between batches of birds, plus the use of footbaths for personnel, help to reduce the incidence.

A disease as yet unnamed (S. enteriditis)

This is very important, not because it causes big losses in poultry, but because the organism infects the ovary and hens lay infected eggs which can cause food poisoning in humans. This disease is now fairly well controlled in most countries through testing and elimination of reactors. There are also vaccines available.

Symptoms No clear symptoms.

Transmission Vertical through hatching egg.

Horizontal through egg-eating and possibly through droppings.

Treatment Recommended not to treat but to eradicate.

Prevention Breeders should be blood-tested using an agglutination test.

Arizona disease (S. arizonae *also known as* Arizona hinshawi)

Symptoms Important in turkeys and to a less extent chickens. In young birds there is diarrhoea, listlessness, sometimes nervousness. In older birds there can be paralysis of legs. Mortality can reach 25%.

Transmission Horizontal:

- in the hatcher (from outside of shell);
- through the droppings (into feed and water);
- from infected equipment.

Treatment Furazolidone is commonly used but eradication is the real answer.

Prevention The organism is very resistant to disinfectants and fumigants (which is why it can be present on the outside of hatching eggs after fumigation). Fumigate at double strength.

Fowl cholera (Pasteurella multocida)

Symptoms In the acute form there are rapid deaths (up to 50%), with 12–18 weeks of age being a very susceptible stage. In the chronic form there is swelling of wattles and internal organs can be affected.

Transmission Horizontal, entry by respiratory tract or digestive tract.

Diagnosis Bacteria are isolated and can be cultured in the laboratory.

Treatment Sulfa drugs in drinking water are fairly effective.

Prevention A live vaccine is available and can be given by wing web but aim for eradication (a blood test is available).

Infectious coryza (Hemophilus paragallinarum)

Symptoms This is a persistent but non-fatal disease of the upper respiratory tract with sneezing, discharge from nostrils and swelling of the face. Organism can only live 5–6 h outside bird.

Transmission Horizontal through air and drinking water.

Diagnosis Symptoms plus laboratory tests.

Treatment Sulfa drugs are fairly effective.

Prevention Isolation from other poultry, and use all-in, all-out management.

Vibrionic hepatitis (Campylobacter fetus)

Symptoms Birds have pale, withered, scaly combs, show a drop in egg production, and watery green diarrhoea. A swollen liver and thickened bile duct are evident at *post-mortem* examination.

Transmission Horizontal through the droppings and so in the feed and on equipment and from room to room on people's feet.

Diagnosis Sick birds should be sent to the pathology laboratory, where diagnosis is by isolation of organism from bile.

Treatment Furazolidone in feed gives quite good results. Injection of streptomycin is also effective.

Prevention Stressed birds seem more susceptible – so avoid stress. Normal sanitary precautions will stop spread.

Coliform infections (Escherichia coli)

Coli enteritis

Symptoms The organism multiplies and causes lesions in the upper digestive tract. There can be blood in droppings similar to coccidiosis plus listlessness.

Coli septicaemia

Symptoms This is often the next stage of coliform infection. The organisms enter the blood stream and infect internal organs.

Air-sac infection

Symptoms Eventually *E. coli* reach the air sacs and cause an infection there. The birds cough and wheeze and production falls.

Transmission Mainly horizontal:

- in the hatcher, infected shells etc;
- through the droppings (into feed and water);
- from infected dust (into lungs);
- from infected feed.

Diagnosis Bacteria are isolated and cultured in the laboratory.

Treatment Furazolidone and tetracycline can be useful if disease is caught at early stage. Once air-sacs are infected, treatment is not effective.

Prevention *E. coli* infections are a sign of dirty surroundings, so treatment should be accompanied by a clean-up campaign. The usual cleaning, disinfecting and fumigating plus all-in, all-out management will do much to prevent coliform infections.

Omphalitis or navel infection (E. coli, Staphylococcus, Pseudomonas, *and others*)

Symptoms This is a disease of hatching chicks, which seem weak, huddle together, have watery diarrhoea, and an infected open navel. It may be accompanied by 10% mortality.

Transmission Horizontal transmission in hatcher. This disease is **very** infectious.

Diagnosis Send suspect chicks to pathology laboratory for diagnosis. They will identify which organism is responsible.

Treatment No effective treatment. There is little spread of infection once chicks are out of the hatcher.

Prevention The seat of this infection is always the hatcher. If an outbreak occurs, the hatcher must be thoroughly cleaned and fumigated with a fumigant at three times normal strength. Hatching eggs should be fumigated at twice normal strength until infection is eradicated.

Malignant oedema or gangrenous dermatitis (Clostridium septicum)

Symptoms Disease of broilers particularly towards end of the growing period. There is gangrene of muscle and skin so that birds 'fall apart' whilst still alive. Massive mortality (up to 50%) is common.

Transmission Horizontal.

Diagnosis Fairly obvious but send suspect birds to laboratory for diagnosis. Although *Clostridium septicum* is the usual organism, *Staphylococcus aureus* can also cause the disease and treatments differ depending on the bacterium that is involved.

Treatment Penicillin works quite well if the main organism is *Clostridium*. The synthetic penicillin ampicillin is better if *Staphylococcus* is the main organism.

Prevention This disease can be associated with dirty conditions (but not always). Using litter more than once can increase problem. The disease sometimes appears as a secondary infection after the birds have been weakened by, say, an outbreak of gumboro disease.

Necrotic enteritis (Clostridium welchii)

Symptoms This disease is more usually found in broilers. Birds fail to thrive. Mortality commonly reaches 5–10%.

Transmission Horizontal.

Diagnosis Small intestine grossly inflamed and distended. Send suspect birds to laboratory for confirmation of diagnosis.

Treatment Penicillin works quite well.

Prevention This disease can be associated with dirty conditions (but not always). Thorough disinfection between batches of birds can reduce the incidence.

Mycoplasma diseases

MG (Mycoplasma gallisepticum) *or*
PPLO (pleuro-pneumonia-like-organism) or
CRD (chronic respiratory disease)

Symptoms This is a respiratory disease affecting the whole respiratory tract particularly the air sacs. Young chicks show sniffling, sneezing and rattling. It is not a killer itself, however, it is often followed by secondary infections particularly with coliforms which make symptoms worse and can lead to 30% mortality. Adult birds have a few symptoms – inactivity, drop in production – but low mortality.

Transmission Vertical through the hatching egg – this is important.

Horizontal:

- through air within a room;
- on feet, clothing, feed and equipment between rooms.

Diagnosis Suspect birds can be diagnosed in a pathology laboratory. There is an agglutination test available.

Treatment Should only be regarded as a temporary solution. Tylosin is an antibiotic with specific activity against MG.

Prevention Control can be by vaccination (usually layers) or eradication (usually broilers). Eradication is centred on identifying broiler breeder hens reacting to a blood test, and eliminating them. However, eradication is difficult because MG is **very** infectious.

MS (Mycoplasma synoviae)

Symptoms Although this is a respiratory disease, the respiratory symptoms are slight and easily missed. What causes the problem is that the organism tends to move to the synovial fluid and the hock and foot pad joints are often affected and become swollen and inflamed. This is mainly a disease of growing birds, particularly 6–14 weeks of age, which become lame and lose their appetites. In older birds there is a drop in egg production and lameness.

Transmission Vertical through the hatching egg.

Horizontal:
- through air within a room;
- on feet, clothing, feed and equipment between rooms.

Diagnosis Suspect birds can be diagnosed in a pathology laboratory. There is an agglutination test available.

Treatment Oxytetracycline in feed can be useful, but aim for eradication.

Prevention Eradication by identifying breeder hens reacting to a blood test and eliminating them. Also, hatching eggs can be heat treated to 46°C before incubation. This kills the organism and only lowers hatchability slightly.

Viral diseases

Infectious bronchitis (IB)

Symptoms This is a disease of domestic fowl only. In chicks there is wheezing and sneezing and perhaps a nasal discharge. Birds gasp for breath. Typically it starts very suddenly and spreads very quickly with up to 50% mortality. In a flock it is likely that all birds will be affected and those that recover will have poor performance in adult life. It is often followed by secondary infections particularly by the coliforms. In adult birds, there are few respiratory symptoms. There is however a huge drop in egg production and a dramatic decrease in egg quality. Soft-shelled, misshapen and wrinkled eggs are very characteristic and albumen quality is poor. Many birds become internal layers.

Transmission Horizontal:
- through air within a room;
- on feet, clothing, feed and equipment between rooms.

Diagnosis Diagnosis is difficult and is often done by eliminating other possibilities. Agglutination tests for antibodies are available.

Treatment No treatment.

Prevention There are several vaccines, mostly attenuated, available:
- Broilers – at day-old, spray vaccine into mouth or eye (ocular).
- Layers – at 2 and 6 weeks give a water-borne or ocular vaccine.
- Breeders – at 1, 10 and 30 weeks then every 10–20 weeks during the laying cycle, give a water-borne or ocular vaccine.

Newcastle disease (ND)

Symptoms A very infectious disease affecting all poultry and some wild birds. There are different forms depending on where in the body the virus strikes. The main symptoms are one of the following:
1. respiratory difficulty;
2. nervous disorders ('twisted necks' and 'tumblers');
3. reduced egg production and quality.

Transmission Horizontal:
- through air within a room;
- on feet, clothing, feed and equipment between rooms.

Diagnosis The nervous symptoms give an accurate diagnosis, otherwise it is difficult. Pathology laboratory diagnosis is possible.

Treatment No treatment.

Prevention The usual method is to try to keep completely free from this disease. However, if it gets into the area, then it is wise to vaccinate, since transfer from other sites is very easy. The vaccination program is complicated – so take advice.

Fowl pox

Symptoms There are two forms of the disease:
1. Dry pox (scabs) on comb, wattles, eyes and ear-lobes.
2. Wet pox in mouth, trachea and respiratory tract which eventually cause suffocation. This often follows dry pox.

Transmission Horizontal. The skin must be broken for the virus to enter. This can happen in two ways:
1. Birds pecking each other during fighting.
2. Mosquitos can transmit the disease.

Transmission is therefore usually slow.

Diagnosis The lesions are very symptomatic. If in doubt, a pathology laboratory will take some material from an infected bird and inject it into the face of another bird. If the typical pox develop, then the disease is fowl pox.

Treatment No treatment.

Prevention If fowl pox is a problem, then there are vaccines available. However, vaccines are not used routinely.

Infectious laryngotracheitis (ILT or LT)

Symptoms A very severe respiratory disease usually in chickens over 6 weeks old. The infected birds gasp for breath. There is often haemorrhaging in the respiratory tract and blood can be coughed up. Mortality varies but can reach 30%.

Transmission Horizontal:
- through air within a room;
- on feet, clothing, feed and equipment between rooms.

Diagnosis Can only be diagnosed in a lab.

Treatment No treatment.

Prevention There is now a very good attenuated vaccine which gives good immunity. Vaccinate at 6 and 16 weeks using ocular route.

Gumboro disease or infectious bursal disease (IBD)

Symptoms Affects chicks aged 20–60 days. Birds are listless, nervous, sleepy, with a whitish diarrhoea which causes them to peck at their vents. Mortality is variable. The problem is that the virus damages the cells in the Bursa responsible for proper working of the immune system. Organism can live several months outside bird – so important to clean and disinfect between batches.

Transmission Horizontal through droppings.

Diagnosis Can only be diagnosed in laboratory.

Treatment No treatment.

Prevention If IBD is a problem in an area, then the usual method is to vaccinate breeders which pass on antibodies in their eggs and this gives protection to the chicks at least for the first part of the vulnerable period.

Avian encephalomyelitis (epidemic tremors)

Symptoms Mainly a disease of chicks between 6 and 21 days. They show nervous symptoms including quivering, which is very obvious if the chick is held in the palm of the hand, and paralysis. Many chicks lie on their sides.

Mortality is high because chicks cannot get to food or water. Adult birds which become infected show few symptoms but lay infected eggs.

Transmission Vertical in the hatching egg. Horizontal through the droppings.

Treatment No treatment.

Prevention Vaccination of breeders is the answer. Their immunity should be checked regularly as they pass on antibodies to their chicks and this gives good protection.

Marek's disease

Symptoms A tumour-causing virus which is present in most chickens worldwide, but does not always cause tumours. Sometimes tumours enlarge and cause death. The virus can infect the bursa of Fabricius and reduce birds' immunity to other diseases.

Transmission Horizontal. This virus has a unique method of transfer – it lodges in the feather follicles and then gets into the air on skin debris and feather particles. It floats around and is inhaled by other birds. The infected dust and debris can be carried around on feet, clothes, etc.

Diagnosis Tumours are very symptomatic.

Treatment No treatment.

Prevention Several vaccines are available, all derived from herpes virus turkey (HVT).

Avian influenza (bird flu)

Symptoms A contagious infection caused by the influenza virus type A, which can affect most bird species, including all poultry species and occasionally some mammalian species. Avian influenza can be classified into two categories, low pathogenic (LPAI) and high pathogenic (HPAI) forms, based on the severity of the illness caused in birds. Avian influenza is a reportable disease. The LPAI form commonly causes only mild symptoms (ruffled feathers, a drop in egg production) and may easily go undetected. The HPAI form spreads very rapidly through poultry flocks, causes disease affecting multiple internal organs, and has a mortality that can approach 100%, often within 48h. The great concern is that the H5N1 strain of this virus has been known to infect human beings with a very severe form of influenza with a high mortality rate.

Transmission Horizontal. The main route of transmission is probably as an aerosol but other routes may be possible.

Diagnosis Laboratory diagnosis is required.

Treatment No treatment.

Prevention No vaccines are available yet for avian influenza.

Parasitic diseases

Other important infectious diseases of chickens are caused by coccidia. These are protozoa that live in the intestinal tract and can cause great damage there. There are several species of coccidia that infect chickens and all belong to the group *Eimeria*. The 3 most important ones are *E. tenella*, *E. necatrix* and *E. acervulina*. The diseases are generally called 'coccidiosis' no matter which organism is responsible.

Coccidia have a complex life history spent partly in the chicken and partly outside it. Coccidiosis is spread by single-celled bodies known as oocysts. These are passed in the droppings, but are not infectious. They must first go through a process called sporulation, which requires correct conditions of temperature, moisture and air and takes 2–4 days. If the sporulated oocyst is eaten by a chicken it ends up in the intestines where it multiplies in the gut wall and causes damage. Eventually after 4–7 days, more oocysts are produced and expelled in the droppings and the whole cycle starts again.

The amount of damage is closely related to the number of oocysts present and if only a few are present then little damage is caused. However, if the bird goes on ingesting more and they keep multiplying, very soon there can be millions present – and then the bird has a big problem. If the numbers build up slowly, then the bird can develop immunity. However, this seldom happens under the artificial conditions found in a laboratory and numbers usually build up very quickly.

Coccidiosis (Eimeria *species*)

Symptoms Bloody droppings, ruffled feathers, paleness (anaemia due to blood loss) loss of appetite, poor growth, poor production, diarrhoea. The different species of coccidia produce different lesions in different parts of the intestine.

Transmission Through droppings – but of course infected material can be carried on feet, equipment etc, and so be spread from room to room.

Diagnosis Bloody droppings and characteristic lesions in gut are usually enough for diagnosis. A pathology laboratory can identify the species involved.

Treatment and prevention There are lots of good coccidiostats available, which can be added to the feed. However, some of them are very specific to some species of coccidia, so it is advisable to get a laboratory identification. Also, coccidia can develop resistance to a particular coccidiostat, so it sometimes helps to rotate coccidiostats from time to time. Birds on the floor will be at biggest risk (ie, most young birds, all broilers, some layer replacements and all breeders). A coccidiostat is usually fed to broilers at a rate to completely suppress coccidia since there is no time for broilers to develop immunity. With replacement birds (layers and breeders) another strategy is employed. A coccidiostat is fed at full strength for the first 5–6 weeks. It is then gradually withdrawn so that the birds get a very mild coccidiosis. They then slowly develop an immunity and in time the coccidiostat can be withdrawn completely. Another approach is to use a so-called 'vaccine'. This is a material which contains a limited number of oocysts and is fed to chicks at about 10–12 days of age. The idea is that the numbers of oocysts are small and immunity will build up. Obviously a coccidiostat should not be used with this approach. **Warning** – Some coccidiostats are **very** toxic to other classes of livestock. For example, monensin at normal poultry dosages causes acute heart failure in horses and dogs.

There are some other parasitic diseases of poultry caused by various round and flat worms, but these are unlikely to be a problem in the laboratory. There are also various species of lice that parasitise the skin of domestic fowl, but these are unlikely to be a problem in the laboratory. However, mites can be a serious problem, particularly the common red mite, *Dermanyssus gallinae*. Every effort should be made to keep laboratory facilities free of red mite since an infestation can cause birds extreme distress and major blood loss, and the mite is very difficult to eradicate because of resistance to all permitted arachnicides. Precautions would include an all-in, all-out policy and allowing only hatching eggs or day-old chicks into the facility.

Metabolic disorders

The implementation of good biological security and the use of vaccines have resulted in control of most of the infectious diseases of chickens. Non-infectious diseases are now of more importance to the poultry industry, and these diseases, usually referred to as metabolic disorders, will no doubt be evident in the laboratory, particularly if modern, high-producing strains of chicken are used. The most important ones are sudden death syndrome, ascites, fatty liver and kidney syndrome, and various skeletal disorders in broiler chickens, and liver haemorrhagic syndrome and osteoporosis in laying hens. Most of these disorders have a multifactorial aetiology and are therefore complex. They are mentioned here, simply to warn laboratory managers of their existence. If morbidity due to metabolic disorders is suspected, then more detailed texts such as Saif *et al.* (2003) and Leeson *et al.* (1995) should be consulted.

Abnormal behaviour

The occurrence of abnormal behaviour is often a sign that birds are suffering. As mentioned previously, the laboratory manager should be able to recognise behavioural signs of disease. In addition to this, some other behavioural symptoms of suffering are fairly easy to recognise. Severe frustration is often characterised by stereotyped back-and-forward pacing and increased aggression (Duncan & Wood-Gush 1971, 1972). Lack of a suitable nesting place is the most likely cause of severe frustration. Severe food restriction often leads to stereotyped pecking at the feeder or some other aspect of the environment (Savory 1989).

Occasionally some strains of chickens in some circumstances will show panic or hysteria. These may be defined as excessive and inappropriate flight–fright reactions, panic having some external trigger and hysteria without an apparent cause (Mills & Faure 1990). Both panic and hysteria seem to have complex aetiologies. However, since they are often associated with large group size, they are unlikely to occur in the laboratory.

Further reading

The primary breeding companies produce 'Management Guides' for each of their hybrids. These set out the management conditions that will optimise the productivity of that particular strain. Laboratories using these hybrids should always ensure that they have the relevant guide. In addition, there are several excellent text books on poultry management and husbandry such as Sainsbury (1992) and Bell and Weaver (2002) which should be used to expand this text. The welfare implications of different commercial husbandry systems are dealt with in some detail by Appleby *et al.* (2004) and this should also be studied.

References

Abrahamsson, P., Tauson, R. and Appleby, M.C. (1996) Behaviour health and integument of four hybrids of laying hens in modified and conventional cages. *British Poultry Science*, **37**, 521–540

Appleby, M.C. and Hughes, B.O. (1995) The Edinburgh modified cage for laying hens. *British Poultry Science*, **36**, 707–718

Appleby, M.C., Mench, J.A. and Hughes, B.O. (2004) *Poultry Behaviour and Welfare*. CAB International, Wallingford

Axelsson, M., Dang, Q., Pitsillides, K. *et al.* (2007) A novel, fully implantable, multichannel biotelemetry system for measurement of blood flow, pressure, ECG, and temperature. *Journal of Applied Physiology*, **102**, 1220–1228

Bell, D.D. and Weaver, W.D. (eds) (2002) *Chicken Meat and Egg Production*, 5th edn. Springer, New York

Blokhuis, H.J. (1986) Feather pecking in poultry: Its relation with ground pecking. *Applied Animal Behaviour Science*, **16**, 63–67

Blokhuis, H.J. and Arkes, J.G. (1984) Some observations on the development of feather pecking in poultry. *Applied Animal Behaviour Science*, **12**, 145–157

Canadian Council on Animal Care (1993) Euthanasia. In: *Guide to the Care and Use of Experimental Animals*, Vol. **2**. pp 141–153. CCAC, Ottawa

Close, B., Banister, K., Baumans, V. *et al.* (1996) Recommendations for euthanasia of experimental animals. Part 1. *Laboratory Animals*, **30**, 293–316

Close, B., Banister, K., Baumans, V. *et al.* (1997) Recommendations for euthanasia of experimental animals. Part 2. *Laboratory Animals*, **31**, 1–32

Collias, N.E., Collias, E.C., Hunsaker, D. *et al.* (1966) Locality fixation mobility and social organization within an unconfined population of Red Jungle Fowl. *Animal Behaviour*, **14**, 550–559

Danbury, T.C., Weeks, C.A., Chambers, J.P. *et al.* (2000) Self-selection of the analgesic drug Carprofen by lame broiler chickens. *Veterinary Record*, **146**, 307–311

Decuypere, E. and Bruggeman, V. (2007) The endocrine interface of environmental and egg factors affecting chick quality. *Poultry Science*, **86**, 1037–1042

Dove, W.F. (1935) A study of individuality in the nutritive instincts and of the causes and effects of variation in the selection of food. *American Naturalist*, **69**, 469–544

Duncan, I.J.H. (1980) The ethogram of the domesticated hen. In: *The Laying Hen and Its Environment*. Ed. Moss, R., pp. 5–18. Martinus Nijhoff, The Hague

Duncan, I.J.H. (1981) Telemetry. In: *First European Symposium on Poultry Wefare*. Ed. Sørenson L.Y., pp. 15–21. Danish Branch of the World's Poultry Science Association, Køge

Duncan, I.J.H. (1990) Reactions of poultry to human beings. In: *Social Stress in Domestic Animals*. Eds Zayan, R. and Dantzer, R., pp. 121–131. Kluwer Academic, Dordrecht

Duncan, I.J.H. and Filshie, J.H. (1980) The use of radiotelemetry devices to measure temperature and heart-rate in the domestic fowl. In: *A Handbook on Biotelemetry and Radio Tracking*. Eds Amlaner, C.J. and Macdonald, D.W., pp. 579–588. Pergamon Press, London

Duncan, I.J.H., Filshie, J.H. and McGee, I.J. (1975) Radiotelemetry of avian shank temperature using a thin film hybrid microcircuit. *Medical and Biological Engineering*, **13**, 544–550

Duncan, I.J.H. and Kite, V.G. (1989) Nest site selection and nest building behaviour in domestic fowl. *Animal Behaviour*, **37**, 215–231

Duncan, I.J.H., Slee, G.S., Seawright, E. *et al.* (1989) Behavioural consequences of partial beak amputation (beak trimming) in poultry. *British Poultry Science*, **30**, 479–488

Duncan, I.J.H. and Wood-Gush, D.G.M. (1971) Frustration and aggression in the domestic fowl. *Animal Behaviour*, **19**, 500–504

Duncan, I.J.H. and Wood-Gush, D.G.M. (1972) Thwarting of feeding behaviour in the domestic fowl. *Animal Behaviour*, **20**, 444–451

Etches, R.J. (1996) *Reproduction in Poultry*. CAB International, Wallingford

European Commission (2007) Commission recommendations of 18 June 2007 on guidelines for the accommodation and care of animals used for experimental and other scientific purposes. Annex II to European Council Directive 86/609. See 2007/526/EC. http://eurlex.europa.eu/LexUriServ/site/en/oj/2007/l_197/l_19720070730en00010089.pdf (accessed 13 May 2008)

Fasenko, G.M. (2007) Egg storage and the embryo. *Poultry Science*, **86**, 1020–1024

Filshie, J.H., Duncan, I.J.H. and Clark, J.S.B. (1980) Radiotelemetry of the avian electrocardiogram. *Medical, Biological and Engineering Computing*, **18**, 633–637

Follensbee, M.E., Duncan, I.J.H. and Widowski, T.M. (1992) Quantifying nesting motivation of domestic hens. *Journal of Animal Science*, **70**, 50 (Abstract)

Gentle, M.J., Hughes, B.O., Fox, A. *et al.* (1997) Behavioural and anatomical consequences of two beak trimming methods in 1- and 10-d-old domestic chicks. *British Poultry Science*, **38**, 453–463

Gentle, M.J., Waddington, D., Hunter, L.N. *et al.* (1990) Behavioural evidence for persistent pain following partial beak amputation in chickens. *Applied Animal Behaviour Science*, **27**, 149–157

Howlett, J.C. (2008) Local anesthesia and analgesia. In: *Avian Medicine*. Ed. Samour, J., pp. 151–153. Mosby, Elsevier, Edinburgh

Hughes, B.O. and Black, A.J. (1976) The influence of handling on egg production, egg shell quality and avoidance behaviour in hens. *British Poultry Science*, **17**, 135–144

Hulet, R.M. (2007) Managing incubation: Where are we and why? *Poultry Science*, **86**, 1017–1019

Humane Slaughter Association (2001) *Practical slaughter of poultry. A guide for small producers*, 2nd edn. Humane Slaughter Association, Herts

Joint Working Group on Refinement (2001) Laboratory birds: Refinements in husbandry and procedures. Fifth Report of the BVAAWF/FRAME/RSPCA/UFAW Joint Working Group on Refinement. *Laboratory Animals*, **35** (Suppl. 1), S1–S163

Jones, R.B. and Faure, J.M. (1981) The effects of regular handling on fear responses in the domestic chick. *Behavioural Processes*, **6**, 135–143

Jordan, F.T.W. (*Ed.*) (1990) *Poultry Diseases*, 6th edn. Bailliere Tindall, London

Kjaer, J.B. and Sørensen, P. (1997) Feather pecking in White Leghorn chickens – a genetic study. *British Poultry Science*, **38**, 333–341

Kjaer, J.B. and Vestergaard, K.S. (1999) Development of feather pecking in relation to light intensity. *Applied Animal Behaviour Science*, **65**, 243–254

Lawton, M.P.C. (2008) Anaesthesia and soft tissue surgey. In: *Avian Medicine*. Ed. Samour, J., pp. 135–151. Mosby, Elsevier, Edinburgh

Leeson, S. and Summers, J.D. (1997) *Commercial Poultry Nutrition*, 2nd edn. University Books, Guelph

Leeson, S., Diaz, G. and Summers, J.D. (1995) *Poultry Metabolic Disorders and Mycotoxins*. University Books, Guelph

Lewis, P. and Morris, T. (2006) *Poultry Lighting: The Theory and Practice*. Northcot, Andover

Malleau, A.E., Duncan, I.J.H., Widowski, T.M. *et al.* (2007) The importance of rest in young domestic fowl. *Applied Animal Behaviour Science*, **106**, 52–69

McBride, G., Parer, I.P. and Foenander, F. (1969) The social organization and behaviour of the feral domestic fowl. *Animal Behaviour Monographs*, **2**, 125–181

Mills, A.D. & Faure, J.-M. (1990) Panic and hysteria in domestic fowl: A review. In: *Social Stress in Domestic Animals*. Eds Zayan, R. and Dantzer, R., pp. 248–272. Kluwer, Dordrecht

Muir, W.M. and Craig, J.V. (1998) Improving animal well-being through genetic selection. *Poultry Science*, **77**, 1781–1788

Murphy, L.B. and Duncan, I.J.H. (1978) Attempts to modify the responses of domestic fowl towards human beings. II. The effect of early experience. *Applied Animal Ethology*, **4**, 5–12

Olsson, I.A.S. and Keeling, L.J. (2002) The push-door for measuring motivation in hens: laying hens are motivated to perch at night. *Animal Welfare*, **11**, 11–19

Saif, Y.M., Barnes, H.J., Glisson, J.R. *et al.* (Eds.) (2003) *Diseases of Poultry*, 11th edn. Blackwell Publishing, Oxford

Sainsbury, D. (1992) *Poultry Health and Management*, 3rd edn. Blackwell Publishing, Oxford

Savory, C.J. (1989) Stereotyped behaviour as a coping strategy in restricted-fed broiler breeder stock. In: *Third European Symposium on Poultry Welfare*. Eds Faure J.-M. and Mills A.D., pp. 261–264. World's Poultry Science Association, Tours

Schaeffer, D.O. (1994) Miscellaneous species: anesthesia and analgesia. In: *Research Animal Anesthesia, Analgesia and Surgery*. Eds Smith, A.C. and Swindle, M.M., pp. 129–136. Scientists Center for Animal Welfare, Greenbelt, Maryland

Siegel, P.B., Haberfield, A., Mukherjee, T.K. *et al.* (1992) Jungle fowl – domestic fowl relationships: a use of DNA fingerprinting. *World's Poultry Science Journal*, **48**, 147–155

Sinn, L. (1994) Anesthesiology. In: *Avian Medicine: Principles and Application*. Eds. Ritchie, B.W., Harrison, G.J. and Harrison, L.R., pp. 1066–1080. Wingers Publishing Inc, Lake Worth

Tauson, R. (1980) Cages: how could they be improved? In: *The Laying Hen and Its Environment*. Ed. Moss, R., pp. 269–299. Martinus Nijhoff, The Hague

Tauson, R. (1985) Mortality of laying hens caused by differences in cage design. *Acta Agriculturæ Scandinavica*, **35**, 165–174

Tauson, R. and Abrahamsson, P. (1994) Foot and skeletal disorders in laying hens. Effects of perch design hybrid housing system and stocking density. *Acta Agriculturæ Scandinavica Section A Animal Science*, **44**, 110–119

Whittow, G.C. (1986) Regulation of body temperature. In: *Avian Physiology*, 4th edn. Ed. Sturkie, P.D., pp. 221–252. Springer Verlag, New York

Wood-Gush, D.G.M. (1959) A history of the domestic chicken from antiquity to the 19th century. *Poultry Science*, **38**, 321–326

Wood-Gush, D.G.M. (1971) *The Behaviour of the Domestic Fowl*. Heinemann Educational Books Ltd, London

42 The Japanese quail

Kimberly M. Cheng, Darin C. Bennett, and Andrew D. Mills[1]

Biological overview

The Japanese quail (*Coturnix japonica*) is a small, chubby, brown-coloured terrestrial migratory bird (Wetherbee 1961). The species is indigenous to East Asia (Latitude 17°N to 55°N) and is sympatric with the common quail (*Coturnix coturnix*) in their breeding range in Mongolia (Wakasugi 1984). Their habitat is in grasslands, croplands, riversides, alpine meadows and grass steppes (Long 1981).

The Japanese quail belongs to the order Galliformes, family Phasianidae, genus *Coturnix*, and was previously considered to be a sub-species of the common quail (see Crawford 1990). It was given full species status in 1983 (American Ornithologists' Union 1983; Howard & Moore 1984) because no interbreeding has been observed between the common quail and the Japanese quail in areas where the two species are sympatric. Barilani *et al.* (2005), however, have suggested that natural hybridisation is a possibility on the basis of mtDNA and nuclear DNA analyses of a small sample of five birds. In captivity, hybridisation is possible but difficult (Derégnaucourt *et al.* 2002), and only after some failed attempts (Lepori 1964; Pala & Lissia-Frau 1966; Moreau & Wayne 1968). The Japanese quail (Old World quail) should not be confused with Bobwhite quail (*Colinus virginianus*), a species in the family Odotophonidae (New World quail). Both species have been domesticated and used as food and as research animals.

Japanese quail were originally introduced to North America by the US Fish and Wildlife Service as game birds in 1870, and releases continued into the late 1950s (Standford 1957). Most of the birds released were domestic birds imported from Japan. All stocks released in North America failed to establish and perished within 1 year. However, release attempts in the 1940s on the Hawaiian Islands were successful. Populations survived on Kauai, Molokai, Lanai, Maui and Hawaii (Peterson 1961) and have been regularly hunted (Munro 1960). Although the populations originated from released domestic birds, they are now considered wild.

Domestication and origin of domestic and laboratory lines

The first records of domestic Japanese quail were from twelfth century Japan and it appears that the species was domesticated there during the eleventh century, or imported from China in an already domesticated form (Chang *et al.* 2005), at about that time (Howes 1964, Crawford 1990). Japanese quail were originally kept for their song (Howes 1964) and it has been inferred that lines of quail with particular call types were bred for use in song contests (Taka-Tsukasa 1935; Wakasugi 1984).

Between 1910 and 1941, the Japanese selected quail for increased egg production and by 1940, a thriving industry existed (Howes 1964; Wakasugi 1984). However, all lines of song-type quail and the majority of egg production lines were lost during World War II. Following the war, the quail industry was rebuilt from the few remaining domesticated birds available, possibly with the addition of domesticated lines from Korea, China and Taiwan and quail captured in the wild (Howes 1964; Wakasugi 1984). All present day laboratory and commercial lines of Japanese quail appear to have been derived from this post-war population (Crawford 1990).

General biology

Morphology

The wild-type natal plumage of Japanese quail is the same in both sexes (Cheng & Kimura 1990). Chicks have tawny coloured heads with small black patches above the beak. A buff stripe bordered by black stripes runs along the top of the head and there are four dark brown stripes on the back. The back and wings are pale brown (Cheng & Kimura 1990). Juvenile plumage is present at 3–4 weeks of age and full adult plumage is present at about 6 weeks of age. The species is sexually dimorphic in adult plumage (Figure 42.1). In both sexes, body plumage is predominantly brown (Wetherbee 1961; Kawahara 1967, 1973) but it is highly variable in terms of shades of brown and some of the markings on the breast and the throat (Cheng & Kimura 1990). Females have pale-coloured breast feathers which are speckled with dark-coloured spots whereas males have uniform dark rufous breast and cheek feathers. Furthermore, males may develop a white collar while females have cream coloured feathers on the cheeks and do not develop white collars (Urbanski 1984). With domestication came the development of many strains with various plumage colour and pattern (Cheng & Kimura 1990).

Domestic quail reach sexual maturity at 4–5 weeks of age, depending on the lighting schedule. Females enter into full

[1]Deceased

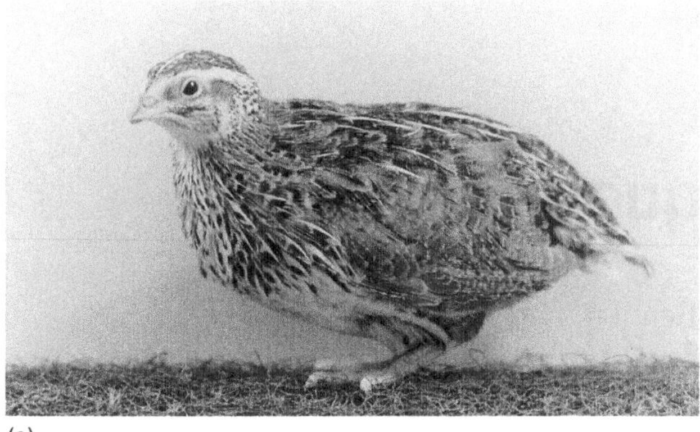

(a)

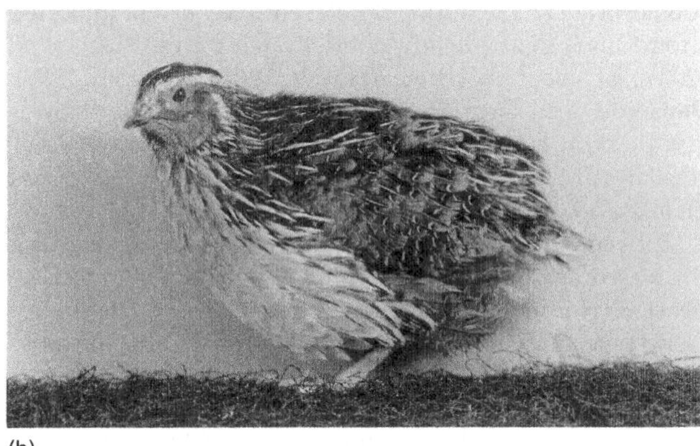

(b)

Figure 42.1 Wild-type plumage of female (a) and male (b) adult Japanese quail. Pictures reproduced by permission of the UBC Quail Genetic Resource Centre.

lay at about 6 weeks of age (see also Gerken & Mills 1993). Quail eggs are variably mottled. The background colour of shells varies from white through to pale brown or blue. The shell colour pigments are porphyrin and biliverdin (Poole 1965). Shell colour, mottling pattern, size and shape vary considerably between females but are consistent for and unique to a given female (Jones *et al.* 1964). Eggs weight varies between 8 and 13 g depending on the strain of the bird (see below).

Size range and lifespan

Adult wild males and females weigh about 90 and 100 g, respectively (Kawahara 1967), and unselected domestic males and females weigh about 100 and 120 g, respectively. There is considerable variability in body weight between different genetic strains of quail (Gerken & Mills 1993). Some domestic strains that have been selectively bred for meat production weigh as much as 300 g at 6 weeks of age (Cheng & Nichols 1992).

The domestic Japanese quail is notable for its rapid growth rate (Figure 42.2). Chicks weigh between 8 and 12 g at hatching. They double this weight by 5 days of age and triple it by 8 days of age (Lucotte 1974). By 5–6 weeks of age, birds may weigh 160–250 g depending on sex and strain (Gerken & Mills 1993).

There appear to be no reports concerning the lifespan of wild quail. Under artificial husbandry conditions,

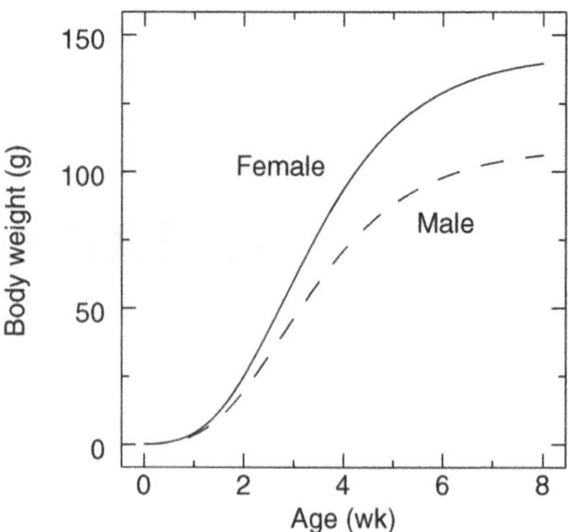

Figure 42.2 Growth curve for male (dashed line) and female (solid line) domestic Japanese quail from hatching to 8 weeks of age (data from Aggrey (2003)).

reported lifespan varied depending on breeds, rearing conditions (e.g. continuous lighting) and nutrition factors. In most cases, life was terminated artificially and the reported lifespan may mean productive lifespan (eg, see Table 42.1 and Gerken & Mills 1993). Woodard & Abplanalp (1971) reported that males live longer (more than 5 years) than females (less than 4 years). In the authors' laboratory, a male that was kept as a mascot lived for 8 years before being euthanased because of the development of skin tumours.

Social organisation

Studies of social organisation in wild Japanese quail appear to be limited to those by Taka-Tsukasa (1935), and opportunistic observations of wild quail have produced conflicting reports (Kawahara 1967; Dement'ev *et al.* 1967). It has been reported that the birds live in pairs during the breeding season but gather in large flocks during migration and in the winter (Crawford 1990). Observations of feral Japanese quail in Hawaii indicate that males are territorial, and mating and nesting take place within these territories (Schwartz & Schwartz 1949). Members of a pair remain in close proximity before and during the egg-laying period (which implies mate guarding and thus the possibility of extra-pair copulations (McKinney *et al.* 1983)). Dement'ev *et al.* (1967) reported that the species is polygamous. Kawahara (1967) noted that males and females live in pairs during the breeding season. On the basis of such evidence and studies of other *Coturnix* species, Kovach (1975) concluded that the mating system of wild Japanese quail is in a transitional state between polygamy and monogamy. However, one of the few studies with captive quail (Orcutt & Orcutt 1976) indicated that males and females formed strong pair bonds, and that males were monogamous and courted only their own female. There is also evidence that Japanese quail are able to recognise the calls of a pair-bonded mate (Guyomarc'h 1974). Crowing rate increases in males visually separated from females, and crowing intensity increases with rises in ambient noise levels (Potash 1972, 1975). Crowing patterns of pair-bonded males differ from those of unmated males (Potash 1975). Potash (1975) argued that crowing by males and cricket calls by females serve the function of contact calls when a bonded pair is out of sight of each other. Nichols *et al.* (1992) studied captive Japanese quail in outdoor flight pens and confirmed that males were paired with one female for the whole breeding season. Females also paired with only one male during the breeding season. Nichols (1991) concluded that wild Japanese quail are monogamous with some opportunistic forced extra-pair copulations by the male.

Under simulated natural conditions in outdoor flight pens, domestic quail males are serially monogamous with significantly higher frequencies of extra-pair copulations compared to wild males (Nichols 1991). With higher density rearing in floor-pens or cages, they become promiscuous. Cheng *et al.* (1989a) observed that the cloacal foam gland in domestic males is much more prominent than that of wild males. Adkins-Regan (1995) suggested that the enlarged foam gland of the domestic males '*hints at a genetically non-monogamous mating system*'.

The common courtship displays performed by wild males include zig-zag dancing, leading, tidbitting, strutting and squatting (Eynon 1968; Nichols 1991). The male initiates sexual behaviour by strutting towards the female. During strutting, the male stretches himself such that his beak, body, head and neck are parallel to the ground, erects his body feathers and walks on his claws and digits with a characteristic stiff-legged gait. Under simulated natural conditions, domestic males also perform these displays but with significantly less frequency and with less specific contexts (Nichols 1991). An indication of female acceptance of the male could be solicitation of copulation by the female. A female would walk in front of her suitor and crouch, inviting the male to mount her (Nichols 1991). A mated pair also keeps in close vocal contact with each other, giving very quiet calls as they move around together. Under husbandry conditions, the role of the female in courtship and mating appears to be minimal (Kovach 1975). Sefton and Siegel (1973) reported that male courtship displays were rare. The male approaches the female, grabs her head or neck feathers and attempts to mount her without any additional courtship or display behaviour (Farris 1964, 1967; Wilson & Bermant 1972). Cheng (unpublished data) observed mating behaviour of domestic quail using two-male, six-female mating groups in 2.5 × 3.1 m indoor floor-pens. Under this situation, a male could dominate the other male and attempt to keep the subordinate male from mating with the females. Often the subordinate male would dash into a group of females and perform zig-zag dancing, and the females responded by scattering in different directions, crouching and hopping up in the air. The subordinate male, and sometimes both males, would start to grab and mount females. During mounting, the male 'grabs' the head or neck feathers of the female, positions himself on the back of the female, spreads his wings and begins treading. The copulatory response sequence results in ejaculation in about half of these cases. On those occasions, the male brings his cloaca down and underneath the female, establishes cloacal contact and ejaculates. The male releases his grip on the female and dismounts immediately after ejaculation. Following dismounting, both the male and the female may show ruffling and shaking of the feathers. While males mount females regardless of the females' receptivity (Lucotte 1974), the type of female's reaction significantly influenced the latency of the male's grab, mount and cloacal contact responses and also determined the efficiency of the male's copulatory behaviour (Domjan & Nash 1988).

Under husbandry conditions Japanese quail form dominance hierarchies. Although the nature of these hierarchies has not been extensively studied, they appear to be of the peck order type and confer priority of access to resources (Otis 1972; Nol *et al.* 1996). In group-housed birds, subordinate birds show ambivalent behaviour (Edens *et al.* 1983). This ambivalent behaviour comprises aspects of both aggressive and submissive behaviour and is an attempt to displace dominant birds from feeders or drinkers. Furthermore, under conditions of deprivation, levels of aggression increase as distance from the food source decreases, and dominance relationships change from a peck order system to a peck dominance system.

Domestic males do not respond well to disruption of established hierarchies. If birds are introduced into established groups, they are likely to be attacked. Attacks are more likely if a stranger is introduced into the home cage of other birds. As a consequence, it is unwise to mix groups of birds or to introduce replacement birds into groups where hierarchies have been established.

Reproduction

Reproduction in Japanese quail is strongly dependent on the lighting regimen. Wild birds breed in spring and summer. However, in the laboratory, birds can be maintained in breeding condition all year if they are kept on day lengths of 12 h or more. If birds are kept on short day lengths (6 h or less) sexual development is delayed or inhibited. Social factors as well as photoperiod influence the onset of sexual maturity. The sound of male vocalisations can speed female sexual development (Guyomarc'h & Guyomarc'h 1984) and males housed with females show faster sexual development than males housed alone (Delville *et al.* 1984). If birds are transferred from long to short day lengths the gonads regress and reproduction ceases (Sachs 1967). However, some females will lay eggs under short photoperiods or even under continuous darkness (Noble 1972; Stein & Bacon 1976).

If the photoperiod is sufficiently long, sperm production commences at around 4 weeks of age (Mather & Wilson 1964; Ottinger & Brinkley 1978; Ottinger & Brinkley 1979a) and sperm are present in large numbers in the vas deferens and testes by 35 days of age (Ottinger 1978). Males begin crowing at about 2 weeks of age, show cloacal gland development (Cheng *et al.* 1989b) at about 4 weeks of age and begin mating attempts. Completed copulations may occur only a few days later (Ottinger & Brinkley 1979b).

Male fertility starts to decline as early as 15 weeks of age (Ottinger 1991). Old males have lower fertility than younger males (Ottinger *et al.* 1983; Woodard & Abplanalp 1967) and males kept on a chronic long day length photoperiod develop more age-related abnormalities in testes and sperm than males kept on shorter day length photoperiods (Eroschenko *et al.* 1977). Advanced age adversely affects sexual behaviour in male quail (see reviews by Ottinger 1983; 1991).

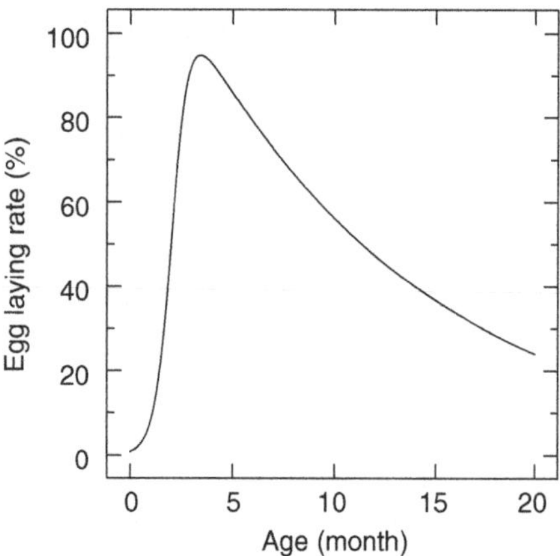

Figure 42.3 Hen-day egg laying rate as a function of age in domestic Japanese quail (data from Minvielle *et al.* (2000)).

Egg production declines with age (Figure 42.3) and eggs from older females (post 20 weeks) have low hatchability and fertility even though older females are more sexually receptive than younger females (Woodard & Abplanalp 1967). Wild females in their first breeding season display little sexual activity until late in the season and are usually not successful in laying a clutch until their second breeding season (Nichols 1991). Keeping females on chronic long photoperiods shortens their reproductive life presumably because of the physiological demands associated with high egg production.

Table 42.1 Standard biological data for the Japanese quail. Modified from Cooper (1987) and Mills *et al.* (1999).

Parameter	*Value*
Body weight (g)	
1 day	6–8
Adult male	100–130
Adult female	120–160
Organ weight (% body weight)	
Liver	1.95
Heart	0.91
Kidney	0.73
Testes	2.88
Performance and longevity	
Egg weight (g)	9–10
Egg number/100 bird days	80–90
Age at sexual maturity (days)	38–42
Lifespan (months)	24–26
Blood pressure (mmHg)	
Systolic	
Adult male	158.1 ± 4.6[1]
Adult female	156.1 ± 4.7[1]
Diastolic	
Adult male	151.8 ± 4.7[1]
Adult female	146.9 ± 4.2[1]
Heart rate (beats/min)	
Adult male	530.7 ± 17.7[1]
Adult female	489.5 ± 17.1[1]

[1] mean ± se

Breeds, strains and genetics

A wide variety of plumage colour mutants exist (Cheng & Kimura 1990; Butkauskas 2001) and various strains have been selected for physiological and behavioural traits. Details of existing known mutations, gene nomenclature, mutations, physical linkage maps and specific genetic lines can found in Cheng and Kimura (1990), Cheng and Nichols (1992) and Somes (1984).

The karyotype of the Japanese quail consists of seven pairs of macrochromosomes (including the sex chromosomes) and 32 pairs of microchromosomes. The integrated linkage map has been published by Kayang *et al.* (2006).

Standard biological data

There is a paucity of recent information concerning common physiological parameters in present-day strains of Japanese quail. Tables 42.1 and 42.2 show physiological and baseline haematological and clinical chemistry data, respectively. However, these tables should be considered only a guideline since present-day laboratory and domestic strains may be physiologically different because of selection for other traits, such as body weight or increased egg production.

Quail as food animals

Japanese quail have been farmed in many parts of the world. Due to their small body size, fast growth, high rate of egg production and ease of management, they are a practical solution to the problem of animal protein shortage in developing countries and an alternative to chicken in developed countries (Shanaway 1994). Under commercial production systems, quail can be marketed at about 5 weeks of age with an average weight of about 215 g. A feed conversion ratio (feed/gain) ratio of 3.5 is not as efficient as that of broiler chickens (Hoffmann 1990). However, the strength of the Japanese quail is in egg production. Domestic quail hens start egg-laying at about 5 weeks of age, eggs are about 10 g each, and a hen can produce 280–300 eggs in a year (Minvielle 1998). The feed conversion (feed/egg) ratio of 3.3 makes the Japanese quail the champion species in converting feed into eggs (Shanaway 1994).

In the past four decades, commercial quail farming has developed in many parts of the world, particularly in Japan, China, Korea, India, Italy, France (Bessei 1977; Minvielle 1998), Spain, Hungary, Poland, Estonia, Russia, Czech Republic, Slovakia (Baumgartner 1993), Saudi Arabia, South-eastern United States, Brazil (Murakami & Ariki 1998) and Chile.

Quail as laboratory animals

The Japanese quail's small size, inexpensive rearing requirements, rapid maturation and adaptability to a wide range of husbandry conditions have made it popular as a laboratory

Table 42.2 Haematological and clinical chemistry values for adult domestic Japanese quail (mean ± se). Data from Nirmalan and Robinson (1971) and Faqi *et al.* (1997).

Parameter	*Normal value*	
	Adult male	*Laying females*
Erythrocytes (10^6/mm^3)	4.14 ± 0.07	3.81 ± 0.14
Packed cell volume (%)	53.1 ± 0.8	46.9 ± 1.3
Haemoglobin (g/100 ml)	15.8 ± 0.2	14.3 ± 0.5
Mean corpuscular volume (μm^3)	127.0 ± 2.0	124.0 ± 2.0
Mean corpuscular haemoglobin (ng)	38.5 ± 0.1	37.7 ± 0.7
Mean corpuscular haemoglobin concentration (%)	29.6 ± 0.3	30.4 ± 0.4
Reticulocytes (%)	7.0 ± 0.5	6.1 ± 0.4
Thrombocytes (10^3/mm^3)	117.0 ± 9.0	132.0 ± 17.0
Total leucocytes (10^3/mm^3)	19.7 ± 0.7	23.1 ± 1.0
Heterophils (%)	20.8 ± 1.9	21.8 ± 1.8
Eosinophils (%)	2.5 ± 0.04	4.3 ± 1.5
Basophils (%)	0.4 ± 0.1	0.2 ± 0.1
Lymphocytes (%)	73.6 ± 2.1	71.6 ± 1.6
Monocytes (%)	2.7 ± 0.3	2.1 ± 0.3
Glucose (mmol/l)	18.1 ± 0.8	17.5 ± 1.6
Uric acid (mmol/l)	455 ± 198	426.5 ± 276
Total cholesterol (mmol/l)	5.3 ± 0.4	3.1 ± 0.8
Bilirubin (μmol/l)	0.7 ± 0.05	0.8 ± 0.1
ASAT (U/l)	127.3 ± 10	130.4 ± 18.3
ALAT (U/l)	4.7 ± 1.1	4.3 ± 1.1
γ-GT (U/l)	4.7 ± 1.1	4.3 ± 1.1
Cholinesterase (kU/l)	3.9 ± 0.7	2.8 ± 0.4
Creatinine (μmol/l)	35.4 ± 9.3	29.7 ± 6.1
Protein (g/l)	25.0 ± 1.0	33.6 ± 4.6
Albumin (g/l)	10.7 ± 1.4	16.5 ± 3.6
Phosphate (mmol/l)	1.2 ± 0.3	1.9 ± 0.4
Calcium (mmol/l)	2.3 ± 0.1	4.0 ± 1.3
Magnesium (mmol/l)	1.0 ± 0.04	1.2 ± 0.1
Iron (μmol/l)	12.5 ± 0.4	21.0 ± 2.8

animal for studies of behaviour, development, genetics, growth, endocrinology, nutrition, physiology, pharmacology and toxicology (Landsdown *et al.* 1970; Padgett & Ivey 1959; Wilson *et al.* 1959; Reese & Reese 1962). Since quail have been used as a model organism in many research studies, there is an abundance of background information available. Additionally, numerous mutations are known (Cheng & Kimura 1990) and several strains have been developed for use in research (Marks 1978; Shih *et al.* 1983; Hazard *et al.* 2005; Minvielle *et al.* 2007).

Japanese quail have been used extensively as a research model in neuroendocrinology. Since they have prominent and clearly defined sex differences in their behaviour (Ottinger 1989), they have been particularly useful in studies on the endocrine and neural mechanisms that control sexual differentiation and reproductive behaviour (Balthazart & Ball 1998; Balthazart *et al.* 2003; Ball & Balthazart 2004). Gonadotropin-inhibitory hormone, which directly acts on the pituitary to inhibit gonadotropin release, was first discovered in quail (Tsutsui *et al.* 2000). Since much is known about their hormonal regulation of sexual development and behaviour, Japanese quail are often used as model species for avian toxicology tests (Ottinger *et al.* 2002; Scanes & McNabb 2003). They are a key model for examining the effects of endocrine-disrupting chemicals (Halldin *et al.* 1999; Ottinger *et al.* 2001, 2002). Because of their early maturation and short generation time, quail are best suited for testing trans-generational effects of chemicals (Ottinger *et al.* 2002; Kamata *et al.* 2006). For similar reasons the quail has been a popular model for studying avian genetics (eg, Yang *et al.* 1999; Aggrey 2003; Minvielle *et al.* 1999; Piao *et al.* 2003; Suda & Okamoto 2003; Kim *et al.* 2007).

The species has been of particular value in studies of photoperiodism and the hormonal control of sexual behaviour (Mills *et al.* 1997). Quail are strongly photoperiodic and been used to examine how circadian rhythms are entrained in birds and the role of melatonin in various physiological processes (Underwood 1994; Cheng *et al.* 1994; Underwood & Edmonds 1995; Ohta *et al.* 1989; Moore & Siopes 2000, 2003; Fu *et al.* 2002; Houdelier *et al.* 2002; Nakahara *et al.* 2003).

Furthermore, Japanese quail have many characteristics and behaviour patterns in common with the domestic chicken (*Gallus gallus domesticus*). They have been used to test the nutritive value of various feedstuffs for chickens (eg, Kaya *et al.* 2003; Elangovan *et al.* 2003), and are increasingly being used as model of that species for studies of applied animal ethology related to animal welfare (Gerken & Petersen 1987; Gerken & Mills 1993; Mills & Faure 1990; Odeh *et al.* 2003).

Although Japanese quail have been, and continue to be, a useful laboratory species, Minvielle (2004) reported that their popularity as a research model, as measured by the number of published papers, had declined between 1992 and 2002. His analysis showed that only 115–120 papers per year were published on Japanese quail in 2001–2002. The authors searched BIOSIS Previews for research papers published between 2003 and 2006 on Japanese quail, and found that the number had increased to an average of 154 papers per year. Like Minvielle (2004), they found that the number of papers published on Japanese quail is small in comparison to those published on other laboratory species like rats and mice. However, given the significance of many of the studies outlined above, solely counting the number of published studies on quail may not be a good reflection of their importance as a research model.

Although the amount of research involving Japanese quail has been considerable, the species has largely been used as a model or for comparative purposes, and little attention has been paid to the bird itself (Cheng & Kimura 1990).

Sources of supply (conservation status)

In those countries where quail are farmed for meat or eggs, it may be possible to obtain birds from commercial suppliers. However, one has to be aware that the quality and genetic background of birds from commercial suppliers may vary. This may compromise comparison of results from different experiments or the potential to obtain consistent results from long-term studies. Other sources of supply are laboratories or research stations that maintain breeding populations. In North America, birds of known genetic history and lines selected for particular traits such as atherosclerosis resistance or susceptibility used to be maintained by the Quail Genetic Resource Centre at the University of British Columbia. Because of budgetary problems, the Centre was closed in 2003 and the quail populations have been transferred to and are maintained by the Agassiz Poultry Research Centre (Agriculture and Agri-Food Canada, 6947 #7 Highway, P.O. Box 1000, Agassiz, British Columbia V0M 1A0, Canada). In Europe, The French National Institute for Agricultural Research (INRA) (Department of Animal Genetics, 78352 Jouy-en-Josas, France), and in Asia, The Japan National Institute for Environmental Sciences (NIES) (16-2 Onogawa, Tsukuba Ibaraki, 305-8506, Japan), are both involved in quail research and maintain conservation populations and specialised lines.

Laboratory management and breeding

General husbandry

Different strains of domestic quail differ greatly in their husbandry requirement. The information provided in this section is generic in nature. Researchers working with particular strains of quail may need to modify their husbandry practice accordingly. Management information can usually be obtained from the organisation from which the birds were obtained. Other sources of information include Ottinger and Rattner (1999) and Randall and Bolla (2007).

Housing

Quail can be housed in facilities as diverse as battery cages or outdoor aviaries. The type of housing used will be determined by the nature of the research, statutory requirements, welfare considerations and other factors. Although battery cages have frequently been used, the Joint Working Group on Refinement (JWGR) recommended that, when it is not possible to keep the birds in outdoor aviaries, indoor pens were more suitable than cages, and that if cages have to be used these should be modified to improve the quality of the space they provide (JWGR 2001b). In that report, information on cage sizes used in common practice is also presented together with recommendation for best practice. The European Commission has provided updated housing guidelines (European Commission 2007) which provide advice on rearing, enrichment and housing. These guidelines also recommend pens rather than cages and that housing systems should allow for the provision of substrate for scratching, pecking and dustbathing, nest boxes and cover whenever possible. In European agricultural research where the housing condition has to be similar to that of commercial farms, the standards laid down by the European Union Directive 98/58/EC and Council Directive 1999/74/EC should be followed (see also Table 42.3). General recommendations adopted under the Council of Europe Convention for The Protection of Farm Animals (ETS No 87)[2] and general and species-specific recommendations under The Protection of Vertebrate Animals used for Experimental and other Scientific Purposes (ETS No 123) should also be consulted. In the UK, in circumstances in which Japanese quail are not defined as domestic poultry under the legislative framework, the housing condition guidelines encompassed within the Wildlife and Countryside Act may have to be followed. In the following sections the authors provide a description of some commercially available caging systems. These are not intended to be descriptions of the ideal as there has been little research in this area, and further research into optimal quail housing is required.

Table 42.3 Space allowances for domestic Japanese quail (modified from JWGR (2001b), European Commission (2007)).

Parameter	*Body mass (g)*	
	Up to 150	*Over 150*
Minimum enclosure size (m^2)	1.0	1.0
Area per bird: pair housed (m^2)	0.5	0.6
Area per bird: group housed (m^2)	0.10	0.15
Minimum height (cm)	20	30
Minimum length of feeding trough (cm)	4	4

Breeding facilities

Because domestic quail hens do not take to nest boxes readily and eggs laid on the floor are easily soiled and broken, difficult to collect and impossible to pedigree, cages are by far the most practical system for the housing of breeder or layer stock. Even though Buchwalder and Wechsler (1997) have found that quail may use solid-sided nest boxes with a small entrance, no further research has been carried out to facilitate housing breeding quail in floor pens as an alternative to conventional battery cages. New non-cage housing requirements for farmed poultry will come into effect in Europe in 2012.

A lighting regimen of 16–18h of light and 6–8h of dark is usually sufficient to maintain a bird in good breeding condition.

Brooding facilities

Deep litter floor pens can be used to house birds from hatching to the end of their lives. Deep litter systems can range in size from entire rooms to small boxes mounted on wheels.

[2]http://www.coe.int/t/e/legal_affairs/legal_co-operation/biological_safety%2C_use_of_animals/farming/A_texts_documents.asp#TopOfPage

Heat is provided by lamps, gas burners or radiant heaters suspended above the floor. Wood shavings are the most frequently used floor covering.

Chicks can be kept in wooden boxes until they are 2–3 weeks of age. Typical boxes measure 40 cm × 65 cm × 30 cm (w × d × h). When there is no place to hide, quail will jump upwards with tremendous force in a flight response when startled. If cage height exceeds 30 cm, it will allow the quail to pick up momentum in the flight response and which may result in severe head injuries (Gerken & Mills 1993). For this reason, ceilings can be of soft material. However, the soft material should be: (1) non-porous and washable; (2) non-flammable; and (3) not obstruct ventilation. Brooding boxes with soft ceilings are not commercially available. Heat and light can be provided by an infra-red lamp suspended over one end of the box. Temperature directly under the heat source should be 37 °C, allowing the chicks to find their comfort zone as they move towards the other end of the box. The floor of the boxes should be covered with wood shavings or some other form of litter. After 2 weeks, the heat source is no longer needed if the room temperature is maintained within the 18–26 °C range. At this age, the juveniles can also be moved to deep litter floor pens.

Chicks and juvenile birds have also been kept in commercial battery brooder cages (Figure 42.4). As their name suggests, battery brooder cages are arranged in batteries mounted on metal frames. Heat is provided from radiant heaters which are usually built into the roof of the cage. Light and additional heat can be provided by lamps mounted on the ceiling of the cage. In most commercial brooder cages, the heat source can be controlled by a thermostat. At hatching quail chicks require an ambient temperature of 37 °C. After 3 days the temperature can be reduced to 35 °C. Thereafter, the temperature can be progressively reduced by 5 °C per week until 25 °C.

Battery brooder cages can be of different sizes but usually measure at least 100 cm × 75 cm × 16–20 cm (w × d × h). Cage roofs are made of solid metal sheeting. Cage sides are made of 1 cm^2 (or smaller) wire mesh or solid metal sheeting. The cage fronts usually serve as hinged doors and are usually made out of vertical wire grill. If trough feeders are attached to the front of the cage, then the space between the bars should be large enough to allow the birds to reach the feeder easily but not so large as to allow chicks to escape. Similar provisions should be made for access to drinkers if these are located outside of the cage. The vertical distance between tiers of cages should be sufficient to allow easy collection and removal of droppings. Obviously, there must be an impervious separation between each tier of cages so as to prevent faeces falling from one level to another. Droppings can be collected on sheets of paper, pull out trays or moving belts.

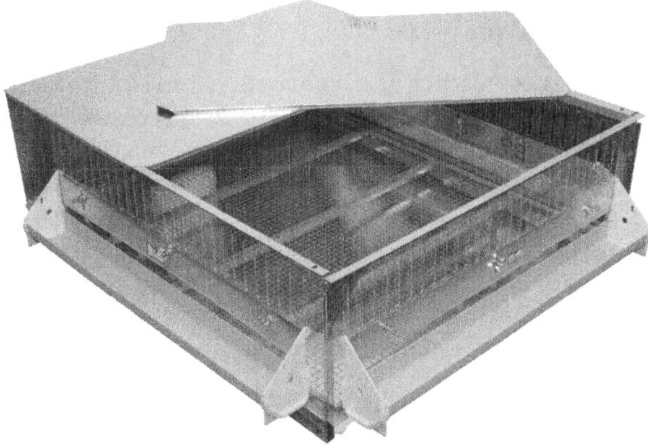

Figure 42.4 Box brooder for Japanese quail chicks. Reproduced with permission of GQF Manufacturing Company.

Cage floors of 1 cm^2 mesh have been used, which allow for the passage of the droppings from the cage. However, this mesh size is too large to support the feet of chicks under 1 week of age. Therefore, for chicks of less than 1 week of age, the cage floor should be lined with sheets of paper or fine mesh plastic mesh (0.2 cm^2). Some droppings will pass through plastic mesh of this size and with reasonable stocking densities, a single sheet of plastic mesh can be left in place from hatching to about 10 days of age when it is no longer required. Paper sheets, pull out trays or moving belts should be cleaned before there is excessive accumulation of droppings. In this context, it is important to remember that droppings will not be evenly distributed over the cage floor but will be concentrated in the areas around feeders and drinkers.

Feeders for young chicks must not have high (<2 cm) sides or the birds may not be able to reach the food. Petri dishes make excellent feeders for chicks from hatching to 4 or 5 days of age when food spillage becomes an important problem. From hatching onwards it is usual to present food in both petri dishes and some other form of feeder so that the chicks are familiar with these other feeders when the petri dishes are removed. In brooder and battery cages food is usually presented in feeders attached to the front of the cage. These feeders can be simple troughs or more complicated 'back-well feeders'.

The appropriate type of drinker varies with the husbandry system. In small cages and boxes, cage-bird drinkers can be used (one per five birds). When birds are housed in deep-litter pens, or boxes, plastic 0.5 l gravity-fed bell drinkers are probably the most appropriate for chicks and sub-adult birds. However, for small chicks it may be advisable to fit drinkers with a grill or rubber ring to reduce the available watering area or some chicks may drown. An alternative solution is to partially fill the drinker with pebbles. Bell drinkers should be placed on wooden sheets to prevent them becoming clogged with litter. However, this is only a partial solution to clogging and drinkers should be inspected daily and cleaned out when necessary.

Irrespective of the type of housing system used, chicks less than 2 weeks old should be kept under continuous illumination at a minimum of 20 lux light intensity. This is of particular importance when birds are kept in large deep litter pens with a single heat source such as a gas burner. Under such conditions, if a period of darkness occurs, chicks will disperse from beneath the heat source and may die. There is no evidence that quail suffer from being kept under UV-deficient lighting (Smith *et al.* 2005).

Rearing and holding facilities

Juvenile and adult birds can best be housed in deep litter floor pens. They can also be kept in colony or pedigree battery cages that do not have internal sources of heating or lighting (Figure 42.5). Commercial colony cages for adults can often be sub-divided into smaller cages for one to three birds.

Floor pens have to be custom built. They can be of various dimensions depending on the number of birds to be housed and other research requirements. Readers should consult JWGR (2001b) and also see Chapter 41 on domestic fowl.

Like brooder cages, adult cages can be of different sizes. However, commercially available colony cages normally measure 100 cm × 50 cm × 16–20 cm (w × d × h) and pedigree cages suitable for up to three or four birds measure 25 cm × 50 cm × 20 cm (w × d × h).

Pedigree and colony cages usually have roofs made of solid metal sheeting. If the cage roof is not solid metal sheeting but of wire mesh, it is advisable to hang soft, wide plastic strips vertically from the cage roof half way down the cage for birds to hide behind. This will minimise their flight response and head injuries. The material used for making these strips should be able to withstand high pressure or steam cleaning without turning brittle. Cages with soft mesh netting roofs are not commercially available, but can be custom installed. However, soft mesh netting roofs have the disadvantages that they are flammable, not easily cleaned and disinfected, there is a risk of birds tangling or strangling themselves in a flight response, and they may not easily used with rack cage systems. Cage sides are made of 1 cm^2 or smaller wire mesh or solid metal sheeting. Cage floors are made of 1–2 × 1 cm mesh to allow the passage of droppings. The cage floors should be sloping so as to allow eggs to roll out. As for brooder cages, the cage fronts are usually hinged and serve as the cage doors. The cage fronts and backs should be made from wire grill with 2.5 cm spaces between the bars to allow birds to reach food and water easily. Adult cages are mounted on metal frames and arranged in batteries with an impervious separation between tiers. The vertical distance between tiers should be sufficient to allow easy collection and removal of droppings. Again, as for brooder cages, droppings can be collected on sheets of paper, pull out trays or moving belts.

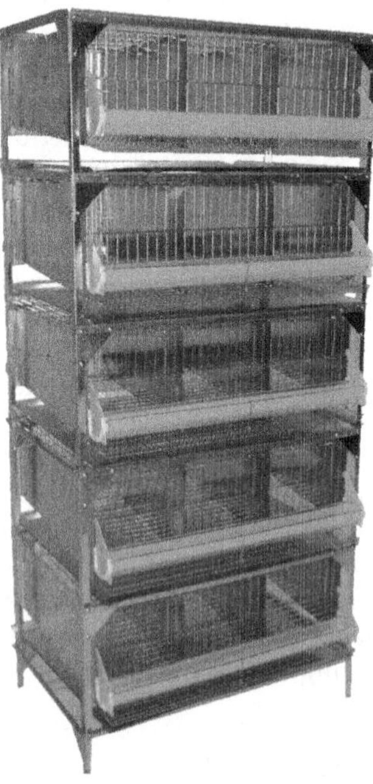

Figure 42.5 Battery breeding cages for adult Japanese quail. Reproduced with permission of GQF Manufacturing Company.

Domestic quail grow rapidly and reach adult size in 4 weeks. Therefore, stocking densities should be predetermined at hatching or should decrease with the age of the birds, until they reach adult size. Strain, breed and line differences in body weight may confound this problem. Lucotte (1974) suggested that stocking densities should be 250 birds/m^2 during the first week after hatching and 175 birds/m^2 during the and third weeks after hatching. However, sex ratio and body weight may require that these estimates be modified. Current recommendations suggest that adult birds should not be kept at stocking densities greater than 40–45 birds/m^2, thus providing each birds with 225–250 cm^2 of space (National Research Council (NRC) 1996; National Advisory Committee for Laboratory Animal Research 2004; see also Table 42.3).

In deep litter systems, food can be provided in hoppers which require less maintenance than other feeder types. Quail have high nutritional requirements throughout their lives, particularly during the growing period, so it is important that the feeding space provided is adequate (see Table 42.3). In large deep litter systems, continuous-flow bell drinkers can be used for juvenile and adult birds. These drinkers can be suspended at a height within easy access by the birds but sufficiently high to minimise clogging with litter. Alternatively, cup or nipple drinkers can be installed. Colony cages and pedigree cages are usually equipped with cup or nipple drinkers (one per five birds).

Although juvenile birds readily adapt to changes in drinker type, this is not the case in adult birds. Birds which have been raised with bell drinkers may not recognise nipple or cup drinkers and *vice versa*. Therefore, when birds are transferred from one type of husbandry system to another, it is important to ensure that the animals find the drinkers.

From 3–6 weeks of age birds should be kept under a lighting regimen of 8 h light to 16 h darkness. If this is not the case females may enter into lay too early, giving rise to reproductive problems (see later in this chapter). Adult birds can be kept on photoperiods of 12–18 h.

Environmental provisions

Quail do not readily use conventional nest boxes (see Buchwalder & Wechsler (1997) for a discussion of the improvement of nest box design and usage) but do use litter for dust-bathing. Enriching the environment of chicks by providing coloured objects and other 'toys' reduces fear and aggressive responses in later life (Jones *et al.* 1991; JWGR 2001b). Providing soft background music and human conversations from radio stations may lessen fear responses elicited by human entering the room.

Social grouping

Male quail react vigorously to the presence of unfamiliar males (Selinger & Bermant 1967) and rearing males in pairs and then interchanging pair members leads to an increase in the frequency of aggressive interactions relative to that observed in the original pairs (Edens *et al.* 1983; Edens 1987). Further, birds that have been left in their 'home' cages are more aggressive than birds that have been transferred to an unfamiliar cage (Edens *et al.* 1983). Therefore, once groups have been established it is inadvisable to attempt to mix groups or introduce new animals into established groups.

In groups where the male:female ratio is high, misdirected head grabs by males (particularly if the female is not receptive) may result in head wounds and eye damage or loss. Under such circumstances, frequent attempts at mounting may result in wounds and, in extreme cases, the death of the females.

Where possible, housing of females in single-sex groups is desirable on welfare grounds. However, this is not the case for males. In all male groups, or in groups where the male:female ratio is high, homosexual copulation attempts are frequent (Wilson & Bermant 1972). This leads to subordinate males suffering feather loss and injuries similar to those sustained by females in mixed-sex groups. In breeding flocks, the ratio of males to females is usually kept at 1:4 to avoid repeated mounting by males leading to injury of the females.

Sexing

Day-old chicks can be vent sexed (examination of the cloaca) (Homma *et al.* 1966) but accuracy is difficult to achieve in practice, except perhaps in Japan where hatcheries hire professional sexers to sex the chicks. However, by the time the chicks are 3–4 weeks old they can be sexed on the basis of plumage colour (Figure 42.1). Researchers working with strains that have plumage colour other than the wild type can identify males at 4 weeks of age by the protruding foam gland above the cloaca (Cheng *et al.* 1989b).

Identification

Individual birds can be identified by means of leg bands or wing tags. The use and application of split rings and wing tags is described in JWGR (2001b). Wing bands and tags are readily available from commercial suppliers. Both bands and tags can be placed on birds of any age. However, the banding and tagging of chicks present certain difficulties. Leg bands, which are suitable for small chicks, do not have a diameter sufficient to accommodate the leg of juvenile or adult birds and must be replaced with larger ones when the birds are 1–2 weeks of age. Wing tags can be left in place throughout the life of the birds but only if they are correctly placed in the propatagium (the membrane or fold of skin in front of the humeral and radio-ulnar parts of the wing). However, in chicks the propatagium is very small and there is a risk that some tags will be placed in the muscles of the wing. If this is the case, then the tag will progressively become imbedded in the musculature of the wing as the bird grows. Therefore, birds should be inspected at 1–2 weeks of age and any incorrectly placed tags replaced. #5 Fingerling tags are suitable for quail chicks and aluminium chick wing bands are suitable for adult quail. Ear tags for mice may also be suitable for the wing tagging of chicks and adults. Transponder microchips could be used as an alternative to leg bands or wing tags. However, these are relatively expensive and do not appear to have been widely used.

In pedigree breeding systems, where two or more hens are kept with a male, egg colour, size and shape can be used to identify which of the hens laid them. These parameters vary greatly between individuals but are extremely consistent within individuals over a 3 week period (Lucotte,1974; Cheng, personal observations).

Hygiene

Good hygiene is essential at all stages of husbandry. Incubators and hatchers should be cleaned and disinfected after each use. Rooms, cages, feeders and drinkers must be kept clean and disinfected after each cycle of use. When birds are kept in cages, dropping collectors should be changed or cleaned on a weekly basis. As far as possible, cages floors should be kept free from droppings. In deep litter floor pens, litter should be topped up weekly, with a total clean out and replacement every 2 months. If breeding birds are kept in deep litter floor pens, a cleaning schedule has to be carefully planned because the cleaning procedure will disrupt egg laying.

Where possible, the buildings used to house quail should be emptied periodically and cleaned and disinfected before being used again.

Health monitoring, quarantine and barrier systems

Birds should be carefully inspected at least once daily and any birds showing signs of sickness or injury should be examined and treated appropriately and any dead birds removed. From hatching to 6 weeks of age, the mortality rate should be less than 5%. During breeding, the mortality rate should be less than 2%. Disease may be indicated by reduced egg output, morbidity and emaciation (see also section on disease). If animals are introduced to existing stock from an external source (this should be avoided if at all possible), it is very important that the source flock is disease free. It is better to bring in fumigated eggs or chicks than adult birds. If chicks or adult birds are brought in from external sources, they should be kept in quarantine for a period of 5–6 weeks. Contact between quail and other birds (particularly game birds) should be avoided. Access to housing facilities should be restricted to persons who have not been in contact with other birds for 72 h. It is prudent to provide disinfectant footbaths and protective clothing for workers and, for biosecurity reasons, visitors should not be allowed into the husbandry unit. Rodents and insects should be prevented from access to buildings housing quail.

Transport

It is advisable not to ship quail less than 2 weeks old, but if unavoidable, chicks are best transported in commercially available cardboard chick boxes (46 cm × 31 cm × 15 cm) with a floor lining of wood shavings. The boxes should have air

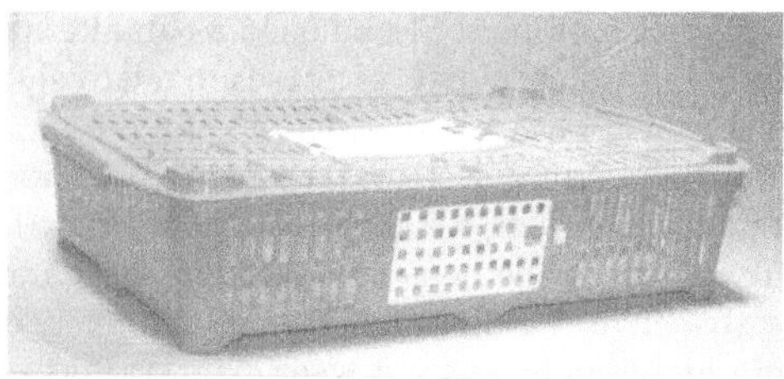

Figure 42.6 Specially designed shipping crate for adult Japanese quail. The crate has openings on the top and the side to facilitate the introduction and removal of birds. Reproduced with permission of KUHL Corporation.

holes of a size sufficient to allow adequate ventilation but small enough to prevent the chicks from escaping. When transporting chicks, it is important to ensure that the ambient temperature is suitable (35–30 °C, depending on the age of the chicks) and the time in transit be kept to less than 4h. Adults should be transported in crates with solid floors and mesh or grill walls and roofs (65 cm × 52 cm × 19 cm for 20 birds). Specially designed crates can be purchased (Figure 42.6). For shipping adults over long distances, it is recommended that a cut open apple be attached to the inside of the crate for birds to peck at to obtain moisture. Time in transit should be limited to less than 8h unless drinking water can be applied every 4h. Information on the transport of laboratory animals is given by Laboratory Animal Science Association (LASA 2005) and IATA[3] (see also Chapter 13).

Breeding

Condition of adults

The reproductive status of both male and female quail can be determined from behavioural, hormonal, neuro-anatomical and morphological parameters (for details and references see Mills *et al.* 1997). However, in practical terms, behavioural and morphological measures are the most easy to apply. Age of sexual maturity can be manipulated by photoperiod. Birds kept under short photoperiod will not become sexually mature. Birds kept under long photoperiod will become sexually mature at 4–5 weeks of age. At sexual maturity, the cloacal diameter of females and the protodeal (foam) gland of males increases. These anatomical changes and the beginning of sexual behaviour are reliable indicators of sexual maturity.

Breeding systems

The main criteria for the selection of breeding stock are that the birds are in good physical condition and meet the requirements of any selection criteria. However, it should be remembered that quail are extremely susceptible to inbreeding depression. According to Lucotte (1974) the hatchability of eggs falls to near zero after three generations of brother × sister mating. No full-sib mating inbred line has been maintained for more than eight generations (Kim *et al.* 2007). Therefore it is important to avoid consanguineous matings. To achieve this in small populations, it is important to maintain pedigree records for breeding stock.

At least three methods exist for the management of breeding birds. Each of these has particular advantages and disadvantages but there is a clear order of preference on both welfare and husbandry grounds.

1. Birds can be housed in small cages containing one male and two or three females. Under such conditions, males do not usually damage the females, the method is not labour intensive and it is possible to pedigree offspring or identify birds which are not reproducing well.
2. Males and females may be kept in individual cages and the males introduced into the cages of the females at intervals of 2–3 days since females are fertile for 3–9 days after a single insemination (Reddish *et al.* 1996). Males are introduced into the female cages in the morning for a period of 15–30 minutes. This is a sufficiently long period for copulation to take place but short enough to prevent the males from injuring the females. However, this method is extremely labour intensive although it permits one male to be mated to a relatively large number of females.
3. Males and females may be kept together in colony cages containing 5–10 males and 20–40 females. This is not labour intensive but the males may fight or attempt to copulate with one another, the mating of individual females is irregular and the parents of chicks cannot be identified. This method is probably the least satisfactory method for the management of breeding birds.

In the authors' laboratory, they keep two males with four females as a unit in a breeding cage and keep 24 cages (total of 48 males and 96 females) for propagating their random-bred population. They have found this arrangement much more satisfactory than the colony cages.

Techniques for the artificial insemination (AI) of Japanese quail have been developed (Marks & Lepore 1965), but fertility by AI is highly variable. AI is seldom used in practice because it is difficult to obtain semen that is not contaminated with foam or cloacal products (Buxton & Orcutt 1975). In addition, the volume of semen collected per male is between 3.9 and 6.9 µl (Marks & Lepore 1965) whereas an inseminating dose of 2.5–15 µl is required to achieve acceptable fertility levels. Furthermore, quail lay at the end of the photoperiod (late afternoon). Inseminating the female when there is a hard-shell egg in her oviduct will result in very poor fertility. The best time to inseminate after the egg is laid would be in the dark. For these reasons, reproduction of Japanese quail is usually by natural mating rather than by artificial insemination.

Incubation of the eggs

The nest of the Japanese quail, like those of most gallinaceous species, is little more than a simple scrape on the ground with a rim of dry grass or similar material (Kawahara 1967; Nichols 1991). In the wild or in aviaries, quail hens choose to nest in secluded sites within areas containing rough grasses and scattered shrubs (Taka-Tsukasa 1935;

[3] http://www.iata.org

Kawahara 1967; Nichols 1991; Schmid & Wechsler 1997). However, little is known about the nesting behaviour of wild birds although it appears that nest-building and incubation are carried out exclusively by the female (Schwartz & Schwartz 1949; Orcutt & Orcutt 1976; Nichols 1991).

In deep litter floor pens, natural incubation of eggs is not practical because quail hens do not readily become broody. Even with nest boxes provided, her nest-building and incubation behaviour is disrupted or not expressed because of close proximity and disturbance from other birds in the pen (Nichols 1991). Eggs can be incubated by bantam hens or pigeons but by far the most practical method is artificial incubation.

Eggs which are intended for incubation should be collected daily. Collection is usually carried out in the morning since most eggs will have been laid at the end of the previous day. Quail eggs have thin and fragile shells and they therefore should be handled carefully during collection and subsequent manipulations. After collection, the eggs should be stored on cardboard or specially designed polystyrene or foam-rubber trays for quail eggs. Eggs should be stored at 10–15 °C in a well ventilated room (with a relative humidity of about 40%). Turning stored eggs at regular intervals may help to maintain hatchability. Storage time from collection to setting should be less than 7 days for maximum fertility and should not exceed 14 days since extended storage increases the incidence of embryonic abnormalities (Sittman *et al.* 1971). Further, there is a fall in hatchability from 10 days onwards (Kraszewska-Domanska & Pawluczuk 1977). Before setting, eggs should be inspected and any that are dirty, cracked, under- or over-sized, or with shell abnormalities (soft or under or over pigmented) eliminated.

Artificial incubators are of two types – horizontal or vertical. The major difference between these two types of incubators is that horizontal incubators have a single fixed shelf for eggs whereas vertical incubators have several tiers of shelves which can be inclined up to an angle of 45%. Most horizontal incubators are simple in design and can be purchased cheaply. However, they may have low capacity and relatively poor stability of incubation temperature and humidity. More sophisticated horizontal incubators for research use are also available. Vertical incubators have higher capacity and better controlled temperature and humidity than the simple horizontal incubators. Popular models for incubating quail eggs can be obtained from commercial incubator companies.

Incubation conditions for quail eggs are similar to those for chicken eggs, but because quail eggs are much smaller than chicken eggs they are more sensitive to temperature and humidity fluctuations during incubation. In vertical incubators temperature should be between 37.5 °C and 38 °C. In simple horizontal incubators, where heat loss to the environment tends to be greater than in vertical incubators, the temperature should be set at 39 °C. This higher temperature is used to compensate for the greater temperature fluctuations inherent in these incubators. In both types of incubator, humidity should be 40–50%.

Incubation lasts 16–18 days. Under normal incubation conditions, there are peaks in embryonic mortality during the first 3 days of incubation and during the last 2 days of incubation (Figure 42.7).

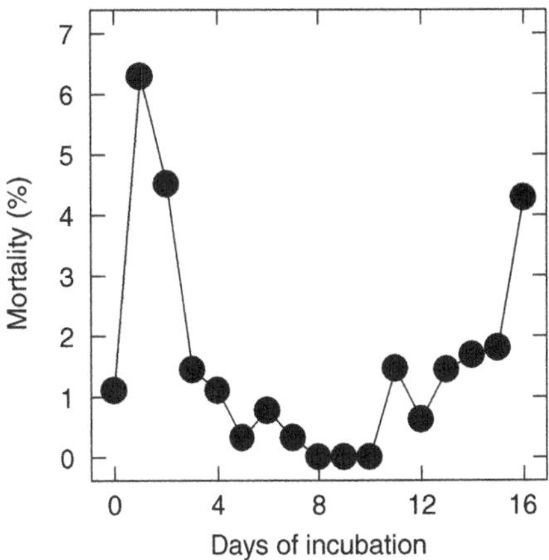

Figure. 42.7 Daily embryonic mortality during incubation of Japanese quail eggs (modified from Mills *et al.* (1999)).

Hatching of young

On day 14 of incubation, eggs should be prepared for hatching by transferring them to a hatcher apparatus or arranging them in hatcher trays in the incubator. Eggs should be placed on their sides and should not be turned thereafter. The temperature should be increased to 40 °C and the humidity increased to 70–80%. Eggs hatch between days 16 and 18 of incubation with most chicks hatching on day 17 (Lucotte 1974). However, these values may vary slightly depending on incubation conditions. For example, Wilson *et al.* (1961) found that the time from setting of eggs to external pipping was about just under 16 days, the time from pipping to hatching about 10 h and the time from hatching to complete drying of the down about 5 h.

Within batches the time of hatching of quail chicks is synchronised to some degree. This synchronisation of hatching is partially the result of communication between embryos by means of a vocalisation known as clicking which accompanies each air intake (Kovach 1975). Clicking by advanced embryos accelerates hatching in retarded embryos and vice versa (Vince 1966, 1968; Vince & Cheng 1970). Hatchability is therefore better when eggs are put close together in the hatching tray.

The young

Quail chicks are nidifugous (precocial) and do not necessarily require parental care post hatching. Provided that the rearing environment is adequate (see earlier) they have no other specific requirements. In 1974 Lucotte suggested that a mortality rate of 10–15% during the first weeks after hatching should not be considered excessive but with modern management systems it should be considerably less. In the authors' laboratory, quail mortality rate has been below 5% for the last 25 years. The greatest mortality occurs due to 'starve out' on the third and fourth days after hatching when the nutrients from the yolk sack (vitellus) have been depleted and some chicks may fail to adapt to external sources for water and nourishment. It is important to monitor closely at this time.

Table 42.4 Nutrient requirements of Japanese quail (NRC, 1994). Dietary requirements are on a per kg diet basis, assuming 90% dry matter.

Nutrient	*Unit*	*Diets*	
		Starting and growing	*Breeding*
Metabolisable energy	kcal/kg	2900	2900
Protein and amino acids			
Protein	%	24.0	20.0
Arginine	%	1.25	1.26
Glycine + serine	%	1.15	1.17
Histidine	%	0.36	0.42
Isoleucine	%	0.98	0.90
Leucine	%	1.69	1.42
Lysine	%	1.30	1.00
Methionine	%	0.50	0.45
Methionine + cystine	%	0.75	0.70
Phenylalanine	%	0.96	0.78
Phenylalanine + tyrosine	%	1.80	1.40
Threonine	%	1.02	0.74
Tryptophan	%	0.22	0.19
Valine	%	0.95	0.92
Fat			
Linoleic acid	%	1.0	1.0
Macrominerals			
Calcium	%	0.8	2.5
Cholorine	%	0.14	0.14
Magnesium	mg/kg	300	500
Non-phytate phosphorus	%	0.3	0.35
Potassium	%	0.4	0.4
Sodium	%	0.15	0.15
Trace minerals			
Copper	mg/kg	5	5
Iodine	mg/kg	0.3	0.3
Iron	mg/kg	120	60
Manganese	mg/kg	60	60
Selenium	mg/kg	0.2	0.2
Zinc	mg/kg	25	50
Fat-soluble vitamins			
A	IU/kg	1650	3300
D3	ICU/kg	750	900
E	IU/kg	12	25
K	mg/kg	1	1
Water-souluble vitamins			
B12	mg/kg	0.003	0.003
Biotin	mg/kg	0.3	0.15
Choline	mg/kg	2000	1500
Folacin	mg/kg	1	1
Niacin	mg/kg	40	20
Pantothenic acid	mg/kg	10	15
Pyridoxine	mg/kg	3	3
Riboflavin	mg/kg	4	4
Thiamin	mg/kg	2	2

Feeding and water

Dietary requirements

Quail chicks have very high requirements for dietary protein and amino acids early in life but these requirements diminish as the birds age. Recommended nutrient levels for growing and breeding birds are shown in Table 42.4. In the case of laying hens, although food intake is low (20–30g/day), the ratio of egg weight to body is high (approximately 5%) and it is particularly important to ensure a high intake of protein and sulphur amino acids.

Table 42.5 Food consumption of sample lines of Japanese quail at different ages.

Age (wk)	*Food consumption (g/day)*	
	Random-bred line[1]	*Commercial meat lines*[2]
1		6.8
2	10.2	13.7
3	13.0	15.7
4	17.5	19.8
5		23.5

[1] Data from Farrell *et al.* (1982).
[2] Data from Güler *et al.* (2005) and Hyánkova *et al.* (1997).

Natural and laboratory diets

Wild quail are omnivorous and have a diet composed of small seeds, insects and spiders (Kawahara 1967). Table 42.5 shows the food consumption of birds up to 5 weeks of age. The metabolisable energy value of diets should be in the range of 2600–3200 kcal/kg (Shim & Vohra 1984). In commercial operations where maximising production is a premium, it is usual to provide the birds with 'starter' diets until they are 21 days of age, with 'grower diets' from 3–6 weeks of age and 'breeder or layer' diets thereafter. In laboratory operations, the authors found that using a commercial turkey starter diet (26% protein) fortified with extra calcium (2.5%) is satisfactory for feeding quail of all ages. The diet comes in 'crumble' form (crumbled pellets) and has to be ground to a dry mash for feeding newly hatched chicks to 2 weeks old. Thereafter, the diet can be fed as crumbles. Specially prepared diets for quail may be available from some feed companies. Some commercial game bird diets can also be used for quail. Diet with high wheat content should be avoided, as the feed will become glutinous when moistened and will stick to the toes of the birds and ball up. Advice on quail nutrition in the tropics is available online[4].

For nutritional physiology studies, commercial diets may not provide the background consistency of the feed ingredients and the precise level of various nutrients needed. In this situation, a synthetic diet (Table 42.6) may be used.

Water

Clean drinking water must be provided at all times. Water consumption (Table 42.7) increases with age (Farrell *et al.* 1982; Visser *et al.* 2000), and is greater in lines selected for increased body mass (Visser *et al.* 2000). Drinking rates of adults increase as salinity of their drinking water increases, but quail do not tolerate salinities greater than isotonic (150 mM NaCl; Roberts & Hughes 1983).

[4] http://www.thatquailplace.com/quail/coturn1.htm

Table 42.6 Formula for a synthetic basal diet for laboratory Japanese quail. This diet is used at the UBC Quail Genetic Resource Centre for nutrition research projects.

Ingredient	*Amount (g/kg diet)*
Soya protein flour (50% protein)	340
Corn starch	400
Limestone	50
Mineral premix	5
Monofos	30
Sucrose	20
Alphacel	70
Vitamin premix	5
D-L methionine	4
Choline chloride	0.8
Tallow	50
Vegetable oil	30

Table 42.7 Water consumption of domestic Japanese quail at different ages.

Age (wk)	*Water intake[1] (ml/day)*	*Water flux[2] (g/day)*	
		C strain[3]	*P strain[4]*
1		18.0	21.0
2	23.3	23.7	30.7
3	26.2	29.7	27.1
4	30.0		
7		40.9	62.1

[1] Farrell *et al.* (1982).
[2] Visser *et al.* (2000).
[3] Random bred line (body mass at 7 wk of age = 184 g).
[4] Rapid growth line (body mass at 7 wk of age = 294 g).

Laboratory procedures

Handling and capture

Quail chicks are very small and must be handled very gently. They should be picked up using only the thumb and forefinger and held in the palm of the hand. When frightened or presented with unfamiliar stimuli, quail frequently injure themselves during the expression of escape behaviour. Therefore, care should be taken to minimise disturbances and staff and visitors should wear clothing with colours familiar to the birds. When birds are caught, they should be held so that their wings are pinned against the body and their legs hang freely. If birds are held by the legs or in such a manner that they can flap their wings, there is a high risk of bone breakage.

Physiological monitoring

Recording of body temperature

Methods for the measurement of body temperature of Japanese quail are similar to those used for domestic chickens. Yousef *et al.* (1966) studied the temperature of the hypothalamus, rectum and skin under different environmental conditions. The temperatures observed had the following ranges: hypothalamus 42.7–42.8 °C, rectum 42.0–42.2 °C and skin 39.0–39.8 °C. McNabb and McNabb (1977) describe the measurement of heat transfer across the skin and feather pelts in young birds. Woodard and Mather (1964) have described circadian rhythms in body temperature and Woodard and Wilson (1972) have measured body temperature in relation to oviposition. For further information concerning body temperature in Japanese quail see Wilson (1972).

Collection of blood samples

Blood samples can be taken from the jugular or brachial veins. The blood volume of quail is approximately 7 ml/100 g body weight (Nirmalan & Robinson 1971) and 0.5 ml blood/100 g body weight can be safely withdrawn. Arora (1979) suggested 0.5 mm diameter (25 G) needles for obtaining blood from the jugular vein and 0.46 mm diameter (26 G) needles for obtaining blood from the brachial vein (see also JWGR 1993). Arora (1979) suggested that for ease of collection, safety and for repeated sampling, the jugular vein was the most suitable site. However, repeated bleeding is not advisable.

Administration of medicines

Dosing and injection procedures

The jugular vein is the most suitable site for intravenous injections. Intramuscular injection should be made in the pectoral muscles. Subcutaneous injections should be placed under the skin of the neck. Intra-coelomic injections are sometimes used to administer anaesthetics, but care should be taken not to place the injection into the air sacs.

Liquids can be administered orally by direct intubation of the crop using a standard 12–16 G gavage needle (bulbous tipped 100 mm long) (Ichilcik & Austin 1978). If doses do not need to be precise, it is possible to incorporate compounds into the diet or drinking water.

Although quail are not specifically dealt with, detailed information on the procedures involved in the administration of substances to animals can be found in JWGR (2001a).

Anaesthesia

There has been limited research into appropriate anaesthetics for use in quail but knowledge of the principles of avian anaesthesia have developed considerably in recent years. The report of the Joint Working Group on Refinement (JWGR 2001b) provides a useful introduction and source of information on anaesthesia and analgesia. Currently, inhalational anaesthesia is the preferred method for anesthetising birds in many cases. The gas anaesthetic of choice is isoflurane (Carpenter 2000) due to its rapid induction, rapid recovery and minimal myocardial depressant effects. Concentrations have not been set for quail, but the recommended minimum concentration for isoflurane use in birds is 0.5–3%. Although now not often recommended, injectable anesthetics can be used when inhalation anesthesia is unavailable (Paul-Murphy and Fialkowshi 2001). However, as many injectable anesthetics are no longer recommended, a veterinarian should be consulted before they are considered. Paul-Murphy and Fialkowshi (2001) summarise the various injectable drugs and dosages that have been used in birds. Further valuable information on avian anaesthesia is provided in Chapter 44 on pigeons and doves.

Euthanasia

Methods of euthanasia for birds are reviewed in the Report of the Joint Working Group on Refinement (JWGR 2001b). Quail are usually killed by cervical dislocation or lethal injection. For a small bird like the quail, cervical dislocation is often the preferred method. However, it should be noted that unless the brainstem is destroyed in the process, brain function may persist for some seconds. A suitable agent for lethal injection is sodium pentobarbital. The dose rate for intra-coelomic injection is 6 ml/kg body weight of a 6% solution (Mills *et al.* 1999). See Chapter 44 for further information on euthanasia of birds.

Common welfare problems

Causes of mortality

The highest rates of mortality are usually seen during the first week post-hatching (Löliger & Schubert 1966; Zucker *et al.* 1967; Lucotte 1974). Careful management (control of temperature, pre-heating of husbandry units and avoidance of draughts) and correct nutrition are important in reducing early mortality. Under proper management, mortality should be less than 5%.

In adult male birds, traumatic injury is the most frequently cited cause of death. Infections of the reproductive organs following prolapse of the uterus, or shell gland, are a common cause of death in adult females (Ernst & Coleman 1966; Löliger & Schubert 1966; Nagarajan *et al.* 1991; Woodard *et al.* 1973). Woodard & Abplanalp (1971) estimated that approximately 1% of female birds died from injury or prolapse of the shell gland during each week of their study. However, such mortality can be reduced or prevented by delaying the onset of sexual maturity through manipulation of the photoperiod. The authors found that the frequency of prolapse varied among different strains. If the female can be taken out of egg production (put under a short lighting scheme) when prolapse is first observed, and housed individually to avoid pecking by other birds, the prolapse can generally recover. Prolapses that occur for more than 24 h are difficult to revert.

Other reported causes of mortality in quail include head injuries and emaciation and careful measures should be taken to avoid these. Emaciation appears to occur for a variety of reasons including social competition (Löliger & Schubert 1966; Zucker *et al.* 1967; Benoff & Rice 1980; Edens *et al.* 1983) and mechanical difficulties in reaching drinkers and feeders.

Disease

Prophylaxis

Good hygiene and barrier systems which prevent infection from outside sources are the most important aspects of prophylaxis in Japanese quail. Good ventilation and husbandry (see earlier in this chapter) are important for the prevention of aspergillosis. Fumigation of eggs before incubation may help prevent the transmission of diseases from one generation to the next. Vaccination is not widely practised. With the exception of quail pox vaccine, no vaccines have been developed for quail. However, adult (5 week old) birds can be vaccinated against Newcastle disease using chicken vaccines (Lima *et al.* 2004). Chicken vaccine against avian encephalomyelitis (AE) is also effective in adult quail. Many commercially produced feeds contain antibiotics and anticoccidials to prevent diseases and coccidiosis. It is generally advised not to vaccinate quail unless there is a disease outbreak in the area.

Signs of disease

The quail is an extremely disease-resistant species. Although it is susceptible to the majority of diseases found in gallinaceous birds, quail appear to have a much greater resistance to these pathogens than do domestic fowl (Farrow *et al.* 1975). Where disease and excessive mortality do occur they are frequently a consequence of management failures in high-density production flocks. Many of the symptoms of disease in quail (reduced egg output, morbidity, mortality and emaciation) are common to a wide range of infections. Furthermore, infected birds do not always present obvious clinical symptoms and it is important that specialist help for diagnosis, treatment and control be sought if outbreaks of disease are suspected.

Common diseases

Japanese quail are susceptible to the majority of diseases found in gallinaceous birds. A list of some of these diseases is given in Table 42.8.

Abnormal behaviour

Feather pecking, cannibalism and head-banging (caused by the birds jumping and striking their heads on the cage roof) are the most frequently cited behavioural causes of injury in Japanese quail (see Gerken & Mills 1993). Ways to minimise these behaviour patterns have been mentioned in previous sections of this chapter. Females kept in battery cages show pre-laying restlessness similar to that observed in some strains of domestic chickens (Gerken & Mills 1993) and birds of both sexes show vacuum dust-bathing behaviour (Gerken 1983). In deep litter floor pens, at higher than recommended stocking densities, and when eggs are not collected daily, egg eating has been observed in some flocks of birds. Stereotyped behaviour can be induced experimentally (Kostal *et al.* 1992) but its incidence under other conditions is unknown.

Table 42.8 Natural and experimentally induced diseases of the Japanese quail. Modified from Mills *et al.* (1999).

Disease	*Reference*
Aspergillosis	Ghori and Edgar (1973)
Avian encephalomyelitis	Hill and Raymond (1962)
Coronavirus	Mills *et al.* (1999)
Campylobacteriosis	Marumya and Katasube (1988)
Erysipelas	Panigrahy and Hall (1977)
Fowl typhoid	Pomeroy and Nagaraja (1991)
Hexamitiasis	McDougald (1991)
Infectious coryza	Reece *et al.* (1981)
Influenza	Easterday and Hinshaw (1991)
Lymphoid leucosis	Payne *et al.* (1991)
Marek's disease	Kenzy and Cho (1969)
Mycoplasmosis (*Mycoplasma gallisepticum*)	Yoder (1991)
Mycoplasmosis (*Mycoplasma synoviae*)	Bencina *et al.* (1987)
Nematode parasites	Ruff (1991)
Newcastle disease	Alexander (1991)
Paratyphoid (salmonellosis)	Mills *et al.* (1999)
Pullorum disease (salmonellosis)	Snoeyenbos (1991)
Quail bronchitis	Mills *et al.* (1999)
Reticuloendtheliosis	Theilen *et al.* (1966)
Staphylococcosis	Skeeles (1991)
Thrush (mycosis of the digestive tract)	Chute (1991)
Ulcerative enteritis (quail disease)	Mills *et al.* (1999)
Pox virus	Mills *et al.* (1999)
Inclusion body hepatitis (adenovirus)	Mills *et al.* (1999)

Reproductive problems

The main reproductive problem observed in quail is prolapse of the shell gland (Woodard & Abplanalp 1971). The condition is most frequently seen in young birds at the start of lay. Its incidence is greatly increased if birds are brought in lay early by keeping them on long photoperiods (eg, 16L:8D) as juveniles.

Acknowledgements

This chapter is written based on a manuscript submitted by Andrew Mills for the previous edition of this book. The authors would like to dedicate this chapter to Andrew. They also thank Cathleen Nichols (UBC Quail Genetic Resource Centre) for valuable inputs and Dr Chris Harvey-Clarke (UBC Animal Care Centre) for reviewing an earlier draft of this manuscript.

References

Adkins-Regan, E. (1995) Predictors of fertilization in the Japanese quail, *Coturnix japonica. Animal Behaviour*, **50**, 1405–1415

Aggrey, S.E. (2003) Dynamics of relative growth rate in Japanese quail lines divergently selected for growth and their control. *Growth Development and Aging*, **67**, 47–54

Alexander, D.J. (1991) Newcastle disease and other paramyxovirus infecetions. In: *Diseases of Poultry*. Eds Calnek B.W., Barnes H.J., Beard C.W. *et al.*, pp. 496–519. Wolfe Publications Ltd, London

American Ornithologist's Union (1983) *Check-list of North American Birds*. Allen Press Incorporated, Kansas

Arora, K.L. (1979) Blood sampling and intravenous injections in Japanese quail (*Coturnix coturnix japonica*). *Laboratory Animal Science*, **29**, 114–118

Ball, G.F. and Balthazart, J. (2004) Hormonal regulation of brain circuits mediating male sexual behavior in birds. *Physiology and Behavior*, **83**, 329–346

Balthazart, J., Baillien, M., Charlier, T.D. *et al.* (2003) The neuroendocrinology of reproductive behavior in Japanese quail. *Domestic Animal Endocrinology*, **25**, 69–82

Balthazart, J. and Ball, G.F. (1998) New insights into the regulation and function of brain estrogen synthase (aromatase). *Trends in Neurosciences*, **21**, 243–249

Barilani, M., Derégnaucourt, S., Gallego, S. *et al.* (2005) Detecting hybridization in wild (*Coturnix c. coturnix*) and domesticated (*Coturnix c. japonica*) quail populations. *Biological Conservation*, **126**, 445–455

Baumgartner, J. (1993) Japanese quail: genetics, breeding, and production. In: *Proceedings of the 10th International Symposium on Current Problems in Avian Genetics*, Nitra, Slovakia. pp. 11

Bencina, D.T., Tadina, T. and Dorrer, D. (1987) Mycoplasma species isolated from six avian species. *Avian Pathology*, **16**, 653–664

Benoff, F.H. and Rice, D.H. (1980) Social dominance and productivity in caged female Japanese quail. *Poultry Science*, **59**, 424–427

Bessei, W. (1977) Quail breeding in France. *Deutsche Geflugelwirtschaft und Schweineproduktion*, **29**, 4–5

Buchwalder, T. and Wechsler, B. (1997) The effect of cover on the behaviour of Japanese quail. *Applied Animal Behaviour Science*, **54**, 335–343

Butkauskas, D. (2001) *Genetic diversity and reproductive traits of Japanese quail*. PhD Dissertation, Institute of Ecology, Lithuania

Buxton, J.R. and Orcutt, F.S. (1975) Enzymes and electrolytes in the semen of Japanese quail. *Poultry Science*, **54**, 1556–1566

Carpenter, N.A. (2000) Anseriform and galliform therapeutics. *Veterinary Clinics of North America: Exotic Animal Practice*, **3**, 1–17

Chang, G.B., Chang, H., Liu, X.P. *et al.* (2005) Developmental research on the origin and phylogeny of quails. *World's Poultry Science Journal*, **61**, 105–111

Cheng, K.M., Hickman, A.R. and Nichols, C.R. (1989b) Role of the proctodeal gland foam of male Japanese quail in natural copulations. *Auk*, **106**, 279–286

Cheng, K.M., and Kimura, M. (1990) Mutations and major variants in Japanese quail. In: *Developments in Animal and Veterinary Sciences, Vol. 22. Poultry Breeding and Genetics*. Ed. Crawford, R.D., pp. 333–362. Elsevier, Amsterdam

Cheng, K.M., McIntyre, R.F. and Hickman, A.R. (1989a) Proctodeal gland foam enhances competitive fertilization in domestic Japanese quail. *Auk*, **106**, 287–291

Cheng, K.M. and Nichols, C.R. (1992) Japanese quail (*Coturnix japonica*): conservation and management of genetic resources in Canada. *Gibier Faune Sauvage*, **9**, 667–676

Cheng, K.M., Pang, C.S., Wang, Z.P. *et al.* (1994) A comparison of ^{125}I iodomelatonin binding sites in testes and brains of heavy meat-type Japanese quail with a random bred strain. *Journal of Heredity*, **85**, 136–139

Chute, H.L. (1991) Thrush (Mycosis of the digestive tract). In: *Diseases of Poultry*. Eds Calnek B.W., Barnes H.J., Beard C.W. *et al*., pp. 335–337. Wolfe Publications Ltd, London

Cooper, D.M. (1987) The Japanese quail. In: *UFAW Handbook on the Care and Management of Laboratory Animals*, 6th edn. Ed Poole T.B., pp. 678–686. UFAW, Potters Bar

Crawford, R.D. (1990) Origins and history of poultry species. In: *Developments in Animal and Veterinary Sciences, Vol. 22. Poultry Breeding and Genetics*. Ed. Crawford, R.D., pp. 1–41. Elsevier, Amsterdam

Delville, Y., Sulon, J., Hendrick, J.C. *et al*. (1984) Effect of the presence of females on the pituitary-testicular activity in male Japanese quail (*Coturnix coturnix japonica*). *General Comparative Endocrinology*, **55**, 295–305

Derégnaucourt, S., Guyomarc'h, J.C. and Aebischer, N.J. (2002) Hybridization between European *Coturnix c. coturnix* and Japanese *Coturnix c. japonica* quail. *Ardea*, **90**, 15–21

Dement'ev, G.P., Gladkov, N.A., Isakov, Y.A. *et al*. (1967) In: *Birds of the Soviet Union*. Israel Program for Scientific Translation, Jerusalem

Domjan, M. and Nash, S. (1988) Stimulus control of social behaviour in male Japanese quail, *Coturnix coturnix japonica*. *Animal Behaviour*, **36**, 1006–1015

Easterday, B.C. and Hinshaw, V.S. (1991) Influenza. In: *Diseases of Poultry*. Eds Calnek B.W., Barnes H.J., Beard C.W. *et al*., pp. 531–551. Wolfe Publications Ltd, London

Edens, F.W. (1987) Agonistic behaviour and neurochemistry in grouped Japanese quail. *Comparative Biochemistry and Physiology Series A*, **86**, 473–480

Edens, F.W., Bursian, S.J. and Holladay, S.D. (1983) Grouping in Japanese quail. 1. Agonistic behaviour during feeding. *Poultry Science*, **62**, 1647–1651

Elangovan, A.V., Verma, S.V.S., Sastry, V.R.B. *et al*. (2003) Laying performance of Japanese quail fed on different seed meals in diet. *Indian Journal of Animal Nutrition*, **19**, 244–250

Ernst, R.A. and Coleman, T.H. (1966) The influence of floor space on growth, egg production, fertility and hatchability of *Coturnix coturnix japonica*. *Poultry Science*, **45**, 437–440

Eroschenko, V.P., Wilson, W.O. and Siopes, T.D. (1977) Function and histology of testes from aged coturnix maintained on different photoperiods. *Journal of Gerontology*, **32**, 279–285

European Commission (2007) Commission recommendations of 18 June 2007 on guidelines for the accommodation and care of animals used for experimental and other scientific purposes. Annex II to European Council Directive 86/609. See 2007/526/EC. http://eurlex.europa.eu/LexUriServ/site/en/oj/2007/l_197/l_19720070730en00010089.pdf (accessed 13 May 2008)

Eynon, A.E. (1968) *The agonistic and sexual behaviour of captive Japanese quail (Coturnix coturnix japonica)*. PhD Thesis, University of Wisconsin

Faqi, A.S., Solecki, R., Pfeil, R. and Hilbig, V. (1997) Standard values for reproductive and clinical chemistry parameters of Japanese quail. *Deutsche Tierärztliche Wochenschrift*, **104**, 167–169

Farrell, D.J., Atmamihardja, S.I. and Pym, R.A.E. (1982) Calorimetric measurements of the energy and nitrogen metabolism of Japanese quail. *British Poultry Science*, **23**, 375–382

Farris, H.E. (1964) *Behavioral development, social organization and conditioning of courting behavior in Japanese quail Coturnix coturnix japonica*. PhD dissertation, Michigan State University

Farris, H.E. (1967) Classical conditioning of courting behaviour in the Japanese quail, *Coturnix coturnix japonica*. *Journal of the Experimental Analysis of Behaviour*, **10**, 213–217

Farrow, W.M., Scmitt, M.W. and Groupe, J. (1975) Responses of isolator – derived Japanese quail and quail cell cultures in selected animal viruses. *Journal of Clinical Microbiology*, **2**, 419–424

Fu, Z., Inaba, M., Noguchi, T. and Kata, H. (2002) Molecular cloning and circadian regulation of cryptochrome genes in Japanese quail (*Coturnix coturnix japonica*). *Journal of Biological Rhythms*, **17**, 14–27

Gerken, M. (1983). Untersuchungen zur genetischen Fundierung und Beeinflubarkeit von Verhaltensmerkmalen des Geflügels, durchgeführt in einem Selektionexperiment auf Staubbadedeverhalten bei der japenishcen Wachtel (Coturnix coturnix japonica) Thesis. Rheinsche Freidrich Wilhelms Universität, Bonn

Gerken, M. and Mills, A.D. (1993) Welfare of domestic quail. In: *Proceedings of the Fourth European Symposium on Poultry Welfare*. Eds Savory, C.J. and Hughes, B.O., pp. 158–176. UFAW, Potters Bar

Gerken, M. and Petersen, J. (1987) Bidirectional selection for dust-bathing activity in Japanese quail (*Coturnix coturnix japonica*). *British Poultry Science*, **28**, 23–37

Ghori, H.M. and Edgar, S.A. (1973) Comparative susceptibility of chickens, turkeys and Coturnix quail to aspergillosis. *Poultry Science*, **52**, 2311–2315

Güler, T., Ertaş, O.N., Çiftçi, M. *et al*. (2005) The effect of coriander seed (*Coriandrum sativum* L.) as diet ingredient on the performance of Japanese quail. *South African Journal of Animal Science*, **35**, 260–266

Guyomarc'h, C. and Guyomarc'h, J.C. (1984) The influence of social factors on the onset of egg production in Japanese quail (*Coturnix coturnix japonica*). *Biology of Behaviour*, **9**, 333–342

Guyomarc'h, J.C. (1974) *Les vocalisations des Gallinacés – Structure des Sons et des Répertoires. Ontogenèse Motrice et Acquisition de Leur Sémantique (Volumes 1 and 2)*. Thèse de Docteur d'État (Série C, N° d'ordre 198, N° de série 56), Université de Rennes

Halldin, K., Berg, C., Brandt, I. *et al*. (1999) Sexual behavior in Japanese quail as a test end pint for endocrine disruption: Effects of in ovo exposure to ethinylestradiol and diethylstilbestrol. *Environmental and Health Perspectives*, **107**, 861–866

Hazard, D., Couty, M., Faure, J.M. *et al*. (2005) Relationship between hypothalamic-pituitary-adrenal axis responsiveness and age, sexual maturity status, and sex in Japanese quail selected for long or short duration of tonic immobility. *Poultry Science*, **84**, 1913–1919

Hill, R.W. and Raymond, R.G. (1962) Apparent natural infection of Coturnix hens with the virus of avian encephalomytis. Case report. *Avian Diseases*, **6**, 226–227

Hoffmann, E. (1990) *Coturnix Quail*. Cannings, Nova Scotia

Homma, K., Siopes, T.D., Wilson, W.O. *et al*. (1966) Identification of sex of day old quail (*Coturnix coturnix japonica*) by cloacal examination. *Poultry Science*, **45**, 469–472

Houdelier, C., Guyomarc'h, C., Lumineau, S. *et al*. (2002) Circadian rhythms of oviposition and feeding activity in Japanese quail: effects of cyclic administration of melatonin. *Chronobiology International*, **19**, 1107–1119

Howard, R. and Moore, A. (1984) *A complete checklist of the birds of the World*, revised edition. Macmillan, London

Howes, J.R. (1964) Japanese quail as found in Japan. *Quail Quarterly*, **1**, 19–30

Hyánkova, L., Dŭdkova, L., Knížetova, H. *et al*. (1997) Responses in growth, food intake and food conversion efficiency to different dietary protein concentrations in meat-type lines of Japanese quail. *British Poultry Science*, **38**, 564–570

Ichilcik, R. and Austin, J. (1978) The Japanese quail (*Coturnix coturnix japonica*) as a laboratory animal. *Journal of the South African Veterinary Association*, **49**, 203–207

Joint Working Group on Refinement (1993) Removal of blood from laboratory mammals and birds. First Report of the BVA/FRAME/RSPCA/UFAW Joint Working Group on Refinement. *Laboratory Animals*, **27**, 1–22

Joint Working Group on Refinement (2001a) Refining procedures for the administration of substances. Report of the BVAAWF/FRAME/RSPCA/UFAW Joint Working Group on Refinement. *Laboratory Animals*, **35**, 1–41

Joint Working Group on Refinement (2001b) Laboratory birds: refinements in husbandry and procedures. Fifth report of the BVAAWF/FRAME/RSPCA/UFAW Joint Working Group on Refinement. *Laboratory Animals*, **35**, 1–163

Jones, R.B., Mills, A.D. and Faure, J.M. (1991) Genetic and experiential manipulation of fear related behaviour in Japanese quail chicks (*Coturnix coturnix japonica*). *Journal of Comparative Psychology*, **105**, 15–24

Jones, J.W., Maloney, M.A. and Gilbreath, J.C. (1964) Size, shape and color pattern as criteria for identifying *Coturnix* eggs. *Poultry Science*, **43**, 1292–1294

Kamata, R., Takahashi, S., Shimizu, A. *et al.* (2006) Avian transgenerational reproductive toxicity test with in ovo exposure. *Archives of Toxicology*, **80**, 846–856

Kawahara, T. (1967) Wild Coturnix quail in Japan. *Quail Quarterly*, **4**, 62–63

Kawahara, T. (1973) Comparative study of quantitative traits between wild and domestic Japanese quail (*Coturnix coturnix japonica*). *Experimental Animals*, **22**, 139–150

Kaya, S., Erdogan, Z. and Erdogan, S. (2003) Effect of different dietary levels of Yucca schidigera powder on the performance, blood parameters and egg yolk cholesterol of laying quails. *Journal of Veterinary Medicine Series A*, **50**, 14–17

Kayang, B.B., Fillon, V., Inoue-Murayama, M. *et al.* (2006) Integrated maps in quail (*Coturnix japonica*) confirm the high degree of synteny conservation with chicken (*Gallus gallus*) despite 35 million years of divergence. *BMC Genomics*, **7**, 101–118

Kenzy, S.G. and Cho, B.R. (1969) Transmission of classical Marek's disease by affected and carrier birds. *Avian Diseases*, **13**, 211–214

Kim, S.H., Cheng, K.M., Ritland, C. *et al.* (2007) Inbreeding in Japanese quail estimated by pedigree and microsatellite analyses. *Journal of Heredity*, **98**, 378–381

Kostal, L., Vyboh, P., Bilcik, B. *et al.* (1992) Stereotyped pacing in Japanese quail: the role of endogenous opioids. *Journal of Animal Science*, **70**, 24

Kovach, J.K. (1975) The behaviour of quail. In: *The Behaviour of Domestic Animals*, 3rd edn. Ed. Hafez, E.S.E., pp. 437–453. Bailliere Tindall, London

Kraszewska-Domanska, B. and Pawluczuk, B. (1977) The effect of periodic warming of stored quail eggs on their hatchability. *British Poultry Science*, **18**, 531–533

Landsdown, A.B.G., Crees, S.J. and Wilder, R.G. (1970) The Japanese quail: its suitability for embryonic and reproductive investigations. *Journal of the Institute of Animal Technology*, **21**, 71–77

Laboratory Animal Science Association (2005) Guidance on the transport of laboratory animals. Report of the Transport Working Group established by LASA. *Laboratory Animals*, **39**, 1–39

Lepori, N.G. (1964) Primi dati sugli ibridi di *Coturnix c. japonica* X *Coturnix c. coturnix* ottenuti in allevamento. *Rivista Italiana di Ornithologia*, **34**, 192–198

Lima, F.S., Santin, E., Paulillo, A.C. *et al.* (2004) Evaluation of different programs of Newcastle disease vaccination in Japanese quail (Coturnix coturnix japonica). *International Journal of Poultry Science*, **3**, 354–356

Löliger, H.C. and Schubert, H.J. (1966) Spontanerkrankungen bei japanischen Wachteln (*Coturnix coturnix japonica*). *Celler Jahrbuch*, **15**, 42–43

Long, J.L. (1981) *Introduced birds of the world*. Universe Books, New York

Lucotte, G. (1974) *Elevage de la caille*. Vigot Frères, Paris

Marks, H.L. (1978) Long term selection for four-week body weight in Japanese quail under different nutritional environments. *Theoretical and Applied Genetics*, **52**, 105–111

Marks, H.L. and Lepore, H.D. (1965) A procedure for artificial insemination of Japanese quail. *Poultry Science*, **44**, 1001–1003

Marumya, S. and Katasube, Y. (1988) Intestinal colonization of *Campylobacter jejeuni* in young Japanese quails (*Coturnix coturnix japonica*). *Japanese Journal of Veterinary Science*, **50**, 569–572

Mather, F.B. and Wilson, W.O. (1964) Post-natal testicular development in Japanese quail. *Poultry Science*, **43**, 860–864

McDougald, L.R. (1991) Other diseases of the intestinal tract. In: *Diseases of Poultry*. Eds Calnek B.W., Barnes H.J., Beard C.W. *et al.*, pp. 804–813. Wolfe Publications Ltd, London

McKinney, F., Derrickson, S.R. and Mineau, P. (1983) Forced copulation in waterfowl. *Behaviour*, **86**, 250–294

McNabb, F.M.A. and McNabb, R.A. (1977) Skin and plumage changes during the development of thermoregulatory ability of Japanese quail chicks. *Comparative Biochemistry and Physiology*, **58A**, 163–166

Mills, A.D. and Faure, J.M. (1990) Diviergierende selektion für soziale motivation und tonische immobilitätswort bei der Japenischen wachtel (*Coturnix coturnix japonica*). In: Proceedings of the 7th Leipziger Tierzuchtsymposien. Ed Wussow, J., pp. 87–101. Karl Marx Universistät, Leipzig

Mills, A.D., Domjan M., Crawford L.L. *et al.* (1997) The behaviour of the Japanese or domestic quail *Coturnix japonica*. *Neuroscience and Biobehavioural Reviews*, **21**, 261–281

Mills, A.D., Faure, J.M. and Rault, P. (1999) The Japanese quail. In: *UFAW Handbook on the Care and Management of Laboratory Animals*, 7th edn. Ed. Poole T.B., pp. 697–713. Blackwell Publishing, Oxford

Minvielle, F. (1998) Genetics and breeding of Japanese quail for production around the world. In: Proceedings of the 6th World's Poultry Science Association Asian Pacific Poultry Congress, Nagoya, Japan. pp. 122–127

Minvielle, F. (2004) The future of Japanese quail for research and production. *World's Poultry Science Journal*, **60**, 500–507

Minvielle, F., Grossmann, R. and Gourichon, D. (2007) Development and performances of a Japanese quail line homozygous for the diabetes insipidus (di) mutation. *Poultry Science*, **86**, 249–254

Minvielle, F., Monvoisin, J.-L., Costa, J. *et al.* (1999) Changes in heterosis under within-line selection or reciprocal recurrent selection: An experiment on early egg production in Japanese quail. *Journal of Animal Breeding and Genetics*, **116**, 363–377

Minvielle, F., Monvoisin, J.-L., Costa, J. *et al.* (2000) Long-term egg production and heterosis in quail lines after within-line or reciprocal recurrent selection for high early egg production. *British Poultry Science*, **42**, 150–157

Moore, C.B. and Siopes, T.D. (2000) Effects of lighting conditions and melatonin supplementation on the cellular and humoral immune responses in Japanese quail *Coturnix coturnix japonica*. *General and Comparative Endocrinology*, **119**, 95–104

Moore, C.B. and Siopes, T.D. (2003) Melatonin enhances cellular and humoral immune responses in the Japanese quail (*Coturnix coturnix japonica*) via an opiatergic mechanism. *General and Comparative Endocrinology*, **131**, 258–263

Moreau, R.E. and Wayne, P. (1968) On the Palearctic quails. *Ardea*, **56**, 209–226

Munro, G.C. (1960) *Birds of Hawaii*. Charles E. Tuttle, Rutland, Vermont

Murakami, A.E. and Ariki, J. (1998) *Produção de Codorna Japonesas*. Jaboticabal, Funep, Brazil

Nagarajan, S., Narahari, D., Jayaprasad, I.A. *et al.* (1991) Influence of stocking density and layer age on production traits and egg quality in Japanese quail. *British Poultry Science*, **32**, 243–248

Nakahara, K., Kawan, O.T., Shiota, K. *et al.* (2003) Effects of microinjection of melatonin into various brain regions of Japanese quail on locomotor activity and body temperature. *Neuroscience Letters*, **345**, 117–120

National Advisory Committee for Laboratory Animal Research (2004) *Guidelines on the Care and Use of Animals for Scientific Purposes.* NACLAR, Singapore

National Research Council (1994) *Nutrient Requirements of Poultry.* National Academy Press, Washington, DC

National Research Council (1996) *Guide for the Care and Use of Laboratory Animals.* National Academy Press, Washington, DC

Nichols, C.R. (1991) *A comparison of the reproductive and behavioural differences in feral and domestic Japanese quail.* Unpublished MSc Thesis, University of British Columbia

Nichols, C.R., Robinson, C.A.F. and Cheng, K.M. (1992) Influence of domestication on fecundity and reproductive behaviour in Japanese quail, *Coturnix japonica. Gibier Faune Sauvage,* **9**, 743–756

Nirmalan, G.P. and Robinson, G.A. (1971) Hematology of Japanese quail (*Coturnix coturnix japonica*). *British Poultry Science,* **12**, 475–481

Noble R. (1972) The effects of estrogen and progesterone on copulation in female quail (*Coturnix coturnix japonica*) housed in continuous dark. *Hormones and Behavior,* **3**, 199–204

Nol, E., Cheng, K.M. and Nichols, C.R. (1996) Heritability and phenotypic correlations of behaviour and dominance rank of Japanese quail. *Animal Behaviour,* **52**, 813–820

Odeh, F.M., Cadd, G.G. and Satterlee, D.G. (2003) Genetic characterization of stress responsiveness in Japanese quail. 1. Analyses of line effects and combining abilities by diallel crosses. *Poultry Science,* **82**, 25–30

Ohta, M., Kadota, C. and Konishi, H. (1989) A role of melatonin in the initial stage of photoperiodism in the Japanese quail. *Biology of Reproduction,* **40**, 935–941

Orcutt, F.S. and Orcutt, A.B. (1976) Nesting and parental behavior in domestic common quail. *Auk,* **93**, 135–141

Otis, R.E. (1972) *Social organisation in the Japanese quail (Coturnix coturnix japonica): Appetitive and consummatory components.* Unpublished PhD dissertation, Michigan State University

Ottinger, M.A. (1978) *The relationship of testosterone, sex-related behaviour and morphology during the sexual maturation of the male Japanese quail.* Unpublished PhD Dissertation, University of Maryland

Ottinger, M.A. (1989) Sexual differentiation of neuroendocrine systems and behavior. *Poultry Science,* **68**, 979–989

Ottinger, M.A. (1983) Sexual behavior and endocrine changes during reproductive maturation and ageing in the avian male. In: *Hormones and Behavior in Higher Vertebrates.* Eds Balthazart, J., Prove, E. and Giles, R., pp. 350–367. Springer-Verlag, Berlin

Ottinger, M.A. (1991) Neuroendocrine and behavioral determinants of reproductive ageing. *Critical Reviews in Poultry Biology,* **3**, 131–142

Ottinger, M., Abdelnabi, M., Henry, P. *et al.* (2001) Neuroendocrine and behavioral implications of endocrine disrupting chemicals in quail. *Hormones and Behavior,* **40**, 234–247

Ottinger, M., Abdelnabi, M., Quin, M. *et al.* (2002) Reproductive consequences of EDCs in birds. What do laboratory effects mean in field species? *Neurotoxicology and Teratology,* **24**, 17–28

Ottinger, M.A. and Brinkley, H.J. (1978) Testosterone and sex related behavior and morphology: relationship during maturation and in the adult Japanese quail. *Hormones and Behavior,* **11**, 175–182

Ottinger, M.A. and Brinkley, H.J. (1979a) Testosterone and sex physical characteristics during the maturation of the male Japanese quail. *Biology of Reproduction,* **20**, 905–909

Ottinger, M.A. and Brinkley, H.J. (1979b) The ontogeny of crowing and copulatory behaviour in Japanese quail (*Coturnix coturnix japonica*). *Behavioural Processes,* **4**, 43–51

Ottinger, M.A., Duchala, C.S. and Mason, M. (1983) Age-related reproductive decline in the male Japanese quail. *Hormones and Behavior,* **17**, 197–207

Ottinger, M.A. and Rattner, B.A. (1999) Husbandry and care of quail. *Poultry and Avian Reviews,* **10**, 117–120

Padgett, C.A. and Ivey, W.D. (1959) Coturnix quail as a laboratory research animal. *Science,* **129**, 267–268

Pala, M. and Lissia-Frau, A.M. (1966) Ricerche sulla sterilita degli ibridi tra la quaglia giaponese (*Coturnix c. japonica*) e la quaglia europea (*Coturnix c. coturnix*). *Rivista Italiana di Ornithologia,* **36**, 4–9

Panigrahy, B. and Hall, C.F. (1977) An outbreak of erysipelas in *Coturnix* quails. *Avian Diseases,* **21**, 708–710

Paul-Murphy, J. and Fialkowshi, J. (2001) Injectable Anesthesia and Analgesia of Birds. In: *Recent Advances in Veterinary Anesthesia and Analgesia: Companion Animals.* Eds Gleed, R.D. and Ludders, J.W. Electronic publication, International Veterinary Information Service, Ithaca, New York (http://www.ivis.org)

Payne, L.N., Purchase, H.G. and Barnes, H.J. (1991) Lymphoid leukosis. In: *Diseases of Poultry.* Eds Calnek B.W., Barnes H.J., Beard C.W. *et al.*, pp. 386–439. Wolfe Publications Ltd, London

Peterson, R.T. (1961) *A Field Guide to Western Birds.* Houghton Mifflin Co, Boston

Piao, J., Shimogiri, T., Maeda, Y. and Okamoto, S. (2003) Analysis of genetic traits by AFLP in the Japanese quail lines selected for large and small body weight. *Japanese Poultry Science,* **40**, J13–J20

Poole, H.K. (1965) Spectophotometric identification of egg shell pigments and time of superficial pigment deposition in the Japanese quail. *Proceedings of the Society for Experimental Biology and Medicine,* **119**, 547–551

Pomeroy, B.S. and Nagaraja, K.V. (1991) Fowl typhoid. In: *Diseases of Poultry.* Eds Calnek B.W., Barnes H.J., Beard C.W. *et al.*, pp. 87–89. Wolfe Publications Ltd, London

Potash, L.M. (1972) Noise-induced changes in calls of the Japanese quail. *Psychonomic Science,* **26**, 252–254

Potash, L.M. (1975) An experimental analysis of the use of location calls by Japanese quail, *Coturnix coturnix japonica. Behaviour,* **54**, 153–179

Randall, M., and Bolla, G. (2007) Raising Japanese quail. *Primefact 602.* NSW Department of Primary Industries, Australia

Reddish, J.M., Kirby J.D. and Anthony N.B. (1996) Analysis of poultry fertility data. 3. Analysis of the duration of fertility in naturally mating Japanese quail. *Poultry Science,* **75**, 135–139

Reece, R.L., Barr D.A. and Owen A.C. (1981) The isolation of of *Haemophilus paragallium* from Japanese quail. *Australian Veterinary Journal,* **57**, 350–351

Reese, E.P. and Reese, T.W. (1962) The quail *Coturnix coturnix* as a laboratory animal. *Journal of the Experimental Analysis of Behaviour,* **5**, 265–270

Roberts, J.R. and Hughes, M.R. (1983) Glomerular filtration rate and drinking rate in Japanese quail, Coturnix coturnix japonica, in response to acclimation to saline water. *Canadian Journal of Zoology,* **61**, 2394–2398

Ruff, M.D. (1991) Nematodes and Acanthocephalans. In: *Diseases of Poultry.* Eds Calnek B.W., Barnes H.J., Beard C.W. *et al.*, pp. 731–763. Wolfe Publications Ltd, London

Sachs, B.D. (1967) Photoperiodic control of the cloacal gland of the Japanese quail. *Science,* **157**, 201–203

Schmid, I. and Wechsler, B. (1997) Behaviour of Japanese quail kept in semi-natural aviaries. *Applied Animal Behaviour Science,* **55**, 103–112

Scanes, C.G. and McNabb, F.M.A. (2003) Avian models for research in toxicology and endocrine disruption. *Avian and Poultry Biology Reviews,* **14**, 21–52

Schwartz, C.W. and Schwartz, E.R. (1949) *A Reconnaissance of the Game Birds in Hawaii.* Hawaii Board of Commissioners of Agriculture and Forestry, Hilo, Hawaii

Sefton, A.E. and Siegel, P.B. (1973) Mating behavior of Japanese quail. *Poultry Science,* **52**, 1001–1007

Selinger, H.E. and Bermant, G. (1967) Hormonal control of aggressive behaviour in Japanese quail (*Coturnix coturnix japonica*). *Behaviour*, **28**, 255–268

Shanaway, M.M. (1994) *Quail Production System – A Review*. Food and Agriculture Organization of the United Nations, Rome

Shih, J.C.H., Pullman. E.P. and Kao, K.J. (1983) Genetic selection, general characterization, and histology of atherosclerosis-suscptible and -resistant Japanese quail. *Atherosclerosis*, **49**, 41–53

Shim, K.F. and Vohra, P.A. (1984). A review of the nutrition of the Japanese quail. *World's Poultry Science Journal*, **40**, 261–274

Sittman, K., Abplanalp, H. and Abbott, U.K. (1971) Extended storage of quail, chicken and turkey eggs. 2. Embryonic abnormalities and the inheritance of twinning in quail. *Poultry Science*, **50**, 714–722

Skeeles, J.K. (1991) Staphylococcossis. In: *Diseases of Poultry*. Eds Calnek B.W., Barnes H.J., Beard C.W. *et al.*, pp. 293–299. Wolfe Publications Ltd, London

Smith, E.L., Greenwood, V.J., Goldsmith, A.R. *et al.* (2005) Effect of supplementary ultraviolet lighting on the behaviour and corticosterone levels of Japanese quail chicks. *Animal Welfare*, **14**, 103–109

Snoeyenbos, G.H. (1991) Pullorum disease. In: *Diseases of Poultry*. Eds Calnek B.W., Barnes H.J., Beard C.W. *et al.*, pp. 73–86. Wolfe Publications Ltd, London

Somes, R.G. (1984) International registry of poultry genetic stocks. *Bulletin of Storrs Agricultural Experimental Station, University of Connecticut*, **469**, 1–96

Standford, J.A. (1957) A Progress Report of coturnix quail investigations in Missouri. Twenty-second North American Wildlife Conference, 316–359

Stein, G.S. and Bacon, W.L. (1976) Effect of photoperiod upon age and maintenance of sexual development in female *Coturnix coturnix japonica*. *Poultry Science*, **55**, 1214–1218

Suda, Y. and Okamoto, S. (2003) Long term selection for small body weight in Japanese quail II: Changes in reproductive traits from 60 to 65th generations. *Journal of Poultry Science*, **40**, 30–38

Taka-Tsukasa, N. (1935) *Coturnix coturnix japonica* Teminick et Schlegel. In: *The Birds of Nippon*, Vol **1**. pp. 204–238. Whitherby, London

Theilen, G.H., Zeigel, R.F. and Twiehaus, M.J. (1966) Biological studies with REV (strain T) that induces reticuloendothelosis in turkeys, chickens and Japanese quail. *Journal of the National Cancer Institute*, **37**, 731–743

Tsutsui, K., Saigoh, E., Ukena, K. (2000) A novel avian hypothalamic peptide inhibiting gonadotrophin release. *Biophysical Research Communications*, **275**, 661–667

Urbanski, H.F. (1984) Episodic release of LH in gonadectomized male Japanese quail. *Journal of Endocrinology*, **100**, 209–212

Underwood, H. (1994) The circadian rhythm of thermoregulation in Japanese quail. I. Role of the eyes and pineal. *Journal Comparative Physiology A*, **175**, 639–653

Underwood, H. and Edmonds, K. (1995) The circadian rhythm of thermoregulation in Japanese quail. III. Effects of melatonin administration. *Journal Biological Rhythms*, **10**, 284–298

Vince, M.A. (1966) Artificial acceleration of hatching in quail embryos. *Animal Behaviour*, **14**, 389–394

Vince, M.A. (1968) Retardation as a factor in the synchronization of hatching. *Animal Behaviour*, **16**, 332–335

Vince, M.A. and Cheng, R. (1970) The retardation of hatching in Japanese quail. *Animal Behaviour*, **18**, 210–214

Visser, G.H., Boon, P.E. and Meijer, H.A.J. (2000) Validation of the doubly labelled water method in Japanese quail Coturnix c. japonica chicks: is there an effect of growth rate? *Journal of Comparative Physiology*, **170**, 365–372

Wakasugi, N. (1984) Japanese quail. In: *Evolution of Domestic Animals*. Ed. Mason, J.L., pp. 319–321. Longman, London

Wetherbee, D.K. (1961) Investigations in the life history of the common coturnix. *American Midland Naturalist*, **65**, 168–186

Wilson, M.I. and Bermant, G. (1972) An analysis of social interactions in Japanese quail, *Coturnix coturnix japonica*. *Animal Behaviour*, **20**, 252–258

Wilson, W.O. (1972) A review of the physiology of Coturnix (Japanese) quail. *World's Poultry Science Journal*, **28**, 413–423

Wilson, W.O., Abbott, U.K. and Abplanalp, H. (1959) Developmental and physiological studies with a new pilot animal for poultry – *Coturnix* quail. *Poultry Science*, **38**, 1260–1261

Wilson, W.O., Abbott, U.K. and Abplanalp, H. (1961) Evaluation of *Coturnix* (Japanese quail) as a pilot animal for poultry. *Poultry Science*, **40**, 651–657

Woodard. A.E. and Abplanalp, H. (1967) The effects of mating ratio and age on fertility and hatchability in Japanese quail. *Poultry Science*, **46**, 383–388

Woodard, A.E. and Abplanalp, H. (1971) Longevity and reproduction in Japanese quail maintained under stimulatory lighting. *Poultry Science*, **50**, 688–692

Woodard, A.E., Abplanalp, H., Wilson, W.O. *et al.* (1973) *Japanese Quail Husbandry in the Laboratory*. University of California, Davis, California

Woodard, A.E. and Mather, F.B. (1964) Effect of photoperiod on the cyclic patterns of body temperature in the quail. *Nature*, **203**, 422–423

Woodard, A.E. and Wilson, W.O. (1972) Behavioral patterns associated with oviposition in Japanese quail and chickens. *Journal of Interdisciplinary Cycle Research*, **1**, 173–180

Yang, N., Dunnington, E.A. and Siegel, P.B. (1999) Heterosis following long-term bidirectional selection for mating frequency in male Japanese quail. *Poultry Science*, **78**, 1252–1256

Yoder, H.W. Jr (1991) Mycoplasmosis. In: *Diseases of Poultry*. Eds Calnek B.W., Barnes H.J., Beard C.W. *et al.*, pp. 196–212. Wolfe Publications Ltd, London

Yousef, M.K., McFarland, L.Z. and Wilson W.O. (1966) Ambient temperature effects on hypothalmic, rectal and skin temperature in coturnix. *Life Sciences*, **5**, 1887–1896

Zucker, H., Gropp J., Peh J. *et al.* (1967) Erfahrungen mit der japanischen Wachtel (*Coturnix coturnix japonica*) als Labortier sowie einige Ergebnisse von Nährstoffbedarfsuntersuchungen. *Tierärztl Umschauft*, **22**, 416–423

43 The zebra finch

Ruedi G. Nager and Graham Law

Biological overview

Natural history

The zebra finch is a small passerine from the family *Estrildidae* (weaver finches), a group that is found in the Old World tropics and Australasia. All estrildids are similar in structure and habits, but vary widely in plumage colour and patterns. Within the estrildid finches, the zebra finch has occasionally been placed in the genus *Poephila*, but morphological, behavioural and genetic characteristics set it clearly apart from *Poephila* (Christidis 1987) into its own genus *Taeniopygia*, the name of which is based on the zebra finch's earliest name.

The zebra finch is abundant and widespread in the wild and there are two subspecies. The first of these, the Australian zebra finch *Taeniopygia guttata castanotis* (Gould 1837), has a range that covers most of the continental arid and semi-arid zones of Australia only avoiding the cool moist south and the tropical far north. The second subspecies, the Lesser Sundas zebra finch *T. g. guttata* (Vieillot 1817), lives on the Lesser Sundas and neighbouring islands north of Australia. *T. g. guttata* is smaller, the male having a smaller chest-band and less barring on the throat and upper breast compared with *T. g. castanotis*. Zebra finches are sexually dimorphic, the males having a more ornate plumage and a redder bill than females (Figure 43.1).

Zebra finches inhabit arid open steppes that provide grass seeds for food, accessible surface water for drinking and scattered bushes and trees for nesting and roosting. They are adapted for feeding on a large variety of grass-seeds and rely much more on these for food than the other estrildines. Zebra finches usually take ripened seeds from the ground, but also take half-ripe seeds from the heads of standing grasses; and this is what they feed their young on almost exclusively in the wild. Despite their tropical and subtropical distribution, zebra finches tolerate low temperatures, as in the wild they can be exposed to low overnight temperatures.

Size range and lifespan

There are clear morphological differences among different breeding stocks of zebra finches. Among a sample of 18 captive populations, zebra finches in European laboratories were found to be the largest (mean body mass: 16.1 g, range 13.7–18.6 g, n = 10), presumably due to selection for large body size by the European aviculturists and Australian captive birds were the smallest (mean: 12.1 g, range 11.9–12.4 g, n = 2) and similar in size to wild birds. North American birds were intermediate in size (mean: 14.4 g; range 13.7–15.2 g, n = 6; information on body mass from Forstmeier *et al.* (2007)). Domesticated females are also skeletally larger, but take longer to reach adult skeletal size compared to wild birds; no such differences were found for domesticated males compared to wild birds (Zann 1996).

In the wild, there is an initial steep decline in numbers between fledging (day 15–20) and nutritional independence (day 35) when 68.5% of fledglings are lost (Zann 1996). Zann reported high offspring mortality at his field sites with only 9% of eggs leading to young surviving to breeding age. Mature free-living birds have an annual mortality of between 72 and 96%, but can occasionally live for up to 5 years; and there is no difference in the survival rates between males and females (Zann 1996). In captivity, domesticated males typically live about 3 years and females about 2 years, although under optimal conditions, the potential lifespan of domesticated zebra finches is 5–7 years (Burley 1985; own unpublished data); the oldest recorded bird in captivity reached 17 years. Among captive, domesticated birds annual mortality in females is higher than in males throughout their lives (Burley 1985).

Social organisation

The zebra finch is a gregarious species forming feeding flocks of a few hundred individuals when not breeding. During breeding, they nest in colonies ranging from just a few pairs up to 40–50 pairs and territoriality is confined to the nest itself (Zann 1996). Zebra finches can form pair bonds any time during the year when conditions are favourable for breeding and, once paired, develop a strong pair bond (Butterfield 1970). The pair bond is maintained through a series of calls that allow them to recognise and locate their mate (Zann 1996). Mates are selected on the basis of colour and song, and patterns of choice are similar in artificial choice chambers and free-choice aviary situations (Collins & ten Cate 1996; Zann 1996). Due to high mortality rates in the wild there is frequent formation of new pairs, but even when the pair mate has survived birds have never been observed to re-pair with their previous mate. No bird has

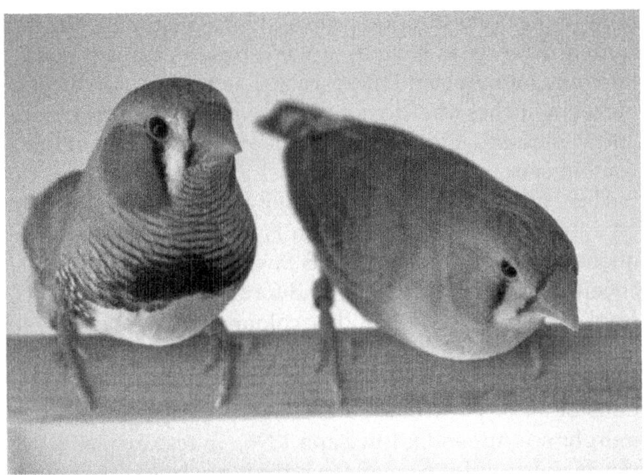

Figure 43.1 Male and female wild-type zebra finches. Females have a grey back, whitish undersides and a white cheek patch bordered by a black stripe. Males are more ornate with reddish brown cheek patches, chestnut brown flanks with white spots and a black and white barred chest. Legs are orange in both sexes, but males have a deeper red bill while females' bills are more orange. (Photo: G. Law.)

been observed with more than one mate at any one time and only the two parents attend the nest (Zann 1996). In the wild, intraspecific brood parasitism is common with 10.9% of offspring and 36% of broods usually containing one or more parasitic eggs, whereas extra-pair paternity is less common with 2.4% of offspring and 8% of broods affected (Birkhead *et al.* 1990) and hence the attending parents may not always be the genetic parents of all of young they rear. Thus zebra finches are socially, but not genetically monogamous.

Biological data

Nestlings of domesticated zebra finches weigh 0.6–0.9g at hatching. Over the first 10 days they gain 0.4–0.7g/day in body mass and about 1mm/day in tarsus length (Skagen 1988; Martins 2004), but this varies with sex, size of the adult stock birds and food levels (Boag 1987). Typical rectal temperature of healthy birds during the day is 41.8°C (Conover & Messmer 1996). Haematolological values for wild and captive zebra finches are given in Ewenson *et al.* (2001), with healthy captive zebra finches typically having a heterophil:lymphocyte ratio of 0.17. Birkhead *et al.* (2006) give a mean haematocrit of 51.2 (standard deviation = 3.58) for male captive zebra finches.

Reproduction

Zebra finches are opportunistic breeders that breed whenever favourable conditions occur, regardless of time since the last breeding event and photoperiodicity (Zann 1996). This allows them to respond to the unpredictable arrival of favourable conditions and to breed rapidly at any time of year. The hatching of eggs coincides with the appearance of ripening grass seeds (Zann *et al.* 1995). Wild zebra finches in unpredictable habitat maintained a high level of reproductive readiness (large gonad size and high level of circulating gonadotrophins) and more males showed readiness to breed than females (Perfito *et al.* 2007). Wild zebra finches in a predictable habitat, where breeding occurs during approximately the same months each year, changed reproductive readiness consistently between the breeding and non-breeding state. When non-breeding birds from the predictable environment were taken into the laboratory they were able to activate their reproductive axis quickly (Perfito *et al.* 2007). This suggests that there is constant activation of gonads without a refractory period and that they can rapidly respond to the presence of favourable breeding conditions. Along with this high reproductive readiness or 'hypersexuality' goes an early reproductive maturity in young birds; birds as young as 62–67 days old (median age of birds breeding in the same breeding season in which they hatched: 95 and 92 days for males and females, respectively) have been seen to breed in the wild (Zann 1996). 'Hypersexuality' distinguishes zebra finches from other small passerines and is presumably an adaptation to the unpredictable arid conditions in Australia. However, some aspects of this trait have declined in domesticated zebra finches, which show slower sexual development than wild females; domesticated females lay eggs only as early as 90 days old (Sossinka 1972a).

Zebra finches typically lay a clutch of five white eggs (range two to seven eggs) that measure about 1.5 × 1cm, laying one egg each day in the wild and captivity. Each egg takes about 4 days of rapid follicle growth before it is laid (Houston *et al.* 1995). In the wild, parents usually start to incubate on the last or penultimate egg so that hatching occurs over 24–48h. In captivity, parents start incubation much earlier during laying and clutches hatch far more asynchronously than in the wild. Both sexes incubate, although only the female has a brood patch (Zann 1996). Incubation takes between 11 and 14 days from the day the last egg has been laid. Zebra finches are altricial, the chicks depending on their parents for food and warmth. Young are fed by both sexes, with parents transferring seeds from their crop to the chick's crop. Chicks that have not been fed can easily be spotted as the crop of fed chicks bulges and seeds can be seen through the skin of the crop. Parents may brood their young for the first few days, and can feed their chicks several times during one nest attention bout; therefore, the number of nest visits is a poor measure of parental feeding effort.

Normal behaviour

Males sing a complex courtship song but females do not sing. Zann (1996) estimates a foraging time of 2–4h and that about 4g of seeds per day is needed for wild zebra finches to meet their daily requirements. In search of food, individual zebra finches can range over an area up to at least 1km around the nest during breeding and are highly mobile, deserting an area when conditions become unfavourable (Zann 1996). The lack of genetic differentiation of populations up to 2000km apart (Forstmeier *et al.* 2007) supports the view that populations can range over such large distances. Non-breeding zebra finches often roost in old breeding nests or purpose-built nests (Zann 1996). As another adaptation to their arid and semi-arid habitat, zebra finches have an unusually slow moult for passerines and females moult more slowly than males. Arid conditions in the wild and intense breeding activity in captivity slow the moult.

Sources and supplies

Zebra finches used in research laboratories are derived from *Taeniopygia guttata castanotis* and have been domesticated for more than a century. In Europe, zebra finches were frequently bred in captivity by the late 1800s, but large numbers of zebra finches were still being imported from Australia until World War I, and in the 1950s further small numbers of birds that had been domesticated in Australia were imported (Sossinka 1970). In 1960, the Australian government implemented export bans on all native wildlife. Currently, zebra finches in research laboratories worldwide have presumably been domesticated for more than a century without any significant input of wild zebra finches and are genetically clearly distinct from the wild stock (Forstmeier *et al.* 2007). Domestication has altered a number of behavioural and other traits resulting in larger body size and delayed female sexual maturity in domesticated zebra finches (see earlier in this chapter) as well as in changes to the structure of distance calls and duration of song phrases (eg, Sossinka 1970; Slater & Clayton 1991; Zann 1996).

Many research laboratories maintain their own breeding stocks derived from larger stocks of aviculturists. Compared to wild birds, all captive populations have lost genetic variability, but all populations still show substantial genetic variability at 12 highly polymorphic microsatellite markers, suggesting that they were unlikely to have experienced severe genetic bottlenecks (Forstmeier *et al.* 2007). There is significant genetic and morphological differentiation among captive populations between Australia, Europe and North America with further differences between regions, in particular in Europe (Zann 1996; Forstmeier *et al.* 2007). It is clear that there have been regional differences in the directions of the domestication process, which might have arisen from differences in sources of wild stock, in climatic conditions and in show standards for size (Zann 1996). Researchers on zebra finches thus do not use a genetically uniform stock and it is essential to give information on the origin of birds used in every study.

There are many colour morphs of zebra finches. The wild type or grey morph is shown in Figure 43.1. The most frequently found colour mutant is fawn. This morph was discovered in wild birds in 1927 and formed the breeding stock from which many of the other colour morphs were developed (Zann 1996). Aviculturists have bred about 30 main morphs mainly for show competitions and most are mutations of all or particular parts of the plumage (for a list of morphs see Appendix 1 in Zann 1996). In research laboratories mainly wild-type and fawn birds are used. The colour mutation fawn is sex-linked and this has been used in the past to sex very young offspring (Birkhead *et al.* 1989; Kilner 1998). Imprinting studies have shown a strong effect of plumage colour on mate choice (eg, Immelmann *et al.* 1978) and this needs to be considered in studies on sexual selection and mate selection. Ideally, one would want to have birds of the same colour morph, but this is difficult to achieve since most colour mutations are recessive and unexpected colour morphs may appear in later generations.

Use in research

The zebra finch is widely studied by biologists in the laboratory and field. It is one of the most popular caged birds in the world. It is hardy, easy to keep and one of the most readily bred aviary birds. Zebra finches are inexpensive to buy. They are widely used in research with the number of publications steadily increasing each year, reaching over 100 publications per year in recent years (Figure 43.2). Research using zebra finches focuses mainly on the neural basis of song learning, but also sexual selection, development of sexual preferences and physiological studies such as endocrinology and toxicity testing.

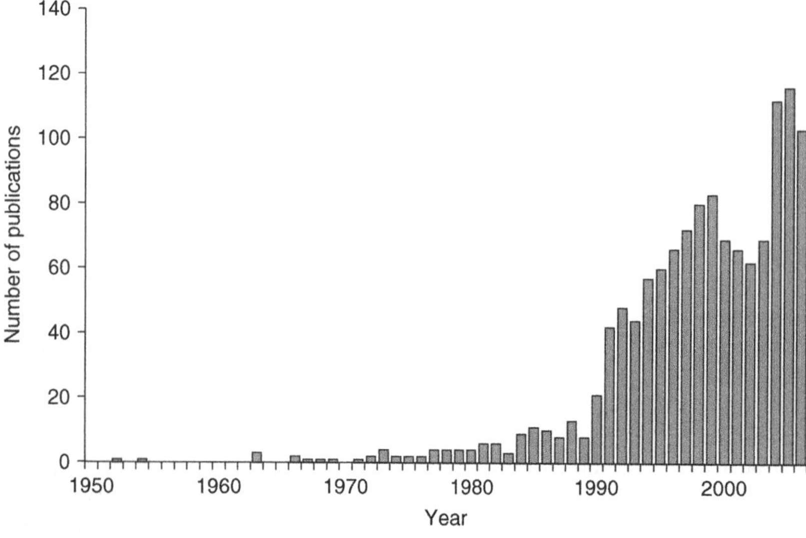

Figure 43.2 The number of publications per year containing 'zebra finch' in the title, keywords or abstract is steadily increasing (searched on Web of Knowledge 24 October 2007).

The zebra finch genome was the second avian genome to be sequenced to 6X coverage in 2007, using initially one male bird from a North American captive breeding population (University of California in Los Angeles, UCLA). The availability of extensive genomic information is likely to be a great catalyst for further studies of the species.

General husbandry

Although zebra finches are one of the most commonly used experimental bird species, it is surprising that very little work has been conducted on their welfare. The following account is based on 'good practice' advice from a number of laboratories and organisations (eg, Joint Working Group on Refinement (JWGR) 2001) who have many years of experience in working with this species. In most cases, however, there are no systematic scientific studies to evaluate the impact of common husbandry practices on the birds' welfare. Future work into the welfare of captive zebra finches is needed to refine guidelines for their husbandry.

Enclosure

Enclosures for captive animals need to allow as much natural behaviour to be performed as possible (Young 2003). In the wild, zebra finches regularly flock in trees and forage on the ground and therefore require the space to carry out such movements. In the wild, the birds are highly sociable, maintaining close contact to each other and hence in captivity can be maintained at higher densities than many other species. The size of the enclosure needs to take these needs of the birds into consideration.

The size of the enclosure and the layout of the enclosure furnishings should be organised to maximise space for movement. The size of aviary should be such as to permit birds to perform horizontal flight and, if space is limited, width can be compromised in order to defend sufficient length for free flight. Spacing of the perches should be such as to encourage the maximum flight distances possible, while satisfying the need for a comfortable roost. Due to their social nature, zebra finches can be kept at relatively high densities in large flight cages or aviaries. For scientific reasons, it may be necessary to hold birds under standardised conditions in smaller cages either individually or in pairs. Although the effect of separation from conspecifics on isolated zebra finches has not been studied, many sources recommend minimising the time zebra finches are not kept with others (eg, JWGR 2001).

Zebra finches can be kept in standard cages with solid sides on all but the front. It is recommended that cages should be made of an easy-to-clean material to provide a hygienic environment for the birds. Cages can be stacked or mounted on wall brackets. Zebra finches can also be kept in aviaries constructed with a frame of steel or treated wood and covered with wire mesh of ≤10 mm width or vertical bars not more than 12 mm apart. Aviaries can be indoors. Zebra finches in the wild, however, experience a wide range conditions and can be exposed to freezing temperatures (Meijer *et al.* 1996). Thus they can also be kept outdoors throughout the year provided they have sufficient protection from wind and rain such as shrubs and access to an indoor area with supplemental heating in winter (JWGR 2001).

Table 43.1 Minimum enclosure dimensions and space allowances for zebra finches as good practice recommended by the BVA(AWF)/FRAME/RSPCA/UFWA Joint Working Group (JWGR 2001) and the European Commission (2007).

	Minimum enclosure area (m²)	*Minimum height (m)*	*Minimum number of feeders*
Single bird or breeding pair	0.5	0.3–0.4[1]	
Up to 6 birds	1	1	2
7–12 birds	1.5	2	2
13–20 birds	2	2	3
Per each additional bird above 20	0.05	2	1 per 6 birds

[1] BVA(AWF)/FRAME/RSPCA/UFAW joint working group report (JWGR 2001) recommends a minimum height of 0.3 m whereas the European Commission (2007) recommends 0.4 m

There are hardly any data on the effects of enclosure size on the welfare of zebra finches. In a study involving very small numbers, Jacobs *et al.* (1995) found reduced activity, in a number of behaviours, in cages with an area of 0.11 m^2 compared to cages with an area of 0.22 m^2 (the latter cage size is approximately current practice). There is a large gap in our understanding of the effects of enclosure size on zebra finch behaviour and physiology. Nonetheless, several organisations have provided guidelines on what they consider best practice for space requirements of groups of various sizes (summarised in Table 43.1) and these may become legally binding in a number of countries.

Environmental provisions and enrichments

Zebra finches normally feed on the ground and therefore require solid flooring. The floor can be covered with a paper liner or some substrate, such as bark chips, wood shavings, hemp core or sand which gives the birds a softer and more varied substrate and makes foraging for spilled seeds more challenging. Bark chips have the advantage that they maintain a hygienic floor litter, but do not work well under the dry conditions usually encountered in laboratory bird rooms. Floor substrate should produce as little dust as possible under the conditions usually encountered in bird rooms in order to keep dust levels low for the benefit of the birds and of the staff working with the birds.

Wild zebra finches spend much time perching in trees. Perches of a variety of diameters and at different heights should therefore be provided. In captivity, they prefer to perch high up in the cage and to approach the food by moving to progressively closer perches. Care needs to be taken not to overcrowd the space with perches that would restrict the birds' flight movements. Furthermore, care should be taken not to place perches over food and water dishes to prevent fouling. Often doweling rods (ca. 0.5 cm in diameter) are provided as perches, but these are not recommended as they are too hard. Sandpaper perch covers should not be used as they can abrade the feet and provide a route for infection. Softer wood or a variety of natural branches (apple, aspen, birch, cactus wood, cherry, elm, maple, mountain ash, pear, pine, poplar and willow) are good alternative perches. Natural branches in a range of diameters (0.5–2 cm), which are often less rigid than artificial perches, allow the muscles of the feet and body involved in balance to be properly exercised and help to keep the claws in good trim. There are also artificial perches that are not of a constant diameter and are attached to the cage wall at only one side giving them the springiness of a natural branch. Perches that sway when the birds land and take off, as well as commercially available swings designed for zebra finches, help mimic the movement of trees in the wild and cause the birds to exercise a variety of muscles and use the wings for balance. Zebra finches like to sit close together and therefore perches and swings should be of sufficient length to allow at least two birds to sit on them. Perches need to be replaced, or cleaned where possible, possibly every 6 weeks to provide a hygienic environment (see Hygiene section).

Zebra finches will use both sand and water baths, sometimes using the bowl communally. In the authors' experience, baths once a week help to keep their plumage in good condition. Baths are usually provided for a few hours per day, water should be 0.5–1 cm deep and if size allows, a flat stone can be placed in the water bath, to help prevent the bath tipping over. Since zebra finches are prolific nest builders and also build roosting nests outside the breeding season, provision of some nest material to non-breeding birds may help provide good sensory stimulation. Jacobs *et al.* (1995), using a very small sample size, suggested that simple enrichments such as a larger number of perches, twigs, sand and water baths may result in increased frequency of a number of behaviours. Zebra finches with little opportunity for exercise can become obese (Birkhead *et al.* 2006).

An obvious way to stimulate captive birds is to increase foraging time and, like many other animals, they will work for food even if it is freely available (contra freeloading). Zebra finches can be provided with additional sprays of *Panicum* millet and these can be placed so that the birds need to increase their effort to feed from them. Seed spillage or intentional scatter feeding on the ground can encourage natural foraging behaviour (JWGR 2001). Mixing seeds with husks also increases foraging time and effort, but birds provided with mixtures with the highest husks:seed ratio for their entire lifetime had low foraging efficiencies (effectively starving) and produced small and few broods as well as having a poor survival (Lemon & Barth, 1992; Lemon 1993), therefore extreme caution is needed when applying this feeding method.

Feeding and watering

In the wild, zebra finches forage on a wide variety of seed types and sizes (Zann 1996). Captive birds do best on a diet of foreign finch seed mixes (largely millet and canary seeds). Food can be provided in feeders mounted on the cage wall or in petri dishes provided on the ground but the latter result in a lot of seed spillage. The daily requirement for seed by domesticated zebra finches under standard laboratory conditions is about 3 g. Seeds should be provided in at least two feeders per cage and, if birds are kept in social groups, provisioning of several dishes is recommended (see Table 43.1) to avoid monopolisation of the food by dominant birds at the expense of subordinates. To assist the breakdown of seeds in the gizzard it is essential that birds are given fine oyster shell and other grit, and this should be available separate from the seeds, so that the birds can control their intake.

To balance the diet, zebra finches should, once or twice a week, be given good-quality greens such as dandelion leaves, the darker outer leaves of lettuce, chickweed, spinach, watercress or vegetables (eg, grated carrots, cucumbers) and fruits (eg, apples, oranges and bananas). Several vegetables and fruits may have to be tried to see what appeals to the individual finches. Greens, vegetables and fruits form an important source of dietary carotenoids that positively influence the bird's health and affect bill coloration (Blount *et al.* 2003a; McGraw *et al.* 2003). Sprouted seeds should also be given to birds to satisfy the need for greens. In order to germinate the seeds, normal finch mix can be soaked in clean water, thoroughly rinsed after 24 h and then soaked in water again. After 48 h rinse again, drain thoroughly and place on paper towels in a flat tray in a warm and dark place. Depending on temperatures, seeds will sprout in 24–36 h and sprouting of over 60% indicates that the seeds are relatively fresh. The sprouted seeds can be fed at any stage but are best in the first 36 h. Zebra finches also like soaked seeds (seeds are soaked for a day in clean water and rinsed) and live insect prey, such as mealworms or cricket nymphs (again one may need to try different live insects to see what appeals the individual finches). Birds should always also have access to some form of calcium as this is an essential mineral. A good source of calcium is cuttlefish bones, positioned so that the birds have access to the softer side. These have the additional benefit of helping to keep the birds' bill in good trim. Other good sources of calcium are crushed sea shells or domestic chicken egg shells (it is recommended to microwave domestic chicken egg shells for a few minutes to kill any bacteria that may pose a health risk) or commercially available calcium supplements can be provided in the drinking water.

Any potential deficits in the diet can be corrected with supplements. Supplements can be added in liquid form to the birds' drinking water or in powder form to the grit. Because finches remove the husk from all seeds before consumption, any food additives on the seed surface are likely to be discarded before eating. Protein-rich foods such as cooked domestic chicken eggs or commercially available protein supplements, live insect prey and greens should be provided regularly but in small amounts and in several separate dishes to prevent birds overeating protein-rich food that can cause diarrhoea.

Special attention should be paid to diet during breeding. Egg formation is a very demanding process both in nutrients and energy requirements. Protein is of paramount importance in egg formation. Zebra finch females use protein stored in muscle tissue to contribute to egg formation and build these stores up over several weeks prior to breeding. Females fed *ad libitum* with a protein-enriched diet from 2 weeks before breeding produced larger eggs, larger clutches and had a higher breeding success than birds on a control diet (Selman & Houston 1996). Good sources of protein are boiled chicken's eggs or commercial protein supplements. Dietary calcium is also important for egg formation. Females with *ad libitum* calcium (calcareous grit, cuttlefish bone and fine oyster shell) provided regularly throughout pre-breeding and breeding laid eggs with stronger shells compared to females on a calcium-deficient diet (Reynolds 2001). Calcium may also be given as a supplement in drinking water and the manufacturer's guidelines should be checked for proper dosage. Pre-laying females supplemented with carotenoids mixed into their drinking water and with carotenoid intakes raised to the upper range of that which their normal seed diet provides, formed eggs with higher carotenoid content in the yolk. This was found to result in higher hatching and fledging success and in more brightly coloured males compared to offspring from females on a control diet (McGraw *et al.* 2005). Rearing and conditioning supplements and greens and fruits are a good source for additional carotenoids.

The quality of the rearing diet affects growth and development. Compared to nestlings on a diet of mixed seeds with *ad libitum* low-protein (7%) commercial conditioning food, nestlings on a mixed seed diet enriched with high-protein (34%) commercial conditiong food and 1 g of minced hard-boiled hen's egg per day per family, grew faster and reached larger adult size (Boag 1987). Compared to nestlings that received 1.5 g of conditioning food per family once a week (conditioning food is the main source of dietary antioxidants), during their first 15 days of life, nestlings that received daily 1.5 g of conditioning food per family had higher plasma levels of antioxidants in adulthood, which have beneficial effects on the birds' health, bill coloration and immune functions (Blount *et al.* 2003a, 2003b) and had a greater reproductive performance as an adult (Blount *et al.* 2006).

Zebra finches should have access to clean drinking water on a daily basis. Birds would naturally drink from open water surfaces on the ground, but they also easily accept commercially available drinking bottles. The latter can be mounted externally to the cage, which will reduce stress to the birds at water changes. When switching from one kind of water container to another, both should be provided for a while. Although, in captivity, zebra finches (providing they are healthy) can survive several months without water on a diet of dry seed, this can result in severe bill deformation and poor plumage (Sossinka 1972b).

Social housing

Zebra finches are gregarious birds during both the breeding and the non-breeding season, and therefore can be kept in high densities in large aviaries (see Enclosure section). When introducing unfamiliar birds, or regrouping birds, the groups need to be carefully monitored for social compatibility, unusual weight loss or signs of pecking. Whilst breeding in groups, care should be taken that an excess of nesting sites are provided as birds will compete for and actively and aggressively defend these. Breeding in several smaller aviaries may be preferable to breeding all together in one large aviary to minimise levels of aggression. In breeding populations, male-biased sex ratios may cause social instabilities which could result in more aggressive behaviours, weight loss, reduced body condition and poorer immune functions, as have been for example observed in other captive finches (Greives *et al.* 2007).

Identification and sexing

The most common method to individually mark zebra finches is to use split leg rings. If coloured leg rings are required for individual identification it is important to be aware that the colour of the rings may have profound effects on their social behaviour, mate attractiveness, longevity and offspring sex ratio (Burley *et al.* 1982; Burley 1986, 1988; Swaddle & Cuthill 1994; Cuthill *et al.* 1997); although not all studies have confirmed these effects (see eg, Hunt *et al.* 1997; Rutstein *et al.* 2004, 2005). In some studies, females preferred males with red leg rings and with symmetrical arrangements of multiple colours and disliked males with green leg rings and with asymmetrical arrangements of multiple colours and the same colour preferences were found for captive and recently caught wild females. Males most prefer females with black leg rings and least prefer females with light-blue colour rings. Zebra finches do not appear to distinguish between un-ringed birds and those with orange leg rings. Ring colour also affects intra-sexual dominance interactions with red-ringed males being socially dominant over green-ringed males. Hence, it is best to use colours that have less impact on the birds' behaviour and where different colours are unavoidable, to provide a sufficient number of different food sources to avoid dominant birds monopolising the food (JWGR 2001).

The zebra finch is sexually dimorphic and from 2–3 months of age the sexes can readily be distinguished on the basis of plumage markings (Figure 43.1) and the fact that only the male sings. In addition, males have a redder beak colour, whereas the beak of females is more orange, which may help to determine sex in pure white colour varieties. Before reaching the mature plumage, the sexes may be distinguished by using certain varieties where colour inheritance is sex-linked (Birkhead *et al.* 1989; Kilner 1998) or by taking a small drop of blood or a growing feather to use in a molecular sex determination (Griffiths *et al.* 1996).

Physical environment

Zebra finches can withstand a wide range of temperatures (but it is important that extremes are avoided). The flight areas of outdoor aviaries should be protected from wind and driving rain in the winter months and suitably shaded areas provided for the summer. Hessian sacking or other garden centre windbreak materials can be used around bird flights to provide protection. Various species of dense shrubs in the outside flight areas, avoiding poisonous varieties, have been used to provide zebra finches with shelter and a secure retreat. Outside the breeding season, zebra finches are known to protect themselves from lower night temperatures by building nests. Birds kept indoors do well when the temperature is maintained between 20 and 25 °C, and it may be worth considering a slightly reduced night-time temperature where the heating system allows.

It is unlikely that minor fluctuations in relative humidity levels would stress captive zebra finches. Humidity levels between 40 and 80% are typically recommended, and colonies have been maintained at ca. 40–55% for many years without mishap.

Most zebra finch colonies are kept at cycles of between 14h:10h and 12h:12h of light:dark. Provision of shorter days a few weeks before breeding may increase the percentage of birds breeding (see Perfito *et al.* 2007). Lights should gradually fade on and off at the start and end of each day avoiding sudden changes from dark to light and *vice versa*. Light levels should be of an appropriate brightness and as bird vision works well in light levels suitable for humans, around 500 lux should suffice. Light levels that are constantly low (below 20 lux) can cause the birds to become stressed. The visual system of birds differs from that of humans in the way that birds perceive light in the UV range and in that they have a higher temporal resolution. The latter means that captive birds may perceive the flicker emitted from conventional low-frequency fluorescent lights (100 Hz in Europe, 120 Hz in the USA). The flicker rate of the light can affect female mate choice behaviour in captive birds, possibly due to non-specific stress effects or impaired discrimination ability of visual signals (Evans *et al.* 2006). Therefore the type of fluorescent tubes needs to be carefully chosen. High-frequency fluorescent tubes (>30 kHz) that mimic the daylight spectrum (ie, with some UV component) are preferable. It is also worth considering whether there needs to be an emergency lighting system in case of power failures, as birds will not forage in the dark.

Adequate air circulation is essential to prevent accumulation of dust and gases (eg, carbon dioxide, ammonia); in the authors' bird rooms there are about 13–15 air changes per hour. This is for the benefit of the birds but also the health of staff working in these rooms. This should be achieved without causing draughts. Bird house ventilation ducts should be fitted with filters of a suitable size to remove fine dust and dander before venting outside. The build-up of feathers and dust on ventilation ducts can be remedied by regular vacuuming.

Birds should not be housed near any equipment that emits low frequency vibrations and white noise. Environmental white noise can erode the strong pair bond in zebra finches, with females subjected to this challenge showing no greater preference for their chosen male than for strangers; presumably because the noise prevents the female from hearing the calls that allow her to recognise and locate her mate (Swaddle & Page 2006). Playback of conspecific vocalisation showed that it influences the breeding schedule and clutch size in zebra finch colonies presumably through social stimulation (Waas *et al.* 2005). Playing music may be an acceptable method for managing the auditory environment by masking potential auditory stressors, helping them feel more settled when unexpected sounds occur or introducing auditory stimulation, but more research in this area is required (reviewed in Patterson-Kane & Farnworth 2006). If playing music in bird rooms it is suggested to use classical or easy listening music played not above a conversational level (about 60 dB) and only during the birds' active periods (Patterson-Kane & Farnworth 2006). The potential positive and negative effects of playing music, however, need to be carefully monitored when introducing it.

Hygiene

Hygiene measures in the bird room should take account of both birds, and the people working in the facility. Access to the unit should be restricted to essential staff and protective clothing, masks, footwear/shoe covers and hand-washing facilities should be used to create a viable barrier.

The accommodation should be cleaned and sanitised before each batch of birds arrives, and should be decontaminated when all the stock is exchanged. Internal bird flights and cages should have the substrates regularly changed; the length of time between changes will depend on the stocking density. Waste substrate and seed from birdcages should, where possible, be vacuumed with low-noise vacuum cleaners fitted with high-efficiency particulate air (HEPA) filters, which help avoid the displacement of fine dust particles into the air. Perches should be removed and washed in disinfectant. Perches can then be rinsed in fresh water and left to dry before re-use. Cage walls and wire need periodic cleaning. All food, water and grit containers should be regularly sterilised. Floors and walls of the bird laboratory room should be cleaned and disinfected.

Health monitoring, quarantine and barrier systems

Occasionally individuals need to be singly housed in a 'hospital cage' because of illness or injury. A 'hospital cage' should contain a heat source that the bird can move towards or away from. A good heat source is a 25 W tungsten bulb with a temperature of about 24 °C. Hospital cages can be provided within the same room, but if there is concern about a contagious disease, the bird needs to be kept in isolation with separate air ventilation or appropriate filters to protect the stock. Hospital cages should provide a good supply of food and fresh water in shallow dishes on the floor for easier access.

All staff should be aware of the normal behaviour of zebra finches and able to recognise when they are ill and need attention (see Health section). All birds entering the unit should be health screened and should be quarantined for at least 28 days before being added to stock (long enough for many common diseases to manifest themselves). Quarantine, health screening and monitoring protocols should be agreed with the attending veterinarian. All deaths must be recorded and, where there is a cause of concern, *post-mortem* examinations should be undertaken to identify the cause whenever possible.

Breeding

Zebra finches breed readily throughout the year in indoor aviaries. Captive birds as young as 3 months are physiologically ready to breed, but for best results they should be at least 6–9 months old. For best breeding results, birds older than 4 years, particularly females, should be avoided. Little is known about variation in breeding success in relation to the birds' age and experience (but see Williams & Christians 2003). Under the relatively constant environmental temperature of captive breeding facilities, productivity may show seasonal variation with day length, more clutches being produced in summer and autumn (Boruszewska *et al.* 2007).

For best breeding results, young birds should be allowed to express mate choice, choosing their own partners from a small mixed-sex group. If particular pairings are required, most male/female couples in good condition will breed when placed in the same cage. Pair bond formation between unfamiliar birds can start immediately after introduction where the males performs a characteristic courtship dance and direct song towards the female and the female carries out an acceptance posture (for more details see Zann 1996). A sure sign of an established pair bond is when the male and female sit close to and preen each other.

Captive birds need to be provided with suitable nesting sites. Different types of nesting sites are available from wicker baskets, half coconut shells, to re-usable wooden or single-use cardboard nest boxes. Commercially available nest boxes typically have linear dimensions of at least 10 cm and an entrance hole of at least 4 cm diameter. Nest boxes mounted externally to the aviary mesh are convenient since the nest can be checked with minimal disturbance to the breeding birds. Birds need to be provided with suitable nesting material, but not in great excess. Usually the birds will start to build a nest almost immediately. Coconut fibre is a good nesting material. On a foundation platform, males and females together build an enclosed nest chamber (Figure 43.3), but when offered nest boxes they often build much less complex structures. The inside of the nest chamber is lined with some softer material. In captivity, feathers, cotton wool, fine sisal string or moss can be used. It is important that there is no risk of the birds getting their toes caught in the nesting material. When using nest boxes, the bottom of the nest box can be filled with floor substrate to allow the bird to sit level with the entrance hole. Provision of nest material should stop once the clutch is complete as otherwise birds may continue to add nest material over the eggs and lay another clutch on top ('sandwich clutches').

The onset of breeding can be promoted by provision of soaked seeds, and greens and/or spraying a fine mist of water over the birds, but these measures are not essential. Also, good nutrition will affect the birds' breeding behaviour (see Feeding and watering section). Usually within a week, the nest is finished and the females start laying. In captivity, around the time when the third egg is laid or even earlier, the birds start sitting on the eggs and this onset of incubation is earlier than in wild birds, resulting in a larger hatching asynchrony than in wild birds. Both sexes help to incubate the eggs and keep them covered for close to 100% of the time (Gorman & Nager 2003; Gorman *et al.* 2005). After approximately 2 weeks of incubation, the eggs will start to hatch. The newly hatched nestlings are blind and only have a few areas of soft down. At hatching a rearing food (see Feeding and watering section) should be provided together with the regular seed mixture.

Like most estrildines, zebra finch nestlings are slow developers and they spend longer in the nest and take longer to reach adult weight than other granivorous species, such as fringillids and ploceines (Zann 1996). Nestling zebra finches are very hardy and 4–5-day-old chicks can endure periods of up to 36 h without food and warmth, presumably entering some form of torpor. Nestlings are fed by both parents and store seeds in their crop; the crop of newly hatched nestlings (day 0) is empty and parents only start feeding the next day. First only the right side of the crop is filled and only later when larger quantities need to be stored, the left side of the crop also fills. Nestlings start to make soft begging calls from the third day onwards, feathers start to break through by 6–7 days and eyes open fully by day 10–11. Nestlings can be individually marked using non-toxic pens on the skin and tufts of down, and marks may need to be renewed regularly. From around 8 or 9 days old, nestlings can be ringed with leg rings. To avoid birds leaving the nest prematurely, regular nest checks should be stopped when the birds are about 2 weeks old. When the birds are around 18 days old, they will leave the nest for the first time. Around day 35 the

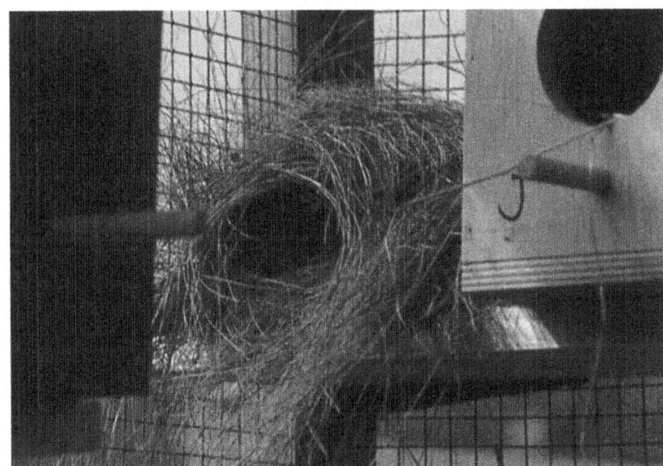

Figure 43.3 Zebra finches build nests when suitable nest support and nest material are available (nest on the left). Similar nests can be built inside nest boxes, which might be more suitable for outdoor aviaries and, when mounted from the outside, minimise disturbance to the breeding birds. (Photo: R. Nager.)

birds will become independent and feed independently, although they will continue to beg for a while longer. Around this time the bill colour starts to change from black to a lighter colour (which will eventually turn orange or red) and the post-juvenile moult into the adult plumage begins.

For best breeding results, birds should be kept at lower densities than in standard holding accommodation, and should be maintained in an equal sex ratio and with an excess of nest sites provided. When zebra finches breed in groups, both extra-pair paternity and intra-specific brood parasitism can occur (Birkhead *et al.* 1990). Under good conditions, zebra finches may breed continuously; but it is best not to allow them to produce more than two successive broods before a period of non-breeding. At the end of breeding, the nest should be removed. If two successive clutches are desired, young need to be removed from the cage when independent. If they are left with the parents, they may interrupt the next clutch and the parents may chase off the young birds and pluck their feathers. If a particular behavioural study, for example on song learning, requires that young are raised by females alone, this is possible. In this case it is best to delay removing the male until day 5 as there is no evidence for memorising the father's song before that age, and a reduction of the brood size can be considered (Royle *et al.* 2002). Zebra finches can also be raised from the egg stage onwards by Bengalese finches. Both inter-specific cross-fostering and female-only rearing will affect the behavioural development of the chicks. If pairs fail to feed their chicks at first, particularly first-time breeders, the nestlings can be helped through that period by some hand feeding.

It is important to keep detailed records on the breeding activity of individual birds and pairs. This prevents breeding between close relatives, allows the elimination of poor breeders and efficient rotation of the stock used in breeding. Several pedigree software packages are now available for this purpose, such as ZooEasy or LaoTzu's Animal Register.

Laboratory procedures

Handling

If specific individuals need to be captured and handled on a regular basis, it may be preferable to keep them in small cages where they are more easily and rapidly captured. This is less stressful to the individual bird as well as for other birds in the group. In large cages, a bird net with padded edges will be required to catch birds. Switching off the light can help to catch the bird more quickly in the dark. Once in the hand, birds should be kept with the back inside the palm of the hand, its head between the index and second finger and the wings gently closed against its sides so that the bird's chest remains free.

Training and habituation for procedures

Zebra finches are believed not to habituate easily to handling and, compared to many other cage birds, they do not become very tame and are not as inquisitive. Nonetheless, zebra finches will work for food, and can learn to respond to light and colour cues and to discriminate between different songs and sounds. Rewarding zebra finches after disturbance is an effective and simple way to improve their habituation to handling (Collins *et al.* 2008). Suitable rewards are small pieces of fruit, salad and live insect prey. Providing cover, eg, by an opaque cloth over part of the cage, where birds can take refuge when humans are present, however, can lead to increased fearfulness over time (Collins *et al.* 2008).

Monitoring methods

Body temperature can be recorded using small temperature probes (<0.5 mm wide) that are carefully inserted into the rectum. Blood for haematological, hormonal and biochemical analyses can be collected from three points: right jugular vein, ulnar vein and the medial metatarsal vein. As these are all superficial veins they can be punctured with a sterile needle or lancet and anaesthesia is not necessary. Blood collection should only be carried out by trained and experienced staff. Bleeding can be stopped by pressure from a swab. The vein, in particular the jugular vein, may be more easily recognisable in a well exercised bird with small fat deposits, which would reduce the duration of handling the bird. The quantity of blood that can be safely collected from healthy individuals is limited to 10% of circulating blood volume (which is about 0.1 ml for a 16 g zebra finch) and less if the same bird is re-sampled in less than 3–4 weeks (maximum of 1% of circulating blood volume or 0.01 ml for a 16 g zebra finch per 24 h) (Morton *et al.* 1993). There are non-destructive methods to collect a sample of the crop content (Zann & Straw 1984) and of semen (Pellatt & Birkhead 1994).

Administration of substances

Some drugs can be mixed with food or drinking water. Since zebra finches usually remove the husk of the seeds before ingesting them it is unlikely that they would ingest any drugs on the outside of the seed, unless de-husked seed is used. These methods can be useful for administering substances to a large number of birds, but do not permit accurate control of dosage. Suitably-sized oesophageal tubes can be used for individual birds, which allows for more accurate dosing. Injections in small passerines like the zebra finch are difficult and hazardous. Subcutaneous and intramuscular injections can be given with a 27 G needle and a 1 ml insulin syringe, but great caution is necessary. A small amount of alcohol with 10% glycerine is normally used to prepare the site before injection. When the needle is removed, a dry cotton-tipped applicator is placed over the site to apply gentle pressure and stop any bleeding.

Anaesthesia and analgesia

General anaesthesia can be achieved using gaseous or injectable anaesthetics. Gaseous anaesthetics have the advantage that dosage is easily changed during the procedure, and recovery can be extremely rapid. They require special equipment for precision delivery. The most commonly used gaseous anaesthetic for birds is isoflurane. This agent has proved safe and extremely useful in many avian species and it is the recommended choice for anaesthesia. Ketamine has been used as an injectable anaesthetic in birds, but recovery is often troublesome, with the bird flapping and thrashing due to involuntary excitement. Hence, ketamine should be mixed with an equal volume of xylazine, which has strong muscle relaxing as well as weak analgesic properties. The reader should refer to specialised textbooks on avian anaesthesia (eg, Samour 2000) for drug dosages, methods of delivery and monitoring of anaesthesia.

Euthanasia

Zebra finches can be euthanased by overdose of gaseous or injectable anaesthetic. Exposure to a rising concentration of carbon dioxide in an enclosed chamber has also been used but the humaneness of this method is controversial. Birds can also be killed by neck dislocation by an experienced person but this may not be ideal as evidence from studies in poultry indicate that this does not always lead to immediate loss of brain function. See also Chapter 17.

Common health and welfare problems

Health

Zebra finches can be affected by a range of infectious and non-infectious diseases (see Dorrestein 1996; Jones & Slater 1999). An ill bird is normally less active than usual, and may sit in a corner in a huddled position, fluffed up, and with dull, slit or closed eyes. It is best to place ill birds in a hospital cage (see Health monitoring, quarantine and barrier systems section) and to seek prompt veterinary attention. If a contagious disease is suspected, ill birds should be immediately isolated. A summary of common infectious diseases of the zebra finch is given in Table 43.2. It is important to remember that some of these diseases can affect humans and due care is essential. Ectoparasites such as feather lice and

Table 43.2 Some infectious diseases of zebra finches

Disease	*Comments*
Viral	
Avian pox	Uncommon. Conjunctivitis, blepharitis. Self-limiting but may be fatal. Common in some species. Torticollis, depression, weight loss
Paramyxovirus	Severe pancreatitis on *post-mortem*
Papovavirus	Common in some aviaries. Deaths amongst nestlings and young birds, developmental abnormalities, beak deformities. Hepatocellular necrosis on histopathology
Bacterial	
Enterobacteriaceae	*E. coli* septiceaemia can be a problem in new shipments (stress-related). *Citrobacter, Salmonella* and *Yersinia* have also been reported
Mycobacteria	Tuberculosis (usually due to atypical *M. avium*) can affect finches, but it is not commonly encountered
Campylobacter	More common in tropical finches such as the Bengalese. Inactivity, yellow droppings and high mortality amongst fledglings. Can be treated with appropriate antibiotics
Chlamydophila (Psittacosis)	Rare. Conjunctivitis, debilitation, diarrhoea. May see hepatomegaly on *post-mortem*
Pseudomonas	Usually associated with poor hygiene. Foul-smelling diarrhoea
Fungal	
Gastric yeast	*Macrorhabdus ornithogaster* (formerly Megabacteria) is commonly found in finches. Not too clear whether it can be a primary pathogen but it can certainly result in a chronic, debilitating condition. Affected birds are fluffed up, constantly hungry and progressively lose condition
Candida	Associated with poor hygiene and unbalanced diets. Crop candidiasis is seen as a distended, thickened crop with a white covering of the mucosa. Can also cause diarrhoea and moulting problems
Parasitic	
Protozoans	Various coccidian species can affect finches. *Isospora serine* (atoxoplasmosis) causes debilitation, diarrhoea and sometimes neurological signs, but is not very common. Other *Isospora* species (causing diarrhoea and weight loss) are more frequently encountered. Trichomoniasis causes respiratory symptoms, regurgitation and emaciation. *Cochlosoma* is not uncommon in Bengalese finches and can cause problems in other varieties. *Toxoplasma* can also be found in finches
Helminths	Both tapeworms and roundworms can be a problem but they are rare in well managed aviaries and tend to be associated with the feeding of live food
Arthropods	*Cnemidocoptes* mites can cause abnormal crusting and deformities on the base of the beak. Air sac mites (*Sternostoma tracheacolum*) can cause respiratory signs but are rare in finches

mites are a potential health problem in bird rooms. They can spread quickly and have an adverse effect on the birds' condition. Infected birds should be isolated and treated, and the affected bird housing should be isolated and thoroughly cleaned with compounds that are safe to use around birds.

Bald patches in the plumage could indicate presence of a pathogen or be the result of abnormal behaviour (see next section). Claws and beaks may overgrow, although they should usually be maintained naturally by the inclusion of a whole cuttlefish bone in the aviary. If claws grow too long or the beak overgrows, then the bird should be caught and these appendages trimmed with a nail clipper taking care not to clip too much. Birds that have been ringed should be monitored to ensure that their legs have not outgrown the ring, which could result in swelling of the foot, gangrene and necrosis.

Breeding females can become egg bound. This may occur for a variety of reasons (eg, a calcium deficiency, low environmental temperature, fatigue, oversized egg, etc) but the result is that the bird is unable to pass the egg through the oviduct. Affected females become hunched and fluffed up and immediate veterinary treatment is essential.

Readers may refer to Rosskopf and Woerpel (1996), Tully *et al.* (2000) or Chitty and Lierz (2008) for further information on epidemiology, diagnosis, treatment and prevention of diseases in birds.

Behaviour

The most common abnormal behaviour observed in caged zebra finches is feather pecking resulting in bald patches in their plumage. This can be caused by self-harm, by other individuals or by environmental conditions. If persistent feather peckers are identified they may need to be removed from the group. Environmental conditions that could trigger feather pecking are overcrowding and a shortage of nest materials for breeding birds.

Breeding birds can produce 'sandwich clutches' (see Breeding section) when too much nesting material is provided for too long. Females may also lay a large number of eggs on the cage floor and in most cases don't incubate the eggs. In both cases, females will have an increased egg formation effort, which is costly to the female, without any breeding output.

Acknowledgements

The authors thank Dr Michael Wilkinson (Deputy Named Veterinary Surgeon, University of Glasgow) for compiling the list of infectious diseases of zebra finches in Table 43.2.

References

Birkhead, T.R., Hunter, F.M. and Pellatt, J.E. (1989) Sperm competition in the zebra finch, *Taeniopygia guttata*. *Animal Behaviour*, **38**, 935–950

Birkhead, T.R., Burke, T., Zann, R.A. *et al.* (1990) Extra-pair paternity and intra-specific brood parasitism in wild zebra finches *Taeniopygia guttata*, revealed by DNA fingerprinting. *Behavioural Ecology and Sociobiology*, **27**, 315–324

Birkhead, T.R., Pellatt, E.J., Matthews, I.M. *et al.* (2006) Genic capture and the genetic basis of sexually selected traits in the zebra finch. *Evolution*, **60**, 2389–2398

Blount, J.D., Metcalfe, N.B., Birkhead, T.R. *et al.* (2003a) Carotenoid manipulation of immune function and sexual attractiveness in zebra finches. *Science*, **300**, 125–127

Blount, J.D., Metcalfe, N.B., Arnold, K.E. *et al.* (2003b) The effect of pre-breeding diet on reproductive output in zebra finches. *Proceedings of the Royal Society of London Series B-Biological Sciences*, **263**, 1585–1588

Blount, J.D., Metcalfe, N.B., Arnold, K.E. *et al.* (2006) Effects of neonatal nutrition and adult reproduction in a passerine bird. *Ibis*, **148**, 509–514

Boag, P. (1987) Effects of nestling diet on growth and adult size of Zebra Finches (*Poephila guttata*). *Auk*, **104**, 155–166

Boruszewska, K., Witkowski, A. and Jaszczak, K. (2007) Selected growth and development traits of the Zebra Finch (*Poephila guttata*) nestlings in amateur breeding. *Animal Science Papers and Reports*, **25**, 97–110

Burley, N. (1985) Leg-band colour and mortality patterns of captive breeding populations of zebra finches. *Auk*, **102**, 647–651

Burley, N. (1986) Comparison of band colour preferences of two species of estrildid finches. *Animal Behaviour*, **34**, 1732–1741

Burley, N. (1988) Wild zebra finches have band-colour preferences. *Animal Behaviour*, **36**, 1235–1237

Burley, N., Krantzberg, G. and Radman, P. (1982) Influence of colour banding on the conspecific preferences of zebra finches. *Animal Behaviour*, **30**, 444–455

Butterfield, P.A. (1970) The pair bond in the zebra finch. In: *Social Behaviour in Birds and Mammals*. Ed. Cook, J.H., pp. 149–278. Academic Press, London

Collins, S.A. and ten Cate, C. (1996) Does beak colour affect female preference in zebra finches? *Animal Behaviour*, **52**, 105–112

Collins, S.A., Archer, J.A. and Barnard, C.J. (2008) Welfare and mate choice in zebra finches: effects of handling regime and presence of cover. *Animal Welfare*, **17**, 11–17

Conover, M.R. and Messmer, T.A. (1996) Consequences for captive Zebra Finches of consuming tall Fescue seeds infected with the endophytic fungus *Acremonium coenophialum*. *Auk*, **113**, 492–495

Chitty, J. and Lierz, M. (2008) *BSAVA Manual of Raptors, Pigeons and Passerine Birds*. Blackwell Publishing, Oxford

Christidis, L. (1987) Phylogeny and systematics of estrildine finches and their relationship to other seed-eating passerines. *Emu*, **87**, 119–123

Cuthill, I.C., Hunt, S., Cleary, C. *et al.* (1997) Colour bands, dominance, and body mass regulation in male zebra finches (*Taeniopygia guttata*). *Proceedings of the Royal Society of London Series B – Biological Sciences*, **264**, 1093–1099

Dorrestein, G.M. (1996) Medicine and surgery of canaries and finches. In: *Diseases of Cage and Aviary Birds*, 3rd edn. Eds Rosskopf, W.J. and Woerpel, R.W., pp. 915–927. William and Wilkins, Baltimore

European Commission (2007) Commission recommendations of 18 June 2007 on guidelines for the accommodation and care of animals used for experimental and other scientific purposes. Annex II to European Council Directive 86/609/EEC. http://eurlex.europa.eu/LexUriServ/site/en/oj/2007/l_197/l_19720070730en00010089.pdf (accessed 13 June 2008)

Evans, J.E., Cuthill, I.C. and Bennett, A.T.D. (2006) The effect of flicker from fluorescent lights on mate choice in captive birds. *Animal Behaviour*, **72**, 393–400

Ewenson, E.L., Zann, R.A. and Flannery, G.R. (2001) Body condition and immune response in wild zebra finches: effects of capture, confinement and captive-rearing. *Naturwissenschaften*, **88**, 391–394

Forstmeier, W., Segelbacher, G., Mueller, J.C. *et al.* (2007) Genetic variation and differentiation in captive and wild zebra finches (*Taeniopygia guttata*). *Molecular Ecology*, **16**, 4039–4050

Gorman, H.E. and Nager, R.G. (2003) State-dependent incubation behaviour in the zebra finch. *Animal Behaviour*, **65**, 745–754

Gorman, H.E., Arnold, K.E. and Nager, R.G. (2005) Incubation effort in relation to male attractiveness in zebra finches (*Taeniopygia guttata*). *Journal of Avian Biology*, **36**, 413–420

Greives, T.J., Casto, J.M. and Ketterson, E.D. (2007) Relative abundance of males to females affects behaviour, condition and immune function in a captive population of dark-eyed juncos *Junco hyemalis*. *Journal of Avian Biology*, **38**, 255–260

Griffiths, R., Daan, S. and Dijkstra, C. (1996) Sex identification in birds using two CHD genes. *Proceedings of the Royal Society of London Series B – Biological Sciences*, **263**, 1251–1256

Houston, D.C., Donnan, D. and Jones, P.J. (1995) The source of nutrients required for egg production in zebra finches *Poephila guttata*. *Journal of Zoology*, **235**, 469–483

Hunt, S., Cuthill, I.C., Swaddle, J.P. *et al.* (1997) Ultraviolet vision and band-colour preferences in female zebra finches, *Taeniopygia guttata*. *Animal Behaviour*, **54**, 1383–1392

Immelmann, K., Kalberlah, H.-H., Rausch, P. *et al.* (1978) Sexuelle Prägung als möglicher Faktor innerartlicher Isolation beim Zebrafinken. *Journal für Ornithologie*, **119**, 197–212

Jacobs, H., Smith, N., Smith, P. *et al.* (1995) Zebra finch behaviour and effect of modest enrichment of standard cages. *Animal Welfare*, **4**, 3–9

Jones, A.E., Slater, P.J.B. (1999) The zebra finch. In: *The UFAW Handbook on the Care and Management of Laboratory Animals*, 7th edn. Ed. Poole, T.B., pp. 722–730. UFAW, Potters Bar

Joint Working Group on Refinement (2001) Laboratory birds: Refinements in husbandry and procedures. Fifth Report of the BVAAWF/FRAME/RSPCA/UFAW Joint Working Group on Refinement. *Laboratory Animals*, **35** (Suppl. 1), S1–S163

Kilner, R. (1998) Primary and secondary sex ratio manipulation by zebra finches. *Animal Behaviour*, **56**, 155–164

Lemon, W.C. (1993) The energetics of lifetime reproductive success in the zebra finch *Taeniopygia guttata*. *Physiological Zoology*, **66**, 946–963

Lemon, W.C. and Barth, R.H. (1992) The effects of feeding rate on reproductive success in the zebra finch, *Taeniopygia guttata*. *Animal Behaviour*, **44**, 851–857

Martins, T.L.F. (2004) Sex-specific growth rates in zebra finch nestlings: a possible mechanism for sex ratio adjustment. *Behavioral Ecology*, **15**, 174–180

McGraw, K.J., Gregory, A.J., Parker, R.S. *et al.* (2003) Diet, plasma carotenoids, and sexual coloration in zebra finch (*Taeniopygia guttata*). *Auk*, **120**, 400–410

McGraw, K.J., Adkins-Regan, E. and Parker, R.S. (2005) Maternally derived carotenoid pigments affect offspring survival, sex ratio, and sexual attractiveness in a colourful songbird. *Naturwissenschaften*, **92**, 375–380

Meijer, T., Rozman, J., Schulte, M. *et al.* (1996) New findings in body mass regulation in zebra finches (*Taeniopygia guttata*) in response to photoperiod and temperature. *Journal of Zoology*, **240**, 717–734

Morton, D.B., Abbot, D., Barclay, R. *et al.* (1993) Removal of blood from laboratory mammals and birds. *Laboratory Animals*, **27**, 1–22

Patterson-Kane, E.G. and Farnworth, M.J. (2006) Noise exposure, music, and animals in the laboratory: a commentary based on laboratory animal refinement and enrichment forum (LAREF) discussions. *Journal of Applied Animal Welfare Science*, **9**, 327–332

Pellatt, E.J. and Birkhead, T.R. (1994) Ejaculate size in zebra finches *Taeniopygia guttata* and a method for obtaining ejaculates from passerine birds. *Ibis*, **136**, 97–106

Perfito, N., Zann, R.A., Bentley, G.E. *et al.* (2007) Opportunism at work: habitat predictability affects reproductive readiness in free-living zebra finches. *Functional Ecology*, **21**, 291–301

Reynolds, S.J. (2001) The effects of low dietary calcium during egg-laying on eggshell formation and skeletal calcium reserves in the zebra finch *Taeniopygia guttata*. *Ibis*, **143**, 205–215

Rosskopf, W.J. and Woerpel, R.W. (1996) *Diseases of Cage and Aviary Birds*, 3rd edn. William and Wilkins, Baltimore

Royle, N.J., Hartley, I.R. and Parker, G.A. (2002) Sexual conflict reduces offspring fitness in zebra finches. *Nature*, **416**, 733–736

Rutstein, A.N., Gilbert, L., Slater, P.J.B. *et al.* (2004) Mate attractiveness and primary resource allocation in the zebra finch. *Animal Behaviour*, **68**, 1087–1094

Rutstein, A.N., Gorman, H.E., Arnold, K.E. *et al.* (2005) Sex allocation in response to paternal attractiveness in the zebra finch. *Behavioral Ecology*, **16**, 763–769

Samour, J. (2000) *Avian Medicine*. Mosby, London

Selman, R.G. and Houston, D.C. (1996) The effect of pre-breeding diet on reproductive output in zebra finches. *Proceedings of the Royal Society of London Series B – Biological Sciences*, **263**, 1585–1588

Skagen, S.K. (1988) Asynchronous hatching and food limitation: a test of Lack's hypothesis. *Auk*, **105**, 78–88

Slater, P.J.B. and Clayton, N.S. (1991) Domestication and song learning in zebra finches *Taeniopygia guttata*. *Emu*, **91**, 126–128

Sossinka, R. (1970) Domestikationserscheinungen beim Zebrafinken *Taeniopygia guttata castanotis* (Gould). *Zoologisches Jahrbuch Systematik*, **97**, 455–524

Sossinka, R. (1972a) Besonderheiten in der sexuellen Entwicklung des Zebrafinken *Taeniopygia guttata castanotis* (Gould). *Journal für Ornithologie*, **113**, 29–36

Sossinka, R. (1972b) Langfristiges Durstvermögen wilder und domestizierter Zebrafinken (*Taeniopygia guttata castanotis* Gould). *Journal für Ornithologie*, **113**, 418–426

Swaddle, J.P. and Cuthill, I.C. (1994) Preferences for symmetric males by female zebra finches. *Nature*, **367**, 165–166

Swaddle, J.P. and Page, L.C. (2006) High levels of environmental noise erode pair preferences in zebra finches: implications for noise pollution. *Animal Behaviour*, **74**, 363–368

Tully, T.N., Lawton, M.P.C. and Dorrestein, G.M. (2000) *Avian Medicine*. Butterworth-Heinemann, Oxford

Waas, J.R., Colgan, P.W. and Boag, P.T. (2005) Playback of colony sound alters the breeding schedule and clutch size in zebra finch (*Taeniopygia guttata*) colonies. *Proceedings of the Royal Society of London Series B – Biological Sciences*, **272**, 383–388

Williams, T.D. and Christians, J.K. (2003) Experimental dissociation of the effects of diet, age and breeding experience on primary reproductive effort in zebra finches *Taeniopygia guttata*. *Journal of Avian Biology*, **34**, 379–386

Young, R.L. (2003) *Environmental Enrichment for Captive Animals*. Blackwell Publishing, Oxford

Zann, R.A. (1996) *The Zebra Finch. A Synthesis of Field and Laboratory Studies*. Oxford University Press, Oxford

Zann, R.A., Morton, S.R., Jones, K.R. *et al.* (1995) The timing of breeding by zebra finches in relation to rainfall in central Australia. *Emu*, **95**, 208–222

Zann, R.A. and Straw, B. (1984) A non-destructive method to determine the diet of seed-eating birds. *Emu*, **84**, 40–41

44 Pigeons and doves

Anthony McGregor and Mark Haselgrove

Biological overview

General biology

Doves and pigeons make up the family Columbidae within the order Columbiformes. While there is no scientific distinction between the terms dove and pigeon, in practice 'dove' tends to be used for smaller species, such as turtle doves and collared doves, and 'pigeon' for larger species, such as the wood pigeon. There are currently 313 known species (Cramp 1986) within the order Columbiformes, over 300 of which are Columbidae. The majority of these species are arboreal. However, they are found within most habitats and there are both cliff- and ground-nesting species. Species vary greatly in size and in plumage colour. The smallest species measure little more than 150 mm in length, while the largest can reach up to 850 mm (Goodwin 1983). Their diet consists mostly of fruit or seeds, although invertebrates are consumed by some species that otherwise specialise as fruit or seed eaters. A common feature among species is bi-parental care, in which both sexes incubate eggs, produce crop milk and provision young. In addition, all species drink water by sucking it up without lifting their heads.

The most commonly used species for research purposes is probably the domestic pigeon, and the various varieties bred from it (eg, White Carneaux). The rock pigeon (*Columba livia*) is thought to be the ancestor of all domestic and feral pigeons. The other common species used in research is the Barbary dove (*Streptopelia risoria*), also known as the ringdove, although Hutchison (1999) points out that, in fact, this is a domesticated variety of the African collared dove (*Streptopelia roseogrisea*). There is little sexual dimorphism between the sexes (but see below for differences in behaviour) and individual pigeons have been recorded as living for 30 years (Hutchison, 1999). Biological data are provided in Table 44.1.

Social organisation

Feral pigeons are colonial breeders and forage in flocks (Cramp 1986). Aggressive competition for food and partners is often observed where they occur in high densities (Murton *et al.* 1974; Johnston 1992). Although the feral (domestic) pigeon is socially monogamous, frequent pair copulation and intense mate guarding by males suggest a degree of sperm competition (Lovell-Mansbridge 1995). However, when male partners are experimentally removed, females showed no tendency to approach other males or to engage in extra-pair copulations (Lovell-Mansbridge & Birkhead 1998). Higher levels of aggression from cuckolded males may have selected against extra-pair copulations. For example, pair bond structure in females paired with aggressive males is poorer, leading to delayed breeding in these pairs (Erickson and Zenone 1976), which subsequently affects reproductive fitness. Alternatively, Trivers (1972) suggested that one cost of cuckoldry is the withdrawal of parental care by the male. In pigeons and doves, where bi-parental care is important not only in provisioning young, but also in producing crop milk, the cost of extra-pair copulations for the female is potentially high.

Reproduction

Many aspects of reproductive behaviour and endocrinology have been studied in the Barbary dove and the main findings are summarised briefly here.

Courtship and pair bonding

The male Barbary dove expends considerable time, energy and physical resources on its own offspring, participating in both the incubation of the eggs and in rearing chicks by producing crop milk for feeding the offspring. This resource provisioning by the male is mediated by the synchrony of breeding behaviour in male–female pairs, since reproduction is successful only when the male's physical condition is synchronised with egg laying. The purpose of courtship behaviour, therefore, is to bring about the synchronisation of the physical condition of the pair (Lehrman 1965; Lovari & Hutchison 1975).

Courtship behaviour in the male Barbary dove is characterised by a transition from initial aggressive interactions (chasing, bowing and kah-calls) to nest-orientated behaviour (nest display and cooing), and changes in hormonal states accompany these behaviours. There is a change from testosterone-driven aggressive behaviour to oestrogen-dependent nest-orientated behaviour as courtship progresses (Hutchison 1999). Since the male dove has no oestrogen circulating in the plasma, testosterone is converted to

Table 44.1 Standard biological data (Hutchison 1999).

	Body weight	*Body temperature (cloacal)*	*Resting respiration rate*
Pigeon	350–550 g	40–41 °C (104–105.8 °F)	25–30/min
Dove	130–180 g	40–41 °C (104–105.8 °F)	40–42/min

oestrogen by the enzyme aromatase in the preoptic area and hypothalamus (Hutchison 1991).

Hutchison (1999) notes that courtship patterns in doves and pigeons perform a number of functions, such as identification of sex and reproductive condition of females. The initial aggressive courtship by the male consists of chasing, with the body horizontal, and a kah-call, and may alternate with bowing (in doves) or head nodding (in pigeons). In doves, the male will lift his head, inflate the crop and coo as the head is lowered towards the floor. The feet are stamped between bow–coos. In pigeons, depending on the species, the beak can nearly touch the ground or the breast, and in some types, crests may be fanned out or the tail fanned. The pupil of the eye contracts in both doves and pigeons showing the iris. If the male meets another male, the encounter may result in wing-boxing. However, if opposite sexes meet, the female will alternate between retreating from and approaching the male, and this leads to nesting activity, attempted mating and full copulation 1–2 days after pairing.

Nest building, ovulation and incubation

Both doves and pigeons build rudimentary nests consisting of a few twigs with grass or hay collected by the male and placed in the nest by the female. The female Barbary dove increases wing-flipping (vibration of the wings) when sitting on the nest 4–5 days before egg laying. This behaviour in turn stimulates the male to bring nesting material to the female.

The time course of the transitions in male courtship behaviour has retarding or accelerating effects on the female's ovarian development. Persistent aggressive courtship patterns by the male are associated with a delay in egg laying and nest soliciting in the female. However, provisioning of nesting material by the male accelerates the female's ovulation.

In both pigeons and doves, females lay two eggs. The first egg is usually laid in the afternoon, with incubation occurring immediately afterwards. Incubation behaviour is performed by both sexes, although the male usually incubates in the mid-afternoon (Hutchison 1999). Ovulation involves the hormone prolactin, but in the Barbary dove at least, progesterone mediates the initiation of incubation behaviour and egg-laying in the female. During incubation, prolactin levels increase and the milk cells lining the crop begin to proliferate to form crop milk in readiness for hatching of the young. Young are fed with crop milk within the first hour of hatching. The crop milk becomes mixed with seeds as the young get older.

Breeds and supply

Barbary doves have probably been domesticated for centuries and are available as caged birds throughout the world. The wild-type African collared dove (*Streptopelia roseogrisea*) is slightly smaller than the Barbary dove and is confined to Northern Africa, south of the Sahara, and western central and south western Arabia, occurring in acacia thorn scrub. The collared dove (*Streptopelia decaocto*), which has recently spread across the north-west of Europe into Britain, is occasionally used as a laboratory bird. It is slightly larger than a Barbary dove and with darker coloration. The courtship and incubation behaviour are very similar to those of the Barbary dove.

There are over 200 breeds of domesticated pigeons, and within each breed there may be a number of colours and markings. In pigeons there are four main colours: red, black, blue and brown, and many plumage types: fantails, feathered feet and crests. 'Croppers' have the ability to inflate the crop, while 'tumblers and rollers' tumble and roll while in full flight. Because of the genetic variety available, checks should be made to ensure that the strain or breed selected does not show abnormal behaviour when selecting a strain for use in the laboratory.

Barbary doves and especially different strains of pigeons are available from bird dealers, while a useful source of domestic pigeons is pigeon racers. As they are domesticated species, there is no need to obtain free-living birds. In fact, obtaining pigeons from the wild may import diseases into the laboratory.

Uses in the laboratory

The pigeon is the standard avian animal when comparison between mammals and other phyla are made in physiology and anatomy; it has a similar status to the 'white rat' in laboratory studies. Pigeons have been used extensively in visual and auditory physiological research (eg, Granda & Maxwell 1979; Erichsen *et al.* 1982). Particularly important in some of these studies is the strong lateralisation of brain function that occurs in birds (eg, Güntürkün *et al.* 1998). The sensory basis of mechanisms that allow the domestic (homing) pigeon (*Columba livia*) to display the remarkable ability to return to its loft from unfamiliar sites has been studied extensively over the past 50 years (eg, Papi 1992; Bingman 1998; Wallraff 2001). The pigeon is known to use olfaction, magnetic fields and the position of the sun in the sky for long-range homing (Walcott 1996). Less well studied are the mechanisms behind homing in the birds' familiar area. Visual landmarks are thought to be important (eg, Braithwaite & Guilford 1991; Wallraff *et al.* 1993), and how the pigeon learns and uses information about landmarks is becoming clearer (eg, Biro *et al.* 2004). The other major laboratory use for pigeons is in experimental psychology in studying visual discrimination, cognition and learning. Pavlovian and instrumental conditioning tasks in conditioning chambers are used extensively with pigeons in experimental psychology (eg, Haselgrove *et al.* 2005; McGregor *et al.* 2006). In addition, pigeons have been valuable in work on toxicology.

Since the 1960s, the endocrine basis of the reproductive behaviour of the Barbary dove has been studied. More recently neuroendocrine studies have focused on the androgen-metabolising brain enzymes, the aromatase system (Hutchison 1991) which forms oestrogen in brain neurones. Brain aromatase levels providing oestrogen for nesting behaviour are high in doves and are regulated by environmental as well as endocrine factors. The male dove has provided a model for studying this system. The control of prolactin secretion and its role in maintaining incubation behaviour and crop milk production is also being extensively studied in the Barbary dove (Lea & Sharp 1991; Horseman & Buntin 1995).

Because the domestic pigeon and the Barbary dove are the most commonly used species in the laboratory, the following sections on Laboratory management and breeding and Common welfare problems will be primarily concerned with this species. Where other species are discussed, this will be made clear in the text.

Laboratory management and breeding

General husbandry

Housing

Indoor

The European Commission (2007) has recently produced updated guidelines on minimum standards of housing that include the housing of pigeons (see also the revised Appendix A to the European Convention for the Protection of Vertebrate Animals used for Experimental and other Scientific Purposes (Council of Europe 2006) and Joint Working Group on Refinement (JWGR 2001a)). If pigeons or doves are to be housed indoors, it is recommended that both the quantity and quality of space provided is sufficient to allow the bird to engage in a range of behaviours including, if possible, flight. Pigeons housed either individually, or in pairs in small cages are often unable to extend their wings fully. Such housing, therefore, should not be considered appropriate for long-term housing. Wherever possible, pigeons and doves should be housed in an aviary large enough to permit flight. JWGR (2001a) recommends pens (7 m × 3 m × 3 m high) or tunnel aviaries (20 m × 7 m × 3.5 m high). If the provision of an aviary is not possible, access to a room in which exercise flights can be conducted is recommended during the morning and/or late afternoon. There is a circadian rhythm in bird activity, with more calling and feeding in the morning than the afternoon. Long, narrow pens (eg, 2 m × 1 m) can also be recommended as these permit short flights.

In laboratory cages, there is a build-up of white 'dust' (keratinised scales) from the feathers and skin of doves and pigeons. Cages should be cleaned at least once a week: wiping with a damp cloth removes this dust. In addition, it is essential to have frequent air changes – fans bringing fresh air into the laboratory, and extraction fans to clear laboratories of dust. Wolfensohn and Lloyd (2003) recommend at least 10 air changes per hour, although the UK Home Office recommends 15–20 (Home Office 1989).

Outdoor

If pigeons and doves are to be housed in an outdoor aviary, then consideration must be given to the provision of ventilated, but draught-proof, covered shelters. If necessary, a supplementary heater may be used. The environmental provisions and enrichments described in the next section outline some of the steps that may be taken to further enhance this environment.

Environmental provision and enrichment

Nesting facilities, nesting material and perches (allow 20 cm per dove, 30 cm per pigeon) are necessary in cages when birds are paired and in aviaries. In aviaries, shelving on which the birds can display courtship can be provided. A flat tray with clean water for bathing will be used frequently by both sexes. Pigeons also seem to enjoy a shower, and a fine mist of warm water can be sprayed at individual birds with a commercial plant sprayer. If birds are caged indoors, it is advisable to use 'daylight' strip lighting controlled by a time clock. Fourteen hours of light will induce and maintain sexual activity and breeding behaviour. Birds housed in cages can benefit from the provision of toys such as bells and mirrors that can be hung from the cage by chains.

Social grouping

Doves and pigeons can be maintained as single-sex colonies, but usually the sexes are mixed to prevent excessive aggression. It is advisable to monitor groups closely when first acquired to ensure that birds do not bully or injure others. If housed in pairs, males should not be caged together as they may fight.

Laboratory feeding and dietary requirements

Food can be provided either in open bowls or in hoppers attached to the side of the cage or aviary. Since some birds consume preferred foods selectively, it is essential that food hoppers are replenished each day with fresh food. Females can be discouraged from nesting in the food trays by providing covered nesting boxes positioned well away from the food. Foraging can be encouraged by scattering seed upon the floor. In addition, hand feeding provides an excellent method to habituate the birds to contact with humans, which is desirable if the birds are to be handled regularly.

Domestic pigeons and many doves are omnivourous (JWGR 2001a; Redrobe 2002). Consequently, vegetable proteins alone will not provide sufficient nutrients and amino acids for these birds. Thus, a supplement such as turkey starter crumbs or chick-rearing meal should be given. Grains commonly fed to pigeons are kaffir corn, maple peas, hemp, maize, vetch, millet, wheat, oats and barley. Some green food, chick-rearing meal, shell, grit and salt are usually given. Kaffir corn, wheat, maize, millet, finely ground oyster shells and starter turkey crumbs can be fed to doves. Turkey crumbs typically contain vitamins A, D_3 and E supplements, ash, methionine, copper(II) sulphate, lasalocid sodium and may contain dimetridazole to control protozoal diseases. If starter turkey crumbs are not used, vitamin supplements should be used. Adult pigeons require approximately 28 g of food per day, and pigeons which have only limited exercise should not be fed *ad libitum* otherwise they tend to become overweight. Body condition can be monitored by regular weighing.

Minerals play an important role in bone growth and eggshell formation, and are an essential supplement. Calcium and phosphorus are required in relatively large quantities and can be given as crushed shells, for example crushed oyster shell, or as powdered or liquid supplements added to the water (although it may be hard to meet daily requirements in this way). It is also usual to consider a vitamin supplement, as sufficient vitamins do not occur in cereals and legumes. Insoluble grit plays a key role in the digestive process of the pigeon and dove as it is stored in the gizzard and used to grind and break down seeds and other fibrous matter before chemical digestion.

Water

Fresh water should be provided daily. To prevent the birds fouling the water, the containers should either be covered or, if the birds are housed in a cage, the container should be mounted on the outside of the cage. Some birds do not drink when first caged individually. This problem can be avoided by provided the water in see-through reservoirs. Birds which still refrain from drinking can be encouraged to do so by gently immersing their beaks in the water.

Identification and sexing

Individual birds can be identified for life if ringed at fledging with numbered and/or coloured, split plastic rings. Although the males of some strains of pigeon have distinctive colouring (eg, red chequers, mealies and silvers, which show black flecking), in general, the plumage of the male and female pigeon or dove will have the same form throughout the lifespan of the bird, making sexing a difficult task. In the domestic pigeon, the eyes of the young male are more widely spaced than in the female. In adults the male may be more heavily built than the female and the head rounder with larger wattles and ceres than the female who will tend to have a slighter build and a flatter head.

Hutchison (1999) suggests that domestic pigeons can also be sexed by their behaviour. Males strut, bob up and down and emit a double 'coo', while females emit only a single coo. In addition, males turn 360° circles, fan out their tails and drag them along the floor whilst courting a female. At about a year old, once doves and pigeons are sexually mature, the sex of the birds can be determined using observations of courtship behaviour. Each bird is placed in a cage with a known sexually active male. If the unsexed bird is female, it will retreat from the sexually active male and, usually after 5 minutes, the known sexually active male will display nest soliciting and the female will approach the male. If the unsexed bird is a male, aggressive courtship behaviour (chasing, bowing, pecking, kah-calls and wing-boxing) will be displayed. However, it is important to note that identification of sex by either observation of behaviour or external anatomy requires considerable experience before these criteria can be used with any degree of accuracy, and even then, should not be regarded as an entirely accurate method of identification. More reliable methods of sexing doves and pigeons before the birds are sexually mature include DNA sexing by commercial laboratories (using a blood sample or tissue from a growing feather), or by visually examining the gonads by laparotomy under general anaesthesia.

Transport and quarantine

Information on the transport of laboratory animals has been provided by Laboratory Animal Science Association (2005). The Live Animals Regulations Manual (2007/2008) provides comprehensive information concerning international regulations for air transportation of animals, and is available from the international air traffic association website[1]. For establishments in the UK, transport of non-human vertebrates within Europe must comply with regulations set out by The Department for Environment, Food and Rural affairs[2] and the Home Office code of practice (Home Office, 1989). See also Chapter 13 on transport.

Providing there is adequate ventilation, pigeons and doves may be transported for short distances in wicker baskets or in cardboard boxes. It is not advisable to give them water continuously as the plumage may become damaged. After a journey of 1–2 h birds should be given food and water. Upon arrival in the laboratory, it is recommended that incoming birds should be health checked by a vet and any treatments and disease control procedures necessary should be undertaken (eg, to control internal and external parasites).

Breeding

Condition of adults

A 14 h light/10 h dark regime induces sexual activity in adult male and female doves. If, however, artificial light is not used to induce sexual activity, it is best to pair doves in February or March in northern latitudes. To reduce aggression in the male, it is advisable to introduce the female to a male who has already established a perching and nesting site. Doves and pigeons can form pair bonds and mate for life, therefore separating breeding pairs may cause distress. However, if the birds are kept in an aviary, breeding can be unsuccessful due to competition for the females from intruder males. Placing pairs in separate cages prevents this interference and allows the behaviour of the pair to be monitored. When the birds are sexually active and behaviourally compatible, egg-laying should occur about 10–12 days after pairing. However, if no eggs are laid within 20 days then the birds should be paired with different partners. Pigeons should be allowed to rest and should not be bred all year round. In particular, they should be allowed to moult normally in the autumn.

[1] http://www.iata.org

[2] http://www.defra.gov.uk

Nesting and incubation

When birds are paired, nesting material (straw and twigs), as well as earthenware nesting bowls or papier maché nest pans, should be provided. Filling the nesting bowl with sand or newspaper prevents cracking of the eggs. The male sits for shorter periods, usually in the afternoon. Earthenware pans should be disinfected between broods.

Hatching

Hatching occurs 14 days after the beginning of the incubation period, in the dove. In pigeons, hatching occurs after 17 or 18 days of incubating. If pairs are compatible, about three to four broods are produced on normal day length during the reproductive season, which is until the end of September in northern latitudes. Maintained on artificial light, pairs will produce young at about 2-monthly intervals for 1–2 years.

The young

Squabs are incapable of locomotion and do not leave the nest for the first 8–10 days. Both the male and female produce crop milk to feed the young for approximately 10–12 days after hatching. The crop milk, as mentioned earlier, becomes mixed with seeds as the young get older. The parents then continue to feed the squabs grain, until fledging occurs at between 21 and 24 days. Young birds should not be allowed to breed until they are at least 36 weeks old. Squabs must be able to grip the substrate with their feet to prevent 'splayleg'. Birds that hatch with splayed legs, or develop them, will never walk, and must be humanely killed. It is usual to leave the parents with the young for the first month. The young birds are then ringed and caged.

Reproductive problems

Egg binding may be caused by calcium deficiency, infection or malformation of the oviduct, or soft-shelled or broken eggs. Egg binding can be very serious and signs may include depression, droopy wings, abdominal straining and weakness or paralysis of one or both legs. A hard swelling can usually be felt in the lower abdomen. A lukewarm bath may help the egg pass. Soft-shelled eggs are almost always due to a deficiency of calcium in the diet. During breeding, pigeons and doves have a particularly high requirement for calcium, which should be freely available. Females that continually lay soft-shelled eggs should not be used for breeding.

Laboratory procedures

Handling

Pigeons and doves can easily lose feathers if they are improperly handled. To avoid this, quickly grasp the bird from behind around its body and wings (Figure 44.1a). An inexperienced handler may have to use both hands used at first, but with practice, an adult pigeon or dove can be both caught and held with one hand, leaving the other hand free to open wings, check feather condition, etc (Figure 44.1b). Avoid pointing the cloaca towards the person, as the bird may choose to defecate, particularly if it is not habituated to humans. Pigeons housed in an aviary or in large groups can be caught with a net, and dimming the lights can ease capture. However, if the birds are accustomed to hand feeding, pigeons and doves will fly to the hand. A number of pigeons can be transported a short distance (such as

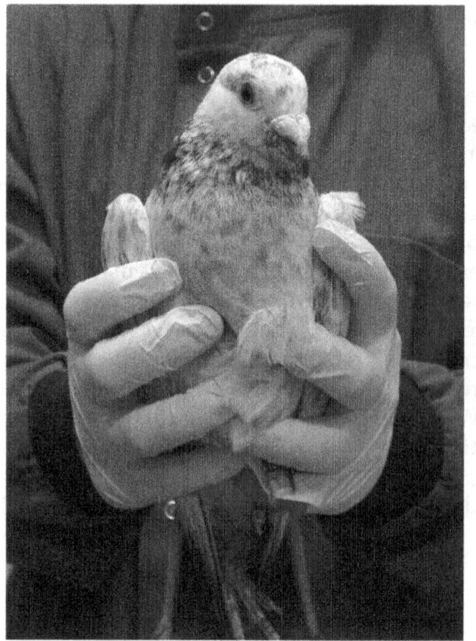

(a)

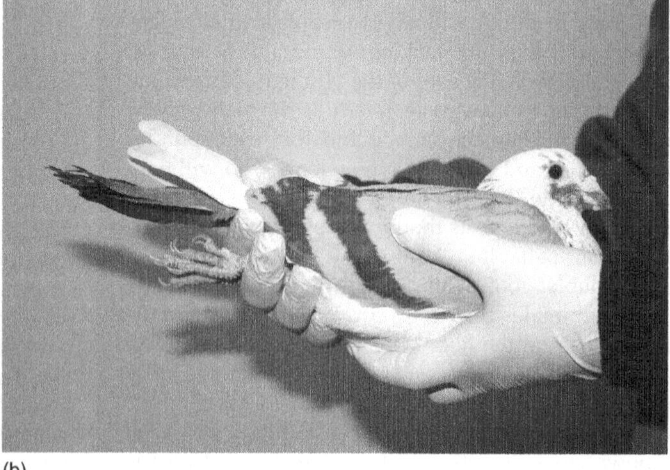

(b)

Figure 44.1 (a) An experimenter handling an adult pigeon, using two hands. (b) Holding a smaller bird, giving the handler more freedom.

between an aviary/holding room and a nearby laboratory) at the same time by gently placing them head first into individual measuring jugs. The pigeon will typically remain in the jug without attempting to escape.

Behavioural training

Pigeons are frequently used in experiments designed to investigate the psychology of learning and memory. Usually, they are housed individually or in pairs before tests in conditioning chambers in which visual or (less frequently) auditory stimuli are presented to the bird, along with food reward. Prior to the tests the animal is caught, placed in either an cloth bag, or plastic jug for weighing before being placed into a dark, or dimly illuminated chamber. Before training begins, there is usually a period during which the bird settles.

A less stressful procedure for housing, weighing and testing pigeons in the laboratory has been described by Huber (1994). The pigeons are, in this case, housed in outdoor aviaries with perches, a pigeon loft for nesting and hatching eggs, water, but no food. They enter the experimental chamber directly from the outdoor aviary through connecting channels to obtain food. After an acclimatisation phase of several days, the birds enter the channels daily. The animals are weighed automatically on a scale in the floor at the rear of the chamber.

Recording body temperature

Temperature may be taken by inserting, to a depth of not more than 2cm, a cloacal thermometer, or thermister into the cloaca. The average body temperature of the dove and pigeon is 40–41 °C (Hutchison 1999).

Collection of blood sample

In adult birds, blood samples may be collected from the brachial vein, which runs parallel to the external aspect of the humerus, on the underside of the wing. Puncture immediately above the elbow joint is not recommended, as haemostasis can be difficult to achieve at this site. Application of pressure with the thumb at the proximal humerus can help to raise the vein, making it clearly visible. Once the route of the vein is located, feathers can be parted by lightly wiping the injection area with cotton wool soaked in surgical spirit. The blood volume in birds in general is approximately 7ml/100g body weight. For a single sample, 0.5ml/100g of body weight can be drawn safely (see also JWGR 1993).

Administration of substances

As with the collection of blood, it is not necessary to pluck the feathers when administering substances by injection. Lightly wiping the injection site with surgical spirit and parting the feathers will provide sufficient access to the skin.

- Oral administration. Solid or liquid oral preparations are best administered in the drinking water or in the feed. However, oral gavage may be necessary for unpalatable substances, or under conditions in which a precise dose is necessary. Take care to avoid the trachea when inserting a tube or substance into the oesophagus. The trachea in the pigeon is located behind the tongue and should be identified before carrying out the procedure. Catheters to be inserted into the oesophagus should be lubricated to avoid damage to either the oesophagus or the pharynx. This procedure requires two people, and firm but gentle restraint of the bird. Sharman *et al.* (2001) recommend a maximum oral dosing volume of 10ml/kg.
- Subcutaneous injection. The most common site for subcutaneous injection is under the loose skin in the back of the neck. The maximum dose is 2–5ml/kg (Sharman *et al.* 2001).
- Intravenous injection. Frequently used sites include the ulna, right jugular and medial metatarsal veins. One should aim to use the smallest gauge needle possible for injecting pigeons and doves intravenously. Sharman *et al.* (2001) recommend that the injected volume be no more than 5ml/kg. It is essential to ensure that the bird is adequately restrained.
- Intramuscular injection. Intramuscular injections can be given into the pectoral muscles. Pigeons possess a renal system that can move the blood flow from the lower extremities to the central circulation. Injection into the thigh muscle, therefore, is not recommended as drugs may be eliminated quickly by the kidneys. Intramuscular injections are painful and can affect mobility. They can also result in death of living tissue (necrosis), it is therefore preferable to administer substances subcutaneously, wherever possible. Intramuscular administration of large volumes should be divided between different injection sites, and the total dose should not exceed 0.05ml/kg (Sharman *et al.* 2001). Care must be exercised so as to not inject into blood vessels. This can be achieved by refraining from inserting the needle too deeply and, prior to depressing the plunger, withdrawing it slightly to check for signs of blood.
- Intraperitoneal injection. Substances should not normally be administered to pigeons or doves by intraperitoneal injection as the substance can easily enter the air sacs and disrupt their function.

Further guidance and recommendations of the administration of substances to birds can be found in Harrison and Harrison (1986); Richie *et al.* (1994); Sharman *et al.* (2001); JWGR (2001b).

Anaesthesia and analgesia

Anaesthesia

The inhalant anaesthetic, isoflurane, has become the preferred agent for both short and long anaesthesia due to its reliability and the rapid recovery from its effects. Prior to anaesthesia, the pigeon must be fasted for 6–8h to empty its crop and minimise regurgitation. Ophthalmic ointment should be applied to the eyes to prevent the drying of the corneas.

Induction of anaesthesia can be achieved with either a face mask, or an induction chamber at 4% isoflurane, and 1–2 l/min flow. Once induction has occurred, anaesthesia should be maintained using endotracheal intubation if the bird is over 100 g (Redrobe, 2002; Wolfensohn & Lloyd, 2003). Redrobe (2002) recommends flushing with oxygen every 5 minutes to prevent hypercapnia. Air exchange is very efficient in birds, and the depth of anaesthesia can change rapidly when using gas inhalants. However, maintenance anaesthesia may be set initially at 2–3% isoflurane and 1–2 l/min flow. Responses should be monitored to maintain a light to medium depth of anaesthesia, and concentration of isoflurane adjusted accordingly. The relationships between responsivity and the depth of anaesthesia were reported by Abou-Madi (2001), and a selection of these are shown in Table 44.2. Birds lose heat rapidly during anaesthesia and a heated blanket may not provide sufficient thermal support to prevent a decrease in body temperature. A heat lamp may be employed during surgery, but care must be taken not to overheat the bird. Body temperature should be monitored with a rectal thermometer.

Wolfensohn and Lloyd (2003) state the importance of flushing with oxygen at the end of anaesthesia to prevent reabsorption of anaesthetic. Warmth and subcutaneous fluids should be provided during recovery from anaesthesia. The wings can be controlled during recovery by wrapping the bird in a towel, taking care not to restrict breathing. The bird should be monitored during recovery in a dark, or dimly lit, quiet area. A smooth recovery can be produced by administering analgesics immediately after surgery, but they can also be administered preoperatively for a smoother induction. Indications of pain in birds can include agitation and restlessness, loss of weight, appetite and variations in the preening of a painful site. Opioids (eg, butorphanol, 1–4 mg/kg subcutaneously) and non-steroidal anti-inflammatory drugs (eg, carprofen, 5 mg/kg, or meloxicam, 0.2 mg/kg) can be administered as analgesics.

Table 44.2 Levels of anaesthesia (after Abou-Madi, 2001).

Response	*Light anaesthesia*	*Medium anaesthesia*	*Deep anaesthesia*
Voluntary blinking	Slow or absent	Slow or absent	Absent
Muscle relaxation	Moderate–good	Good	Absent
Breathing pattern	Rapid and deep	Slow, deep, regular	Slow, shallow
Palpebral reflex[a]	Present or slow	Slow, intermittent	Absent
Pedal reflex[b]	Present or slow	Slow, intermittent	Absent

[a] The palpebral reflex can be elicited by running the finger along the eyelashes.

[b] The pedal reflex can be elicited by squeezing the toes between the thumb and forefinger.

Euthanasia

Injectable agents such as sodium pentobarbital can be administered intravenously into the medial metatarsal vein to bring about death (150 mg/kg). Injection may also be given intrahepatically, with the injection site under the sternum along the ventral midline. However, intracoelomic injection should be avoided because the crysallisation of barbiturate drugs may cause pain and distress to the animal. Cousquer and Parsons (2007) provide excellent details on locating the medial metatarsal vein and other advice on euthanasia.

Exposure to carbon dioxide is widely used for the euthanasia of mammals, but its applicability to birds remains controversial as exposure to the gas can result in distress in some animals (JWGR 2001a), and there are other satisfactory alternatives (see 2006 report by the Animal Procedures Committee[3]). The authors' observations, however, suggest that a rising concentration of carbon dioxide introduced into an induction chamber does not result in any noticeable aversive response in the pigeon. Whichever method is used, death must be confirmed with dislocation of the neck.

Common welfare problems

Health and disease

Prevention of disease

In outdoor aviaries or lofts, primary prophylaxis may be aided if wild birds such as sparrows, pigeons and wild doves are prevented from entering or perching on top of aviaries. When contact with wild birds is limited, doves and pigeons are usually free of infectious disease, particularly if they are sourced from a reputable supplier. Transmission of endoparasites occurs where there is poor hygiene, overcrowding and warm, moist conditions. Therefore, as secondary prophylactic measures, keep drinking water clean and remove faeces weekly, so as to break the life cycles of these parasites.

Health monitoring and signs of disease

Hygiene is of prime importance since infections can spread rapidly from one bird to another. Clinical signs of disease are not always obvious. One useful method of monitoring the health of birds is to keep regular records of the weights of individual birds. Birds may initially be examined in the cage or on a perch. Redrobe (2002) lists criteria for monitoring health in the perching bird: can it perch?; are its feathers ruffled?; is it alert and responsive?; is its respiration normal?; is there feather loss, or a change in quality of feathers, beak and nails?; is the bird standing with equal weight on both legs and are the wings held at equal lengths? The authors would also recommend observation for changes in faeces. Abnormalities in any of these factors may indicate problems with the bird's health.

[3] http://www.apc.gov.uk/reference/schedule-1-report.pdf

Feeding is a good time for health monitoring. If hand feeding, the opportunity may be taken to inspect the feathers which, in a healthy bird, should feel silky to the touch. Redrobe (2002 p. 171) lists common clinical conditions that may be detected when the animal is being handled.

Later signs of illness include the bird remaining in a moribund state on the perch or floor of the aviary, crouched with feathers fluffed out and head down. Birds in this state will not respond to a loud noise such as clapped hands.

More specific information on the diseases most likely to occur in captive pigeons and doves, their diagnosis, and appropriate treatments follows (Davis *et al.* 1971; Keymer 1991). A particularly good source of information on disease and pathologies in pigeons is Cousquer and Parsons (2007). Other sources include Nepote (1999), Redrobe (2002), Rupiper (1998a, 1998b) and Tudor (1991).

Endoparasitic infections

The following may occur in pigeons:

1. *Trichomonas gallinae* is a flagellated protozoan which causes 'canker', 'diphtheria' or , particularly in falconry, 'frounce'. The domestic pigeon is considered the primary host of *T. gallinae*, although it also occurs naturally in a wide variety of species. Infection is spread from parents to squabs during feeding, and through contamination of the drinking water. There are thought to be more than 20 strains of *T. gallinae*, varying in virulence, which infect domestic pigeons. The immune response associated with the disease includes yellow round lesions on the epithelium of the mouth, oesophagus and crop, with accompanying diarrhoea and loss of appetite (Hutchison 1999). However, as Frank[4] points out, with breeders and racers at least, the widespread use of antibiotics in the 1970s and 1980s led to the near eradication of those strains that produce these symptoms. In addition, milder strains of *T. gallinae* are thought to enhance immunity against more virulent strains, making detection of the presence of *T. gallinae* by presence of symptoms more difficult. However, in the most virulent strain (Jones' Barn) death occurs in almost 96% of infected non-immune birds, through the necrosis of liver and other internal organs[5]. Therefore, if infection is suspected treatment is necessary. Infection may be confirmed by a swab taken from the crop lining and the contents inspected under magnification. Hutchison (1999) recommends treatment with dimetridazole 500mg/l in the drinking water for 7 days. However, others have questioned the efficacy of nitroimidazole class drugs in eradicating *T. gallinae* from pigeons (eg, Munoz *et al.* 1998), while others have called for higher doses for nitroimidazoles for effective treatment (Franssen & Lumeij 1992). Cousquer and Parsons (2007) point out that carnidazole (Spartrix: Harkers) is the only licenced nitroimidazole available in the UK. Administer 10mg tablets for 5 days.
2. Roundworms (*Ascaridia columbae*) and hairworms (*Capillaria columbae* and *C. longicollis*) may infect the duodenum and upper part of the small intestine. *A. columbae* average about 2–6cm in length and 1mm in thickness, and reproducing worms are generally detectable by visible ova in the faeces. In severe infections the gut wall may be thinned and transparent, and may occasionally rupture. *Capillaria* species. are smaller, at around 2.5cm in length and much more slender than *A. columbae*. Ova in the faeces may only be detected with microscopy. In both infections, birds are likely to lose weight chronically, develop diarrhoea and suffer a general loss of condition. For *A. columbae*, Hutchison (1999) recommends treatment with piperazine citrate dissolved in the drinking water at a dosage rate of 2g/l given for 2–3 days, with administration of liquid paraffin to facilitate elimination of the worms. However, piperazine is considered an older treatment and worms may now be resistant to its effects. It is more common to treat both worm infections with levamisole hydrochloride or fenbendazole at 20mg/kg of bodyweight. Walker[6], however, points out the negative side effects of these treatments, such as vomiting and loss of condition, and recommends avermectins such as moxidectin at 10mg/l of drinking water.
3. Coccidia are a widespread and important group of protozoa, causing the problematic coccidiosis condition in poultry, sheep, dogs, cattle and rabbits. Coccidiosis is most commonly caused by parasites of the genus *Eimeria*. Species in this genus are unusual in having a high degree of host-specifity. In pigeons *Eimeria labbeana* and *E. columbarum* are most common, and affect pigeons at 3–4 months of age most severely. Many birds have a low level of the disease, but affected birds have a greenish diarrhoea, and become emaciated and stunted. Diagnosis is through the number of oocysts present in the faeces and is necessary to distinguish the symptoms from those of salmonellosis, trichomoniasis, worm infestation and gut infection. Treat with sodium sulphadimidine, 15ml of the solution in 4.5l of drinking water. This should be given in the place of the normal drinking water for 5 consecutive days.

Ectoparasites

Ectoparasites, such as ticks, mites and lice may result in feather loss, anaemia, and the stunted growth of squabs. Therefore affected birds should be inspected for the causal organisms.

Some species of lice such as the long feather louse, *Columbicola columbae*, and coccyx louse, *Campanulotes bidentatus*, are common and may cause irritation and damage to the feathers, but feed only from feather dust after attaching themselves to the feather shaft. Very small feather mites such as *Falculifer rostratis* may cause irritation if present in large numbers. If anaemia accompanies skin irritation then the red mite, *Dermanyssus gallinae*, may be suspected. It should be noted that these mites do not breed on the birds

[4]Frank, K.H. (2005) Canker! http://www.albertaclassic.net/trichomonas/trichomonas.php

[5]Chalmers, G. (2005) Canker revisited. http://www.albertaclassic.net/trichomonas/trichomonas.php

[6]Walker, C. (2005, Sept, 14) Parasitic control. http://www.auspigeonco.com.au/Articles/Parasite_control.html

but in cracks and crevices from which they emerge at night. Moxidectin, used for worm infestations, has the advantage of killing any blood-sucking mite. The cage or aviary should be sprayed at the same time as treatment to the bird. Bromocyclen in the form of a dusting powder may be used as a general treatment for most lice and mites. An alternative is a synthetic pyrethroid such as permethrin, sprayed directly on to the bird at 10–20 ml/l of water.

Bacterial and viral diseases

Below is a non-exhaustive list of diseases that may occur in pigeons. Cousquer and Parsons (2007) and Redrobe (2002) discuss a wider range of less common diseases.

1. Salmonellosis, also known as paratyphoid, is usually caused by *Salmonella typhimurium* and is the most common bacterial infection of pigeons. The organisms can be transmitted in the faeces, crop milk or infected eggs. Clinical signs of infection are extremely variable. Young pigeons often show stunted growth, are underweight and listless, and are affected by diarrhoea. Affected adults may lose weight and develop diarrhoea and swelling of the joints. Swelling and necrosis of the inner eye, known as panophthalmitis, may occur. Isolation and identification of the *Salmonella* micro-organisms, usually from faeces or blood, is the only certain means of identifying presence of the disease. In the UK positive tests for *Salmonella* must be reported, under the Animal Health Act (1981)[7], to a local Veterinary Laboratories Agency (VLA) laboratory in England and Wales and to the local Divisional Veterinary Manager in Scotland. Because *Salmonella* is a zoonosis, the risk of a pigeon infecting humans should not be underestimated and strict hygiene measures are essential in handling infected birds. Hutchison (1999) notes that treatment is unlikely to be satisfactory, since a proportion of birds in a loft are likely to remain carriers after treatment, with the result that the disease may flare up again. She does, however, recommend chlortetracycline in the drinking water, made up fresh each day, at 120 mg or more per litre, for 5–7 days. However, more recent advice from Cousquer and Parsons (2007) recommends that the most severely affected birds be culled and the remainder treated with an antimicrobial, to be determined by culture and sensitivity tests, for 10–14 days.
2. *Chlamydophila psittaci*, formerly known as *Chlamydia psittaci*, is an intracellular bacterium that causes ornithosis in pigeons and respiratory psittacosis in humans. In pigeons it can be associated with other diseases such as trichomoniasis, pox and herpes virus infections. Symptoms in birds include diarrhoea, weight loss and egg infection, and may only appear if the animals are under stress. Humans that have come into contact with infected birds may show influenza-like symptoms that may indicate psittacosis, which may develop into pneumonia. Therefore if human and pigeon symptoms coincide ornithosis may be suspected. Infection is spread through inhalation or ingestion of nasal discharges or through faeces. The currently favoured treatment is doxycycline or a chlortetracycline-medicated feed. If antibiotics are not available, or ineffective, the birds should be killed and a thorough disinfection of the aviary and cages should be carried out before restocking.
3. Newcastle disease is rare in pigeons. However, there is a strain which occurs in pigeons called avian paramyxovirus type 1 (APMV-1). According to Wallis (1983) the pigeon strain of APMV-1 causes green watery diarrhoea, clearly audible upper respiratory sounds and some sneezing. This may be followed by lack of coordination, twitching and paralysis of the legs. In the UK, occurrences of APMV-1 and Newcastle disease must be reported, under the Animal Health Act (1981), to a local DEFRA office. Amendments to the Act in 2002 and under the Avian Influenza and Newcastle Disease (England and Wales) Order (2003)[8] extended previous powers to protect the public from outbreaks of Newcastle disease in poultry. There is no treatment. Inactivated and live vaccines are now freely available for use under veterinary supervision, although only healthy pigeons should be vaccinated.
4. Pigeon pox or so-called diphtheria is common especially in young birds. The incubation period is usually 1 week. Squabs are infected by their parents. Mosquitoes and other blood-sucking parasites may also play a role in transmission. Therefore prevention may be facilitated by a clean cage or aviary. Swellings develop on unfeathered areas of the body, particularly around the eyes, beak and legs. Affected birds lose weight and a few young birds may die following spread of the virus to the mouth and throat. Removal of scabs or swellings is not recommended because this is likely to spread infection by releasing viral particles. An infected pigeon is not dangerous to humans. Pigeon pox may occur in doves. There is no treatment, and with care, birds will recover. Vaccination is recommended in previously infected populations.
5. Avian influenza has received high media coverage since the zoonotic nature of the deadly H5N1 strain was discovered in Hong Kong in 1997. On that occasion six people died from contact with infected chickens. However, it has been widely reported that should the H5N1 strain mutate to allow transmission between humans then a pandemic, killing millions, would be likely (Webster & Walker 2003). H5N1 is only one strain of many that vary in their pathogenicity. Low pathogenic avian influenza (AI) infection does not always produce clinical symptoms. However, in the UK, AI is a notifiable disease under the Animal Health Act (1981) and associated amendments, and must be reported to a local DEFRA Animal Health Office if suspected. In birds, clinical signs include respiratory illness, swollen head and loss of appetite. In poultry, high pathogenic AI causes multiple organ failure, rapid death within 48 h, and is spread through a population very quickly. The disease is spread though contact or faeces, and is not airborne. However, there is little evidence that pigeons are a major factor in the spread of the disease.

[7] http://www.opsi.gov.uk/RevisedStatutes/Acts/ukpga/1981/cukpga_19810022_en_1

[8] http://www.opsi.gov.uk/si/si2003/20031734.htm

Perkins and Swayne (2002) showed that pigeons were resistant to the Hong Kong strain that killed poultry and waterfowl so readily (but see Klopfleisch *et al.* (2006) for evidence of artificial H5N1 inoculation effects in pigeons). In addition, with low pathogenic AI, pigeons are not thought to shed viruses post-inoculation (Panigrahy *et al.* 1996). However, AI has a high mutation rate, and the situation for pigeons may change very quickly. The best recommendation is to keep laboratory pigeons under cover and out of contact with wild birds.

Vitamin deficiency

Vitamin A deficiency may occur in caged doves and pigeons, especially young birds kept on a deficient diet with no green food or yellow seeds such as maize that contain carotene, the precursor of vitamin A. Symptoms include 'rattling' respiratory sounds, resulting from degeneration of mucous membranes in the mouth, and eye infections. Affected birds will lose weight and may move in an uncoordinated way. Birds should be given an oral preparation of vitamin A.

Risks to humans

Health and hygiene

Handlers should wear appropriate protective clothing at all times, to avoid potential health risks from handling birds. The authors recommend the use of disposable examination gloves and a face mask as a minimum. Cuts and grazes should be covered, and hands and arms washed thoroughly with disinfectant after handling.

Sources of allergens for bird handlers

Humans may develop pigeon-breeders disease, a form of hypersensitivity pneumonitis caused by inhalation of antigens of pigeon (or dove) origin. It is characterised by a diffuse inflammation of the lower respiratory tract. T-lymphocytes recognise a wide range of proteins from pigeons and can induce T-cell proliferation. It has also been found that feather mites are a source of allergens for pigeon handlers, with allergic rhinitis being the most common reaction. Dry skin may also occur.

Acknowledgements

The authors would like to thank Claire Richardson for helpful comments, and Jemma Dopson and Guillem Esber for providing the photographs for Figure 44.1.

References

Abou-Madi, N. (2001) Avian Anesthesia. *Veterinary Clinics of North America: Exotic Animal Practice*, **4**, 147–167

Bingman, V.P. (1998) Spatial representation and homing pigeon navigation. In: *Spatial Representation in Animals*. Ed. Healy, S., pp. 69–85. Oxford University Press, Oxford

Biro, D., Meade, J. and Guilford, T. (2004) Familiar route loyalty implies visual pilotage in the homing pigeon. *Proceedings of the National Academy of Sciences of the USA*, **101**, 17440–17443

Braithwaite, V. A. and Guilford, T. (1991) Viewing familiar landscapes affects pigeon homing. *Proceedings of the Royal Society B – Biological Sciences*, **245**, 183–186

Council of Europe (2006) Multilateral Consultation of Parties to the European Convention for the Protection of Vertebrate Animals used for Experimental and other Scientific Purposes (ETS 123) Appendix A. *Cons 123 (2006) 3*. Available from URL: http://www.coe.int/t/e/legal_affairs/legal_co-operation/biological_safety,_use_of_animals/laboratory_animals/2006/Cons123(2006)3AppendixA_en.pdf (accessed 31 July 2008)

Cousquer, G. and Parsons, D. (2007) Veterinary care of the racing pigeon. *In Practice*, **29**, 344–355

Cramp, S. (1986) *Handbook of the Birds of Europe, the Middle East and North Africa. The Birds of the Western Palearctic*, Vol. IV. Oxford University Press, Oxford

Davis, J.W., Anderson, R.C., Karstad, L. *et al.* (1971) *Infectious and Parasitic Diseases of Wild Birds*. The Iowa State University Press, Ames

Erickson, C.J. and Zenone, P.G. (1976) Courtship differences in male ring doves: avoidance or cuckoldry? *Science*, **192**, 1353–1354

Erichsen, J.T., Karten, H.J., Eldred, W.D. *et al.* (1982) Localization of substance P-like and enkephalin-like immunoreactivity within preganglionic terminals of the avian ciliary ganglion: light and electron microscopy. *Journal of Neuroscience*, **2**, 994–1003

European Commission (2007) Commission recommendations of 18 June 2007 on guidelines for the accommodation and care of animals used for experimental and other scientific purposes. Annex II to European Council Directive 86/609. See 2007/526/EC. http://eurlex.europa.eu/LexUriServ/site/en/oj/2007/l_197/l_19720070730en00010089.pdf (accessed 13 May 2008)

Franssen, F.F. and Lumeij, J.T. (1992) In vitro nitroimidazole resistance of *Trichomonas gallinae* and successful therapy with an increased dosage of ronidazole in racing pigeons (*Columba livia domestica*). *Journal of Veterinary Pharmacology and Therapeutics*, **15**, 409–415

Goodwin, D. (1983) *Pigeons and Doves of the World*. Comstock Publishing Associates, a division of Cornell University Press, Ithaca

Granda, A.M. and Maxwell, J.H. (1979) *Neural Mechanisms of Behavior in the Pigeon*. Plenum Press, New York

Güntürkün, O., Hellmann, B., Melsbach, G. *et al.* (1998) Asymmetries of representation in the visual system of pigeons. *NeuroReport*, **9**, 4127–4130

Harrison, G.J. and Harrison, L. (1986) *Clinical Avian Medicine and Surgery*. WB Saunders, Philadelphia

Haselgrove, M., George, D.N. and Pearce, J.M. (2005) The discrimination of structure: III. Representation of spatial relationships. *Journal of Experimental Psychology. Animal Behavior Processes*, **31**, 433–448

Home Office (1989) *Code of Practice for the Housing and Care of Animals Used in Scientific Procedures*. HMSO, London. Available from URL: http://scienceandresearch.homeoffice.gov.uk/animal-research/publications-and-reference/publications/code-of-practice/code-of-practice-housing-care/ (accessed 17 November 2009)

Horseman, N.D. and Buntin, J.D. (1995) Regulation of pigeon cropmilk secretion and parental behaviors by prolactin. *Annual Review of Nutrition*, **15**, 213–238

Huber, L. (1994) Amelioration of laboratory conditions for pigeons (*Columba livia*). *Animal Welfare*, **3**, 321–324

Hutchison, J.B. (1991) How does the environment influence the behavioural action of hormones? In: *The Development and Integration of Behaviour: Essays in honour of Robert Hinde.* Ed Bateson, P., pp. 149–170. Cambridge University Press, Cambridge

Hutchison, R.E. (1999) Doves and Pigeons. In: *The UFAW Handbook on the care and Management of Laboratory Animals Volume 1: Terrestrial Vertebrates,* 7th edn. Ed Poole, T., pp. 714–721. Blackwell Publishing, Oxford

Johnston, R.F. (1992) The rock dove. In: *The Birds of North America,* Vol. 13. Eds Poole, A., Stettenheim, P. and Gill, F., pp. 1–16. The Academy of Natural Sciences and Washington DC, The American Ornithologists' Union, Philadelphia

Joint Working Group on Refinement (1993) Removal of blood from laboratory mammals and birds. First Report of the BVA/FRAME/RSPCA/UFAW Joint Working Group on Refinement. *Laboratory Animals,* **27**, 1–22

Joint Working Group on Refinement (2001a) Laboratory birds: Refinements in husbandry and procedures. Fifth Report of the BVAAWF/FRAME/RSPCA/UFAW Joint Working Group on Refinement. *Laboratory Animals,* **35** (Suppl. 1), S1–S163

Joint Working Group on Refinement (2001b) Refining procedures for the administration of substances. Report of the BVAAWF/FRAME/RSPCA/UFAW Joint Working Group on Refinement. *Laboratory Animals,* **35**, 1–41

Keymer, I.F. (1991) Pigeons. In: *Manual of Exotic Pets.* Eds Beynon, P.H. and Cooper, J.E., pp. 180–202. British Small Animal Veterinary Association, Cheltenham

Klopfleisch, R., Werner, O., Mundt, E. *et al.* (2006) Neurotropism of highly pathogenic avian influenza virus A/chicken/Indonesia/2003 (H5N1) in experimentally infected pigeons (*Columba livia f. domestica*). *Veterinary Pathology,* **43**, 463–470

Laboratory Animal Science Association (2005) Guidance on the transport of laboratory animals. Report of the Transport Working Group established by LASA. *Laboratory Animals,* **39**, 1–39

Lea, R.W. and Sharp, P.J. (1991) Effects of presence of squabs upon plasma concentrations of prolactin and LH and length of time of incubation in ringdoves on 'extended' incubatory patterns. *Hormones and Behavior,* **25**, 275–282

Lehrman, D.S. (1965) Interaction between internal and external environments in the regulation of the reproductive cycle of the ring dove. In: *Sex and Behavior.* Ed Beach, F.A., pp. 55–380. John Wiley & Sons, New York

Lovari, S. and Hutchison, J.B. (1975) Behavioural transitions in the reproductive cycle of barbary doves (*Streptopelia risoria*). *Behaviour,* **53**, 126–150

Lovell-Mansbridge, C. (1995) *Sperm competition in the feral pigeon, Columba livia.* Ph.D. thesis, University of Sheffield

Lovell-Mansbridge, C. and Birkhead, T.R. (1998) Do female pigeons trade pair copulations for protection? *Animal Behaviour,* **56**, 235–241

McGregor, A., Saggerson, A., Pearce, J.M. *et al.* (2006) Blind imitation in pigeons, *Columba livia. Animal Behaviour,* **72**, 287–296

Munoz, E., Castella, J. and Gutierrez, J.F. (1998) In vivo and in vitro sensitivity of *Trichomonas gallinae* to some nitroimidazole drugs. *Vetinary Parasitology,* **78**, 239–246

Murton, R.K., Thearle, R.J.P. and Coombs, C.F.B. (1974) Ecological studies of the feral pigeon *Columba livia* var. III Reproduction and plumage polymorphism. *Journal of Applied Ecology,* **122**, 841–854

Nepote, K. (1999) Pigeons as laboratory animals. *Poultry and Avian Biology Reviews,* **10**, 109–115

Papi, F. (1992) *Animal Homing.* Chapman-Hall, London

Panigrahy, B., Senne, D.A., Pedersen, J.C. *et al.* (1996) Susceptibility of pigeons to avian influenza. *Avian Diseases,* **40**, 600–604

Perkins, L.E. and Swayne, D.E. (2002) Pathogenicity of a Hong Kong-origin H5N1 highly pathogenic avian influenza virus for emus, geese, ducks, and pigeons. *Avian Diseases,* **46**, 53–63

Redrobe, S. (2002) Pigeons. In: *Manual of Exotic Pets,* 4th edn. Eds Meredith, A. and Redrobe, S., pp. 168–178. British Small Animal Veterinary Association, Gloucester

Richie, B.W., Harrison, G.J. and Harrison, L.R. (1994) *Avian Medicine: Principles and Applications.* Wingers Publishing Inc., Lake Worth

Rupiper, D.J. (1998a) Diseases that affect race performance of homing pigeon. Part I: Husbandry, diagnostic strategies, and viral diseases. *Journal of Avian Medicine and Surgery,* **12**, 70–77

Rupiper, D.J. (1998b) Diseases that affect race performance of homing pigeons. Part II: Bacterial, fungal, and parasitic diseases. *Journal of Avian Medicine and Surgery,* **12**, 138–148

Sharman, I., Morton, D.B., Verschoyle, R. *et al.* (2001) Refining procedures for the administration of substances. *Laboratory Animals,* **35**, 1–41

Trivers, R.L. (1972) Parental investment and sexual selection. In: *Sexual Selection and the Descent of Man, 1871–1971.* Ed. Campbell, B., pp. 136–179. Aldine-Atherton, Chicago

Tudor, D.C. (1991) *Pigeon Health and Disease.* The Iowa State University Press, Ames

Walcott, C. (1996) Pigeon homing – observations, experiments and confusions. *Journal of Experimental Biology,* **199**, 21–27

Wallraff, H.G. (2001) Navigation by homing pigeons: updated perspective. *Ethology, Ecology and Evolution,* **13**, 1–48

Wallraff, H.G., Kiepenheuer, J. and Streng, A. (1993) Further experiments on olfactory navigation and non-olfactory pilotage by homing pigeons. *Behavioral Ecology and Sociobiology,* **32**, 387–390

Wallis, A.S. (1983) Paramyxovirus infection. Virus Report. *The Racing Pigeon* 22nd July, p. 1010

Webster, R.G. and Walker, E.J. (2003) The world is teetering on the edge of a pandemic that could kill a large fraction of the human population. *Scientific American,* **91**, 122–129

Wolfensohn, S. and Lloyd, M. (2003) *Handbook of Laboratory Animal Management and Welfare.* Blackwell Publishing, Oxford

45 The European starling

Melissa Bateson and Lucy Asher

Biological overview

General biology

The European starling (*Sturnus vulgaris* L.), henceforth the starling, is a medium-sized song-bird with a length of about 20 cm, belonging to the family Sturnidae, sub-order Oscines, order Passeriformes. Starlings are native to most of temperate Europe and western Asia. Northeastern populations migrate in autumn, with some birds over-wintering in Iberia and Africa. Starlings were introduced to Australia (late 1800s), New Zealand (1862), North America (1891) and South Africa (1890); the species is currently estimated to inhabit 30% of the earth's land area, excluding Antarctica (Feare 1984).

Use in research

Benefits

Starlings are a readily available and robust species, settling fast in captivity and usually remaining in good health. Their gregarious nature allows group housing at relatively high densities, and they have simple dietary requirements. For many experimental purposes starlings are an ideal size, being large enough to handle easily, but small enough to allow natural behaviour such as flight in captivity (eg, Witter *et al.* 1994). Being naturally inquisitive, starlings are easy to train on operant tasks using autoshaping procedures (eg, Bateson & Kacelnik 1995). Starlings can readily be brought into breeding condition by manipulation of day length, and will both sing and court in captivity (eg, Heimovics & Riters 2006; Meaden 1979). However, they are hard to breed in captivity.

Types of research

Due to the range of benefits outlined above, starlings are currently among the most popular passerine bird species used in laboratory-based biological research (Asher & Bateson 2008). They were first used for studies on avian infectious diseases over 25 years ago (Cooper & Needham 1981; Cooper 1987), and are currently a widely used model species in many areas of behavioural research including foraging decisions, mate choice and social learning (eg, Fernandez-Juricic *et al.* 2004). Starlings have been useful subjects for the neurobiology of both hearing and song learning/production (eg, Langemann & Klump 2001). They have also been important for understanding the environmental (photoperiod and temperature) control of breeding and moult and endocrine control of reproduction and the stress response (eg, Dawson 2001; Nephew & Romero 2003). Visual and auditory discrimination testing have been performed on starlings (eg, Swaddle & Ruff 2004) and studies of flight mechanisms and aerodynamics (eg, Ward *et al.* 2004). The widespread use of starlings in laboratory experiments has led to a recent increase in research on the laboratory welfare of this species (eg, Maddocks S.A. *et al.* 2002; Matheson *et al.* 2008).

Size range and lifespan

Basic biometric data for free-living British starlings are shown in Table 45.1. It is important to realise that the mass of individual birds will vary depending on time of day (a bird can lose 10 g on a long winter night (Tait 1973)), season (birds can be as much as 15 g heavier in winter than summer), current diet (birds eating more plant food will have a longer gut (Al-Joborae 1979)), and cage size (birds will lose flight muscle in smaller cages). In studies where control of weight is important, birds should be weighed at the same time of day (preferably before it is light in the morning when the gut is empty), and baseline weights should be established immediately prior to the start of a study (eg, Barnett *et al.* 2007).

Free-living adult starlings (ie, at least 1 year of age) have an average annual survival rate of around 45%, with most birds dying during the annual breeding season. However, survival should be much higher in captivity where birds are protected from starvation, hypothermia, predation and certain diseases. Maximum recorded longevities for free-living birds vary between 15 years 3 months (North America) and 21 years (Germany) (Klimkiewicz 2007).

Social organisation

Starlings do not have a strong social structure, but are gregarious throughout the year, tending to form larger and denser feeding flocks in winter. They form communal roosts in winter that can comprise up to one million birds.

Dominance hierarchies are established in captive flocks, with males dominant to females and adults to juveniles. Birds may jockey to defend preferred perching positions or feeding sites, and fighting involving grappling with feet and bill stabbing can occasionally occur. During the breeding season birds will defend a territory immediately around the nest site with males chasing away other males up to 10 m from the nest. Both monogamous and polygamous mating systems have been reported. Pair bonding does not occur until the weeks immediately before laying. Both sexes feed the young.

Reproduction

Starlings are cavity nesters and are usually colonial breeders with nests as little as 1 m apart. Females breed at 1 year of age, males not till 2 years. In England, first clutches are initiated between early April and late May (Joys & Crick 2004). Eggs are pale blue or white-spotted and 30 mm × 21 mm and 7 g (BTO Nest Record Scheme data). They hatch asynchronously, with the last egg hatching up to 24 h after others. Basic reproductive data are shown in Table 45.2. Chicks grow fast, reaching their adult weight within two weeks of hatching.

Starlings go through a complete moult once each year, following breeding, with juveniles moulting their distinct grey–brown, spotless, plumage at the same time. New feathers are tipped with white or buff giving a spotted appearance that is less apparent by the following breeding season as the pale feather tips wear off.

Table 45.1 Biometric data for free-living British starlings (British Trust for Ornithology 2005). Cells show: mean ± sd (range).

Variable	*Male*	*Female*	*Juvenile*
Wing length (mm)	132.6 ± 3.1 (135–137)	129.5 ± 3.3 (132–135)	130.2 ± 4.2 (122–136)
Mass (g)	86.95 ± 9.97 (76.00–100.0)	82.50 ± 9.27 (72.00–95.00)	81.83 ± 7.59 (70.00–95.00)

Table 45.2 Reproductive data for starlings.

Variable	*Mean ± sd*	*Range*
Clutch size (number of eggs)	4.60 ± 0.94	2–9
Incubation (days)	12.38 ± 1.61	10–16
Fledging (days)	20.50 ± 3.25	15–26

Normal behaviour

Starlings are opportunistic and adaptable foragers, but forage predominantly on the ground in open areas of short grass. They are adapted for terrestrial foraging with powerful legs for walking and a strong, pointed bill for probing into the substrate to locate soil invertebrates. Probing behaviour involves the bird pushing its closed bill into the soil, opening its bill to create a hole whilst rotating its eyes forwards to gain binocular vision of the contents of the hole (Figure 45.1). Hawking of flying insects has also been observed. Starlings often feed up to 20 miles from their winter roost sites, and have relatively long and pointed wings adapted for fast flight across open country. Starlings can be tame and approachable in gardens, but are generally more wary in rural areas.

Starlings are highly vocal, with both sexes singing, except in the breeding season when only the males sing. They have a complex song, incorporating mimicry, and are open-ended learners extending their repertoire throughout life.

Sources

The vast majority of starlings used in laboratory research are caught from the wild either as adults or juveniles (Asher & Bateson 2008). The advantage of juveniles is that they are easier to catch and may adapt to captivity better. However, they also typically have higher parasite loads, and are more prone to developing symptoms of avian pox following capture. A number of methods can be used to catch starlings. Walk-in traps and funnel traps can be very successful, especially if live decoy birds are used. However, the ethical and legal considerations of the latter strategy need to be carefully considered. Mist nets and baited spring-loaded whoosh nets have also been used successfully. Adult birds can easily be captured roosting in nest boxes prior to the start of the breeding season.

Hand raising chicks is extremely time-consuming, but can be achieved successfully provided chicks are at least 4 days old at the time they are taken from the nest. Hand raising chicks of less than 4 days is reported to be unsuccessful.

Captive breeding is generally unsuccessful (but see Meaden 1979). Starlings will attempt to breed if housed in mixed-sex aviaries with nest boxes. However, the chicks usually die soon after hatching due to the lack of availability of appropriate food. A possible solution to this problem is

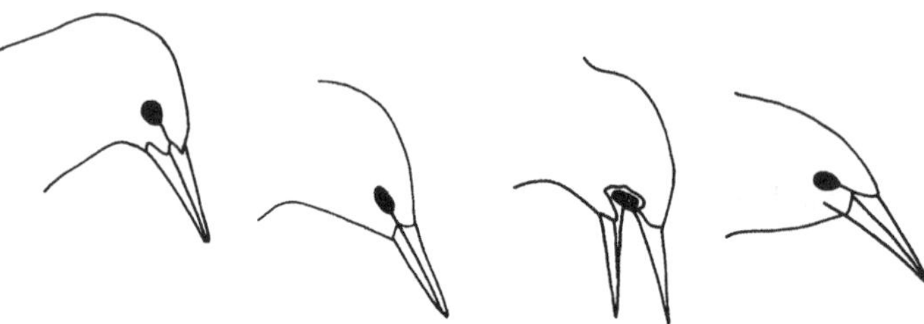

Figure 45.1 Distinctive probing behaviour of a starling. From left to right the bird searches for indication of a prey item; lowers its head pushing its closed bill into the soil; it opens its bill to create a hole whilst rotating its eyes forwards; then raises its head to complete the movement. Reproduced from *The Starling* by Feare, Christopher (1984), by permission of Oxford University Press (www.oup.com).

to use a large portable aviary that can be moved around natural pasture during the night so that a constant supply of fresh invertebrates is always available to the birds.

Conservation status

The International Union for the Conservation of Nature and Natural Resources places the starling in the category of Least Concern. However, the number of starlings has fallen rapidly in the UK since the early 1980s (Robinson *et al.* 2005) leading to upgrading of the species' UK conservation listing to Red (>50% population decline). Starlings are rated as SPEC category 3 (declining) in Europe. In the UK, starlings are protected under the Wildlife and Countryside Act 1981, which makes it illegal to intentionally kill, injure or take a starling, or to take, damage or destroy an active nest or its contents. In England, a licence is required from Natural England to catch and hold starlings. In the USA, starlings are not protected under American wildlife conservation laws due to their status as both an introduced species and an agricultural pest.

Laboratory management

General husbandry

Enclosures

Captive starlings are successfully kept in a wide variety of enclosures of different sizes and shapes. Where possible, group housing in large, outdoor aviaries is always preferable. Advantages include reduced feather damage, greater space and lower maintenance, but individuals are less easy to inspect and capture. Where birds have to be kept in smaller cages, a minimum space requirement of 1 m^3 for a singly housed bird was recommended by the Joint Working Group on Refinement (JWGR 2001b). However, this latter volume was not chosen on the basis of any scientific evidence, and represents a much larger cage than the median of 0.42 m^3 revealed by a review of current practice with this species (Asher & Bateson 2008). Within the volume range of 0.14–1.00 m^3 measurements of stereotypic behaviour patterns show that the environmental enrichment present in a cage may be more important in determining starling welfare than cage volume (Asher 2007). Thus, while larger cages are preferable if all else is equal, there is currently little evidence to suggest that welfare of birds is significantly greater in cages of 1.00 m^3 volume than in smaller cages down to 0.14 m^3. At all volumes, long-shaped cages that allow for flight are preferable to squarer cages or taller cages (Asher *et al.* 2009).

Environmental provisions

Cages should be equipped with adequate perches for all birds so as to reduce competition (Boogert *et al.* 2006). Plenty of high perches should be provided because birds will tend to spend most of their time on the highest perch available. In aviaries it is advantageous to have some moving perches since this will help maintain agility. In smaller cages, particularly when birds are singly housed, perches should be fixed because birds seem more fearful of moving items in this environment. Perches of varying thicknesses and textures (natural branches are ideal) will help maintain healthy claws and feet and provide a variety of substrates for bill-wiping (Witter & Cuthill 1992). Perches should not be located directly over food and water dishes to avoid fouling and possible spread of pathogens.

Bathing is probably important for feather maintenance (Brilot *et al.* 2009) and appears to be a strong behavioural need in this species. Starlings will attempt to bathe in their drinking water unless suitable baths are provided. Trays of bathing water at least 20 cm in diameter and not more than 3 cm deep should be provided, and will need to be replaced daily due to fouling.

Nest boxes should not be provided in mixed-sex aviaries because they are likely to provoke aggressive nest defence and may encourage unsuccessful breeding attempts.

Environmental enrichment

Provision of environmental enrichment reduces the incidence of behavioural stereotypies in starlings, and may be more important in determining the welfare of caged starlings than cage size *per se* (Asher 2007; Bateson & Matheson 2007). Starlings will choose to work for food by searching for it in a substrate such as sand even if the same food is freely available (Inglis & Ferguson 1986; Bean *et al.* 1999). This contra-freeloading behaviour may suggest a behavioural need to perform natural foraging techniques (Kacelnik 1987), which can be met in captivity by providing a substrate for starlings to probe. Ideally the entire floor of the enclosure should be covered with a substrate such as bark chippings, but if this is not possible, trays of bark chips or turf should be provided that are large enough not to allow aggressive defence by a single bird (Gill 1995; Gill *et al.* 1995).

Protective foliage cover in the form of evergreen trees or branches is likely to reduce perceived predation risk in starlings and may be important in reducing anxiety (Lazarus & Symonds 1992) and encouraging birds to use other available enrichment.

Feeding/watering

Starlings are omnivores eating both animal (predominantly insects and their larvae, but also other non-insect invertebrates) and plant material (soft fruits in autumn and seeds and cereals in autumn and winter) at all times of year. In captivity starlings can be kept indefinitely on commercial poultry or game bird starter crumbs or dry cat or dog food, provided the protein content is at least 30%. This diet should be provided *ad libitum* and can be supplemented with live invertebrates (eg, mealworms) and low-sucrose fruit such as apple pieces, cherries and grapes; the Sturnidae are unable to digest sucrose (Avery *et al.* 1995). Live insect prey can be placed in the probing substrate to encourage natural foraging behaviour. Insoluble grit does not appear to be required by starlings.

Drinking water should be available at all times, and should be changed at least once a day. Use of gravity dispensers for both food and water will help to reduce fouling.

An adequate number of feeders and water bottles should be provided to reduce aggressive interactions.

Social housing

Captive starlings prefer to be in proximity to conspecifics (Vasquez & Kacelnik 2000), and can be housed at relatively high densities as long as adequate roosting perches and food dishes are provided so that all birds can use these simultaneously (Boogert *et al.* 2006). Groups of 4–12 birds are recommended. It is better to keep several birds together in a larger cage, even if this is at a reduced space per bird.

It is feasible to house starlings individually for experimental purposes; however, if possible auditory and visual contact with other birds should be maintained.

Identification and sexing

Individual identification

Starlings can be individually identified with leg rings (bands) of either plastic or aluminium. Ring size 'C' (diameter 4.3 mm, weight 0.14 g) is usually appropriate for a starling. Split plastic rings are fitted with the tool provided with them, whereas metal rings will require specialist ringing pliers (Redfern & Clark 2001). Rings should be large enough to move freely on the starling's leg but not too large to fall over its foot. Rings are available printed with numbers and also in a range of colours to aid identification of birds without the need for catching. Up to two rings can be accommodated on each leg if a large range of colour combinations is required.

Sexing

Starlings are sexually dimorphic and can be accurately sexed from external features alone (see Table 45.3). Juveniles can be more difficult to sex based on plumage; however, 98% can be correctly classified based on iris colour alone (Smith *et al.* 2005a).

Physical environment

Temperature and humidity

Starlings can withstand a wide range of temperatures and humidity as evidenced by their geographic distribution, and will thrive in outdoor aviaries (in the UK climate) provided that some shelter is available. Inside it is typical to maintain laboratory temperatures at 14–20°C; however, deviations from this range are unlikely to cause problems. Ambient temperature is known to affect foraging decisions (Bateson 2002) and fat storage (Cuthill *et al.* 2000).

Photoperiod

Photoperiod is extremely important in starlings because, like other temperate-zone species, they use the shape of the annual change in day length to control the time of breeding and moult (Dawson 2007). The short days of winter render birds photosensitive such that when days lengthen, the neuroendocrine changes leading to gonadal maturation and breeding are stimulated. Starlings held on 11 L:13 D will retain mature gonads indefinitely. Prolonged exposure (>30 days) to long days results in a photorefactory phase, gonadal regression and finally moult. In starlings held on 13 L:11 D the gonads will remain regressed indefinitely and birds will never come into breeding condition. Moult duration can be reduced from 119 days for birds held on constant long days of 18 L:6 D to 92 days by gradually reducing day length by 1 h/week from 18 L:6 D to 12 L:12 D; however this acceleration is bought at the expense of reduced final feather quality (Dawson 2004). Following a period of long days, photosensitivity in starlings can be reinstated by a period of 25–35 days of 8 L:16 D (Goldsmith & Nicholls 1984).

For birds housed indoors, either the daily transition between light and dark should be gradual in order to allow

Table 45.3 Sexually dimorphic features in starlings.

Variable	*Male*	*Female*	*Accuracy in juveniles?**
Colour of base of bill	Grey–blue	Salmon pink	100%, but only in the breeding season (when males have yellow bills)
Lightness of iris colour relative to dark chocolate brown pupil	Either dim ring, visible with careful observation or so dark as to be indistinguishable from pupil	Either much lighter with a highly distinct ring or lighter with a clear ring	98% classified correctly using this feature alone
Throat and chest feather length	Mostly long and thin	Range from 50% long and thin, 50% short and wide to mostly short and wide	93–94%
Throat and chest feather tip shape	Range from 50% round, 50% V-shaped to mostly V-shaped	Mostly rounded	81–89%
Mass	Heavier: ≥78 g	Lighter: <78 g	70–72%
Tarsus length	Longer: ≥29.3 mm	Shorter: <29.3 mm	65-67%
Speckling (density of pale feather tips)	Fewer to no spots	More spots	Not a useful trait in juveniles

*Figures are taken from an analysis in Smith *et al.* (2005a).

birds to find a roosting site for the night, or a dim nightlight should be provided.

Quality of light

The frequency at which a flickering light source is perceived as continuous is believed to be higher in birds than in humans (>100 Hz vs. 50–60 Hz), leading to concern that starlings may be able to perceive the flicker from conventional low-frequency fluorescent lights (100 Hz in Europe and 120 Hz in the USA) and cathode ray tube monitors. In preference tests, starlings prefer high-frequency (>30 kHz) over low-frequency (100 Hz) lighting, indicating that they can detect a difference (Greenwood *et al.* 2004). Myoclonus is induced in starlings exposed to fluorescent lighting and cathode ray tube monitors flickering below 150 Hz (Smith *et al.* 2005b). Birds are less active and have higher basal corticosterone levels under low frequency lighting, suggesting that they may find it more stressful (Smith *et al.* 2005c). Starlings also show changes in mate choice in low- and high-frequency lighting, becoming less consistent in the preferences in low-frequency conditions (Evans *et al.* 2006). It is therefore recommended that, if natural light is not available, rooms are lit with high-frequency fluorescent lights.

Most birds, including starlings, have an additional retinal cone type tuned to UV wavelengths meaning that if they are housed in laboratories without UV light they may be deprived of visual information usually available to them in the outside world. There is some evidence to suggest that starlings may prefer a light environment containing UV (Greenwood *et al.* 2002), and that being housed in a UV-deficient light environment causes higher basal corticosterone levels and changes in behaviour (Maddocks A.A. *et al.* 2002). It is therefore recommended that starlings are housed in rooms with full-spectrum lighting.

Hygiene

The main disadvantage of starlings as an experimental animal is the large quantities of droppings (faeces and urates) they produce. The floor covering will need to be replaced daily in smaller cages, but in larger aviaries less frequent cleaning will be necessary. Cleaning can be stressful for birds, particularly those in cages, but stress can be reduced if husbandry is conducted as quietly as possible, ideally by a familiar person, at a similar time each day (Rich & Romero 2005). It may also help if birds are provided with cover in which they can hide.

Starlings can carry human pathogens and there is therefore a potential risk of infection from their droppings. However, a recent analysis on bacteria present in free-living starling droppings showed that most did not belong to the specific types most often found in humans. The authors concluded that starlings are unlikely to present a major source of infection for humans (Gautsch *et al.* 2000). Nevertheless, appropriate precautions should be taken by humans working with this species. Some laboratories routinely screen incoming starlings for common pathogens including *Salmonella*, *Yersinia* and coccidia.

Health monitoring and quarantine

Quarantine

Recently acquired starlings should be kept isolated from existing laboratory stock for at least 2 weeks to establish as far as is possible that birds are free from infectious diseases and to allow screening for zoonoses and treatment for parasites (see later in this chapter).

Bill and claw trimming

Starlings' claws and bills are adapted for walking and probing in soil and can become overgrown in captivity where they are not naturally abraded. Provision of rough wooden or sandpaper-covered perches can help (Cuthill *et al.* 1992), but usually birds will need to be caught and their bills and claws trimmed with nail clippers every few months. Overgrowth of the upper mandible will result in feeding and preening problems. It is important to check regularly that leg rings have not become too tight (see also Dietary related health problems).

Laboratory procedures

Handling

Capture by hand is possible in smaller cages. Since birds will not fly in the dark it is often easier to turn off the room lights and use a small torch to locate birds. In larger cages or outdoor aviaries a net (with padded edges) will be necessary. Birds will usually fly towards the light, and an indoor aviary can easily be emptied by turning off the lights and allowing the birds to fly into an adjacent lit room. Starlings can be trained to enter a small transport cage by reinforcing this behaviour with a preferred treat such as mealworms. Cotton drawstring bags are ideal for transporting starlings short distances. A recommended procedure for holding a starling is shown in Figure 45.2.

Training procedures

Captive starlings can rapidly be habituated to familiar humans if human visits are associated with beneficial con-

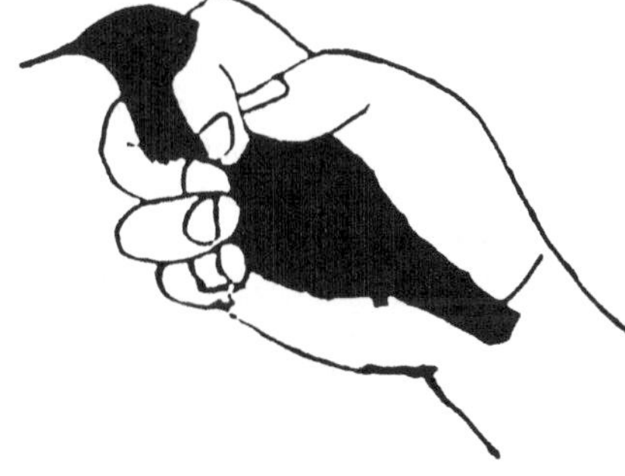

Figure 45.2 A recommended way to hold a starling: the bird's head is held between the index and middle finger with its back in the palm of the hand. The ring finger, little finger and thumb rest across the bird's closed wings to prevent them from flapping.

sequences such as provision of mealworms or water baths. It is not unusual for well habituated birds to take mealworms directly from humans. However, if birds are to be released to the wild, consideration should be given as to the possible adverse consequences of extensive habituation to humans.

Starlings can be easily trained to perform responses including hopping on perches, flying through mazes, probing holes through paper, going through push-doors, pecking lids off wells/dishes, and pecking illuminated keys or touchscreens. Pecking illuminated keys for food reward can be trained using standard auto-shaping procedures (for details see Bateson and Kacelnik 1995). Other behaviour patterns such as hopping between perches or using their feet to remove the stopper from a food container will need to be trained by gradual shaping with positive reinforcement.

Birds will learn to work for preferred treats such as mealworms without prior food deprivation. However, if birds are being reinforced with their normal diet it may be necessary to restrict their food intake, either by removing *ad libitum* food a few hours prior to the training session, or by feeding a restricted daily ration. If the latter approach is adopted, it is important to monitor birds by daily weighing (eg, Barnett *et al.* 2007). Birds maintained at 90–95% of their free-feeding mass will typically work well in operant experiments, and greater weight reduction is not recommended in this species. Given the possible temporal variation in free-feeding mass (see earlier), new baselines will always need to be established immediately prior to the start of an experiment.

Monitoring methods

Weighing

Birds can be weighed either by catching and placing in a cloth bag or clear plastic cone, or by training birds to come to a balance in their cage for mealworms. The balance can either be connected to a computer or read directly (a video camera or binoculars can be used for this in the case of shy birds).

Removal of blood

For a general review of procedures for removal of blood from laboratory birds (specifically chickens) see JWGR (1993). Recommended procedures for removal of blood from chickens should be extrapolated to starlings with extreme caution due to the large size difference between the species. Ideally, advice should be sought from researchers with first-hand experience with either starlings or another similarly sized bird species. In starlings, small blood samples (of the order of 0.05–0.1ml) are most easily taken from the alar (ie, wing or brachial) vein. Use of the jugular vein is not recommended due to the risks of accidentally puncturing the nearby carotid artery. Use of alcohol for site preparation is not recommended, because it causes cooling, and the consequent vasoconstriction can make the alar vein hard to locate. Up to four 0.1 ml samples have been taken in a 60-minute period (with no subsequent resampling) without problems.

Administration of substances

For general principles and summaries for specific protocols see JWGR (2001a). The easiest injection site on a starling is the pectoral muscle (the largest muscle in the body), but care should be taken, especially if repeated injections are required, because damage to this muscle can cause impairment of flight (Cooper 1983). For substances that can be administered by mouth, feeding birds injected mealworms should be considered as a low-stress approach (eg, Barnett *et al.* 2007).

Anaesthesia

Starlings can be successfully anaesthetised for up to 2–3h with inhalation agents. Isofluorane, for example, is used at 5% for induction and 1.5–2.5% for maintenance (eg, Bee & Klump 2004). Injectable agents can also be used (Cooper 1987).

Euthanasia

Alternatives to euthanasia should be considered where possible. It is common practice (and indeed sometimes a requirement of licensing bodies such as Natural England) to release wild-caught starlings following research that does not involve any invasive procedures. Ideally, birds should be given a period (eg, 2 weeks) in a large aviary to build-up and exercise their flight muscles prior to release either near the site of original capture, or at another location frequented by wild starlings.

For general principles of euthanasia, see Chapter 17 and Close *et al.* (1996). A summary of methods of euthanasia appropriate specifically for birds is provided by Close *et al.* (1997). A range of different procedures is used for euthanasing starlings, the most common being cervical dislocation and concussion by striking the head on a hard surface followed by cervical dislocation. The latter methods have the advantage of being quick but require confidence on the part of the handler. Overdose of anaesthetic (eg, pentobarbital injected intraperitoneally) is also possible.

Common welfare problems

Health

This chapter is not the appropriate place to present a full review of all the health problems that can occur in starlings, and for more information readers should consult an avian veterinary text (eg, Altman *et al.* 1997; Ritchie *et al.* 1997; Rupley 1997). The internet is also a source of useful sites aimed at pet owners containing health advice specific to starlings. Here we present the most common health problems reported in a questionnaire sent to researchers in both

Europe and North America with extensive experience keeping starlings in the laboratory.

Dietary related health problems

Hyperkeratosis characterised by raised overgrown scales on feet and legs, overgrown beak and nails and poor feather condition is common in captive starlings (Figure 45.3). In extreme cases scales can grow over the leg rings. Hyperkeratosis appears to be caused by diets that are too low in protein, as is the case for some poultry foods and softbill diets designed for fruit-eating Mynahs. It is important to check the protein content of the basic diet used for starlings (see Feeding/watering section for details).

Haemochromatosis, also known as iron storage disease, is a cause of mortality in some of the Sturnidae when they are kept in captivity, and could be related to dietary factors influencing the bioavailability of iron (Sheppard & Dierenfeld 2002). Cause of death appears to be heart failure or liver disease. Recent feeding experiments with European starlings suggest that a diet containing 34–125 ppm of iron is optimal for preventing accumulation of iron in the liver. Alternatively, adding a phytate (inositol), tannic acid, or both to readily available food stuffs may be a practical alternative to feeding low-iron diets (Olsen *et al.* 2006). However, despite the evidence that European starlings will accumulate iron in their organs, there is no evidence that birds fed long-term on the basic diets recommended earlier in the chapter commonly develop iron storage disease. Therefore, the authors conclude that concerns about haemochromatosis in European starlings are probably exaggerated.

Parasites and infectious diseases

Parasites and infectious diseases are not thought to be a major cause of mortality in free-living starling populations (Feare 1984), and captive starlings rarely have disease problems if husbandry is good. However, the species is host to a wide range of parasites with infection rates in free-living birds being higher in juveniles than adults and peaking in the summer, and it is good practice to treat incoming birds for endo and ectoparasites.

Ectoparasites include feather lice, ticks and mites. These can be vectors of disease in addition to producing clinical signs of anaemia, feather loss and skin lesions. Ectoparasites can be treated with ivermectin applied topically to the back of the neck. Starlings are recorded hosts of many endoparasites including nematodes, trematodes, cestodes and acanthocephalans. The gapeworm (*Syngamus trachea*) is a long red nematode that attaches to the trachea of birds. The worms cause bleeding in the throat and can block the trachea. Starlings infected with gapeworm can often be heard coughing. Nematode worms in starlings can be treated with the following drugs: fenbendazole (by addition to feed), flubendazole (by addition to feed), ivermectin (by mouth) and levamisole (by addition to drinking water).

Avian pox is a viral disease that produces wart-like lesions on the bird's head, particularly around the eyes and the base of the bill. Badly affected birds may need to be euthanased, but most usually recover without treatment. It is common for birds to develop the disease shortly after capture from the wild. Juvenile starlings seem particularly susceptible to pox, but survivors appear to become immune, and captive adults rarely develop the disease.

Aspergillosis is a common fungal infection of starlings causing clinical signs ranging from mild debility to sudden death. It is usually secondary to immunosuppression from chronic stress or other primary diseases, and can also occur in the presence of high concentrations of the fungus in the environment. Clinical diagnosis of aspergillosis is difficult and prognosis is poor.

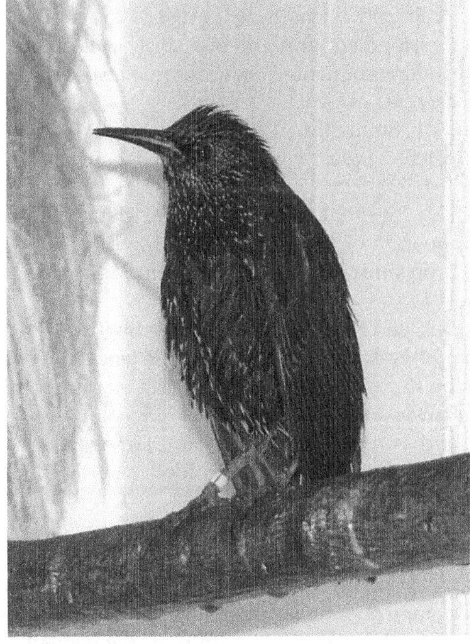

Figure 45.3 A laboratory starling with hyperkeratosis. Note the poor feather condition and specifically the heavy, overgrown bill and thickened scaley legs.

Behavioural

The most frequently reported abnormal behaviour pattern exhibited by caged starlings is the somersaulting or flipping stereotypy (although incidences of stereotypy are relatively low compared with other captive birds). This appears to be most common in birds housed in small barren cages, and can be reduced by adding enrichment to the cage or returning victims to a larger aviary.

Aggression and persistent harassment can occasionally become a problem in some group-housed birds. This will sometimes result in feather loss. In such cases birds should be carefully monitored and separated if necessary.

Polydypsia leading to watery diarrhoea occasionally occurs in captive starlings. This can be caused by birds trained on operant schedules erroneously associating their own drinking with reinforcement with food. Removing the bird from the operant schedule and adding oat flakes to the diet may help.

Feather damage, including complete loss of the tail, is common in birds housed in wire mesh cages. Although this is unsightly, it is unlikely to be a welfare problem unless birds are about to be released, in which case it could affect flight performance.

Further reading

Asher and Bateson (2008) provide a recent review of current practice in laboratory husbandry of European starlings. Feare (1984) is the best general source on the biology of European starlings although is mainly focused on free-living birds. Meaden (1979) provides details of captive care and breeding of many European bird species including the starling, and Perrins (1994) is a good review of general biological information, especially geographical distributions and song.

References

Al-Joborae, F. (1979) *The influence of diet on the gut morphology of the starling (Sturnus vulgaris).* DPhil Thesis, Oxford University

Altman, R.B., Clubb, S.L., Dorrenstein, D.M. *et al.* (1997) *Avian Medicine and Surgery.* Saunders, Philadelphia

Asher, L. (2007) The welfare of captive European starlings (Sturnus vulgaris). PhD Thesis, Newcastle University

Asher, L. and Bateson, M. (2008) Use and husbandry of captive European starlings (*Sturnus vulgaris*) in scientific research: a review of current practice. *Laboratory Animals*, **42**, 111–126

Asher, L., Davies, G.T.O., Bertenshaw, C.E. *et al.* (2009) The effects of cage size and shape on the welfare of captive European starlings (*Sturnus vulgaris*). *Applied Animal Behaviour Science*, **116**, 286–294

Avery, M.L., Decker, D.G., Humphrey, J.S. *et al.* (1995) Colour, size, and location of artificial fruits affect sucrose avoidance by Cedar Waxwings and European Starlings. *Auk*, **12**, 436–444

Barnett, C.A., Bateson, M. and Rowe, C. (2007) State-dependent decision making: educated predators strategically trade-off the costs and benefits of consuming aposematic prey. *Behavioural Ecology*, **18**, 645–651

Bateson, M. (2002) Context-dependent foraging preferences in risk sensitive starlings. *Animal Behaviour*, **64**, 251–260

Bateson, M. and Kacelnik, A. (1995) Preferences for fixed and variable food sources: variability in amount and delay. *Journal of the Experimental Analysis of Behavior*, **63**, 313–329

Bateson, M. and Matheson, S.M. (2007) Performance on a categorisation tasks suggests that removal of environmental enrichment induces 'pessimism' in captive European starlings (*Sturnus vulgaris*). *Animal Welfare*, **16**, 33–36

Bean, D., Mason, G.J. and Bateson, M. (1999) Contrafreeloading in starlings: testing the information hypothesis. *Behaviour*, **136**, 1267–1282

Bee, M.A. and Klump, G.M. (2004) Primitive auditory stream segregation: a neurophysiological study in the songbird forebrain. *Journal of Neurophysiology*, **92**, 1088–1104

Boogert, N.J., Reader, S.M. and Laland, K.N. (2006) The relation between social rank, neophobia and individual learning in starlings. *Animal Behaviour*, **72**, 1229–1239

Brilot, B. O., Asher L. and Bateson, M. (2009) Water bathing in European starlings improves escape flight performance. *Animal Behaviour*, **78**, 801–807

British Trust for Ornithology (2005) *Ringing Scheme Data.* Thetford, BTO

Close, B., Banister, K., Baumans, V. *et al.* (1996) Recommendations for euthanasia of experimental animals Part 1 Report of a Working Party. *Laboratory Animals*, **30**, 293–316

Close, B., Banister, K., Baumans, V. *et al.* (1997) Recommendations for euthanasia of experimental animals Part 2 Report of a Working Party. *Laboratory Animals*, **31**, 1–32

Cooper, J.E. (1983) Pathological studies on the effects of intramuscular injections in the starling (*Sturnus vulgaris*). Sonderdruck aus Verhandlungsbericht des 25 Internationalen Symposiums über die Erkrankungen der Zootiere, Wien. Akademie-Verlag, Berlin

Cooper, J.E. (1987) European wild birds. In: *The UFAW Handbook on the Care and Management of Laboratory Animals*, 6th edn. Ed Poole, T.B., pp. 709–715. Longman, Essex

Cooper, J.E. and J.R. Needham (1981) The starling (*Sturnus vulgaris*) as an experimental model for staphylococcal infection of the avian foot. *Avian Pathology*, **10**, 273–279

Cuthill, I.C., Maddocks, S.A., Weall, C.V. *et al.* (2000) Body mass regulation in response to changes in feeding predictability and overnight energy expenditure. *Behavioural Ecology*, **11**, 189–195

Cuthill, I.C., Witter, M. and Clarke, L. (1992) The function of bill-wiping. *Animal Behaviour*, **43**, 103–115

Dawson, A. (2001) The effects of a single long photoperiod on the induction and dissipation of reproductive photorefractoriness in European starlings. *General and Comparative Endocrinology*, **121**, 316–324

Dawson, A. (2004) The effects of delaying the start of moult on the duration of moult, primary feather growth rates and feather mass in Common Starlings *Sturnus vulgaris*. *Ibis*, **146**, 493–500

Dawson, A. (2007) Seasonality in a temperate zone bird can be entrained by near equatorial photoperiods. *Proceedings of the Royal Society B*, **274**, 721–725

Evans, J.E., Cuthill, I.C. and Bennett, A.T.D. (2006) The effect of flicker from fluorescent lights on mate choice in captive birds. *Animal Behaviour*, **72**, 393–400

Feare, C. (1984) *The Starling.* Oxford University Press, Oxford

Fernandez-Juricic, E., Siller, E. and Kacelnik, A. (2004) Flock density, social foraging, and scanning: an experiment with starlings. *Behavioural Ecology*, **15**, 371–379

Gautsch, S., Odermatt, P., Burnens, A.P. *et al.* (2000) The role of starlings (*Sturnus vulgaris*) in the epidemiology of potentially human bacterial pathogens. *Schweizer Archiv fur Tierheilkunde*, **142**, 165–172 (in German)

Gill, E.L. (1995) Environmental enrichment for captive starlings. *Animal Technology*, **45**, 89–93

Gill, E.L., Chivers, R.E., Ellis, S.C. *et al.* (1995) Turf as a means of enriching the environment of captive starlings (*Sturnus vulgaris*). *Animal Technology*, **46**, 97–102

Goldsmith, A.R. and Nicholls, T.J. (1984) Prolactin is associated with the development of photorefractoriness in intact, castrated and testosterone-implanted starlings. *General and Comparative Endocrinology*, **54**, 247–255

Greenwood, V.J., Smith, E.L., Cuthill, I.C. *et al.* (2002) Do European starlings prefer light environments containing UV? *Animal Behaviour*, **64**, 923–928

Greenwood, V.J., Smith, E.L., Goldsmith, A.R. *et al.* (2004) Does the flicker frequency of fluorescent lighting affect the welfare of captive European starlings? *Applied Animal Behaviour Science*, **86**, 145–149

Heimovics, S.A. and Riters, L.V. (2006) Breeding-context-dependent relationships between song and cFOS labeling within social behavior brain regions in male European starlings (*Sturnus vulgaris*). *Hormones and Behavior*, **50**, 726–735

Inglis, I.R. and Ferguson, N.J.K. (1986) Starlings search for food rather than eat readily available food. *Animal Behaviour*, **34**, 614–616

Joys, A.C. and Crick, H.Q.P. (2004) *Breeding Periods for Bird Species in England.* British Trust for Ornithology, Thetford

Joint Working Group on Refinement (1993) Removal of blood from laboratory mammals and birds. First Report of the BVA/FRAME/RSPCA/UFAW Joint Working Group on Refinement. *Laboratory Animals*, **27**, 1–22

Joint Working Group on Refinement (2001a) Refining procedures for the administration of substances. Report of the BVAAWF/

FRAME/RSPCA/UFAW Joint Working Group on Refinement. *Laboratory Animals*, **35**, 1–41

Joint Working Group on Refinement (2001b) Laboratory birds: Refinements in husbandry and procedures. Fifth Report of the BVAAWF/FRAME/RSPCA/UFAW Joint Working Group on Refinement. *Laboratory Animals*, **35** (Suppl. 1), S1–S163

Kacelnik, A. (1987) Information primacy or preference for familiar foraging techniques? A critique of Inglis and Ferguson. *Animal Behaviour*, **35**, 925–926

Klimkiewicz, M.K. (2007) *Longevity Records of North American Birds. Version 2007.1.* Patuxent Wildlife Research Center. Bird Banding Laboratory, Laurel

Langemann, U. and Klump, G.M. (2001) Signal detection in amplitude-modulated maskers. I. Behavioural auditory thresholds in a song bird. *European Journal of Neuroscience*, **13**, 1025–1032

Lazarus, J. and Symonds, M. (1992) Contrasting effects of protective and obstructive cover on avian vigilance. *Animal Behaviour*, **43**, 519–521

Maddocks, A.A., Goldsmith, A.R. and Cuthill, I.C. (2002) Behavioural and physiological effects of absence of ultraviolet wavelengths on European starlings *Sturnus vulgaris*. *Journal of Avian Biology*, **33**, 103–106

Maddocks, S.A., Bennett, A.T.D. and Cuthill, I.C. (2002) Rapid behavioural adjustments to unfavourable light conditions in European starlings (*Sturnus vulgaris*). *Animal Welfare*, **11**, 95–101

Matheson, S.M., Asher, L. and Bateson, M. (2008) Larger enriched cages are associated with 'optimistic' response biases in captive European starlings (*Sturnus vulgaris*). *Applied Animal Behaviour Science*, **109**, 374–383

Meaden, F. (1979) *A Manual of European Bird Keeping*. Blandford Press, Poole, Dorset

Nephew, B.C. and Romero, L.M. (2003) Behavioral, physiological and endocrine responses of starlings to acute increases in density. *Hormones and Behavior*, **44**, 222–232

Olsen, G.P., Russell, K.E., Dierenfeld, E. *et al.* (2006) Impact of supplements on iron abosrption from idets containing high and low iron concentrations in the European starling (*Sturnus vulgaris*). *Journal of Avian Medicine and Surgery*, **20**, 67–73

Perrins, C.M. (1994) *Handbook of the birds of Europe the Middle East and North Africa. The Birds of the Western Palaearctic*. Oxford University Press, Oxford

Redfern, C.P.F. and Clark, J.A. (2001) *Ringers' Manual*. BTO, Thetford

Rich, E.L. and Romero, L.M. (2005) Exposure to chronic stress downregulates corticosterone responses to acute stressors. *American Journal of Physiology: Regulatory Integrative and Comparative Physiology*, **288**, R1628–R1636

Ritchie, B.W., Harrison, G.L. and Harrison, L.R. (1997) *Avian Medicine: Principles and Application*. Wingers, Lake Worth

Robinson, R.A., Siriwardena, G.M. and Crick, H.Q.P. (2005) Status and population trends of Starlings *Sturnus vulgaris* in Great Britain. *Bird Study*, **52**, 252–260

Rupley, A.E. (1997) *Manual of Avian Practice*. Saunders, Philadelphia

Sheppard, C. and Dierenfeld, E. (2002) Iron storage disease in birds: Speculation on etiology and implications for captive husbandry. *Journal of Avian Medicine and Surgery*, **16**, 192–197

Smith, E.L., Cuthill, I.C., Griffiths, R. *et al.* (2005a) Sexing starlings *Sturnus vulgaris* using iris colour. *Ringing and Migration*, **22**, 193–197

Smith, E.L., Evans, J.E. and Parraga, C.A. (2005b) Myoclonus induced by cathode ray tube screens and low-frequency lighting in the European starling (*Sturnus vulgaris*). *The Veterinary Record*, **157**, 148–150

Smith, E.L., Greenwood, V.J., Goldsmith, A.R. *et al.* (2005c) Effect of repetitive visual stimuli on behaviour and plasma corticosterone of European starlings. *Animal Biology*, **55**, 245–258

Swaddle, J.P. and Ruff, D.A. (2004) Starlings have difficulty in detecting dot symmetry: Implications for fluctuating asymmetry. *Behaviour*, **141**, 29–40

Tait, M.J. (1973) Winter food and feeding requirements of the starling. *Bird Study*, **20**, 226–236

Vasquez, R.A. and Kacelnik, A. (2000) Foraging rate versus sociality in the starling *Sturnus vulgaris*. *Proceedings of the Royal Society B*, **267**, 157–164

Ward, S., Moller, U., Rayner, J.M.V. *et al.* (2004) Metabolic power of European starlings *Sturnus vulgaris* during a flight in a wind tunnel, estimated from heat transfer modelling, doubly labelled water and mask respirometry. *Journal of Experimental Biology*, **207**, 4291–4298

Witter, M.S. and Cuthill, I.C. (1992) Strategic perch choice for bill-wiping. *Animal Behaviour*, **43**, 1056–1058

Witter, M.S., Cuthill, I.C. and Bonser, R.H.C. (1994) Experimental investigations of mass-dependent predation risk in the European starling, *Sturnus vulgaris*. *Animal Behaviour*, **48**, 201–222

Reptiles and Amphibia

46 Terrestrial reptiles: lizards, snakes and tortoises

John E. Cooper

Introduction

I am grateful to my friend and former teacher, Dr Roger Avery, for permitting me to base some of this chapter on his original, excellent, text in the previous edition of the Handbook.

There are four orders and approximately 7000 extant species of reptiles (class Reptilia). The majority of these are lizards and snakes (order Squamata). There are more than 40 species in the order Chelonia that can be regarded as terrestrial; these are called 'tortoises' in Europe, Australasia and elsewhere but in North America they are usually referred to as 'turtles', a term which there encompasses also marine and freshwater aquatic chelonians, but in the UK (and elsewhere) refers only to the marine species. There are just over 20 species of crocodiles, alligators, caimans and their allies (order Crocodylia), and two species of lizard-like tuataras (order Rhynchocephalia), neither of which is dealt with in this chapter.

Much has been published in recent years, in various languages, concerning the husbandry and captive care of reptiles. This is critically relevant to laboratory management. General information about the biology, restraint and treatment of reptiles can be found in various texts. For instance, useful, succinct, summaries for lizards are provided by Schumacher (2003), for snakes by Mitchell (2003) and for chelonians by Raphael (2003). This chapter does not attempt to provide details of the husbandry of individual species. Instead, this chapter outlines and explains the general biological principles underlying successful reptile husbandry.

Many of the requirements of reptiles, and the husbandry techniques appropriate for successfully maintaining them in captivity, are significantly different from those of mammals or birds. With a few exceptions (see, eg, Thorogood & Whimster 1979; Wisniewski 1992), relatively little has been published specifically on the laboratory management of terrestrial reptiles: therefore it is often necessary (and wise) to extrapolate from the experiences of those who successfully keep and breed these species in private collections or in zoos. While some of the accounts tend to be anecdotal, others are based on sound observation and study – see, eg, Divers (1995), Frye (1993), Harling (1993, 1994), Langerwerf (1990, 1991), Rose (1992), Sheriff (1988), Sweeney (1993) and Townson (1994).

Biological overview

Anatomy

Reptiles are vertebrate animals that show considerable variation in morphology, especially modifications to limbs, vertebral column and pectoral and pelvic girdles (Davis 1981). There are snakes with vestiges of hindlimbs and lizards that are leg-less; an example of the latter are members of the family Amphisbaenidae (Schumacher 2003). Some indication of the complexity of structures in the cephalic region of squamate reptiles (snakes and lizards) is given in Figure 46.1. The integument of all reptiles is particularly important in terms of biology and health and is therefore discussed in detail in the next section.

The integument

In almost all reptile species the outer layer of the skin, the epidermis, is thickened (see Figure 46.1) and highly keratinised to form plate-like scales (Figures 46.2 and 46.3), which in places overlap one another (imbrication) (Cooper 2006). The surface of the epidermis is lost periodically, a process known as ecdysis or sloughing, and is replaced by growth of new cells from deeper layers. In snakes, the entire skin is shed, usually in one piece, including the keratinous 'spectacle', which covers the eye. Changes in the spectacle, characterised by an opacity or translucency, are a sign that sloughing is imminent. In lizards the skin is lost in small portions and the process takes place more or less simultaneously over the entire surface of the body. In other reptiles shedding tends to be piecemeal.

Sloughing (shedding) is an important physiological event (Maderson 1965). When reptiles are kept in laboratories it is important that detailed records of sloughing are maintained as a change in frequency, or a failure of/difficulty in shedding (dysecdysis), may indicate ill-health. It is good practice to retain shed skins, in a sealed plastic bag, so that they can be examined in the laboratory as part of routine health monitoring (see section on health) (Figure 46.4).

The 'shell' of terrestrial chelonians consists in most cases of bone, sometimes cartilage, that is covered with connective tissue and highly keratinised stratified squamous epithelium. It is well innervated and sensitive to trauma and

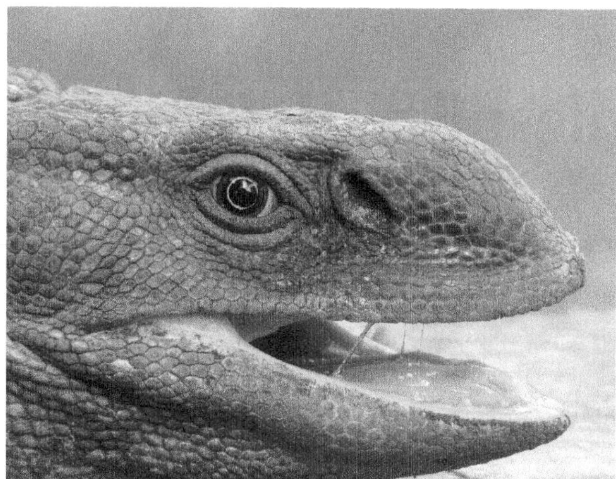

Figure 46.1 Head of a monitor lizard (*Varanus* sp.), illustrating the detailed scalation. The animal has a clear, shiny, eye, usually indicative of health.

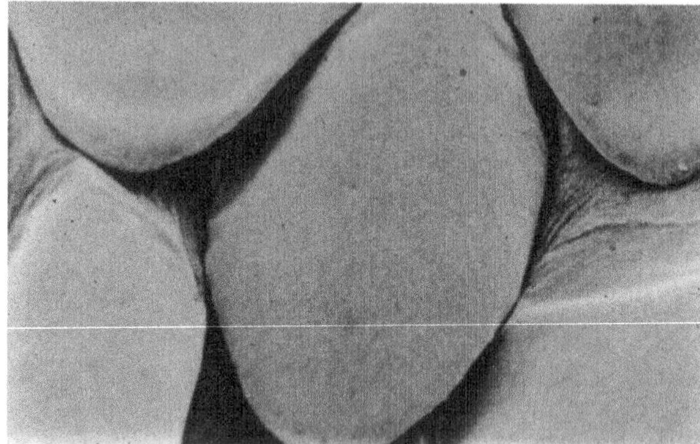

Figure 46.2 A low-power scanning electron microscope view of the skin of a skink, showing the overlapping scales.

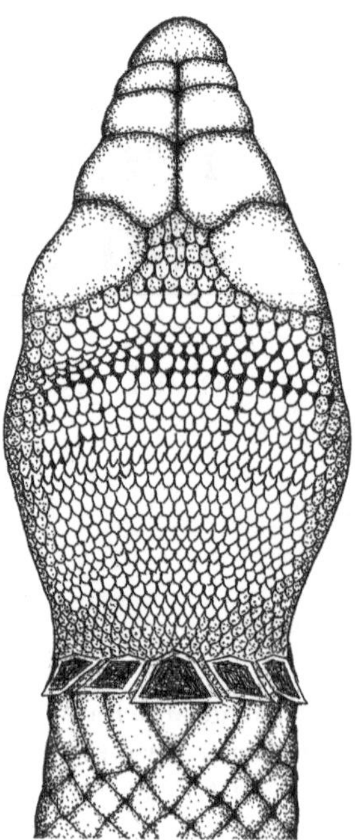

Figure 46.3 Line drawing of *Lacota viridis* head (drawn courtesy of the Edward Elkan Memorial Collection).

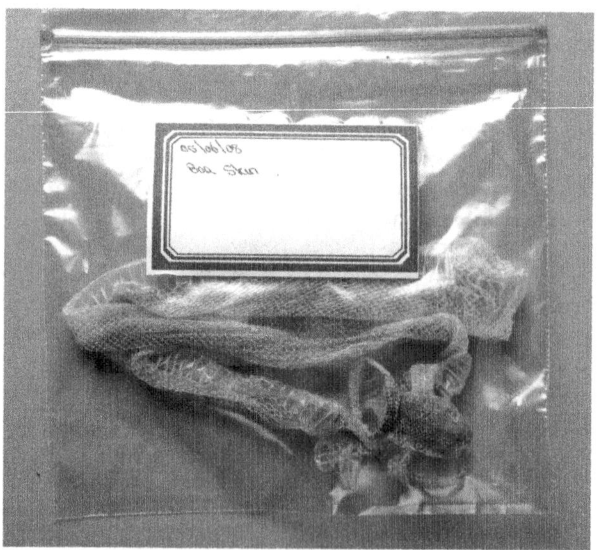

Figure 46.4 A sloughed (shed) skin from a boa constrictor. Regular and complete sloughing is usually a sign of good health in snakes. Under laboratory conditions the sloughing cycle should be monitored and shed skins carefully preserved, in sealed plastic bags, so that they can be examined for parasites and evidence of disease. (Photo: Richard Spence.)

painful stimuli. The care of, and veterinary attention to, chelonians can be very specialised (McArthur *et al.* 2004a).

Ectothermy and behavioural thermoregulation

Reptiles are ectothermic animals and, apart from rare exceptions, such as brooding pythons, cannot control their body temperature by internal means. This can have profound effects on their health and welfare, especially in captivity where environmental features are usually dictated by the keeper of the animal. The amount of heat produced by reptiles is small and because they have no insulation (hair or feathers) it can be rapidly lost. Without some external source of heat, the body temperature of a reptile will approximate to its immediate surroundings. Many species of reptiles adjust their behaviour to take advantage of external heat sources, usually either direct sunlight or sun-warmed substrates such as rocks, sand or (less frequently) water (Figure 46.5). Typically, a reptile will lie in the sun ('basking') until its body temperature rises to a threshold level ('upper thermoregulatory set point') at which metabolic rate is optimal and it will begin to perform other kinds of behaviour such as searching for food, courtship and mating and defensive aggression (Schieffelin & Queiroz 1991).

Basking often involves distinct postures, such as flattening and positioning the body so that the maximum surface area is exposed to solar radiation. When the animal stops basking, these postures are no longer maintained. If it remains in the sun, it may nevertheless drop in temperature because the rate of heat gain has been reduced. If it moves

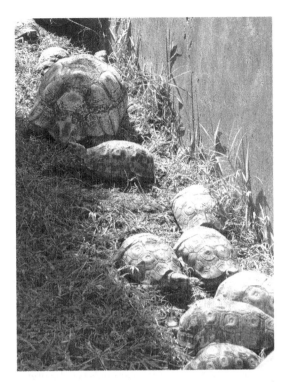

Figure 46.5 A mixed group of leopard (*Testudo pardalis*) and hinge-back (*Kinixys belliana*) tortoises in an outdoor pen. This sort of management is popular in the tropics because it is inexpensive and provides natural sunlight (note how the tortoises are thermoregulating in the sunlit area). It offers environmental enrichment but may predispose animals to damage and predation.

into the shade, for example while feeding, it will cool. In both cases a second threshold temperature ('lower thermoregulatory set point') will be reached, and the animal will seek sunlight and resume basking. In small lizards, the rates of heat loss and heat gain are rapid, and as they move from sun to shade and back again, they are often called 'shuttling heliotherms'. This method of maintaining a relatively high body temperature by basking to gain heat (and in very hot environments, actively seeking to cool by spending long periods in the shade or panting) is termed 'behavioural thermoregulation'. It is a major key to understanding many aspects of reptile biology, including how best to provide suitable conditions in captivity.

The actual threshold temperatures (Firth & Turner 1982) vary from species to species, and sometimes amongst individuals of the same species, depending upon various factors (Huey 1982). The mean temperatures recorded in active animals (mean activity temperature (MAT); Pough & Gans 1982) will thus fluctuate. More than 500 species of reptiles for which MATs or similar thermoregulatory data are available were listed in Avery (1982), Meek and Avery (1988) and Peterson *et al.* (1993). Another term used by herpetologists is 'preferred optimum temperature zone' (POTZ) or 'preferred optimum temperature range' (POTR) and published data are available on the POTZ for numerous species of reptile, some of which may be kept in laboratories (Rossi 2006).

It is important under laboratory conditions to ensure that the temperature of different areas in the reptile's environment is properly monitored and recorded. Maximum and minimum thermometers are the basic tools but digital thermography is increasingly being used (Fleming *et al.* 2003). Thermostats are an important item in any reptile house and should be pulse-proportional so as to regulate energy flow to the heat source.

Behavioural interactions

Many species of reptile are territorial, and when group housed they may form dominance hierarchies. In nature, animals with low status can usually flee to alternative locations. This option is not available in a small cage, and low-status individuals may be subject to chronic stress (see later) and sustain physical injury. They may be excluded from basking, feeding or retreat sites, and as a consequence fail to thrive. It follows that great care must be exercised if potentially territorial reptiles are kept together in cages. There are, however, measures that can be taken to reduce agonistic interactions. Enriching the environment by increasing complexity and installing refugia (see later) can ensure that individuals encounter one another less frequently, and may actually reduce territory size in some species, eg *Anolis aeneus* (Eason & Stamps 1991). Providing multiple basking and feeding sites and non-communal retreats may also minimise aggression.

Special senses

Most reptiles other than snakes have colour vision and some can sense the near ultraviolet (UV) (Fleishman *et al.* 1993). All chelonians and many lizards have a parietal eye (pineal organ) situated at the top of the head which is connected to the pineal organ. This has a lens and a retina, but because it lies beneath the scales, cannot form an image. It responds to the wavelength and intensity of light and seems to be concerned with rhythmic behaviour, seasonal reproductive cycles and thermoregulation.

All terrestrial reptiles can respond to vibrations (an important consideration in the positioning of cages as proximity to electrical and other equipment may have adverse effects), and many can hear. Few reptiles vocalise, an exception being some species of gecko. Even the sounds made by copulating tortoises may serve as communication (Galeotti *et al.* 2005).

There are other aspects of reptile senses that differ from those in mammals. Direct olfaction is not well developed, but lizards and snakes have forked tongues, the tips of which can be inserted into the paired organs of Jacobson at the top of the palate. This provides a kind of 'touch–smell' sense, and enables the animals to obtain detailed information about the immediate environment and to make extensive use of communication by pheromones. Such communication is often important in mediating social behaviour (Mason 1992; Alberts *et al.* 1994a) and physiology (Alberts *et al.* 1994b). The 'touch–smell' sense may also enable reptiles to detect the presence of other species, including potential predators and possible prey. Discrimination using this sense can be subtle. Many snakes can use chemical cues to follow the 'trails' of prey, and this is particularly important for those venomous species that track envenomated victims until they die – so-called 'strike-induced chemosensory searching'. Pythons and some other snakes have small pits on the side of the head that are sensitive to infrared radiation, and enable them to sense the presence of warm-blooded prey.

UV radiation can be important in social behaviour (Fleishman *et al.* 1993). There is evidence, for example, that secretions from the femoral glands of some desert iguanas selectively absorb longwave UV radiation; deposits from these glands left in the environment will be very obvious to another individual (Alberts 1989; Alberts *et al.* 1994a). Chin glands in certain chelonians may play a similar role (Alberts *et al.* 1994b).

Size and lifespan

Adult reptiles range in size from lizards that measure 40 mm or less in length and weigh less than 1 g, to snakes that are more than 9 m in length (eg, *Python reticulatus*, *Eunectes murinus*). The largest lizards (*Varanus komodoensis*) reach 3 m in length, and have a body mass of up to 160 kg.

In general, smaller reptiles live for shorter periods than do larger ones. Small lizards characteristically have a maximum longevity of 10 years; larger lizards may live for more than 30 years. Pythons and boas can also live for more than three decades, but the potential longevity of most other snakes is not known. Small species of tortoise have a life-expectancy of 20 years; larger species more than 100. Reptiles are likely to survive longer in captivity than they would in the wild.

Hibernation and aestivation

Some species of reptile hibernate, others will undergo periods of aestivation when environmental conditions are hot, dry and adverse.

The physiology of hibernation (brumation) is complex and some examples draw attention to the remarkable resilience of certain reptile species to hypoxia (Jackson 2002).

There is much published advice on how best to prepare reptiles, mainly tortoises, for hibernation (see, eg, McArthur *et al.* 2004a). Under laboratory conditions, however, these and other species are usually kept awake during the cold months and not allowed to hibernate (see, eg, Arbour *et al.* 2007), apparently without any adverse effects on health and welfare.

Sex determination and reproduction

Most reptile species (all chelonians and crocodilians, most lizards and some snakes) lay eggs. Some lizards and certain snakes, particularly but not exclusively those that inhabit cold climates (eg the European common lizard, *Lacerta vivipara)* or high altitudes where incubation of eggs may be retarded (eg certain Central African chameleons) produce live young. In such taxa the eggs are retained in the oviducts until the young are ready for independent existence. Reptiles that produce live young are usually termed 'viviparous' or 'live-bearing' but the word 'ovoviviparous' is sometimes also used.

Fertilisation, in reptiles, is internal, and may follow elaborate courtship behaviour (Hernandez-Divers 2001). Male lizards and snakes have two intromittent organs, the hemipenes: chelonians have one hemipenis (phallus).

Some species of reptiles are sexually dimorphic, showing distinct colour, markings, size or anatomical features such as the presence of femoral pores in certain lizards (Schumacher 2003).

Distinguishing the sex of monomorphic species or (of almost all) juvenile reptiles, can be difficult but various methods can be used (Denardo 2006a). In snakes scale counts often help (male snakes usually have a longer tail, with more subcaudal scales, than do females) and even a sloughed skin can be used to determine this (Cooper & Cooper 2007) (Figure 46.4).

'Cloacal probing', using a slender, blunt object of suitable size, is the most frequently employed technique for the sexing of snakes and the larger lizards. If the probe cannot be advanced when gently directed caudally from the cloaca, the animal is female. In males the probe will enter a sulcus which contains an invaginated hemipenis (Frye 1991). Probing is used routinely by herpetologists but the technique needs to be properly learned if damage to animals is to be prevented. Probing is often taught using a freshly dead reptile.

As discussed in more detail in the section on reproduction, sex determination in some species, such as sea turtles, is temperature-dependent (Ewert *et al.* 1994), and this has to be borne in mind when incubating eggs under laboratory conditions. Egg-laying female reptiles usually bury their eggs in soil or sand, or lay them in crevices in rock or bark. Eggs of most species are oval or round in shape and are surrounded by a shell, which may be hard as a result of impregnation with calcium salts, or soft and leathery. In nature the site at which the eggs are laid is important. Protection from predators is necessary but the temperature will affect the rate of development and, in some species, the sex of the offspring. Relative humidity is also relevant. If it is too low, the eggs will dehydrate; if too high, they will drown or become infected by fungi or bacteria.

Laboratory management

General

Reptiles are adept at escaping from cages and enclosures. Many species climb or burrow and, by flattening their bodies, can squeeze through small holes or cracks.

The Council of Europe has provided recommendations for minimum housing standards for reptiles used in research (Council of Europe 2006). Some reptiles can be kept satisfactorily in large aquaria, wooden cages with a glass panel or open-topped wooden or fibreglass containers. Certain species appear to require such cages to be only very simply furnished in order to thrive – a *'clinical habitat'* (Varga 2004) that lends itself well to laboratory research. Others need more specialised accommodation, and may thrive better if the internal construction and 'furnishing' of the cage bear some relationship to their normal environment – a *'natural-*

istic habitat' (Varga 2004). Thus, sand-burrowing lizards (eg, *Chalcides ocellatus*) remain in far better condition if they have sand in which to burrow, as do arboreal species when provided with branches on which they can climb, for example most *Anolis* lizards. Species that are 'sit-and-wait' predators (eg, many species of snakes and geckos), and herbivorous reptiles, usually need little space. Some species, such as most lizards in the families Lacertidae and Teiidae, will be restricted by smaller cages. In these, they often spend much of their time trying to get out, possibly suggesting that a motivation to range is being thwarted. This has been linked with poor welfare in mammals (Clubb & Mason 2003). The immediate action should be to provide such species with more space but it is important to realise that, in contrast to the situation in other taxa, scientific data on the significance of escape-like behaviour in reptiles is sadly lacking.

Handling and restraint

Competent handling and restraint are as important for reptiles as they are for other species of laboratory animals. Training of staff is highly desirable and in some countries, such as the UK, may be mandatory before appropriate licences are issued. Inexperienced research workers can learn much from herpetologists.

Smaller lizards and snakes can usually be rested, or restrained gently, on the hand for routine inspection or movement from one cage to another. Many species of snake will support themselves if allowed to move from hand to hand. When restraint of snakes and lizards is necessary, they should be grasped firmly behind the head while supporting the body. Support is particularly important for snakes and legless lizards which become damaged or stressed if they are allowed to 'dangle'. Guidance on handling venomous snakes is provided in Locke (2008). Care must be taken with lizards to ensure that the tail is not grasped or pinned, since certain species can spontaneously shed it (autotomy) (Bellairs & Bryant 1985). Some geckos are particularly fragile; they not only shed their tails extremely readily but their skin is only loosely attached, so that it easily tears away from the underlying tissue.

Large lizards, such as iguanas and monitors, have a powerful, possibly toxic (see later), bite and can also inflict damage with their tail and claws. It is a wise precaution to use leather gloves when handling them.

Chelonians can usually be handled by grasping the 'shell' (carapace and plastron) and land tortoises, in contrast to many species of terrapin and turtle, rarely bite. Restraint of tortoises in order to carry out procedures is less easy. It may be possible to grasp the animal's head but sometimes light anaesthesia is required to facilitate this and other investigative techniques.

Training and habituation of captive reptiles can facilitate handling and thereby minimise stress to both animal and personnel.

Species used in the laboratory

Reptiles of various species are kept in laboratories. Table 46.1 lists some that are used widely for research, and which are relatively easy to obtain, maintain and breed. Most of them and certain others can be obtained as captive-bred animals. A very few species of captive-bred terrestrial reptile are produced commercially specifically for research purposes – *Anolis carolinensis*, for example. Other species that are not listed are regularly bred in captivity as part of conservation projects or for the pet trade.

Whenever possible, reptiles for research should be captive-bred and obtained from reliable sources. On occasion, however, animals need to be taken from the wild – either because they are not available as captive-bred specimens or because the research is specifically concerned with free-living reptiles – for example, reintroduction or translocation conservation projects.

It is essential to adhere to relevant legislation. Even common and widespread species of reptile may be covered by national laws, requiring (for example) a licence to take them from the wild or to retain them in captivity. Special legislation may apply to venomous snakes and lizards. International regulations may also be relevant, in particular the Convention on the International Trade in Endangered Species of Wild Fauna and Flora (CITES). Many species are covered by this Convention which controls 'trade' (movement) of live and dead organisms and their derivatives, including blood samples and tissues for DNA analysis (Cooper *et al.* 2006).

Reptiles and other ectothermic vertebrates have played a significant part in scientific research. Cooper (1977) reviewed the role of such species and stressed that they can serve as useful models for studies on the origin and aetiology of human diseases.

Some indication of the value of terrestrial reptiles in research is given in Table 46.1. Lizards have been extensively used in studies of biological rhythms and seasonal cycles (Underwood 1992), control mechanisms for reproductive cycles and comparative endocrinology (Moore & Lindsey 1992), neuroethology (Crews & Gans 1992), regeneration processes (Bellairs & Bryant 1985), brain chemistry, neuropeptide neurotransmitters (Reiner 1992), evolutionary aspects of exercise physiology (Garland 1994) and growth and longevity (Roitberg & Smirina 2006).

Vipers, mambas and cobras are frequently kept in laboratories for the production of venom, or to study the pathological effects of such toxins. The pit organs of some vipers and pythons have been widely studied.

Tortoises have been used in studies of sensory physiology, leading to a better understanding of pain in these animals (Rosenberg 1972) and contributing to the development of what would appear to be more humane methods for euthanasia (Cooper *et al.* 1984; UFAW/World Society for the Protection of Animals (WSPA) 1989, WSPA 1994). Tortoises are popular subjects for research on *Salmonella* and other bacterial pathogens (eg, Arbour *et al.* 2007).

In many parts of the world lizards, snakes and tortoises are kept in laboratories for teaching students and for simple, non-invasive, studies on nutrition, growth or reproduction. All such animals deserve the highest level of care. An important prerequisite is an understanding of the natural history and biology of the species. For some there may be extensive published information – *Iguana iguana*, for example (Jacobson 2003). For others, data may be sparse or largely anecdotal.

Table 46.1 Some terrestrial reptile species that are frequently kept in laboratories.

Scientific name	Common English name	Studies for which the species is commonly used	Reference
Lizards			
Anolis carolinensis	American anole	A wide range of physiological topics, especially neuroethology and colour change	Harling (1994)
Chalcides ocellatus	Eyed or ocellated skink	A wide range of physiological topics	Wisniewski (1992)
Chamaeleo spp.	Chameleons	Colour change, sensorimotor coordination of eyes and tongue	Townson (1994)
Eublepharis macularius	Leopard gecko	Skin grafts, temperature-dependent sex determination	Thorogood & Whimster (1979), Wisniewski (1992)
Gekko gecko	Tokay gecko	Eye and brain	Wisniewski (1992)
Iguana iguana	Common or green iguana	Metabolism and physiology	Frye (1993), Divers (1995)
Podarcis muralis and *P. sicula* (and other small lacertid lizards)	European wall lizards	Neurotransmitters, physiology of endogenous rhythms, endocrinology	Langerwerf (1990; 1991), Harling (1993) Townson (1994)
Pogona spp.	Bearded dragons	Endocrinology	Sheriff (1988)
Tiliqua spp.	Blue-tongued skinks	A wide range of physiological topics	Rose (1992), Townson (1994)
Snakes			
Elaphe spp.	Corn and rat snakes	A wide range of physiological topics	Bartlett (1993)
Lampropeltis spp.	King snakes	A wide range of physiological topics	Edwards (1991)
Thamnophis spp.	Garter snakes	Various; especially muscle physiology, reproductive endocrinology, physiology of hibernation	Sweeny (1993)
Tortoises			
Terrapene carolina	Carolina box turtle	Sensory physiology	
Testudo graeca and *T. hermanni*	European tortoises	Physiology of the pineal and associated organs	Jackson (1991), British Chelonia Group (undated)

Temperature and thermoregulation

Many nocturnal geckos and lizards and snakes from the leaf litter or lower levels of tropical rain forests do not routinely thermoregulate. Ideally, they require air temperatures that equate with their natural environments. However, during the day some species warm themselves by (for example) pressing themselves on to the warm rock under which they live and then use the heat obtained to help sustain them at night. Most species of reptile do, however, need to thermoregulate and this can be accommodated under laboratory conditions by providing a diversity of substrate temperatures, using heating pads, lamps or other sources of surface warmth. The provision of radiant heat from a small tungsten bulb enables many species to bask in the light and heat, treating it as though it is natural sunshine. Sources of heat that produce only infrared radiation, such as ceramic bulbs, are usually, but not necessarily, less suitable as they do not provide light, which many basking reptiles use as a cue to prompt thermoregulation. Larger incubator bulbs that give out yellow light are suitable for bigger reptiles (but not those which emit visible light mostly in the red part of the spectrum). The bulb should be positioned so that the animal can approach close enough to be able to warm fairly readily, but not so near that it will burn (Mader 2006a) either from the infrared radiation itself or from a substrate that has been heated by the radiation.

Care must be taken that laboratory cages do not become too hot. There must be areas that are sufficiently cool to enable the reptiles to lose heat as well as to gain it. This can often be achieved by placing the bulb(s) at one end of the cage. The heat should not be switched on for too long; 8–10 h per day is ideal for most species. The longer there is heat provided, the more protracted the period for which the reptile maintains its activity temperature and the greater its metabolic expenditure. Various papers, mainly relating to studies on captive and free-living European common lizards (*Lacerta vivipara*), describe research that is relevant to the care of this and possibly other species under laboratory conditions (Avery 1984, 1994). Avery (1984) has suggested that relatively short daily exposure to radiant heat minimises the risk of respiratory disease caused by the bacterium *Aeromonas*, whilst Guillette *et al.* (1995) postulated that the daily period for which radiant heat is available may affect the immune system.

The air temperature when the heating bulb is switched off may be allowed to vary: this corresponds to the situation in all but the most stable of tropical climates. There is often a tendency to keep the background temperature too high and this may be deleterious for species from desert or montane environments, where high solar radiation during the day can be followed by cool nights. Successful captive husbandry and breeding in environments in which temperatures were carefully controlled and monitored was reported in relation to the Malagasy panther chameleon, *Chamaeleo pardalis* (Ferguson 1994). Similar data are required for other species and those who keep reptiles under laboratory conditions are in a particularly strong position to carry out the necessary studies.

Light

Light appears to be less important to reptiles than is heat. In general, natural light (in which the greatest energy is in the blue part of the spectrum) usually results in better survival, growth and reproduction than does artificial light (which usually peaks in the yellow), although the reasons for this are not fully understood (Gehrmann 2006). There is some evidence that the duration of the daily photoperiod may be an important factor, controlling reproductive cycles in many species (Avery 1994), and this must be taken into account by those wishing to breed reptiles in captivity.

Ultraviolet radiation

The importance of UV radiation for many species of reptiles has already been emphasised. When exposure to natural sunshine is not practicable, artificial UV radiation must be supplied. A wide range of fluorescent tubes that will provide this are available commercially. While both middle (UV-b) (290–320 nm) and long (UV-a) (315–400 nm) wavelength UV appear to be important to reptiles, it is the former that is of prime importance in converting vitamin D; UV-a is believed to be more of value in encouraging recognition of food and mates (Rossi 2006). It remains true, however, that despite many reports of UV radiation resulting in improved reproduction in captive reptiles (mainly lizards), most studies remain empirical (Gehrmann 1994).

There are several important considerations when using UV sources:

1. UV emission from fluorescent tubes usually decreases with time; the tubes have a relatively short useful life.
2. Exposure must be direct: normal glass blocks UV radiation.
3. The intensity of UV radiation declines rapidly, so the tubes must be close to the animals.
4. Broad-spectrum tubes (designed to mimic daylight or sunlight) are of limited usefulness.
5. Tubes designed to improve plant growth (which have peak emission in the blue part of the spectrum) usually emit little UV radiation.
6. Fluorescent and mercury vapour sunlamps, sometimes used for tanning in humans, emit a wide range of UV wavelengths, but may damage the retinae or skin of both reptiles and laboratory personnel. They are best avoided.

Relative humidity

Laboratory environments often have drier air than the microhabitats of free-living reptiles. This may prove deleterious, even to desert species, as these spend much of their natural lives in humid burrows. The relative humidity in rooms housing reptiles, or in individual cages, can be increased in many ways. Spraying the inside of cages with water from a mist nozzle is effective but, unless it is automated, can be labour-intensive. One very simple measure is to furnish cages with living plants, transpiration will then add water to the local atmosphere. High humidity zones can be created within the cage by the use of 'humidity boxes', usually made of plastic (Rossi 2006). On a larger scale, dripper systems and waterfalls can be used.

Various diseases of the skin, scales, the shell in tortoises, and the respiratory system, may be induced or exacerbated by too high or too low humidity (Cooper 2006). In the case of the latter, Gram-negative bacteria such as *Aeromonas* and *Pseudomonas* and certain fungi are likely to multiply excessively under damp conditions (Frye 1991).

Limited data are available on the humidity requirements of reptiles: much of the available information is based upon observational and anecdotal evidence. This is another field which would benefit from input from those who work with reptiles in the laboratory.

Ventilation and air changes

Optimum ventilation for laboratory reptiles can be difficult to achieve. Too little ventilation results in inadequate diffusion of oxygen into, and carbon dioxide out of, a cage and can also increase humidity, leading to condensation. Too much ventilation, on the other hand, can make it difficult to control the temperature and keep the relative humidity high. The optimum ventilation for a particular cage design must sometimes be determined by trial and error; there is increasingly a tendency to specify the number of air changes in order to conform with research protocols and, ostensibly, to promote health and welfare. These are not necessarily the most appropriate for a given species (Cooper & Williams 1995).

Environmental enrichment

Many species of terrestrial reptiles can be kept successfully in relatively plain cages; provided that the space is adequate for reasonable movement, such containment seems to satisfy their behavioural requirements although there is an absence of research in this area. As discussed earlier, however, some species thrive better in cages or enclosures that mimic the natural environment (Figure 46.5). The welfare of the reptile is likely to be enhanced if accommodation is appropriate to the species (Varga 2004).

There are many species of reptile that clearly benefit from environmental enrichment. When, for example, small European lacertid lizards are kept in plain unfurnished cages, they tend to spend long periods motionless, often basking at length beneath the bulb that is provided for thermoregulation. Creating an area of spatial diversity, even simply by adding a number of wooden blocks, results in a dramatic change in behaviour. The lizards then bask for only relatively short periods, interspersing this with periods of movement (presumably looking for food) amongst the blocks, behaviour that is much closer to that seen in the field (Avery 1994).

Training and habituation

Training and habituation of reptiles is possible to a limited degree. It may facilitate procedures and reduce risks to staff. For example, lizards can be taught to feed at the same location each day. Snakes can learn by association and some species, eg, iguanas, recognise cause and effect relationships. Habituation has been studied in some reptiles (Xavier *et al.* 2006) but needs further research.

The importance of 'good stockmanship' cannot be overemphasised. Those who tend captive reptiles, especially technicians, should exhibit an empathy with their charges and, preferably, have personal experience of herpetology.

Refugia (hiding places)

Most species of reptiles, like almost all metazoan animals, have periods of the day when they are active. When they are not active, they seek some kind of refuge – in burrows, under rocks or in crevices, high in trees, or amongst dense vegetation (many terrestrial chelonians). Failure to provide a refuge for captive reptiles may be stressful (Hernandez-Divers 2001). The problem appears never to have been systematically investigated.

In contrast to physiological measures of stress, which have received some preliminary study (Guillette *et al.* 1995; Kreger & Mench 1993), there is as yet no totally reliable behavioural means of defining or measuring stress in the diverse species of reptile (Greenberg 1995; Warwick *et al.* 1995). Captive reptiles should always be provided with a refuge that mimics places where they would hide in nature. Given a choice, snakes prefer an opaque refuge to one with transparent walls, although the latter are more convenient from the standpoint of the reptile-keeper (Chiszar *et al.* 1987). It is best not to disturb individuals in the refuge except in extreme necessity. For similar reasons, as a general rule, it is preferable not to alter the internal arrangements of a cage once an individual has become familiar with it, especially under laboratory conditions where standardisation of procedures is so important. This is because many reptiles learn the immediate topography of their enclosure and can become stressed when it alters (Chiszar *et al.* 1995). On the other hand, many herpetologists and veterinarians would argue that a novel environment can encourage chemosensory behaviour and thereby promote welfare. The relationships between refugia and other elements of cage design are important. Small lacertids such as European wall lizards (*Podarcis muralis*), for example, behave more naturally if one or more of the refuges is placed near to their basking places (Avery, unpublished observations).

Hygiene

It is usually a basic tenet of captive management of animals that cages should be cleaned regularly in order to minimise build-up of parasites or other pathogens. This can be particularly important where infections might compromise research. Hygiene is also important to reduce the risk of spread of zoonotic infections. However, there are indications that cage-cleaning for certain reptiles should not be too frequent. Some of the chemicals in faeces can act as pheromones and may be used for communication. Some snakes, for example, thrive less well in clean cages than in cages containing some faeces and leaving a small amount of faecal material in a cage every time it is cleaned reduces the incidence of escape behaviour (Chiszar *et al.* 1980). In contrast, certain species of gecko avoid contact with their own faeces, probably to mimimise exposure to parasites (Brown *et al.* 1998).

Disinfection of cages should be preceded by through cleaning. The choice of a disinfectant is important. Some can be toxic, especially to small reptiles. Disinfectants have different modes of action (Slomka-McFarland 2006). Under circumstances where quality disinfectants are unavailable or prohibitively expensive, hot water is an easy and cheap alternative, preferably followed by drying in the sun or in a hot-air oven.

There is evidence for some mammalian species that irregular husbandry can be a stressor. While there are few equivalent unequivocal data for reptiles, consideration should be given to regular cleaning routines.

Diet and feeding

Reptiles as a class eat a variety of foods though many species have narrow food preferences. Lizards are predominantly carnivorous (a few species are herbivorous), and snakes are almost entirely carnivorous. Chelonians vary: as a general rule, terrestrial species (land tortoises) are primarily vegetarian while freshwater aquatic species (terrapins) are carnivorous. Calvert (2004) provides a useful and succinct review of the nutrition of captive reptiles.

Reptiles have relatively low metabolic rates and high net food-conversion efficiencies. Over-feeding is often as much of a problem as under-feeding, and can lead to a range of pathological conditions (see later). Small and medium-sized lizards, and most chelonians, need feeding daily. Large lizards and many snakes should be fed less frequently: some large snakes probably feed in nature less than once per week or once per month. The essential requirements are a regime and diet that will ensure the maintenance of bodyweight in non-breeding adults, and normal growth by juveniles. Many reptiles cease feeding spontaneously from time to time, especially just prior to skin-shedding.

Many insectivorous and carnivorous reptiles feed only on items that are moving. Live vertebrates should not be used as food unless there is no alternative (see later) and even invertebrates should be used in a way that is sensitive to the fact that they too are living animals. There are many methods to simulate the movement of non-living prey: these include placing them in a Petri dish on an automatic shaker, or employing tongs to shake the prey, or dragging the food item around the vivarium so as to create a scent trail for the snake/lizard to follow.

Some snakes refuse to feed in captivity. They can be force-fed (Cooper & Jackson 1981), often now referred to as 'assisted feeding', but it is preferable to try to coax them to feed spontaneously first. One technique, often successful with pythons and boas, is to condition them always to feed in the same place, which may be marked with scent of potential prey from time to time to reinforce the association. Other ruses include hiding the food in a tube or another unexpected location.

Most authorities concur that the diets of captive reptiles should be as varied as possible, as this helps to reduce nutritional disorders that are so commonly encountered in captivity (Frye 1991, 1994, 1996; Calvert 2004). This injunction applies to herbivorous as well as insectivorous or carnivorous species. Because tortoises, iguanas and other herbivorous reptiles feed with apparent relish on soft leaves and fruits, it is sometimes not appreciated that their diets in nature are usually very varied, and often include insects, molluscs and other invertebrates which may be swallowed deliberately or accidentally and usefully contribute to the animal's nutrient intake.

Insectivorous reptiles will often take only living prey. Invertebrates can be purchased from dealers who breed the animals for the pet trade or propagated within the laboratory animal facility. It is important to ensure that such animals are from a reliable source and health checks on them may be advisable as they can be a source of infection, including iridoviruses that can affect both invertebrates and reptiles (Marschang *et al.* 2005).

The most commonly used cricket is *Acheta domestica*, but species that do not stridulate are increasingly becoming available and are often preferable in animal houses. Crickets that are not eaten within a few hours should be removed as they are nocturnal and are likely to nibble the appendages of lizards if allowed to remain in the cage and increase the risk of autoinfection with parasites. There may also be an ethical issue as far as the crickets are concerned.

Mealworms and are larvae of the beetle *Tenebrio molitor* are easy to breed, although other species are increasingly becoming available, including 'giant mealworms' which are suitable for larger species of reptiles. They should not form a major part of the diet of the diet of any reptiles, however, because they contain far too high a concentration of phosphorus ions relative to calcium ions. Sooner or later, reptiles fed a diet of mealworms succumb to disorders caused by mineral imbalance (Frye 1991, 1996). Many reptile keepers 'preload' or 'gutload' mealworms and other invertebrates with calcium, and sometimes other minerals, vitamins and plant material, by adjusting their diet immediately prior to using them as food. Finke *et al.* (2005) evaluated four dry commercial gut-loading products for improving the calcium content of crickets.

Invertebrate prey can also be dusted externally with minerals to increase dietary intake but care must be taken to ensure that the invertebrate is ingested quickly as some species, especially crickets, quickly groom and remove the dust.

An increasingly large range of dietary supplements is available commercially, some formulated specifically for reptiles. They all contain vitamin D and calcium; some are very finely ground, so that the particles adhere readily to the cuticle of invertebrate prey. Almost all captive reptiles need dietary supplementation: the only possible exceptions are those kept in large, open outdoor enclosures, with exposure to natural sunlight and a varied diet. In some studies and locations (eg, the tropics) it may be acceptable to allow the reptiles to eat insects that have flown into the enclosure from outside.

Many reptiles are susceptible in captivity to mineral deficiencies or imbalances. These may result from a faulty diet (Calvert 2004) or from insufficient exposure to appropriate ultraviolet radiation. There are four main reasons why problems associated with calcium arise so commonly:

1. Inadequate calcium in the diet.
2. Calcium: phosphorus ratio is too low.
3. A dietary deficiency of vitamin D_3.
4. Inadequate exposure to UV radiation, which in many species is necessary for dermal synthesis of cholecalciferol, the metabolic precursor of vitamin D. It is important to note that it is UV-b light in the range 290–320 nm, that is of prime importance in converting vitamin D. The amount of UV-b that is available to the reptile can be measured using an appropriate meter.

The value of natural (solar) lighting must not be overlooked. In many reptile collections in the tropics, including some used for research purposes, sunlight is the only source of UVB-b and the animals appear to fare very well.

Mineral deficiencies or imbalances can give rise to osteodystrophic disorders (Frye 1991), referred to by Mader (2006b) as the '*metabolic bone diseases*'. These are characterised by a range of skeletal lesions, fibrous osteodystrophy (Figure 46.6), impaired locomotion and, in chelonians, abnormalities of the carapace. Problems of mineral imbalances may also occur in larger reptiles fed on day-old chicks or rodents, especially when neonatal rodent pups ('pinkies') are used.

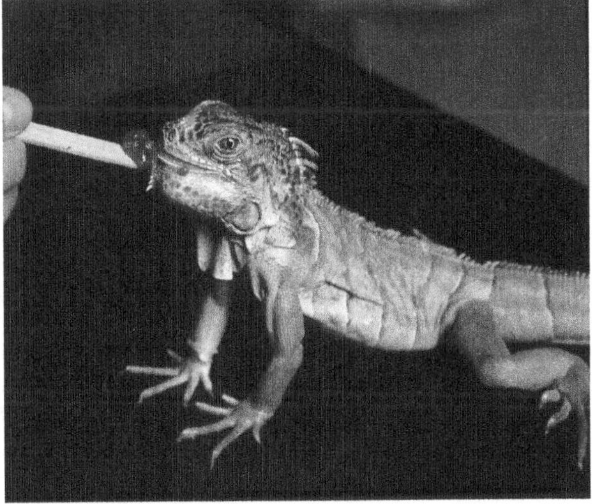

Figure 46.6 A green iguana (*Iguana iguana*) with metabolic bone disease. The swelling of the lower jaw is a sign of fibrous osteodystrophy. A balanced diet will usually prevent the development of this condition under laboratory conditions.

Various vitamin deficiencies are recognised or suspected in captive reptiles. Hypovitaminosis A was the first to be properly described and documented. In chelonians it can produce characteristic ocular lesions. Other effects may include retarded healing of wounds and predisposition to infectious diseases (Cooper *et al.* 1980). Studies have been carried out on the vitamin A requirements of some species – chameleons, for example (Abate *et al.* 2003).

It is not only a deficiency of vitamin A that can cause disease in captive reptiles. Hypervitaminosis A may result from excessive administration resulting in skin lesions (Cooper 2006).

In nature, most vertebrate prey is taken alive. The question of whether it is acceptable to feed living mammalian or avian prey to snakes and large lizards in captivity raises important ethical and sometimes legal issues. Many large reptiles will feed on dead animals; others quickly learn to do so. It is the animal that persistently refuses to feed on anything but living prey which creates a dilemma. Some authorities take the view that feeding living prey may be acceptable as a last resort (if the predator would otherwise starve to death) but that the prey animal should be removed from the cage immediately if the predator takes no interest in it, in the interests of both predator and prey. There are also legal considerations; however, in the UK, for example, the offering of live prey is not, *per se*, illegal but may provide grounds for a criminal action.

How much to feed laboratory reptiles is an important consideration (see earlier). Condition scores play a crucial part in monitoring nutritional status (see later).

Underfeeding will result in weight loss, 'poverty lines' and weakness. However, such findings can also be the result of providing an adequate but unsuitable diet, or because a reptile is unwell and unable to feed, or is unwilling to do so on account of stressors, including territorial or other aggression. Too low an ambient temperature or other adverse environmental factors may also be a cause of decreased feeding behaviour and food intake.

Over-feeding of captive reptiles can result in a range of pathological changes, including hepatic lipidosis (Divers & Cooper 2000). Some information on food intake of captive snakes in relation to body weight is provided by Kirkwood and Gili (1994).

Laboratory reptiles should always be provided with water. Dehydration can rapidly prove fatal in reptiles, in part because it leads to renal damage and the development of visceral gout (Figure 46.7). Some species will use water for bathing as well as for drinking. Snakes may immerse themselves in water when sloughing is imminent. How water is presented is important. Some lizards and chelonians will drown if they fall into a water container from which they are unable to escape. Chameleons will not usually drink from a waterbowl: they should be provided with water in the form of drops on foliage, using a spray.

Recognition and marking

The marking for identification of captive reptiles is important both for scientific and legal reasons (Cooper & Cooper 2007). It has long been recognised that many individual reptiles can be identified by a combination of their size, colour, pattern and, in certain lizards, the state of the tail (since this may have been broken off in the past, and be at various stages of regrowth). It is possible to build up databases of sets of pictures of individuals – eg, of the plastral markings of tortoises.

When individual reptiles cannot be recognised visually, it may be necessary to mark them. Methods for snakes were reviewed by Lang (1992). Clipping ventral scales is simple and effective, but the animal must usually be handled in order to see the marks. Implanted transponder tags, commonly termed microchips, are routinely used in zoos and in the pet trade in many countries and may be a legal requirement for certain species as part of enforcing legislation – eg, for tortoises that are traded in the European Union under EC Regulations 338/97 & 865/2006 (Cooper & Cooper 2007). Transponders hare also regularly used in field studies (Germano & Williams 1993). There are correct and incorrect methods of implanting microchips, most dictated by factors such as practicability and welfare, some by legal regulations. A useful review insofar as reptiles are concerned is to be found at the website of the British Veterinary Zoological Society[1].

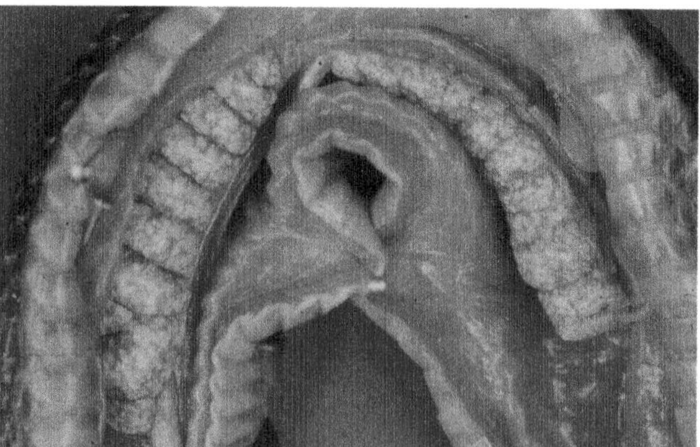

Figure 46.7 *Post-mortem* appearance of a Jamaican boa (*Epicrates subflavus*). The kidneys are white as a result of deposition of urates (visceral gout), possibly because of dehydration.

Welfare and welfare assessment

As a general rule, the application of the Five Freedoms will do much to promote the welfare of captive reptiles (Rayment-Dyble 2004). As with all species that are kept in the laboratory, the assessment of welfare of reptiles is of great importance. Over 20 years ago, guidelines for the recognition of pain, distress and discomfort in laboratory mammals were first formulated in the UK (Morton & Griffiths 1985). Little comparable advice appears to have been devised for laboratory reptiles, although very general criteria/guide-

[1]http://bvzs.org.uk

lines for recognising pain, distress and discomfort have been developed by WSPA (1994) and Warwick *et al.* (1995).

Some reptile behaviour is considered to be associated with stressors and stress (Hernandez-Divers 2001). Stereotypy, for example, is well recognised in captive reptiles: it has received little scientific attention in these species in contrast to the situation in domesticated mammals and birds (Mason & Rushen 2006).

There are limited data on the physiological effects of handling and restraining some species of reptile (eg, Kreger & Mench 1993). Chelonians readily defaecate when handled or contained and, indeed, these 'stress faeces' (Josseaume 2002) are used in some research studies.

A useful review of current thinking concerning stress in reptiles can be found in Denardo (2006b), and Hernandez-Divers (2001) provided a very useful introduction to reptile ethology, including examples of normal and abnormal behaviour patterns. Interactions between stress and other aspects of reptile metabolism were discussed by Guillette *et al.* (1995).

In summary, there is an urgent need for more research on the welfare of reptiles and the formulation of protocols to aid research workers, animal technicians and laboratory animal veterinarians.

Reproduction

General considerations

Breeding reptiles in captivity demands care and attention to detail, and is usually time-consuming (Wright 2004). Many species require either a natural seasonal regime of temperature and photoperiod (and occasionally also rainfall), or artificial regimes that mimic seasonality (Chiszar *et al.* 1994). Most temperate species require the 'priming' effects of cool-induced hibernation or quiescence in order to promote breeding, eg, *Lacerta vivipara* (Gavaud 1991). Social behaviour often has a modulating effect on the development of reproductive condition, for example in *Anolis* lizards. Successful reproduction may depend on the correct social context (Hernandez-Divers 2001). In the leopard gecko (*Eublepharis macularius*), for example, females will lay only if sexually mature males are present. In the American anole (*Anolis carolinensis*) courtship displays by males facilitate ovarian growth in females, whereas aggressive interactions, which may occur if more than one male is present, may inhibit ovarian development (Crews *et al.* 1994).

Most reptiles are oviparous. Under laboratory conditions the eggs should be removed immediately after laying, because they need a carefully controlled environment for successful development. In addition, the hatchlings may be eaten by the adults. Gecko eggs, however, should not be removed, because they are laid in such a way that they adhere to hard surfaces such as rocks or the walls of a cage. They can be protected by taping a small plastic container over them until they hatch. Temperature, substrate, substrate moisture and relative humidity of the surrounding atmosphere are particularly important. Unlike the eggs of birds, reptile eggs should not be moved or turned during incubation.

Role of temperature

All reptile species have an optimum temperature for incubation of their eggs. This is usually lower than the mean activity temperatures maintained by adults. Eggs incubated at temperatures that lie outside the optimum have lower levels of hatching success, and may be associated with developmental abnormalities (see later).

There are many species of reptiles in which the sex of an embryo depends not on sex chromosomes but on the temperature during the early stages of incubation (Table 46.2). Three general patterns are seen (Lance 1994):

1. Higher temperatures produce males, lower temperatures produce females; this applies in many species of lizards and in alligators.
2. The opposite effect: higher temperatures produce females, lower temperatures produce males eg, in many chelonians.
3. Intermediate temperatures produce males, higher and lower temperatures produce females. This occurs in the leopard gecko (*Eublepharis macularius*), the snapping turtle (*Chelydra serpentina*) and some crocodiles.

In most of the species that show temperature-dependent sex determination (TSD), the transition from production of one sex to production of the other takes place within a comparatively narrow range of temperatures (intersexes are rare). In American alligators (*Alligator mississippiensis*), however, intermediate temperatures result in the production of a mixture of males and females. The actual temperatures that are important for producing changes in the sex ratio vary from species to species, and sometimes geographically within a species. Fluctuating temperatures may produce different results from constant temperatures. Table 46.2 lists lizard species shown to exhibit TSD. Because of the com-

Table 46.2 Lizards, terrestrial chelonians and crocodilians that have unequivocally been shown to have temperature-dependent sex determination (TSD). There are many other species which are likely to have TSD. Most reptile species have not been studied in sufficient detail to know whether their sex determination is genetic, environmental or temperature-dependent. The data in this table are mostly from Ewert *et al.* (1994), Lang and Andrews (1994) and Viets *et al.* (1994).

Lizards	*Agama agama, A. caucasia* *Dipsosaurus dorsalis* *Eublepharis macularius* *Gekko japonicus* *Hemitheconyx caudicinctus* *Tarentola boettgeri* *Phelsuma madagascariensis*
Chelonians (terrestrial species)	*Testudo graeca, T. hermanni* *Terrapene ornata*
Crocodilians	*Alligator mississipiensis, A. sinensis* *Caiman crocodilus* *Crocodylus palustris, C. johnstoni, C. moreletti, C. niloticus, C. porosus, C. siamensis* *Gavialis gangeticus* *Paleosuchus trigonatus*

plexity of responses, no attempt has been made to provide crucial temperatures. The implications of TSD for the breeding of those reptile species in which it occurs are profound; in management programmes for sea turtles, sexing by endoscopy is increasingly being used to ensure an even mix of sexes when juvenile animals are returned to the sea.

Substrate

The eggs of many reptiles may be incubated on damp tissue paper, *Sphagnum* moss, peat, sand, polystyrene foam or other substrates. The medium most frequently used, however, is vermiculite. Made primarily for insulating buildings, vermiculite is cheap, relatively non-toxic and absorbent; it contains sufficient air-filled spaces among the granules that diffusion of air can readily take place. Whatever medium is employed, it should be used only once. There has been much discussion about the extent to which eggs should be buried in the substrate. Packard and Phillips (1994) recommended that eggs of species with flexible shells should be half-buried; those with rigid shells should be placed in small depressions at the surface of the medium.

Health and diseases

The aim in captivity is to provide reptiles with good welfare, of which physical health is a vital component. Under laboratory conditions it is particularly important to establish health profiles for the animals so as to help ensure consistency of research results, to detect early signs of disease and to promote welfare (see later). The diagnosis and treatment of reptile diseases are primarily the remit of the veterinarian, preferably one with experience of reptile medicine and surgery (Frye 1994). A useful table of differential diagnoses is to be found in an Appendix to the BSAVA Manual of Reptiles (Girling & Raiti 2004). The animal technician and research worker, who are familiar with the behaviour and natural history of the species, have an important part to play in health monitoring.

Health monitoring

Health monitoring involves the regular and routine investigation of live reptiles, *post-mortem* examination of any animals that die or have to be culled, and laboratory studies on samples from live reptiles, dead reptiles and their environment. Relatively little has been published on the health monitoring of laboratory reptiles but methods used for lizards, snakes, chelonians and other species in zoological collections and conservation programmes (Woodford 2001) can be usefully adapted. Cooper (1989) wrote a paper specific to laboratory reptiles and amphibians.

The exclusion of infectious disease is facilitated by the use of quarantine, whereby incoming reptiles are kept separately prior to their introduction to the colony. During this period the animals should be screened for pathogens and, if possible, health monitored. Subsequently, as in other fields of laboratory animal science, there is a need to maintain the reptiles' status by having efficient barrier systems, with rules to which all staff adhere.

An essential aspect of monitoring the health and, to a certain extent, the welfare of captive reptiles is the assessment of body condition. This is not always easy or straightforward; for example, some reptiles go through normal, cyclical, periods of fat deposition or loss. Essentially, however, body condition scoring (BCS) implies that laboratory reptiles are weighed and measured on a regular basis. How these data are processed may depend on the species: formulae are available for Mediterranean tortoises (eg, Jackson 1991; Hailey 2000; Willemser & Hailey 2002).

Newer books do not necessarily supersede older works. Often the latter contain sound, basic information which can be of great value to research workers and animal technicians. Scientific literature about reptile diseases goes back to the seminal work of Reichenbach-Klinke and Elkan (1965): although now over 40 years old, their book remains a useful guide to some aspects, especially parasite identification. More recent publications that provide up-to-date information on medical and surgical treatment include Frye (1991) and Mader (2006c). It is important to remember that not all relevant texts are in English. For example, excellent sources of information on lizards, snakes and tortoises are the relevant chapters in the German work *Krankheiten der Heimtier* (Gabrisch & Zwart 2005).

The effects of captivity on health

Captivity imposes physical, behavioural and physiological constraints on reptiles. Confinement in a relatively small space, often in close contact with others of the same species, can precipitate infectious or non-infectious disease and compromise welfare (Arena & Warwick 1995). This is an important ethical, often legal, consideration when reptiles are kept in laboratories. Examples of health problems that are due to, or exacerbated by, captivity are given later, under Non-infectious diseases.

The influence of temperature on health

The immune responses of reptiles, both humoral (production of antibodies) and cellular, are temperature-dependent and therefore less effective at lower temperatures (Guillette *et al.* 1995). Some species respond to bacterial (and perhaps other) infections, or the introduction of bacterial pyrogens, by spontaneously seeking higher body temperatures the so-called '*behavioural fever*' (Ramos *et al.* 1993). For these reasons, many authorities suggest that sick reptiles undergoing treatment should be kept warm or assisted in doing so by providing a temperature gradient and given the opportunity to maintain high body temperatures by basking for longer periods than usual (Frye 1991).

As mentioned elsewhere, adverse or fluctuating temperatures can affect the survival and health of neonatal reptiles. An increased prevalence of developmental abnormalities may be indicative of such a situation (Figure 46.8).

Non-infectious diseases

Reptiles kept in the laboratory are particularly prone to non-infectious disease, largely because they are confined in captivity and therefore more likely to encounter physical insults. The latter include trauma (physical damage to rostrum (Figure 46.9) or limbs, often associated with cage design or insensitive management), electrocution (from poorly maintained electrical circuits), burns (from proximity to badly positioned bulbs or heaters) and drowning (deep water containers from which lizards and chelonians, is particular, cannot escape). Non-infectious insults can readily lead to infectious disease – for example, a wound may become infected with bacteria.

One of the most common problems in captive reptiles is damage to the rostrum, caused by the animals colliding with the walls of the cage or enclosure, especially when they are trying to escape (a behaviour that can develop into a stereotypy). Attempts to reduce the incidence of such lesions include giving individuals as large a cage as is practicable, providing refugia (see above) and avoiding disturbance and stress whenever possible. Painting or otherwise marking vertical glass surfaces so that they are opaque can also sometimes reduce the incidence of collisions. Some materials are particularly damaging, eg, wire mesh, which should be screened with protective partitions made from other materials. Treatment is by cleaning the wound (Frye 1991) followed by standard medication and prevention of further trauma. Burns, usually caused by an animal being able to get to close to the hot surface of a bulb or heating pad, can also be treated (Mader 2006a). In lizards and snakes, that shed their skins regularly, the area of the burn can become a site of incomplete ecdysis and a focus for infection.

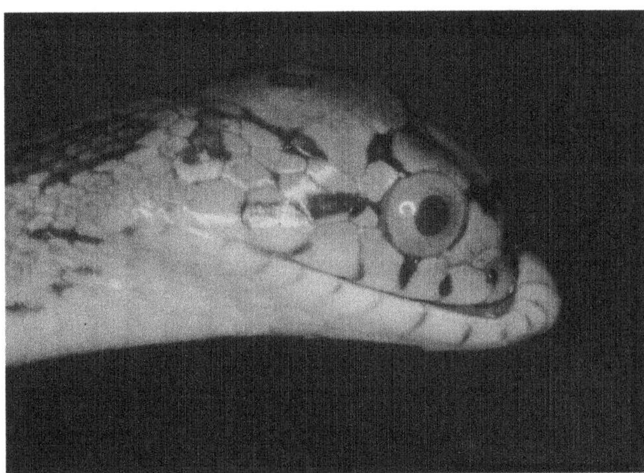

Figure 46.8 A developmental abnormality, an undershot jaw and hydrocephalus, in a captive-bred king snake (*Lampropeltis* sp.). Such anomalies can have a genetic aetiology, often associated with inbreeding, or follow temperature fluctuations during incubation.

Chelonians in captivity often have overgrowth of the highly keratinised edges to the mouth, because the diet is softer then that in the wild. Treatment is by burring the beak back to normal anatomy, and prevention by ensuring that the diet is as varied as possible and contains harder material, such as fibrous plants. Overgrowth of the claws, also caused by insufficient abrasion, may occur in chelonians and large lizards.

Snakes in captivity often fail to slough properly (dysecdysis – see earlier). There can be many reasons for this, including poor health, malnutrition, dehydration and endocrine imbalances caused by failure to provide the correct photothermal stimuli that cue seasonal cycles of reproduction and activity (Avery 1994). A dysecdytic snake can be helped to shed by soaking for about an hour in warm water.

Other non-infectious diseases include poisoning, genetic/congenital/developmental abnormalities and metabolic dosorders associated with old age and/or dietary imbalances. Poisoning can result from overdosage of medical agents, prolonged exposure to toxins (eg, insecticidal preparations) or ingestion of toxic material in the food (Fitzgerald & Vera 2006). Developmental abnormalities may be present at birth (congenital) or appear later in life. They may or may not have an underlying genetic basis. Environmental factors may play a part in producing some abnormalities, especially during incubation of eggs. All such anomalies should be investigated and documented and specimens retained for study (Bellairs 1981; Cooper *et al.* 1998).

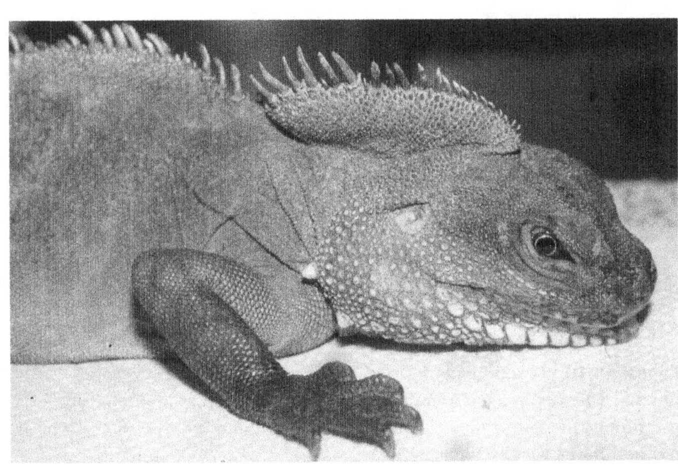

Figure 46.9 Chronic damage to the rostrum of a water dragon (*Physignathus* sp.) due to repeated rubbing on the glass sides of its cage.

Infectious diseases

Many infectious agents can cause morbidity (ill-health) or mortality (death) in captive reptiles. While some organisms appear to be frank pathogens, many others are opportunists that take advance of an injured or immunocompromised animal. Host–parasite relations are still poorly understood in reptiles but knowledge of these is often the key to the prevention or control of infectious disease. Experimental work on reptiles is yielding useful information about inflammatory and other responses in reptiles (Tucunduva *et al.* 2001).

Bacteria

Numerous pathological conditions in captive reptiles are caused by bacteria, especially Gram-negative species such as *Aeromonas* and *Pseudomonas* (Cooper & Jackson 1981). Pneumonia, often coupled with a septicaemia, is one such example. Necrotic stomatitis ('mouth rot') is another; it is not a single disease entity, but a syndrome that may be caused by a wide range of bacteria (Cooper & Sainsbury 1994). Necrotic dermatitis ('scale rot') shows a similar pattern, as does 'shell rot' in chelonians. 'Blister disease' of snakes and lizards, characterised by fluid-filled vesicles on the skin, is often a result of a non-infectious factor, adverse humidity: the lesions can quickly become secondarily infected by bacteria.

Subcutaneous abscesses are often seen in lizards and snakes and are usually due to bacteria (Figure 46.10). The pus of reptiles is semisolid, often laid down over several weeks in concentric layers, and needs to be removed surgically.

Salmonella is of particular importance under laboratory conditions because of the zoonotic risk (see later). The genus consists of over 2400 serotypes, a number of which (some termed 'Arizona' – *S. enterica arizonae*) may be isolated from captive reptiles, including those kept for research purposes, and may cause pathological lesions and clinical signs of disease (Cambre *et al.* 1980; Onderka & Finlayson 1985; Gene & Loeschner 2002).

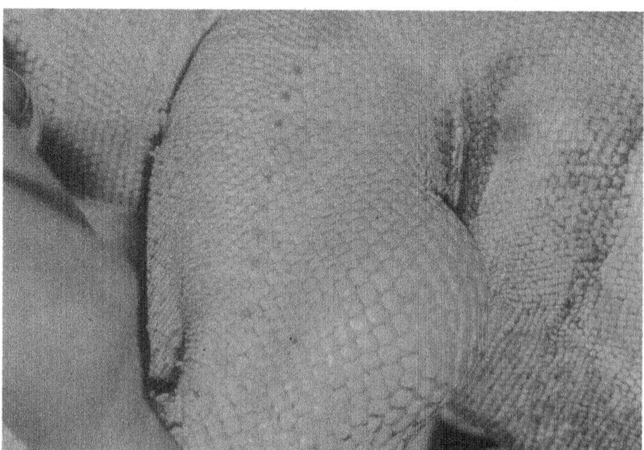

Figure 46.10 A subcutaneous abscess in the hindlimb of a green iguana. The pus in such a case is likely to be semi-solid and needs to be removed surgically. This is a male animal and the row of femoral pores is very apparent.

Many other bacteria may cause disease in captive reptiles (Cooper 1999) including *Neisseria* species, especially *N. iguanae* (Plowman *et al.* 1987; Barrett *et al.* 1994) and *Mycobacterium* species (Soldati *et al.* 2004).

Any breach in the skin may permit the ingress of bacteria which can then cause a localised infection, such as an abscess or cellulitis, possibly followed by bacteraemia and septicaemia, often with fatal results (Cooper 1999).

Most bacterial diseases may be treated with standard antibiotics following sensitivity testing and appropriate palliation (Rees Davies & Klingenberg 2004; Carpenter 2005; Mader 2006c). Reliable pharmacokinetic data are available on a number of antibacterial agents such as enrofloxacin (Young *et al.* 1997).

The eggs of reptiles may be infected with and may spread bacterial and other diseases. The *post-mortem* examination of reptile eggs was detailed by Cooper (2004).

Fungi

Austwick and Keymer (1981) provided a useful earlier review of mycotic infections of reptiles. Reports in recent years include those by Nichols *et al.* (1999), Bertelsen *et al.* (2005) and Paré and Sigler (2006). Fungal infections appear to be less prevalent in terrestrial reptiles than in aquatic species but the pattern is not straightforward, particularly as 'new' organisms, such as the *Chrysosporium* anamorph of *Nannizziopis vriesii* (CANV), become recognised as important emerging pathogens of reptiles (Paré & Sigler 2006).

Mycotic infections need to be diagnosed early, using a variety of clinical and laboratory techniques (Cooper 2006), as they are often difficult to treat successfully (Frye 1991).

Viruses

The importance of viral infections in reptiles began to be appreciated over 25 years ago (Clark & Lunger 1981). Since then great advances have been made, with a range of viruses recognised as causes of disease, in various parts of the world (Gravendyck *et al.* 1998; Marschang *et al.* 2002). A number of these are potentially important in the laboratory maintenance of terrestrial reptiles:

- paramyxoviruses, primarily in snakes but also in lizards (Jacobson *et al.* 2001);
- herpesviruses, in lizards, snakes and chelonians (Jacobson 2007);
- eastern equine encephalitis virus (EEEV) (Essbauer & Ahne 2001; Hernandez-Divers 2006);
- adenoviruses in lizards (Wellehan *et al.* 2004; Julian & Durham 1982);
- poxviruses (or pox-like viruses) in lizards and other reptiles (Stauber & Gogolewski 1990; Jacobson & Telford 1990; Gal *et al.* 2003);
- ranaviruses in tortoises, occasionally lizards and snakes (Essbauer & Ahne 2001; Just *et al.* 2001);
- erythrocytic viruses ('pirhemocyton' or 'toddia') in various reptiles (Paperna & Dematos 1993);

- papillomaviruses, mainly in lizards (Cooper *et al.* 1982; Raynaud & Adrian 1976);
- reoviruses of various reptiles (Gravendyck *et al.* 1998; Drury *et al.* 2002);
- Iridoviruses, possibly acquired from invertebrate prey (Marschang *et al.* 2005).

Captive reptiles can be screened serologically for certain viruses – for example, ophidian paramyxovirus (OPMV) and herpesviruses of chelonians (Mader 2006c). These and other tests, such as polymerase chain reaction (PCR), should be considered an important part of excluding infectious disease from laboratory colonies of snakes, lizards and chelonians.

Stomatitis associated with virus infections in tortoises have been successfully treated but the general rule in laboratory animal work should be to exclude such pathogens by obtaining reptiles from 'clean' captive-bred sources and by quarantining and screening incoming stock. The serological testing of snakes for evidence of paramyxovirus infection and PCR testing of chelonians for herpesviruses are two such examples.

Protozoa

Keymer (1981) provided an excellent review of protozoa of reptiles and Barnard and Upton (1994) produced a practical '*veterinary guide*' to many of these species. It should be noted that some intestinal protozoa are beneficial – for example, ciliates that aid digestion in tortoises and large herbivorous lizards (Troyer 1982).

Haematozoa (blood-borne protozoa) are not uncommonly seen in terrestrial reptiles, both in wild (free-living) and captive animals. Their classification remains uncertain, as does the understanding of their significance (Davies & Johnston 2000). Their presence in blood smears should be noted during routine health monitoring. Smears should be examined on two occasions, at least 14 days apart, during any quarantine period.

Entamoeba invadens has a direct life cycle, with cysts being passed in faeces. Meerovitch (1958, 1961) elucidated the life stages of this protozoon. She concluded that the parasite is usually a commensal in chelonians, where it ingests plant polysaccharides. In snakes *E. invadens* proves pathogenic because they are carnivorous and, in the absence of plant ingesta, the *Entamoeba* obtains its polysaccharide requirements from intestinal mucosal secretions, rendering the gut wall susceptible to invasion. It follows that, in laboratories, herbivorous and carnivorous/omnivorous reptiles should not be kept together and strict hygiene must be practised when moving from one reptile species to another.

The coccidian parasite *Cryptosporidium* is increasingly a problem in reptile collections – eg, in leopard geckos (Deming *et al.* 2008) – and is difficult to treat. It can be zoonotic (McArthur *et al.* 2004b).

Helminths and pentastomids

All of the major groups of parasitic worms are found in reptiles. Tapeworms (Cestoda) and flukes (Trematoda) are not usually a major problem in captive reptile husbandry, especially in the laboratory, as they require the appropriate intermediate host as part of their life cycle. The same is true of pentastomids which, although worm-like in appearance, are in fact highly modified arthropods. The life cycles of pentastomids are complex, and, depending on the species of parasite, a reptile may be a definitive or an intermediate host. Most infections of reptiles with pentastomes are asymptomatic (Greiner & Mader 2006).

In comparison, many species of nematodes have direct life cycles and these worms can increase rapidly under suitable conditions. A range of clinical signs and pathological lesions may be seen in infected reptiles. Treatment of the affected animal must be coupled with hygiene and other measures in order to prevent re-infection. Parasitic worms are readily treated with various anthelmintics but care must always be taken as adverse sequelae sometimes result. Ivermectin can be toxic to chelonians (Frye 1991) and should be employed with appropriate caution in all reptile species. Treatment during quarantine, coupled with microscopical examination of faeces, will help to limit and control nematode infestations in laboratory reptiles.

Ticks and mites

Ticks and other ectoparasites of reptiles can be pathogenic in their own right, causing local or systemic disease, or they may transmit other organisms (Burridge 2001). Ticks (Figure 46.11) can be removed with forceps, but care must be taken that the mouthparts do not remain because they may become a focus for infection with bacteria and other pathogens. Certain acaricides, such as permethrins, are effective in control but, as with all treatment under laboratory conditions, may be contra-indicated in reptiles that are part of an experimental procedure.

Mites, especially the 'snake mite', *Ophionyssus natricis*, can be the cause of ill-health or death in laboratory reptiles. Parasitic mites feed on blood, and can transmit viruses, spirochaetes, rickettsiae, bacteria and protozoa. The parasites and their eggs can survive in crevices in the environment for long periods.

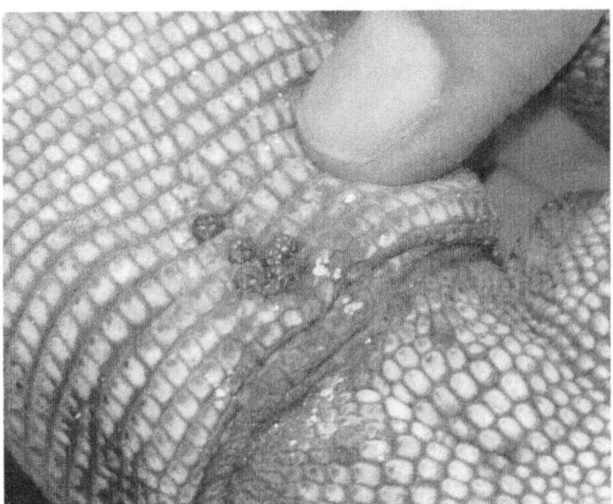

Figure 46.11 Cloacal region of a monitor lizard, showing the presence of tightly-attached *Amblyomma* ticks.

Small and medium-sized reptiles can be treated for mites by isolating them for 24h in a small cage with a strip of, for example, dichlorvos (Vapona) or trichlorfon, placed out of reach of the animal. However, care must be taken to avoid over-exposure and resultant toxicity, usually characterised by nervous signs. Alternatively, fipronil wipes can be used or ivermectin can be administered topically or by injection. Large reptiles can be treated with proprietary (dog and cat) flea sprays (Frye 1991) Under laboratory conditions, where the use of drugs that have a systemic effect may be contra-indicated, mites can be killed by painting the reptile with vegetable oil, which is then blotted off (Espinosa *et al.* 1998) or trapped with sticky tape and removed.

Routine treatment and quarantine of incoming animals will help to prevent the introduction of mites to a laboratory animal facility. Scrupulous attention to hygiene is then necessary to prevent treated animals from becoming re-infected.

Health and physiological monitoring

Standard veterinary procedures for reptiles are applicable to those that are kept for research. Imaging is practicable using radiography, ultrasonography, magnetic resonance imaging (MRI) and computed tomography (CT) scanning (Anderson *et al.* 2000; Raiti 2004).

Collection of samples and laboratory investigations

Samples may need to be taken from reptiles for research purposes, for health monitoring or for diagnostic purposes. Samples can be of many types. Some, such as faeces, can be collected without handling the reptile, while others, such as blood, will necessitate invasive techniques. The most appropriate methods will depend on many factors, including the temperament, size and anatomy of the reptile. Veterinary texts provide useful guidance (see, for example, Hernandez-Divers *et al.* 2004a).

Blood sampling can be an important part of research procedures involving reptiles. It is also a useful adjunct to health monitoring. Specific papers relating to laboratory work are available – eg, on blood sampling of lizards (Brown 2007) – while other texts refer more to pet, zoo and wild animals. Sampling sites depend upon the species and the requirements but include withdrawing blood from a vein (jugular, caudal/coccygeal, brachial, abdominal or subcarapacial), heart orbital sinus or via a toe-nail clip. An excellent review of methods, with clear photographs, is to be found in Hernandez-Divers (2006). However, in order to perfect techniques specific training is necessary, preferably under the supervision of an experienced veterinarian.

The amount of blood and frequency of sampling are important considerations in experimental work where regular bleeding may be part of the research protocol. In some countries, quantity and frequency may be stipulated in regulations designed to promote welfare. Where this is not the case, a general rule is not, on any one occasion, to remove a sample of blood that is more than 1% of the body weight of the animal. The author's personal guideline for repeat bleeding is to restrict the volume to 0.7% (ie 7ml of blood per kilogram body weight) and to take this amount from the reptile no more frequently than once a week.

Reference values

Reference values for blood parameters are available for some species (see, for example, Mader 2006c). These usually include both haematological and biochemical figures. There is a need to expand these databases and those scientists and laboratory animal veterinarians who need to take blood samples from reptiles for other purposes should, whenever possible, prepare smears and carry out haematological and biochemical analyses. Such information is not just of scientific importance: it can also enhance health monitoring and assist in the assessment of welfare.

Laboratory investigation of samples taken from reptiles are covered by a number of authors for example, bacteriology by Cooper (1999), haematology and cytology by Campbell and Ellis (2007) and haematology alone by Diethelm and Stein (2006).

Methods of treatment

Terrestrial reptiles may need to be treated with medicinal agents either as part of an experiment or for health reasons. Supportive care is always important and useful information is to be found in texts directed at veterinary nurses/technicians (Cooper *et al.* 2003; McBride & Hernandez-Divers 2004; Mitchell 2004). Emergency and critical care have been covered by a number of authors, eg, of chelonians by Norton (2005). Techniques for dosing and injection procedures are described in various publications (eg, Rees Davies & Klingenberg 2004). The dose and the frequency of administration of some agents may need to be based on allometric scaling (Mayer *et al.* 2006).

Telemetry

Telemetry is a well established procedure in field studies on reptiles and both invasive and non-invasive techniques for attaching a transmitter can be adapted to laboratory research (eg, Ferrell *et al.* 2005).

Surgical procedures

Both experimental and therapeutic surgery may be carried out on laboratory reptiles. These do not differ significantly from those employed in veterinary practice (Hernandez-Divers 2004a). Under laboratory conditions it is particularly important to minimise invasive techniques. Endoscopy, for example, can be used very successfully in reptiles and often reduces the need to perform traumatic, painful or stressful procedures (Brearley *et al.* 1991; Hernandez-Divers 2004a, 2004b).

Anaesthesia and analgesia

Anaesthetic methods for reptiles have advanced dramatically in recent years and much has been published in both books and journals (Redrobe 2004; Mosley 2005). Awareness of the susceptibility of reptiles to painful stimuli has prompted studies on analgesia (Greenacre *et al.* 2005). This information is of great relevance to the use of reptiles in research where procedures may be performed that may cause pain.

Euthanasia

Laboratory reptiles may need to be killed at the end of an experiment, or on welfare grounds because of injury, disease, or old age. Some nations may have local regulations regarding acceptable techniques. Euthanasia of terrestrial reptiles presents special problems (UFAW/WSPA 1989; Cooper 2004), on account of the low metabolic rates of many and the ability of some species to tolerate hypoxia for long periods (Jackson 2002). Useful resumés of methods of euthanasia for reptiles are given by WSPA (1994), British Veterinary Zoological Society (BVZS) (2003), Baier (2006) and Reilly (2001).

Decapitation and cervical dislocation are no longer standard methods, because of concerns that the animal may continue to be aware of painful stimuli for a period after the process. Nevertheless, in the UK, Schedule I of the Animals (Scientific Procedures) Act 1986 continues to permit the use of decapitation so long as it is followed immediately by physical destruction of the brain. Freezing is also no longer advocated by most authorities, again on welfare grounds. The exception is dropping small reptiles (of 1 cm maximum diameter) into liquid nitrogen (BVZS 2003). Other methods that are now considered unacceptable (BVZS 2003) include drowning, overdose of anaesthetic agents by certain routes and use of neuromuscular blockers.

The currently preferred techniques, where practicable, are an overdose of either an appropriate volatile agent, such as isoflurane, or of a barbiturate given by injection (Cooper 2004).

Zoonoses and other health hazards

Any laboratory animal can present a hazard to those who work with or tend it. The dangers may be infectious, physical or toxic. Pathogenic bacteria that may be transmitted from reptiles to humans include *Salmonella*, *Leptospira*, *Mycobacterium* and *Cryptosporidium* (Frye 1991; Johnson-Delaney 2006). *Salmonella* is always considered a particular hazard, although it is not easy to quantify the dangers, partly because so many serotypes or strains may be involved (Burnham *et al.* 1998).

Under laboratory conditions it is important to draw-up proper risk assessments (see next section). A useful summary of precautions, including reference to the BVZS Guidelines, was provided by Redrobe (2002). Handling animals using appropriate techniques (see Handling and restraint) will lessen the likelihood of physical injury.

A number of species of snake and two species of lizard have traditionally been considered venomous. However, recent research (Fry *et al.* 2006) on monitor lizards and iguanids indicates that other species have saliva which may cause tissue damage (in addition to infection) if the animal bites. It is important, therefore, to be aware of the identity of any snake or lizard that is to be kept in the laboratory. If in doubt, advice should be sought and full precautions put into place.

Details of techniques for keeping and handling venomous squamates are not included here: useful guidelines are provided by Boyer *et al.* (2003), Boyer (2004) and Whitaker and Gold (2006). These animals should be managed only by trained personnel and a proper risk assessment carried out. Venomous species should be handled with appropriate equipment, such as tongs or a snake-hook (Locke 2008). In order to restrain venomous snakes for radiography or injection, they may be induced to enter a rigid transparent plastic tube (Mader 2006c; Locke 2008), of a diameter equivalent to that of the snake. Once the snake is inside, the ends can be closed with bungs. For injection, tubes have small holes drilled at appropriate points so that a needle can be inserted. This technique should not be used for narrow-bodied venomous species such as kraits or mambas, as these may succeed in turning around within the tube.

Risk assessment

In any work involving laboratory reptiles it is important to carry out a risk assessment. There are five important steps:

1. identify the hazards (anything that may cause harm, such as the animals themselves, chemicals or electricity);
2. decide who might be harmed and how;
3. evaluate the risks (the chance, high or low, that somebody could be harmed and state what precautions are to be taken);
4. record the findings and implement them;
5. review the above and update as necessary.

More information may be found on the (UK) Health and Safety Executive website.

Other legal considerations

The importance of adhering to relevant legislation when keeping reptiles was emphasised earlier. In many countries reptiles are covered by laws that regulate the use of animals in research. Other statutes may also be relevant, including those concerning conservation of endangered species, welfare, dangerous wild animals and zoonoses (Cooper *et al.* 2006). Where there is no legislation controlling the maintenance and use of terrestrial reptiles for research, it is wise to use and follow established codes of practice. Sometimes specific guidelines are available for example, those produced for field research on reptiles in Canada (Canadian Council on Animal Care (CCAC) 2003) and the USA (ASIH/HL/SSAR 1987); if this is not the case or the guidelines are inappropriate, the researchers (in collaboration with others) should formulate and use their own.

Acknowledgements

My wife, Margaret E. Cooper, advised on the sections on legislation and risk assessment. Dr Adrian Hailey, Miss Kristel-Marie Ramnath and Mr Sean Wensley commented on an early draft of this contribution. Miss Nicole Theroulde typed the original manuscript and the Library of the Faculty of Medical Sciences, The University of the West Indies, helped with the references. Two anonymous referees made helpful comments. I am indebted to them all.

References

Abate, A.L., Coke, R., Ferfuson, G. *et al.* (2003) Chameleons and vitamin A. *Journal of Herpetological Medicine and Surgery*, **13**, 23–31

Alberts, A.C. (1989) Ultraviolet visual sensitivity in desert iguanas: implications for pheromone detection. *Animal Behaviour*, **38**, 129–137

Alberts, A.C., Jackintell, L.A. and Phillips, J.A. (1994a) Effects of chemical and visual exposure to adults on growth hormones, and behaviour of juvenile green iguanas. *Physiology and Behaviour*, **55**, 987–992

Alberts, A.C., Rostal, D.C. and Lance, V.A. (1994b) Studies on the chemistry and social significance of chin gland secretions in the desert tortoise, *Gopherus agassizii*. *Herpetological Monographs*, **8**, 116–124

Anderson, C.L., Kabalka, G.W., Layne, D.G. *et al.* (2000) Noninvasive high field MRI brain imaging of the garter snake, *Thamnophis sirtalis*. *Copeia*, **1**, 265–269

Arbour, E.K., Chacra, N.A., Gali-Mouhtaseb, H. *et al.* (2007) Performance, bacterial shedding and microbial drug resistance in two tortoise species. *Veterinary Record*, **161**, 62–65

Arena, P.C. and Warwick, C. (1995) Miscellaneous factors affecting health and welfare. In: *Health and Welfare of Captive Reptiles*. Eds Warwick, C., Frye, F.L. and Murphy, J.B., pp. 263–283. Chapman and Hall, London

ASIH/HL/SSAR (1987) *Guidelines for Use of Live Amphibians and Reptiles in Field Research*. USA. http://iacuc.ucsd.edu/PDF_References/ASIH-HL-SSAR%20Guidelines%20for%20Use%20of%20Live%20Amphibians%20and%20Reptiles.htm (accessed 03 January 2009)

Austwick, P.K.C. and Keymer, I.F. (1981) Fungi and actinomycetes. In: *Diseases of the Reptilia*. Eds Cooper, J.E. and Jackson, O.F., pp. 193–231. Academic Press, London

Avery, R.A. (1982) Field studies of body temperatures and thermoregulation. In: *Biology of the Reptilia 12. Physiology C. Physiological Ecology*. Eds Gans C. and Pough F.H., pp. 93–166. Academic Press, London

Avery, R.A. (1984) Physiological aspects of lizard growth: the role of thermoregulation. *Symposia of the Zoological Society of London*, **52**, 407–424

Avery, R.A. (1994) The effects of temperature on captive amphibians and reptiles. In: *Captive Management and Conservation of Amphibians and Reptiles*. Eds Murphy, J.B., Adler, K. and Collins, J.T., pp. 47–51. Society for the Study of Amphibians and Reptiles, Ithaca, New York

Baier, J. (2006) Reptiles. In: *Guidelines for Euthanasia of Nondomestic Animals*. pp. 42–45. American Association of Zoo Veterinarians, Florida

Barnard, S.M. and Upton, S.J. (1994) *A Veterinary Guide to the Parasites of Reptiles, Vol 1: Protozoa*. Krieger, Florida

Barrett, S.J., Schlater, L.K., Montali, R.J. *et al.* (1994) A new species of Neisseria from iguanid lizards, *Neisseria iguanae* sp. nov. *Letters in Applied Microbiology*, **18**, 200–202

Bartlett, R.D. (1993) Comments on the *obsoleta*-complex rat snakes of Florida (with mention of three extralimital forms). *Tropical Fish Hobbyist*, **41**, 120–137

Barten, S.L. (2006) Reference sources for reptile clinicians. In: *Reptile Medicine and Surgery*, 2nd edn. Ed. Mader, D.R., pp. 9–13. Saunders Elsevier, St. Louis

Bellairs, A.d'A. (1981) Congenital and developmental diseases. In: *Diseases of the Reptilia*. Eds Cooper, J.E. and Jackson, O.F., pp. 469–485. Academic Press, London

Bellairs, A. d'A and Bryant, S.V. (1985) Autotomy and regeneration in reptiles. In: *Biology of the Reptilia, Development B, volume 15*. Eds Gans, C. and Billett, F., pp. 301–410. John Wiley and Sons, New York

Bertelsen, M.F., Crawshaw, G.J., Sigler, L. *et al.* (2005) Fatal cutaneous mycosis in tentacled snakes (*Erpeton tentaculatum*) caused by the *Chrysosporium* anamorph of *Nannizziopsis vriesii*. *Journal of Zoo and Wildlife Medicine*, **36**, 82–87

Boyer, D.M. (2004) Special considerations for venomous reptiles. In: *BSAVA Manual of Reptiles*, 2nd edn. Eds Girling, S.J. and Raiti, D., pp. 357–362. British Small Animal Veterinary Association, Gloucester

Boyer, D.M., Ettling, J., Flanagan, J.P. *et al.* (2003) Venomous reptile handling. *Journal of Herpetological Medicine and Surgery*, **13**, 23–37

Burnham, B.R., Atchley, D.H., De Fusco, R.P. *et al.* (1998) Prevalence of fecal shedding of *Salmonella* organisms among captive green iguanas and potential public health implications. *Journal of the American Veterinary Medical Association*, **214**, 48–50

Brearley, M.J., Cooper, J.E. and Sullivan, M. (1991) *Colour Atlas of Small Animal Endoscopy*. Mosby, London

British Chelonia Group (undated) *Care Sheet: Mediterranean Tortoises Testudo graeca and T. hermanni*. British Chelonia Group, Chippenham. http://www.britishcheloniagroup.org.uk (accessed 26 January 2009)

British Veterinary Zoological Society (2003) *Guidelines for Acceptable Methods of Euthanasia for Zoo, Exotic Pet and Wildlife Species. No. 1: Reptiles*. BVZS, London

Brown, C. (2007) Blood sample collection in lizards. *Lab Animal Europe*, **36**, 23–24

Brown, S.G., Gomes, F. and Miles, F.L. (1998) Faeces avoidance behaviour in unisexual and bisexual geckos. *Herpetological Journal*, **8**, 169–172

Burridge, M.J. (2001) Ticks (*Acari: Ixodidae*) spread by the international trade in reptiles and their potential roles in dissemination of diseases. *Bulletin of Entomological Research*, **91**, 3–23

Calvert, I. (2004) Nutrition. Nutritional problems. In: *BSAVA Manual of Reptiles*, 2nd edn. Eds Girling, S.J. and Raiti, D., pp. 18–39 and pp. 289–308. British Small Animal Veterinary Association, Gloucester

Cambre, R.C., Green, D.E., Smith, E.E. *et al.* (1980) Salmonellosis and Arizonosis in the reptile collection at the National Zoological Park. *Journal of the American Veterinary Medical Association*, **177**, 800–803

Campbell, T.W. and Ellis, C.K. (2007) *Avian and Exotic Animal Hematology and Cytology*. Blackwell Publishing, Oxford

Canadian Council on Animal Care (2003) *Guidelines on the Care and Use of Wildlife*. CCAC, Ottawa

Carpenter, J.W. (2005) *Exotic Animal Formulary*, 3rd edn. Elsevier Saunders, Philadelphia

Chiszar, D., Radcliffe, C.W., Boyer, T. *et al.* (1987) Cover-seeking behaviour in red spitting cobras (*Naja mossambica pallida*): effects of tactile cues and darkness. *Zoo Biology*, **6**, 161–167

Chiszar, D., Smith, H.M. and Carpenter, C.C. (1994) An ethological approach to reproductive success in reptiles. In: *Captive Management and Conservation of Amphibians and Reptiles*. Eds Murphy, J.B., Adler, K. and Collins, J.T., pp. 147–173. Society for the Study of Amphibians and Reptiles, Ithaca, New York

Chiszar, D., Tomlinson, W.T., Smith, H.M. *et al.* (1995) Behavioural consequences of husbandry manipulations: indicators of arousal, quiescence and environmental awareness. In: *Health and Welfare of Captive Reptiles*. Eds Warwick, C., Frye, F.L. and Murphy, J.B., pp. 186–204. Chapman and Hall, London

Chiszar, D., Wellborn, S., Wand, M.A. *et al.* (1980) Investigatory behaviour in snakes. II. Cage cleaning and the induction of defecation in snakes. *Animal Learning and Behaviour*, **8**, 505–510

Clark, H. F. and Lunger, P.D. (1981) Viruses. In: *Diseases of the Reptilia*. Eds Cooper, J.E. and Jackson, O.F., pp. 136–164. Academic Press, London

Clubb, R. and Mason, G. (2003) Captivity effects on wide-ranging carnivores. *Nature*, **425**, 473–474

Cooper, J.E. (1977) Diseases of lower vertebrates and biomedical research. *Laboratory Animals*, **11**, 119–123

Cooper, J.E. (1989) Health monitoring and quality control of reptiles and amphibians kept for biomedical research. Proceedings of the Third International Colloquium on the Pathology of Reptiles and Amphibians, Florida, pp. 4–7

Cooper, J.E. (1999) Reptilian microbiology. In: *Laboratory Medicine. Avian and Exotic Pets*. Ed. Fudge, A.M., pp. 223–227. Saunders, Philadelphia

Cooper, J.E. (2004) Humane euthanasia and *post-mortem* examination. In: *BSAVA Manual of Reptiles*, 2nd edn. Eds Girling, S.J. and Raiti, D., pp. 168–183. British Small Animal Veterinary Association, Gloucester

Cooper, J.E. (2006) Dermatology. In: *Reptile Medicine and Surgery*, 2nd edn. Ed. Mader, D.R., pp. 196–216. Saunders Elsevier, St. Louis

Cooper, J.E. and Cooper, M.E. (2007) *Introduction to Veterinary and Comparative Forensic Medicine*. Blackwell Publishing, Oxford

Cooper, J.E., Dutton, C.J. and Allchurch, A.F. (1998) Reference collections: their importance and relevance to modern zoo management and conservation biology. *Dodo*, **34**, 159–166

Cooper, J.E., Dutton, C.J. and Belle, J. (2003) Exotic pets and wildlife. In: *Jones's Animal Nursing*. Eds Lane, D.R. and Cooper, B., pp. 265–308. Elsevier, Oxford

Cooper, J.E., Ewbank, R. and Rosenberg, M.E. (1984) Euthanasia of tortoises. *Veterinary Record*, **115**, 635

Cooper, J.E., Gschmeissner, S. and Holt, P.E. (1982) Viral particles in a papilloma from a green lizard (*Lacerta viridis*). *Laboratory Animals*, **16**, 12–13

Cooper, J.E. and Jackson, O.F. (Eds) (1981) *Diseases of the Reptilia*. Academic Press, London

Cooper, M.E., Lewbart, G.A. and Lewbart, D.T. (2006) Laws and regulations. European and American. In: *Reptile Medicine and Surgery*, 2nd edn. Ed. Mader, D.R., pp. 1031–1050. Saunders Elsevier, St Louis

Cooper, J.E., McClelland, M.H. and Needham, J.R. (1980) An eye infection in laboratory lizards associated with an *Aeromonas* sp. *Laboratory Animals*, **14**, 149–151

Cooper, J.E. and Sainsbury, A.W. (1994) Review: oral diseases of reptiles. *Herpetological Journal*, **4**, 117–125

Cooper, J.E. and Williams, D.L. (1995) Veterinary perspectives and techniques in husbandry and research. In: *Health and Welfare of Captive Reptiles*. Eds Warwick, C., Frye, F.L. and Murphy, J.B., pp. 98–111. Chapman and Hall, London

Council of Europe (2006) Multilateral Consultation of Parties to the European Convention for the Protection of Vertebrate Animals used for Experimental and other Scientific Purposes (ETS 123) Appendix A. *Cons 123 (2006) 3*. Available from URL: http://www.coe.int/t/e/legal_affairs/legal_co-operation/biological_safety,_use_of_animals/laboratory_animals/2006/Cons123(2006)3AppendixA_en.pdf (accessed 31 July 2008)

Crews, D., Bergeron, J.M., Bull, J.J. *et al.* (1994) Temperature-dependent sex determination in reptiles: proximal mechanisms, ultimate outcomes, and practical applications. *Developmental Genetics*, **15**, 297–312

Crews, D. and Gans, C. (1992) The interaction of hormones, brain and behavior: an emerging discipline in herpetology. In: *Biology of the Reptilia 18. Physiology E*. Eds Gans C. and Crews D., pp. 1–23. Chicago University Press, Chicago

Davies, A.J. and Johnston, M.R.L. (2000) The biology of some intraerythrocytic parasites of fishes, amphibia and reptiles. *Advances in Parasitology*, **45**, 1–107

Davis, P.M.C. (1981) Anatomy and physiology. In: *Diseases of the Reptilia*. Eds Cooper, J.E. and Jackson, O.F., pp. 9–73. Academic Press, London

Deming, C., Greiner, E. and Uhl, E.W. (2008) Prevalence of *Cryptosporidium* infection and characteristics of oocyst shedding in a breeding colony of leopard geckos. (*Eublepharis macularius*). *Journal of Zoo and Wildlife Medicine*, **39**, 600–607

Denardo, D. (2006a) Reproductive biology. In: *Reptile Medicine and Surgery*, 2nd edn. Ed. Mader, D.R., pp. 376–390. Saunders Elsevier, St. Louis, Missouri

Denardo, D. (2006b) Stress in captive reptiles. In: *Reptile Medicine and Surgery*, 2nd edn. Ed. Mader, D.R., pp. 119–123. Saunders Elsevier, St. Louis, Missouri

Diethelm, G. and Stein, G. (2006) Hematologic and blood chemistry values in reptiles. In: *Reptile Medicine and Surgery*, (ed D.R. Mader), 2nd edn. pp. 1103–1118. Saunders Elsevier, St. Louis, Missouri

Divers, S.J. (1995) The green iguana (*Iguana iguana*): a guide to successful captive management. *British Herpetological Society Bulletin*, **51**, 7–26

Divers, S.J. and Cooper, J.E. (2000) Reptile hepatic lipidosis. *Seminars in Avian and Exotic Pet Medicine*, **9**, 153–164

Drury, S.E.N., Gough, R.E. and Welchman, D. de. B. (2002) Isolation and identification of a reovirus from a lizard, *Uromastyx hardwickii*, in the United Kingdom. *Veterinary Record*, **151**, 637–638

Eason, P.K. and Stamps, J.A. (1991) The effect of visibility on territory size and shape. *Behavioural Ecology*, **3**, 166–172

Edwards, J. (1991) It's just the beginning – my experience with Florida kingsnakes. *Snake Breeder*, **8**, 3–4

Espinosa, R.E., Tracey, C.R. and Tracey, C.R. (1998) A safe single-application procedures for eradicating mites on reptiles. *Herpetological Review*, **29**, 35–36

Essbauer, S. and Ahne, W. (2001) Viruses of lower vertebrates. *Journal of Veterinary Medicine Series B*, **48**, 403–475

Ewert, M.A., Jackson, D.R. and Nelson, C.E. (1994) Patterns of temperature-dependent sex determination in turtles. *Journal of Experimental Zoology*, **270**, 3–15

Ferguson, G.W. (1994) Old World chameleons in captivity: growth, maturity and reproduction of Malagasy *Chamaeleo pardalis*. In: *Captive Management and Conservation of Amphibians and Reptiles*. Eds Murphy, J.B., Adler, K. and Collins, J.T., pp. 323–331. Society for the Study of Amphibians and Reptiles, Ithaca, New York

Ferrell, S.T., Marlar, A.B., Alberts, A.C. *et al.* (2005) Surgical technique for permanent intracoelomic radiotransmitter placement in anegada iguanas (*Cyclura pinguis*). *Journal of Zoo and Wildlife Medicine*, **36**, 712–715

Finke, M.D., Dunham, S.U. and Kwabi, C.A. (2005) Evaluation of four dry commercial gut loading products for improving the calcium content of crickets, *Acheta domesticus*. *Journal of Herpetological Medicine and Surgery*, **15**, 7–12

Firth, B.T. and Turner, J.S. (1982) Sensory, neuronal and hormonal aspects of thermoregulation. In: *Biology of the Reptilia 12. Physiology C. Physiological Ecology*. Eds Gans, C. and Pough, F.M., pp. 213–274. Academic Press, London

Fitzgerald, K.T. and Vera, R. (2006) Reported toxicities in reptiles. In: *Reptile Medicine and Surgery*, 2nd edn. Ed. Mader, D.R., pp. 1068–1080. Saunders Elsevier, St. Louis

Fleishman, L.J., Loew, E.R. and Leal, M. (1993) Ultraviolet vision in lizards. *Nature*, **365**, 397

Fleming, G.J., Isaza, R., Spire, M.F. *et al.* (2003) The use of digital thermography for environmental evaluation of reptile enclosures. *Journal of Herpetological Medicine and Surgery*, **13**, 38–42

Fry, B.G., Vidal, N., Norman, J.A. *et al.* (2006) Early evolution of the venom system in lizards and snakes. *Nature*, **439**, 584–588

Frye, F.L. (1991) *Biomedical and Surgical Aspects of Captive Reptile Husbandry*. Krieger, Florida

Frye, F.L. (1993) *Iguanas: A Guide to their Biology and Captive Care*. Krieger, Florida

Frye, F.L. (1994) *Reptile Clinician's Handbook*. Krieger, Florida

Frye, F.L. (1996) *A Practical Guide for Feeding Captive Reptiles*, 2nd edn. Krieger, Florida

Gabrisch, K. and Zwart, P. (2005) *Krankheiten der Heimtiere*. Schlütersche, Hannover

Gal, J., Dobos-Kovacs, M. and Sos, E. (2003) Nodular dermatitis of emerald swift (*Sceloporus malachiticus*) kept in captivity. *Magyar Allatorvosok Lapja*, **125**, 44–48

Galeotti, P., Sacchi, R., Fasola, M. *et al.* (2005) Do mounting vocalizations in tortoises have a communication function? A comparative analysis. *Herpetological Journal*, **15**, 61–71

Garland, T. (1994) Phylogenetic analyses of lizard endurance capacity in relation to body size and body temperature. In: *Lizard Ecology: Historical and Experimental Perspectives*. Eds Vitt L.J. and Pianka, E.R., pp. 237–259. Princetown University Press, Princetown

Gavaud, J. (1991) Role of cryophase temperature and therophase duration in thermoperiodic regulation of the testicular cycle in the lizard *Lacerta vivipara*. *Journal of Experimental Zoology*, **260**, 239–246

Gehrmann, W.B. (1994) Light requirements of captive amphibians and reptiles. In: *Captive Management and Conservation of Amphibians and Reptiles*. Eds Murphy, J.B., Adler, K. and Collins, J.T., pp. 53–59. Society for the Study of Amphibians and Reptiles, Ithaca, New York

Gehrmann, W.H. (2006) Artificial lighting. In: *Reptile Medicine and Surgery*, 2nd edn. Ed. Mader, D.R., pp. 1081–1084. Saunders Elsevier, St. Louis, Missouri

Gene, L. and Loeschner, U. (2002) *Salmonella enterica* in reptiles of German and Austrian origin. *Veterinary Microbiology*, **84**, 79–91

Germano, D.J., and Williams, D.F. (1993) Field evaluation of using passive integrated transponder (PIT) tags to permanently mark lizards. *Herpetological Review*, **24**, 54–56

Girling, S.J. and Raiti, P. (Eds) (2004) *BSAVA Manual of Reptiles*. British Small Animal Veterinary Association, Gloucester

Gravendyck, M., Ammermann, P., Marschang, R.E. *et al.* (1998) Paramyxoviral and reoviral infections of iguanas on Honduran Islands. *Journal of Wildlife Diseases*, **34**, 33–38

Greenacre, C., Paul-Murphy, J., Sladky, K.K. *et al.* (2005) Reptile and amphibian analgesia. *Journal of Herpetological Medicine and Surgery*, **15**, 24–29

Greenberg, N. (1995) Ethologically informed design in husbandry and research. In: *Health and Welfare of Captive Reptiles*. Eds Warwick, C., Frye, F.L. and Murphy, J.B., pp. 239–262. Chapman and Hall, London

Greiner, E.C. and Mader, D.R. (2006) Parasitology. In: *Reptile Medicine and Surgery*, 2nd edn. Ed. Mader, D.R., pp. 343–363. Saunders Elsevier, St Louis

Guillette, L.J., Cree, A. and Rooney, A.A. (1995) Biology of stress: interactions with reproduction, immunology and intermediary metabolism. In: *Health and Welfare of Captive Reptiles*. Eds Warwick, C., Frye, F.L. and Murphy, J.B., pp. 32–81. Chapman and Hall, London

Hailey, A. (2000) Assessing body mass condition in the tortoise, *Testudo hermanni*. *Herpetological Journal*, **10**, 57–61

Harling, R. (1993) Successfully keeping and breeding *Podarcis pityusensis* in indoor vivaria. *British Herpetological Society Bulletin*, **44**, 38–40

Harling, R. (1994) The successful keeping and breeding of *Anolis carolinesis*. *British Herpetological Review*, **27**, 71–72

Hernandez-Divers, S.J. (2001) Clinical aspects of reptile behavior. *Veterinary Clinics of North America Exotic Animal Practice*, **4**, 599–612

Hernandez-Divers, S.J. (2004a) Surgery: principles and techniques. In: *BSAVA Manual of Reptiles*, 2nd edn. Eds Girling, S.J. and Raiti, D., pp. 147–167 British Small Animal Veterinary Association, Gloucester

Hernandez-Divers, S.J. (2004b) Endoscopic renal valuation and biopsy in chelonians. *Veterinary Record*, **154**, 73–80

Hernandez-Divers, S.J. (2006) Diagnostic techniques. In: *Reptile Medicine and Surgery*, 2nd edn. Ed. Mader, D.R., pp. 490–532. Elsevier Saunders, St. Louis, Missouri

Hernandez-Divers, S.J., Cooper, J.E. and Cooke, S.W. (2004a) Diagnostic techniques and sample collection in reptiles. *Compendium on Continuing Education of the Practicing Veterinarian*, **26**, 470–483

Hernandez-Divers, S.J., Stahls, Hernandez-Divers, S.M. *et al.* (2004b) Coelomic endoscopy of the green iguana (*Iguana iguana*). *Journal of Herpetological Medicine and Surgery*, **14**, 10–18

Huey, R.B. (1982) Temperature, physiology and ecology of reptiles. In: *Biology of the Reptilia 12. Physiology C Physiological Ecology*. Eds Gans, C. and Pough, F.H., pp. 25–91. Academic Press, London

Jackson, O.F. (1991) Reptiles. Part 1. Chelonians. In: *Manual of Exotic Pets*. Eds Beynon, P.H. and Cooper, J.E., pp. 221–243. British Small Animal Veterinary Association, Cheltenham

Jackson, D.C. (2002) Hibernating without oxygen: physiological adaptations of the painted turtle, *Chrysemys picta*. *Journal of Physiology*, **543**, 731–737

Jacobson, E.R. (2003) *Biology, Husbandry and Medicine of the Green Iguana*. Krieger, Melbourne, Florida

Jacobson, E.R. (2007) *Infectious Diseases and Pathology of Reptiles*. Taylor and Francis, New York

Jacobson, E.R. and Telford, S.R. (1990) Chlamydial and poxvirus infections of circulating monocytes of a flap-necked chameleon. *Journal of Wildlife Diseases*, **26**, 572–577

Jacobson, E.R., Origgi, F., Pessier, A.P. *et al.* (2001) Paramyxovirus infection in caiman lizards *(Draecaena guianensis)*. *Journal of Veterinary Diagnostic Investigation*, **13**, 143–151

Johnson–Delaney, C.A. (2006) Reptile zoonoses and threats to public health. In: *Reptile Medicine and Surgery*, 2nd edn. Ed. Mader, D.R., pp. 1017–1030. Saunders Elsevier, St. Louis Missouri

Josseaume, B. (2002) Faecal collector for field studies of digestive responses in forest tortoises. *Hepetological Journal*, **12**, 169–172

Julian, A.F. and Durham, P.J.K. (1982) Adenoviral hepatitis in a female bearded dragon *(Amphibolurus barbatus)*. *New Zealand Veterinary Journal*, **30**, 59–60

Just, F., Essbauer, S., Ahne, W. *et al.* (2001) Occurrence of an invertebrate iridescent-like virus (Iridoviridae) in reptiles. *Journal of Veterinary Medicine. Series B*, **48**, 685–694

Keymer, I.F. (1981) Protozoa. In: *Diseases of the Reptilia*. Eds Cooper, J.E. and Jackson, O.F., pp. 235–290. Academic Press, London

Kirkwood, J.K. and Gili, C. (1994) Food consumption in relation to bodymass in some snakes in captivity. *Research in Veterinary Science*, **57**, 35–38

Kreger, M.D. and Mench, J.A. (1993) Physiological and behavioral effects of handling and restraint in the ball python (*Python regius*) and the blue-tongued skink (*Tiliqua scincoides*). *Applied Animal Behaviour Science*, **38**, 323–336

Lance, V.A. (1994) Environmental sex determination in reptiles: pattern and process. *Journal of Experimental Zoology*, **270**, 1–127

Lang, M. (1992) A review of techniques for marking snakes. *Smithsonian Herpetological Information Service*, **90**, 1–19

Lang, J.W. and Andrews, H.V. (1994) Temperature-dependent sex determination in crocodilians. *Journal of Experimental Zoology*, **270**, 28–44

Langerwerf, B.A.W.A. (1990) The successful breeding of lizards from temperate regions. In: *Care and Breeding of Captive Reptiles*. Eds Townson, S., Millichamp, N.J., Lucas, D.G.D. *et al*., pp. 20–35. British Herpetological Society, London

Langerwerf, B.A.W.A. (1991) A large scale lizard breeding facility in Alabama. *British Herpetological Society Bulletin*, **36**, 43–46

Locke, B. (2008) Venomous snake restraint and handling. *Journal of Exotic Pet Medicine*, **17**, 273–284

Mader, D.R. (2006a) Thermal burns. In: *Reptile Medicine and Surgery*, 2nd edn. Ed. Mader, D.R., pp. 916–923. Saunders Elsevier, St. Louis, Missouri

Mader, D.R. (2006b) Metabolic bone diseases. In: *Reptile Medicine and Surgery*, 2nd edn. Ed. Mader, D.R., pp. 841–851. Saunders Elsevier, St. Louis, Missouri

Mader, D.R. (Ed.) (2006c) *Reptile Medicine and Surgery*. Saunders Elsevier, St Louis, Missouri

Maderson, P.F.A. (1965) Histological changes in the epidermis of snakes during the sloughing cycle. *Journal of Zoology, London*, **146**, 98–113

Marschang, R.E., Donahoe, S., Manvell, R. *et al.* (2002) Paramyxovirus and reovirus infections in wild-caught Mexican lizards (*Xenosaurus* and *Abronia* spp.). *Journal of Zoo and Wildlife Medicine*, **33**, 317–321

Marschang, R.E., Papp, T., Weinmann, N. *et al.* (2005) Invertebrate iridoviruses in lizards. Proceedings of the *Association of Reptilian and Amphibian Veterinarians*, **14**

Mason, R.T. (1992) Reptilian pheromones. In: *Biology of the Reptilia 18. Physiology E Hormones, Brain and Behavior*. Eds Gans C. and Crews D., pp. 114–128. Chicago University Press, Chicago

Mason, G. and Rushen, J. (2006) *Stereotypic Animal Behaviour: Fundamentals and Applications to Welfare*, 2nd edn. CAB International, Wallingford

Mayer, J., Kaufman, G. and Pokras, M. (2006) Allometric scaling. In: *Reptile Medicine and Surgery*, 2nd edn. Ed. Mader, D.R., pp. 419–427. Saunders Elsevier, St. Louis, Missouri

McArthur, S.D., Wilkinson, R.J. and Meyer, J. (2004a) *Medicine and Surgery of Tortoises and Turtles*. Blackwell Publishing, Oxford

McArthur, S., McLellan, L. and Brown, S. (2004b) Gastrointestinal system. In: *BSAVA Manual of Reptiles*, 2nd edn. Eds Girling, S.J. and Raiti, D., pp. 210–229. British Small Animal Veterinary Association, Gloucester

McBride, M. and Hernandez-Divers, S.J. (2004) Nursing care of lizards. *Veterinary Clinics of North American Exotic Animal Practice*, **7**, 375–396

Meek, R. and Avery, R.A. (1988) Thermoregulation in chelonians. *Herpetological Journal*, **1**, 253–259

Meerovitch, E. (1958) Some biological requirements on host-parasite relations of *Entamoeba invadens*. *Canadian Journal of Zoology*, **36**, 513–523

Meerovitch, E. (1961) Infectivity and pathogenicity of polyxenic and monoxenic *Entamoeba invadens* to snakes kept at normal and high temperatures and natural history of reptile amoebiasis. *Journal of Parasitology*, **47**, 791–794

Mitchell, M. (2003) Ophidia (snakes). In: *Zoo and Wild Animal Medicine*, 5th edn. Eds Fowler, M.E. and Miller, R.E., pp. 82–93. Saunders, St Louis

Mitchell, M.A. (2004) Snake care and husbandry. *Veterinary Clinics of North America Exotic Animal Practice*, **7**, 42–446

Moore, M.C. and Lindsey, J. (1992) The physiological basis of behavior in male reptiles. In: *Biology of the Reptilia 18. Physiology E*. Eds Gans C. and Crews D., pp. 70–113. Chicago University Press, Chicago

Morton, D.B. and Griffiths, P.H. (1985) Guidelines on the recognition of pain, distress and discomfort in experimental animals and an hypothesis for assessment. *Veterinary Record*, **116**, 431–436

Mosley, C.A.E. (2005) Anesthesia and analgesia in reptiles. *Seminars in Avian and Exotic Pet Medicine*, **14**, 243–262

Nichols, D.K., Weyant, R.S., Lamirande, E.W. *et al.* (1999) Fatal mycotic dermatitis in captive brown tree snakes (*Boiga irregularis*). *Journal of Zoo and Wildlife Medicine*, **30**, 111–118

Norton, T.M. (2005) Chelonian emergency and critical care. *Seminars in Avian and Exotic Pet Medicine*, **14**, 106–130

Onderka, D.K. and Finlayson, M.C. (1985) Salmonellae and salmonellosis in captive reptiles. *Canadian Journal of Comparative Medicine*, **49**, 268–270

Packard, G.C. and Phillips, J.A. (1994) The importance of the physical environment for the incubation of reptile eggs. In: *Captive Management and Conservation of Amphibians and Reptiles*. Eds Murphy, J.B., Adler, K. and Collins, J.T., pp. 195–208. Society for the Study of Amphibians and Reptiles, Ithaca, New York

Paperna, I. and Dematos, A.P.A. (1993) Erythrocytic viral-infections of lizards and frogs – new hosts, geographical locations and description of the infection process. *Annales de Parasitologie Humaine et Comparée*, **68**, 11–23

Paré J.A. and Sigler, L. (2006) Fungal diseases. In: *Reptile Medicine and Surgery*, 2nd edn. Ed. Mader, D.R., pp. 217–226. Saunders Elsevier, St. Louis, Missouri

Peterson, C.R., Gibson, A.R. and Dorcas, M.E. (1993) Snake thermal ecology: the causes and consequences of body-temperature variation. In: *Snakes: Ecology and Behavior*. Eds Seigel, R.A. and Collins, J.T., pp. 241–314. McGraw-Hill, New York

Plowman, C.A., Montali, R.J. Phillips, L.G. *et al.* (1987) Septicemia and chronic abscesses in iguanas (*Cyclura cornuta* and *Iguana iguana*) associated with a *Neisseria* species. *Journal of Zoo Animal Medicine*, **18**, 86–93

Pough, F.H. and Gans, C. (1982) The vocabulary of reptilian thermoregulation. In: *Biology of the Reptilia 12. Physiology C Physiological Ecology*. Eds Gans, C. and Crews, D., pp. 17–23. Academic Press, London

Raiti, P. (2004) Non-invasive imaging. In: *BSAVA Manual of Reptiles*, 2nd edn. Eds Girling, S.J. and Raiti, D., pp. 87–102. British Small Animal Veterinary Association, Gloucester

Ramos, A.B., Don, M.T. and Muchlinski, A.E. (1993) The effect of bacteria infection on mean selected body temperature in the common agama, *Agama agama*: a dose-response study. *Comparative Biochemistry and Physiology A*, **105**, 479–484

Raphael, B.L. (2003) Chelonians (turtles, tortoises). In: *Zoo and Wild Animal Medicine*, 5th edn. Eds Fowler, M.E. and Miller, R.E., pp. 48–58. Saunders, St Louis

Rayment-Dyble, L.J. (2004) Introduction: reptiles as pets. In: *BSAVA Manual of Reptiles*, 2nd edn. Eds Girling, S.J. and Raiti, D., pp. 1–5. British Small Animal Veterinary Association, Gloucester

Raynaud, A. and Adrian, M. (1976) Cutaneous lesions of papillomatous structure associated with viruses in green lizard, (*Lacerta viridis* Laur). *Comptes Rendus Hebdomadaires des Seances de l' Academie des Sciences Serie D*, **283**, 845–847

Redrobe, S. (2002) Reptiles and disease – keeping the risks to a minimum. *Journal of Small Animal Practice*, **43**, 471–472

Redrobe, S. (2004) Anaesthesia and analgesia. In: *BSAVA Manual of Reptiles*, 2nd edn. Eds Girling, S.J. and Raiti, D., pp. 131–146. British Small Animal Veterinary Association, Gloucester

Rees Davies, R. and Klingenberg, R.J. (2004) Therapeutics and medication. In: *BSAVA Manual of Reptiles*, 2nd edn. Eds Girling, S.J. and Raiti, D., pp. 115–130. British Small Animal Veterinary Association, Gloucester

Reichenbach-Klinke, H. and Elkan, E. (1965) *The Principal Diseases of Lower Vertebrates*. Academic Press, London

Reiner, A.J. (1992) Neuropeptides in the nervous system. In: *Biology of the Reptilia 17. Neurology C.* Eds Gans, C. and Ulinski, P.S., pp. 587–739. Chicago University Press, Chicago

Reilly, J.S. (2001) *Euthanasia of Animals Used for Scientific Purposes.* Australian and New Zealand Council for the Care of Animals in Research and Teaching. Adelaide University, Adelaide

Roitberg, E.S. and Smirina, E.M. (2006) Age, body size and growth of *Lacerta agilis boemica* and *L. strigata*: a comparative study of two closely related lizard species based on skeleton-chronology. *Herpetological Journal*, **16**, 133–148

Rose, T.A. (1992) Husbandry and successful breeding of the New Guinea blue-tongued skink. *Association for the Study of Reptiles and Amphibians Monograph*, **2**, 22–28

Rosenberg, M.E. (1972) Excitation and inhibition of motorneurones in the tortoise. *Journal of Physiology*, **221**, 715–730

Rossi, J.V. (2006) General husbandry and management. In: *BSAVA Manual of Reptiles*, 2nd edn. Eds Girling, S.J. and Raiti, D., pp. 25–41. Saunders Elsevier, St. Louis

Sheriff, D. (1988) The inland bearded dragon, *Pogona vitticeps*, and its maintenance and breeding in captivity. *Royal Zoological Society of Scotland Annual Report*, **76**, 49–55

Schieffelin, C.D. and de Queiroz, A. (1991) Temperature and defense in the common garter snake: warm snakes are more aggressive than cold snakes. *Herpetologica*, **47**, 230–237

Schumacher, J. (2003) Lacertilia (lizards, skinks, geckos) and amphisbaenids (worm lizards). In: *Zoo and Wild Animal Medicine*, 5th edn. Eds Fowler, M.E. and Miller, R.E., pp. 73–81. Saunders, St Louis, Missouri

Slomka-McFarland, E. (2006) Disinfectants for the vivarium. In: *Reptile Medicine and Surgery*, 2nd edn. Ed. Mader, D.R., pp. 1055–1087. Saunders Elsevier, St. Louis, Missouri

Soldati, G., Lu, Z.H., Vaughan, L. *et al.* (2004) Detection of Mycobacteria and Chlamydiae in granulomatous inflammation of reptiles: a retrospective study. *Veterinary Pathology*, **41**, 388–397

Stauber, E. and Gogolewski, R. (1990) Poxvirus dermatitis in a tegu lizard (*Tupinambis teguixin*). *Journal of Zoo and Wildlife Medicine*, **21**, 228–230

Sweeney, R. (1993) *Garter Snakes: Their Natural History and Care in Captivity.* Blandford, London

Thorogood, J. and Whimster, I.W. (1979) The maintenance and breeding of the leopard gecko, *Eublepharis macularius*, as a laboratory animal. *International Zoo Yearbook*, **19**, 74–78

Townson, S. (1994) *Breeding Reptiles and Amphibians.* British Herpetological Society, London

Troyer, K. (1982) Transfer of fermentative microbes between generations of a herbivorous lizard. *Science*, **216**, 540–542

Tucunduva, M., Borelli, P. and Silva, J.R.M.C. (2001) Experimental study of induced inflammation in the Brazilian boa (*Boa constrictor constrictor*). *Journal of Comparative Pathology*, **125**, 174–181

UFAW/WSPA (1989) *Euthanasia of Amphibians and Reptiles.* Report of a Joint UFAW/WSPA Working Party UFAW, Potters Bar/WSPA, London

Underwood, H. (1992) Endogenous rhythms. In: *Biology of the Reptilia 18. Physiology E.* Eds Gans C. and Crews D., pp. 229–297. Chicago University Press, Chicago

Varga, M. (2004) Captive maintenance and welfare. In: *BSAVA Manual of Reptiles*, 2nd edn. Eds Girling, S.J. and Raiti, D., pp. 6–17. British Small Animal Veterinary Association, Gloucester

Viets, B.E., Ewert, M.A., Talent, L.G. *et al.* (1994) Sex-determining mechanisms in squamate reptiles. *Journal of Experimental Zoology*, **270**, 45–56

Warwick, C., Frye, F.L. and Murphy, J.B. (1995) *Health and Welfare of Captive Reptiles.* Chapman and Hall, London

Wellehan, J.F.X., Johnson, A.J., Harrach, B. *et al.* (2004) Detection and analysis of six lizard adenoviruses by consensus primer PCR provides further evidence of a reptilian origin for the atadenoviruses. *Journal of Virology*, **78**, 13366–13369

Whitaker, B.R. and Gold, B.S. (2006) Working with venomous species: emergency protocols. In: *Reptile Medicine and Surgery*, 2nd edn. Ed. Mader, D.R., pp. 1051–1061. Saunders Elsevier, St. Louis, Missouri

Willemser, R.E. and Hailey, A. (2002) Body mass condition in Greek tortoises: regional and interspecific variation. *Herpetological Journal*, **12**, 105–114

Wisniewski, P.J. (1992) Maintenance and breeding of some lizards from arid areas under laboratory conditions. *Association for the Study of Reptiles and Amphibians Monograph*, **2**, 49–53

Woodford, M.H. (2001) *Quarantine and Health Screening Protocols for Wildlife prior to Translocating and Release into the Wild.* OIE, Paris

Wright, K.M. (2004) Breeding and neonatal care. In: *BSAVA Manual of Reptiles*, 2nd edn. Eds Girling, S.J. and Raiti, D., pp. 40–50. British Small Animal Veterinary Association, Gloucester

WSPA (1994) *Pain Assessment and Euthanasia of Ectotherms.* Scientific Advisory Panel Report 09/90, revised 02/94. World Society for the Protection of Animals, London

Xavier, G., Winne, C. and Fedewa, L. (2006) Ontogeny of anti-predator behavioural habituation in cottonmouths. *Ethology*, **112**, 608–615

Young, L.A., Schumacher, J., Papich, M.G. and Jacobson, E.R. (1997) Disposition of enrofloxacin and its metabolite ciprofloxacin after intramuscular injection in juvenile Burmese pythons (*Python molurus bivittatus*). *Journal of Zoo and Wildlife Medicine*, **28**, 71–79

Other sources of information

Herpetological societies exist in many countries of the world. Most publish newsletters, members' information sheets, journals or bulletins, often in different languages and many have their own websites.

The British Chelonia Group produces *Care Sheets.* relating to most of the species of terrestrial chelonians likely to be found in captivity. These are obtainable from the British Chelonian Group[2].

Journals published in English (and, where appropriate, the associations that publish them) that are of particular relevance to the care and use of reptiles include the *Herpetological Journal* (British Herpetological Society), *Applied Herpetology*, *Copeia* (American Society of Ichthyologists and Herpetologists), *Herpetological Review* (American Society of Ichthyologists and Herpetologists) and *Journal of Herpetological Medicine and Surgery* (Association of Amphibian and Reptilian Veterinarians (ARAV)).

There are numerous websites that provide advice on the care of reptiles in captivity. Some but not all of the information given is sound. A useful list of reference sources for reptile clinicians, albeit with a strong North American slant, was given by Barten (2006). Some websites refer to legislation that affects the keeping and use of reptiles: see Cooper *et al.* (2006).

[2]http://www.britishcheloniagroup.org.uk/

47 Aquatic reptiles

Simon Tonge

Biological overview

General biology

Aquatic reptiles include representatives from all the major orders of reptiles. Most of the truly aquatic squamates (snakes and lizards) are highly venomous snakes of the family Elapidae and are not suitable for laboratory use, so their maintenance will not be considered further in this chapter. Many other squamates are at least partially aquatic but their husbandry does not differ, at least in the laboratory context, from other more terrestrial taxa so their husbandry is considered elsewhere in this volume. Crocodilians and testudines comprise the bulk of the aquatic reptiles, but the former are generally unsuitable for laboratory usage, when adult, due to their great size and the risks they present to those handling and servicing them.

There are 22 extant species of crocodilians (crocodiles, alligators and caimans) found throughout the tropical, and in some subtropical, areas of the globe. The best current sources of information on crocodilian biology are the Crocodilian Specialist Group website[1] and its subsequent links; also see Trutnau and Sommerlad (2006) and Ross (1989). The species are all rather similar externally, and details of their laboratory maintenance are similarly uniform.

Aquatic testudines are found throughout the temperate and tropical marine and freshwater habitats of the world. Marine turtles are large and highly specialised, belonging to two families. They are not suitable for laboratory usage and are therefore not discussed further in this chapter. Further information on facilities and life support issues relating to aquatic species in general have been provided in Chapters 1 and 4 of Poole (1999).

Freshwater turtles (henceforth referred to as terrapins) comprise nine families and approximately 209 species (Iverson 1992) within two suborders (Cryptodira and Pleurodira) of the order, Testudines. New species are still occasionally described (eg, see Cann & Legler 1994; McCord & Pritchard 2002). Within the constraints of the basic testudine body plan, terrapins show a huge range of morphological variation, from highly adapted, strictly aquatic forms with 'soft' shells, such as the Fly River turtle (*Carettochelys insculpta*), through to secondarily terrestrial species such as the eastern box turtle (*Terrapene carolina*). Some specialisations are quite bizarre, such as the worm-like tongue lure of the alligator snapper (*Macroclemmys temmincki*) or the leaf-like appendages on the neck and body of the matamata (*Chelus fimbriatus*).

[1]http://www.flmnh.ufl.edu/cnhc/

Size range and lifespan

Some crocodilians can grow to 7 m or more. Only the very smallest juveniles under 1 m in length can be maintained satisfactorily in the laboratory. Terrapins vary enormously in size. The largest species is probably the giant Asiatic soft shell (*Chitra indica*), which may reach up to 1.8 m in carapace length, and weigh perhaps 200 kg or more. By contrast, Reeve's terrapin (*Chinemys reevesi*) reaches only 12 cm and a weight of 150 g.

Little is known of the lifespan of terrapins or crocodilians, but, in view of their ectothermy and relatively slow growth rates, it is likely that many species live up to 70 years or more, once an individual has achieved the critical size where it is relatively invulnerable to predation. Most species either lay one large clutch of relatively small eggs per annum or several smaller clutches of larger ones, but, in both cases, the majority of hatchlings probably die within their first year of life, mostly as a result of predation.

Social organisation

Social behaviour in most terrapins is poorly understood, but ranges from the apparently solitary snappers (Chelydridae) to the highly social sliders (Emydidae), though whether these animals are truly social is something of a moot point as they may simply be gathering at a scarce resource such as a suitable basking site.

Some species are exclusively aquatic, emerging from water only to lay eggs or to move between ephemeral water bodies. Examples of these species include softshells (Trionychidae): the Fly River turtle (*Carettochelys insculpta*), the matamata (*Chelus fimbriatus*) and snappers, Chelydridae. Many more species are partially aquatic, spending a good deal of their time, at least during the day, basking out of the water on rocks, logs or stream banks. Most of the emydid terrapins, including the sliders and cooters (*Trachemys* spp. and *Pseudemys* spp.) fall into this category, along with kinosternids and many chelids. A final category includes those species that have deserted the water and live exclusively on land. The American box turtles (*Terrapene* spp.) are the best known examples, though there are probably several Asian species, mostly in the genus *Cuora*, that have similar life-styles but which are very poorly known.

Bonin *et al.* (2006) provides the most comprehensive modern review of recent testudines, and should be consulted for a description and brief notes on the biology of particular species. Other important works include those by Pritchard (1979) and Harless and Morlock (1979).

All crocodilians are strictly aquatic, except when basking or nesting. Males are usually territorial and may hold harems in the breeding season. Juvenile crocodilians are not territorial and can usually be kept at high density.

Sources of supply (conservation status)

One hundred and forty species of Testudines (66% of the total) are currently listed as threatened with extinction (International Union for Conservation of Nature and Natural Resources (IUCN) 2007) and many are very poorly known biologically. However, some species are amongst the best known and most familiar of all reptiles, for example, the red-eared slider (*Trachemys scripta elegans*).

Relations between humans and testudines have been predominantly disastrous for the reptiles. The decline in turtle and terrapin populations over the last two decades has been shocking, mirroring the decline and extinction of many tortoise species a century before. Many species are threatened by direct consumption for food or medicinal purposes, or the taking of eggs, for example, the giant arrau (*Podocnemis expansa*) in South America or tuntong (*Batagur baska*) in Asia. More insidious threats to terrapins are habitat destruction, pollution, the diversion of rivers and lakes and incidental by catch by fisheries. Many species have naturally small ranges (such as the western swamp terrapin, (*Pseudemydura umbrina*) in Australia) and are vulnerable to even minor habitat alteration, because of their narrow ecological niches.

For laboratory purposes, the most commonly used species is the red-eared slider, which is bred commercially in the United States for sale to the pet trade. Juvenile specimens are still available from pet stores but not as widely as was once the case. Occasionally, juvenile softshells (Trionychidae) turn up in shipments of tropical fish, but most species of terrapin are not available commercially.

Ten of the 23 species of crocodilian are listed as threatened (IUCN 2007) but a number of species, for example, the American alligator (*Alligator mississippiensis*) are now farmed for their hides or meat, and are readily available commercially.

Uses in the laboratory

Because of their relatively expensive (though not complex) requirements in captivity, and the lack of biological information available, terrapins and crocodilians are not widely used experimentally. Studies that have been undertaken include those on heart rate (Bethea 1972), gut passage time (Parmenter 1981), respiratory rate (Jackson 1971), gas uptake (Bagatto & Henry 1999), heat exchanges during diving (Glidewell *et al.* 1981), heart rate during diving (Belkin 1964) and radionuclide uptake (Peters & Brisbin 1996; Bickham *et al.* 1988; Hinton *et al.* 1992). In addition, more broad-based studies have included environmental sex determination (Yntema 1981; Georges & McInnes 1998), the effects of incubation temperature (Pina *et al.* 2007), behavioural studies (Cloudsley-Thompson 1982) and the construction of heating and cooling curves (Spray & May 1972).

Laboratory management and breeding

General husbandry

The great variety of terrapin form and function means that for every 'rule' given in an account of how to maintain them in captivity, it will be usually possible to find a species or individual that is the exception. However, for laboratory purposes, a relatively limited subset of species, mostly emydids, are likely to be used, so it is probable that the following account will cover most species likely to be encountered. If in doubt, refer to the specialised literature contained in such journals as *Sauria*, *The Vivarium*, *Bulletin of the British Herpetological Society* and *Salamandra*; see also Highfield (1996). Recent recommendations can be found in European Commission (2007).

Housing

The geographical origin of the taxon in question will determine whether the species is kept indoors or outdoors. However, many species from subtropical areas, such as the southern USA, are perfectly capable of withstanding colder weather if kept outdoors further north. They can, therefore, be kept in small ponds, lakes or reservoirs, but extreme care should be taken to ensure that escape is not possible. Accidentally introduced terrapins can cause damage to native invertebrate, fish and amphibian faunas. When kept outdoors, terrapins require access only to deep, unfrozen water in winter, in order to hibernate satisfactorily. Some species, eg, box turtles (*Terrapene* spp.) may not, normally, hibernate in water and will need to be provided with soft soil or leaf litter into which they can burrow. Those species that do not normally hibernate will need to be maintained indoors during winter.

The pond or lake should be surrounded by a solid wall or fence, which will act as a partial sun-trap, thus creating a more suitable microclimate by allowing the terrapins to bask and regulate their own body temperatures. Terrapins can climb, to a certain extent, so wire mesh barriers should exceed 60 cm in height and should be sloped inwards to form an overhang. Approximately 30–50% of the enclosure should be land area and the water depth should shelve gently to allow the animals to emerge easily. The land area should include areas of soil, sand or peat (or a mixture) to a depth of 20–30 cm, to allow the females to lay eggs when the substrate temperature is high enough.

In most laboratories, terrapins will be maintained indoors and, for ease of maintenance, vivarium conditions should be as simple as possible without compromising animal welfare.

Vivaria can be constructed of glass, metal, plastic or fibreglass, the main consideration being that the surface should be smooth, easily sterilised and waterproof. They should be of an appropriate size, a 'rule of thumb' being that the water area should be at least three times as long, in all dimensions, as the largest inhabitant, and should be sufficient to hold all the vivarium occupants in the water at the same time, with space for them to move freely. Likewise, the land area should be large enough for all the vivarium occupants to be out of the water at the same time (Figure 47.1).

Water depth should not be uniform but should enable the terrapins to immerse themselves completely, and most species will make use of water depths that allow them to swim freely. Juveniles especially need some access to deep water in order to learn to regulate their buoyancy properly. Many species are most comfortable lying on the floor of the vivarium, with their necks extended to the water surface and their eyes protruding out of the water. Comfort and security are also enhanced if the substrate at the bottom of the tank is dark in colour enhancing crypsis.

Land : water ratios in vivaria are usually in the region of 30 : 70. The terrapins should be provided with metal or wooden rungs to assist emergence from the water onto the land (Figure 47.2). In the wild, many terrapins prefer to emerge on to rocks or branches completely surrounded by water in order to facilitate escape from predators.

Maintenance of juvenile crocodilians is very similar to that of terrapins, although allowance must be made for the extra size of the animals and the consequent need to maintain only like-sized animals together. Crocodilians are also agile climbers so vivaria should have a suitable lid.

Environmental provisions

Most crocodilians and terrapins require a background temperature in the region of 22–27 °C during the day. At this temperature, they will be active and some feeding will occur. They should also be given access to a basking source positioned over the land area of their vivarium. Traditionally an infrared bulb of an appropriate wattage has been used,

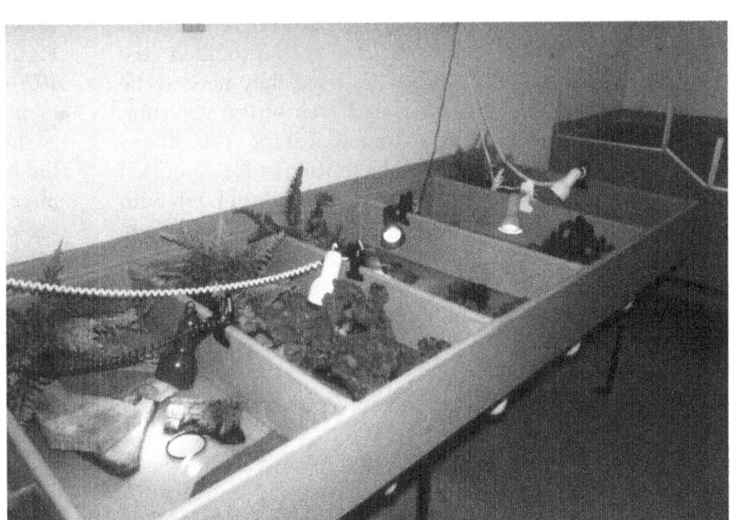

Figure 47.1 Vivaria for rearing juvenile terrapins. The construction is wood covered with fibreglass. Note multiple hiding places and moveable spotlights.

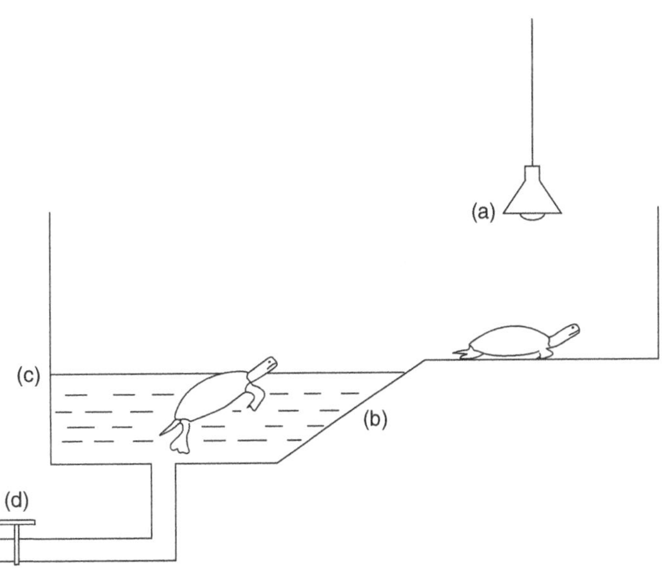

Figure 47.2 Cross-section of suggested enclosure for terrapins: (a) heat lamp; (b) ramp; (c) water level; (d) drainage valve.

but bulbs that also emit high levels of ultraviolet-b (UV-b) radiation as well as heat are preferred. This should provide a temperature of approximately 35 °C at its warmest point. The temperature gradient thus created will allow the animals to maintain their own preferred body temperatures and will improve feeding rates. For those species that do not normally emerge from water to bask, such as softshells (Trionychidae), the water should be heated to about 26 °C. This can be done using thermostatically controlled aquarium heaters that are well protected from the animals.

Many temperate species hibernate during the winter but this does not appear to be obligatory for normal physiological functions in many of those species. Where hibernation is allowed or desired, it should be done at a temperature of about 5 °C, either under water or in damp leaf litter. Some species are capable of surviving lower temperatures, even below freezing (Storey *et al.* 1993) but this is neither normal nor recommended. Temperature fluctuations and desiccation should be avoided.

As with most diurnal animals, crocodilians and terrapins are affected by both the quantity (photoperiod and intensity) and quality (wavelength) of light. Natural daylight is the preferred source of light, though if this is filtered through glass, a source of UV light should also be provided (see section on disease). If UV tubes are used they need to be suspended 15–20 cm above the land area of the vivarium (see also Chapter 46), which is impractical for crocodilians hence the preference for high UV-b emitting bulbs described earlier; in any case, these produce higher levels of UV-b with consequent benefit for the animals' vitamin D3 metabolism. A wide variety of UV light sources is available (Gehrmann 1987; Baines *et al.* 2005). Photoperiod and temperature are the major cues for the initiation of reproduction in temperate-region species, but both they and tropical species can be kept perfectly well using 12:12 h day:night ratio. If reproduction is desired, some fluctuation in photoperiod may be required.

Over the last decade, captive animal husbandry has made great strides in the provision of enriched environments for mammals and birds. Less work has been carried out on reptiles and there is a perception that they are more limited behaviourally and therefore less 'in need' of enrichment. This is unlikely to be completely true as many reptiles have been shown to have complex behavioural repertoires. Nevertheless, given that many reptiles, including terrapins and crocodilians, are solitary, 'sit and wait' predators it is unlikely that elaborate enrichment devices are either necessary or effective. If the physical environment is hygienic and complex (in terms of hiding and basking places), the correct social groupings are applied and the diet is diverse and behaviourally stimulating it is unlikely that any further enrichment is required.

Social grouping

Most terrapins are aggressive to conspecifics to some degree. In softshell and snapping turtles, the level of aggression is usually such that maintenance of more than one animal per vivarium becomes problematic. Most emydids, kinosternids and chelids are more amenable and can be kept in groups. However, where adult animals are concerned, fighting may occur when animals of the same sex are housed together during the breeding season.

Hatchling crocodilians can be maintained in small vivaria in groups but, with adequate feeding, growth occurs rapidly, and it will become necessary to 'thin' the group in all but the largest vivaria. Crocodile farms maintain high stocking densities (up to 4000 crocodilians in an enclosure measuring 18 m × 90 m metres (Ross *et al.* 1989).

Identification and sexing

Terrapins are quite easy to identify individually. Many of them have variable markings on their plastral scutes, which can be photographed or even photocopied to provide a semi-permanent record. These markings change with age so regular updating of the photograph or photocopy may be required. Temporary numbering can be applied to the carapace using non-toxic paint, marker pens, nail varnish or even typing correction fluid.

More permanent marking can be achieved using notches filed into the marginal scutes of the carapace. Care needs to be taken not to file too deeply and thereby damage the underlying bony plate. A typical scute code is shown in Figure 47.3 (Swingland 1978; Honegger 1979; Plummer 1979). Microchip transponders can also be used and the usual place of insertion in both crocodilians and testudines is subcutaneously in the left inguinal region at the base of the hindlimb. Crocodilians are usually identifiable visually but can be marked with notches in tail scutes or with a small tag placed in the webbing between the toes.

Distinguishing between the sexes of most species of terrapins is normally fairly straightforward. In many species, there is a sexual dimorphism in size – females usually, though not exclusively, being larger. In males, the tail is often longer than in the female, sometimes up to twice the length. The tails also differ in shape, being tapered and long

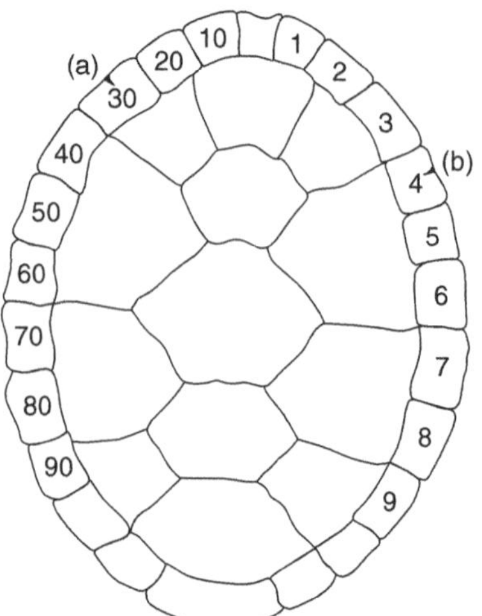

Figure 47.3 Diagram of chelonian carapace, showing suggested method of marking for identification. Right-hand marginal scutes are numbered 1–9 (units). Left-hand marginal scutes are numbered 10–90 (tens). This example shows notching at (a) and (b), indicating no. 34.

in the male and short and somewhat triangular in the female. However, without some experience and lacking animals for comparative purposes, this technique can be confusing. In box terrapins, it can be impossible if the individuals concerned shut the posterior plastral hinge! In some species, there is minor variation in the degree of concavity of the plastron, eg, *Terrapene coahuila* (personal observation), but this is rarely as pronounced as it is in some tortoise species. Finally, some species show other sexually dimorphic traits, such as the presence of long nails on the forelimbs in male *Trachemys scripta* (Gibbons & Lovich 1990) which are used in courtship, or differences in colour between the sexes, as in *Batagur baska* (Pritchard 1979).

Sexing crocodilians is very difficult with animals of less than 1 m in length. For older animals, physical examination of the cloaca (using a finger) to detect the male's penis, is an accurate technique but requires training and experience.

Physical environment and hygiene

The water area should include some furnishings, such as pipes, slates on bricks and half flower pots, under which the animals can hide. The vivarium should either have a drain or be of easy access with a siphon. The main constraint on good management of terrapins in particular is water hygiene. They are messy feeders and the vivarium may need cleaning after every feed. This can rapidly become an onerous and time-consuming task if the keeping system is poorly designed. Generally, the floor of the vivarium should be kept free of substrate but, for some softshells, the provision of fine gravel allows them to bury themselves, which is more natural behaviour. The presence of gravel affects the ease of cleaning and, in those circumstances, consideration should be given to providing permanent, aquarium-type filtration. For details of appropriate filtration, see Poole (1999) and specialist aquarium publications.

When permanent filtration systems are not being used water changes should occur as often as necessary to maintain hygiene. The vivarium will need to be stripped down completely at regular intervals. It should be scrubbed with a proprietary cleanser such as F10 (Health and Hygiene Pty, South Africa) to kill any pathogens and to remove algal build-up. The disinfectant should be removed by thorough rinsing. Very frequent water changes may result in cooler water temperatures than are desirable for some species, if the water input is directly from the mains supply without some sort of pre-warming, which is why filtration systems are preferable. It should also be noted that mains water can be variable in quality.

Health monitoring

It is highly likely that newly acquired terrapins and crocodilians will be carrying parasites and potentially harmful bacteria in their guts, so they should be subjected to the usual faecal bacteriology and parasitology screening before being mixed with animals already on site. Wild-caught animals, in particular, should also be screened for external parasites such as ticks, which can be removed manually. Many reptiles carry *Salmonella* spp. asymptomatically and cases of salmonellosis in humans have purportedly been traced back to terrapins kept as pets (Arvy 1998). Therefore, normal hygiene precautions should be performed after handling. The use of gloves, when cleaning out, is possibly advantageous in this regard.

When reptiles are fed correctly and kept in a low-stress environment, medical problems are rare; most problems are ultimately related to poor environment, diet or stress.

Transport

Sympathetic and sensitive methods of transportation should be used. Most species of terrapin, and all crocodilians, can be transported in strong, ventilated, wooden boxes with a suitable lining of moisture-retaining material such as hay, moss or foam padding for insulation and to cushion against shocks. There is a suggestion in the literature (International Air Transport Association (IATA) 2007) that those species, such as softshells, that risk desiccation when out of water for long periods, can be transported the same way, but with a thin layer of petroleum jelly applied to the shell, if the journey is not longer than 4–6 h, but this technique does not appear to be widely used. For longer journeys, some sort of supplemental watering may be required. Small softshells can be transported in plastic bags in the same way as tropical fish. Care should be taken to ensure that tropical species are not subjected to temperatures below 10 °C. This may preclude shipment at certain times of the year. Care should also be taken to ensure that crates are not left in direct sunshine or exposed to temperatures over 30 °C for long periods. A suitable design for a crate for air freight can be found in the IATA Live Animal Regulations (2007).

Breeding

Reproduction in crocodilians is diverse and fascinating, involving complex social behaviours, environmental sex determination and parental care. However, as it is not part of laboratory maintenance, it will not be discussed here.

Some species of terrapin breed readily in captivity; others have never been bred. It is unwise to extrapolate directly between species, and what works for one species may not work for another. Nevertheless, some general trends are apparent. Like most reptiles, the timing of reproduction is controlled by a combination of temperature, photoperiod and humidity, the details of which depend on the local environment to which each species, or population, is adapted.

Mating systems

Some species exhibit quite elaborate courtship behaviour (eg, the red-eared slider, *Trachemys scripta elegans*) before mating (Gibbons 1990) but, in others, brute force appears to be used to subdue the female. Biting and butting, or ramming, are the primary means by which this is achieved. Vivaria in which breeding terrapins are held should be large enough to allow full expression of this behaviour (proper courtship in *T. scripta*, for example, cannot occur if the water is too shallow) and should allow the female to be able to gain respite from the attentions of the male. Sex ratios of parity, or slightly female-biased, should be used. If too many males are present, they may spend too much time fighting between themselves or harass the female to the point where they cause her physical harm. However, apparently brutal behaviour leading to obvious injuries appears to be normal in many species, and the females recover.

Nesting

Terrapins may be quite secretive when nesting. Oviposition may occur at night in many species and is usually completed, at least in small (<1 kg) species, within 1 h. It is often preceded by much restless pacing by the female, apparently looking for a suitable site. She will often choose the warmest part of an enclosure, perhaps directly under a spotlight, but will often dig trial holes and then not lay. Eggs scattered on the surface of the vivarium or laid in the water are usually an indication that the nesting facilities provided are inadequate in some way. It is rarely apparent exactly how the nesting area is deficient! A nesting area of damp sand, peat, or a mixture of the two, with a depth of up to 30 cm, and a substrate temperature of 25 °C or more should be provided. Excavation occurs with the hind feet in most species, an exception being the highly endangered Australian chelid, *Pseudemydura umbrina*, which uses its forelimbs.

In emydids, oviposition usually occurs about 60 days after mating, but the pattern is less clear in other families. Clutch sizes vary from a single, large egg in many chelids and pelomedusids, to more than 100 in *Podocnemis expansa*. There is a positive correlation between body size and clutch size. Eggs may be spherical or almost cylindrical in shape, and are normally brittle-shelled.

In situations where terrapins are maintained outdoors, careful searching may be necessary to find all nests. Eggs should be removed from the nesting area as soon as possible after laying. They should be set in a moistened medium, such as peat or vermiculite, with about two thirds of the egg buried. If peat is used, the medium should be moist, but not wet, to the touch. Conventional wisdom has it that the eggs should not be turned or rotated, as this may damage the embryo, but this may be unnecessary (Gad 1988). The eggs should be incubated at a temperature between 28 and 32 °C. In some species, the sex of the hatchling is determined by the temperature at which the egg is incubated (Yntema & Mrosovsky 1979; Vogt & Bull 1982): 30 °C produces both males and females, but, at higher temperatures, predominantly females are produced, while more males occur at lower temperatures. There is speculation that laying females may deliberately select nest sites at a particular temperature, in order to produce either males or females. However, other species, eg, *Elusor macrurus*, do not show temperature-dependent sex determination (Georges & McInnes 1998).

Emydid eggs usually take 60–90 days to hatch, depending upon the incubation temperature and possibly other factors, as yet unknown. Eggs laid by species from other families may take longer, possibly including a period of embryonic diapause. Some take significantly shorter periods; for example, *Terrapene coahuila* takes a mean of 46.3 days (Cerda & Waugh 1992) at 29–31.5 °C.

Early development

After pipping, the infant should be left in the incubation chamber until the yolk sac has been completely absorbed. This may take 1–3 days, during which time the hatchling will bury into the substrate and be invisible. Once the yolk sac has been absorbed, the infant can be transferred to a rearing vivarium. This should be similar to the adults' vivarium, but with smaller water depths sufficient to allow the infant to right itself, should it fall on its back, but not too deep that it may risk drowning, and there should be ample provision of hiding places.

Management of juvenile terrapins is similar to that of adults. Similar diets are used for both, though foodstuffs must be more finely chopped. Weight and length should be monitored at regular intervals, at least monthly, and any specimens that are lagging behind the rest should be isolated and given individual attention. It is inadvisable to leave juveniles in the same vivarium as adults, as predation may occur.

Feeding

Natural and laboratory diets

Correct nutritional regimes for terrapins are still a matter of some controversy. Little experimental work has been carried out on the topic, and much of the literature is based on hearsay and/or personal experience, rather than scientific investigation (but see Stancel *et al.* 1998; McRoberts & Hopkins 1998).

The majority of terrapins are predatory animals to some degree. Some species are specialised, such as the big-headed terrapin (*Platysternon megacephalum*) and have not fared particularly well in captivity, while others, such as sliders (*Trachemys* spp.), have an extremely catholic diet. Some exhibit a form of ontogenetic dietary shift, usually becoming more herbivorous with age (Clark & Gibbons 1969). For the majority of species, there is little information on diet in the wild.

Box 47.1 lists dietary items that have been used to feed terrapins. The list is not exhaustive; there are certainly others that have been used subject to local availability. Wild terrapins will feed on almost any animal (alive or dead) that they can overpower, often attacking in groups and developing a feeding frenzy. This is one advantage of keeping terrapins in groups, as this behaviour often stimulates reluctant feeders. Terrapins are unsophisticated predators, biting hard and then ripping prey with the forelimbs. This is one reason why they are messy feeders. Another is due to the rapid disintegration of food items that are not patent, for example, some gelatine-based mixtures, proprietary dog foods, etc.

The author's particular preference is to use whole animal carcases, usually rodents, fish and chicks. The former are available in a large range of sizes, from tiny pinkies to large, adult rats, and provide bone and roughage though

Box 47.1 Foodstuffs used to feed terrapins

Lean meat (diced); chopped liver:
Useful as 'treats' but poor Ca:P ratio precludes regular use. Patency is improved by cooking. Liver is particularly messy
Rodents, chicks (whole or chopped):
Excellent, palatable food. Good Ca:P ratio. Fairly patent; chicks can be messy if the internal yolk sac is large
Insects (giant mealworms, mealworms, crickets, locusts, waxmoth larvae):
Good 'treat' value, especially when fed live. Poor Ca:P ratio but good roughage content
Molluscs and crustaceans (prawns, crab meat, snails, mussels):
Fairly palatable; poor Ca:P ratio unless the shells are included; useful 'treats'. Expensive
Other animal foodstuffs (dry dog food, earthworms, tinned fish):
Fairly palatable; poor patency (fish) or low Ca:P ratio (worms) preclude frequent use
Plants (lettuce, grated vegetables, water plants):
Good Ca:P ratios; fairly palatable; good roughage. Can be offered *ad libitum*
Other foodstuffs mentioned in the literature but not used by the author:
Herrings, sprats, hard-boiled egg, trout pellets, tinned cat and dog food, cockles, lobster meat, squid, tubifex, mosquito larvae, mackerel, commercial terrapin diet

they are often high in both fat and protein so should not be relied upon exclusively. Most terrapins will also avidly pursue live insects, which can also be used to stimulate reluctant feeders. A most important aspect of feeding is to provide variety, as this has great behavioural and nutritional benefit.

Some keepers place vitamin or mineral supplements on food before feeding but, as most terrapins can, or will, feed only in water, the benefits of this practice are dubious. A varied diet of whole animals will provide the majority of the vitamin and mineral needs for most species of terrapin. As with most reptiles, calcium metabolism is of critical importance to health, and an extra calcium supplement to most terrapins is diced or flaked cuttlebone, placed in water.

For those species that are herbivorous a diet of green vegetables, with high calcium content, such as dandelions, chicory, endive, pak choi and watercress, should be offered with the occasional 'treat' fruit such as mango, apple, pear etc.

Crocodilians are exclusively carnivorous. Most species that are suitable for laboratory use will feed very well on laboratory rodents, day-old chicks, or whole freshwater fish and all their nutritional needs will be catered for. Dietary 'treats', such as live insects, can be offered occasionally, for behavioural enrichment. Feeding of live vertebrates, such as fish or frogs, although it may have some benefits, is not essential and is illegal in some areas of the world. Even where it is technically legal it is a dubious practice ethically.

Laboratory procedures

Handling

It is advisable to be cautious when handling terrapins. Some are completely docile, withdrawing into their shell until handling ceases. Others are highly irritable, administering painful bites frequently and rapidly, whilst struggling vigorously. In general, the handler should always be aware of the orientation of the animal and the head should always be pointed away from the handler. Some pleurodires have enormously long necks and are capable of reaching almost round to their rear feet, eg, *Chelodina oblonga*, so care must be taken to keep fingers well out of the way.

Small cryptodire terrapins can be safely picked up by holding the sides of the carapace from above, the legs and neck being too short to reach the fingers. Larger specimens need to be held from behind to avoid the head and forelimbs. However, it should be borne in mind that the hindlimbs are also powerful and can cause loss of grip, as well as scratching the handler. With softshells, the problem is exacerbated because of the slippery carapace, in which case, a damp cloth may be useful. Some terrapins are too heavy and aggressive to be handled by a single person. Terrapins should never be held far above a substrate as they do wriggle or bite without warning, and there is a risk of their being dropped and injured. As a general rule handling should be kept to a minimum and the animals should not be unnecessarily inverted as this is stressful.

Handling crocodilians is not to be undertaken lightly. Even hatchlings can give painful bites, and animals over 1 m in length should always be regarded as dangerous. Small (less than 0.5 m) specimens can be seized from behind (never laterally), grasping the back of the head and then using the other hand to hold the pelvis at the base of the tail. Once held the mouth should be taped shut to remove the bite risk. For details of how to capture larger specimens, see Wise (1994).

Physiological monitoring

Chelonians and crocodilians are ectotherms, so relatively little information about the physiological status of the animal can be gained from monitoring the body temperature. Critical thermal maxima for most species occur in the region of 34–38 °C. Information about body temperatures is obtained by insertion of a thermal probe into the cloaca, but this is not safely possible in hatchling or small juvenile specimens.

Obtaining blood samples is relatively straightforward. Most crocodilians and chelonians have venous sinuses in the post-occipital region, from which blood can be obtained using an appropriately sized needle (Bennett 1986). The jugular vein is another potential site if the terrapin can be induced to protrude its neck from the shell, and the caudal vein can be productive in larger specimens. In very small chelonians, direct cardiopuncture, via a plastral suture, may be the only practical way of obtaining blood (Frye 1991) though this is not without risk to the animal so should only be used as a last resort.

Urine may be ejected spontaneously on handling, but otherwise may be obtained by placing the terrapin in a dry, plastic tank, and waiting.

Administration of medicines and euthanasia

Most bacteria that are pathogenic to reptiles are gram-negatives such as *Pseudomonas* sp. or *Aeromonas* sp. These are usually secondary infections to some other illness or injury and can be treated using antibiotics, but care must be taken to ensure that supportive therapy, such as rehydration and adequate ambient temperatures (30–32 °C), are also in place. Comparatively few antibiotics have been tested in reptiles and some are known to have nephrotoxic effects. Therefore, injection sites should always be in the anterior part of the body, intramuscularly or subcutaneously in the forelimbs. The venous sinuses behind the cranium are also potential sites. Dose rates of 2.5–10 mg/kg for gentamicin are given in Frye (1991), which also contains a very full discussion of antibiotic therapy in general.

Terrapins and crocodilians can be anaesthetised using standard, injectable anaesthetic drugs such as ketamine hydrochloride, propofol or saffan. Volant, inhalant drugs such as isoflurane cannot safely be used to induce anaesthesia but can maintain it provided that this is supported by suitable ventilation. This should only be done under veterinary supervision. Hypothermia should not be used for anaesthetic purposes as there is no evidence that this reduces the animal's sensitivity to pain, merely its ability to move away from it.

Terrapins and crocodilians are tough animals that can be difficult to kill in the laboratory context. Insertion into a freezing environment, or the use of volant anaesthetics such as chloroform have been used in the past, but these are now regarded as either ineffective or potentially painful. The only method of euthanasia now considered acceptable is injection with an overdose of an anaesthetic agent such as pentobarbital followed by pithing to ensure destruction of the brain (Baier 2006).

Common welfare problems

Disease

General veterinary medicine for reptiles is discussed in Mader (2006) and much detailed information on testudines is in McArthur *et al.* (2004). The main constraint on terrapin welfare is adequate water hygiene, as discussed previously. Most other problems are related to inadequate nutrition, lighting or physical environment. For example, necrotic dermatitis ('shell rot') can occur and is often traceable to some sort of inadequate husbandry. It is usually treatable with an appropriate antibiotic. Respiratory diseases, potentially leading to pneumonia, are not uncommon, particularly in terrapins, and can be difficult to treat. If access to adequate levels of heat and UV light are not sufficient to treat the condition then veterinary assistance will be required. Improvements in the quality of available diets have meant that terrapin diseases that caused difficulties in the past are no longer such a problem.

Vitamin A deficiency (hypovitaminosis A) is probably the most common illness observed in terrapins. It is often found in juveniles after the age of about 6 months. The most obvious manifestation is a swelling of the tissues around the eyes and the airways.

Hyperkeratinosis is also sometimes visible. It is a result of inadequate diet, usually the persistent feeding of red meat. It is fairly easily treated, using multivitamin drops administered orally, and by the addition of supplemental items to the diet, such as earthworms, fish and fresh aquatic vegetation. In the past, some veterinarians have over-reacted to this condition and initiated regular injections of vitamin A as a prophylactic. This should not be necessary if the diet is adequate.

Vitamin B deficiency occurs due to the destructive activity of the enzyme thiaminase, which occurs in frozen fish and molluscs. Chronic nervous system abnormalities can occur, such as nervous tremors, postural abnormalities and blindness. They are easily treated with an injection of thiamin hydrochloride.

Metabolic bone disorders caused by imbalances in the calcium content of the diet are very common and can lead to spectacular shell deformities, which are untreatable (Stancel *et al.* 1998). The imbalances in the calcium content may be a function of poor calcium levels in the diet but can also be caused by a poor calcium:phosphorus ratio. The feeding of large quantities of red meat or insects is a typical cause. Correct calcium:phosphorus ratios are in the range of 1:1 to 2:1. Whole neonate mice are a good source of dietary calcium (Barten 1988). Even if adequate calcium:phosphorus ratios are present in the diet, it is possible that metabolic bone disease may still occur, as vitamin D_3 is required by reptiles in order to metabolise calcium. They can manufacture vitamin D_3 endogenously if given sufficient exposure to a source of UV radiation at about 290–310 nm wavelength. Natural sunlight has this in abundance, but terrapins maintained indoors will require an artificial source.

As a rule, most terrapins are tough, adaptable creatures that cope well with captive management conditions. Those species that are exceptions should not be considered for laboratory use.

Reproductive problems

The most common reproductive complication is egg retention (dystocia). The cause of this is often behavioural, perhaps an inability to find or identify a suitable nesting site. Signs include lethargy, reluctance to walk and unsteadiness on the hindlimbs. It is difficult to identify, as it can only be confirmed by X-ray, and can be life-threatening. If warm water enemas and lubrication fail to work, the alternatives are injection with oxytocin (2–10 mg/kg) (Hoggard 2000), following a course of calcium borogluconate injections (10 mg/kg) (Highfield 1996) or surgical removal (Frye 1991).

References

Arvy, C. (1998) Salmomelloses humaines lieus aux tortues: une revue de probleme et de son evolution. *Bulletin de la Societe Herpetologique de France*, **84**, 25–31

Bagatto, B. and Henry, R.P. (1999) Exercise and forced submergence in the pond slider (*Trachemys scripta*) and softshell (*Apalone ferox*): influence on bimodal gas exchange, diving behaviour and blood acid-base status. *Journal of Experimental Biology*, **202**, 267–278

Baier, J. (2006) Reptiles. In: *Guidelines for Euthanasia of Non-domestic Animals*. American Association of Zoo Veterinarians, Florida

Baines, F., Beveridge, A. and Lane, R. (2005) Looking at UVB in a new light. A four part study of ultra-violet light in reptile husbandry. *Herptile*, **30**, 148–172

Barten, S.L. (1988) Herp health and husbandry hints. Calcium metabolism when feeding herps pinky mice. *Bulletin of the Chicago Herpetological Society*, **23**, 14–15

Belkin, D.A. (1964) Variations in heart rate during voluntary diving in the turtle, *Pseudemys concinna*. *Copeia*, 321–330

Bennett, J.M. (1986) A method for sampling blood from hatchling loggerhead turtles. *Herpetological Review*, **17**, 43

Bethea, N.J. (1972) Effects of temperature on heart rate and rates of cooling and warming in *Terrapene ornata*. *Comparative Biochemistry and Physiology* (A), **41**, 301–305

Bickham, J.W., Hanks, B.G., Smolen, M.J. *et al.* (1988) Flow cytometric analysis of the effects of low level radiation exposure on natural populations of slider turtles (*Pseudemys scripta*). *Archives of Environmental Contamination and Toxicology*, **17**, 837–841

Bonin, F., Devaux, B. and Dupre, A. (2006) *Turtles of the world*. A and C Black, London

Cann, J. and Legler, J. M. (1994) The Mary River tortoise: a new genus and species of short-necked chelid from Queensland. *Chelonian Conservation and Biology*, **1**, 81–96

Cerda, A. and Waugh, D. (1992) Status and management of the Mexican box terrapin, *Terrapene coahuila*, at the Jersey Wildlife Preservation Trust. *Dodo Journal of the Wildlife Preservation Trusts*, **28**, 126–142

Clark, P.B. and Gibbons, J.W. (1969) Dietary shift in the turtle, *Pseudemys scripta*, from youth to maturity. *Copeia*, **4**, 704–706

Cloudsley-Thompson, J.W. (1982) Rhythmic activity in young red-eared terrapins (*Pseudemys scripta elegans*). *British Journal of Herpetology*, **6**, 188–193

European Commission (2007) Commission recommendations of 18 June 2007 on guidelines for the accommodation and care of animals used for experimental and other scientific purposes. Annex II to European Council Directive 86/609 See 2007/526/EC. http://eurlex.europa.eu/LexUriServ/site/en/oj/2007/l_197/l_19720070730en00010089.pdf (accessed 13 May 2008)

Frye, F.L. (1991) *Reptile Care. An Atlas of Diseases and Treatments. Vols I and II*. T.F.H. Publications, New Jersey

Gad, J. (1988) Drehversuche an Schildkröteneiern im Hinblick auf Schildanomalien hier bei *Sternotherus odoratus*. *Salamandra*, **25**, 109–111

Gehrmann, W.H. (1987) Ultraviolet irradiances of various lamps used in animal husbandry. *Zoo Biology*, **6**, 117–127

Georges, A. and McInnes, S. (1998) Temperature fails to influence hatchling sex in another genus and species of chelid turtle *Elusor macrurus*. *Journal of Herpetology*, **32**, 596–598

Gibbons, J.W. (Ed.) (1990) *Life History and Ecology of the Slider Turtle*. Smithsonian Institution Press, Washington, DC

Gibbons, J.W. and Lovich, J.C. (1990) Sexual dimorphism in turtles with emphasis on the slider turtle, *Trachemys scripta*. *Herpetological Monographs*, **4** 1–29

Glidewell, J.R., Beitinger, T.L. and Fitzpatrick, L.C. (1981) Heat exchange in submerged red-eared turtle (*Chrysemys scripta*). *Comparative Biochemistry and Physiology* (A), **70**, 141–143

Harless, H. and Morlock, H. (1979) *Turtles: Perspectives and Research*. John Wiley & Sons, New York

Highfield, A.C. (1996) *Practical Encyclopedia of Keeping and Breeding Tortoises and Freshwater Turtles*. Carapace Press, Tortoise Trust, England

Hinton, T.G., Whicker, F.W., Pinder, J.E. III *et al.* (1992) Comparative kinetics of ^{47}Ca, ^{90}Sr and ^{226}Ra in the freshwater turtle, *Trachemys scripta*. *Journal of Environmental Radioactivity*, **16**, 25–47

Hoggard, C. (2000) The use of oxytocin in gravid aquatic turtles. *Wildlife Rehabilitation*, **18**, 15–24

Honegger, R. E. (1979) Marking reptiles and amphibians for future identification. *International Zoo Yearbook*, **19**, 14–22

International Air Transport Association (2007) *Live Animals Regulations 2007*, 34th edn. IATA, Montreal

International Union for Conservation of Nature and Natural Resources (2007) IUCN Red List *www.iucnredlist.org*

Iverson, J.B. (1992) *A Revised Checklist with Distribution Maps of the Turtles of the World*. Privately printed, Richmond, Indiana

Jackson, D.C. (1971) The effects of temperature on ventilation in the turtle *Pseudemys scripta elegans*. *Respiration Physiology*, **12**, 131–140

Mader, D.R. (2006) *Reptile Medicine and Surgery*. Elsevier, Philadelphia

McArthur, S., Wilkinson, R. and Meyer, J. (2004) *Medicine and Surgery of Tortoises and Turtles*. Blackwell Publishing, Oxford

McCord, W.P. and Pritchard, P.C.H. (2002) A review of the softshell genus *Chitra* with the description of new taxa from Myanmar and Indonesia (Java). *Hamadryad*, **27**, 11–56

McRoberts, S.P. and Hopkins D.T. (1998) The effects of dietary vitamin C on growth rates of juvenile slider turtles (*Trachemys scripta elegans*). *Journal of Zoo and Wildlife Medicine*, **29**, 419–422

Parmenter, R.R. (1981) Digestive turnover rates in freshwater turtles: the influence of temperature and body size. *Comparative Biochemistry and Physiology*, **70A**, 235–238

Peters, E.C. and Brisbin, I.L. (1996) Environmental influences on the ^{137}Cs kinetics of the yellow-bellied turtle (*Trachemys scripta*). *Ecological Monographs*, **66**, 115–136

Pina, C.L., Larriera, A., Medina, M. *et al.* (2007) Effects of incubation temperature on the size of *Caiman latirostris* at hatching and after one year. *Journal of Herpetology*, **41**, 205–210

Plummer, M.V. (1979) Collecting and marking. In: *Turtles. Perspectives and Research*. Eds Harless, H. and Morlock, H., pp. 45–60. John Wiley & Sons, New York

Poole, T. (ed) (1999) *The UFAW Handbook on the Care and Management of Laboratory Animals*, 7th edn., vol. 2. Blackwell Publishing, Oxford

Pritchard, P.C.H. (1979) *Encyclopedia of Turtles*. T.F.H. Publications, New Jersey

Ross, C.A. (Ed.) (1989) *Crocodiles and Alligators*. Merehurst Press, London

Ross, C.A., Blake, D.K. and Onions, J.T.V. (1989) Farming and ranching. In: *Crocodiles and Alligators*. Ed. Ross, C.A., pp. 202–214. Merehurst Press, London

Spray, D.C. and May, M.L. (1972) Heating and cooling rates in four species of turtles. *Comparative Biochemistry and Physiology*, **41A**, 507–522

Stancel, C.F., Dierenfeld, E.S. and Schoknecht P.A. (1998) Calcium and phosphorous supplementation decreases growth but does not induce pyramiding in young red-eared sliders (*Trachemys scripta elegans*). *Zoo Biology*, **17**, 17–24

Storey, K.B., Layne, J.R., Cutwa, M.M. *et al.* (1993) Freezing survival and metabolism of box turtles. *Copeia*, 628–634

Swingland, I. R. (1978) Marking reptiles. In: *Animal Marking: Recognition Marking of Animals in Research*. Ed. Stonehouse, B., 119–141. Macmillan, London

Trutnau, L. and Sommerlad, R. (2006) *Crocodilians: their Natural History and Captive Husbandry*. Edition Chimaira, Frankfurt-am-Main

Vogt, R.C. and Bull, J.J. (1982) Temperature controlled sex determination in turtles: ecological and behavioural aspects. *Herpetologica*, **38**, 156–164

Wise, M. (1994) Techniques for the capture and restraint of captive crocodilians. In: *Captive Management and Conservation of Amphibians and Reptiles*. Eds Murphy, J.B., Adler, K. and Collins, J.T., pp. 401–405. Society for the Study of Amphibians and Reptiles, St Louis

Yntema, C.L. (1981) Characteristics of gonads and oviducts in hatchlings and young of *Chelydra serpentina* resulting from three incubation temperatures. *Journal of Morphology*, **167**, 297–304

Yntema, C. L. and Mrosovsky, N. (1979) Incubation temperature and sex ratio in hatchling loggerhead turtles: a preliminary report. *Marine Turtle Newsletter*, **11**, 17–28

48 Amphibians, with special reference to *Xenopus*

Richard Tinsley

Biological overview

Amphibians occupy a curious place in the perceptions of many biologists. They are often regarded as a 'minor group', intermediate between fish that are successful in water and the reptiles, birds and mammals that overcame the constraints of life on land; they are considered to represent a tentative experiment in the conquest of land, condemned to an unsatisfactory dependence on damp conditions for survival. In fact, amphibians are highly successful in particular environments with approximately the same number of species as mammals. Many of the specialisations assumed characteristic of higher tetrapod vertebrates are found to be well developed in amphibians (Tinsley 1995). Thus, the immune system has been shown, in an intensively studied anuran such as *Xenopus laevis*, to have virtually all the components found in mammals. Other adaptations of amphibians are unique amongst tetrapod vertebrates.

Amphibians are abundant locally, especially in the tropics but also elsewhere. A visitor from another planet arriving in the Sonoran desert of North America on the first night of the summer rains could be misled into concluding that anurans are the dominant form of vertebrate life in areas that, by day, seem largely uninhabited. On nights when spawning occurs there may be hundreds of toads of half a dozen different species in newly formed ephemeral ponds only a few metres in diameter. Indeed, it is during periods of breeding – in water – that the abundance of amphibians resident in the surrounding area becomes apparent.

Amphibians are exceptional amongst vertebrates in using the skin as a respiratory surface (in addition, in most species, to the lungs and buccal cavity). This has profound implications for many aspects of biology. The skin is a delicate layer that, typically, is kept moist for respiration by extensive mucus secretion; it is highly permeable and well supplied with blood vessels. Amphibians are able to absorb water rapidly through the skin. The kidneys cannot concentrate urine to conserve water. Nitrogenous wastes are eliminated primarily as urea (or ammonia in some amphibians) in very dilute urine. Together, these features prevent measures to restrict water loss. Most amphibians lose water by continuous evaporation from the skin and this confines them to relatively moist environments. The urinary bladder serves as an important water store: this water can be resorbed into the body during dehydration (a process impossible in higher tetrapods).

Amphibians are ectothermic, with body temperature dependent on the external environment, but they can regulate temperature both behaviourally and by evaporative cooling. At very low temperatures, amphibians enter a state of torpor: they seek refuges, their metabolic rate slows, and all physiological requirements are reduced. For small animals in a cool temperate climate, ectothermy may be a distinct advantage: metabolic needs correspond with food availability. In winter, hibernating amphibians do not need to eat until favourable conditions (and prey) return. By contrast, many small mammals need to eat more when cold to maintain constant body temperature even when food is scarce.

All amphibians are carnivorous as juveniles and adults but the larval (tadpole) stage has a wide range of food types including vegetation, microscopic particles and aquatic prey. The diet of post-metamorphic amphibians is primarily composed of small invertebrates but may include young of the same or other amphibian species. With few exceptions, prey capture occurs on land involving terrestrial and aerial targets. Vision is the predominant sense for most species. It is used to detect prey, with movement triggering a feeding response. Prey size appears to be the main determinant of food intake – usually anything that can be taken into the mouth and swallowed. There is typically no overlap in food types (and hence competition) between the tadpole (in water) and the metamorphosed juveniles and adults (on land).

There is much variation in the abilities of amphibians to tolerate dry conditions but almost all return to water to breed. Amphibians (especially anurans) have entirely different juvenile and adult forms. The tadpole is essentially fish-like, and transforms into a tetrapod juvenile that is usually adapted for life on land. This process of metamorphosis is unique amongst vertebrates: the juvenile stage is redesigned and reconstructed out of the components that made up the larva.

Amphibians evolved from fish ancestors in the late Devonian period. The radiation that followed in the Carboniferous, Permian and Triassic led to an abundance of species and a worldwide distribution. However, all these lines became extinct and fossils of present-day amphibians, the Lissamphibia, appear first in the Triassic but then diversify in the Jurassic. Curiously, there is no overlap in the fossil record between the extinct groups that represent 'The Age of the Amphibians' and the ancestors of modern extant taxa. Timescales are impressive: the first amphibians evolved

380–360 million years ago (mya) and were abundant for around 120 million years. Subsequent to the extinction of these groups, the morphology of the oldest anuran fossils was already equivalent to that of modern representatives: thus, the pipids (the family to which *Xenopus* belongs) have fossils in the Cretaceous (125 mya) very similar to present species. However, the major diversification of anurans is relatively recent with genera such as *Bufo* appearing in the Paleocene (60 mya) and *Rana* in the Eocene (50 mya). Remarkably, this evolution is roughly contemporaneous with that of the mammals.

There are three orders of Lissamphibians. Apoda (alternatively called Caecilia or Gymnophiona) comprise about 170 species. Urodela (alternatively called Caudata) – newts and salamanders – comprise about 540 species. Anura (or Salientia or Batrachia) – frogs and toads – have about 5200 species (Stuart *et al.* 2008). They are easily distinguished: apodans have no limbs or limb girdles and are worm-like, burrowing in tropical soils; urodeles have a long tail and their limbs are more or less of equal length; anurans have a very short vertebral column, no tail, and hindlimbs are typically longer than the forelimbs, adapted for jumping.

Over the past 20 years, there have been reports of declining amphibian populations. Comprehensive data have been compiled documenting both their diversity and threats to their survival (Stuart *et al.* 2008). At least 43% of all species are declining in population numbers and about one third (32%) of the world's species are classified as threatened. At least 34 species have become extinct since their recognition scientifically, nine since 1980, but over 100 others have uncertain status. Data on the causes of decline show that habitat loss represents the greatest threat, followed by pollution. Current concerns about disease focus on the chytrid fungus *Batrachochytrium dendrobatidis*, considered responsible for dramatic population declines in many regions worldwide. The survey also shows that many species are declining for unknown reasons and this increases concerns that amphibians may be sensitive indicators of wider fundamental changes affecting biodiversity.

Uses in the laboratory

Biologists have long recognised that amphibians offer important advantages for laboratory investigation. Major advances in fundamental knowledge of physiology and biochemistry were first made with studies on amphibians, and subsequently these animals were used in research fields including embryology and endocrinology, genetics and immunology. For the past 30 years, one species – *Xenopus laevis* – has become one of the most intensively used of all 'laboratory animals' (alongside the mouse and chick) in developmental, cell and molecular biology (Gurdon 1996).

Reproduction is exceptional amongst tetrapod vertebrates in that mating of one male and female anuran may generate several thousand offspring that are siblings of one another. This is an advantage for laboratory studies that require replicate groups of animals with limited (brother/sister) genetic variability: such replication is impossible with the typically small clutch sizes of higher tetrapods including birds and mammals.

Factors affecting the use of amphibians in the laboratory

In contrast to many 'lab animals', amphibians are often caught in the wild as adults before maintenance in the laboratory; these animals are accustomed to natural environmental conditions and have specific behaviours, especially predator avoidance, that influence their responses to laboratory regimens.

Amphibians are typically secretive animals, generally dispersed and more-or-less solitary in natural habitats and often encountered in large numbers only when breeding. Most species are nocturnal and their activity is strongly influenced by temperature and moisture availability. Not surprisingly, transfer to laboratory conditions may result in significant stress.

Many factors affecting the welfare of wild animals brought into the laboratory relate to their state and experience in the wild prior to capture. Season of the year is particularly important with respect to the physiology of amphibians beginning laboratory maintenance. In temperate regions, amphibians (especially frogs, species of *Rana*) caught during reproduction in spring may not have fed significantly for many months (since before hibernation). Typically, these animals have survived on stored fat reserves designed to meet reduced metabolic needs during hibernation at low temperatures. Following this, reserves may be near to exhaustion. In the wild, feeding may be relatively intensive post-breeding as temperatures rise in late spring/summer. Prey intake serves to restore physiological condition, including lipid reserves, and to prepare the gonads (in late summer/autumn) for the following year's reproduction. Laboratory maintenance that does not allow for this energy intake and increased metabolism may leave amphibians in a progressively weakening condition, ultimately so that they are unfit to be used in research. Thus, following collection in spring, frogs may be kept alive for several months at low temperatures with little or no food intake, but their stamina may be limited, especially if brought to higher temperatures for laboratory investigations.

Seasonal conditions in the natural habitat may strongly influence 'fitness for purpose' of wild-caught amphibians used for egg production (*Xenopus*, for instance). Thus, *X. laevis* at the Cape, South Africa (the origin of most laboratory supplies) breeds from early spring to mid/late summer, typically September to February. Females may spawn up to three times during this period, so a proportion of adults brought into laboratories worldwide for oocyte 'harvesting' may have gravid ovaries fully prepared for ovulation whilst others may have depleted ovaries following recent natural spawning. These animals may be accustomed to natural water temperatures close to those typically experienced in laboratories (ie, around 20 °C). On the other hand, adult *X. laevis* collected during April–July (late autumn/winter at the Cape) may be taken from water at low temperatures (around 10 °C), unprepared for immediate spawning, and transfer to laboratory temperatures may represent a shock. These natural seasonal cycles may explain part of the variation in physiological state of *X. laevis* when employed in laboratory research immediately after importation. This variation is avoided when *X. laevis* is maintained under appropriate laboratory conditions (especially regarding temperature and food supply) for a period (at least 1 but preferably 2 months) after importation and before laboratory use. On the other hand, the use of lab-raised *X. laevis* in research eliminates these problems altogether.

Workers concerned with the maintenance of amphibians are familiar with instances where animals die suddenly or after a period of deterioration where it seems that 'nothing can be done' to alleviate ill-health. As a result, infectious diseases are much feared. The perception of vulnerability is enhanced by the fact that amphibians live naturally in damp, dark conditions favouring microbial growth and have a delicate, naked skin that seems to offer poor protection against pathogens. However, amphibians have occupied the equivalents of their present niches for over 100 million years, through periods of enormous environmental change – including the catastrophes linked with the extinction of the dinosaurs. Hence, we might anticipate profound and very successful specialisations. The delicate skin is equipped with glands that secrete over 50 different chemicals, many with protective functions including antibiotic action. Understanding the factors influencing the health of amphibians requires recognition of responses to unfavourable conditions, the effects of stress and the circumstances that can lead to infection and disease.

Approaches to laboratory maintenance

One approach to the maintenance of amphibians in the laboratory is to provide environmental conditions closely matching those of natural habitats. With information on the ecology of a particular species, it is usually feasible to provide an aquarium or terrarium in which major habitat characteristics – including appropriate substrate, water supply, temperature, humidity, illumination, vegetation and cover – are reproduced at a scale sufficient to ensure well-being. Where there are specialist needs, for instance maintenance of rare species requiring critical environmental conditions, this approach may require the resources typically employed in zoos and conservation centres. For large-scale maintenance, simplified systems are often employed that are designed to achieve a cost-effective balance between numbers of animals maintained and the requirements for technician time, environmental control and feeding. For these, the aim is to provide essential needs in a 'minimalist' environment, without attempting to simulate natural habitat conditions. The major problem for amphibian maintenance is that, in most cases, there are no universally accepted methods for optimum husbandry. In particular, there have been few quantitative experimental studies producing data enabling laboratory 'users' to compare outcomes. Recommendations are often anecdotal and reflect the personal preferences of laboratory staff. Whilst experience often provides the best guide (in the absence of controlled experimental data) to high welfare standards, recent surveys of laboratory protocols reveal wide disparity in maintenance practices, including some that would be judged intuitively as inappropriate (Major & Wassersug 1998). There is a clear need for specific guidelines that will improve the care of laboratory-maintained amphibians so that they can retain near-normal activity and physiological condition.

The approach of this chapter is, first, to use three examples to show how information on natural habitat conditions of an amphibian species can be linked to the design of maintenance procedures and, second, to discuss a range of techniques enabling the reader to make informed judgements according to his/her specific requirements. The successive editions of the UFAW Handbooks include detailed accounts of management approaches for amphibians, including comprehensive directions for urodeles. However, the anuran genus most widely used in laboratory research worldwide – *Xenopus* – has had relatively brief coverage so far in the UFAW Handbooks. So, this chapter ends with a special focus on this 'model organism'. The recommendations are based on the author's 40 years of experience of laboratory and field research involving *Xenopus* species and many of the suggestions reflect personal practice.

Alongside this, the author has also selected *Rana* species to illustrate the husbandry of anurans from a mesic environment (ie, damp terrestrial conditions) and, as an extreme contrast, the challenge of laboratory maintenance of a desert specialist, *Scaphiopus couchii*. The intention here is to show that, 'starting from scratch', it is possible to use knowledge of physiology and ecology 'in the wild' to design effective procedures for laboratory maintenance.

The best assurance of optimum care is to have laboratory personnel with a natural sympathy for living amphibians, able to recognise the behaviour patterns and other indicators that reflect good health and absence of stress. They should also possess a thorough knowledge of the 'natural history' of the species.

The following guidelines relate to anuran species that illustrate a range of needs for laboratory management. For urodeles that have general requirements related to those of mesic anurans, readers are referred to earlier editions of the UFAW Handbook (for instance, Verhoeff de Fremery *et al.* 1987; Halliday 1999).

Husbandry of anurans from mesic environments, *Rana* spp.

Ecological and physiological considerations

Species of *Rana* are typically adapted for life in habitats where vegetation provides cover, relatively high humidity, protection from major temperature changes and concealment from predators. Populations are often established near water bodies and a common escape response by a frog on land is to jump into water. While feeding is generally terrestrial, frogs may rehydrate in water. Most activity is nocturnal, corresponding with greatest availability of invertebrate prey, decreased water loss by dehydration and reduced exposure to predators. Frogs are often observed to carry relatively large populations of parasites. For wild-caught animals maintained in the laboratory, these parasites may have implications for health (affecting use in research) and for disease transmission to other individuals.

Laboratory maintenance

It is difficult to envisage effective and humane husbandry procedures other than the simulation, as far as possible, of semi-natural conditions. Most attempts at 'minimalist' accommodation are associated with significant stress and deterioration in condition. There should be no place in current laboratory practices for approaches intended simply to keep amphibians 'alive' until their intended use in research. Thus, it was formerly not unusual for frogs, caught after hibernation when stored reserves are low, to be kept at low temperature without feeding (or with little food intake). Where this approach was accompanied by continuous low-level mortality, it provided clear indication both of the inappropriateness of conditions and of the likelihood of poor performance of surviving animals in subsequent experimental procedures.

Some husbandry handbooks recommend a solid substrate (glass, plastic, metal, ceramic tiles) and a continuous flow of water, designed to wash away faecal material. These conditions are optimal for observation, but not for the well-being of the amphibian. Provision of live prey (crickets, mealworms etc) is difficult when these may become trapped in water and die. Light levels are often too high and frogs tend to huddle together creating a risk of skin damage from urination. Even when given refuges, frogs rarely show natural behaviour patterns. Laboratory aquarium design and size must avoid circumstances where the natural startle response – to jump – will result in collision with tank walls etc.

Appropriate maintenance conditions need to be relatively large scale, with a choice between areas with water and 'land' which has numerous refuges, vegetation, and a substrate of damp soil or seedling compost. Contamination of the soil with faeces (and hence microbial pathogens and parasite infective stages) may be addressed by removing the surface layer and replacing it with fresh sterilised soil, probably at weekly intervals. As with other amphibians that naturally seek concealment, provision of secluded refuges as part of optimum maintenance may conflict with the needs (and legal requirement) for daily inspection to check well-being.

Parasites requiring intermediate hosts such as snails and arthropods are not normally transmitted during laboratory maintenance, so burdens of trematodes (commonly in the lungs and alimentary tract) will not increase. However, the lung nematode *Rhabdias bufonis* has a direct life cycle with infective larvae passed in faeces and re-invading by skin penetration. This and other nematodes infecting the intestine and rectum may increase during laboratory maintenance. Smyth and Smyth (1980) provide a comprehensive account of parasites infecting frogs.

Husbandry of an anuran from an arid environment, *Scaphiopus couchii*

Ecological and physiological considerations

The example chosen for this section, the spadefoot toad *Scaphiopus couchii*, illustrates important principles regarding the laboratory maintenance of amphibians. First, successful laboratory procedures can be devised even for species with highly specialised environmental requirements; but, a detailed knowledge of ecology and physiology is essential to understand these needs. Second, laboratory conditions may be required that diverge significantly from those experienced naturally: the design of procedures may require an innovative approach to achieve appropriate circumstances for feeding, growth and optimum welfare. While this case study represents a relatively extreme example of anuran lifestyle, the experience of laboratory management is equally useful for other anuran species.

Scaphiopus couchii is abundant in the deserts of the southwestern USA and northern Mexico. It might be expected that amphibians would be excluded from such areas of extreme aridity because of their limitations for terrestrial life including highly permeable skin, inability to concentrate excretory products, and the need for breeding and early development to occur in water. However, in most hot deserts, there are periodic weather patterns that, often very briefly, provide conditions favourable for life. The key for survival by many desert organisms includes a fast response to these favourable conditions and a life style geared to rapid growth, reproduction and accumulation of reserves enabling survival through the next period of hostile conditions (Tinsley 1999). *Scaphiopus couchii* escapes the most arid conditions for over 10 months each year by burrowing up to a metre below the desert surface. During this long period, the toads do not feed and rely on stored energy reserves for survival at low metabolic rate. Activity is prompted by heavy rainfall, which typically occurs in July and August in the Sonoran Desert. Spadefoot toads emerge immediately at the onset of torrential rain, triggered not by moisture but by the low frequency vibrations of rainfall on the soil surface. They breed on the first night when there is sufficient water to create temporary ponds. Typically, spawning is restricted to a single night each year (during darkness, 21.00h to 04.00h) but, if there are subsequent heavy rains, spawning may be repeated on two or three further nights. After this, activity is directed towards intensive feeding, but this occurs only on nights when the soil surface is reasonably moist, after rain. In southeast Arizona, *S. couchii* probably has a maximum of 20 nights each year when conditions are suitable for foraging. In between these, the toads bury themselves in shallow burrows to avoid the desert heat. In late August, conditions become dry again and, from late September onwards, relatively cold. Spadefoot toads excavate deep burrows for hibernation where they are buffered from the major temperature and moisture extremes at the surface. Digging is a backwards 'shuffle' using the thickened protuberances on the feet – the 'spades' of their common name. The process does not produce a tunnel; instead, the soil collapses in on the burrowing toad, which remains completely surrounded by soil during dormancy.

To meet spadefoot toads' needs in the laboratory, it is essential to understand the nature of their environmental constraints and specialisations. The skin of *S. couchii* is one of its major adaptations. This is delicate and permeable and might be thought to be the wrong covering for any desert animal. However, *S. couchii* is able to use its skin to take up moisture from the soil when buried beneath the surface. As moisture levels decline, the skin is able to absorb water against an increasing concentration gradient, assisted by accumulation in the tissues of nitrogenous wastes as urea which increases osmotic potential. *Scaphiopus couchii* does not produce a cocoon to isolate itself from the environment as do some other arid-adapted anurans: the skin remains in intimate contact with the soil. Paradoxically, the toads cannot control water influx through the skin and if they are maintained in soil which is too wet they become waterlogged and die. The urinary bladder serves as a major water store: the weight of dilute urine in the bladder may amount to 50% of a toad's total body weight.

Although daytime temperatures on the desert surface exceed 50 °C in summer, average temperature at a depth of 5 cm (the level of shallow burrows) is around 35 °C, dropping to around 22 °C at night. On damp nights when *S. couchii* emerges to feed, surface temperatures vary from 18 to 24 °C. During the period of hibernation, surface temperatures fall below freezing and there may be snow; at the depth of the deep burrows, soil temperatures show reduced extremes but are still below 15 °C for 6–7 months each year, and below 10 °C for 3–5 months (Tocque & Tinsley 1991).

These desert conditions severely restrict the period each year during which *S. couchii* can obtain nutrients for growth, for storage of reserves to sustain hibernation and for production of gonadal products for breeding in the following year. Studies on feeding ecology show that *S. couchii* may be so efficient that it can, exceptionally, survive for 1 year on a single meal (albeit one equal to 55% of the toad's body weight and consisting of lipid-rich termites). Field data of Tocque *et al.* (1995) recorded that opportunities for such an energy-rich diet are limited to the start of the activity season; much of total prey intake comprises hard-bodied invertebrates (especially beetles, ants, crickets and spiders) that have lower calorific values but may provide other essential nutrients.

Laboratory maintenance

With these ecological and physiological characteristics, *S. couchii* requires a carefully designed laboratory maintenance system. Animals can be kept successfully on a semi-natural temperature cycle: 25 °C during the period of active feeding, growth and storage of reserves, followed by simulated dormancy during which temperatures reduce gradually to 15 and 10 °C, and then rise again towards the next activity period. Soil composition is important: *S. couchii* remain in good condition in a loose friable soil consisting of sterilised loam, peat and sand in the ratio 7:3:2 (this may be obtained as a commercial potting compost in some countries). The soil should be kept moist when the animals are active; optimum water content is best achieved by mixing water a little at a time into the soil using the hands. The degree of wetness should not result in soil sticking to the hands. This mixing process provides aeration and prevents growth of moulds. Horticultural seedling composts with a high degree of organic material (including peat) may become too spongy and wet for the sensitive water uptake mechanism of the toad's skin.

During the laboratory 'activity' period, *S. couchii* will burrow to a depth of 10–15 cm, but at the start of hibernation (induced by reducing temperatures) toads burrow to greater depths. Hibernating toads can be maintained singly in plastic tubes (10 cm diameter sections of water pipe) containing soil 25–30 cm deep. The base can be sealed with a lid that is perforated to allow diffusion of moisture. If groups of tubes are stored vertically in a soil-filled tank, the surrounding soil provides insulation and can be watered at intervals so that moisture rises up inside the tubes. The tops of the tubes should be covered to prevent excessive moisture loss but finely perforated to allow air circulation.

Attempts to feed *S. couchii* during the 'activity' period by simulating semi-natural conditions are not successful. If groups of toads are maintained in tanks of soil on a 12 h light: 12 h dark photoperiod, and prey items (crickets, mealworms etc) are added during darkness, most toads remain buried and do not feed. Meanwhile, the prey animals seek refuge and become inaccessible. Entirely unnatural procedures work well in ensuring good food intake. Toads should be gently removed from the soil and transferred singly into plastic aquaria (approx 40 cm × 25 cm basal area) with secure lids, a pre-weighed quantity of prey organisms added, and left undisturbed in dim light. *Scaphiopus couchii* quickly adapts to this unnatural regime and begins prey capture immediately, feeding to satiation generally within an hour. After this, toads should be rinsed with clean water to remove urine that might burn the delicate skin and then returned to soil into which they promptly burrow until the next meal. The feeding periods provide the opportunity to check soil moisture and to re-mix it prior to return to the tube or tank. At the end of a 'feeding season' (perhaps 15–20 meals), the soil should be replaced with fresh sterile compost to exclude risks of infection from faecal material produced between meals.

Procedures involving individual maintenance and feeding allow detailed records of food intake (with prey items that remain after feeding weighed and subtracted from the weight initially offered), body weight increase, etc. Experiments reported by Tocque *et al.* (1995) showed that body weight increased in proportion to weight of food ingested over a 'feeding season' of 6–8 weeks (more than would occur in the wild). This relationship remained whether the toads were fed once or four times a week. Weight increase was greater at 20–24 °C than at 31–33 °C, presumably because a greater proportion of the energy intake was used in maintaining higher metabolic rate at higher temperatures. In these experiments, adult toads given 24 meals could eat a total weight of food equivalent to twice their own body weight and could increase in weight by around 100%. The nutritional quality of food significantly influences body weight gain and fat body accumulation: toads amassed very large fat reserves (up to 14% of their body weight) when fed with lipid-rich mealworms compared with those fed crickets (fat bodies up to 10% toad body weight). However, whilst ensuring energetic needs for hibernation, a lipid-rich diet does not enable good growth (in terms of protein deposition and bone formation). For this, crickets should be fed on a high-protein diet to boost nutrient value and dusted with mineral and vitamin supplements. In the wild, these nutrients would presumably be supplied by the wide diversity of prey organisms (and their gut contents) (Figure 48.1).

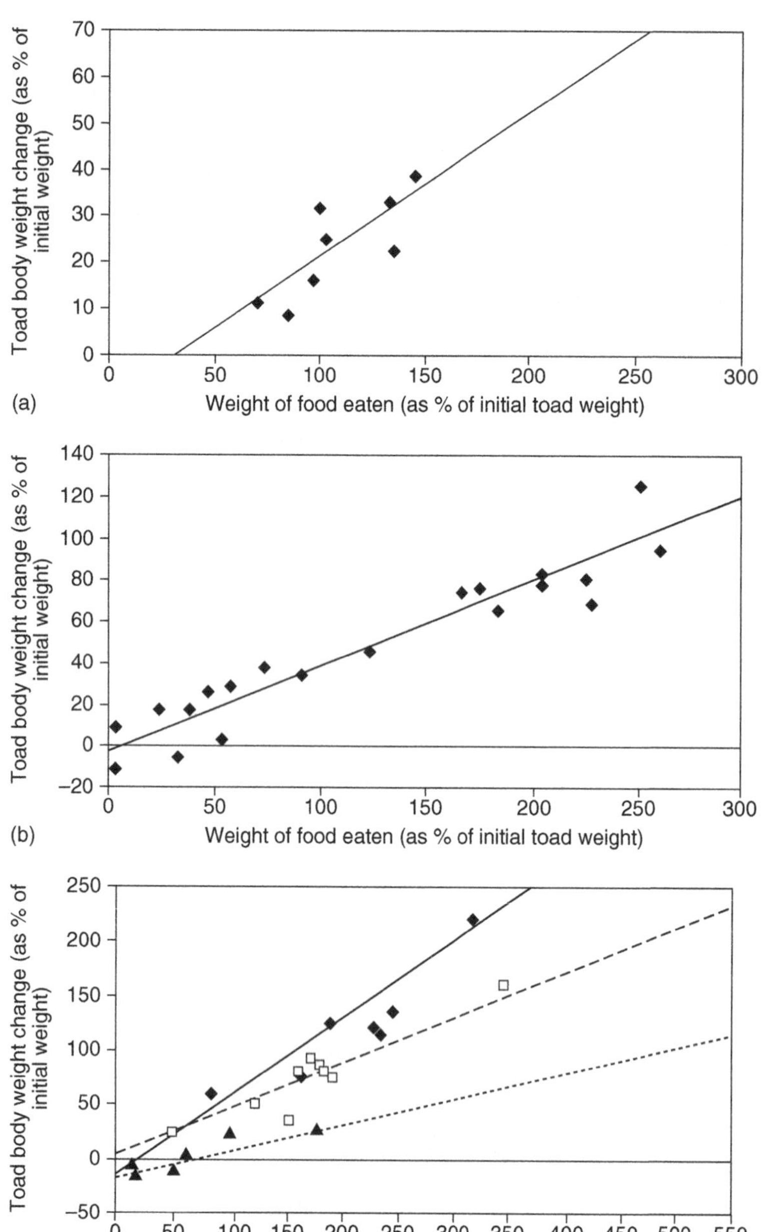

Figure 48.1 Body growth (weight increase) of *Scaphiopus couchii* in alternative laboratory regimens, with varying food intake, frequency and quality. Toad weight change (shown in relation to original weight for each individual), (a) after 16 meals in 51 days at 20 °C; (b) 6 or 24 meals in 42 days at 24 °C (ie, toads fed once or 4 times per week: 6 meals were equivalent to <100% of toad weight); (c) 28 meals in 56 days at 25 °C with crickets (solid diamonds), mealworms (open squares) or woodlice (solid triangles). Adapted from Tocque *et al.* (1995), which provides full details of relationships. Data from these procedures, modified for different amphibian species, are valuable for assessing the effectiveness of laboratory protocols for maintaining body condition and growth.

These findings confirm the exceptional capacity of *S. couchii* to convert energy intake into growth, and to accumulate reserves for hibernation. In laboratory maintenance, the ability to measure food intake and body weight increase provides assurance that animals will then survive a period of starvation, at low temperatures, matching the 9–10 month dormancy in the desert.

At the end of this long dormancy, *S. couchii* can be roused by simulating natural events: the drumming of heavy rainfall. If an electric motor (fan heater or hair dryer) is placed on the soil surface, the vibrations transmitted through the soil will prompt emergence. In one instance in the author's laboratory, animals that had been dormant for 9 months, buried in 30 cm of soil, reached the surface in 7 minutes after initiation of vibrations.

Maintenance regimens such as this require changes to the normal health inspection requirements. If *S. couchii* are disturbed regularly to confirm health during hibernation, they will die because of the repeated switching between low and high metabolic rate and associated consumption of reserves.

Husbandry of an anuran from an aquatic environment, *Xenopus*

Ecological and physiological considerations

Xenopus species occur in most kinds of water bodies in sub-Saharan Africa, especially still waters of swamps, ponds and streams. They are strongly associated with man-made habitats including dams, flooded pits, ditches and wells. They tend to be less common, or absent, from rivers or lakes especially those with well established fish communities. In general, *Xenopus* species prefer cloudy water and areas of vegetation where they are hidden from aerial predators once below the surface. Information on ecology, including habitat conditions and water chemistry, is reviewed by Tinsley *et al.* (1996).

There are currently 18 species of *Xenopus* (together with a series of other distinct forms not yet named) (see Evans *et al.* 2008). These are of major genetic and evolutionary interest because they form a polyploid series with two species groups: one with chromosome numbers of 20 and 40 (generally given a separate genus name, *Silurana*), and the other with 36, 72 and 108 chromosomes (*Xenopus*). *Xenopus* (or *Silurana*) *tropicalis* has increasing application in laboratory research as the only diploid species ($2n = 20$); all others with higher ploidy levels evolved through allopolyploidisation – genome duplication associated with hybridisation between species (Evans 2008).

There are broad distinctions between the species on the basis of geographical distribution and habitat type, but it is difficult to determine niche separation at a fine scale: in some areas up to four different species can be found in the same ponds. However, the two species most commonly employed in laboratory research, *laevis* and *tropicalis*, are ecologically distinct. *Xenopus laevis* is a generalist savannah species occurring in a wide range of habitats from the Cape, South Africa, to Sudan, but typically occupying relatively cooler areas in each region. A succession of subspecies corresponds generally with latitudinal zones within this range. Most laboratory research has been based on *X. laevis laevis* from South Africa but even within this subspecies there is evidence of significant evolutionary divergence. The form occurring in the winter rainfall area of the western Cape is distinct from that in the summer rainfall area further north (Measey & Channing 2003). Fortunately, this should not cause confusion for existing research findings because worldwide export of *X. laevis* has been from populations around the Cape.[1]

Xenopus (or *Silurana*) *tropicalis* is strictly limited to lowland tropical forest in West Africa, from Nigeria to Senegal. It is not found outside the canopy of tropical forest (indeed, in areas when the forest margin is cut back, *X. tropicalis* also contracts its distribution). This suggests a strict requirement for shade, but perhaps also a requirement for relative uniformity of conditions including temperature (where ponds are not exposed to fluctuations in sunshine). Water temperature in natural habitats is typically around 25 °C (Tinsley *et al.* 1996). These species characteristics provide an important guide for laboratory welfare.

X. laevis has been released into the wild and has established self-maintaining populations outside Africa (Tinsley & McCoid 1996). The current list of locations includes Europe (UK, France, Portugal, Italy), North America (many areas but most abundantly in California), South America (Chile), Ascension Island, Indonesia and Japan. Many of the localities have a Mediterranean climate equivalent to that at the Cape, but the diversity of habitat conditions confirms the adaptability of *X. laevis*. This adaptability has contributed to its success as a 'model organism' in laboratory research.

Xenopus laevis is normally very robust with the potential to survive more than 20 years in the laboratory. Animals in the laboratory are protected from many natural mortality factors, but successive recaptures of individually marked *X. laevis* in an introduced population in Wales show that they can also live 20 years in the wild (Tinsley *et al.* 1996 and subsequent unpublished records). Long-term laboratory experience has shown that *Xenopus* species can spawn successfully after 15 years of laboratory maintenance.

Xenopus is unusual in feeding underwater and, in contrast to most terrestrial-feeding amphibians, *Xenopus* may feed communally on larger prey items. Prey is located by sight, odour and by vibrations detected by the lateral line sense organs; this correlates with the preference for still water. The diet may include carrion and contrasts with the situation for most amphibians where, if there is no movement, a potential food item is not recognised. Both tadpoles and post-metamorphs of *Xenopus* feed in the same environment but there is no overlap in diet since the tadpoles are filter-feeders. However, post-metamorphic *Xenopus* may feed on tadpoles. This habit allows very efficient exploitation of energy sources, especially in newly formed habitats where food chains are not well established: the tadpoles feed on phytoplankton which gains energy directly from sunlight, and the adults trap this source of nutrients by cannibalism on the typically very large tadpole populations. *Xenopus* species communicate by specialised vocalisations, maintain territories underwater and have dominant/subordinate hierarchy; they are capable of complex learning and long-term memory (Elepfandt 1996a, 1996b). Above all, they are cryptic and nocturnal.

X. laevis exported from South Africa for laboratory research are caught as adults, after at least 3 years (probably up to 10 years) in natural habitats. The conditions to which they are transferred are often totally at variance with their previous experience. Nocturnal animals accustomed to the security of cloudy water are likely to experience stress in high-density populations in clear, shallow water, illuminated from all sides (and even below), with frequent disturbance and a lack of refuges.

Laboratory maintenance

Aquarium conditions

Laboratory environmental conditions reflecting the preferred habitats of *Xenopus* in the wild can be provided by a dark-sided aquarium with light coming primarily from above, water depth at least 50 cm, a partial surface covering, refuges and still water without appreciable circulation or disturbance.

This combination of features can be achieved with aquaria with thick glass walls and a substrate of rounded gravel ('pea gravel') in which sections of drain pipes or plant pots

[1]*Note: Xenopus* is variously described in the literature as a frog or a toad but these popular terms do not have strict scientific relevance and *Xenopus* is actually distant from both 'divisions'. Although the use of a genus name alone is not accepted scientifically, the name *Xenopus* will be used as an informal designation in this account for the species of *Xenopus* and *Silurana*.

are partially embedded as refuges. A 'three-dimensional' environment can be created with leafy plants (plastic foliage is easier to 'maintain' at low light levels and to wash/sterilise). An appropriate water surface covering can be provided by natural growth of duckweed (*Lemna* spp.) where there is good illumination, including daylight, or by floating synthetic material cut to resemble lily pads. 'Furnished' aquaria of this type can provide relatively stable environments if the bottom gravel supports a culture of bacteria that de-nitrify metabolic and digestive wastes. To maintain equilibrium in water quality, it is essential that the animals are not over-fed (avoiding breakdown of uneaten food in the gravel). This form of management works well with 'chunky' food items (ox-heart, meal worms etc) that are ingested intact, without creating debris during 'capture'. It is impractical with reconstituted, pellet-type food which disintegrates if not eaten quickly. Food input requires judgment (ideally direct observation to note the amount of food that will be eaten within 30–60 minutes). Animals fed to satiation with a single meal each week will maintain optimum physiological condition (with good gonad and fat body development). The complexity of setting up 'semi-natural' habitats such as this is off-set by ease of maintenance: the frequency of water changes can be judged visually by noting water clarity and the build-up of anoxic sediment in the gravel. With good management, water changes may be at 4–6-month intervals (shorter intervals if algal blooms occur in response to sunlight). Water changes require the removal of animals to temporary holding tanks whilst the aquarium is emptied completely and cleaned. The gravel should be thoroughly washed and re-introduced together with a small quantity of the original sediment from which the population of de-nitrifying bacteria can re-establish. Under these semi-natural conditions, animals appear not to be disturbed by movements adjacent to the tank and they can easily be checked for health and well-being. This approach works well for small populations of rare species, especially those sensitive to disturbance.

Whilst these aquarium conditions attempt to achieve optimum welfare by simulating natural habitat conditions, the systems found in some laboratories represent a marked contrast. In some cases, *X. laevis* are maintained in transparent aquaria that allow entry of light from all directions (including above and below), a featureless substrate without refuges, and water depth less than 10 cm. Under these conditions, *Xenopus* may locate themselves in a 'heap', resulting from their attempts to hide underneath each other. The rationale for such systems is that animals can be seen easily, aquaria can be kept clean, and feeding and water changing can be efficient. However, environmental design promoting optimum physiological condition of *Xenopus* requires careful evaluation.

Water depth

When undisturbed, *Xenopus* spend long periods at the water surface, with nostrils exposed to the air. This has been taken to suggest that maximum water depth should allow animals to stand on the tank bottom and reach the surface 'in comfort'; but the assumption is probably anthropocentric. Animals adjust their buoyancy in deep water with the air capacity of their lungs so that they can 'hang' from the surface without effort. In the wild, *X. laevis* rarely occurs in shallow water: greater depths are preferred probably because of increased protection from predation. It has long been established (Alexander & Bellerby 1938; Bellerby & Hogben 1938) that shallow water and overcrowding lead to ovary regression. In the laboratory, deep water increases the three-dimensional structure of the aquarium habitat and, in conjunction with plants and other enrichment, allows greater subdivision of the space for groups of *Xenopus*. On this basis, water depth of at least 30 cm, preferably 50 cm, is recommended. (In the author's view, the recent European recommendations (Council of Europe 2006, European Commission 2007) in which minimum water depth is approximately the same as snout–vent length is too low.)

Population density

For animals taken from the wild, it seems intuitive that the lowest practicable density (consistent with laboratory constraints) should be advisable. Recommendations in the literature based on volume of water per animal need to take account of associated parameters. If *X. laevis* is maintained at low density in a clear featureless tank, individuals will tend to huddle in a group, furthest from direct light or external movement, and may actually experience the effects of high density. Environmental enrichment creating subdivision of the habitat has an important influence on density. Water volume/animal must also take account of water quality, and hence frequency of water changes and type of diet.

Some guidelines in the literature omit consideration of body size (but presumably relate specifically to fully grown adults). Recommendations on the volume of water to be provided per animal vary (see Reed 2005a). As a general guide, 2 l/animal is too restrictive for adult *X. laevis*, while 12 l/animal (as recommended by the Council of Europe (2006) and European Commission (2007)) may be impractical for large-scale maintenance. Very fast growth rates of juvenile *X. laevis* (with sexual maturity in less than 10 months post-metamorphosis) can be achieved at relatively high density (1.5–2 l/animal at 40–50 mm snout–vent length) if feeding is intensive. This outcome may not necessarily indicate good conditions; instead, it may parallel the fast growth characteristics of intensively reared animals in agriculture and aquaculture.

Tank design

Tanks with darkened sides and a black base provide conditions resembling those in natural habitats but inspection of animals is difficult. *Xenopus* in thick glass-walled aquaria do not appear to react to minor movements lateral to the tank. Tank materials that are smooth and impervious include various plastics, glass and stainless steel, but moulded constructions with rounded junctions between the tank sides and base are easier to clean than the angular joins between glass sheets. 'Food grade' plastics avoid risks of leaching of toxic chemicals. Surfaces should never be cleaned with abrasive materials: the roughened surface may be more easily colonised by micro-organisms.

Xenopus are adept at exploiting any opportunity to escape. They can jump at least their own body length above the water surface, so tanks should have secure, well fitting lids. However, animals should not be able to reach the lid as this can cause nasal trauma; so tank design should allow for height of walls at least 20 cm above the water surface. Solid lids should have air holes. However, in large scale establishments, such tank design has major implications for space needs. Laboratories equipped with semi-automated systems typically find that adult animals maintain excellent condition with water depth 15 cm, density 3 l/animal, and lids only 5 cm above the surface. The key factor may relate to origin: *X. laevis* raised from metamorphosis in such systems adapt well and show no signs of stress; animals caught as adults from the wild are more likely to find such restrictions stressful.

Environmental enrichment

Provision of refuges within the aquarium environment simulates habitat conditions in the natural environment. Various studies (eg, Brown & Nixon 2004) have shown that, when given a choice of secluded or exposed areas, laboratory-maintained *X. laevis* prefer cover. This may be provided by sections of plastic pipe (including water pipes around 100 mm diameter), plastic aquarium foliage etc. It might be expected that this should reduce stress. However, in tanks with appropriate refuges, *X. laevis* remain much more sensitive to disturbance and are startled more easily than animals maintained without cover. Hilken *et al.* (1995) recorded poorer growth in *X. laevis* given shelter compared with those without; this was attributed to greater shyness. There are potential problems where provision of refuges conflicts with the need for periodic inspection to ensure well-being. There is also the possibility of increased stress created by competition within groups of *X. laevis* over utilisation of refuges. The provision of refuges requires further research and evaluation.

Temperature

Information on the ecology of *X. laevis* is necessary to appreciate the thermal limits of this 'laboratory amphibian'. At the Cape, South Africa, *X. laevis* experiences a Mediterranean climate with temperatures below 10 °C in winter and above 25 °C in summer. Records from the various introduced populations in the northern hemisphere show a tolerance of wider extremes. In the eastern USA, animals overwinter beneath the ice of frozen ponds; in Arizona, *X. laevis* occurs in ponds whose summer temperatures reach 30 °C (close to the thermal maximum). In addition to longer-term seasonal variations in temperature, *Xenopus* naturally experience short-term fluctuations determined by habitat conditions including thermal differences between pond areas exposed to sun and in deep shade. Temperature records in ponds inhabited by introduced *X. laevis* in the UK show an annual cycle between 4 and 24 °C, and short-term changes (especially in spring and autumn) of up to 8 °C over 5 days. In these UK populations, *X. laevis* typically experience temperatures below 10 °C for over 6 months (October to March), but they still show fast growth rates, excellent condition and successful breeding. Experience from the author's laboratory shows that *X. laevis* can adapt to long-term maintenance (up to 2 years) at 10 and 15 °C and can be maintained for more limited periods at 5 °C. Although spawning appears to be optimal at around 20 °C, *X. laevis* can spawn in water at 15 °C and the tadpoles can develop to metamorphosis at this temperature that is low relative to conditions in South Africa.

It is clear that *X. laevis* can adapt to a wide range of temperatures, but this is not reflected simply in increased or decreased activity and metabolic rate. There is evidence of behavioural, physiological and immunological changes that represent acclimation to extremes of temperature. Thus, locomotor performance of *X. laevis* acclimated to low temperature is significantly greater at low temperatures than that of animals acclimated to high temperature (Wilson *et al.* 2000). Haematological profiles change in relation both to oxygen-carrying capacity of the blood and to the mechanisms of immune defence. All aspects of laboratory maintenance must take account of profoundly altered physiological characteristics at different temperatures. The functioning of the immune response of *Xenopus* (as in other ectotherm vertebrates) is temperature dependent (Robert & Ohta 2009). At temperatures below about 18 °C, *X. laevis* are progressively immunosuppressed, so special care is necessary to prevent infection. At low temperatures (including 10 °C), *X. laevis* are relatively quiescent and will not tolerate the frequent disturbance typically associated with water changes. (Thus, long-term maintenance is best achieved with stable aquarium systems including a gravel substrate where water changes are necessary only at several month intervals.) Food supply should be proportional to temperature, corresponding with respective metabolic needs. *Xenopus laevis* may remain in good condition in long-term maintenance at 25 °C but they require increased food supply to fuel higher metabolic rate and more frequent water changes to remove waste products.

Laboratory maintenance at different temperatures must also take account of rate of change. Thermal acclimation requires time for physiological changes to occur. Green *et al.* (2003) attributed deaths of *X. laevis* in a laboratory colony to thermal shock following direct transfer from 16 to 23 °C. However, there are no established data for rates of change that are tolerated. Changes of about 5 °C over 2–5 days would accord with conditions experienced naturally; but, for greater changes, animals should be allowed time to acclimate at intermediate temperatures. Animals should not be transferred directly from a tank of water at one temperature to another at higher or lower temperature: they should be moved in water at their original temperature to new conditions where this water then warms or cools gradually. Alternatively, with thermostatically controlled heater/chiller units, settings should be changed by only about 2 °C per day. Jackson and Tinsley (1998) transferred *X. laevis* through a thermocline from 20 °C to 6 °C, leaving animals for about 2 weeks between each 2 °C change.[2]

[2]Note: Reed (2005a) was in error in stating that a 2–5 °C temperature change could cause thermal shock and mortality. The reference miscited (actually Green *et al.* 2003) gave this finding for other amphibian species, not for *X. laevis*.

As with other aspects of *Xenopus* biology, approaches to management of laboratory temperatures should take account of other stressors related to maintenance. Thus, transfer between temperatures may have no ill-effects for animals in good physiological condition in a stress-free environment, but may precipitate illness in animals maintained in suboptimal conditions.

It is generally accepted that optimum temperature conditions for *X. laevis* fall within 18–22 °C. Hilken *et al.* (1995) found no significant differences in growth of *X. laevis* maintained at 19, 22 or 24 °C. The immune system is most effective above 20 °C. Recommendations in the literature for maintenance at lower temperatures than these (including 15 or 16 °C) may lead to risks of pathogenic infection. Researchers primarily interested in egg production should note that spawning in the Cape, S. Africa is triggered by temperatures at or over 20 °C (although oocytes may have developed at lower temperatures in the period preceding spawning). The field and laboratory evidence reported here confirms that *X. laevis* will adapt to temperatures throughout the range 15–25 °C, but on either side of the central band of about 19–22 °C animals will be more vulnerable to co-occurring stress.

Diet and feeding frequency

While there is much debate in publications about optimal environmental conditions for maintaining *Xenopus* species, there is relatively little discussion about diets. Although some laboratories advocate specific preferences, a range of alternative diets appears to satisfy nutritional requirements. A 'scientific' approach suggests the advantages of commercially formulated composite diets (including regulated quantities of proteins, fats, carbohydrates, minerals, trace elements, etc). Certainly, *X. laevis* will grow rapidly on high-protein diets and reach sexual maturity in only about 8 months post-hatching. Although it is counterintuitive, the author has maintained *X. laevis* for over 15 years exclusively on bovine muscle (ox heart), without vitamin or other supplements. In vertebrate taxa, such diets often lead to bone disease due to lack of calcium but no nutritional deficiencies were evident in the *X. laevis*, and females spawned prolifically when aged 12–15 years. Other diets are reviewed by Reed (2005a). Live food such as *Tubifex* carries risks of infection while the gut contents of prey such as earthworms produce significant water contamination.

Some accounts of *X. laevis* maintenance protocols put emphasis on the presumed benefits of a so-called 'feeding frenzy'. Certainly, animals that are stimulated to feed simultaneously avoid the outcome where some that are slow to react may miss a meal. This seems to accord with circumstances in nature where one or a few individuals finding food may trigger searching behaviour by others in the vicinity. A 'frenzy' can be advantageous in the wild when *Xenopus* encounter a food source, including carrion, that is too big for an individual to ingest alone. A group of *Xenopus* can quickly shred a large food item by repeated scratching with the sharp hindfoot claws. However, the author is not convinced that this behaviour is an advantage in the laboratory. When two or more individuals attempt to ingest the same food item, the violent struggles and kicking with the claws are potentially damaging. Pieces of food (eg, cubes of meat) should be small enough to be swallowed quickly, avoiding simultaneous 'capture' by other individuals. In practice, *X. laevis* become conditioned to a regular feeding routine and all individuals respond together when food is given, so a 'frenzy' does not improve intake.

Different authorities advocate feeding *X. laevis* at a variety of frequencies. Young post-metamorphs certainly require frequent feeding: their gut size may limit food intake per meal and significant gaps between meals may affect growth. Fast-growing juveniles benefit from two to three feeds per week and fastest development to maturity can be achieved with daily feeding. However, fully grown adults can maintain excellent condition and develop ripe ovaries with a single meal per week. The key to this regimen is that all animals in a tank should be fed to satiation avoiding competitive effects that might induce differences in growth rate and size. Satiation can be achieved by providing a sufficient quantity of food so that some always remains uneaten at the end of a session. Otherwise there can be no assurance that some individuals are not under-fed (or unfed). In relatively large-scale maintenance, a meal appropriate to each population can be added to the aquarium, which is then inspected about an hour later; if all food has been eaten, more can be added until just a few items remain. This slight excess can be removed (with a net) at the end of the day, avoiding fouling of the water. This process of matching food supply to need is more difficult with a pellet-type diet where uneaten food disintegrates relatively quickly and an excess leads to greater water fouling.

Water changes

Mains tap water intended as drinking water should meet the maintenance needs of *X. laevis*, but supply pipes must not contaminate the water with metals such as copper and lead: heavy metal contamination can have serious effects on oocyte quality. Water must be dechlorinated (most simply by allowing it to stand for 12–24 h) but where water supplies are treated with chloramines these can be removed with commercial aquarium agents containing sodium thiosulphate.

For *X. laevis* maintained in 'fill-and dump' systems, there are two alternative approaches to the feeding/water change sequence. Where animals are fed once weekly and the water is also changed once per week, some lab regimens advocate feeding on the day before the water change. Alternatively, the water change may be carried out first and the animals are then fed (usually immediately afterwards). In the first case, maximum water pollution in the weekly cycle occurs on the day after feeding: a combination of accumulated waste from the previous week (including faeces) and debris from the recent feeding process, including fragments of uneaten food. All this is removed and the animals begin the next week with clean water, which becomes progressively more contaminated until the next feed/water change. In the second case, maximum pollution (lowest water quality) occurs in the period preceding feeding but ingestion of food takes place in clean water. The start of the inter-change week may then have debris resulting from feeding but faecal material does not begin to accumulate for several days. The advantage of this latter sequence is that food intake avoids re-ingestion of faeces, shed skin and other debris with the meal. Both approaches appear to work well and good-quality oocytes may be obtained from females. One disadvantage of the first 'feed-then-change' sequence is that animals experience the major disturbance of the water change on the day after feeding and this may provoke regurgitation. If the change is delayed by a further day or two, the animals remain in poor-quality water for longer. In practice, *X. laevis* readily become conditioned to the change-then-feed sequence: with repetition, they begin to search for food as soon as they are transferred to clean water. This means that the meal is eaten more efficiently and there is less debris. It has the further advantage that animals are undisturbed (for a week) after food intake and digestion does not experience the disruption inherent in water changes.

Feeding with commercial formulations (pellets) leads to more rapid deterioration in water quality (especially from disintegration of uneaten pellets), so more frequent water changes may be necessary.

Water change procedures must ensure that animals are transferred to water at the same temperature. The smoothest changes are achieved by direct transfer of animals from one tank to a duplicate, limiting disturbance to the moment of transfer. For a series of tank changes, the just-vacated tank can then be cleaned out, refilled and used to receive the animals from the next tank to be changed, and so on. This minimises disturbance but incurs the risk that any infection established in one tank is transferred between groups. An alternative approach is to transfer animals from their aquarium to a temporary 'holding' tank; the original container is washed, re-filled and the same animals are returned to it. Animals and tanks always remain together, but this method increases the disturbance to the animals during temporary holding and successive transfers.

At no point in the transfer process should animals be left in very shallow water or, even worse, be left in their original tank whilst the old water is drained out and new water poured in. Rapid decrease in water depth (equivalent to disappearance of the natural habitat), and temporary exposure of animals out of water is highly stressful.

Transfer of animals may be by net but this should have a mesh size sufficient to prevent carrying over debris from dirty to clean water. Animals should not be transferred in groups in a net such that they fall on top of each other. For experienced laboratory workers, it is often most efficient and least disruptive to transfer animals gently by hand. Using naked hands (without plastic gloves) provides a check on the condition of each animal: roughening of *Xenopus* skin and decrease in slipperiness (reduced mucus secretion) give early warning of poor health (see later in this chapter).

To reduce risks of infection, tanks should be washed between water changes and the sides and bottom wiped; this also removes growths of algae. Rinsing with clean water before refilling will wash away parasite eggs (if natural infections are present). Basic maintenance protocols associated with water changes etc should incorporate rigorous commonsense hygiene measures. Nets, cleaning cloths etc should be washed thoroughly (ideally with hot water) between uses. Most pathogens affecting *X. laevis* do not survive complete drying: there are no resistant stages (but the capillarid skin nematode is an exception). So, tanks, aquaria, holding containers, nets, cloths, etc should be dried thoroughly between uses (with aquaria propped upside-down to drain completely). Containers (including plastic aquaria) must not be stacked with moisture trapped inside.

Increasingly, laboratories that keep *Xenopus* are adopting automated or semi-automated systems in which racks of aquaria are maintained with recirculating water, controlled for water chemistry, temperature and other parameters. Purpose-built systems provide a standardised design that removes many of the uncertainties considered in the previous sections and achieves greater uniformity in conditions without the cyclical changes in water quality inherent in static, 'fill-and-dump' regimens (Figure 48.2). With these systems, some laboratories employ every-day feeding with pellet-type diets and achieve fast growth rates (equivalent to those in 'intensive rearing' in agricultural production).

Recirculation and continuous flow systems that are little modified from those designed for tropical fish may have racks of relatively small translucent tanks in which animals

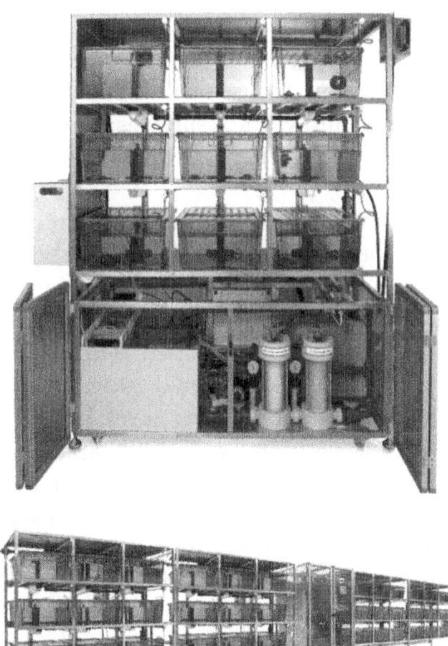

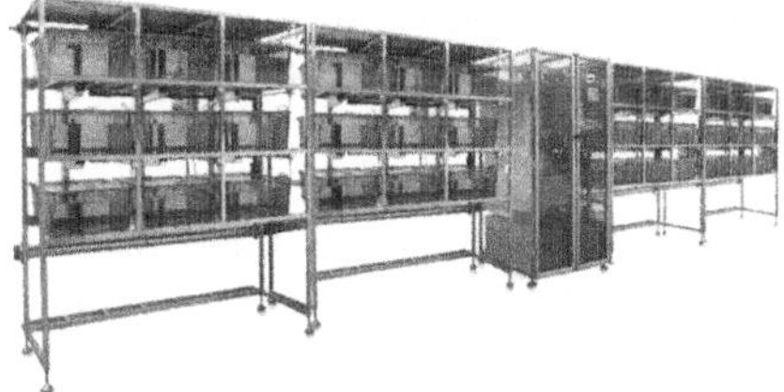

Figure 48.2 Example of purpose-designed, automated aquarium housing for laboratory-maintained *Xenopus* species, providing comprehensive environmental control including temperature, pH, conductivity, and regulating water quality with continuous circulation and filtration. In this design, each tank contains 27 l of water (depth 12 cm) and is intended for up to nine adult *X. laevis*; 10% of the water is replaced each day and passed through biological, mechanical and charcoal filters before UV sterilisation. Racks of tanks may be self-contained (upper image) or joined together in series with a central water treatment and environmental control unit (lower image). Photographs courtesy of Techniplast, Italy.

are exposed to all-round light. Such conditions are likely to be stressful. Improvements include 'smoked' plastic tanks with opaque bases. The choice between manual or automated husbandry systems has more to do with costs (including installation and servicing), technician workload, space and other resources, than the condition of the animals.

Reproduction, rearing of tadpoles

One of the major advantages of *Xenopus* for laboratory research derives from the ease with which these amphibians can be bred in captivity at any time of year. In the wild, age at sexual maturity is generally 2 years for males and 3 years for females; but, with intensive growth in the laboratory, *X. laevis* can reach maturity at about 6 months post-metamorphosis (Tinsley & Kobel 1996). Males in mating condition develop black nuptial gloves on the inner surface of the arms to help grip the female; in receptive females, the cloacal labia become pink. Acoustic communication is well developed in the *Xenopus* species and males and females have a repertoire of vocalisations based on clicks. The male advertisement call is a continuous trilling made by the larynx without any visible movement. Amplexus is inguinal (around the waist). Egg production in the laboratory under hormonal stimulation typically results in deposition of eggs *en masse* on the bottom of an aquarium tank. Under natural conditions, eggs are released singly or in small groups during slow swimming by the mating pair, and the eggs are stuck to vegetation and vertical surfaces: eggs are not deposited on the pond bottom where they would encounter anoxic conditions.

Under optimum conditions, spawning can occur spontaneously in the laboratory at around 20–22 °C, but it is usually induced by injection of human chorionic gonadotrophin (hCG). Females should have been well fed for several weeks and should be plump and pear shaped, reflecting an enlarged ovary. Males should have nuptial gloves (these can be induced by isolating the male for a week before spawning). Typically, two injections are given 48 h apart: a primer to bring animals into mating condition and a final dose to stimulate spawning. Male and female are kept separate after the primer and put together after the final injection. Doses are related to body size but, for adult *X. laevis*, the primer may be 50 IU for males and 100 IU for females, and final doses 100 IU and 300 IU respectively. The aquarium tank in which spawning occurs should be fitted with a false platform of plastic (not wire) netting through which eggs can settle avoiding risk of being eaten by the parents.

To avoid damage to spawn, the adults should be removed from the tank and eggs left *in situ* until they hatch. Larvae break free after about 48 h (at 22 °C) and attach to a vertical surface until remaining yolk is absorbed. The tadpoles are filter-feeders, sieving microscopic particles from the water whilst hovering head-down at an angle of 45° with the tip of the tail flicking continuously. In the wild, tadpoles of *X. laevis* form large schools, all orientated in the same direction and swimming in unison. Under these natural conditions, body length (head to tail tip) typically exceeds 90 mm, but in the laboratory maximum body size is considerably less.

Tadpoles may be fed a range of diets including finely powdered plant material (nettle powder, algae), commercial fish food, finely ground pellets intended for post-metamorphic *X. laevis*, and milk (which produces a droplet suspension of appropriate size for filtration). Feeding frequency should allow the suspension to be cleared between meals. The amount of food required increases with development; material that settles to the tank bottom can support an infusorial culture that adds to the food supply. Large aquaria may become relatively stable with water changes needed at intervals of a few weeks but, with intensive feeding, once-weekly changes may be required. Water quality can be maintained with gentle aeration but *X. laevis* tadpoles also breathe air, visiting the surface about every 30 minutes in normoxic water. A study of factors affecting growth and developmental rates of *X. laevis* tadpoles (Warren 2008) found no significant differences in growth rates in populations maintained in a range of different laboratory conditions. Parameters measured included feeding frequency, aquarium design and materials, water surface cover and even population densities (within the range cited by many laboratories). These findings emphasise that the adaptability of *X. laevis*, well known for the adults, also includes the tadpoles.

Laboratory procedures

Handling

The slippery skin of *X. laevis* makes capture by predators – and handling by laboratory workers – difficult. The powerful hindlimbs and sharp claws may deter inexperienced handlers. Practice is required so that attempts to pick up animals are neither too tentative nor too rough. The hand should be positioned palm down above the animal so that its head is facing the handler's wrist. The index finger should be moved between the animal's hindlimbs and flexed forward beneath its abdomen. Then the thumb and remaining fingers can be closed around the animal's flanks. The animal can then be lifted above the water surface with its body held gently but firmly against the palm of the hand and its legs hanging between thumb and forefinger on one side and forefinger and middle finger on the other. In this position, the animal is unable to bring its hindlimbs forward to push itself away or scratch the handler. In routine maintenance, *X. laevis* becomes accustomed to this procedure (and so do the handlers), so that animals can be transferred between adjacent containers in a few seconds, without struggling.

Small individuals may be more agile and it is often better to catch these with two hands enclosing the animal in the cupped palms and avoiding gaps between the fingers through which it may squeeze. *Xenopus* should not be held in a position where, if they do escape from the hands, they may fall to the floor. For further manipulation, animals should be held immediately above an uncluttered bench surface where escape would not cause injury. Temporary immobilisation is best achieved by holding the animal in soft paper towelling: the dampness of the animal after removal from water prevents skin abrasion and the soft paper towelling facilitates appropriate grip. Instructions in some laboratory manuals to handle *X. laevis* with a rough cloth are best avoided: restraint relying on a rough surface may risk skin damage, and a cloth used for a succession of animals becomes slime-covered and could transfer infection. Paper towelling can be discarded after a single use.

Administration of substances

For injection (for instance, with hormones to stimulate spawning), *X. laevis* can be held securely by the extended hindlimbs if these are gripped together in soft paper towelling just posterior to the pelvis. There must be no possibility that one or both legs can be brought forward, allowing the animal to push itself out of the restraint. The abdomen and anterior of the animal can then be rested on the bench surface (on damp paper towel) with the hindlimbs immobilised within a 'wrapping' of paper towelling. In this position, an injection can be given without risk of movement that could lead to injury. Gonadotrophic and other hormones are typically introduced into the dorsal lymph sac; fluid in this large subdermal space is quickly transported into the general circulation and hence around the body. Injection directly through the skin of the back can lead to leakage so it is more efficient to introduce the hypodermic needle very superficially (almost horizontally) through the skin of the dorsal thigh and then forwards through the septum that separates the lymph spaces of upper leg and back. Injected fluid can then be expelled into the dorsal lymph sac with reduced risks both of loss through the perforation and of entry of potential infections. The needle should meet only very fine superficial capillaries so the procedure should not produce bleeding or bruising.

Monitoring

For measurement of weight and length (to record growth rates and other indices of condition), it is least stressful to weigh animals in a container of water on a top pan balance. Measurement of body length (typically the distance from the tip of the nose to the cloaca: snout–vent length) in *X. laevis* is prone to errors created by the sliding pelvis. The forward-directed iliac processes of the pelvic girdle articulate with the sacral vertebrae by means of a sliding joint (resembling the sliding seat of some rowing boats). This adaptation, enabling the animal to shorten or lengthen its spine by up to 15%, is effective in rapid escape movements and also burrowing in mud. Accurate snout–vent length data require *Xenopus* to be measured in a relaxed 'standard' position (without the legs being contracted up to the body, reducing length, nor extended too fully, increasing length). With practice, this can be done in a few seconds with animals transferred quickly from water to damp paper towel on a flat surface. A flexible transparent ruler is most efficient; callipers should be avoided because of the risk of injury if the animal moves suddenly. It is difficult to reduce variation between successive measurements of the same individual to <2 mm but, even with this error, valuable data on growth and condition can be compiled.

Identification and marking techniques

Individual identification of amphibians may be valuable in laboratory maintenance to follow growth rates, breeding history etc under specific husbandry regimens. Older established techniques that include removal of combinations of digits are no longer acceptable and, in *Xenopus*, cut toes re-grow.

In laboratory populations, with limited numbers of individuals, photographs of skin patterns provide an effective, although sometimes laborious, means of individual recognition. However, with large populations in the wild, the unknown extent of pattern variation may make this impractical. Use of other methods, including applications of dyes and other distinguishing marks (summarised by Halliday (1999)), depends on the skin of the species. In many amphibians, the skin is too delicate to tolerate dye injection.

Xenopus laevis is unusual in having a relatively tough skin and marks applied to the white ventral belly skin are easy to see. The author's field studies based on populations of several thousand individuals have confirmed the effectiveness of several methods and the lack of ill-effects when employed carefully. Introduction of dye (typically alcian blue) with a pressure injector (a 'panjet') produces discrete spots that have remained visible for over 20 years (in very long-lived *X. laevis*). Freeze-branding using metal numbers and digits produces dark, easily-read figures on the white belly skin that are permanent (over 15 years in marked natural populations) and have never been found to cause skin damage or infection. In the UK, this procedure requires a Home Office licence. Currently, introduction of PIT tags (passive integrated transponders) beneath the skin does not require a licence. The cylindrical tags (approximately 5 mm long, 1 mm diameter) produce a unique signal that can be read with a portable scanner. However, the process of insertion seems questionable on welfare grounds. The needle injectors work effectively on the thick skin and subcutaneous muscle of mammalian species where the point of insertion in elastic tissues closes as the needle is withdrawn. However, in amphibians, including *X. laevis* that has relatively inelastic skin, the perforation can remain open producing a risk of infection and sometimes loss of the tag.

A recent development that exploits the natural distinction between dorsal pigment patterns and avoids the labour-intensive comparison of photographs involves digital imaging and machine vision techniques (Figure 48.3).

Safety considerations

There are no records of transfer of infection from *Xenopus* species to humans (although extra caution is needed in cases of antibiotic-resistant bacteria). Commonsense hygiene measures should be adopted when handling *Xenopus* and aquarium water. Hand creams that might irritate amphibian skin should not be used. Some workers use gloves but these reduce sensitivity in handling: information on the animal's condition from its skin texture is missed. Latex and nitrile gloves cause high mortality in amphibian tadpoles includ-

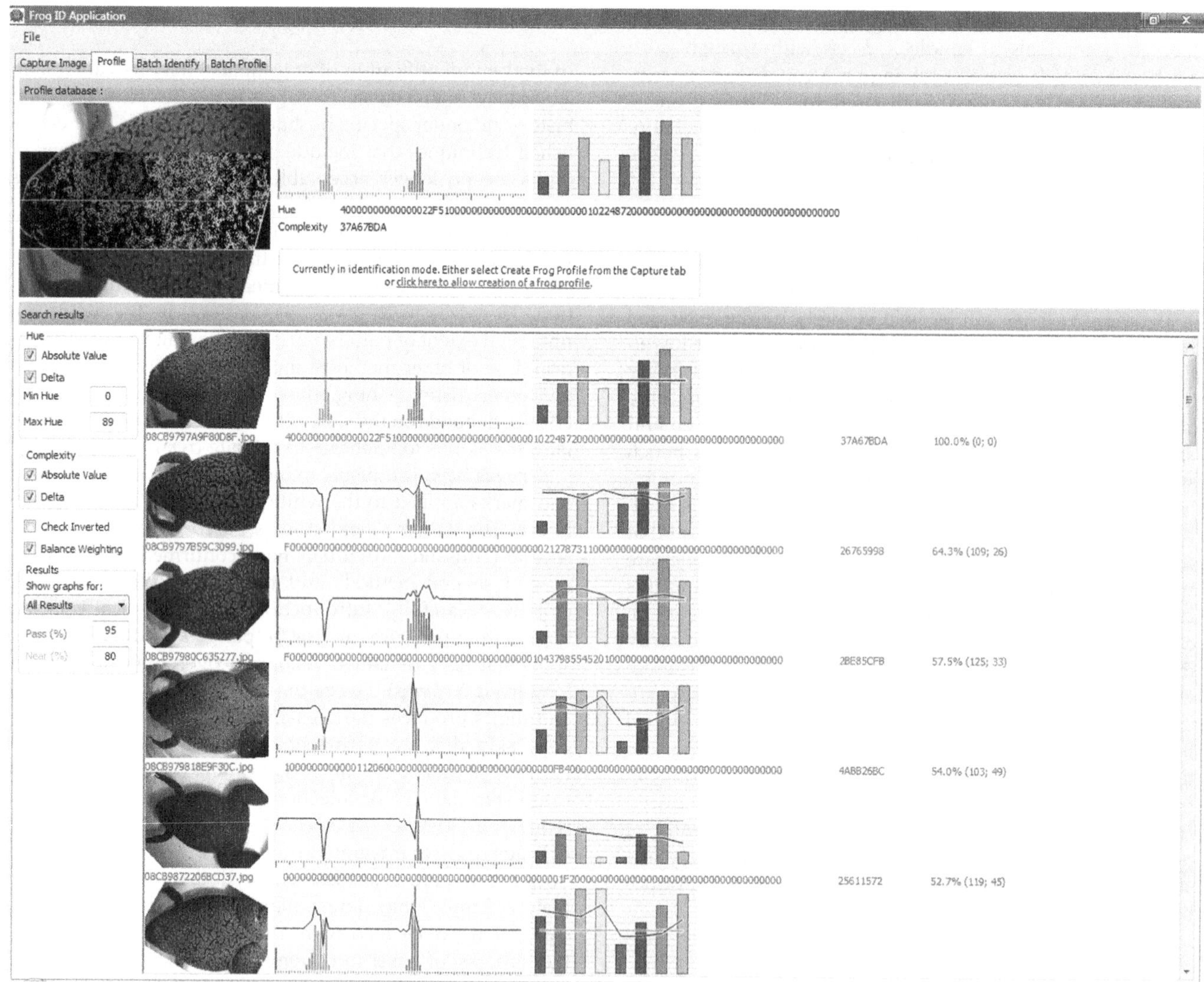

Figure 48.3 Illustration of an approach for individual identification of *Xenopus* based on dorsal pigment patterns. Images are analysed in two ways. First, by using edge detection techniques to count the number of transitions from light to dark in eight separate regions of the dorsal surface, representing texture. Second, by analysing the variety of hues in the skin pigmentation; hue is examined at 110000 distinct points over the back of the animal and allocated to one of 90 bands covering the visible spectrum. The histograms show the counts within the hue bands which are converted to a single hexadecimal digit to create a 90-character hue profile. (Images and explanation courtesy of Professor Matt Guille, European *Xenopus* Resource Centre, University of Portsmouth, UK.)

ing *X. laevis* and unwashed vinyl gloves are also toxic (Cashins *et al*. 2008). There is currently no evidence for negative effects on juveniles or adults but the lethality in tadpoles suggests the need for caution.

Skin secretions of the *Xenopus* species (like those of many amphibians) are toxic. Workers handling *X. laevis* must avoid transfer of mucus to their eyes (if irritated, eyes should be washed with copious amounts of water). Animals stressed by rough handling may discharge a milky exudate from the body surface. This is highly toxic, intended to deter predators, and has an acrid odour. The secretions coalesce to form glutinous strands that are difficult to remove from surfaces to which they stick. This secretion is toxic to the animals themselves: *X. laevis* that acquire a covering of thick white secretion, develop paralysis and die within about 10 minutes. The effects spread to others in the same tank. If recognised quickly, the symptoms can be prevented by transferring affected animals to clean water and gently removing the glutinous secretion with a succession of pieces of paper towelling. Production of the exudates stops when animals are calmed and they can recover in a series of changes of clean water; but all containers, surfaces etc must be thoroughly washed to remove chemical traces that might affect other *Xenopus* or handlers. This extreme defence reaction (equivalent to a 'last resort') may be encountered in *X. laevis* recently caught in the wild, but it is rare in animals habituated to laboratory conditions. Most disastrously, it may occur during transport if animals are crowded and/or subjected to unfavourable conditions (see Transport section).

Anaesthesia

MS222 (tricaine methane sulphonate) is the most effective anaesthetic, administered by immersion of the animal in a 0.05–0.10% solution. MS222 forms an acidic solution in water and should be buffered to pH7 with sodium bicarbonate. Adult *X. laevis* left in MS222 for about 10 minutes after loss of reflexes will take 20–30 minutes to recover when transferred to clean, preferably flowing, water (but times vary with factors including body size and temperature). During anaesthesia and recovery, animals should be propped with nostrils above the water surface and, if out of water, should be kept wet with damp tissue.

Euthanasia

Amongst several alternative methods (Reed 2005a, 2005b), an overdose of MS222 (generally 2–3 g/litre of water, buffered to ph7) is most effective and humane. After unconsciousness, time to death is variable (commonly more than 1 h); *X. laevis* anaesthetised for less than this time should be double-pithed to ensure destruction of brain and spinal cord tissue. Where perfusion might wash out MS222, barbiturate overdose (injected into the dorsal lymph sac) may be recommended.

Transport

Problems that may affect *Xenopus* during transport include exposure to unfavourable environmental conditions (especially heat, poor water quality, restricted access to air); stress from overcrowding; and physical damage from movement within containers. It is essential that containers are not exposed to sun during transport. Animals should not be fed for 3–4 days prior to travelling to reduce fouling of the water.

Xenopus laevis are sometimes transported over long and short distances with minimal water in insulated boxes packed with damp moss or sponge. The lightness of the packaging reduces cost but the method increases the risk of stress or injury. Although *X. laevis* will tolerate emersion from water in a damp environment, they continue to excrete ammonia that can cause severe skin burns. Without water, the animals are also more vulnerable to temperature fluctuations and to injury from erratic movements of the container.

It is better to transport *Xenopus* in clean water deep enough to cover all individuals. Addition of sterile sponge reduces waves and provides a more stable covering for submerged animals. Polystyrene boxes that are waterproof (sometimes lined with polythene sheeting) provide insulation; it is essential that air holes cannot become blocked. In relatively shallow boxes, *Xenopus* may jump and hit their heads, incurring injuries ('red nose' symptoms) and subsequent bacterial infection.

For transport over shorter distances between laboratories, typically by road where there may be reduced constraints on weight and volume, it is best to house animals in relatively deep water (around 30 cm) in a tall container (where the lid is above jumping height): securely covered bins are ideal. Travel should be at a time of day avoiding high temperatures (including exposure to sunshine through vehicle windows); air conditioning may be advisable.

Some suppliers expect mortalities during transport; however, there should be no deaths if animals are in good condition and appropriately packed and transported.

Quarantine

Reports of outbreaks of severe disease (including that caused by the nematode *Pseudocapillaroides xenopodis*, see Parasites section) in animals maintained in laboratories for over a year without symptoms, indicate the need for extended quarantine periods. In practice, maintenance of *X. laevis* in separate tanks provides some restriction on spread of infection. Nevertheless, animals newly imported from the wild should be kept in separate accommodation (with separate nets, cleaning equipment etc) for at least several months.

Welfare issues

Health and disease

In response to unfavourable conditions or poor health, *X. laevis* may adopt a 'hunched' posture with fore- and hindlimbs held close to the body and the head depressed. Skin texture is an important indicator of well-being: it should have a glossy appearance and slippery feel (reflecting effective mucus production), but in ill-health may feel relatively rough and 'dry'. In healthy animals, the process of moulting involves separation of large sheets of outer keratinised skin which are typically pushed into the mouth with the forelimbs and eaten. When animals are unhealthy or stressed, the outer skin is shed into the water in small fragments. In chronic ill-health, there may be pinpoint haemorrhages visible on the white skin of the belly and legs.

The older literature provides detailed accounts of a range of pathological conditions affecting *Xenopus* including degenerative diseases, neoplasms and microbial infections (described from a medical perspective by Dr Edward Elkan and others). These conditions are rare and tend to illustrate three related principles (Tinsley 1995). First, *X. laevis* may carry a range of pathogens without the development of disease until there is a physiological check, caused by malnutrition, temperature change or other environmental stress; until this point, the condition may apparently be controlled and it becomes overtly pathogenic only following the additional precipitating factor. Second, once disease has become established, pathogenesis may develop to an extreme degree before *X. laevis* exhibits obvious ill-effects. Commonly, in tuberculosis of the lungs, liver or gut, a considerable part of the organ may become non-functional before illness and death occur. Reichenbach-Klinke and Elkan (1965) observed that such '*crippling injuries and disease would have killed warm-blooded animals at a much earlier stage*'. Third, in the overcrowded conditions of laboratory maintenance, one animal may develop severe disease (tuberculosis, for instance) and die, whilst others in the same aquarium remain unaffected. These observations suggest that immune defences are normally highly effective in the control of microbial disease.

In contrast to these chronic conditions, a variety of microbial pathogens may cause acute disease leading rapidly to high mortality, including severe generalised sepsis attributable to haemolytic bacteria, particularly *Aeromonas hydrophila*. Little is known of the influence of these infections in wild *Xenopus* populations: virtually all experience derives from lethal outbreaks under the unnatural conditions of laboratory maintenance.

The concerns of export authorities about spread of disease, and of receiving laboratories about introduction of infections, now result in routine treatment for infection in wild-caught *X. laevis*. Whilst the principle is commendable, the effectiveness is currently uncertain. For parasitic worms, the optimum drugs and dosages are generally not known and imported *X. laevis* may still arrive at their destinations with parasitic infections. For bacterial infections, there is the major concern that uncontrolled antibiotic use may select for resistance leading to the export of pathogenic infections that cannot be controlled in the receiving laboratory. Personal experience of this includes a consignment of over 400 *X. laevis* from the Cape that showed symptoms on arrival in the UK of pathogenic *Aeromonas hydrophila* infection. The bacterial strain had resistance to some of the most important antibiotic groups – the beta lactams (penicillins), quinolones (oxolinic acid, ciprofloxacin and enrofloxacin), potentiated sulphonamides (co-trimoxazole) and the tetracyclines. Despite control and treatment efforts over a period of 6 months, all animals died or were culled. The unsuccessful control of this infection suggests that outbreaks of such severity are best managed by early culling, not least to prevent spread to established populations within laboratories. Many laboratories have experience of other devastating epidemics (including the skin nematode *Pseudocapillaroides xenopodis*), indicating the need for careful attention to the disease risks of laboratory maintenance of *Xenopus*. Wider implications include the potential for international spread of antibiotic resistant bacteria and establishment of exotic infections in waterways in distant countries.

For relatively minor skin infections and abrasions, the strong immune defences of *Xenopus* are often the best means of recovery. Affected animals should be transferred to clean water at frequent intervals (preferably daily), so that skin healing is not hampered by elevated ammonia or bacterial populations, and animals should be maintained in isolation, free of disturbance. Feeding may be minimal and should be restricted to food taken immediately by the animal, with uneaten food removed to prevent chemical and bacterial contamination of the water. In cases where this natural recovery is effective, the improvement is visible over a few days to 1 week, with progressive reduction in areas of damaged skin. If there is deterioration, antibiotic treatment may be required (under direction from a vet). If there is severe pathology and visible distress, recovery is often unlikely and euthanasia may be necessary to reduce suffering. Strict hygiene is essential to prevent pathogen spread to other groups of *Xenopus* (especially with nets, tanks and tank-cleaning materials): sterilisation of containers in bleach should be followed by repeated rinsing in clean water which is left to stand for at least 24 h.

Xenopus laevis is naturally infected by a chytrid fungus, *Batrachochytrium dendrobatidis*. Infection leads to epidermal damage but in *X. laevis* this appears normally to be relatively minor. Current evidence is that, both in the wild and in laboratory populations, a few percent of *X. laevis* show detectable infection and this may be related to immune status (influenced by factors such as temperature and stress). Major concerns are not for the health of *X. laevis* but for the risk of spread to other susceptible amphibian species, including the possibility of environmental contamination via drainage water.

Parasites

Xenopus species carry a richer assemblage of parasites than most other anurans – over 25 genera from seven invertebrate groups infecting almost every organ of the body. This spectrum appears to reflect a dual origin: some of the parasites are characteristic of those found in anurans, reflecting a common evolutionary origin, and some are related to those typical of fish, reflecting an ecological origin through shared diet, habitats etc. Almost all are strictly host-specific to *Xenopus* so they do not normally represent a hazard to other amphibians. References to studies on these parasites are listed in Tinsley (1995, 1996) (for earlier work) and Jackson & Tinsley (2001) (for later accounts) (Figure 48.4).

Workers in *Xenopus* laboratories may encounter worms passed into the water from recently imported wild-caught *X. laevis*, but their significance requires evaluation. For parasites with indirect life cycles that require specific intermediate hosts, there are generally no risks of transmission in the laboratory. These parasites, present at the time of capture, gradually decline and are not replaced. Thus, although potentially worrying to non-specialists, occasional expulsion of gut parasites, including tapeworms (*Cephalochlamys namaquensis*), nematodes (*Camallanus* and *Batrachocamallanus* species) and several species of digenean flukes, has little importance for health and welfare. Parasites with indirect life cycles employing *Xenopus* species as an intermediate host may occur in large numbers, including *Tylodelphylus xenopodis* in the pericardium and echinostome metacercariae in the eyelids. Pathological effects are rare (reviewed by Tinsley 1996). However, all these worms may represent a confounding factor if present in *Xenopus* used in controlled experiments (for instance, on growth rates or physiological characteristics).

Those parasites that have direct life cycles (with only a single host species in the life cycle) have the potential to increase in laboratory conditions and need precautions. One helminth parasite of *X. laevis*, the nematode *Pseudocapillaroides xenopodis*, is notorious for lethal pathogenic effects in laboratory populations. Affected animals develop roughened skin, become anorexic, emaciated and die. The worms burrow throughout the epidermis causing severe damage. Parasite reproduction involves deposition of embryonated eggs within the epidermal tunnels, so infective larvae hatch already in their final habitat leading to a progressive increase in worm burdens. Host-to-host transfer is assumed to occur by skin penetration, through existing abrasions or intact skin. However, the circumstances leading to epidemics in laboratory populations are not clear-cut. Reports in the literature describe outbreaks in *X. laevis* that had been imported from South Africa more than a year before the appearance

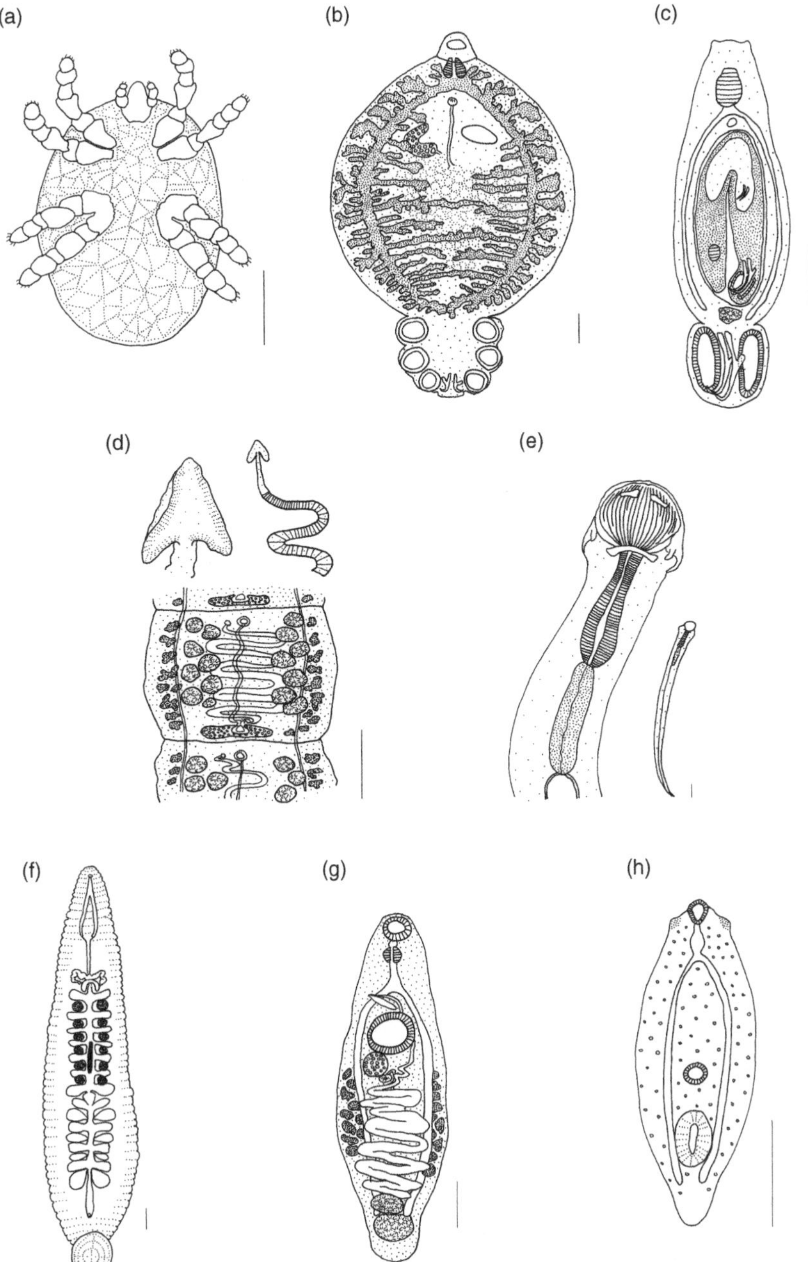

Figure 48.4 Selected parasites of *Xenopus laevis*. (a) *Xenopacarus africanus* (acarine mite; nasal and eustachian passages). Reproduction occurs within the host and heavy infections may accumulate in laboratory *Xenopus* populations. Larval stages are white; digestion of host blood produces black pigmentation as the mites develop. (b) *Protopolystoma xenopodis* (monogenean platyhelminth; urinary bladder and kidneys): blood-feeding flukes with a direct life cycle; eggs are released with urine, a swimming larva hatches and invades the host via the cloaca. Infections can transmit in laboratory maintenance if sediment is allowed to accumulate in aquaria (see text). (c) *Gyrdicotylus gallieni* (monogenean platyhelminth; membranes of the oral cavity). An offspring develops to maturity within the uterus of the parent worm and may, in turn, contain a further developing embryo *in utero* before its birth. This method of reproduction, with progeny emerging directly at the site of infection, produces rapid increase in parasite numbers; host-to-host transfer of worms occurs by contact. (d) *Cephalochlamys namaquensis* (tapeworm, intestine): infections can be detected when mature segments are passed in the water; arrowhead-shaped scolices may also be expelled as a result of host stress or hormone treatment. Worms present in wild-caught *Xenopus* are gradually lost in laboratory maintenance and are not replaced. (e) Several species of camallanid nematodes attach by a chitinized buccal capsule to the wall of the oesophagus, stomach and intestine. As in the tapeworm (d), the life cycle requires a copepod intermediate host and transmission does not normally occur in laboratory maintenance. (f) *Marsupiobdella africana* (leech; external skin): this species is unique amongst leeches in brooding up to 50 offspring in a ventral pouch; when developed, the young emerge through a mid-ventral pore and attach to *Xenopus*, feeding on blood from epidermal capillaries. (g) *Oligolecithus elianae* (digenean platyhelminth; intestine). This and three other species of digeneans occurring in the gut (stomach, intestine, gall bladder and rectum respectively) all have complex life cycles with a snail intermediate host; they do not transmit in laboratory populations of *Xenopus*. (h) *Tylodelphylus xenopodis* (digenean platyhelminth; pericardial cavity): larvae may be detected only at host dissection; worms released from the pericardial membranes sometimes occur on the surface of the ovaries. Infections result from skin penetration by larvae from snail intermediate hosts in natural habitats, so there is no laboratory transmission. Related trematodes, all requiring transfer to a predator of *Xenopus* to complete their life cycles, occur in the body cavity, lateral line system and eyelids. The pathogenic nematode, *Pseudocapillaroides xenopodis*, is not shown. Fine thread-like worms may be found in teased fragments of skin examined as fresh, wet preparations under the microscope. Eggs hatch within epidermal tunnels created by adult worms; parasite burdens accumulate within individual hosts and transmit by contamination. Anthelmintic treatment and strict hygiene are necessary for control (see text). For references to parasite infections, see text. All scale bars = 250 μm.

of symptoms. So, wild-caught laboratory populations may harbour individuals carrying pre-existing low-level, asymptomatic infection. There is evidence for the role of a thymus-dependent immune response in protecting against development of disease; overt symptoms may follow factors that cause immunosuppression, such as reduction in water temperature (Tinsley 1995). Once infection becomes apparent, no spontaneous cures occur. However, the infection can be treated with anthelmintic drugs, including thiabendazole and ivermectins (either by injection or addition to aquarium water). The infective eggs are highly resistant and can be transferred between aquaria on nets and, possibly, the hands of laboratory workers. In parallel with control of infection in the host, it is essential to eliminate all potential sources of re-infection by disinfection of equipment, aquaria and associated surfaces with bleach (followed by thorough rinsing to eliminate traces of chemicals).

Occasionally, *X. laevis* are imported with infections of the leech, *Marsupiobdella africana*. Wounds produced by blood-feeding may become a site for bacterial infection, but the leeches are easily removed with a dilute salt bath. There are also two monogeneans (*Protopolystoma xenopodis* and *Gyrdicotylus gallieni*) and an acarine mite (*Xenopacarus africanus*) that have direct life cycles with the potential for multiplication during laboratory maintenance. However, for all three there is direct or indirect evidence that primary infection leads to an immune response that eliminates the parasites (Tinsley 1996). In laboratory colonies where different populations of *X. laevis* are maintained separately from one another, infection would eventually die out after a period reflecting the lifespan of the original infection: around 4 months for *G. gallieni* but over 2 years for *P. xenopodis*. However, if new imports of *X. laevis* or successive generations of laboratory-produced animals are mixed with previously established populations in the laboratory, the naïve individuals will provide susceptible reservoirs for infection that could persist for long periods.

Transmission by *G. gallieni* and *X. africanus* involves transfer of established parasites from host to host – by reattachment of parasites dislodged into the water or by direct contact between hosts. However, *Protopolystoma xenopodis*, in the urinary bladder, produces eggs that pass out with the urine, develop for about 3 weeks in the sediment, and hatch to release a swimming ciliated larva that invades the next host via the cloaca. Juvenile worms develop in the kidneys for 2–3 months before migrating to the bladder, maturing, and beginning egg production. This life cycle is easily controlled in the laboratory when parasite eggs are removed during routine water changes or by continuous inflow/outflow of water. Detailed studies on *P. xenopodis* show that burdens in the urinary bladder and kidneys are very strictly regulated (reviewed by Tinsley 2005). Despite continuous transmission in the wild, the numbers of worms present at sexual maturity is low (mean <2 adult parasites per host). So, although these parasites feed on blood, there is strict limitation on the extent of blood loss. However, juvenile infections in the host kidneys are potentially more serious. A major part of the host response occurs in the kidneys (a highly immunogenic site in amphibians), but repeated invasion by infective stages may produce a continuous 'rolling' population of parasites. Even though these may be killed within about 1 month post-infection, they are nevertheless responsible for continual low-level pathology including disruption of kidney tissue, blood-feeding and stimulation of inflammatory and other anti-parasitic responses. As with the other parasites, the presence of *P. xenopodis* could represent a confounding factor in controlled experiments.

The risk of pathogenic disease is increased by the husbandry procedure of partial water changes. Where routine maintenance involves removal of half or even three quarters of the old water in an aquarium tank and replacement with clean water, the layer of sediment may allow parasite eggs to complete development, hatch and reinfect the occupants of the tank. It is essential, with 'fill and dump' maintenance, that the aquarium tanks are emptied, rinsed and refilled with a complete change of clean water. At around 20 °C, weekly water changes prevent transmission of *Protopolystoma xenopodis* but infrequent water changes risk auto-infection. Therefore, wild-caught *X. laevis* potentially still carrying their natural parasite infection, should not be maintained in tanks with a gravel or sand substrate where parasite eggs may accumulate.

Thus, there is direct and indirect evidence for low-level infections of all the important pathogens of *X. laevis*, including *Aeromonas* and other bacterial infections, chytrid fungus, the skin-infecting nematode and the monogeneans, in most groups of wild-caught imported animals but that infections are kept in check by highly effective immune responses. The potential exists for severe disease but only when immunity is compromised by stress and other factors. Overt pathology is rare but sporadic infections may be important in laboratory research as a confounding factor in controlled experiments. This highlights two general principles: first, the importance of ensuring optimum conditions that eliminate stress; and second, the desirability of employing purpose-bred, laboratory-reared animals for most research use, rather than *Xenopus* caught in the wild.

Behavioural considerations

Semi-natural conditions are recommended for small-scale maintenance of *Xenopus* species caught in the wild and required for breeding, especially rare species. However, this approach is impractical for large-scale laboratory maintenance of *Xenopus*. Semi-natural conditions require careful management (to regulate food input, monitor water quality etc). They are also less suitable for achieving fast growth rates by juveniles for which it is better to provide an excess of food with more frequent feeding and, hence, water changes.

There have been many attempts to produce a 'compromise' between simulation of natural habitat conditions and sterile 'battery farm' systems. In general, these have been guided by a commonsense, intuitive approach that recognises the need for adequate space, water depth, refuges etc for reduction in stress, whilst achieving ease of feeding and water changes together with reduction in labour (time and cost). The literature includes a range of experimental approaches that attempt to quantify the benefits of specific maintenance regimens assessed by growth rates, ovary condition, etc. However, it is still difficult to find a consensus supported by experimental data. Frustratingly, attempts to compare different environmental parameters have often not found significant differences in the animals. Three aspects may be important. First, there is typically very marked variation in growth and condition of animals in experimental trials (eg, Hilken *et al.* 1995). Recent studies (Tinsley in prep) have shown large differences in growth rates, maturation time, etc between different sibships of *X. laevis* maintained under the same conditions. So, it is possible that genetic effects may have confounded some published trials. Second, *X. laevis* is highly adaptable, even to regimens that are apparently inferior. In these situations, general health (including growth rate) may be indistinguishable from that of animals in more favourable conditions but ill-effects may be subtle, perhaps affecting the quality of oocytes. Third, animals provided with conditions that exclude all (or almost all) stressors may suffer extreme stress when they are disturbed for routine maintenance. As a result, these animals may show suboptimal attributes determined by brief but significant stress even though the investigator designed their maintenance to be 'optimal'.

As an illustration of potential confounding effects of husbandry, *X. laevis* in open tanks seem not to adapt to overhead movements (including shadows). This response corresponds with the direction of major risk in the wild from aerial predators. Indeed, when housed in tanks with lids the animals typically show great alarm when a tank lid is lifted for visual inspection and this is made worse if there are vibrations when the lid is lowered. The stress created by periodic overhead disturbance may outweigh the benefits of intended 'optimum' conditions operating for the majority of each day.

Hence efforts to provide conditions intended to reduce stress by simulating natural conditions may actually result in greater overall effects of stress. This dilemma is illustrated when we consider the alternative sources of laboratory populations of *Xenopus*. In the case of wild-caught adults, attempts to provide aquarium conditions resembling those in natural habitats reflect a recognition that these animals will have spent at least 3 years 'in nature' with behavioural patterns adapted to stresses including predator avoidance. Features such as refuges may inhibit adaptation to laboratory conditions. Where laboratory-maintained *X. laevis* have been raised in captivity throughout life, their experience relates to these artificial conditions. For these animals, refuges that increase sensitivity to periodic disturbance may be unnecessary as long as other aspects of aquarium design (for instance, freedom from overhead movements) remove overall stress.

This discussion points to the conclusion that, for the most demanding research needs, especially in molecular, cell and developmental biology, the use of wild-caught animals generates behavioural and welfare problems for laboratory maintenance that are best avoided by the use of purpose-bred populations.

Concluding remarks

The use of amphibians as a major 'laboratory animal', in research and teaching, was formerly motivated by the belief that amphibians (especially frog populations) are an abundant, easily caught, relatively inexpensive source of live vertebrate material for practical exercises. However, in most cases now, large-scale capture of frogs is not sustainable (especially where populations are threatened by human activities), physiological condition is often poor (especially because of inappropriate maintenance or holding facilities) and large-scale use can no longer be justified. This conclusion is inescapable on the grounds of conservation, ethics, welfare and cost, but use of amphibians may be additionally unjustified on scientific grounds where the reliability of results may be compromised by poor condition or stamina.

However, laboratory use of *Xenopus laevis* differs in important respects. Populations in the areas of supply are abundant; animals occur in huge numbers in man-made habitats. There are no major conservation concerns. It is ironic that this species which is exploited for scientific needs is, at the same time, favoured by human activities especially the creation of water supplies for agricultural and domestic use. The export of *X. laevis* from South Africa, principally the Cape, has been very successful in meeting a major research need. Research based on the *Xenopus* species continues to contribute to major advances in biomedical and fundamental science.

However, there are growing concerns about wider aspects of laboratory use based on wild-caught animals. In the case of *X. laevis*, it is anomalous that very demanding research should be based on animals that have spent their lives in the natural environment, prior to being caught and transported to the artificial conditions of a laboratory. These animals exhibit unavoidable variation reflecting their experience of seasonal changes in environmental conditions, food supply and stress over several years. They will have been exposed to natural parasite and microbial infections and, despite attempted treatment, often reach laboratories still carrying transmissible infections. There is now a greater concern that *X. laevis* established in introduced populations outside Africa are becoming part of the international trade. Currently, this is the case for populations that were introduced in Chile in the 1970s and are now exported to laboratories elsewhere in the world. Transport of these creates a risk of worldwide transfer of additional pathogenic infection from a continent where *X. laevis* is not native. All these considerations suggest that it is an anachronism that wild-caught animals should be employed in modern laboratory research.

It is likely that a series of separate pressures – relating to cost, welfare, legal regulations and disease risks – will combine to replace wild-caught *Xenopus* species. However, *Xenopus* will continue to be a very important model system for advancing understanding in molecular, cell and developmental biology and use is almost certain to expand in the future. It is appropriate that this should increasingly be based on laboratory-raised animals. This shift in practice will also reduce concerns about stress, especially the inevitable problems associated with transfer of animals adapted to natural conditions to the artificial restrictions of laboratory maintenance.

Acknowledgements

Research on *Xenopus* has been supported by grants from the Natural Environment Research Council and the Biotechnology and Biological Sciences Research Council, most recently BB/C506272/1 and BB/D523051/1 from BBSRC, which I gratefully acknowledge.

References

Alexander, S.S. and Bellerby, C.W. (1938) Experimental studies on the sexual cycle of the South African clawed toad (*Xenopus laevis*). *International Journal of Experimental Biology*, **15**, 74–81

Bellerby, C.W. and Hogben, L. (1938) Experimental studies on the sexual cycle of the South African clawed toad (*Xenopus laevis*). III. *Journal of Experimental Biology*, **15**, 91–100

Brown, M.J. and Nixon, R.M. (2004) Enrichment for a captive environment – the *Xenopus laevis*. *Animal Technology and Welfare*, **3**, 87–95

Council of Europe (2006) Multilateral Consultation of Parties to the European Convention for the Protection of Vertebrate Animals used for Experimental and other Scientific Purposes (ETS 123) Appendix A. *Cons 123 (2006) 3*. Available from URL: http://www.coe.int/t/e/legal_affairs/legal_co-operation/biological_safety,_use_of_animals/laboratory_animals/2006/Cons123(2006)3AppendixA_en.pdf (accessed 31 July 2008)

Cashins, S.D., Alford, R.A. and Skerratt, L.F. (2008) Lethal effect of latex, nitrile, and vinyl gloves on tadpoles. *Herpetological Review*, **39**, 298–301

Elepfandt, A. (1996a) Sensory perception and the lateral line system in the clawed frog, *Xenopus*. In: *The Biology of Xenopus*. Eds Tinsley, R.C. and Kobel, H.R., pp. 97–120. The Zoological Society of London, Clarendon Press, Oxford

Elepfandt, A. (1996b) Underwater acoustics and hearing in the clawed frog, *Xenopus*. In: *The Biology of Xenopus*. Eds Tinsley, R.C. and Kobel, H.R., pp. 177–193. The Zoological Society of London, Clarendon Press, Oxford

European Commission (2007) Commission recommendations of 18 June 2007 on guidelines for the accommodation and care of animals used for experimental and other scientific purposes. Annex II to European Council Directive 86/609. See 2007/526/EC. http://eurlex.europa.eu/LexUriServ/site/en/oj/2007/l_197/l_19720070730en00010089.pdf (accessed 13 May 2008)

Evans, B.J. (2008) Genome evolution and speciation genetics of allopolyploid clawed frogs (*Xenopus* and *Silurana*). *Frontiers of Bioscience*, **13**, 4687–4706

Evans, B.J., Carter, T.F., Tobias, M.L. *et al.* (2008) A new species of clawed frog (genus *Xenopus*) from the Itombwe Massif, Democratic Republic of the Congo: implications for DNA barcodes and biodiversity conservation. *Zootaxa*, **1780**, 55–68

Green, S.L., Moorhead, R.C. and Bouley, D.M. (2003) Thermal shock in a colony of South African clawed frogs (*Xenopus laevis*). *Veterinary Record*, **152**, 336–337

Gurdon, J.B. (1996) Introductory comments: *Xenopus* as a laboratory animal. In: *The Biology of Xenopus*. Eds Tinsley, R.C. and Kobel, H.R., pp. 3–8. The Zoological Society of London, Clarendon Press, Oxford

Halliday, T. (1999) Amphibians. In: *The UFAW Handbook on the Care and Management of Laboratory Animals*, Vol 2, 7th edn. Ed. Poole, T., pp. 90–102. Blackwell Publishing, Oxford

Hilken, G., Dimigen, J. and Iglauer, F. (1995) Growth of *Xenopus laevis* under different laboratory rearing conditions. *Laboratory Animals*, **29**, 152–162

Jackson, J.A. and Tinsley, R.C. (1998) Effects of temperature on oviposition rate in *Protopolystoma xenopodis* (Monogenea: Polystomatidae). *International Journal of Parasitology*, **28**, 309–315

Jackson, J.A. and Tinsley, R.C. (2001) Host-specificity and distribution of cephalochlamydid cestodes: correlation with allopolyploid evolution of pipid anuran hosts. *Journal of Zoology*, **254**, 405–419

Major, N. and Wassersug, R.J. (1998) Survey of current techniques in the care and maintenance of the African Clawed Frog (*Xenopus laevis*). *Contemporary Topics*, **37**, 57–60

Measey, G.J. and Channing, A. (2003) Phylogeography of the genus *Xenopus* in southern Africa. *Amphibia-Reptilia*, **24**, 321–330

Reed, B.T. (2005a) *Guidance on the Housing and Care of the African Clawed Frog Xenopus laevis*. Research Animals Department, RSPCA, Horsham

Reed, B. (2005b) African Clawed Frog – *Xenopus*. In: *Manual of Animal Technology*. Ed. Barnett, S.W., pp. 85–93. Blackwell Publishing, Oxford

Reichenbach-Klinke, H. and Elkan, E. (1965) *The Principal Diseases of Lower Vertebrates. Book II Diseases of Amphibians*. T.F.H. Publications, New Jersey

Robert, J. and Ohta, Y. (2009) Comparative and developmental study of the immune system in *Xenopus*. *Developmental Dynamics*, **238**, 1249–1270

Smyth, J.D. and Smyth, M.M. (1980) *Frogs as host-parasite systems I*. Macmillan Press, London

Stuart, S.N., Hoffmann, M., Chanson, J.S. *et al.* (2008) *Threatened Amphibians of the World*. Lynx Edicions, Barcelona, Spain; IUCN, Gland, Switzerland; and Conservation International, Arlington

Tinsley, R.C. (1995) Parasitic disease in amphibians: control by the regulation of worm burdens. *Parasitology*, **111**, S153–S178

Tinsley, R.C. (1996) Parasites of *Xenopus*. In: *The Biology of Xenopus*. Eds Tinsley, R.C. and Kobel, H.R., pp. 233–261. The Zoological Society of London, Clarendon Press, Oxford

Tinsley, R.C. (1999) Parasite adaptation to extreme conditions in a desert environment. *Parasitology*, **119**, S31–S56

Tinsley, R.C. (2005) Parasitism and hostile environments. In: *Parasitism and Ecosystems*. Eds Thomas, F., Renaud, F. and Guégan, J.-F., pp. 85–112. Oxford University Press, Oxford

Tinsley, R.C. and Kobel H.R. (1996) *The Biology of Xenopus*. The Zoological Society of London, Clarendon Press, Oxford

Tinsley, R.C. and McCoid, M.J. (1996) Feral populations of *Xenopus* outside Africa. In: *The Biology of Xenopus*. Eds Tinsley, R.C. and Kobel, H.R., pp. 81–94. The Zoological Society of London, Clarendon Press, Oxford

Tinsley, R.C., Loumont, C. and Kobel, H.R. (1996) Geographical distribution and ecology. In: *The Biology of Xenopus*. Eds Tinsley, R.C. and Kobel, H.R., pp. 35–59. The Zoological Society of London, Clarendon Press, Oxford

Tocque, K. and Tinsley, R.C. (1991) The influence of desert temperature cycles on the reproductive biology of *Pseudodiplorchis americanus*. *Parasitology*, **103**, 111–120

Tocque, K., Tinsley, R.C. and Lamb, T. (1995) Ecological constraints on feeding and growth of *Scaphiopus couchii*. *Herpetological Journal*, **5**, 257–265

Verhoeff de Fremery, R., Griffin, J. and Macgregor, H.C. (1987) Urodeles (newts and salamanders). In: *The UFAW Handbook on the Care and Management of Laboratory Animals*, 6th edn. Ed. Poole, T.B., pp. 759–772. Longman, Harlow

Warren, A.G. (2008) *Environmental effects on the growth and development of Xenopus laevis tadpoles: towards improved laboratory welfare*. Unpublished PhD Thesis. University of Bristol

Wilson, R.S., James, R.S. and Johnston, I.A. (2000) Thermal acclimation of locomotor performance in tadpoles and adults of the aquatic frog *Xenopus laevis*. *Journal of Comparative Physiology B: Biochemical, Systematic and Environmental Physiology*, **170**, 117–124

Fish

49 Fish

James F. Turnbull and Iain Berrill

Introduction

The central theme of this chapter is the diversity of fish. An understanding of the nature of this diversity, and its implications for the needs of different species in captivity, will help care staff and researchers to be better equipped to care for and conduct experiments with fish. In a single chapter it is not possible to provide detailed advice on the husbandry of all species that might be used in research. Instead, we will provide detailed information for some of the more common species including, rainbow trout (*Oncorhynchus mykiss*), Atlantic salmon (*Salmo salar*) and zebrafish (*Danio rerio*). Other examples will be used, including Atlantic cod (*Gadus morhua*) and the guppy (*Poecilia reticulata*) where these species illustrate diversity.

What is a fish?

Fish inhabit a vast range of habitats and ecological niches. From the smallest vertebrate *Paedocypris progenetica* which matures at less than 8 mm (Kottelat *et al.* 2006) to one of the largest, the whale shark (*Rhincodon typus*), reaching lengths of over 12 m (Colman 1997). It has been estimated that almost half of all known vertebrates are fish. There are around 28 000 extant species of fish; the majority (>96%) are the bony fishes (Osteichthyes), with the cartilaginous sharks and rays (Chondrichthyes) representing less than 4% and the jawless lampreys and hagfish (Agnatha) less than 1% (Potts 1999a; Nelson 2006). The term teleost is frequently used when referring to bony fish, this is a common form of the infraclass Teleostei within the class Actinopterygii (ray finned fishes) subclass Neopterygii. Cyclostome is another term used, which, although not a formal classification, is commonly used to refer to the lamprays and hagfish. The class Pisces is no longer used since any clade containing fish also contains tetrapods. A reasonable definition of fish would be aquatic vertebrates that rely, at least in part, on gills for respiration in the adult form.

In addition to species diversity fish can also be highly adaptable, even within sibling groups. They have the capacity to exhibit various behavioural, anatomical and physiological adaptations to environmental cues. Many of the fixed characteristics of mammals and birds are more flexible in fish; not even gender is genetically determined in some species of fish, with individuals changing from functional males to females sequentially or in response to their social or physical environment.

Fish welfare

The study of fish welfare is still in its infancy. Experiments that have allowed us to understand the basic coping mechanisms or explore preferences in terrestrial animals have not yet been replicated in fish. This would seem to pose an insurmountable challenge when attempting to provide guidance on the care and welfare of fish. However, the thriving aquaculture industry, which relies on healthy and productive fish and the wealth of high-quality science conducted using live fish, testifies to the ability of fish keepers to take care of fish despite this lack of scientific information. This chapter will attempt to provide a basic understanding of the care of fish kept for experimental purposes but can in no way replace familiarity with the fish under your care. Provision of training for personnel taking care of fish is essential as are appropriate resources, health and contingency plans. More detailed descriptions can be found in other texts such as the previous edition of this handbook (Potts *et al.* 1999).

Although there is an ongoing scientific debate regarding the ability of fish to suffer pain (eg, Rose 2002, 2007; Sneddon *et al.* 2003; Chandroo *et al.* 2004a, 2004b; Braithwaite & Boulcott 2007), various national legislation, regulation and guidelines (Canadian Council on Animal Care 2005; Home Office 2006; Council of Europe 2006) provide protection for fish used for experimental or other scientific purposes. In Europe, for example, fish are protected from the time that they are capable of independent feeding on the assumption that they are capable of experiencing pain, suffering and distress (European Directive 86/609 implemented within the UK by The Animals (Scientific Procedures) Act 1986). Therefore the capacity of fish to suffer will not be discussed further here.

The subject of fish welfare is discussed by Huntingford *et al.* (2006), in a book on the subject edited by the late Edward Branson (2008) and in a dedicated special edition of Diseases of Aquatic Organisms which is open access[1].

[1] http://www.int-res.com/abstracts/dao/v75/n2/

Biological overview

General biology

The ecological niches occupied by fish include most of the water on the planet from small freshwater puddles or pools to oceans, from the sea bed (benthic) to open waters (pelagic). The fish occupying these niches range from those with limited capacity to adapt to those that are highly adaptable. Some (eg, Atlantic cod) have limited capacity to adapt to changing salinity (stenohaline) whereas others, eg, Asian sea bass (*Lates calcarifer*), are highly adaptable (euryhaline).

Fish can be predatory carnivores, omnivorous or herbivorous. The vast majority of fish are ectothermic with their internal temperature close to that of the surrounding environment. Consequently, all biological processes are temperature dependent. This means that growth, inflammation, healing, reproduction, metabolism, excretion of chemicals and many other physiological processes are not just a function of time but a function of time and temperature. Ectothermy requires much less energy than homeothermy for an equivalent sized animal. Unlike birds and mammals, ectotherms do not have to constantly feed a demanding metabolism and can survive on relatively little feed and use available feed to grow very efficiently. Many salmonids in commercial culture facilities will achieve a food conversion ratio (weight of feed consumed to wet weight of fish produced) of less than one. Fish can also be naturally anorexic for periods of time.

Many fish demonstrate plasticity where a single group of siblings will adopt a variety of behavioural and physiological strategies. For example, young freshwater Atlantic salmon may undergo smoltification (pre-adaptation to the marine environment) in the first year of life or only after 2 or more years, dependent on available food resources.

Life cycles and reproduction

There is considerable diversity in the life history strategies of different species. However, it is possible to simplify most life history strategies as follows. After external fertilisation, embryos develop within the egg. They hatch and rely on the yolk sac until they are able to ingest and digest external sources of food. The exception may be some of the live-bearing species, where nutrients are passed between the mother and embryo. Following first feeding, fish develop into juveniles, in some species, such as flatfish, undergoing dramatic metamorphosis; and then become reproductively mature adults. Some species may include a habitat switch during their life, often as part of their reproductive cycle. For example adult eels (*Anguilla anguilla*) reside in fresh water, but migrate to the sea to reproduce (catadromous) whereas Atlantic salmon mostly grow in the sea but reproduce in fresh water (anadromous). As with so many aspects of their biology, there is considerable species diversity in fish reproduction.

One method of categorising reproduction is through the level of protection provided by adults for their embryos before and after fertilisation (eg, Balon 1990). Reproductive styles range from fish that are non-guarding pelagic spawners, producing a large number of small ova requiring a long larval period (eg, Atlantic cod), through to live-bearing fish, in which a relatively small number of eggs are fertilised and develop within the female and are released as fry capable of independent feeding (eg, guppies).

Reproduction in fish might occur during specific spawning seasons (eg, rainbow trout), or throughout the year (eg, captive-reared zebrafish). Environmental signals play an important role in cueing both the seasonal and daily timing of reproduction. Photoperiod is one of the most important environmental signals influencing reproduction (Bromage *et al.* 1991) but other variables may also be of importance, eg, temperature (Gillet & Dubois 2007).

Under some culture conditions, maturation and reproduction may be considered beneficial, for example to maintain a specific strain of fish. However, maturation can lead to traits that may be considered undesirable in laboratory systems. In many species, maturation leads to changes in behaviour and, most notably, increased aggression. Male Siamese fighting fish (*Betta splendens*) will fight to the death when reproductively mature, and so should be housed singly. Maturation may also be considered detrimental as it may be linked to a decrease in immunocompetence and an increase in susceptibility to pathogens (Suzuki *et al.* 1997; Skarstein *et al.* 2001). Maturation often also results in a reduction in growth as energy is diverted into gonadal development (eg, Lester *et al.* 2004).

Where maturation is detrimental it may be appropriate to use sterile fish. The production of triploid fish, which have three sets of chromosomes instead of two, is one of the most practical ways of producing sterile fish (reviewed by Piferrer *et al.* 2009). Triploids are typically produced using a thermal, pressure or chemical shock applied to embryos during a specific stage in early development. While the use of sterile triploid fish might protect against the negative effects of sexual reproduction, there is currently a lack of information regarding the physiology of triploids. Therefore, it may not always be appropriate to extrapolate from results obtained with triploids to diploid populations.

To illustrate the diversity, we now describe the fish life history strategies of four species reared in captivity. Of these, three lay eggs: a tropical freshwater species (ie, zebrafish), a temperate freshwater species (ie, rainbow trout) and a temperate marine species (ie, Atlantic cod); the fourth is a tropical fresh- to brackish water live bearer (ie, the guppy).

Zebrafish (*Danio rerio*)

The zebrafish is one of the most widely used models of vertebrate development (Spence *et al.* 2008) and it is commonly used in genetic and toxicological studies (Home Office 2006). It is a small, omnivorous cyprinid (rarely exceeding 40mm in length). In the wild, it inhabits slow-moving water bodies in the south-eastern Himalayan region. Breeding in captivity can occur all year round, although in the wild it is more seasonal, possibly linked to changes in food availability (Spence *et al.* 2006). Zebrafish mature at between 3 and 4 months of age and they are then able to reproduce every 2–3 days. They produce between 100 and 200 relatively large eggs (0.7mm diameter), which are fertilised externally and afforded no further parental care. Indeed, in captivity, zebrafish can be voracious predators of their own eggs (Andrews 2000). Following fertilisation, development is rapid and at a standard rearing temperature of 28.5 °C embryos hatch after 48–72 h. Three to four days later the embryos inflate their swim bladder and begin feeding on fine particulate food. Gonads initially develop as ovaries, with testes differentiating after 5–7 weeks. Zebrafish live for 3.5 years on average, with the oldest individuals reaching 5.5 years (Gerhard *et al.* 2002).

For more detailed descriptions of zebrafish development, ecology and culture see Kimmel *et al.* (1995), Westerfield (2000), Lawrence (2007) and Spence *et al.* (2008).

Rainbow trout (*Oncorhynchus mykiss*)

The rainbow trout is a carnivorous salmonid, which inhabits oxygen-rich waters. Its native distribution covers the pacific coast of North America, but humans have distributed it widely and it is now farmed throughout the world (Hershberger 1992). They are also used in experimental and toxicological studies (Home Office 2006). Previously it was commonly classified as *Salmo gairdneri* but has been confirmed as *Oncorhynchus mykiss.*

In the wild, maturation in rainbow trout (like all salmonids) is stimulated by a decreasing photoperiod, but spawning times can vary greatly between strains (Bromage & Cumaranatunga 1988). Under natural photoperiod in temperate regions, hatchery strains spawn in late autumn and winter, with a broodstock population producing eggs over a 6–8-week period (Bromage *et al.* 1992); individual salmonids produce a single batch of eggs in a season. However, eggs and milt are available throughout the year due to the use of photoperiod manipulation. When spawning occurs in the wild, eggs (3–6 mm diameter) are deposited and fertilised in gravel nests called redds, covered with gravel and left to incubate. Outside their native range they do not normally spawn naturally. For example in the UK there are only one or two naturally spawning populations, despite the wide distribution of potentially fertile rainbow trout throughout the country. In captivity, eggs and milt are manually stripped from the adults, and artificially fertilised.

Following fertilisation embryos take approximately 300 degree days (ie, the average daily temperature in degrees Celsius multiplied by time in days) to hatch and a further 200 degree days to reach first feeding (Bromage 1995). After hatching, growth can be rapid, depending on the temperature, with males typically maturing in their 2nd year and females in their 3rd year. Rainbow trout live for between 5 and 6 years and can reach weights of over 10 kg.

Atlantic cod (*Gadus morhua*)

The Atlantic cod is an omnivorous, demersal (living on or near the sea bed) soft-finned fish belonging to the family Gadidae, that is found throughout the North Atlantic Ocean and the European coast, through to the Barents sea (Cohen *et al.* 1990). The commercial culture of this species is still in a relatively early stage of development and predominantly occurs in Norway.

The Atlantic cod is a batch spawner with each female producing several batches of eggs within the spawning season, which occurs between November and September, varying between sub-populations and location (Cohen *et al.* 1990). In captivity, photoperiod manipulation allows fish to be spawned throughout the year (Norberg *et al.* 2004). In the wild, Atlantic cod spawn pelagically and in captivity they spawn and fertilise their eggs naturally. Atlantic cod are highly fecund, producing many small eggs (1.0–1.5 mm), up to 4.30×10^5 eggs/kg of fish (Hansen *et al.* 2001). Following fertilisation, hatching takes approximately 250 h, after which first feeding takes a further 3 days at 7 °C (Hall *et al.* 2004), although these times vary depending on strain and temperature. At hatch, the embryos are poorly developed, requiring a 2.5 month pelagic larval period (Cohen *et al.* 1990) after which they become demersal. Cod then grow and reach sexual maturity after 2 years at the earliest (Karlsen *et al.* 1995; Olsen *et al.* 2004). Atlantic cod can live for 20 years and reach lengths of up to 2 m (Cohen *et al.* 1990).

Guppy (*Poecilia reticulata*)

The guppy is an omnivorous fish belonging to the viviparous family Poeciliidae. It is a popular aquarium fish but it is also used in a range of scientific studies (Home Office 2006). In the wild guppies are found in a range of brackish and freshwater habitats in South America (notably Trinidad, Venezuela and Barbados). It is a live-bearing fish, with internal fertilisation and development of embryos. Males have a modified anal fin, the 'gonopodium', which transfers sperm into the female. Females are able to store sperm and use it to fertilise several batches of eggs. Once fertilised embryos take 3–5 weeks to develop before being released by the female. In that time they will rely solely on yolk as a nutrient source: they do not receive any additional nutrients from their mother. Females are able to produce batches of juveniles at approximately 4 week intervals throughout the year with no specific spawning season. In captivity 20–200 juveniles are produced in each batch, although in the wild this number is lower. Following release by the female, juveniles are capable of independent feeding and are afforded no further parental care. Cannibalism by parents is common. Males reach sexual maturity after 2 months, at approximately 19 mm, and females after 3 months, at approximately 25 mm. Adult male guppies reach a maximum size of 35 mm and females 60 mm.

Detailed information on the biology, ecology and culture of guppies can be found in Axelrod and Schultz (1990), Magurran *et al.* (1995) and Andrews (2000).

Biological data

To monitor a culture system, feeding, behaviour, water quality and health should all be recorded. Fortunately only a relatively small number of species are kept in the laboratory (see Ostrander 2000), however, even these species exemplify the complexity and plasticity of fish. Inter-individual variability in fish is generally greater than in terrestrial animals and the inherent plasticity of fish is demonstrated by the variability of normal values for the majority of haematological parameters (see Wedemeyer 1996). For this reason haematology and clinical biochemistry is much less useful in fish.

Growth rates are determined not only by rate of feeding, but also by social cues, environmental conditions, genetic factors and physiological states such as reproductive condition. Growth charts are available for commercial production, mostly supplied by feed companies and combined with suggested feeding rates. In some cases these are more complex than simple tables and may be based on multiple regression models. The determinants of fish growth can be complex. In Atlantic salmon, growth in the sea is determined by the size of the fish (bigger fish have higher daily weight gain) but also by daylight, with temperature having a relatively minor role. Salmon grow faster during periods of decreasing day length and during longer days, therefore the period of most rapid growth is usually June to September in the northern hemisphere (Metcalfe 1994).

Since most growth and feeding charts are developed for commercial systems they can be used as a starting point but must be adapted for use in experimental systems, since the aim in most cases is not necessarily to achieve rapid cost-effective growth. Accurate and accessible records are necessary to ensure you can develop a prediction of normal growth and feeding in your systems. This can be developed into predictive models to allow early detection of deviations from expected performance.

Normal behaviour

Fish are capable of creating complex social and internal environmental models (reviewed in Braithwaite 2006). Male Siamese fighting fish are able to judge the performance of other fish from observing fights. This is not simply recognition of the winner and loser but a true evaluation of the relative fighting abilities. In some cases the observer will act aggressively to both winner and loser, in others respond aggressively to only the loser or respond submissively to both (Oliveira *et al.* 1998). This is thought to represent a process of comparing his own abilities with those of the observed combatants. Some fish are also able to develop complex spatial maps, a goby (*Bathygobius soporator*) can create a model of the topography of the shore line at high tide which allows it to escape from a rock pool to other pools and eventually back to the sea at low tide, when it is impossible for it to see its destination (Aronson 1971).

Commonly observed behaviours in captivity include feeding, predator avoidance, exploration, social interactions and reproduction. In experimental systems it is preferable to avoid any form of behaviour that can be damaging to the fish. For example, reproduction and territoriality, which are often associated with increased aggression.

Many species of fish, such as salmonids and tilapia, establish territories if provided with the opportunity. However, such behaviour can result in unequal access to food and injury through fighting. Potentially territorial species can often be encouraged to adopt a less damaging shoaling strategy through manipulation of the water flow and number of individuals in the tanks (Christiansen *et al.* 1992). Since aggression is often a feature of competition for resources, avoiding defensible food resources and visual cues, which identify territories, can also reduce aggression. This may result in a conflict of priorities when attempting to provide environmental enrichment. Aggression can also be influenced by the size distribution in the tank. This is not simply a matter of maintaining uniform size, since the presence of larger obviously dominant individuals can suppress overall aggression (Adams *et al.* 2000). There is also evidence in salmonids that the removal of dominant individuals from small populations can result in increased levels of aggression (Adams *et al.* 1998).

Predator avoidance is most obviously seen in tanks of salmonids with bright overhead light and no access to cover. In these conditions, fish will crowd together swimming rapidly from group to group or crowd into any shade. Such behaviour may be indicative of poor welfare, however this area requires further study.

In experimental or commercial facilities, the behaviours that will be observed are dependent on the nature of the tank or husbandry unit, the number and density of fish and the clarity of the water. Frequently, observation is limited to the times when the tank lid is lifted to feed the fish or clean the tank. The behaviour of fish at this time can in no way be considered to be resting or normal behaviour. They may either show an escape response or rise to the surface in anticipation of feeding, depending on the nature of the disturbance and their previous experience. Although over time there may be a reduced response to disturbance we do not fully understand the consequence of such adaptation. The degree of habituation to any form of human interference is species dependent. Sea bass (*Dicentrachus labrax*), if frequently disturbed, may become very difficult to stress since they appear to interpret any form of human presence as a prelude to feeding (M. Pavlidis, personal communication). Under commercial conditions underwater video equipment is used to monitor fish behaviour, especially in large production units, allowing observation of their undisturbed behaviour.

Often the best conditions for observing fish are not the most suitable for the fish under observation. Clear water in glass tanks can be stressful for some species, particularly those more suited to living in dimly lit or turbid water.

Sources, supply and conservation status

Many of the commonly used laboratory species are available from captive-bred stocks. However, some species, particularly marine fish, must be collected from the wild. The capture of wild fish for experimental purposes is covered in the previous edition of this handbook (Andrews 1999; Potts 1999b). For ethical reasons, no fish that is collected using unsustainable methods or from endangered species or populations should be used in experiments, except where those experiments are directly related to their conservation. At the time of writing only 86 out of the 5000 species of animals protected against over-exploitation through international trade by CITES were fish. Protected species include the whale shark and the common or European eel (*Anguilla anguilla*). None of the protected species are commonly used for experimental purposes.

The sources and previous history of the fish are extremely important for experimental populations. Uncontrolled genetic variability can lead to unacceptable levels of error. However, the plasticity of many fish species means that even in relatively genetically homogeneous populations there is considerable variability. This is compounded by the influence of previous experience. For example, a study examined two populations of rainbow trout selected for either a low level of cortisol response (proactive and socially dominant) or a high cortisol response to a standardised confinement stressor. When they were deprived of food during a long transportation the fish switched roles, the low responders becoming subordinate (Ruiz-Gomez *et al.* 2008). Other work has shown that other relatively small changes in the early rearing environment can result in substantial difference in the behaviour of fish in later life (Braithwaite & Salvanes 2005). Therefore, it is important that wherever possible fish with known genetic make-up and rearing history should be used. In many cases this is most easily achieved by breeding on site. Where this is not possible unknown variability in the population should be controlled for in experimental designs.

Individual fish, in common with many animals, demonstrate an inherent tendency to be proactive or reactive. Even in well studied species, separating individuals into these two categories is still problematic and it is generally only possible to identify those individuals exhibiting extremes of pro- or reactive nature. Recent work has demonstrated that the causes or effects of these strategies influence all processes down to the level of gene transcriptions (MacKenzie *et al.* 2009). Assuming that individuals from a genetically homogeneous population of fish with similar previous experience are uniform in their responses may lead to increased error and significant effects being masked.

There are clonal lines of fish available and these provide potential experimental populations with no genetic variability, eg, tilapia (Sarder *et al.* 1999).

Transportation

Any procedure that involves handling or disturbance of fish should usually be preceded by a period of starvation. This period is necessary for several reasons. Immediately following feeding, fish have an increased oxygen demand associated with digestion; this specific oxygen demand necessitates increased oxygen supply. Similarly, the excretion of ammonia via the gills increases after feeding and by using a period of starvation the level of ammonia excreted into the relatively small volume of transport water can be reduced. In addition, if the digestive tract is empty there is less chance the fish will regurgitate or defecate in the water. The length of time that they should be starved is dependent on the digestive transit time, which in turn is related to body size and the temperature. Generally small fish, <400 g, would be starved for 24 h and larger fish for 48 h.

Wherever possible, fish should be transported in water even for very short period of time (<1 minute). Many commercial farms now use fish pumps rather than nets to move fish. During transportation, oxygen levels must be maintained and stocking densities kept to a level that will avoid excess deterioration of the water quality over the duration of the transport. Typical densities used for commercial transportation of trout range from 40–150 kg/m^3 (unpublished data). Commercial fish transporters recommend that the fish should not be disturbed during transportation unless absolutely necessary. Therefore, there should be a remote method of monitoring dissolved oxygen, and water should not be exchanged during transportation under normal circumstances.

On a small scale, fish can be transported in sealed plastic bags. Usually two bags, one within the other, would be used to reduce the risk of breaking, especially with fish with spiny fin rays such as tilapia or many species of catfish. The inner bag should be one third filled with water from the tank the fish are kept in (provided that is of high quality) and the remainder of the bag filled with oxygen. The neck of the bag can be twisted and bent over before being tied with cable ties or castration rings (Figure 49.1). If small fish are being transported the corners of the bag may be tied off to provide a rounded rather than pointed corner to avoid fish becoming trapped and suffering from hypoxia.

During any transportation, temperature fluctuations should be kept to a minimum. In order to maintain steady temperature, bags may be packed in polystyrene boxes (Figure 49.2) and should not be transported during periods of high temperatures. For larger groups of fish, transportation tanks are used which have an opening in the top and a drain for releasing fish and water at the bottom, and are usually insulated.

On arrival at the destination the fish should be acclimatised to the new environment. Acclimatisation is not only for temperature but also water quality including pH. Even adaptable species have a limited capacity to adapt rapidly and therefore every effort should be made to ensure that the transportation water conditions are similar to the receiving conditions. In some cases this may require the originating water to be adjusted slowly over a period of several days to reduce any rapid changes following transportation, for example pH or salinity. Under normal circumstances the bags should be floated on the new water until temperature has equilibrated (30–60 minutes). Either during this time or

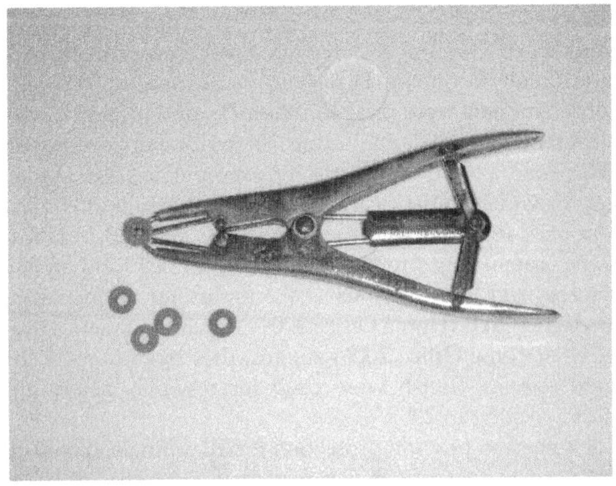

Figure 49.1 Elastic castration rings and applicator, an easy way of sealing fish transport bags.

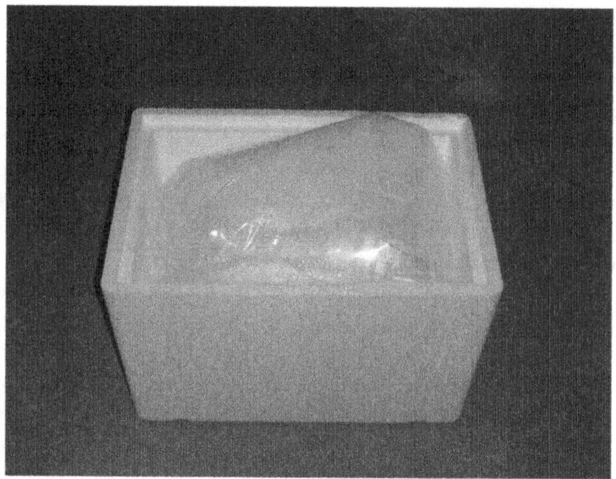

Figure 49.2 Fish transportation bags about to be sealed in a polystyrene box.

subsequently some of the recipient water should be mixed with that in the bag to avoid any rapid changes in water chemistry. Acclimatising fish on arrival is always a compromise. Fish should not be confined in the bag for longer than necessary and if they have already had a long transportation it may be necessary to aerate the bag during the acclimatisation period. In some circumstances if the water quality has deteriorated to a dangerous level, as may happen if some fish have died during transportation, then the need for acclimatisation may be secondary to the urgent need for clean water. Under such circumstances the surviving fish should be separated from the dead fish and placed in clean water of similar temperature as soon as possible.

Fish should be closely monitored after transportation for signs of ill-health or damage since moving fish can result in disruption of the social structure and result in social stress, aggression and damage (Adams *et al.* 1998).

The International Air Transport Association's Live Animals Regulations (LAR) Manual 2008/2009, contains details of transporting fish and is available from the IATA website[2].

Use in research

Estimates of the number of fish used for research worldwide are difficult to obtain. However, in Europe in 2005, 12.1 million animals were used for research, of which 15% were cold-blooded animals, including fish (European Commission 2007). Taking the UK as a specific example, in 2008, the last year for which statistics are available, 0.605 million live fish were used for scientific procedures. This equated to 17% of all the animals used for experiments in the UK and an 85% increase from the previous year, continuing an increasing trend since 2001 (Home Office 2009). Previous statistics from the UK (Home Office 2006) suggest that more than 13 different species of fish were used for research, safety and efficacy testing in 2005.

The need to provide protection for all animals, including fish, used in scientific experiments has led to the development of guidelines on appropriate rearing conditions and animal care (eg, Canadian Council on Animal Care 2005; Council of Europe 2006).

General husbandry

Enclosures

Fish are cultured commercially in a wide range of systems and environments, from temperate to tropical and fresh to salt water, in tanks, ponds and cages using semi-natural waters. Although the majority of experimental work is conducted in purpose-built facilities, some also occur on a range of commercial scale sites.

Various systems employ different degrees of water exchange and treatment. Systems can rely entirely on water exchange to maintain the environment or rely entirely on water treatment. The extent of water exchange and treatment has been used to define static, flow-through and recirculation systems. Many experimental systems would employ some form of water filtration or treatment combined with replacement of a proportion of the water. Systems with relatively small amounts of filtration and only occasional replacement of water, such as many simple ornamental fish tanks, are often described as static systems. Semi-closed systems, where water is circulated from each tank through a filter are often referred to as recirculation systems. Filtration systems typically include a mechanical filter, to remove particulate matter, and a biological filter to remove harmful ammonia and nitrite, converting them into less toxic nitrate. Some recirculation systems may also include chemical filters (eg, activated carbon) to improve water quality and also protein skimmers, which remove excess protein from the water. Recirculation systems typically require a low rate of water replenishment. Other systems referred to as flow-through rely primarily on exchange of water to maintain the environmental conditions. The rate of exchange can vary from total replacement in less than an hour to very slow partial replacement over days or weeks.

All systems used to rear fish have several common key functions, they must provide appropriate water, allow feeding, cleaning, waste disposal and necessary access to the fish. In many cases these functions conflict (eg, feeding systems may restrict access to the fish, or interfere with cleaning) and the range of enclosures or systems used is not just determined by the various species or the purpose for which the fish are kept but also an attempt to produce a manageable system.

Environmental provisions

It may seem facetious to say that water is important for fish but it is easy to forget the range of functions water serves for fish. Obviously it is the medium in which they live and which supports their weight. It also supplies oxygen to them, dilutes and removes toxic waste, carbon dioxide and all other excretory products. Fish can also absorb soluble minerals such as calcium directly from the water. Water also has many other physical properties including velocity,

[2]http://www.iata.org/index.htm

turbulence, opacity, colour and many chemical properties resulting from substances carried or dissolved in it. Maintaining adequate water supply is the central and essential aspect of caring for fish. In recirculation systems the water filtration and treatment systems may require as much effort to maintain as the fish. Many recirculation systems rely on biological filtration consisting of a large biomass of organisms exposed to a constant flow of water through a physical substrate. Treatment with chemicals damaging to the biological filter or failure of the water flow can result in collapse of the filter and catastrophic deterioration in the water quality.

The requirements of the species and life stage of the fish can vary dramatically, depending upon their natural habitat. Salmonids require very clean water and high levels of dissolved oxygen while some catfish (eg, *Clarius* spp.) appear to prefer turbid water and as air breathers are largely independent of dissolved oxygen.

In any aquatic system the loading (ratio of fish to water for dilution/removal of toxic waste metabolites) of the system is related to its vulnerability or susceptibility to failure. Typically problems deteriorate more rapidly in systems with higher biomass of fish to water volume. Often, but not in every case, an increase in loading of the system is associated with increasing complexity or sophistication of the system. Again the more complex the system the more likely there will be system failures. Vulnerable systems require more regular and detailed monitoring, higher levels of staff competence, more effective contingency planning and resources to deal with problems. For all these reasons it is not possible to recommend a single water quality monitoring protocol.

Many fish in simple tank or pond systems at ambient temperature, with regular water changes, and adequate aeration, require very little monitoring above regular observation of the fish. The most common form of monitoring is that of temperature with many tropical fish kept in temperate regions supplied with combined heater thermostats. Complex recirculation systems with high loading rates or sensitive species may require additional automated monitoring and in some cases automated manipulation of oxygen and other parameters.

Regular monitoring of the rearing system is required for any fish used in controlled experiments. Ideally, such parameters as water level, temperature, pH and dissolved oxygen should be monitored twice daily. In large systems with many units on a common filtration or water supply it may only be possible to monitor a limited number of positions in the system. How such monitoring is conducted depends on the scale of the system, for systems holding large numbers of salmonids or any marine species there would normally be automated temperature, dissolved oxygen and water level monitoring, linked to at least an alarm system and perhaps to an automated oxygenation system.

For small systems with either heavy loading rates or sensitive species it is possible to monitor a large number of parameters with inexpensive test kit technologies. These would usually be supplemented with an electronic dissolved oxygen meter and perhaps an electronic pH meter. With all electronic systems regular calibration is essential, although more recent technologies greatly reduce the necessity for calibration (eg, LED-based oxygen probes).

The ability to alter the nature of the incoming water is dependent on the supply and the volume used. The most common manipulation is that of temperature. This may be expensive if the deviation from ambient is substantial, and cooling water may be more costly than heating. The cost of changing water temperature is so great that the main function of some recirculation systems is to conserve heat. Another common and essential manipulation is the removal of chlorine from domestic water supplies. Chlorinated water can be very harmful to the gills of fish and vigorous aeration or filtration through activated charcoal is essential.

No single set of criteria is suitable for all species of fish and much of the available information relates to salmonids. Many species are capable of adapting to a wide range of environmental parameters; however, there is very little understanding of either the welfare implications or the consequences of such adaption other than acute toxic effects. Adaptive capacity is dependent on species and the animals' past experience, but can be remarkable; for example, freshwater phases of salmon are easily able to adapt to temperatures from close to 0 °C up to 20 °C. Different species have different pH requirements, with salmonids performing best around pH 7, while the Japanese *Tribolodon hakonensis* lives in water from pH 3.4–3.8 (Hirata *et al.* 2003) and the African lake Magadi tilapia (*Oreochromis alcalicus grahami*) survives in a lake at pH 10 (Randall *et al.* 1989).

Any attempt to define appropriate water quality levels for fish is constrained by lack of data and the complex interaction of water quality parameters. There is very little evidence for the effect of water quality on functional or feeling-based aspects of fish welfare of even the most commonly studied species, most of the information relates to effects of water quality on survival or growth. The stability of the fish's natural environment affects its capacity to adapt to changes. Fish from the deep ocean such as Atlantic halibut (*Hippoglossus hippoglossus*), especially in the larval stages, require very constant conditions, whereas fish adapted to rock pools may be capable of withstanding sudden and extreme fluctuations in salinity and temperature. The ability to adapt may be function specific so that while fish may survive a wide range of conditions they may not be able to reproduce outside a limited environmental range. Some life stages and very young or old fish may be less able to cope with fluctuations in environmental conditions and the rate at which conditions change often has a significant effect on the ability of fish to cope with new environmental conditions.

Water quality parameters can be grouped into those largely determined by the water supply (acidity, alkalinity, hardness, temperature, conductivity and heavy metal concentration), those largely determined by the practices in the fish-keeping facility (oxygen, ammonia, carbon dioxide and nitrite) and those that are a product of the source water and the management (nitrate, suspended solids and supersaturation).

Table 49.1 is a guide to the levels of various parameters that have been found to be safe for fish health and productivity. A recent review of water quality and welfare of farmed trout deals with this topic in considerably more

Table 49.1 Suggested water quality parameters for commonly used species of fish.

Species	*O_2 (mg/l)*	*Temp (°C)*	*pH*	*Ammonia (NH_3)*	*Source(s)*
Arctic charr (*Salvelinus alpinus*)	>6.5	<15	6.5–8.5	<0.015	Johnston (2002)
Carp (*Cyprinus carpio*)	5–12	8–25	7.0–8.5	<0.1	Horváth *et al.* (2002)
Channel catfish (*Ictalurus punctatus*)	>5.0	24–30	6.3–7.5	<0.12	Landau (1992) Stickney (1993a)
Guppy (*Poecilia reticulata*)	>4	18–28	7.0–8.0	<0.2	Wedemeyer (1996) Mills *et al.* (1999) Andrews (2000) www.fishbase.org
Rainbow trout (*Oncorhynchus mykiss*)	>5	7–18	6.5–9.0	<0.0125	McLarney (1998) MacIntyre *et al.* (2008)
Salmonids (general)	>5	>0–20	6.0–9.0	<0.0125	Bromage and Shepherd (1992) Wallace (1993)
Sea bass (*Dicentrarchus labrax*)	6–9	14–20	7.9–8.2		Pillay and Kutty (2005)
Tilapia (general)	3.0–8.0	25–30	6.5–9.0	<0.24	Stickney (1993b) Hussain (2004)
Zebrafish (*Danio rerio*)	>4	18–29	6.0–8.0	<0.2	Wedemeyer (1996) Mills *et al.* (1999) Andrews (2000) www.fishbase.org

detail (MacIntyre *et al.* 2008). Table 49.1 contains an indication of appropriate water quality levels for common species.

Photoperiod is the most regularly periodic of variables and conveys a lot of information to fish, it is therefore very important to consider in long-term experiments. The length of daylight and the change in day length experienced by fish control many processes in temperate species including reproduction, smoltification (pre-adaptation to salt water in young salmon) and, in marine Atlantic salmon, can have a greater influence on growth than temperature (Metcalfe 1994).

Bright illumination can also be stressful for fish and should be avoided, with many species seeking shade or cover when exposed to bright lights. Although fish have no eyelids to protect the sensitive photoreceptors they do have other protective mechanisms and, unlike mammals, the photoreceptors of fish can regenerate. However, continuous high-intensity light can result in damage to the eyes of fish (Vihtelic *et al.* 2006).

Many species of fish may show a fright response to rapid changes in illumination (for example when aquarium lights are switched on). This can be stressful to the fish and may result in injury, for example if the fish strikes the tank walls or another fish as a result of the fright response. Dimmer switches used on any lighting system that illuminates rearing systems can minimise this problem. Currently, there is little information regarding the effects of the spectral composition of light on fish, although this area is the focus of current research.

Fish are very sensitive to vibrations, through their lateral line system and in some cases inner ears. Any vibration transmitted through the water can have an effect on fish and where possible should be kept to a minimum. However, some disturbance through observation and routine husbandry is unavoidable. Although inevitable, vibrations and other forms of disturbance are rarely uniform throughout the experimental facilities and should be controlled for in experiments (Adams *et al.* 2007). Predictable disturbance appears to be less stressful for fish and therefore routine care and feeding should be conducted on a regular and consistent timetable.

The practical procedures for establishing a fish-keeping facility are very diverse depending on the nature of the system (tanks, ponds, cages), the type of fish (species and life stage) and the purpose for which they are kept. More detailed practical descriptions can be found in other texts such as the previous edition of this handbook (Potts *et al.* 1999), and for example, cage aquaculture (Beveridge 2004), aquaria (Scott 1997), intensive aquaculture (Shepherd and Bromage 1992) and many other species specific texts.

Environmental enrichment

We know that even relatively simple environmental enrichment can have a significant effect on the behaviour and development of Atlantic cod (Braithwaite & Salvanes 2005). However, the effects of environmental enrichment are species specific (Williams *et al.* 2009) and for many species there is a lack of robust information on the benefits of various environmental enrichments (Kihslinger & Nevitt 2006; Brydges & Braithwaite 2009). It is also possible that some forms of enrichment may be detrimental through providing cues for territorial behaviour or by causing physical harm. Objects in the tank may also make it harder to clean without disturbing the fish and can also provide areas for parasites such as *Ichthyophthirius multifiliis* to reproduce (Shinn *et al.* 2003). Water flow could be considered as a form of environmental enrichment over static conditions.

Some fish such as wrasse (eg, *Ctenolabrus rupestris*) seek out shelter and have to be provided with pipes or similar structures to hide in (Sayer *et al.* 1996). Some form of substrate is also essential for larval salmonids or alevins to prevent them crowding and/or becoming overactive, prematurely exhausting the energy supplies in yolk.

Feeding

Fish, as ectotherms, require significantly less food to survive and grow than homeotherms of equivalent size. Fish are adapted to periods of shortage rather than excess and can be naturally anorexic. While there is little evidence to suggest that short periods of food deprivation have any significant adverse effect on the welfare of fish it is known that overfeeding has many adverse effects, both physiological and environmental.

Fresh feeds may be required by some adult wild-captured fish but the quality and disease risk make such feeds unsuitable under most conditions. Under no circumstance should closely related fish species or fish from similar ecosystems be fed to each other since this is associated with a higher disease risk. Other animals such as snails or zooplankton can also be intermediate hosts for parasitic infections.

It is essential that the specific requirements of the species and life stage are catered for (see Conklin 2000). The majority of hatching embryos initially rely on a yolk sac. This supplies the developing larvae with energy until they are capable of independent feeding. The size of the yolk sac and the rate it is depleted depend on the species and on the incubation temperature. Atlantic cod larvae, for example, reach first feeding 3 days after hatching at 7 °C (Hall *et al.* 2004), whereas rainbow trout may take 20 days at 10 °C (Bromage 1995). Access to sufficient food (in term of quantity and nutritional content) when larvae are ready to feed is critical to development and survival. Food should be made available some time before the complete absorption of yolk. For Atlantic cod, food is made available immediately after hatching to avoid significant mortality (A. Davie, personal communication). The type of food given to first-feeding fry also varies between species. Larvae that are small and poorly developed are often given a suitably sized live food source (eg, *Artemia* or rotifers). Some larger, well developed larvae may be fed directly on a commercially available formulated diet. Even in species such as salmonids, which have no particular need for live food, first feeding is still a critical time when food must be made available in an appropriate manner or the fish will not successfully achieve independent feeding and will eventually die. Species that require live feed at the start of their life usually require to be weaned onto more easily managed feed (eg, commercial pellets). First feeding of demanding species and especially provision of specialist live feeds such as algae cultures or rotifers requires considerable technical expertise, since the production of live feed is the culture of an additional organism equally or more challenging than the fish themselves (see Conklin 2000).

There is often a tendency to use what is easily available and that is often trout pellets, goldfish or tropical ornamental fish food. Although this can be a reasonable solution, in some cases it is inappropriate: feeding trout feed to tilapia or carp can result in nutritional pathologies including liver damage due to the very high lipid content. In general fish have a requirement for high-quality unsaturated lipids in their diets in order to retain membrane integrity especially at lower temperatures. Many species are also highly susceptible to oxidised or rancid fats in the diet. Therefore, it is important not only to source the correct type of feed, but also to store it correctly to avoid oxidation of the high proportion of polyunsaturated lipids. Storage should be for a minimum of time and in cool dry conditions. Incorrectly stored food not only runs the risk of rancidity but will probably have dangerously low levels of the more labile micronutrients eg, vitamin C. If stored under damp conditions, feed with high lipid content is also prone to contamination with the fungus *Aspergillus fluviatus*. This fungus produces aflatoxins, which in high concentrations can result in liver failure and at lower doses can result in liver tumours.

Provision of social housing

Some species of fish are so aggressive that they cannot be kept in groups, eg, snakeheads (*Channa* spp.). Such territoriality can often be overcome in large groups where the fish revert to shoaling behaviour. Other fish have tightly fixed social structures. Clown fish (eg, *Amphiprion ocellaris*) are hermaphrodite: the largest individual in the population is female and if she is removed a smaller immature male will become female. However, if two mature females are mixed in a small tank where they are unable to establish separate territories they will fight, often resulting in the death of one individual. Reproduction in many species requires particular types of housing. In both Siamese fighting fish and three-spined sticklebacks males and females must be separated following spawning to avoid harm to the female and fry. This is a strategy also used in other species. In species such as tilapia, fish can be brought into spawning condition if they can see a suitable member of the opposite sex. However, keeping them together as a pair can result in injuries due to their aggressive courting behaviour. A simple solution is to keep them in aquaria with a dividing transparent partition.

Fish are often housed in mixed species groups for display purposes and under these circumstances it is essential that the fish have compatible environmental and social habits. Housing a piscivorous snakehead (eg, *Channa striata*) with any other fish of similar or smaller size will generally result in one large snakehead and few if any other survivors. One type of mixed species group is the use of 'dither fish'. When keeping some shy species, for example discus (*Symphysodon* spp.), shoals of small fish that spend time in the open can result in bolder behaviour from the larger discus. Similar cross-species behaviour is seen in birds and mammals (Barlow 1968).

Many people have claimed that limiting the stocking density or biomass of fish per unit volume is a means to protect the welfare of fish. However, the relationship between stocking density and fish welfare is complex (Turnbull *et al.* 2008). Stocking density is only indirectly related to fish welfare, and is mediated through and confounded by water quality, social interactions, feed availability and other factors. Both good and bad welfare can be observed over a range of stocking densities and low stocking densities can result in territorial behaviour and increased aggression. Therefore suggesting or dictating specific stocking density guidelines can be misleading. Any recommendation for stocking density to protect welfare would have to take account of many other parameters and could not be a simple table of density for given species at specific sizes.

Identification

A variety of methods have been used for identifying fish, and the choice is largely dependent on the purpose for which they will be used. However, as a general principle the least invasive method that is practical should be used. The methods can be grouped into body mutilations, or implanting visual or electronic tags. The first type of identification includes fin clipping and freeze branding. Fin clipping is the removal of part or all of a fin, usually to identify a population. This technique has been used for identifying hatchery-reared fish after restocking. The removal of even a small amount of fin can have an adverse effect on the swimming ability of the fish (Horak 1969; Deitricht & Cunjak 2006). For this reason the adipose fin was often removed from salmonids. Although this fin was thought to have little mechanical function its size and coloration, especially in mature male brown trout (*Salmo trutta*), would suggest that it may have some signalling or display function (I Semple, personal communication). The other method of body mutilation is freeze branding, which damages the pigments cells providing some form of identification.

There are a large number of methods for either injection or inserting a simple coloured compound or small tags for identification (Figure 49.3). The coloured compounds can either be injected or forced into the skin as a high pressure jet, as with the panjet system (Deitricht & Cunjak 2006). Several brightly coloured elastomers (Hartman & Janney 2006) are also available for identifying fish (Olsen & Vøllestad 2001). A combination of colours and location can be used to provide a range of identifications.

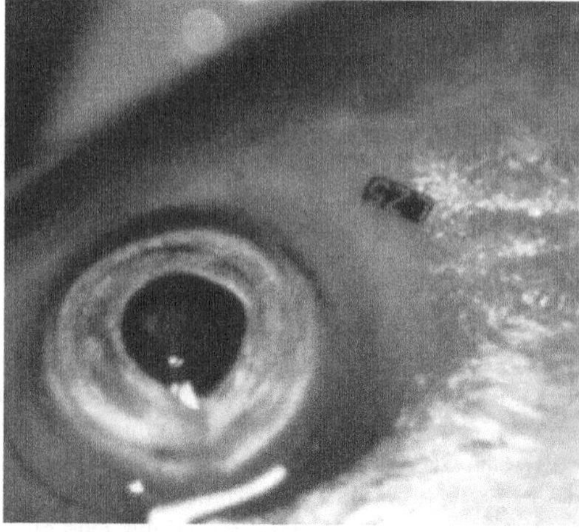

Figure 49.3 Fish tag inserted by needle with an identification number.

It is usually necessary to handle fish to check for the identification mark and confirm identity when using fin clipping and coloured spots as marking techniques. There are also passive integrated transponder (PIT) tags, which contain and transmit a unique identification code in response to a radio signal from a reader. Although these readers do not penetrate water for any great distance they can be used for identifying fish passing through an area of shallow or narrow water without touching them. There are also various other tags from coded wire tags to those containing monitoring and data-logging functions.

When applying any form of tag it is essential to anaesthetise the fish and hold them on a soft wet surface; the time out of water should be kept to a minimum. Any operative should practise the techniques under supervision and initially on dead fish until competent.

Health management

The health status of fish used in research is crucially important since in many cases the health of the experimental animals can have a more significant effect on the outcome of the experiment than the treatment under study. In addition to outbreaks of introduced infections, some pathogens are endemic in cultured and wild populations of fish such as *Mycobacterium* spp. infections in zebrafish and *Flavobacterium psychrophilum* in trout. Therefore, health management is much more than just keeping infections out of a system. It concerns all aspects of the construction and management of the system and should be a central consideration when establishing any fish-holding facility. Strategies to avoid introducing infections and to control them if they do occur are essential. Health management also has financial implications: if a disease occurs, resources must be available to deal with it. In the event of a disease problem it may be necessary to seek advice from, and send samples to, experts in the field and the necessary contingency funds must be available.

Every population of fish for experimental purposes should have a veterinary health plan, developed with the named veterinary surgeon. This should be a comprehensive plan including data recording, staff training, health and safety and any other statutory data requirements. The nature of the plan will be dependent on the business of the unit (eg, experimental research, environmental monitoring, toxicological studies, breeding of animals for other purposes etc). The plan must essentially be a part of a process that ensures effective implementation. In the UK, the Fish Veterinary Society[3] can be contacted to identify veterinary surgeons with expertise in fish health management.

In general terms, health management can be divided in to three main areas: (1) general prevention; (2) monitoring; and (3) response to problems. In some cases, fish will be kept with the purpose of exposing them to adverse conditions, disease-causing agents or introducing harmful genetic traits. This section, however, concentrates on maintaining optimal health and productivity in stock fish. All aspects of disease prevention and control should be discussed with the

[3]http://www.fishvetsociety.org.uk/

named veterinary surgeon and included in the veterinary health plan. In this section the subject is discussed in enough detail to allow a non-specialist to obtain an overview of the subject.

General prevention of disease

All management and husbandry systems should be designed to maintain the health of the fish. Key points include:

- only handling when necessary and in the least stressful and harmful way;
- maintaining as near optimal physical and social environment as possible;
- not only supplying the necessary feed but also delivering it in a way appropriate to the fish;
- ensuring a sound breeding strategy.

Biosecurity (or keeping infections out) should always be a central concern. In terms of introducing infections, introductions of new fish are the largest risk. Any introduction of stock into the system has an associated risk, since even the most stringent testing cannot be perfect due to the limitations of the tests, subclinical or carrier states of diseases and occasionally the large sizes of the populations involved. Sampling aquatic populations and issues of test limitations are discussed in detail elsewhere (Cameron 2002). The capacity to quarantine introduced fish should be planned into every system. There is no rational general recommendation for length of quarantine, although a figure of 3 weeks is often quoted. In reality the length of the quarantine period is related to the risk of introducing a serious pathogen. Where there has been a substantial investment in the existing stock, introductions should be avoided altogether or at very least be limited to disinfected eggs or second-generation of quarantined fish. Where this is not possible a trial introduction should be attempted to identify any potential problems.

Other sources of infections include the water, especially if it is from a natural water body, contains fish or potential intermediate hosts. Incoming water may be treated or filtered but only in low throughput systems. In systems open to the environment, intermediate hosts for multihost pathogens, eg, snails and piscivorous birds, may introduce infections. Control of intermediate hosts and predators can be difficult and may require the welfare of fish under your care to be balanced against the welfare of wild and perhaps endangered species.

Processed feed has not been the source of many infections in animals but the spread of bovine spongiform encephalopathy ('mad cow disease') in mammals demonstrates that there may be unexpected risks. Equipment should not be shared between establishments where possible, but if sharing cannot be avoided good disinfection practices are essential (ie, clean, disinfect and dry). People should also be discouraged from moving between establishments in quick succession or at least discouraged from using the same clothing and footwear. Footbaths are frequently cited as a means to remind people of the need for biosecurity. It is debatable whether a poorly maintained footbath has any such effect and many are not well maintained. Again, if the population at risk is valuable it is better to keep people out where possible.

Biosecurity overlaps with hygiene (or preventing infections spreading within establishments). As with biosecurity the largest risk is movement of fish. Where possible populations of fish should not be mixed and certainly different age groups should be kept separate. Water can also present a risk within establishments and can spread infections through systems reusing the same water. In the case of flow-through systems, which reuse water in a cascade, it is preferable to have younger fish in the first use water and older fish in the subsequent use water. Water can also spread infections through aerosol or splashes. Bacterial and viral infection can easily spread by this route (Wooster & Bowse 1996). There are also pathogenic fungal spores that can spread through the air, eg, *Phoma herbarum* (Ross *et al.* 1975). Individual units (systems with separate water supplies) should be supplied with separate nets and cleaning equipment. The cost of separate equipment is minimal and the alternative of cleaning and disinfecting between each use is so time consuming that eventually a busy person will not do it effectively or at all. Personnel should be discouraged from moving between separate units when possible, especially when they contain different age groups, for example hatchery and on-growing units.

A key aspect of controlling the spread of infections is using a compartmentalised system. Although some textbooks suggest that systems for zebrafish should run on a central reservoir and filtration system, keeping a large number of valuable animals (eg, genetically modified fish) on a single recirculating system is a very high-risk strategy. A common health problem in zebrafish is *Mycobacterium* spp. infections; these are easily spread through water and once established are difficult to eradicate. Compartmentalisation of the system reduces the risk of the infection spreading and also provides the opportunity to eradicate the infection through identification and removal of infected stocks, followed by thorough disinfection and fallowing. Even in the absence of a specific infectious threat, a compartmentalised system allows parts of the system to be occasionally emptied and thoroughly disinfected. The risk of infectious disease is greatly reduced by using an all-in all-out stocking policy rather than continually adding and removing stock without the option to fallow the system.

The spread of some infectious diseases can also be limited through the use of vaccination. In temperate commercial aquaculture facilities the majority of fish are vaccinated against at least one infectious disease. Currently there are vaccines available against several of the major bacterial pathogens and in some parts of the world against viral infections. The majority of vaccines are administered by intraperitoneal injection; further details can be found in Sommerset *et al.* (2005).

Health monitoring

Monitoring health comprises the detection of problems (surveillance) and the identification of those problems (diagnosis). Wherever possible, protocols for monitoring health and welfare should be species-specific; it is often not appropriate to provide generic guidelines covering all species of fish (Johansen *et al.* 2006). Detecting a problem in the earliest stages requires familiarity with the normal behaviour, feeding and appearance. For example being aware of normal feed response, fish coloration, ventilation rates, position in the tank, swimming activity, body condition and responsiveness to for example human presence or nets. In small animals such as guppies or zebrafish, fin clamping or holding the fins close to the body is often an early sign of stress or poor health. Clinical signs or evidence of disease detectable to the unaided senses may be useful to detect problems. Unfortunately they are seldom adequate to identify the specific cause of the problem. The reasons are that fish have a far more limited capacity to express clinical signs than mammals and birds, secondly individual pathogens can result in dramatically different clinical syndromes, thirdly different pathogens can produce similar clinical presentations and finally even within a single disease outbreak there will be variability in the presentation between individuals.

A further challenge is the difficulty of conducting clinical examinations: you cannot easily palpate a fish, its temperature is not informative and there is no movement of gasses within the body to create any sounds worth listening to. Neither is it easy to observe the normal behaviour of fish in many systems. Given all these limitations what can a fish keeper do to monitor the health of the fish and obtain a diagnosis in the face of a disease outbreak?

As has been frequently mentioned throughout this chapter, familiarity with the normal appearance and behaviour of the fish under your care is crucial in order to detect the earliest signs of deviation from normality. Some time spent observing the fish should be a normal part of a keeper's job description. Records are also important and these should be based on sound data, stored in a manner enabling them to be easily accessed, analysed and regularly checked for deviations from expected values. Records can be valuable for the daily management of the system but also to retrospectively investigate problems. Those responsible for measuring and recording data should appreciate the importance and the task should be proportionate to the benefit. Recording excessive amounts of apparently useless data is very demotivating and can result in poor data or failure to record any data at all.

Records should include environmental data, feeding records, details of stock number and movements allowing the origin of fish to be tracked through the system. Although batches may have to be mixed it should be easy to identify the originating populations. Records should also record fish growth and reproduction information. Finally, all health data should be recorded including evidence of ill-health, samples taken, diagnoses or evidence of pathogens and any treatments. There will also be a statutory requirement to record and display data relating to experiments, health and safety.

Diagnosis is a complex term that has been variously defined but may be considered as identifying the nature or cause of some phenomenon (disease) or distinguishing one disease from another. In the discipline of aquatic veterinary studies, diagnosis is constrained by the lack of informative clinical signs, and the limited capacity to conduct clinical examination. There is also a lack of true diagnostic tests, although there are several pathogen identification tests (falsely called diagnostic tests by some). While these tests may have a role in the control of notifiable pathogens and when eradicating pathogens from a husbandry system, they are of little value in the control of endemic diseases. Many of the common aquatic pathogens are endemic. For example, on some trout farms there may be four or five endemic pathogens. The task when controlling diseases is usually to determine the cause of the disease problem; identifying the presence of a pathogen is at best only part of this process. Most of our truly diagnostic techniques are related to histopathology or the examination of fresh tissue preparations. Histopathology is one of the only disciplines available for fish that can identify the nature of the disease process and provide strong evidence for the nature of any associated pathogen. Despite the power of histopathology, it has to be combined with all other clinical and laboratory evidence to reach a diagnosis. Achieving a diagnosis requires specialist and lengthy training; however, the person in charge of fish should have a sufficient understanding to provide the necessary information when seeking advice and should be able to take samples for diagnosis and pathogen identification (see below).

Response to a problem

When a health problem occurs there can be rapid deterioration and, therefore, advice should be sought at the earliest possible stage. Once a diagnosis is achieved a course of action has to be decided. This requires an understanding of the nature of the husbandry system, the purpose of the system (what are the fish used for), the disease and available treatments. Again, identifying the appropriate course of action is a specialist task but it is important to know that treatment with therapeutic substances is not always the most appropriate course of action. For severe diseases that are difficult or impossible to treat, eradication may be the best option. In some cases an understanding of the natural history of the disease may provide an opportunity to avoid transmission of the infectious agent. In other cases it may not be possible or necessary to do anything at all.

Following a disease outbreak there should be a detailed discussion with the veterinary surgeon and the veterinary health plan should be amended where necessary.

Breeding

Given the diversity of reproductive styles (eg, Huet 1994; Andrews 2000; Westerfield 2000) it is not possible to provide details of breeding for all commonly cultured species. Here we provide an overview of the general principles of breeding fish, which apply to a wide range of species.

Reproduction is energetically demanding (Jonsson *et al.* 1991; Okuda, 2001), due to the investment in gametes and associated behaviour. The condition of the parents can influence fertilisation, hatching and survival of offspring (eg, Laine & Rajasilta 1999; Saillant *et al.* 2001; Donelson *et al.* 2008). In some species reproduction leads to fatal exhaustion and in others survival depends on their condition at spawning (Hutchings 1994; Okuda 2001). Therefore, under laboratory conditions it is important to ensure that fish are in good condition prior to spawning and that following spawning they are given sufficient time to recover fully before they reproduce again.

Environmental cues, including photoperiod, temperature and pressure, have been shown to influence reproduction. For many seasonally spawning fish it is now possible to manipulate the timing of reproduction by artificially controlling the photoperiod, and to a lesser extent temperature. However, we have very little understanding of the welfare implications of such manipulations.

Most fish held in captivity exhibit some degree of reproductive dysfunction (reviewed by Zohar & Mylonas 2001). In the most extreme cases, this might involve a complete absence of reproduction in captivity, eg, European eel (*Anguilla anguilla*). However, two common dysfunctions occur in females and are relatively easy to address. Firstly, in some species, although females are able to produce and ovulate eggs normally they are unable to release them into the water (eg, rainbow trout). To alleviate this problem, mature females can be manually 'stripped' of eggs. Pressure is applied to the abdominal region of the fish in order to gently force the eggs out. Eggs will then be fertilised by the fish keeper using sperm gathered by stripping males. Secondly, in some species eggs may develop normally in the female but final oocyte maturation, ovulation and release into the water do not occur. This problem is often addressed using hormone treatment. Currently agonists of gonadotropin-releasing hormone (GnRHa) are the preferred substances for inducing final maturation in fish (Zohar & Mylonas 2001). GnRHa has been found to be effective in inducing final maturation over a range of concentrations (eg, Arabaci *et al.* 2004; Vermeirssen *et al.* 2004; Corriero *et al.* 2007), although levels are typically <100 µg/kg of fish. Commercial hormone induction products (ie, injections and sustained-release pellets) are now available to rapidly stimulate maturation 60–238 h post treatment (Marino *et al.* 2003); such treatments are only effective in relatively mature fish, however, not in immature fish. As well as inducing final maturation, GnRHa may be used to synchronise maturation in males and females and to increase milt (sperm) output in males, which is often necessary in captive-reared fish.

Following the fertilisation of eggs, the fish keeper must provide suitable care for the developing embryos and fry. These life stages are sensitive and it is important to ensure that optimal, species-specific rearing conditions are provided. The environmental requirements of fish change throughout their life and those of embryonic and juvenile stages may be different from those of their parents (Ishimatsu *et al.* 2004; Imsland *et al.* 2005), from subtle differences to the change from fresh to salt water seen in some salmonids.

Cannibalism can occur when fish are bred in captivity. This can take the form of adults eating eggs and juveniles (eg, zebrafish; Andrews 2000) or sibling fry cannibalising one another (eg, Atlantic cod; Puvenandran *et al.* 2008). The tendency for cannibalism varies between species as do the methods to control it, which include separating adults and eggs/fry, maintaining high feeding rates, adjusting stocking densities and introducing refuges (Andrews 2000; Kestemont *et al.* 2003; Al-Hafedh & Ali 2004).

Laboratory procedures

Handling

Fish vary in their ability to withstand handling, but capture and handling are undoubtedly stressful (Mazeaud *et al.* 1977; Billard *et al.* 1981; Pickering *et al.* 1982; Barton & Iwama 1991; Pickering 1992; Wendelaar Bonga 1997). Handling fish appropriately is not only important for their health and welfare but can also improve the outcome of experiments by reducing another source of variability (Pottinger & Calder 1995).

Fish skin is very different from that of terrestrial animals. The epithelium is relatively thin, unstratified and consists of live cells with no keratinisation. The surface layer has a complex pattern, which is species specific (Figure 49.4). This pattern increases surface area and may have the effect of retaining the superficial layer of mucus. The mucus is continually produced from the mucous cells in the epidermis and is continually sloughed off. The scales are contained within pockets of dermis extending up into the epidermis and therefore removal of a scale creates a wound extending in to the vascular tissue. The loss of a scale is **not** equivalent to losing hair or the ends of claws. Although some species have relatively tough skin, many including salmonids have very delicate skin. Physical handling must be kept to a minimum and any abrasive or dry surfaces must be avoided, they should only come in contact with soft, non-abrasive wet surfaces. This means that nets should be soft, knot-less and placed in the water prior to handling. The mesh size of the nets should also be small enough to avoid parts of the fish protruding through the net and being damaged. Fish should be handled with wet hands or wet gloved hands and kept moist even during brief periods of air exposure since this is highly stressful in most species (eg, Sloman *et al.* 2001; Lankford *et al.* 2006). In warm conditions, with rapid airflow, fish skin can desiccate very rapidly and, when the temperature is below freezing, can freeze very rapidly.

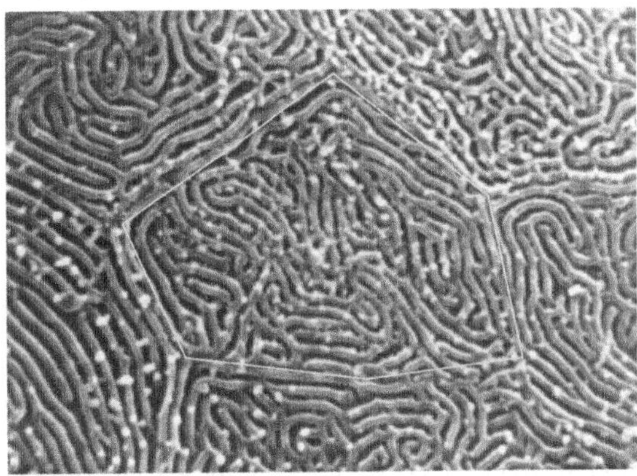

Figure 49.4 Scanning electron microscope photograph of the superficial epidermis on the ventral flank of a rainbow trout. (A single cell is outlined.)

As previously mentioned, fish should be starved prior to any form of handling and any air exposure should be kept to a minimum. Where possible fish should be encouraged into a container and then removed from the tank in water (Brydges *et al.* 2009). Capturing a specific individual can be difficult; this is especially true when capturing larger fish in larger tanks or any fish in tanks containing objects or structures. Capturing larger fish is often easier using two nets with which to corral the fish. Capturing is a skill that requires practice and inexperienced people can spend a lot of time chasing a fish, which can be very stressful and potentially damaging for it.

Fish can generally be weighed in water by first measuring the weight of the container and water. There are numerous references to blotting fish dry prior to weighing, it is doubtful whether this is a justifiable process. It is damaging and the small amount of water removed probably represents less error than the content of the gut and water in the mouth and opercular cavity. If individual or groups of fish are weighed in a net then the total weight in the net should not be too heavy or fish at the bottom can suffer injury from crushing.

Occasionally fish may have to be held in temporary containers, such as when administering anaesthetic. While adequate aeration in such vessels is essential, excessive aeration can disturb the fish and even damage them. The need for anaesthesia when handling fish is dependent on the species of fish and its previous experiences. Some may be easily handled with little or no signs of distress or attempts to escape, for example some flatfish may be handled quite easily, even out of water, providing their eyes are covered. Others, for example salmonids, may be severely stressed by even the gentlest handling. Once again the necessity for anaesthesia requires an assessment based on familiarity with the fish.

Training/habituation for procedures

There is evidence for poorer functional welfare resulting from disturbance but also complex interaction between other aspects of the environment such as stocking density and disturbance. It would appear that in some circumstances occasional disturbance can have greater detrimental effects than more regular exposure to mild disturbance (Adams *et al.* 2007). Fish can also be rapidly trained to use self-feeding systems (Alanara 1996) and will anticipate any form of feeding through visual cues (Stien *et al.* 2007).

Monitoring methods

Fish present the keeper with many challenges since they are difficult to observe in all but glass display aquaria. The position of fish can be tracked through video analysis software (Kane *et al.* 2004), or PIT tags (see section on identification) can be used to identify individuals and also determine their location in larger tanks or flumes but these techniques have limited application. Tanks that are suitable for easy observation may subject the fish to visual disturbance and affect their behaviour. There is no doubt that the effects of disturbance are complex and we have a very poor understanding of the consequences of adaptation to disturbance. Therefore in many experimental systems monitoring is confined to observation of feeding response, obvious aspects of group behaviour and gross signs of disease, occasionally combined with destructive sampling.

Monitoring the condition of fish in larger populations and in systems where they cannot be easily observed is more problematic. Growth and food conversion ratio are very useful indicators of the health of the population but monitoring these obviously involves disturbance and handling which may not be appropriate under some circumstances. Other important signs of good health include, 'normal' swimming, feeding, response to disturbance and appearance for that population. It may not seem to be very useful to say 'normal', however, it is not possible to identify generic appearance across species, husbandry systems or even between apparently similar populations. Variability is probably the result of inherent population dynamics, genetic and epigenetic variability.

It has been suggested that evaluation of reflex responses as described by Davis and Ottmar (2006) might be used to monitor the health and welfare of fish. However, the stimuli used to evaluate reflexes were in themselves stressors, including lifting the lid of the tank or striking the side. Non-invasive methods for monitoring fish are not well developed and this is an area requiring urgent attention.

Although clinical biochemistry and haematology have relatively little value for monitoring the health of fish, blood samples are taken for a variety of reasons. Blood samples can be obtained from fish in a variety of ways. In most cases with fish over 10 cm in length, blood is collected from the caudal vessels, which lie under the spine. In some cases the fish may be killed prior to blood sampling. With a typical fusiform fish such as the trout, it should be placed on its side with the ventral surface facing towards the operator. The needle should be inserted on or close to the mid-line behind the anal fin angled slightly forward towards the ventral aspect of the spine. Once the needle touches the spine, negative pressure should be applied to withdraw blood, the needle may need to be repositioned in order to puncture one of the blood vessels (Figure 49.5). Other techniques may be used for fish with other shapes such as flat fish or laterally compressed fish. With these, it is easier to obtain a sample by inserting the needle in the flank below the level of the spine and then directing the needle up towards the ventral spine. Provided it complies with national or local regulatory guidelines fish may be blood sampled under anaesthesia and then allowed to recover; however, the volume of blood removed should not exceed 1% of the weight of the fish. Blood samples may also be obtained through cardiac puncture and from other vessels, however, such techniques require specialist training and often require euthanasia. Obtaining blood samples from very small fish can be difficult via venepuncture and therefore they may be killed and the tail cut off at the caudal peduncle. Blood can then be collected from the severed vessels, with a capillary tube or small syringe and needle. This technique has the disadvantage that extravascular fluids contaminate the blood.

Since the health of fish is a major aspect of their welfare, destructive sampling for health checks is a normal part of

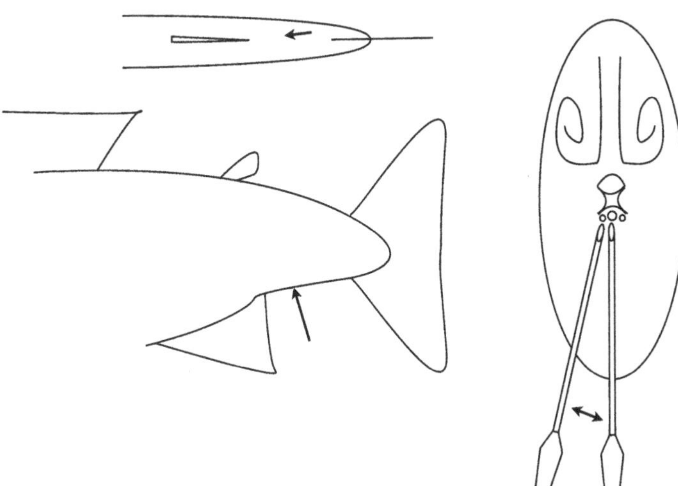

Figure 49.5 Insertion point for needle when blood sampling a typical fusiform fish.

the husbandry of many fish populations. Although the necessity and exact nature of the sampling would be part of the veterinary health plan, some basic principles are an important part of training for fish keepers since samples may have to be taken at very short notice.

Fish, unlike warm blooded animals, will often increase in temperature after death and, due to enzyme systems designed to function over wide temperature ranges, autolysis occurs very rapidly even in fish that are cooled after death. Therefore, the most important principal of sampling is to use very recently killed fish, even a 5 minute delay can result in changes in the gills rendering diagnosis more complex (Ferguson 2006). In the majority of cases fish suffering from clinical disease or those to be sampled for other purposes should be killed and then immediately sampled. Fish that are already dead can only be used for a limited number of specific purposes.

One has to be practised in order to take a full set of samples from a single fish before autolytic changes set in and the number and range of samples that can be collected are dependent upon the size of the fish. Once the fish is killed it should be kept moist in the water from which it was removed since many parasites are most easily detected by their movement and either desiccation or chlorinated water will kill them.

Prior to collecting samples, a brief examination of the external appearance should be conducted paying attention to the eyes, gills and vent and ensuring both sides are examined. Fresh preparations can then be made from the skin or gills, although interpretation requires some training. To examine the mucus on the body surface a scalpel blade should be gently scraped over the surface of the fish especially behind fins. The areas behind fins are protected and are therefore a site preferred by parasites (Figure 49.6). The resulting material should primarily consist of mucus with epithelial cells. If there are scales in the material then the scraping was too vigorous and deep. The accumulated material should be transferred to a glass slide, a drop of the water in which the fish was kept added and a cover slip placed on top. This can be examined under the microscope once the other samples have been collected. It may be easier to observe the cells and any parasites by lowering the condenser on the microscope. A sample of gill should be taken for examination. Part or all of one of the gill arches should be removed and placed on a wet Petri dish or a glass slide. A group of the primary lamellae should be removed above the level of the bifurcation (Figure 49.7). The freed primary lamellae should then be placed on a glass slide with a drop of water (as before). When the cover slip is placed over the tissue it may be necessary to move it in order to observe the secondary lamellae. Again the preparation can be examined under the microscope at the end of sampling, ensuring that the preparation does not dry out in the mean time.

Once external examination or sampling has been carried out, in fish over 5–7 cm in length the body surface is opened to expose the internal organs and take samples for bacteriology and histopathology.

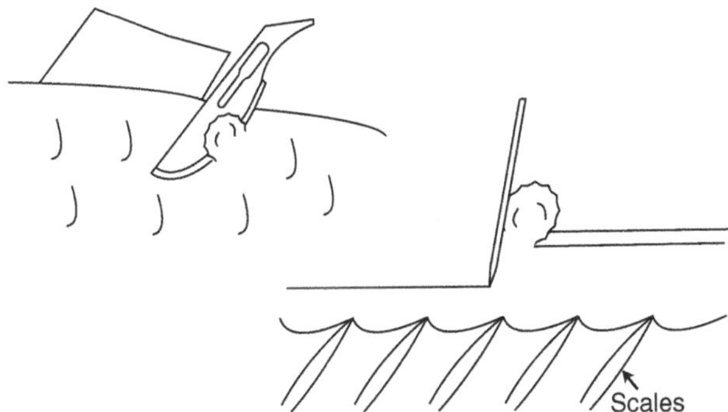

Figure 49.6 Diagram of process to collect superficial scraping from a fish avoiding deeper tissues and scales.

Bacteriology

Petri dishes containing solid medium (agar) are used to provide a large surface of media for the cultivation of bacteria and fungi. The agar used for most common fish pathogens is tryptone soya agar (TSA) and incubation temperatures are usually as close as possible to the temperature of the water from which the fish were sampled (Frerichs & Miller 1993; Inglis *et al.* 1993). Inoculation of an agar plate is often carried out using the streak plate technique. This involves

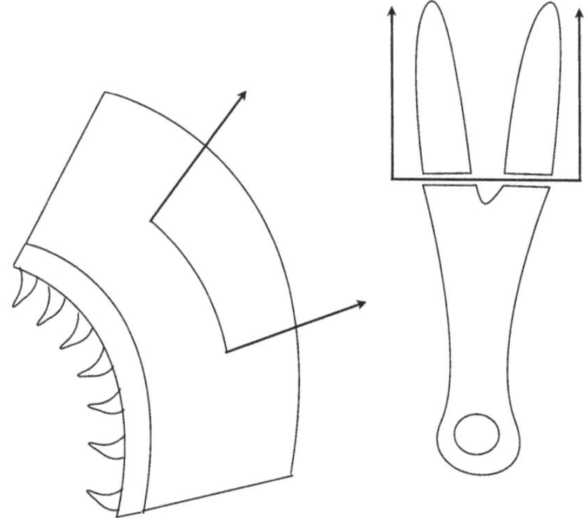

Figure 49.7 Diagram of process to collect superficial fresh preparation from the gills.

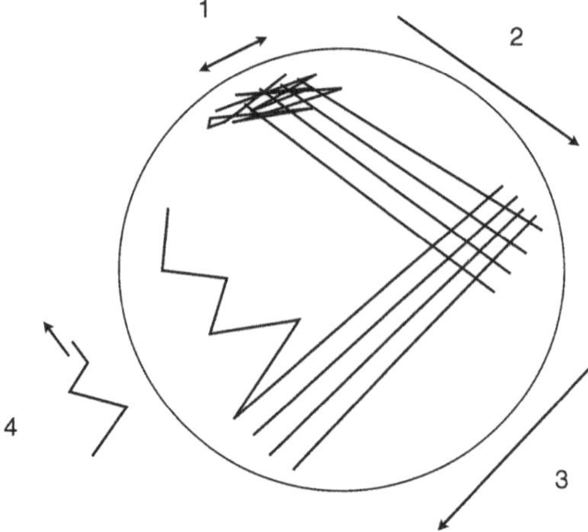

Figure 49.8 Diagram of plate streaked for bacterial recovery.

diluting the sample, eg, kidney material, by smearing it across the surface of the agar. Organisms present in the samples will be separated and after suitable incubation each organism (or at least attached group) present will give rise to a colony. Although this colony contains many millions of organisms they will have all originated from one, and therefore all organisms in one colony should be identical.

For typical fusiform fish >5–7 cm long:

1. Using a scalpel blade, carefully make an incision through the body wall in the mid-ventral line at the base of the pelvic fins.
2. Using scissors or scalpel blade extend the incision anteriorly and posteriorly to expose the internal organs. Take care not to puncture any part of the intestinal tract.
3. Hold or pin back or remove the side of the body wall.
4. Carefully move the alimentary tract to one side to expose the swim bladder.
5. Carefully peel back the swim bladder to reveal the kidney.
6. Note any abnormalities.
7. Sterilise a bacteriological loop by heating and allow to cool (touch edge of an uninoculated area of medium to ensure coolness) or use a disposable loop.
8. (Sterilise a scalpel blade and use this to make a small incision in the kidney.) – Optional
9. Insert a sterile loop into the kidney and remove a small portion of kidney using the loop, taking care not to touch the loop on any other part of the fish.
10. Inoculate the sample on a segment of the surface of the culture medium. This is known as the 'well'.
11. Sterilise the loop, allow it to cool.
12. Spread part of the sample over about one quarter of the plate by making three to four parallel streaks with the loop.
13. Repeat streaking procedure as shown (Figure 49.8), sterilising and cooling the loop or using a new disposable loop between each step. By using this method organisms can be cultured in the laboratory and individual colonies selected. This process is essential since it is impossible to carry out bacterial identification on mixed cultures. Care should be taken to ensure that plates used for this purpose are not contaminated by water droplets from condensation. Avoid unnecessary exposure of the agar surface to potential contamination from the environment throughout the procedure.
14. Label underside (not lid) of the plate using a waterproof marker, writing only round the edge, and incubate at a suitable temperature.
15. Material from other organs, eg, liver, spleen, heart, can be taken if any abnormality is evident.

For smaller fish it may be possible to open the abdomen and insert a very small loop or straight wire avoiding the gut. Whole fish homogenates can be used but are difficult to interpret since the bacteria from the gut, skin and gills are mixed with the tissues.

Samples for histopathology

Samples for histology must be taken as soon as possible after death and fixed immediately, preferably in neutral buffered formalin, which may be cooled for improved preservation if the ambient temperature is high. Neutral buffered formalin consists of:

- 40% formaldehyde 100 ml
- $NaH_2PO_4.H_2O$ 4 g
- $NaHPO_4$ 6 g
- Tap water 900 ml

The organs sampled depend on the nature of the problem but in most cases most of the major organs are sampled (eg, gill, skin including muscle around lateral line, heart, liver, pancreas/gut, spleen and kidney). The samples should be sufficiently small to allow the fixative to penetrate rapidly through the tissue. Therefore one of the dimensions of the tissue removed should be less than 7.5 mm. The tissues should be placed in at least one part tissue to ten parts fixative. Small fish may be killed and placed directly into fixative or preferably the abdomen opened and then placed in fixative. The tissue can be kept in formalin for prolonged periods but they should be stored in such a way as to avoid any portion of the tissues remaining out of the fixative.

Administration of substances

Substances, whether for experimental or therapeutic purposes, can be administered in food, by injection or by immersion. Anyone treating fish should be trained before undertaking any treatments and the nature of the treatment should be agreed with the veterinary surgeon. There are, however, some general precautions and considerations that anyone taking care of fish should be aware of.

In-feed administration

When administering a substance in food there are several major considerations. The substance has to be evenly mixed with the feed, fixed to the surface to avoid leaching prior to consumption and any unpalatable tastes masked. The medicated feed then has to be fed to the fish in sufficient quantities and sufficiently regularly to maintain levels in all the fish in the population. If the substance is being administered for therapeutic purposes it is important to realise that any fish suffering from clinical disease are probably inappetant and therefore the treatment will only be taken by those that are not yet ill. The use of veterinary medicines and the mixing of medicated feed may be covered by national legislation and advice should be sought from the veterinary surgeon responsible.

Immersion

There are various forms of immersion administration (dip, bath or flush) which can be used depending on the system and the purpose of the treatment. As with any form of handling fish should be starved for 24–48h prior to treatment and the general health of the fish should be checked. Fish are commonly treated with formalin to remove skin parasites. Formalin is a reducing agent and will reduce the available oxygen in the water. If the fish have concurrent gill pathology the formalin treatment without very careful monitoring of the oxygen levels could result in the fish dying from hypoxia.

Calculating the dose of chemical for administration is simple arithmetic but it is still easy to misplace a decimal point or make some other simple error and therefore two people should calculate the dose independently. It is also worth having a system to quickly and easily make a rough estimate. For example, one cubic metre is 1 tonne of water or 1000 litres or 1 million ml. Therefore a dose of 150 parts per million (ppm) will be 150ml of the chemical in 1 cubic metre.

There are many things that can change unpredictably and therefore if a large number or expensive fish are being treated then it is wise to conduct a trial therapy on a small number of fish in the water and chemical that will be used. Trial therapies are particularly important for inexperienced staff but can avoid mistakes by even the most experienced staff.

Normally, the volume of the system to be treated would be reduced to minimise the amount of chemical that has to be used and therefore the amount that has to be disposed of. Disposal must be in accordance with all relevant legislation and compliant with the discharge consents for the premises. In flow-through systems the water inflow would be turned off to avoid dilution of the chemical. In recirculation systems the effect of the chemical on any biofiltration must be considered before any treatment. Even in systems without specifically designed biofilters there will be a large biomass of microorganisms on all wet surfaces. If the chemical treatment kills these organisms they will decompose leading to the release of nutrients and a decline in water quality. The ability to treat the fish for minor parasitic infections while protecting the biofilter should be designed into the system. This may necessitate removal of the fish from the system. However, in some cases the pathogens may be able to survive in the filter and in these cases the only option is to sterilise the system and re-start the filter system.

Some of the chemicals that might be used, including anaesthetics, may be held in a pre-prepared stock solution. Storage conditions are important since evaporation or deterioration in the chemical can result in an over- or underdose. The chemical would normally be premixed in a container with some of the water from the system so that it can be rapidly and evenly dispersed through the tank. Some of the substances that may be administered will also be irritants, which may necessitate an alternative route of administration or diluent.

At all times adequate dissolved oxygen levels should be maintained, through aeration, oxygenation or agitation of the water. The combination of confinement and the effects of the treatments may stress the fish increasing their oxygen demand.

At the end of the treatment the water in flow-through systems should be turned back on and the discharge water run to waste in accordance with legislation. Following a treatment all the details should be recorded and the efficacy of the treatment confirmed by the collection of further samples.

If a treatment causes the fish excessive stress or injury they may become lethargic, hyperactive or gasp at the surface of the water. The priorities are to reduce the concentration of the chemical and ensure adequate oxygen supply. In circular tanks it is necessary to ensure that diluting the chemical does not also result in increased directional flow, which may be fatal for already stressed fish. In most tanks the inlet would be arranged to create a directional flow by angling the pipe round the circumference of the tank. If the treatment has to be terminated then the pipe should be directed vertically down into the tank to increase the water exchange without increasing the water velocity (Figure 49.9).

Anaesthesia/analgesia

Anaesthesia is defined as the blocking of all sensation, whereas analgesia is the blocking of the conscious sensation of pain. It has been shown that fish respond to noxious stimuli and it is believed that they are able to experience pain although this is still the subject of debate (see section on fish welfare). However, it is necessary to use anaesthetics or analgesics whenever any laboratory procedure might result in significant pain or distress. Here the discussion is focused on anaesthetics, which are more widely used in fish. There is a range of methods for anaesthetising fish, but here

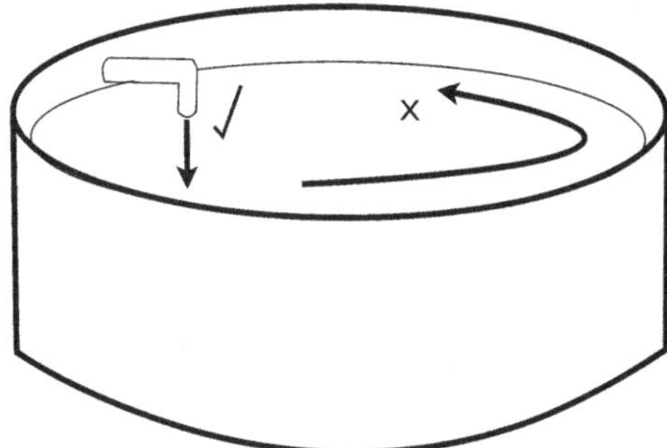

Figure 49.9 In the case of a treatment causing the fish distress the chemical should be diluted as rapidly as possible but avoiding increasing the directional flow in the tank.

an overview of only on the most widely used approaches is provided. For more detailed information see Burka *et al.* (1997) and Ross and Ross (2008).

In fish, anaesthetics may be used for two purposes: to alleviate pain during procedures and to restrain fish, often for routine tasks such as weighing. Anaesthetics can be applied to fish by injection or via ventilation through the gills. Injections are only occasionally used for surgical or lengthy procedures. Their use requires considerable expertise and specialised training. This section will focus on the more widely used methods, the most common of which involves immersing fish in water containing anaesthetic, which is taken into the body via the gills.

Various anaesthetic compounds are available for use with fish, the most common being tricaine methane sulphonate (MS 222). MS 222 is the only anaesthetic licensed for use on fish in the UK and approved by the US Food and Drug Administration. It is highly soluble and can be used in either fresh or salt water. However, when MS 222 is dissolved in the water it reduces the pH, which can be harmful to fish. Therefore working solutions should be buffered to a pH of between 7.0 and 7.5 using sodium bicarbonate or Tris-buffer. Benzocaine is another widely used anaesthetic, which is often considered a less expensive alternative to MS 222. However, it is relatively insoluble in water and must be prepared in acetone or ethanol prior to use. Other anaesthetics include clove oil, 2-phenoxyethanol, metomidate, quinaldine and quinaldine sulphate. Doses necessary to induce anaesthesia vary between compounds and also between different species and due to biotic and abiotic factors such as temperature, life stage and fish size (Hoskonen & Pirhonen 2004).

While it is necessary to consider the aversive properties of an anaesthetic there is a lack of research in this area[4].

The main issues associated with anaesthetising fish using immersion methods are discussed here. Other more specialised and less commonly used techniques are described by Ross and Ross (2008).

Prior to anaesthetising fish, it is recommended that they are starved for 24–48h. The tanks, air supply, nets etc used to anaesthetise fish should be set up in advance of handling any fish. They should be located in a convenient position close to the tanks where the fish are held and where any procedures will be conducted. The system should include a static water tank (not flow-through) for anaesthetising the fish and a separate tank with very low or no directional flow in which fish will recover before to being returned to their normal tank. Fish should not be allowed to recover in their normal tank as other fish might be aggressive towards them and any directional water flow may disorientate them resulting in superficial damage. Each tank should be appropriately sized for the species concerned. Tanks should be filled with water from the normal rearing tanks and gently aerated, since vigorous aeration can be stressful or disorientating. It must be possible to see the fish in the tanks but bright lights should be avoided. Water in the anaesthetic and recovery baths must be replaced if there is any evidence of deterioration in water quality. The keeper should give due consideration to hygiene and biosecurity before anaesthetising any fish.

Due to the variability in the responses of different fish to anaesthetics, published doses should be used only as a guide. Initially, the water should be dosed with a concentration of anaesthetic at the lower end of the calculated range. Then one fish should be placed into the anaesthetic bath and monitored until it is anaesthetised. More anaesthetic can be added if necessary or the concentration diluted if anaesthesia occurs too rapidly. Once a suitable concentration of anaesthetic is achieved, more fish may be anaesthetised at a time. However, the anaesthesia bath (and the recovery tank) must not become over-stocked as this may lead to deterioration in water quality or it may become difficult to monitor the fish adequately.

Different levels of anaesthesia are classified in four stages ranging from light sedation (stage 1) to medullary collapse (stage 4). The level of anaesthesia achieved can be assessed by monitoring the behaviour of the fish. Behavioural changes might range from reduced swimming activity in stage 1 anaesthesia (light sedation), to a loss of equilibrium and altered ventilation rate during stage 2 (light to deeper anaesthesia), through to a total loss of reactivity and a very low respiratory rate in stage 3 (surgical anaesthesia) (Burka *et al.* 1997; Ross & Ross 2008).

Following anaesthesia, recovered fish should display normal ventilation and swimming behaviour, and be responsive to stimuli. However, some effects of anaesthesia (eg, changes in physiology or blood chemistry) can persist for a significant time after recovery, in some cases for several hours. Fish should therefore be monitored regularly in the hours and days following anaesthesia. Personnel should also be aware that anaesthesia can result in side effects which might influence their experimental results.

Finally, prior to undertaking anaesthesia users must consider all personal and environmental health and safety implications. Anaesthetic compounds can have broad, sometimes unknown, effects on animals and man (including possible effects through the food chain). The physical process of anaesthetising fish presents further risks to health and safety. Therefore anaesthesia of fish must be conducted in compliance with institutional, regional and national guidelines and legislation.

[4]http://www.apc.gov.uk/reference/apc_supplementary_review_schedule_1.pdf

Euthanasia

Euthanasia requires an appropriate humane killing method and any handling or restraint should have as little adverse effect on the animals as possible (see Chapter 17 for general principles of euthanasia). Most of the information relating to the humane killing of fish is in the context of slaughter of farmed fish (Robb & Kestin 2002; van de Vis & Kestin 2003; Lines & Kestin 2005) and there is relatively little evidence for the most humane method in the wide range of circumstances where experimental fish have to be euthanased.

The two techniques recommended in the UK for humane killing of research fish are concussion and destruction of the brain prior to the regaining of consciousness, and overdose of a suitable anaesthetic. However, whilst an overdose of anaesthetic is considered a humane method for killing fish, it also requires that death is confirmed or assured. This can be through confirmation of permanent cessation of the circulation, destruction of the brain, dislocation of the neck, exsanguination (ie, fatal blood loss), the onset of rigor mortis or instantaneous destruction of the body in a macerator. The choice of method to confirm or assure death will depend on any subsequent sample collection, for example if brain tissue is required it is not appropriate to destroy the brain to assure death.

Problems that can occur whilst killing fish include those associated with dealing with fish which have heavily armoured heads making them difficult to effectively concuss and differing susceptibility to anaesthesia, eg, air breathers. An attempt should be made to maximise the dose of the anaesthetic to reduce the time to loss of sensibility but avoiding irritant or aversive nature of the anaesthetic. Large numbers of fish or very small fish can also be a problem since concussion may not be feasible and following anaesthetic overdose it may be difficult to confirm death in a short period of time. Large fish can also pose a problem since capture and restraint prior to killing may be difficult and stressful for the fish. While adding anaesthetic to the water where the fish are kept may avoid the stress of handling it may not be possible where only some individuals need to be killed or in recirculation systems.

Other methods that have been proposed are maceration, chilling (which raises welfare concerns) and electrical stunning[5]. Although electrical stunning is now widely used in trout farming (Lines & Kestin 2005) at this point there is insufficient data to support the use of the other techniques in fish for experimental purposes.

Common welfare problems

Any discussion of fish welfare is constrained by a lack of information regarding the preferences expressed by fish. The majority of relevant work to date has focused on functional aspects of welfare. The welfare of fish was discussed by Huntingford *et al.* (2006), Branson (2008) and a special edition of *Disease of Aquatic Organisms*[6].

When evaluating the welfare of fish it is often not appropriate to extrapolate from terrestrial animals since fish are a diverse group of cold-blooded animals, do not have the same constant need for food and can be naturally inappetant for protracted periods; most live in a three-dimensional environment, may exhibit shoaling behaviour and many aspects are inherently adaptable.

We have little information with which to assess the welfare implications of the various behaviours observed in fish, unless they result in damage such as escape behaviour, hyperactivity or aggression. The majority of welfare issues could be summarised as injury through handling, predators, conspecifics or self-inflicted through contact with solid objects. Infections are common and fish suffer from the same range of pathogens as humans or animals (viruses, rickettsia, bacteria, fungi, protozoa and a wide range of metazoan parasites). Fish suffer from pathology as a result of inappropriate water quality or feed. They may also suffer from genetic manipulation intentionally introducing harmful traits or from careless breeding strategies. Detailed descriptions of the pathologies and disease can be found in Ferguson (2006) and Roberts (2001).

Despite the lack of information, practical experience and adherence to basic principles of health management can avoid many of the most obvious welfare problems observed in captive fish; we hope this chapter provides at least a useful starting point and have attempted to include reference to useful review texts or those containing useful specific information.

References

Adams, C.E., Huntingford, F.A., Turnbull, J.F. *et al.* (2000) Size heterogeneity can reduce aggression and promote growth in Atlantic Salmon parr. *Aquaculture International*, **8**, 543–549

Adams, C.E., Huntingford, F.A., Turnbull, J.F. *et al.* (1998) Alternative competitive strategies and the cost of food acquisition in juvenile Atlantic salmon. *Aquaculture*, **167**, 17–26

Adams, C., Turnbull, J.F., Bell, A. *et al.* (2007) Multiple determinants of welfare in farmed fish: stocking density, disturbance and aggression in salmon. *Canadian Journal of Fisheries and Aquatic Science*, **64**, 336–344

Alanara, A. (1996) The use of self-feeders in rainbow trout (*Oncorhynchus mykiss*) production. *Aquaculture*, **145**, 1–20

Al-Hafedh, Y.S. and Ali, S.A. (2004) Effects of feeding on survival, cannibalism, growth and feed conversion of African catfish, *Clarias gariepinus* (Burchell) in concrete tanks. *Journal of Applied Ichthyology*, **20**, 225–227

Andrews, C. (1999) Freshwater fish. In: *The UFAW Handbook on the Care and Management of Laboratory Animals, Volume 2: Amphibious and Aquatic Vertebrates and Advanced Invertebrates*, 7th edn. Ed. Poole, T., pp. 36–67. Blackwell Publishing, Oxford

Andrews, C. (2000) *Guide to Fish Breeding*, 1st edn. Interpet Publishing, Surrey

Arabaci, M., Diler, I. and Sari, M. (2004) Induction and synchronisation of ovulation in rainbow trout, *Oncorhynchus mykiss*, by administration of emulsified buserelin (GnRHa) and its effects on egg quality. *Aquaculture*, **237**, 475–484

Aronson, L.R. (1971) Further studies on orientation and jumping behaviour in the Gobiid fish, *Bathygobius soporator*. *Annals of the New York Academy of Sciences*, **188**, 378–392

Axelrod, H.R. and Schultz, L.P. (1990) *Handbook of Tropical Aquarium Fishes*, 4th edn. T.F.H. Publications Inc, Maidenhead

[5]http://www.apc.gov.uk/reference/apc_supplementary_review_schedule_1.pdf

[6]http://www.int-res.com/abstracts/dao/v75/n2/

Balon, E.K. (1990) Epigenesis of an epigeneticist: the development of some alternative concepts on the early ontogeny and evolution of fishes. *Guelph Ichthyology Reviews*, **1**

Barlow, G.W. (1968) Dither – a way to reduce undesirable fright behavior in ethological studies. *Zeitschrift fur Tierpsychologie*, **25**, 315–318

Barton, B.A. and Iwama, G.K. (1991) Physiological changes in fish from stress in aquaculture with emphasis on the response and effects of corticosteroids. *Annual Reviews in Fish Diseases*, **1**, 3–26

Beveridge, M. (2004) *Cage Aquaculture*, 3rd edn. Blackwell Publishing, Oxford

Billard, R., Bry, C. and Gillet, C. (1981) Stress, environment and reproduction in teleost fish. In: *Stress and Fish*, 1st edn. Ed. Pickering, A.D., pp. 85–108. Academic Press, London

Braithwaite, V.A. (2006) Cognitive ability in fish. *Fish Physiology*, **24**, 1–37

Braithwaite, V.A. and Boulcott, P. (2007) Pain perception, aversion and fear in fish. *Diseases of Aquatic Organisms*, **75**, 131–138

Braithwaite, V.A. and Salvanes, A.G. (2005) Environmental variability in the early rearing environment generates behaviourally flexible cod: implications for rehabilitating wild populations. *Proceedings of the Royal Society Series B: Biological Sciences*, **272**, 1107–1113

Branson, E. (2008) *Fish Welfare*, 1st edn. Blackwell Publishing, Oxford

Bromage, N. (1995) Broodstock management and seed quality – general considerations. In: *Broodstock Management and Egg and Larval Quality*, 1st edn. Eds Bromage, N. and Roberts, R.J., pp. 1–24. Blackwell Publishing, Oxford

Bromage, N. and Cumaranatunga, R. (1988) Egg production in the rainbow trout. In: *Recent Advances in Aquaculture*, Vol. 3, 1st edn. Eds Muir, J.F. and Roberts, R.J., pp. 63–138. Croom Helm Ltd, London

Bromage, N., Jones, J., Randall, C. *et al.* (1992) Broodstock management, fecundity, egg quality and the timing of egg production in the rainbow trout (*Oncorhynchus mykiss*). *Aquaculture*, **100**, 141–166

Bromage, N., Porter, M. and Randall, C. (1991) The environmental regulation of maturation in farmed finfish with special reference to the role of photoperiod and melatonin. *Aquaculture*, **197**, 63–98

Bromage, N. and Shepherd, J. (1992) Fish, their requirements and site evaluation. In: *Intensive Fish Farming*, 2nd edn. Eds Shepherd, J. and Bromage, N., pp. 17–49. Blackwell Publishing, Oxford

Brydges, N.M. and Braithwaite, V.A. (2009) Does environmental enrichment affect the behaviour of fish commonly used in laboratory work? *Applied Animal Behaviour Science*, **118**, 137–143

Brydges, N.M., Boulcott, P., Ellis, T. *et al.* (2009) Quantifying stress responses induced by different handling methods in three species of fish. *Applied Animal Behaviour Science*, **116**, 295–301

Burka, J.F., Hammell, K.L., Horsberg, T.E. *et al.* (1997) Drugs in salmonid aquaculture – a review. *Journal of Veterinary Pharmacology and Therapeutics*, **20**, 333–349

Cameron, A. (2002) *Survey Toolbox for Aquatic Animal Diseases. A Practical Manual and Software Package*. ACIAR Monograph No. 94. Australian Centre for International Agricultural Research, Canberra

Canadian Council on Animal Care (2005) *Guidelines on: the Care and Use of Fish in Research, Teaching and Testing*. Canadian Council on Animal Care, Ontario, Canada

Chandroo, K.P., Duncan, I.J.H. and Moccia, R.D. (2004a) Can fish suffer? Perspectives on sentience, pain, fear and stress. *Applied Animal Behaviour Science*, **86**, 225–250

Chandroo, K.P., Yue, S. and Moccia, R.D. (2004b) An evaluation of current perspectives on consciousness and pain in fishes. *Fish and Fisheries*, **5**, 281–295

Christiansen, J.S., Svendsen, Y.S. and Jobling, M. (1992) The combined effects of stocking density and sustained exercise on the behaviour, food intake, and growth of juvenile Arctic charr (*Salvelinus alpinus* L.). *Canadian Journal of Zoology*, **70**, 115–122

Cohen, D.M., Inada, T., Iwamato, T. *et al.* (1990) FAO species catalogue, Vol. 10. Gadiform fishes of the world (Order Gadiformes). An annotated and illustrated catalogue of cods, hakes, grenadiers and other gadiform fishes known to date. *FAO Fisheries Synopsis*, **125**, 10

Colman, J.G. (1997) A review of the biology and ecology of the whale shark. *Journal of Fish Biology*, **51**, 1219–1234

Conklin, D.E. (2000) Diet. In: *The Laboratory Fish*, 1st edn. Ed. Ostrander G.K., pp. 65–77. Academic Press, London

Corriero, A., Medina, A., Mylonas, C.C. *et al.* (2007) Histological study of the effects of treatment with gonadotropin-releasing hormone agonist (GnRHa) on the reproductive maturation of the captive-reared Atlantic bluefin tuna (*Thunnus thynnus* L.). *Aquaculture*, **272**, 675–686

Council of Europe (2006) Multilateral Consultation of Parties to the European Convention for the Protection of Vertebrate Animals used for Experimental and other Scientific Purposes (ETS 123) Appendix A. *Cons 123 (2006) 3*. Available from URL: http://www.coe.int/t/e/legal_affairs/legal_co-operation/biological_safety,_use_of_animals/laboratory_animals/2006/Cons123(2006)3AppendixA_en.pdf (accessed 31 July 2008)

Davis, M.W. and Ottmar, M.L. (2006) Wounding and reflex impairment may be predictors for mortality in discarded or escaped fish. *Fisheries Research*, **82**, 1–6

Dietricht, J.P. and Cunjak, R.A. (2006) Evaluation of the impacts of carlin tags, fin clips, and panjet tattoos on juvenile Atlantic salmon. *North American Journal of Fisheries Management*, **26**, 163–169

Donelson, J.M., McCormick, M.I. and Munday, P.L. (2008) Parental condition affects early life-history of a coral reef fish. *Journal of Experimental Marine Biology and Ecology*, **360**, 109–116

European Commission (2007) *Fifth Report on the Statistics on the Number of Animals Used for Experimental and Other Scientific Purposes in the Member States of the European Union*. Report from the Commission to the Council and European Parliament. Brussels, Belgium

Ferguson, H.W. (2006) *Systemic Pathology of Fish: A Text and Atlas of Normal Tissues in Teleosts and Their Responses in Disease*, 2nd edn. Scotian Press, London

Frerichs, G.N. and Millar, S.D. (1993) *Manual for the Isolation and Identification of Fish Bacterial pathogens*, 1st edn. Pisces Press, Stirling

Gerhard, G.S., Kauffman, E.J., Wang, X. *et al.* (2002) Life spans and senescent phenotypes in two strains of Zebrafish (*Danio rerio*). *Experimental Gerontology*, **37**, 1055–1068

Gillet, C. and Dubois, J.P. (2007) Effect of water temperature and size of females on the timing of spawning of perch *Perca fluviatilis* L. in Lake Geneva from 1984 to 2003. *Journal of Fish Biology*, **70**, 1001–1014

Hall, T.E., Smith, P. and Johnston, I.A. (2004) Stages of embryonic development in the Atlantic cod *Gadus morhua*. *Journal of Morphology*, **259**, 255–270

Hansen, T., Karlsen, Ø., Taranger, G.L. *et al.* (2001) Growth, gonadal development and spawning time of Atlantic cod (*Gadus morhua*) reared under different photoperiods. *Aquaculture*, **203**, 51–67

Hartman, K.J. and Janney, E.C. (2006) Visual implant elastomer and anchor tag retention in largemouth bass. *North American Journal of Fisheries Management*, **26**, 665–669

Hershberger, W.K. (1992) Genetic variability in rainbow trout populations. *Aquaculture*, **100**, 51–71

Hirata, T., Kaneko, T., Ono, T. *et al.* (2003) Mechanism of acid adaptation of a fish living in a pH 3.5 lake. *The American Journal of*

Physiology – Regulatory, Integrative and Comparative Physiology, **284**, 1199–1212

Home Office (2006) *Animals (Scientific Procedures) Inspectorate Annual Report 2005*. Home Office, London

Home Office (2009) *Statistics of Scientific Procedures on Living Animals – Great Britain 2008*. Home Office, London

Horak, D.L. (1969) The effect of fin removal on stamina of hatchery-reared rainbow trout. *Progressive Fish Culturist*, **31**, 217–220

Horváth, L., Tamás, G. and Seagrave, C. (2002) *Carp and Pond Fish Culture*, 2nd edn. Fishing News Books, Oxford

Hoskonen, P. and Pirhonen, J. (2004) Temperature effects on anaesthesia with clove oil in six temperate-zone fishes. *Journal of Fish Biology*, **64**, 1136–1142

Huet, M. (1994) *Textbook of Fish Culture: Breeding and Cultivation of Fish*, 2nd edn. Fishing News Books, Oxford

Huntingford, F.A., Adams, C., Braithwaite, V.A. *et al.* (2006) Current understanding on fish welfare: a broad overview. *Journal of Fish Biology*, **68**, 332–372

Hussain, M.G. (2004) *Farming of Tilapia – Breeding Plans, Mass Seed Production and Aquaculture Techniques*, 1st edn. Momin Offset Press, Dhaka

Hutchings, J.A. (1994) Age-specific and size-specific costs of reproduction within populations of brook trout, *Salvelinus fontinalis*. *Oikos*, **70**, 12–20

Imsland, A.K., Foss, A., Folkvord, A. *et al.* (2005) The interrelation between temperature regimes and fish size in juvenile Atlantic cod (*Gadus morhua*): effects on growth and feed conversion efficiency. *Fish Physiology and Biochemistry*, **31**, 347–361

Inglis, V.B., Roberts, R.J. and Bromage, N.R. (1993) *Bacterial Diseases of Fish*, 1st edn. Blackwell Publishing, Oxford

Ishimatsu, A., Kikkawa, T., Hayashi, M. *et al.* (2004) Effects of CO_2 on marine fish: larvae and adults. *Journal of Oceanography*, **60**, 731–741

Johansen, R., Needham, J.R., Colquhoun, D.J. *et al.* (2006) Guidelines for health and welfare monitoring of fish used in research. *Laboratory Animals*, **40**, 323–340

Johnston, G. (2002) *Arctic Charr Aquaculture*, 1st edn. Fishing News Books, Oxford

Jonsson, N., Jonsson, B. and Hansen, L.P. (1991) Energetic cost of spawning in male and female Atlantic salmon (*Salmo salar* L.). *Journal of Fish Biology*, **39**, 739–744

Kane, A.S., Salierno, J.D., Gipson, G.T. *et al.* (2004) A video-based movement analysis system to quantify behavioral stress responses of fish. *Water Research*, **38**, 3993–4001

Karlsen, Ø., Holm, J.C. and Kjesbu, O.S. (1995) Effects of periodic starvation on reproductive investment in first-time spawning Atlantic cod (*Gadus morhua*). *Aquaculture*, **133**, 159–170

Kestemont, P., Jourdan, S., Houbart, M. *et al.* (2003) Size heterogeneity, cannibalism and competition in culture predatory fish larvae: biotic and abiotic influences. *Aquaculture*, **227**, 333–356

Kihslinger, R.L. and Nevitt, G.A. (2006) Early rearing environment impacts cerebellar growth in juvenile salmon. *The Journal of Experimental Biology*, **209**, 504–509

Kimmel, C.B., Ballard, W.W., Kimmel, S.R. *et al.* (1995) Stages of embryonic development of the zebrafish. *Developmental Dynamics*, **203**, 253–310

Kottelat, M., Britz, R., Hui, T.H. *et al.* (2006) *Paedocypris*, a new genus of Southeast Asian cyprinid fish with a remarkable sexual dimorphism, comprises the worlds smallest vertebrate. *Proceedings of the Royal Society B – Biological Sciences*, **273**, 895–899

Laine, P. and Rajasilta, M. (1999) The hatching success of Baltic herring eggs and its relation to female condition. *Journal of Experimental Marine Biology and Ecology*, **237**, 61–73

Landau, M. (1992) *Introduction to Aquaculture*, 1st edn. John Wiley & Sons, New York

Lankford, S.E., Adams, B.M., Adams, T.E. *et al.* (2006) Using specific antisera to neutralize ACTH in sturgeon: a method for manipulating the interrenal response during stress. *General and Comparative Endocrinology*, **147**, 384–390

Lawrence, C. (2007) The husbandry of zebrafish (*Danio rerio*): a review. *Aquaculture*, **269**, 1–20

Lester, N.P., Shuter, B.J. and Abrams, P.A. (2004) Interpreting the von Bertalanffy model of somatic growth in fishes: the cost of reproduction. *Proceedings of the Royal Society of London B – Biological Sciences*, **271**, 1625–1631

Lines, J. and Kestin, S. (2005) Electric stunning of trout: power reduction using a two-stage stun. *Aquacultural Engineering*, **32**, 483–491

MacIntyre, C., Ellis, T., North, B.P. *et al.* (2008) The influences of water quality on the welfare of farmed trout: a review. In: *Fish Welfare*, 1st edn. Ed. Branson, E., pp. 150–178. Blackwell Publishing, Oxford

MacKenzie, S., Ribas, L., Pilarczyk, M. *et al.* (2009) Screening for coping style increases the power of gene expression studies. *PLoSONE* 4, **e5314**, 1–5

Magurran, A.E., Seghers, B.H., Shaw, P.W. *et al.* (1995) The behavioural diversity and evolution of guppy, *Poecilia reticulata*, populations in Trinidad. *Advances in the Study of Behavior*, **24**, 155–202

Marino, G., Panini, E., Longobardi, A. *et al.* (2003) Induction of ovulation in captive-reared dusky grouper, *Epinephelus marginatus* (Lowe, 1834), with a sustained-release GnRHa implant. *Aquaculture*, **219**, 841–858

Mazeaud, M.M., Mazeaud, F. and Donaldson, E.M. (1977) Primary and secondary effects of stress in fish: some new data with a general review. *Transaction of the American Fisheries Society*, **106**, 201–212

McLarney, W. (1998) *Freshwater Aquaculture: A Handbook for Small Scale Fish Culture in North America*, 2nd edn. Hartley and Marks Publishers Inc, Vancouver, British Columbia

Metcalfe, N.B. (1994) The role of behaviour in determining salmon growth and development. *Aquaculture Research*, **25**, 67–76

Mills, D., Sands, D. and Scott, P.W. (1999) *Guide to Tropical Aquarium Fishes*, 1st edn. Interpet Publishing, Surrey

Nelson, J.S. (2006) *Fishes of the World*, 4th edn. John Wiley & Sons, London

Norberg, B., Brown, C.L., Halldorsson, O. *et al.* (2004) Photoperiod regulates the timing of sexual maturation, spawning, sex steroid and thyroid hormone profiles in the Atlantic cod (*Gadus morhua*). *Aquaculture*, **229**, 451–467

Okuda, N. (2001) The costs of reproduction to males and females of a paternal mouthbrooding cardinalfish *Apogon notatus*. *Journal of Fish Biology*, **58**, 776–787

Oliveira, R.F., McGregor, P.K. and Latruffe, C. (1998) Know thine enemy: fighting fish gather information from observing conspecific interactions. *Proceedings of the Royal Society of London Series B – Biological Sciences*, **265**, 1045–1049

Olsen, E.M., Knutsen, H., Gjøsæter, J. *et al.* (2004) Life-history variation among local populations of Atlantic cod from the Norwegian Skagerrak coast. *Journal of Fish Biology*, **64**, 1725–1730

Olsen, E.M. and Vøllestad, L.A. (2001) An evaluation of visible implant elastomer for marking age-0 brown trout. *North American Journal of Fisheries Management*, **21**, 967–970

Ostrander, G.K. (2000) *The Laboratory Fish*, 1st edn. Academic Press, London

Pickering, A.D. (1992) *Stress and Fish*, 1st edn. Academic Press, London

Pickering, A.D., Pottinger, T.G. and Christie, P. (1982) Recovery of brown trout, *Salmo trutta* L., from acute handling stress: a time course study. *Journal of Fish Biology*, **20**, 229–244

Piferrer, F., Beaumont, A., Falguière, J-C. *et al.* (2009) Polyploid fish and shellfish: Production, biology and applications to aquaculture for performance improvement and genetic containment. *Aquaculture*, **293**, 125–156

Pillay, T.V.R. and Kutty, M.N. (2005) *Aquaculture: Principles and Practises*, 2nd edn. Blackwell Publishing, Oxford

Pottinger, T.G. and Calder, G.M. (1995). Physiological stress in fish during toxicological procedures: a potentially confounding factor. *Environmental Toxicology and Water Quality*, **10**, 135–146

Potts, G.W. (1999a) Introduction to fish. In: *The UFAW Handbook on the Care and Management of Laboratory Animals, Volume 2: Amphibious and Aquatic Vertebrates and Advanced Invertebrates*, 7th edn. Ed. Poole, T., pp. 25–35. Blackwell Publishing, Oxford

Potts, G.W. (1999b) Marine fish. In: *The UFAW Handbook on the Care and Management of Laboratory Animals, Volume 2: Amphibious and Aquatic Vertebrates and Advanced Invertebrates*, 7th edn. Ed. Poole, T., pp. 68–89. Blackwell Publishing, Oxford

Potts, G.W., Aiken, A. and Andrews, C. (1999) Life support systems for aquatic research centres. In: *The UFAW Handbook on the Care and Management of Laboratory Animals, Volume 2: Amphibious and Aquatic Vertebrates and Advanced Invertebrates*, 7th edn. Ed. Poole, T., pp. 5–21. Blackwell Publishing, Oxford

Puvenandran, V., Laurel, B.J. and Brown, J.A. (2008) Cannibalism of Atlantic cod *Gadus morhua* larvae and juveniles on first-week larvae. *Aquatic Biology*, **2**, 113–118

Randall, D.J., Wood, C.M., Perry, S.F. *et al.* (1989) Urea excretion as a strategy for survival in a fish living in a very alkaline environment. *Nature*, **337**, 165–166

Robb, D.F.H. and Kestin, S.C. (2002) Methods used to kill fish: field observations and literature reviewed. *Animal Welfare*, **11**, 269–282

Roberts, R.J. (2001) *Fish Pathology*, 3rd edn. W.B. Saunders, Philadelphia

Rose, J.D. (2002) The neurobehavioural nature of fishes and the question of awareness and pain. *Reviews in Fisheries Science*, **10**, 1–38

Rose, J.D. (2007) Anthropomorphism and mental welfare of fishes. *Diseases of Aquatic Organisms*, **75**, 139–154

Ross, L.G. and Ross, B. (2008) *Anaesthetic and Sedative Techniques for Aquatic Animals*, 3rd edn. Blackwell Publishing, Oxford

Ross, A.J., Yasutake, W.T. and Leek, S. (1975) *Phoma herbarum*, a fungal plant saprophyte, as a fish pathogen. *Journal of the Fisheries Research Board of Canada*, **32**, 1648–1652

Ruiz-Gomez, M. de L., Kittilsen, S., Höglund, E. *et al.* (2008) Behavioural plasticity in rainbow trout (*Oncorhynchus mykiss*) with divergent coping styles: When doves become hawks. *Hormones and Behavior*, **54**, 534–538

Saillant, E., Chatain, B., Fostier, A. *et al.* (2001) Parental influence on early development in the European sea bass. *Journal of Fish Biology*, **58**, 1585–1600

Sarder, M.R.I., Penman, D.J., Myers, J.M. *et al.* (1999) Production and propagation of fully inbred clonal lines in the Nile tilapia (*Oreochromis niloticus* L.). *The Journal of Experimental Zoology*, **284**, 675–685

Sayer, M.D.J., Treasurer, J.W. and Costello, M.J. (1996) *Wrasse: Biology and Use in Aquaculture*, 1st edn. Fishing News Books, Oxford

Scott, P.W. (1997) *The Complete Aquarium*, 1st edn. Dorling Kindersley Publishers Ltd, London

Shepherd, J. and Bromage, N. (1992) *Intensive Fish Farming*, 1st edn. Blackwell Publishing, Oxford

Shinn, A.P., Wootten, R., Côté, I. *et al.* (2003) The efficacy of selected bath and oral chemotherapeutants against *Ichthyophthirius multifiliis* Fouquet, 1876 (Ciliophora: Ophyroglenidae) infecting rainbow trout (*Oncorhynchus mykiss* Walbaum). *Diseases of Aquatic Organisms*, **55**, 17–22

Skarstein, F., Folstad, I. and Liljedal, S. (2001) Whether to reproduce or not: immune suppression and costs of parasites during reproduction in the Arctic charr. *Canadian Journal of Zoology*, **79**, 271–278

Sloman, K.A., Taylor, A.C., Metcalfe, N.B. *et al.* (2001) Stress from air emersion fails to alter chloride cell numbers in the gills of rainbow trout. *Journal of Fish Biology*, **59**, 186–190

Sneddon, L.U., Braithwaite, V.A. and Gentle, M.J. (2003) Do fishes have nociceptors? Evidence for the evolution of a vertebrate sensory system. *Proceedings of the Royal Society of London B – Biological Sciences*, **270**, 1115–1121

Sommerset, I., Krossøy, B., Biering, E. *et al.* (2005) Vaccines for fish in aquaculture. *Expert Reviews*, **4**, 89–101

Spence, R., Fatema, M.K., Reichard, M. *et al.* (2006) The distribution and habitat preferences of the zebrafish in Bangladesh. *Journal of Fish Biology*, **69**, 1435–1448

Spence, R., Gerlach, G., Lawrence, C. *et al.* (2008) The behaviour and ecology of the zebrafish, *Danio rerio*. *Biological Reviews*, **83**, 13–34

Stickney, R.R. (1993a) Channel catfish. In: *Culture of Nonsalmonid Freshwater Fishes*, 2nd edn. Ed. Stickney, R.R., pp. 33–79. CRC Press, Boca Raton

Stickney, R.R. (1993b) Tilapia. In: *Culture of Nonsalmonid Freshwater Fishes*, 2nd edn. Ed. Stickney, R.R., pp. 81–115. CRC Press, Boca Raton

Stien, L.H., Bratland, S., Austevoll, I. *et al.* (2007) A video analysis procedure for assessing vertical fish distribution in aquaculture tanks. *Aquacultural Engineering*, **37**, 115–124

Suzuki, Y., Otaka, T., Sato, S. *et al.* (1997) Reproduction related immunoglobulin changes in rainbow trout. *Fish Physiology and Biochemistry*, **17**, 415–421

Turnbull, J.F., North, B.P., Ellis, T. *et al.* (2008) Stocking density and the welfare of farmed salmonids. In: *Fish Welfare*, 1st edn. Ed. Branson, E., pp. 111–118. Blackwell Publishing, Oxford

van de Vis, H. and Kestin, S. (2003) Is humane slaughter of fish possible for industry? *Aquaculture Research*, **34**, 211–220

Vermeirssen, E.L.M., Mazorra de Quero, C., Shields, R.J. *et al.* (2004) Fertility and motility of sperm from Atlantic halibut (*Hippoglossus hippoglossus*) in relation to dose and timing of gonadotrophin-releasing hormone agonist implant. *Aquaculture*, **230**, 547–567

Vihtelic, T.S., Soverly, J.E., Kassen S.C. *et al.* (2006) Retinal regional differences in photoreceptor cell death and regeneration in light-lesioned albino zebrafish. *Experimental Eye Research*, **82**, 558–575

Wallace, J. (1993) Environmental considerations. In: *Salmon Aquaculture*, 1st edn. Eds Heen K., Monahan, R.L. and Utter, F., pp. 127–143. Fishing News Books, Oxford

Wedemeyer, G.A. (1996) *Physiology of Fish in Intensive Aquaculture*, 1st edn. Chapman and Hall, London

Wendelaar Bonga, S.E. (1997) The stress response in fish. *Physiological Reviews*, **77**, 591–625

Westerfield, M. (2000) *The Zebrafish Book. A Guide for the Laboratory Use of Zebrafish (Danio rerio)*, 4th edn. University of Oregon Press, Eugene

Williams, T.D., Readman, G.D. and Owen, S.F. (2009) Key issues concerning environmental enrichment for laboratory-held fish species. *Laboratory Animals*, **43**, 107–120

Wooster, G.A. and Bowse, P.R. (1996) The aerobiological pathway of a fish pathogen: survival and dissemination of *Aeromonas salmonicida* in aerosols and its implications in fish health management. *Journal of the World Aquaculture Society*, **27**, 7–14

Zohar, Y. and Mylonas, C.C. (2001) Endocrine manipulations of spawning in cultured fish: from hormones to genes. *Aquaculture*, **197**, 99–136

Cephalopoda

50 Cephalopoda

Bernd U. Budelmann

Note: This short chapter has not been written to stand on its own. It is an update of Peter Boyle's Chapter 7 in the 7th edition of the UFAW Handbook, which was published in 1999 and is reprinted after this update. Consequently, for details and earlier references the reader should consult that chapter as the authoritative text. In addition, some key literature on cephalopods published earlier (but not mentioned in that chapter) has been added. For an easy follow-up and comparison, the updates given below use (sub)headings similar to those of the earlier chapter. This chapter update is dedicated to the memory of Peter Boyle.

Introduction

Cephalopods are the only invertebrate animal group included in this edition of the Handbook, however information on decapod crustaceans is available in the 7th edition of the Handbook. Invertebrates are not generally protected in animal welfare legislation, although certain species are included in some national legislation (eg, UK, New Zealand & Australian Capital Territories, and some Scandinavian countries). The UK, at the time of writing, includes one species, *Octopus vulgaris,* in its legislation on the use of animals in research. However, there is debate within Europe (unresolved at the time of writing) as to whether some, all or no cephalopods (as well as decapod crustacea) should be included in a new European Directive on research using animals (see also Chapter 8 on legislation).

Cephalopods belong to the phylum Mollusca and thus are close relatives to gastropods and bivalves. Although the cephalopod body design conserved some typical molluscan features, it developed a level of complexity, and especially a sophisticated nervous system and sense organs, that in several aspects reach vertebrate standards (Budelmann 1995). The cephalopod nervous system is certainly the most advanced of any invertebrate nervous system and this complexity correlates well with the animals' (in general) very active, fast moving predatory life styles and sophisticated behaviours (Bullock and Horridge 1965; Budelmann 1995; Hanlon & Messenger 1996). Not surprisingly then, beginning in the 1930s with J.Z. Young's rediscovery of the giant axon and the subsequent early understanding of the processes involved in nerve impulse conduction and transmission (Adelman & Gilbert 1990), cephalopods have become fascinating and valuable invertebrate model systems for comparative vertebrate research. However, in such comparisons a number of limitations apply (see below, nervous system). It is important that these limitations should be understood because of the recent increased interest in this animal group from media and laymen that is sometimes combined with a tendency for 'over-interpretation' of the fascinating behaviours that cephalopods show.

The class Cephalopoda comprises two sub-classes: Nautiloidea (*Nautilus*) and Coleoidea (octopuses, cuttlefish and squids). The latter two are often referred to as 'decapods' but care should be taken as this term is also commonly used for the order of crustaceans that includes crabs, lobsters, prawns, etc). Nautiloids and coleoids show significant differences with regard to their anatomy, physiology and behaviour (for example, nautiluses have a much less sophisticated nervous system and sensory outfit; they show no colour change and have a much simpler behavioural repertoire; and they are scavengers and thus seem to have a well developed chemosensory system for food detection). These differences between nautiloids and coleoids, however, unfortunately are often not considered in the literature when the term 'cephalopod(s)' is applied. The term as used often refers to the coleoid cephalopods only (that is, to the octopuses, cuttlefish and squids) and, therefore, great care must be taken in the use, interpretation and generalisation of the 'cephalopod' data described.

Cephalopod biology

A number of comprehensive monographs has become available that cover almost all aspects of cephalopod biology, from palaeobiology (Landman *et al.* 1996, 2007), evolution, systematics, identification, and biogeography (Clarke 1986; Guerra 1992; Sweeney *et al.* 1992; Payne *et al.* 1998; Voss *et al.* 1998; Norman 2000; Capua 2004; Jereb & Roper 2005), to gross and microscopic anatomy (Mangold 1989; Budelmann *et al.* 1997; Nixon & Young 2003), physiology (Abbott *et al.* 1995), ecology, fisheries and culture (Boucaud-Camou 1991; Boyle & Rodhouse 2005; Chotiyaputta *et al.* 2005), age determination (Jereb *et al.* 1991), behaviour (Hanlon & Messenger 1996; Nixon & Young 2003; Borelli & Fiorito 2008) and diseases (Hanlon & Forsythe 1990; Hochberg 1990). Some more recent data are summarised below.

Habitat and distribution

An excellent monograph is now available on many aspects of cephalopod ecology and fisheries, including: cephalopod biodiversity and zoogeography; life cycle, growth and reproduction; population ecology; cephalopods as prey and predators; fishing methods and scientific sampling; fishery resources; fisheries oceanography; and assessment and management (Boyle & Rodhouse 2005).

Locomotion

The cephalopod musculature lacks a skeletal support system and, instead, operates on the principle of a muscular hydrostat, similar to the 'mechanism' of an elephant trunk or the human tongue (Kier & Smith 1985; Smith & Kier 1989). This allows cephalopod (specifically octopod) arms a great range of movement. Over the past more than 10 years, significant progress has been made in understanding the nervous control of cephalopod arm movements; this ultimately could inspire completely new strategies for the control of highly flexible robotic arms (Gutfreund *et al.* 1996, 1998; Matzner *et al.* 2000; Sumbre *et al.* 2001, 2005; Walker *et al.* 2005; Yekuteli *et al.* 2005a, 2005b, 2007).

Shell and buoyancy

The neutral buoyancy of many squids is achieved by storing ammonia in body tissue. The various mechanisms for storage (in coelomic cavities, vacuoles, or gelatinous outer layers) have been reviewed in support for the argument that ammoniacal squids have evolved as a polyphyletic animal group (Voight *et al.* 1994).

Respiration and circulation

Water temperature, pH and oxygen supply are critical factors in cephalopod culture and breeding. Recently, the cuttlefish (*Sepia officinalis*) has served as a valuable model system for understanding the mechanisms of thermal tolerance in ectothermic animals (Melzner *et al.* 2006, 2007).

Nervous system

The cephalopod nervous system is the most highly evolved of all invertebrate nervous systems. On the other hand and despite that level of complexity, the overall organisation of its central part (the brain) is fundamentally different from that of the vertebrate nervous system and, therefore, any direct comparison between the two has serious limitations. This, however, neither excludes careful comparison of basic brain functions, nor weakens the great value of the cephalopod nervous system in comparative research. Details of the anatomy of the cephalopod central nervous system are available for *Nautilus* (Young 1965), *Octopus* (Young 1971; Budelmann & Young 1985; Plän 1987) and *Loligo* (Young 1974, 1976, 1977, 1979; Messenger 1979; Budelmann & Young 1987); recent overviews are given in Budelmann (1995), Budelmann *et al.* (1997), Nixon and Young (2003) and Williamson and Chrachri (2004).

In addition to their highest level of complexity, cephalopod brains are also the largest of all the invertebrate brains; their brain:body weight ratio exceeds that of many fishes and reptiles (Packard 1972). This is not too surprising, however, since cephalopods lack an internal skeleton and lack joints, and thus lack a 'simple' antagonistic muscle control of movements. Consequently, about half of the volume of the brain of coleoid cephalopods consists of the relatively large motoneurons that form the sub-oesophageal mass of the brain; this area includes the motoneurons that expand all the chromatophore organs in the skin (for a summary of the numbers of nerve cells in the various parts of the *Octopus* brain, see Budelmann 1995). On the other hand, the comparatively large size and complexity of the brains of octopuses, cuttlefish and squids are the basis for the animals' large repertoire of fascinating behaviours, including various forms of learning and short- and long-term memory (Hanlon & Messenger 1996; Hochner *et al.* 2003; Borelli & Fiorito 2008). Ultimately, these make coleoid cephalopods, especially shallow-water octopods, cuttlefish and squids, the only invertebrate species with which humans can directly interact ('communicate') in a back and forth manner and beyond a simple reflex-like (re)action on the animals' side.

Octopuses, cuttlefish and squids are often considered the most 'intelligent' invertebrate species (whichever way intelligence is defined). The web-based Wikipedia summarises this issue quite well:

> *Cephalopod intelligence has an important comparative aspect in our understanding of intelligence, because it relies on a nervous system fundamentally different from that of vertebrates. ... The scope of cephalopod intelligence is controversial ... Classical conditioning of cephalopods has been reported, and one study (Fiorito and Scotto 1992) even concluded that octopuses practice observational learning. However, the latter idea is strongly disputed, and doubt has been shed on some other reported capabilities as well. In any case, impressive spatial learning capacity, navigational abilities, and predatory techniques remain beyond question.*

Other impressive behaviours that can be added to this list are cephalopod mating and social behaviours, including social recognition (Hanlon & Messenger 1996; Boal *et al.* 2000; Dickel *et al.* 2000; Karson *et al.* 2003; Boal 2006; Alves *et al.* 2008; Borelli & Fiorito 2008).

Powerful techniques have now successfully been applied to cephalopod brains to the study of their anatomy and function (Budelmann *et al.* 1995): three-dimensional magnetic resonance imaging of brain pathways (Quast *et al.* 2001) and individual neurons (Gozansky *et al.* 2003); brain slice recordings (Williamson & Budelmann 1991); recordings from intact animals with implanted electrodes (Bullock & Budelmann 1991); and mapping of metabolic brain activity (Novicki *et al.* 1992). With these modern neurophysiological techniques cephalopods have become an increasingly valuable invertebrate model system for comparative vertebrate research, such as the evolution of learning and memory and other higher brain functions (Hochner *et al.* 2006). Recently, laterality in the brain (Byrne *et al.* 2002, 2004, 2006), play behaviour (Kuba *et al.* 2006), personality (Sinn & Moltschaniwskyj 2005), sleep (Brown *et al.* 2006) and complex phenomena, such as consciousness and suffering in cephalopods, have been discussed (Mather 2001, 2008).

Sense organs

Cephalopods have a sophisticated sensory outfit that includes all major sense organs, such as photoreceptors (including extra-ocular photoreceptors), distance and contact chemoreceptors, and various mechanoreceptors (including equilibrium receptor organs, a lateral line analogue system and a neck proprioceptive organ) (Budelmann 1996). Knowledge about touch, pressure and muscle proprioceptors is limited, and it still remains to be seen whether cephalopods have electroreceptors and are sensitive to pain. For a comprehensive summary on cephalopod sense organs, see Budelmann *et al.* (1997).

Eyes and vision

The cephalopod and vertebrate lens eyes are a textbook example of analogy (convergent evolution) between an invertebrate and a vertebrate sensory system. Recent advances have been made in understanding visual processing (Chrachri & Williamson 2003, 2004, 2005; Chrachri *et al.* 2005; Douglas *et al.* 2005), and the role of polarised vision (Saidel *et al.* 1983; Shashar *et al.* 1998, 2002; Boal *et al.* 2004; Saidel *et al.* 2005; Mäthger & Hanlon 2006). In addition, in the squid *Lolliguncula* a dorsal light reflex has been described (Preuss & Budelmann 1995a) and in cuttlefish a countershading reflex (Ferguson *et al.* 1994).

Equilibrium receptor organs

A tremendous body of data has accumulated over the past 40 years on the anatomy, ultrastructure and physiology of the cephalopod equilibrium receptor organs (statocysts), which include sophisticated receptor systems for the detection of linear (gravity) and angular accelerations (Budelmann *et al.* 1987; for summaries, see Budelmann 1990; Budelmann *et al.* 1997; for the *Nautilus* statocyst, see Neumeister & Budelmann 1997). Special emphasis has been paid to the similarities between the structure and function of the cephalopod and vertebrate hair cells (eg, Budelmann & Williamson 1994; Budelmann 2000), including their ion channels and efferent innervation (Williamson 1995) and transmitter and transmitter-like substances; the latter include nitric oxide (Tu & Budelmann 2000) and cannabinoids (Tu & Budelmann, unpublished). Cephalopod statocysts are known to drive a sophisticated control system for compensatory eye movements; part of its central organisation resembles that of the vertebrate vestibulo-oculomotor reflex pathway and involves four (*Nautilus*), seven (octopods), or 13–14 (cuttlefish and squids) extra-ocular eye muscles (Budelmann & Young 1984, 1993; Neumeister & Budelmann 1997).

Epidermal lines

The epidermal lines (formerly known as 'Drüsenlinien') that occur on the head and arms of at least some of the coleoid species are analogous to the fish and aquatic amphibian lateral line systems (Budelmann & Bleckmann 1988; Budelmann *et al.* 1997).

Neck proprioceptive organ

Similar to the vertebrate neck muscle proprioceptors, cuttlefish and squid have groups of epidermal hair cells on their neck that serve as a proprioceptive neck organ for the control of the position of the head relative to the body (Preuss & Budelmann 1995b).

Vibration receptors and hearing

Cephalopods are sensitive to vibrational stimuli via statocyst receptors and sense local water movements with their lateral line analogue system (Budelmann & Bleckmann 1988; Williamson 1988; Packard *et al.* 1990; Bleckmann *et al.* 1991; Komak *et al.* 2005). On the other hand, there is much confusion regarding cephalopods ability to 'hear'. Ultimately, this is a semantic issue since the answer depends on the definition of underwater sound and underwater hearing (Budelmann 1992). In conventional terms, cephalopods cannot hear because they do not have a receptor system that is specialised for the detection of the pressure wave of underwater sound.

Maintenance, culture and laboratory procedures

With the growing interest in cephalopods for research and commercial mariculture, as well as their popularity in public and private displays, knowledge about the maintenance, culture and proper laboratory procedures is of increased importance (Oestmann *et al.* 1997; Sykes *et al.* 2006; Dunlop & King 2008). For advice on optimising the survival of hatchling cuttlefish and squid, see Forsythe *et al.* (1994), Vidal *et al.* (2002a, 2002b) and Sykes *et al.* (2003). With regard to culture density, recent cuttlefish data show that lower stocking density results in better growth (Domingues *et al.* 2003; Correia *et al.* 2005), as does higher water temperature (25°C compared to 17°C; Forsythe *et al.* 2002). On the other hand, lower temperature (15°C compared to 27°C) extends the life cycle (Domingues *et al.* 2002). For the development of memory in cuttlefish, an enriched environment is crucial during their second and/or third months of life (Dickel *et al.* 2000). Crowding of adult cuttlefish should be avoided since it stimulates aggression (Boal *et al.* 1999).

Not surprisingly, the quality and composition of food has been proven to be critical for good growth and survival. Adult cuttlefish show much better growth rates when fed with live or thawed natural prey than when fed with an artificial diet (Domingues *et al.* 2005). Shrimp-based food pellets, although less palatable, produce maintenance growth, whereas a highly palatable fish-based surimi diet (mimicking the meat of lobster, crab and other shellfish) results in poor survival (Castro *et al.* 1993). When fed with live mysid shrimp, grass shrimp, or fish fry, young cuttlefish showed best growth during the first week after hatching when fed with mysid shrimp, and thereafter when fed with grass shrimp; cuttlefish fed with fish fry showed lowest growth rates at all times (Domingues *et al.* 2004). When prey is maintained for feeding juvenile cuttlefish, prey starvation should be avoided (Correia *et al.* 2009). Although *Sepia* shows an innate food preference, early familiarisation with other food can override this preference (Darmaillacq *et al.* 2006). For the importance of certain elements (including copper and strontium) in the food of octopus, cuttlefish and squid, see Koueta *et al.* (2002) Villanueva and Bustamente (2006) and Iglesias *et al.* (2007).

A comprehensive monograph is now available on invertebrate medicine that includes a chapter on cephalopods (Lewbart 2006) and ethical and welfare considerations for working with cephalopods have recently been summarised (Mather & Anderson 2007; Moltschaniwskyj *et al.* 2007).

Occupational health hazards

Many octopus and, particularly, cuttlefish and squid species may bite, specifically when stressed, disturbed or improperly handled. Their sharp, parrot-like beaks can inflict significant wounds and the saliva can have a variety of toxic effects. The tetrodotoxin-like venom of the Australian blue-ringed octopod (*Hapalochlaena maculosa*) can be lethal to humans (Williamson *et al.* 1996, for a review).

Cannibalism

Cannibalism is well known in octopuses, cuttlefish and squids when held in captivity. Obvious reasons include a too high stocking density and an inadequate amount of food and shelter. Specifically, when food supply is limited and feeding *ad libitum* becomes a problem, larger animals may prey upon smaller ones when kept is the same tank. In addition, sexual cannibalism has been described in an octopus species on a coral reef (Hanlon & Forsythe 2008).

Autophagy

Some data (other than anecdotal) are now available on autophagy (self eating) in *Octopus vulgaris.* They suggest that it is caused by either a substance that is released by the animals themselves or, more likely, by viruses or bacteria; stress may contribute to this behaviour but does not seem to be its primary cause (Budelmann 1998).

Further information and reading

A large number of references to the literature on cephalopods are available from the library service of the Smithsonian Institution Research Information System at http://sirismm.si.edu/siris/siris-cephalopod.htm.

The following web pages provide very useful information regarding all major aspects of cephalopod biology, supply and maintenance, rearing, culture and breeding and laboratory procedures (with regard to the scientific accuracy, however, general caution must be taken because of its lack of peer review):

Tree of Life – Cephalopods: http://tolweb.org/cephalopoda
Association of Zoos & Aquariums: http://www.aza.org
The Cephalopod Page: http://www.thecephalopodpage.org
The National Resource Center for Cephalopods: http://www.cephalopod.org
Cephbase: http://www.cephbase.com
The Octopus News Magazine Online: http://www.tonmo.com

References

Abbott, N.J., Williamson, R. and Maddock, L. (Eds) (1995) *Cephalopod Neurobiology.* Oxford University Press, Oxford

Adelman, W.J. and Gilbert, D.L. (1990) Electrophysiology and biophysiscs of the squid giant axon. In: *Squid as Experimental Animals.* Eds Gilbert, D., Adelman, H. and Arnold, J., pp. 93–132. Plenum Press, New York

Alves, C., Boal, J.G. and Dickel, L. (2008) Short distance navigation in cephalopods: a review. *Cognitive Processing*, **9**, 239–247

Bleckmann, H., Budelmann, B.U. and Bullock, T.H. (1991) Peripheral and central nervous responses evoked by small water movements in a cephalopod. *Journal of Comparative Physiology A*, **168**, 247–257

Boal, J.G. (2006) Social recognition: a top down view of cephalopod behavior. *Vie et Milieu*, **56**, 69–79

Boal, J.G., Hylton, R.A., Gonzalez, S.A. *et al.* (1999) Effects of crowding on the social behavior of cuttlefish (*Sepia officinalis*). *Contemporary Topics in Laboratory Animal Science*, **38**, 49–55

Boal, J.G., Dunham, A., Williams, K. *et al.* (2000) Experimental evidence for spatial learning in octopuses. *Journal of Comparative Psychology*, **114**, 246–252

Boal, J.G., Shashar, N., Grable, M. *et al.* (2004) Behavioral evidence for intraspecific signals with achromatic and polarized light by cuttlefish (*Mollusca: Cephalopoda*). *Behaviour*, **141**, 837–861

Borelli, L. and Fiorito, G. (2008) Behavioral analysis of learning and memory in cephalopods. In: *Learning and Memory: A Comprehensive Reference* (Ed. Byrne, J.H.), Vol. I. Ed. Menzel, R., pp. 605–627. Elsevier, Amsterdam

Boucaud-Camou, E. (Ed.) (1991) *The Cuttlefish.* Centre de Publications de l'Université de Caen, Caen

Boyle, P. and Rodhouse, P. (2005) *Cephalopods: Ecology and Fisheries.* Blackwell Publishing, Oxford

Brown, E.R., Piscopo, S., De Stefano, R. *et al.* (2006) Brain and behavioural evidence for rest-activity cycles in *Octopus vulgaris. Behavioural Brain Research*, **172**, 355–359

Budelmann, B.U. (1990) The statocysts of squid. In: *Squid as Experimental Animals.* Eds Gilbert, D., Adelman, H. and Arnold, J., pp. 421–439. Plenum Press, New York

Budelmann, B.U. (1992) Hearing in non-arthropod invertebrates. In: *The Evolutionary Biology of Hearing.* Eds Webster, B., Fay, R.R. and Popper, A.N., pp. 141–155. Springer, New York

Budelmann, B.U. (1995) The cephalopod nervous system: What evolution has made of the molluscan design. In: *The Nervous System of Invertebrates: An Evolutionary and Comparative Approach.* Eds Breidbach, O. and Kutsch, W., pp. 115–138. Birkhäuser Verlag, Basel

Budelmann, B.U. (1996) Active marine predators: The sensory world of cephalopods. *Marine and Freshwater Behavior and Physiology*, **27**, 59–75

Budelmann, B.U. (1998) Autophagy in *Octopus. South African Journal of Marine Science*, **20**, 101–108

Budelmann, B.U. (2000) Kinociliary mechanoreceptors in the equilibrium receptor organs of cephalopods. In: *Cell and Molecular Biology of the Ear*. Ed. Lim, D.J., pp. 3–17. Kluwer/Plenum Press, New York

Budelmann, B.U. and Bleckmann, H. (1988) A lateral line analogue in cephalopods: water waves generate microphonic potentials in the epidermal head lines of *Sepia* and *Lolliguncula*. *Journal of Comparative Physiology A*, **164**, 1–5

Budelmann, B.U. and Williamson, R. (1994) Directional sensitivity of hair cell afferents in the *Octopus* statocyst. *Journal of Experimental Biology*, **187**, 245–259

Budelmann, B.U. and Young, J.Z. (1984) The statocyst-oculomotor system of *Octopus vulgaris*: Eye muscles, eye muscle nerves, statocyst nerves, and the oculomotor centre in the central nervous system. *Philosophical Transactions of the Royal Society London B*, **306**, 159–189

Budelmann, B.U. and Young, J.Z. (1985) Central pathways of the nerves of the arms and mantle of *Octopus*. *Philosophical Transactions of the Royal Society London B*, **310**, 109–122

Budelmann, B.U. and Young, J.Z. (1987) Brain pathways of the brachial nerves of *Sepia* and *Loligo*. *Philosophical Transactions of the Royal Society London B*, **315**, 345–352

Budelmann, B.U. and Young, J.Z. (1993) The oculomotor system of decapod cephalopods: eye muscles, eye muscle nerves, and the oculomotor neurons in the central nervous system. *Philosophical Transactions of the Royal Society London B*, **340**, 93–125

Budelmann, B.U., Bullock, T.H. and Williamson, R. (1995) Cephalopod brains: promising preparations for brain physiology. In: *Cephalopod Neurobiology*. Eds Abbott, N.J., Williamson, R. and Maddock, L., pp. 399–413. Oxford University Press, Oxford

Budelmann, B.U., Sachse, M. and Staudigl, M. (1987) The angular acceleration receptor system of *Octopus vulgaris*: morphometry, ultrastructure, and neuronal and synaptic organization. *Philosophical Transactions of the Royal Society London B*, **315**, 305–343

Budelmann, B.U., Schipp, R. and von Boletzky, S. (1997) Cephalopoda. In: *Microscopic Anatomy of Invertebrates, Vol. 6A, Mollusca II*, Eds Harrison, F.W. and Kohn, A., pp. 119–414. Wiley-Liss, New York

Bullock, T.H. and Budelmann, B.U. (1991) Sensory evoked potentials in unanesthetized unrestrained cuttlefish: a new preparation for brain physiology in cephalopods. *Journal of Comparative Physiology A*, **168**, 141–150

Bullock, T.H. and Horridge, G.A. (1965) *Structure and Function of the Nervous Systems of Invertebrates*. Freeman, San Francisco

Byrne, R.A., Kuba, M.J. and Griebel, U. (2002) Lateral asymmetyry of eye use in *Octopus vulgaris*. *Animal Behaviour*, **64**, 461–468

Byrne, R.A., Kuba, M.J. and Meisel, D.V. (2004) Lateralized eye use in *Octopus vulgaris* shows antisymmetrical distribution. *Animal Behaviour*, **68**, 1107–1114

Byrne, R.A., Kuba, M., Meisel, D.V. *et al.* (2006) Does *Octopus vulgaris* have preferred arms? *Journal of Comparative Psychology*, **120**, 198–204

Castro, B.G., DiMarco, F.P., DeRusha, R.H. *et al.* (1993) The effects of surimi and pelleted diets on the laboratory survival, growth and feeding rate of the cuttlefish *Sepia officinalis* L. *Journal of Experimental Marine Biology and Ecology*, **170**, 241–252

Capua, D. (2004) *I Cefalopodi dell coste e dell 'arcipelago Toscano: Systematica, anatomia, fisiologia e sfruttamento delle specie presenti nel Mediterraneo*. ConchBooks, Hackenheim

Chotiyaputta, C., Hatfield, E.M.C. and Lu, C.C. (eds) (2005) *Cephalopod Biology, Recruitment and Culture*. Phuket Marine Biological Center Research Bulletin No. 66, Phuket

Chrachri, A. and Williamson, R. (2003) Modulation of spontaneous and evoked EPSCs and IPSCs in in optic lobe neurons of cuttlefish *Sepia officinalis* by the neuropeptide FMRF-amide. *European Journal of Neuroscience*, **17**, 1–11

Chrachri, A. and Williamson, R. (2004) Cholinergic and glutamatergic spontaneous and evoked excitatory postsynaptic currents in optic lobe neurons of cuttlefish, *Sepia officinalis*. *Brain Research*, **1020**, 178–187

Chrachri, A. and Williamson, R. (2005) Dopamin modulates synaptic activity in the optic lobes of cuttlefish, *Sepia officinalis*. *Neuroscience Letters*, **377**, 152–157

Chrachri, A., Nelson, L. and Williamson, R. (2005) Whole-cell recording of light-evoked photoreceptor responses in a slice preparation of the cuttlefish retina. *Visual Neuroscience*, **22**, 359–370

Clarke, M.R. (Ed.) (1986) *A Handbook for the Identification of Cephalopod Beaks*. Clarendon Press, Oxford

Correia, M., Domingues, P.M., Sykes, A. *et al.* (2005) Effects of culture density on growth and broodstock management of the cuttlefish, *Sepia officinalis* (Linnaeus, 1758). *Aquaculture*, **245**, 163–173.

Correia, M., Palma, J., Kirakowski, T. and Andrade J.P. (2009) Effects of prey nutritional quality on the growth and survival of juvenile cuttlefish, *Sepia officinalis* (Linnaeus, 1758). *Aquaculture Research*, **39**, 869–876

Darmaillacq, A.S., Chichery, R., Shashar, N. and Dickel, L. (2006) Early familiarization overrides innate prey preference in newly hatched *Sepia officinalis* cuttlefish. *Animal Behaviour*, **71**, 511–514

Dickel, L., Boal, J.G. and Budelmann, B.U. (2000) Effect of early experience on learning and memory in cuttlefish. *Developmental Psychobiology*, **36**, 101–110

Domingues, P.M., Sykes, A. and Andrade, J.P. (2002) The effects of temperature in the life cycle of two consecutive generations of the cuttlefish *Sepia officinalis* (Linnaeus, 1758), cultured in the Algarve (South Portugal). *Aquaculture International*, **10**, 207–220

Domingues, P., Poirier, R., Dickel, L. *et al.* (2003) Effects of culture density and live prey on growth and survival of juvenile cuttlefish, *Sepia officinalis*. *Aquaculture International*, **11**, 225–242

Domingues, P., Sykes, A., Sommerfield, A. *et al.* (2004) Growth and survival of cuttlefish (*Sepia officinalis*) of different ages fed crustaceans and fish. Effects of frozen and live prey. *Aquaculture*, **229**, 239–254

Domingues, P.M., DiMarco, F.P., Andrade, J.P. *et al.* (2005) Effect of artificial diets on growth, survival and condition of adult cuttlefish, *Sepia officinalis* Linnaeus, 1758. *Aquaculture International*, **13**, 423–440

Douglas, R.H., Williamson, R. and Wagner, H.J. (2005) The pupillary response of cephalopods. *Journal of Experimental Biology*, **208**, 261–265

Dunlop, C. and King, N. (2008) *Cephalopods: Octopuses and Cuttlefish for the Home Aquarium*. tfh Publications, Neptune City

Ferguson, G.P., Messenger, J.B. and Budelmann, B.U. (1994) Gravity and light influence the countershading reflexes of the cuttlefish *Sepia officinalis*. *Journal of Experimental Biology*, **191**, 247–256

Fiorito, G. and Scotto, P. (1992) Observational learning in *Octopus vulgaris*. *Science*, **256**, 545–547

Forsythe, J.W., DeRusha, R.H. and Hanlon, R.T. (1994) Growth, reproduction and life-span of *Sepia officinalis* (Cephalopoda, Mollusca) cultured through seven consecutive generations. *Journal of Zoology*, **233**, 175–192

Forsythe, J.W., Lee, P.G., Walsh, L.S. *et al.* (2002) The effects of crowding on growth of the European cuttlefish, *Sepia officinalis* Linnaeus, 1758 reared at two temperatures. *Journal of Experimental Marine Biology and Ecology*, **269**, 173–185

Gozansky, E.K., Ezell, E.L., Budelmann, B.U. *et al.* (2003) Magnetic resonance histology: in situ single cell imaging of receptor cells in an invertebrate (*Lolliguncula brevis*, Cephalopoda) sense organ. *Magnetic Resonance Imaging*, **21**, 1019–1022

Guerra, A. (1992) Mollusca, Cephalopoda. In: *Fauna Iberica*, Vol. **1**. Ed. Ramos, M.A., pp. 1–327. Museo Nacional de Ciencias Naturales CSIC, Madrid

Gutfreund, Y., Flash, T., Yarom, Y. *et al.* (1996) Organization of octopus arm movements: a model system for studying the control of flexible arms. *Journal of Neuroscience*, **16**, 7297–7307

Gutfreund, Y., Flash, T., Fiorito, G. *et al.* (1998) Patterns of arm muscle activation involved in octopus reaching movements. *Journal of Neuroscience*, **18**, 5976–5987

Hanlon, R.T. and Forsythe, J.W. (1990) Diseases of mollusca: cephalopoda. 1.1 Diseases caused by microorganisms. In: *Diseases of Marine Animals*, Vol. 3. Ed. Kinne, O., pp. 23–46. Biologische Anstalt Helgoland, Hamburg

Hanlon, R. and Forsythe, J. (2008) Sexual cannibalism by *Octopus cyanea* on a Pacific coral reef. *Marine and Freshwater Behavior and Physiology*, **41**, 19–28

Hanlon, R.T. and Messenger, J.B. (1996) *Cephalopod Behaviour*. Cambridge University Press, Cambridge

Hochberg, F.G. (1990) Diseases of mollusca: cephalopoda. 1.2 Diseases caused by protistans and metazoans. In: *Diseases of Marine Animals*, Vol. **3**. Ed. Kinne, O., pp. 47–227. Biologische Anstalt Helgoland, Hamburg

Hochner, B., Brown, E., Langella, M. *et al.* (2003) A learning and memory area in the *Octopus* brain manifests a vertebrate-like long-term potentiation. *Journal of Neurophysiology*, **90**, 3547–3554

Hochner, B., Shomrat, T. and Fiorito, G. (2006) The octopus: a model for a comparative analysis of the evolution of learning and memory. *Biological Bulletin*, **210**, 308–317

Iglesias, J., Sánchez, F.J., Bersano, J.G.F. *et al.* (2007) Rearing of *Octopus vulgaris* paralarvae: Present status, bottlenecks and trends. *Aquaculture*, **266**, 1–15

Jereb, P. and Roper, C.F.E. (Eds) (2005) *Cephalopods of the World, an Annotated and illustrated Catalogue of Cephalopod Species Known to Date*, Vol. 1. tfh Publicatios, Neptune City

Jereb, P., Ragonese, R. and von Boletzky, S. (1991) *Squid Age Determination using Statoliths*. Note Techniche e Reprints dell'Istituto di Technologia della Pesca e del Pescato. Special Publication 1. Mazara del Vallo, Italy

Karson, M.A., Boal, J.G. and Hanlon, R. (2003) Experimental evidence for spatial learning in cuttlefish (*Sepia officinalis*). *Journal of Comparative Psychology*, **117**, 149–155

Kier, W.M. and Smith, K.K. (1985) Tongues, tentacles and trunks: the biomechanics of movement in muscular-hydrostats. *Zoological Journal of the Linnean Society*, **83**, 307–324

Komak, S., Boal, J.G., Dickel, L. *et al.* (2005) Behavioural responses of juvenile cuttlefish (*Sepia officinalis*) to local water movements. *Marine and Freshwater Behavior and Physiology*, **38**, 117–125

Kuba, M.J., Byme, R.A., Meisel, D.V. *et al.* (2006) When do octopuses play? Effects of repeated testing, object type, age, and food deprivation on object play in *Octopus vulgaris*. *Journal of Comparative Psychology*, **120**, 184–190

Koueta, N., Boucaud-Camou, E. and Noel, B. (2002) Effect of enriched natural diet on survival and growth of juvenile cuttlefish *Sepia officinalis* L. *Aquaculture*, **203**, 293–310

Landman, N.H., Davis, R.A. and Mapes, R.H. (Eds) (2007) *Cephalopods Present and Past: New Insights and Fresh Perspectives*. Springer, Heidelberg

Landman, N.H., Tanabe, K. and Davis, R.A. (Eds) (1996) *Ammonioid Palaeobiology*. Plenum Press, New York

Lewbart, G.A. (Ed.) (2006) *Invertebrate Medicine*. Blackwell Publishing, Iowa

Mangold, K. (Ed.) (1989) Céphalopodes. In: *Traité de Zoologie*, Vol. **5**(4). Ed. Grassé, P.P., pp. 1–804. Masson, Paris

Mather, J.A. (2001) Animal suffering: An invertebrate perspective. *Journal of Applied Animal Welfare Science*, **4**, 151–156

Mather, J.A. (2008) Cephalopod consciousness: Behavioural evidence. *Consciousness and Cognition*, **17**, 37–48

Mather, J.A. and Anderson, R.C. (2007) Ethics and invertebrates: a cephalopod perspective. *Diseases of Aquatic Organisms*, **75**, 119–129

Mäthger, L.M. and Hanlon, R. (2006) Anatomical basis for camouflaged polarized light communication in squid. *Biological Letters*, **2**, 494–496

Matzner, H., Gutfreund, Y. and Hochner, B. (2000) The neuromuscular system of the flexible arm of the octopus: physiological characterization. *Journal of Neurophysiology*, **83**, 1315–1328

Melzner, F., Bock, C. and Pörtner, H.O. (2006) Critical temperatures in the cephalopod *Sepia officinalis* investigated using in vivo 31P NMR spectroscopy. *Journal of Experimental Biology*, **209**, 891–906

Melzner, F., Mark, F.C. and Pörtner, H.O. (2007) Role of blood-oxygen transport in thermal tolerance of the cuttlefish, *Sepia officinalis*. *Integrative Comparative Biology*, **47**, 645–655

Messenger, J.B. (1979) The nervous system of *Loligo*. IV. The peduncle and olfactory lobes. *Philosophical Transactions of the Royal Society London B*, **285**, 275–309

Moltschaniwskyj, N.A., Hall, K., Lipinski, M.R. *et al.* (2007) Ethical and welfare considerations when using cephalopods as experimental animals. *Reviews in Fish Biology and Fisheries*, **17**, 455–476

Neumeister, H. and Budelmann, B.U. (1997) Structure and function of the *Nautilus* statocysts. *Philosophical Transactions of the Royal Society London B*, **352**, 1565–1588

Nixon, M. and Young, J.Z. (2003) *The Brains and Lives of Cephalopods*. Oxford University Press, Oxford

Norman, M. *(2000) Cephalopods: A World Guide*, 2nd edn. ConchBooks, Hackenheim

Novicki, A., Messenger, J.B., Budelmann, B.U. *et al.* (1992) (^{14}C) Deoxyglucose labelling of functional activity in the cephalopod central nervous system. *Proceedings of the Royal Society of London B*, **249**, 7–82

Oestmann, D.J., Scimeca, J.M., Forsythe, J.W. *et al.* (1997) Special considerations for keeping cephalopods in laboratory facilities. *Contemporary Topics in Laboratory Animal Science*, **36**, 89–93

Packard, A. (1972) Cephalopods and fish: the limits of convergence. *Biological Review*, **47**, 241–307

Packard, A., Karlsen, H.E. and Sand, O. (1990) Low frequency hearing in cephalopods. *Journal of Comparative Physiology A*, **166**, 501–505

Payne, A.I.L., Lipinski, M.R., Clarke, M.R. *et al.* (Eds) (1998) Cephalopod: Biodiversity, Ecology and Evolution. *South African Journal of Marine Science*, **20**, 143–151

Plän, T. (1987) *Functional neuroanatomy of sensory-motor lobes of the brain of Octopus vulgaris*. PhD thesis, University of Regensburg

Preuss, T. and Budelmann, B.U. (1995a) A dorsal light reflex in a squid. *Journal of Experimental Biology*, **198**, 1157–1159

Preuss, T. and Budelmann, B.U. (1995b) Proprioceptive hair cells on the neck of the squid *Lolliguncula brevis*: a sense organ in cephalopods for the control of head-to-body position. *Philosophical Transactions of the Royal Society London B*, **349**, 153–178

Quast, M.J., Neumeister, H., Ezell, E.L. *et al.* (2001) MR microscopy of cobalt-labeled nerve cells and pathways in an invertebrate brain (*Sepia officinalis*, Cephalopoda). *Magnetic Resonance in Medicine*, **45**, 575–579

Saidel, W.M., Lettvin, J.Y. and MacNichol, E.F. (1983) Processing of polarized light by squid photoreceptors. *Nature*, **304**, 534–536

Saidel, W.M., Shashar, N., Schmolesky, M.T. *et al.* (2005) Discriminative responses of squid (*Loligo pealeii*) photoreceptors to polarized light. *Comparative Biochemistry and Physiology*, **142**, 340–346

Shashar, N., Hanlon, R.T. and Petz, A.D. (1998) Polarization vision helps detect transparent prey. *Nature*, **393**, 222–223

Shashar, N., Milbury, C.A. and Hanlon, R. (2002) Polarization vision in cephalopods: neuroanatomical and behavioral features that illustrate aspects of form and function. *Marine and Freshwater Behavior and Physiology*, **35**, 57–68

Sinn, D.L. and Moltschaniwskyj, N.A. (2005) Personality traits in dumpling squid (*Euprymna tasmanica*): context-specific traits and their correlation with biological characteristics. *Journal of Comparative Psychology*, **129**, 99–110

Smith, K.K. and Kier, W.M. (1989) Trunks, tongues and tentacles: moving with skeletons of muscle. *American Scientist*, **77**, 28–35

Sumbre, G., Gutfreund, Y., Fiorito, G. *et al.* (2001) Control of octopus arm extension by a peripheral motor program. *Science*, **293**, 1845–1848

Sumbre, G., Fiorito, G., Flash, T. *et al.* (2005) Motor control of the octopus flexible arm. *Nature*, **433**, 595–596

Sweeney, M.J., Roper, C.F.E., Mangold, K.M. *et al.* (Eds) (1992) 'Larval' and juvenile cephalopods: a manual for their identification. *Smithsonian Contributions to Zoology*, **513**, 1–282

Sykes, A.V., Domingues, P.M., Correia, M. *et al.* (2006) Cuttlefish culture – state of the art and future trends. *Vie et Milieu*, **56**, 129–137

Sykes, A.V., Domingues, P.M., Loyd, M. *et al.* (2003) The influence of culture density and enriched environments on the first stage culture of young cuttlefish, *Sepia officinalis* (Linnaeus, 1758). *Aquaculture International*, **11**, 531–544

Tu, Y. and Budelmann, B.U. (2000) Inhibitory effect of cyclic guanosine 3′,5′-monophosphate (cGMP) on the afferent resting activity in the cephalopod statocyst. *Brain Research*, **880**, 65–69

Vidal, E.A.G., DiMarco, F.P., Wormuth, J.H. *et al.* (2002a) Optimizing rearing conditions of hatchling loliginid squid. *Marine Biology*, **140**, 117–127

Vidal, E.A.G., DiMarco, F.P., Wormuth, J.H. *et al.* (2002b) Influence of temperature and food availability on survival, growth and yolk utilization in hatchling squid. *Bulletin of Marine Science*, **71**, 915–931

Villanueva, R. and Bustamente, P. (2006) Composition in essential and non-essential elements of early stages of cephalopods and dietary effects on the elemental profiles of *Octopus vulgaris* paralarvae. *Aquaculture*, **261**, 225–240

Voight, J.R., Pörtner, H.O. and O'Dor, R.K. (1994) A review of ammonia-mediated buoyancy in squids (*Cephalopoda: Teuthoidea*). *Marine and Freshwater Behavior and Physiology*, **25**, 193–203

Voss, N.A., Vecchione, M., Toll, R.B. *et al.* (eds) (1998) Systematics and biogeography of cephalopods. *Smithsonian Contributions to Zoology*, **586**, 1–599

Walker, I.D., Dawson, D.M., Flash, T. *et al.* (2005) Continuum robot arms inspired by cephalopods. *Proceedings of SPIE*, **5804**, 303–314

Williamson, J.A., Fenner, P.J., Burnett, J.W. *et al.* (eds) (1996) *Venomous and Poisonous Animals: A Medical and Biological Handbook*. University of New South Wales Press, Sydney

Williamson, R. (1988) Vibration sensitivity in the statocysts of the Northern octopus, *Eledone cirrosa*. *Journal of Experimental Biology*, **134**, 451–454

Williamson, R. (1995) The statocysts of cephalopods. In: *Cephalopod Neurobiology*. Eds Abbott, N.J., Williamson, R. and Maddock, L., pp. 503–520. Oxford University Press, Oxford

Williamson, R. and Budelmann, B.U. (1991) Convergent inputs to octopus oculomotor neurones demonstrated in a brain slice preparation. *Neuroscience Letters*, **121**, 215–218

Williamson, R. and Chrachri, A. (2004) Cephalopod neural networks. *Neurosignals*, **13**, 87–98

Yekuteli, Y., Mitelman, R., Hochner, B. *et al.* (2007) Analyzing octopus movements using three dimensional reconstruction. *Journal of Neurophysiology*, **98**, 1775–1790

Yekuteli, Y., Sagiv-Zohar, R., Aharonov, R. *et al.* (2005a) Dynamic model of the octopus arm. I. Biomechanics of the octopus reaching movement. *Journal of Neurophysiology*, **94**, 1443–1458

Yekuteli, Y., Sagiv-Zohar, R., Hochner, B. *et al.* (2005b) Dynamic model of the octopus arm. II. Control of reaching movements. *Journal of Neurophysiology*, **94**, 1459–1468

Young, J.Z. (1965) The central nervous system of *Nautilus*. *Philosophical Transactions of the Royal Society London B*, **249**, 1–25

Young, J.Z. (1971) *The Anatomy of the Nervous system of Octopus vulgaris*. Clarendon Press, Oxford

Young, J.Z. (1974) The central nervous system of *Loligo*. I. The optic lobe. *Philosophical Transactions of the Royal Society London B*, **267**, 263–302

Young, J.Z. (1976) The nervous system of *Loligo*. II. Suboesophageal centres. *Philosophical Transactions of the Royal Society London B*, **274**, 101–167

Young, J.Z. (1977) The nervous system of *Loligo*. III. Higher motor centres: the basal supraoesophageal lobes. *Philosophical Transactions of the Royal Society London B*, **276**, 351–398

Young, J.Z. (1979) The nervous system of *Loligo*. V. The vertical lobe complex. *Philosophical Transactions of the Royal Society London B*, **285**, 311–354

Cephalopods
Reproduced from the 7th Edition

Peter R. Boyle

General introduction

The popular perception of the cephalopods is represented by the coastal octopus, cuttlefish and squid. These large and active molluscs have a complicated behavioural repertoire. Living in diverse marine habitats they show a wide range of behavioural expression during prey capture, feeding and reproduction. Many parallels with vertebrate behaviour patterns can be recognised, such as hunting, sexual display, attention, conflict and concealment behaviours. In the laboratory, numerous experimental studies have described their remarkable capabilities of sensory discrimination, especially of visual stimuli. They have demonstrated that true learning occurs and is likely to be an integral part of the normal life of an octopus. These qualities of behavioural complexity, sensory discrimination and learning in cephalopods bear comparison with those of many lower vertebrates, and provide ample cause for considering their welfare in the laboratory for humane and scientific reasons.

The anatomy and physiology of cephalopods are very different from those of the vertebrates, so that it is necessary to include considerably more information about their general biology than for the vertebrate subgroups. Historically cephalopods have been considered as difficult animals to keep in captivity, and only relatively recently has much critical attention been given to the necessary handling and maintenance conditions. With even the most commonly held species we are still on a steep learning curve and guidance can be given here only on the general requirements. Precise details will usually have to be left to the judgement of the person responsible and will be to some extent determined by individual experience.

Since 1991, when the UFAW Handbook on the Care and Management of Cephalopods in the Laboratory (Boyle 1991) was first published, the legal position concerning experimental studies on cephalopods in the UK has been altered by the addition of *Octopus vulgaris* to the list of species covered by the *Laboratory Animals (Scientific Procedures) Act 1986* (Home Office 1986a). The effect of this change is that no procedures likely to cause recognisable pain or suffering may be carried out on *Octopus vulgaris* in the UK without valid Personal and Project Licences issued by the Home Office. This species, *Octopus vulgaris,* is the first invertebrate animal for which formal licensing procedures are required in the UK, and the legal position may change in the future simply by the inclusion of additional species to the list covered by the 1986 Act. The European Union, and possibly other countries, are also considering legislation in this area, and consultation with the relevant authorities will be advisable before commencing any work on cephalopods likely to fall within its scope.

As members of the phylum Mollusca, the cephalopods share certain basic features of their body organisation with the gastropods, bivalves and other molluscs. Molluscs typically produce a hard calcareous shell to protect the body, but the shell originally present in the cephalopods is greatly reduced or lost in the modern forms, as it is in some other molluscan lines, such as many marine gastropods and the terrestrial slugs. The radula, a ribbon of chitinous teeth which functions in gastropods and chitons as a versatile feeding organ for rasping or scraping, is one of the most characteristic molluscan features. It is present, too, in all cephalopods, although its role in feeding may be subsidiary to other structures. Standard invertebrate texts (Russell-Hunter 1979; Barnes 1980; Brusca & Brusca 1990; Willmer 1990) and molluscan reviews (Solem 1974; Yonge & Thompson 1976; Wilbur, 1983–1988; Boyle 1981b, 1987b) will give access to the general features of molluscan organisation and the special points of comparison between cephalopods and other molluscs.

Cephalopods are generally large animals; however, some species attain only very small adult body sizes such as the pygmy octopus (*Octopus joubini*) at 30g total body weight or 40mm mantle length (ML) (Hanlon 1983). Others reach exceptionally large sizes such as *Octopus dofleini*, commonly over 50kg in weight (Hartwick 1983), and the occasional specimens of the giant squid (*Architeuthis* sp.) which have been reliably estimated at 450kg or 18m length overall (Roper & Boss 1982). Typically, however, specimens required for laboratory use will be in the size range 0.25–2.5kg in weight, and thus require substantial space provision and water flow. They are also active and mobile animals. Squids swim constantly by jet propulsion or hover midwater using lateral fins. The octopuses, although generally bottom-dwelling, are very exploratory and prone to escape from tanks. All cephalopods are voracious predators, and with few exceptions will take only living prey. These characteristics of size, activity and predatory habits mean that cephalods impose many more demands on aquarium space and resources than other molluscs.

Human interest in, and relationship to, cephalopods is of long standing. The classical civilisations of the Mediterranean had a good knowledge of the various types. Representations of octopus, squid and cuttlefish are commonly found on glazed pots and mosaics of the Greeks and Romans. Aristotle (ca. 330 BC) gave clear descriptions of many aspects of their biology, including details of the specialised mating of the octopus. From mediaeval times to the end of the nineteenth century, however, cephalopods were more likely to be regarded with awe and suspicion as hostile sea creatures capable of sinking ships and drowning sailors. Many of these stories probably resulted from fearfully exaggerated accounts of rare encounters with giant squids. Lane (1957), and to a lesser extent Cousteau and Diolé (1973) provide popular introductions to the general biology of cephalopods and fascinating insights into their interactions with people.

In modern times, numerous aspects of cephalopod biology have been the subject of laboratory research, and cephalopod material has proved exceptionally valuable for studying basic properties of nerve function. Commercial fisheries are operating on a substantial scale and currently about 3 million tonnes are caught annually. Pilot trials to assess mariculture potential have also taken place. These interests have led to a series of review books and workshops in recent years which form the basis for further reading in the cephalopod literature (Messenger & Nixon 1977; Wells 1978; Roper *et al.* 1983; Boyle 1983a, 1987a; Hanlon 1988a; Okutani *et al.* 1993; Boyle & Boletzky 1996; Hanlon & Messenger 1996). Detailed knowledge of their biology and the availability of animals in captivity are still restricted to a few species studied at a relatively small number of institutions. Insights into their life in the wild are even more limited, but are rapidly being improved through the use of underwater video by divers and from submersible vehicles. Although some generalisations about their biology and requirements are possible, these are based on a narrow range of studies and there is much to learn.

We should remember that the majority of cephalopods are offshore and deepwater animals. Probably their range of behaviour patterns and levels of sensory discrimination and activity are quite different from those of their coastal and surface-dwelling relatives. The inclusion of the class Cephalopoda, though, into the remit of this *Handbook* must show that generally more attention is being given to the requirements of invertebrates in captivity. While this may lead to greater demands on the scientists and technicians who need to maintain the variety of animal types currently held for laboratory work, the encouragement to maximise their health and survival must have positive benefits both to the animals concerned and the resulting research.

Cephalopod biology

Evolution and classification

Cephalopods as a molluscan class arose early in the Silurian period with distinctive, heavy, external shells (ectocochleate) and are well represented in the fossil record. Some of these shells were very large, reaching 2 m across in the case of coiled forms or as straight shells as much as 10 m long (Lehmann 1981). Over 10 000 species are described from fossils, mainly in the subclasses Nautiloidea and Ammonoidea. These early types are represented today only by a few species of the single genus *Nautilus* (Figure 50.1). The remaining nautiloids and all of the ammonoids are extinct.

Modern cephalopods, in which the shell remnant is greatly modified or absent completely, appeared relatively recently and all belong to the subclass Coleoidea (Figure 50.1). In Table 50.1 a synopsis of the classification of living subclasses of cephalopods and the main orders of Coleoidea is given, together with a brief description of their characteristic features. The accepted terminology of the external features of cephalopods and diagrammatic representations of the internal anatomy of *Nautilus* and each of the three common living cephalopod types are shown in Figures 50.2–50.5.

Approximately 650 species of living cephalopods are known (Voss 1977a), a small fraction of the total fossil fauna. The number of species is very unevenly distributed among genera and families. As Voss (1977a) points out, the two genera *Octopus* and *Sepia* are each credited with over 100 species. A few other coastal genera may have an appreciable number of species, for example *Loligo*, but the remainder are scattered throughout a large number of diverse families of mainly deep-sea distribution. This situation has given rise to the speculation that the original cephalopod fauna may have become restricted to the relatively unfavourable habitats of the deep sea (mesopelagic) through competition with the teleost fishes. Only when the lighter, faster, more active coleoid forms evolved were they able to reinvade the more productive coastal and upwelling marine zones. Many of the characteristics of common cephalopods can be interpreted in terms of competition and parallel evolution with fish (Packard 1972). The practical consequences of this situation are that most of our knowledge of cephalopod biology has been gained from relatively few types which, although common and available, may not be particularly representative of the full range.

Habitat and distribution

Cephalopods are exclusively marine. The squid *Lolliguncula brevis* of the Gulf of Mexico is one of the very few species known to tolerate sea water of lowered salinity (>24 parts per thousand) but cephalopods generally must be regarded as stenohaline.

The few species of *Nautilus* have distributions in the Indo-Pacific region. *N. macromphalus* lives in deep water off the reef edge. Although most common in water of 300–500 m, they are caught in traps between 600 m and the surface (Ward 1983). They are relatively sluggish animals, relying on the strength of their shell for protection against predators. In the aquarium, eggs are laid attached to a hard substrate, and in the field the adults are found to have been eating benthic crustacea; both of these observations suggest that their normal life is close to the bottom. In recent years, there has been considerable interest in these animals as representatives of a mainly extinct type, and much success in keeping them in aquaria. They are subject to significant fishing pressure in certain localities, and there is some concern for conservation. Ward (1987) gives a comprehen-

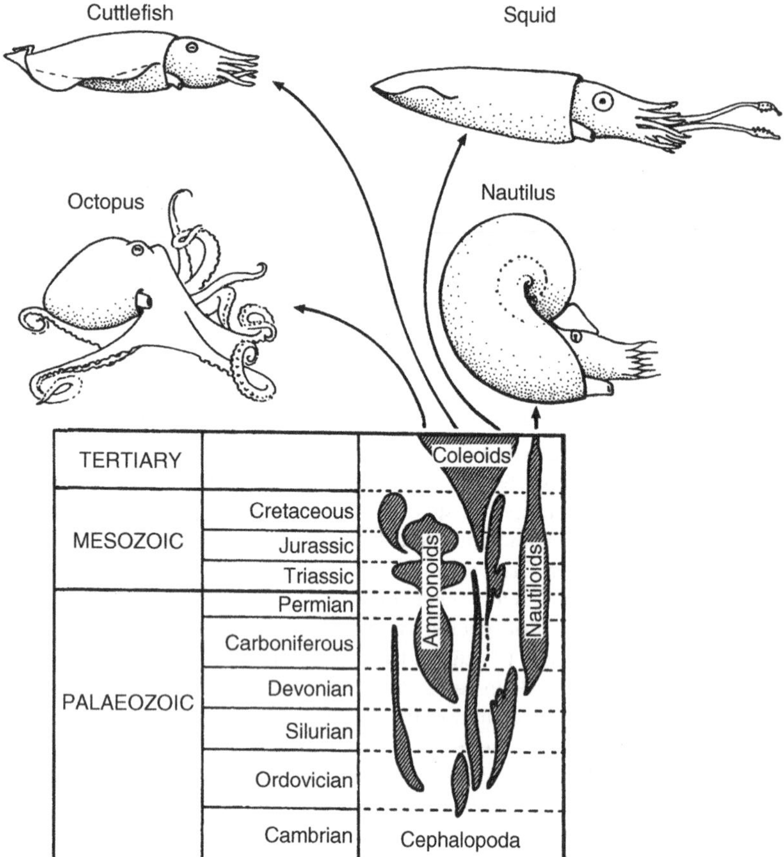

Figure 50.1 Diagrammatic representation of the evolution and radiation of the modern cephalopod types (partly from Packard 1972; Boyle 1981b).

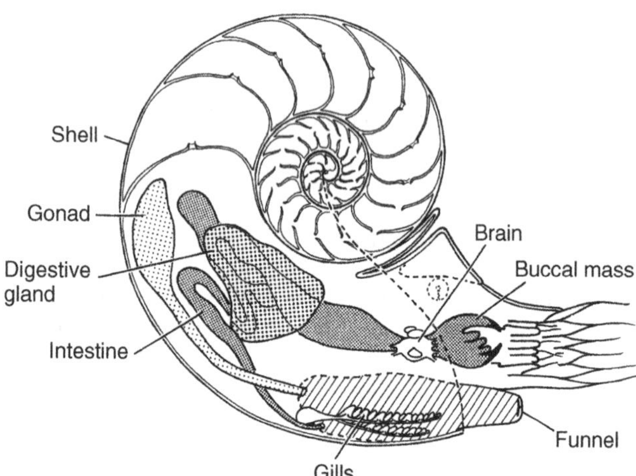

Figure 50.2 Generalised anatomy of *Nautilus*.

sive account of their biology, and a range of scientific studies is reviewed in Saunders and Landman (1987) and O'Dor *et al.* (1993).

The octopuses (Order Octopoda) are represented by a number of families, only one of which is bottom-dwelling (Table 50.1). It is this family, the Octopodidae which, nevertheless, includes all of the common species and those suitable for laboratory work. Coastal octopuses are common and have worldwide distribution. They are epibenthic, living on or close to the bottom. Normally, they are associated with stony or rocky habitats where they can both shelter and find a wide range of invertebrate food sources. In fact, many octopus species also live widely distributed over mud or sandy bottoms. By reason of their natural use of holes and crevices, octopuses are by far the most adaptable and amenable cephalopods to hold in captivity.

Cuttlefishes (order Sepioidea) are also characteristic of coastal water. Like octopuses they are active, bottom-dwelling predators which, instead of hiding amongst stones and rocks, are able to bury themselves in the sediment using lateral fins to excavate a depression and to flick sand over their dorsal surface. The best known genus, *Sepia*, the cuttlefish, is also able to 'hover' above the surface, achieving neutral buoyancy from the gas space enclosed in the shell remnant, the 'cuttlebone'. They are widely kept in aquarium conditions. Cuttlefish are common in coastal waters of most temperate and tropical zones, but are not found anywhere in American continental waters (Voss 1977a). They are often loosely referred to as 'squids', but this is inaccurate and the term 'squid' should be confined to members of the order Teuthoidea unless qualified as 'sepioid squid'.

The true squids (order Teuthoidea) are a very large and diverse assemblage of families which differ widely in habitat and distribution. Two suborders are recognised (Table 50.1), both of which include species of importance to commercial fisheries. The Myopsida are typified by squids of the genus *Loligo*. They are relatively inshore squid, sometimes of great seasonal abundance, laying egg masses attached to the

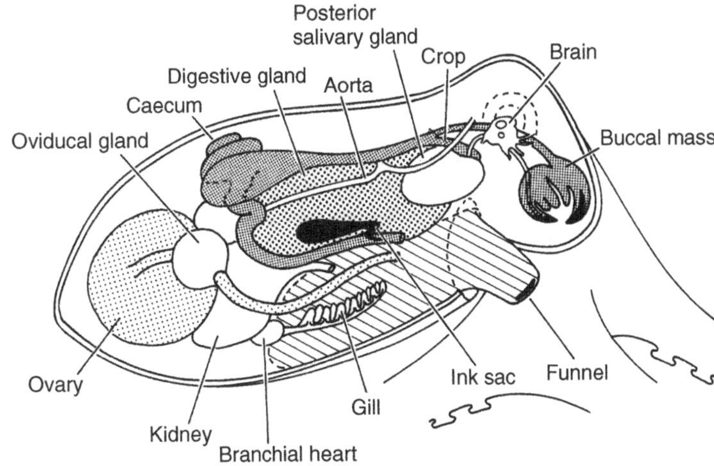

Figure 50.3 Generalised anatomy of a female octopus.

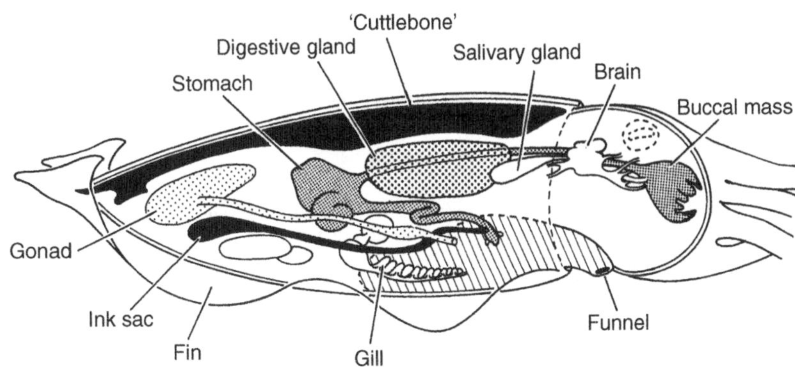

Figure 50.4 Generalised anatomy of cuttlefish.

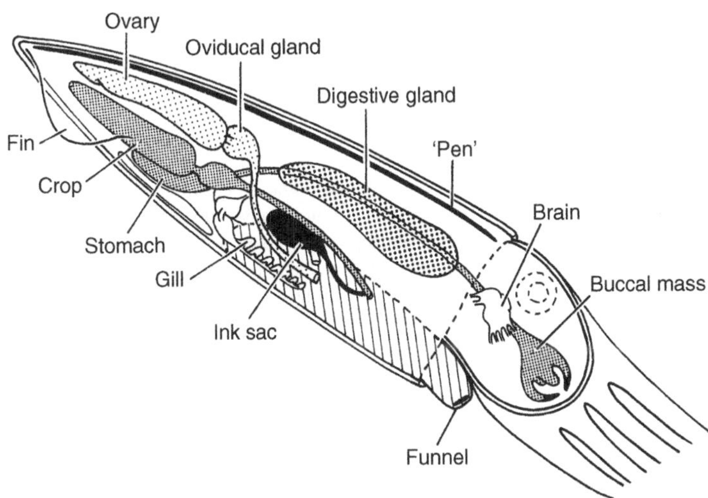

Figure 50.5 Generalised anatomy of squid.

bottom and completing their life cycle in coastal water. The Oegopsida includes a great many families ranging from obscure deepwater species whose biology is almost unknown, to genera such as *Todarodes* and *Illex* which are characteristic of areas of nutrient-rich upwellings such as the edges of the continental shelf. The oegopsids are migratory over large distances, apparently laying large, amorphous, neutrally buoyant egg masses, and completing their whole life cycle in oceanic water. The squids also are active predators, hunting fish and crustacea in the water column and on the bottom. This leads to large populations spreading over the continental shelf zones in annual feeding migrations where they may be subjects of important commercial fisheries (Okutani *et al.* 1993). Due to their active lifestyle, rapid swimming and substantial space requirements, there are relatively fewer opportunities for keeping squid alive and healthy in laboratory conditions although some, such as the Caribbean Reef squid (*Sepioteuthis sepioidea*) (Moynihan & Rodaniche 1982), family Loliginidae, are increasingly held in laboratory and public aquaria.

Table 50.1 Synoptic classification of the class Cephalopoda, listing subclasses, orders and suborders of recent forms and some common genera.*,†

Class Cephalopoda
All marine molluscs; bilateral symmetry; well developed coelom; primitively a chambered, external shell, reduced in modern forms. Radula enclosed within chitinous mandibles; ring of prehensile appendages surround the mouth; 1 or 2 pairs of gills; water circulation in mantle cavity expelled through ventral funnel tube for jet propulsion. Centralised nervous system: highly organised sense organs; complex behaviour. Sexes separate; fertilisation internal; sperm contained in complex spermatophores; eggs large and yolky; direct development (no veliger)

Subclass Nautiloidea
Caphalopods with heavy external chambered shells which may be straight or coiled. Appeared in the Cambrian period and became very numberous in species and individuals throughout warm seas. All now extinct except for one family, the Nautilidae, with restricted distribution in the Indo-Pacific Oceans. Typically for ectocochleate cephalopods the body occupies the terminal chamber of the shell which also acts as a buoyancy organ. Retraction of body into shell displaces water from mantle cavity for jet propulsion. Two pairs of gills and nephridia; head with numerous unsuckered appendages
Nautilus (fam. Nautilidae)

Subclass Ammonoidea
Chambered external shells, usually coiled and with complex septa and sutures separating the chambers. Very numerous from the Devonian to the Cretaceous periods but now all extinct

Subclass Coleoidea
Modern forms, Devonian period to present. Shell internal and reduced. Muscular fins (absent in incirrate octopods) and muscular mantle forming a sac enclosing the viscera. One pair of gills and kidneys; large mantle cavity; ink sac typically present; skin containing pigment organs, chromatophores, variably expanded by neuromuscular control

Order Belemnoidea
Internal shell straight and with a solid posterior portion; commonly fossilised; all extinct

Order Sepiolidea
Calcareous chambered shell present internally and functioning as a buoyancy organ in some (*Spirula, Sepia*); shell greatly reduced to a purely organic pen in others (Sepiolidae, Idiosepiidae); 8 suckered arms, 2 long tentacles with suckered club; suckers pedunculate with horny rims. Includes cuttlefish and sepiolids
Sepia (fam. Sepiidae)
Sepiola (fam. Sepiolidae)
Euprymna (fam. Sepiolidae)
Sepietta (fam. Sepiolidae)

Order Teuthoidea
Shell reduced to chitinous 'pen' (gladius) lying dorsally. Elongate body usually finned; 8 suckered arms, 2 long tentacles with suckered club; suckers pedunculate and with horny rims, some with hooks. Squids

Suborder Myopsida
(with transparent corneal membrane)
Loligo (fam. Loliginidae)

Suborder Oegopsida
(without corneal covering), a large assemblage with many families
Gonatus (fam. Gonatidae)
Illex (fam. Ommastrephidae)
Todarodes (fam. Ommastrephidae)
Dosidicus (fam. Ommastrephidae)
Teuthowenia (fam. Cranchiidae)

Order Octopoda
Internal shell drastically reduced and split into two lateral rods. 8 arms only with non-pedunculate suckers. Globular body with or without fins. Octopuses
Suborder Cirrata (arms bearing cirri)
Deepwater forms with fins
Suborder Incirrata (no cirri)
A large group with several pelagic families, without cirri and fins. The common octopods dealt with in this volume all belong to the only benthic family
Octopus (fam. Octopodidae)
Eledone (fam. Octopodidae)
Bathypolypus (fam. Octopodidae)

Order Vampyromorpha
8 long arms united by a swimming web, 2 small tendril-like arms in dorso-lateral position

*For a full list of recent genera refer to Voss (1977b).
†Reproduced from Boyle (1983a).

Locomotion

All cephalopods make use of a form of 'jet propulsion' in addition to other forms of locomotion. This is achieved by the rapid expulsion of water from the mantle cavity, forcing the animal to move in the opposite direction through the water in a series of jerks.

In *Nautilus* alone, jetting is achieved by the muscular retraction of the body into the terminal chamber of the shell, which displaces water through a fold in the edge of the mantle cavity. In the coleoids, the mantle cavity is enclosed by a flexible muscular wall. There are several orientations of muscle fibres within the mantle musculature (Ward & Wainwright 1972) which drive the regular inhalent and exhalent ventilatory movements. When water is expelled forcibly, the relatively small cross-sectional area of the funnel gives the jet considerable force and propels the animal in the opposite direction. Maximum velocities for jet propulsion of up to 0.35 m/s have been estimated from laboratory data (Trueman 1975). In the field, swimming speeds of over 20 knots (37 km/h) are known for squid (Trueman & Packard 1968; Packard 1969). The funnel of the coleoids is also capable of being directed backwards as well as forwards, and from side to side, giving considerable manouevrability. Generally, the coastal octopods and sepiids (*Sepia*) swim only when actively escaping or making hunting attacks. The squids, though, are negatively buoyant in the water column and swim continually. Lateral fins in sepioids and squid have an important role in maintaining or controlling orientation during locomotion. Delicate undulatory movements of fins alone are also used for small movements or during hovering.

The normal locomotion of octopods on the bottom is a fast relaxed scrambling or slower, exploratory walking, using the arms and suckers. Muscle orientations in the arms are very complicated (Keir 1982) and, coupled with the hydrostatic spaces provided by the vascular system, permit an unparalleled range of movement. The suckers, which are present along the full length of each arm as a single (*Eledone*) or double row (*Octopus*), can exert a powerful holding force on substrate or prey, up to 100 times body weight (Trueman & Packard 1968). The strength and speed with which arms and suckers can be used make the octopus both a powerful predator and a potentially difficult animal to catch and handle.

Shell and buoyancy

The shell of *Nautilus* is divided into a series of chambers by calcareous septa or partitions (Figure 50.2). Sections of the fossil ammonites and nautiloids also show a series of internal partitions, and it is presumed that the role of the shell in *Nautilus* is similar to that in the fossil groups. The shell is heavily calcified and protects the animal from predatory attacks by large fish. Evidence from broken and repaired shells, in both modern nautiloids (Saunders *et al.* 1987; Ward 1987) and fossil ammonites (Lehmann 1981), points to an important role for the shell, albeit not always completely effective, in defence against their predators.

The body of *Nautilus* occupies only the last and largest chamber of the shell. With growth, the shell enlarges at the free edges and internal partitions form successively. The space enclosed by the internal partitions of the shell is partly gas space and partly fluid-filled. The gas is a mixture closely related to the composition of air and contained at a pressure of around 0.7–0.9atm (Denton 1974). This gas space is normally sufficient to reduce the average density of the *Nautilus* to that of the surrounding sea water (relative density 1.025–1.029). In other words, the positive buoyancy contributed by the gas space just balances the sinking tendency of the animal's tissues and the heavy shell. Since the rigid shell resists the hydrostatic pressure of the surrounding water, the pressure and volume of the contained gas space is independent of depth. *Nautilus* can therefore remain neutrally buoyant throughout its depth range without making significant changes to the mass of the contained gas. A strand of living tissue, the siphuncle, connects the body of the animal to the fluid columm contained in the chambers and allows minor adjustments of the gas space to be made by alterations in the osmotic differential between the body fluids and chamber fluid (Denton & Gilpin-Brown 1966). The physiology of the cephalopod buoyancy system differs profoundly from that of the teleost fish (Denton & Gilpin-Brown 1973; Denton 1974).

All the modern cephalopods (Coleoidea) have lost the external shell and its protective functions. Instead they rely on their abilities to alter the pattern and texture of the skin to disguise themselves to an extraordinary degree, and on rapid locomotion for escape. Remnants of the ancestral shell remain. In sepioids such as the cuttlefish (*Sepia*) and the open-ocean sepiolid (*Spirula*), the internal chambered shell also functions as a buoyancy device (Denton & Gilpin-Brown 1961a, 1961b, 1971; Denton & Taylor 1964) allowing *Sepia* to 'hover' motionless before darting forward to strike a prey organism.

The squids have no gas-filled spaces and most of the surface-living 'muscular' forms need to swim continually. The shell is reduced further to a chitinous rod, the 'pen' or gladius, lying dorsally in the mantle which gives rigidity during the convulsive contraction phase. A number of deep-water forms achieve neutral buoyancy by reduction in the protein content of their tissues and accumulation of a low-density solution of ammonium chloride (Denton *et al.* 1969). Octopuses have no significant remnant of the shell, although possibly it is represented by chitinous 'stylets' located in the mantle on either side. These occur where the head retractor muscles insert into the mantle musculature and where they form an anchorage point for the muscles.

Feeding and digestion

All cephalopods actively catch and eat live prey. A very wide range of prey items has been recorded (for reviews see Boletzky & Hanlon 1983; Nixon 1987; Rodhouse & Nigmatullin 1996). Generally, sepioids take crustacea living on or near the bottom, while squid eat mostly crustacea and fish. In both these groups hunting is essentially visual (Messenger 1968, 1977). The cephalopod manoeuvres into a position from which it can strike at the prey by very rapid extension of a pair of tentacles coupled with a rapid jet-propelled forward lunge. These tentacles are suckered only at the tips (tentacular clubs), unlike the eight arms which are usually suckered along their full length. Once trapped, the prey is drawn in towards the mouth and bitten into by the chitinous beaks (mandibles). Bite-sized pieces of flesh are swallowed. Squid feeding in a shoal of fish will often only take one or a few bites before releasing one and catching another (Bradbury & Aldrich 1969).

Octopods feed on a greater variety of prey species, and their diet is probably determined as much by prey availability as predator preference (Ambrose 1983, 1984). Large crustacea such as lobsters and crabs are taken, and octopuses may be significant predators on commercial crustacean fisheries (Boyle *et al.* 1986). Molluscs, worms, fish and other groups are also frequent in the normal diet, but not commonly fed in the aquarium. Octopus prey is also located visually (Wells 1962, 1978) but chemical cues also probably have a role (Wells 1963; Boyle 1983c, 1986a; Chase & Wells 1986).

After capture by an octopus, crustacean and molluscan prey are dealt with in a lengthy and complicated way. Characteristically, flesh is removed from the exoskeleton or shell very cleanly (Arnold & Arnold 1969; Wodinsky 1969; Altman & Nixon 1970). Partly this could be due to delicate movements of the beaks, radula and suckers, but it is generally accepted that octopuses also use secretions from the posterior salivary glands to immobilise the prey and probably to loosen tissues by extracellular enzymic digestion (Nixon 1979, 1980, 1984; Boyle & Knobloch 1981; Nixon & Boyle 1982; Grisley & Boyle 1987; Boyle 1990; Grisley *et al.* 1996).

After ingestion, the already fragmented meal enters a rather short digestive tract consisting of a crop, stomach, caecum and intestine. Some digestion takes place within the lumen of the gut, but most digestion and absorption take place in the large digestive gland (Boucaud-Camou *et al.* 1976; Boucher-Rodoni & Mangold 1977; Boucaud-Camou & Boucher-Rodoni 1983; Boucher-Rodoni *et al.* 1987). Entry into the gland of food particles and the egress of excretory material into the gut lumen occur through a pair of short ducts connecting the digestive gland to the junction of the stomach and caecum. Long strings of pigmented faeces (the residues of the digestive process, usually pink–brown depending on diet composition) bound by mucus, are released from the anus into the exhalent water flow.

Excretion

Digestive excretion occurs by the release of pigmented material from digestive gland cells into the lumen of the gut (Boucher-Rodoni *et al.* 1987). Excretion from the blood system occurs via excretory tissue surrounding the lateral venae cavae (Schipp & Boletzky 1975). The main venous return from the anterior part of the body, the anterior vena cava, divides into two lateral venae cavae before entering the branchial heart of each side. The excretory cells (kidney tissues) are grouped into flocculent masses (renal appendages) sited on fine diverticulae of the lateral venae cavae. The urine is formed, probably by ultrafiltration and secretion, into a coelomic pericardial space, from which it drains into the mantle cavity through a short duct and renal papilla. Little is known about the composition and flow of urine.

A remarkable feature of the excretory organs of many cephalopods is their infestation by minute organisms, the dicyemid mesozoans. The relationship is apparently symbiotic, causing no harmful effect to the host and providing the only known habitat for the mesozoans.

Respiration and circulation

Respiratory exchange with the environment occurs through well vascularised gills suspended in the mantle cavity. In *Nautilus* there are two pairs of gills, but in all the coleoids there is only a single pair (dibranchiate). Due to the orientation of gills within the lumen of the cavity, water flows between the lamellae of each gill in the opposite direction to the flow of blood through the tissue, a countercurrent system which maximises the exchange of gases (Wells & Wells 1982).

Measurements of metabolic rates of cephalopods vary widely. This is partly because of the wide range of species and temperatures which are compared, and because of the inherent difficulty of obtaining a non-active or routine value for oxygen consumption in these animals. Figures collected by O'Dor and Wells (1987) and Wells and Clarke (1996) from many sources suggest routine oxygen consumptions mostly in the range 100–500 mlO_2/kg/h for squid and 10–100 mlO_2/kg/h for octopuses. The smaller number of estimates for sepioids and *Nautilus* fall within the octopus range. Two factors substantially increase the metabolic rate. Swimming or other violent movements rapidly increase metabolic rate to two to three times the resting value as do the energy demands of digestion in the 6–8 h following a meal (O'Dor 1982; Wells *et al.* 1983a, 1983b, 1983c).

Oxygenated cephalopod blood is blue-coloured due to the presence of the copper-containing respiratory pigment haemocyanin. This high molecular weight compound (>10^6 daltons) is in solution and not contained within specialised cells as is the case with the vertebrate erythrocyte. The circulatory system is a complex arrangement of vessels (arteries, veins and sinuses) through which the blood is driven by several contractile elements (Figure 50.6).

Venous return blood mostly collects into the anterior vena cava. This divides into two lateral venae cavae (surrounded by kidney tissue) supplying blood to the contractile branchial heart of either side, from which the gill is supplied. The lateral venae cavae and gills are also contractile and probably contribute as much to movement of the blood as do the branchial hearts themselves (Smith & Boyle, 1983). From the gill, oxygenated blood enters the auricle of each side and into the heart (systemic heart). This powerful contractile organ is capable of high systolic pressures. It pumps blood out to the tissues mainly through the aorta, but with lesser flows through the abdominal and genital arteries.

Nutrition and energy

Cephalopod growth rates, in captivity and in the field, are high. Figures for aquarium growth of many cephalopod species (mostly octopods) have been collected by Forsythe and Van Heukelem (1987). At small sizes (<10g) instantaneous growth rates (percentage increase in body weight per day) are around 4–6%, ranging up to a maximum of 12% (*Sepia subaculeata*). At body weights up to 100g, growth rates are lower but commonly in the range 2–4%. In part, these growth rates result from a very high gross growth efficiency (the conversion of food intake to growth). Many authors record growth efficiency values for octopuses in the range 40–60% with extremes of 20–80% on a wet-weight basis.

O'Dor and Wells (1987) and Wells and Clarke (1996) have summarised information on the nutritional requirements and energy requirements for cephalopods. They point out that, even on a calorific basis, the growth efficiency of cephalopods is only slightly less than the wet-weight figures suggest. The diet of cephalopods is highly proteinacious, low in carbohydrates and lipid. In addition, there is some evidence that cephalopods are hardly able to absorb and metabolise lipid. They apparently operate very largely a protein economy in which proteins are the principal energy source as well as providing the basic requirements for growth.

All studies of growth and lifespan suggest that cephalopods of all types (except *Nautilus*) are surprisingly short-lived, perhaps 1–2 years being the average range of lifespan for most of the better known species. In terms of food

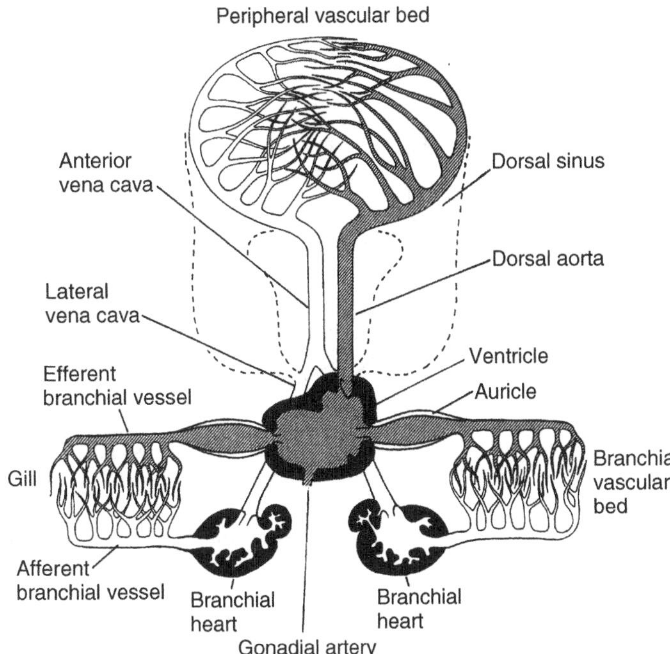

Figure 50.6 Generalised cephalopod circulatory system (after Smith & Boyle 1983).

requirements, O'Dor and Wells (1987) calculate that octopods probably consume 2.5–3 times their body weight over a lifetime. Squid, in contrast, are calculated to need as much as four times their body weight during the first 9 months (O'Dor *et al.* 1980). Their consumption is inevitably higher due to the energy demands of a more active lifestyle and leads to interesting speculations over the fuelling by cannibalism of the long migrations undertaken by many squid species (O'Dor 1988).

Nervous system

The central nervous system of all cephalopods is a more or less compact mass of nerve cells. This, the brain, is located between the eyes and is enclosed in a tough cartilaginous cranium. For *Octopus* there are an estimated $1–2 \times 10^8$ nerve cells. A great deal of information is available on the neuroanatomy of the system (Young 1971; Wells 1978) and the division of function between the many lobes.

In general terms, the suboesophageal areas of the brain are concerned with the control of groups of muscles. There are clear divisions of function between various lobes, and each of these areas can be identified as lower or intermediate motor centres. Groups of muscles known to be controlled from centres in the suboesophageal brain include those of the arms, mantle, head, funnel, fins and chromatophores. These divisions of function were established largely by stimulation experiments (Boycott 1961) coupled with the results of nerve sections and degeneration (Young 1971). Higher motor centres, which coordinate the actions of several groups of muscles, are located in lateral and supraoesophageal areas of the brain. Some regions are allocated to receptor information and analysis. Most notable of these are the optic lobes, large ganglionic masses located laterally on each side of the brain and receiving large numbers of small optic nerves. Many of the features of the neural organisation of cephalopods bear comparison with those of the vertebrates (Young 1967, 1971; Packard 1972; Hanlon & Messenger 1996).

In addition to the brain is a series of peripheral ganglionic masses. These are very extensive and contain enormous numbers of nerve cells with functions restricted to the organ systems where they are located. For example, there are an estimated 3×10^8 in the nerve cords of the arms alone. The main ganglionic masses in a typical octopod are shown in Figure 50.7. It is important to note that this degree of peripheral nervous organisation confers some degree of local autonomy of movement. Thus, certain movements of the arms (Rowell 1963, 1966), mantle (Gray 1960; Wilson 1960b; Boyle 1976) and buccal mass (Boyle *et al.* 1979a, 1979b) take place in isolation from the central nervous system.

Of great interest to physiologists is the giant fibre system of the squid, a connected assembly of single fibres with diameters of up to almost 1 mm (Young 1939; Martin 1977). Mediating the rapid escape response, the giant fibre system provides simplified nervous transmission from the brain (first- and second-order giant cells) to the stellate ganglion, and from there to the mantle musculature (third-order giant fibres). The significance of this system to the behaviour of squid seems to be threefold (Bullock & Horridge 1965): it is a simple method of triggering a supremely important evasive reaction; use of giant fibres gives an appreciable gain in the speed of reaction; and gradation of the fibre diameter of the third-order giants allows differential rates of conduction and synchronous contraction of the full length of the mantle. The 'giant fibre' commonly referred to is the third-order giant which runs the furthest distance of the mantle. The exceptional size of these fibres has allowed many important advances to be made in understanding the basic properties of nervous transmission (see Tasaki 1989).

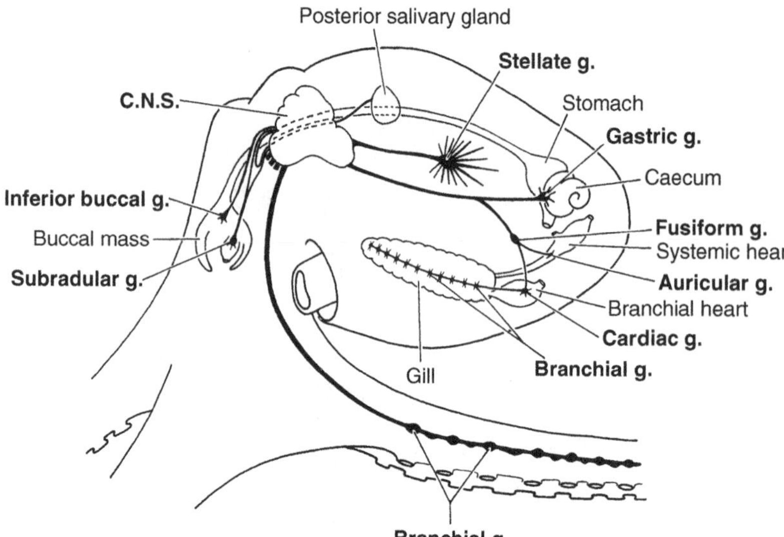

Figure 50.7 Sketch plan of the principal ganglionic masses (g) of an octopus (from Boyle 1986b).

Sense organs

The skin of cephalopods, particularly of the suckers and lips, is liberally supplied with receptor cells responsive to tactile and chemical stimuli. Octopuses are responsive to a very light touch on almost any part of the surface, and may be taught to discriminate between objects which differ only in the quality of surface texture (Wells & Wells 1957; Wells 1964a, 1964b). Mechanically sensitive cells are known also to be located within the blocks of somatic muscle (Alexandrowicz 1960; Graziadei 1965; Boyle 1976), where they are presumed to play a role in providing the sensory feedback necessary for the control of movement. Chemical senses are also thought to be associated with dispersed single cell receptors.

Discrimination between objects can be made on the basis of chemical differences (Wells 1963; Wells *et al.* 1965) and responses to waterborne chemical stimuli have been described in octopuses (MacGinitie & MacGinitie 1968; Joll 1977; Boyle 1983c, 1986a; Chase & Wells 1986).

Cephalopods have large camera-type eyes placed laterally and dorsally. There is a highly refractile spherical lens which focuses light onto a retina of receptive cells (*Nautilus* operates on the different principle of the 'pinhole' camera). General accounts of cephalopod behaviour, and experimental studies on prey capture (Messenger 1968, 1977), confirm the importance of visual input to cephalopods. There are also well known examples of the role played by visual stimuli in sexual recognition by *Sepia* (Tinbergen 1939; Corner & Moore 1981). Visual acuity is high (Packard 1969) but, rather surprisingly, and after a history of uncertainty, octopuses have been shown to be colour-blind (Messenger 1979).

Colour and texture

The pigmentation of cephalopod skin is contained within unique cellular chromatophore organs. These consist of an intracellular, elastic sac which contains the pigment, into which is inserted a series of 25 or so muscle fibres arranged radially (Cloney & Florey 1968). When these muscles contract, the pigment sac is expanded and imparts its colour to the skin surface. When the radial chromatophore muscles relax, the elasticity of the pigment sac causes it to retract to its smallest size. The pigment area is then too small to provide skin colour and the animal appears white by reflection from the muscle surface. The coloured appearance of the cephalopod skin is extended and complicated by the presence of chromatophores of different pigment hues, and by static reflecting bodies deeper in the skin (iridophores, leucophores) which can produce additional colours by differential reflection (Packard & Sanders 1969).

Much attention has been given to the neural mechanism underlying control and coordination of the chromatophores (Florey 1969; Florey & Kriebel 1969; Packard & Sanders 1969; Packard 1973, 1982; Boyle & Dubas 1981; Dubas & Boyle 1985; Hanlon 1982, 1988b). The patterns produced have been classified and related to cryptic or display functions (Packard & Hochberg 1977; Moynihan & Rodaniche 1982; Hanlon & Hixon 1980; Roper & Hochberg 1988; Hanlon & Messenger 1988; Hanlon 1988b). The cryptic functions of pattern display are usually enhanced by modifications to the outline and texture of the octopus by superficial skin muscles. The review of cephalopod behaviour by Hanlon and Messenger (1996) provides a modern synthetic treatment of information on the uses of colour and texture by cephalopods, together with many original photographs and drawings.

Luminescent organs are known from many mid- and deepwater cephalopod species (Herring 1977). Light production is due to symbiotic bacteria located in pockets at specific sites characteristic of each species, or released into the water as a luminescent cloud. Little is known of the control and activity of these organs, but it is commonly held that they have roles in camouflage and/or intraspecific signalling.

Inking

Typically all coleoids have an ink sac. This is a muscular bladder located ventrally and opening into the exhalent water flow at the base of the funnel. Discharge of ink usually occurs when the cephalopod is being pursued by a predator. It is not dispersed in the water, but tends to form a discrete dark mass. Its role is not as a screen but as an object to hold the attention of a pursuer while the cephalopod makes a rapid change in direction. This manoeuvre is often effective in gaining the extra few seconds necessary to make an escape. In captivity, startled or stressed animals will frequently eject ink.

Reproduction

In cephalopods, the sexes are separate (dioecious), and fertilisation is achieved by direct mating. Reviews of the details of reproduction are available by Arnold and Williams-Arnold (1977), Wells and Wells (1977) and Mangold (1987).

In the male, ripe sperm are packaged into complicated spermatophores and stored in a special spermatophoric (Needham's) sac until mating occurs. The male transfers sperm to the female by passing ripe spermatophores along a muscular groove in one arm which becomes modified for this function (the hectocotylus, hectoctylised arm) at sexual maturity. The course of fertilisation then varies among different cephalopod types. Sperm may be held by the female in special pouches at the base of the arms or within the mantle cavity (sepioids and squid), or enter the female genital tract and lodge in the oviducal glands (*Octopus*), or even pass into the ovary itself (*Eledone*). These mechanisms allow the possibility of opportunistic matings and sperm storage in cephalopods. The longest interval between mating and egg laying was recorded in *Octopus tetricus* at 114 days (Joll 1976). Sexual maturation is under the control of hormone(s) released from small bodies called optic glands located on the optic tract (connecting optic lobes to the brain) (Wells & Wells 1959; O'Dor & Wells 1973, 1975, 1978). At the onset of sexual maturity, there is an apparently rapid process of gonad growth, yolk secretion and ripening of accessory glandular systems. After reproduction, both males and females die. The immediate causes of this apparently universal mortality are not clearly understood, but it is as if the sequence of physical changes brought about by the optic gland hormone(s) cannot be reversed. Some direct evidence for this hypothesis is available from experiments in which the optic glands from mature octopuses were excised; their gonads regressed, while feeding and growth was resumed (Wodinsky 1977; Tait 1986).

These consequences of reproduction clearly have profound importance to the survival and lifespan expected of octopuses in captivity and will be discussed in more detail later.

Supply and maintenance

A standard terminology was adopted by Boletkzy and Hanlon (1983) to describe the various phases of holding cephalopods in captivity.

- *Maintenance* Holding wild-caught late juvenile or adult stages at the same approximate developmental stage for varying periods of time, with no specific intention of growing them to more advanced stages.
- *Rearing* Growing a cephalopod over a certain period of time without reaching production of a second generation.
- *Culture* Growing a cephalopod at least from hatching through the complete life cycle (juvenile and adult stages, sexual maturity, mating and egg laying), to hatching viable young of the first filial (F1) generation.

Although the term culture is also used collectively to refer to the whole process, these aspects of holding cephalopods in the laboratory will be dealt with separately.

Research and display roles

The most common reason for holding cephalopods in captivity is for scientific research into various aspects of their biology. The previous chapter has outlined some of the many special features of these animals, which are far from being fully understood. Active experimental research in the fields of physiology and biochemistry require supplies of healthy animals to the laboratory. Often these are provided at marine stations where there is good access to wild-caught specimens and they need not be held long in the aquarium.

One advanced and specialised area of investigation involves the use of squid giant nerve axons for research into the basic biophysical mechanisms of nerve action. Giant fibres were first described in *Loligo* by Williams (1909) and rediscovered independently in *Sepia* by Young (1934). For the squid or cuttlefish, the giant fibres form part of the rapid escape mechanism which, by simultaneous contraction of mantle and retractor muscles, ensures maximum jet propulsion. For the experimenter these exceptional cells (almost 1 mm in diameter) have allowed great advances to be made on the electrical and chemical properties of nerve. For several decades, preparations of these nerve fibres have been very productive and there is still steady demand for them at laboratories such as Plymouth and Woods Hole (Gilbert *et al.* 1990).

Laboratory research into processes such as growth, reproduction, feeding and metabolism, needs animals to be held in captivity for substantial periods of time. These aspects of biology, central to understanding the life cycle, have recently attracted more interest. This is due to greater recognition of the ecological role of cephalopods as food for higher trophic levels, such as whales and seabirds, as predators themselves on a wide range of other marine species, and as major commercial fisheries worldwide (Clarke 1966). It is these life cycle and metabolic studies which have resulted in more attention being given to the long-term maintenance of cephalopods which, in turn, is relevant to their fisheries exploitation and potential for commercial mariculture.

Public interest in live cephalopods is always high. Many public aquaria find it profitable to keep some on display (Vevers 1962), particularly large species such as *Octopus dofleini* (Anderson 1987). There is also a limited aquarium trade in small octopus species for the home aquarium market, but the practical difficulties of keeping the animals from escaping, of supplying live food, and the naturally short lifespan restrict the circle of customers to the real enthusiasts.

Species held in captivity

Boletzky and Hanlon (1983) collected information on some 45 cephalopod species which had been maintained in open seawater circulation systems. A further eight species could be added which had been kept only in closed (recirculating) systems, and new reports continue to add species which have been successfully maintained (Hanlon & Forsythe 1985; Lipinski 1985; Anderson 1987). At present it is likely that over 60 species have been maintained in laboratory conditions, representing almost 10% of the total number of cephalopod species.

Most of those which have been successfully held in captivity are benthic octopods and sepioids. These orders adapt relatively easily to aquarium conditions, provided water quality is adequately maintained, suitable substrate material is present and appropriate prey are provided. In contrast, few squid species have been kept alive for any period of time. As pelagic animals, adapted to live in open water, they readily dash into the sides of aquarium tanks. Damage to the skin surface resulting from this behaviour is usually the prime cause of early death. Advances have been made in keeping squid species in captivity, but their maintenance is undoubtedly a more demanding and specialised task.

Those species most successfully held in captivity come from a narrow range of coastal genera. Particularly widely kept are the cuttlefish *Sepia* and a range of smaller sepiolids such as *Euprymna*, *Sepiola*, *Sepietta* and *Rossia*. Many species of *Octopus* and other octopod genera, such as *Hapalochlaena* and *Eledone*, are also readily maintained. Of the squids, most attempts to keep laboratory stocks relate to members of the Loliginidae, such as *Sepioteuthis*, *Loligo*, *Lolliguncula* and *Alloteuthis*, although some success has been reported for ommastrephid squid such as *Illex illecebrosus* (O'Dor *et al.* 1977) and *Todarodes pacificus* (Sakurai *et al.* 1993).

In most laboratory situations, the choice of species will be determined by the availability of wild-caught animals. Information regarding the worldwide distribution of cephalopod types is available in Roper *et al.* (1983) and Nesis (1987). Other publications which will be helpful in reviewing the species likely to be amenable for laboratory maintenance in a particular region include Boletzky *et al.* (1971), Arnold *et al.* (1974), Boletzky (1974), Boletzky and Hanlon (1983), Hanlon and Forsythe (1985), Hanlon *et al.* (1983), Lipinski (1985), Yang *et al.* (1986) and Anderson (1987).

Capture methods

All cephalopods have a soft delicate skin surface, easily damaged by any form of mechanical abrasion. They are readily bruised by rough handling, striking against hard objects and excessive muscular stretching. Skin damage, or subcutaneous bruising on any scale, is rarely survived in captivity for more than a few days. It follows that capture of juvenile and adult forms from the wild results in high mortality, and considerable care is needed if viable animals are to be returned to the laboratory.

Benthic octopods and sepioids are commonly obtained by commercial fishing gear. Trawls of various kinds will catch these species along with a wide variety of other organisms. The majority of cephalopods caught by moving gear will be already dead or too damaged to survive; nevertheless, because these commercial gears are readily available they still provide the main source of supply at many laboratories. Despite the disadvantages, many studies on aquarium-maintained octopuses (Mangold & Boletzky 1973; Boyle 1981a), sepioids (Boletzky *et al.* 1971) and squid (Hanlon *et al.* 1983; Hulet *et al.* 1979; Lipinski 1985) have been based on trawl-caught specimens. Commercial trawl gear is generally too large, the hauls of too long duration, and their contents too mixed, to capture cephalopods in good condition. Better results will be obtained using, for example, small beam trawls for short hauls (15–20 minutes).

For octopods, the use of traps or pots is much better. In shallow water, fishermen frequently set lines of earthenware pots on the bottom specifically to capture octopuses. Because of the natural tendency for octopuses to establish 'homes' and because natural shelter is limited, they tend to take up residence in the pots. When the pots are lifted at intervals of 2–3 days the octopuses may be captured undamaged. Although principally a method of artisanal fishing, pot-caught octopuses provide the main supply of specimens at major laboratories such as the Zoological Station, Naples. As active predators, octopuses also tend to enter the traps set commercially for crustacea such as crabs and lobsters. Cephalopod predation on trapped crustacea may be a significant commercial nuisance (Ritchie 1972; Boyle 1986c; Boyle *et al.* 1986), but it also provides a means to capture undamaged octopuses.

A small number of species in warm, temperate and tropical areas useful for laboratory studies may be hand collected on the shore in pools or under rocks. Hand collection underwater by SCUBA diving is also an effective method in certain locations.

Methods for the commercial capture of squid are diverse, highly evolved and vary in different parts of the world. They include the use of bottom and pelagic trawling, seine nets of various types, gill nets, lift nets, traps and wide use of jigging lures, both with and without the use of lights. Specialised reviews such as those of Hamabe *et al.* (1982), Rathjen (1984), Roper *et al.* (1984) and Rathjen and Voss (1987) should be consulted for details. Although some trawl-caught squid may be suitable for maintenance in aquarium conditions (Lipinski 1985) the best specimens will be obtained by the use of jigged lures with barbless hooks operated mechanically or by hand. Fishing at night using strong lights attracts squid to the surface where they see and attack the lures. They may also be caught individually in dip nets from the ship (Hanlon *et al.* 1978, 1983) and in either case these squid will provide the best specimens.

Eggs of octopods, sepioids and myopsid squid are laid in protective capsules and attached to hard surfaces on the bottom, or sometimes on objects such as buoys or ropes. The egg capsules are usually quite hardy, and whether collected by hand or bottom-trawling gear, they can provide useful laboratory material. Alternatively, mature adults brought into the aquarium may spawn there.

Handling and transport

As previously mentioned, every effort must be made to avoid skin damage and bruising. The skin is easily damaged by dry surfaces, and cephalopods of all types must be kept continuously moist and exposed to the air for minimal periods.

Small octopuses and sepioids can be placed temporarily in containers part-filled with sea water, but this must be changed with some regularity if temperature, pH and oxygen content are not to alter substantially. For transport over distances taking more than an hour or two, special arrangements must be made. Small numbers of small individuals may be carried in cool boxes with only sufficient water to cover the animals. To promote individual survival, particularly in the case of larger specimens, each animal should be contained in a polythene bag about one third full of sea water. Air, or better still oxygen, fills the remaining space. The bags are sealed and kept cool. Survival for 8–10 h is easily possible in these conditions.

Animals captured at sea are best held in deck tanks of sea water continuously pumped from the ocean. On entering most harbours it will usually be necessary to stop the pump to avoid contaminated harbour water. Squids can also be held in this way, providing there is sufficient tank space, but some authors (Flores *et al.* 1976; Lipinski 1985), recommend that they are contained individually or in small groups within perforated plastic bags floating in the main tank. Small octopuses, large benthic hatchlings or egg masses can be readily transported by these methods over long distances and shipped as unaccompanied packages on public transport.

Notably in Japan, where the price paid for live marine species at commercial fish markets greatly exceeds that for the freshly dead, methods of bulk live transport have been developed. With total journey times of up to 20 h, before live display at the Tokyo fishmarket, the water conditioning in these transport facilities must be of a very high order. Specialised fish restaurants in Japan may also display live squid species in the short term for inspection by their customers.

Water quality

Sea water aquarium systems are basically of two types. At marine laboratories, close to the sea, an open system may be available, whereas at inland sites a closed or recirculating system is usual, in which a fixed volume of water is pumped from a reservoir through the holding tanks with varying degrees of conditioning. Some laboratories operate an intermediate system in which there is continual replacement of a portion of water volume of a recirculating system. The provision of these systems and the maintenance of water quality are discussed in the 7th edition of the UFAW Handbook (Poole 1999) and extensively covered in specialised works (Spotte 1979a, 1979b; Hawkins 1981) although detailed designs specifically for cephalopods have also been published (Forsythe & Hanlon 1980; Hanlon & Forsythe 1985; Hanlon 1990; Yang *et al.* 1986).

Captured cephalopods should be treated as fish in so far as their requirements for the main parameters of water quality: temperature, salinity (parts per thousand), hydrogen ion concentration (pH), oxygen (O_2), and levels of dissolved nitrogen as ammonia (NH_3), nitrite (NO_2) and nitrate (NO_3). The water temperature should be held close to the ambient. Little is known about temperature acclimatisation in cephalopods, but the experience of most workers suggests that they will survive best if aquarium temperatures are not more than a few degrees different from the environmental water temperature.

Cephalopods are stenohaline, that is, living in a narrow salinity range, close to full strength sea water (34–36 parts per thousand). Only the squid *Lolliguncula brevis* (Hendrix *et al.* 1981) of the Bay of Mexico, is known to tolerate significantly lowered salinities (>24 parts per thousand). The aquarium sea water must be held at around 34–36 parts per thousand. Cephalopods are sensitive to acidity and the pH should be held above 7.5, preferably within the range of open sea water (pH range 7.8–8.2), and low pH levels corrected if necessary by addition of sodium bicarbonate. Dissolved oxygen levels should be maintained close to saturation levels by forced aeration. Squids especially are active swimmers, normally living in fully aerated sea water, although some benthic octopods are quite tolerant of reduced oxygen levels.

As with fish, it is the build-up of nitrogenous excretory products which poses the main problem for closed seawater aquaria. Boletzky and Hanlon (1983) recommend the adoption of Spotte's (1979a) standards: <0.10 mg/l ammonia, <0.10 mg/l nitrite, <20.00 mg/l nitrate. However, higher nitrate concentrations are tolerated by some octopuses, for example *Eledone cirrhosa* (50 mg/l nitrate; Boyle 1981a), *Octopus joubini* and *O. digueti* (100–200 mg/l nitrate; Forsythe, 1984; DeRusha *et al.* 1987). These levels have been measured for relatively few species, and range of tolerance levels is not established.

Space requirements

There are no absolute space requirements for cephalopods. Sedentary benthic species can be held individually in very small enclosures provided there is a sufficient rate of water exchange to maintain water quality (Wells *et al.* 1983b; Boyle 1983c, 1986a). Octopods and sepioids quickly establish themselves in aquarium tanks of modest dimensions. Circular tanks of 1 m diameter (0.6 m deep) will provide adequate space for five to ten sizeable *Eledone cirrhosa* (250–1000g) while tanks of 2 m diameter (0.6 m deep) will house 20–30. Factors such as activity and aggression will also determine the number which can be held together.

In small recirculating systems (2600l) with biological and mechanical filtration, physical adsorption ('protein skimmers') and ultraviolet (UV) sterilisation, Hanlon and Forsythe (1985) were able to hold a maximum octopus biomass of 15 kg. Sustained levels of ammonia–nitrogen and nitrate–nitrogen of up to 0.20 mg/l were tolerated. Nitrate–

nitrogen could be held at 500 mg/l, although it was felt that levels over 100 mg/l were affecting reproductive success. Clearly, the holding capacity of any aquarium system is more related to its ability to control water quality rather than absolute space requirements of the animals.

Squids require more area in which to swim, and some laboratories have provided tanks or raceways of substantial volume to accommodate this activity (Matsumoto 1976; O'Dor *et al.* 1977; Matsumoto & Shimada 1980; Yang *et al.* 1986). In any case, the sides of the tanks need to be marked with a bold contrasting pattern to provide sufficient visual cues for the squid to avoid hitting the boundaries. While octopuses quickly adapt to captivity and will become tame, wild-caught squid remain very nervous animals which must not be exposed to sudden stimuli such as lights, movements and vibration.

Housing and substrate

Squids require no special substrate or housing, but low light intensities and shielding from external disturbance are preferred. The seawater drain should be covered with netting to prevent animals becoming trapped there. Plastic sheeting or netting should cover the top of the tank to prevent the occasional animal jetting out and to reduce visual disturbance from movements round about. Constant diffuse overhead illumination is provided to give 10–15 lux in the middle of the water column (Yang *et al.* 1986). Ideally, glass or plastic underwater observation panels should be let into the sides of the tank. The inside tank walls must be painted with an irregular mottle pattern. Moveable black plastic or net curtains may be used as temporary internal partitions to confine the squid to portions of the tank from which they may be gently caught with a lift net, or where they will be less disturbed by tank cleaning operations.

Cuttlefish and sepiolids also may be kept without special substrate, but they will make use of sediment of the right grade on the tank floor. These animals normally partially cover themselves with sand and will thrive well if this is provided. Octopuses should be given plenty of shelter in the form of earthenware flowerpots, pieces of plastic pipe, etc. They will use these objects as temporary 'homes' or 'dens' from which they will make hunting forays (Boyle 1980; Mather 1980).

Since all cephalopods are carnivorous, uneaten food will quickly decompose and must be promptly and rigorously removed from the tanks. The presence of a clutter of pipes and pots in octopus tanks is a nuisance when cleaning, but this cannot be avoided because the provision of shelter for the octopuses allows a much higher stocking density.

However well housed, octopuses are particularly prone to escape from aquarium tanks, presumably a consequence of exploratory hunting activity. Loose lids are of little value because the octopuses will easily lift them and push their way out of the tank. For large tanks a convenient solution is to line the wall above the water level with soft upholstery foam overlapping the tank rim onto the outer surface. Suckers cannot grip on this surface and so octopuses cannot climb the sides (Boyle 1981a). Small species can be prevented from climbing out by gluing a strip of plastic turf around the inside wall above the water line. The alternative to these methods is the provision of strong, close-fitting lids, firmly fixed to the rim of the tank. The precise design of lids depends on the preference of the aquarium manager and the practicalities of each particular situation. A cheap and effective solution to escape problems, particularly where large and powerful species like *Octopus dofleini* are concerned, is to use fishing net of an appropriate mesh tightly tied under the rim of the tank.

Health hazards

The normal feeding methods of octopuses can pose something of a health hazard to human handlers. Many species of octopus are known to bite with the beaks and to inflict an appreciable wound. More important is the injection into the wound of saliva containing a wide variety of pharmacologically active compounds and having several toxic effects in vertebrates (Halstead 1965).

In the small Australian octopod *Hapalochlaena maculosa* the toxin of the saliva, known as 'maculotoxin', has effects in vertebrates indistinguishable from the puff adder venom tetrodrotoxin in blocking the sodium channels of nerve cell membranes and preventing passage of action potentials (Dulhunty & Gage 1971; Crone *et al.* 1976; Cariello & Zanetti 1977). This species has been the cause of human fatalities (Flecker & Cotton 1955).

Other octopuses have been known to bite human handlers, certainly *Octopus vulgaris*, *O. briareus*, *O. fitchi*, *O. rubescens*, *O. macropus* and *Eledone cirrhosa*. It may be assumed that, given the opportunity, most species will bite. The effects are always painful, often described as like a severe bee sting, and some victims have reported other effects such as pain and partial paralysis extending well beyond the site of the bite. Sensitivity to the toxins may differ between individuals, but clearly it is desirable to avoid these incidents. Fear of being bitten and the natural tendency of the octopus to grip the handler with arms and suckers tend to make the inexperienced person nervous. As far as possible, the octopus should not be allowed to bring the mouth area firmly into contact with exposed skin of the handler or to crawl freely over the skin surface. Some practice and experience is usually necessary before octopuses can be handled firmly but with confidence and safety.

A further potential health hazard may arise from infections of skin lesions of cephalopods. These lesions are not uncommon in wild and laboratory-held animals, although no cases of resulting human infection have been described; R.T. Hanlon (personal communication) reports that potentially pathogenic micro-organisms have been cultured from this source. It is also noted that the occurrence of larval nematodes of the genera *Ascaris* and *Anisakis* in cephalopods could also constitute a human health risk if consumed (Hochberg 1983).

Rearing

The term rearing is taken to include the growth and healthy maintenance of cephalopods for any period of time, short of reaching a second generation, and not specifically to the rearing of hatchlings or juveniles.

Feeding and food supplies

As cephalopods are carnivores and normally exclusively predatory, feeding in captivity requires continuous supplies of live food. No artificial diets are routinely available. The reviews of Boletzky and Hanlon (1983), Nixon (1987) and Rodhouse and Nigmatullin (1996) assemble virtually all the information presently available on the diets of cephalopods in the field and aquarium.

Most octopuses will capture and eat almost any type of crustacean of appropriate size (crabs, shrimps, squat lobsters, etc). Many species, for example *Octopus vulgaris*, *O. bimaculatus* and *O. dofleini*, will also readily take a variety of gastropod or bivalve molluscs. Squid and cuttlefish will catch fish and pelagic crustacea such as euphausids. Apart from the special attention required for hatchlings and small juveniles (Villanueva 1994), policy with provision of food should be to supply a choice of prey from the species range likely to be available in the natural habitat and of a size readily tackled by the cephalopod. Octopuses are certainly capable of killing crustacea of their own size, but as a general guide, suitable prey organisms would be not more than about 10% of the mass of the cephalopod predator.

Like many marine invertebrates, octopuses can survive without food for periods of at least several weeks, but feeding rates of healthy, growing cephalopods are high. For cool temperate, warm water and tropical species, daily rates of food intakes for octopods range from 1–10% of body weight, and up to 15% of body weight for some squid (O'Dor & Wells 1987). Flesh retrieval from crabs is around 50% of the gross body weight. Therefore, to fuel even a 5% feeding rate for a 500g octopus, at least 50g of crab will have to be supplied daily. Except where measured levels of food intake are required, food should be supplied *ad libitum*. Live food supply on this scale places significant demands on collections made in the field, or from commercial supply at high expense. Octopuses will attack and eat dead food, such as pieces of sardine when presented on a thin skewer and moved about. This technique has been regularly used to present rewards in training experiments (Wells 1962). Squid will also take dead food, for example, Bradbury and Aldrich (1969) fed captive *Illex illecebrosus* on dead capelin (*Mallotus villosus*). *Nautilus*, in particular, takes dead food and probably is a regular scavenger in the field (Haven 1972). Despite these exceptions, for most practical purposes, keeping and growing live cephalopods will entail regular supplies of live prey of suitable species.

Growth

High food intakes, coupled with exceptional rates of gross food conversion efficiency, result in very high growth rates. Growth conversion efficiency (that is the growth increment expressed as a percentage of the food intake over the same period), ranges normally between 40% and 60% on a wet-weight basis, or even higher for octopods, and somewhat lower for squid, 25–40% (O'Dor & Wells 1987). This means that for even a relatively slow-growing species such as *Eledone cirrhosa*, 100g of crab meat ingested results in 40g of octopus growth (Boyle & Knobloch 1982).

Various mathematical expressions have been used to describe cephalopod growth (Forsythe & Van Heukelem 1987). Growth in laboratory-held octopuses generally follows two phases: an early phase, best described by an exponential relationship, during which most of the adult size is achieved, followed by a much slower logarithmic growth phase. During the early part of the first phase, maximum instantaneous growth rates (the percentage increase in body weight per day) range from 4–8%. Animals nearing their adult size are more likely to be growing at 1–2% per day or less.

Where field data are available, growth rates are correspondingly high, leading most authors to believe that the aquarium growth performance is not abnormal. There are, however, wide differences between individuals, and many animals brought in from the field will not begin to feed as readily or grow as fast.

Lifespan

The second, slower phase of cephalopod growth marks the onset of sexual maturation and the beginning of the end of its life. The physiological changes associated with the final stages of gonad growth and vitellogenesis do not seem to be reversible. In the field, after spawning, the females die almost without exception, although individual 'spent' animals may linger on for a number of weeks. While many of these animals fall to predators or disease, the basic cause of death seems to be endogenous and associated with breakdown of somatic proteins. Less is known about the male life cycle, but they are generally assumed also to die after the first breeding season. While there may be some exceptional species which will spawn several times in a period of months, such as *Octopus chierchiae*, feeding and growing in the intervening periods (Rodaniche 1984), this pattern of breeding and death means that the survival of individual cephalopods in captivity is naturally limited. The degree to which very large species such as the giant squids (*Architeuthis* sp.) conform to these generalisations is not known, but really large octopods (*O. dofleini*) are estimated to live from 3 to 5 years (Hartwick 1983).

Neither the environmental and ecological influences, nor the immediate physiological factors controlling maturity and death, are properly understood. Clearly the lifespan of individuals in aquarium conditions will be quite short. Estimates of 1–2 years' lifespan are common for the medium-sized cephalopods (Boyle 1983a). In practice, the term of survival in the aquarium will be normally less than a year. Maximum survival periods recorded for representative species held in the aquarium are: *Eledone cirrhosa*, 240–270 days (Boyle & Knobloch 1984b); *Octopus joubini*, 331 days (Forsythe, 1984); *Octopus digueti*, 258 days (DeRusha *et al.* 1987); *Octopus maya*, 229 days for females, 360 days for males (Van Heukelem 1983); *Octopus bimaculoides*, 404 days (Forsythe & Hanlon 1988); *Octopus briareus*, 505 days (R.T.

Hanlon & M.R. Wolterding, personal communication); *Loligo opalescens*, 248 days (Yang *et al.* 1986).

Many cephalopods which reach full maturity in the aquarium apparently will not spawn normally, but this does not seem to prolong survival since such 'egg-bound' females will usually die within a few weeks (Boyle & Knobloch 1983, 1984a). There is some suggestion that aquarium conditions themselves, whether through higher temperatures, lower feeding or growth rates, promote increased gonad growth at smaller sizes (Boyle & Knobloch 1984b).

Damage and disease

Wild-caught cephalopods are particularly prone to mechanical damage. Cuts and abrasions of the skin inflicted by nets or rough handling are a frequent cause of mortality, especially in squids, usually within a few days of capture (Summers & McMahon 1970; Hulet *et al.* 1979). Lesions of the skin may also develop in aquarium-held octopuses, often at the most posterior part of the mantle (Boyle 1981a). Octopuses are more hardy than squid, but they also suffer from rough handling. Internal damage to muscles from bruising shows as conspicuous swellings, coloured blue from leakage of blood containing the copper-based respiratory pigment haemocyanin. Nerve damage may be evident from paralysis of one or several arms, an asymmetrical stance, the head not held level, or patches of skin permanently white where chromatophores are no longer working.

In the field quite major injuries are survived. Healthy individuals are captured which have had several arms amputated and are in the process of regenerating. Multiple healed scars are also frequently found. In the aquarium, however, these cuts, abrasions and lesions rarely heal. The animal becomes infected and dies.

Long-term laboratory-held octopuses have been observed to develop ulcerations on the skin. These spread rapidly in the epidermis, enlarging and deepening to affect the dermis and underlying muscle tissue. Unless quickly treated these ulcerations are invariably fatal within 2–4 days. Thraustochytrid and labyrinthulid fungi have been isolated from skin lesions in *Eledone cirrhosa*, but it is not clear whether these organisms are causal agents or secondary infections (Polglase 1980).

At least five types of bacteria have been isolated from lesions in *Octopus joubini* and *O. briareus* (Hanlon *et al.* 1984), and similar numbers from ulcerated tissue in the squid *Lolliguncula brevis* (Ford *et al.* 1986). In laboratory-reared octopuses, the ulcers developed only in groups of animals in high-density cultures. Individually held animals were not affected. *O. joubini* experimentally infected with *Vibrio alginolyticus* developed skin ulcers within 2 days. Treatment with several antibacterial agents showed that periodic dipping in solutions of nifurpirinol at a range of concentrations was effective in reducing mortality and complete healing was achieved in some animals.

The incidence of infected skin lesions is much higher in intensively reared laboratory animals. Trials have shown that some treatments with antibacterial agents can be effective (Hanlon *et al.* 1984; Forsyth *et al.* 1987), but the methods are still a long way from routine application. In the meantime, skin infections are a potential problem in any intensive system.

Parasitism

Cephalopods carry a wide variety of parasites and symbionts (Overstreet & Hochberg 1975; Hochberg 1982) which include viruses, bacteria, fungi, sporozoans, ciliates, dicyemids (mesozoa), monogeneans, digeneans, cestodes, acanthocephalans, nematodes, polychaetes, hirudineans, branchiurans, copepods and isopods (Hochberg 1983).

Apart from the potentially pathogenic micro-organisms described in the previous section, none of this range of parasites are known to cause special problems in captive cephalopods. However, Hochberg (1983) points out that since larval nematodes of many species, including those of the genera *Ascaris* and *Anisakis*, are known from many cephalopod types, a potential human health risk exists. Squids probably function as intermediate hosts for many nematode life cycles, which are then completed when they are consumed by marine mammals.

In areas of the world where uncooked fish and squid are regularly eaten, anisakiasis can be a human health problem in which ascaridoid nematodes cause ulcers and lesions in the digestive tract. Although no direct evidence implicates squid in its transmission, the parasite load of cephalopods must be considered a risk if the flesh is eaten raw or partially cooked.

Cannibalism

Where cephalopods are held collectively, some cannibalism may occur. Small octopuses may be killed and eaten by larger ones, but the incidence of this behaviour depends very much on the size range of animals held together, the stocking density and provision of adequate food and places of shelter. Suitable husbandry can avoid the problem altogether. In the field, the diet of many cephalopods includes smaller representatives of their own species (Nixon 1987). In certain squids, eg, *Illex illecebrosus*, it appears that during long migratory journeys the smaller members of the shoal form a normal and major component of diet for the larger animals (Squires 1957; O'Dor & Wells 1987).

Animals which are sick or dying are commonly eaten by others in the tank, even while still alive. Injured animals, particularly those with damaged blood or nerve supplies to an arm, will even eat their own necrotic tissue (autophagy). Laboratory-held animals in this condition should always be killed.

Culture and breeding

General considerations

The culture and breeding of cephalopods in laboratory conditions is not widely undertaken. There are many examples of cephalopods raised in captivity from eggs brought in from the field or laid in the aquarium, but regular success requires either specially favourable conditions of open seawater circulation or considerable effort to maintain high-quality closed circulation systems. In either case, apart from the practical difficulties of handling small hatchling animals, the main problem is the supply of sufficient live food of suitable type and size.

On the positive side, except for squids of the family Oegopsidae whose eggs drift freely in the water, cephalopod eggs are large, well protected by egg membranes and easily handled. They are normally attached to hard surfaces. Again with the exception of some oegopsid squids, there are no specialised larval forms which undergo distinct metamorphosis. The hatchling is a miniature adult capable of using its arms and swimming in an essentially adult fashion. In many of the sepioid and octopod species the hatchling is bottom-living immediately. Some species which are benthic as adults have a planktonic juvenile phase of variable duration and the term 'paralarva' has been proposed for these planktonic young (Young & Harman 1988). The review of Boletzky and Hanlon (1983) lists all the cephalopod species for which either maintenance or rearing had taken place at that time and identifies those species with benthic young.

Potentially, these benefits of large size, hardiness and benthic young should be very helpful in developing culture and breeding programmes (Hanlon 1987). Very little is known about the juvenile stages in the field (but see Mangold & Boletzky 1985), so this approach is likely to be increasingly useful for completion of life cycle studies.

Maturation

Maturation in females is largely a process of gonad growth by yolk accumulation. The later stages take place rapidly under the influence of the gonadotrophic hormone(s) from the optic gland. Feeding and growth rates of female octopuses in the aquarium decline quickly with the onset of maturation; they become relatively sluggish and may deposit small numbers of eggs, attaching them to the sides of the tank or other hard objects. At this point the female is seeking a suitable place for egg laying, usually within a pot or tube or under an overhang of stones. The single, median ovary, which originally contributed about 0.25% of body weight has now grown to occupy close to 25%.

Fully mature animals can often be recognised by the white appearance of the ovary through the muscle wall and the changed outline of the mantle. Maturity scales based upon the relative enlargement and appearance of the ovary and other components of the reproductive system have been devised for many species. Where it is necessary to evaluate reproductive condition in living animals, the mantle musculature can be simply inverted to expose the gonad, under anaesthesia, after cutting the mid-ventral septum. This simple operation should cause little stress, and the examination may be repeated on successive occasions. The paired oviducts leading from the ovary will be packed with ripe eggs in the final stage of maturity.

The pattern of maturation is similar in squid, except that the oviduct is single and on the left-hand side. These animals will rarely survive anaesthesia or internal examination and surgery. Assessment of maturity is a matter of external appearance of colour and shape (above), and development of the hectocotylus in males (see Sexing section).

The male system in all cephalopods is more complicated. Ripe sperm from the testis pass into the proximal vas deferens. Here, in specialised glandular areas they are packaged into discrete spermatophores. Finished spermatophores are then stored in a spermatophoric sac. The mature male will usually have ripe spermatophores lodged in the distal portion of the vas deferens, the excurrent duct (incorrectly 'penis'), ready for transfer to a female. Males are sexually mature over a wider range of body size than females, and thus appear ready to mate over a greater portion of their lifespan. The total mass of ripe testis and full spermatophoric sac does not usually contribute such a large proportion of body mass as the female ovary.

Sexing

Males and females may be distinguished externally by the presence of modifications to the arm of the mature male used for sperm transfer during mating. In octopods it is the third right arm (counting from the dorsal mid-line) which becomes thickened; a fold in the skin along the arm develops and the tip usually becomes modified and hook-like. The precise form of this hectocotylised arm or hectocotylus, which in myopsid squid is the fourth left, is often a species characteristic.

In immature animals, or where a more precise assessment of maturity state is required, no alternative to an internal examination is currently in use. Sepioids and teuthoids can only be examined after death, but octopods can be anaesthetised and the mantle sac inverted. In octopods, even the most immature animal can be sexed in this way – the paired oviducts always being distinguishable from the single male excurrent duct; squid are more difficult because both oviduct and excurrent duct are singular, and located on the left side.

Mating

Octopuses frequently mate in aquarium conditions. The usual approach is for the male hectocotylus to be inserted into the mantle cavity of the female. Peristaltic and 'pumping' movements of the male arm transfer spermatophores to the female. In *Octopus vulgaris*, the sperm enters the oviducts and lodges in the oviducal glands (Frösch & Marthy 1975), while in *Eledone cirrhosa* spermatangia (ruptured spermatophores) travel all the way into the ovary (Boyle 1983b). Fertilisation is then truly internal and its timing is essentially determined by the female.

Female sepioids and squid have various methods of holding sperm transferred from the male, in buccal membranes or within the mantle cavity. In oegopsid squid, spermatophores may be held in the buccal membrane of the female (*Todarodes*) or attached to the base of the gills (*Illex*). Mating takes place usually in a 'head to head' position, and in some species (*Loligo opalescens*) there may be dense spawning aggregations.

Mating in cephalopods is always one to one, although each individual may perform a series of matings with different partners. Underwater video observations show that while single male and female pairs are formed at mating, small 'sneaker males' may successfully fertilise the same female during the egg-laying process (Hanlon & Messenger 1996). This paired mating is in sharp contrast to most aquatic molluscs which liberate both male and female gametes into the water. Little is known of the stimuli required for mating. Mature male *Octopus* mate readily with mature females in the same tank. Other species such as *Eledone cirrhosa* are more reticent. *Sepia officinalis* and loliginid squids such as *Sepioteuthis sepioidea* and *Loligo opalescens* are known to exhibit chromatophore displays characteristic of sexual maturity and mating. These presumably function as intraspecific visual signals and, incidentally, are another method of externally distinguishing the sexes (Tinbergen 1939; Corner & Moore 1981; Moynihan & Rodaniche 1982; Hanlon & Messenger 1996).

Egg laying

Many sepioid and octopod species will lay viable eggs in aquarium conditions. Usually this occurs when gravid females, close to egg laying, are brought in from the field, but a number of species, mostly those with large eggs (Hanlon & Forsythe 1985), have successfully laid eggs after long-term rearing.

Sepioids lay small numbers (25–1000) of large eggs (1–10 mm in diameter) usually within a period of a few weeks. They are individually deposited, firmly fixed to a hard substrate, each enclosed in a tough sheath which considerably increases the size of each egg. Octopods may also lay large eggs, ranging in size from about 2 mm in length (*Octopus vulgaris*) up to 12–15 mm (*O. bimaculoides*, *O. briareus*, *Eledone moschata*, *Bathypolypus* spp.) or even larger in some Antarctic species. Estimates for total fecundity in octopods range from minima of 25–50 (*O. joubini*, *O. australis*) to well over 100 000 (*O. vulgaris*, *O. tetricus*, *O. cyanea*). The eggs are in strings, attached usually in the protection of rocks or an overhang. Egg laying is completed in less than a day or may take several weeks. Females of many species are known then to brood the egg mass, blowing sea water over it, keeping the eggs clear of epigrowths and protecting them against predators. This behaviour usually continues until hatching of the juveniles is completed. Myopsid squid (*Loligo*) also lay benthic egg masses in the form of a cluster of finger-like capsules, each containing perhaps 100 eggs. These are commonly retrieved from spawning grounds by trawlers, but may also be laid in the aquarium (Yang *et al.* 1986). Oegopsid squid, in contrast, lay large, diffuse egg masses, neutrally buoyant in the water column, and consequently their eggs are rarely available for culture (but see Balch *et al.* 1985).

Egg masses to be cultured need gentle circulation of clean aerated sea water. Commonly used methods to achieve this include suspending the egg masses in water from threads across the tank, or in containers such as net bags or floating plastic strainers. Direct agitation from stirrers or aeration bubbles should be avoided, and low light levels should be maintained.

Hatchlings

Development time in the egg depends on species and temperature, and ranges from less than 10 to over 100 days. At hatching the developed embryo actively breaks out of the enclosing egg coats using a special hatching gland (Boletzky 1987a).

Hatchlings need to be reared in separate facilities, away from adults and other potential predators. A series of replicated small tanks provide security and are easily managed, although growing squids require increasing space to swim. These early stages are vulnerable to excessive water movement or to strong aeration. Inflow and outflow pipes should be screened with fine mesh net, and aeration arranged so that hatchlings are not exposed to bubble streams.

Hatchlings are immediately active, feeding on the remains of the yolk provision for the egg. After a period of half a day to about a week (depending on species and temperature) they will begin to feed on live food. At this point a variety of appropriately small crustacean food must be supplied, such as *Artemia*, copepods, mysids, shrimps and newly metamorphosed crabs. Those species with particularly large eggs and benthic hatchlings are easier to feed at this stage because of the wider range of acceptable food species. Boletzky (1987b) provides a useful account of juvenile behaviour characteristics, and Vecchione (1987) gives an account of their ecology together with a summary of the early feeding and growth characteristics of a number of species.

Villanueva (1994) has shown that with attention to the size of food organisms required by the hatchlings, easily maintained laboratory cultures of crabs producing larval zoea of appropriate dimensions, can provide continuous food supplies. He found that hatchlings of *Octopus vulgaris* successfully fed and grew on zoea of the crab *Pagurus prideauxi*. Similarly, the squid *Loligo vulgaris* could be reared through the first feeding stages on a diet of *P. prideauxi* zoeae supplemented with those from another crab *Dardanus arrosor*. These practical and controllable methods of live food supply could be a significant step towards more laboratory rearing of cephalopods and reduced dependence on wild-caught animals.

The requirement for high-quality sea water is particularly great for hatchlings. Although mortality in the egg stage is remarkably low, early rearing trials with artificial sea water produced a high proportion of defective juveniles. Particularly problematic was the inability to control orientation, resulting in uncoordinated walking and corkscrewing or somersaulting while swimming. These so called 'spinner' cephalopods were found to have defective statolith production and statocyst development (Colmers *et al.* 1984). The cause of the problem was discovered to be a lack of strontium in the artificial sea water leading to inadequate mineralisation and could be rectified simply by the addition of the correct trace elements (Hanlon *et al.* 1989).

Laboratory procedures

Handling

The general requirements of handling cephalopods captured from the sea have been discussed already (see

'Handling and transport'). Apart from the aspects of mechanical damage by rough handling, or self-inflicted damage from striking the tank walls, little attention has been given to more subtle stress effects.

Marine fish are prone to severe physiological consequences of handling stress (Wardle 1981; Potts 1987). Changes in plasma levels of glucose, catecholamines, corticosteroids and adrenaline or noradrenaline lead to hyperglycaemia, elevated lactic acid levels and osmotic effects which may persist for several weeks. The principal causes of these stress effects seem to be the mechanical handling itself, exposure to air for even short periods, low oxygen levels and higher levels of temperature and ammonia.

Laboratories working with cephalopods select out obviously damaged animals and those behaving abnormally, but little or no allowance has been made for the physiological effects of stress. Twenty-four hours in the aquarium is often considered sufficient time for acclimatisation and, for longer-term studies, animals which are feeding regularly are adequate. For many experimental purposes, animals are used immediately after capture. By comparison with fish it might be assumed that, in cephalopods, with their complex behaviour and neural and hormonal control systems, there will be substantial physiological consequences of capture from the wild and laboratory management. No studies are yet available to give guidance as to the significance of these stresses, although there is some evidence to suggest that long-term residence in aquarium conditions leads to changes in maturity (Boyle & Knobloch 1984b) and enzyme activity (M.S. Grisley & P.R. Boyle, unpublished observations) in *Eledone cirrhosa*. The present tendency is for researchers to use wild-caught animals as soon as possible after capture, allowing perhaps only a 3–5-day period of acclimatisation, and more or less ignoring the possibility of longer-term physiological stress effects. Studies aimed at identifying and defining stress effects are urgently needed.

Octopuses in the laboratory may be handled directly or by hand nets. As far as possible, handling should take place under water. Certainly the skin should never be brought into contact with dry absorbent surfaces. Some species, notably *Octopus vulgaris*, are relatively tough and will stand a much greater degree of handling than more delicate octopods such as *Eledone cirrhosa*. Very large species such as *Octopus dofleini* need special care, coaxing the animal rather than forcing it into buckets or nets for transport to tank or to laboratory.

Identity marking

Identity marking of individuals over a long holding period has been rarely attempted, largely because the soft body and delicate skin are not conducive to the attachment of tags. In the field, individual *Octopus dofleini* have been successfully identified by attaching numbered plastic disks on either side of an arm connected through the musculature by a nickel pin (Hartwick *et al.* 1984). Large-scale capture/recapture tag studies have also been successful in Japanese and South African squid fisheries.

In the laboratory, most workers have relied on keeping octopuses in separate enclosures. Where every individual held collectively in stock tanks has to be identified, subcutaneous injections of coloured latex have been used (Boyle & Knobloch 1982). Under anaesthesia, small amounts of latex containing dye (eosin) are injected beneath the ventral mantle skin to form a series of spots, each 2–3 mm in diameter. Using right and left sides, a relatively small number of dots can be used to provide a coded identification mark. These latex implants are inert: among hundreds of *Eledone cirrhosa* marked in this way only in a very few cases was any local reaction seen and, unlike the direct injection of dye, the implants do not disperse or fade. The disadvantage is that, in most cases, the animals have to be caught and handled before their identity can be read with confidence. The use of small (3.5 mm × 1.5 mm) numbered plastic tags implanted under the skin in chromatophore-free areas has also been evaluated. These implanted tags do not appear to cause any adverse reaction, but may be lost from the entry puncture if not implanted sufficiently firmly, and also require the animal to be handled before the tag can be read. Mutilation tagging is not acceptable.

Anaesthesia

Only anaesthesia by immersion has been used for cephalopods. Anaesthesia by injection has not been attempted. The following techniques apply mainly to octopods and sepioids. Squids will not normally recover from handling or surgery under anaesthesia, but animals in really good condition may be briefly anaesthetised in ethanol (in sea water) for weighing or photography (Hanlon 1982; Hanlon *et al.* 1983).

Octopuses may be readily and reversibly anaesthetised by transfer to a container of sea water containing anaesthetic. Depth of anaesthesia is controlled only by its concentration and the period of immersion. Signs of anaesthesia are the progressive loss of activity and paling of the skin. Ventilatory movements slow down and stop, at which point anaesthesia is considered complete. Thereafter, only local movements of arms and skin will take place, or reflex contraction of the mantle if the stellate ganglion is stimulated, and there is no coordinated or directed activity.

Since fully anaesthetised animals have stopped breathing, they will begin to asphyxiate from that point, even though the heart and circulation may be functioning. This sets a strict limit on the period of time for which an octopus may be held under anaesthesia: 10–20 minutes is considered to be the safe limit before the animal must be returned to clean aerated sea water. Recovery can be assisted by flushing water through the mantle cavity and massaging the musculature; 2–5 minutes should be sufficient for full recovery.

A small variety of anaesthetics has been tried. Originally, urethane (ethyl carbamate) 3% in sea water was used, but is now replaced by ethanol (or industrial methylated ethanol, IMS) 2–2.5% in sea water at ambient temperature. Andrews and Tansey (1981) compared the effects of these chemicals with the use of cold sea water alone (3–5°C) as anaesthetics for *Octopus vulgaris* at Naples. They found all three methods to induce anaesthesia within 2–5 minutes using cessation of respiration and loss of chromatophore tone as the main criteria. The action of cold water is arguably analgesic rather than anaesthetic, probably affecting the animal in a fundamentally different way from urethane or alcohol. They observed that in urethane, and to a lesser extent in alcohol, a proportion of the octopuses tested attempted to climb out of the bucket containing the anaesthetic or inked violently. *Eledone cirrhosa* at the considerably cooler temperatures of Aberdeen, also shows signs of distress in urethane, whereas alcohol appears to cause little stress and inking very rarely occurs.

The traditional anaesthetic for marine invertebrates, magnesium chloride, has been evaluated for its effects on *Octopus vulgaris* and other cephalopods (Messenger *et al.* 1985). Made up as an isotonic solution by mixing 7.5% $MgCl_2{\cdot}6H_2O$ (in distilled water) with an equal volume of sea water, this simple salt was found to be an effective anaesthetic for cephalopods and, importantly, seemed to have minimal traumatic effect. It may be especially useful for animals such as *Sepia* which commonly react to handling by violent inking, and squid (O'Dor & Shadwick 1989).

The use of anaesthetics in cephalopods is at a relatively primitive stage. Little is known of the central effects of these compounds and the parameters of adjustment of anaesthetic type or concentration to cephalopod species and body size. For many types of chronic physiological procedures or long surgical techniques, continuous control over anaesthetic level is clearly desirable, but as yet there have been no attempts to establish methods of continuous and controllable anaesthesia.

Euthanasia

The simplest and most effective way of killing an octopus is terminal anaesthesia. Whichever anaesthetic is used (see Anaesthesia section), respiratory movements stop within 5–10 minutes. If left in the anaesthetic the animal will quickly asphyxiate. Under anaesthesia the brain may then be destroyed to ensure that no recovery is possible.

If it is necessary to kill an octopus without anaesthesia, some skill and practice is required. When the animal is placed on a smooth surface the arms and suckers will adhere. The mantle and viscera of the octopus are then gently pulled to stretch the body. One finger of the other hand can then readily locate the cranium, directly between the eyes. Using a sharp scalpel the brain is first bisected with a cut downwards and forwards. This is immediately followed by lateral cuts on each side to sever the brain from the optic lobes and further transverse cuts disconnect the brain tissue from major peripheral nerves. Squid are usually killed simply by decapitation, cutting between the head and mantle.

Embryological techniques

Numerous zoologists have studied the embryology of cephalopods *in vivo*. The eggs of many species are exceptionally large, and in many cases the details of embryogenesis can be followed through the transparent egg coats. Such investigations are largely outside the scope of this chapter and reviews may be found in Marthy (1978–1979, 1982) and Boletzky (1987a, 1988).

Concluding remarks

Compared to the extent of information and wealth of detail available for laboratory vertebrates, the cephalopods are poorly served. This is due to a combination of factors, largely because they can be still treated as wild animals, only temporarily resident in the laboratory. Also, as invertebrates, little attention is customarily given to the refinements of condition and management so long as survival is adequate for the purpose.

Interest in long-term laboratory-held cephalopods is increasing because of their biological importance as advanced invertebrates bearing comparison with vertebrates, and for their ecological and fishery significance. It is also the case that the health, housing and maintenance of all animals held for scientific purpose is of interest and importance generally. These new influences will progressively improve the levels of handling and maintenance expected for these fascinating invertebrates.

Acknowledgements

I gratefully acknowledge the help with the collection and management of octopuses over many years by staff of the Zoology Department, Aberdeen, especially Tom Craig, Gillian Robertson, Steve Adams, Steve Hoskin and Duncan Wood. Many students and co-workers have contributed to our knowledge and experience of aquarium-held animals here, especially Daniela Knobloch, Peter Smith, Francoise Dubas, Maxine Grisley, Rachel Austin, David Chevis, Lorraine Young, Katharine Kelly and Linda Key.

I am grateful to colleagues for comments on and corrections to the first edition of this article (Boyle 1991).

Further reading

Anderson, R.C. (1987) Cephalopods at the Seattle Aquarium. *International Zoo Yearbook*, **26**, 41–48

Boletzky, S.V. and Hanlon, R.T. (1983) A review of the laboratory maintenance, rearing and culture of cepha-lopod molluscs. *Memoirs of the National Museum of Victoria*, **44**, 147–187

Boyle, P.R. (1987) *Cephalopod Life Cycles*, Vol. 2. Comparative Reviews. Academic Press, London

Clarke, M.R. (1996) The role of cephalopods in the world's oceans. *Philosophical Transactions of the Royal Society of London, Series B*, **351**, 977–1112

Forsythe, J.W. (1984) *Octopus joubini* (Mollusca: Cephalopoda): a detailed study of growth through the full life cycle in a closed seawater system. *Journal of Zoology*, **202**, 393–417

Hanlon, R.T. (1987) Mariculture. In: *Cephalopod Life Cycles*, Vol. 2. Ed. Boyle, P.R., pp. 291–305. Academic Press, London

Hanlon, R.T. and Messenger, J.B. (1996) *Cephalopod Behaviour*. Cambridge University Press, Cambridge

Hanlon, R.T., Hixon, R.F. and Hulet, W.H. (1983) Survival growth and behaviour of the loliginid squids *Loligo plei, Loligo pealei* and *Lolliguncula brevis* (Mollusca Cephalopoda) in closed sea water systems. *Biological Bulletin Marine Biological Laboratory, Woods Hole*, **116**, 637–685

Lane, F.W. (1957) *Kingdom of the Octopus: The Life History of the Cephalopods*. Jarrolds, London

Lipinski, M.R. (1985) Laboratory survival of *Alloteuthis subulata* (Cephalopoda: Loliginidae) from the Plymouth area. *Journal of the Marine Biological Association of the United Kingdom*, **65**, 848–855

Messenger, J.B. and Nixon, M. (1977) The biology of cephalopods. *Symposia of the Zoological Society of London*, **38**, 1–65

Packard, A. (1972) Cephalopods and fish. The limits of convergence. *Biological Reviews of the Cambridge Philosophical Society*, **47**, 241–307

Packard, A. and Saunders, G.D. (1969) What the octopus shows to the world. *Endeavour*, **28**, 92–99

Wells, M. J. (1978) *Octopus. Physiology and Behaviour of an Advanced Invertebrate*. Chapman and Hall, London

References

Alexandrowicz, J.S. (1960) A muscle receptor organ in *Eledone cirrhosa*. *Journal of the Marine Biological Association of the United Kingdom*, **39**, 419–431

Altman, J.S. and Nixon, M. (1970) Use of the beaks and radula by *Octopus vulgaris* in feeding. *Journal of Zoology*, **161**, 25–38

Ambrose, R.F. (1983) *Midden* formation by octopus, the role of biotic and abiotic factors. *Marine Behavior and Physiology*, **10**, 137–144

Ambrose, R.F. (1984) Food preferences, prey availability, and the diet of *Octopus bimaculatus* Verrill. *Journal of Experimental Marine Biology and Ecology*, **77**, 29–44

Anderson, R.C. (1987) Cephalopods at the Seattle Aquarium. *International Zoo Yearbook*, **26**, 41–48

Andrews, P.L.R. and Tansey, E.M. (1981) The effects of some anaesthetic agents in *Octopus vulgaris*. *Comparative Biochemistry and Physiology C*, **70**, 241–247

Arnold, J.M. and Arnold, K.O. (1969) Some aspects of hole boring predation by *Octopus vulgaris*. *American Zoologist*, **9**, 991–996

Arnold, J.M., Summers, W.C., Gilbert, D.C., *et al*. (1974) *A Guide to the Laboratory Use of the Squid Loligo pealei*. Marine Biological Laboratory, Woods Hole Mass

Arnold, J.M. and Williams-Arnold, L.D. (1977) Cephalopods: Decapoda. In: *Reproduction of Marine Invertebrates*, Vol. 4. Eds Giese A.C. and Pearse J.S., pp. 243–290. Academic Press, New York

Balch, N., O'Dor, R.K. and Helm, P. (1985) Laboratory rearing of rhynchoteuthions of the ommastrephid squid *Illex illecebrosus* (Mollusca: Cephalopoda). *Vie et Milieu*, **35**, 243–246

Barnes, R.D. (1980) *Invertebrate Zoology*, 4th edn. W. B. Saunders, Philadephia

Boletzky, S.V. (1974), Élevage de Cephalopodes en aquarium. *Vie et Milieu*, **24**(2-A), 309–340

Boletzky, S.V. (1987a) Embryonic phse. In: *Cephalopod Life Cycles*, Vol. 2. Ed. Boyle, P.R., pp. 5–31. Academic Press, London

Boletzky, S.V. (1987b) Juvenile behaviour. In: *Cephalopod Life Cycles*, Vol. 2. Ed. Boyle, P.R., pp. 45–60. Academic Press, London

Boletzky, S.V. (1988) Cephalopod development and evolutionary concepts. In: *The Mollusca*, Vol. 12. Eds Clarke, M.R. and Trueman, E.R., pp. 185–202. Academic Press, London

Boletzky, S.V., Boletzky, M.V., Frösch, D., *et al*. (1971) Laboratory rearing of Sepiolinae (Mollusca: Cephalopoda). *Marine Biology*, **8**, 82–87

Boletzky, S.V. and Hanlon, R.T. (1983) A review of the laboratory maintenance, rearing and culture of cephalopod molluscs. *Memoirs of the National Museun of Victoria*, **44**, 147–187

Boucaud-Camou, E. and Boucher-Rodoni, R. (1983) Feeding and digestion in cephalopods. In: *The Mollusca*, Vol. 5. Ed. Wilbur, K.M., Part 2. pp. 149–187. Academic Press, London

Boucaud-Camou, E., Boucher-Rodoni, R. and Mangold, K. (1976) Digestive absorption in *Octopus vulgaris* (Cephalopoda: Octopoda). *Journal of Zoology*, **179**, 261–271

Boucher-Rodoni, R., Boucaud-Camou, E. and Mangold, K. (1987) Feeding and Digestion. In: *Cephalopod Life Cycles*, Vol. 2. Ed. Boyle, P.R., pp. 85–108. Academic Press, London

Boucher-Rodoni, R. and Mangold, K. (1977) Experimental study of digestion in *Octopus vulgaris* (Cephalopoda: Octopoda). *Journal of Zoology*, **183**, 505–515

Boycott, B.B. (1961) The functional organization of the brain of the cuttlefish *Sepia officinalis*. *Proceedings of the Royal Society of London, Series B*, **153**, 503–534

Boyle, P.R. (1976) Receptor units responding to movement in the octopus mantle. *Journal of Experimental Biology*, **65**, 1–9

Boyle, P.R. (1980) Home occupancy by male *Octopus vulgaris* in a large seawater tank. *Animal Behaviour*, **28**, 1123–1126

Boyle, P.R. (1981a) Methods for the aquarium maintenance of the common octopus of British waters, *Eledone cirrhosa*. *Laboratory Animals*, **15**, 327–331

Boyle, P.R. (1981b) *Molluscs and Man*. Studies in Biology, No. 134. Edward Arnold, London

Boyle, P.R. (1983a) *Cephalopod Life Cycles*, Vol. **1**. Species Accounts. Academic Press, London

Boyle, P.R. (1983b) *Eledone cirrhosa*. In: *Cephalopod Life Cycles*, Vol. 2. Ed. Boyle, P.R., pp. 365–386. Academic, Press, London

Boyle, P.R. (1983c) Ventilation rate and arousal in the octopus. *Journal of Experimental Marine Biology and Ecology*, **69**, 129–136

Boyle, P.R. (1986a) Responses to water-borne chemicals by the octopus. *Eledone cirrhosa* (Lamarck, 1798). *Journal of Experimental Marine Biology and Ecology*, **104**, 23–30

Boyle, P.R. (1986b) Neural control of cephalopod behaviour. In: *The Mollusca*, Vol. 9. Ed. Wilbur, K.M., Part 2. pp. 1–99. Academic Press, London

Boyle, P.R. (1986c) A descriptive ecology of *Eledone cirrhosa* (Mollusca: Cephalopoda) in Scottish waters. *Journal of the Marine Biological Association of the United Kingdom*, **66**, 855–865

Boyle, P.R. (1987a) *Cephalopod Life Cycles*, Vol. 2. Comparative Reviews. Academic Press, London

Boyle, P.R. (1987b) Molluscan comparisons. In: *Cephalopod Life Cycles*, Vol. 2. Ed. Boyle, P.R., pp. 307–327. Academic Press, London

Boyle, P.R. (1990) Prey handling and salivary secretion in Octopus. In: *Trophic Relationships in the Marine Environment. Proceedings of the 24th European Marine Biological Symposium*. pp. 541–552. Aberdeen University Press, Aberdeen

Boyle, P.R. (1991) *The UFAW Handbook on the Care and Management of Cephalopods in the Laboratory*. UFAW, Potters Bar

Boyle, P.R. and Boletzky, S.V. (1996) Cephalopod populations: definition and dynamics. *Philosophical Transactions of the Royal Society of London, Series B*, **351**, 985–1002

Boyle, P.R. and Dubas, F. (1981) Components of body pattern displays in the octopus *Eledone cirrhosa* (Mollusca: Cephalopoda). *Marine Behaviour and Physiology*, **8**, 135–148

Boyle, P.R., Grisley, M.S. and Robertson, G. (1986) Crustacea in the diet of *Eledone cirrhosa* (Mollusca: Cephalopoda) determined by serological methods. *Journal of the Marine Biological Association of the United Kingdom*, **66**, 867–879

Boyle, P.R. and Knobloch, D. (1981) Hole boring of crustacean prey by the octopus *Eledone cirrhosa* (Mollusca, Cephalopoda). *Journal of Zoology*, **193**, 439–444

Boyle, P.R. and Knobloch, D. (1982) On growth of the octopus *Eledone cirrhosa* (Lamarck). *Journal of the Marine Biological Association of the United Kingdom*, **62**, 277–296

Boyle, P.R. and Knobloch, D. (1983) The female reproductive cycle of the octopus, *Eledone cirrhosa*. *Journal of the Marine Biological Association of the United Kingdom*, **63**, 71–83

Boyle, P.R. and Knobloch, D. (1984a) Male reproductive maturity in the octopus *Eledone cirrhosa* (Cephalopoda: Octopoda). *Journal of the Marine Biological Association of the United Kingdom*, **64**, 573–579

Boyle, P.R. and Knobloch, D. (1984b) Reproductive maturity in fresh and aquarium-held *Eledone cirrhosa* (Cephalopoda: Octopoda). *Journal of the Marine Biological Association of the United Kingdom*, **64**, 581–585

Boyle, P.R., Mangold, K. and Froesch, D. (1979a) The organisation of beak movements in octopus. *Malacologia*, **18**, 423–430

Boyle, P.R., Mangold, K. and Froesch, D. (1979b) The mandibular movements of *Octopus vulgaris*. *Journal of Zoology*, **188**, 53–67

Bradbury, H.E. and Aldrich, F.A. (1969) Observations on feeding of the squid *Illex illecebrosus illecebrosus* (Lesueur, 1821) in captivity. *Canadian Journal of Zoology*, **47**, 913–915

Brusca, R.C. and Brusca, G.J. (1990) *Invertbrates*. Sinauer Associates, Sunderland, Mass

Bullock, T.H. and Horridge, G.A. (1965) *Structure and Function in the Nervous System of Invertebrates*, Vol. 2. pp. 1433–1515. W.H. Freeman, San Francisco

Cariello, C. and Zanetti, L. (1977) α- and β- cephalotoxin: two paralysing proteins from posterior salivary glands of *Octopus vulgaris*. *Comparative Biochemistry and Physiology C*, **57**, 169–173

Chase, R. and Wells, M.J. (1986) Chemotactic behaviour in Octopus. *Comparative Biochemistry and Physiology A*, **158**, 375–381

Clarke, M.R. (1966) The role of cephalopods in the world's oceans. *Philosophical Transactions of the Royal Society of London, Series B*, **351**, 977–1112

Cloney, R.A. and Florey, E. (1968) Ultrastructure of cephalopod chromatophore organs. *Zeitschrift für Zellforshung und Mikroskopishe Anatomie*, **89**, 250–280

Colmers, W.F., Hixon, R.F., Hanlon, R.T., *et al.* (1984) 'Spinner' cephalopods: defects of statocyst suprastructures in an invertebrate analogue of the vestibular apparatus. *Cell and Tissue Research*, **236**, 505–515

Corner, B.D. and Moore, H.T. (1981) Field observations on the reproductive behaviour of *Sepia latemanus*. *Micronesia*, **16**, 235–260

Cousteau, J.Y. and Diolé, P. (1973) *Octopus and Squid*. Cassell, London

Crone, H.D., Leake, B., Jarvis, M.W., *et al.* (1976) On the nature of 'Maculotoxin' a toxin from the blue-ringed octopus (*Hapalochlaena maculosa*). *Toxicon*, **14**, 423–426

Denton, E.J. (1974) On buoyancy and the lives of modern and fossil cephalopods. Croonian Lecture 1973. *Proceedings of the Royal Society of London, Series B*, **185**, 273–299

Denton, E.J. and Gilpen-Brown, J. (1961a) The buoyancy of the cuttlefish. *Journal of the Marine Biological Association of the United Kingdom*, **41**, 319–342

Denton, E.J. and Gilpin-Brown, J. (1961b) The distribution of gas and liquid within the cuttlebone. *Journal of the Marine Biological Association of the United Kingdom*, **41**, 365–381

Denton, E.J. and Gilpin-Brown, J. (1966) On the buoyancy of the pearly nautilus. *Journal of the Marine Biological Association of the United Kingdom*, **46**, 723–729

Denton, E.J. and Gilpin-Brown, J. (1971) Further observations on the buoyancy of *Spirula*. *Journal of the Marine Biological Association of the United Kingdom*, **51**, 363–373

Denton, E.J. and Gilpin-Brown, J. (1973) Flotation mechanisms in modern and ancient cephalopods. *Advances in Marine Biology*, **11**, 197–268

Denton, E.J., Gilpin-Brown, J. and Shaw, T.I. (1969) A buoyancy mechanism found in a cranchid squid. *Proceedings of the Royal Society of London, Series B*, **174**, 271–279

Denton, E.J. and Taylor, D.W. (1964) The composition of gas in the chambers of the cuttlebone of *Sepia officinalis*. *Journal of the Marine Biological Association of the United Kingdom*, **44**, 203–207

DeRusha, R.H., Forsythe, J.W. and Hanlon, R.T. (1987) Laboratory growth, reproduction and life span of the Pacific pygmy octopus, *Octopus digueti*. *Pacific Science*, **41**, 104–121

Dubas F. and Boyle, P.R. (1985) Chromatophore units in *Eledone cirrhosa* (Cephalopoda). *Journal of Experimental Biology*, **117**, 415–431

Dulhunty, A. and Gage, P.W. (1971) Selective effects of an octopus toxin as action potentials. *Journal of Physiology*, **218**, 433–445

Flecker, H. and Cotton, B.C. (1955) Fatal bite from octopus. *Medical Journal of Australia, II*, **42**, 329–331

Flores, E.E.C., Igaraski, S. and Mikami, T. (1976) Studies on squid behaviour in relation to fishing. I. On the handling of squid, *Todarodes pacificus* Steenstrup, for behavioural study. *Bulletin Faculty of Fisheries, Hokkaido University*, **27**, 145–151

Florey, E. (1969) Ultrastructure and function of cephalopod chromatophores. *American Zoologist*, **9**, 429–442

Florey, E. and Kriebel, M.E. (1969) Electrical and mechanical reponses of chromatophore muscle fibres of the squid, *Loligo opalescens*, to nerve stimulation and drugs. *Zeitschrift für Vergleichende Physiologie*, **65**, 98–130

Ford, L.A., Alexander, S.K., Cooper, K.M. *et al.* (1986) Bacterial population of normal and ulcerated mantle tissue of the squid *Lolliguncula brevis*. *Journal of Invertebrate Pathology*, **48**, 13–26

Forsythe, J.W. (1984) *Octopus joubini* (Mollusca: Cephalopoda): a detailed study of growth through the full life cycle in a closed seawater system. *Journal of Zoology*, **202**, 393–417

Forsythe, J.W. and Hanlon, R.T. (1980) A closed marine culture system for rearing *Octopus joubini* and other large-egged benthic octopods. *Laboratory Animals*, **14**, 137–142

Forsythe, J.W. and Hanlon, R.T. (1988) Effect of temperature on laboratory growth, reproduction and life span of *Octopus bimaculoides*. *Marine Biology*, **98**, 369–379

Forsythe, J.W., Hanlon, R.T. and Lee, P.G. (1987) A synopsis of cephalopod pathology in captivity. *Proceedings of the International Association of Aquatic Animal Medicine*, **1**, 130–134

Forsythe, J.W. and Van Heukelem, W.F. (1987) Growth. In: *Cephalopod Life Cycles*, Vol. 2. Ed. Boyle, P.R., pp. 135–156. Academic Press, London

Frösch, D. and Marthy, H.J. (1975) The structure and function of the oviducal gland in octopods (Cephalopoda). *Proceedings of the Royal Society of London, Series B*, **188**, 95–107

Gilbert, D.L., Adelman, W.J., Jr. and Arnold, J.M. (1990) *Squid as Experimental Animals*. Plenum Press, New York

Gray, J.A.B. (1960) Mechanically excitable receptor units in the mantle of the octopus and their connections. *Journal of Physiology*, **153**, 573–582

Graziadei, P. (1965) Muscle receptors in cephalopods. *Proceedings of the Royal Society of London, Series B*, **161**, 392–402

Grisley, M.S. and Boyle, P.R. (1987) Bioassay and proteolytic activity of digestive enzymes from octopus saliva. *Comparative Biochemical Physiology B*, **88**, 1117–1123

Grisley, M.S., Boyle, P.R. and Key, L.N. (1996) Eye puncture as a route of entry for saliva during predation on crabs by the octopus *Eledone cirrhosa* (Lamarck). *Journal of Experimental Marine Biology and Ecology*, **202**, 225–237

Halstead, B.W. (1965) *Poisonous and Venomous Marine Animals of the World*, Vol. 1. pp. 663–770

Hamabe, M., Hamuro, C. and Ogura, M. (1982) *Squid Jigging from Small Boats*. Fishing News Books, Farnham, Surrey

Hanlon, R.T. (1982) The functional organization of chromatophores and iridescent cells in the body patterning of *Loligo plei* (Cephalopoda: Myopsida). *Malacologia*, **23**, 89–119

Hanlon, R.T. (1983) *Octopus joubini*. In: *Cephalopod Life Cycles*, Vol. 2. Ed. Boyle, P.R., pp. 307–327. Academic Press, London

Hanlon, R.T. (1987) Mariculture. In: *Cephalopod Life Cycles*, Vol. 2. Ed. Boyle, P.R., pp. 291–305. Academic Press, London

Hanlon, R.T. (1988a) International symposium on life history, systematics and zoogeography of cephalopods in honor of S. Stillman Berry. *Malacologia*, **29**, 1–307

Hanlon, R.T. (1988b) Behavioral and body patterning characters useful in taxonomy and field identification of cepholopods. *Malacologia*, **29**, 247–264

Hanlon, R.T. (1990) Maintenance, rearing and culture of teuthoid and sepioid squids. In: *Squid as Experimental Animals*. Eds Gilbert, D.L., Adelman, W.J. Jr and Arnold, J.M.. Plenum Press, New York

Hanlon, R.T., Bidwell, J.P. and Tait, R. (1989) Strontium is required for statolith development and thus normal swimming behaviour of hatching cephalopods. *Journal of Experimental Biology*, **141**, 187–195

Hanlon, R.T. and Forsythe, J.W. (1985) Advances in the laboratory culture of octopods for biomedical research. *Laboratory Animal Science*, **35**, 33–40

Hanlon, R.T., Forsythe, J.W., Cooper, K.M. *et al.* (1984) Fatal penetrating skin ulcers in laboratory reared octopuses. *Journal of Invertebrate Pathology*, **44**, 67–83

Hanlon, R.T. and Hixon, R.F. (1980) Body patterning and field observations of *Octopus burryi* Voss, 1950. *Bulletin of Marine Science*, **30**, 749–755

Hanlon, R.T., Hixon, R.F. and Hulet, W.H. (1978) Laboratory maintenance of wild-caught lologinid squids. In: *Fisheries and Marine Service*, Technical Report No. 833, December **1978**, 20.1–20.14

Hanlon, R.T., Hixon, R.F. and Hulet, W.H. (1983) Survival growth and behaviour of the loliginid squids *Loligo plei, Loligo pealei* and *Lolliguncula brevis* (Mollusca, Cephalopoda) in closed sea water systems. *Biological Bulletin Marine Biological Laboratory, Woods Hole*, **116**, 637–685

Hanlon, R.T. and Messenger, J.B. (1988) Adaptive coloration in young cuttlefish (*Sepia officinalis* L.): the morphology and development of body patterns and their relation to behaviour. *Philosophical Transactions of the Royal Society of London, Series B*, **320**, 437–487

Hanlon, R.T. and Messenger, J.B. (1996) *Cephalopod Behaviour*. Cambridge University Press, Cambridge

Hartwick, B. (1983) *Octopus dofleini*. In: *Cephalopad Life Cycles*, Vol. 2. Ed. Boyle, P.R., pp. 277–291. Academic Press, London

Hartwick, E.B., Ambrose, R.F. and Robinson, S.M.C. (1984) Den utilization and movements of tagged *Octopus dofleini*. *Marine Behaviour and Physiology*, **11**, 95–110

Haven, N. (1972) The ecology and behaviour of *Nautilus pompilius* in the Philippines. *Veliger*, **15**, 75–80

Hawkins, A.D. (1981) *Aquarium Systems*. Academic Press, London

Hendrix J.P. Jr., Hulet, W.H. and Greenberg, M.J. (1981) Salinity tolerance and the responses to hypoosmotic stress of the Bay Squid, *Lolliguncula brevis*, a euryhaline cephalopod mollusc. *Comparative Biochemistry and Physiology A*, **69**, 641–648

Herring, P.J. (1977) Luminescence in cephalopods and fish. *Symposia of the Zoological Society of London*, **38**, 127–159

Hochberg, F.G. (1982) The 'Kidneys' of cephalopods: a unique habitat for parasites. *Malacologia*, **23**, 121–134

Hochberg, F.G. (1983) The parasites of cephalopods: a review. *Memoirs of the National Museum of Victoria*, **44**, 108–145

Home Office (1986a) *Laboratory Animals (Scientific Procedures) Act*. Her Majesty's Stationery Office, London

Hulet, W.H., Villoch, M.R., Hixon, R.F. *et al.* (1979) Fin damage in captured and reared squids. *Laboratory Animal Science*, **29**, 528–533

Joll, L.M. (1976) Mating, egg-laying and hatching of *Octopus tetricus* (Mollusca: Cephalopoda) in the laboratory. *Marine Biology*, **36**, 327–333

Joll, L.M. (1977) *The predation of post-caught western rock lobster (Panulirus longipes cygnus) by octopus*. Report No. 29. Department of Fisheries and Wildlife, Western Australia

Keir, W.M. (1982) The functional morphology of the musculature of squid (Loligiidae). Arms and tentacles. *Journal of Morphology*, **172**, 179–192

Lane, F.W. (1957) *Kingdom of the Octopus: The Life History of the Cephalopods*. Jarrolds, London

Lehmann, V. (1981) *The Ammonites: Their Life and Their World* (English edn). Cambridge University Press, Cambridge

Lipinski, M.R. (1985) Laboratory survival of *Alloteuthis subulata* (Cephalopoda: Loliginidae) from the Plymouth area. *Journal of the Marine Biological Association of the United Kingdom*, **65**, 848–855

MacGinitie, G.E. and MacGinitie, N. (1968) *Natural History of Marine Animals*, 2nd edn. McGraw Hill, New York

Mangold, K. (1987) Reproduction. In: *Cephalopod Life Cycles*, Vol. 2. Ed. Boyle, P.R., pp. 157–200. Academic Press, London

Mangold, K. and Boletzky, S.V. (1973) New data on reproductive biology and growth of *Octopus vulgaris*. *Marine Biology*, **19**, 7–12

Mangold, K. and Boletzky, S.V. (1985) Biology and distribution of early juvenile cephalopods. *Vie et Milieu*, **35**(3/4) (special volume)

Marthy, H.J. (1978–1979) Embryologie experimentale chez les Cephalopodes. *Vie et Milieu*, **2829**, 121–142

Marthy, H.J. (1982) The cephalopod egg, a suitable material for cell and tissue interaction studies. In: *Embryonic Development, Part B: Cellular Aspects*. pp. 223–233. Alan R. Liss, New York

Martin, R. (1977) The giant nerve fibre system of cephalopods. Recent structured findings. *Symposium of the Zoological Society of London*, **38**, 261–275

Mather, J. (1980) Social organization and use of space by *Octopus joubini* in a semi-natural situation. *Bulletin of Marine Science*, **30**, 848–857

Matsumoto, G. (1976) Transportation and maintenance of adult squid (*Doryteuthis bleekeri*) for physiological studies, *Biological Bulletin of the Marine Biological Laboratory, Woods Hole*, **150**, 279–285

Matsumoto, G. and Shimada, J. (1980) Further improvement upon maintenance of adult squid (*Doryteuthis bleekeri*) in a small circular and closed-system aquarium tank. *Biological Bulletin of the Marine Biological Laboratory, Woods Hole*, **159**, 319–324

Messenger, J.B. (1968) The visual attack of the cuttlefish *Sepia officinalis*. *Animal Behaviour*, **16**, 342–357

Messenger, J.B. (1977) Prey capture and learning in the cuttlefish, *Sepia*. *Symposia of the Zoological Society of London*, **38**, 347–376

Messenger, J.B. (1979) The eyes and skin of octopus: compensating for sensory deficiencies. *Endeavour*, **3**, 92–98

Messenger, J.B. and Nixon, M. (1977) *The biology of cephalopods*. *Symposia of the Zoological Society of London*, **38**, 1–615

Messenger, J.B., Nixon, M. and Ryan, K.P. (1985) Magnesium chloride as an anaesthetic for cephalopods. *Comparative Biochemistry and Physiology C*, **82**, 203–205

Moynihan, M. and Rodaniche, A.F. (1982) The behaviour and natural history of the Caribbean Reef Squid *Sepioteuthis sepioidea*. With consideration of social, signal and defensive patterns for difficult and dangerous environments. *Advances in Ethology*, **25**, 1–151

Nesis, K.N. (1987) *Cephalopods of the World* (English edn). TFN Publications, Neptune City, NJ

Nixon, M. (1979) Has *Octopus vulgaris* a second radula? *Journal of Zoology*, **187**, 291–296

Nixon, M. (1980) The salivary papilla of *Octopus* as an accessory radula for drilling shells. *Journal of Zoology*, **190**, 53–57

Nixon, M. (1984) Is there external digestion by Octopus? *Journal of Zoology*, **202**, 441–447

Nixon, M. (1987) Cephalopod diets. In: *Cephalopod Life Cycles*, Vol. 2. Ed. Boyle, P.R., pp. 201–219. Academic Press, London

Nixon, M. and Boyle, P. (1982) Hole-drilling in crustaceans by *Eledone cirrhosa* (Mollusca: Cephalopoda). *Journal of Zoology*, **196**, 439–444

O'Dor, R.K. (1982) Respiratory metabolism and swimming performance of the squid, *Loligo opalescens*. *Canadian Journal of Fish and Aquatic Science*, **39**, 580–587

O'Dor, R.K. (1988) The energetic limits on squid distribution. *Malacologia*, **29**, 113–119

O'Dor, R.K., Durward, R.D. and Balch, N. (1977) Maintenance and maturation of squid (*Illex illecebrosus*) on a 15 meter diameter circular pool. *Biological Bulletin of the Marine Biological Laboratory, Woods Hole*, **153**, 322–335

O'Dor, R.K., Durward, R.D., Vesey, E. *et al.* (1980) Feeding and growth in captive squid. *Illex illecebrosus*, and the influence of food availability on growth in the natural population. *International Commission for North Atlantic Fisheries Selected Papers*, No. 6. pp. 15–21

O'Dor, R.K., Forsythe, J., Webber, D.M. *et al.* (1993) Activity levels of *Nautilus* in the wild. *Nature*, **362**, 626–627

O'Dor, R.K. and Shadwick, R.E. (1989) Squid, the olympian cephalopods. *Journal of Cephalopod Biology*, **1**, 33–55

O'Dor, R.K. and Wells, M.J. (1973) Yolk protein synthesis in the ovary of *Octopus vulgaris* and its control by the optic gland gonadotropin. *Journal of Experimental Biology*, **59**, 665–674

O'Dor, R.K. and Wells, M.J. (1975) Control of yolk protein synthesis by octopus ganadotropin *in vivo* and *in vitro*. *General and Comparative Endocrinology*, **27**, 129–135

O'Dor, R.K. and Wells, M.J. (1978) Reproduction versus somatic growth: hormonal control in *Octopus vulgaris*. *Journal of Experimental Biology*, **77**, 15–31

O'Dor, R.K. and Wells, M.J. (1987) Energy and nutrient flow. In: *Cephalopod Life Cycles*, Vol. 2. Ed. Boyle, P.R., pp. 109–133. Academic Press, London

Okutani, T., O'Dor, R.K. and Kubodera, T. (1993) *Recent Advances in Cephalopod Fisheries Biology*. Tokai University Press, Tokyo

Overstreet, R.M. and Hochberg, F.G. (1975) Digenetic trematodes in cephalopods. *Journal of the Marine Biological Association of the United Kingdom*, **55**, 893–910

Packard, A. (1969) Visual actuity and eye growth in *Octopus vulgaris* (Lamarck). *Monitore Zoologica Italie*, **3**, 19–32

Packard, A. (1972) Cephalopods and fish. The limits of convergence. *Biological Reviews of the Cambridge Philosophical Society*, **47**, 241–307

Packard, A. (1973) Chromatophore fields in the skin of octopus. *Journal of Physiology*, **238**, 38–40

Packard, A. (1982) Morphogenesis of chromatophore patterns in cephalopods: are morphological and physiological 'units' the same? *Malacologia*, **23**, 193–201

Packard, A. and Hochberg, F.G. (1977) Skin patterning in *Octopus* and other genera. *Symposia of the Zoological Society of London*, **38**, 191–231

Packard, A. and Sanders, G.D. (1969) What the octopus shows to the world. *Endeavour*, **28**, 92–99

Polglase, J.L. (1980) A preliminary report on the Thraustochytrid(s) and Labyrinthulids(s) associated with a pathological condition in the lesser octopus *Eledone cirrhosa*. *Botanica Marina*, **23**, 69–706

Poole, T. (1999) *The UFAW Handbook on the Care and Management of Laboratory Animals*, Vol. 2, 7th edn. UFAW, Potters Bar

Potts, G.W. (1987) Marine fish. In: *UFAW Handbook on the Care and Management of Laboratory Animals*, 6th edn. Ed. Poole, T.B., pp. 824–847. Longman Scientific and Technical, Harlow

Rathjen, W.F. (1984) *Squid Fishing Techniques*. National Marine Fisheries Service, Gloucester, Mass (Published by Gulf and South Atlantic Fisheries Development Foundation

Rathjen, W.F. and Voss, G.L. (1987) The cephalopod fisheries: a review. In: *Cephalopod Life Cycles*, Vol. 2. Ed. Boyle, P.R., pp. 253–275. Academic Press, London

Ritchie, L.D. (1972) *Octopus predation on pot-caught rock lobster, Hokianga area, N.Z. September–October 1970*. Fisheries Technical Report. No. 81. New Zealand Marine Department

Rodaniche, A.D. (1984) Heteroparity in the lesser striped octopus *Octopus chierchiae* (Jatta, 1889). *Bulletin of Marine Science*, **35**, 99–104

Rodhouse, P.G. and Nigmatullin, Ch.M (1996) Role as consumers. *Philosophical Transactions of the Royal Society of London, Series B*, **351**, 977–1112

Roper, C.F.E. and Boss, K.J. (1982) The giant squid. *Scientific American*, **246**, 82–89

Roper, C.F.E. and Hochberg, F.G. (1988) Behaviour and systematics of cephalopods from Lizard Island, Australia, based on color and body patterns. *Malacologia*, **29**, 153–193

Roper, C.F.E., Lu, C.C. and Hochberg, F.G. (1983) Biology and resource potential of cephalopods. Workshop, Procedures and Recommendations. *Memoirs of the National Museum of Victoria*, **44**, 1–311

Roper, C.F.E., Sweeney, M.J. and Nauen, C.E. (1984) Cephalopods of the World. *FAO Fisheries Synopsis No. 125*, Vol. 3. Food and Agriculture Organization, Rome

Rowell, C.H.E. (1963) Excitatory and inhibitary pathways in the arm of *Octopus*. *Journal of Experimental Biology*, **40**, 257–270

Rowell, C.H.F. (1966) Activity of interneurones in the arm of *Octopus* in response to tactile stimulation. *Journal of Experimental Biology*, **44**, 589–605

Russell-Hunter, W.D. (1979) *A Life of Invertebrates*. Macmillan, New York

Sakurai, Y., Ikeda, Y., Shimizu, M. *et al.* (1993) Feeding and growth of captive adult Japanese common squid *Todarodes pacificus*, measuring initial body size by cold anesthesia. In: *Recent Advance in Cephalopod Fisheries Biology*. Eds Okutani, T., O'Dor, R.K. and Kubodera, T., pp. 467–476. Tokai University Press, Tokyo

Saunders, W.B. and Landman, N.H. (1987) *Nautilus. The Biology and Paleobiology of a Living Fossil*. Plenum Press, New York

Saunders, W.B., Spinosa, C. and Davies, L.E. (1987) Predation in *Nautilus*. In: *Nautilus. The Biology and Paleobiology of a Living Fossil*. Eds Saunders, W.B. and Landman, N.H., pp. 201–212. Plenum Press, New York

Schipp, R. and Boletzky, S.V. (1975) Morphology and function of the excretory organs in dibranchiate cephalopods. *Forschritte der Zoologie*, **23**, 89–111

Smith, P.J.S. and Boyle, P.R. (1983) The cardiac inervation of *Eledone cirrhosa* (Lamarck) (Mollusca: Cephalopoda). *Philosophical Transactions of the Royal Society of London, Series B*, **300**, 493–511

Solem, G.A. (1974) *The Shell Makers*. Wiley-Interscience, New York

Spotte, S. (1979a) *Fish and Invertebrate Culture: Water Management in Closed Systems*, 2nd edn. John Wiley & Sons, New York

Spotte, S. (1979b) *Seawater Aquariums: The Captive Environment*. John Wiley & Sons, New York

Squires, H.J. (1957) Squid, *Illex illecebrosus* (LeSeuer), in the Newfoundland fishing area. *Journal of Fisheries Research and Biology, Canada*, **14**, 693–728

Summers, W.E. and McMahon, J.J. (1970) Survival of unfed squid, *Loligo pealei* in an aquarium. *Biolgical Bulletin of the Marine Biological Laboratory, Woods Hole*, **138**, 389–396

Tait, R.W. (1986) *Aspects physiologiques de la senescence postreproductive chez Octopus vulgaris*. PhD thesis, Université de Paris II

Tasaki, I. (1989) *Physiology and Electrochemistry of Nerve Fibres*. Academic Press, New York

Tinbergen, L. (1939) Zur Fortpflanzungsethologie von *Sepia officinalis*. *Archive Nederland Zoologie*, **3**, 323–364

Trueman, E.R. (1975) *The Locomotion of Soft-Bodied Animals*. Edward Arnold, London

Trueman, E.R. and Packard, A. (1968) Motor performances of some cephalopods. *Journal of Experimental Biology*, **49**, 495–507

Van Heukelem, W.F. (1983) *Octopus maya*, In: *Cephalopod Life Cycles*, Vol. 2. Ed. Boyle, P.R., pp. 311–323. Academic Press, London

Vecchione, M. (1987) Juvenile ecology. In: *Cephalopod Life Cycles*, Vol. 2. Ed. Boyle, P.R., pp. 61–84. Academic Press, London

Vevers, H.G. (1962) Maintenance and breeding of *Octopus vulgaris* in an inland aquarium. *Bulletin de l'Institute Oceanographique*, Special no. **1A**, 125–130

Villanueva, R. (1994) Decapod crab zoeae as food for rearing cephaloped paralarvae. *Aquaclture*, **128**, 143–152

Voss, G.L. (1977a) Present status and new trends in cephalopod systematics. *Symposia of the Zoological Society of London*, **38**, 49–60

Voss, G.L. (1977b) Classification of recent cephalopods. *Symposia of the Zoological Society of London*, **38**, 575–579

Ward, P.D. (1983) *Nautilus macromphalus*. In: *Cephalopod Life Cycles*, Vol. 2. Ed. Boyle, P.R., pp. 11–28. Academic Press, London

Ward, P.D. (1987) *The Natural History of Nautilus*. Allen and Unwin, Boston

Ward, D.F. and Wainwright, S.A. (1972) Locomotory aspects of squid mantle structure. *Journal of Zoology*, **167**, 437–449

Wardle, C.S. (1981) Physiological stress in captive fish. In: *Aquarium Systems*. Ed. Hawkin, A.D., pp. 403–414. Academic Press, London

Wells, M.J. (1962) *Brain and Behaviour in Cephalopods*. Heinemann, London

Wells, M.J. (1963) Taste by touch: some experiments with *Octopus*. *Journal of Experimental Biology*, **40**, 187–193

Wells, M.J. (1964a) Tactile discrimination of surface curvature and shape by *Octopus*. *Journal of Experimental Biology*, **41**, 435–445

Wells, M.J. (1964b) Tactile discrimination of shape by *Octopus*. *Journal of Experimental Psychology*, **16**, 156–162

Wells, M.J. (1978) *Octopus. Physiology and Behaviour of an Advance Invertebrate*. Chapman and Hall, London

Wells, M.J. and Clarke, A. (1996) Energetics: the costs of living and reproducing for an individual cephalopod. *Philosophical Transactions of the Royal Society of London, Series B*, **351**, 1083–1104

Wells, M.J., Freeman, N.H. and Ashburner, M. (1965) Some experiments on the chemotactile sense of octopuses. *Journal of Experimental Biology*, **43**, 553–563

Wells, M.J., O'Dor, R.K., Mangold, K. *et al.* (1983a) Diurnal changes in activity and metabolic rate in *Octopus vulgaris*. *Marine Behaviour and Physiology*, **9**, 275–287

Wells, M.J. O'Dor, R.K., Mangold, K. *et al.* (1983b) Oxygen consumption in movement by *Octopus vulgaris*. *Marine Behavour and Physiology*, **9**, 289–303

Wells, M.J., O'Dor, R.K., Mangold, K. *et al.* (1983c) Feeding and metabolic rate in *Octopus vulgaris*. *Marine Behaviour and Physiology*, **9**, 305–317

Wells, M.J. and Wells, J. (1957) The function of the brain of *Octopus* in tactile discrimination. *Journal of Experimental Biology*, **34**, 131–142

Wells, M.J. and Wells, J. (1959) Hormonal control of sexual maturity in octopus. *Journal of Experimental Biology*, **36**, 1–33

Wells, M.J. and Wells, J. (1977) Cephalopoda: Octopoda. In: *Reproduction of Marine Invertebrates*, Vol. 4. Eds Giese, A.C. and Pearse, J.S., pp. 291–336. Academic Press, New York

Wells, M.J. and Wells, J. (1982) Ventilatory currents in the mantle of cephalopods. *Journal of Experimental Biology*, **99**, 315–330

Wilbur, K.M. (1983–1988) *The Mollusca*. Vols 1–12. Academic Press, London

Williams, L.W. (1909) *The Anatomy of the Common Squid Loligo pealii Lesueur*. American Museum Natural History, New York

Willmer, P. (1990) *Invertebrate Relationships: Patterns in Animal Evolution*. Cambridge University Press, Cambridge

Wilson, D.M. (1960b) Nervous control of movement in cephalopods. *Journal of Experimental Biology*, **37**, 57–72

Wodinsky, J. (1969) Penetration of the shell and feeding on gastropods by *Octopus*. *American Zoologist*, **9**, 997–1010

Wodinsky, J. (1977) Hormonal inhibition of feeding and death in *Octopus*: control by optic gland secretion. *Science*, **198**, 948–951

Yang, W.T., Hixon, R.F., Turk, P.E. *et al.* (1986) Growth, behaviour and sexual maturation of the market squid, *Loligo opalescens* cultured through the life cycle. *Fisheries Bulletin*, **84**, 771–798

Yonge, C.M. and Thompson, T.E. (1976) *Living Marine Molluscs*. Collins, London

Young, J.Z. (1934) The structure of nerve fibres in *Sepia*. *Journal of Physiology*, **83**, 278–288

Young, J.Z. (1939) Fused nervous and synaptic contacts in the giant nerve fibres of cephalopods. *Philosophical Transactions of the Royal Society of London, Series B*, **229**, 465–503

Young, J.Z. (1967) Some comparisons between the nervous system of cephalopods and mammals. In: *Invertebrate Nervous Systems*. Ed. Wiersma, C.A.G., pp. 353–362. University of Chicago Press, Chicago

Young, J.Z. (1971) *The Anatomy of the Nervous System of Octopus vulgaris*. Clarendon Press, Oxford

Young, R.E. and Harman, R.F. (1988) 'Larva', 'paralarva' and 'subadult' in cephalopod terminology. *Malacologia*, **29**, 201–207

Index

Note: page numbers in *italics* refer to figures; those in **bold** to tables or boxes.

Lightning Source UK Ltd.
Milton Keynes UK
UKOW07n0118080315

247412UK00001B/1/P